American
DRUG INDEX

39th Edition

American
DRUG INDEX

1995

39th Edition

NORMAN F. BILLUPS, R.Ph., M.S., Ph.D.

Dean and Professor of Pharmacy
College of Pharmacy
The University of Toledo

Associate Editor

SHIRLEY M. BILLUPS, R.N., L.P.C., M.Ed.

Oncology Nurse
The Toledo Hospital

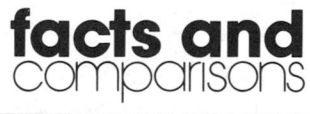

facts and
comparisons

A **Wolters Kluwer** Company

Facts and Comparisons Staff

C. Sue Sewester
publisher

Bernie R. Olin, PharmD
editor-in-chief

Charles E. Dombek, BS, MIM
manager, editorial information systems

L. Douglas Rudder, Jr.
manuscript editor

ISBN 0-932686-32-X
ISSN 0065-8111

Library of Congress Catalog Card Number 55-6286

Printed in the United States of America

Published by
Facts and Comparisons
111 West Port Plaza, Suite 400,
St. Louis, Missouri 63146-3098

Preface

The 39th Edition of the *American Drug Index* (ADI) has been prepared for the identification, explanation and correlation of the many pharmaceuticals available to the medical, pharmaceutical and allied health professions. The need for this index has become even more acute as the variety and number of drugs and drug products have continued to multiply. Hence, the *ADI* should be useful to pharmacists, nurses, healthcare administrators, physicians, medical transcriptionists, dentists, sales personnel, students and teachers in the fields incorporating pharmaceuticals.

Special note to medical transcriptionists: Although all names in the *ADI* appear in bold capitalized type, trade products are easily identifiable by the manufacturer's name in parentheses immediately following the trade name. The names for official products are preceded by a bullet (•) and should appear in lower case in transcription.

The organization of the *ADI* falls into 13 major sections:
Monographs of Drug Products
Common Abbreviations Used in Medical Orders
Common Systems of Weight and Measure
Approximate Practical Equivalents
International System of Units
Normal Laboratory Values
Trademark Glossary
Glossary
Container Requirements for U.S.P. XXIII Drugs
Container and Storage Requirements for Sterile U.S.P.
  XXIII Drugs
Oral Dosage Forms That Should Not Be Crushed
Pharmaceutical Company Labeler Code Index Numbers
Pharmaceutical Manufacturer and Drug Distributor Addresses

MONOGRAPHS: The organization of the monograph section of the *ADI* is alphabetical with extensive cross-indexing. Names listed are generic (also called nonproprietary, public name or common name); brand (also called trademark, proprietary or specialty); and chemical. Synonyms that are in general use also are included. All names used for a pharmaceutical appear in alphabetical order with the pertinent data given under the brand name by which it is made available.

The monograph for a typical brand name product consists of the manufacturer, generic and/or chemical names, composition and strength, pharmaceutical dosage forms available, package size, and use.

Generic names appear in alphabetical order, followed by the corresponding recognition of the drug to the U.S.P. (United States Pharmacopeia), N.F. (National Formulary) and USAN (USP Dictionary of United States Adopted Names and International Drug Names). Each of these official generic names is preceded by a bullet (•) at the beginning of each entry. The information is in accord with the U.S.P. XXIII and N.F. XVIII which became official on January 1, 1995; and the USAN-1995 which became official July 1, 1994.

British Approved Names (B.A.N.) and Veterinary British Approved Names (V.B.A.N.) are also included in this edition.

Because of the multiplicity of brand names used for the same therapeutic agent or the same combination of therapeutic agents, it was apparent that some correlation could be done. As an example of this, please turn to tetracycline HCl. Here under the generic name are listed the various brand names. Following are combinations of tetracycline HCl organized in a manner to point out relationships among the many products. Reference then is made to the brand name or names having the indicated composition. Under the brand name are given manufacturer, composition, available forms, sizes, dosage and use.

The multiplicity of generic names for the same therapeutic agent has complicated the nomenclature of these agents. Examples of multiple generic names for the same chemical substance are (1) parabromdylamine, brompheniramine; (2) acetaminophen, p-hydroxy acetanilid, N-acetyl-p-aminophenol; (3) guaifenesin, glyceryl guaiacolate, glyceryl guaiacol ether, guaianesin, guaifylline, guaiphenesin, guayanesin, methphenoxydiol; (4) pyrilamine, pyranisamine, pyranilamine, pyraminyl, anisopyradamine.

The cross-indexing feature of the *ADI* permits the finding of drugs or drug combinations when only one major ingredient is known. For example, a combination of aluminum hydroxide gel and magnesium trisilicate is available. This combination can be found by looking under the name of either of the two ingredients, and in each case the brand names are given. A second form of cross-indexing lists drugs under various therapeutic and pharmaceutical classes (i.e., antacids, antihistamines, diuretics, laxatives, etc.).

ABBREVIATIONS: The listing of Common Abbreviations used in Medical Orders is included as an aid in interpreting medical orders. The Latin or Greek word and abbreviation are both given with the meaning.

WEIGHT AND MEASURE: Tables containing the Common Systems of Weight and Measure are included to aid the practitioner in calculating dosages in the metric, apothecary and avoirdupois systems, as well as the International System of Units.

CONVERSION FACTORS: A listing of Approximate Practical Equivalents is added as an aid in calculating and converting dosages among the metric, apothecary and avoirdupois systems.

NORMAL LABORATORY VALUES: Tables containing normal reference values for commonly requested laboratory tests are included as a guideline for the health-care practitioner.

TRADEMARK GLOSSARY: An alphabetical listing of trademarked dosage forms and package types is included to aid in the identification of drug products listed in the *ADI.*

GLOSSARY: Commonly used terms are listed and defined as an aid in interpreting the use given for drug monographs included in the *ADI.*

CONTAINER AND STORAGE REQUIREMENTS FOR U.S.P. XXIII DRUGS AND STERILE DRUGS: These sections on container and storage requirements specified by the U.S.P. XXIII for compendial drugs, have been added to aid the practitioner in storing and dispensing.

ORAL DOSAGE FORMS THAT SHOULD NOT BE CRUSHED: This section has been added to alert the health-care practitioner about oral dosage forms that should not be crushed, and to serve as an aid in consulting with patients. Examples of products falling into the "non-crush" category are extended-release, enteric-coated, encapsulated beads, wax matrix, sublingual dosage forms and encapsulated liquid formulations.

LABELER CODE INDEX: The Pharmaceutical Labeler Code Index is presented to aid in tho idontification of drug products. The codes are listed in numerical order followed by the name of the manufacturer.

MANUFACTURER ADDRESSES: The name, address and zip code of virtually every American Pharmaceutical Manufacturer and/or Drug Distributor are listed in alphabetical order in this section. Additionally, a pharmaceutical labeler code number appears before the address of each company as a further aid in the identification of drug products.

Special appreciation and acknowledgment are given to my wife, Shirley, who served again this year as my Associate Editor—and to Dr. Bernie R. Olin, Editor-in-Chief of Facts and Comparisons, for compiling the monograph section of this volume. Special thanks are also extended to the manufacturers who supplied product information, to Dr. Kenneth S. Alexander for organizing the Container and Storage Requirements information, to Dr. John F. Mitchell for the table on Oral Dosage Forms That Should Not Be Crushed, and to Drs. Charles O. Wilson and Tony E. Jones for their earlier contributions to the *ADI*.

Correspondence or communication with reference to a drug or drug products listed in the *American Drug Index* should be directed to Bernie R. Olin, PharmD, Editor-in-Chief, Facts and Comparisons; 111 West Port Plaza, Suite 400; St. Louis, Missouri 63146, or call 1-800-223-0554.

Norman F. Billups, R.Ph., M.S., Ph.D.

Contents

[•] Denotes official name: Generic name or chemical name recognized by the U.S.P., N.F., or USAN.

Monographs

A

A-200 PYRINATE. (SK-Beecham) **Liq.:** Pyrethrins 0.33%, piperonyl butoxide technical 4%, petroleum distillate. Bot. 2 fl oz, 4 fl oz. **Gel:** Pyrethrins 0.33%, piperonyl butoxide technical 4%, petroleum distillate. Tube oz.
Use: Pediculicide.

A.A.A. OINTMENT. (Jenkins) Ammoniated mercury 2%, salicylic acid 1.25%, boric acid 1%, zinc oxide 15%. Jar oz, lb.
Use: Impetigo, nonspecific eczema, minor skin irritations.

AA-HC OTIC. (Schein) Hydrocortisone 1%, acetic acid glacial 2%, propylene glycol diacetate 3%, benzethonium Cl 0.02%, sodium acetate 0.015%, citric acid 0.2%. Soln. Bot. 10 ml.
Use: Otic preparation.

A AND D OINTMENT. (Kenyon) Vitamins A & D in lanolin-petrolatum base. Jar lb.
Use: Emolliont.

A AND D OINTMENT. (Schering) Fish liver oil, cholecalciferol. Tube 1.5 oz, 4 oz. Jar lb.
Use: Emollient.

A & D TABLETS. (Barth's) Vitamins A 10,000 IU, D 400 IU/Tab. Bot. 100s, 500s.
Use: Vitamin supplement.

A AND D VITAMIN CAPSULES. (Lannett) Vitamins A 5000 IU, D 400 IU/Cap. Bot. 500s, 1000s.
Use: Vitamin supplement.

A AND D VITAMIN OINTMENT. (Lannett) Petrolatum-lanolin base. Jar 1 lb, 5 lb.
Use: Emollient.

AAS INFANTIL W/VITAMIN C. (Sanofi Winthrop) Acetylsalicylic acid, vitamin C.
Use: Salicylate analgesic, vitamin C supplement.

AAS TABLETS. (Sanofi Winthrop) Acetylsalicylic acid.
Use: Salicylate analgesic.

• **ABAMECTIN.** USAN.
Use: Antiparasitic.

ABBOKINASE. (Abbott) Urokinase 250,000 IU/5 ml. Lyophilized pow. Vial 5 ml.
Use: Thrombolytic enzyme.

ABBOKINASE OPEN-CATH. (Abbott) Urokinase for catheter clearance 5000 IU/ml. Univial 1 ml.
Use: Thrombolytic enzyme.

ABBOTT AFP-EIA. (Abbott Diagnostics) Enzyme immunoassay for the quantitative measurement of alpha-fetoprotein (AFP) in human serum and amniotic flu-

id. Test kits 100s.
Use: Diagnostic aid.

ABBOTT AFP-EIA MONOCLONAL. (Abbott Diagnostics) Enzyme immunoassay for the quantitative measurement of alpha-fetoprotein (AFP) in human serum and amniotic fluid.
Use: Diagnostic aid.

ABBOTT ANTI-DELTA. (Abbott Diagnostics) Radioimmunoassay for the detection of antibody to delta antigen (HDAg) in human serum or plasma. For research only. Not for use in diagnostic procedures.
Use: Research.

ABBOTT ANTI-DELTA EIA. (Abbott Diagnostics) Enzyme immunoassay for the detection of antibody to hepatitis delta antigen in human serum or plasma. For research only. Not for use in diagnostic procedures.
Use: Research.

ABBOTT β-HCG 15/15. (Abbott Diagnostics) Enzyme immunoassay for the quantitative determination of human chorionic gonadotropin in human serum.
Use: Diagnostic aid.

ABBOTT CA125-EIA. (Abbott Diagnostics) Enzyme immunoassay for the quantitative measurement of cancer antigen (CA) 125 in human serum. For research only. Not for use in diagnostic procedures.
Use: Research.

ABBOTT CEA-EIA MONOCLONAL. (Abbott Diagnostics) Enzyme immunoassay for the quantitative measurement of carcinoembryonic antigen (CEA) in human serum or plasma to aid in the management of cancer patients and assessing prognosis.
Use: Diagnostic aid.

ABBOTT CEA-RIA. (Abbott Diagnostics) Solid phase radioimmunoassay for the quantitative measurement of carcinoembryonic antigen (CEA) in human serum or plasma to aid in the management of cancer patients and assessing prognosis.
Use: Diagnostic aid.

ABBOTT CMV TOTAL AB EIA. (Abbott Diagnostics) Enzyme immunoassay for the detection of antibody to cytomegalovirus in human serum, plasma, and whole blood. Test kits 100s.
Use: Diagnostic aid.

ABBOTT DIAGNOSTIC REAGENTS. (Abbott Diagnostics) A series of diagnostic tests for cancer, cardiovascular, hepatitis, infectious disease and immunol-

ogy, metabolic and digestive disease, OB/GYN, rubella, and thyroid.
Use: Diagnostic aid.

ABBOTT ER-EIA MONOCLONAL. (Abbott Diagnostics) Enzyme immunoassay for the quantitative measurement of human estrogen receptor in tissue cytosol. For research only. Not for use in diagnostic procedures.
Use: Research.

ABBOTT ER-ICA MONOCLONAL. (Abbott Diagnostics) Immunoassay for the detection of estrogen receptor. For research only. Not for use in diagnostic procedures.
Use: Research.

ABBOTT-HB EIA. (Abbott Diagnostics) Enzyme immunoassay for the detection of hepatitis Be antigen and/or antibody to hepatitis Be antigen.
Use: Diagnostic aid.

ABBOTT-HBe TEST. (Abbott Diagnostics) Radioimmunoassay or enzyme immunoassay for detection of hepatitis Be antigen and/or antibody to hepatitis Be antigen. Test kits 100s.
Use: Diagnostic aid.

ABBOTT HIVAB HIV-1 EIA. (Abbott) Enzyme immunoassay for the antibody to human immunodeficiency virus type 1 (HIV-1) in serum or plasma. Test kits 100s, 1000s.
Use: Diagnostic aid.

ABBOTT HIVAG-1. (Abbott) Enzyme immunoassay for the human immunodeficiency virus type 1 (HIV-1) antigens in serum or plasma. Test kits 100s, 1000s.
Use: Diagnostic aid.

ABBOTT HTLV I EIA. (Abbott) To detect antibody to Human T-Lymphotropic Virus Type I in serum or plasma. Test kits 100s.
Use: Diagnostic aid.

ABBOTT HTLV III ANTIGEN EIA. (Abbott Diagnostics) Enzyme immunoassay for the detection of Human T-Lymphotropic Virus Type III (HIV) antigens. For research only. Not for use in diagnostic procedures.
Use: Research.

ABBOTT HTLV III CONFIRMATORY EIA. (Abbott) Enzyme immunoassay for confirmation of specimens found to be positive to antibody to HTLV III. Test kits 100s.
Use: Diagnostic aid.

ABBOTT HTLV III EIA. (Abbott Diagnostics) Enzyme immunoassay for the detection of antibody to Human T-Lymphotropic Virus Type III (HIV) in human serum or plasma. Test kits 1s.
Use: Diagnostic aid.

ABBOTT IgE EIA. (Abbott Diagnostics) Enzyme immunoassay for quantitative determination of IgE in human serum and plasma. Test kits 100s.
Use: Diagnostic aid.

ABBOTT PAP-EIA. (Abbott Diagnostics) Enzyme immunoassay for the measurement of prostatic acid phosphatase (PAP) in serum or plasma.
Use: Diagnostic aid.

ABBOTT RSV-EIA. (Abbott Diagnostics) Enzyme immunoassay for the detection of respiratory syncytial virus (RSV) in nasopharyngeal washes and aspirates.
Use: Diagnostic aid.

ABBOTT SCC-RIA. (Abbott Diagnostics) Radioimmunoassay for the quantitative measurement of squamous cell carcinoma associated antigen in human serum. For research only. Not for use in diagnostic procedures.
Use: Research.

ABBOTT TdT EIA. (Abbott Diagnostics) Enzyme immunoassay for the quantitative measurement of terminal deoxynucleotidyl transferase (TdT), in extracts of human whole blood or isolated mononuclear cells.
Use: Diagnostic aid.

ABBOTT TESTPACK HCG-SERUM. (Abbott Diagnostics) Monoclonal antibody, enzyme immunoassay for the qualitative determination of human chorionic gonadotropin (HCG) in serum. No instrumentation required.
Use: Diagnostic aid.

ABBOTT TESTPAK HCG-URINE. (Abbott Diagnostics) Monoclonal antibody, enzyme immunoassay for the qualitative determination of human chorionic gonadotropin (HCG) in urine. No instrumentation required.
Use: Diagnostic aid.

ABBOTT TESTPACK-STREP A. (Abbott Diagnostics) A rapid screening and confirmatory test for the detection of Group A beta-hemolytic streptococci from throat swabs. No instrumentation required.
Use: Diagnostic aid.

ABBOTT TOXO-G EIA. (Abbott Diagnostics) Enzyme immunoassay for the qualitative and quantitative determination of IgG antibody to toxoplasma gondii in human serum and plasma.
Use: Diagnostic aid.

ABBOTT TOXO-M EIA. (Abbott Diagnostics) Enzyme immunoassay for the qual-

itative determination of IgM antibody to toxoplasma gondii in human serum.
Use: Diagnostic aid.

ABCDG VITAMIN CAPSULES. (Lannett) Vitamins A 5000 IU, D 400 IU, B_1 1 mg, B_2 2 mg, C 30 mg/Cap. Bot. 1000s.
Use: Vitamin supplement.

ABC to Z. (Nature's Bounty) Vitamins A 5000 IU, D 400 IU, E 30 mg, iron 27 mg, B_1 2.25 mg, B_2 2.6 mg, B_3 20 mg, B_5 10 mg, B_6 3 mg, B_{12} 9 mcg, C 90 mg, folic acid 0.4 mg, biotin 45 mcg, vitamin K 25 mcg, zinc 15 mg/Tab. Bot. 100s.
Use: Vitamin/mineral supplement.

• **ABCIXIMAB.** USAN.

ABITREXATE. (International Pharm. Products) Methotrexate sodium 25 mg/ml. Vial 2 ml, 4 ml, 8 ml.
Use: Antineoplastic agent.

• **ABLUKAST SODIUM.** USAN.
Use: Antiallergic; antiasthmatic.

ABORTIFACIENTS.
See: Prostin E 2, Supp. (Upjohn).
Prostin F 2 alpha, Inj. (Upjohn).
Prostin /15 M, Inj. (Upjohn).
20% Sodium Cl, Inj. (Abbott).

ABSORBABLE CELLULOSE COTTON OR GAUZE.
See: Oxidized Cellulose (Various Mfr.).

• **ABSORBABLE DUSTING POWDER,** U.S.P. XXIII.

• **ABSORBABLE GELATIN FILM,** U.S.P. XXIII. Sterile nonantigenic, absorbable, water-insoluble, gelatin film.
Use: Hemostatic, topical.
See: Gelfilm (Upjohn).

• **ABSORBABLE GELATIN SPONGE,** U.S.P. XXIII. Gelatin sponge.
Use: Surgical aid.
See: Gelfoam (Upjohn).

• **ABSORBABLE SURGICAL SUTURE,** U.S.P. XXIII. (Various Mfr.) Surgical Gut, Surgical Catgut, Catgut suture.
Use: Surgical aid.

ABSORBASE. (Carolina Medical) Petrolatum, mineral oil, ceresin wax, wool wax, alcohol. Oint. Tube 114 Gm, 454 Gm.
Use: Ointment and lotion base.

• **ABSORBENT GAUZE,** U.S.P. XXIII.
Use: Surgical aid.

ABSORBENT RUB RELIEF FORMULA. (DeWitt) Green soap 11.64%, camphor 1.63%, menthol 1.63%, pine tar soap 0.87%, wintergreen oil 0.71%, sassafras oil 0.54%, benzocaine 0.48%, capsicum 0.03%, wormwood oil 0.6%, isopropyl alcohol 75%. Bot. 2 oz.
Use: External analgesic.

ABSORBINE ANTIFUNGAL. (W.F. Young) Tolnaftate 1%. **Pow.:** Jar 56.7 g **Cream:** Tube 21.3 g.
Use: Antifungal agent.

ABSORBINE ARTHRITIC PAIN LOTION. (W.F. Young) Bot. 2 oz, 4 oz.

ABSORBINE FOOT POWDER. (W.F. Young) Zinc stearate, parachloroxylenol, aluminum chlorhydroxy, allantonate, benzethonium Cl, menthol. Plastic bot. 3 oz w/shaker top.
Use: Antifungal, external.

ABSORBINE JOCK ITCH. (W.F. Young) Tolnfatate 1%. Pow. Jar 56.7 Gm.
Use: Antifungal agent.

ABSORBINE, JR. (W.F. Young) Wormwood, thymol, chloroxylenol, menthol, acetone, zinc stearate, parachloroxylenol, aluminum chlorhydroxy, allantonate, benzethonium Cl, menthol. Liq. Bot. 1 oz, 2 oz, 4 oz, 12 oz w/applicator.
Use: External analgesic, antifungal.

ABSORBINE JR. ANTIFUNGAL. (W.F. Young) Tolnaftate 1%. Spray Liq. Bot. 59.2 ml, 118.3 ml.
Use: Antifungal agent.

ABSORBINE JR. EXTRA STRENGTH LINIMENT. (W.F. Young) Natural menthol 4%, plant extracts of calendula, enchinacea and wormwood, acetone, chloroxylenol iodine, potassium iodide, thymol, wormwood oil. Lot. Bot. 59 ml, 118 ml.
Uce: Rub or liniment.

ABSORBINE JR. LINIMENT. (W.F. Young) Menthol 1.27%, plant extracts of calendula, enchinacea and artemesia absinthium, iodine, potassium iodide, thymol, oil of artemesia, acetone, chloroxylenol. Lot. Bot. 13 ml, 30 ml, 59 ml, 118 ml, 480 ml.
Use: Rub or liniment.

ABSORBINE JR. LIQUID EXTRA STRENGTH. (W.F. Young) Menthol 4%. Liq. Bot. 59 ml, 118 ml.
Use: Rub or liniment.

ABUSCREEN. (Roche Diagnostics) An immunological and radiochemical assay for morphine and morphine glucuronide in nanogram levels. Utilizes I-125 la beled morphine requiring gamma scintillation equipment. Tests 100s.
Use: Diagnostic aid.

• **ACACIA,** N.F. XVIII. Syr. N.F. XVIII: Acacia senegal, arabic gum. (Penick) Pow. 0.25-1 lb; tears, 0.25-1 lb; whole, 0.25-1 lb.
Use: Demulcent, emulsifier, suspending agent.

• **ACADESINE.** USAN.
Use: Anti-ischemic.

A-CAINE. (A.V.P.) Diperodon HCl 0.25%, pyrilamine maleate 0.1%, phenylephrine HCl 0.25%, bismuth subcarbonate 0.2%, zinc oxide 5%, in cod liver oil and petrolatum base. Oint. Tube 1.25 oz.
Use: Local anesthetic.

A-CAPS. (Drug Industries) Vitamin A 50,000 IU/Cap. Bot. 100s, 500s.
Use: Vitamin A supplement.

• **ACARBOSE.** USAN.
Use: Alpha-glucosidase inhibitor.

A-CASOATE.
See: CASOATE-A.

ACCUPEP HPF. (Sherwood) Hydrolyzed lactalbumin, maltodextrin, MCT oil, corn oil, mono- and diglycerides, vitamins A, B_1, B_2, B_3, B_5, B_6, B_{12}, C, D, E, K, folic acid, Ca, Cl, Cu, Fe, I, Mg, Mn, P, Zn, biotin and choline. Pks. 128 Gm.
Use: Enteral nutritional supplement.

ACCUPRIL. (Parke-Davis) Quinapril 5 mg, 10 mg, 20 mg, 40 mg/Tab. Bot. 90s and UD 100s.
Use: Antihypertensive.

ACCURBRON. (Merrell Dow) Theophylline, anhydrous 10 mg/ml. Bot. pt.
Use: Bronchodilator.

ACCUSENS T TASTE FUNCTION KIT. (Westport) Test for ability to distinguish among salty, sweet, sour and bitter tastants. Kit contains 15 bottles (60 ml) tastants and 30 taste record forms.
Use: Diagnostic aid.

ACCUTANE. (Roche) Isotretinoin 10 mg, 20 mg, or 40 mg/Cap. Bot. UD 100s.
Use: Anti-acne, oral.

A-C-D SOLUTION, U.S.P. Sodium citrate, citric acid and dextrose in sterile pyrogen-free solution.
Baxter: 600 ml bot. with 70 ml, 120 ml, 300 ml soln.; 1000 ml bot. with 500 ml soln.
Cutter: 500 ml bot. with 75 ml, 120 ml soln.; 650 ml bot. with 80 ml, 130 ml soln.
Diamond: (Abbo-Vac) 250 ml, 500 ml.
Use: Anticoagulant for preparation of plasma or whole blood.

A-C-D SOLUTION MODIFIED. (Squibb) Acid citrate dextrose anticoagulant solution modified.
Use: Anticoagulant for use in radiolabeling red blood cells.

• **ACEBUTOLOL.** USAN. (±)-1-(2-Acetyl-4-butyramidophenoxy)-3-isopropylamino-propan-2-ol. (Ives) (±)-N-[3-Acetyl-4-[2-hydroxy-3-[(1-methylethyl)amino]propoxy]-phenyl]butamide.
Use: Beta-adrenergic receptor blocking agent.

See: Sectral, Cap. (Wyeth-Ayerst).

• **ACECAINIDE HYDROCHLORIDE.** USAN.
Use: Cardiac depressant.

• **ACECLIDINE.** USAN. 3-Quinuclidinol acetate (ester). Glaucostat.
Use: Parasympathomimetic.

• **ACEDAPSONE.** USAN. 4′,4″-Sulfonylbis (acetanilide).
Use: Antimalarial; antibacterial (leprostatic).

ACEDOVAL. (Vale) Dover's powder 15 mg, ipecac 1.5 mg, aspirin 162 mg, caffeine anhydrous 8.1 mg/Tab. Bot. 1000s, 5000s.
Use: Analgesic, antispasmodic, antiperistaltic.

ACEFYLLINE PIPERAZINE. Acepifylline. B.A.N.

• **ACEGLUTAMIDE ALUMINUM.** USAN.
Use: Anti-ulcerative.

ACEL-IMUNE. (Lederle) Diphtheria toxoid 7.5 Lf units, tetanus toxoid 5 Lf units, acellular pertussis vaccine 300 hemagglutinating units and aluminum ≤ 0.85 mg/0.5 ml. With formaldehyde ≤ 0.02%, thimersal final concentration of 1:10,000. Vial 5 ml.
Use: Agent for immunization.

• **ACEMANNAN.** USAN.
Use: Antiviral, systemic; immunomodulator; bowel disease, inflammatory, suppressant.

ACEON. (Ortho) Perindopril erbumine 2 mg, 4 mg or 8 mg. Tab. Bot. 100s and UD blister packs.
Use: Antihypertensive.

ACEPHEN. (G&W) **Adult:** Acetaminophen 650 mg/Supp. Box 12s, 100s. **Pediatric:** Acetaminophen 120 mg/Supp. Box 12s, 100s.
Use: Analgesic.

ACEPIFYLLINE. B.A.N. Piperazine theophylline-7-ylacetate. Acefylline Piperazine (I.N.N.). Etophylate.
Use: Spasmolytic.

ACEPROMAZINE. 10(3-Dimethylaminopropyl)-3-acetylphenothiazine maleate. Plegicil. (Wyeth-Ayerst) 1-(1-(Di-methylamino)propyl)-10H-phenothiazin-2-yl)ethanon e(Z)-2-butenedioate.
Use: Tranquilizer.

ACEPROMAZINE. B.A.N. 2-Acetyl-10-(3-di-methylaminopropyl)phenothiazine. Notensil maleate.
Use: Tranquilizer.

• **ACEPROMAZINE MALEATE.** USAN.
Use: Sedative.

ACEROLA-C. (Barth's) Vitamin C 300 mg/Wafer. Bot. 30s, 90s, 180s, 360s.

Use: Vitamin C supplement.
ACEROLA-PLEX. (Barth's) Vitamin C 100 mg, bioflavonoids 50 mg/Tab. Bot. 100s, 500s.
Use: Vitamin supplement.
ACETA. (Century) Acetaminophen 325 mg or 500 mg/Tab. Bot. 100s, 1000s.
Use: Analgesic.
ACETA W/CODEINE. (Century) Acetaminophen 300 mg, codeine phosphate 30 mg/Tab. Bot. 100s, 1000s.
Use: Narcotic analgesic combination.
ACETA ELIXIR. (Century) Acetaminophen 160 mg/5 ml, alcohol 7%. Elix. Bot. 120 ml, 1 gal.
Use: Acetaminophen.
ACETA-GESIC. (Rugby) Acetaminophen 325 mg, phenyltoloxamine citrate/Tab. Bot. 24s, 100s, 1000s.
Use: Analgesic, antihistamine.
• **ACETAMINOPHEN,** U.S.P. XXIII. For Effervescent Oral Soln., Tab., Cap. U.S.P. XXIII. Elix. U.S.P. XXI. N-Acetyl-p-amino-phenol. Acetamide, N-(4-hydroxyphenyl)-. 4'-Hydroxyacetanilide. APAP.
Use: Analgesic, antipyretic.
See: Acephen, Supp. (G&W).
  Aceta, Tab., Elix., Supp. (Century).
  Acetaminophen Uniserts, Supp. (Upsher-Smith).
  Actamin, Tab. (Buffington).
  Actamin Extra, Tab. (Buffington).
  Aminodyne, Elix. (Bowman).
  Anacin-3, Chew. tab., Tab., Elix., Drops (Whitehall).
  Anapap, Tab. (Forest).
  Apap, Cap., Tab. (Various Mfr.).
  Banesin, Tab. (Forest).
  Chlor-A-Tyl (Jenkins).
  Dapa, Tab. (Ferndale).
  Datril 500, Tab. (Bristol-Myers).
  Dolanex, Elix. (Lannett).
  Dorcol, Prods. (Sandoz Consumer).
  Fendon, Tab. (APC).
  G-1 (Hauck).
  Genapap, Chew. tab. (Goldline).
  Genebs, Tab., Cap. (Goldline).
  Halenol, Tab., Elix. (Halsey).
  Lestemp, Elix. (Reid-Rowell).
  Liquiprin, Soln. (SK-Beecham).
  Meda Cap, Cap. (Circle).
  Meda Tab, Tab. (Circle).
  Neopap, Supp. (Webcon).
  Nilprin 7.5, Tab. (AVP).
  Panadol, Chew. tab., Tab., Drops (Glenbrook).
  Panex, Tab. (Hauck).
  Parten, Tab. (Parmed).
  Phenaphen, Cap., Tab. (Robins).
  Proval, Cap., Elix., Drops, Tab. (Reid-Rowell).
  Suppap-120, 325, 650, Supp. (Raway).
  Tapanol Extra Strength, Tab. (Republic).
  Tapar, Tab. (Parke-Davis).
  Temetan, Elix., Tab. (Nevin).
  Tempra, Drops, Syr., (Mead Johnson).
  Ty-Caplets, Tab. (Major).
  Ty-Caps, Cap. (Major).
  Tylenol, Drops, Elix., Liq., Tab., Chew. tab. (McNeil).
  Tylenol Extra-Strength, Tab., Cap. (McNeil).
  Ty-Pap, Supp., Elix. (Major).
  Ty-Tabs, Tab. (Major).
  Valadol, Tab., Liq. (Squibb Mark).
  Valorin, Tab. (Otis Clapp).
ACETAMINOPHEN W/COMBINATIONS
  Aceta w/Codeine, Tab. (Century).
  Akes-N-Pain, Cap. (E. J. Moore).
  Al-Ay Modified, Tab. (Bowman).
  Allerest Headache Strength, Tab. (Pharmacraft).
  Alumadrine, Tab. (Fleming).
  Amaphen, Cap. (Trimen).
  Aminodyne, Elix. (Bowman).
  Anodynos-DHC, Tab. (Berlex).
  Anodynos Forte, Tab. (Buffington).
  Apap w/Codeine, Tab. (Central).
  Arthol, Tab. (Towne).
  Arthralgen, Tab. (Robins).
  Bancaps (Westerfield).
  Banesin-Forte, Tab. (Westerfield).
  Blanex, Cap. (Edwards).
  Bowman Cold, Tab. (Bowman).
  B-Pap, Liq. (Wren).
  BQ Cold, Tab. (Bristol-Myers).
  Bromo-Seltzer, Gran. (Warner-Lambert).
  Capital and Codeine, Susp. (Carnrick).
  Chexit, Tab. (Sandoz Consumer).
  Codalan, Tab. (Lannett).
  Codimal, Tab. (Central).
  Colrex Compound, Elix. (Reid-Rowell).
  Comtrex, Cap., Liq., Tab. (Bristol-Myers).
  Conar-A, Tab., Susp. (Beecham Labs).
  Conex, Preps. (Westerfield).
  Congesprin, Liq., Tab. (Bristol-Myers).
  Contac, Prods. (SK-Beecham).
  Coricidin Sinus Headache, Tab. (Schering).
  Co-Tylenol, Liq., Tab. (McNeil).
  Darvocet-N, Tab. (Lilly).
  Darvocet-N 100, Tab. (Lilly).
  Demerol APAP, Tab. (Sanofi Winthrop).

Dengesic, Tab. (Scott-Alison).
Desa-Hist AT, Tab. (Pharmics).
Dilone, Tab. (Vicks).
Dolene AP-65, Tab. (Lederle).
Drinophen, Cap. (Lannett).
Duoprin, Tab. (Dunhall).
Empracet with Codeine, Tab. (Burroughs Wellcome).
Esgic, Tab. (Gilbert).
Excedrin, Cap., Tab. (Bristol-Myers).
F.C.A.H., Cap. (Scherer).
Fendol, Tab. (Buffington).
Histogesic, Tab. (Century).
Histosal #2, Tab. (Ferndale).
Hycomine Compound, Tab. (Du Pont).
Hydrocet, Cap. (Carnrick).
Kiddies Sialco, Tab. (Foy).
Koryza, Tab. (Forest).
Mapap CF, Tab. (Major).
Maximum Strength Tylenol Flu, Tab. (McNeil-CPC).
Midrin, Cap. (Carnrick).
Myocalm, Tab. (Parmed).
N-D Gesic, Tab. (Hyrex).
Nyquil, Liq. (Vicks).
Ornex, Cap. (SK-Beecham).
Pamprin, Tab. (Chattem Labs.).
Panitol H.M.B., Tab. (Wesley).
Panritis, Tab. (Pan Amer.).
Parafon Forte, Tab. (McNeil).
Partuss-A, Tab. (Parmed).
Partuss T.D., Tab. (Parmed).
Pedric, Elix., Wafer (Vale).
Percogesic, Tab. (DuPont).
Phenaphen #2, #3, #4 (Robins).
Phenaphen-650, Tab. (Robins).
Phrenilin, Tab. (Carnrick).
Phrenilin Forte, Cap. (Carnrick).
Phrenilin w/Codeine, Cap. (Carnrick).
Presalin, Tab. (Hauck).
Proval No. 3, Tab. (Reid-Rowell).
Renpap, Tab. (Wren).
Rentuss, Cap., Syr. (Wren).
Repan, Tab. (Everett).
Rhinex, D. Lay, Tab. (Lemmon).
Rhinidrin, Tab. (Central).
Rhinogesic, Tab. (Vale).
S.A.C. Sinus, Tab. (Towne).
Saleto, Tab. (Hauck).
Saleto-D, Tab. (Hauck).
Salphenyl, Cap., Liq. (Hauck).
Santussin, Preps. (Sandia).
Scotgesic, Cap., Elix. (Scott/Cord).
Scotuss Pediatric Cough, Syr. (Scott/Cord).
Sedacane, Cap. (E. J. Moore).
Sedalgesic, Tab. (Table Rock).
Sedragesic, Tab. (Lannett).
Sialco, Tab. (Foy).
Sinarest, Tab. (Pharmacraft).

Sine-Aid, Tab. (McNeil).
Sine-Off, Prods (SK-Beecham).
Sinubid, Tab. (Warner Chilcott).
Sinulin, Tab. (Carnrick).
Sinus Tab. (Zenith).
Sinutab, Prods. (Warner-Lambert).
Spantuss, Liq. (Arco).
Super-Anahist, Tab. (Warner-Lambert).
Talacen, Cap. (Sanofi Winthrop).
Tega-Code, Cap. (Ortega).
Tegapap, Liq., Tab. (Ortega).
Triaminicin, Tab. (Sandoz Consumer).
Triaprin, Cap. (Dunhall).
Tussagesic, Tab., Susp. (Sandoz Consumer).
Two-Dyne, Tab. (Hyrex).
Tylenol, Preps. (McNeil).
Tylenol with Codeine, Elix., Tab. (McNeil).
Tylox, Cap. (McNeil).
Valihist, Cap. (Clapp).
Vicks Daycare, Liq. (Vicks).
Wygesic, Tab. (Wyeth-Ayerst).
• **ACETAMINOPHEN AND ASPIRIN TABLETS,** U.S.P. XXIII.
Use: Analgesic.
• **ACETAMINOPHEN AND CAFFEINE CAPSULES,** U.S.P. XXIII, Cap., Tab.
• **ACETAMINOPHEN, ASPIRIN AND CAFFEINE,** U.S.P. XXIII, Cap., Tab., U.S.P. XXIII.
Use: Analgesic.
ACETAMINOPHEN BUFFERED.
Use: Analgesic.
See: Bromo-Seltzer (Warner-Lambert).
ACETAMINOPHEN W/CODEINE. (Various Mfr.) **Tab.:** Codeine phosphate 15 mg, acetaminophen 300 mg/Tab. Bot. 100s, 500s, 1000s, UD 100s. Codeine phosphate 30 mg, acetaminophen 300 mg/Tab. **Elix.:** Codeine phosphate 12 mg, acetaminophen 120 mg/5 ml. Bot. 10 ml, 120 ml, 500 ml, pt, gal, UD 5 ml, 12.5 ml, 15 ml (100s).
Use: Narcotic analgesic combination.
• **ACETAMINOPHEN AND CODEINE PHOSPHATE ELIXIR,** U.S.P. XXIII.
Use: Analgesic.
• **ACETAMINOPHEN AND DIPHENHYDRAMINE CITRATE TABLETS,** U.S.P. XXIII.
Use: Analgesic, antihistamine.
• **ACETAMINOPHEN AND PSEUDOEPHEDRINE HYDROCHLORIDE TABLETS,** U.S.P. XXIII.
Use: Analgesic, decongestant.
• **ACETAMINOPHEN ORAL SOLUTION,** U.S.P. XXIII.
Use: Analgesic.

• **ACETAMINOPHEN ORAL SUSPENSION,** U.S.P. XXIII.
Use: Analgesic.

• **ACETAMINOPHEN SUPPOSITORIES,** U.S.P. XXIII.

ACETAMINOPHEN UNISERTS. (Upsher-Smith) Acetaminophen **120 mg or 325 mg/Supp.:** Ctn. 12s, 50s; **650 mg/Supp.:** Ctn. 12s, 50s, 500s.
Use: Analgesic.

ACETAMINOPHENOL.
See: Acetaminophen.

ACETANILID. (Various Mfr.) (Acetylaminobenzene, acetylaniline, antifebrin) N-phenylacetamide cry.
Use: Analgesic.

ACETARSOL.
See: Acetarsone.

ACETARSONE. 3-Acetamido-4-hydroxyphenylarsonic acid. Acetarsol, Acetphenarsine, Amarsan, Dynarsan, Ehrlich 594, Limarsol, Orarsan, Osarsal, Osvarsan, Paroxyl, Stovarsol.

ACETARSONE SALT OF ARECOLINE.
See: Drocarbil.

ACETASOL HC OTIC. (Goldline) Hydrocortisone 1%, acetic acid 2%. Bot. 10 ml.
Use: Otic corticosteroid, anti-Infective.

ACETASOL OTIC. (Goldline) Acetic acid (non-aqueous) 2%. Bot. 5 ml.
Use: Anti infective, otic.

• **ACETAZOLAMIDE,** U.S.P. XXIII B.A.N. N-(5-Sulfamoyl-1,3,4-thiadiazol-2-yl)acetamide. Acetamide, N-[5-(aminosulfonyl)-1,3,4-thiadiazol-2-yl]. (Various Mfr.) **125 mg:** Tab. Bot. 100s; **250 mg:** Tab. Bot. 100s, 1000s, UD 100s.
Use: Carbonic anhydrase inhibitor.
See: Diamox, Tab., Sequels (Lederle).

ACETAZOLAMIDE, ANTICONVULSANTS.
See: Diamox (Lederle)
Acetazolamide (Various Mfr.)
AK-Zol (Akorn)
Dazamide (Major)

• **ACETAZOLAMIDE SODIUM, STERILE,** U.S.P. XXIII.
Use: Carbonic anhydrase inhibitor.
See: Diamox, Inj. (Lederle).

ACET-DIA-MER-SULFONAMIDE. Sulfacetamide, sulfadiazine and sulfamerazine, Susp.
Use: Antibacterial, sulfonamide.

ACETEST REAGENT TABLETS. (Ames) Sodium nitroprusside, disodium phosphate, aminoacetic acid, lactose. Tab. Bot. 100s, 250s.
Use: Diagnostic aid.

• **ACETIC ACID,** U.S.P. XXIII, Glacial, Otic soln., U.S.P. XXIII. Diluted, N.F. XVIII.
Use: Pharmaceutic aid (acidifying agent).

• **ACETIC ACID IRRIGATION,** U.S.P. XXIII. 0.25% soln. (Abbott) 250 ml glass cont.; 250 ml, 1000 ml.
Use: Irrigating solution.

ACETIC ACID OTIC. (Various Mfr.) Acetic acid 2% with propylene glycol diacetate 3%, benzethonium chloride 0.02% and sodium acetate 0.015%. Soln. Bot. 15 ml, 30 ml, 60 ml.
Use: Otic preparation.

ACETIC ACID, POTASSIUM SALT.
Potassium Acetate, U.S.P. XXIII.

ACETICYL.
See: Acetylsalicylic Acid.

ACETILUM ACIDULATUM.
See: Acetylsalicylic Acid (Various Mfr.).

• **ACETOHEXAMIDE,** U.S.P. XXIII. Tab., U.S.P. XXIII. N-(p-acetylphenylsulfonyl)-N′-cyclo-hexylurea. 1-((p-acetylphenyl)sulfonyl)-3-cyclohexylurea. Benzenesulfonamide, 4-acetyl-N-[[cyclohexylamino]carbonyl].
Use: Blood sugar-lowering compound; antidiabetic agent.
See: Dymelor, Tab. (Lilly).

• **ACETOHYDROXAMIC ACID,** U.S.P. XXIII. Tab., U.S.P. XXIII.
Use: Enzyme inhibitor.
See: Lithostat (Mission).

ACETOL.
See: Acetylsalicylic Acid. (Various Mfr.).

ACETOLAX. (Mills) Acetphenylisatin 5 mg, Vitamins B₁ 1 mg, sodium carboxymethyl cellulose 500 mg/Tab. Bulk Pkg. 1000s.
Use: Laxative.

ACETOMEROCTOL. Acetato [2-hydroxy-5-(1,1,-3,3-tetramethylbutyl) phenyl] mercury. Under study.
Use: Antiseptic, topical.

• **ACETONE,** N.F. XVIII.

ACETONE or DIACETIC ACID TEST.
See: Acetest, Tab. (Ames).

ACETOPHEN C.T. GREEN. (Jenkins) Aspirin 3.5 gr, phenacetin 2.5 gr, caffeine 0.25 gr/Tab. Bot. 1000s.

• **ACETOPHENAZINE MALEATE,** U.S.P. XXII. Tab., U.S.P. XXII. 2-Acetyl-10-[3-[4-(-β-hydroxyethyl)-piperazinyl] propyl phenothiazine dimaleate. 10-[3-[4-(2-Hydroxyethyl)-1-piperazinyl]-propyl]-phenothia-zin-2-yl methyl ketone maleate (1:2).
Use: Tranquilizer.
See: Tindal Maleate, Tab. (Schering-

Plough).
ACETOPHENETIDIN. Phenacetin, U.S.P. XXIII. Ethoxyacetanilide.
Use: Analgesic, antipyretic.
ACETORPHINE. B.A.N. O^3-Acetyl-7,8-dihydro-7α[1(R)-hydroxy-1-methylbutyl]-O^6-methyl-6,-14-endoethenomorphine.
Use: Narcotic analgesic.
ACETOSAL.
See: Acetylsalicylic Acid (Various Mfr.).
ACETOSALIC ACID.
See: Acetylsalicylic Acid (Various Mfr.).
ACETOSALIN.
See: Acetylsalicylic Acid (Various Mfr.).
ACETOSULFONE. 4,4'-Diaminodiphenylsulfone-2-N-acetylsulfonamide sodium. (N^1-acetyl-6-sulfanilylmetanilamido) sodium.
• **ACETOSULFONE SODIUM.** USAN.
Use: Antibacterial.
ACETOXYPHENYLMERCURY.
See: Phenylmercuric acetate.
ACETPHENARSINE.
See: Acetarsone, Tab. (City Chemical).
ACETPHENOLISATIN.
See: Oxyphenisatin Acetate Preps.
ACETRIZOATE SODIUM. 3-Acetamido-2,4,6,-triiodobenzoate sodium.
ACETRIZOIC ACID. 3-Acetylamino-2,4,6,-triiodobenzoic acid.
See: Acetrizoate, Sodium.
ACET-THEOCIN SODIUM.
See: Theophylline Sodium acetate (Various Mfr.).
ACETYL ADALIN.
See: Acetylcarbromal (Various Mfr.).
ACETYLAMINOBENZALDEHYDE THIOSEMICARBAZONE-p.
See: p-ACETYLAMINOBENZALDEHYDE THIOSEMICARBAZONE.
ACETYLAMINOBENZENE.
See: Acetanilid (Various Mfr.).
N-ACETYL-p-AMINOPHENOL. Acetaminophen, U.S.P. XXIII.
ACETYLANILINE.
See: Acetanilid (Various Mfr.).
ACETYL-BETA-METHYLCHOLINE CHLORIDE.
ACETYL-BROMO-DIETHYLACETYLCARBAMIDE.
See: Acetylcarbromal (Various Mfr.).
ACETYLCARBROMAL. Acetyladalin, acetylbromodiethylacetylcarbamide. Pow. for manufacturing.
Use: Sedative.
See: Paxarel, Tab. (Circle).
W/Bromisovalum, scopolamine aminoxide HBr.
See: Tranquinal, Tab. (Barnes-Hind).
• **ACETYLCHOLINE CHLORIDE,** U.S.P.

XXIII. For Ophthalmic Soln., U.S.P. XXIII. Ethananinium,2-(acetyloxy)-N, N, N-trimethyl chloride. Choline chloride acetate.
Use: S.C., I.M., I.V. Parasympathomimetic agent, vasodilator. Paroxysmal tachycardia.
See: Miochol Ophthalmic (Iolab).
ACETYLCHOLINE-LIKE THERAPEUTIC AGENTS.
See: Cholinergic agents.
• **ACETYLCYSTEINE,** U.S.P. XXIII. Soln., U.S.P. XXIII. B.A.N. N-Acetyl-L-cysteine.
Use: Mucolytic agent. [Orphan drug]
See: Mucomyst, Soln. (Apothecon).
• **ACETYLCYSTEINE AND ISOPROTERENOL HYDROCHLORIDE INHALATION SOLUTION,** U.S.P. XXIII.
Use: Mucolytic agent.
ACETYLCYSTEINE (FLUMUCIL). (Zambon). Phase I HIV, ARC, AIDS.
Use: Immunomodulator.
ACETYLDIHYDROCODEINONE. Thebacon. B.A.N.
ACETYLIN.
See: Acetylsalicylic Acid (Various Mfr.).
ACETYLMETHADOL, I.N.N. Methadyl acetate. B.A.N.
ACETYLPHENYLISATIN.
See: Oxyphenisatin Acetate.
ACETYLPROCAINAMIDE-N.
Use: Cardiac depressant. [Orphan drug]
ACETYLRESORCINOL.
See: Resorcinol Monoacetate (Various Mfr.).
ACETYLSAL.
See: Acetylsalicylic Acid.
ACETYLSALICYLATE ALUMINUM.
See: Aluminum Aspirin.
• **ACETYLSALICYLIC ACID.** Aspirin, U.S.P. XXIII. Acidum acetylsalicylicum, 2-acetoxybenzoic acid, Acetilum Acidulatum, Acetophen, Acetol, Acetosal, Acetosalic Acid, Acetosalin, Aceticyl, Acetylsal, Acylpryin, Aspro, Helicon, Rhodine, Salacetin, Salcetogen, Saletin.
See: Aspirin Preps. (Various Mfr.).
ACETYLSALICYLIC ACID, ACETOPHENETIDIN AND CAFFEINE.
See: A.P.C., Preps. (Various Mfr.).
ACETYL SULFAMETHOXYPYRIDAZINE. 3-(N-Acetylsulfanilamido)-6-methoxypyridazine.
N^1-ACETYLSULFANILAMIDE. (Albucid; p-Aminobenzenesulfonacetamide; Sulfacet; Sulfacetamide, N-Sulfanilylacetamide).
Use: Sulfonamide therapy.
ACETYL SULFISOXAZOLE. Sulfisoxa-

zole Acetyl, U.S.P. XXIII.

ACETYLTANNIC ACID. Tannic acid acetate.
Use: Antiperistaltic.

AC EYE DROPS. (Walgreen) Tetrahydrozoline HCl 0.05%, zinc sulfate 0.25%. Bot. 0.75 oz.
Use: Decongestant combination, ophthalmic.

ACHES-N-PAIN. (Lederle) Ibuprofen 200 mg. Tab. Bot. 50s.
Use: Nonsteroidal anti-inflammatory drug, analgesic.

ACHLORHYDRIA DETERMINATION.
See: Diagnex Blue, Preps. (Squibb).

ACHLORHYDRIA THERAPY.
See: Acidol (Various Mfr.).
Glutamic Acid HCl (Various Mfr.).
Muripsin, Tab. (Norgine).
Normacid, Tab. (Stuart).

ACHOL. (Enzyme Process) Vitamin A 4000 units, ketocholanic acids 62 mg/Tab. Bot. 100s, 250s.
Use: Vitamin A supplement.

ACHROMYCIN. (Storz Lederle) Tetracycline HCl.
Ophth. Oint.: 10 mg/Gm 1%. Tube 3.75 Gm.
Ophth. Susp.: 1%, Plastic dropper bot. 1 ml, 4 ml.
Use: Antibacterial.

ACHROMYCIN-V. (Lederle) Tetracycline HCl. **Cap: 250 mg:** Bot. 100s, 1000s, UD 10 × 10s, Unit-of-use 12 × 20s, 12 × 28s, 12 × 40s, 12 × 100s; **500 mg:** Bot. 100s, 1000s, Unit-of-use 12 × 20s; UD 10 10s. **Oral Susp:** 125 mg/5 ml w/methylparaben 0.12%, propylparaben 0.03%. Bot. 2 oz, pt.
Use: Antibacterial, tetracycline.

ACID ACRIFLAVINE.
See: Acriflavine HCl (Various Mfr.).

ACID CITRATE DEXTROSE ANTICOAGULANT SOLUTION MODIFIED.
See: A-C-D Solution Modified (Squibb).

ACID CITRATE DEXTROSE SOLUTION.
See: A.C.D. Soln. (Various Mfr.).

ACID HISTAMINE PHOSPHATE.
See: Histamine Phosphate (Various Mfr.).

ACIDIFIERS.
See: Ammonium Cl (Various Mfr.)
pHos-pHaid (Guardian)
K-Phos (Beach)

ACID MANTLE. (Sandoz) Aluminum sulfate, calcium acetate, cetearyl alcohol, glycerin, light mineral oil, methylparaben, sodium lauryl sulfate, synthetic beeswax, white petrolatum, ammonium hydroxide, citric acid. Cream. Jar 120 Gm.
Use: Ointment and lotion base.

ACID MANTLE CREME. (Sandoz Consumer) Aluminum acetate in specially prepared water-soluble hydrophilic cream at pH 4.2. Tube 1 oz, Jar 4 oz, lb.
Use: Prophylactic agent, topical.

ACIDOL.
See: Betaine HCl (Various Mfr.).

ACIDOPHILUS.
See: Bacid (Fisons).
Lactinex (HW&D).
More-Dophilus (Freeda).

ACIDOPHILUS W/PECTIN. (Barth's) *Lactobacillus acidophilus* w/natural citrus pectin 100 mg/Cap. Bot. 100s.
Use: Antidiarrheal.

ACID TRYPAFLAVINE.
See: Acriflavine HCl. (Various Mfr.).

ACIDULATED PHOSPHATE FLUORIDE. (Scherer) Fluoride ion 0.31% in 0.1 molar phosphate. Soln. Bot. 64 oz. (Office Product).
Use: Dental caries preventative.

ACIDULIN. (Lilly) Glutamic acid HCl 340 mg/Pulv. Bot. 100s, 1000s.
Use: Gastric acidifier.

• **ACIFRAN.** USAN.
Use: Antihyperlipoproteinemic.

ACIGLUMIN.
See: Glutamic Acid HCl. (Various Mfr.).

ACI-JEL. (Ortho) Glacial acetic acid 0.92%, ricinoleic acid 0.7%, oxyquinoline sulfate 0.025%, glycerin 5%. Tube 85 Gm w/dose applicator.
Use: Vaginal preparation.

ACINITRAZOLE. B.A.N. 2-Acetamido-5-nitrothiazole, Aminitrozole (I.N.N.).
Use: Treatment of trichomoniasis.
See: Trichorad.
Tritheon.

• **ACITRETIN.** USAN.
Use: Antipsoriatic.

• **ACIVICIN.** USAN.
Use: Antineoplastic.

• **ACLARUBICIN.** USAN.
Use: Antineoplastic.

ACLOPHEN. (Nutripharm) Phenylephrine HCl 40 mg, chlorpheniramine maleate 8 mg, acetaminophen 500 mg/S. R. tab. Dye free. Bot. 100s.
Use: Decongestant, antihistamine, analgesic.

ACLOVATE. (Glaxo) Alclometasone dipropionate 0.05%. Cream or Oint. Tube 15 Gm, 45 Gm.
Use: Anti-inflammatory, topical.

A.C.N. (Person & Covey) Vitamin A 25,000 IU, ascorbic acid 250 mg, niacinamide 25 mg/Tab. Bot. 100s.

Use: Vitamin supplement.
ACNAVEEN. (CooperCare)
See: Aveenobar Medicated (Cooper-Care).
ACNA-VITE. (Cenci) Vitamins A 10,000 IU, C 250 mg, hesperidin 50 mg, niacinamide 25 mg/Cap. Bot. 75s.
Use: Anti-acne, Vitamin supplement.
ACNE-5. (Goldline) Benzoyl peroxide 5%. Bot. oz.
Use: Anti-Acne.
ACNE-10. (Various Mfr.) Benzoyl peroxide 10%. Bot. 30 ml.
Use: Anti-Acne.
ACNE-AID CLEANSING BAR. (Stiefel) Neutral soap of 6.3% surfactant blend. Non-medicated. Bar 112 Gm, 174 Gm.
Use: Skin cleanser.
ACNE-AID CREAM. (Stiefel) Benzoyl peroxide 10%. Tube 54 Gm.
Use: Anti-acne.
ACNEDERM. (Lannett) **Lot.:** Dispersable sulfur 5%, zinc sulfate 1%, zinc oxide 10%, isopropyl alcohol 21%. Bot. 60 ml. **Soap:** Zinc oxide 2%, zinc sulfate 1%, colloidal sulfur 5%. Cake 3.2 oz.
Use: Anti-acne.
ACNE LOTION. (Weeks & Leo) Benzoyl peroxide 10% in odorless, greaseless, vanishing lotion. Bot. 2 oz.
Use: Anti-acne.
ACNO CLEANSER. (Baker/Cummins) Isopropyl alcohol 60%, laureth-23, tetrasodium EDTA. Bot. 240 ml.
Use: Anti-acne.
ACNO LOTION. (Baker/Cummins) Micronized sulfur 3%, salicylic acid 2%. Bot. 120 ml.
Use: Anti-acne.
ACNOMEL. (SK-Beecham) Resorcinol 2%, sulfur 8%, alcohol 11%. Cream Tube 28 Gm.
Use: Anti-acne.
ACNOTEX. (C & M Pharmacal) Sulfur 8%, salicylic acid 2.25%, isopropyl alcohol 22%, acetone. In lotion base. Bot. 60 ml.
Use: Anti-acne.
• **ACODAZOLE HYDROCHLORIDE.** USAN.
Use: Antineoplastic.
ACONIAZIDE. USAN.
Use: Antituberculous agent. [Orphan drug]
ACOTUS. (Whorton) Phenylephrine HCl 5 mg, guaiacol glyceryl ether 100 mg, menthol 1 mg, alcohol by volume 10%/5 ml. Bot. 4 oz, 12 oz, gal.
Use: Decongestant, antitussive.
ACR. (Western Research) Ammonium Cl

7.5 gr/Tab. Handicount 28s (36 bags of 28 tab.).
Use: Diuretic.
ACRIFLAVINE. Euflavine, Gonacrine, Neutroflavine Acriflavine neutral; a mixture of 2, 8-diamino-10-methylacridinium Cl and 2,8-diaminoacridine. (Lilly) Tab. 1.5 gr. Bot. 100s.
Use: Antiseptic.
ACRIFLAVINE HYDROCHLORIDE. (Various Mfr.) Hydrochloride form of acriflavine. Acid acriflavine, acid trypaflavine, flavine, trypaflavine.
National Aniline-Pow., Bot. (1 Gm, 5 Gm, 10 Gm, 25 Gm, 50 Gm). Tab. (1.5 gr). Bot. 50s, 100s.
Use: Antibacterial.
• **ACRISORCIN,** U.S.P. XXII.
Use: Antifungal.
• **ACRIVASTINE.** USAN.
Use: Antihistamine.
• **ACRONINE.** USAN. 3, 12-Dihydro-6-methoxy-3,3,12-trimethyl-7H-pyrano[2,3,-c]acridin-7-one. Under study.
Use: Antineoplastic.
ACT. Dactinomycin, U.S.P. XXIII.
Use: Antineoplastic.
See: Actinomycin D.
ACT. (J & J) **Rinse:** 0.02% (from 0.05% sodium fluoride). **Mint:** Tartrazine, alcohol 8%. **Cinnamon:** Alcohol 7%. Bot. 360 ml, 480 ml.
Use: Dental Rinse.
A-C TABLET. (Century) Aspirin 6 gr, caffeine 0.5 gr/Tab. Bot. 100s, 1000s.
Use: Salicylate analgesic.
ACTACIN TABLETS. (Vangard) Triprolidine HCl 2.5 mg, pseudoephedrine HCl 60 mg/Tab. Bot. 100s, 1000s.
Use: Antihistamine, decongestant.
ACTACIN-C SYRUP. (Vangard) Codeine phosphate 10 mg, triprolidine HCl 2 mg, pseudoephedrine HCl 20 mg, guaifenesin 100 mg/ 5 ml. Bot. pt, gal.
Use: Antitussive, antihistamine, decongestant, expectorant.
ACTAGEN SYRUP. (Goldline) Triprolidine HCl 1.25 mg, pseudoephedrine HCl 30 mg/5 ml. Bot. 120 ml, pt, gal.
Use: Antihistamine, decongestant.
ACTAGEN TABLETS. (Goldline) Triprolidine HCl 2.5 mg, pseudoephedrine HCl 60 mg/Tab. Bot. 100s, 1000s.
Use: Antihistamine, decongestant.
ACTAGEN-C COUGH SYRUP. (Goldline) Triprolidine HCl 1.25 mg, pseudoephedrine HCl 30 mg, codeine phosphate 10 mg/5 ml, alcohol 4.3%. Bot. 120 ml, pt, gal.

Use: Antihistamine, decongestant, anti-
tussive.
ACTAL SUSPENSION. (Sanofi Winthrop)
Aluminum hydroxide.
Use: Antacid.
ACTAL PLUS TABLETS. (Sanofi
Winthrop) Aluminum hydroxide, magne-
sium hydroxide.
Use: Antacid.
ACTAL TABLETS. (Sanofi Winthrop) Alu-
minum hydroxide.
Use: Antacid.
ACTAMIN. (Buffington) Acetaminophen
325 mg/Tab. Dispens-A-Kit 100s, 200s,
500s.
Use: Analgesic.
ACTAMIN EXTRA. (Buffington) Aceta-
minophen 500 mg/Tab. Bot. 100s, 200s,
500s.
Use: Analgesic.
ACTAMIN SUPER. (Buffington) Aceta-
minophen 500 mg, caffeine. Sugar, salt,
and lactose free. Tab. Dispens-A-Kit
500s, Medipak 200s.
Use: Analgesic.
ACTAMINE. (H. L. Moore) **Tab.:** Pseu-
doephedrine HCl 60 mg, triprolidine HCl
2.5 mg. Bot. 100s, 1000s. **Syr.:** Pseu-
doephedrine HCl 30 mg, triprolidine HCl
1.25 mg/5 ml. Bot. 120 ml, pt, gal.
Use: Decongestant, antihistamine.
• **ACTAPLANIN.** USAN.
Use: Growth stimulant.
ACTH-ACTEST GEL. (Forest) Repository
corticotropin 40 units or 80 units/ml. Vial
5 ml.
Use: Corticosteroid.
ACTH. Adrenocorticotropic hormone.
Adrenocorticotropin.
Use: Corticosteroid.
See: Corticotropin, U.S.P.
   Hauck (40 units/ml, 5 ml).
   Forest (40 units or 80 units/ml, 5 ml).
   Parke-Davis (25 units/vial; 40
   units/vial).
   Pharmex (40 units or 80 units/ml, 5
   ml).
ACTH GEL, PURIFIED. (Arcum) 40 or 80
units/ml, vial 5 ml. (Conal) 40 or 80
units/ml, vial 5 ml. (Hart Labs.) 40
units/ml, vial 5 ml. (Bowman) Adrenocor-
ticotropic hormone 40 units, aqueous
gelatin 16%, phenol 0.5%/ml. Vial 5 ml.
Use: Repository corticotropin.
   (Arcum) 40 or 80 units/ml, 5 ml.
   (Bell) 40 or 80 units/ml, 5 ml.
   (Bowman) 40 units/ml, 5 ml.
   (Hyrex) 40 or 80 units/ml, 5 ml.
   (Jenkins) 40 or 80 units/ml, 5 ml.
   (Wesley Pharm.) 40 or 80 units/ml, vial

5 ml.
   (Wyeth-Ayerst) 40 or 80 units/ml or
   Tubex.
ACTHAR. (Armour) Corticotropin for inj.
Vial 25 units, 40 units/vial. (Lyophilized
w/gelatin).
Use: Corticosteroid.
ACTICORT 100 LOTION. (Baker/Cum-
mins) Hydrocortisone 1%. Bot. 60 ml.
Use: Corticosteroid, topical.
ACTIDIL. (Burroughs Wellcome) Triproli-
dine HCl. **Tab.:** 2.5 mg. Bot. 100s. **Syr.:**
1.25 mg/5 ml. Bot. pt.
Use: Antihistamine.
ACTIDOSE. (Paddock) Activated char-
coal. Soln. 25 Gm/120 ml or 50 Gm/240
ml.
Use: Antidote.
ACTIDOSE-AQUA. (Paddock) Activated
charcoal. Aqueous susp. 25 Gm/120 ml
or 50 Gm/240 ml.
Use: Antidote.
ACTIDOSE W/SORBITOL. (Paddock)
Activated charcoal. Liq: 25 Gm in 120 ml
susp. w/sorbitol, 50 Gm in 240 ml susp.
w/sorbitol.
Use: Antidote.
ACTIFED. (Burroughs Wellcome) **Tab.:**
Triprolidine HCl 2.5 mg, pseudoephedrine HCl 60 mg/Tab. Bot. 100s,
1000s, Box 12s, 24s, UD pack 100s.
Cap.: Triprolidine HCl 2.5 mg, pseudoephedrine HCl 60 mg/Cap. Box 10s,
20s. **Syr.:** Triprolidine HCl 1.25 mg,
pseudoephedrine HCl 30 mg/5 ml. Bot.
120 ml, pt.
Use: Antihistamine, decongestant.
ACTIFED ALLERGY. (Burroughs Wellcome) **Daytime:** Pseudoephedrine 30
mg; **Nighttime:** Pseudoephedrine 30
mg, diphenhydramine HCl 25 mg/ Capl.
Pkg. 24 daytime, 8 nighttime.
Use: Decongestant, antihistamine.
ACTIFED 12-HOUR CAPSULES. (Burroughs Wellcome) Triprolidine HCl 5 mg,
pseudoephedrine HCl 120 mg/Cap. Box
10s, 20s.
Use: Antihistamine, decongestant.
ACTIFED PLUS. (Burroughs Wellcome)
Pseudoephedrine HCl 30 mg, triprolidine HCl 1.25 mg, acetaminophen 500
mg/Tab. or Cap. Bot. 20s, 40s.
Use: Decongestant, antihistamine,
analgesic.
ACTIFED SINUS. (Burroughs Wellcome)
Daytime: Pseudoephedrine HCl 30 mg,
acetaminophen 325 mg/Capl. pk. 18s.
Nighttime: Pseudoephedrine HCl 30
mg, diphenhydramine HCl 25 mg. Capl.
pk. 6s.

Use: Decongestant, antihistamine, analgesic.

ACTIFED WITH CODEINE COUGH SYRUP. (Burroughs Wellcome) Codeine phosphate 10 mg, triprolidine HCl 1.25 mg, pseudoephedrine HCl 30 mg/5 ml, alcohol 4.3%. Bot. pt, gal. *Use:* Antitussive, antihistamine, decongestant.

ACTIGALL. (Ciba) Ursodiol (Ursodeoxycholic acid) 300 mg/Cap. Bot. 100s. *Use:* Gallstone solubilizing agent.

ACTIMMUNE. (Genentech) Inteferon gamma-1b 100 mcg (3 million units)/vial. *Use:* Treatment of infections associated with chronic granulomatous disease.

ACTINEX. (Reed & Carnrick) Masoprocol 10%, isostearyl and stearyl alcohol, light mineral oil, parabens, polyethylene glycol 400, propylene glycol and sodium metabisulfate. Cream, Tube 30 Gm. *Use:* Topical drugs, miscellaneous.

ACTINOMYCIN. B.A.N. Antimicrobial substances with antitumor activity produced by *Streptomyces antibioticus* and *Streptomyces chrysomallus.* *Use:* Antineoplastic.

ACTINOMYCIN C. Name previously used for Cactinomycin.

ACTINOMYCIN D. Dactinomycin, U.S.P. XXIII. *Use:* Antineoplastic. *See:* Cosmegen (Merck & Co.).

• **ACTINOQUINOL SODIUM.** USAN. *Use:* Ultraviolet screen.

ACTINOSPECTOCIN. Name previously used for Spectinomycin.

• **ACTISOMIDE.** USAN. *Use:* Cardiac depressant (anti-arrhythmic).

ACTIVASE. (Genentech) Alteplase recombinant. Inj. Vial 20 mg, 50 mg. *Use:* Thrombolytic enzyme.

ACTIVATED ATTAPULGITE. W/Aluminum hydroxide, magnesium carbonate coprecipitate, compressed gel. *See:* Hykasil, Cream (Philips Roxane). W/Polysorbate 80, colloidal sulfur, salicylic acid, propylene glycol. *Use:* Anti-Acne. *See:* Sebasorb Lotion (Summers Labs.).

ACTIVATED CHARCOAL TABLETS. (Cowley) 5 gr/Tab. Bot. 1000s. *Use:* Antidote.

ACTIVATED 7-DEHYDROCHOLESTEROL. *See:* Vitamin D-3 (Various Mfr.).

ACTIVATED ERGOSTEROL. *See:* Calciferol.

• **ACTODIGIN.** USAN. *Use:* Cardiotonic.

ACTOQUINOL SODIUM. 8-Ethoxy-5-quinoline-sulfonic acid sodium salt. *Use:* Ultraviolet screen.

ACTYLATE. (Kinney) Ammonium salicylate 80 mg, potassium salicylate 80 mg, strontium salicylate 80 mg, potassium para-aminobenzoate 0.32 Gm, ascorbic acid 20 mg/Tab. Bot. 100s. *Use:* Rheumatoid arthritis.

ACUCRON. (Seatrace) Acetaminophen 300 mg, salicylamide 200 mg, phenyltoloxamine 20 mg/Tab. Bot. 100s, 1000s, 5000s. *Use:* Analgesic, antihistamine.

ACU-DYNE. (Acme-United) **Douche:** Povidone-iodine. Pkt. 195 ml. **Oint.:** Povidone-iodine. Jar. lb. Pkt. 1.2, 2.7 (100s). **Perineal wash conc:** Available iodine 1%. Bot. 40 ml. **Prep. Soln.:** Povidone-iodine. Bot. 240 ml, pt, qt, gal. Pkt. 30 ml, 60 ml. **Skin Cleanser:** Povidone-iodine. Bot. 60 ml, 240 ml, pt, qt, gal. **Soln, prep. swabs:** Available iodine 1%. Bot. 100s. **Soln, swabsticks:** Povidone-iodine. Pkt. 1 or 3 in 25s. **Whirlpool conc:** Available iodine 1%. Bot. gal. *Use:* Antiseptic, germicide.

ACULAR. (Allergan) Ketorolac tromethamine 0.5% Ophth. Soln. Drop. Bot. 5 ml. *Use:* Nonsteroidal anti-inflammatory agent.

ACUTRIM LATE DAY. (Ciba Consumer) Phenylpropanolamine HCl 75 mg./Tab., precision release Bot. 20s. *Use:* Diet aid.

ACUTRIM MAXIMUM STRENGTH. (Ciba Consumer) Phenylpropanolamine HCl 75 mg./Tab., precision release Bot. 20s, 40s. *Use:* Nonprescription diet aid.

ACUTRIM II MAXIMUM STRENGTH. (Ciba) Phenylpropanolamine HCl 75 mg/Tab. precision release, Bot. 20s, 40s. *Use:* Nonprescription diet aid.

ACUTRIM 16 HOUR. (Ciba Consumer) Phenylpropanolamine HCl 75 mg/Tab., precision release. Bot. 20s, 40s. *Use:* Diet aid.

• **ACYCLOVIR.** U.S.P. XXIII. 9-(2-hydroxyethoxymethyl)-guanine. *Use:* Antiviral. *See:* Zovirax Cap., Oint., Tab. (Burroughs Wellcome).

• **ACYCLOVIR SODIUM.** USAN. *Use:* Antiviral.

ACYLPYRIN.
See: Aspirin.
ADAGEN. (Enzon) Pegademase bovine 250 units/ml. Vial 1.5 ml.
Use: Enzyme (ADA) replacement therapy.
ADALAN LANATABS. (Lannett) Amobarbital 50 mg, homatropine methylbromide 7.5 mg, methamphetamine HCl 10 mg/T.D. Tab. Bot. 100s, 1000s.
Use: Sedative/hypnotic, cycloplegic mydriatic, CNS stimulant.
ADALAT. (Miles Pharm) Nifedipine 10 mg or 20 mg/Cap. Bot. 100s, 300s. UD 100s.
Use: Calcium channel blocking agent.
ADALAT CC. (Miles Pharm.) Nifedipine 30 mg, 60 mg or 90 mg. ER Tab. Bot. 100s, 1000s.
Use: Calcium channel blocking agent.
ADAMANTANAMINE HYDROCHLORIDE. Amantadine HCl. Anti-flu capsule. This drug is thought to protect cells against entry of the flu virus without actually destroying the virus. Also used in the treatment of Parkinson's disease.
See: Symmetrel, Cap., Syr. (Du Pont).
• **ADAPALENE.** USAN.
Use: Antiacne.
ADAPETTES FOR SENSITIVE EYES. (Alcon) EDTA 0.1%, sorbic acid 0.1% Pkg. 15 ml.
Use: Contact lens care.
ADAPIN. (Lotus) Doxepin HCl **10 mg, 75 mg, 100 mg:** Cap. Bot. 100s, 1000s, UD 100s; **25 mg, 50 mg:** Cap. Bot. 100s, 1000s, 5000s, UD 100s; **150 mg:** Cap. Bot. 50s, 100s.
Use: Antidepressant.
• **ADAPROLOL MALEATE.** USAN.
Use: Antihypertensive (β-blocker, ophthalmic).
ADAPT. (Alcon) Povidone, EDTA 0.1%, thimerosal 0.004%. Bot. 15 ml.
Use: Contact lens care.
ADAPT WETTING SOLUTION. (Alcon) Adsorbobase with thimerosol 0.004%, EDTA 0.1%. Soln. Bot. 15 ml.
Use: Hard contact lens care.
• **ADATANSERIN HYDROCHLORIDE** USAN
Use: Anxiolytic, antidepressant.
ADAVITE. (Hudson) Vitamins A 5,000 IU, D 400 IU, E 30 mg, B_1 3 mg, B_2 3.4 mg, B_3 30 mg, B_5 10 mg, B_6 3 mg, B_{12} 9 mcg, C 90 mg, FA 0.4 mg, biotin 35 mcg, beta carotene 1250 IU/Tab. Bot. 100s.
Use: Vitamin/mineral supplement.
ADAVITE. (Nature's Bounty) Vitamins A

5,500 IU, D 400 IU, E 30 mg, B_1 3 mg, B_2 3.4 mg, B_3 30 mg, B_5 10 mg, B_6 3 mg, B_{12} 9 mcg, C 120 mg, folic acid 0.4 mg, biotin 15 mcg. Tab. Bot. 100s.
Use: Vitamin supplement.
ADAVITE-M. (Nature's Bounty) Iron 27 mg, Vitamins A 5,500 IU, D 400 IU, E 30 mg, B_1 3 mg, B_2 3.4 mg, B_3 30 mg, B_5 10 mg, B_6 3 mg, B_{12} 9 mcg, C 120 mg, folic acid 0.4 mg, Cl, Cr, Cu, I, K, Mg, Mn, Mo, Se, Zinc 15 mg, biotin 15 mcg Tab. Bot. 130s.
Use: Vitamin/mineral supplement.
ADC WITH FLUORIDE. (Major) Vitamins A, D and C with fluoride. Dropper bot. 50 ml.
Use: Vitamin/mineral supplement.
ADEECON. (CMC) Vitamins A 5,000 IU, D 1000 IU/Cap. Bot. 1000s.
Use: Vitamin supplement.
ADEFLOR M TABLETS. (Upjohn) Vitamins A 6,000 IU, D 400 IU, B_1 1.5 mg, B_2 2.5 mg, C 100 mg, B_3 20 mg, B_5 10 mg, B_6 10 mg, B_{12} 2 mcg, folic acid 0.1 mg, fluoride 1 mg, calcium 250 mg, iron 30 mg/Tab. Bot. 100s, 500s.
Use: Vitamin supplement, dental caries preventative.
ADEKS. (Scandipharm) Vitamins A 4,000 IU, D 400 IU, E 150 IU, K 150 mcg, C 60 mg, B_1 1.2 mg, B_2 1.3 mg, B_3 10 mg, B_6 1.5 mg, B_{12} 12 mcg, B_6 10 mg, folic acid 0.2 mg, biotin 50 mcg, beta carotene 3 mg, Zn, fructose, sorbitol. Tab. Bot. 60s, 100s.
Use: Vitamin/mineral supplement.
• **ADENINE, U.S.P. XXIII.** 6 Aminopurine.
ADENO TWELVE GEL INJECTION. (Forest Pharm) Adenosine-5-monophosphate 25 mg, methionine 25 mg, niacin 10 mg/ml. Vial 10 ml.
Use: Arthritis, bursitis, tendinitis and other degenerative diseases.
ADENOCARD. (Lyphomed) Adenosine 6 mg/2 ml. Inj. Vial 2 ml.
Use: Antiarrhythmic.
ADENOCREST. (Nutrition) Adenosine-5-monophosphate sodium 25 mg, nicotinic acid as sodium salt 25 mg, gelatin 100 mg, benzyl alcohol 1.5%/ml. Vial 10 ml.
Use: Capillary and arterial vasodilator.
ADENOLIN FORTE. (Lincoln) Adenosine-5-monophosphate 25 mg, methionine 25 mg, niacin 10 mg/ml. Vial 15 ml.
Use: Arthritis, bursitis, tendinitis and other degenerative diseases.
ADENOSINE. (Medco Research)
Use: Treatment of brain tumors. [Orphan drug]
• **ADENOSINE.** USAN. 6-Amino-9-beta-D-

Ribofuranosyl-9H-purine.
Use: Antiarrhythmic.
See: Adenocard (Lyphomed).
ADENOSINE IN GELATIN. (Forest
Pharm) **Forte:** Adenosine-5-monophos-
phate 50 mg/ml. **Super:** Adenosine-5-
monophosphate 100 mg/ml.
Use: Treatment of various vein compli
cations.
**ADENOSINE-5-MONOPHOSPHATE AS
THE SODIUM SALT.**
See: Adenocrest, Amp. (Nutrition).
• **ADENOSINE PHOSPHATE.** USAN. 5-
Adenylic acid. B.A.N. Adenosine-5′-(di-
hydrogen phosphate). Adenosine
monophosphate, AMP.
Use: Nutrient.
See: Cobalasine, Inj. (Keene).
My-B-Den (Miles Pharm).
ADEPSINE OIL.
See: Petrolatum Liquid (Various Mfr.).
ADEQUATE IMPROVED. (Ortega) Calci-
um 125 mg, iron 65 mg, Vitamins A
6,000 IU, D 400 IU, E 25 mg, B_1 1.1 mg,
B_2 1.8 mg, B_3 15 mg, B_6 2.5 mg, B_{12} 5
mcg, C 60 mg, folic acid 1 mg/Tab. Bot.
100s.
Use: Vitamin/mineral supplement.
ADICILLIN. B.A.N. 6-[D(+)-5-Amino-5-
carboxy-valeramido]penicillanic acid.
Penicillin N.
Use: Antibiotic.
• **ADINAZOLAM.** USAN.
Use: Antidepressant, sedative.
• **ADINAZOLAM MESYLATE.** USAN.
Use: Antidepressant, sedative.
ADIPEX-P. (Lemmon) **Cap.:** Phentermine
HCl 37.5 mg. Bot. 100s, 400s. **Tab.:**
Phentermine HCl 37.5 mg. Bot. 100s,
400s, 1000s.
Use: Anorexiant.
• **ADIPHENINE HYDROCHLORIDE.**
USAN. 2-Diethylaminoethyl diphenylac-
etate hydrochloride.
Use: Antispasmodic.
ADIPOST. (Ascher) Phendimetrazine tar-
trate 105 mg/S.R. Cap. Bot. 100s.
Use: Anorexiant.
ADISOL TAB. (Major) Disulfiram **250
mg/Tab:** Bot. 100s. **500 mg/Tab:** Bot.
50s.
Use: Antialcoholic agent.
ADLERIKA. (Last) Magnesium sulfate 4
Gm/15 ml. Bot. 12 oz.
Use: Laxative.
ADLONE. (UAD) Methylprednisolone ac-
etate 40 mg, 80 mg. Vial 5 ml.
Use: Glucocorticoid.
ADOLPH'S SALT SUBSTITUTE.
(Adolph's) Potassium Cl 2480 mg/5 Gm,

silicon dioxide, tartaric acid. Gran. Bot.
99.2 Gm.
Use: Salt substitute.
**ADOLPH'S SEASONED SALT SUBSTI-
TUTE.** (Adolph's) Potassium Cl 1360
mg/5 Gm, silicon dioxide, tartaric acid.
Gran. Bot. 92.1 Gm.
Use: Salt substitute.
ADONIDINE. (City Chem.) Bot. Gm.
Use: Cardiac stimulant.
• **ADOZELESIN.** USAN.
Use: Antineoplastic.
ADR.
Use: Antineoplastic agent.
See: Doxorubicin HCl.
ADRENALIN(E).
See: Epinephrine. (Various Mfr.).
ADRENALIN CHLORIDE SOLUTION.
(Parke-Davis) Epinephrine HCl. Princi-
ple of the medullary portion of
suprarenal glands. **Amp:** 1:1000-1 ml
Epinephrine 1 mg/ml with not more than
0.1% sodium bisulfite as antioxidant.
Amp. 10s. **Steri-Vial 1:1000:** Epineph-
rine 100 mg/ml in isotonic sodium Cl so-
lution with 0.5% chlorobutanol as
preservative and not more than 0.15%
sodium bisulfite as antioxidant. Vial 30
ml. **Soln. 1:1000:** Bot. 30 ml. (Same as
Steri-Vial). **Soln. 1:100:** Each 100 ml
contains 1 Gm epinephrine HCl dissolved in sodium Cl citrate buffer soln
w/phemerol Cl 0.2 mg/ml as preserva-
tive, sodium bisulfite 0.2% as antioxi-
dant. Bot. 0.25 oz.
Use: Sympathomimetic agent.
ADRENALINE HYDROCHLORIDE.
See: Epinephrine Hydrochloride. (Vari-
ous Mfr.).
• **ADRENALONE.** USAN. 3′,4-Dihydroxy-
2-(methylamino)-acetophenone.
Use: Adrenergic (ophthalmic).
ADRENAMINE.
See: Epinephrine (Various Mfr.).
ADRENERGIC AGENTS.
See: Sympathomimetic agents.
ADRENERGIC-BLOCKING AGENTS.
See: Sympatholytic agents.
ADRENINE.
See: Epinephrine (Various Mfr.).
ADRENOCHROMAZONE.
See: Carbazochrome Salicylate.
ADRENOCHROME.
See: Carbazochrome Salicylate.
**ADRENOCHROME MONOSEMICAR-
BAZONE.**
See: Carbazochrome Salicylate.
ADRENOCORTICOTROPIC HORMONE.
ACTH acts by stimulating the endoge-
nous production of cortisone and the fi-

nal result is similar whichever substance is administered. The nature of action of each is unknown. Both are necessary in the metabolism of carbohydrates, protein and fat. They exert profound effects on neuromuscular metabolism.
See: ACTH gel, Inj. (Bowman).
Corticotropin, U.S.P.
Cortigel (Savage).
ADRENOMIST INHALANT AND NEBU-LIZERS. (Nephron) Epinephrine 1%, Bot. 0.5 oz, 1.25 oz.
Use: Bronchodilator.
ADRENUCLEO. (Enzyme Process) Vitamin C 250 mg, d-calcium pantothenate 12.5 mg, bioflavonoids 62.5 mg/Tab. Bot. 100s, 250s.
Use: Vitamin C supplement.
ADRIAMYCIN. (Adria) Doxorubicin HCl 20 mg/vial.
Use: Antineoplastic agent.
ADRIAMYCIN PFS. (Adria) Doxorubicin HCl 2 mg/ml. Inj. Vial: 5 ml, 10 ml, 25 ml.
Use: Antineoplastic agent.
ADRIAMYCIN RDF. (Adria) Doxorubicin HCl. **10 mg:** Methylparaben 1 mg, lactose 50 mg/Vial. Pkg. 10s. **20 mg:** Methylparaben 2 mg, lactose 100 mg/Vial. Pkg. 5s. **50 mg:** Methylparaben 5 mg, lactose 250 mg/Vial. Ctn. 1o. **150 mg:** Methylparaben 15 mg, lactose 750 mg/multi-dose vial. Rapid dissolution formula.
Use: Antineoplastic agent.
ADRIN TABS. (Major) Nylidrin 6 mg or 12 mg/Tab. Bot. 100s, 1000s.
Use: Vasodilator.
ADRUCIL. (Adria) Fluorouracil 50 mg/10 ml. Amp. 10 ml.
Use: Antineoplastic agent.
ADSORBOCARPINE. (Alcon) Pilocarpine HCl 1%, 2% or 4% in adsorbobase, water polymers, polyvinylpyrrolidone. Vial 15 ml.
Use: Miotic.
ADSORBONAC OPHTH. SOLUTION. (Alcon) Sodium Cl 2% or 5% in vehicle of polyvinylpyrrolidone, water-soluble polymers, EDTA 0.1%, thimerosal 0.004%. Dropper Vial 15 ml.
Use: Hyperosmolar preparation.
ADSORBOTEAR. (Alcon) Hydroxyethylcellulose 0.4%, povidone 1.67%, water-soluble polymers, thimerosal 0.004%, EDTA 0.1%. Soln. Bot. dropper 15 ml.
Use: Artificial tears solution.
ADVANCE. (Ross) **Ready-to-Feed infant formula:** (16 cal/fl oz). Can 13 fl oz.
Conc. liq: 32 fl oz.
Use: Enteral nutritional supplement.

ADVANCE FORMULA CENTRUM. (Lederle) Vitamins A 2500 IU, E 30 IU, C 60 mg, B_1 1.5 mg, B_2 1.7 mg, B_3 20 mg, B_5 10 mg, B_6 2 mg, B_{12} 6 mcg, D_2 400 IU, iron 9 mg, biotin 300 mcg, I, Zn, Mn, Cr, Mo/Tab. Bot. 236 ml.
Use: Vitamin/mineral supplement.
ADVANCE PREGNANCY TEST. (Advanced Care) Can be used as early as 3 days after a missed period. Gives results in 30 min. Test kit 1s.
Use: Diagnostic aid.
ADVANCED CARE CHOLESTEROL TEST. (Johnson & Johnson)
Use: At home cholesterol test.
ADVANCED FORMULA TEGRIN. (Block) Coal tar solution USP 7%, alcohol 7%, hydroxypropyl methylcellulose, parabens. Shampoo. Bot. 207 ml.
Use: Antiseborrheic.
ADVIL. (Whitehall) Ibuprofen 200 mg/Tab or Capl. In 8s, 24s, 50s, 100s, 165s, 250s (Tab.).
Use: Nonsteroidal anti-inflammatory drug; analgesic.
ADVIL, CHILDREN'S. (Whitehall) Ibuprofen Susp. 100 mg per 5 ml. Fruit flavor. Liq. Bot. 199 ml, 473 ml.
Use: Nonsteroidal anti-inflammatory drug; analgesic.
ADVIL COLD & SINUS. (Whitehall) Pseudoephedrine HCl 30 mg, ibuprofen 200 mg/Tab. Pkg. 20s. Bot. 48s, 100s.
Use: Decongestant, analgesic.
A.E.R. (Birchwood) Hamamelis water (witch hazel) 50%, glycerin 12.5%, methylparaben, benzalkonium chloride. Pads Jar 40s.
Use: Topical drug, miscellaneous.
AERDIL. (Econo Med) Triprolidine HCl 1.25 mg, pseudoephedrine HCl 30 mg/5 ml. Bot. pt, gal.
Use: Antihistamine, decongestant.
AEROAID. (Graham-Field) Thimerosal 1:1000, alcohol 72%. Spray bot 90 ml.
Use: Antiseptic.
AEROAID MERTHIOLATE. (Health & Medical Techniques) Merthiolate (Lilly) 1:1000, alcohol 72%. Spray bot. 3 oz.
Use: Antiseptic.
AEROBID. (Forest) Flunisolide in an inhaler system. Canister 7 Gm, 100 metered inhalations.
Use: Bronchodilator.
AEROBID M. (Forest) Flunisolide in an inhaler system. Canister 7 Gm, 100 metered inhalations. Menthol flavor.
Use: Bronchodilator.
AEROCAINE. (Health & Medical Techniques) Benzocaine 13.6%, benzethoni-

um Cl 0.5%. Spray bot. 0.5 oz, 2.5 oz.
Use: Local anesthetic.

AEROCELL. (Health & Medical Techniques) Exfoliative cytology fixative spray. Bot. 3.5 oz.
Use: Exfoliative cytology fixative spray.

AERODINE. (Health & Medical Techniques) Povidone-Iodine. Bot. 3 oz.
Use: Antiseptic.

AEROFREEZE. (Health & Medical Techniques) Trichloromonofluoromethane and dichlorodifluoromethane. Aerosol cont. 8 oz. (12s).
Use: Local anesthetic.

AEROLATE-III. (Fleming) Theophylline 65 mg/T.D. Cap. Bot. 100s, 1000s.
Use: Bronchodilator.

AEROLATE SR. & JR. (Fleming) **Cap.:** Theophylline 4 gr for Sr., 2 gr for Jr./Cap. Bot. 100s, 1000s. **Syr.:** 160 mg/15 ml. Bot. pt, gal.
Use: Bronchodilator.

AEROPENT. (Fisons) USAN.
Use: Antibacterial.

AEROPIN.
Use: Cystic fibrosis.
See: Heparin, 2-0-desulfated.

AEROPURE. (Health & Medical Techniques) Isopropanol 7.8%, triethylene glycol 3.9%, essential oils 3%, methyldodecyl benzyl trimethyl ammonium Cl 0.12%, methyldodecylxylene bis (trimethyl ammonium Cl) 0.03%, inert ingredients, 85.15%. Bot. 0.8 oz, 4.5 oz.
Use: Air sanitizer, deodorizer.

AEROSAN. (Ulmer) Aerosol 16.6 oz.
Use: Air sanitizer, deodorizer.

AEROSEB-DEX. (Herbert) Dexamethasone 0.01%, alcohol 65.1%. Aerosol 58 Gm.
Use: Corticosteroid, topical.

AEROSEB-HC. (Herbert) Hydrocortisone 0.5%, alcohol 64.6%. Aerosol 58 Gm.
Use: Corticosteroid, topical.

AEROSEPT. (Dalin) Lidocaine, cetyltrimethylammonium bromide, hexachlorophene. Aerosol 6 oz.
Use: Anesthetic, antiseptic.

AEROSIL. (Health & Medical Techniques) Dimethylpolysiloxane. Bot. 4.5 oz.
Use: Silicone lubricant, protectant.

AEROSOL OT.
See: Docusate Sodium, U.S.P.

AEROSOLV. (Health & Medical Techniques) Isopropyl alcohol, methylene Cl, silicone. Aerosol 5.5 oz.
Use: Adhesive tape remover.

AEROSPORIN STERILE POWDER.
(Burroughs Wellcome) Polymyxin B sulfate 500,000 units/vial. Multidose vial 20

ml.
Use: Antibacterial.

AEROSPORIN SULFATE. (Burroughs Wellcome) Polymyxin B sulfate 50 mg, 500,000 units. **Pow.:** Vial 20 ml. **Otic Soln.:** Bot. 10 ml.
Use: Antibacterial.
See: Polymyxin B sulfate, U.S.P.
W/Bacitracin.
See: Polysporin, Oint. (Burroughs Wellcome).
W/Bacitracin and neomycin sulfate.
See: Neosporin, Oint. and Ophth. Oint. (Burroughs Wellcome).
W/Bacitracin, neomycin, hydrocortisone.
See: Cortisporin, Prep. (Burroughs Wellcome).

AEROTHERM. (Health & Medical Techniques) Benzethonium Cl 0.5%, benzocaine 13.6%. Spray bot. 5 oz.
Use: Local anesthetic.

AEROZOIN. (Health & Medical Techniques) Comp. tr. of benzoin 30%, isopropyl alcohol 44.8%. Spray bot. 3.5 oz.
Use: Skin protectant.

AETHYLIS CHLORIDIUM.
See: Ethyl Cl (Various Mfr.).

AFAXIN CAPSULES. (Sanofi Winthrop) Vitamin A Palmitate 10,000 IU or 50,000 IU/Cap.
Use: Vitamin A supplement.

A-FIL. (GenDerm) Methyl anthranilate 5%, titanium dioxide 5% in vanishing cream base. Tube 45 Gm. Neutral or dark.
Use: Sunscreen.

AFKO-LUBE. (APC) Docusate sodium 100 mg/Cap. Bot. 100s.
Use: Laxative.

AFKO-LUBE LAX. (APC) Docusate sodium 100 mg, casanthranol 30 mg/Cap. Bot. 100s.
Use: Laxative.

AFRIKOL. (Citroleum) Bot. 4 oz.
Use: Sunscreen.

AFRIN. (Schering) Oxymetazoline HCl 0.05%. **Nose Drops:** Drop. Bot. 20 ml. **Nasal Spray:** Reg.: Bot. 15 ml, 30 ml; Menthol: Bot. 15 ml. **Pediatric Nose Drops:** Oxymetazoline HCl 0.025%. Drop. Bot. 20 ml.
Use: Decongestant.

AFRINOL REPETABS. (Schering) Pseudoephedrine sulfate 120 mg/Repeat Action Tab. Box 12s. Bot. 100s, dispensary pack 48s.
Use: Decongestant.

AFTATE. (Plough) Tolnaftate 1%. **Gel:** Tube 15 Gm **Pump Spray Liq.:** 45 ml (with alcohol 83%). **Pow.:** 67.5 Gm, 45

Gm squeeze bot. **Aerosol pow.**: 105 Gm (with alcohol 14% and talc). **Aerosol liq.**: 120 ml (with alcohol 36%).
Use: Antifungal, external.
AFTER BITE. (Tender) Ammonium hydroxide 3.5% in aqueous solution. Penlike dispenser.
Use: Antipruritic, external analgesic.
AFTER BURN. (Tender) Lidocaine 0.5% in aloe vera 98% solution.
Use: Local anesthetic, topical.
• **AGAR,** N.F. XVIII. (Various Mfr.) Agaragar, Bengal Gelatin, Ceylon.
Use: Laxative.
W/Mineral oil.
See: Agoral, Emulsion (Parke-Davis Prods).
Petrogalar (Wyeth-Ayerst).
AGENTS FOR MIGRAINE. Agents used to prevent or cure a headache usually of the recurring type over the region of the external carotid artery.
See: Cafergot, Supp., Tab. (Sandoz).
DHE-45, Inj. (Sandoz).
Gynergen, Amp., Tab. (Sandoz).
Sansert, Tab. (Sandoz).
Wigraine, Tab., Supp. (Organon).
AGGREGATED ALBUMIN.
See: Albumotope-LS (Squibb).
AGOFOLLIN.
See: Estradiol (Various Mfr.).
AGORAL. (Parke Davis) Phenolphthalein 0.2 Gm, mineral oil 4.2 Gm/15 ml in an emulsion containing agar, tragacanth, egg-albumin, acacia, glycerin. Marshmallow and raspberry flavor. Bot. 240 ml, 480 ml.
Use: Laxative.
AGORAL, PLAIN. (Parke-Davis) Emulsion of mineral oil 1.4 Gm/5 ml with agar, tragacanth, egg albumin, acacia, glycerin. Bot. 480 ml.
Use: Laxative.
A/G-PRO. (Miller) Protein hydrolysate 50 gr w/essential and nonessential amino acids 45%, l-lysine 300 mg, methionine 75 mg, Vitamins C, B_6, Fe, Cu, I, Mn, K, Zn, Mg/6 Tab. Bot. 180s.
Use: Nutritional supplement.
AGURIN.
See: Theobromine Sodium Acetate (Various Mfr.).
AH-CHEW. (WE Pharm) Chlorpheniramine maleate 2 mg, phenylephrine HCl 10 mg, methslopolamine nitrate 1.25 mg. Chew. Tab. 100s.
Use: Antitussive combination.
AHF.
See: Antihemophilic factor.
A-HYDROCORT. (Abbott Hospital Prods)

Hydrocortisone sodium succinate. 100 mg or 250 mg/2 ml Univial, with benzyl alcohol; 500 mg/4 ml Univial with benzyl alcohol; 1000 mg/8 ml Univial with benzyl alcohol.
Use: Corticosteroid.
AIDS VACCINE. (MicroGeneSys/Genentech/Immuno AG/NIH/Wyeth-Ayerst) Phase I-III AIDS, HIV prophylaxis and treatment.
Use: Antiviral.
AIRET. (Adams) Albuterol sulfate 0.083%. Soln. for inhalation. Vial.
Use: Bronchodilator.
• **AIR, MEDICAL.** U.S.P. XXIII.
AI-RSA. (Autoimmune, Inc.)
Use: Autoimmune uveitis. [Orphan drug]
AIR & SURFACE DISINFECTANT. (Health & Medical Techniques) Dimethylbenzylammonium Cl 0.33%, o-phenylphenol 0.25%, n-alkyl (50% C-14, 40% C-12, 10% C-16), ethyl alcohol 44.25%. Aerosol 16 oz.
Use: Air sanitizer, deodorizer.
AKARPINE. (Akorn) Pilocarpine HCl 1%, 2% or 4%. Also contains hydroxyethyl cellulose, benzalkonium Cl 0.01%, EDTA 0.01%. Soln. Bot. 15 ml.
Use: Miotic.
AKBETA. (Akorn) Levobunolol HCl 0.25%. Ophthalmic Soln. 5 ml, 10 ml. Levobunolol HCl 0.5%. Soln. Bot. 5 ml, 10 ml, 15 ml.
Use: Glaucoma agent.
AK-CHLOR. (Akorn)**Oint.**:Chloramphenicol 10 mg/Gm, mineral oil, parabens in white petrolatum base. Tube 3.5 Gm.
Soln.: Chloramphenicol 5 mg/ml. Bot. 7.5 ml, 15 ml.
Use: Antibiotic, ophthalmic.
AK-CIDE. (Akorn) **Susp.**: Prednisolone acetate 0.5%, sulfacetamide sodium 10%, phenethyl alcohol 5 mg, benzalkonium chloride 0.25 mg/ml, EDTA. Dropper bot. 5 ml, 15 ml. **Oint.**: Prednisolone acetate 0.5%, sodium sulfacetamide 10%, mineral oil, white petrolatum, lanolin, parabens. Tube 3.5 Gm.
Use: Ophthalmic corticosteroid, anti-infective.
AK-CON. (Akorn) Naphazoline HCl 0.1%, benzalkonium Cl 0.01%, EDTA 0.01%. Soln. Bot. 15 ml.
Use: Vasoconstrictor/mydriatic.
AK-CON-A. (Akorn) Naphazoline HCl 0.025%, pheniramine maleate 0.3%, benzalkonium Cl 0.01%, EDTA. Soln. Bot. 15 ml.
Use: Ophthalmic antihistamine,

decongestant.
AK-DEX. (Akorn) Dexamethasone phosphate (as sodium phosphate). **Oint.:** **0.05% in white petrolatum and mineral oil base with lanolin, parabens, PEG-400. Tube 3.5 Gm. Soln.:** 0.1% with benzalkonium Cl, EDTA. Dropper bot 5 ml.
Use: Corticosteroid, ophthalmic.
AK-DILATE. (Akorn) Phenylephrine HCl 10%. Soln. Bot. 5 ml; 2.5% Bot. 2 ml, 15 ml. Also contains benzalkonium Cl 0.01%, EDTA, sodium bisulfite.
Use: Vasoconstrictor/mydriatic.
AKES-N-PAIN. (E. J. Moore) Acetaminophen 120 mg, salicylamide 210 mg, caffeine 30 mg, calcium gluconate 60 mg/Cap. Bot. 30s.
Use: Analgesic combination.
AKES-N-PAIN RUB. (E. J. Moore) Histamine dihydrochloride, methyl nicotinate, oleoresin capsicum, glycomonosalicylate. Tube 1.25 oz.
Use: Analgesic, external.
AK-FLUOR. (Akorn) Fluorescein sodium. **10%:** Amp. 5 ml, Vial 5 ml; **25%:** Amp. 2 ml, Vial 2 ml.
Use: Ophthalmic diagnostic.
AK-HOMATROPINE. (Akorn) Homatropine HBr 5%, benzalkonium Cl 0.01%, hydroxyethyl cellulose, EDTA. Soln. Bot. 5 ml.
Use: Cycloplegic mydriatic.
AKINETON. (Knoll) Biperiden HCl 2 mg/Tab. Bot. 100s, 1000s.
Use: Antiparkinson agent.
AKINETON LACTATE. (Knoll) Biperiden lactate 5 mg in aqueous 1.4% sodium lactate soln/ml. Amp 1 ml, Box 10s.
Use: Antiparkinson agent.
• **AKLOMIDE.** USAN.
Use: Coccidiostat.
AK-MYCIN. (Akorn) Erythromycin 5 mg/Gm with white petrolatum, mineral oil. Oint. Tube 3.75 Gm.
Use: Anti-infective, ophthalmic.
AK-NACL. (Akorn)**Oint.:**Sodium Cl hypertonic 5%, mineral oil, white petrolatum, anhydrous lanolin. Tube 3.5 Gm. **Soln.:**Sodium chloride, hypertonic 5%. Bot. 15 ml.
Use: Ophthalmic hyperosmolar preparation.
AKNE DRYING LOTION. (Alto) Zinc oxide 12%, urea 10%, sulfur 6%, salicylic acid 2%, benzalkonium Cl 0.2%, isopropyl alcohol 70%, in a base containing menthol, silicon dioxide, iron oxide, perfume. Bot. 3/4 oz, 2.25 oz.
Use: Anti-acne.

AK-NEFRIN. (Akorn) Phenylephrine HCl 0.12%, benzalkonium Cl 0.01%, hydroxyethyl cellulose 0.5%, EDTA. Soln. Bot. 15 ml.
Use: Vasoconstrictor/mydriatic.
AKNE-MYCIN. (Hermal) Erythromycin. **Oint.:** 2%. Tube 25 Gm. **Soln.:** 2%. Bot. 00 ml.
Use: Anti-acne.
AK-NEO-DEX. (Akorn) Dexamethasone sodium phosphate 0.1% and neomycin sulfate 3.5 mg/ml. With EDTA, polysorbate 80, sodium bisulfite, and 0.01% benzalkonium chloride. Ophth. Soln. 5 ml.
Use: Corticosteroid/anti-infective, ophthalmic.
AKNE SCRUB. (Alto) Povidone iodine with polyethylene granules. Bot. 3/4 oz.
Use: Anti-acne.
AKOLINE C.B. (Akorn) Choline bitartrate 111 mg, inositol 111 mg, methionine 28 mg, Vitamins B_1 0.3 mg, B_2 0.3 mg, B_3 3.3 mg, B_5 0.39 mg, B_6 0.3 mg, B_{12} 1.7 mcg, C 100 mg, lemon bioflavonoids complex 100 mg/Cap. Bot. 100s.
Use: Lipotropics with vitamins.
AK-PENTOLATE. (Akorn) Cyclopentolate HCl 1%, benzalkonium Cl 0.01%, EDTA. Soln. Bot. 2 ml, 15 ml.
Use: Cycloplegic mydriatic.
AK-POLY-BAC. (Akorn) Polymyxin B sulfate 10,000 units, bacitracin zinc 500 units/Gm in a white petrolatum and mineral oil base. Oint. Tube 3.5 Gm.
Use: Anti-infective, ophthalmic.
AK-PRED. (Akorn) Prednisolone sodium phosphate 0.125% or 1%, benzalkonium Cl 0.01%, EDTA, hydroxyethyl cellulose, sodium bisulfite. **0.125%:** Soln. Bot w/dropper 5 ml. **0.1%:** Soln. Bot. w/dropper 5 ml, 15 ml.
Use: Corticosteroid, ophthalmic.
AK-RAMYCIN. (Akorn) Doxycycline hyclate 100 mg/Cap. Bot. 50s, 100s, 200s, 250s, 500s, UD 100s.
Use: Anti-infective, tetracycline.
AK-RATABS. (Akorn) Doxycycline hyclate 100 mg/Tab. Bot. 50s.
Use: Anti-infective, tetracycline.
AK-RINSE. (Akorn) Sodium Cl 0.49%, potassium Cl 0.075%, calcium Cl 0.048%, magnesium Cl 0.03%, sodium acetate 0.39%, sodium citrate 0.17%, benzalkonium Cl 0.013%. Soln. Bot. 30 ml, 118 ml.
Use: Ophthalmic irrigation solution.
AK-SPORE. (Akorn) **Oint.:** Polymyxin B sulfate 10,000 units, neomycin (as sulfate) 3.5 mg, bacitracin zinc 400

units/Gm in a white petrolatum and mineral oil base. Tube 3.5 Gm. **Soln.:** Polymyxin B sulfate 10,000 units, neomycin sulfate 1.75 mg, gramicidin 0.025 mg/ml, thimerosal 0.001%, alcohol 0.5%, propylene glycol, polyoxyethylene, polyoxypropylene. Soln. Dropper bot. 2 ml, 10 ml.
Use: Anti-infective, ophthalmic.
AK-SPORE H.C. OPHTHALMIC. (Akorn) **Susp.:** Hydrocortisone 1%, neomycin sulfate 0.35%, polymyxin B sulfate 10,000 units, thimerosal 0.001%, benzalkonium Cl 0.01%, cetyl alcohol, glyceryl monostearate, polyoxyl 40 stearate, propylene glycol, mineral oil. Bot. 7.5 ml. **Oint.:** Hydrocortisone 1%, neomycin sulfate 0.35%, bacitracin zinc 400 units, polymyxin B sulfate 10,000 units in a white petrolatum, mineral oil base. Tube 3.5 g.
Use: Corticosteroid, anti-infective.
AK-SPORE H.C. OTIC. (Akorn) **Susp.:** Hydrocortisone 1%, neomycin sulfate 5 mg, polymyxin B sulfate 10,000 units/ml. Bot. w/dropper 10 ml. **Soln.:** Hydrocortisone 1%, neomycin sulfate 5 mg, polymyxin B sulfate 10,000 units/ml. Bot. w/dropper 10 ml.
Use: Corticosteroid, anti-infective combination.
AK-SULF. (Akorn) **Soln.:** Sodium sulfacetamide 10%, hydroxyethyl cellulose, sodium thiosulfate 0.2%, chlorobutanol 0.2%, parabens. 10%: Dropper Bot. 2 ml, 5 ml, 15 ml; **Oint.:** Sodium sulfacetamide 10%, parabens, petrolatum base. Tube 3.5 Gm.
Use: Anti-infective, ophthalmic.
AK-TAINE. (Akorn) Proparacaine HCl 0.5%, glycerin, chlorobutanol, benzalkonium Cl. Dropper bot. 2 ml, 15 ml.
Use: Local anesthetic, ophthalmic.
AK-TATE. (Akorn) Prednisolone acetate 1%, benzalkonium Cl, EDTA, polysorbate 80, polyvinyl alcohol, hydroxyethyl cellulose. Susp. Dropper bot. 5 ml, 10 ml, 15 ml.
Use: Corticosteroid, ophthalmic.
AKTOB. (Akorn)Tobramycin 0.3%. Soln. Bot. 5 ml.
Use: Anti-infective, ophthalmic.
AK-TRACIN. (Akorn) Bacitracin 500 units/Gm. Oint. Tube 3.5 Gm.
Use: Anti-infective, ophthalmic.
AK-TROL. (Akorn) **Susp.:** Dexamethasone 0.1%, neomycin sulfate equivalent to 0.35% neomycin base, polymyxin B sulfate 10,000 units/ml, hydroxypropyl methylcellulose, polysorbate 20, benza-

lkonium Cl. Bot. w/dropper 5 ml. **Oint.:** Dexamethasone 0.1%, neomycin sulfate equivalent to 0.35% neomycin base, polymyxin B sulfate 10,000 units/Gm, white petrolatum, liquid lanolin, mineral oil, parabens. Tube 3.5 Gm.
Use: Ophthalmic corticosteroid, anti-infective.
AKWA TEARS. (Akorn) **Soln.:** Polyvinyl alcohol, sodium Cl, benzalkonium Cl 0.01%, EDTA. Bot. 15 ml. **Oint.:** White petrolatum, mineral oil, lanolin. Tube 3.5 g.
Use: Artificial tears.
AK-ZOL. (Akorn) Acetazolamide 250 mg/Tab. Bot. 100s, 1000s.
Use: Anticonvulsant, diuretic.
AL-721. (Matrix Laboratories) Phase I/II AIDS, ARC, HIV positive.
Use: Antiviral.
ALA-BATH. (Del-Ray) Bath oil. Bot. 8 oz.
Use: Emollient.
ALA-CORT. (Del-Ray) Hydrocortisone 1%. **Cream:** Tube 1 oz, 3 oz. **Lot.:** Bot. 4 oz.
Use: Corticosteroid.
ALA-DERM. (Del-Ray) Lot. Bot 8 oz, 12 oz.
Use: Emollient.
ALADRINE. (Scherer) Ephedrine sulfate 8.1 mg, secobarbital sodium 16.2 mg/Tab. Bot. 100s.
Use: Decongestant, sedative/hypnotic.
ALAMAG. (Barre) Magnesium-aluminum hydroxide gel. Susp. Bot. pt.
Use: Antacid.
W/Belladonna alkaloid. Susp. Bot. 8 oz.
Use: Antacid.
ALAMAG SUSPENSION. (Goldline) Aluminum hydroxide 225 mg, magnesium hydroxide 200 mg, sorbitol, sucrose, parabens. Bot. 355 ml.
Use: Antacid.
ALAMAG PLUS ANTACID. (Goldline) Magnesium hydroxide 200 mg, aluminum hydroxide 225 mg, simethicone 25 mg/5 ml. Bot. 355 ml.
Use: Antacid.
• **ALAMECIN.** USAN.
Use: Antibacterial.
• **ALANINE,** U.S.P. XXIII. $C_3H_7NO_2$. L-Alanine.
Use: Amino acid.
• **ALAPROCLATE.** USAN.
Use: Antidepressant.
ALA-QUIN 0.5%. (Del-Ray) Hydrocortisone, iodochlorhydroxyquin cream. Tube 1 oz.
Use: Corticosteroid, topical.
ALA-SCALP HP 2%. (Del-Ray) Hydrocortisone lotion. Bot. 1 oz.

Use: Corticosteroid, topical.
ALA-SEB SHAMPOO. (Del-Ray) Bot. 4 oz, 12 oz.
Use: Antiseborrheic.
ALA-SEB T SHAMPOO. (Del-Ray) Bot. 4 oz, 12 oz.
Use: Antiseborrheic.
ALACULF. (Major) Sulfanilamide 15%, aminacrine HCl 0.2%, allantoin 2%. Vaginal Cream Tube w/applicator 120 Gm.
Use: Anti-infective, vaginal.
ALATONE. (Major) Spironolactone 25 mg/Tab. Bot. 100s, 250s, 500s, 1000s, UD 100s.
Use: Antihypertensive.
ALAXIN. (Delta) Oxyethlene oxypropylene polymer 240 mg/Cap. Bot. 100s.
Use: Laxative.
AL-AY. (Bowman) **Green Oblong Tube:** Phenylephrine HCl 5 mg, chlorpheniramine maleate 2 mg, aspirin 162 mg, caffeine 15 mg, aminoacetic acid 162 mg/Tab. Bot. 100s, 1000s. **Dark Green S.C:** Phenylephrine HCl 5 mg, chlorpheniramine maleate 2 mg, acetaminophen 160 mg, caffeine 15 mg/Tab. Bot. 100s, 1000s.
Use: Decongestant, antihistamine, analgesic.
ALAZANINE TRICHLORPHATE. 3-Ethyl-2-[3-(3-ethyl-2-benzothiazolinylidene) propenyl]-benzo-thiazolium 2,4,5-trichlorophenoxide salt with two formula weights of 2,4,5[trichlorophenol].
Use: Anthelmintic.
ALAZIDE TABS. (Major) Spironolactone w/hydrochlorothiazide. Bot. 250s, 1000s.
Use: Antihypertensive.
ALAZINE TABS. (Major) Hydralazine 10 mg, 25 mg or 50 mg/Cap. Bot. 100s, 1000s.
Use: Antihypertensive.
ALBA-DEX. (Pharma-Serv) Dexamethasone phosphate (as sodium phosphate) solution 4 mg/ml, methyl and propyl parabens, sodium bisulfite. Inj. Vial 1 ml, 5 ml, 30 ml.
Use: Corticosteroid.
ALBALON LIQUIFILM. (Allergan America) Naphazoline HCl 0.1%, polyvinyl alcohol 1.4%, benzalkonium Cl 0.004%, edetate disodium, citric acid, sodium citrate, sodium Cl, sodium hydroxide, purified water. Bot. 15 ml.
Use: Vasoconstrictor, ophthalmic.
ALBALON-A LIQUIFILM. (Allergan) Naphazoline HCl 0.05%, antazoline phosphate 0.5%, polyvinyl alcohol 1.4%, benzalkonium Cl 0.004%, edetate disodium, povidone, sodium Cl, sodium acetate, acetic acid and/or sodium hydroxide, purified water. Bot. 5 ml, 15 ml.
Use: Decongestant, ophthalmic.
ALBAMYCIN. (Upjohn) Novobiocin sodium 250 mg/Cap. Bot. 100s.
Use: Anti infective.
ALBAY. (Hollister-Stier) Freeze-dried venom (honeybee) 500 mcg and venom protein (yellow jacket, yellow hornet, white faced hornet, wasp and mixed vespid). Inj. Vial 10 ml.
Use: Allergenic extract.
• **ALBENDAZOLE,** U.S.P. XXIII USAN.
Use: Anthelmintic.
ALBOLENE CREAM. (SK-Beecham) Unscented or scented. Jar 6 oz, 12 oz.
ALBUCID.
See: Sulfacetamide.
ALBUCONN 25% SOLUTION. (Cryosan) Normal serum albumin (human) 12.5 Gm in 50 ml solution for IV administration. Vial 50 ml.
Use: Treatment of plasma or blood volume deficit, acute hypoproteinemia, oncotic deficit.
• **ALBUMIN, AGGREGATED.** USAN.
Use: Diagnostic aid.
• **ALBUMIN, AGGREGATED IODINATED 1 131 SERUM.** USAN.
Use: Radioactive agent.
• **ALBUMIN, CHROMATED Cr 51 SERUM.** USAN. Radio-Chromated Serum Albumin Human.
Use: Radioactive agent.
See: Chromalbin (Squibb).
• **ALBUMIN HUMAN,** U.S.P. XXIII. Normal Human Serum Albumin.
Use: Plasma protein fraction.
See: Proserum 5, Inj. (Merrell Dow).
ALBUMIN HUMAN, 5%. (Immuno-US) Normal serum albumin 5%. Inj. Vial 250 ml.
Use: Plasma protein fraction.
ALBUMIN HUMAN, 25%. (Immuno-US) Normal serum albumin 25%. Inj. Vial 10 ml, 50 ml.
Use: Plasma protein fraction.
• **ALBUMIN, IODINATED I-125 SERUM.** USAN. Radio-iodinated (I-125) Serum Albumin Human.
Use: Diagnostic aid.
• **ALBUMIN, IODINATED I-131 SERUM,** U.S.P. XXIII. Radio-iodinated (^{131}I) Serum Albumin Human. Aggregated Radio-Iodinated (I-131) Albumin Human.
Use: Diagnostic aid.
See: Albumotope-LS (Squibb).
• **ALBUMIN, IODINATED I-131 AGGRE-**

GATED INJECTION, U.S.P. XXIII.
Use: Diagnostic aid.
ALBUMIN, NORMAL SERUM 5%. (Immuno-US) Albumin human 5%. Inj. vial 120 ml.
Use: Plasma protein fraction.
ALBUMIN, NORMAL SERUM 25%. (Immuno-US) Albumin human 25%. Inj. vial 10 ml, 50 ml.
Use: Plasma protein fraction.
ALBUMIN-SALINE DILUENT. (Hollister-Stier) Dilute allergenic extracts and venom products for patient testing and treating. Pre-measured vials 1.8 ml, 4 ml, 4.5 ml, 9 ml, 30 ml. Vial 2 ml, 5 ml, 10 ml, 30 ml.
Use: Diagnostic aid, treatment.
ALBUMINAR-5 AND ALBUMINAR-25. (Armour) Albumin, (human) U.S.P. 5% solution with administration set. Bot. 50 ml, 250 ml, 500 ml, 1000 ml. 25% solution. Vial 20 ml, 50 ml, 100 ml with administration set.
Use: Plasma protein fraction.
ALBUMOTOPE I-131. (Squibb) Albumin, Iodinated I-131 Serum (50 uCi).
Use: Diagnostic aid.
ALBUSTIX REAGENT STRIPS. (Ames) Firm paper reagent strips impregnated with tetrabromphenol blue, citrate buffer and a protein-adsorbing agent. Bot. 50s, 100s.
Use: Diagnostic aid.
ALBUTEIN 5%. (Alpha Therapeutic) Normal serum albumin 5%. Inj. Vial w/IV set: 250 ml, 500 ml.
Use: Plasma protein fraction.
ALBUTEIN 25%. (Alpha Therapeutic) Normal serum albumin 25%. Inj. Vial w/IV set: 50 ml.
Use: Plasma protein fraction.
• **ALBUTEROL.** USAN.
Use: Bronchodilator.
See: Ventolin, Inh. Aerosol (Allen & Hanburys).
• **ALBUTEROL SULFATE.** USAN.
Use: Bronchodilator.
See: Airet, Inhalation soln. (Adams).
Proventil, Tab., Soln., Syr. (Schering).
Ventolin, Inhalation, Soln., Syr., Tab.
(Allen & Hanburys).
Ventolin Rotacaps (Allen & Hanburys).
Volmax, ER Tab. (Muro)
• **ALBUTEROL TABLETS,** U.S.P. XXIII.
Use: Bronchodilator.
• **ALBUTOIN.** USAN. 3-Allyl-5-isobutyl-2-thiohydantoin.
Use: Anticonvulsant.
ALCAINE. (Alcon) Proparacaine HCl 0.5%, glycerin, sodium Cl, benzalkoni-

um Cl. Bot. 15 ml.
Use: Local anesthetic, ophthalmic.
ALCARE. (Vestal) Ethyl alcohol 62%. Foam Bot. 210 ml, 300 ml, 600 ml.
Use: Antiseptic.
ALCLEAR EYE LOTION. (Walgreen) Sterile isotonic fluid. Bot. 8 oz.
Use: Eye irritation relief.
• **ALCLOFENAC.** USAN. 4-Allyloxy-3-chlorophenylacetic acid.
Use: Analgesic, anti-inflammatory.
See: Prinalgin.
• **ALCLOMETASONE DIPROPIONATE.** USAN.
Use: Anti-inflammatory.
See: Aclovate, Cream, Oint. (Glaxo).
• **ALCLOXA.** USAN. Tetrahydroxychloro-[(2- hydroxy-5-oxo-2-imidazolin-4-yl)ureato]-dialuminum.
Use: Astringent, keratolytic.
ALCO-GEL. (Tweezerman) Ethyl alcohol 60%. Tube 60 g, 480 g.
Use: Skin cleanser.
• **ALCOHOL,** U.S.P. XXIII. Ethanol, ethyl alcohol.
Use: Topical anti-infective; pharmaceutic aid (solvent).
• **ALCOHOL, DEHYDRATED,** U.S.P. XXIII.
Use: Solvent, vehicle.
• **ALCOHOL, DEHYDRATED INJECTION,** U.S.P. XXIII.
• **ALCOHOL IN DEXTROSE INJECTION,** U.S.P. XXIII.
• **ALCOHOL, DILUTED,** N.F. XVIII.
Use: Solvent, vehicle.
• **ALCOHOL, RUBBING,** U.S.P. XXIII.
Use: Rubefacient.
ALCOHOL 5% AND DEXTROSE 5%. (Abbott Hospital Prods) Alcohol 5 ml, dextrose 5 Gm/100 ml. Bot. 1000 ml.
Use: Parenteral nutritional supplement.
ALCOJET. (Alconox) Biodegradable machine washing detergent and wetting agent. Ctn. 9 × 4 lb, 25 lb, 50 lb, 100 lb, 300 lb.
Use: Detergent, wetting agent.
ALCOLEC. (American Lecithin) Lecithin w/choline base, cephalin, lipositol. Cap. 100s. Gran. 8 oz, lb.
Use: Nutritional supplement.
ALCONEFRIN 12 AND 50. (PolyMedica) Phenylephrine HCl 0.16% w/benzalkonium Cl. Dropper bot. 30 ml.
Use: Nasal decongestant.
ALCONEFRIN 25. (PolyMedica) Phenylephrine HCl 0.25% w/benzalkonium Cl. Dropper bot. 30 ml. Spray Pkg. 30 ml.
Use: Nasal decongestant.
ALCON ENZYMATIC CLEANING

TABLETS FOR EXTENDED WEAR. (Alcon Lenscare) Pancreatin tablets. Pkg. 12s. *Use:* Contact lens care.

ALCON LENS CASE. (Alcon Lenscare) Two lens cases. Ctn. 12s. *Use:* Contact lens care.

ALCON OPTI-PURE STERILE SALINE SOLUTION. (Alcon Lenscare) Sterile unpreserved saline solution. Aerosol 8 oz. *Use:* Soft contact lens care.

ALCON SALINE SOLUTION FOR SENSITIVE EYES. (Alcon Lenscare) Sodium Cl edetate disodium, sorbic acid 0.1%. Bot. 8 oz, 12 oz. *Use:* Soft contact lens care.

ALCONOX. (Alconox) Biodegradable detergent and wetting agent. Box 4 lb, Container 25 lb, 50 lb, 100 lb, 300 lb. *Use:* Anionic detergent, wetting agent.

ALCOTABS. (Alconox) Tab. Box 6s, 100s. *Use:* Test tube cleaner.

• **ALCURONIUM CHLORIDE.** USAN. Diallyldinortoxiferin dichloride. *Use:* Muscle relaxant. *See:* Alloferin (Roche). Toxiferene (Roche).

ALDACTAZIDE TABLETS. (Searle) Spironolactone and hydrochlorothiazide. **25 mg/25 mg:** Bot. 100s, 500s, 1000s, 2500s, UD 100s. **50 mg/50 mg:** Bot. 100s, UD 32s, UD 100s. *Use:* Antihypertensive.

ALDACTONE TABLETS. (Searle) Spironolactone. **25 mg/Tab.:** Bot. 100s, 500s, 1000s, UD 100s. **50 mg/Tab.:** Bot. 100s, UD 100s. **100 mg/Tab.:** Bot. 100s, UD 100s. *Use:* Antihypertensive.

ALDERLIN HYDROCHLORIDE. Pronethalol, B.A.N.

• **ALDESLEUKIN.** USAN *Use:* Biological response modifier; antineoplastic; immunostimulant. [Orphan drug]

ALDINAMIDE. 2-Carbamoyl pyrazine.

• **ALDIOXA.** USAN. Aluminum dihydroxy allantoinate. Dihydroxy-[(2-hydroxy-5-oxo-2-imidazolin-4-yl)ureato] aluminum. *Use:* Astringent, keratolytic.

ALDOCLOR 150. (Merck & Co.) Methyldopa 250 mg, chlorothiazide 150 mg/Tab. Bot. 100s. *Use:* Antihypertensive.

ALDOCLOR 250. (Merck & Co.) Methyldopa 250 mg, chlorothiazide 250 mg/Tab. Bot. 100s. *Use:* Antihypertensive.

ALDOMET. (Merck & Co.) Methyldopa. **125 mg/Tab.:** Bot. 100s. **250 mg/Tab.:** Bot. 100s, 1000s, UD 100s, Unit-of-use 100s. **500 mg/Tab.:** Bot. 100s, 500s, UD 100s, Unit-of-use 60s, 100s. *Use:* Antihypertensive. W/Chlorothiazide. *See:* Aldoclor, Tab. (Merck & Co.). W/Hydrochlorothiazide. *See:* Aldoril, Tab. (Merck & Co.).

ALDOMET ESTER HYDROCHLORIDE. (Merck & Co.) Methyldopate HCl 250 mg/5 ml, citric acid anhydrous 25 mg, sodium bisulfite 16 mg, disodium edetate 2.5 mg, monothioglycerol 10 mg, sodium hydroxide to adjust pH, methylparaben 0.15%, propylparaben 0.02% w/water for inj. q.s. to 5 ml. Vial 5 ml. *Use:* Antihypertensive.

ALDOMET ORAL SUSPENSION. (Merck & Co.) Methyldopa 250 mg/5 ml, alcohol 1%, benzoic acid 0.1%, sodium bisulfite 0.2%. Bot. 473 ml. *Use:* Antihypertensive.

ALDORIL-15. (Merck & Co.) Methyldopa 250 mg, hydrochlorothiazide 15 mg/Tab. Bot. 100s, 1000s, UD 100s. *Use:* Antihypertensive.

ALDORIL-25. (Merck & Co.) Methyldopa 250 mg, hydrochlorothiazide 25 mg/Tab. Bot. 100s, 1000s, UD 100s. *Use:* Antihypertensive.

ALDORIL D30. (Merck & Co.) Methyldopa 500 mg, hydrochlorothiazide 30 mg/Tab. Bot. 100s. *Use:* Antihypertensive.

ALDOSTERONE. B.A.N. 11β,21-Dihydroxy-3,-20-di-oxopregn-4-en-18-al. Aldocorten. Electrocortin. *Use:* Corticosteroid.

ALDOSTERONE RIA DIAGNOSTIC KIT. (Abbott Diagnostics) Test kits 50s. *Use:* Diagnostic aid.

• **ALENDRONATE SODIUM.** USAN. *Use:* Bone resorption inhibitor.

ALENIC ALKA LIQUID. (Rugby) Aluminum hydroxide 31.7 mg, magnesium carbonate 137.3 mg, sodium alginate, EDTA, sodium 13 mg. Bot. 355 ml. *Use:* Antacid.

ALENIC ALKA TABLETS. (Rugby) Aluminum Hydroxide 80 mg, magnesium trisilicate 20 mg, sodium bicarbonate, calcium stearate, sugar. Chew Tab. Bot. 100s. *Use:* Antacid.

ALENIC ALKA TABLETS, EXTRA STRENGTH. (Rugby) Aluminum hydroxide 160 mg, magnesium carbonate 105 mg, sodium 29.9 mg. Chew. Tab.

Bot. 100s.
Use: Antacid.
• **ALENTEMOL HYDROBROMIDE.** USAN
Use: Antipsychotic.
ALERSULE CAPSULES. (Misemer)
Chlorpheniramine maleate 8 mg,
phenylephrine HCl 20 mg/Cap. Bot.
100s.
Use: Antihistamine, decongestant.
ALERT-PEP. (Approved) Caffeine 200
mg/Cap. Bot. 16s.
Use: CNS stimulant.
• **ALETAMINE HYDROCHLORIDE.** USAN.
Use: Antidepressant.
ALEVE. (Procter & Gamble) Naproxen
sodium 220 mg (naproxen base 200 mg
with sodium 20 mg) Tab. Bot. 24s, 50s,
100s.
Use: Nonsteroidal anti-inflammatory
agent.
• **ALEXIDINE.** USAN. 1,1'-Hexamethyl-
enebis[5-(2-ethylhexyl) biguanide].
Use: Antibacterial.
ALFA INTERFERON-2A.
See: Roferon A (Roche).
ALFA INTERFERON-2B.
See: Intron A (Schering).
ALFA INTERFERON-N3.
See: Alferon N (Purdue Frederick).
ALFENTA. (Janssen) Alfentanil 0.5
mg/ml. Amp. 2 ml, 5 ml, 10 ml, 20 ml.
Use: Narcotic analgesic, anesthetic.
• **ALFENTANIL HYDROCHLORIDE.**
USAN.
Use: Analgesic, narcotic; anesthetic.
See: Alfenta, Inj. (Janssen).
ALFERON N. (Purdue Frederick) Interfer-
on alfa-n3 5 mIU/vial. Vial 1 ml.
Use: Antineoplastic agent.
• **ALFUZOSIN HYDROCHLORIDE.** USAN.
Use: Antihypertensive.
ALGEL. (Faraday) Magnesium trisilicate
0.5 Gm, aluminum hydroxide 0.25
Gm/Tab. Bot. 100s. Susp. Bot. gal.
Use: Antacid.
• **ALGELDRATE.** USAN.
Use: Antacid.
ALGEMIN. (Thurston) Macrocystis
pyrifera alga. Pow. Jar 8 oz. Tab. Bot.
300s.
Use: Dietary aid.
ALGENIC ALKA IMPROVED TABLETS.
(Rugby) Aluminum hydroxide 240 mg,
magnesium hydroxide 100 mg/Chew.
Tab. Bot. 100s, 500s.
ALGENIC ALKA LIQUID. (Rugby) Alu-
minum hydroxide 31.7 mg/ml, magne-
sium carbonate 137 mg/ml, sodium algi-
nate, sorbitol. Bot. 355 ml.
Use: Antacid.

Use: Antacid.
• **ALGESTONE ACETONIDE.** USAN. 16α,-
17α-Isopropylidenedioxypregn-4-ene-
3,20-dione.
Use: Progestin.
• **ALGESTONE ACETOPHENIDE.** USAN.
(R)-16α, 17-Dihydroxypregn-4-ene-
3,20-dione cyclic acetal with acetophe-
none.
Use: Progestin.
ALGEX LINIMENT. (Approved) Menthol,
camphor, methylsalicylate, eucalyptus.
Bot. 4 oz.
Use: External analgesic.
ALGIN.
See: Sodium Alginate, N.F. XVIII.
ALGIN-ALL. (Barth's) Sodium alginate
from kelp. Tab. Bot. 100s, 500s.
• **ALGINIC ACID,** N.F. XVIII.
Use: Pharmaceutic aid (tablet binder,
thickening agent).
ALGINIC ACID. W/Aluminum hydroxide
dried gel, magnesium trisilicate, sodium
bicarbonate.
Use: Antacid.
See: Gaviscon Foamtabs (Marion).
• **ALGLUCERASE.** Glucocerebrosidase-
beta-glucosidase.
Use: Enzyme replacement therapy. [Or-
phan drug]
See: Ceredase (Genzyme).
• **ALGRELDRATE.** USAN.
Use: Antacid.
**ALIDINE DIHYDROCHLORIDE OR
PHOSPHATE.** Anileridine, N.F.
• **ALIFLURANE.** USAN.
Use: Anesthetic.
ALIKAL POWDER. (Sanofi Winthrop)
Sodium bicarbonate, tartaric acid pow-
der.
Use: Antacid.
ALIMENTUM. (Ross) Casein hy-
drolysate, sucrose, tapioca starch, MCT
(fractionated coconut oil), safflower oil,
soy oil. Qt ready-to-use.
Use: Enteral nutritional supplement.
• **ALIPAMIDE.** USAN. 4-Chloro-3- sul-
famoylbenzoic acid 2,2-dimethylhy-
drazide.
Use: Diuretic, antihypertensive.
ALIPAMIDE. B.A.N. 4-Chloro-2′,2-di-
methyl-3-sulfamoylbenzohydrazide.
Use: Diuretic.
ALISOBUMAL.
See: Butalbital, U.S.P. XXIII.
• **ALITAME.** USAN.
Use: Sweetener.
**ALKALINIZERS, MINERALS AND ELEC-
TROLYTES.**
See: Polycitra (Willen).

Oracit (Carolina Medical Products).
Bicitra (Willen).
**ALKALINIZERS URINARY TRACT
PRODUCTS.**
See: Sodium Bicarbonate (Various
Mfr.).
Urocit-K (Mission).
Citrolith (Beach Pharm.).
Polycitra (Willen).
Bicitra (Willen).
ALKALOL. (Alkalol Co.) Thymol, euca-
lyptol, menthol, camphor, benzoin,
potassium alum, potassium chlorate,
sodium bicarbonate, sodium Cl, sweet
birch oil, spearmint oil, pine and cassia
oil, alcohol 0.05%. Bot. pt. Nasal douche
cup pkg. 1s.
Use: Eyes, nose, throat and all inflamed
mucous membranes.
ALKA-MED LIQUID. (Blue Cross) Alu-
minum hydroxide 200 mg, magnesium
hydroxide 200 mg/ 5 ml. Bot. 8 oz.
Use: Antacid.
ALKA-MED TABLETS. (Blue Cross)
Magnesium hydroxide, aluminum hydroxide. Bot. 60s.
Use: Antacid.
ALKA-MINTS. (Miles) Calcium carbonate
850 mg/Chew. tab. Carton 30s.
Use: Antacid.
ALKA-SELTZER. (Miles) Heat treated
sodium bicarbonate 1916 mg, citric acid
1000 mg, aspirin 325 mg, sodium 567
mg/Tab. Bot. 36s.
Use: Effervescent antacid, analgesic.
**ALKA-SELTZER, ADVANCED FORMU-
LA.** (Miles) Heat treated sodium bicar-
bonate 465 mg, citric acid 900 mg, ac-
etaminophen 325 mg, potassium bicarbonate 300 mg, calcium carbonate 280
mg/Tab. Foil pack 36s.
Use: Effervescent antacid, analgesic.
**ALKA-SELTZER EFFERVESCENT,
GOLD TABLETS.** (Miles) Heat treated
sodium bicarbonate 958 mg, citric acid
832 mg, potassium bicarbonate 312 mg,
sodium 311 mg/Tab. Bot. 20s, 36s.
Use: Effervescent antacid, analgesic.
ALKA-SELTZER, EXTRA STRENGTH.
(Miles) Aspirin 500 mg, heat treated
sodium bicarbonate 1985 mg, citric acid
1000 mg, sodium 588 mg/Tab. Bot. 12s,
24s.
Use: Effervescent antacid, analgesic.
**ALKA-SELTZER FLAVORED EFFER-
VESCENT ANTACID-ANALGESIC.**
(Miles) Aspirin 325 mg, sodium bicarbonate 1700 mg, citric acid 1000 mg,
phenylalanine 9 mg, sodium 506 mg, aspartame, lemon-lime flavor. Tab. Bot.

24s.
Use: Effervescent antacid, analgesic.
ALKA-SELTZER PLUS. (Miles) Chlorpheniramine maleate 2 mg, phenylpropanolamine bitartrate 24 mg, aspirin
324 mg, sodium 506 mg/Tab. Foil pack
20s, 36s.
Use: Antihistamine, decongestant, analgesic.
**ALKA-SELTZER PLUS NIGHT-TIME
COLD TABLETS.** (Miles) Phenylpropanolamine bitartrate 24 mg, diphenhydramine citrate 38 mg, aspirin 324
mg, sodium 506 mg. Tab. 20s, 36s.
Use: Decongestant, antihistamine,
analgesic.
**ALKA-SELTZER PLUS SINUS
ALLERGY.** (Miles) Phenylpropanolamine bitartrate 24.08 mg,
brompheniramine maleate 2 mg, aspirin
500 mg, aspartame, phenylalanine 9
mg/Tab. Bot. 16s, 32s.
Use: Decongestant, antihistamine,
analgesic.
**ALKA-SELTZER SPECIAL EFFERVES-
CENT ANTACID.** (Miles) Heat treated
sodium bicarbonate 958 mg, citric acid
832 mg, potassium bicarbonate 312 mg,
sodium 284 mg/Tab. Foil pack 12s, 20s,
36s.
Use: Effervescent antacid.
ALKA-SELTZER TABLETS. (Miles) Aspirin 325 mg, citric acid 1000 mg, phenylalanine 9 mg, sodium 506 mg/Tab. Bot.
24s.
Use: Effervescent antacid, analgesic.
ALKA-SELTZER W/ASPIRIN. (Miles)
Sodium bicarbonate 1916 mg, citric acid
1000 mg, aspirin 325 mg and sodium
567 mg. 17.2 mEq acid neutralizing capacity. Foil pack 8s, 12s, 24s, 26s and
36s.
Use: Effervescent antacid, analgesic.
ALKERAN. (Burroughs Wellcome) Mel-
phalan 2 mg/Tab. Bot. 50s.
Use: Antineoplastic agent.
ALKETS. (Roberts Hauck) Calcium car-
bonate 500 mg, dextrose, peppermint
flavor. Chew. Tab. Bot. 36s, 96s, 150s.
Use: Antacid.
**ALKYLBENZYLDIMETHYLAMMONIUM
CHLORIDE.** Benzalkonium Cl, N.F.
XVIII.
W/Methylrosaniline Cl, polyoxyethyle-
nenonylphenol, polyethylene glycol tert-
dodecylthioether.
See: Hyva, Tab. (Holland-Rantos).
•**ALLANTOIN.** USAN.
Use: Emollient.
See: Cutemol, (Summers).

W/Aminacrine, sulfanilamide.
See: Par Cream (Parmed).
Vagidine, Cream (Elder).
Vagitrol, Cream (Syntex).
W/Balsam, Lano-sil, silicone.
See: Balmex Med. Lot. (Macsil).
W/Camphor, menthol, tincture benzoin.
See: Siltex, Oint. (E. J. Moore).
W/p-Chloro-m-xylenol.
See: Cebum, Shampoo (Dermik).
W/Coal tar extract, hexachlorophene, glycerin, lanolin.
See: Pso-Rite, Cream (DePree).
W/Coal tar in cream base.
See: Tegrin Cream (Block Drug).
W/Coal tar solution, isopropyl myristate, psorilan.
See: Psorelief, Soln. (Quality Generics).
W/Dienestrol, sulfanilamide, aminacrine HCl.
See: AVC/Dienestrol Cream, Supp. (Marion Merrell Dow).
W/Hydrocortisone.
See: Tarcortin, Cream (Reed & Carnrick).
W/Nitrofurazone.
See: Eldezol, Oint. (Elder).
W/Pramoxine HCl, benzalkonium Cl.
See: Perifoam, Aerosol (Reid-Rowell).
W/Resorcinol, hexachlorophene, menthol.
See: Tackle, Gel. (Colgate-Palmolive).
W/Salicylic acid, sulfur.
See: Neutrogena Disposables (Neutrogena).
W/Sulfanilamide, 9-aminoacridine HCl.
Nil Vaginal Cream (Century).
Vagisan, Creme (Sandia).
Vagisul, Creme (Sheryl).
W/Sulfisoxazole, Aminoacridine.
Use: Topically, aid in the promotion of granulation.
See: Vagilia, Cream, Supp. (Lemmon).
W/Tarbonis.
See: Sebical, Shampoo (Reed & Carnrick).
W/Vitamins A, D.
See: A-D Dressing (LaCrosse).
ALLAY. (LuChem) Acetaminophen 650 mg, hydrocodone bitartrate 7.5 mg/ Cap. Bot. 100s.
Use: Narcotic analgesic combination.
ALLBEE C-800. (Robins) Vitamins E 45 IU, C 800 mg, B$_1$ 15 mg, B$_2$ 17 mg, niacin 100 mg, B$_6$ 25 mg, B$_{12}$ 12 mcg, pantothenic acid 25 mg/Tab. Bot. 60s.
Use: Vitamin supplement.
ALLBEE C-800 PLUS IRON. (Robins) Vitamins E 45 IU, C 800 mg, B$_1$ 15 mg, B$_2$ 17 mg, niacin 100 mg, B$_6$ 25 mg, B$_{12}$ 12 mcg, pantothenic acid 25 mg, iron 27

mg, folic acid 0.4 mg/Tab. Bot. 60s.
Use: Vitamin/mineral supplement.
ALLBEE W/VITAMIN C. (Robins) Vitamins B$_1$ 15 mg, B$_6$ 5 mg, B$_2$ 10.2 mg, niacin 50 mg, pantothenic acid 10 mg, C 300 mg/Cap. Bot. 30s, 100s, 1000s. Disco pack 10x100s.
Use: Vitamin supplement.
ALLBEE-T. (Robins) Vitamins B$_1$ 15.5 mg, B$_2$ 10 mg, B$_6$ 8.2 mg, pantothenic acid 23 mg, niacin 100 mg, C 500 mg, B$_{12}$ 5 mcg/Tab. Bot. 100s, 500s.
Use: Vitamin supplement.
ALLBEX. (Approved) Vitamins B$_1$ 5 mg, B$_2$ 2 mg, B$_6$ 0.25 mg, calcium pantothenate 3 mg, niacinamide 20 mg, ferrous sulfate 194.4 mg, inositol 10 mg, choline 10 mg, B$_{12}$ (concentrate) 3 mcg/Cap. Bot. 100s, 1000s.
Use: Vitamin/mineral supplement.
ALL-DAY B-COMPLEX. (Barth's) Vitamins B$_{12}$ 25 mcg, B$_1$ 7 mg, B$_2$ 14 mg, niacin 4.67 mg, B$_6$, pantothenic acid, folic acid, choline, aminobenzoic acid, inositol, biotin, Mg, Mn, Cu/Cap. Bot. 30s, 90s, 180s, 360s.
Use: Vitamin/mineral supplement.
ALL-DAY-C. (Barth's) Vitamin C 200 mg/Cap. or 500 mg/Tab. with rose hip extract. Bot. 30s, 90s, 180s, 360s.
Use: Vitamin supplement.
ALL-DAY IRON YEAST. (Barth's) Iron 20 mg, Vitamins B$_1$ 2 mg, B$_2$ 4 mg, niacin 0.57 mg/Cap. Bot. 30s, 90s, 180s.
Use: Vitamin/mineral supplement.
ALL-DAY-VITES. (Barth's) Vitamins A 10,000 IU, D 400 IU, B$_1$ 3 mg, B$_2$ 6 mg, niacin 1 mg, C 120 mg, B$_{12}$ 10 mcg, E 30 IU/Cap. Bot. 30s, 90s, 180s, 360s.
Use: Vitamin supplement.
ALLEGRON. Nortriptyline.
Use: Antidepressant.
ALLENT. (Ascher) Pseudoephedrine HCl 120 mg, brompheniramine maleate 12 mg. Slow-release cap. Bot. 100s.
Use: Decongestant, antihistamine.
ALLERBEN INJECTION. (Forest) Diphenhydramine 10 mg/ml. Vial 30 ml.
Use: Antihistamine.
ALLERCHLOR INJECTION. (Forest) Chlorpheniramine maleate 10 mg/ml. Vial 30 ml.
Use: Antihistamine.
ALLER-CHLOR. (Rugby) Chlorpheniramine maleate. **Tab.:** 4 mg. Bot. 24s, 100s, 1000s. **Syr.:** 2 mg/5 ml. Bot. 4 oz, pt, gal.
Use: Antihistamine.
ALLERCON. (Parmed) pseudoephedrine HCl 60 mg, triprolidine HCl 2.5 mg/Tab.

Bot. 100s and 1000s.
Use: Decongestant, antihistamine.
ALLERCREME SKIN. (Owen/Galderma)
Mineral oil, petrolatum, lanolin, lanolin
oil, lanolin alcohols, glycerin, tri-
ethanolamine, cetyl alcohol, stearic acid,
parabens. Lot. Bot. 240 ml.
Use: Emollient.
ALLERCREME ULTRA EMOLLIENT.
(Owen/Galderma) Mineral oil, petrola-
tum, lanolin, lanolin alcohol, lanolin oil,
glycerin, glyceryl stearate, PEG-100
stearate, squalane, cetyl alcohol, sorbi-
tan laurate, quaternium-15, parabens.
Cream Bot. 60 Gm.
Use: Emollient.
ALLERDEC CAPSULES. (Towne)
Phenylpropanolamine HCl 25 mg, chlorpheniramine maleate 1 mg, pyrilamine
maleate 5 mg/Cap. Bot. 25s, 50s.
Use: Decongestant, antihistamine.
ALLEREST. (Ciba Consumer) **Tab.:**
Phenylpropanolamine HCl 18.7 mg,
chlorpheniramine maleate 2 mg/Tab.
Sleeve Pack 24s, 48s. Bot. 72s. **Chew.
Tab. for Children:** Phenylpropanolamine HCl 9.4 mg, chlorpheniramine maleate 1 mg/Tab. Sleeve Pack
24s. **Eye Drops:** Naphazoline HCl
0.012%, benzalkonium Cl 0.01%, disodium edetate 0.1% w/boric acid, sodium
borate. Bot. 0.5 oz. **Headache Strength
Tab.:** Acetaminophen 325 mg, phenylpropanolamine HCl 18.7 mg, chlorpheniramine maleate 2 mg/Tab. Sleeve Pack
24s. **Nasal Spray:** Oxymetazoline HCl
0.05%. Bot. 0.5 oz.
Use: Decongestant, antihistamine;
analgesic (Headache strength Tab
only).
ALLEREST 12-HOUR CAPLETS. (Pharmacraft) Phenylpropanolamine HCl 75
mg, chlorpheniramine maleate 12
mg/Capl. Pkg. 10s.
Use: Decongestant, antihistamine.
ALLEREST 12-HOUR CAPSULES.
(Pharmacraft) Phenylpropanolamine
HCl 75 mg, chlorpheniramine maleate 8
mg/Cap. Sleeve pak 10s.
Use: Decongestant, antihistamine.
ALLEREST, CHILDREN'S. (Fisons)
Phenylpropanolamine HCl 94 mg, chlor-
pheniramine maleate 6 mg. Chew. Tab.
Bot. 24s.
Use: Pediatric decongestant, antihista-
mine.
ALLEREST MAXIMUM STRENGTH.
(Fisons) Pseudoephedrine 30 mg, chlor-
pheniramine maleate 2 mg/Tab. Bot.
24s, 48s, 72s.

Use: Decongestant, antihistamine.
ALLEREST NO DROWSINESS. (Phar-
macraft) Pseudoephedrine 30 mg, ac-
etaminophen 325 mg/Tab. Bot. 20s.
Use: Decongestant, analgesic.
ALLEREST SINUS PAIN FORMULA.
(Pharmacraft) Acetaminophen 500 mg,
phenylpropanolamine HCl 18.7 mg,
chlorpheniramine maleate 2 mg/Tab.
Sleeve pack 20s.
Use: Analgesic, decongestant, antihist-
amine.
ALLERFRIN. (Rugby) **Tab.:** Pseu-
doephedrine HCl 60 mg, triprolidine HCl
2.5 mg. Bot. 24s, 100s, 1000s. **Syr.:**
Pseudoephedrine HCl 30 mg, triproli-
dine HCl 1.25 mg. Bot. 120 ml, pt.
Use: Decongestant, antihistamine.
ALLERFRIN OTC SYRUP. (Rugby)
Pseudoephedrine 30 mg, triprolidine
1.25 mg. Syr. Bot. Pt.
Use: Decongestant, antihistamine.
ALLERFRIN W/CODEINE. (Rugby)
Pseudoephedrine HCl 30 mg, triprolidine HCl 1.25 mg, codeine phosphate
10 mg, alcohol 4.3%. Syr. Bot. 120 ml,
pt, gal.
Use: Decongestant, antihistamine, antitussive.
ALLERGAN ENZYMATIC. (Allergan) Papain, sodium Cl, sodium carbonate,
sodium borate, edetate disodium. Kits
12s, 24s, 36s, 48s.
Use: Soft contact lens care.
**ALLERGAN HYDROCARE CLEANING &
DISINFECTING SOLUTION.** (Allergan)
tris(2-hydroxyethyl)tallow ammonium Cl
0.013%, thimerosal 0.002%, bis(2-hy-
droxyethyl)tallow ammonium Cl, sodium
bicarbonate, dibasic, monobasic and anhydrous sodium phosphate, hydrochloric acid, propylene glycol, polysorbate
80, special soluble polyhema. Bot. 4 oz,
8 oz, 12 oz.
Use: Soft contact lens care.
**ALLERGAN HYDROCARE PRESERVED
SALINE SOLUTION.** (Allergan) Sodium
Cl, sodium hexametaphosphate, sodium
hydroxide, boric acid, sodium borate,
EDTA 0.01%, thimerosal 0.001%. Bot. 8
oz, 12 oz.
Use: Soft contact lens care.
ALLERGEN EAR DROPS. (Goldline)
Benzocaine 1.4%, antipyrine 5.4%, glycerin, oxyquinoline sulfate. Bot. 0.5 oz.
Use: Otic preparation.
ALLERGENIC EXTRACTS. (Center) Al-
lergenic extracts of pollen, mold, house
dust, inhalants, epidermals, insects in
saline 0.9% and phenol 0.4% up to 1:10

w/v or 40,000 PNU/ml in sets or vials up to 30 ml.
Use: Diagnosis of specific allergies, relief of allergic symptoms.

ALLERGENIC EXTRACTS. (Hollister-Stier) Allergenic extracts of pollens, foods, inhalants, epidermals, fungi, insects, miscellaneous antigens.
Use: Diagnosis of specific allergies, relief of allergic symptoms.

ALLERGEX. (Hollister-Stier) Silicones, polyethylene and triethylene glycol, antioxidants, mineral oil concentrate. Bot. pt. Aerosol pt.
Use: Control of house dust allergens.

ALLERGY. (Parmed) Chlorpheniramine maleate 4 mg/Tab. Bot. 24s, 100s.
Use: Antihistamine.

ALLERGY COLD. (Geneva) Pseudoephedrine HCl 60 mg, triprolidine HCl 2.5 mg/Tab. Bot. 100s.
Use: Decongestant, antihistamine.

ALLERGY DROPS. (Bausch & Lomb) Naphazoline HCl 0.012%, PEG 300 0.2%. Bot. 0.5 oz.
Use: Mydriatic/vasoconstrictor.

ALLERGY PREPARATIONS.
See: Antihistamine Preparations.

ALLERGY RELIEF MEDICINE.
Use: Decongestant, antihistamine.
See: A.R.M. Caplets (SK-Beecham).

ALLERGY-SINUS COMTREX. (Bristol-Myers) Pseudoephedrine HCl 30 mg, chlorpheniramine maleate 2 mg, acetaminophen 500 mg/Capl. or Tab. Bot. 50s, UD 24s.
Use: Decongestant, antihistamine, analgesic.

ALLERGY TABLETS. (Weeks & Leo) Phenylpropanolamine HCl 37.5 mg, chlorpheniramine 4 mg/Tab. Bot. 30s.
Use: Decongestant, antihistamine.

ALLERID. (Murdock) Pseudoephedrine HCl 60 mg/Cap. Bot. 30s.
Use: Decongestant.

ALLERMAX. (Pfeiffer) Diphenhydramine HCl 50 mg/Cap. Pkg. 20s.
Use: Antihistamine.

ALLERPHED SYRUP. (Great Southern) Pseudoephedrine HCl 30 mg, triprolidine HCl 1.25 mg/5 ml. Syr. Bot. 120 ml.
Use: Decongestant, antihistamine.

ALLERSONE. (Hauck) Hydrocortisone 0.5%, diperodon HCl 0.5%, zinc oxide 5%, sodium lauryl sulfate, propylene glycol, cetyl alcohol, petrolatum, methyl and propyl parabens. Oint. Tube 15 Gm.
Use: Corticosteroid, topical.

ALLERSULE FORTE. (Misemer) Phenylephrine HCl 20 mg, chlorpheni-

ramine maleate 8 mg, methscopolamine nitrate 2.5 mg/Cap. Bot. 100s.
Use: Decongestant, antihistamine, anticholinergic.

ALLETORPHINE. B.A.N. N-Allyl-7,8-dihydro-7α-(1(R)-hydroxy-1-methylbutyl)-0^6-methyl-6,14-endoethenonormorphine. N-Allylnoretorphine.
Use: Analgesic.

ALL-NITE COLD FORMULA. (Major) Pseudoephedrine HCl 10 mg, doxylamine succinate 1.25 mg, dextromethorphan HBr 5 mg, acetaminophen 167 mg/5 ml. Liq. Bot. 177 ml.
Use: Decongestant, antihistamine, antitussive, analgesic.

• **ALLOBARBITAL.** USAN. 5,5-Diallylbarbituric acid.
Use: Hypnotic.
W/Acetaminophen, salicylamide, caffeine.
See: Allylvon, Cap. (Elder).
W/Aspirin, acetaminophen, aluminum aspirin.
See: Allylgesic, Tab. (Elder).
W/Ergotamine tartrate.
See: Allylgesic w/Ergotamine, Cap. (Elder).

ALLOBARBITONE.
See: Diallylbarbituric Acid (Various Mfr.).

ALLOMETHADIONE. (I.N.N.) Aloxidone. B.A.N.

• **ALLOPURINOL,** U.S.P. XXIII. Tablets, U.S.P. XXIII. 1 H-Pyrazolo-[3, 4-d] pyrimidin-4-ol.
Use: Antigout, xanthine oxidase inhibitor.
See: Lopurin, Tab. (Boots Pharm).
Zyloprim, Tab. (Burroughs Wellcome).

• **ALLOPURINOL RIBOSIDE.** USAN.
Use: Antiprotozoal. [Orphan drug]

• **ALLOPURINOL SODIUM.** USAN.
Use: Ex vivo preservation of cadaveric kidneys for transplantation; antineoplastic. [Orphan drug]

ALLPYRAL. (Miles Pharm) Allergenic extracts, alum-precipitated. For subcutaneous inj. pollens, molds, epithelia, house dust, other inhalants, stinging insects.
Use: Diagnosis of specific allergies, relief of allergic symptoms.

ALLYLBARBITURIC ACID. Allylisobutylbarbituric acid, butalbital. Tab. (Various Mfr.).
Use: Sedative.
W/A.P.C.
See: Anti-Ten, Tab. (Century).
Fiorinal, Cap., Tab. (Sandoz).
Salipral, Tab. (Kenyon).

Tenstan (Standex).
W/Acetaminophen, homatropine methyl-
bromide.
See: Panitol H.M.B., Tab. (Wesley).
W/Acetaminophen, salicylamide, caffeine.
See: Renpap, Tab. (Wren).
ALLYLESTRENOL. 17a-Allyl-17b-hy-
droxy-4-estrene.
ALLYL-ISOBUTYLBARBITURIC ACID.
See: Allyl Barbituric Acid.
ALLYLISOPROPYLMALONYLUREA.
See: Aprobarbital.
ALLYL ISOTHIOCYANATE, Oil of mus-
tard. (Various Mfr.).
Use: Counterirritant in neuralgia.
4-ALLYL-2-METHOXYPHENOL.
Eugenol, U.S.P. XXIII.
N-ALLYLNOROXYMORPHONE HCl.
Naloxone Hydrochloride, U.S.P. XXIII.
ALLYLOESTRENOL. B.A.N. 17α-Ally-
loestr-4-en-17β-ol. Gestanin.
Use: Progestational steroid.
ALLYLPRODINE. B.A.N. 3-Allyl-1-
methyl-4-phenyl-4-propionyloxypiperi-
dine.
Use: Analgesic.
**5-ALLYL-SEC-BUTYLBARBITURIC
ACID.**
See: Talbutal.
ALMACONE. (Rugby) **Chew tab.:** Alu-
minum hydroxide 200 mg, magnesium
hydroxide 200 mg, simethicone 20
mg/Bot. 100s, 1000s. **Liq.:** Aluminum
hydroxide 200 mg, magnesium hydrox-
ide 200 mg, simethicone 20 mg, sodium
0.75 mg/5 ml. Bot. 360 ml, gal.
Use: Antacid.
**ALMACONE II DOUBLE STRENGTH
LIQUID.** (Rugby) Aluminum hydroxide
400 mg, magnesium hydroxide 400 mg,
simethicone 40 mg/5 ml. Bot. 360 ml,
gal.
Use: Antacid.
• **ALMADRATE SULFATE.** USAN. Aluminum magnesium hydroxide-oxide-sul-
fate-hydrate.
Use: Antacid.
• **ALMAGATE.** USAN.
Use: Antacid.
ALMAGUCIN. Gastric mucin, dried aluminum hydroxide gel, magnesium trisilicate.
Use: Antacid.
ALMA-MAG #4 IMPROVED. (Rugby) Alu-
minum hydroxide 200 mg, magnesium
hydroxide 200 mg, simethicone 25
mg/Chew. tab. Bot. 100s, 1000s.
Use: Antacid.
ALMA-MAG LIQUID IMPROVED. (Rugby) Aluminum hydroxide 200 mg, mag-

nesium hydroxide 200 mg, simethicone
25 mg/5 ml. Bot. 360 ml.
Use: Antacid.
ALMATRI. (Robinson) Aluminum hydrox-
ide gel 4 gr, magnesium trisilicate 7.5
gr/Tab. Bot. 100s, 1000s, Bulk pack
5000s.
Use: Antacid
ALMEBEX PLUS B12. (Dayton) Vitamins
B$_1$ 1 mg, B$_2$ 2 mg, B$_3$ 5 mg, B$_6$ 0.4 mg,
B$_{12}$ 5 mcg, choline 33 mg/5 ml, alcohol
5%. Pt. (with B$_{12}$ in separate container).
Use: Vitamin supplement.
• **ALMOND OIL,** N.F. XVIII.
Use: Pharmaceutical aid (emollient and
perfume).
ALMORA. (Forest) Magnesium gluconate
0.5 Gm/Tab. Pkg. 100s.
Use: Mineral supplement.
ALNYTE. (Mayer) Scopolamine aminox-
ide HBr 0.2 mg, salicylamide 250
mg/Tab. Pkg. 16s.
Use: Anticholinergic, analgesic.
ALOCASS LAXATIVE. (Western Re-
search) Aloin 0.25 gr, cascara sagrada
0.5 gr, rhubarb 0.5 gr, ginger $^1/_{32}$ gr, pow-
dered extract of belladonna gr/Tab. Bot.
1000s. Pak 28s.
Use: Laxative.
ALODOPA-15 TABLETS. (Major) Hy-
drochlorothiazide 15 mg, methyldopa
250 mg. Bot. 100s.
Use: Antihypertensive.
ALODOPA-25 TABLETS. (Major) Hy-
drochlorothiazide 25 mg, methyldopa
250 mg. Bot. 100s.
Use: Antihypertensive.
• **ALOE,** U.S.P. XXIII.
Use: See Compound Benzoin Tincture.
ALOE GRANDE CREME. (Gordon) Aloe,
vitamins E 1500 IU, A 100,000 units/oz
in cream base. Jar 2.5 oz.
Use: Emollient.
ALOE VERA ACTIVE PRINCIPLE.
See: Alvagel, Oint. (Kenyon).
ALOE VESTA. (Vestal Labs) Solution of
sodium C14-16 olefin sulfonate, ampho-
teric 2, propylene glycol, aloe vera gel,
TEA-COCO hydrolyzed protein with sor-
bitol, DMDM hydantoin, cetethyl mor-
pholinium ethosulfate, citric acid. Bot.
120 ml, 240 ml, gal.
Use: Perianal hygiene.
• **ALOFILCON A.** USAN.
Use: Contact lens material (hy-
drophilic).
ALOIN. (Baker, J.T.) A mixture of crys-
talline pentosides from various aloes.
Bot. oz.
Use: Laxative.

W/Ox bile (desiccated), phenolphthalein, cascara sagrada extract, podophyllin.
See: Bilgon (Reid-Rowell).

ALOMIDE. (Alcon) Lodoxamide tromethamine 0.1%. Soln. Drop-tainers 10 ml.
Use: Antiallergy agent, ophthalmic.

• **ALONIMID.** USAN.
Use: Sedative.

ALOPHEN PILLS. (Warner-Lambert Consumer) Phenolphthalein 60 mg/Tab. Bot. 100s.
Use: Laxative.

ALOTONE. (Major) Triamcinolone 4 mg/Tab. Bot. 100s.
Use: Corticosteroid.

• **ALOVUDINE.** USAN.
Use: Antiviral.

ALOXIDONE. B.A.N. 3-Allyl-5-methyloxa- zolidine-2,4-dione. Allomethadione (I.N.N.) Malidone.
Use: Anticonvulsant.

ALOXIPRIN. B.A.N. Polymoric condonca- tion product of aluminum oxide and O- acetylsalicylic acid. Palaprin.
Use: Antirheumatic.

• **ALPERTINE.** USAN.
Use: Antipsychotic.

L-ALPHA-ACETYL-METHADOL (LAAM). (Biodevelopment)
Use: Treatment of heroin addicts. [Or- phan drug]

• **ALPHA AMYLASE.** USAN. A concentrat- ed form of alpha amylase produced by a strain of nonpathogenic bacteria.
Use: Digestive aid.
See: Kutrase, Cap. (Kremers-Urban). Ku-Zyme, Cap. (Kremers-Urban).

ALPHA-AMYLASE W-100. W/Proteinase W-300, cellase W-100, lipase, estrone, testosterone, vitamins, minerals.
Use: Digestive aid.
See: Geramine, Tab. (Brown).

ALPHA₁-ADRENERGIC BLOCKERS.
Use: Antihypertensive.
See: Cardura (Roerig).

ALPHA₁ANTITRYPSIN (RECOMBINANT DNA ORIGIN).
Use: Supplementation therapy for alpha₁ antitrypsin deficiency in the ZZ phenotype population. [Orphan drug]

ALPHA-1-PROTEINASE INHIBITOR.
Use: Treatment of Alpha-1-antitrypsin deficiency. [Orphan drug]

ALPHA/BETA-ADRENERGIC BLOCKER.
See: Normodyne (Schering). Trandate (Allen & Hanburys).

ALPHACETYLMETHADOL. B.A.N. α-4- Dimethylamino-1-ethyl-2,2- diphenylpentyl acetate.
Use: Analgesic.

ALPHA-CHYMOTRYPSIN.
See: Alpha Chymar, Vial (Armour). Zolyse, Vial (Alcon).

ALPHADERM. (Lemmon) Hydrocorti- sone 1%. Cream 30 Gm, 100 Gm.
Use: Corticosteroid, topical.

ALPHA-D-GALACTOSIDASE.
Use: Antiflatulent.

ALPHADOLONE. B.A.N. 3α,21-Dihy- droxy-5α- pregnane-11,20-dione.
Use: Anesthetic component.

ALPHA-E. (Barth's) d-Alpha tocopherol.
50 IU or 100 IU: Cap. Bot. 100s, 500s, 1000s. **200 IU:** Cap. Bot. 100s, 250s. **400 IU:** Cap. Bot. 100s, 250s, 500s.
Use: Vitamin E Supplement.

ALPHA-ESTRADIOL. Known to be beta- estradiol.
See: Estradiol (Various Mfr.).

ALPHA-ESTRADIOL BENZOATE.
See: Estradiol benzoate (Various Mfr.).

ALPHA FAST. (Eastwood) Bath oil. Bot. 16 oz.
Use: Emollient.

ALPHA-FETOPROTEIN W/TC-99M. USAN.
Use: Diagnostic aid.

ALPHA-GALACTOSIDASE.
See: Aspergillus niger enzyme.

ALPHA-GALACTOSIDASE A.
Use: Fabry's disease. [Orphan drug]

ALPHA-GALACTOSIDE A. USAN.
Use: Treatment of Fabry's disease.

ALPHA-HYPOPHAMINE.
See: Oxytocin Inj.

ALPHA INTERFERON-2A.
See: Roferon-A (Roche).

ALPHA INTERFERON-2B.
See: Intron A (Schering).

ALPHA-KERI. (Westwood) **Therapeutic Bath:** Mineral oil, lanolin oil, PEG 4 di laurate, benzophenone-3, D & C green #6, fragrance. Bot. 4 oz, 8 oz, 16 oz. **Spray:** 5 oz. **Cleansing Bar:** Bar con- taining sodium tallowate, sodium co- coate, water, mineral oil, fragrance, PEG-75, glycerin, titanium dioxide, lano- lin oil, sodium Cl, BHT, EDTA, D & C green #5, D & C yellow # 10. 120 g.
Use: Emollient.

ALPHAMEPRODINE. B.A.N. α-3-Ethyl-1- methyl-4-propionyloxypiperidine.
Use: Analgesic.

ALPHAMETHADOL. B.A.N. α-6-Di- methyl-amino-4,4-diphenylheptan-3-ol.

Use: Analgesic.

ALPHAMUL. (Lannett) Castor oil 60% w/v, emulsifying agent. Bot. 3 fl oz, gal.
Use: Laxative.

ALPHA-METHYLDOPA. Name previously used for Methyldopa.

ALPHANINE. (Alpha Therapeutic) Purified heat-treated/solvent preparation of coagulation Factor IX from human plasma. With ≥ 50 units Factor IX per mg protein, < 5 units each Factor II and Factor VII per 100 IU Factor IX and < 20 units Factor X per 100 IU Factor IX. In single-dose vials with diluent, double-ended needle and microaggregated filter. Powder for injection.
Use: Prevention and control of bleeding in Factor IX deficiency.

ALPHANINE SD. (Alpha Therapeutic) Purified, solvent detergent treated preparation of Factor IX derived from human plasma, ≥ 50 units Factor IX per mg protein, < 5 units each Factor II (prothrombin) and Factor VII (proconvertin) per 100 IU Factor IX, < 20 units Factor X (Stuart-Prower factor) per 100 IU Factor IX. Inj. In a single-dose vial with 10 ml diluent, double-ended needle and microaggregate filter.
Use: Prevention and control of bleeding in Factor IX deficiency due to hemophilia B.

ALPHA-PHENOXYETHYL PENICILLIN, POTASSIUM.
See: Phenethicillin Potassium.

ALPHAPRODINE. B.A.N. U.S.P. XXI. α-1,3-Dimethyl-4-phenyl-4-propionyloxypiperidine.
Use: Analgesic.

ALPHASONE ACETOPHENIDE. Name previously used for Algestone acetonide.

ALPHA-TOCOPHEROL.
See: Dalfatol, Cap. (Reid-Rowell).
Tocopherol, Alpha (Various Mfr.).

dl-ALPHA-TOCOPHEROL SUCCINATE.
See: DAlpha-E, Cap. (Alto).

ALPHATREX. (Savage) **Cream and Oint.:** Betamethasone dipropionate 0.05%. Tube 15 Gm, 45 Gm. **Lot.:** Betamethasone dipropionate 0.05%. Bot. 60 ml.
Use: Corticosteroid, topical.

ALPHA VEE-12. (Schlicksup) Hydroxocobalamin 1000 mcg/ml. Vial 10 ml.
Use: Vitamin B_{12} supplement.

ALPHAXALONE. B.A.N. 3α-Hydroxy-5α-pregnane-11,20-dione.
Use: Anesthetic component.

ALPHA-ZETA. (Parmed) Fe 27 mg, vitamins A 5,000 IU, D 400 IU, E 30 IU, B_1 2.25 mg, B_2 2.6 mg, B_3 20 mg, B_5 10 mg, B_6 3 mg, B_{12} 9 mcg, C 90 mg, FA 0.4 mg, biotin 45 mcg, Ca, Cl, Cr, Cu, I, K, Mg, Mn, Mo, P, Se, Zn/Tab. Bot. 30s.
Use: Vitamin supplement with iron.

ALPHOSYL. (Reed & Carnrick) Allantoin 1.7%, special crude coal tar extracts 5%. **Lot.:** Bot. 8 fl oz. **Cream:** 2 oz.
Use: Antipruritic.

• **ALPIDEM.** USAN.
Use: Antianxiety agent (anxiolytic).

• **ALPRAZOLAM,** U.S.P. XXIII. Tab., U.S.P. XXIII. 8-Chloro-1-methyl-6-phenyl-4H-s-triazolo (4,3-α)(1,4)benzodiazepine.
Use: Management of anxiety disorders.
See: Xanax, Tab. (Upjohn).

ALPRAZOLAM. (Various Mfr.) Alprazolam **0.25 mg, 0.5 mg, 1 mg:** Tab. Bot. 30s, 100s, 500s, 1000s, UD 100s; **2 mg:** Tab. Bot. 100s, 500s.
Use: Management of anxiety disorders.

ALPRAZOLAM. (Roxane) **Oral soln.:** Alprazolam 0.5 mg/5 ml, sorbitol, saccharin. Bot. 500 ml, UD 2.5 ml, UD 5 ml, UD 10 ml. **Intensol soln.:** Alprazolam 1 mg/ml. Bot. 30 ml with dropper.
Use: Management of anxiety disorders.

ALPRENOLOL. B.A.N. 1-(2-Allylphenoxy)-3-iso-propylaminopropan-2 ol. Betaptin hydrochloride.
Use: Beta-adrenergic receptor blocking agent.

• **ALPRENOLOL HYDROCHLORIDE.** USAN.
Use: Anti-adrenergic.

• **ALPRENOXIME HYDROCHLORIDE.** USAN.
Use: Antiglaucoma agent.

• **ALPROSTADIL,** U.S.P. XXIII. Inj., U.S.P. XXIII. (11α, 13E,15S)-11,15 dihydroxy-9-oxoprost-13-en-1-oic acid.
Use: Palliative therapy to maintain patency of the ductus arteriosus in neonates with congenital heart defects.
See: Prostin VR, Inj. (Upjohn).

ALRAMUCIL. (Alra) Psyllium. Pow. effervescent Pkg. 30s.
Use: Laxative.

ALREDASE. (Wyeth-Ayerst).
Use: Aldose reduction inhibitor.

• **ALRESTATIN SODIUM.** USAN.
Use: Enzyme inhibitor.

ALSEROXYLON-ALKAVERVIR. A mixture of partially purified extracts of Rauwolfia serpentina and Veratrum viride.

ALSORB GEL. (Standex) Magnesium and aluminum hydroxide. Colloidal Susp.
Use: Antacid.

ALSORB GEL, C.T. (Standex) Calcium carbonate 2 gr, glycine 3 gr, magnesium trisilicate 3 gr/Tab.
Use: Antacid.
ALTACE. (Hoechst-Roussel/Upjohn) Ramipril 1.25 mg, 2.5 mg, 5 mg or 10 mg/Cap. Bot. 100s, UD 100s.
Use: Antihypertensive.
• **ALTANSERIN TARTRATE.** USAN.
Use: Serotonin antagonist.
ALTEPLASE. U.S.P. 23, Injection, U.S.P. 23. Tissue plasminogen activator; tPA.
Use: Thrombolytic.
See: Activase.
ALTERNAGEL. (J & J-Merck) Aluminum hydroxide 600 mg/5 ml. Liq. Bot. 150 ml, 360 ml.
Use: Antacid.
ALTHIAZIDE. USAN. 3-Allylthiomethyl-3-4-dihydro-6-chloro-7-sulfamoyl-1,2,4-benzothiadiazine-1-dioxide.
Use: Hypotensive, diuretic.
ALTRACIN. USAN.
Use: Antibiotic.
• **ALTRETAMINE.** USAN.
Use: Antineoplastic. [Orphan drug]
See: Hexalen (US Bioscience)
ALU-CAP. (3M Pharm) Aluminum hydroxide gel 400 mg/Cap. Bot. 100s.
Use: Antacid.
AL-U-CREME. (MacAllister) Aluminum hydroxide equivalent to 4% aluminum oxide. Susp. Bot. pt, gal.
Use: Antacid.
ALUDROX. (Wyeth-Ayerst) Aluminum hydroxide gel 307 mg, magnesium hydroxide 103 mg/5 ml. Susp. Bot. 355 ml
Use: Antacid.
ALUKALIN. Activated kaolin.
Use: Antidiarrheal.
See: Lusyn, Tab. (Pennwalt).
ALULEX. (Lexington) Magnesium trisilicate 3.25 gr, aluminum hydroxide gel 3.5 gr, phenobarbital 1/8 gr, homatropine methylbromide gr/Tab. Bot. 100s.
Use: Agent for peptic ulcer.
• **ALUM,** U.S.P. XXIII. Sulfuric acid, aluminum ammonium salt (2:1:1), dodecahydrate. Sulfuric acid, aluminum potassium salt (2:1:1), dodecahydrate.
Use: Astringent.
• **ALUM, AMMONIUM,** U.S.P. XXIII.
Use: Astringent.
• **ALUM, POTASSIUM,** U.S.P. XXIII.
Use: Astringent.
ALUMADRINE. (Fleming) Acetaminophen 500 mg, phenylpropanolamine HCl 25 mg, chlorpheniramine maleate 4 mg/Tab. Bot. 100s, 1000s.

Use: Analgesic, decongestant, antihistamine.
ALUMATE-HC. (Dermco) Hydrocortisone 1/8%, 0.25%, 0.5% or 1%. Cream % Pkg. 4 oz. 0.25% Pkg. 1 oz. 0.5% Pkg. 0.5 oz, 1 oz. 1% Pkg. 0.5 oz.
Use: Corticosteroid, topical.
ALUMATE MIXTURE. (Schlicksup) Aluminum hydroxide gel, milk of magnesia/5 ml. Bot. 12 oz, gal.
Use: Antacid.
ALUMA HYDRATED POWDER.
W/Activated attapulgite, pectin.
Use: Antidiarrheal.
See: Polymagma, Plain, Tab. (Wyeth-Ayerst).
• **ALUMINA, MAGNESIA, AND CALCIUM CARBONATE TABLETS,** U.S.P. XXIII.
Use: Antacid.
• **ALUMINA, MAGNESIA, CALCIUM CARBONATE, AND SIMETHICONE TABLETS,** U.S.P. XXIII.
• **ALUMINA, MAGNESIA, AND CALCIUM CHLORIDE ORAL SUSPENSION,** U.S.P. XXIII.
Use: Antacid.
• **ALUMINA AND MAGNESIA ORAL SUSPENSION,** U.S.P. XXIII.
Use: Antacid.
• **ALUMINA AND MAGNESIA TABLETS,** U.S.P. XXIII.
Use: Antacid
• **ALUMINA, MAGNESIA AND SIMETHICONE,** U.S.P. XXIII, Susp., Tab., U.S.P. XXIII.
Use: Antacid, antiflatulent.
ALUMINA, MAGNESIA AND SIMETHICONE SUSPENSION. (Roxane) Aluminum hydroxide 213 mg, magnesium hydroxide 200 mg, simethicone 20 mg, parabens, sorbitol/5 ml. Susp. Bot. UD 15, 30 ml.
Use: Antacid.
• **ALUMINA AND MAGNESIUM CARBONATE ORAL SUSPENSION,** U.S.P. XXII.
Use: Antacid.
• **ALUMINA, MAGNESIUM CARBONATE, AND MAGNESIUM OXIDE TABLETS,** U.S.P. XXIII.
Use: Antacid.
• **ALUMINA AND MAGNESIUM TRISILICATE ORAL SUSPENSION,** U.S.P. XXIII.
Use: Antacid.
• **ALUMINA AND MAGNESIUM TRISILICATE TABLETS,** U.S.P. XXIII.
Use: Antacid.
ALUMINETT. (Lannett) Aluminum hydroxide 10 gr/Tab. Bot. 1000s.

Use: Antacid.
ALUMINOSTOMY. (Richards Pharm.)
Aluminum pow. 18%, zinc oxide, zinc
stearate in a bland water repellent oint-
ment. Jar 2 oz, 6 oz, lb.
Use: Skin protectant.
ALUMINUM.
See: Aluminostomy (Richards Pharm.).
ALUMINUM ACETATE.
Use: Astringent.
See: Acid Mantle Creme (Sandoz Con-
sumer).
Buro-Sol pow. (Doak).
W/Phenol, zinc oxide, boric acid, eucalyp-
tol, ichthammol.
See: Lanaburn, Oint. (Lannett).
W/Salicylic acid, boric acid.
• **ALUMINUM ACETATE TOPICAL SOLU-
TION,** U.S.P. XXIII. (Various Mfr.).
Burow's Solution.
Use: Astringent.
See: Bluboro Powder (Herbert).
Buro-Sol Powder Conc. (Doak).
Burotor, Emul. (Torch).
Domeboro, Pow. (Miles Pharm).
**ALUMINUM AMINOACETATE, DIHY-
DROXY.**
See: Dihydroxy aluminum aminoac-
etate (Various Mfr.).
ALUMINUM CARBONATE BASIC.
Use: Antacid.
See: Basaljel, Susp. (Wyeth-Ayerst).
• **ALUMINUM CARBONATE, DRIED BA-
SIC, GEL,** U.S.P. XXIII, Cap., Tab.,
U.S.P. XXIII.
Use: Antacid.
• **ALUMINUM CARBONATE GEL, BASIC,**
U.S.P. XXIII.
Use: Antacid.
See: Basaljel, Preps (Wyeth-Ayerst).
**ALUMINUM CHLORHYDROXY ALLAN-
TOINATE.**
See: Alcloxa (Schuylkill).
• **ALUMINUM CHLORIDE,** U.S.P. XXIII.
Aluminum Cl hexahydrate.
Use: Astringent.
W/Oxyquinoline sulfate, benzalkonium Cl.
See: Alochor Stypic (Gordon Labs.).
**ALUMINUM CHLORIDE
HEXAHYDRATE.**
Use: Astringent.
See: Drysol (Person & Covey).
• **ALUMINUM CHLOROHYDRATE.** U.S.P.
23, Solution, U.S.P. 23.
Use: Anhidrotic.
See: Ostiderm, Lot., Roll-On (Pedinol).
• **ALUMINUM CHLOROHYDREX.** USAN.
Use: Astringent.
ALUMINUM CLOFIBRATE. B.A.N. Di-[2-
(4-chlorophenoxy)-2-methylpropionato]

hydroxyaluminum.
Use: Treatment of arteriosclerosis.
**ALUMINUM DIHYDROXYAMINOAC-
ETATE.**
See: Dihydroxy Aluminum Aminoac-
etate, U.S.P. XXIII. (Various Mfr.).
ALUMINUM GLYCINATE, BASIC.
See: Dihydroxy Aluminum Aminoac-
etate, U.S.P. XXIII.
W/Aspirin, Magnesium carbonate.
See: Bufferin, Tab. (Bristol-Myers).
• **ALUMINUM HYDROXIDE GEL,** U.S.P.
XXIII. Aqueous susp. of aluminum hy-
droxide equivalent to 4% aluminum ox-
ide.
Use: Antacid.
See: Alterna GEL, Liq. (J & J-Merck).
Alu-Cap, Cap. (3M Pharm).
Al-U-Creme, Susp. (MacAllister).
Aluminett, Tab. (Lannett).
Alu-Tab, Tab. (3M Pharm).
Amphojel, Susp., Tab. (Wyeth-Ayerst).
Dialume, Cap. (RPR).
Nutrajel (Cenci).
W/Aminoacetic acid, magnesium trisili-
cate.
See: Maracid-2, Tab. (Marin).
W/Aminophylline.
See: Asmadrin, Tab. (Jenkins).
W/Belladonna extract, magnesium hydrox-
ide.
See: Trialka, Liq., Tab. (Commerce).
W/Calcium carbonate.
See: Alkalade, Susp., Tab. (DePree).
W/Calcium carbonate, magnesium car-
bonate, magnesium trisilicate.
See: Marblen, Susp., Tab. (Fleming).
W/Clioquinol, methylcellulose, atropine
sulfate, hyoscine HBr, hyoscyamine sul-
fate.
See: Enterex, Tab. (Person & Covey).
W/Dicyclomine HCl, magnesium hydrox-
ide, methylcellulose.
See: Triactin Liq., Tab. (Norwich).
W/Gastric mucin, magnesium glycinate.
See: Mucogel, Liq., Tab. (Inwood).
W/Kaolin, pectin.
See: Metropectin, Liq. (Pennwalt).
W/Magnesium carbonate.
See: Algicon, Tab. (Rorer Consumer).
Estomul-M Liq., Tab. (Riker).
W/Magnesium carbonate, calcium carbon-
ate, amino-acetic acid.
See: Glycogel Tab., Susp. (Central).
W/Magnesium hydroxide.
See: Alsorb Gel (Standex).
Aludrox, Susp., Tab. (Wyeth-Ayerst).
Delcid, Liq. (Merrell Dow).
Kolantyl, Gel, Wafer (Merrell Dow).
Maalox, Susp. (Rhone-Poulenc Ror-

er).
Mylanta, Tab. (Stuart).
Mylanta II, Tab. (Stuart).
Neutralox, Susp. (Lemmon).
WinGel, Liq., Tab. (Sanofi Winthrop
    Consumer Products).
W/Magnesium hydroxide, aspirin.
    See: Ascriptin, Tab. (Rhone-Poulenc
    Rorer).
    Ascriptin Extra Strength, Tab. (Rorer
    Consumer).
    Calciphen, Tab. (Westerfield).
    Cama, Tab. (Dorsey).
    Cama Inlay-Tab. (Sandoz Consumer).
W/Magnesium hydroxide, belladonna ex-
    tract
W/Magnesium hydroxide, calcium carbon-
    ate.
    See: Camalox, Susp. (Rhone-Poulenc
    Rorer).
W/Magnesium hydroxide, glycine, magne-
    sium trisilicate, belladonna extract.
W/Magnesium hydroxide and simethicone.
    See: DI-GEL, Liq. (Plough).
    Maalox Plus, Susp. (Rhone-Poulenc
    Rorer).
    Mylanta, Liq. (Stuart).
    Mylanta-II, Liq. (Stuart).
    Silain-Gel, Liq., Tab. (Robins).
    Simeco, Liq. (Wyeth-Ayerst).
W/Magnesium trisilicate.
    See: Antacid G, Tab. (Walgreen).
    Antacid Tablets, Tab. (Panray).
    Arcodex Antiacid, Tab. (Arcum).
    Gacid, Tab. (Arcum).
    Malcogel, Susp. (Upjohn).
    Malcotabs (Upjohn).
    Manalum, Tab. (Paddock).
    Trisogel, Pulv., Susp. (Lilly).
W/Paregoric, kaolin (colloidal), bismuth
    subcarbonate, pectin, aromatics.
    See: Kapinal, Tab. (Jenkins).
W/Phenindamine tartrate, phenylephrine
    HCl, aspirin, caffeine, magnesium car-
    bonate.
    See: Dristan, Tab. (Whitehall).
W/Phenol, zinc oxide, camphor, eucalyp-
    tol, ichthammol.
    See: Almophen, Oint. (Bowman).
W/Prednisolone.
    See: Fernisolone-B (Ferndale).
    Predoxine, Tab. (Hauck).
W/Sodium salicylate, acetaminophen, vita-
    min C.
    See: Gaysal-S., Tab. (Geriatric).
ALUMINUM HYDROXIDE GEL. (Various
    Mfr.) 320 mg/5 ml. Susp. Bot. 360 ml,
    480 ml, UD 15 and 30 ml.
    Use: Antacid.
ALUMINUM HYDROXIDE GEL, CON-

CENTRATED. (Various Mfr.) 600 mg/5
    ml. Liq. Bot. 30 ml, 180 ml, 480 ml.
    Use: Antacid.
ALUMINUM HYDROXIDE GEL, CON-
    CENTRATED. (Roxane) Susp. 450
    mg/5 ml: Bot. 500 ml, UD 30 ml; 675
    mg/5 ml: Bot. 180 ml, 500 ml, UD 20 ml
    and 30 ml.
    Use: Antacid.
• ALUMINUM HYDROXIDE GEL, DRIED,
    U.S.P. XXIII. Tab. U.S.P. XXIII.
    Use: Antacid.
    See: Amphojel, Tab. (Wyeth-Ayerst).
• ALUMINUM HYDROXIDE GEL, DRIED,
    CAPSULES, U.S.P. XXIII.
    Use: Antacid.
ALUMINUM HYDROXIDE GEL, DRIED
    W/COMBINATIONS.
    Use: Antacid.
    See: Aludrox, Susp., Tab. (Wyeth-Ay-
    erst).
    Alurex, Tab. (Rexall).
    Banacid, Tab. (Buffington).
    Camalox, Tab. (Rhone-Poulenc Ror-
    er).
    Delcid, Liq. (Merrell Dow).
    Eulcin, Tab. (Leeds).
    Fermalox, Tab. (Rhone-Poulenc Ror-
    er).
    Gas-Eze, Tab. (E. J. Moore).
    Gaviscon, Foamtab (Marion).
    Gelusil, Preps. (Parke-Davis).
    Kolantyl, Wafers (Merrell Dow).
    Maalox, Tab. (Rhone-Poulenc Rorer).
    Maalox Plus, Tab. (Rhone-Poulenc
    Rorer).
    Magnatril, Tab., Susp. (Lannett).
    Malcotabs, Tab. (Upjohn).
    Mylanta, Tab., Liq. (Stuart).
    Mylanta II, Tab., Liq. (Stuart).
    Phencaset Improved, Tab. (Elder).
    Presalin, Tab. (Hauck).
    Silmagel, Tab. (Lannett).
    Spasmasorb, Tab. (Hauck).
ALUMINUM HYDROXIDE GLYCINE.
    See: Dihydroxy aluminum aminoac-
    etate.
ALUMINUM HYDROXIDE MAGNESIUM
    CARBONATE.
    Use: Antacid.
    See: Aloxine (Forest).
    DI-GEL, Tab. (Plough).
    Magnagel, Susp., Tab. (Hauck).
W/Aminoacetic acid, calcium carbonate.
    See: Eugel, Tab., Liq. (Reid-Rowell).
W/Dicyclomine HCl, magnesium trisilicate,
    methylcellulose.
    See: Triactin, Liq., Tab. (Norwich).
W/Magnesium trisilicate.
    See: Escot, Cap. (Reid-Rowell).

W/Magnesium trisilicate, bismuth alumi-
nate.
See: Escot, Cap. (Reid-Rowell).
• **ALUMINUM MONOSTEARATE,** N.F.
XVIII. Aluminum, dihydroxy(octade-
canoato-O-)-,Dihydroxy (stearato)alu-
minum.
ALUMINUM OXIDE
See: Epi-Clear Scrub Cleanser
(Squibb).
ALUMINUM PASTE. (Paddock) Metallic
aluminum 10%. Oint. Jar lb.
Use: Topical combination, miscella-
neous.
ALUMINUM PHENOSULFONATE.
See: AR-EX Cream Deodorant (Ar-Ex).
• **ALUMINUM PHOSPHATE GEL,** U.S.P.
XXIII. Aluminum phosphate 4.15%.
Use: Antacid.
See: Phosphaljel, Susp. (Wyeth-Ay-
erst).
• **ALUMINUM
SESQUICHLOROHYDRATE.** USAN.
Use: Anhidrotic.
**ALUMINUM SODIUM CARBONATE HY-
DROXIDE.**
See: Dihydroxyaluminum Sodium Car-
bonate.
• **ALUMINUM SUBACETATE TOPICAL
SOLUTION,** U.S.P. XXIII. (Various Mfr.)
Aluminum acetate basic solution, alu-
minum subacetate solution.
Use: Astringent wash.
• **ALUMINUM SULFATE,** U.S.P. XXIII.
Use: Pharmaceutic necessity for prepa-
ration of aluminum subacetate solu-
tion.
• **ALUMINUM ZIRCONIUM OC-
TACHLOROHYDRATE,** U.S.P. 23.
• **ALUMINUM ZIRCONIUM OC-
TACHLOROHYDREX GLY,** U.S.P. 23.
• **ALUMINUM ZIRCONIUM PEN-
TACHLOROHYDRATE,** U.S.P. 23.
• **ALUMINUM ZIRCONIUM PEN-
TACHLOROHYDRATE GLY,** U.S.P. 23.
• **ALUMINUM ZIRCONIUM TETRA-
CHLOROHYDRATE,** U.S.P. 23.
• **ALUMINUM ZIRCONIUM TETRA-
CHLOROHYDREX GLY,** U.S.P. 23.
Use: Anhidrotic.
• **ALUMINUM ZIRCONIUM TRICHLORO-
HYDRATE.** U.S.P. 23.
• **ALUMINUM ZIRCONIUM TRICHLORO-
HYDREX GLY,.** U.S.P. 23.
Use: Anhidrotic.
ALUPENT. (Boehringer Ingelheim)
Metaproterenol sulfate. **Metered dose
inhaler:** 225 mg in 15 ml. **Tab.:** 10 mg or
20 mg. Bot. 100s. **Syr.:** 10 mg/5 ml. Bot.
pt. **Inhalant Soln.:** 0.4%: 2.5 ml UD vial.

0.6%: 2.5 ml UD vial. **5%:** Bot. 10 ml, 30
ml UD.
Use: Bronchodilator.
ALURATE. (Roche) Aprobarbital 40 mg/5
ml. Alcohol 20%. Elix. Bot. pt.
Use: Sedative/hypnotic.
ALUREX. (Rexall) Magnesium-aluminum
hydroxido. **Susp.:** (200 mg 150 mg/5
ml) Bot. 12 oz. **Tab:** (400 mg-300 mg)
Box 50s.
Use: Antacid.
ALU-TAB. (3M Pharm) Aluminum hydrox-
ide gel 500 mg/Tab. Bot. 250s.
Use: Antacid.
ALVAGEL. (Kenyon) Aloe vera active
principle 55% in ointment base. Tube 2
oz, 4 oz.
Use: Skin protectant.
ALVEDIL CAPS. (Luly-Thomas) Theo-
phylline 4 gr, pseudoephedrine HCl 50
mg, butabarbital 15 mg/Cap. Bot. 100s.
Use: Bronchodilator, decongestant,
sedative/hypnotic.
• **ALVERINE CITRATE.** USAN. N-ethyl-
3,3'-diphenyl dipropylamine citrate.
Use: Anticholinergic.
See: Spacolin, Tab. (Philips Roxane).
• **ALVIRCEPT SUNDOTOX. USAN.**
Use: Antiviral agent.
AL-VITE. (Drug Industries) Vitamins A
10,000 IU, D_3 400 IU, E 25 IU, C 200
mg, B_1 20 mg, B_2 10 mg, B_6 6 mg, calci-
um pantothenate 20 mg, niacinamide
100 mg, B_{12} w/intrinsic factor concen-
trate 0.5 units/Tab. Bot. 100s, 500s.
Use: Vitamin/mineral supplement.
ALZAPAM. (Major) Lorazepam 0.5 mg, 1
mg or 2 mg/Tab. Bot. 100s, 500s.
Use: Antianxiety agent.
AMA. (Wampole-Zeus) Antimitochondrial
antibodies test by IFA. Test 48s.
Use: Diagnostic aid.
• **AMACETAM SULFATE.** USAN.
Use: Cognition adjuvant.
AMACID. (Kenyon) An acid protein hy-
drolysate prepared from casein and lac-
talbumin by special process which re-
tains l-tryptophan and other essential
amino acids. Bot. 4 oz, pt, gal.
AMACODONE. (Trimen) Hydrocodone
bitartrate 5 mg, acetaminophen 500
mg/Tab. Bot. 100s.
Use: Narcotic analgesic combination.
• **AMADIMONE ACETATE.** USAN.
Use: Progestin.
AMANOZINE HYDROCHLORIDE. 2-
Amino-4-anilino-s-triazine HCl.
AMANTADINE. B.A.N. 1-Adaman-
tanamine.

Use: Antiviral agent, treatment of Parkinson's disease.
See: Symadine, Cap. (Solvay). Symmetrel, Cap. (Du Pont).

• AMANTADINE HYDROCHLORIDE, U.S.P. XXIII. Caps., Syr., U.S.P. XXIII. 1-Adamantanamine HCl. Tricylo(3.3.1.1^{3,7})decan-1-amine, HCl. (Various Mfg.) **Cap.:** 100 mg. Bot. 100s, 250s, 500s, UD 100s. **Syrup:** 50 mg/5 ml Bot. pint.
Use: Antiviral agent, treatment of Parkinson's disease.
See: Symmetrel, Cap., Syr. (DuPont).

AMAPHEN. (Trimen) Butalbital 50 mg, caffeine 40 mg, acetaminophen 325 mg/Cap. Bot. 100s.
Use: Sedative/hypnotic, analgesic.

AMAPHEN W/CODEINE #3. (Trimen) Codeine phosphate 30 mg, acetaminophen 325 mg, caffeine 40 mg, butalbital 50 mg Cap. Bot. 100s.
Use: Narcotic analgesic combination, sedative/hypnotic.

AMARANTH. 3-Hydroxy-4-[(4-sulfo-1-naphthyl)azo]-2,7-naphthalene-disulfonic acid trisodium salt. F.D. and C. Red No. 2.
Use: Color (Not for internal use).

AMARSAN.
See: Acetarsone.

AMAZONE. 1:4-Benzoquinone amidinohydrazine thiosemicarbazone hydrate. Iversal.

AMBAZONE. B.A.N. 1,4-Benzoquinone amidinohydrazone thiosemicarbazone.
Uso: Antiseptic.

AMBENONIUM CHLORIDE. N,N′-bis-(2-Diethyl aminoethyl) oxamide bis-2-chlorobenzyl Cl. [Oxalylbis (iminoethylene)] bis [(o-chlorobenzyl)-diethylammonium] dichloride. B.A.N. NN-Di-[2-(N-2-chlorobenzyldiethylammonio) ethyl] oxamide dichloride.
Use: Cholinergic for treatment of myasthenia gravis.
See: Mytelase, Cap. (Sanofi Winthrop).

AMBENOXAN. B.A.N. 2-(2-Methoxyethoxyethyl-aminomethyl)-1,4-benzodioxan.
Use: Muscle relaxant.

AMBENYL COUGH SYRUP. (Forest) Codeine phosphate 10 mg, bromodiphenhydramine HCl 12.5 mg/5 ml, alcohol 5%. Bot. 4 oz, pt, gal.
Use: Antitussive, antihistamine.

AMBENYL-D LIQUID. (Forest) Guaifenesin 100 mg, pseudoephedrine HCl 30 mg, dextromethorphan HBr 15 mg/10 ml, alcohol 9.5%. Bot. 4 oz.

Use: Expectorant, decongestant, antitussive.

AMBERLITE, I.R.P.-64. (Rohm and Haas). Polacrilin.

AMBERLITE, I.R.P.-88. (Rohm and Haas). Polacrilin potassium.

AMBI 10 CREAM. (Kiwi Brands) Benzoyl peroxide 10%, bentonite carbomer 940, glyceryl stearate, parabens, PEG, PPG. Cream. Tube 28.3 Gm.
Use: Anti-acne.

AMBI 10 SOAP. (Kiwi Brands) Triclosan, sodium tallouate, PEG-20, titanium dioxide. Soap, Bar 99 Gm.
Use: Therapeutic skin cleanser.

AMBIEN. (Searle) Zolipidem tartrate 5 mg, 10 mg/Tab. Bot. 100s, 500s, UD 100s.
Use: Sedative, hypnotic.

AMBI SKIN TONE. (Kiwi Brands) Hydroquinone, padimate O, sodium metabisulfate, parabens, EDTA, vitamin E. Cream. Tube 57 Gm, 28.4 Gm.
Use: Topical drug, miscellaneous.

• AMBOMYCIN. USAN. Isolated from filtrates of *Streptomyces ambofaciens.*
Use: Antineoplastic.

AMBROSIACEAE POLLENS. (Parke-Davis) Ragweed and related pollens.
See: Allergenic extracts.

• AMBRUTICIN. USAN.
Use: Antifungal.

AMBUCAINE. Ambutoxate HCl.

AMBUCETAMIDE. 2-(di-n-Butylamino)-2-(p-methoxyphenyl)acetamide

AMBUCETAMIDE. B.A.N. α-Dibutylamino-4-methoxyphenylacetamide.
Use: Antispasmodic.

• AMBUPHYLLINE. USAN. Theophylline compound with 2-amino-2-methyl-1-propanol. Bufylline.
Use: Diuretic, smooth muscle relaxant.

• AMBUSIDE. USAN. 5-Allylsulfamoyl-2-chloro-4-(3-hydroxybut-2-enylideneamino)benzenesulfonamide.
Use: Diuretic.
See: Novohydrin.

AMBUTONIUM BROMIDE. Ethyl-dimethylammonium(3-carbamyl-3,3-diphenyl propyl)-ethyl dimethylammonium bromide.
Use: Antispasmodic.

AMBUTONIUM BROMIDE. B.A.N. (3-Carbamoyl-3,3-diphenylpropyl)ethyl-dimethylammonium bromide.
Use: Antispasmodic.

AMBUTOXATE HYDROCHLORIDE. 2-Diethylaminoethyl-4-amino-2-butoxybenzoate HCl. Ambucaine.

AMC. (Schlicksup) Ammonium Cl 7.5 gr/Tab. Bot. 1000s.
Use: Diuretic, expectorant.

AMCILL. (Parke-Davis) **Cap.:** Ampicillin trihydrate 250 mg or 500 mg/Cap. Bot. 100s, 500s, UD pkg 100s. **Oral Susp.:** 125 mg or 250 mg/5 ml. Bot. 100 ml, 200 ml.
Use: Antibacterial, penicillin.

• **AMCINAFAL.** USAN. 9-Fluoro-11β, 16α,17,21-tetrahydroxypregna-1,4-diene-3, 20-dione cyclic 16, 17-acetal with 3-pentanone.
Use: Anti-inflammatory agent.

• **AMCINAFIDE.** USAN. (R)-9-Fluoro-11β, 16α,17,21-tetrahydroxypregna-1, 4-diene-3,20-dione cyclic 16,17-acetal with acetophenone.
Use: Anti-inflammatory agent.

• **AMCINONIDE,** U.S.P. XXIII. Cream, Oint., U.S.P. XXIII.
Use: Glucocorticoid.
See: Cyclocort, Cream, Oint. (Lederle).

AMCORT. (Keene) Triamcinolone diacetate 40 mg/ml. Vial 5 ml.
Use: Corticosteroid.

• **AMDINOCILLIN.** USAN. 6-β-amidinopenicillanic acid.
Use: Antibacterial.

AMEBAN.
See: Carbarsone.

AMEBICIDES.
See: Acetarsone (Various Mfr.).
  Aralen HCl, Inj. (Sanofi Winthrop).
  Aralen Phosphate, Tab. (Sanofi Winthrop).
  Carbarsone, Pulv., Tab. (Lilly).
  Chiniofon, Tab. (Various Mfr.).
  Chloroquine Phosphate, Tab. (Various Mfr.).
  Diiodohydroxyquin (Various Mfr.).
  Diodoquin, Tab. (Searle).
  Emetine HCl (Various Mfr.).
  Flagyl, Tab. (Searle).
  Humatin, Kapseal, Syr. (Parke-Davis).
  Yodoxin, Tab. (Glenwood).

AMECHOL.
Use: Diagnostic aid.
See: Methacholine Cl.

• **AMEDALIN HYDROCHLORIDE.** USAN. 3-Methyl-3-[3-(methylamino)propyl]-1-phenyl-2-indolinone monohydrochloride.
Use: Antidepressant.

• **AMELTOLIDE.** USAN.
Use: Anticonvulsant.

AMEN. (Carnrick) Medroxyprogesterone acetate 10 mg/Tab. Bot. 50s, 100s, 1000s.

Use: Progestin.

AMERICAINE AEROSOL. (Ciba) Benzocaine 20% in a water-soluble vehicle. Bot. 0.67 oz, 2 oz, 4 oz.
Use: Local anesthetic.

AMERICAINE ANESTHETIC LUBRICANT. (Ciba) Benzocaine 20%, benzethonium Cl 0.1% in a water-soluble polyethylene glycol base. Foil pack 2.5 Gm, Pkg. 144s. Tube oz.
Use: Local anesthetic.

AMERICAINE FIRST AID BURN OINTMENT. (Ciba) Benzocaine 20%, benzethonium Cl 0.1% in a water-soluble polyethylene glycol base. Tube 0.75 oz.
Use: Local anesthetic.

AMERICAINE HEMORRHOIDAL OINTMENT. (Ciba) Benzocaine 20%, benzethonium Cl 0.1% in a water-soluble polyethylene glycol base. Tube oz w/rectal applicator.
Use: Local anesthetic.

AMERICAINE OTIC. (Ciba) Benzethonium Cl 0.1%, benzocaine 20% in a water-soluble base of 1% (w/w) glycerin, polyethylene glycol 300. Bot. 0.5 oz.
Use: Otic preparation.

AMES DEXTRO SYSTEM LANCETS. (Ames) Sterile disposable lancet. Box 100s.
Use: Diagnostic aid.

AMESEC. (Whitby) Theophylline 104 mg, aminophylline 130 mg, ephedrine HCl 25 mg/Cap. Bot. 100s.
Use: Bronchodilator.

AMESEC CAPSULES. (Glaxo) Aminophylline 130 mg, ephedrine HCl 25 mg/Cap. Bot. 100s, 500s.
Use: Bronchodilator.

• **AMESERGIDE.** USAN.
Use: Serotonin antagonist.

• **AMETANTRONE ACETATE.** USAN.
Use: Antineoplastic.

AMETAZOLE. B.A.N. 3-(2-Aminoethyl)pyrazole. Betazole (I.N.N.). Histalog, hydrochloride.
Use: To stimulate gastric secretion in diagnostic tests.

A-METHAPRED UNIVIAL. (Abbott Hospital Prods) Methylprednisolone sodium succinate. **40 mg/ml:** Pkg. 1s, 25s, 50s, 100s; 125 mg/2 ml Pkg. 1s, 5s, 25s, 50s, 100s; **500 mg/4 ml:** Pkg. 1s, 5s, 25s, 100s; **1000 mg/8 ml:** Pkg. 1s, 5s, 25s 100s.
Use: Corticosteroid.

AMETHOCAINE HYDROCHLORIDE.
Use: Local anesthetic.
See: Tetracaine HCl.

AMETHOPTERIN.

Use: Antineoplastic.
See: Methotrexate (Lederle).
AMFECLORAL. B.A.N. α-Methyl-
N(2,2,2-trichloroethylidene)-phenethy-
lamine.
Use: Appetite suppressant.
• **AMFENAC SODIUM.** USAN.
Use: Anti-inflammatory.
• **AMFILCON A.** USAN.
Use: Contact lens material (hy-
drophilic).
• **AMFLUTIZOLE.** USAN.
Use: Treatment of gout.
AMFODYNE.
See: Imidecyl iodine.
• **AMFONELIC ACID.** USAN. 7-Benzyl-1-
ethyl-4-oxo-1,8-naphthyridine-3-car-
boxylic acid.
Use: Central nervous system stimulant.
AMGENAL COUGH SYRUP. (Goldline)
Bromodiphenhydramine HCl 12.5 mg,
codeine phosphate 10 mg/5 ml, alcohol
5%. Bot. 120 ml, pt, gal.
Use: Antihistamine, antitussive.
AMIBIARSON.
See: Carbarsone (Various Mfr.).
AMICAR. (Lederle) Aminocaproic acid.
Syr.: 25%. Bot. pt. **Inj.:** 250 mg/ml. Vial
20 ml, 96 ml. **Tab.:** 500 mg. Bot. 100s.
Use: Antifibrinolytic agent.
• **AMICYCLINE.** USAN.
Use: Antibacterial.
AMIDATE. (Abbott Hospital Prods) Etomi-
date 2 mg/ml, propylene glycol 35%.
Single dose Amp 20 mg/10 ml or 40
mg/20 ml;Abboject syringe 40 mg/20
ml .
Use: General anesthetic.
AMIDEPHRINE. B.A.N. 3-(1-Hydroxy-2-
methylaminoethyl)methanesulfo-
nanilide. Dricol.
Use: Vasoconstrictor, nasal deconges-
tant.
• **AMIDEPHRINE MESYLATE.** USAN.
Use: Adrenergic.
AMIDOFEBRIN.
See: Aminopyrine (Various Mfr.).
AMIDONE HYDROCHLORIDE.
Use: Narcotic agonist analgesic.
See: Methadone HCl (Various Mfr.).
AMIDOPYRAZOLINE.
See: Aminopyrine (Various Mfr.).
AMIDOTRIZOATE, SODIUM.
See: Diatrizoate sodium.
AMIDOTRIZOIC ACID. Diatrizoic Acid.
B.A.N.
• **AMIFLOXACIN.** USAN.
Use: Antibacterial.
• **AMIFLOXACIN MESYLATE.** USAN.
Use: Antibacterial.

• **AMIFOSTINE.** USAN.
Use: Chemoprotectant; radioprotectant.
AMIGEN. (Baxter) Protein hydrolysate.
5%: Bot. 500 ml, 1000 ml; **10%:** Bot. 500
ml, 1000 ml. **5% w/dextrose 5%:** Bot.
500 ml, 1000 ml. **5% w/dextrose 5%, al-
cohol 5%:** Bot. 1000 ml. **5% w/fructose
10%:** Bot. 1000 ml. **5% w/fructose
12.5%, alcohol 2.4%:** Bot. 1000 ml.
Use: Nutritional supplement.
AMIGESIC. (Amide) Salsalate 500
mg/Cap or Tab. Salsalate 75 mg/capl.
Bot. 100s, 500s.
Use: Salicylate analgesic.
• **AMIKACIN,** U.S.P. XXIII.
Use: Antibacterial.
• **AMIKACIN SULFATE,** U.S.P. XXIII.
Use: Antibacterial.
• **AMIKACIN SULFATE INJECTION,** U.S.P.
XXIII. 0-3-Amino-3-deoxy-α-D-glucopy-
ranosyl(1-6)-0-[6-amino-6-deoxy-α-D-
glucopyranosyl(1-4)]-N-[(S)-4-amino- 2-
hydroxyl-1-oxobutyl]-2-deoxy-D-strepta-
mine sulfate.
Use: Antibacterial.
See: Amikin, Inj. (Bristol).
AMIKIN. (Bristol) Amikacin sulfate inj. Vial
100 mg, 500 mg, 1 Gm, disposable sy-
ringes 500 mg.
Use: Anti-infective.
AMILORIDE. B.A.N. N-Amidino-3,5-di-
amino-6 chloropyrazine 2-carboxamide.
Use: Diuretic.
See: Midamor, Tab. (Merck & Co.).
W/Hydrochlorthiazide.
See: Moduretic, Tab. (Merck & Co.).
• **AMILORIDE HYDROCHLORIDE,** U.S.P.
XXIII. Tab., U.S.P. XXIII. Pyrazinecar-
boxamide,3,5-diamino-N-(ami-noimi-
nomethyl)-6-chloro-, monochloride.
Use: Diuretic, antihypertensive.
See: Midamor, Tab. (Merck & Co.).
**AMILORIDE HCl SOLUTION FOR IN-
HALATION.** (Glaxo)
Use: Cystic fibrosis. [Orphan drug]
• **AMILORIDE HYDROCHLORIDE AND
HYDROCHLORTHIAZIDE TABLETS,**
U.S.P. XXIII.
Use: Diuretic, antihypertensive.
See: Moduretic, Tab. (Merck & Co.).
AMIN-AID INSTANT DRINK POWDER.
(Kendall McGaw) Essential amino acids,
maltodextrin, sucrose, partially hydro-
genated soybean oil, lecithin, mono-
diglycerides. Packet 162 Gm.
Use: Enteral nutritional supplement.
AMINA-21. (Miller) L-form amino acids
600 mg/Cap. Bot. 100s, 300s.
Use: Tissue repair.

• **AMINACRINE.** F.D.A. 9-Aminoacridine.
Use: Anti-infective, topical.
• **AMINACRINE HYDROCHLORIDE.**
USAN. 9-Aminoacridine hydrochloride.
Use: Anti-infective, topical.
W/Dienestrol, sulfanilamide, allantoin.
See: AVC/Dienestrol Cream, Supp.
(Merrell Dow).
Use: Bacteriostatic agent.
W/Oxyquinoline benzoate.
See: Triva, Vaginal Jelly (Boyle).
W/Sulfanilamide, allantoin.
See: AVC, Cream, Supp. (Merrell Dow).
Femguard Vaginal Cream (Reid-Row-
ell).
Sulfem Vaginal Cream (Federal
Pharm.).
Vagidine, Cream (Elder).
Vagitrol, Cream, Supp. (Lemmon).
AMIN-AID. (American McGaw) Instant
drinks, puddings.
Use: Enteral nutritional supplement.
AMINARSONE.
See: Carbarsone (Various Mfr.).
AMINE RESIN.
See: Polyamine Methylene Resin.
AMINESS. (Clintec) Essential amino
acids. 10 Tab. = adult amino acid MDR.
Jar 300s.
Use: Parenteral nutitional supplement.
AMINESS 5.2%. (Clintec) Amino acids
and electrolytes, Inj.
Use: Parenteral nutritional supplement.
AMINICOTIN.
Use: Vitamin supplement.
See: Nicotinamide (Various Mfr.).
AMINOACETIC ACID. Glycerine, U.S.P.
XXIII. (Various Mfr.). (Glycine, glycocoll)
available as elix., pow., tab.
Use: Myasthenia gravis, irrigating solu-
tion.
W/Aluminum hydroxide, magnesium hy-
droxide, calcium carbonate.
See: Eugel, Tab., Liq. (Reid-Rowell).
W/Calcium carbonate.
See: Antacid pH, Tab. (Towne).
Eldamint, Tab. (Elder).
W/Calcium carbonate, aluminum hydrox-
ide, magnesium carbonate.
See: Glytabs, Tab. (Pharmics).
W/Calcium carbonate, magnesium car-
bonate, bismuth subcarbonate, dried
aluminum hydroxide gel.
See: Buffer-Tabs (Forest).
W/Magnesium trisilicate, aluminum hy-
droxide.
See: Maracid-2, Tab. (Marin).
W/Phenylephrine HCl, pyrilamine maleate,
acetylsalicylic acid, caffeine.

See: Al-Ay, Tab. (Bowman).
W/Phenylephrine HCl, chlorpheniramine
maleate, acetaminophen, caffeine.
See: Codimal, Tab. (Central).
**AMINOACETIC ACID & CALCIUM CAR-
BONATE.**
W/Lysine.
See: Lycolan, Elix. (Lannett).
AMINO ACID & PROTEIN PREP.
See: Aminoacetic Acid, U.S.P. XXIII.
Glutamic Acid.
Histidine HCl.
Lysine.
Phenylalanine.
Thyroxine.
AMINO ACIDS.
Use: Amino acid supplement.
See: Aminosol, Soln. (Abbott).
Aminosyn, Soln. (Abbott).
W/Estrone, testosterone, vitamins, miner-
als.
See: Geramine, Tab., Inj. (Brown).
W/Vitamin B_{12}.
See: Stuart Amino Acids and B_{12}, Tab.
(Stuart).
AMINO ACID COMBINATIONS.
See: Dequasine (Miller).
NeuRecover-LT (NeuroGenesis).
NeuroSlim (NeuroGenesis/Matrix).
NeuRecover-DA (NeuroGenesis/Ma-
trix).
NeuRecover-SA (NeuroGenesis/Ma-
trix).
Herpetrol (Alva).
A/G-Pro (Miller).
Jets (Freeda).
PDP Liquid Protein (Wesley Pharm.).
AMINO ACID DERIVATIVES.
See: Carnitor (Sigma-Tau).
L-Carnitine (Various Mfr.).
VitaCarn (Kendall McGaw).
AMINO-MIN-D CAPSULES. (Tyson) Ca
250 mg, D 100 IU, Fe 7.5 mg, Zn 5.6
mg, Mg, I, Mn, Cu, K, Cr, Se, betaine
HCl, glutamic acid HCl. Cap. Bot. 100s.
Use: Vitamin/mineral supplement.
AMINOACRIDINE.
Use: Bacteriostatic agent.
See: 9-aminoacridine.
9-AMINOACRIDINE HCl. (Various Mfr.).
Aminacrine HCl.
Use: Anti-infective, vaginal.
See: Vagisec Plus (J. Schmid).
W/Hydrocortisone acetate, tyrothricin,
phenylmercuric acetate, polysorbate-80,
urea, lactose.
See: Aquacort, Vaginal Supp. (Web-
con).
W/Iodoquinol.
See: Vagitric, Oint. (Elder).

W/Phenylmercuric acetate, tyrothricin, urea, lactose.
See: Trinalis, Vaginal Supp. (Webcon).
W/Polyoxyethylene nonyl phenol, sodium edetate, docusate sodium.
See: Vagisec Plus, Supp. (Schmid).
W/Pramoxine HCl, acetic acid, parachlorometa-xylenol, methyl-dodecylbenzyltrimethyl ammonium Cl.
See: Drotic No. 2, Drops (Ascher).
W/Sulfanilamide, allantoin.
See: AVC Cream, Supp. (Merrell Dow).
Nil Vaginal Cream (Century).
Par Cream (Parmed).
Vagisan, Creme (Sandia).
Vagisul, Creme (Sheryl).
W/Sulfisoxazole, allantoin.
See: Vagilia, Cream (Lemmon).
p-AMINOBENZENE-SULFONY-LACETYLIMIDE.
See: Sulfacetamide.
• **AMINOBENZOATE POTASSIUM,** U.S.P. XXIII. Cap., for Oral Soln., Tab., U.S.P. XXIII.
Use: Analgesic.
See: Potaba, Pow., Tab. (Glenwood).
W/Hydrocortisone, ammonium salicylate, ascorbic acid.
See: Neocylate sodium free, Tab. (Central).
W/Potassium salicylate.
See: Pabalate-SF, Tab. (Robins).
W/Potassium salicylate, ascorbic acid.
See: Pabalan, Tab. (Lannett).
• **AMINOBENZOATE SODIUM,** U.S.P. XXII.
Use: Analgesic.
See: PABA sodium, Tab. (Various Mfr.).
W/Phenobarbital, colchicine salicylate, Vitamin B₁, aspirin.
See: Doloral, Tab. (Alamed).
W/Salicylamide, ascorbic acid.
See: Sylapar, Tab. (Forest).
W/Salicylamide, sodium salicylate, ascorbic acid, butabarbital sodium.
See: Bisalate, Tab. (Allison Lab).
W/Sodium salicylate.
See: Pabalate, Tab. (Robins).
Salpara, Tab. (Reid-Rowell).
• **AMINOBENZOIC ACID,** U.S.P. XXIII. Gel, Topical Soln., U.S.P. XXIII. Benzoic acid, 4-amino. PABA. Available as Cap., Bot., Pow., Soln., Tab. Massengill Soln. (10%) Bot. pt.
Use: Topical protectant (sunscreening agent).
See: Pabafilm (Owen/Galderma).
Pabanol, Lot. (Elder).
W/Mephenesin, salicylamide.
See: Sal-Phenesin, Tab. (Marion).

W/Sodium salicylate, ascorbic acid.
See: Nucorsal, Tab. (Westerfield).
AMINOBENZOIC ACID, PARA.
See: PARA-AMINOBENZOIC ACID.
p-AMINOBENZOIC ACID, SALTS.
See: p-Aminobenzoate potassium and p-Aminobenzoate sodium.
• **AMINOCAPROIC ACID,** U.S.P. XXIII. Syr., Inj., Tab., U.S.P. XXIII. 6-Aminohexanoic acid.
Use: Antifibrinolytic, hemostatic.
See: Amicar, Syr., Tab., Vial (Lederle).
• **AMINOCAPROIC ACID.** USAN. 6-Aminohexanoic acid. Amicar. Epsikapron.
Use: Inhibitor of fibrinolytic activity.
AMINOCARDOL.
Use: Bronchodilator.
See: Aminophylline. (Various Mfr.).
AMINO CERV. (Milex) Urea 8.34%, sodium propionate 0.5%, methionine 0.83%, cystine 0.35%, inositol 0.83%, benzalkonium Cl 0.000004%, buffered to pH 5.5. Tube with applicator 2.75 oz.
Use: Vaginal preparation.
AMINODYNE COMPOUND. (Bowman) Acetaminophen 2.5 gr, aspirin 3.5 gr, caffeine 0.5 gr/Tab. Bot. 100s, 1000s.
Use: Analgesic combination.
2-AMINOETHANETHIOL. USAN.
Use: Nephropathic cystinosis.
AMINO-ETHYL-PROPANOL.
See: Aminoisobutanol.
W/Bromotheophyllin.
See: Pamabrom (Various Mfr.).
AMINOFEN. (Dover) Acetaminophen 325 mg/Tab. Sugar, lactose and salt free. UD Box 500s.
Use: Analgesic.
AMINOFEN MAX. (Dover) Acetaminophen 500 mg/Tab. Sugar, lactose and salt free. UD Box 500s.
Use: Analgesic.
AMINOFORM.
Use: Anti-infective, urinary.
See: Methenamine (Various Mfr.).
AMINOGEN. (Christina) Vitamin B complex, folic acid. Amp. 2 ml Box 12s, 24s, 100s. Vial 10 ml.
Use: Vitamin B supplement.
• **AMINOGLUTETHIMIDE,** U.S.P. XXIII. Tab., U.S.P. XXIII. 2-(p-Aminophenyl)-2-ethylglutarimide.
Use: Treatment of Cushing's syndrome.
See: Cytadren (Ciba).
• **AMINOHIPPURATE SODIUM,** U.S.P. XXIII. Inj., U.S.P. XXIII. Glycine, N-(4-aminobenzoyl), monosodium salt. Monosodium p-aminohippurate. (Merck & Co.) 2 Gm/10 ml. Amp. 10 ml, 50 ml.
Use: I.V., diagnostic aid for renal

plasma flow.
• **AMINOHIPPURIC ACID,** U.S.P. XXII.
Glycine, N-(4-aminobenzoyl)-.
Use: Diagnostic aid (renal function de-
termination).
AMINOISOBUTANOL. 2-Amino-2-
methylpronanol-1.
See: Butaphyllamine.
Pamabrom for combinations.
AMINOISOMETRADINE. DL-2-Amino-4-
(methylthio) butyric acid.
See: Methionine.
AMINOMETRADINE. B.A.N. 1-Allyl-6-
amino-3-ethyl-pyrimidine-2,4-dione.
Mictine.
Use: Diuretic.
AMINONAT. Protein hydrolysates (oral).
AMINONITROZOLE. N-(5-Nitro-2-thia-
zolyl) acetamide.
Use: Antitrichomonal.
AMINO-OPTIC-C. (Tyson) Lemon
bioflavonoids 250 mg, rutin, hesperidin,
vitamin C and rose hips powder 1000
mg/SR Tab. Bot. 100s.
Use: Vitamin supplement.
AMINO-OPTI-E. (Tyson) 165 mg/Cap.
Bot. 100s.
Use: Vitamin E supplement.
AMINOPENTAMIDE SULFATE. 4-(Di-
methylamino)-2,2-diphenylvaleramide
sulfate.
Use: Anticholinergic.
AMINOPHYLLIN. (Searle) Trademark for
Aminophylline. **100 mg/Tab.** Bot. 100s,
1000s, UD 100s. **200 mg/Tab.** Bot.
100s, 1000s, UD 100s.
Use: Bronchodilator.
AMINOPHYLLIN INJECTION. (Searle)
Trademark for Aminophylline. Amp. **250
mg:** 10 ml; 25s, 100s; **500 mg:** 20 ml;
25s, 100s.
Use: Bronchodilator.
• **AMINOPHYLLINE,** U.S.P. XXIII. Enema,
Inj., Supp., Tab., U.S.P. XXIII. Theo-
phylline compound w/ethylenediamine
(2:1). (Aminocardol, Ammophyllin, Car-
dophyllin, Carena, Diophyllin, Geno-
phyllin, Ionphylline, Metaphyllin,
Phyllindon, Teholamine, Theophyldine.).
Use: Smooth muscle relaxant (bron-
chodilator).
See: Aminodur, Dura-Tab. (Berlex).
Lixaminol, Elix. (Ferndale).
Phyllocontin, Tab. (Purdue Frederick).
Rectalad-Aminophylline (Wallace).
Somophyllin Oral Liq. (Fisons).
Somophyllin Rectal Soln. (Fisons).
AMINOPHYLLINE COMBINATIONS.
Amesec, Cap. (Glaxo).
Amphedrine Compound, Cap. (Lan-

nett).
Asmadrin (Jenkins).
Asminorel, Tab. (Reid-Rowell).
B.M.E., Elix. (Brothers).
Bronchovent, Tab. (Mills).
Lixaminol AT/5 ml (Ferndale).
Mudrane GG-2, Tab. (Poythress).
Orthoxine and Aminophylline, Cap
(Upjohn).
Quinamm, Tab. (Merrell Dow).
Quinite, Tab. (Reid-Rowell).
Strema, Cap. (Foy).
• **AMINOPHYLLINE INJECTION,** U.S.P.
XXIII. (Abbott) Amp. 250 mg/10 ml, 500
mg/20 ml; Fliptop vial 10 mg/20 ml, 20
mg/50 ml.
Use: Bronchodilator.
• **AMINOPHYLLINE INJECTION,** U.S.P.
XXIII. Theophylline ethylenediamine.
Amp. 3¾ gr, 7.5 gr (Various Mfr.).
Use: Smooth muscle relaxant.
• **AMINOPHYLLINE SUPPOSITORIES,**
U.S.P. XXIII. 3⅜ gr, 7.5 gr (Various Mfr.).
Use: Smooth muscle relaxant.
• **AMINOPHYLLINE TABLETS,** U.S.P. XXI-
II. Plain or enteric coated 1.5 gr, 3 gr
(Various Mfr.).
Use: Smooth muscle relaxant.
AMINOPHYLLINE-PHENOBARBITAL.
(Robinson) Aminophylline 1.5 gr, pheno-
barbital 0.25 gr or 0.5 gr/Tab. Bot. 100s,
1000s, Bulk Pack 5000s. Aminophylline
3 gr, phenobarbital 0.25 gr or 0.5 gr/Tab.
Bot. 100s, 1000s, Bulk Pack 5000s.
Use: Bronchodilator, sedative/hypnotic.
**AMINOPHYLLINE WITH PHENOBARBI-
TAL COMBINATIONS.**
Amodrine, Tab. (Searle).
Mudrane, Tab. (Poythress).
Mudrane GG, Tab. (Poythress).
AMINOPREL. (Pasadena) L-lysine 60
mg, dl-methionine 15 mg, hydrolyzed
protein 750 mg, iron 2 mg, Cu, I, K, Mg,
Mn, Zn. Cap. Bot. 180s.
Use: Nutritional supplement.
AMINOPROMAZINE. (I.N.N.). Pro-
quamezine. B.A.N.
AMINOPTERIN SODIUM. B.A.N. Sodium
N-[4-(2,4-diaminopteridin-6-
ylmethyl)aminobenzoyl]-L-glutamate.
Sodium N-[p-[[2,4,-(diamino-6-
pteridinyl)methyl]amino]benzoyl]-L-glu-
tamate.
Use: Antineoplastic agent.
4-AMINOPYRIDINE. USAN.
Use: Relief of symptoms of multiple
sclerosis. [Orphan drug]
AMINOPYRINE. Amidofebrin, Amidopy-
razoline, Anafebrina, Novamidon,
Pyradone. Dimethylamino-phenyl-di-

methylpyrazolone.
Use: Antipyretic, analgesic.
See: Dipyrone, Vial (Maurry).
AMINOQUIN NAPHTHOATE.
See: Pamaquine Naphthoate.
4-AMINOQUINOLINE DERIVATIVES.
Use: Antimalarial.
See: Aralen HCl (Sanofi Winthrop).
Chloroquine Phosphate (Various Mfr.).
Plaquenil Sulfate (Sanofi Winthrop).
8-AMINOQUINOLINE DERIVATIVES.
Use: Antimalarial.
See: Primaquine Phosphate, U.S.P.
Primaquine Phosphate (Sanofi
Winthrop).
• **AMINOREX.** USAN. 2-Amino-5-phenyl-2-
oxazoline.
Use: Appetite suppressant.
See: Apiquel fumarate.
AMINOSALICYLATE CALCIUM, U.S.P.
XXI. Cap., Tab., U.S.P. XXI. Calcium 4-
Aminosalicylate (1:2) trihydrate. (Du-
mas-Wilson) 7.5 gr, Bot. 1000s.
Use: Tuberculosis therapy.
W/Isoniazid, pyridoxine HCl.
See: Calpas-Inah-6, Tab. (Amer. Chem.
& Drug).
AMINOSALICYLATE POTASSIUM.
Monopotassium 4-aminosalicylate.
Use: Antibacterial (tuberculostatic).
See: Paskalium, Tab., Pow. (Glen-
wood).
• **AMINOSALICYLATE SODIUM,** U.S.P.
XXIII. Tab., U.S.P. XXIII. Aminosalicylate
sodium Benzoic acid, 4-amino-2-hy-
droxy-, monosodium salt, dihydrate.
Monosodium 4 amino salicylate dihy
drate.
Use: Tuberculostatic, Crohn's disease.
[Orphan drug]
See: Neopasalate, Tab. (Mallinckrodt).
P.A.S., Pow. (Century).
Pasara Sodium, Pow., Tab. (Dorsey).
Pasdium, Tab. (Kasar).
AMINOSALICYLATE, SODIUM, PARA.
See: PARA-AMINOSALCYLATE SODI-
UM.
AMINOSALICYLATE, SODIUM, PARA.
See: PARA-AMINOSALCYLATE SODI-
UM.
AMINOSALICYLIC ACID, PARA.
See: PARA- AMINOSALCYLIC ACID.
4-AMINOSALICYLIC ACID.
Use: Treatment of ulcerative colitis in
patients intolerant to sulfasalazine.
4-AMINOSALICYLIC ACID.
Use: Ulcerative colitis. [Orphan drug]
p-AMINOSALICYLIC ACID SALTS.
See: Aminosalicylate Calcium.
Aminosalicylate Potassium.

Aminosalicylate Sodium.
AMINOSIDINE.
Use: *Mycobacterium avium* complex.
[Orphan drug]
See: Gabbromicina.
AMINOSYN. (Abbott Hospital Prods)
Crystalline amino acid solution. **3.5%:**
1000 ml; **5%:** Container 250 ml, 500 ml,
1000 ml; **7%:** 500 ml; 7% kit (cs/3);
8.5%: Single dose container 500 ml,
1000 ml. **10%:** 500 ml, 1000 ml.
W/Dextrose.
W/Electrolytes.
7%: 500 ml; **8.5%:** 500 ml.
Use: Parenteral nutritional supplement.
AMINOSYN. (Abbott) Crystalline
amino acid infusion. **8.5%:** 500 ml, 1000
ml; **10%:** 500 ml, 1000 ml.
Use: Parenteral nutritional supplement.
AMINOSYN-HBC 7%. (Abbott) Crystalline amino acid infusion for high metabolic stress. 500 ml, 1000 ml.
Use: Parenteral nutritional supplement.
AMINOSYN M 3.5%. (Abbott) Crystalline
amino acid infusion with electrolytes.
1000 ml.
Use: Parenteral nutritional supplement.
AMINOSYN-PF. (Abbott) Crystalline
amino acid infusions for pediatric use.
7%: 250 ml, 500 ml; **10%:** 1000 ml.
Use: Parenteral nutritional supplement.
AMINOSYN-RF. (Abbott) Crystalline
amino acid infusion for renal failure patients. **5.2%:** 300 ml.
Use: Parenteral nutritional supplement.
AMINOSYN II, (Abbott) Crystalline amino
acid infusion. **3.5%:** 1000 ml; **5%:** 1000
ml; **7%:** 500 ml; **8.5%:** 500 ml, 1000 ml;
10%: 500 ml, 1000 ml.
W/Dextrose:
3.5% in 5% dextrose: 1000 ml; **3.5% in
25% dextrose:** 1000 ml; **5% in 25%
dextrose:** 1000 ml.
W/Dextrose and electrolytes.
3.5% in 5% dextrose: 1000 ml; **3.5% in
25% dextrose:** 1000 ml; **4.25% in 10%
dextrose:** 1000 ml; **4.25% in 25%
dextrose:** 1000 ml.
W/Electrolytes.
7%: 1000 ml; **8.5%:** 1000 ml; **10%:** 1000
ml.
Use: Parenteral nutritional supplement.
AMINOSYN II M. (Abbott) Crystalline
amino acid infusion with maintenance
electrolytes, 10% dextrose. Soln. 1000
ml.
Use: Parenteral nutritional supplement.
AMINO-THIOL. (Marcen) Sulfur 10 mg,
casein 50 mg, sodium citrate 5 mg, phenol 5 mg, benzyl alcohol 5 mg/ml. Vial

10 ml, 30 ml.
Use: Treatment of arthritis, neuritis.
AMINOTRATE PHOSPHATE. Trolnitrate
phosphate.
See: Triethanolamine, Preps.
AMINOXYTROPINE TROPATE HCI. At-
ropine-N-oxide HCl.
• **AMIODARONE.** USAN.
Use: Antiarrhythmic agent. [Orphan
drug]
AMIODARONE HYDROCHLORIDE.
Use: Antiarrhythmic agent.
See: Cordarone, Tab. (Wyeth-Ayerst).
AMIPAQUE. (Sanofi Winthrop) Metriza-
mide 18.75%/20 ml Vial.
Use: Radiopaque agent.
AMIPHENAZOLE. B.A.N. 2,4-Diamino-5-
phenyl-thiazole.
Use: Respiratory stimulant.
AMIPHENAZOLE HCI. 2,4-Diamino-5-
phenylthiazole HCl. Daptazole.
• **AMIPRILOSE HYDROCHLORIDE.**
USAN.
Use: Antibacterial, antifungal, anti-in-
flammatory, antineoplastic, antiviral,
immunomodulator.
• **AMIQUINSIN HYDROCHLORIDE.**
USAN. 4-Amino-6,7-dimethoxyquinoline
hydrochloride monohydrate. Under
study.
Use: Antihypertensive.
AMISOMETRADINE. B.A.N. 6-Amino-
1,2-methylallyl-3-methylpyrimidine-2,4-
dione. Rolicton.
Use: Diuretic.
AMI-TEX LA. (Amide) Phenyl-
propanolamine HCl 75 mg, guaifenesin
400 mg/tab. Bot. 100s, 500s, 1000s.
Use: Decongestant, expectorant.
AMITIN. (Thurston) Vitamin C 200 mg,
lemon bioflavonoid 100 mg, niacinamide
60 mg, methionine 100 mg/Tab. Bot.
100s, 500s.
Use: Vitamin supplement.
AMITONE. (Menley & James) Calcium
carbonate 350 mg/Chew. Tab. Bot.
100s.
Use: Antacid.
• **AMITRAZ.** USAN.
Use: Scabicide.
AMITRIPTYLINE. B.A.N. 3-(3-Dimethy-
lamino-propylidene)dibenzo[a,d]cyclo-
hepta-1,4-diene. Amitriptyline hy-
drochloride. Laroxyl, Lenitzol, Saroten,
Tryptizol.
Use: Antidepressant.
See: Elegen-G, Tab. (Grafton).
• **AMITRIPTYLINE HYDROCHLORIDE.**
U.S.P. XXIII. Inj., Tab. U.S.P. XXIII.
10,11-dihydro-N, N-dimethyl-5H-diben-

zo[a,d]cycloheptene-D^5,-propylamine
hydrochloride.
Use: Antidepressant.
See: Amitril, Tab. (Parke-Davis).
Elavil HCl, Tab., Inj. (Merck & Co.).
Emitrip, Tab. (Major).
Endep, Tab. (Roche).
W/Chlordiazepoxide.
See: Limbitrol, Tab. (Roche).
W/Perphenazine.
See: Etrafon, Prods. (Schering).
Triavil, Tab. (Merck & Co.).
AMLODIPINE.
Use: Calcium channel blocking agent.
See: Norvasc (Pfizer).
• **AMLODIPINE BESYLATE.** USAN.
Use: Anti-anginal; antihypertensive.
See: Norvasc (Pfizer).
• **AMLODIPINE MALEATE.** USAN.
Use: Antianginal, antihypertensive.
AMMENS MEDICATED POWDER. (Bris-
tol-Myers) Boric acid 4.55%, zinc oxide
9.10%, talc, starch. Can 6.25 oz, 11 oz.
Use: Skin protectant.
AMMOIDIN. Methoxsalen.
Use: Psoralen.
AMMONIA. Aromatic Ammonia Spirit,
U.S.P. XXIII. Strong soln., N.F. XVIII.
(Lilly) 0.4 ml; pt; Aspirols 0.4 ml Pkg.
12s. (Burroughs-Wellcome). Vaporoles
5.41 min in crushable glass capsule.
Box 12s, 100s (Glenwood) Amp 0.33 ml.
Box 10s.
Use: Source of ammonia for fainting
spells.
• **AMMONIA N 13.** USAN.
Use: Diagnostic radiopharmaceutical.
• **AMMONIA SOLUTION, STRONG,** N.F.
XVIII.
Use: Pharmaceutic aid (source of am-
monia).
• **AMMONIATED MERCURY,** U.S.P. XXIII.
Oint., Ophth. Oint., U.S.P. XXIII. (Vari-
ous Mfr.).
Use: Anti-infective, topical.
See: Mercuronate 5% Oint. (Bowman).
W/Salicylic acid.
See: Emersal, Lot. (Medco).
AMMONIUM BENZOATE.
Use: Urinary antiseptic.
• **AMMONIUM CARBONATE,** N.F. XVIII.
Use: Source of ammonia.
• **AMMONIUM CHLORIDE,** U.S.P. XXIII.
Inj., Delayed Release Tab., U.S.P. XXIII.
Delayed Release Tab.: (Various Mfr.)
Plain or E.C. (5 gr or 7.5 gr). **Inj.:** (Cut-
ter) 120 mEq/30 ml Vial.
Use: Diuretic, expectorant, alkalosis.
See: Nodema, Tab. (Towne).

AMMONIUM CHLORIDE, ENSEALS.
(Lilly) Ammonium Cl. Tab. Enseal 7.5 gr.
Bot. 100s.
Use: Urinary acidifier.
AMMONIUM MANDELATE. Ammonium
salt of mandelic acid. Syr. 8 Gm/fl oz.
Bot. pt, gal.
Use: Urinary antiseptic, oral.
• **AMMONIUM MOLYBDATE,** U.S.P. XXIII.
Inj., U.S.P. XXIII.
AMMONIUM NITRATE.
See: Reditemp-C, Cold Pack (Wyeth-
Ayerst).
• **AMMONIUM PHOSPHATE,** N.F. XVIII.
Phosphoric acid diammonium salt. Di-
ammonium phosphate.
AMMONIUM TETRATHIOMOLYBDATE.
Use: Treatment of Wilson's disease.
[Orphan drug]
AMMONIUM VALERATE.
Use: Sedative.
AMMOPHYLLIN.
Use: Bronchodilator.
See: Aminophylline, U.S.P. XXIII. (Vari-
ous Mfr.).
AMMORID. (Kinney) Benzethonium Cl,
zinc oxide in a lanolin absorption base.
Oint. Tube 2 oz.
Use: Dermatologic agent.
AMMORID DIAPER RINSE. (Kinney)
Methylbenzethonium Cl 5%, deionizing
and buffering agents in dry powder form,
readily soluble in water. Bot. 240 Gm.
Use: Skin protectant.
• **AMOBARBITAL,** U.S.P. XXII. Tab., U.S.P.
XXII. Elix., U.S.P. XXI. (Various Mfr.). 5-
Ethyl-5-isoamylbarbituric acid.
Use: Hypnotic of intermediate duration.
See: Amytal, Elix., Pulv. (Lilly).
AMOBARBITAL W/COMBINATIONS.
Amodex, Cap. (Forest).
Bronchovent, Tab. (Mills).
Dextrobar, Tab. (Lannett).
Ectasule, Cap. (Fleming).
Obalan Lanatabs, Tab. (Lannett).
Obe-Slim, Tab. (Jenkins).
Trimex, Cap. (Mills).
• **AMOBARBITAL SODIUM,** U.S.P. XXIII.
Cap., Sterile, XXII. (Various Mfr.)
2,4,6(1H,3H,5H)-Pyrimidinetrione, 5-
ethyl-5-(3-me-thylbutyl)-, monosodium
salt. Sodium 5-ethyl-5-isopentylbarbitu-
rate.
Cap. **1 gr:** Bot. 100s, 500s; **3 gr:** Bot.
100s, 500s, 1000s. (Various Mfr.).
Pow. Bot. 15 Gm, 30 Gm. (Lannett).
Tab. **30 mg:** Bot. 100s; **50 mg:** Bot.
100s; **100 mg:** Bot. 100s. (Lilly).
Vial 250 mg, 500 mg. (Lilly).
Use: Hypnotic of intermediate duration,

sedative.
See: Amytal sodium (Lilly).
W/Ephedrine HCl, theophylline, chlor-
pheniramine maleate.
See: Theo-Span, Cap. (Scrip).
W/Secobarbital sodium.
See: Amsee, Tab. (Kenyon).
Compobarb, Cap. (Vitarine).
Dusotal, Cap. (Harvey).
Lanabarb, Cap. (Lannett).
Tuinal, Cap. (Lilly).
**AMOBARBITAL-EPHEDRINE CAP-
SULES.** (Lannett) Amobarbital 50 mg,
ephedrine sulfate 25 mg/Cap. Bot. 500s,
1000s.
Use: Sedative/hypnotic combination.
AMOCAL JR. (Jenkins) Pyrilamine
maleate 3 mg, phenylephrine HCl 1 mg,
tartar emetic 1/136 gr, benzoic acid gr,
ipecac pow. gr, ammonium Cl 0.5 gr,
iodized calcium gr, licorice extract 1
gr/Tab. Bot. 1000s.
Use: Antihistamine, decongestant.
AMO-DERM. (I ligh) Mineral abrasive,
lecithin soap base, 3,4,4'-trichlorocar-
banilide 1%, allantoin 2%. Pkg. Bar 3.5
oz.
Use: Skin cleanser.
AMO ENDOSOL. (Allergan) Sodium chloride 0.64%, potassium chloride 0.075%,
calcium chloride dihydrate 0.048%,
magnesium chloride hexahydrate
0.03%, sodium acetate trihydrate
0.39%, sodium citrate dihydrate 0.17%.
Soln. Bot. 18 ml, 500 ml.
Use: Physiological irrigating solution.
AMO ENDOSOL EXTRA. (Allergan) Part
I: water for injection with sodium chloride
7.14 mg, potassium chloride 0.38 mg,
calcium chloride dihydrate 0.154 mg,
magnesium chloride hexahydrate 0.2
mg, dextrose 0.92 mg/ml. Part II:
Lyophilized powder containing sodium
bicarbonate 1081 mg, sodium phosphate anhydrous 216 mg, glutathione
disulfide 95 mg. Soln. Bot. 515 ml.
Use: Ophthalmic irrigation solution.
• **AMODIAQUINE,** U.S.P. XXIII. 7-Chloro-
4-(3-diethyl-aminomethyl-4-hydrox-
yanilino)quinoline.
Use: Antimalarial.
• **AMODIAQUINE HYDROCHLORIDE,**
U.S.P. XXIII. Tab., U.S.P. XXIII. 4-(7-
Chloro-4-quinolylamino)-α-(Diethylamino)-o-cresol-di-HCl.
Use: Antimalarial.
AMODOPA. (Major) Methyldopa 125 mg,
250 mg or 500 mg. **125 mg:** 100s, UD
100s. **250 mg:** 100s, 1000s, UD 100s.
500 mg: 100s, 500s, UD 100s.

Use: Antihypertensive.
AMOL. Mono-n-amyl-hydroquinone ether.
See: B-F-I, Pow. (Calgon).
AMOLINE. (Major) Aminophylline 100 mg or 200 mg/Tab. Bot. 100s, 1000s, UD 100s.
Use: Bronchodilator.
AMONIDRIN. (Forest) Ammonium Cl 200 mg, guaifenesin 100 mg/Tab. Bot. 1000s.
Use: Expectorant.
AMOPYROQUIN HYDROCHLORIDE. 4-(7-Chloro-4-quinolylamino)-a-1-pyrrolidyl-o-cresoldihydrochloride.
See: Propoquin.
• **AMOROLFINE.** USAN.
Use:
AMOSAN. (Oral-B) Sodium perborate. Single-dose packet box 20s, 40s.
Use: Mouth and gum product.
AMOSECO. (Robinson) Secobarbital, amobarbital. Bot. 100s, 1000s.
Use: Sedative/hypnotic.
AMOTRIPHENE. 2,3,3-Tris(p-methoxyphenyl)-N,N-dimethylallylamine, 3-Dimethylamino-1,1.2-tris(4-methoxyphenyl)-1-propene HCl.
Use: Coronary vasodilator.
AMO VITRAX. (Allergan) Sodium hyaluronate 30 mg/ml. Inj. Disp. syringe 0.65 ml.
Use: Viscoelastic agent, ophthalmic.
• **AMOXAPINE.** USAN. 2-Chloro-II-(I-piperazinyl)dibenz[b,f][1,4]oxazepine.
Use: Antidepressant.
See: Asendin, Tab. (Lederle).
• **AMOXAPINE TABLETS,** U.S.P. XXIII.
Use: Antidepressant.
• **AMOXICILLIN.** U.S.P. XXIII. Cap., Oral Susp., For Susp., Tab., U.S.P. XXIII. 6-[D-(-)2-Amino-2-(p-hydroxyphenyl)acetamido]-3,3-dimethyl-7-oxo-4-thia-1-azabicy-clo[3.2.0]heptane-2-carboxylic acid.
Use: Antibiotic.
See: Amoxil, Preps. (Beecham Labs).
Polymox, Preps. (Bristol).
Sumox, Preps. (Reid-Rowell).
• **AMOXICILLIN AND CLAVULANATE POTASSIUM FOR ORAL SUSPENSION,** U.S.P. XXIII.
Use: Antibiotic, inhibitor (β-lactamase).
See: Augmentin (Beecham Labs).
• **AMOXICILLIN AND CLAVULANATE POTASSIUM TABLETS,** U.S.P. XXIII.
Use: Antibiotic, inhibitor (β-lactamase).
See: Augmentin (Beecham Labs).
• **AMOXICILLIN INTRAMAMMARY INFU-**

SION, U.S.P. XXIII.
Use: Antibiotic.
AMOXICILLIN TRIHYDRATE.
Use: Antibiotic.
See: Amoxil Chew. Tab. (Beecham Labs).
Polymox, Cap., Susp. (Bristol).
Trimox, Preps. (Squibb Mark).
Utimox, Cap, Susp. (Parke-Davis).
Wymox, Cap, Liq. (Wyeth-Ayerst).
W/Clavulanate Potassium.
See: Augmentin, Tab., Chew. tab., Pow. for susp. (Beecham Labs).
AMOXIL. (Beecham Labs) Amoxicillin.
Cap.: 250 mg. Bot. 100s, 500s, UD 10 × 10; 500 mg Bot. 50s, 500s. UD 10 × 10;
Pow. for Oral Susp.: 125 mg or 250 mg/5 ml. Bot. 80 ml, 100 ml, 150 ml, UD 5 ml.
Use: Antibacterial, penicillin.
AMOXIL CHEWABLE TABLETS.
(Beecham Labs) Amoxicillin trihydrate. 125 mg or 250 mg/Tab. Bot. 60s.
Use: Antibacterial, penicillin.
AMOXIL PEDIATRIC DROPS. (Beecham Labs) Amoxicillin 50 mg/ml. Bot. 15 ml, 30 ml.
Use: Antibacterial, penicillin.
D-AMP. (Dunhall) Ampicillin trihydrate 500 mg. Cap. Bot. 100s.
Use: Antibacterial, penicillin.
AMP. Adenosine Phosphate. USAN.
Use: Nutrient.
AMPERIL. (Geneva) Ampicillin trihydrate 250 mg or 500 mg/Cap. Bot. 100s, 500s.
Use: Antibacterial, penicillin.
• **AMPHECLORAL.** USAN. α-Methyl-N-(2,2,2- trichloroethylidene) phenethylamine.
Use: Sympathomimetic.
AMPHEDRINE COMPOUND CAPSULES. (Lannett) Aminophylline-ephedrine compound. Bot. 1000s.
Use: Agent for varicose veins.
See: Cobalasine (Keene).
AMPHENIDONE. I-(m-Aminophenyl)-2-(IH)-pyridone.
Use: CNS stimulant.
AMPHETAMINE COMPLEX.
See: Biphetamine 12 1/2 (Pennwalt).
Biphetamine 20 (Pennwalt).
AMPHETAMINE HYDROCHLORIDE.
Racemic amphetamine HCl, methylphenethylamine HCl, dl-1-phenyl-2-aminopropane HCl, dl-methylphenethylamine HCl, racemic desoxynorephedrine HCl. **Amp:** 20 mg/ml, 1 ml (Various Mfr.). **Cap:** (Various Mfr.).
Use: Vasoconstrictor, CNS stimulant.
AMPHETAMINE, LEVO.

Use: CNS stimulant.
See: Levamphetamine.
AMPHETAMINE PHOSPHATE. Monobasic dl-a-methyl-phenethylamine phosphate. Monobasic racemic amphetamine phosphate.
Use: CNS stimulant.
• **AMPHETAMINE PHOSPHATE, DEXTRO,** U.S.P. XXIII. Tab., U.S.P. XXIII. Dextroamphetamine phosphate. (Various Mfr.).
Use: CNS stimulant.
AMPHETAMINE PHOSPHATE, DIBASIC, Racemic amphetamine phosphate. **Cap:** 5 mg or 10 mg. **Tab:** 5 mg or 10 mg. (Various Mfr.).
Use: CNS stimulant.
AMPHETAMINES.
See: Amphetamine Sulfate, Tab. (Lannett).
Biphetamine, Cap. (Pennwalt).
Desoxyn, Tab. (Abbott).
Desoxyn Gradumets, Long-acting tab. (Abbott).
Dexampex, Cap., Tab. (Lemmon).
Dexedrine, Elix., Tab., S.R. Cap. (SKF).
Dextroamphetamine Sulfate, Tab., S.R. Cap. (Various Mfr.).
Ferndex, Tab. (Ferndale).
Methampex, Tab. (Lemmon).
Obetrol, Tab. (Obetrol).
• **AMPHETAMINE SULFATE,** U.S.P. XXIII. Tab., U.S.P. XXIII. dl-a-Methyl phenethylamine sulfate. (Racemic or dl form). **Cap.:** 5 mg or 10 mg (Various Mfr.). **Tab.:** 5 mg or 10 mg (Various Mfr.). **Vial:** 20 mg/ml (Various Mfr.).
Use: CNS stimulant.
AMPHETAMINE SULFATE, DEXTRO.
Use: CNS stimulant.
See: Dextroamphetamine Sulfate, U.S.P. XXIII.
AMPHETAMINE WITH DEXTROAMPHETAMINE AS RESIN COMPLEXES.
Use: Appetite depressant.
See: Biphetamine, Cap. (Pennwalt).
AMPHOCAPS. (Blue Cross) Ampicillin 250 mg or 500 mg/Cap. Bot. 100s.
Use: Antibacterial, penicillin.
AMPHOJEL. (Wyeth-Ayerst) Aluminum hydroxide gel **Susp.:** 320 mg/5 ml. Bot. 355 ml; **Tab.:** 300 mg or 600 mg. Bot. 100s.
Use: Antacid.
• **AMPHOMYCIN.** USAN. An antibiotic produced by *Streptomyces canus.* Amphocortrin.
Use: Anti-infective.
See: Ecomytrin.

AMPHOTERICIN.
Use: Antifungal.
See: Fungizone, Preps. (Squibb).
• **AMPHOTERICIN B,** U.S.P. XXIII. Cream, Inj., Lot., Oint., U.S.P. XXIII. B.A.N. A polyene antibiotic substance obtained from cultures of *Streptomyces nodosus.*
Use: Antifungal.
See: Amphotericin B (Lyphomed). Fungizone, Preps. (Squibb).
W/Tetracycline and K metaphosphate.
See: Mysteclin-F, Preps. (Squibb).
AMPHOTERICIN B. (Lyphomed) Polyene antibiotic obtained from cultures of *Streptomyces nodosus.* Inj. 50 mg/15 ml.
Use: Antifungal.
AMPHOTERICIN B LIPID COMPLEX. (B-M Squibb)
Use: Treatment of cryptococcal meningitis. [Orphan drug]
• **AMPICILLIN,** U.S.P. XXIII. Cap., Pow. for Oral Susp., Soln. Pow., Pow. for Sterile Susp., Tab., U.S.P. XXIII. 6[(D)-α-aminophenyl-acetamido] penicillanic acid. 6-(D-2-amino-2-phenylacetamido)-3, 3-dimethyl-7-oxo-4-thia-1-azabicyclo [3.2.0] heptane-2-carboxylic acid.
Use: Antibiotic.
See: Omnipen, Preps. (Wyeth-Ayerst). Polycillin, Preps. (Bristol). Principen, Preps. (Squibb Mark). Totacillin, Preps. (Beecham Labs).
W/Probenecid.
See: Polycillin-PRB, UD (Bristol). Principen W/Probenecid Cap. (Squibb).
• **AMPICILLIN AND PROBENECID.** Cap., Oral Susp., U.S.P. XXIII.
Use: Antibiotic.
See: Principen w/Probenecid (Squibb). Polycillin PRB (Bristol). Probanpacin (Various Mfr.).
• **AMPICILLIN SODIUM STERILE,** U.S.P. XXIII.
Use: Antibiotic.
See: Omnipen-N, Inj. (Wyeth-Ayerst). Polycillin-N (Bristol Labs). Totacillin-N, Vial (Beecham Labs).
AMPICILLIN SODIUM/SULBACTAM SODIUM.
Use: Antibacterial, penicillin.
See: Unasyn (Roerig).
AMPICILLIN TRIHYDRATE. Cap., Oral Susp. Marketed by various manufacturers.
Use: Antibacterial, penicillin.
See: Amcil, Cap., Susp. (Parke-Davis). D-Amp, Cap., Susp. (Dunhall). Marcillin, Cap., Susp. (Marnel).

Omnipen, Cap., Susp. (Wyeth-Ayerst).
Polycillin Preps. (Bristol).
Principen, Cap., Susp. (Squibb).
Totacillin, Cap., Susp. (Beecham
Labs).
AMPLIGEN. (HEM Pharmaceutical)
Phase II/III HIV.
Use: Immunomodulator.
AMPROTROPINE PHOSPHATE. 2-Di-
ethylamino-2,2-dimethylpropyl tropate.
• **AMPYZINE SULFATE.** USAN.
Use: Stimulant (Central).
• **AMQUINATE.** USAN.
Use: Antimalarial.
• **AMRINONE.** USAN.
Use: Cardiotonic.
See: Inocor Lactate Inj. (Sanofi
Winthrop).
AMRINONE LACTATE.
See: Inocor (Sanofi Winthrop).
• **AMSACRINE.** USAN.
Use: Antineoplastic agent. [Orphan
drug]
AMSEE. (Kenyon) Amobarbital sodium ³/₄
gr, secobarbital sodium gr/Cap. Bot.
100s, 1000s.
Use: Sedative/hypnotic.
AMSEE #2. (Kenyon) Amobarbital sodi-
um 1.5 gr, secobarbital sodium 1.5
gr/Cap. Bot. 100s, 1000s.
Use: Sedative/hypnotic.
AM-TUSS ELIXIR. (T.E. Williams)
Codeine phosphate 10 mg, phenyle-
phrine HCl 10 mg, phenylpropanolamine
HCl 5 mg, prophenpyridamine maleate
12.5 mg, guaifenesin 44 mg, fluid extract
of ipecac 0.17 min., citric acid 60 mg,
sodium citrate 197 mg/5 ml, alcohol 5%.
Bot. pt, gal.
Use: Antitussive, decongestant, antihis-
tamine, expectorant.
AMVISC. (Iolab) **Inj.:** Sodium hyaluronate
12 mg/ml. Disp. syringe 0.5 ml, 0.8 ml.
Use: Viscoelastic agent.
AMVISC PLUS. (Iolab) **Inj.:** Sodium
hyaluronate 16 mg/ml. Disp. syringe: 0.5
ml, 0.8 ml.
Use: Viscoelastic agent.
AM-WAX. (Amlab) Urea, benzocaine,
propylene glycol, glycerin. Bot. 10 ml.
Use: Otic preparation.
AMYL. Phenyl phenol, phenyl mercuric
nitrate.
See: Lubraseptic Jelly (Guardian).
α**AMYLASE.**
W/Calcium carbonate, glycine, belladonna
extract.
See: Trialka, Tab. (Commerce).
W/Pancreatin, protease, lipase.
See: Dizymes, Cap. (Recsei).

W/Pepsin, homatropine methyl bromide, li-
pase, protease, bile salts.
See: Digesplen, Tab., Elix. (Med. Prod.
Panamericana).
W/Pepsin, pancreatin, ox bile extract.
See: Gourmase, Cap. (Reid-Rowell).
W/Phenobarbital, belladonna, pepsin,
amylase, pancreatin, ox bile extract.
See: Gourmase-PB, Cap. (Reid-Row-
ell).
• **AMYLENE HYDRATE,** N.F. XVIII. Tertiary
amyl alcohol. Tert-pentyl alcohol. 2-
Methyl-2-butanol. (Various Mfr.).
Use: Pharmaceutic aid (solvent).
• **AMYL NITRITE,** U.S.P. XXIII. Inhalant,
U.S.P. XXIII. Isoamyl nitrite. Isopentyl ni-
trite. Burroughs Wellcome Vaporole 0.18
ml or 0.3 ml. Box 12s. Lilly Aspirols 0.3
ml. Box 12s.
Use: Inhalation, coronary vasodilator in
angina pectoris.
W/Sodium nitrite, sodium thiosulfate.
See: Cyanide Antidote Pkg. (Lilly).
AMYLOLYTIC ENZYME.
W/Butabarbital sodium, belladonna ex-
tract, cellulolytic enzyme, proteolytic en-
zyme, lipolytic enzyme, iron ox bile.
See: Butibel-Zyme, Tab. (McNeil).
W/Calcium carbonate, glycine, proteolytic
and cellulolytic enzymes.
See: Co-Gel, Tab. (Arco).
W/Cellulolytic, proteolytic and lipolytic en-
zymes, hyoscyamine sulfate.
See: Converspaz, Tab. (Ascher).
W/Lipase, proteolytic, cellulolytic enzymes,
phenobarbital, hyoscyamine sulfate, at-
ropine sulfate.
See: Arco-Lipase Plus, Tab. (Arco).
W/Proteolytic, cellulolytic, lipolytic en-
zymes, iron, ox bile.
See: Spaszyme, Tab. (Dooner).
W/Proteolytic enzyme, d-sorbitol.
See: Kuzyme, Cap. (Kremers-Urban).
W/Proteolytic, cellulolytic, lipolytic en-
zymes.
See: Arco-Lase, Tab. (Arco).
Zymme, Tab. (Scrip).
W/Proteolytic enzyme (Papain), homat-
ropine methylbromide, d-sorbitol.
See: Converzyme, Liq. (Ascher).
W/Proteolytic enzyme, lipolytic enzyme,
cellulolytic enzyme, belladonna extract.
See: Mallenzyme Improved, Tab.
(Hauck).
AMYTAL SODIUM. (Lilly) Amobarbital
sodium. Pow. for Inj.: 15 Gm, 30 Gm.
Vial: 250 mg/vial or 500 mg/vial. Traypak
10s, 25s.
Use: Sedative/hypnotic.
ANA. (Wampole-Zeus) Antinuclear anti-

bodies test by IFA. Test 54s.
Use: Diagnostic aid.
ANA HEp-2. (Wampole-Zeus) Antinuclear antibodies test by IFA. Tests 60s.
Use: Diagnostic aid.
ANABOLIC AGENTS. These agents stimulate constructive processes leading to retention of nitrogen and increasing the body protein.
See: Adroyd, Tab. (Parke-Davis).
Anabolin-IM, Vial (Alto).
Anadrol, Tab. (Syntex).
Anavar, Tab. (Searle).
Android, Tab. (Brown).
Androlone, Vial (Keene).
Crestabolic, Vial (Nutrition).
Deca-Durabolin, Amp., Vial (Organon).
Dianabol, Tab. (Ciba).
Di Genik, Vial (Savage).
Drolban, Vial (Lilly).
Durabolin, Amp., Vial (Organon).
Halotestin, Tab. (Upjohn).
Hybolin, Vial (Hyrex).
Maxibolin, Elix., Tab. (Organon).
Nandrobolic, Vial (Forest Pharm).
Ora-Testryl, Tab. (Squibb).
Os-Cal-Mone, Tab. (Marion).
Winstrol, Tab. (Sanofi Winthrop).
W/Vitamins and minerals
See: Dumogran, Tab. (Squibb).
ANABOLIN. (Alto) Nandrolone phenpropionate 50 mg, benzyl alcohol 2%, sesame oil q.s./ml. Vial 2 ml.
Use: Anabolic steroid.
ANABOLIN-IM. (Alto) Nandrolone phenpropionate 50 mg, benzyl alcohol 2%, sesame oil q.s./ml. Vial 2 ml.
Use: Anabolic steroid.
ANABOLIN LA-100. (Alto) Nandrolone decanoate 100 mg/ml. Vial 2 ml.
Use: Anabolic steroid.
ANACAINE. (Gordon) Benzocaine 10%. Jar oz, lb.
Use: Local anesthetic.
ANACIN TABLETS. (Whitehall) Aspirin 400 mg, caffeine 32 mg. **Tab.:** Tin 12s, bot. 30s, 50s, 100s, 200s. **Cap.:** Bot. 30s, 50s, 100s.
Use: Analgesic.
ANACIN MAXIMUM STRENGTH. (Whitehall) Aspirin 500 mg, caffeine 32 mg/ Tab. Bot. 12s, 20s, 24s, 40s, 72s, 150s.
Use: Analgesic.
ANADROL-50. (Syntex) Oxymetholone 50 mg/Tab. Bot. 100s.
Use: Anabolic steroid.
ANAFEBRINA.
See: Aminopyrine (Various Mfr.).
ANAFER. (British Drug House) Ferrous sulfate 200 mg, vitamin C 10 mg, mena-

dione as diacetyl derivative 1.5 mg/Tab. Bot. 100s, 1000s.
Use: Vitamin/mineral supplement.
ANAFRANIL. (Ciba) Clomipramine HCl 25 mg, 50 mg or 75 mg/Cap. Bot. 100s, UD 100s.
Use: Antidepressant.
• **ANAGESTONE ACETATE.** USAN. 17-Hydroxy-6α-methylpregn-4-en-20-one acetate.
Use: Progestin.
See: Anatropin (Ortho).
• **ANAGRELIDE HYDROCHLORIDE.** USAN.
Use: Antithrombotic. [Orphan drug]
ANA-GUARD EPINEPHRINE. (Hollister Stier/Miles) Epinephrine 1:1000, chlorobutanol < 5 mg and sodium bisulfite 1.5 mg per ml. In 1 ml syringes designed to deliver 2 doses of 0.3 ml each.
Use: Insect sting treatment.
ANAIDS. (Forest) Calcium carbonate 300 mg, sodium phenobarbital 9 mg/Tab. Bot. 1000s.
Use: Antacid combination.
• **ANAKINRA.** USAN.
Use: Antiinflammatory.
ANA-KIT. (Hollister-Stier) Syringe, epinephrine 1.1000 in 1 ml, four Chloramine tablets, each 2 mg chlorpheniramine maleate; two sterilized swabs, tourniquet, instructions/kit.
Use: Emergency kit.
ANALBALM IMPROVED FORMULA. (Central) Methyl salicylate 10%, menthol 1.25%, camphor 3%. Liq. Bot. **Green:** 4 oz, gal. **Pink:** 4 oz, pt, gal.
Use: Counter-irritant.
ANALEPTICS. Usually a term applied to agents with stimulant action, particularly on the central nervous system. See also central nervous system stimulants.
See: Amphetamine salts (Various Mfr.).
Caffeine (Various Mfr.).
Cylert, Tab. (Abbott).
Dextroamphetamine salts (Various Mfr.).
Dopram, Vial (Robins).
Ephedrine Salts (Various Mfr.).
Methamphetamine salts (Various Mfr.).
Ritalin HCl, Tab. (Ciba).
Sodium Succinate (Various Mfr.).
ANALGESIA CREME. (Rugby) Trolamine sulfate 10%. Cream, Tube 85 Gm.
Use: Rubs and liniment.
ANALGESIC BALM. (Various Mfr.) Menthol w/methyl salicylate in a suitable base.
Use: Counter-irritant.

A.P.C., 1.5 oz, lb.
Fougera, oz.
Horton & Converse, oz, lb.
Lilly, oz.
Musterole (Plough).
Stanlabs, oz, pt.
Wisconsin, 1 lb, 5 lb.
ANALGESIC LIQUID. (Weeks & Leo) Triethanolamine salicylate 20% in an alcohol base. Bot. 4 oz.
Use: External analgesic.
ANALGESIC LOTION. (Weeks & Leo) Methyl nicotinate 1%, methyl salicylate 10%, camphor 0.1%, menthol 0.1%. Bot. 4 oz.
Use: External analgesic.
ANALGESIC OINTMENT "LANNETT". (Lannett) Camphor, menthol syn., methyl salicylate in lanolin petrolatum base. Tube oz, Jar 1 lb, 5 lb.
Use: External analgesic.
ANALGESICS.
See preparations of: Acetanilid-type, Antipyrine-type, Aspirin, Salicylamide.
ANALGIC-C. (Kenyon) Salicylamide 250 mg, acetaminophen 250 mg, ascorbic acid 25 mg/Tab. Bot. 100s, 1000s.
Use: Analgesic combination.
ANALPRAM-HC. (Ferndale Labs) Hydrocortisone acetate 1%, pramoxine HCl 1%. Cream Tube 30 Gm.
Use: Topical corticosteroid, local anesthetic.
ANALVAL TABLETS. (Vale) Aspirin 227 mg, acetaminophen 162 mg, caffeine 32 mg/Tab. Bot. 1000s.
Use: Analgesic combination.
ANAMINE. (Mayrand) Pseudoephedrine HCl 30 mg, chlorpheniramine maleate 2 mg/5 ml. Syr. Bot. 473 ml.
Use: Decongestant, antihistamine.
ANAMINE HD SYRUP. (Mayrand) Phenylephrine HCl 5 mg, chlorpheniramine maleate 2 mg, hydrocodone bitartrate 1.67 mg. 10 ml tid or qid.
Use: Decongestant, antihistamine, antitussive.
ANAMINE T.D. CAPSULES. (Mayrand) Chlorpheniramine maleate 8 mg, pseudoephedrine HCl 120 mg/T.D. Cap. Bot. 100s.
Use: Antihistamine, decongestant.
ANANAIN, COMOSAIN.
Use: Burn treatment. [Orphan drug]
See: Vianain (Genzyme).
ANAPLEX HD SYRUP. (Medi-Plex) Hydrocodone bitartrate 1.7 mg, phenylephrine HCl 5 mg, chlopheniramine maleate 2 mg. Bot. 120 ml, 480 ml.
Use: Antitussive, decongestant, antihis-

tamine.
ANAPROX. (Syntex) Naproxen sodium 275 mg (naproxen base 250 mg with sodium 25 mg)/Tab. Bot. 100s, 500s. UD 100s.
Use: Nonsteroidal anti-inflammatory agent.
ANAPROX DS. (Syntex) Naproxen sodium 550 mg (naproxen base 500 mg with sodium 50 mg)/Tab. Bot. 100s, 500s, UD 100s.
Use: Nonsteroidal anti-inflammatory agent.
ANAREL. Guanadrel sulfate.
• **ANARITIDE ACETATE.** USAN.
Use: Antihypertensive, diuretic. [Orphan drug]
ANAROL. (Kenyon) Acetaminophen 120 mg/5 ml. Bot. 4 oz.
Use: Analgesic.
ANASPAZ. (Ascher) l-Hyoscyamine sulfate 0.125 mg/Tab. Bot. 100s, 500s.
Use: Anticholinergic, antispasmodic.
ANATRAST. (Lafayette Pharm.) GI contrast agent, 100% paste. Tube 500 Gm.
ANATUSS DM. (Mayrand) **Syrup:** Guaifenesin 100 mg, pseudoephedrine HCl 30 mg, dextromethorphan HBr 10 mg/5 ml. Bot. 480 ml; **Tab.:** Guaifenesin 400 mg, pseudoephedrine HCl 60 mg, dextromethorphan HBr 20 mg. Bot. 100s.
Use: Antitussive, expectorant, decongestant.
ANATUSS LA. (Mayrand)Guaifenesin 400 mg, pseudoephedrine HCl 120 mg. Tab. Bot. 100s.
Use: Expectorant, decongestant.
ANATUSS SYRUP. (Mayrand) Dextromethorphan HBr 15 mg, phenylpropanolamine HCl 25 mg, guaifenesin 100 mg/10 ml. Bot. 120 ml, 480 ml.
Use: Antitussive, decongestant, expectorant.
ANATUSS TABS. (Mayrand) Guaifenesin 100 mg, acetaminophen 325 mg, dextromethorphan HBr 15 mg, phenylpropanolamine HCl 25 mg/Tab. Bot. 100s, 500s.
Use: Expectorant, analgesic, antitussive, decongestant.
ANATUSS W/CODEINE. (Mayrand) **Syr.:** Phenylpropanolamine HCl 25 mg, codeine phosphate 10 mg, guaifenesin 100 mg/5 ml. Bot. 120 ml, 480 ml. **Tab.:** Phenylpropanolamine HCl 25 mg, codeine phosphate 10 mg, guaifenesin 100 mg, acetaminophen 300 mg. Bot. 100s.
Use: Decongestant, antitussive, expec-

torant, analgesic (Tab.).
ANAVAR. (Searle) Oxandrolone 2.5
mg/Tab. Bot. 100s.
Use: Anabolic steroid.
ANAYODIN.
See: Chiniofon.
• **ANAZOLENE SODIUM.** USAN. 4-[(4-
Anilino-5-sulfo-1-naphthyl)azo]-5-hy-
droxy-2,7-naphthalenedisulfonic acid
trisodium salt. (2) C.I. acid blue 92
trisodium salt. Sodium Anoxynaph-
thonate. B.A.N.
Use: Diagnostic aid.
See: Coomassie Blue (Wyeth-Ayerst).
ANBESOL BABY GEL. (Whitehall) Ben-
zocaine 7.5%. Tube 0.25 oz.
Use: Local anesthetic.
ANBESOL GEL. (Whitehall) Benzocaine
6.3%, phenol 0.5%, alcohol 70%. Tube
7.2 Gm.
Use: Local anesthetic, topical combination.
ANBESOL LIQUID. (Whitehall) Benzocaine 6.3%, phenol 0.5%, povidone-iodine 0.04%, alcohol 70%. Bot. 9 ml, 22
ml.
Use: Local anesthetic topical combination.
ANBESOL MAXIMUM STRENGTH.
(Whitehall) **Gel:** Benzocaine 20%, alcohol 60%, carbomer 934P, polyethylene
glycol, saccharin. Tube 7.2 Gm. **Liq.:**
Benzocaine 20%, alcohol 60%, saccharin, polyethylene glycol. Bot. 9 ml.
Use: Local anesthetic.
ANCEF. (SK-Beecham) Cefazolin sodium. **Vial:** Equivalent to 250 mg, 500 mg
or 1 Gm of cefazolin. **Multi Pack:** 500
mg or 1 Gm/Pack. 25s. **Bulk Vial:** 5 Gm,
10 Gm. **Piggyback Vial:** 500 mg or 1
Gm/100 ml. **Minibag:** 1 Gm/50 ml w/5%
dextrose inj. (D5W). 500 mg/50 ml D5W.
Use: Antibacterial, cephalosporin.
ANCID TABLET AND SUSPENSION.
(Sheryl) Calcium aluminum carbonate,
di-amino acetate complex. Tab. 100s.
Susp. pt.
Use: Antacid.
ANCOBON. (Roche) Flucytosine 250 mg
or 500 mg/Cap. Bot. 100s.
Use: Anti-infective.
• **ANCROD.** USAN. An active principle ob-
tained from the venom of the Malayan
pit viper *Agkistrodon rhodostoma*.
Use: Anticoagulant. [Orphan drug]
See: Arvin.
ANDESTERONE SUSPENSION. (Lin-
coln) Estrone 2 mg, testosterone 6
mg/ml. Vial 15 ml. **Forte:** Estrone 1 mg,
testosterone 20 mg/ml. Inj. Vial 15 ml.

Use: Estrogen, androgen combination.
ANDREST 90-4. (Seatrace) Testosterone
enanthate 90 mg, estradiol valerate 4
mg/ml. Vial 10 ml.
Use: Androgen, estrogen combination.
ANDRO 100. (Forest) Testosterone 100
mg/ml. Vial 10 ml.
Use: Androgen.
depANDRO 100. (Forest) Testosterone
cypionate in cottonseed oil 100 mg/ml,
benzyl alcohol. Vial 10 ml.
Use: Androgen.
depANDRO 200. (Forest) Testosterone
cypionate in cottonseed oil 200 mg/ml,
benzyl benzoate, benzyl alcohol. Vial 10
ml.
Use: Androgen.
ANDROCUR. Cyproterone acetate (Orphan Drug).
Use: Hirsutism, severe.
Sponsor: Berlex.
ANDRO-CYP 100. (Keene) Testosterone
cypionate 100 mg/ml. Vial 10 ml.
Use: Androgen.
ANDRO-CYP 200. (Keene) Testosterone
cypionate 200 mg/ml. Vial 10 ml.
Use: Androgen.
ANDRO-ESTRO 90-4. (Rugby) Estradiol
valerate 4 mg, testosterone enanthate
90 mg/ml with chlorobutanol in sesame
oil. Inj. Vial. 10 ml.
Use: Estrogen, androgen combination.
ANDRO FEM. (Pasadena Research)
Testosterone cypionate 50 mg, estradiol
cypionate 2 mg, chlorobutanol 0.5%,
cottonseed oil/ml. Vial 10 ml.
Use: Androgen, estrogen combination.
dep ANDROGYN. (Forest) Testosterone
cypionate 50 mg, estradiol cypionate 2
mg/ml, chlorobutanol, cottonseed oil.
Vial 10 ml.
Use: Androgen, estrogen combination.
ANDROGENS. Substances which pos-
sess masculinizing activities.
See: Methyltestosterone.
Testosterone.
Testosterone cyclopentylpropionate.
Testosterone enanthate.
Testosterone heptanoate.
Testosterone phenylacetate.
Testosterone propionate.
ANDROGEN-ESTROGEN THERAPY.
See: Dienestrol with Methyltestos-
terone.
Estradiol Esters with Methyltestos-
terone.
Estradiol Esters with Testosterone.
Estrogenic Substance, Conjugated
with Methyltestosterone.

Estrogenic Substance Mixed with Methyltestosterone.
Estrogenic Substance Mixed with Testosterone.
Estrone with Testosterone.
Gynetone, Tab. (Schering).
ANDROGEN HORMONE INHIBITOR.
Soo: Procoar (MSD).
ANDROGYN L.A. (Forest) Testosterone enanthate 90 mg, estradiol valerate 4 mg/ml in sesame oil. Vial 10 ml.
Use: Androgen, estrogen combination.
ANDROID-10 and 25. (Brown) Methyltestosterone 5 mg/Buccal Tab., 10 mg/Tab. or 25 mg/Tab. Bot. 60s.
Use: Androgen.
ANDRO L.A. 200. (Forest) Testosterone enanthate 200 mg/ml in cottonseed oil with chlorobutanol. Inj. vial 10 ml.
Use: Androgen.
ANDROLAN AQUEOUS. (Lannett) Testosterone 25 mg, 50 mg or 100 mg/ml. Susp. Vial 10 ml.
Use: Androgen.
ANDROLAN IN OIL. (Lannett) Testosterone propionate 25 mg, 50 mg or 100 mg/ml in oil. Vial 10 ml.
Use: Androgen.
ANDROLIN. (Lincoln) Testosterone 100 mg/ml. Vial 10 ml.
Use: Androgen.
ANDROLONE. (Keene) Nandrolone phenpropionate 25 mg/ml in sesame oil. Vial 5 ml.
Use: Anabolic steroid.
ANDROLONE-D 200. (Keene) Nandrolone decanoate w/benzyl alcohol, 200 mg/ml. Inj. Vial 1 ml.
Use: Anabolic steroid.
ANDRONAQ-50. (Central) Testosterone 50 mg/ml, sodium carboxymethylcellulose, methylcellulose, povidone, DSS, thimerosal. Inj. Vial. 10 ml.
Use: Androgen.
ANDRONAQ LA. (Central) Testosterone cypionate 100 mg, benzyl alcohol 0.9% in cottonseed oil. Vial 10 ml. Bot. 12s.
Use: Androgen.
ANDRONATE 100. (Pasadena Research) Testosterone cypionate 100 mg/ml with benzyl alcohol in cottonseed oil. Vial 10 ml.
Use: Androgen.
ANDRONATE 200. (Pasadena Research) Testosterone cypionate 200 mg/ml with benzyl alcohol, benzyl benzoate in cottonseed oil. Vial 10 ml.
Use: Androgen.

ANDROPOSITORY 100. (Rugby) Testosterone enanthate 100 mg/ml in sesame oil with chlorobutanol. Inj. Vial 10 ml.
Use: Androgen.
ANDROSTANAZOLE.
See: Stanozolol.
ANDROSTANE-17-(beta)-ol-3-one.
See: Stanolone.
ANDROSTANOLONE. (I.N.N.)
Stanolone.
ANDROSTENOPYRAZOLE. Anabolic steroid; pending release.
ANDROTEST P.
See: Testosterone propionate.
ANDRYL 200. (Keene) Testosterone enanthate 200 mg/ml. Vial 10 ml.
Use: Androgen.
ANDYLATE FORTE. (Vita Elixir) Acetaminophen 3 gr, salicylamide 3 gr, caffeine 0.25 gr/Tab.
Use: Analgesic combination.
ANDYLATE RUB. (Vita Elixir) Methylnicotinate, methylsalicylate, camphor, dipropyleneglycol salicylate, oil of cassia, oleoresin of capsicum, oleoresin of ginger.
Use: External analgesic.
ANDYLATE TABLETS. (Vita Elixir) Sodium salicylate 10 gr/Tab.
Use: Salicylate analgesic.
ANECAL CREAM. (Lannett) Benzocaine 3%, calamine 5%, zinc oxide 5%. Jar lb.
Use: Local anesthetic, antiseptic, skin protectant.
ANECTINE. (Burroughs Wellcome) Succinylcholine Cl. Soln. 20 mg/ml. Multidose Vial 10 ml. Sterile Pow. Flo-Pak 500 mg or 1000 mg. Box 12s.
Use: Muscle relaxant.
ANEFRIN NASAL SPRAY, LONG ACTING. (Walgreen) Oxymetazoline HCl 0.05%. Bot. 0.5 oz.
Use: Nasal decongestant.
ANELEP-O.D. (Trimen) Phenytoin 250 mg/Cap. Bot. 100s.
Use: Anticonvulsant.
ANERGAN 25. (Forest) Promethazine HCl 25 mg/ml. Vial 10 ml.
Use: Antihistamine.
ANERGAN 50. (Forest) Promethazine HCl 50 mg/ml. Vial 10 ml.
Use: Antihistamine.
ANERTAN.
See: Testosterone propionate.
ANESTACON. (PolyMedica) Lidocaine HCl 20 mg/ml. Bot. 15 ml, 240 ml.
Use: Local anesthetic.
ANESTHESIN. Ethyl-p-aminobenzoate.
Use: Local anesthetic.
See: Benzocaine, U.S.P. XXIII.

ANETHAINE.
See: Tetracaine HCl.
• **ANETHOLE,** N.F. XVIII. p-Propeny-
lanisole. Benzene, 1-methoxy-4-(1-
propenyl).
Use: Flavor.
ANEURINE HYDROCHLORIDE.
See: Thiamine HCl, Preps. (Various
Mfr.).
ANEXSIA. (Boehringer Mannheim) Hy-
drocodone bitartrate 5 mg, aceta-
minophen 500 mg/Tab. Bot. 100s,
1000s.
Use: Narcotic analgesic combination.
ANEXSIA 5/500 TABLETS. (Boehringer
Mannheim) Hydrocodone bitartrate 5
mg, acetaminophen 500 mg/Tab. Bot.
100s.
Use: Narcotic analgesic combination.
ANEXSIA 7.5/650. (Boehringer
Mannheim) Hydrocodone bitartrate 7.5
mg, acetaminophen 650 mg/Tab. Bot.
100s, 1000s.
Use: Narcotic analgesic combination.
ANGEL SWEET. (Garrett) Vitamins A and
D-$_2$. Cream 90 Gm.
Use: Skin protectant.
ANGEN. (Davis & Sly) Estrone 2 mg,
testosterone 25 mg/ml Aqueous susp.
Vial 10 ml.
Use: Estrogen, androgen combination.
ANGERIN. (Kingsbay) Nitroglycerin 1
mg/Cap. Bot. 60s.
Use: Coronary vasodilator.
ANGEX. (Janssen) Lidoflazine.
Use: Coronary vasodilator.
ANGIJEN GREEN. (Jenkins) Pentaery-
thritol tetranitrate 10 mg or 20 mg/Tab.
Bot. 1000s.
Use: Antianginal.
ANGIJEN S.C. SALMON. (Jenkins) Pen-
taerythritol tetranitrate 10 mg, phenobar-
bital 8 mg/Tab. Bot. 1000s.
Use: Antianginal, sedative/hypnotic.
ANGIJEN NO. 1. (Jenkins) Pentaerythri-
tol tetranitrate 20 mg, phenobarbital 15
mg/Tab. Bot. 1000s.
Use: Antianginal, sedative/hypnotic.
ANGIL. (Kenyon) Pentaerythritol tetrani-
trate 10 mg, mephobarbital 0.25 gr, phe-
nobarbital 1/8 gr/Tab. Bot. 100s, 1000s.
Use: Antianginal, sedative/hypnotic.
ANGIO-CONRAY. (Mallinckrodt) Iothalamate sodium 80% (48% iodine), EDTA.
Inj. Vial 50 ml.
Use: Radiopaque agent.
• **ANGIOTENSIN AMIDE.** USAN. 1-L-as-
paraginyl-5-L-valyl angiotensin octapeptide. 1L-asparagine-5-L-Valine angiotensin.

Use: Vasoconstrictor.
See: Hypertensin (Ciba).
**ANGIOTENSIN CONVERTING ENZYME
INHIBITORS.**
Use: Antihypertensive.
See: Accupril, Tab. (Parke-Davis).
Altace (Hoechst-Roussel).
Capoten, Tab. (Squibb).
Lotensin, Tab. (Ciba).
Monopril, Tab. (Mead Johnson).
Prinivil, Tab. (Merck & Co.).
Vasotec, Tab. (Merck & Co.).
Vasotec I.V., Inj. (Merck & Co.).
Zestril, Tab. (Stuart).
ANGIOVIST 282. (Berlex) Diatrizoate
meglumine 60% (iodine 28%). Vial 50
ml, 100 ml or 150 ml. Box 10s.
Use: Radiopaque agent.
ANGIOVIST 292. (Berlex) Diatrizoate
meglumine 52%, diatrizoate sodium 8%
(iodine 29.2%). Vial 30 ml, 50 ml or 100
ml. Box 10s.
Use: Radiopaque agent.
ANGIOVIST 370. (Berlex) Diatrizoate
meglumine 66%, diatrizoate sodium
10%, (iodine 37%). Vial 50 ml, 100 ml,
150 ml or 200 ml. Box 10s.
Use: Radiopaque agent.
ANHYDROHYDROXYPROGESTERONE.
Ethisterone.
• **ANIDOXIME.** USAN. 3-Diethylaminopro-
piophenone-O-(p-methoxyphenylcar-
bamoyl)oxime.
Use: Analgesic.
See: Bamoxine (U.S.V. Pharm.).
A-NIL. (Vangard) Codeine phosphate 10
mg, bromodiphenhydramine HCl 3.75
mg, diphenhydramine HCl 8.75 mg, am-
monium Cl 80 mg, potassium guaiacolsulfonate 80 mg, menthol 0.5 mg/5 ml,
alcohol 5%. Bot. pt. gal.
Use: Antitussive, expectorant.
• **ANILERIDINE HYDROCHLORIDE,**
U.S.P. XXIII. Tab., U.S.P. XXIII. 1-(4-
aminophenethyl)-4-phenylisonipecotic
acid ethyl ester.
Use: Analgesic.
See: Leritine HCl, Tab. (Merck & Co.).
• **ANILOPAM HYDROCHLORIDE.** USAN.
Use: Analgesic.
ANIMAL SHAPES. (Major) Vitamin A
2500 IU, D 400 IU, E 15 IU, C 60 mg, B$_1$
1.05 mg, B$_2$ 1.2 mg, B$_3$ 13.5 mg, B$_6$ 1.05
mg, B$_{12}$ 4.5 mcg, folic acid 0.3 mg.
Chew. Tab. Bot. 250s.
Use: Vitamin supplement.
ANIMAL SHAPES + IRON. (Major) Vita-
min A 2500 IU, D 400 IU, E 15 IU, C 60
mg, B$_1$ 1.05 mg, B$_2$ 1.2 mg, B$_3$ 13.5 mg,
B$_6$ 1.05 mg, B$_{12}$ 4.5 mcg, folic acid 0.3

mg, iron 15 mg. Chew. Tab. Bot. 250s.
Use: Vitamin and iron supplement.
ANION EXCHANGE RESINS.
See: Polyamine-Methylene Resin.
• **ANIRACETAM.** USAN.
Use: Mental performance enhancer.
• **ANIROLAC.** USAN.
Use: Anti-inflammatory, analgesic.
• **ANISE OIL,** N.F. XVIII.
Use: Flavor.
ANISINDIONE.
See: Miradon (Schering).
ANISOPYRADAMINE.
See: Pyrilamine Maleate.
• **ANISOTROPINE.** F.D.A. Tropine 2-propy-
lvalerate.
• **ANISOTROPINE METHYLBROMIDE.**
USAN. Octatropine Methylbromide,
B.A.N. 2-Propyl-pentanoyl tropinium
methylbromide. 8-Methyltropinium bro-
mide 2 Propylvalerate.
Use: Anticholinergic.
See: Valpin 50, Tab. (Du Pont).
• **ANISTREPLASE.** USAN.
Use: Fibrinolytic, thrombolytic.
See: Eminase (Beecham).
• **ANITRAZAFEN.** USAN.
Use: Anti-inflammatory.
ANODYNON.
See: Ethyl Cl.
ANODYNOS. (Buffington) Aspirin 420.6
mg, salicylamide 34.4 mg caffeine 34.4
mg/Tab. Sugar, lactose and salt free.
Dispens-A-Kit 500s, Bot. 100s, 500s,
Medipak 200s.
Use: Analgesic combination.
ANODYNOS-DHC TABLETS. (Forest)
Hydrocodone bitartrate 5 mg, aceta-
minophen 500 mg/Tab. Bot. 100s.
Use: Narcotic analgesic combination.
ANODYNOS FORTE. (Buffington) Chlor-
pheniramine maleate, phenylephrine
HCl, salicylamide, acetaminophen, caf-
feine/Tab. Sugar, lactose and salt free.
Dispens-A-Kit 500s, Bot. 100s.
Use: Antihistamine, decongestant, anal-
gesic.
ANOQUAN. (Hauck) Butalbital 50 mg,
caffeine 40 mg, acetaminophen 325
mg/Cap. Bot. 100s, 1000s.
Use: Sedative/hypnotic, analgesic.
ANOREX. (Dunhall) Phendimetrazine 35
mg/Tab. Bot. 100s.
Use: Anorexiant.
ANOREXIGENIC AGENTS. Appetite de-
pressants.
See: Amphetamine Preps.
Didrex, Tab. (Upjohn).
Plegine, Tab. (Wyeth-Ayerst).
Preludin HCl (Boehringer Ingelheim).

Sanorex, Tab. (Sandoz).
Tenuate (Merrell Dow).
Tepanil, Tab. (Riker).
Wilpo, Tab. (Dorsey).
ANOVLAR. Norethindrone plus ethinyl
estradiol.
Use: Oral contraceptive.
• **ANOXOMER.** USAN.
Use: Pharmaceutic aid.
ANOXYNAPHTHONATE SODIUM. Ana-
zolene Sodium.
ANSAID. (Upjohn) Flurbiprofen 50 mg or
100 mg. Tab. 100s, 500s, UD 100s.
Use: Nonsteroidal anti-inflammatory
agent.
ANSPOR. (SK-Beecham) Cephradine (a
semisynthetic cephalosporin) **Cap.:** 250
mg. Bot. 100s, UD 100s; 500 mg. Bot.
20s, 100s, UD 100s. **Oral Susp.:** 125
mg or 250 mg/5 ml. Bot. 100 ml.
Use: Antibacterial, cephalosporin.
ANSWER. (Carter Products) Reagent in-
home pregnancy test kit for urine test-
ing. Test kit box 1s.
Use: Diagnostic aid.
ANSWER 2. (Carter Products) Reagent
in-home pregnancy test kit for urine test-
ing. Test kit box 2s.
Use: Diagnostic aid.
ANSWER OVULATION. (Carter) Home
test to predict time of ovulation. In 6 day
test kits.
Use: Ovulation prediction.
ANSWER PLUS. (Carter Products)
Reagent in-home pregnancy test kit for
urine testing. Test kit box 1s.
Use: Diagnostic aid.
ANSWER PLUS 2. (Carter Products)
Reagent in-home pregnancy test kit for
urine testing. Test kit box 2s.
Use: Diagnostic aid.
ANSWER QUICK & SIMPLE. (Carter)
Reagent in-home kit for urine testing.
Test kit box 1s.
ANTABUSE. (Wyeth-Ayerst) Disulfiram.
250 mg/Tab. Bot. 100s; **500 mg/Tab.**
Bot. 50s, 1000s.
Use: Antialcoholic agent.
ANTACID. (Walgreen) Calcium carbonate
500 mg/Tab. Bot. 75s.
Use: Antacid.
ANTACID #2. (Richlyn) Calcium carbon-
ate 5.5 gr, magnesium carbonate 2.5
gr/Tab. Bot. 100s.
Use: Antacid.
ANTACID M LIQUID. (Walgreen) Alu-
minum oxide 225 mg, magnesium hy-
droxide 200 mg/5 ml. Bot. 12 oz, 26 oz.
Use: Antacid.
ANTACID NO. 6. (Bowman) Calcium car-

bonate 0.42 Gm, glycine 0.18 Gm/Tab.
Bot. 100s.
Use: Antacid.
ANTACID RELIEF TABLETS. (Walgreen)
Dihydroxyaluminum sodium carbonate
334 mg/Tab. Bot. 75s.
Use: Antacid.
ANTACIDS. Drugs that neutralize excess
gastric acid.
See: Alka-Seltzer, Tab. (Miles).
Alka-Seltzer Plus, Tab. (Miles).
Alka-Seltzer Special Effervescent
Antacid, Tab.(Miles).
Alka-2 Chewable Antacid, Tab. (Miles).
Aluminum Hydroxide Gel (Various
Mfr.).
Aluminum Hydroxide Gel w/Combina-
tions (Various Mfr.).
Aluminum Hydroxide Gel Dried (Vari-
ous Mfr.).
Aluminum Hydroxide Gel Dried
w/Combinations (Various Mfr.).
Aluminum Hydroxide Magnesium Car-
bonate, Tab. (Various Mfr.).
Aluminum Phosphate Gel (Wyeth-Ay-
erst).
Aluminum Proteinate, Tab. (Reid-Row-
ell).
Amitone, Tab. (Smith-Kline Beecham).
Calcium Carbonate, Precipitated (Vari-
ous Mfr.).
Calcium Carbonate Tab. (Various
Mfr.).
Carbamine (Key Pharm.).
Ceo-Two, Supp. (Beutlich).
Chooz, Gum Tab. (Schering-Plough).
Citrocarbonate, Liq. (Upjohn).
Dicarbosil, Tab. (Arch).
Di-Gel, Liq., Tab. (Schering-Plough).
Dihydroxyaluminum Aminoacetate
(Various Mfr.).
Dihydroxyaluminum Sodium Carbon-
ate Tab. (Warner-Lambert).
Magaldrate, Tab., Susp. (Wyeth-Ay-
erst).
Magnesium Carbonate (Various Mfr.).
Magnesium Glycinate, Tab. (Various
Mfr.).
Magnesium Hydroxide (Various Mfr.).
Magnesium Oxide, Tab., Cap. (Various
Mfr.).
Magnesium Trisilicate (Various Mfr.).
Neutralox, Susp. (Lemmon).
Oxaine, Susp. (Wyeth-Ayerst).
Ratio, Tab. (Adria).
Rolaids, Tab. (Warner-Lambert).
Romach, Tab. (ROR Pharmacal).
Sodium Bicarbonate, Inj., Tab. (Vari-
ous Mfr.).
Tums, Tab. (Smith-Kline Beeecham).

ANTACID SPECIAL NO. 1. (Jenkins)
Magnesium carbonate 3 gr, calcium car-
bonate 2 gr, bismuth subcarbonate 1 gr,
cerium oxalate 0.5 gr/Tab. Bot. 1000s.
Use: Antacid.
ANTACID SUSPENSION. (Geneva) Alu-
minum hydroxide 225 mg, magnesium
hydroxide 200 mg/5 ml. Bot. 360 ml.
Use: Antacid.
ANTACID TABLETS. (Goldline) Calcium
carbonate 500 mg/Chew. tab. Bot. 150s.
Use: Antacid.
ANTACID EXTRA STRENGTH. (Various
Mfr.) Calcium carbonate 750 mg/Tab.
Bot. 96s.
Use: Antacid.
ANTACID W/PHENOBARBITAL.
(Archer-Taylor) Magnesium hydroxide
0.3 Gm, calcium carbonate 9.3 Gm, at-
ropine 0.2 mg, phenobarbital 8 mg/Tab.
Bot. 1000s.
Use: Antacid, sedative/hypnotic.
ANTA-GEL. (Halsey) Aluminum hydrox-
ide 200 mg, magnesium hydroxide 200
mg, simethicone 20 mg/5 ml. Bot. 12 oz.
Use: Antacid, antiflatulent.
**ANTAGONISTS OF CURARIFORM
DRUGS.**
See: Neostigmine Methylsulfate.
Tensilon Cl (Roche).
ANTASTAN.
See: Antazoline Hydrochloride, U.S.P.
XXIII.
ANTAZOLINE. B.A.N. N Phenylbenzy-
lamino-methyl-2-imidazoline.
Use: Antihistamine.
ANTAZOLINE HYDROCHLORIDE. An-
tastan. 2(N-Benzylanilinomethyl)-2-imi-
dazoline HCl.
See: Arithmin, Tab. (Lannett).
• **ANTAZOLINE PHOSPHATE,** U.S.P. XXI-
II. 2-[(N-Benzylanilino)methyl]-2-imida-
zoline dihydrogen phosphate.
Use: Antihistamine.
See: Arithmin, Inj. (Lannett).
W/Naphazoline, boric acid, phenylmer-
curic acetate, sodium Cl, sodium carbon-
ate anhydrous.
See: Vasocon-A Ophthalmic, Soln.
(Smith, Miller & Patch).
W/Naphazoline HCl, polyvinyl alcohol.
See: Albalon-A Liquifilm, Ophth. Soln.
(Allergan).
ANTAZOLINE-V. (Rugby) Naphazoline
HCl 0.05%, antazoline phosphate 0.5%,
PEG 8000, polyvinyl alcohol, EDTA,
benzalkonium chloride 0.01%. Soln.
Drop. Bot. 5 ml, 15 ml .
Use: Ophthalmic decongestant combi-
nation.

ANTERIOR PITUITARY.
See: Pituitary, Anterior.
ANTHELMINTIC. A remedy for worms.
See: Antiminth, Susp. (Roerig).
Atabrine, Tab. (Sanofi Winthrop).
Betanaphthol Benzoate (Various Mfr.).
Biltricide, Tab. (Miles Pharm).
Carbon Tetrachloride (Various Mfr.).
Gentian Violet (Various Mfr.).
Jayne's PW Vermifuge (Glenbrook).
Jayne's RW, Tab. (Glenbrook).
Mintezol, Tab., Susp. (Merck & Co.).
Niclocide, Chew. tab. (Miles Pharm.).
Piperazine Preps. (Various Mfr.).
Povan, Tab., Susp. (Parke-Davis).
Terramycin (Various Mfr.).
Tetrachloroethylene.
Vansil, Cap. (Pfipharmecs).
Vermox, Chew tab., Oral Susp. (Merck & Co.).
• **ANTHELMYCIN.** USAN.
Use: Anthelmintic.
ANTHELVET. Tetramisole HCl.
ANTHRA-DERM. (Dermik) Anthralin 0.1%, 0.25%, 0.5% or 1% in petrolatum ointment base. Tube 1.5 oz.
Use: Antipsoriatic.
• **ANTHRALIN,** U.S.P. XXIII. Cream, Oint., U.S.P. XXIII. 1,8,9-Anthracenetriol. Cignolin, Dithranol, Dihydroxy-Anthranol.
Use: Treatment of psoriasis.
See: Anthra-Derm Oint. (Dermik)
Drithocreme, Cream (Dermik).
Dritho-Scalp, Cream (Dermik).
Lasan, Cream, Oint. (Stiefel)
W/Mineral oil.
See: Lasan Pomade (Stiefel).
ANTHRALIN PASTE 0.2%. (Durel) Anthralin 0.2%, salicylic acid 0.2%, paraffin 5%, Lassar's paste q.s. Jar oz, lb.
Use: Enzyme metabolism inhibitor.
ANTHRALIN POMADE 0.4%. (Durel) Anthralin 0.4%, salicylic acid 0.4%, sodium lauryl sulfate 2.1%, cetyl alcohol 21.9%, mineral oil q.s. Bot. 1 oz, 4 oz.
Use: Enzyme metabolism inhibitor.
• **ANTHRAMYCIN.** USAN.
Use: Antineoplastic agent.
ANTHRAQUINONE OF CASCARA.
See: Cascara Sagrada, Prods.
• **ANTI-A BLOOD GROUPING SERUM.**
U.S.P. XXIII.
Use: Diagnostic aid (blood in vitro).
• **ANTI-B BLOOD GROUPING SERUM.**
U.S.P. XXIII.
Use: Diagnostic aid (blood in vitro).
ANTIACID. (Hillcrest North) Aluminum hydroxide, magnesium trisilicate, calcium carbonate/Tab. Bot. 100s.
Use: Antacid.

ANTIALCOHOLIC.
See: Disulfiram (Various Mfr.).
Antabuse (Wyeth-Ayerst).
ANTI-ALLERGY TABLET. (Walgreen)
Phenylpropanolamine HCl 18.7 mg,
chlorpheniramine maleate 2 mg/Tab.
Bot. 24s.
Use: Decongestant, antihistamine.
ANTIANDROGEN.
See: Eulexin (Schering).
ANTIASTHMATIC COMBINATIONS.
See: Cromolyn Sodium, Cap. (Various Mfr.).
Decadron Respihaler, Aerosol. (Merck & Co.).
Ephedrine HCl (Various Mfr.).
Ephedrine Sulfate (Various Mfr.).
Isoephedrine HCl (Various Mfr.).
Isoetharine (Sanofi Winthrop).
Isoetharine HCl (Sanofi Winthrop).
Isoetharine Mesylate (Sanofi Winthrop).
Isoproterenol HCl (Various Mfr.).
Isoproterenol Sulfate (Various Mfr.).
Methoxyphenamine HCl (Various Mfr.).
Phenylephrine HCl (Various Mfr.).
Phenylpropanolamine HCl (Various Mfr.).
Pseudoephedrine HCl (Various Mfr.).
Racephedrine HCl (Various Mfr.).
ANTIASTHMATIC INHALANT.
See: AsthmaHaler (Smith-Kline Beecham).
AsthmaNefrin, Soln. (Smith-Kline Beecham).
ANTIBACTERIAL SERUMS.
See: Hypertussis Serum.
Influenzae Antihaemophilus Type B Serum.
ANTIBASON.
See: Methylthiouracil (Various Mfr.).
ANTIBIOTIC. (Parnell) **Otic susp.:**
Polymyxin B sulfate 10,000 units, neomycin (as sulfate) 3.5 mg, hydrocortisone 10 mg/ml, thimerosal 0.01%. Bot. 10 ml w/dropper. **Otic soln.:** Polymyxin B sulfate 10,000 units, neomycin (as sulfate) 3.5 mg, hydrocortisone 10 mg/ml. Bot. 10 ml w/dropper.
Use: Antibiotic, anti-inflammatory.
ANTIBIOTICS.
See: Amoxicillin (Various Mfr.).
Amphotericin B (Squibb).
Ampicillin (Various Mfr.).
Ampicillin Sodium (Various Mfr.).
Ampicillin Trihydrate (Various Mfr.).
Bacitracin (Various Mfr.).
Benzathine Penicillin G (Various Mfr.).
Carbenicillin Disodium, Inj., (Various

Mfr.).
Carbenicillin Indanyl Sodium, Tab.
(Roerig).
Cefadroxil (Bristol, Mead Johnson).
Cefazolin Sodium, Vial (Various Mfr.).
Cephalexin (Lilly).
Cephalexin Monohydrate, Pulv., Susp.
(Lilly).
Cephalothin, Sodium, Vial (Lilly).
Chloramphenicol (Various Mfr.).
Chloramphenicol Sodium Succinate,
Inj. (Various Mfr.).
Clindamycin (Upjohn).
Cloxapen, Cap. (Beecham Labs).
Colistimethate Sodium, Inj. (Parke-
Davis).
Colistin Sulfate, Ophth., Susp. (Vari-
ous Mfr.).
Demeclocycline (Lederle).
Demethylchlortetracycline HCl (Leder-
le).
Dicloxacillin, Cap., Susp. (Various
Mfr.).
Doxycycline (Various Mfr.).
Erythromycin (Various Mfr.).
Erythromycin Ethylsuccinate (Abbott,
Ross).
Erythromycin Lactobionate for Inj. (Ab-
bott).
Erythromycin Stearate, Tab. (Various
Mfr.).
Flucytosine, Cap. (Roche).
Gentamicin Sulfate (Schering-Plough).
Griseofulvin, Tab., Susp. (Various
Mfr.).
Griseofulvin Microcrystalline, Tab.,
Cap. (Various Mfr.).
Hetacillin (Bristol-Myers).
Kanamycin Sulfate, Cap., Inj. (Bristol-
Myers).
Ledercillin VK, Prods. (Lederle).
Lincomycin (Upjohn).
Methacycline HCl, Cap., Syr. (Wal-
lace).
Methicillin Sodium, Vial, Pow. (Various
Mfr.).
Minocycline, Cap. (Lederle).
Nafcillin Sodium, Vial, Cap., Pow.
(Wyeth-Ayerst).
Nalidixic Acid, N.F.
NegGram, Prods. (Sanofi Winthrop).
Neomycin Sulfate, Tab., Soln. (Various
Mfr.).
Novobiocin (Various Mfr.).
Novobiocin Calcium (Upjohn).
Novobiocin Sodium, Cap. (Upjohn).
Nystatin (Various Mfr.).
Oxacillin, Sodium (Various Mfr.).
Oxytetracycline (Pfizer).
Paromomycin, Cap., Syr. (Parke-

Davis).
Penicillin G, Potassium (Various Mfr.).
Penicillin G, Potassium w/Comb. (Vari-
ous Mfr.).
Penicillin G, Procaine (Various Mfr.).
Penicillin G, Procaine w/Comb. (Vari-
ous Mfr.).
Penicillin G, Sodium (Various Mfr.).
Penicillin V Potassium (Various Mfr.).
Phenethicillin Potassium, Tab., Pow.,
Soln. (Various Mfr.).
Phenoxymethyl Penicillin (Various
Mfr.).
Polymyxin B Sulfate (Various Mfr.).
Primaxin, Inj. (Merck & Co.).
Rifampin, Cap. (Various Mfr.).
Seromycin, Pulv. (Lilly).
Sodium Cloxacillin, Cap., Soln. (Bris-
tol-Myers)
Streptomycin Sulfate (Various Mfr.).
Tetracycline (Various Mfr.).
Tetracycline HCl (Various Mfr.).
Tetracycline Phosphate Complex (Var-
ious Mfr.).
Triacetyloleandomycin (Various Mfr.).
Troleandomycin, Cap., Susp. (Various
Mfr.).
Vancomycin HCl (Lilly)

ANTICHOLINERGIC AGENTS. Parasym-
patholytic agents.
See: Akineton (Knoll).
Antrenyl Bromide (Ciba).
Artane HCl (Lederle).
Atropine Preps.
Banthine Bromide (Searle).
Belladonna Preps.
Cantil Preps. (Merrell Dow).
Cogentin (Merck & Co.).
Daricon, Tab. (Beecham Labs).
Dicyclomine HCl (Various Mfr.).
Disipal (Riker).
Donabarb Sr., Cap. (Elder).
Homatropine methylbromide.
Hybephen, Prods. (Beecham Labs).
Kemadrin, Tab. (Burroughs Well-
come).
Kinesed, Tab. (Stuart).
L-Hyoscyamine, Tab. (Kremers-Ur-
ban).
Murel, Amp. (Wyeth-Ayerst).
Norflex, Inj., Tab. (Riker).
Oxyphencyclimine HCl (Various Mfr.).
Pagitane HCl, Tab. (Lilly).
Pamine Bromide, Tab., Soln. (Upjohn).
Panparnit HCl.
Parsidol HCl, Tab. (Parke-Davis).
Pathilon (Lederle).
Phenoxene HCl (Marion Merrell Dow).
Prantal Methylsulfate, Tab. (Schering-
Plough).

Pro-Banthine Bromide, Preps. (Searle).
Robinul, Tab., Inj. (Robins).
Scopolamine methylbromide.
Scopolamine methylbromide HBr.
Tral, Preps. (Abbott).
Trihexyphenidyl HCl (Various Mfr.).
Trocinate, Tab. (Poythress).
Valpin 50, Tab. (DuPont).
Valpin 50-PB, Tab. (DuPont).
• **ANTICOAGULANT CITRATE DEXTROSE SOLUTION,** U.S.P. XXIII.
Use: Anticoagulant for storage of whole blood.
See: A.C.D. Solution. (Various Mfr.).
• **ANTICOAGULANT CITRATE PHOSPHATE DEXTROSE ADENINE SOLUTION,** U.S.P. XXIII.
Use: Anticoagulant for storage of whole blood.
• **ANTICOAGULANT CITRATE PHOSPHATE DEXTROSE SOLUTION,** U.S.P. XXIII.
Use: Anticoagulant for storage of whole blood.
• **ANTICOAGULANT HEPARIN SOLUTION,** U.S.P. XXIII.
Use: Anticoagulant for storage of whole blood.
ANTICOAGULANTS.
See: Acenocoumarin.
Anisindione.
Bishydroxycoumarin (Various Mfr.).
Calciparine, Inj. (American Critical Care).
Coumadin, Amp., Tab. (DuPont).
Depo-Heparin, Sodium (Upjohn).
Dicumarol (Various Mfr.).
Dipaxin, Tab. (Upjohn).
Diphenadione.
Eridione, Tab. (Eric, Kirk & Gary).
Ethyl Biscoumacetate, Tab.
Hedulin, Tab. (Merrell Dow).
Heparin, Sodium (Various Mfr.).
Liquaemin Sodium, Vial (Organon).
Liquamar, Tab. (Organon).
Miradon, Tab. (Schering-Plough).
Panheprin, Amp., Vial (Abbott).
Panwarfin, Tab. (Abbott).
Phenindione, Tab. (Various Mfr.).
Warfarin (Various Mfr.).
• **ANTICOAGULANT SODIUM CITRATE SOLUTION,** U.S.P. XXIII. Anticoagulant (plasma and blood, fractionation).
ANTICONVULSANTS. Agents that inhibit muscular spasms originating in the central nervous system.
See: Amytal Sodium, Amp. (Lilly).
Celontin, Cap. (Parke-Davis).
Depakene, Liq., Tab. (Abbott).

Dilantin, Preps. (Parke-Davis).
Gemonil, Tab. (Abbott).
Glutamic Acid (Various Mfr.).
Magnesium sulfate.
Mephobarbital.
Mesantoin, Tab. (Sandoz).
Milontin, Cap. (Parke-Davis).
Paradione, Cap., Soln. (Abbott).
Peganone, Tab. (Abbott).
Phenobarbital (Various Mfr.).
Phenurone, Tab. (Abbott).
Phenytoin, Susp., Tab. (Various Mfr.).
Phenytoin Sodium, Cap. (Various Mfr.).
Tegretol, Tab. (Geigy).
Tridione, Cap., Dulcet, Soln., Tab. (Abbott).
Valium, Tab. (Roche).
Zarontin, Cap., Syr. (Parke-Davis).
ANTI-CYTOMEGALOVIRUS MONOCLONAL ANTIBODIES. USAN.
Use: Treatment of cytomegalovirus.
ANTIDEPRESSANTS.
See: Adapin, Cap. (Lotus).
Amitid, Tab. (Squibb).
Amitriptyline HCl (Various Mfr.).
Aventyl HCl, Pulv., Liq. (Lilly).
Deaner, Tab. (Riker).
Deprol, Tab. (Wallace).
Desipramine HCl, Cap., Tab. (Various Mfr.).
Effexor, Tab. (Wyeth-Ayerst).
Elavil Tab., Inj. (Merck & Co.).
Imipramine HCl, Amp., Tab. (Various Mfr.).
Imipramine Pamoate, Cap. (Geigy).
Marplan, Tab. (Roche).
Monoamine oxidase inhibitors.
Nardil, Tab. (Parke-Davis).
Niamid, Tab. (Pfizer).
Norpramin, Preps. (Merrell Dow).
Pamelor, Cap., Liq. (Sandoz).
Parnate Sulfate, Tab. (SK-Beecham).
Paxil, Tab. (SK-Beecham).
Pertofrane, Cap. (USV).
Presamine, Tab. (USV).
Protriptyline HCl (Merck & Co.).
Prozac, Liq., Pulv. (Dista).
Ritalin, Tab., Vial (Ciba).
Sinequan, Cap. (Pfizer).
Tofranil, Amp., Tab. (Geigy).
Tofranil-PM, Cap. (Geigy).
Triavil, Tab. (Merck & Co.).
Vivactil, Tab. (Merck & Co.).
Wellbutrin, Tab. (Burroughs Wellcome).
Zoloft, Tab. (Roerig).
ANTIDIARRHEALS.
See: Attapulgite, Activated (Various Mfr.).

Cantil, Liq., Tab. (Merrell Dow).
Coly-Mycin S, Oral Susp., (Parke-
Davis).
Corrective Mixture, Liq. (Beecham
Labs).
Corrective Mixture with Paregoric, Liq.
(Beecham Labs).
DIA-Quel Liq. (Inter. Pharm. Corp.).
Diasorb, Liq., Tab. (Columbia).
Diastay, Tab. (Elder).
Diastop, Liq. (Elder).
Diatrol, Tab. (Otis Clapp).
Donnagel, Chew. Tab., Liq., Susp.
(Wyeth-Ayerst).
Donnagel-PG (Robins).
Furoxone Liq., Tab. (Eaton).
Homapin, Preps. (Mission).
Infatol Pink, Liq. (Scherer).
K-C, Susp. (Century).
K-Pek, Susp. (Rugby).
Kaodene Non-Narcotic, Liq. (Pfeiffer).
Kaolin (Various Mfr.).
Kaolin Colloidal (Various Mfr.).
Kaomin, Pow. (Lilly).
Kaopectate, Preps (Upjohn).
Kao-Spen, Susp. (Century).
Kapectolin (Various Mfr.)
Lactinex, Tab., Gran. (Hynson, West-
cott & Dunning).
Lactobacillus acidophilus & bulgaricus
mixed culture, Tab. (Hynson, West-
cott & Dunning).
Lactobacillus acidophilus, viable cul-
ture (Various Mfr.).
Lomotil, Liq., Tab., (Searle & Co.).
Milk of Bismuth (Various Mfr.).
Mycifradin Sulfate, Soln., Tab. (Up-
john).
Palsorb Improved, Liq. (Hauck).
Paocin, Susp. (Massengill).
Paregel, Liq. (Ferndale).
Parelixer, Liq. (Purdue-Frederick).
Parepectolin, Susp. (Rhone-Poulenc
Rorer).
Pectocel, Susp. (Lilly).
Pektamalt, Susp. (Warren-Teed).
Pepto-Bismol, Liq., Tab. (Norwich).
Rheaban, Capl. (Pfizer).
Sorboquel, Tab. (Schering-Plough).
ANTIDIURETICS.
See: Pitressin, Amp. (Parke-Davis).
Pitressin Tannate In Oil, Amp. (Parke-
Davis).
Pituitary Post. Inj. (Various Mfr.).
ANTIEMETIC/ANTIVERTIGO AGENTS.
See: Antinauseants Supprettes
"WANS" (Webcon).
Atarax, Tab., Syr. (Roerig).
Bendectin, Tab. (Merrell Dow).
Bucladin-S, Softab Tab. (Stuart).

Cesamet, Cap. (Lilly).
Compazine, Preps. (SK-Beecham).
Dramamine, and Dramamine-D,
Preps. (Searle).
Emecheck, Liq. (Savage).
Emesert, Rectal Insert (American Criti-
cal Care).
Emetrol, Liq. (Rhone-Poulenc Rorer).
Marezine, Preps. (Burroughs Well-
come).
Marinol, Cap. (Roxane).
Meclizine HCl, Tab. (Various Mfr.).
Mepergan, Inj. (Wyeth-Ayerst).
Naus-A-Tories, Supp. (Table Rock).
Nausetrol, Syr. (Medical Chemicals).
Phenergan, Preps. (Wyeth-Ayerst).
Prochlorperazine, Supp. (G & W
Labs).
Pyridoxine HCl, Preps. (Various Mfr.).
Thorazine, Preps. (SK-Beecham).
Tigan, Preps. (Beecham Labs).
Torecan Amp., Supp., Tab. (Sandoz).
Trilafon, Preps. (Schering-Plough).
Vistaril, Cap., Susp., Soln. (Pfizer).
Zofran, Inj. (Glaxo).
ANTIEPILEPSIRINE. USAN.
Use: Anticonvulsant. [Orphan drug]
ANTIEPILEPTIC AGENTS.
See: Anticonvulsants.
ANTIESTROGEN. Tamoxifen citrate.
Use: Hormone for cancer therapy.
See: Nolvadex (Zeneca).
Tamoxifen (Barr).
ANTIFEBRIN.
See: Acetanilid (Various Mfr.).
ANTIFLATULENTS.
See: Di-Gel, Prods. (Schering-Plough).
Silain, Tab., Gel (Robins).
Simethicone Prods.
ANTIFOAM A COMPOUND. (Merrell
Dow).
Use: Antiflatulent.
See: Simethicone, U.S.P. XXIII.
ANTIFOLIC ACID.
See: Methotrexate, Tab. (Lederle).
ANTIFORMIN. Sodium hypochlorite in
sodium hydroxide 7.5%, available chlo-
rine 5.2%; may be colored with meta
cresol purple.
Use: Antiseptic, germicide.
ANTIFUNGAL AGENTS.
See: Fungicides.
• **ANTIHEMOPHILIC FACTOR,** U.S.P. XXI-
II. Human antihemophilic factor. (Hyland
& Alpha Therapeutics) Antihemophilic
Factor, human. Method for Syringe Ad-
ministration 10 ml 450 A.H.F. or 300
A.H.F. units/Pkg. W/Syringe 30 ml or
900 A.H.F. units/Pkg.
Use: Antihemophilic.

See: AlphaNine, Inj. (Alpha Therapeutic).
Hemofil, Vial (Hyland).
Humate-P, Inj. (Armour).
Koate HP, Inj. (Miles).
Koate-HS, Vial (Cutter).
Koate-HT, Vial (Cutter).
KoaCNate, Inj. (Miles).
Monoclate-P, Inj. (Armour).
Mononine, Inj. (Armour).
Profilate HP. Inj. (Alpha Therapeutic).
Recombinate, Inj. (Hyland).

ANTIHEMOPHILIC FACTOR, HUMAN.
Use: Treatment of Von Willebrand's disease. [Orphan drug]
See: Humate P.

ANTIHEMOPHILIC FACTOR (PORCINE)
HYATE: C. (Porton) Freeze-dried concentrate of Antihemophilic Factor, 400 to 700 porcine units of Factor VIII:C. Pow. for inj. Vials.
Use: Antihemophilic product.

ANTIHEMOPHILIC FACTOR (RECOMBINANT).
Use: Prophylaxis/treatment of bleeding in hemophilia A. [Orphan drug]
See: Kogenate.

ANTIHEPARIN. Protamine Sulfate.

ANTIHISTAMINE CREAM. (Towne)
Methapyrilene HCl 10 mg, pyrilamine maleate 5 mg, allantoin 2 mg, diperodon HCl 2.5 mg, benzocaine 10 mg, menthol 2 mg/Gm. Cream Jar 2 oz.
Use: Antihistamine, topical.

ANTIHISTAMINES.
See: Actidil, Tab., Syr. (Burroughs Wellcome).
Ambodryl, Kapseal (Parke-Davis).
Benadryl HCl, Preps. (Parke-Davis).
Chlorpheniramine Maleate (Various Mfr.).
Chlorpheniramine Maleate w/Comb. (Various Mfr.).
Clistin, Elix., Tab. (McNeil).
Co-Pyronil, Pulv., Susp. (Lilly).
Diafen, Tab. (Riker).
Dimetane, Preps. (Robins).
Diphenhydramine HCl (Various Mfr.).
Diphenylpyraline HCl (Various Mfr.).
Disophrol, Prods. (Schering-Plough).
Doxylamine Succinate (Merrell Dow).
Drixoral, Prods. (Schering-Plough).
Forhistal Maleate, Syr., Tab. (Ciba).
Inhiston, Tab. (Plough).
Novahistine LP, Tab. (Merrell Dow).
Optimine, Prods. (Schering-Plough).
PBZ, Tab. (Geigy).
PBZ-SR, Tab. (Geigy).
Periactin, Syr., Tab. (Merck & Co.).
Promethazine HCl (Various Mfr.).

Prophenpyridamine Maleate (Various Mfr.).
Pyrilamine Maleate (Various Mfr.).
Tripelennamine HCl (Various Mfr.).
Triprolidine HCl (Various Mfr.).

ANTIHYPERLIPIDEMICS.
See: Atromid-S, Cap. (Wyeth-Ayerst).
Choloxin, Tab. (Flint).
Cholybar, Bar. (Parke-Davis).
Clofibrate, Cap. (Various Mfr.).
Colestid, Gran (Upjohn).
Lopid, Cap., Tab. (Parke-Davis).
Lorelco, Tab. (Merrell Dow).
Lovastatin.
Mevacor, Tab. (Merck & Co.).
Pravachol, Tab. (Bristol-Myers Squibb).
Questran, Pow. (Bristol-Myers U.S. Pharm.).
Zocor, Tab. (Merck & Co.).

ANTIHYPERTENSIVES.
See: Hypertension Therapy.

ANTI-INHIBITOR COAGULANT COMPLEX.
Use: Antihemophilic agent.
See: Autoplex T. (Hyland Therapeutic).
Feiba VH. (Immuno-U.S.).

ANTI-ITCH CREAM. (Spencer-Mead)
Burow's solution 5%, phenol 0.5%, menthol 0.5%, camphor 1% in washable base. Tube oz.
Use: Antipruritic, counter-irritant.

ANTI-J5MAB. USAN.
Use: Antibiotic.

ANTILEPROTICS.
Use: Local anesthetic, antipruritic.
See: Hansen's disease.

ANTILERGE. (Metz) Chlorpheniramine maleate 8 mg, phenylephrine HCl 12 mg/Tab. Bot. 30s.
Use: Antihistamine, decongestant.

ANTILEUKEMIA.
See: Antineoplastic agents.

ANTILIRIUM. (Forest) Physostigmine salicylate 2 mg/2 ml. Amp. Box. 12s.
Use: Antidote.

ANTIMALARIAL AGENTS.
See: Amodiaquin HCl.
Aralen HCl, Inj. (Sanofi Winthrop).
Aralen Phosphate (Sanofi Winthrop).
Aralen Phosphate w/Primaquine (Sanofi Winthrop).
Atabrine HCl, Tab. (Sanofi Winthrop).
Chloroguanide HCl.
Daraprim Tab. (Burroughs Wellcome).
Hydroxychloroquine Sulfate.
Paludrine HCl, Tab. (Wyeth-Ayerst).
Pamaquine Naphthoate.
Plaquenil Sulfate, Tab. (Sanofi Winthrop).

Plasmochin Naphthoate.
Primaquine Phosphate, Tab. (Sanofi Winthrop).
Pyrimethamine.
Quinacrine HCl, Tab.
Quinine Salts (Various Mfr.).
Quinine Sulfate (Various Mfr.).
Totaquine, Pow.
ANTIME. (Rand) Pentaerythritol tetranitrate 30 mg or 80 mg/Cap. Bot. 60s, 500s.
Use: Smooth muscle relaxant.
ANTIME FORTE. (Rand) Pentaerythritol tetranitrate 30 mg, secobarbital 50 mg/Cap. Bot. 60s, 500s.
Use: Smooth muscle relaxant, sedative/hypnotic.
ANTIMELANOMA ANTIBODY XMMME-001-DTPA 111 INDIUM. (Xoma)
Use: Diagnostic aid for melanoma metastasis. [Orphan drug]
ANTIMELANOMA ANTIBODY XMMME-001-RTA. USAN.
Use: Treatment of stage III melanoma. [Orphan drug]
ANTIMINTH. (Pfizer Laboratories) Pyrantel pamoate 250 mg/5 ml. Bot. 60 ml.
Use: Anthelmintic.
• **ANTIMONY POTASSIUM TARTRATE,** U.S.P. XXIII. Antimonate (2-),bis[u-[2,3-dihydroxybutanedioato(4-)-0,0:0,0]] dipotassium, trihydrate, stereoisomer. Dipotassium bis[u-tar-trato(4-)] diantimonate (2-) trihydrate. Tartar emetic. (Various Mfr.).
Use: Schistosomiasis, leishmaniasis, expectorant, emetic.
W/Cocillana, euphorbia pilulifera, squill, senega.
See: Cylana, Syr. (Bowman).
W/Guaifenesin, codeine phosphate.
See: Cheracol, Syr. (Upjohn).
W/Guaifenesin, dextromethorphan HBr.
See: Cheracol-D, Syr. (Upjohn).
W/Paregoric, glycyrrhiza fluid extract.
See: Brown Mixture (Lilly).
W/Thenylpyramine HCl, ammonium Cl, sodium citrate, menthol, aromatics.
See: Histacomp, Syr., Tab. (Approved Pharm.).
ANTIMONY PREPARATIONS.
See: Antimony Potassium Tartrate (Various Mfr.).
Antimony Sodium Thioglycollate (Various Mfr.).
Tartar Emetic (Various Mfr.).
• **ANTIMONY SODIUM TARTRATE,** U.S.P. XXIII.
ANTIMONY SODIUM THIOGLYCOLLATE. (Various Mfr.).

Use: Schistosomiasis, leishmaniasis, filariasis.
• **ANTIMONY TRISULFIDE COLLOID.** USAN.
Use: Pharmaceutic aid.
ANTIMONYL POTASSIUM TARTRATE.
See: Antimony Potassium Tartrate, U.S.P. XXIII.
ANTI-MY9-BLOCKED RICIN. USAN.
Use: Leukemia treatment.
ANTINAUSEANTS.
See: Antiemetic/antivertigo agents.
ANTINEOPLASTIC AGENTS.
See: Adriamycin, Vial (Adria).
Alkeran, Tab. (Burroughs Wellcome).
Blenoxane, Amp. (Bristol).
Cosmegen, Inj. (Merck & Co.).
Cytosar, sterile (Upjohn).
Cytoxan, Tab., Vial (Mead Johnson).
Dicorvin, Tab. (Amfre-Grant).
Drolban, Inj. (Lilly).
Elspar, Inj. (Merck & Co.).
Emcyt, Cap. (Pharmacia).
Estinyl, Tab. (Schering-Plough).
Estradurin, Inj. (Wyeth-Ayerst).
5-Fluorouracil, Amp. (Roche).
FUDR, Vial (Roche).
Hexalen (US Bioscience)
Hydrea, Cap. (Squibb).
Idamycin (Adria).
Leukeran, Tab. (Burroughs Wellcome).
Lysodren, Tab. (Calbio).
Matulane, Cap. (Roche).
Medroxyprogesterone Acetate Tab., Vial (Various Mfr.).
Megace, Tab. (Mead Johnson).
Mercaptopurine, Tab. (Burroughs Wellcome).
Methosarb, Tab. (Upjohn).
Methotrexate, Tab. (Lederle).
Methotrexate Sodium, Vial (Lederle).
Meticorten, Tab. (Schering-Plough).
Mithracin, Vial (Pfizer).
Mustargen, Inj. (Merck & Co.).
Myleran, Tab. (Burroughs Wellcome).
Nolvadex, Tab. (Zeneca).
Oncovin, Amp. (Lilly).
Progynon, Pellets, Susp. (Schering-Plough).
Purinethol, Tab. (Burroughs Wellcome).
TACE, Cap. (Merrell Dow).
Tamoxifen, Tab. (Barr).
Teslac, Tab., Vial (Squibb).
Thioguanine, Tab. (Burroughs Wellcome).
Thio-Tepa, Vial (Lederle).
Triethylene Melamine, Tab. (Lederle).
Uracil Mustard, Cap. (Upjohn).
Velban, Amp. (Lilly).

Vercyte, Tab. (Abbott).
ANTI-OBESITY AGENTS.
See: Thyroid.
Amphetamine Preps. (Various Mfr.).
Dextroamphetamine Preps. (Various Mfr.).
Diethylpropion HCl.
Fastin, Cap. (Beecham Labs)
Ionamin, Cap. (Pennwalt).
Levo-Amphetamine.
Methamphetamine Preps. (Various Mfr.).
Plegine, Tab. (Wyeth-Ayerst).
Preludin, Tab. (Boehringer Ingelheim).
Sanorex, Tab. (Sandoz).
Statobex, Tab. (Lemmon).
Tenuate, Tab. (Merrell Dow).
Tepanil, Tab. (Riker).
ANTIOX. (Mayrand) Vitamin C 120 mg, vitamin E 100 IU, beta carotene 25 mg. Cap. Bot. 60s.
Use: Vitamin supplement.
ANTI-OXIDANT. (Murdock) Vitamins A 5000 IU, E 134 mg, C 90 mg, zinc 15 mg, selenium 100 mg, glutathione 30 mg. Cap. Bot. 90s.
Use: Vitamin/mineral supplement.
ANTIOXIDANT FORMULA. (Life's Finest) Vitamins E 134 mg, C 250 mg, selenium 100 mcg. Cap. Bot. 100s, 200s, 250s.
Use: Vitamin supplement.
ANTI-PAK COMPOUND. (Lowitt) Phenylephrine HCl 5 mg, salicylamide 0.23 Gm, acetophenetidin 0.15 gr, caffeine 0.03 Gm, ascorbic acid 50 mg, hesperidin complex 50 mg, chlorprophen-pyridamine maleate 2 mg/Tab. Bot. 30s, 100s.
Use: Decongestant, analgesic, antihistamine combination.
ANTI PAN T LYMPHOCYTE MONO-CLONAL ANTIBODY.
Use: Aid in eliminating mature T-cells from bone marrow grafts. [Orphan drug]
See: Anti-T Lymphocyte Immunotoxin XMMLY-H65-RTA.
ANTIPARASYMPATHOMIMETICS.
See: Parasympatholytic agents.
ANTI-PELLAGRA VITAMIN.
See: Nicotinic acid.
ANTI-PERNICIOUS ANEMIA PRINCIPLE.
See: Vitamin B_{12}.
ANTIPHLOGISTINE. (Denver) Medicated poultice. Jar 5 oz, lb. Tube 8 oz. Can 5 lb.
ANTIPROTOZOAN AGENTS.
See: Antimony Preps.
Arsenic Preps.

Bismuth Preps.
Chiniofon (Various Mfr.).
Diiodohydroxyquinoline.
Emetine HCl (Various Mfr.).
Furazolidone.
Iodocholohydroxyquinoline.
Iodohydroxyquinoline Sulfonate Sodium
Levofuraltadone.
Ornidyl (Marion Merrell Dow).
Quinoxyl.
Suramin Sodium.
• **ANTIPYRINE,** U.S.P. XXIII. 2,3-Dimethyl-1-phenyl-3-pyrazolin-5-one. (Various Mfr.) Analgesine, anodynine, dimethyloxyquinazine, oxydimethylquinizine, parodyne, phenazone, phenylone, pyrazoline, sedatine.
Use: Analgesic, antipyretic. [Orphan drug]
W/Benzocaine, chlorobutanol.
See: G.B.A., Drops (Scrip).
W/Carbamide, benzocaine, cetyldimethyl-benzylammonium HCl.
See: Auralgesic, Liq. (Elder).
W/Phenylephrine HCl, benzocaine.
See: Tympagesic, Liq. (Adria).
W/Pyrilamine maleate, phenylephrine, benzalkonium.
See: Prefrin-A Ophthalmic (Allergan).
• **ANTIPYRINE AND BENZOCAINE OTIC SOLUTION,** U.S.P. XXIII.
Use: Local anesthetic.
See: Auro Ear Drops (Commerce).
Lanaurine, Drops (Lannett).
Pyrocaine Eardrop, Liq. (Med. Chem.).
• **ANTIPYRINE, BENZOCAINE AND PHENYLEPHRINE HYDROCHLORIDE OTIC SOLUTION,** U.S.P. XXIII.
Use: Local anesthetic, decongestant eardrop.
ANTIRABIES SERUM. (Sclavo) Antirabies serum, equine origin (ARS) 125 IU/ml with m-Cresol 0.3%. Inj. Vial 1000 units.
Use: Rabies prophylaxis.
ANTIRHEUMATIC PREPARATIONS.
See: p-Aminobenzoic Acid and salts (calcium, potassium, sodium).
Ammonium Salicylate.
Colchicine, Preps.
Gentisate Sodium.
Gold Sodium Thiosulfate, Preps. (Various Mfr.).
Myochrysine, Inj. (Merck & Co.).
Salicylamide, Preps.
Sodium Salicylate.
Solganal, Vial (Schering-Plough).
ANTIRICKETTSIAL AGENTS.
See: p-Aminobenzoic Acid (Various

Mfr.).
p-Aminobenzoate Sodium (Various
　Mfr.).
Aureomycin, Preps. (Lederle).
Chloromycetin, Preps. (Parke-Davis).
Rocky Mountain Spotted Fever Serum
　(Rabbit), Vial (Lederle).
Terramycin, Preps. (Pfizer).
ANTISCORBUTIC VITAMIN.
See: Ascorbic Acid.
ANTISEPTIC, CHLORINE, ACTIVE.
See: Antiseptic, N-Chloro Compounds,
　Hypochlorite Preps.
ANTISEPTIC, DYES.
See: Acriflavine (Various Mfr.).
　Aminoacridine HCl.
　Bismuth Violet, Preps. (Table Rock).
　Brilliant Green.
　Crystal Violet.
　Fuchsin.
　Gentian Violet (Various Mfr.).
　Methylrosaniline Cl (Various Mfr.).
　Methyl Violet.
　Pyridium, Tab. (Parke-Davis).
　Serenium, Tab. (Squibb).
ANTISEPTIC, MERCURIALS.
See: Mercresin (Upjohn).
　Merthiolate, Preps. (Lilly)
　Phenylmercuric Acetate (Various Mfr.).
　Phenylmercuric Borate (Various Mfr.).
　Phenylmercuric Nitrate (Various Mfr.).
　Phenylmercuric Picrate (Various Mfr.).
　Thimerosal.
**ANTISEPTIC, N-CHLORO
COMPOUNDS.**
See: Chloramine-T (Various Mfr.).
　Chlorazene, Pow., Tab. (Badger).
　Dichloramine-T (Various Mfr.).
　Halazone, Tab. (Abbott).
ANTISEPTIC, PHENOLS.
See: Anthralin (Various Mfr.).
　Bithionol.
　Coal Tar Products (Various Mfr.).
　Creosote (Various Mfr.).
　Cresols (Various Mfr.).
　Guaiacol (Various Mfr.).
　Hexachlorophene (Various Mfr.).
　Hexylresorcinol (Various Mfr.).
　Methylparaben (Various Mfr.).
　o-Phenylphenol (Various Mfr.).
　Oxyquinoline Salts (Various Mfr.).
　Parachlorometaxylenol (Various Mfr.).
　Phenol (Various Mfr.).
　Picric Acid (Various Mfr.).
　Propylparaben (Various Mfr.).
　Pyrogallol (Various Mfr.).
　Resorcinol (Various Mfr.).
　Resorcinol Monoacetate (Various
　Mfr.).
　Thymol (Various Mfr.).

Trinitrophenol (Various Mfr.).
ANTISEPTICS.
See: Furacin, Preps. (Eaton).
　Iodine Products.
　Mercurials.
　N-Chloro Compounds.
　Phenols.
　Surface-Active Agents.
**ANTISEPTIC, SURFACE-ACTIVE
AGENTS.**
See: Bactine, Preps. (Miles).
　Benzalkonium Cl (Various Mfr.).
　Benzethonium Cl (Various Mfr.).
　Ceepryn (Merrell Dow).
　Cpacol Preps. (Merrell Dow).
　Cetylpyridinium Cl (Various Mfr.).
　Diaparene Cl, Preps. (Glenbrook).
　Methylbenzethonium Cl (Various Mfr.).
　Zephiran Cl, Preps. (Sanofi Winthrop).
ANTISPAS. (Keene) Dicyclomine HCl 10
mg/ml. Vial 10 ml.
Use: Antispasmodic.
ANTISPASMODIC ELIXIR. (Various Mrf.)
Atropine sulfate 0.0194 mg, scopo-
lamine HBr 0.0065 mg, hyoscyamine
HBr or SO_4 0.1037 mg, phenobarbital
16.2 mg/ml w/alcohol 23%. Elix. Bot.
120 ml, pt, gal and UD 5 ml.
Use: Anticholinergic/antispasmodic,
　sedative/hypnotic.
ANTISPASMODICS. Usually refers to
agents that combat the muscarinic effect
of liberated acetylcholine. Relief of
smooth muscle spasms. Parasympa-
tholytic agents.
See: Anticholinergic Agents.
　Spasmolytic Agents.
ANTISPASMODIC CAPSULES. (Lem-
mon) Phenobarbital 16.2 mg,
hyoscyamine sulfate 0.1037 mg, at-
ropine sulfate 0.0194 mg, scopolamine
HBr 0.0065 mg/Cap. Bot. 1000s.
Use: Sedative/hypnotic, anticholiner-
　gic/antispasmodic.
ANTISTEREPTOLYSIN-O. Titration pro-
cedure.
See: Also (Wampole Labs).
ANTISTERILITY VITAMIN.
See: Vitamin E.
**ANTI-T LYMPHOCYTE IMMUNOTOXIN
XMMLY-H65-RTA.** (Xoma)
See: ANTI PAN T LYMPHOCYTE
　MONOCLONAL ANTIBODY.
ANTI-TAC, HUMANIZED. (Hoffman-
LaRoche)
Use: Prevention of acute renal allograft
　rejection. [Orphan drug]
ANTI-TAP-72 IMMUNOTOXIN.
Use: Treatment of metastatic colorectal
　cancer adenocarcinoma. [Orphan

drug]

ANTI-TEN. (Century) Allylisobutylbarbituric acid ¾ gr, aspirin 3 gr, phenacetin 2 gr, caffeine gr/Tab. Bot. 100s, 1000s. *Use:* Sedative, analgesic, CNS stimulant.

ANTITHROMBIN III CONCENTRATE IV. *Use:* Prophylaxis/treatment of thromboembolic episodes in AT-III deficiency. [Orphan drug]

ANTITHROMBIN III HUMAN. *Use:* Thromboembolic agent. [Orphan drug] *See:* ATnativ (Hyland).

ANTI-THYMOCYTE SERUM. *Use:* Prevention of allograft rejection. [Orphan drug]

ANTITHYROID AGENTS. *See:* Iothiouracil Sodium.
Methimazole.
Methylthiouracil (Various Mfr.).
Propylthiouracil (Various Mfr.).
Tapazole, Tab. (Lilly).

ANTITOXINS. *See:* Botulism Antitoxin.
Diphtheria Antitoxin.
Gas Gangrene Antitoxin.
Tetanus Antitoxin.

ANTITRYPSIN, ALPHA 1. *See:* Prolastin (Cutter).

ANTITUBERCULOSIS AGENTS. *See:* Aminosalicylates (Na, Ca, K) (Various Mfr.).
Benzapas, Pow., Tab. (Dorsey).
Calcium Benzoylpas (Various Mfr.).
Capastat Sulfate, Amp. (Lilly).
Cycloserine, Pulv. (Lilly).
Diasone Sodium, Tab. (Abbott).
Dihydrosteptomycin (Various Mfr.).
Isoniazid (Various Mfr.).
Myambutol, Tab. (Lederle).
Natri-Pas, Pow., Tab. (Glenwood).
Niadox, Tab. (Barnes-Hind).
Niconyl, Tab. (Parke-Davis).
P.A.S. Acid, Tab. (Kasar).
Pasara Sodium, Pow., Tab. (Dorsey).
Pasdium, Tab. (Kasar).
Pyrazinamide, Tab. (Lederle).
Rifadin, Cap. (Merrell Dow).
Rimactane, Cap. (Ciba).
Seromycin, Pulv. (Lilly).
Streptomycin (Various Mfr.).
Trecator-SC, Tab. (Wyeth-Ayerst).
Triniad, Tab. (Kasar).
Uniad, Tab. (Kasar).
Uniad-Plus 5,10, Tab. (Kasar).

ANTI-TUSS. (Century) Guaifenesin 100 mg/5 ml. Bot. 4 oz, gal. *Use:* Expectorant.

ANTI-TUSS D.M. (Century) Guaifenesin 100 mg, dextromethorphan HBr 15 mg/5 ml. Bot. 4 oz, pt, gal. *Use:* Expectorant, antitussive.

ANTI-TUSSIVE. (Canright) Dextromethorphan HBr 10 mg, potassium guaiacol sulfonate 125 mg, terpin hydrate 100 mg, phenylpropanolamine HCl 12.5 mg, pyrilamine maleate 12.5 mg/Tab. Bot. 60s. *Use:* Antitussive, expectorant, decongestant, antihistamine.

ANTITUSSIVE COUGH SYRUP. (Weeks & Leo) Chlorpheniramine 2 mg, phenylephrine HCl 5 mg, dextromethorphan 15 mg, ammonium Cl 50 mg/5 ml. *Use:* Antihistamine, decongestant, antitussive, expectorant.

ANTITUSSIVE COUGH SYRUP WITH CODEINE. (Weeks & Leo) Chlorpheniramine maleate 2 mg, phenylephrine HCl 5 mg, codeine phosphate 10 mg, ammonium Cl 50 mg/5 ml. Bot. 4 oz. *Use:* Antihistamine, decongestant, antitussive, expectorant.

ANTITUSSIVE-DECONGESTANT. *See:* St. Joseph Cough Syrup for Children (Schering-Plough).
Tussend, Tab., Liq. (Merrell Dow).

• **ANTIVENIN (CROTALIDAE) POLYVALENT,** U.S.P. XXIII. Polyvalent crotaline antivenin. Rattlesnake antivenin for four species of pit vipers. *Use:* Passive immunizing agent for treatment of rattlesnake bite.

• **ANTIVENIN (LATRODECTUS MACTANS),** U.S.P. XXIII. (Merck & Co.) Black widow spider antivenin. Each vial contains not less than 6000 antivenin units. Thimerosal (mercury derivative) 1:10,000 added as preservative. Vial 2.5 ml. *Use:* Treatment of black widow spider bites.

• **ANTIVENIN (MICRURUS FULVIUS),** U.S.P. XXIII. (Wyeth-Ayerst) Lyophilized antivenin of animal origin (*Micrurus fulvius*) with phenol 0.25% and thimerosal 0.005% as preservatives. Bacteriostatic water w/phenylmercuric nitrate 1:10,000 as preservative. Combination package. Vial 10 ml. *Use:* Bites of North American coral snake and Texas coral snake.

ANTIVENIN, CROTALIDAE, POLYVALENT. (Wyeth-Ayerst) Antivenin Crotalidae, Polyvalent, U.S.P. XXIII. (*Crotalidae*) Rattlesnake, copperhead and moccasin antitoxic serum. Pkg. Comb w/Phenol 0.25%, thimerosal 0.005% as preservatives. One disposable syringe,

10 ml of bacteriostatic water for inj. w/preservative phenyl mercuric nitrate 0.001%; one applicator vial iodine tincture. Normal horse serum 1:10, as sensitivity testing material w/preservatives thimerosal 0.005% and phenol 0.35%.
Use: Bites of crotalid snakes of the United States.

ANTIVENIN, POLYVALENT CROTALID (OVINE) FAB.
Use: Bites of North American crotalid snakes. [Orphan drug]
See: Crotab (Therapeutic Antibodies).

ANTIVERT. (Roerig) Meclizine HCl 12.5 mg, 25 mg or 50 mg/Tab., 25 mg/Chew. Tab. **12.5 mg:** Bot. 100s, 1000s, UD 100s; **25 mg:** Bot. 100s, 1000s, UD 100s. **50 mg:** Bot. 100s. **Chew. tab.:** Bot. 100s, 500s.
Use: Antiemetic/antivertigo.

ANTIVIRAL AGENTS.
See: Cytovene, Inj. (Syntex).
Famvir, Tab. (SK-Beecham).
Foscavir, Inj. (Astra).
Hivid, Tab. (Roche).
Retrovir, Preps. (Burroughs Wellcome).
Symmetrel, Cap., Syr. (DuPont).
Videx, Pow., Tab. (Bristol-Myers Squibb).
Vira-A, Inj. (Parke-Davis).
Virazole, Pow. for Reconstitution for aerosol (ICN).
Zerit, Cap. (B-M Squibb).
Zovirax, Cap, Inj. (Burroughs Wellcome).

ANTIXEROPHTHALMIC VITAMIN.
See: Vitamin A.

ANTRIZINE TABS. (Major) Meclizine 12.5 mg, 25 mg or 50 mg/Tab. **12.5 mg:** 100s, 500s, 1000s. **25 mg:** 100s, 500s, 1000s, UD 100s. **50 mg:** 100s.
Use: Antiemetic/antivertigo.

ANTROCOL. (Poythress) Atropine sulfate 0.195 mg, phenobarbital 16 mg/Tab. or Cap. Tab. Bot, 100s. Cap. Bot. 100s, 500s.
Use: Anticholinergic/antispasmodic, sedative/hypnotic.

ANTROCOL ELIXIR. (Poythress) Atropine sulfate 0.039 mg, phenobarbital 3 mg, alcohol 20%/5 ml. Bot. oz. w/dropper. Bot. pt.
Use: Anticholinergic/antispasmodic, sedative/hypnotic.

ANTRYPOL. Suramin.
Use: CDC anti-infective agent.

ANTURANE. (Ciba) Sulfinpyrazone, U.S.P. **100 mg/Tab.:** Bot 100s. **200 mg/Cap.:** Bot. 100s.

Use: Agent for gout.

ANUCAINE. (Calvin) Procaine 50 mg, butyl-p-aminobenzoate 200 mg, benzyl alcohol 265 mg in sweet almond oil/5 ml. Amp. 5 ml. Box 6s, 24s, 100s.
Use: Anorectal preparation.

ANUCORT-HC. (G&W Labs) Hydrocortisone acetate 25 mg in a hydrogenated vegetable oil base. Supp. Box 12s, 24s, 100s.
Use: Anorectal preparation.

ANUJECT. (Hauck) Procaine. Soln. Vial 5 ml or 10 ml.
Use: Anorectal preparation.

ANULAN SUPPOSITORIES. (Lannett) Bismuth resorcin compound, bismuth subgallate, zinc oxide, boric acid, balsam Peru. Supp. Box 12s.
Use: Anorectal preparation.

ANUMED. (Major) Bismuth subgallate 2.25%, bismuth resorcin compound 1.75%, benzyl benzoate 1.2%, zinc oxide 11%, balsam Peru 1.8% in a hydrogenated vegetable oil base. Supp. Box 12s.
Use: Anorectal preparation.

ANUMED HC. (Major) Bismuth subgallate 2.25%, bismuth resorcin compound 1.75%, benzyl benzoate 1.2%, balsam Peru 1.8%, zinc oxide 11%. Supp. Box 12s.
Use: Anorectal preparation.

ANUPREP HC. (Great Southern) Hydrocortisone acetate 25 mg. Supp. Box 12s.
Use: Anorectal preparation.

ANUPREP HEMORRHOIDAL. (Great Southern) Bismuth subgallate 2.25%, bismuth resorcin compound 1.75%, benzyl benzoate 1.2%, peruvian balsam 1.8% and zinc oxide 11% in a hydrogenated vegetable oil base. Supp. Box 12s, 24s.
Use: Anorectal prepration.

ANUSOL. (Parke-Davis Prods) Bismuth subgallate 2.25%, bismuth resorcin compound 1.75%, balsam Peru 1.8%, zinc oxide 11%, benzyl benzoate 1.2%, in hydrogenated vegetable oil/Supp. Box 12s, 24s, 48s.
Use: Anorectal preparation.

ANUSOL-HC 2.5%. (Parke-Davis) Hydrocortisone 2.5%, benzyl alcohol, petrolatum, EDTA. Cream Tube 30 Gm.
Use: Corticosteroid, topical.

ANUSOL HC 1. (Parke-Davis) Hydrocortisone 1%, diazolidinyl urea, parabens, mineral oil, sorbitan sesquioleate, white petrolatum. Oint. Tube 21 Gm.
Use: Corticosteroid, topical.

ANUSOL OINTMENT. (Parke-Davis

Prods) Balsam Peru 18 mg, zinc oxide 110 mg/Gm, benzyl benzoate 1.2%, pramoxine HCl 1% in a mineral oil glyceryl stearate and water base. Tube 1 oz, 2 oz.
Use: Anorectal preparation.

ANUSOL-HC. (Parke-Davis Prods) Hydrocortisone acetate 25 mg/Supp. Box 12s, 24s.
Use: Anorectal preparation.

ANXANIL. (Econo Med) Hydroxyzine HCl 25 mg/Tab. Bot. 100s.
Use: Antianxiety agent.

AORACILLIN-B. (Vita Elixir) Penicillin G 200,000 units or 500,000 units/Tab. Bot. 50s.
Use: Antibacterial, penicillin.

AOSEPT. (Ciba Vision) Hydrogen peroxide 3%, sodium Cl 0.85%, phosphonic acid, phosphate buffer. Soln. Bot. 120 ml, 237 ml, 355 ml, 480 ml.
Use: Contact lens care.

APACET. (Parmed) Acetaminophen 80 mg/Chew. tab. Bot. 100s.
Use: Analgesic.

• **APALCILLIN SODIUM.** USAN.
Use: Antibacterial.

APAP.
See: Acetaminophen.

APATATE LIQUID. (Kenwood) Vitamins B_1 15 mg, B_{12} 25 mcg, B_6 0.5 mg/5 ml. Liq. Bot. 4 oz, 8 oz.
Use: Vitamin supplement.

APATATE TABLETS. (Kenwood) Vitamins B_1 15 mg, B_{12} 25 mcg, B_6 0.5 mg/Tab. Bot. 50s.
Use: Vitamin supplement.

• **APAZONE.** USAN. 5-(Dimethylamino)-9-methyl-2-propyl-1H-pyrazolo[1,2,-a][1,2,4] benzotriazine-1,-3(2H)-dione.
Use: Anti-inflammatory agent.

A.P.C. (Various Mfr.) Aspirin, phenacetin, caffeine. Cap., Tab.
Use: Analgesic combination.
See: A.S.A. Compound, Preps. (Lilly).
P.A.C. Compound, Cap., Tab. (Upjohn).
Pan-APC, Tab. (Panray).
Phensal, Tab. (Merrell Dow).
W/Codeine phosphate. (Various Mfr.).
See: Anexsia w/Codeine, Tab. (Beecham Labs).
Anexsia D, Tab. (Beecham Labs).

A.P.C. W/GELSEMIUM COMBINATIONS.
See: Aidant, Tab. (Noyes).
Ansemco, No. 2, Tab. (Elder).
Asphac-G, Tab. (Central).
Valacet, Tab. (Vale).

APCOGESIC. (Apco) Sodium salicylate 5 gr, colchicine 1/320 gr, calcium carbon-

ate 65 mg, dried aluminum hydroxide gel 130 mg, phenobarbital ⅛ gr/Tab. Bot. 100s.
Use: Agent for gout, sedative/hypnotic.

APCOHIST. (APC) Phenylpropanolamine HCl 25 mg, chlorpheniramine maleate 1 mg/Tab. Bot. 100s.
Use: Decongestant, antihistamine.

APCORETIC. (APC) Caffeine anhydrous 100 mg, ammonium Cl 325 mg/Tab. Bot. 90s.
Use: Diuretic.

AP CREME. (T.E. Williams) Hydrocortisone 0.5%, iodochlorhydroxyquin 3%. Tube oz.
Use: Corticosteroid, antifungal (topical).

APF. (Whitehall).
Use: Salicylate analgesic.
See: Arthritis Pain Formula. (Whitehall).

APHCO HEMORRHOIDAL COMBINATION. (APC) Combination package of Aphco Hemorrhoidal Ointment 1.5 oz tube, Aphco Hemorrhoidal Supp. Box 12s, 1000s.
Use: Anorectal preparation.

APHEN TABS. (Major) Trihexyphenidyl 2 mg or 5 mg/Tab. Bot. 250s, 1000s.
Use: Antiparkinson agent.

APHRODYNE. (Star) Yohimbine HCl 5.4 mg/Tab. Bot. 100s, 1000s.
Use: Alpha-adrenergic blocking agent.

APICILLIN. D-(-)-α-Aminobenzyl penicillin.
See: Ampicillin.

APIQUEL FUMARATE. Aminorex. B.A.N.

A.P.L. (Wyeth-Ayerst) Chorionic Gonadotropin for Injection. Dry form, package vial 1s containing 5000 U.S.P. units, 10,000 U.S.P. units or 20,000 U.S.P. units, sterile diluent, w/benzyl alcohol, phenol, lactose.
Use: Chorionic gonadotropin therapy.

APLISOL. (Parke-Davis) Tuberculin purified protein derivative diluted 5 units/0.1 ml, polysorbate 80, potassium and sodium phosphates, phenol. Vial 1 ml (10 tests), 5 ml (50 tests).
Use: Diagnostic aid.

APLITEST. (Parke-Davis) Purified tuberculin protein derivative buffered with potassium and sodium phosphates, phenol 0.5%/single-use, multipuncture unit. 25s.
Use: Diagnostic aid.

APOMORPHINE HCl. (Britannia Pharm)
Use: Antiparkinson agent. [Orphan drug]

APORPHINE-10, 11-DIOL HYDROCHLORIDE.
See: Apomorphine HCl.

APPEDRINE. (Thompson Medical) Phenylpropanolamine HCl 25 mg, multivitamins, caffeine 100 mg/Tab.
Use: Diet aid.
APPETITE-DEPRESSANTS.
See: Anorexiants.
APPG.
See: Penicillin G, Procaine, Aqueous.
APRACLONIDINE HYDROCHLORIDE.
Use: Agent for glaucoma.
See: Iopidine (Alcon).
• **APRACLONIDINE OPHTHALMIC SOLUTION,** U.S.P. XXIII.
APRAZONE. (Major) Sulfinpyrazone.
Cap.: 200 mg. Bot. 100s, 500s, 1000s.
Tab.: 100 mg. Bot. 100s.
Use: Agent for gout.
APRESAZIDE. (Ciba) **25/25:** Hydralazine HCl 25 mg, hydrochlorothiazide 25 mg/Cap. **50/50:** Hydralazine HCl 50 mg, hydrochlorothiazide 50 mg/Cap. **100/50:** Hydralazine 100 mg, hydrochlorothiazide 50 mg/Cap. Bot. 100s.
Use: Antihypertensive.
APRESODEX. (Rugby) Hydrochlorothiazide 15 mg, hydralazine HCl 25 mg. Tab. Bot. 100s, 1000s.
Use: Antihypertensive.
APRESOLINE. (Ciba) Hydralazine HCl.
Amp.: 20 mg w/propylene glycol, methyl and propyl parabens/ml. Pkg. 5s. **Tab.:** 10 mg Bot. 100s, 1200s; 25 mg or 50 mg Bot. 100s, 1000s; 100 mg Bot. 100s. Consumer pack 100s.
Use: Antihypertensive.
W/Serpasil.
See: Serpasil Prods., Preps. (Ciba).
APRESOLINE-ESIDRIX. (Ciba) Hydralazine HCl 25 mg, hydrochlorothiazide 15 mg/Tab. Bot. 100s.
Use: Antihypertensive.
• **APRINDINE.** USAN. 3-[N-(Indan-2-yl)-N-phenylamino]propyldiethylamine. (Lilly) N-(2,3-Dihydro-1H-inden-2-yl)-N′,N-diethyl-N-phenyl-1,3-propanediamine.
Use: Antiarrhythmic.
APROBARBITAL. 5-Allyl-5-isopropylbarbituric acid, Allylisopropylmalonylurea. Pow.
Use: Sedative/hypnotic.
See: Alurate, Elix. (Roche).
APROBEE W/C. (Approved) Vitamins B_1 15 mg, B_2 10 mg, B_6 5 mg, niacinamide 50 mg, calcium pantothenate 10 mg, C 250 mg/Cap. or Tab. **Cap.:** Bot. 100s, 1000s. **Tab.:** Bot. 50s, 100s, 1000s.
Use: Vitamin supplement.
APRODINE. (Major) **Tab.:** Pseudoephedrine HCl 60 mg, triprolidine HCl 2.5 mg. Bot. 24s, 100s, 1000s, UD 100s.

Syr.: Pseudoephedrine HCl 30 mg, triprolidine HCl 1.25 mg/15 ml. Bot. 120 ml, pt.
Use: Decongestant, antihistamine.
APRODINE W/C. (Major) Pseudoephedrine HCl 30 mg, triprolidine HCl 1.25 mg, codeine phosphate 10 mg. Syr. Bot. pt, gal.
Use: Decongestant, antihistamine.
• **APROTININ.** USAN. A polypeptide proteinase inhibitor.
Use: Enzyme inhibitor (proteinase). [Orphan drug]
See: Trasylol.
APROZIDE 25/25 CAPSULES. (Major) Hydralazine 25 mg, hydrochlorothiazide 25 mg/Cap. Bot. 100s, 250s.
Use: Antihypertensive.
APROZIDE 50/50 CAPSULES. (Major) Hydrochlorothiazide 50 mg, hydralazine 50 mg/Cap. Bot. 100s, 250s.
Use: Antihypertensive.
A.P.S. Aspirin, phenacetin and salicylamide.
APSAC. Thrombolytic enzyme.
See: Eminase (Beecham).
• **APTAZAPINE MALEATE.** USAN.
Use: Antidepressant.
APTOCAINE. B.A.N. 2-Pyrrolidin-1-ylpropiono-o-toluidide.
Use: Local anesthetic.
See: Pirothesin HCl.
APYRON.
See: Magnesium acetylsalicylate.
AQ-4B. (Western Research) Trichlormethiazide 4 mg/Tab. Bot. 1000s.
Use: Diuretic.
AQUA-BAN. (Thompson Medical) Caffeine 100 mg, ammonium Cl 325 mg/Tab. Bot. 60s.
Use: Diuretic.
AQUA-BAN PLUS. (Thompson Medical) Ammonium Cl 650 mg, caffeine 200 mg, iron 6 mg/Tab. Bot. 30s.
Use: Diuretic, CNS stimulant, mineral supplement.
AQUABASE. (Vale) Cetyl alcohol, propylene glycol, sodium lauryl sulfate, white wax, purified water. Jar lb.
Use: Hydrophilic ointment base.
AQUACARE CREAM. (Herbert) Urea 2%, benzyl alcohol, carbomer 934, cetyl esters wax, fragrance, glycerin, oleth-3 phosphate, petrolatum, phenyl dimethicone, water, sodium hydroxide. Tube 2.5 oz.
Use: Emollient.
AQUACARE/HP. (Herbert) Urea 10%, benzyl alcohol. **Cream:** Tube 2.5 oz. **Lot.:** Bot. 8 oz, 16 oz.

Use: Emollient.

AQUACARE LOTION. (Herbert) Benzyl alcohol, oleth-3 phosphate, phenyl dimethicone, fragrance. Bot. 8 oz.
Use: Emollient.

AQUACHLOR. (Geneva) Chlortetracycline.
Use: Antibacterial, tetracycline.

AQUACHLORAL. (PolyMedica) Chloral hydrate, polyethylene glycol, spreading agent. Supp. 5 gr, 10 gr. Strip 12s.
Use: Sedative/hypnotic, rectal.

AQUA-CILLIN 250. (Kenyon) Crystalline penicillin G potassium 3 million units buffered w/sodium citrate/60 ml vial.
Use: Antibacterial, penicillin.

AQUACILLIN G. (Geneva) Penicillin G.
Use: Antibacterial, penicillin.

AQUACYCLINE. (Geneva) Tetracycline HCl.
Use: Antibacterial, tetracycline.

AQUADERM. (C & M Pharmacal) Purified water, glycerin 25%, salicylic acid 0.1%, octoxynol-9 0.03%, FD&C; Red #40 0.0001%. Bot. 2 oz.
Use: Emollient.

AQUADERM. (Baker Commins). Octyl methoxycinnamate 7.5%, oxybenzone 6%. SPF 15. Cream 105 g.
Use: Sunscreen.

AQUAFLEX ULTRASOUND GEL PAD. (Parker) Clear, solid, flexible, moist, standoff gel pad for use where transducer movement is impeded by bony or irregular body surfaces. 2 cm × 9 cm.
Use: Ultrasound agent.

AQUAFUREN. (Geneva) Nitrofurantoin.
Use: Anti-infective, urinary.

AQUAKAY.
See: Menadione (Various Mfr.).

AQUA LACTEN LOTION. (Herald Pharmacal) Demineralized water, urea, petrolatum, propylene glycol monostearate, sorbitan monostearate, lactic acid. Bot. 8 oz.
Use: Emollient.

AQUAMEPHYTON INJECTION. (Merck & Co.) Phytonadione 2 mg/ml or 10 mg/ml, vitamin K-1, w/polyoxyethylated fatty acid derivative 70 mg, dextrose 37.5 mg, benzyl alcohol 0.9%, water for injection q.s. to 1 ml. Inj. Amp. 1 mg/0.5 ml Box 25s; 10 mg/1 ml Box 6s, 25s. Vial 10 mg/ml 2.5 ml, 5 ml.
Use: Prothrombogenic

AQUA MIST. (Faraday) Nasal spray. Squeeze Bot. 20 ml.

AQUAMYCIN. (Geneva) Erythromycin.
Use: Antibacterial.

AQUANIL. (Sig) Mersalyl 100 mg, theo-phylline (hydrate) 50 mg, methylparaben 0.18%, propylparaben 0.02%. Vial 10 ml.
Use: Diuretic, bronchodilator.

AQUANINE. (Geneva) Quinine HCl.
Use: Antimalarial.

AQUAOXY. (Geneva) Oxytetracycline HCl.
Use: Antibacterial, tetracycline.

AQUAPHENICOL. (Geneva) Chloramphenicol.
Use: Anti-infective.

AQUAPHILIC OINTMENT. (Medco Lab) Hydrated hydrophilic oint. Jar 16 oz.
Use: Emollient, ointment base.

AQUAPHILIC OINTMENT WITH CARBAMIDE 10% and 20%. (Medco Lab) Stearyl alcohol, white petrolatum, sorbitol, propylene glycol, sodium lauryl sulfate, lactic acid, methylparaben, propylparaben.
Use: Prescription compounding, emollient.

AQUAPHOR NATURAL HEALING. (Beiersdorf) Petrolatum, mineral oil, mineral wax, woolwax alcohol, panthenol, glycerin, chamomile essense. Oint. Tube 52.5 Gm.
Use: Ointment and lotion base.

AQUAPHOR. (Beiersdorf) Cholesterolized anhydrous petrolatum ointment base. Tube 1.75 oz, 3.25 oz, 16 oz, Jar 5 lb, Bar 3 oz.
Use: Water-miscible ointment base.
See: Eucerin, Emulsion (Duke).

AQUAPHOR ANTIBIOTIC. (Beiersdorf) 10,000 units polymyxin B sulfate and 500 units bacitracin zinc/g in a cholesterolized ointment base. Oint. Tube 15 g.
Use: Topical anti-infective.

AQUAPHYLLIN SYRUP. (Ferndale) Theophylline anhydrous 80 mg/15 ml UD pk. 15 ml, 30 ml. Bot. 16 oz, gal.
Use: Bronchodilator.

AQUAPOOL CONCENTRATE. (Parker) Color additive for hydrotherapy to control foaming. Bot. pt, gal.

AQUASITE. (Ciba Vision) PEG-400 0.2%, dextran 70 0.1%, polycarbophil, NaCl, EDTA, sodium hydroxide. Preservative free. Soln. Single-use vials 0.6 ml.
Use: Artificial tears.

AQUASOL A. (Armour) Water-miscible Vitamin A. **Inj.:** 50,000 U.S.P. units/ml. Vial 2 ml Box 10s. **Cap.:** 25,000 U.S.P. units/Cap. Bot. 100s. 50,000 U.S.P. units/Cap. Bot. 100s, 500s. **Drops:** 5000 U.S.P. units/0.1 ml. Bot. 30 ml w/dropper.
Use: Vitamin A supplement.

AQUASOL E. (Armour) Vitamin E. **Cap.:** 73.5 mg Bot. 100s; 400 IU Bot. 30s. **Drops:** 50 mg/ml Bot. 12 ml, 30 ml w/dropper.
Use: Vitamin E supplement.
AQUASONIC 100. (Parker) Water-soluble, viscous, contact medium gel for ultrasonic transmission. Bot. 250 ml, 1 L, 5 L.
Use: Ultrasound agent.
AQUASONIC 100 STERILE. (Parker) Water-soluble, sterile gel for ultrasonic transmission. Overwrapped Foil Pouches 15 Gm, 50 Gm.
Use: Ultrasound agent.
AQUASULF. (Geneva) Triple sulfa tablet.
Use: Anti-infective.
AQUATAR THERAPEUTIC TAR GEL. (Herbert) Coal tar extract (BioTar) 2.5% w/DEA oleth-3 phosphate, glycerin, imidurea, methylparaben, mineral oil, oleth-3, oleth-10, oleth-20, poloxamer 407, polysorbate 80, propylparaben, purified water. Tube 3 oz.
Use: Antipruritic, keratoplastic, antipsoriatic.
AQUATENSEN. (Wallace) Methyclothiazide 5 mg/Tab. Bot. 100s, 500s.
Use: Diuretic, antihypertensive.
AQUAVITE. (Geneva) Soluble multivitamin.
Use: Vitamin supplement.
AQUAZIDE. (Western Research) Trichlormethiazide 4 mg/Tab. Bot. 100s.
Use: Antihypertensive, diuretic.
AQUAZIDE H. (Western Research) Hydrochlorothiazide 50 mg/Tab. Bot. 1000s.
Use: Diuretic.
AQUAZOL. (Geneva) Sulfisoxazole.
Use: Anti-infective.
AQUEOUS ALLERGENS. (Miles Pharm).
Use: Hyposensitizing agents.
AQUEST. (Dunhall) Estrone 20,000 IU. 2 mg/ml. Vial 10 ml or 30 ml.
Use: Estrogen.
AQUEX TABLETS. (Lannett) Trichlormethiazide 4 mg/Tab. Bot. 100s. 1000s.
Use: Diuretic.
AQUINONE.
See: Menadione, U.S.P. XXIII.
AQUOL BATH OIL. (Lamond) Vegetable oil, olive oil. Bot. 4 oz, 6 oz, 16 oz, qt, gal.
Use: Emollient, antipruritic.
AR-121. (Argus) Phase I/II HIV.
Use: Antiviral.
ARA-A.
See: Vidarabine.
ARA-C.

See: Cytarabine.
ARALEN HYDROCHLORIDE. (Sanofi Winthrop) Chloroquine HCl 50 mg/ml. Amp 5 ml. Box 5s.
Use: Antimalarial, amebicide.
ARALEN PHOSPHATE. (Sanofi Winthrop) Chloroquine phosphate 500 mg/Tab. Bot. 25s.
Use: Antimalarial, amebicide.
ARALEN PHOSPHATE W/PRIMAQUINE PHOSPHATE. (Sanofi Winthrop) Aralen phosphate 500 mg, primaquine phosphate 79 mg/Tab. Bot. 100s.
Use: Antimalarial.
ARALIS TABLETS. (Sanofi Winthrop) Glycobiarsol, chloroquine phosphate.
Use: Amebicide.
ARAMINE. (Merck & Co.) Metaraminol bitartrate (equivalent to metaraminol) 10 mg/ml, sodium Cl 4.4 mg, water for injection q.s. ad. 1 ml, methylparaben 0.15%, propylparaben 0.02%, sodium bisulfite 0.2%. Vial 10 ml.
Use: Treatment of acute hypotension.
• **ARANOTIN.** USAN.
Use: Antiviral.
• **ARBAPROSTIL.** USAN.
Use: Antisecretory.
ARBOLIC. (Burgin-Arden) Methandriol dipropionate 50 mg/ml. Vial 10 ml.
Use: Anabolic steroid.
ARBON. (Forest) Iron 18 mg, Vitamins A 5000 IU, D 400 IU, E 30 IU, B_1 1.5 mg, B_2 1.7 mg, B_3 20 mg, B_5 10 mg, B_6 2 mg, B_{12} 6 mcg, C 60 mg, folic acid 0.4 mg, Ca, Cu, I, Mg, P, Zn. Bot. 100s, 1000s.
Use: Vitamin/mineral supplement.
ARBON PLUS. (Forest) Iron 27 mg, Vitamins A 5000 IU, D 400 IU, E 30 IU, C 90 mg, folic acid 400 mcg, B_1 2.25 mg, B_2 2.6 mg, niacinamide 20 mg, B_6 3 mg, B_{12} 9 mcg, pantothenic acid 10 mg, biotin 150 mcg, calcium 162 mg, phosphorus 125 mg, iodine 150 mcg, magnesium 100 mg, copper 3 mg, manganese 7.5 mg, potassium 7.5 mg, zinc 22.5 mg/Tab. Bot. 100s.
Use: Vitamin/mineral supplement.
ARBUTAL. (Arcum) Butalbital ³/₄ gr, phenacetin 2 gr, aspirin 3 gr, caffeine gr/Tab. Bot. 100s, 1000s.
Use: Sedative/hypnotic, analgesic.
• **ARBUTAMINE HYDROCHLORIDE.** USAN.
Use: Cardiac stimulant.
ARCET. (EconoMed) Butalbital 50 mg, acetaminophen 325 mg, caffeine 40 mg/Tab. Bot. 100s.
• **ARCLOFENIN.** USAN.

Use: Diagnostic aid for hepatic function determination.

ARCOBAN TABLETS. (Arcum) Meprobamate 400 mg/Tab. Bot. 50s, 1000s.
Use: Antianxiety agent.

ARCOBEE W/C. (Nature's Bounty) Vitamins B_1 15 mg, B_2 10.2 mg, B_3 50 mg, B_5 10 mg, B_6 5 mg, C 300 mg, tartrazine. Cap. Box UD 100s.
Use: Vitamin supplement.

ARCOBEX EXTRA STRENGTH CAPS. (Arcum) Vitamins B_1 100 mg, B_2 2 mg, B_6 5 mg, niacinamide 125 mg, panthenol 10 mg, B_{12} 30 mcg, benzyl alcohol 1%, genistic acid ethanolamide 2.5%/ml. Vial 30 ml.
Use: Vitamin B supplement.

ARCOCILLIN. (Arcum) Crystalline penicillin G potassium 400,000 units/Tab. Bot. 100s, 1000s. Pow. 400,000 units/5 ml. Bot. 80 ml.
Use: Antibacterial, penicillin.

ARCODEX ANTACID TABLETS. (Arcum) Magnesium trisilicate 500 mg, aluminum hydroxide 250 mg/Tab. Bot. 100s, 1000s.
Use: Antacid.

ARCO-LASE. (Arco) Trizyme 38 mg (amylase 30 mg, protease 6 mg, cellulase 2 mg), lipase 25 mg/Tab. Bot. 50s.
Use: Digestive aid.

ARCO-LASE PLUS. (Arco) Phenobarbital 8 mg, hyoscyamine sulfate 0.1 mg, atropine sulfate 0.02 mg, trizyme 38 mg, lipase 25 mg/Tab. Bot. 50s.
Use: Sedative/hypnotic, digestive aid.

ARCOSTERONE. (Arcum) Methyltestosterone. **Oral:** 10 mg or 25 mg/Tab. Bot. 100s, 1000s. **Sublingual:** 10 mg/Tab. Bot. 100s, 1000s.
Use: Androgen.

ARCO-THYROID. (Arco) Thyroid 1.5 gr/Tab. Bot. 1000s.
Use: Thyroid hormone.

ARCOTINIC. (Arco) Iron 106 mg, liver fraction 200 mg, Vitamin C 250 mg Tab. Bot. 100s.
Use: Vitamin/mineral supplement.

ARCOTRATE. (Arcum) Pentaerythritol tetranitrate 10 mg/Tab. **No. 2:** Pentaerythritol tetranitrate 20 mg/Tab. **No. 3:** Pentaerythritol tetranitrate 20 mg, phenobarbital 1/8 gr/Tab. Bot. 100s, 1000s.
Use: Antianginal.

ARCOVAL IMPROVED. (Arcum) Vitamin A palmitate 10,000 IU, D 400 IU, thiamine mononitrate 15 mg, B_2 10 mg, nicotinamide 150 mg, B_6 5 mg, calcium pantothenate 10 mg, B_{12} 5 mcg, C 150 mg, E 5 IU/Cap. Bot. 100s, 1000s.
Use: Vitamin supplement.

ARCUM R-S. (Arcum) Reserpine 0.25 mg/Tab. Bot. 100s, 1000s.
Use: Antihypertensive.

ARCUM V-M. (Arcum) Vitamin A palmitate 5000 IU, D 400 IU, B_1 2.5 mg, B_2 2.5 mg, B_6 0.5 mg, B_{12} 2 mcg, C 50 mg, niacinamide 20 mg, calcium pantothenate 5 mg, iron 18 mg/Cap. Bot. 100s, 1000s.
Use: Vitamin/mineral supplement.

A-R-D. (Birchwood) Anatomically shaped dressing. Dispenser 24s.
Use: Rectal counter-irritant, antipruritic.

ARDEBEN. (Burgin-Arden) Diphenhydramine HCl 10 mg, chlorobutanol 0.5%. Inj. Vial 30 ml.
Use: Antihistamine.

ARDECAINE 1%. (Burgin-Arden) Lidocaine HCl 1%. Inj. Vial 30 ml.
Use: Local anesthetic.

ARDECAINE 2%. (Burgin-Arden) Lidocaine HCl 2%. Inj. Vial 30 ml.
Use: Local anesthetic.

ARDECAINE 1% W/EPINEPHRINE. (Burgin-Arden) Lidocaine HCl 1%, epinephrine. Inj. Vial 30 ml.
Use: Local anesthetic.

ARDECAINE 2% W/EPINEPHRINE. (Burgin-Arden) Lidocaine HCl 2%, epinephrine. Inj. Vial 30 ml.
Use: Local anesthetic.

ARDEFEM 10. (Burgin-Arden) Estradiol valerate 10 mg/ml. Vial 10 ml.
Use: Estrogen.

ARDEFEM 20. (Burgin-Arden) Estradiol valerate 20 mg/ml. Vial 10 ml.
Use: Estrogen.

ARDEFEM 40. (Burgin-Arden) Estradiol valerate 40 mg/ml. Vial 10 ml.
Use: Estrogen.

ARDEPARIN SODIUM.. USAN.
Use: Anticoagulant.

ARDEPRED SOLUBLE. (Burgin-Arden) Prednisolone 20 mg, niacinamide 25 mg, disodium edetate 0.5 mg, sodium bisulfite 1 mg, phenol 5 mg/ml. Vial 10 ml.
Use: Corticosteroid combination.

ARDERONE 100. (Burgin-Arden) Testosterone enanthate 100 mg/ml. Vial 10 ml.
Use: Androgen.

ARDERONE 200. (Burgin-Arden) Testosterone enanthate 200 mg/ml. Vial 10 ml.
Use: Androgen.

ARDEVILA TABLETS. (Sanofi Winthrop) Inositol hexanicotinate.
Use: Vasodilator.

ARDIOL 90/4. (Burgin-Arden) Testos-

terone enanthate 90 mg, estradiol valer-
ate 4 mg/ml. Vial 10 ml.
Use: Androgen/estrogen combination.
ARDUAN. (Organon) Pipecuronium Br 10
mg/10 ml. Vial.
Use: Neuromuscular blocking agent.
ARECOLINE ACETARSONE SALT.
See: Drocarbil.
AREDIA. (Ciba) Pamidronate disodium
30 mg. Lyophilized inj. Vial.
Use: Treatment of hypercalcemia.
AR-EX PRODUCTS. (Ar-Ex) A series of
hypo-allergenic products for sensitive
skin including:
Skin Care Products:
Body Lotion.
Chap Cream.
Cleansing Cream.
Cold Cream.
Cream For Dry Skin.
Enriched Night Cream.
Eye Cream.
Moisture Cream.
Moicturo Lotion.
Personal Care Products:
Bath Oil.
Bath Soap.
Cream Deodorant.
Roll-On Deodorant.
Safe Suds (liquid detergent).
Shampoo.
Soap.
Cosmetics and Eye Make-up:
Brush-On.
Disappear (blemish stick).
Eye Make-Up Remover Pads.
Eye Pencil.
Face and Compact Powder.
Foundation Lotion.
Lip Gloss.
Lipstick.
Mascara.
ARFONAD. (Roche) Trimethaphan cam-
sylate 50 mg/ml, sodium acetate
0.013%. Amp. 10 ml. Box 10s.
Use: Vasodilator.
ARGESIC. (Econo Med) Methyl salicylate
and triethanolamine in a nongreasy van-
ishing cream base. Jar 60 Gm.
Use: External analgesic.
ARGESIC-SA. (Econo Med) Disalicylic
acid 500 mg/Tab. Bot. 100s.
• **ARGININE,** U.S.P. XXIII. $C_6H_{14}N_4O_2$. L-
Arginine.
Use: Ammonia detoxicant, diagnostic
aid (pituitary function determination).
ARGININE BUTYRATE.
Use: Treatment of sickle cell disease
and beta-thalassemia. [Orphan drug]
• **ARGININE GLUTAMATE.** USAN. L(+)-

arginine salt of L(+)-glutamic acid.
Use: Aid in ammonia intoxication due to
hepatic failure.
See: Modumate (Abbott).
• **ARGININE HYDROCHLORIDE,** U.S.P.
XXIII. Inj., U.S.P. XXIII.
Use: Ammonia detoxicant.
ARGIPRESSIN. B.A.N. 8-Argininevaso-
pressin.
Use: Antidiuretic hormone.
• **ARGIPRESSIN TANNATE.** USAN.
Use: Antidiuretic.
ARGYN.
See: Mild Silver Protein (Various Mfr.).
ARGYROL S.S. 20%. (Iolab) Mild silver
protein 20%. Dropperette 1 ml. Box 12s.
Use: Anti-infective, ophthalmic.
ARIDOL. (MPL) Pamabrom 52 mg, pyril-
amine maleate 30 mg, homatropine
methylbromide 1.2 mg, hyoscyamine
sulfate 0.10 mg, scopolamine HBr 0.02
mg, methamphetamine HCl 1.5 mg/Tab.
Bot. 100s.
Use: Diuretic, anticholinergic/antispas-
modic, CNS stimulant.
• **ARILDONE.** USAN.
Use: Antiviral.
**ARIS PHENOBARBITAL REAGENT
STRIPS.** (Ames) Box 25s.
Use: Diagnostic aid.
ARIS PHENYTOIN REAGENT STRIPS.
(Ames) Box 25s.
Use: Diagnostic aid.
ARISTOCORT. (Lederle) Triamcinolone.
Tab.: 1 mg Bot. 50s; 2 mg Bot. 100s; 4
mg Bot. 30s, 100s; 8 mg Bot. 50s. **Syr.:**
Diacetate (w/methylparaben 0.08%,
propylparaben 0.02%) 2 mg/5 ml. Bot. 4
oz.
Use: Corticosteroid.
ARISTOCORT A CREAM. (Fujisawa) Tri-
amcinolone acetonide w/emulsifying
wax, isopropyl palmitate, glycerin, sor-
bitol, lactic acid, benzyl alcohol. **0.025%
w/Aquatain:** Tube 15 Gm, 60 Gm. **0.1%:**
Tube 15 Gm, 60 Gm, Jar 240 Gm. **0.5%:**
Tube 15 Gm.
Use: Corticosteroid.
**ARISTOCORT ACETONIDE, SODIUM
PHOSPHATE SALT.** (Lederle)
Use: Corticosteroid.
See: Aristocort Preps.
Sodium Phosphate Triamcinolone
Acetonide.
ARISTOCORT A OINTMENT. (Fujisawa)
Triamcinolone acetonide 0.1%. Tube 15
Gm, 60 Gm.
Use: Corticosteroid.
ARISTOCORT A OINTMENT. (Fujisawa)
Triamcinolone acetonide 0.1%. Tube 15

Gm, 60 Gm.
Use: Corticosteroid.
ARISTOCORT CREAM. (Fujisawa) Triamcinolone acetonide w/emulsifying wax, polysorbate 60, mono and diglycerides, squalane, sorbitol soln., sorbic acid, potassium sorbate. **LP: 0.025%:** Tube 15 Gm, 60 Gm, Jar 240 Gm, 480 Gm; **H: 0.1%:** Tube 15 Gm, 60 Gm, Jar 240 Gm, 480 Gm; **HP: 0.5%:** Tube 15 Gm, Jar 240 Gm.
Use: Corticosteroid.
ARISTOCORT FORTE. (Lederle) Triamcinolone diacetate 40 mg/ml. Vial 1 ml, 5 ml.
Use: Corticosteroid.
ARISTOCORT INTRALESIONAL. (Lederle) Triamcinolone diacetate 25 mg/ml. Vial 5 ml.
Use: Corticosteroid.
ARISTOCORT OINTMENT. (Fujisawa) Triamcinolone acetonide. **R: 0.1%:** Tube 15 Gm, 60 Gm, Jar 240 Gm. **HP: 0.5%:** Tube 15 Gm, Jar 240 Gm.
Use: Corticosteroid.
ARISTO-PAK. (Lederle) Triamcinolone 4 mg/Tab. 16s.
Use: Corticosteroid.
ARISTOSPAN INTRA-ARTICULAR. (Lederle) Triamcinolone hexacetonide 20 mg/ml micronized susp., polysorbate 80 0.4% w/v, sorbitol soln. 64% w/v, water q.s., benzyl alcohol 0.9% w/v. Vial 1 ml, 5 ml.
Use: Corticosteroid.
ARISTOSPAN INTRALESIONAL. (Lederle) Triamcinolone hexacetonide 5 mg/ml, polysorbate 80 0.2% w/v, sorbitol soln. 64% w/v, water q.s., benzyl alcohol 0.9% w/v. Vial 5 ml.
Use: Corticosteroid.
ARITHMIN INJECTABLE. (Lannett) Antazoline phosphate 100 mg/2 ml. Amp. 12s, 100s.
Use: Antihistamine.
ARITHMIN TABLETS. (Lannett) Antazoline HCl 100 mg or 200 mg/Tab. Bot. 100s.
Use: Antihistamine.
ARLACEL 83. (ICI Americas) Sorbitan Sesquioleate.
Use: Surface-active agent.
ARLACEL 165. (ICI Americas) Glyceryl monostearate, PEG-100 stearate nonionic self-emulsifying.
Use: Surface-active agent.
ARLACEL C. (ICI Americas) Sorbitan Sesquioleate. Mixture of oleate esters of sorbitol and its anhydrides.
Use: Surface-active agent.

ARLAMOL E. (ICI Americas) Polyoxypropylene (15), stearyl ether, BHT 0.1%.
Use: Emollient.
ARLATONE 507. (ICI Americas) Padimate O.
Use: Sunscreen.
ARLIDIN. (Rhone-Poulenc Rorer) Nylidrin HCl 6 mg or 12 mg/Tab. Bot. 100s, 1000s, UD 100s.
Use: Vasodilator.
ARLIX. (Hoechst) Piretanide HCl.
Use: Diuretic, antihypertensive.
ARM-A-MED ISOETHARINE HCl. (Astra) Soln. for nebulization: Isoetharine 0.125%, sodium metabisulfite, glycerin. Bot. UD 4 ml.
Use: Bronchodilator.
ARM-A-MED METAPROTERENOL SULFATE. (Armour) Soln. for nebulization: Metaproterenol sulfate 0.4% or 0.6% with sodium Cl, EDTA. Vial UD 2.5 ml for use with IPPB device.
Use: Bronchodilator.
ARM-A-VIAL. (Armour) Sterile water, sodium Cl 0.45% or 0.9%. Box 100s. Plastic vial 3 ml, 5 ml.
Use: Electrolyte.
ARMOUR THYROID. (Rorer) Desiccated animal thyroid glands (active thyroid hormones): T-4 thyroxine, T-3 thyronine 0.25 gr, 0.5 gr, 1 gr, 1.5 gr, 2 gr, 3 gr, 4 gr or 5 gr/Tab. Bot. 100s, 1000s, Handy Hundreds, Carton Strip 100s.
Use: Thyroid hormone.
A.R.M. TABLETS. (SK-Beecham) Chlorpheniramine maleate 4 mg, phenylpropanolamine HCl 25 mg/Tab. Pkg. 20s, 40s.
Use: Antihistamine, decongestant.
• **AROMATIC AMMONIA SPIRIT,** U.S.P. XXIII (Lilly) Bot. 16 oz. Aspirols 0.4 ml. Box 12s.
Use: Source of ammonia for fainting spells.
See: Ammonia.
AROMATIC AMMONIA VAPOROLE. (Burroughs Wellcome) Inhalant. Vial 5 min. Box 10s, 12s, 100s.
Use: Respiratory/CNS stimulant.
• **AROMATIC ELIXIR,** N.F XVII. (Lilly) Alcohol 22%. Bot. 16 fl. oz.
Use: Flavored vehicle.
ARNICA TINCTURE. (Lilly) Arnica 20% in alcohol 66%. Bot. 120 ml, 480 ml.
Use: External analgesic.
AROPAX. A serotonin reuptake inhibitor for depression.
See: Paxil (SK-Beecham).
• **ARPRINOCID.** USAN.

Use: Coccidiostat.
ARS. Rabies prophylaxis product.
See: Antirabies serum (Sclavo).
ARSECLOR.
See: Dichlorophenarsine HCl (Various Mfr.).
ARSENIC COMPOUNDS.
Use: Rarely employed in modern medicine; there are no longer any official compounds.
See: Acetarson.
Arsphenamine.
Carbarsone (Various Mfr.).
Dichlorophenarsine HCl.
Ferric Cacodylate.
Glycobiarsol.
Neoarsphenamine.
Oxophenarsine HCl.
Sodium Cacodylate (Various Mfr.).
Tryparsamide.
ARSENOBENZENE.
See: Arsphenamine.
ARSENPHENOLAMINE.
See: Arsphenamine.
ARSOBOL. Melarsoprol (Mel B).
Use: CDC anti-infective agent.
ARSPHENAMINE. 3, 3′-diamino-4, 4 dihydroxy-arsenobenzene dihydrochloride. Arsenobenzene, arsenobenzol, arsenphenolamine, Ehrlich 606, salvarsan.
Use: Formerly used as antisyphilitic.
ARSTHINOL. Cyclic (hydroxymethyl)ethylene-3-acetamido-4-hydroxydithiobenzenearsonite.
Use: Antiprotozoal.
ARTANE. (Lederle) Trihexyphenidyl HCl.
Elix.: 2 mg/5 ml w/methylparaben 0.08%, propylparaben 0.02%, Bot. pt.
Tab.: 2 mg or 5 mg, Bot. 100s, 1000s, UD 10×10 in 10s. **Sequel:** 5 mg Bot. 60s, 500s.
Use: Anti-parkinson agent.
ARTARAU. (Archer-Taylor) Rauwolfia serpentina 50 mg or 100 mg/Tab. Bot. 100s, 1000s.
Use: Antihypertensive.
ARTA-VI-C. (Archer-Taylor) Multivitamins with Vitamin C 100 mg/Tab. Bot. 100s.
Use: Vitamin supplement.
ARTAZYME. (Archer-Taylor) Bot. 13 ml.
Use: Autolyzed proteolytic enzyme.
• **ARTEGRAFT.** USAN. Arterial graft composed of a section of bovine carotid artery that has been subjected to enzymatic digestion with ficin and tanned with dialdehyde starch.
Use: Prosthetic aid (arterial).
ARTERENOL.
See: Norepinephrine bitartrate.

ARTERIAL GRAFT. (Johnson & Johnson) Bovine origin.
Use: Arterial grafting.
ARTHA-G. (T.E. Williams) Salsalate 750 mg/Tab. Bot. 120s.
Use: Salicylate analgesic.
ARTHRALGEN. (Robins) Salicylamide 250 mg, acetaminophen 250 mg/Tab. Bot. 30s, 100s, 500s.
Use: Analgesic.
ARTHRICARE DAYTIME FORMULA. (Commerce) Menthol 1.25%, methyl nicotinate 0.25%, capsaicin 0.025%, with aloe vera gel, carbomer 940, DMDM hydantoin, glyceryl stearate SE, myristyl propionate, propylparaben, triethanolamine. Cream. Jar 90 Gm.
Use: Topical analgesic for arthritis.
ARTHRICARE DOUBLE ICE. (Commerce) Menthol 4%, camphor 3.1%, with aloe vera gel, carbomer 940, dioctyl sodium sulfosuccinate, propylene glycol, triethanolamine. Gel. Jar 90 Gm.
Use: Topical analgesic for arthritis.
ARTHRICARE ODOR FREE RUB. (Commerce) Menthol 1.25%, methyl nicotinate 0.25%, capsaicin 0.025%, aloe vera gel, carbomer 940, DMDM hydantoin, emulsifying wax, glyceryl stearate SE, isopropyl alcohol, myristyl propionate, propylparaben, triethanolamine. Oint. Jar 90 Gm.
Use: Rub and liniment.
ARTHRICARE TRIPLE MEDICATED. (Commerce) Methylsalicylate 30%, menthol 1.25%, methyl nicotinate 0.7%, dioctyl sodium sulfosuccinate, hydroxypropylmethylcellulose, isopropyl alcohol, propylene glycol. Gel. Tube 3 oz.
Use: Topical analgesic.
ARTHRITEN MAXIMUM STRENGTH. (Alva-Amco) Acetaminophen 250 mg, magnesium salicylate 250 mg, caffeine anhydrous 32.5 mg/Tab. Bot. 40s.
Use: Nonnarcotic analgesic combination.
ARTHRITIC PAIN LOTION. (Walgreen) Triethanolamine salicylate 10%. Bot. 6 oz.
Use: External analgesic.
ARTHRITIS BAYER TIMED RELEASE ASPIRIN. (Glenbrook) Aspirin 650 mg/TR Tab. Bot. 30s, 72s, 125s.
Use: Salicylate analgesic.
ARTHRITIS HOT CREME. (Thompson) Methyl salicylate 15%, menthol 10%, glyceryl stearate, carbomer 934, lanolin, PEG-100 stearate, propylene glycol, trolamine, parabens. Cream Jar 90 Gm.
Use: Rub and liniment.

ARTHRITIS PAIN FORMULA. (Whitehall) Aspirin 486 mg, aluminum hydroxide gel 20 mg, magnesium hydroxide 60 mg/Tab. Bot. 40s, 100s, 175s.
Use: Analgesic combination.
ARTHRITIS PAIN FORMULA, ASPIRIN FREE. (Whitehall) Acetaminophen 500 mg/Tab. Bot. 30s, 75s.
Use: Analgesic.
ARTHRITIS VACCINES.
See: Streptococcus Vaccine (Lilly).
ARTHROPAN LIQUID. (Purdue Frederick) Choline salicylate 870 mg/5 ml. Bot. 8 oz, 16 oz.
Use: Analgesic.
ARTHROTRIN TABLETS. (Whiteworth) Enteric coated aspirin 325 mg/Tab. Bot. 100s.
Use: Salicylate analgesic.
ARTICULOSE-50. (Seatrace) Prednisolone acetate 50 mg/ml. Vial 10 ml, 30 ml.
Use: Corticosteroid.
ARTICULOSE L. A. (Seatrace) Triamcinolone diacetate 40 mg/ml. Vial 5 ml.
Use: Corticosteroid.
ARTIFICIAL TANNING AGENT.
See: QT, Prods. (Schering-Plough).
Sudden Tan, Prods. (Schering-Plough).
ARTIFICIAL TEAR INSERT.
See: Lacrisert (Merck & Co.).
ARTIFICIAL TEARS. (Various Mfr.) Benzalkonium Cl 0.01%, EDTA, NaCl. May also contain polyvinyl alcohol. Sol. Bot. 15 ml or 30 ml.
Use: Lubricant, ophthalmic.
ARTIFICIAL TEARS. (Rugby) **Soln.:** Polyvinyl alcohol 1.4%, EDTA, chlorobutanol. Bot. 15 ml. **Oint.:** White petrolatum, mineral oil, lanolin. Tube 3.5 Gm.
Use: Lubricant, ophthalmic.
ARTIFICIAL TEARS PLUS. (Various Mfr.) Polyvinyl alcohol 1.4%, povidone 0.6%, chlorobutanol 0.5%, NaCl. Soln. Bot. 15 ml.
Use: Lubricant, ophthalmic.
ARTIFICIAL TEARS PLUS. (Rugby) Polyvinyl alcohol 1.4%,povidone 0.6% and chlorobutanol 0.5% in an aqueous solution. Ophth. soln. Bot. 15 ml.
Use: Lubricant, ophthalmic.
• **ARTILIDE FUMARATE.** USAN.
Use: Cardiac depressant (antiarrhythmic).
ARTRA BEAUTY BAR. (Schering-Plough) Triclocarban 1% in soap base. Cake 3.6 oz.
Use: Skin cleanser.
ARTRA SKIN TONE CREAM. (Schering-Plough) Hydroquinone 2%. Oint. Tube 1 oz. (normal only), 2 oz, 4 oz.
Use: Skin bleaching agent.
AS-101. (Wyeth-Ayerst) Phase I/II ARC, AIDS.
Use: Immunomodulator. [Orphan drug]
5-ASA. Mesalamine.
See: Asacol (Procter & Gamble Pharm.).
Rowasa (Solvay).
ASA. (Wampole-Zeus) Anti-skin antibodies test by IFA. Test 48s.
Use: Diagnostic aid.
A.S.A. (Lilly) Aspirin. Acetylsalicylic acid.
Enseal: 5 gr or 10 gr. Bot. 100s, 1000s.
Supp.: 5 gr or 10 gr. Pkg. 6s, 144s.
Use: Salicylate analgesic.
ASACOL. (Procter & Gamble Pharm.) Mesalamine 400 mg/Tab. DR Bot. 100s.
Use: Anti-inflammatory.
ASAFETIDA, EMULSION OF. Milk of Asafetida.
ASALCO NO. 1. (Jenkins) Acetylsalicylic acid 3.5 gr, acetophenetidin 2.5 gr, caffeine 0.5 gr/Tab. or Cap. Bot. 1000s.
Use: Analgesic.
ASAPED TABLETS. (Sanofi Winthrop) Acetylsalicylic acid.
Use: Analgesic.
ASAWIN TABLETS. (Sanofi Winthrop) Acetylsalicylic acid.
Use: Analgesic.
A.S.B. (Femco) Calcium carbonate, magnesium carbonate, bismuth subcarbonate, sodium bicarbonate, kaolin. Pow., Can 3 oz. Tabs. 50s.
Use: Antacid.
ASBRON G. (Sandoz) **Tab.:** Theophylline sodium glycinate 300 mg, guaifenesin 100 mg. Bot. 100s. **Elix.:** Theophylline sodium glycinate 300 mg, guaifenesin 100 mg, alcohol 15%/15 ml. Bot. pt.
Use: Bronchodilator, expectorant.
ASCLEROL. (Spanner) Liver injection crude (2 mcg/ml) 50%, Vitamins B_1 20 mg, B_2 3 mg, B_6 1 mg, B_{12} 30 mcg, niacinamide 100 mg, panthenol 2.8 mg, choline Cl 20 mg, inositol 10 mg/ml. Multiple dose vial 10 ml.
Use: Vitamin supplement.
ASCORBATE SODIUM. Antiscorbutic vitamin.
• **ASCORBIC ACID,** U.S.P. XXIII. Inj., Oral Soln., U.S.P. XXIII. Tab., U.S.P. XXIII. 3-Oxo-L-gulofuranolactone (enol form). Antiscorbic vitamin; Vitamin C.
Cap.: (Various Mfr.) 25 mg, 100 mg, 250 mg, 500 mg. **Inj.:** (Various Mfr.) Amp. (100 mg/ml) 1 ml, 2 ml, 5 ml; (200 mg/ml) 5 ml, (500 mg) 2 ml, 5 ml, 10

ml, 30 ml, (250 mg/ml) 10 ml; (1000 mg/ml) 10 ml. **Tab.**: (Various Mfr.) 50 mg, 100 mg, 250 mg, 500 mg. **Chew. Tab.**: (Various Mfr.) 100 mg, 250 mg, 500 mg. **SR Tab.**: (Various Mfr.) 500 mg, 1500 mg. **SR Cap.**: (Various Mfr.) 4 Gm/5 ml. **Soln.**: (Various Mfr.) 35 mg/0.6 ml or 100 mg/ml.
Use: Vitamin C supplement.
See: Ascorbajen, Tab. (Jenkins).
Ascorbicap, Cap. (ICN).
Ascorbineed, Cap. (Hanlon).
C-Caps 500 (Drug Industries).
Cecon, Soln. (Abbott).
Cenolate, Amp. (Abbott).
Cetane, Cap., Vial (Forest).
Cevalin, Tab., Amp. (Lilly).
Cevi-Bid, Cap. (Geriatric).
Ce-Vi-Sol, Drops (Mead Johnson).
C-Syrup-500 (Ortega).
Neo-Vadrin, Preps. (Scherer).
Solucap C, Cap. (Jamieson-McK-ames).
Sunkist Vitamin C, Capl., Chow. Tab. (Ciba).
Tega-C Tab. (Ortega).
• **ASCORBIC ACID INJECTION,** U.S.P. XXIII.
Use: Vitamin C supplement.
See: Cevalin, Amp. (Lilly).
ASCORBIC ACID SALTS.
See: Bismuth Ascorbate.
Calcium Ascorbate.
Sodium Ascorbate.
ASCORBICAP. (ICN) Ascorbic acid 500 mg/S.R. Cap. Bot. 50s.
Use: Vitamin C supplement.
ASCORBIN/11. (Pasadena Research) Lemon bioflavonoids 110 mg, Vitamin C 1 Gm, rose hips powder 50 mg, rutin 25 mg/S.R. Tab. Bot. 100s.
Use: Vitamin supplement.
ASCORBINEED. (Hanlon) Vitamin C 500 mg/T-Cap. Bot. 100s.
Use: Vitamin C supplement.
ASCORBOCIN POWDER. (Paddock) Vitamin C 500 mg, niacin 500 mg, B_1 50 mg, B_6 50 mg, d-α-tocopheryl, polyethylene glycol 1000 succinate 50 IU, lactose/3 Gm. Bot. lb.
Use: Vitamin supplement.
• **ASCORBYL PALMITATE,** N.F. XVIII.
L-Ascorbic acid 6-palmitate.
Use: Preservative, antioxidant.
ASCORVITE S.R.. (Vitarine) Vitamin C 500 mg/S.R. Cap.
Use: Vitamin C supplement.
ASCRIPTIN. (Rorer Consumer) Aspirin 325 mg, magnesium hydroxide 50 mg, aluminum hydroxide 50 mg/Tab. Bot.

50s, 100s, 225s, 500s.
Use: Analgesic, antacid.
ASCRIPTIN A/D. (Rorer) Acetylsalicylic acid 325 mg with magnesium hydroxide 75 mg, aluminum hydroxide and calcium carbonate 75 mg/Capsule shape coated tabs. Bot. 225s.
Use: Analgesic.
ASCRIPTIN EXTRA STRENGTH. (Rhone-Poulenc Rorer) Aspirin 500 mg with magnesium hydroxide 80 mg, aluminum hydroxide and calcium carbonate 80 mg. Capsule shape coated tabs. Bot. 50s.
Use: Analgesic.
ASENDIN. (Lederle) Amoxapine. **25 mg/Tab.**: Bot. 100s; **50 mg/Tab.**: Bot. 100s, 500s, UD 100s; **100 mg/Tab.**: Bot. 100s, UD 100s; **150 mg/Tab.**: Bot. 30s.
Use: Antidepressant.
ASEPTICHROME.
See: Merbromin (Various Mfr.).
ASLUM. (Drug Products) Carbolic acid 1%, aluminum acetate, ichthammol, zinc oxide, aromatic oils in a petrolatum-stearin base. Tube oz. Jar lb.
Use: Astringent, dressing.
ASMA. (Wampole-Zeus) Anti-smooth muscle antibody test by IFA. Test 48.
Use: Diagnostic aid.
ASMADRIN. (Jenkins) Aminophylline 4 gr, aluminum hydroxide gel, dried, 4 gr, ephedrine HCl ⅜ gr, "trio-bar" 0.25 gr (representing 33% each of pentobarbital sodium, butabarbital sodium, phenobarbital sodium)/Tab. Bot. 100s.
ASMALIX. (Century) Theophylline 80 mg, alcohol 20%/15 ml. Bot. qt, gal.
Use: Bronchodilator.
ASMATEX. (Kenyon) Chlorpheniramine 1.25 mg, phenylephrine HCl 2.5 mg, acetylsalicylic acid 150 mg buffered w/aluminum and magnesium hydroxide/Tab. Bot. 100s.
Use: Antihistamine, decongestant.
ASMA-TUSS. (Blue Cross) Phenobarbital 4 mg, theophylline 15 mg, ephedrine sulfate 12 mg, guaifenesin 50 mg/5 ml. Bot. 4 oz.
Use: Bronchodilator.
ASOLECTIN. (Associated Conc.) Chemical lecithin 25%, chemical cephalin 22%, inositol phosphatides 16%, soybean oil 2.5%, other miscellaneous sterols and lipids 34.5%.
Use: Diet supplement.
• **ASPARAGINASE.** USAN. L-asparagine amidohydrolase.
Use: Antineoplastic agent.
See: Elspar, Inj. (Merck & Co.).

• **ASPARTAME,** N.F. XVIII. 3-Amino-N-(α-methoxycarbonyl-phenethyl)succinamic acid. L-Aspartyl-L-phenyl-alanine methyl ester.
Use: Sweetening agent.
• **ASPARTIC ACID.** USAN. Aspartic acid; aminosuccinic acid.
Use: Management of fatigue.
• **ASPARTOCIN.** USAN.
Use: Antibacterial.
A-SPAS. (Hyrex) Dicyclomine HCl 10 mg/ml. Vial 10 ml.
Use: Antispasmodic.
ASPERCIN. (Otis Clapp) Aspirin 325 mg/Tab. Sugar, caffeine, lactose, and salt free. Safety pack 500s.
Use: Salycylate analgesic.
ASPERCIN EXTRA. (Otis Clapp) Aspirin 500 mg/Tab. Sugar, caffeine, lactose, and salt free. Safety pack 500s.
Use: Salicylate analgesic.
ASPERCREME. (Thompson Medical) Triethanolamine salicylate 10% in cream base.
Use: External analgesic.
ASPERGILLUS NIGER ENZYME. Alphagalactosidase.
See: Beano, Tab. (AK-Pharma).
ASPERGILLUS ORYZAE ENZYME. Diastase.
See: Taka-Diastase, Preps. (Parke-Davis).
ASPERGUM. (Schering-Plough) Aspirin 227.5 mg/1 Gum. Tab. Orange or Cherry flavor. Box 16s, 40s.
Use: Salicylate analgesic.
ASPERKINASE. Proteolytic enzyme mixture derived from aspergillus oryzae.
• **ASPERLIN.** USAN.
Use: Antibacterial, antineoplastic agent.
ASPERMIN. (Buffington) Aspirin 325 mg/Tab. Sugar, caffeine, lactose, and salt free. Dispens-A-Kit 500s.
Use: Salicylate analgesic.
ASPERMIN EXTRA. (Buffington) Aspirin 500 mg/Tab. Sugar, caffeine, lactose, and salt free. Dispens-A-Kit 500s.
Use: Salicylate analgesic.
ASPIRBAR. (Lannett) Phenobarbital 0.25 gr, aspirin 10 gr/Tab. Bot. 1000s.
Use: Sedative/hypnotic, salicylate analgesic.
ASPIR-D COMPOUND CAPSULES. (Lannett) Cap. Bot. 100s.
• **ASPIRIN,** U.S.P. XXIII. Cap., Supp., Tab., U.S.P. XXIII. A.S.A., Acetophen, Acetol, Acetosal, Acetosalin, Aceticyl, Acetylin, Acetylsal, Empirin, Saletin. Acetylsalicylic acid, Benzoic acid, 2-(acetyloxy)-.,

Salicyclic acid acetate.
Use: Analgesic, antipyretic, antirheumatic. Prophylactic to reduce risk of death or non-fatal MI in patients with a previous infarction or unstable angina pectoris (FDA Drug Bull, Dec. 1985).
See: A.S.A., Preps. (Lilly).
Aspergum, Gum, Tab. (Schering-Plough).
Aspirjen Jr., Tab. (Jenkins).
BC Tablets (Block Drug).
Buffinol, Tab. (Otis Clapp).
Ecotrin, Tab. (SK-Beecham).
Empirin, Tab. (Burroughs Wellcome).
Halfprin 81, EC Tab. (Kramer).
Measurin, Tab. (Sanofi Winthrop).
Norwich Aspirin, Tab. (Norwich Eaton).
St. Joseph, Prods. (Schering-Plough).
• **ASPIRIN, ALUMINA, AND MAGNESIA TABLETS,** U.S.P. XXIII.
Use: Analgesic, antacid.
• **ASPIRIN, ALUMINA, AND MAGNESIUM OXIDE TABLETS,** U.S.P. XXIII.
Use: Analgesic, antacid.
ASPIRIN-BARBITURATE COMBINATIONS.
Use: Analgesic, sedative/hypnotic.
See: Amytal w/Acetylsalicylic acid, Cap. (Lilly).
Aspirbar, Tab. (Lannett).
Axotal, Tab. (Warren-Teed).
Brogesic, Tab. (Brothers).
Buff-A Comp., Cap., Tab. (Mayrand).
Cefinal, Tab. (Alto).
Doloral, Tab. (Alamed).
Fiorinal, Cap., Tab. (Sandoz).
Palgesic, Tab., Cap. (Pan Amer.).
Salibar Jr., Tab. (Jenkins).
Sedalgesic, Tab. (Table Rock).
• **ASPIRIN, CAFFEINE AND DIHYDROCODEINE CAPSULES,** U.S.P. XXIII.
Use: Analgesic.
ASPIRIN W/CODEINE No. 2. (Halsey) Codeine phosphate 15 mg, aspirin 325 mg Tab. Bot. 100s, 1000s.
Use: Narcotic analgesic.
ASPIRIN W/CODEINE No. 3. (Halsey) Codeine phosphate 30 mg, aspirin 325 mg Tab. Bot. 100s, 1000s.
Use: Narcotic analgesic.
ASPIRIN W/CODEINE No. 4. (Halsey) Codeine phosphate 60 mg, aspirin 325 mg Tab. Bot. 100s, 1000s.
Use: Narcotic analgesic.
• **ASPIRIN, CODEINE, PHOSPHATE ALUMINA, AND MAGNESIA TABLETS,** U.S.P. XXIII.
Use: Analgesic.

• **ASPIRIN AND CODEINE PHOSPHATE TABLETS,** U.S.P. XXIII.
Use: Analgesic.

• **ASPIRIN DELAYED-RELEASE CAPSULES,** U.S.P. XXIII.
Use: Analgesic.

• **ASPIRIN DELAYED-RELEASE TABLETS,** U.S.P. XXIII.
Use: Analgesic.
See: Bayer Low Adult Strength (Sterling Health).

ASPIRIN, ENTERIC COATED.
Use: Analgesic.
See: A.S.A., Preps. (Lilly).
Ecotrin, Tab. (SK-Beecham).

ASPIRIN FREE ANACIN MAXIMUM STRENGTH. (Whitehall) Acetaminophen 500 mg. **Capl., Gel Capl.:** Bot. 100s; **Tab.:** Bot. 60s.
Use: Analgesic.

ASPIRIN FREE ANACIN P.M. (Robins) Diphenhydramine HCl 25 mg, acetaminophen 500 mg/Tab. Bot. 20s.
Use: Nonprescription sleep aid.

ASPIRIN-FREE BAYER SELECT ALLERGY SINUS. (Sterling Health) Pseudoephedrine HCl 30 mg, chlorpheniramine maleate 2 mg, acetaminophen 500 mg. Cap. Bot. 16s.
Use: Nonnarcotic analgesic combination.

ASPIRIN-FREE BAYER SELECT HEAD & CHEST COLD. (Sterling Health) Pseudoephedrine HCl 30 mg, dextromethorphan HBr 10 mg, guaifenesin 100 mg, acetaminophen 325 mg. Cap. Bot. 16s.
Use: Nonnarcotic analgesic combination.

ASPIRIN-FREE BAYER SELECT HEADACHE. (Sterling Health) Acetaminophen 500 mg, caffeine 65 mg. Cap. Bot. 50s.
Use: Nonnarcotic analgesic combination.

ASPIRIN FREE EXCEDRIN. (Bristol-Myers) Acetaminophen 500 mg, caffeine 65 mg/Tab., Capl. Bot. 24s, 50s, 100s.
Use: Analgesic.

ASPIRIN-FREE EXCEDRIN DUAL. (B-M Squibb) Acetaminophen 500 mg, calcium carbonate 111 mg, magnesium carbonate 64 mg, magnesium oxide 30 mg/Capl. Bot. 100s.
Use: Nonnarcotic analgesic combination.

ASPIRIN FREE PAIN RELIEF. (Hudson) Acetaminophen 325 mg/Tab. Bot. 100s.
Use: Analgesic.

ASPIRIN W/O.T.C. COMBINATIONS.
See: Alka Seltzer, Tab. (Miles).
Alka Seltzer Plus, Tab. (Miles).
A.P.C., Tab., Cap. (Various Mfr.).
A.S.A. Comp., Cap., Tab. (Lilly).
Ascriptin, Tab. (Rhone-Puolenc Rorer Consumer).
Ascriptin A/D, Tab. (Rhone-Puolenc Rorer Consumer).
Ascriptin, Extra Strength, Tab. (Rhone-Puolenc Rorer Consumer).
Ascriptin Codeine, Tab. (Rhone-Puolenc Rorer).
Bayer Aspirin Preps. (Glenbrook).
Bayer Prods. (Glenbrook).
BC Powder (Block Drug).
Buffaprin, Tab. (Buffington).
Bufferin, Tab. (Bristol Myers).
Buffinol, Tab. (Otis Clapp).
Cama, Tab. (Sandoz Consumer).
Capathyn, Cap. (Scrip).
Damason, Preps. (Mason).
Emagrin, Tab. (Otis Clapp).
Excedrin, Cap., Tab. (Bristol-Myers).
4-Way, Tab., Spray (Bristol-Myers).
Liquiprin, Tab. (Mitchum-Thayer).
Midol, Cap., Spray (Glenbrook).
PAC, Cap., Tab. (Upjohn).
Pap, Cap. (Zenith).
Presalin, Tab. (Hauck).
Saleto, Preps. (Hauck).
Salocol, Tab. (Hauck).
Sine-Off Tablets (Menley & James).
Stanback, Pow., Tab. (Stanback).
St. Joseph Cold Tablets For Children (Schering-Plough).
Trigesic, Tab. (Squibb).
Vanquish, Cap. (Glenbrook).

ASPIRIN & OXYCODONE. (Various Mfr.) Oxycodone HCl 4.5 mg, oxycodone terephthalate 0.38 mg, aspirin 325 mg/Tab. Bot. 100s, 500s, 1000s, UD 25s.
Use: Narcotic analagesic combination.

ASPIRIN PLUS. (Walgreen) Aspirin 400 mg, caffeine 32 mg/Tab. Bot. 100s.
Use: Nonnarcotic analgesic combination.

ASPIRIN SALTS.
See: Calcium Acetylsalicylate.

• **ASPIRIN TABLETS, BUFFERED,** U.S.P. XXIII.
Use: Salicylate Analgesic.

ASPIRIN UNISERTS. (Upsher-Smith) Aspirin 125 mg, 300 mg or 650 mg/supp. Ctn. 12s, 50s.
Use: Salicylate Analgesic.

ASPIRJEN JR.. (Jenkins) Aspirin 2.5 gr/Tab. Bot. 1000s.
Use: Salicylate analgesic.

ASPIRTAB. (Dover) Aspirin 325 mg/Tab. Sugar, lactose, and salt free. UD Box 500s.
Use: Salicylate analgesic.
ASPIRTAB MAX. (Dover) Aspirin 500 mg/Tab. Sugar, lactose, and salt free. UD Box 500s.
Use: Analgesic.
ASPOGEN. Dihydroxyaluminum aminoacetate.
ASPRO.
See: Acetylsalicylic acid.
ASTARIL TABLETS. (Sanofi Winthrop) Theophylline anhydrous, ephedrine sulphate.
Use: Bronchodilator.
• **ASTEMIZOLE.** USAN.
Use: Antihistamine.
See: Hismanal, Tab. (Janssen).
ASTEROL. 6-(2-Diethylaminoethoxy)-2-dimethylaminobenzothiazole dihydrochloride. Diamthazole Dihydrochloride, B.A.N.
Use: Antifungal.
ASTHMAHALER. (SK-Beecham) Epinephrine bitartrate 0.3 mg/ml in an inert propellant. Oral inhaler, 15 ml with mouthpiece; 15 ml refills.
Use: Bronchodilator.
ASTHMALIXIR. (Reese) Theophylline 45 mg, ephedrine sulfate 36 mg, guaifenesin 150 mg, phenobarbital 12 mg/ 15 ml. Alcohol 19%. Bot.
Use: Bronchodilator, expectorant, sedative/hypnotic.
ASTHMANEFRIN. (Menley & James) Racepinephrine HCl 2.25%. Soln. Nebulizer 15 ml, 30 ml.
Use: Sympathomimetic.
ASTHMANEFRIN SOLUTION & NEBULIZER. (SK-Beecham) Racepin (racemic epinephrine) as HCl equivalent to epinephrine base 2.25%, chlorobutanol 0.5%. Bot. 0.5 fl oz. With sodium bisulfite. Bot. 1 fl oz.
Use: Bronchodilator.
• **ASTIFILCON A.** USAN.
Use: Contact lens material (hydrophilic).
ASTRAMORPH PF. (Astra) Morphine sulfate 0.5 mg/ml or 1 mg/ml preservative free. Amp. 10 ml, Vial 10 ml.
Use: Narcotic analgesic.
ASTROGLIDE. (BioFilm) Purified water, glycerin, propylene glycol, polyquaternium #5 and parabens. Vaginal gel. Bot 70.5 oz. Travel pks. 3 ml.
Use: Vaginal lubricant.
• **ASTROMICIN SULFATE.** USAN.
Use: Antibacterial.

ASTRO-VITES. (Faraday) Vitamins A 3500 IU, D 400 IU, C 60 mg, B_1 0.8 mg, B_2 1.3 mg, niacinamide 14 mg, B_6 1 mg, B_{12} 2.5 mcg, folic acid 0.05 mg, pantothenic acid 5 mg, iron 12 mg/Tab. Bot. 100s, 250s.
Use: Vitamin/mineral supplement.
AST/SGOT REAGENT STRIPS. (Amoo) Seralyzer reagent strip. A quantitative strip test for asparate transaminase/serum glutamic oxaloacetic transaminase in serum or plasma. Bot. Strip 25s.
Use: Diagnostic aid.
ASUPIRIN. (Suppositoria) Aspirin 60 mg, 120 mg, 200 mg, 300 mg, 600 mg or 1.2 Gm/Supp. Box 12s, 100s, 1000s.
Use: Salicylate analgesic.
A.T. 10.
See: Dihydrotachysterol.
ATABEE TD. (Defco) Vitamins C 500 mg, B_1 15 mg, B_2 10 mg, B_6 2 mg, nicotinamide 50 mg, calcium pantothenate 10 mg/Cap. Bot. 30s, 1000s.
Use: Vitamin supplement.
ATABRINE HYDROCHLORIDE. (Sanofi Winthrop) Quinacrine HCl 100 mg Tab. Bot. 100s.
Use: Antimalarial, anthelmintic.
ATARAX. (Roerig) Hydroxyzine HCl.
Tab.: 10 mg or 25 mg Bot. 100s, 500s, UD 10 × 10s, Unit-of-use 40s; 50 mg Bot. 100s, 500s, UD 10 × 10s; 100 mg Bot. 100s, UD 10 × 10s. **Syr.:** 10 mg/5 ml, alcohol 0.5%. Bot. pt.
Use: Antianxiety agent.
W/Ephedrine sulfate, theophylline.
See: Marax, Tab., Syr. (Roerig).
W/Penta-erythrityltetranitrate.
See: Cartrax, Tab. (Roerig).
ATARAXIC AGENTS.
See: Tranquilizers.
ATARVET. Acepromazine.
ATENOLOL. USAN. 4-(2-Hydroxy-3-isopropylaminopropoxy) phenylacetamide.
Use: Beta-adrenergic blocking agent.
See: Tenormin, Tab. (Stuart).
• **ATEVIRDINE MESYLATE.** USAN.
Use: Antiviral (reverse transcriiptase inhibitor).
ATGAM. (Upjohn) Lymphocyte immune globulin, antithymocyte globulin 250 mg protein (50 mg/ml). Amp. 5 ml.
Use: Management of allograft rejection in renal transplant patients.
ATHLETE'S FOOT OINTMENT. (Walgreen) Zinc undecylenate 20%, undecylenic acid 5%. Tube 1.5 oz.
Use: Antifungal, external.
• **ATIPAMEZOLE.** USAN.

Use: Antiadrenergic.

• **ATIPROSIN MALEATE.** USAN.
Use: Antihypertensive.

ATIVAN INJECTION. (Wyeth-Ayerst) Lorazepam in 2 mg/ml or 4 mg/ml. Vial 1 ml, 10 ml/2 ml Tubex (w/1 ml fill). Pkg. 10s.
Use: Antianxiety agent.

ATIVAN TABLETS. (Wyeth-Ayerst) Lorazepam 0.5 mg, 1 mg or 2 mg/Tab. Bot. 100s, 500s, 1000s, Redipak 25s.
Use: Antianxiety agent.

• **ATLAFILCON A.** USAN.
Use: Contact lens natural (hydrophilic).

ATNATIV. (Hyland) Antithrombin III (human), lyophilized powder/500 IU. Inj. Bot. 50 ml w/10 l sterile water.
Use: Thromboembolic agent.

• **ATOLIDE.** USAN. 2-Amino-4'-(diethylamino)-o-benzotoluidide. Under study.
Use: Anticonvulsant.

ATOLONE. (Major) Triamcinolone 4 mg/Tab. Bot. 100s, Uni-Pak 16s.
Use: Corticosteroid.

• **ATORVASTATIN CALCIUM.** USAN.
Use: HMG-CoA reductase inhibitor; antihyperlipidemic.

• **ATOSIBAN.** USAN.
Use: Antagonist, oxytocin.

• **ATOVAQUONE.** USAN.
Use: Antiprotozoal. [Orphan drug]
See: Mepron (Burroughs Wellcome).

ATOZINE TABS. (Major) Hydroxyzine HCl 10 mg, 25 mg or 50 mg/Tab; **10 and 25 mg:** Bot. 100s, 250s, 1000s, UD 100s; **50 mg:** Bot. 100s, 250s, 500s, UD 100s.
Use: Antianxiety agent.

ATPEG. (ICI Americas) Polyethylene glycol available as 300, 400, 600 or 4000.
Use: Surfactant, humectant.

• **ATRACURIUM BESYLATE.** USAN.
Use: Skeletal muscle relaxant.
See: Tracrium (Burroughs Wellcome).

ATRIDINE. (Interstate) Triprolidine 2.5 mg, pseudoephedrine HCl 60 mg/Tab. Bot. 100s, 1000s
Use: Antihistamine, decongestant.

ATROCAP. (Freeport) Atropine sulfate 0.06 mg, hyoscyamine sulfate 0.3 mg, hyoscine hydrobromide 0.02 mg, phenobarbital 50 mg/T.R. Cap. Bot. 1000s.
Use: Sedative/hypnotic, anticholinergic/antispasmodic.

ATROCHOLIN TABLETS. (Glaxo) Dehydrocholic acid 130 mg/Tab. Bot. 100s.
Use: Laxative.

ATROFED. (Genetco) Pseudoephedrine HCl 60 mg, triprolidine HCl 2.5 mg. Tab.

Bot. 24s, 100s, 1000s.
Use: Antihistamine, decongestant.

ATROHIST LA. (Adams) Pseudoephedrine HCl 120 mg, brompheniramine maleate 4 mg, phenyltoloxamine citrate 50 mg/SR Tab with atropine sulfate 0.0242 mg available for immediate release. Bot. 100s.
Use: Decongestant, antihistamine.

ATROHIST SPRINKLE. (Adams) Pseudoephedrine HCl 120 mg, brompheniramine maleate 2 mg, phenytoloxamine citrate 25 mg/SR Cap. Bot. 100s.
Use: Decongestant, antihistamine.

ATROMID-S. (Wyeth-Ayerst) Clofibrate 500 mg/Cap. Bot. 100s.
Use: Antihyperlipidemic.

ATROPEN AUTO-INJECTER. (Survival Technology) Atropine sulfate, phenol 2 mg. In prefilled automatic injection device.
Use: For toxic exposure to organophosphorus or carbamate insecticides.

ATROPHYSINE. (Lannett) Physostigmine salicylate 0.6 mg, atropine sulfate 0.6 mg/ml. Vial 30 ml.
Use: Antispasmodic.

• **ATROPINE,** U.S.P. XXIII. 1αH, 5αH-Tropan-3α-ol dl-Tropate (Ester) (dl-Hyoscyamine) Tropyltropate.
Use: Anticholinergic.
See: Atropine Combinations.

ATROPINE-1. (Optopics) Atropine sulfate 1% soln. Bot. 2, 5, 15 ml.
Use: Cycloplegic mydriatic.

ATROPINE-CARE. (Akorn) Atropine sulfate 1%, benzalkonium Cl 0.01%, hydroxypropyl methylcellulose. Soln. Bot. 2 ml, 5 ml, 15 ml.
Use: Cycloplegic mydriatic.

ATROPINE AND DEMEROL INJECTION. (Sanofi Winthrop) Atropine sulfate 0.4 mg, meperidine HCl 50 mg or 75 mg/Carpuject.
Use: Preoperative sedative.

ATROPINE-HYOSCINE-HYOSCYAMINE COMBINATIONS. (See also Belladonna Products)
See: Barbella, Tab., Elix. (Forest).
    Barbeloid, Tab. (Vale).
    Bar-Don, Tab., Elix. (Warren-Teed).
    Belakoids TT, Tab. (Philips Roxane).
    Belbutal No. 2 Kaptabs. (Churchill).
    Brobella-P.B., Tab. (Brothers).
    Buren, Tab. (Ascher).
    Donnacin, Elix., Tab. (Pharmex).
    Donnagel, Susp. (Robins).
    Donnamine, Elix., Tab. (Tennessee Pharm.).

Donnatal, Cap., Elix., Tab. (Robins).
Donnatal #2, Tab. (Robins).
Donnatal Extentabs, Tab. (Robins).
Donnazyme, Tab. (Robins).
Eldonal, Preps. (Canright).
Haponal, Cap. (Jenkins).
Hyatal, Elix. (Winsale).
Hybophon, Prop. (Boocham Labs).
Hyonal, Preps. (Paddock).
Hyonatol B, Preps. (Bowman).
Hytrona, Tab. (Webcon).
Kinesed, Tab. (Stuart).
Koryza, Tab. (Forest).
Maso-Donna, Elix., Tab. (Mason).
Nilspasm, Tab. (Parmed).
Sedamine, Tab. (Dunhall).
Sedapar, Tab. (Parmed).
Seds, Tab. (Pasadena Research).
Spabelin, Elix. (Arcum).
Spasdel, Cap. (Marlop).
Spasloids, Tab. (G.F. Harvey).
Spasmolin, Tab. (Bell).
Spasquid, Elix. (Geneva).
Uriseptin, Tab. (Blaine).
Urogesic, Tab. (Edwards).
ATROPINE METHYLNITRATE. (Various Mfr.) dl-Hyoscyamine methylnitrate.
See: Harvatrate, Tab. (Forest Pharm.).
Thitrate W.P., Tab. (Blaine).
W/Hyoscine HBr, hyoscyamine sulfate, amobarbital sodium.
See: Amocine, Tab. (Hauck).
W/Methenamine mandelate and phenylazodiaminopyridine HCl.
See: Uritral, Cap. (Central).
W/Phenobarbital and dihydroxyaluminum aminoacetate.
See: Atromal, Tab. (Blaine).
Harvatrate A, Tab. (Forest Pharm.).
ATROPINE-N-OXIDE HCl.
See: Atropine Oxide HCl.
• **ATROPINE OXIDE HYDROCHLORIDE.**
USAN. Atropine N-oxide HCl.
Use: Anticholinergic.
See: X-Tro (Xttrium).
• **ATROPINE SULFATE,** U.S.P. XXIII. Inj., Ophth., Oint., Ophth. Soln., Tab, U.S.P. XXIII. (Various Mfr.) Benzeneacetic acid, α-(hydroxymethyl)-8-methyl-8-azabicyclo-[3.2.1.]oct-3-yl ester, endo-(±)-, sulfate (2:1) (salt), monohydrate. l-αH, 5-α-H-Tropan-3-α-ol (±)-tropate (ester), sulfate (2:1) (salt) monohydrate. **Pediatric Inj.:** 0.05 mg/ml 5 ml Abboject. **Tab, Hypodermic:** 0.3 mg, 0.4 mg and 0.6 mg/Tab. Bot. 100s. **Tab, Oral:** 0.4 mg/Tab. Bot. 100s. **Inj.:** 0.1 mg/ml 5 ml and 10 ml Abboject 0.3 mg/ml. Vial 1 ml; 0.4 mg/ml. Amp. 1 ml, vial 20 ml; 0.8 mg/ml. Amp. 1 ml, dosette 0.5 ml; 1

mg/ml. Amp., vial 1 ml, syringe 10 ml; 1.2 mg/ml. Vial 1 ml syringe.
Lyophilized: Lyopine (Hyrex). **Ophth. Oint:** 0.5% Tube 3.5 Gm.; 1% Tube 3.5 Gm., UD 1 Gm. **Ophth. Soln:** 0.5% Bot. 1 ml, 5 ml; 1% Bot. UD 1 ml, 2 ml, 5 ml, 15 ml; 2% Bot. 1 ml, 2 ml; 3% Bot. 5 ml.
Use: Anticholinergic, antidote to cholinesterase inhibitors.
See: Atropine-1, Soln., (Optopics).
Atropine Care, Soln., (Akorn).
Atropine Sulfate S.O.P., Oint., (Allergan).
Atropisol, Soln., (Iolab).
Isopto-Atropine (Alcon).
Lyopine, Inj. (Hyrex).
Parasympatholytic and antispasmodic.
Sal-Tropine (Hope Pharm.).
W/Ephedrine sulfate.
See: Enuretrol, Tab. (Berlex).
ATROPINE SULFATE/EDROPHONIUM CHLORIDE. Anticholinesterase muscle stimulant.
See: Enlon-Plus (Anaquest).
ATROPINE SULFATE AND MEPERIDINE HCl.
See: Atropine and Demerol. (Sanofi Winthrop.).
ATROPINE SULFATE AND MORPHINE SULFATE.
See: Morphine and Atropine Sulfates. (Beecham Labs).
ATROPINE SULFATE S.O.P.. (Allergan) 0.5%, 1%. Oint. Tube 3.5 g.
Use: Cycloplegic mydriatic.
ATROPINE SULFATE W/PHENOBARBITAL.
See: Antrocol, Tab., Cap. (Poythress).
Arco-Lase Plus, Tab. (Arco).
Barbeloid, Tab. (Vale).
Briabell, Tab. (Briar).
Brobella-P.B., Tab. (Brothers).
Donnatal, Cap., Extentab, Tab., Elix. (Robins).
Donnatal #2, Tab. (Robins).
Haponal, Cap. (Jenkins).
Hyatal Elix. (Winsale).
Palbar No. 2, Tab. (Hauck).
Seds, Tab. (Pasadena Research).
Spabelin, Elix. (Arcum).
Spasdel, Cap. (Marlop).
Spasmolin, Tab. (Kenyon).
Stannitol (Standex).
ATROPISOL. (Iolab) Atropine sulfate soln. **Dropperette:** 0.5%, 1% or 2%. 1 ml Box 12s. **Dropper Bot.:** 1%. 5 ml. **Bot.:** 1%. 15 ml.
Use: Cycloplegic mydriatic.
ATROSED. (Freeport) Atropine sulfate

0.0195 mg, hyoscine HBr 0.0065 mg, hyoscyamine sulfate 0.104 mg, phenobarbital 0.25 gr/Tab. Bot. 1000s, 5000s.
Use: Anticholinergic/antispasmodic, sedative/hypnotic,.
ATROSEPT. (Geneva Generics) Methenamine 40.8 mg, phenyl salicylate 18.1 mg, atropine sulfate 0.03 mg, hyoscyamine 0.03 mg, benzoic acid 4.5 mg, methylene blue 5.4 mg/Tab. Bot. 100s, 1000s.
Use: Urinary anti-infective.
ATROVENT. (Boehringer Ingelheim) Ipratropium bromide 18 mcg/dose. Inhalation aerosol 15 ml.
Use: Bronchodilator.
A/T/S. (Hoechst-Roussel) Erythromycin 2%. Gel. Tube 30 Gm.
Use: Anti-acne.
A/T/S TOPICAL SOLUTION. (Hoechst) Erythromycin 2% topical soln. Bot. 60 ml w/applicator.
Use: Anti-acne.
AT-SOLUTION. (Sanofi Winthrop) Dihydrotachysterol solution.
Use: Hypocalcemic tetany.
ATTAIN LIQUID. (Shorwood). Sodium caseinate, calcium caseinate, maltodextrin, corn oil, soy lecithin. Can 250 ml and 1000 ml closed system.
Use: Enteral nutritional supplement.
ATTAPULGITE, ACTIVATED.
Use: Antidiarrheal.
See: Quintess, Susp. (Lilly).
W/Pectin, hydrated alumina powder.
See: Polymagma Plain Tab. (Wyeth-Ayerst).
W/Polysorbate 80, salicylic acid, propylene glycol.
See: Sebasorb Lot. (Summer).
ATTENUVAX. (Merck & Co.) Measles virus vaccine, live, attenuated w/neomycin 25 mcg/Vial. Single-dose vial w/diluent. Pkg. 1s, 10s.
Use: Agent for immunization.
W/Meruvax.
See: M-R-Vax-II, Vial (Merck & Co.).
W/Mumpsvax, Meruvax.
See: M-M-R II, Vial (Merck & Co.).
ATUSS HD. (Atley) Hydrocodone bitartrate 2.5 mg, phenylephrine HCl 5 mg, chlorpheniramine maleate 2mg/5ml. Liq. Bot. 473 ml.
Use: Antitussive, decongestant, antihistamine.
ATUSSIN-D.M. EXPECTORANT. (Amfre-Grant) Chlorpheniramine maleate 2 mg, phenylephrine HCl 5 mg, phenylpropanolamine HCl 5 mg, guaifenesin 100 mg, dextromethorphan HBr 15 mg/5

ml Syr. Bot. 4 oz, pt, gal.
Use: Antihistamine, decongestant, expectorant, antitussive.
W/Pentobarbital sodium, 2-diethylaminoethyl diphenyl-acetate HCl, aluminum hydroxide.
See: Spasmasorb, Tab. (Hauck).
AUGMENTED BETAMETHASONE DIPROPIONATE. Corticosteroid, topical.
See: Diprolene (Schering).
AUGMENTIN CHEWABLE TABLETS. (Beecham Labs) **125:** Amoxicillin 125 mg, clavulanic acid 31.25 mg/Tab. Ctn. 30s. **250:** Amoxicillin 250 mg, clavulanic acid 62.5 mg/Tab. Ctn. 30s.
Use: Antibacterial, penicillin.
AUGMENTIN ORAL SUSPENSION. (Beecham Labs) **125:** Amoxicillin 125 mg, clavulanic acid (as potassium salt) 31.25 mg/5 ml. Bot. 75 ml, 150 ml. **250:** Amoxicillin 250 mg, clavulanic acid (as potassium salt) 62.5 mg/5 ml. Bot. 75 ml, 150 ml.
Use: Antibacterial, penicillin.
AUGMENTIN TABLETS. (Beecham Labs) Amoxicillin trihydrate 250 mg or 500 mg, clavulanic acid (as potassium salt) 125 mg/Tab. **250:** Bot. 30s, UD 100s. **500:** Bot. 30s, 100s.
Use: Antibacterial, penicillin.
AURAL ACUTE. (Saron) Polymyxin B sulfate 10,000 units, neomycin sulfate 5 mg, hydrocortisone 10 mg/10 ml, alcohol 0.1%.
Use: Corticosteroid combination.
AURALGAN OTIC SOLUTION. (Wyeth-Ayerst) Antipyrine 54 mg, benzocaine 14 mg/ml w/oxyquinoline sulfate in dehydrated glycerin (contains not more than 0.6% moisture). Bot. w/dropper 15 ml.
Use: Otic preparation.
AURALGESIC. (Wesley) Carbamide 10%, antipyrine 5%, benzocaine 2.5%, cetyldimethylbenzylammonium HCl 0.2%. Bot. 0.5 oz.
Use: Otic preparation.
• **AURANOFIN.** USAN.
Use: Antirheumatic.
AUREOMYCIN PREPARATIONS. (Storz Lederle) Chlortetracycline HCl.
Ophth. Oint.: 1% (10 mg/Gm) Tube 0.125 oz.
Topical Oint.: 3% (30 mg/Gm) in white petrolatum, anhydrous lanolin base. Tube 0.5 oz, 1 oz.
Use: Anti-infective.
AUREOQUIN DIAMATE. Name previously used for Quinetolate.
AURINOL EAR DROPS. (Various)

Chloroxylenol and acetic acid, w/benzalkonium chloride and glycerin. Soln. Bot. 15 ml.
Use: Otic preparation.
AUROCAINE. (Republic) Carbamide, glycerin, propylene glycol with chlorobutanol 0.5%. Bot. 15 ml.
Use. Otic preparation.
AUROCAINE 2. (Republic) Boric acid in isopropyl alcohol 2.75%. Soln. Bot. 30 ml.
Use: Otic preparation.
AUROCEIN. (Christina) Gold naphthyl sulfhydryl derivative. 5% or 12.5% Amp. 10 ml.
Use: Antirheumatic agent.
AURO-DRI. (Commerce) Boric acid 2.75% in isopropyl alcohol. Bot. oz.
Use: Otic preparation.
AURO EAR DROPS. (Commerce) Carbamide peroxide 6.5% in a specially prepared base. Bot. 15 ml.
Use: Otic preparation.
AUROLATE. (Pasadena) Gold sodium thiomalate 50 mg, benzyl alcohol 0.5%/ml. Inj. Vial 2 ml, 10 ml.
Use: Antirheumatic agent.
AUROLIN.
See: Gold sodium thiosulfate.
AUROPIN.
See: Gold sodium thiosulfate.
AUROSAN.
See: Gold sodium thiosulfate.
AUROTHIOBLYCANIDE. 2-Mercaptoacetanilide S-gold (1+) salt.
Use: Antirheumatic agent.
AUROTHIOGLUCOSE INJECTION.
See: Sterile aurothioglucose suspension.
AUROTHIOMALATE, SODIUM.
See: Gold Sodium Thiomalate, U.S.P. XXIII.
AUROTO OTIC. (Barre) Benzocaine 1.4%, antipyrine 5.4%, glycerin and oxyquinoline sulfate/Soln. Bot. 15 ml w/dropper.
Use: Otic preparation.
AUSAB. (Abbott Diagnostics) Radioimmunoassay or enzyme immunoassay for detection of antibody to hepatitis B surface antigen. Test kit 100s.
Use: Diagnostic aid.
AUSAB EIA. (Abbott Diagnostics) Enzyme immunoassay for the detection of antibody to hepatitis B surface antigen.
Use: Diagnostic aid.
AUSCELL. (Abbott Diagnostics) Reverse passive hemagglutination test for hepatitis B surface antigen. Test kit 110s, 450s, 1800s.

Use: Diagnostic aid.
AUSRIA II-125. (Abbott Diagnostics) Radioimmunoassay for detection of hepatitis B surface antigen. Test kit 100s, 500s, 600s, 700s, 800s, 900s, 1000s.
Use: Diagnostic aid.
AUSZYME II. (Abbott Diagnostics) Enzyme immunoassay for detection of hepatitis B surface antigen (HBsAg) in human serum or plasma. Test kit 100s, 500s.
Use: Diagnostic aid.
AUSZYME MONOCLONAL. (Abbott Diagnostics) Qualitative third generation enzyme immunoassay for the detection of hepatitis B surface antigen (HBsAg) in human serum or plasma.
Use: Diagnostic aid.
AUTOANTIBODY SCREEN. (Wampole-Zeus) Autoantibody screening system. To screen serum for the presence of a variety of autoantibodies. Test 48s.
Use: Diagnostic aid.
AUTOLET KIT. (Ames) Automatic blood letting spring-loaded device to obtain capillary blood samples from fingertips, earlobes or heels.
Use: Diagnostic aid.
AUTOLYMPHOCYTE THERAPY; ALT. (Callcor)
Use: Treatment of renal cancer. [Orphan drug]
AUTOPLEX. (Hyland) Anti-inhibitor coagulant complex prepared from pooled human plasma. Vial 30 ml.
Use: Diagnostic aid.
AUTOPLEX T. (Hyland) Dried anti-inhibitor coagulant complex. With a maximum of heparin 2 units and polyethylene glycol 2 mg per ml reconstituted material. Inj. Vial with diluent and needles.
Use: Diagnostic aid.
AUTRINIC. Intrinsic factor concentrate.
Use: To increase absorption of Vitamin B_{12}.
AUXOTAB ENTERIC 1 & 2. (Colab) Rapid identification of enteric bacteria and *pseudomonas.* Test contains capillary units with selective biochemical reagents.
Use: Diagnostic aid.
AVAIL. (SK-Beecham) Elemental iron 18 mg, vitamin A 5000 IU, D 400 IU, E 30 mg, B_1 2.25 mg, B_2 2.55 mg, B_3 20 mg, B_6 3 mg, B_{12} 9 mcg, C 90 mg, folic acid 0.4 mg, Ca, Cr, I, Mg, Se and zinc 22.5 mg/Tab. Bot. 60s, 100s.
Use: Vitamin/mineral supplement.
AVALGESIC LOTION. (Various Mfr.) Methyl salicylate, menthol, camphor,

methyl nicotinate, dipropylene glycol salicylate, oil of cassia, oleoresins capsicum and ginger. Bot. 120 ml, pt, gal.
Use: External analgesic.
A-VAN. (Stewart-Jackson) Dimenhydrinate 50 mg/Cap. Bot. 100s.
Use: Antivertigo agent.
AVC CREAM. (Marion Merrell Dow) Sulfanilamide 15% in a water-miscible base of propylene glycol, stearic acid, diglycol stearate to acid pH. Tube 4 oz. w/applicator.
Use: Anti-infective, vaginal.
AVC SUPPOSITORIES. (Marion Merrell Dow) Sulfanilamide 1.05 Gm in a base made from polyethylene glycol 400, polysorbate 80, polyethylene glycol 3350, glycerin, inert glycerin-gelatin covering. Box 16s w/inserter.
Use: Anti-infective, vaginal.
AVEENO ANTI-ITCH. (Rydelle) Calamine 3%, pramoxine HCl, camphor 0.3% in a base of glycerin, distearyldimonium chloride, petrolatum, oatmeal flour, isopropyl palmitate, cetyl alcohol, dimethicone and sodium chloride. Cream 30 Gm, Lotion 120 ml
Use: Antipruritic.
AVEENOBAR MEDICATED. (Rydell) Aveeno colloidal oatmeal 50%, sulfur 2%, salicylic acid 2%, in soap-free cleansing bar. Formerly Acnaveen. Bar 3.5 oz.
Use: Antipruritic.
AVEENOBAR OILATED. (Rydell) Vegetable oils, lanolin derivative, glycerine 29%, aveeno colloidal oatmeal 30% in soap-free base. Formerly Emulave. Bar 3 oz.
Use: Emollient.
AVEENOBAR REGULAR. (Rydell) Colloidal oatmeal 50%, anionic sulfonate, hypo-allergenic lanolin. Formerly Aveeno Bar. Bar 3.2 oz, 4.4 oz.
Use: Skin cleanser.
AVEENO BATH. (Rydell) Colloidal oatmeal. Box 1 lb, 4 lb.
Use: Emollient.
AVEENO CLEANSING BAR. (Rydelle) Sulfur 2%, salicylic acid 2%, colloidal oatmeal 50%, mild surfactant. Soap Bar 105 Gm.
Use: Anti-acne.
AVEENO COLLOIDAL OATMEAL. (Rydell) Colloidal oatmeal. Box 1 lb, 4 lb.
Use: Emollient.
AVEENO DRY. (Rydelle) Dry skin formula, soap free, emollient colloidal oatmeal, vegetable oils, lanolin derivative and glycerin 29% in mild surfactant

base. Cleansing bar 90 Gm.
Use: Skin cleansers.
AVEENO LOTION. (Rydell) Colloidal oatmeal in aqueous lotion base. Bot. 6 oz.
Use: Emollient.
AVEENO MOISTURIZING CREAM. (Rydelle) Colloidal oatmeal, glycerin, petrolatum, dimethicone, phenylcarbinol. Cream Tube 120 Gm.
Use: Emollient.
AVEENO NORMAL. (Rydelle) Normal to oily skin formula, soap free. Colloidal oatmeal 50%, lanolin derivative and mild surfactant. Cleansing bar 96 Gm, 132 Gm.
Use: Skin cleanser.
AVEENO OILATED. (Rydelle) Aveeno colloidal oatmeal impregnated with 35% liquid petrolatum, refined olive oil. Box 8 oz, 2 lb.
Use: Emollient.
AVEENO SHOWER & BATH. (Rydelle) Colloidal oatmeal, 5% mineral oil, glyceryl stearate, PEG 100 steasrate, laureth-4, benzyl alcohol, silica benzaldehyde. Oil. Bot. 240 ml.
Use: Emollient
AVENTYL HCl. (Lilly) Nortriptyline HCl. **Liq.:** Equivalent to 10 mg base/5 ml in alcohol 4%. Bot. 16 fl. oz. **Pulv.:** Equivalent to 10 mg base or 25 mg base/Cap. Bot. 100s, 500s, Blisterpak 10 × 10s.
Use: Antidepressant.
AVERTIN. Tribromoethanol (Various Mfr.).
• **AVILAMYCIN.** USAN.
Use: Antibacterial.
AVINAR. Uredepa.
Use: Antineoplastic agent.
AVITENE. (Shionogi) Hydrochloric acid salt of purified bovine corium collagen. **Fibrous Form:** Jar 1 Gm, 5 Gm. **Web Form:** Blister Pak. Sheets of 70 mm × 70 mm, 70 mm 35 mm.
Use: Topical hemostat.
• **AVOBENZONE.** USAN.
Use: Sunscreen.
AVONIQUE. (Geneva) Vitamins A 4000 IU, D 400 IU, B_1 1 mg, B_2 1.2 mg, B_6 2 mg, B_{12} 2 mcg, calcium pantothenate 5 mg, B_3 10 mg, C 30 mg, calcium 100 mg, phosphorous 76 mg, iron 10 mg, manganese 1 mg, magnesium 1 mg, zinc 1 mg.
Use: Vitamin/mineral supplement.
• **AVOPARCIN.** USAN.
Use: Antibacterial.
A.V.P. CILLIN TABS AND POWDER FOR SYRUP. (A.V.P.) Potassium penicillin G. **Syr.:** (400,000 units) 250 mg/5 ml. Bot.

80 ml. **Tab.**: 250 mg. Bot. 100s.
Use: Antibacterial, penicillin.
A.V.P. NATAL-FA. (A.V.P.) Vitamins A
5000 IU, elemental iron 200 mg, ferrous
fumarate 65 mg, calcium 165 mg, phosphorus 75 mg, C 100 mg, B_6 10 mg, folic
acid 1 mg/Tab. Bot. 100s.
Use: Vitamin/mineral supplement.
• **AVRIDINE.** USAN.
Use: Antiviral.
AWAKE. (Walgreen) Caffeine 100
mg/Tab. Bot. 36s.
Use: CNS stimulant.
AXEROPHTHOL.
See: Vitamin A.
AXID. (Lilly) Nizatidine 150 mg or 300
mg/Cap. Bot. 30s, 60s.
Use: H_2 antagonist.
AXON THROAT SPRAY. (McKesson)
Bot. 5 Gm.
Use: Throat preparation.
AXOTAL. (Adria) Butalbital 50 mg, aspirin
650 mg/Tab. Bot. 100s, 500s.
Use: Sedative/hypnotic, salicylate analgesic.
AXSAIN.
See: Zostrix (GenDerm).
AXSINATE. (Lannett) Styramate 200 mg,
salicylamide 210 mg, acetophenetidin
150 mg, caffeine 30 mg/Tab. Bot. 50s.
Use: Analgesic.
AYDS APPETITE SUPPRESSANT CANDY. (Jeffrey Martin) Benzocaine 5 mg in
chewy candy base w/25 cal./Cube. Ctn.
12s, 48s, 96s.
Use: Diet aid.
AYGESTIN. (Wyeth-Ayerst) Norethindrone acetate 5 mg/Tab. Bot. 50s, Cycle
pack 10s.
Use: Progestin.
AYR SALINE NASAL DROPS. (Ascher)
Sodium Cl 0.65% adjusted with phosphate buffers to proper tonicity and pH
to prevent nasal irritation. **Drops:** Bot.
20 ml. **Mist:** Bot. 50 ml.
Use: Moisture replenisher.
• **AZABON.** USAN.
Use: Stimulant.
• **AZACITIDINE.** USAN.
Use: Antineoplastic.
• **AZACONAZOLE.** USAN.
Use: Antifungal.
AZA-CR. NCI Investigational agent.
See: Azacitadine.
AZACTAM FOR INJECTION. (Squibb) L-arginine 780 mg/Gm aztreonam. **Single
dose 15 ml vial:** 500 mg/Vial Pkg. 10s,
25s. 1 Gm/Vial Pkg. 10s, 25s. 2 Gm/vial
Pkg. 10s, 25s. **Single dose 100 ml IV infusion bottle w/ball bands:** 500

mg/Bot. Pkg. 10s. 1 Gm/vial Pkg. 10s. 2
Gm/vial Pkg. 10s.
Use: Antibacterial.
AZACYCLONOL. B.A.N. α-4-Piperidyl-benzhydrol. Frenquel HCl.
Use: Tranquilizer.
AZACYCLONOL HCl. Alpha, alpha-diphonyl 1 piperidino methanol HCl.
5-AZA-2 DEOXYCYTIDINE. USAN.
Use: Treatment of acute leukemia.
AZALINE TABS. (Major) Sulfasalazine
500 mg/Tab. Bot. 100s, 500s, 1000s.
Use: Agent for ulcerative colitis.
AZALOMYCIN. B.A.N. A mixture of related antibiotics produced by *Streptomyces hygroscopicus var. azalomyceticus.*
Use: Antibacterial.
• **AZALOXAN FUMARATE.** USAN.
Use: Antidepressant.
AZAMETHONIUM BROMIDE. B.A.N. 3-Methyl-3-azapentamethylenedi(ethyl-dimethylammonium bromide). Pendiomide.
Use: Ganglionic blocking agent.
AZAMETHONIUM BROMIDE. (Ciba) 3-Methyl-3-azapentamethylenebis (ethyl-dimethyl-ammonium) dibromide. Pendiomide, Pentamin.
Use: Ganglionic blocking agent.
• **AZANATOR MALEATE.** USAN.
Use: Bronchodilator.
• **AZANIDAZOLE.** USAN.
Use: Antiprotozoal.
AZAPETINE. B.A.N. 6-Allyl-5,7-dihydrodibenz-[c,e]azepine. Ilidar phosphate.
Use: Vasodilator.
AZAPETINE PHOSPHATE. 6-Allyl-6,7-dihydro-5H-dibenz(c,e)azepine, azephine.
AZAPROPAZONE. B.A.N. 5-Dimethylamino-9-methyl-2-propyl-1H-pyrazolo[1,2-α][1,2,4]-benzotriazine-1,3(2H)-dione.
Use: Analgesic, anti-inflammatory.
• **AZARIBINE.** USAN. 2-β-D-Ribofuranosyl-1,2,4-triazine-3,5-(2H,4H)dione2,3',5-triacetate. 6-Azauridine 2,3,5-triacetate. Triazure.
Use: Treatment of psoriasis.
• **AZAROLE.** USAN.
Use: Immunoregulator.
• **AZASERINE.** USAN.
Use: Antifungal.
• **AZATADINE MALEATE,** U.S.P. XXIII. 5-H-Benzo (5-6) cyclohepta (1,2-b) pyridine, 6,11-dihydro-11-(1-methyl-4-piperidylidene)-5H-benzo(5,6)-cyclohepta (1,2-b) pyridine maleate (1:2).
Use: Antihistamine.

See: Optimine, Tab. (Schering-Plough).
Trinalin, Tab. (Schering-Plough).
• **AZATHIOPRINE,** U.S.P. XXIII. Tab.,
U.S.P. XXIII. (Burroughs Wellcome) 6-
(1-Methyl-4-nitroimidazol-5-ylthio)
purine. IH-Purine, 6-[(I-methyl-4-nitro-IH-
imidazol-5-yl)thio]-.6-[(I-Methyl-4-ni-
troimidazolyl-5-)thio]purine.
Use: Anti-leukemic compound.
See: Imuran, Inj., Tab. (Burroughs Well-
come).
AZATHIOPRINE. B.A.N. 6-(1-Methyl-4-ni-
troimidazol-5-ylthio)purine.
Use: Antimetabolite.
AZATHIOPRINE SODIUM, U.S.P. XXIII.
Use: Anti-leukemic compound.
5-AZC.
See: Azacitidine.
AZDONE. (Central) Hydrocodone bitar-
trate 5 mg, aspirin 500 mg/Tab. Bot.
100s, 1000s.
Use: Narcotic analgesic combination.
• **AZELASTINE HYDROCHLORIDE.**
USAN.
Use: Antiallergic, antiasthmatic.
• **AZEPINDOLE.** USAN.
Use: Antidepressant.
• **AZETEPA.** USAN. PP-Diaziridin-1-yl-N-
ethyl-1,3,4-thiadiazol-2-ylphosphi-
namide.
Use: Antimetabolite.
3-AZIDO-2, 3 DIDEOXYURIDINE. USAN
Use: Treatment of AIDS.
AZIDOCILLIN. B.A.N. 6-[D( )-α-Azi-
dophenyl-acetamido]penicillanic acid.
Use: Antibiotic.
AZIDOTHYMIDINE.
See: Zidovudine.
AZIDOURIDINE. (Berlex) Phase I HIV
positive symptomatic, ARC, AIDS.
Use: Antiviral.
• **AZIPRAMINE HYDROCHLORIDE.**
USAN.
Use: Antidepressant.
• **AZITHROMYCIN.** USAN.
Use: Antibacterial.
See: Zithromax (Pfizer).
AZLIN. (Miles Pharm) Azlocillin sodium.
Vial 2 Gm, 3 Gm, 4 Gm.
Use: Antibacterial; penicillin.
• **AZLOCILLIN.** USAN.
Use: Antibacterial.
See: Azlin, Inj. (Miles).
• **AZLOCILLIN SODIUM, STERILE,** U.S.P.
XXIII.
Use: Antibacterial.
AZMA-AID. (Purepac) Theophylline 118
mg, ephedrine 24 mg, phenobarbital 8
mg/Tab. Bot. 100s, 250s, 1000s.
Use: Bronchodilator.

AZMACORT INHALER. (Rhone-Puolenc
Rorer) Triamcinolone acetonide ≈ 100
mcg delivered from the collapsible ex-
pansion chamber activator. Canister 20
Gm, contains triamcinolone acetonide
60 mg w/oral adapter.
Use: Bronchodilator.
AZO-100. (Scruggs) Phenylazodi-
aminopyridine HCl 100 mg/Tab. Bot.
100s, 1000s.
Use: Urinary tract analgesic.
• **AZOCONAZOLE.** USAN.
Use: Antifungal.
AZODYNE.
W/Sulfadiazine, sulfamethizole.
See: Suladyne, Tab. (Stuart).
AZODYNE HCl.
See: Pyridium, Tab. (Parke Davis).
AZO-GAMAZOLE TABS. (Major) Bot.
100s, 1000s.
Use: Urinary anti-infective.
AZO GANTANOL. (Roche) Sulfamethox-
azole 500 mg, phenazopyridine HCl 100
mg/ Tab. Bot. 100s, 500s.
Use: Urinary anti-infective.
AZO GANTRISIN. (Roche) Sulfisoxazole
500 mg, phenazopyridine HCl 50
mg/Tab. Bot. 100s, 500s.
Use: Urinary anti-infective.
• **AZOLIMINE.** USAN.
Use: Diuretic.
AZO NEGACIDE TABLETS. (Sanofi
Winthrop) Nalidixic acid, phenazopyri-
dine HCl.
Use: Urinary anti-infective.
• **AZOSEMIDE.** USAN.
Use: Diuretic.
AZO-STANDARD. (PolyMedica)
Phenazopyridine HCl 100 mg/Tab. Bot.
360s.
Use: Urinary anti-infective.
AZOSTIX REAGENT STRIPS. (Ames)
Bromthymol blue, urease, buffers. Col-
orimetric test for blood urea nitrogen lev-
el. Bot 25 strips.
Use: Diagnostic aid.
AZO-SULFISOXAZOLE. (Forest Pharm.)
Sulfisoxazole 500 mg, phenazopyridine
HCl 50 mg/Tab. Bot. 100s, 1000s.
Use: Urinary anti-infective.
AZO-SULFISOXAZOLE. (Richlyn) Sul-
fisoxazole 500 mg, phenazopyridine HCl
50 mg/Tab. Bot. 1000s.
Use: Urinary anti-infective.
• **AZOTOMYCIN.** USAN. Antibiotic isolated
from broth filtrates of *Streptomyces am-
bofaciens.*
Use: Antineoplastic agent.
AZO-URIZOLE. (Jenkins) Sulfisoxazole
0.5 Gm, phenazopyridine HCl 50

mg/Tab. Bot. 1000s.
Use: Urinary anti-infective.
AZOVAN BLUE. Tetrasodium salt of 4:4'-di-[7-(1-amino-8-hydroxy-2:4-disulpho)-naphthylazo]-3:3-bitolyl.
See: Evans Blue Dye, Amp. (City Chemical; Harvey).
AZOVAN BLUE. B.A.N. Tetrasodium salt of 4,4'-di-(8-amino-1-hydroxy-5,7-disulfo-2-naphthylazo)-3,3-bitolyl.
Use: Diagnostic aid.
AZO WINTOMYLON. (Sanofi Winthrop) Nalidixic acid, phenazopyridine HCl.
Use: Urinary anti-infective.
AZT.
See: Zidovudine.
AZT-P-ddl. (Baker Norton) Phase I AIDS.
Use: Antiviral.
• **AZTREONAM,** U.S.F. XXIII. Inj.
Use: Antimicrobial.
See: Azactam, Vial (Squibb).
AZULFIDINE ORAL SUSPENSION. (Pharmacia) Sulfasalazine 250 mg/5 ml. Bot. pt.
Use: Agent for ulcerative colitis.
AZULFIDINE TABLETS and EN-TABS. (Pharmacia) Sulfasalazine (salicylazosulfapyridine) 500 mg/Tab or En-tab. Bot. 100s, 500s, UD 100s, 1000s.
Use: Agent for ulcerative colitis.
• **AZUMOLENE SODIUM.** USAN.
Use: Relaxant.
AZURESIN. B.A.N. Prepared from carbacrylic cation exchange resin and azure A dye (3-amino-7-dimethylaminophenazathionium Cl). Diagnex Blue. (Squibb UK).
Use: Diagnostic aid.

B

B$_1$. Thiamine HCl.
B$_2$. Riboflavin.
B$_3$. Niacinamide.
B$_6$. Pyridoxine HCl.
B$_6$ 50. (Western Research) Vitamin B$_6$ 50 mg/Tab. Bot. 1000s.
Vitamin B$_6$ supplement.
B$_{12}$. Cyanocobalamin.
B50. (Nature's Bounty) Vitamins B$_1$ 50 mg, B$_2$ 50 mg, B$_3$ 50 mg, B$_5$ 50 mg, B$_6$ 50 mg, B$_{12}$ 50 mcg, folic acid 0.1 mg, d-biotin 50 mcg, PABA 50 mg, choline bitartrate 50 mg, inositol 50 mg, lecithin/Tab. Bot. 100s.
Use: Vitamin/mineral supplement.
B50 TIME RELEASE. (Nature's Bounty) Vitamins B$_1$ 50 mg, B$_2$ 50 mg, B$_3$ 50 mg, B$_5$ 50 mg, B$_6$ 50 mg, B$_{12}$ 50 mcg, folic

acid 0.1 mg, d-biotin 50 mcg, PABA 50 mg, choline bitartrate 50 mg, inositol 50 mg, lecithin/Tab. Bot. 100s.
Use: Vitamin/mineral supplement.
B100. (Nature's Bounty) Vitamins B$_1$ 100 mg, B$_2$ 100 mg, B$_3$ 100 mg, B$_5$ 100 mg, B$_6$ 100 mg, B$_{12}$ 100 mcg, folic acid 0.1 mg, d-biotin 100 mcg, PABA 100 mg, choline bitartrate 100 mg, inositol 100 mg, lecithin. Tab. Bot. 100s.
Use: Vitamin/mineral supplement.
B125. (Nature's Bounty) Vitamins B$_1$ 125 mg, B$_2$ 125 mg, B$_3$ 125 mg, B$_5$ 125 mg, B$_6$ 125 mg, B$_{12}$ 125 mcg, folic acid 0.1 mg, d-biotin 125 mcg, PABA 125 mg, choline bitartrate 125 mg, inositol 125 mg, lecithin. Tab. Bot. 100s.
Use: Vitamin/mineral supplement.
B150. (Nature's Bounty) Vitamins B$_1$ 150 mg, B$_2$ 150 mg, B$_3$ 150 mg, B$_5$ 150 mg, B$_6$ 150 mg, B$_{12}$ 150 mcg, folic acid 0.1 mg, d-biotin 150 mcg, PABA 150 mg, choline bitartrate 150 mg, inositol 150 mg, lecithin. Tab. Bot. 100s.
Use: Vitamin/mineral supplement.
B & A. (Eastern Research) Sodium bicarbonate, potassium, aluminum, borax. Hygenic pow. Jar. 8 oz, 5 lb.
Use: Vaginal preparation.
B.A. GRADUAL. (Federal) Theophylline 260 mg, pseudoephedrine HCl 50 mg, butabarbital 15 mg/Gradual. Bot. 50s, 1000s.
Use: Bronchodilator, decongestant, sedative/hypnotic.
BABEE TEETHING. (Pfeiffer) Benzocaine 2.5%, cetalkonium Cl 0.02%, alcohol 20%, hamamelis water, propylene glycol, sodium benzoate, urea, menthol, camphor. Soln. Bot. 15 ml.
Use: Local anesthetic.
BABY ANBESOL. (Whitehall) Benzocaine 7.5%, carbomer 934, EDTA, glycerin, polyethylene glycol, saccharin. Gel Tube 7.2 Gm.
Use: Mouth and throat product.
BABY COUGH SYRUP. (Towne) Ammonium Cl 300 mg, sodium citrate 600 mg/oz w/citric acid. Bot. 4 oz.
Use: Antitussive.
BABY ORAJEL. (Del) Benzocaine 7.5%. Gel. Tube 9.45 g.
Use: Mouth and throat product.
BABY ORAJEL NIGHTTIME FORMULA. (Del) Benzocaine 10%, saccharin, sorbitol, alcohol free. Gel. Tube 5.3 g.
Use: Mouth and throat product.
BABY ORAGEL TEETH & GUM CLEANSER. (Del) Poloxamer 407 2%, simethicone 0.12%, parabens, saccha-

rin, sorbitol. Gel Tube 14.2 Gm.
Use: Mouth and throat product.
BAC. Benzalkonium Cl.
B-A-C #3. (Mayrand) Codeine phosphate
30 mg, aspirin 325 mg, caffeine 40 mg,
butalbital 50 mg/Tab. Bot. 100s.
Use: Analgesic combination.
• **BACAMPICILLIN HYDROCHLORIDE,**
U.S.P. XXIII. for Oral Soln., Tab., U.S.P.
XXIII.
Use: Antibiotic.
See: Spectrobid (Roerig).
BACCO-RESIST. (Vita Elixir) Lobeline
sulfate 1/64 gr.
Use: Antismoking lozenge.
BACID. (Ciba) A specially cultured strain
of human *Lactobacillus acidophilus,*
sodium carboxymethylcellulose 100 mg,
sodium 0.5 mEq/Cap. Bot. 50s, 100s.
Use: Antidiarrheal.
BACIGUENT ANTIBIOTIC OINTMENT.
(Upjohn) Bacitracin 500 units/Gm. Oint.
Tube 0.5 oz, 1 oz, 4 oz.
Use: Anti-infective, external.
• **BACITRACIN,** U.S.P. XXIII. Oint., Ophth.,
Oint., Sterile, U.S.P. XXIII. B.A.N. An an-
tibiotic produced by a strain of *Bacillus
subtilis.*
　Available forms (Various Mfr.).
　Diagnostic Tabs.
　Oint.
　Ophthalmic Oint.
　Soluble Tab.
　Systemic Use, Vial.
　Topical Use, Vial.
　Troche.
　Vaginal Tab.
Use: Antibacterial. [Orphan drug]
See: AK-Tracin, Oint. (Akorn).
　Baciquent, Oint. (Upjohn).
W/Neomycin sulfate.
See: Bacimycin, Oint. (Merrell Dow).
　Bacitracin-Neomycin, Oint., Ophth.
　Oint. (Various Mfr.).
W/Neomycin, polymyxin B sulfate.
See: Baximin, Oint. (Quality Generics).
　BPN Ointment (Norwich Eaton).
　Mycitracin, Oint., Ophth. Oint. (Up-
john).
　Neosporin, Oint., Ophth. Oint.,
　Aerosol, Pow. (Burroughs Well-
come).
　Neo-Thrycex, Oint. (Commerce).
　P.B.N., Oint. (Jenkins).
　Tigo, Oint. (Burlington).
　Tri-Biotic Oint. (Burgin-Arden).
　Tri-Biotic, Oint. (Standex).
　Tri-Bow Oint. (Bowman).
　Triple Antibiotic Oint. (Kenyon,
Towne).

W/Neomycin sulfate, polymyxin B sulfate,
diperodon HCl.
See: Epimycin A, Oint. (Delta).
　Mity-Mycin, Oint. (Solvay).
W/Neomycin sulfate, polymyxin B sulfate,
hydrocortisone acetate.
See: Neopolycin-HC, Oint., Ophth. Oint.
　(Merrell Dow).
W/Polymyxin B sulfate.
See: Polysporin, Oint., Ophth. Oint.
　(Burroughs Wellcome).
W/Polymyxin B sulfate and neomycin sul-
fate.
See: Trimixin, Oint. (Hance).
W/Polymyxin B sulfate, neomycin sulfate
and hydrocortisone-free alcohol.
See: Biotic-Ophth. W/HC, Oint. (Scrip).
　Cortisporin, Preps. (Burroughs Well-
come).
• **BACITRACIN METHYLENE DISALICY-
LATE,** U.S.P. XXIII. Soluble, Soluble
Pow., U.S.P. XXIII.
Use: Antibiotic.
BACITRACIN-NEOMYCIN OINTMENT.
(Various Mfr.) Neocyin sulfate equivalent
to 3.5 mg base, bacitracin 500 units/Gm.
Topical Oint. Tube 0.5 oz, 1 oz, Ophth.
Oint. 1/8 oz.
Use: Anti-infective, external.
**BACITRACIN/NEOMYCIN/POLYMYXIN
B OINTMENT.** (Various Mfr.) Polymyxin
B sulfate 10,000 units/g, neomycin sul-
fate 3.5 mg/g, bacitracin zinc 400
units/g. Tube 3.5 g.
Use: Antibiotic, ophthalmic.
• **BACITRACIN AND POLYMYXIN B SUL-
FATE,** U.S.P. XXIII. Topical Aerosol.
Use: Antibiotic.
See: Polysporin Spray (Burroughs Well-
come).
• **BACITRACIN ZINC,** U.S.P. XXIII. Sterile,
Soluble Pow., U.S.P. XXIII. (Upjohn)
Sterile pow. 10,000 units, 50,000
units/Vial.
Use: Antibiotic.
W/Neomycin sulfate, polymyxin B sulfate.
See: AK-Spore Ophth. Oint. (Akorn).
　Neomixin, Oint. (Hauck).
　Neosporin, Prods. (Burroughs Well-
come).
　Neotal, Oint. (Hauck).
　Ocutricin Ophth. Oint. (Bausch &
Lomb).
　Triple Antibiotic Ophth. Oint. (Various
Mfr.)
W/Neomycin sulfate, polymyxin B, benza-
lkonium Cl.
See: Biotres, Oint. (Central Pharmacal).
W/Neomycin sulfate, polymyxin B sulfate,
hydrocortisone acetate.

See: Biotres HC, Cream (Central).
Coracin, Oint. (Hauck).
W/Polymyxin B sulfate, neomycin sulfate.
See: Ophthel, Ophth. Oint. (Elder).
BACITRACIN ZINC/NEOMYCIN SUL-FATE/POLYMYXIN B SULFATE/HY-DROCORTISONE. (Various Mfr.) Hydrocortisone 1%, neomycin sulfate 0.35%, bacitracin zinc 400 units, polymyxin B sulfate 10,000 units in a white petrolatum and mineral oil base. Tube 3.5 g.
Use: Antibiotic, corticosteroid, ophthalmic.
• **BACITRACIN ZINC OINTMENT,** U.S.P. XXIII. Bacitracin zinc in an anhydrous ointment base.
Use: Antibiotic.
• **BACITRACIN ZINC AND POLYMYXIN B SULFATE OINTMENT,** U.S.P. XXIII. Ophth. Oint., U.S.P. XXIII.
Use: Antibiotic.
BACIT-WHITE. (Whiteworth) Bacitracin. Oint. Tube 0.5 oz, 1 oz.
Use: Anti-infective, external.
BACKACHE MAXIMUM STRENGTH RE-LIEF. (B-M Squibb) Magnesium salicylate anhydrous (as tetrahydrate) 467 mg. Capl. Bot. 24s, 50s.
Use: Salicylate analgesic.
• **BACLOFEN.** USAN. 4-Amino-3-(4-chlorophenyl) butyric acid.
β-Aminomethyl-p-chlorohydrocinnamic acid. 10 mg or 20 mg/**Tab.** Bot. 100s, UD 100s; 10 mg/20 ml or 10 mg/5 ml/**Intrathecal.** Single-use amps 1 amp refill kit (10 mg/20 ml), 2 or 4 amp refill kit (10 mg/5 ml).
Use: Muscle relaxant.
See: Lioresal, Tab. (Geigy).
Baclofen, Tab. (Vitarine).
BACLOFEN, L-BACLOFEN.
Use: Treatment of muscle spasticity.
[Orphan drug]
See: Neuralgon.
BACMIN. (Marnel) Iron 27 mg, A 5000 IU, E 30 IU, C 500 mg, B_1 20 mg, B_2 20 mg, B_3 100 mg, B_5 25 mg, B_6 25 mg, B_{12} 50 mcg, biotin 0.15 mg, folic acid 0.8 mg, Cr, Cu, Mg, Mn, Zn. Tab. Bot. 100s.
Use: Vitamin/mineral supplement.
BAC-NEO-POLY OINTMENT. (Burgin-Arden) Bacitracin 400 units, neomycin sulfate 5 mg, polymyxin B sulfate 5000 units/Gm. Tube 0.5 oz.
Use: Anti-infective, external.
BACTAL SOAP. (Whittaker General) Triclosan 0.5% and anhydrous soap 10%. Liq. 240 ml, 1/2 gal.
Use: Antiseptic soap.

BACTERIOSTATIC SODIUM CHLORIDE. (Various Mfr.) Sodium Cl 0.9%. Also contains benzyl alcohol or parabens. Inj. Bot. 10 ml, 20 ml, 30 ml.
Use: Parenteral diluent.
• **BACTERIOSTATIC WATER FOR INJEC-TION.** U.S.P. XXIII. (Abbott) 30 ml. Multiple-dose Fliptop Vial (plastic)
Use: Pharmaceutic acid for diluting and dissolving drugs for injection.
BACTERIURIA TESTS. In vitro diagnostic aids.
See: Microstix-3 Strips (Ames).
Uricult (Medical Technology).
Isocult for Bacteriuria (SmithKline Diagnostics).
BACTICORT. (Rugby) Hydrocortisone 1%, neomycin sulfate equivalent to 0.35% neomycin base, polymyxin B sulfate 10,000 units/ml, benzalkonium Cl, cetyl alcohol, glyceryl monostearate, mineral oil, polyoxyl 40 stearate, propylene glycol. Ophth. Soln. Bot. 7.5 ml.
Use: Ophth. corticosteroid, anti-infective.
BACTIGEN GROUP A STREPTOCOC-CUS. (Wampole) Latex agglutination slide test for the qualitative detection of group A streptococcal antigen directly from throat swabs. Test kit 60s.
Use: Diagnostic aid.
BACTIGEN GROUP A STREPTOCOC-CUS WITH FAST TRAK SLIDES. (Wampole) Latex agglutination slide test for qualitative detection of group A streptococcal antigen directly from throat swabs. Test 24s. Test kit 48s.
Use: Diagnostic aid.
BACTIGEN GROUP B STREPTOCOC-CUS. (Wampole) Latex agglutination slide test for the qualitative detection of group B streptococcus antigen in urine, cerebrospinal fluid and serum. Test kit 15s.
Use: Diagnostic aid.
BACTIGEN H. INFLUENZAE. (Wampole) Rapid latex agglutination slide test for the qualitative detection of *Hemophilus influenzae,* type b antigen in cerebrospinal fluid, serum and urine. Test kit 15s, 30s.
Use: Diagnostic aid.
BACTIGEN MENINGITIS PANEL. (Wampole) Rapid latex agglutination slide test for the qualitative detection of *Hemophilus influenzae* type b, *Neisseria meningitidis* A/B/C/Y/W135 and Streptococcus pneumoniae antigens in cerebrospinal fluid, serum and urine. Test kit 18.

Use: Diagnostic aid.
BACTIGEN N. MENINGITIDIS.
(Wampole) Rapid latex agglutination slide test for the qualitative detection of *Neisseria meningitidis,* serogroups A/B/C/Y/W135 antigens in cerebrospinal fluid, serum and urine. Test kit 15s, 30s.
Use: Diagnostic aid.
BACTIGEN SALMONELLA-SHIGELLA.
(Wampole) Latex agglutination slide test for the qualitative detection of *Salmonella* or *Shigella* from cultures. 96s.
Use: Diagnostic aid.
BACTIGEN S. PNEUMONIAE.
(Wampole) Rapid latex agglutination slide test for the qualitative detection of *Streptococcus pneumoniae* antigens in cerebrospinal fluid, serum and urine. Test kit 15s, 30s.
Use: Diagnostic aid.
BACTINE ANTISEPTIC/ANESTHETIC FIRST AID SPRAY. (Miles) Benzalkonium Cl 0.13%, lidocaine 2.5%. **Squeeze Bot.:** 2 oz, 4 oz. **Liq.:** 16 oz. **Aerosol:** 3 oz.
Use: Antiseptic, anesthetic.
BACTINE FIRST AID ANTIBIOTIC.
(Miles) Polymyxin B sulfate 5,000 units, bacitracin 500 units, neomycin sulfate 5 mg/Gm in mineral oil, white petrolatum. Oint. Tube 15 Gm.
Use: Anti-infective, external.
BACTINE FIRST AID ANTIBIOTIC PLUS ANESTHETIC. (Miles) Polymyxin B sulfate 5,000 units, neomycin 3.5 mg/Gm, bacitracin 400 units, diperodon HCl 10 mg, in mineral oil and white petrolatum. Oint. Tube 15 Gm.
Use: Topical antibiotic.
BACTINE HYDROCORTISONE SKIN CREAM. (Miles) Hydrocortisone 0.5%. Tube 0.5 oz.
Use: Corticosteroid.
BACTINE MAXIMUM STRENGTH. (Miles Inc.) Hydrocortisone 1%, glycerin, mineral oil, methylparaben, white petrolatum. Cream tube 30 Gm.
Use: Corticosteroid, topical.
BACTOCILL. (Beecham Labs) Oxacillin sodium. **Cap.:** 250 mg or 500 mg Bot. 100s. **Vial:** (w/dibasic sodium phosphate 40 mg, methylparaben 3.6 mg, propylparaben 0.4 mg, sodium 3.1 mEq/Gm) 500 mg, 1 Gm, 2 Gm or 4 Gm/Vial; 10s. Piggyback vial 1 Gm, 2 Gm; 25s. Bulk pharm pkg 10 Gm; Box 25s.
Use: Antibacterial; penicillin.
BACTOSHIELD. (Amsco) **Foam:** Chlorhexidine gluconate 4%, isopropyl alcohol 4%. Can 180 ml. **Soln.:**

Chlorhexidine gluconate, isopropyl alcohol 4%. Bot. 960 ml.
Use: Pre-operative skin preparation/cleanser.
BACTOSHIELD 2. (Amsco) Chlorhexidine glyconate 2%, isorpropyl alcohol 4%. Soln. Bot. 960 ml.
Use: Pre-operative skin preparation/cleanser.
BACTRIM. (Roche) Sulfamethoxazole 400 mg, trimethoprim 80 mg/Tab. Bot. 100s, 500s, Teledose 100s, Prescription Pak 40s.
Use: Anti-infective combination.
BACTRIM DS. (Roche) Trimethoprim 160 mg, sulfamethoxazole 800 mg/Tab. Bot. 100s, 500s, Tel-E-Dose 100s, Prescription Pak 20s.
Use: Anti-infective combination.
BACTRIM IV INFUSION. (Roche) Sulfamethoxazole 400 mg, trimethoprim 80 mg/5 ml. Amp. Box 10 × 5 ml. Vials Box 10 × 5 ml, 10 × 10 ml. Multidose vials. Box 1 30 ml.
Use: Anti-infective.
BACTRIM PEDIATRIC SUSPENSION.
(Roche) Trimethoprim 40 mg, sulfamethoxazole 200 mg/5 ml. Bot. 100 ml, 480 ml.
Use: Anti-infective combination.
BACTRIM SUSPENSION. (Roche) Sulfamethoxazole 200 mg, trimethoprim 40 mg/5 ml. Bot. 16 oz.
Use: Anti-infective.
BACTROBAN. (Beecham) Mupirocin 2% in a polyethylene glycol base. Oint. Tube 15 Gm.
Use: Anti-infective, external.
BACTURCULT. (Wampole) A urinary bacteria culture medium diagnostic urine culture system for urine collection, bacteriuria screening and presumptive bacterial identification. Test kit 10s, 100s.
Use: Diagnostic aid.
BAFIL CREAM. (Scruggs) Hydrocortisone 0.5%, clioquinol 3%, lidocaine 3%, pH adjusted to 6. Tube oz.
Use: Corticosteroid, antifungal, local anesthetic.
BAIN DE SOLEIL ALL DAY FOR KIDS SPF 30. (Procter & Gamble) Ethylhexyl p-methoxycinnamate, 2-ethylhexyl-2 cyano-3, 3 diphenyl acrylate, oxybenzone, titanium dioxide, stearyl alcohol, tocopheryl acetate, EDTA. PABA free. Waterproof. Lot. Bot. 120 ml.
Use: Sunscreen.
BAIN DE SOLEIL ALL DAY WATERPROOF SUNBLOCK. (Procter & Gamble) SPF 15, 30. Ethylhexyl p-

methoxycinnamate, 2-ethylhexyl-2 cyano-3, 3-diphenyl acrylate, oxybenzone, titanium dioxide, stearyl alcohol, vitamin E, EDTA. Lot. Bot. 120 g.
Use: Sunscreen.

BAIN DE SOLEIL ALL DAY WATER-PROOF SUNFILTER. (Procter & Gamble) SPF 4, 8, 2-ethylhexyl 2-cyano-3, 3 diphenyl acrylate, ethylhexyl p-methoxycinnamate, titanium dioxide, stearyl alcohol, vitamin E, EDTA. Lot. Bot. 120 ml.
Use: Sunscreen.

BAIN DE SOLEIL BODY SILKENING CREME. (Procter & Gamble) Padimate O, ethylhexyl p-methoxycinnamate, oxybenzone, benzyl alcohol. Waterproof cream. Bot. 94 Gm.
Use: Sunscreen.

BAIN DE SOLEIL BODY SILKENING SPRAY. (Procter & Gamble) Padimate O, oxybenzone, ethylhexyl p-methoxycinnamate. Waterproof lotion. Bot. 240 ml.
Use: Sunscreen.

BAIN DE SOLEIL BODY SILKENING STICK. (Procter & Gamble) Padimate O, ethylhexyl p-methoxycinnamate, oxybenzone, dioxybenzone. Stick 53 Gm.
Use: Sunscreen.

BAIN DE SOLEIL FACE CREME. (Procter & Gamble) Padimate O, ethylhexyl p-methoxycinnamate, oxybenzone. Waterproof cream. Bot. 60 Gm.
Use: Sunscreen.

BAIN DE SOLEIL KIDS SPORT. (Procter & Gamble) SPF 25. Ethylhexyl-p-methoxycinnamate, 2-ethylhexyl-2 cyano-3, 3-diphenyl acrylate, titanium dioxide, PVP/eicosene copolymer, dimethicone, cyclomethicone, triethanolamine, glyceryl tribehenate, tocopheryl acetate, carbomer, EDTA, DMDM hydantoin. PABA free. Waterproof, all day protection. Lot. Bot. 120 ml.
Use: Sunscreen.

BAIN DE SOLEIL LIP PROTECTEUR. (Procter & Gamble) Ethylhexyl p-methoxycinnamate, oxybenzone, 2-ethylhexyl salicylate, oleyl alcohol, petrolatum. PABA free lip balm, 3 Gm.
Use: Sunscreen.

BAIN DE SOLEIL MEGATAN. (Procter & Gamble) Ethylhexyl p-methoxycinnamate, 2-ethylhexyl salicylate, lanolin, cocoa butter, palm oil, aloe, DMDM hydantoin, xanthan gum, shea butter, EDTA. Lot. Bot. 120 ml.
Use: Sunscreen.

BAIN DE SOLEIL ORANGE GELEE SPF 4. (Procter & Gamble) Ethylhexyl p-methoxycinnamate, 2-ethylhexyl salicylate. PABA free. Gel Tube 93.75 g.
Use: Sunscreen.

BAIN DE SOLEIL SPF 8 + COLOR. (Procter & Gamble) Octyl methoxycinnamate, octocrylene, mineral oil, cetyl alcohol, EDTA. Lot. Bot. 118 ml.
Use: Sunscreen.

BAIN DE SOLEIL SPF 15 + COLOR. (Procter & Gamble) Octyl methoxycinnamate, octocrylene, oxybenzone, mineral oil, cetyl alcohol, EDTA. Lot. Bot. 118 ml.
Use: Sunscreen.

BAIN DE SOLEIL SPF 30 + COLOR. (Procter & Gamble). Octocrylene, octyl methoxycinnamate, oxybenzone, mineral oil, cetyl alcohol, EDTA. Lot. Bot. 118 ml.
Use: Sunscreen.

BAIN DE SOLEIL SPORT. (Procter & Gamble). SPF 15. 2-ethylhexyl 2-cyano-3, 3 diphenyl acrylate, ethylhexyl-p-methoxycinnamate, titanium dioxide, dimethicone, cyclomethicone, panthenol, tocopheryl acetate, carbomer, EDTA, DMDM hydantoin. PABA free. Waterproof, sweatproof, all day protection. Lot. Bot. 180 ml.
Use: Sunscreen.

BAIN DE SOLEIL TROPICAL DELUXE SPF 4. (Procter & Gamble) Ethylhexyl p-methoxycinnamate, 2-ethylhexyl salicylate, cetyl alcohol, EDTA. PABA free. Waterproof. Lot. Bot. 240 ml.
Use: Sunscreen.

BAIN DE SOLEIL UNDER EYE. (Procter & Gamble) Ethylhexyl p-methoxycinnamate, oxybenzone, 2-ethylhexyl salicylate. Stick 1.5 Gm.
Use: Sunscreen.

BAKERS BEST. (Scherer) Water, alcohol 38%, propylene glycol, extract of capsicum, glycerin, boric acid, Tween 80, diethylphthalate, rose oil, pyrilamine maleate, glacial acetic acid, Uvinul MS 40, hexetidine, benzalkonium Cl 50%, sodium hydroxide 76%. Bot. 8 oz.
Use: Antipruritic, antiseborrheic.

BALANCED B$_{100}$. (Fibertone) Vitamins B$_1$ 100 mg, B$_2$ 100 mg, B$_3$ 100 mg, B$_5$ 100 mg, B$_6$ 100 mg, B$_{12}$ 100 mcg, folic acid 0.1 mg, PABA 100 mg, inositol 100 mg, d-biotin 100 mcg/SR Tab. Bot. 50s,
Use: Vitamin/mineral supplement.

BALANCED SALT SOLUTION. (Various Mfr.) Sodium Cl 0.64%, potassium Cl, 0.075%, calcium Cl 0.036%, magnesium Cl 0.03% in sodium acetate-sodi-

um citrate buffer system. Soln. Drop-
tainer 15 ml, 30 ml, 300 ml, 500 ml.
Use: Intraocular irrigant.
BALDEX OPHTHALMIC OINTMENT.
(Bausch & Lomb) Dexamethasone
phosphate 0.05%. 3.75 Gm.
Use: Corticosteroid, ophthalmic.
BALDEX OPHTHALMIC SOLUTION.
(Bausch & Lomb) Dexamethasone
phosphate 0.01%. Dropper bot 5 ml.
Use: Corticosteroid, ophthalmic.
BAL IN OIL. (Hynson, Westcott & Dun-
ning) 2,3-dimercaptopropanol 100 mg,
benzyl benzoate 210 mg, peanut oil 680
mg/ml. Amp. 3 ml Box 10s.
Use: Antidote.
BALMEX BABY POWDER. (Macsil) Spe-
cially purified balsam Peru, zinc oxide,
starch, calcium carbonate. Shaker top
can. 4 oz.
Use: Adsorbent, emollient.
BALMEX EMOLLIENT LOTION. (Macsil)
Fraction of lanolin, allantoin, specially
purified balsam Peru, silicone in a non-
mineral oil base. Bot. 6 fl. oz.
Use: Emollient.
BALMEX OINTMENT. (Macsil) Specially
purified balsam Peru, Vitamins A and D,
zinc oxide, bismuth subnitrate in a base
w/silicone. Tube 1 oz, 2 oz, 4 oz. Jar lb.
Use: Emollient.
BALNEOL. (Solvay) Water, mineral oil,
propylene glycol, glyceryl stearate,
PEG-100 stearate, PEG-40 stearate,
laureth-4, PEG-4-dilaurate, lanolin oil,
sodium acetate, carbomer-934, tri-
ethanolamine, methylparaben, docusate
sodium, acetic acid, fragrance. Bot. 120
ml.
Use: Anorectal preparation.
BALNETAR. (Westwood) Tar equivalent
to 2.5% coal tar, U.S.P. Bot. 8 oz.
Use: Bath dermatological.
BALSAN. Specially purified balsam Peru.
See: Balmex Prods. (Macsil).
• **BAMBERMYCINS.** USAN.
Use: Antibacterial.
BAMETHAN B.A.N. 2-Butylamino-1-(4-
hydroxyphenyl)ethanol.
Use: Vasodilator.
• **BAMETHAN SULFATE.** USAN. α-[(Buty-
lamino) methyl]-p-hydroxybenzyl alcohol
sulfate.
Use: Vasodilator.
BAMIFYLLINE. B.A.N. 8-Benzyl-7-[2-(N-
ethyl-2-hy- droxy-ethylamino)ethyl]theo-
phylline. Trentadil HCl.
Use: Bronchodilator.
BAMIFYLLINE HYDROCHLORIDE.
USAN. 8-Benzyl-7-[2-[ethyl (2-hydrox-

yethyl) amino]ethyl]-theophylline HCl.
Use: Bronchodilator.
BAMIPINE. B.A.N. 4-(N-Benzylanilino)-1-
methyl-piperidine.
Use: Antihistamine.
• **BAMNIDAZOLE.** USAN.
Use: Antiprotozoal.
BANACID TABLETS. (Buffington) Mag-
nesium trisilicate 220 mg. Bot. 100s,
200s, 500s.
Use: Antacid.
BANADYNE-3. (Norstar) Lidocaine 4%,
menthol 1%, alcohol 45%. Soln. Bot. 3
ml.
Use: Relief of cold sores, fever blisters.
BANALG. (Forest) Menthol, camphor,
methyl salicylate, eucalyptus oil in a
greaseless base. Regular liniment and
hospital strength. Bot. 2 oz, pt, gal.
Use: External analgesic.
**BANALG HOSPITAL STRENGTH LINI-
MENT.** (Forest) Methyl salicylate 14%,
menthol 3%. Bot. 60 ml.
Use: External analgesic.
BANATIL. (Trimen) Butabarbital 32.4 mg,
hyoscyamine sulfate 0.25 mg, scopo-
lamine methylnitrate 0.05 mg, atropine
sulfate 0.086 mg/D.R. Tab. Bot. 100s.
Elix. pt.
Use: Sedative/hypnotic, anticholiner-
gic/antispasmodic.
BANCAP HC. (Forest) Acetaminophen
500 mg, hydrocodone bitartrate 5
mg/Cap. Bot. 100s, 500s, UD 100s.
Use: Narcotic analgesic combination.
• **BANDAGE, ADHESIVE,** U.S.P. XXIII.
Use: Surgical aid.
• **BANDAGE, GAUZE,** U.S.P. XXIII.
Use: Surgical aid.
BANEX CAPSULES. (LuChem) Phenyl-
propanolamine HCl 45 mg, phenyle-
phrine HCl 5 mg, guaifenesin 200 mg.
Bot. 100s, 500s.
Use: Decongestant, expectorant.
BANEX-LA TABLETS. (LuChem)
Phenylpropanolamine HCl 75 mg,
guaifenesin 400 mg. Bot. 100s, 500s.
Use: Decongestant, expectorant.
BANFLEX. (Forest) Orphenadrine citrate
30 mg/ml. Inj. Vial 10 ml.
Use: Skeletal muscle relaxant.
BANGESIC. (H.L. Moore) Menthol, cam-
phor, methyl salicylate, eucalyptus oil in
non-greasy base. Bot. 2 oz, gal.
Use: External analgesic.
BANOCIDE.
See: Diethylcarbamazine Citrate,
U.S.P.
BANOPHEN. (Major) Pseudoephedrine
HCl 60 mg, diphenhydramine HCl 25

mg. Cap. Bot. 24s.
Use: Antihistamine.
BANSMOKE. (Thompson) Benzocaine 6 mg, corn syrup, dextrose, lecithin, sucrose. Gum Pack 24s.
Use: Smoking deterrent.
BANTHINE. (Schiapparelli Searle) Methantheline bromide 50 mg/Tab. Bot. 100s.
Use: Anticholinergic.
BANTRON BRAND SMOKING DETERRENT TABLETS. (Jeffrey Martin) Magnesium carbonate 129.6 mg, lobeline sulfate 2 mg, tribasic calcium phosphate 129.6 mg/Tab. Carton 18s, 36s.
Use: Smoking deterrent.
BARBASED. (Major) **Tab.:** Butabarbital 0.25 gr or 0.5 gr/Tab. Bot. 1000s. **Elix.:** Butabarbital- 30 mg/5 ml, alcohol 7%. Bot. 480 ml.
Use: Sedative/hypnotic.
BARBATOSE NO. 2 TABLETS. (Vale) Barbital 64.8 mg/Tab. w/hyoscyamus sulfate, passiflora, valarian. Bot. 1000s.
Use: Sedative.
BARBELLA ELIXIR. (Forest) Phenobarbital 0.25 gr, hyoscyamine sulfate 0.1037 mg, atropine sulfate 0.0194 mg, scopolamine HBr 0.0065 mg, alcohol 23%/5 ml. Bot. 4 oz, gal.
Use: Sedative/hypnotic, anticholinergic/antispasmodic.
BARBELLA TABLETS. (Forest) Phenobarbital 16.2 mg, atropine sulfate 0.0194 mg, hyoscyamine sulfate 0.1037 mg, hyoscine HBr 0.0065 mg/Tab. Bot. 100s, 1000s, 5000s.
Use: Sedative/hypnotic, anticholinergic/antispasmodic.
BARBELOID. (Vale) Phenobarbital 16.2 mg, hyoscyamine sulfate 0.1037 mg, atropine sulfate 0.0194 mg, scopolamine HBr 0.0065 mg/Tab. Bot. 100s, 1000s.
Use: Sedative/hypnotic, anticholinergic/antispasmodic.
BARBENYL.
See: Phenobarbital.
BARBIDONNA. (Wallace) **Elix.:** Phenobarbital 21.6 mg, hyoscyamine sulfate 0.174 mg, atropine sulfate 0.034 mg, scopolamine HBr 0.01 mg, alcohol 15%/5 ml. Bot. pt. **Tab.:** Phenobarbital 16 mg, hyoscyamine sulfate 0.1286 mg, atropine sulfate 0.025 mg, scopolamine HBr 0.0074 mg/Tab. Bot. 100s, 500s.
Use: Sedative/hypnotic, anticholinergic/antispasmodic.
BARBIDONNA NO. 2. (Wallace) Phenobarbital 32 mg, hyoscyamine sulfate 0.1286 mg, atropine sulfate 0.025 mg,

scopolamine HBr 0.0074 mg/Tab. Bot. 100s.
Use: Sedative/hypnotic, anticholinergic/antispamodic.
BARBINAL CAPSULES. (Forest) Phenobarbital 0.5 gr, acetophenetidin 2 gr, aspirin 3 gr, hyoscyamus 0.25 gr/Cap. Bot. 100s, 500s.
Use: Sedative/hypnotic, analgesic combination, anticholinergic/antispasmodic.
BARBINAL NO. 3. (Forest) Phenobarbital 0.25 gr, codeine phosphate 0.5 gr, acetophenetidin 2 mg, aspirin 3 gr, hyoscyamine sulfate 0.031 mg/Cap. Bot. 100s, 500s.
Use: Sedative/hypnotic, analgesic combination, anticholinergic/antispasmodic.
BARBIPHENYL.
See: Phenobarbital.
BARBITAL. Barbitone, Deba, Dormonal, Hypnogene, Malonal, Sedeval, Uronal, Veronal, Vesperal, diethylbarbituric acid, diethylmalonylurea.
Use: Sedative/hypnotic.
W/Aspirin, caffeine, niacinamide.
See: Mentran, Tab.(Pasadena Research).
BARBITAL SODIUM. Barbitone Sodium, diethylbarbiturate monosodium, diethylmalonylurea sodium, Embinal, Medinal, Veronal Sodium.
Use: Sedative/hypnotic.
BARBITONE.
See: Barbital.
BARBITONE SODIUM.
See: Barbital Sodium.
BARBITURATE-ASPIRIN COMBINATIONS.
See: Aspirin-Barbiturate Combination.
BARBITURATES, INTERMEDIATE DURATION.
See: Butabarbital (Various Mfr.).
Butethal (Various Mfr.).
Diallylbarbituric Acid (Various Mfr.).
Lotusate, Cap. (Sanofi Winthrop).
Vinbarbital. (Various Mfr.).
BARBITURATES, LONG DURATION.
See: Barbital (Various Mfr.).
Mebaral, Tab. (Sanofi Winthrop).
Mephobarbital (Various Mfr.).
Phenobarbital (Various Mfr.).
Phenobarbital Sodium (Various Mfr.).
BARBITURATES, SHORT DURATION.
See: Amobarbital (Various Mfr.).
Amobarbital Sodium (Various Mfr.).
Butalbital (Various Mfr.).
Butallylonal (Various Mfr.).
Cyclobarbital (Various Mfr.).

Cyclopal.
Pentobarbital Salts (Various Mfr.).
Sandoptal.
Secobarbital (Various Mfr.).
BARBITURATES, TRIPLE.
See: Butseco, S.C.T., Tab. (Bowman).
Ethobral, Cap. (Wyeth-Ayerst).
**BARBITURATES, ULTRASHORT DURA-
TION.**
See: Hexobarbital.
Neraval.
Pentothal Sodium, Amp. (Abbott).
Surital Sodium, Amp., Vial (Parke-
Davis).
Thiopental Sodium (Various Mfr.).
BARC GEL. (Commerce) Pyrethrins
0.18%, piperonyl butoxide technical
2.2%, petroleum distillate 4.8% in gel
base. Tube oz.
Use: Pediculicide.
BARC LIQUID. (Commerce) Pyrethrins
0.18%, piperonyl butoxide technical
2.2%, petroleum distillate 5.52%. Bot. 2
oz.
Use: Pediculicide.
**BARC NON-BODY LICE CONTROL
SPRAY.** (Commerce) Resmethrin-5-
(phenylmethyl)-3-furanyl] methyl-2, 2-di-
methyl-3-(2-methyl-1-propanyl) cyclopropanecarboxylate. Spray can 5 oz.
Use: Pediculicide.
BARICON. (Lafayette) Barium sulfate
95% pow. for susp. In UD 340 Gm.
Use: Gastrointestinal contrast agent.
BARIDIUM. (Pfeiffer) Phenazopyridine
HCl 100 mg/Tab. Bot. 32s.
Use: Urinary analgesic.
BARI-STRESS M. (Barre) Vitamins B_1 10
mg, B_2 10 mg, niacinamide 100 mg, C
300 mg, B_6 2 mg, B_{12} 4 mcg, folic acid
1.5 mg, calcium pantothenate 20
mg/Cap or Tab. **Cap.:** Bot. 30s, 100s,
1000s. **Tab.:** Bot. 100s, 1000s.
Use: Vitamin/mineral supplement.
• **BARIUM HYDROXIDE LIME,** U.S.P. XXI-
II.
Use: Carbon dioxide absorbant.
BARIUM SULFATE PREPARATION.
See: Baroflave, Pow. (Lannett).
Barotrast, Pow., Cream (Barnes-
Hind).
Fleet.
Raybar, Susp. (Fleet).
Redi-Flow, Susp. (Berlex).
Rugar, Susp. (McKesson).
BARLEVITE. (Barth's) Vitamins B_6 0.6
mg, B_{12} 3 mcg, pantothenic acid 0.6 mg,
D 3 IU, l-lysine 20 mg/0.6 ml. 100-Day
Supply.
Use: Vitamin/mineral supplement.

• **BARMASTINE.** USAN.
Use: Antihistamine.
**BARNES-HIND CLEANING AND SOAK-
ING SOLUTION.** (Barnes-Hind) Clean-
ing and buffering agents, benzalkonium
Cl 0.01%, disodium edetate 0.2%. Bot.
1.2 oz, 4 oz.
Use: Hard contact lens care.
**BARNES-HIND WETTING & SOAKING
SOLUTION.** (Barnes-Hind) Polyvinyl al-
chohol, povidone, hydroxyethyl cellu-
lose, octylphenoxy (oxyethylene)
ethanol, benzalkonium Cl, edetate dis-
odium. Bot. 4 oz.
Use: Hard contact lens care.
BARNES-HIND WETTING SOLUTION.
(Barnes-Hind) Polyvinyl alcohol, edetate
disodium 0.02%, benzalkonium Cl
0.004%. Bot. 35 ml, 60 ml.
Use: Hard contact lens care.
BAROBAG, EMPTY. (Lafayette) Dispos-
able enema kit.
Use: Barium enema.
BARO-CAT. (Lafayette) Barium sulfate
1.5% susp. 300 ml, 900 ml.
Use: Gastrointestinal contrast agent.
BAROFLAVE POWDER. (Lannett) Barium sulfate for diagnostic X-ray use. Bot.
5 lb, Fibre drum 25 lb.
Use: Gastrointestinal contrast agent.
BAROPHEN. (Various Mfr.) **Elix.:** At-
ropine sulfate 0.0194 mg, scopolamine
HBr 0.0065 mg, hyoscyamine HBr or
SO_4 0.1037 mg, phenobarbital 16.2
mg/5 ml w/alcohol 23%. Elix. Bot. 120
ml, pt, gal.
Use: Anticholinergic/antispasmodic,
sedative/hypnotic.
BAROS. (Lafayette) Sodium bicarbonate
460 mg (sodium 126 mg) and tartaric
acid 420 mg/Gm with simethicone. Plastic amp. 3 Gm.
Use: Diagnostic aid.
BAROSET. (Lafayette) Air contrast stom-
ach. Unit-of-use kit. Case 12s.
Use: Radiopaque agent.
BAROSMIN.
See: Diosmin.
BAROSPERSE. (Lafayette) Barium sulfate 95%, suspending agent. Susp. 25
lb.
Use: Radiopaque agent.
BAROSPERSE 110. (Lafayette) Barium
sulfate 95%. Susp. 900 Gm.
Use: Radiopaque agent.
W/Iron. Ferric pyrophosphate 250 mg/5 ml
plus Barovite liquid formula.
BARTONE. (Rand) Phenobarbital 16.2
mg, scopolamine HBr 0.0065 mg, at

ropine sulfate 0.0194 mg, hyoscyamine sulfate 0.1037 mg/Tab. or 5 ml. **Tab.:** Bot. 100s, 1000s. **Elix.:** Pt, gal. *Use:* Sedative/hypnotic, anticholinergic/antispasmodic.

BASA. (Freeport) Acetylsalicylic acid 324 mg/Tab. Bot. 1000s. *Use:* Salicylate analgesic.

BASALJEL. (Wyeth-Ayerst) Aluminum carbonate gel. **Susp.:** Equivalent to aluminum hydroxide 400 mg/5 ml. Bot. 355 ml. **Cap.:** Equivalent to 608 mg dried aluminum hydroxide gel or 500 mg aluminum hydroxide. Bot. 100s, 500s. **Tab.:** Equivalent to 608 mg dried aluminum hydroxide gel or 500 mg aluminum hydroxide. Bot. 100s. *Use:* Antacid.

BASIC ALUMINUM AMINOACETATE. *See:* Dihydroxyaluminum Aminoacetate.

BASIC ALUMINUM CARBONATE. *See:* Basaljel, Susp. (Wyeth-Ayerst).

BASIC ALUMINUM GLYCINATE. *See:* Dihydroxyaluminum aminoacetate.

BASIC BISMUTH CARBONATE. *See:* Bismuth Subcarbonate.

BASIC BISMUTH GALLATE. *See:* Bismuth Subgallate (Various Mfr.).

BASIC BISMUTH NITRATE. *See:* Bismuth Subnitrate (Various Mfr.).

BASIC BISMUTH SALICYLATE. *See:* Bismuth Subsalicylate.

BASIC FUCHSIN. *See:* Carbol-Fuchsin Topical Soln., U.S.P. XXIII.

BASIS, GLYCERIN SOAP. (Beiersdorf) **Bar:** Tallow, coconut oil, glycerin. **Sensitive:** Bar 90 Gm, 150 Gm. **Normal to dry:** Bar 90 Gm, 150 Gm. *Use:* Therapeutic skin cleanser.

BASIS, SUPERFATTED SOAP. (Beiersdorf) **Bar:** Sodium tallowate, sodium cocoate, petrolatum, glycerin, zinc oxide, sodium Cl, titanium dioxide, lanolin, alcohol, beeswax, BHT, EDTA. Bar 99 Gm, 225 Gm. *Use:* Therapeutic skin cleanser.

BATANOPRIDE HYDROCHLORIDE. USAN. *Use:* Antiemetic.

BATELAPINE MALEATE. USAN. *Use:* Antipsychotic.

BAYER 8-HOUR TIMED-RELEASE ASPIRIN. (Glenbrook) Aspirin 10 gr (650 mg) /T.R. Tab. Bot. 30s, 72s, 125s. *Use:* Salicylate analgesic.

BAYER 205. *See:* Suramin Sodium. (No Mfr. current ly listed.).

BAYER 2502. *See:* Nifurtimox. (No Mfr. currently listed.).

BAYER ASPIRIN, GENUINE. (Glenbrook) Aspirin 325 mg/Tab. Bot. 50s, 100s, 200s, 300s. Pkg. 12s, 24s. *Use:* Salicylate analgesic.

BAYER ASPIRIN, MAXIMUM. (Glenbrook) Aspirin 500 mg/Tab. Bot. 30s, 60s, 100s. *Use:* Salicylate analgesic.

BAYER BUFFERED ASPIRIN. (Sterling Health) Buffered aspirin 325 mg. Tab. Bot. 100s. *Use:* Salicylate analgesic.

BAYER CHILDREN'S CHEWABLE ASPIRIN. (Glenbrook) Aspirin 1.25 gr (81 mg) /Tab. Bot. 30s. *Use:* Salicylate analgesic.

BAYER CHILDREN'S COLD TABLETS. (Glenbrook) Phenylpropanolamine HCl 3.125 mg, aspirin 1.25 gr (81 mg)/Tab. Bot. 30s. *Use:* Decongestant, salicylate analgesic.

BAYER COUGH SYRUP FOR CHILDREN. (Glenbrook) Phenylpropanolamine HCl 9 mg, dextromethorphan HBr 7.5 mg/5 ml w/alcohol 5%. Bot. 3 oz. *Use:* Decongestant, antitussive.

BAYER LOW ADULT STRENGTH. (Sterling Health) Aspirin 81 mg. Delayed release. Tab. bot. 120s. *Use:* Salicylate analgesics.

BAYER PLUS EXTRA STRENGTH. (Sterling Health) Aspirin 500 mg buffered with calcium carbonate magnesium carbonate, magnesium oxide. Cap. Bot. 30s, 60s. *Use:* Salicylate analgesic with antacid buffers.

BAYER SELECT MAXIMUM STRENGTH BACKACHE. (Sterling Health) Magnesium salicylate tetrahydrate 580 mg. Capl. bot. 24s, 50s. *Use:* Salicylate analgesic.

BAYER SELECT MAXIMUM STRENGTH HEADACHE. (Sterling Health) Acetaminophen 500 mg, caffeine 65 mg/Cap. Bot. 50s. *Use:* Nonnarcotic analgesic combination.

BAYER SELECT CHEST COLD. (Sterling Health) Dextromethorphan HBr 15 mg, acetaminophen 500 mg. Caplets in Pkg. 16s. *Use:* Antitussive, analgesic.

BAYER SELECT FLU RELIEF. (Sterling

Health) Acetaminophen 500 mg, pseudoephedrine HCl 30 mg, dextromethorphan HBr 15 mg, chlorpheniramine maleate 2 mg. Capl. Blister-pack 16s.
Use: Antitussive combination.
BAYER SELECT HEAD COLD (Sterling Health) Pseudoephedrine HCl 30 mg, acetaminophen 500 mg. Capl. Pkg. 16s.
Use: Decongestant combination.
BAYER SELECT NIGHTTIME COLD. (Sterling Health) Acetaminophen 500 mg, pseudoephedrine HCl 30 mg, dextromethorphan HBr 15 mg, triprolidine HCl 1.25 mg. Capl. Blister-pack 16s.
Use: Antitussive combinations.
BAYER SELECT MAXIMUM STRENGTH MENSTRUAL. (Sterling Health) Acetaminophen 500 mg, pamabrom 25 mg/Capl. Bot. 50s.
Use: Nonnarcotic analgesic combination.
BAYER SELECT MAXIMUM STRENGTH NIGHT TIME PAIN RELIEF. (Sterling Health) Acetaminophen 500 mg, diphenhydramine HCl/Tab. Bot. 24s, 50s.
Use: Nonnarcotic analgesic combination.
BAYER SELECT MAXIMUM STRENGTH SINUS RELIEF. (Sterling Health) Acetaminophen 500 mg, pseudoephedrine HCl 30 mg/Tab.. Bot. 24s, 50s.
Use: Nonnarcotic analgesic combination.
BAYER SELECT PAIN RELIEF FORMULA. (Sterling Health) Ibuprofen 200 mg/Cap. Bot. 50s.
Use: Nonnarcotic anti-inflammatory agent.
BAYER THERAPY CAPLETS. (Glenbrook) Aspirin, 325 mg, enteric coated. Tab. Bot. 50s, 100s.
Use: Analgesic.
BAYLOCAINE 2% Viscous. (Bay Labs) Lidocaine 2% w/sodium carboxymethylcellulose. Soln. Bot. 100 ml.
Use: Local anesthetic.
BAYLOCAINE 4%. (Bay Labs) Lidocaine 4% w/methylparaben. Soln. Bot. 50 ml, 100 ml.
Use: Local anesthetic.
BAYPRESS. Type II calcium channel blocking agent.
See: Nitrendipine.
BC-1000. (Solvay) Vitamins B_1 50 mg, B_2 5 mg, B_{12} 1000 mcg, B_6 5 mg, d-panthenol 6 mg, niacinamide 125 mg, ascorbic acid 50 mg, benzyl alcohol 1%/ml. Vial 10 ml.
Use: Vitamin supplement.
BC ARTHRITIS STRENGTH. (Block) As-

pirin 742 mg, salicylamide 222 mg, caffeine 36 mg/Pow. Bot. 6s, 24s, 50s.
Use: Nonnarcotic analgesic combination.
B-C-BID CAPSULES. (Geriatric) Vitamins B_1 15 mg, B_2 10 mg, B_6 5 mg, niacinamide 50 mg, calcium pantothenate 10 mg, C 300 mg, B_{12} 5 mcg /Cap. Bot. 30s, 100s, 500s.
Use: Vitamin/mineral supplement.
BC COLD POWDER NON-DROWSY FORMULA. (Block) Phenylpropanolamine HCl 25 mg, aspirin 650 mg, lactose. Pkg. 6s, 24s.
Use: Decongestant combination.
B COMPLEX-150. (Nion) B_1 150 mg, B_2 150 mg, B_3 150 mg, B_5 150 mg, B_6 150 mg, B_{12}150 mg, FA 0.4 mg, biotin 150 mcg, PABA 100 mg, choline bitartrate 150 mg, inositol 150 mg. SR Tab. Bot. 30s.
Use: Vitamin/mineral supplement.
B-COMPLEX ELIXIR. (Nion) B_1 2.3 mg, B_2 1 mg, B_3 6.7 mg, B_6 0.3 mg, alcohol 10%, sorbitol. Elix. Bot. 240 ml.
Use: Vitmin/mineral supplement.
• **BCG VACCINE,** U.S.P. XXIII. (Various Mfr.) Prepared from a Glaxo culture of a Danish strain of BCG bacillus. Amp. ml.
Use: Immunization against tuberculosis.
See: Theracys (Connaught).
BC MULTI SYMPTOM COLD POWDER PACKETS. (Block) Pheylpropanolamine HCl 25 mg, chlorpheniramine maleate 4 mg, aspirin 650 mg, lactose. Pow. Pck. 6s, 24s.
Use: Decongestant, antihistamine, analgesic.
BCNU. 1,3-bis(2-Chloroethyl)-1-nitrosourea.
Use: Antineoplastic agent.
See: BiCNU, Inj. (Bristol).
BCO. (Western Research) Vitamins B_1 10 mg, B_2 2 mg, B_6 1.5 mg, B_{12} 25 mcg, niacinamide 50 mg/Tab. Bot. 1000s.
Use: Vitamin supplement.
B-COM. (Century) Vitamins B_1 3 mg, B_2 3 mg, B_6 0.5 mg, niacinamide 20 mg, calcium pantothenate 5 mg, B_{12} 1 mcg, desiccated liver (undefatted) 60 mg, debittered brewer's dried yeast 60 mg/Cap. Bot. 100s, 1000s.
Use: Vitamin/mineral supplement.
B-COMPLEX 2. (Kenyon) Vitamins B_1 3 mg, B_2 3 mg, B_6 0.5 mg, calcium pantothenate 5 mg, niacinamide 20 mg, dried yeast N.F. 60 mg/Cap. Bot. 100s.
Use: Vitamin supplement.
B-COMPLEX NO. 5. (Pharmex) Vitamins

B_1 100 mg, B_2 2 mg, B_6 4 mg, panthenol 10 mg, niacinamide 100 mg, benzyl alcohol 1%, propylparaben 0.02%, methylparaben 0.18%/ml. Vial 30 ml.
Use: Vitamin supplement.

B-COMPLEX 25-25 INJ. (Forest) Niacinamide 100 mg, Vitamins B_1 25 mg, B_2 1 mg, B_6 2 mg, pantothenic acid 2 mg/ml. Vial 30 ml.
Use: Vitamin supplement.

B-COMPLEX "50". (Vitaline) Vitamins B_1 50 mg, B_2 50 mg, B_3 50 mg, B_4 50 mg, B_5 50 mg, B_6 50 mg, B_{12} 50 mcg, FA 0.1 mg, PABA 30 mg, inositol 50 mg, biotin 50 mcg, choline bitartrate 50 mg. Reg. or TR tabs. Bot. 90s, 1000s.
Use: Vitamin supplement.

B-COMPLEX 100. (Kenyon) Vitamins B_1 100 mg, B_2 2 mg, B_6 4 mg, d-panthenol 4 mg, niacinamide 100 mg/ml. Vial 30 ml.
Use: Vitamin supplement.

B COMPLEX #100. (Medical Chem) Vitamins B_1 100 mg, B_2 2 mg, B_6 4 mg, d-panthenol 4 mg, niacinamide 100 mg/ml. Vial 30 ml.
Use: Vitamin supplement.

B COMPLEX 100. (Rabin-Winters) Vitamins B_1 100 mg, B_2 2 mg, B_6 2 mg, niacinamide 125 mg, panthenol 10 mg/ml. Vial 30 ml.
Use: Vitamin supplement.

B-COMPLEX 100/100. (Sandia) Vitamins B_1 100 mg, B_2 2 mg, B_6 2 mg, niacinamide 100 mg/ml. Inj. Vial 30 ml.
Use: Vitamin supplement.

B COMPLEX AND B_{12}. (Nature's Bounty) Vitamins B_1 7 mg, B_2 14 mg, B_3 4.5 mg, B_{12} 25 mcg, protease 10 mg/Tab. Bot. 90s.
Use: Vitamin supplement.

B COMPLEX CAPSULES. (Arcum) Vitamins B_1 1.5 mg, B_2 2 mg, niacinamide 10 mg, B_6 0.1 mg, calcium pantothenate 1 mg, desiccated liver 70 mg, dried yeast 100 mg/Cap. Bot. 100s, 1000s.
Use: Vitamin/mineral supplement.

B COMPLEX CAPSULES J.F. (Bryant) Vitamins B_1 1 mg, B_2 0.3 mg, nicotinic acid 0.3 mg, B_6 0.25 mg, desiccated liver 0.15 Gm, yeast powder, dried 0.15 Gm/Cap. Bot. 100s, 1000s.
Use: Vitamin/mineral supplement.

B COMPLEX INJECTION WITH VITAMIN C.
Use: Vitamin supplement.
See: Cplex Cap. (Arcum).

B COMPLEX WITH B_{12} CAPSULES. (Bryant) Vitamins B_1 2 mg, B_2 2 mg, B_6 0.5 mg, niacinamide 10 mg, B_{12} 2 mcg,

biotin 10 mcg, calcium pantothenate 1.5 mg, choline dihydrogen citrate 40 mg, inositol 30 mg, desiccated liver 1 gr, brewer's yeast 3 gr/Cap. Bot. 100s, 1000s.
Use: Vitamin/mineral supplement.

B-COMPLEX WITH VITAMIN C AND B_{12}-10,000. (Lyphomed) Vitamins B_1 20 mg, B_2 3 mg, B_3 75 mg, B_5 5 mg, B_6 5 mg, B_{12} 1000 mcg, C 100 mg. Covial. 10 ml multiple dose.
Use: Vitamin supplement.

B-COMPLEX + C. (Nature's Bounty) Vitamins C 200 mg, B_1 10 mg, B_2 10 mg, B_3 50 mg, B_5 10 mg, B_6 5 mg/Tab. Bot. 100s.
Use: Vitamin supplement.

BC POWDER. (Block) Aspirin 650 mg, salicylamide 195 mg, caffeine 32 mg/Pow. Pkg. 2s, 6s, 24s, 50s.
Use: Salicylate analgesic.

BC POWDER, ARTHRITIS STRENGTH. (Block) Aspirin 742 mg, salicylamide 222 mg, caffeine 36 mg/Powder. Pkg. 6s, 24s, 50s.
Use: Salicylate analgesic.

BC TABLETS. (Block) Aspirin 325 mg, salicylamide 95 mg, caffeine 16 mg/Tab. Bot. 12s, 50s, 100s.
Use: Salicylate analgesic.

BC-VITE. (Drug Industries) Vitamins B_1 25 mg, B_2 5 mg, B_3 50 mg, B_5 10 mg, B_6 1 mg, B_{12} 2 mcg, C 150 mg/Tab. Bot. 100s, 500s.
Use: Vitamin supplement.

B-C WITH FOLIC ACID. (Geneva Marsam) Vitamins B_1 15 mg, B_2 15 mg, B_3 100 mg, B_5 18 mg, B_6 4 mg, B_{12} 5 mcg, C 500 mg, folic acid 0.5 mg/Tab. Bot. 100s.
Use: Vitamin/mineral supplement.

B-C W/FOLIC ACID PLUS. (Geneva) Fe 27 mg, A 5000 IU, E 30 IU, B_1 20 mg, B_2 20 mg, B_3 100 mg, B_5 25 mg, B_6 25 mg, B_{12} 50 mcg, C 500 mg, FA 0.8 mg, biotin 0.15 mg, Cr, Cu, Mg, Mn, Zn. Tab. Bot. 100s.
Use: Vitamin/mineral supplement.

B-DAY TABLETS. (Barth's) Vitamins B_1 7 mg, B_2 14 mg, niacin 4.67 mg, B_{12} 5 mcg/Tab. Bot. 100s, 500s.
Use: Vitamin B supplement.

B-D GLUCOSE. (Becton Dickinson) Glucose 5 Gm. Chew. Tab. Bot. 36s.
Use: Glucose elevating agent.

BDEP.
See: Benzathine Penicillin G.

B-DOX. (Lannett) Vitamins B_1 100 mg, B_6 100 mg/ml. Vial 10 ml.
Use: Vitamin B supplement.

B DOZEN. (Standex) Vitamin B_{12} 25 mcg /Tab. Bot. 1000s.
Use: Vitamin B supplement.
B-DRAM w/C COMPUTABS. (Dram) Vitamins B_2 10 mg, B_6 5 mg, nicotinamide 50 mg, calcium pantothenate 20 mg, B_1 5 mg/Tab. Bot. 100s.
Use: Vitamin supplement.
BEANO. (AK Pharma) alpha-D-galactosidase derived from *Aspergillus niger*, a fungal source in carrier of water and glycerol. Liq. Bot. 75 serving size at 5 drops per dose. Tab. Pkg. 12s. Bot. 30s, 100s.
Use: Antiflatulent.
BEBATAB NO. 2. (Freeport) Belladonna $1/6$ gr, phenobarbital 0.25 gr/Tab. Bot. 1000s.
Use: Anticholinergic/antispasmodic, sedative/hypnotic.
• **BECANTHONE HYDROCHLORIDE.** USAN.
Use: Antischistosomal.
BECAUSE. (Schering) Nonoxynol 9 8%. Vaginal foam. Bot. 10 Gm (6 dose contraceptor unit).
Use: Spermicide.
BECEEVITE CAPSULES. (Blue Cross) Vitamins C 300 mg, B_1 15 mg, B_2 10 mg, niacin 50 mg, B_6 5 mg, pantothenic acid 10 mg/Tab. Bot. 100s.
Use: Vitamin supplement.
BE-CE FORTE. (Kenyon) Vitamins B_1 15 mg, B_2 10 mg, niacinamide 80 mg, B_6 20 mg, d-panthenol 23 mg, C 100 mg/2 ml. Vial 20 ml.
Use: Vitamin supplement.
BECLAMIDE. B.A.N. N-Benzyl-3-chloropropionamide.
Use: Anticonvulsant.
BECLOMETHASONE. B.A.N. 9α-Chloro-11β, 17α, 21-trihydroxy-16β-methyl-pregna-1, 4-diene-3,20-dione.
9α-Chloro-16β-methylprednisolone.
Use: Corticosteroid.
• **BECLOMETHASONE DIPROPIONATE.** USAN.
Use: Corticosteroid.
See: Beclovent Inhalation Aerosol (Allen & Hanburys).
Beconase Nasal Inhaler (Allen & Hanburys).
Beconase AQ Nasal Spray (Allen & Hanburys).
Vancenase Nasal Inhaler (Schering).
Vanceril Inhaler (Schering).
• **BECLOMYCIN DIPROPIONATE,** U.S.P. XXIII.
Use: Corticosteroid.
BECLOVENT INHALATION AEROSOL.

(Allen & Hanburys) Beclomethasone dipropionate 42 mcg/actuation. Aerosol canister (16.8 Gm) containing 200 metered inhalations. Canister 16.8 Gm w/oral adapter. Refill canister 16.8 Gm.
Use: Corticosteroid.
BECOMJECT-100. (Mayrand) B_1 100 mg, B_2 2 mg, B_3 100 mg, B_5 2 mg, B_6 2 mg. Inj. Vial 30 ml.
Use: B vitamin, parenteral.
BECOMP-C. (Cenci) Vitamins C 250 mg, B_1 25 mg, B_2 10 mg, nicotinamide 50 mg, B_6 2 mg, calcium pantothenate 10 mg, hesperidin complex 50 mg/Cap. Bot. 100s, 500s.
Use: Vitamin supplement.
BECONASE AQ NASAL SPRAY. (Allen & Hanburys) Beclomethasone dipropionate 42 mcg/metered spray. Pump aerosol bot. 25 Gm (200 metered inhalations) w/nasal adapter.
Use: Corticosteroid.
BECONASE INHALATION AEROSOL. (Allen & Hanburys) Beclomethasone dipropionate 42 mcg /actuation. Aerosol canister (16.8 Gm) containing 200 metered inhalations. Canister 16.8 Gm w/nasal adapter.
Use: Corticosteroid.
BECOTIN-T. (Dista) Vitamins B_1 15 mg, B_2 10 mg, B_6 5 mg, niacinamide 100 mg, pantothenic acid 20 mg, B_{12} 4 mcg, C 300 mg/Tab. Bot. 100s, 1000s, Blister pkg. 10 × 10s.
Use: Vitamin supplement.
BEDOCE. (Lincoln) Crystalline anhydrous vitamin B_{12} 1000 mcg/ml Vial 10 ml.
Use: Vitamin B_{12} supplement.
BEDOCE-GEL. (Lincoln) Vitamin B_{12} 1000 mcg/ml in 17% gelatin soln. Vial 10 ml.
Use: Vitamin B_{12} supplement.
BEDSIDE CARE. (Sween) Bot. 8 oz, gal.
Use: Non-rinsing shampoo, body wash.
BEECEEVITES CAPSULES. (Halsey)
Use: Vitamin supplement.
BEECHWOOD CREOSOTE.
See: Creosote, N.F.
BEE-FORTE W/C. (Rugby) Vitamins B_1 25 mg, B_2 12.5 mg, B_3 50 mg, B_5 10 mg, B_6 3 mg, B_{12} 2.5 mcg, C 250 mg/Cap. Bot. 100s.
Use: Vitamin supplement.
BEEF PEPTONES. (Sandia) Water soluble peptones derived from beef 20 mg/2 ml. Inj. Vial 30 ml.
Use: Nutritional supplement.
BEELITH. (Beach) Pyridoxine HCl 20 mg, magnesium oxide 600 mg/Tab. Bot.

100s.
Use: Vitamin/mineral supplement.
BEEPEN-VK. (Beecham Labs) Penicillin VK. **Tab.:** 250 mg. Bot. 1000s; 500 mg. Bot. 500s. **Oral Susp.:** 125 mg/5 ml Bot. 100 ml, 200 ml; 250 mg/5 ml Bot. 100 ml, 200 ml.
Use: Antibacterial: penicillin
BEEPEN-VK. (SK Beecham) Penicillin V potassium 125 mg/5 ml, saccharin, sucrose. Pow. 100 ml, 200 ml.
Use: Antibacterial natural penicillin.
BEE-THI. (Burgin-Arden) Cyanocobalamin 1000 mcg, thiamine HCl 100 mg in isotonic soln. of sodium Cl/ml. Vial 10 ml, 20 ml.
Use: Vitamin B supplement.
BEE-T-VITES. (Rugby) Vitamins B_1 15 mg, B_2 10 mg, B_3 100 mg, B_5 20 mg, B_6 5 mg, B_{12} 4 mcg, C 300 mg/Tab. Bot. 100s.
Use: Vitamin supplement.
BEE-TWELVE 1000. (Burgin-Arden) Cyanocobalamin 1000 mcg /ml. Vial 10 ml, 30 ml.
Use: Vitamin B supplement.
BEE-ZEE. (Rugby) Vitamins E 45 mg, B_1 15 mg, B_2 10.2 mg, B_3 100 mg, B_5 25 mg, B_6 10 mg, B_{12} 6 mcg, C 600 mg, zinc 22.5 mg/Tab. Bot. 60s.
Use: Vitamin/mineral supplement.
BEFERRIC. (Kenyon) Ferric ammonium citrate 500 mg, vitamins B_1 12 mg, B_2 6 mg, B_6 0.6 mg, folic acid 0.5 mg, calcium pantothenate 6 mg, niacinamide 15 mg, magnesium 1 mg, cobalt 0.1 mg, zinc 2 mg/fl oz. Bot. 4 oz.
Use: Vitamin/mineral supplement.
BEHEPAN.
See: Vitamin B_{12}.
BELATOL NO. 1; NO. 2. (Cenci) **No. 1:** Belladonna leaf extract 1/8 gr, phenobarbital 0.25 gr/Tab. 100s, 1000s. **No. 2:** Belladonna leaf extract gr, phenobarbital 0.5 gr/Tab. Bot. 100s, 1000s.
Use: Anticholinergic/antispasmodic, sedative/hypnotic.
BELATOL ELIXIR. (Cenci) Phenobarbital 20 mg, belladonna 6.75 min./5 ml w/alcohol 45%. Elix. Bot. pt, gal.
Use: Sedative/hypnotic, anticholinergic/antispasmodic.
BELBUTAL NO. 2 KAPTABS. (Churchill) Phenobarbital 32.4 mg, hyoscyamine sulfate 0.1092 mg, atropine sulfate 0.0215 mg, hyoscine HBr 0.0065 mg/Tab. Bot. 100s.
Use: Sedative/hypnotic, anticholinergic/antispasmodic.
BELDIN. (Blue Cross) Diphenhydramine

HCl 12.5 mg/5 ml w/alcohol 5%. Bot. gal.
Use: Antitussive.
BELEXAL. (Vale) Vitamins B_1 1.5 mg, B_2 2 mg, B_6 0.167 mg, calcium pantothenate 1 mg, niacinamide 10 mg/Tab. w/brewer's yeast. Bot. 1000s, 5000s.
Use: Vitamin supplement.
BELEXON FORTIFIED IMPROVED. (APC) Liver fraction No. 2 3 gr, yeast extract 3 gr, vitamins B_1 5 mg, B_2 6 mg, niacinamide 10 mg, calcium pantothenate 2 mg, cyanocobalamin 1 mcg, iron 10 mg/Cap. Bot. 100s.
Use: Vitamin/mineral supplement.
BELFER. (Forest) Vitamins B_1 2 mg, B_2 2 mg, B_{12} 10 mcg, B_6 2 mg, C 50 mg, iron 17 mg/Tab. Bot. 100s.
Use: Vitamin/mineral supplement.
• **BELFOSDIL.** USAN.
Use: Antihypertensive (calcium channel blocker).
BELGANYL. CDC anti-infective agent.
See: Surmarin.
BELIX ELIXIR. (Blue Cross) Diphenhydramine HCl 12.5 mg/5 ml. Bot. 118 ml.
Use: Antihistamine.
BELLADONNA ALKALOIDS.
Use: Anticholinergic/antispasmodic. W/Combinations.
See: Accelerase-PB, Cap. (Organon).
Belphen Timed Cap. (Robinson).
Coryztime, Cap. (Elder).
Decobel, Lanacap (Lannett).
Fitacol Stankap (Standex).
Nilspasm, Tab. (Parmed).
Ultabs, Tab. (Burlington).
Urised, Tab. (Webcon).
U-Tract, Tab. (Bowman).
Wigraine, Tab., Supp. (Organon).
Wyanoids, Supp. (Wyeth-Ayerst).
BELLADONNA ALKALOIDS W/PHENOBARBITAL. (Various Mfr.) Atropine sulfate 0.0194 mg, scopolamine HBr 0.0065 mg, hyoscyamine HBr or SO_4 0.1037 mg, phenobarbital 16.2 mg/Tab. Bot. 20s, 1000s, UD 100s.
Use: Anticholinergic/antispasmodic, sedative/hypnotic.
• **BELLADONNA EXTRACT,** U.S.P. XXIII. (Lilly) 15 mg (0.187 mg belladonna)/Tab.
Use: Intestinal antispasmodic.
BELLADONNA EXTRACT COMBINATIONS.
Use: Anticholinergic/antispasmodic.
See: Amobell, Cap. (Bock).
Amsodyne, Tab. (Elder).
B & O Supprettes (Webcon).
Belap, Tab. (Lemmon).
Bellafedrol A-H, Tab. (Lannett).

Bellkatal, Tab. (Ferndale).
Butibel, Tab., Elix. (McNeil).
Gelcomul, Liq. (Commerce).
Hycoff Cold, Cap. (Saron).
Lanothal, Pills (Lannett).
Phebe (Western Research).
Rectacort, Supp. (Century).
• **BELLADONNA LEAF,** U.S.P. XXIII.
Use: Intestinal antispasmodic.
W/Phenobarbital and benzocaine.
Use: Anticholinergic.
See: Gastrolic, Tab. (Hauck).
**BELLADONNA PRODUCTS AND PHE-
NOBARBITAL COMBINATIONS.**
Use: Anticholinergic/antispasmodic,
sedative/hypnotic.
See: Accelerase-PB, Cap. (Organon).
Alised, Tab. (Elder).
Atrocap, Cap. (Freeport).
Atrosed, Tab. (Freeport).
Bebatab, Tab. (Freeport).
Belap, Tab., Elix. (Lemmon).
Belatol, Tab., Elix. (Cenci).
Bellergal, Tab., Spacetab. (Dorsey).
Bellkatal, Tab. (Ferndale).
Bellophen, Tab. (Richlyn).
B-Sed, Tab. (Scrip).
Chardonna, Tab. (Rhone-Poulenc
Rorer).
Donabarb, Tab., Elix. (Elder).
Donnafed Jr., Tab. (Jenkins).
Donnatal, Tab., Extentab, Cap., Elix.
(Robins).
Donnatal #2, Tab. (Robins).
Donnazyme, Tab. (Robins).
Gastrolic, Tab. (Hauck).
Hypnaldyne, Tab. (North American
Pharm).
Kinesed, Tab. (Stuart).
Mallenzyme, Tab. (Hauck).
Medi-Spas, Elix. (Medical Chemicals).
Phenobarbital and Belladonna, Tab.
(Lilly).
Sedapar, Tab. (Parmed).
Spabelin, Tab. (Arcum).
Spabelin No. 2, Tab. (Arcum).
Spasnil, Tab. (Rhode).
• **BELLADONNA TINCTURE,** U.S.P. XXIII.
(Lilly) Bot. 4 oz, 16 oz.
Use: Intestinal antispasmodic.
BELLAFEDROL A-H TABLETS. (Lan-
nett) Pyrilamine maleate 12.5 mg, chlor-
pheniramine maleate 1 mg, phenyle-
phrine HCl 2.5 mg, belladonna extract 6
mg/Tab. Bot. 100s, 500s, 1000s.
Use: Antihistamine, decongestant, anti-
cholinergic/antispasmodic.
BELLAFOLINE. (Sandoz) Levorotatory
alkaloids of belladonna. **0.25 mg/Tab.:**
Bot. 100s. **0.5 mg/ml.:** Amp 1 ml.

Use: Anticholinergic/antispasmodic.
BELLANEED. (Hanlon) Belladonna, phenobarbital 16 mg/Cap. Bot. 100s.
Use: Anticholinergic/antispasmodic,
sedative/hypnotic.
BELL/ANS. (C.S. Dent) Sodium bicarbonate 520 mg, sodium content 144
mg/Tab. Bot. 30s, 60s.
Use: Antacid.
BELLASTAL. (Wharton) Atropine sulfate
0.0194 mg, scopolamine HBr 0.0065
mg, hyoscyamine HBr or SO_4 0.1037
mg, phenobarbital 16.2 mg Cap. Bot.
1000s.
Use: Anticholinergic/antispasmodic.
BELLERGAL-S. (Sandoz) Ergotamine
tartrate 0.6 mg, bellafoline 0.2 mg, phe-
nobarbital 40 mg, tartrazine/SR Tab.
Bot. 100s.
Use: Anticholingergic/antispasmodic,
sedative/hypnotic.
• **BELOXAMIDE.** USAN.
Use: Antihyperlipoproteinemic.
BEL-PHEN-ERGOT S. (Goldline) Pheno
barbital 40 mg, ergotamine tartrate 0.6
mg, l-alkaloids of belladonna 0.2 mg.
Tab. Bot. 100s.
BELPHEN TIMED CAPS. (Robinson)
Belladonna alkaloids, phenobarbital.
T.D. Cap. Bot. 100s, 500s, 1000s.
Use: Anticholinergic/antispasmodic,
sedative/hypnotic.
• **BEMARINONE HYDROCHLORIDE.**
USAN.
Use: Cardiotonic (positive inotropic, va-
sodilator).
BEMEGRIDE. B.A.N. 3-Ethyl-3-methyl-
glutarimide.
Use: Medullary respiratory stimulant.
• **BEMESETRON.** USAN.
Use: Antiemetic.
BEMINAL 500. (Wyeth Ayerst) Vitamins
B_1 25 mg, B_2 12.5 mg, niacinamide 100
mg, B_6 10 mg, calcium pantothenate 20
mg, C 500 mg, cyanocobalamin 5
mcg/Tab. Bot. 100s.
Use: Vitamin supplement.
BEMINAL FORTE W/VIT. C. (Wyeth-Ay-
erst) Vitamins B_1 25 mg, B_2 12.5 mg,
niacinamide 50 mg, B_6 3 mg, calcium
pantothenate 10 mg, C 250 mg, B_{12} 2.5
mcg/Cap. Bot. 100s.
Use: Vitamin supplement.
BEMINAL STRESS PLUS IRON. (Wyeth-
Ayerst) Vitamins B_1 25 mg, B_2 12.5 mg,
B_3 100 mg, B_5 20 mg, B_6 10 mg, B_{12} 25
mcg, folic acid 400 mcg, C 700 mg, E 45
IU, iron 27 mg. Dye-free. Tab. Bot. 60s.
Use: Vitamin/mineral supplement.
BEMINAL STRESS PLUS ZINC. (Wyeth-

Ayerst) Vitamins B_1 25 mg, B_2 12.5 mg, B_3 100 mg, B_5 20 mg, B_6 10 mg, B_{12} 25 mcg, C 700 mg, E 45 IU, zinc 45 mg/Tab. Bot. 60s, 250s.
Use: Vitamin/mineral supplement.
●**BEMITRADINE.** USAN.
Use: Antihypertensive, diuretic.
●**BEMORADAN.** USAN.
Use: Cardiotonic.
BENACEN. (Cenci) Probenecid 0.5 Gm/Tab. Bot. 100s, 1000s.
Use: Agent for gout.
BENACOL. (Cenci) Dicyclomine HCl 20 mg/Tab. Bot. 100s, 1000s.
Use: Anticholinergic/antispasmodic.
BENACTYZINE. B.A.N. 2-Diethylaminoethyl benzilate.
Use: Tranquilizer.
BENACTYZINE HYDROCHLORIDE. 2-Diethylaminoethyl benzilate HCl.
Use: Tranquilizer.
W/Meprobamate.
See: Deprol, Tab. (Wallace).
BENACTYZINE/MEPROBAMATE. Psychotherapeutic combination.
See: Deprol (Wallace).
BENA-D-10. (Seatrace) Diphenhydramine HCl 10 mg/ml. Vial 30 ml.
See: Antihistamine.
BENA-D-50. (Seatrace) Diphenhydramine HCl 50 mg/ml. Vial 10 ml.
Use: Antihistamine.
BENADRYL. (Parke-Davis) Diphenhydramine HCl.
Cap.: 25 mg. Bot. 100s, 1000s, UD 100s.
Cream: 1%. Tube 1 oz.
Elix. (w/alcohol 14%): 12.5 mg/5 ml. Bot. 4 oz, pt, gal, UD 5 ml 100s.
Kapseal: 50 mg. Bot. 100s, 1000s, UD 100s.
Spray: 1%. Bot. 2 oz.
Tab.: 25 mg. Bot. 100s.
Use: Antihistamine.
BENADRYL-25 CAPSULES. (Parke-Davis) Diphenhydramine HCl 25 mg/Cap. Box 24s.
Use: Antihistamine.
BENADRYL COLD LIQUID. (Parke-Davis) Pseudoephedrine HCl 10 mg, diphenhydramine HCl 8.3 mg, acetaminophen 167 mg, alcohol 10%, saccharin. Liq. Bot. 180 ml.
Use: Decongestant.
BENADRYL COUGH PREPARATION.
See: Benylin Cough Syrup (Parke-Davis).
BENADRYL DECONGESTANT CAPSULES. (Parke-Davis) Diphenhydramine HCl 25 mg, pseudoephedrine

HCl 60 mg/Cap. Box 24s.
Use: Antihistamine, decongestant.
BENADRYL DECONGESTANT ELIXIR. (Parke-Davis) Diphenhydramine HCl 5 ml, pseudoephedrine HCl 30 mg/5 ml /alcohol 5%. Bot. 4 oz.
Use: Antihistamine, decongestant.
BENADRYL ELIXIR. (Parke-Davis) Diphenhydramine HCl 12.5 mg/5 ml w/alcohol 14%. Bot. 4 oz, pt, gal, UD (5 ml) 100s.
Use: Antihistamine.
BENADRYL INJECTION. (Parke-Davis) Diphenhydramine HCl.
Amp: 50 mg/ml. Amp. 1 ml. Box 10s.
Steri-Dose: 50 mg/ml, pH adjusted w/HCl or sodium hydroxide. Amp. 1 ml. Box 10s. Disposable syringe 1 ml.
Steri-Vial: 10 mg/ml. Phemerol benzethonium Cl as germicidal agent. pH adjusted w/sodium hydroxide or HCl 10 ml, 30 ml. (50 mg/ml) 10 ml.
Use: Antihistamine.
BENADRYL MAXIMUM STRENGTH. (Parke-Davis) **Cream:** Diphenhydramine HCl 2% and parabens in a greaseless base in 15 Gm. **Non-aerosol spray:** Diphenhydramine HCl 2%, alcohol 85% in 60 ml.
Use: Topical antihistamine.
BENADRYL MAXIMUM STRENGTH 2%. (Parke-Davis) **Cream:** Diphenhydramine HCl 2%, parabens. 15 Gm. **Spray, non-aerosol: Diphenhydramine HCl 2%, alcohol 85%. 60 ml.**
Use: Topical antihistamine-containing preparation.
BENADRYL PLUS. (Parke-Davis) Pseudoephedrine 30 mg, diphenhydramine 12.5 mg, acetaminophen 500 mg/Tab. 24s.
Use: Decongestant, antihistamine, analgesic.
BENADRYL PLUS NIGHTTIME. (Parke-Davis). Pseudoephedrine 30 mg, diphenhydramine 25 mg, acetaminophen 500 mg/ 5 ml. 180 ml, 300 ml.
Use: Decongestant, antihistamine, analgesic.
BENAHIST 10. (Keene) Diphenhydramine 10 mg/ml. Vial 30 ml.
Use: Antihistamine.
BENAHIST 50. (Keene) Diphenhydramine 50 mg/ml. Vial 10 ml.
Use: Antihistamine.
BEN-ALLERGIN-50. (Mayrand) Diphenhydramine HCl 50 mg/ml w/chlorobutanol. Inj. Vial 10 ml.
Use: Antihistamine.

BENANEERIN HYDROCHLORIDE. 3-(2-Aminoethyl)-1-benzyl-5-methoxy-2-methylindole HCl.
BENANSERIN HYDROCHLORIDE. 3-(2-Aminoethyl)-1-benzyl-5-methoxy-2-methylindole monohydrochloride.
Use: Serotonin antagonist.
BENAPEN.
See: Benethamine.
BENAPHEN CAPS. (Major) Diphenyhdramine 25 mg or 50 mg/Cap. Bot. 100s, 1000s.
Use: Antihistamine.
BENAPRYZINE. B.A.N. 2-(N-Ethylpropylamino)-ethyl benzilate.
Use: Treatment of Parkinsonism.
• **BENAPRYZINE HYDROCHLORIDE.** USAN.
Use: Anticholinergic.
BEN-AQUA. (Syosset) **Gel:** Benzoyl peroxide 5% or 10% w/polyoxyethylene laurylether. Tube 45 Gm, 120 Gm.
Use: Anti-acne.
BENASE. (Ferndale) Proteolytic enzymes extracted from Carica papaya 20,000 units enzyme activity. Tab. Bot. 1000s.
Use: Reduction of edema, relief of episiotomy.
BENAT-12. (Hauck) Cyanocobalamin 30 mcg, liver injection 0.5 ml, vitamins B_1 10 mg, B_2 2 mg, niacinamide 50 mg, d-panthenol 1 mg, B_6 1 mg/ml, benzyl alcohol 4%, phenol 0.5%. Vial 10 ml.
Use: Vitamin/mineral supplement.
• **BENAZEPRIL HYDROCHLORIDE.** USAN.
Use: ACE inhibitor.
See: Lotensin (Ciba-Geigy).
• **BENAZEPRILAT.** USAN.
Use: ACE inhibitor.
• **BENDACALOL MESYLATE.** USAN.
Use: Antihypertensive.
• **BENDAZAC.** USAN. [I-Benzyl-(H-indazol-3yl)oxy] acetic acid.
Use: Anti-inflammatory.
BENDROFLUAZIDE. B.A.N. 3-Benzyl-3,4-dihydro-6-trifluoromethylbenzo-1,2,4-thiadiazine-7-sulfonamide 1,1-dioxide. Bendroflumethiazide (I.N.N.).
Use: Diuretic.
• **BENDROFLUMETHIAZIDE,** U.S.P. XXIII. Tab., U.S.P. XXIII. 3-Benzyl-3:4-dihydro-7-sulphamoly-6-tri-fluoromethylbenzo-1:2:4-thiadiazine 1:1-dioxide. 6-(Trifluoromethyl)-2H-1,2,4-benzothiadiazine-7-sulfonamide 1, 1-dioxide.
Use: Diuretic, antihypertensive.
See: Naturetin, Tab. (Squibb).
W/Potassium Cl.

See: Naturetin W-K, Tab. (Squibb).
W/Rauwolfia serpentina.
See: Rauzide, Tab.
W/Rauwolfia serpentina, potassium Cl.
See: Rautrax-N, Tab. (Squibb).
Rautrax-N Modified, Tab. (Squibb).
BENEMID. (Merck & Co.) Probenecid 0.5 Gm/Tab. Bot. 100s, 1000s, UD 100s.
Use: Agent for gout.
W/Colchicine.
See: Colbenemid, Tab. (Merck & Co.).
BENEPHEN ANTISEPTIC MEDICATED POWDER. (Halsted) Methylbenzethonium Cl 1:1800, magnesium carbonate in cornstarch base. Shaker can 3.56 oz.
Use: Deodorant, antiseptic.
BENEPHEN ANTISEPTIC OINTMENT W/COD LIVER OIL. (Halsted) Methylbenzethonium Cl 1:1000, water-repellent base of zinc oxide, cornstarch. Tube 1.5 oz, jar lb.
Use: Antiseptic.
BENEPHEN ANTISEPTIC VITAMIN A & D CREAM. (Halsted) Methylbenzethonium Cl 1:1000, cod liver oil w/vitamins A and D in petrolatum and glycerin base. Tube 2 oz, jar lb.
Use: Antiseptic.
BENEPRO TABS. (Major) Probenecid 500 mg/Tab. Bot. 100s, 1000s.
Use: Agent for gout.
BENETHAMINE PENICILLIN. B.A.N. N-Benzyl-phenethylammonium 6-phenylacetamidopenicillanate. N-Benzylphenethylamine salt of benzylpenicillin.
Use: Antibiotic.
BENGAL GELATIN.
See: Agar.
BEN-GAY CHILDREN'S VAPORIZING RUB. (Leeming) Camphor, menthol, w/oils of turpentine, eucalyptus, cedar leaf, nutmeg, thyme in stainless white base. Jar 1.125 oz.
Use: External analgesic.
BEN-GAY EXTRA STRENGTH BALM. (Leeming) Methylsalicylate 30%, menthol 8%. Jar 3.75 oz.
Use: External analgesic.
BEN-GAY EXTRA STRENGTH SPORTS BALM. (Leeming) Methylsalicylate 28%, menthol 10%. Tube 1.25 oz, 3 oz.
Use: External analgesic.
BEN-GAY GEL. (Leeming) Methylsalicylate 15%, menthol 7%, alcohol 40%. Tube 1.25 oz, 3 oz.
Use: External analgesic.
BEN-GAY GREASELESS OINTMENT. (Leeming) Methylsalicylate 18.3%, menthol 16%. Tube 1.25 oz, 3 oz, 5 oz.

Use: External analgesic.
BEN-GAY LOTION. (Leeming) Methylsalicylate 15%, menthol 7% in lotion base. Bot. 2 oz, 4 oz.
Use: External analgesic.
BEN-GAY ORIGINAL. (Leeming) Methyl salicylate 18.3% and menthol 16%. Oint. Tube. 37.5 Gm, 90 Gm, 150 Gm.
Use: Topical analgesic.
BEN-GAY OINTMENT. (Leeming) Methylsalicylate 15%, menthol 10% in ointment base. Tube 1.25 oz, 3 oz, 5 oz.
Use: External analgesic.
BEN-GAY SPORTSGEL. (Leeming) Methylsalicylate, menthol, alcohol 40%. Tube 1.25 oz, 3 oz.
Use: External analgesic.
BENOJECT. (Mayrand) Diphenhydramine HCl 50 mg/ml. Vial 10 ml.
Use: Antihistamine, anticholinergic.
BENOQUIN. (Elder) Monobenzone 20% in cream base. Tube 35 Gm, 453.6 Gm.
Use: Treatment of vitiligo.
BENORAL CAPSULES. (Sanofi Winthrop) Benorylate.
Use: Analgesic, antipyretic.
BENORAL SUSPENSION. (Sanofi Winthrop) Benorylate.
Use: Analgesic, antipyretic.
BENORAL TABLETS. (Sanofi Winthrop) Benorylate.
Use: Analgesic, antipyretic.
•**BENORTERONE.** USAN. 17 β-Hydroxy-17- methyl-β-norandrost-4-en-3-one.
Use: Antiandrogen.
BENORYLATE. B.A.N. 4-Acetamidophenyl O-acetylsalicylate.
Use: Analgesic.
•**BENOXAPROFEN.** USAN. 2-(2-p-Chlorophenyl-benzoxazol-5-yl)propionic acid.
Use: Anti-inflammatory, analgesic.
•**BENOXINATE HYDROCHLORIDE,** U.S.P. XXIII. Ophth. Soln., U.S.P. XXIII. 2-(Diethylaminoethyl)4-amino-3-butoxybenzoate HCl.
Use: Ophth. anesthesia.
See: Fluress (Pilkington Barnes-Hind).
BENOXYL LOTION. (Stiefel) Benzoyl peroxide 5% or 10% in mild lotion base. Bot. 1 oz, 2 oz.
Use: Anti-acne.
•**BENPERIDOL.** USAN. 1-[fb]1-[3-(4-Fluorobenzoyl)-propyl]-4-piperidylbenzimidazolin-2-one.
Use: Tranquilizer.
See: Anquil.
•**BENSALAN.** USAN. 3,5-Dibromo-N-(p-bromobenzyl)salicylamide. Under study.

Use: Germicide.
•**BENSERAZIDE.** USAN. DL-2-Amino-3-hydroxy-2'-(2,3,4-trihydroxybenzyl)propionohydrazide.
Use: Treatment of Parkinson's disease.
BENSULFOID. (E.C. Robins/Poythress) Colloidal sulfur 33%.
Use: Prescription compounding.
W/Phenobarbital.
See: Solfoton, Tab. or Cap. (Poythress).
BENSULFOID CREAM. (E.C. Robins/Poythress) Sulfur 8%, resorcinol 2%, alcohol 10%. 15 Gm.
Use: Anti-acne.
•**BENTAZEPAM.** USAN.
Use: Sedative.
BENTICAL. (Lamond) Bentonite, zinc oxide, zinc carbonate, titanium dioxide. Bot. 4 oz, 6 oz, 8 oz, 16 oz, 32 oz, 0.5 gal, gal.
Use: Bland lotion.
•**BENTIROMIDE.** USAN.
Use: Diagnostic aid.
See: Chymex, Soln. (Adria).
•**BENTONITE,** N.F. XVIII.
Use: Pharmaceutical aid (suspending agent).
•**BENTONITE MAGMA,** N.F. XVIII.
Use: Pharmaceutical aid (suspending agent).
•**BENTONITE, PURIFIED,** N.F. XVIII.
Use: Pharmaceutical aid.
BENTRAC 25, 50. (Kenyon) Diphenhydramine HCl 25 mg or 50 mg/Cap. Bot. 100s.
Use: Antihistamine.
BENTRAC-ELIXIR. (Kenyon) Diphenhydramine HCl 10 mg/4 ml. Alcohol 14%. Bot. 4 oz.
Use: Antihistamine.
BENTRAC EXPECTORANT. (Kenyon) Diphenhydramine HCl 80 mg, ammonium Cl 12 gr, sodium citrate 5 gr, chloroform 2 gr, menthol 1/10 gr, alcohol 5%/fl oz. Bot. 4 oz.
Use: Antitussive, expectorant.
BENTYL. (Lakeside) Dicyclomine HCl.
Cap.: 10 mg. Bot. 100s, 500s, UD 100s.
Tab.: 20 mg. Bot. 100s, 500s, 1000s, UD 100s. **Syr.:** 10 mg/5 ml. Bot. pt. **Inj.:** 10 mg/ml. Amp. 2 ml, syringe 2 ml. Vial 10 ml (also contains chlorobutanol).
Use: Anticholinergic/antispasmodic.
•**BENURESTAT.** USAN.
Use: Enzyme inhibitor.
BENYLIN COUGH SYRUP. (Parke-Davis) Diphenhydramine HCl 12.5 mg, alcohol 5%. Bot. 4 oz, 8 oz, UD 5 ml, 10 ml. Box 100s.
Use: Antitussive.

BENYLIN DECONGESTANT LIQUID.
(Parke-Davis) Pseudoephedrine HCl 30
mg, diphenhydramine HCl 12.5 mg, al-
cohol 5%, saccharin. Bot. 120 ml.
Use: Decongestant, antihistamine.
BENYLIN DM COUGH SYRUP. (Parke-
Davis) Dextromethorphan HBr 10 mg/5
ml, alcohol 5%. Bot. 4 oz, 8 oz.
Use: Antitussive.
BENYLIN DME. (Parke-Davis) **Liq.:** Dex-
tromethorphan HBr 5 mg, guaifenesin
100 mg, alcohol 5%, saccharin, men-
thol. Bot. 240 ml.
Use: Antitussive, expectorant.
BENYLIN EXPECTORANT LIQUID.
(Warner-Lambert) Dextromethorphan
HBr 5 mg, guaifenesin 100 mg, alcohol
5%, saccharin, menthol, sucrose. Bot.
Liq. 118, 236 ml.
Use: Antitussive, expectorant.
BENZA. (Century) Benzalkonium Cl
1:5000 and 1:750. Bot. 2 oz, 4 oz.
Use: Antiseptic, germicide.
BENZAC 5 & 10. (Owen/Galderma) Ben-
zoyl peroxide 5% or 10% w/polyoxyeth-
ylene lauryl ether 6%, alcohol 12%.
Tube 60 Gm, 90 Gm.
Use: Anti-acne.
BENZAC w 2.5, 5 & 10. (Owen/Galder-
ma) Benzoyl peroxide **2.5%:** Tube 60
Gm, 90 Gm; **5%:** Tube 60 Gm or **10%:**
Tube 60 Gm, gel in water base w/car-
bomer 940.
Use: Anti-acne.
BENZAC AC. (Owen/Galderma) Benzoyl
peroxide 2.5%, 5% or 10% and EDTA in
water base. Gel. Tube. 60 Gm.
Use: Anti-acne.
BENZAC AC WASH. (Owen/Galderma)
Benzoyl peroxide 2.5%, 5%, 10%, glyc-
erin, carbomer 940. Liq. Bot. 240 ml.
Use: Anti-acne.
BENZAC w WASH. (Owen/Galderma)
Benzoyl peroxide 5% or 10% in vehicle
of sodium C14-16 olefin sulfonate, car-
bomer 940, purified water. **5%:** Bot. 4 oz,
8 oz. **10%:** Bot. 8 oz.
Use: Anti-acne.
BENZAGEL. (Dermik) Benzoyl peroxide
5% or 10% in gel base of water, car-
bomer 940, alcohol 14%, sodium hy-
droxide, docusate sodium, fragrance.
Tube 1.5 oz, 3 oz.
Use: Anti-acne.
• **BENZALDEHYDE,** N.F. XVIII. Cpd. Elix.,
N.F. XVIII.
Use: Pharmaceutic aid (flavor).
• **BENZALKONIUM CHLORIDE,** N.F. XVI-
II. Soln., N.F. XVIII. Alkyldimethylbenzy-
lammonium Cl. Zephirol. Soln. 1:5000.

ammonium, alkyldimethyl(phenyl-
methyl)-, Cl.
Use: Surface antiseptic, antimicrobial
preservative.
See: Benz-All, Liq. (Xytrium).
Econopred, Susp. (Alcon).
Eye-Stream (Alcon).
Germicin, Soln. (Consolidated Mid.).
Hyamine 3500 (Rohm & Haas).
Otrivin Spray (Geigy).
Ultra Tears (Alcon).
Zalkon Conc., Liq. (Gordon).
Zephiran Chloride Preps. (Sanofi
Winthrop).
W/Aluminum Cl, oxyquinoline sulfate.
See: Alochor Styptic, Liq. (Gordon).
W/Bacitracin zinc, polymyxin B, neomycin
sulfate.
See: Biotres, Oint. (Central).
W/Benzocaine, benzyl alcohol.
See: Aerocain, Oint. (Aeroceuticals).
W/Benzocaine, orthohydroxyphenyl-mer-
curic Cl, parachlorometaxylenol.
See: Unguentine, Aerosol (Norwich).
W/Berberine HCl, sodium borate, phenyle-
phrine HCl, sodium Cl, boric acid.
See: Ocusol, Eye Lotion, Drops (Nor-
wich).
W/Boric acid, potassium Cl, sodium car-
bonate anhydrous, disodium edetate.
See: Swim-Eye, Drops (Savage).
W/Chlorophyll.
See: Mycomist, Spray Liq. (Gordon).
W/Hydrocortisone.
See: Barseb Thera-Spray, Soln.
(Barnes-Hind).
W/Diperodon HCl, carbolic acid, ichtham-
mol, thymol, camphor, juniper tar.
See: Boro Oint. (Scrip).
W/Disodium edetate, potassium Cl, isoton-
ic boric acid.
See: Dacriose (Smith, Miller & Patch).
W/Epinephrine.
See: Epinal, Soln. (Alcon).
W/Epinephrine bitartrate, pilocarpine HCl,
mannitol.
See: E-Pilo Ophth., Preps. (Smith,
Miller & Patch).
W/Ethoxylated lanolin, methylparaben,
hamamelis water, glycerin.
See: Mediconet, clothwipes.
(Medicone).
W/Gentamicin sulfate, disodium phos-
phate, monosodium, phosphate, sodium
Cl.
See: Garamycin Ophth. Soln., Preps.
(Schering).
W/Hydroxypropyl methylcellulose.
See: Isopto Plain & Tears (Alcon).
W/Hydroxypropyl methylcellulose, disodi-

um edetate.
See: Goniosol (Smith, Miller & Patch).
W/Isopropyl alcohol, methyl salicylate.
See: Cydonol Massage Lotion (Gordon).
W/Lidocaine, phenol.
See: Unguentine, spray (Norwich).
W/Methylcellulose.
See: Tearisol (Smith, Miller & Patch).
W/Methylcellulose, phenylephrine HCl.
See: Efricel % (Professional Pharmacal).
W/Oxyquinolin sulfate, distilled water.
See: Oxyzal Wet Dressing, Soln. (Gordon).
W/Phenylephrine, pyrilamine maleate, antipyrine.
See: Prefrin-A, Ophth. (Allergan).
W/Pilocarpine HCl, epinephrine bitartrate, mannitol.
See: E-Pilo Ophth., Preps. (Smith, Miller & Patch).
W/Polymyxin B, neomycin sulfate, zinc bacitracin.
See: Biotres, Oint. (Central).
W/Polyoxyethylene ethers.
See: Ionax, Aerosol Can (Owen/Galderma).
W/Polyvinyl alcohol.
See: Contique Artificial Tears (Alcon).
W/Pramoxine HCl, allantoin.
See: Perifoam, Aerosol (Solvay).
W/Pramoxine HCl, hydrocortisone, parachlorometaxylenol, acetic acid.
See: My Cort Otic #2, Ear Drops (Scrip).
Steramine Otic, Drops. (Mayrand).
W/Pramoxine HCl, hydrocortisone, parachlorometaxylenol, acetic acid, propylene glycol.
See: Otostan H.C. (Standex).
W/Pyrilamine maleate, pheniramine maleate, chlorpheniramine maleate, menthol.
See: Trigelamine, Oint. (E.J. Moore).
W/Sodium borate, sodium bicarbonate, sodium Cl.
See: Zalkon Wet Dressing, Liq. (Gordon).
W/Tripelennamine HCl, methapyrilene.
See: Didelamine, Cream (Commerce).
W/Zinc oxide, urea, sulfur, salicylic acid, isopropyl alcohol in a base containing menthol, silicon dioxide, iron oxide and perfume.
See: Akne Drying Lotion, Bot. (Alto).
BENZ-ALL. (Xttrium) Benzalkonium Cl 12.9%. Bot. 10 ml, 40 ml. 15s.
Use: Germicidal concentrate with anti-rust factor.

BENZALOIDS. (Jenkins) Benzocaine 5 mg, cal. iodized 12 mg, eucalyptol 0.35 mg, methenamine 6.5 mg, menthol 0.2 mg/Loz. Bot. 1000s.
BENZAMYCIN TOPICAL GEL. (Dermik) Erythromycin 3%, benzoyl peroxide 5%. Jar 23.3 Gm.
Use: Anti-acne.
BENZASHAVE. (Medicis) Benzoyl peroxide 5% or 10%, with mineral oil, triethanolamine, diisopropyl dimerate, PEG-15, cocamine, carbomer 940, aloe vera, diazolidinyl urea, parabens. Tube. Shaving cream. 113.4 Gm.
Use: Anti-acne and treatment of ingrown hair.
BENZATHINE PENICILLIN. B.A.N. NN'-Dibenzylethylenedi(ammonium 6-phenylacetamido-penicillanate). NN-Dibenzylethylenediamine di-(benzylpenicillin).
Use: Antibiotic.
• **BENZATHINE PENICILLIN G,** U.S.P. XXIII. Oral Susp. Sterile, Tab., U.S.P. XXIII. N,N'-Dibenzylethylenediamine di(benzylpenicillin) Benzethacil. 3,3-Dimethyl-7-oxo-6-(2-phenylacetamido)-4-thia-1-azabicyclo [3.2.0] heptaine-2-carboxylic acid compound with N,N-Dibenzylethylene-diamine (2:1). Dibencil, Penidural.
Use: Antibiotic.
See: Permapen, Disp. Syringe (Roerig). Isoject Permapen, Aq. Susp. (Pfizer).
W/Procaine penicillin G.
See: Bicillin P.A.B., Disp. Syr. (Wyeth-Ayerst).
BENZAZOLINE HYDROCHLORIDE.
See: Tolazoline HCl.
• **BENZBROMARONE.** USAN.
Use: Uricosuric.
BENZCHLORPROPAMID.
Used in Europe under:
Nydrane.
Posedrine.
BENZ-EASE. (Novocol) Benzocaine, oil of clove, oxyquinoline benzoate. Oint. Tube 0.25 oz, 6s, 36s.
Use: Anesthetic, antiseptic, adhesive.
BENZEDREX INHALER. (SK-Beecham) Propylhexedrine 250 mg, menthol and lavender oil. Single plastic tube 12s.
Use: Nasal decongestant.
BENZEHIST. (Pharmex) Diphenhydramine HCl 10 mg/ml. Vial 30 ml.
Use: Antihistamine.
BENZENE HEXACHLORIDE, GAMMA.
See: Lindane U.S.P. XXIII.
BENZESTROL. 4,4'-(1,2-Diethyl-3-methyltrimethylene) diphenol.

BENZETHACIL. Dibenzylethylenedi-
amine dipenicillin G DBED.
See: Penicillin G Benzathine, U.S.P.
XXIII.
BENZETHIDINE. B.A.N. Ethyl 1-(2-ben-
zyloxyethyl)-4-phenylpiperidine-1-car-
boxylate.
Use: Narcotic analgesic.
•**BENZETHONIUM CHLORIDE,** U.S.P.
XXIII. Tincture, Topical Soln., U.S.P.
XXIII. Benzyldimethyl [2-[2-[p-(1,1,3,3-
tetramethylbutyl)phenoxy]ethoxy]ethyl]a
mmonium Cl.
Use: Surface antiseptic, antimicrobial
preservative.
See: Ammorid Diaper Rinse, Oint. (Kin-
ney).
Hyacide, Soln. (Niltig).
Hyamine 1622 (Rohm & Haas).
Phemerol Chloride, Soln., Tr. (Parke-
Davis).
Phemithyn, Liq. (Davis & Sly).
W/Benzocaine.
See: Americaine, Oint., Aerosol (Arnar-
Stone).
Dermoplast, Spray (Wyeth-Ayerst).
W/Nonyl phenoxypolyoxyethylene ethanol.
See: Dalkon Foam (Robins).
Emko Pre-Fil, Foam (Emko).
W/Zinc oxide.
See: Ammorid, Oint. (Kinney).
BENZETHONIUM CHLORIDE. B.A.N.
Benzyldimethyl-2-[fb]2-[4-(1,1,3,3-
tetramethylbutyl)-phenoxy]ethoxyethy-
lammonium Cl.
Use: Antibacterial.
•**BENZETIMIDE HYDROCHLORIDE.**
USAN. (1)2-(I-Benzyl-4-piperidyl)-2-
phenylglutarimide monohydrochloride.
Use: Anticholinergic.
BENZHEXOL. B.A.N. 1-Cyclohexyl-1-
phenyl-3- piperidinopropan-1-ol. Tri-
hexyphenidyl (I.N.N.).
Use: Treatment of Parkinson's disease.
**alpha-BENZHYDROL HYDROCHLO-
RIDE.** Diphenylhydroxy-carbinol.
BENZIDE. (Canright) Benzthiazide 50
mg/Tab. Bot. 100s, 1000s.
Use: Diuretic, antihypertensive.
•**BENZILONIUM BROMIDE.** USAN. 1-Eth-
yl-3-pyrrolidinyl benzilate ethylbromide.
Use: Anticholinergic.
BENZILONIUM BROMIDE. B.A.N. 3-
Benziloyloxy-1, 1-diethylpyrrolidinium
bromide.
Use: Inhibition of gastric secretion.
BENZINDAMINE HYDROCHLORIDE.
Benzydamine hydrochloride.
•**BENZINDOPYRINE HYDROCHLORIDE.**
USAN. 1-Benzyl-3-[2-(4-pyridyl)-ethyl]

indole HCl. Pyrbenzindole.
Use: Tranquilizer.
BENZIODARONE. B.A.N. 2-Ethyl-3-4-hy-
droxy-3,5-di-iodobenzoyl-benzofuran.
Use: Coronary vasodilator.
BENZOATE AND PHEYLACETATE.
USAN.
Use: Treatment of hyperammonemia.
[Orphan drug]
BENZO-C. (Freeport) Benzocaine 5 mg,
cetalkonium Cl 5 mg, ascorbic acid 50
mg/Troche. Bot. 1000s, cello-packed
boxes 1000s.
Use: Local anesthetic.
•**BENZOCAINE,** U.S.P. XXIII. Cream,
Oint., Otic Soln., Topical Aerosol, Topical
Soln., U.S.P. XXIII. Ethyl-p-aminoben-
zoate. Anesthesin, orthesin, parathesin.
Use: Local anesthetic.
See: BanSmoke, Gum (Thompson).
W/Combinations.
See: Aerotherm, Oint. (Aeroceuticals).
Aerocaine, Oint. (Aeroceuticals).
Americaine, Oint., Aerosol (American
Critical Care).
Anacaine, Oint. (Gordon).
Anecal, Cream (Lannett).
Aura-Aid, Liq. (E.J. Moore).
Auralgan, Otic Drops (Wyeth-Ayerst).
Auralgesic, Liq. (Elder).
Benadex, Oint. (Fuller).
Benzo-C, Troche (Freeport).
Benzocol, Oint. (Hauck).
Benzodent, Oint. (Vicks).
Biscolan, Supp. (Lannett).
Boilaid, Oint. (E.J. Moore).
Bonal Itch Cream, Cream (E.J.
Moore).
Bowman Drawing Paste, Oint. (Bow-
man).
Boil-Ease Anesthetic Drawing Salve
(Commerce).
Burn Gon, Oint. (E.J. Moore).
20-Cain Burn Relief, (Alto).
Calamatum, Preps. (Blair).
Cpacol, Troches (Merrell Dow).
Cetacaine, Preps. (Cetylite).
Chiggerex, Oint. (Scherer).
Chiggertox, Liq. (Scherer).
Chloraseptic Children's Lozenges
(Norwich Eaton).
CPI Hemorrhoidal, Supp. (Century).
Culminal, Cream (Culminal).
D.D.D. Cream (Campana).
Dent's Dental Poultice (C.S. Dent).
Dent's Lotion, Jel (C.S. Dent).
Dent's Toothache Gum (C.S. Dent).
Derma Medicone (Medicone).
Derma Medicone-HC (Medicone).
Dermoplast, Spray (Wyeth-Ayerst).

Detane, Gel (Del).
Diplan, Cap. (Solvay).
Dulzit, Cream (Commerce).
Epinephricaine, Oint. (Upjohn).
Erase, Supp. (LaCrosse).
E.R.O. Forte, Liq. (Scherer).
Extend, Tab. (E.J. Moore).
Foille, Preps. (Carbisulphoil).
Formula 44 Cough Control Discs, Loz.
(Vicks).
Fung-O-Spray (Scrip).
G.B.A. Drops (Scrip).
Hemocaine, Oint. (Hauck).
Hurricaine, Liq. or Gel (Beutlich).
Isodettes Loz. (SK-Beecham).
Jiffy, Drops (Block Drug).
Kanalka, Tab. (Lannett).
Kankex, Liq. (E.J. Moore).
Lanaurine, Drop. (Lannett).
Lanazets, Loz. (Lannett).
Listerine Cough Control Lozenges
(Warner-Lambert).
Medicone Dressing (Medicone).
Meditrating Throat Lozenge, Loz.
(Vicks).
My-Cort Drops (Scrip).
Myringacaine, Liq. (Upjohn).
Nilatus, Loz. (Bowman).
Off-Ezy Corn Remover, Liq. (Com-
merce).
Oracin, Loz. (Vicks).
Oradex-C, Troche (Commerce).
Ora-Jel, Gel. (Commerce).
Pain-Eze, Oint. (E.J. Moore).
Pazo, Oint., Supp. (Bristol-Myers).
Pyrogallic Acid Oint. (Gordon).
Rectal Medicone (Medicone).
Rectal Medicone-HC, Supp.
(Medicone).
Rectal Medicone Unguent (Medicone).
Ridupois Capsule (Elder).
Rite-Diet, Cap. (E.J. Moore).
Robitussets, Troche (Robins).
Salicide, Oint. (Gordon).
Scrip, Preps. (Scrip).
Sepo, Loz. (Otis Clapp).
Solarcaine, Lot. (Schering).
Soretts, Loz. (Lannett).
Spec-T Sore Throat-Cough Suppres-
sant Loz. (Squibb).
Spec-T Sore Throat-Decongestant
Loz. (Squibb).
Sucrets Cold Decongestant Lozenge
(Calgon).
Sucrets Cough Control Lozenge (Cal-
gon).
Tanac, Liq. (Commerce).
Tympagesic, Liq. (Adria).
Tyro-Loz, Loz. (Kenyon).
Unguentine Aerosol (Norwich).

Vicks Cough Silencers, Loz. (Vicks).
Vicks Formula 44 Cough Control
Discs, Loz. (Vicks).
Vicks Medi-Trating Throat Lozenges,
Loz. (Vicks).
Vicks Oracin, Loz. (Vicks).
BENZOCHLOROPHENE SODIUM. The
sodium salt of ortho-benzyl-para-
chlorophenol.
BENZOCOL. (Hauck) Benzocaine 5%.
Tube Cream. Bot. 30 Gm. Jar lb.
Use: Local anesthetic.
BENZOCTAMINE. B.A.N. N-Methyl-9,10-
ethanoanthracene-9(10H)-methylamine.
Use: Tranquilizer.
• **BENZOCTAMINE HYDROCHLORIDE.**
USAN. N-Methyl-9,10-ethanoan-
thracene-9(10H)-methylamine HCl.
Use: Muscle relaxant, sedative.
BENZODENT. (Vicks Products) Benzo-
caine 20%, eugenol 0.4%, hydrox-
yquinoline sulfate 0.1% in an adhesive
ointment base. Tube 0.25 oz, 1 oz.
Use: Local anesthetic.
BENZODEPA. USAN.
Benzyl[bis(aziridinyl)-phosphinyl] carba-
mate.
Use: Antineoplastic.
BENZOIC ACID. (Various Mfr.) Pkg. 0.25
lb, 1 lb.
Use: Fungistatic, fungicidal.
W/Boric acid, zinc oxide, zinc stearate.
See: Ting, Cream, Pow. (Pharmacraft).
W/Salicylic acid.
See: Whitfield's Oint. (Various Mfr.).
BENZOIC ACID, 2-HYDROXY. Salicylic
Acid, U.S.P. XXIII.
• **BENZOIC AND SALICYLIC ACIDS OINT-
MENT,** U.S.P. XXIII.
Use: Antifungal (topical).
See: Whitfield's Oint. (Various Mfr.).
• **BENZOIN,** U.S.P. XXIII. Tincture, Com-
pound, U.S.P. XXIII.
Use: Topical protectant, expectorant.
See: Arcum—Bot. 2 oz, 4 oz, pt, gal.
Lilly—Bot. 4 fl oz, pt.
Rals—Aerosol 12 oz.
Stanlabs—Bot. 2 oz, 4 oz, pt, Com-
pound. Bot. 1 oz, 4 oz, pt.
W/Methyl salicylate, guaiacol.
See: Methagul, Oint. (Gordon).
W/Podophyllum resin.
See: Podoben, Liq. (Maurry).
W/Polyoxyethylene dodecanol, aromatics.
See: Vicks Vaposteam, Liq. (Vicks).
BENZOIN SPRAY. (Morton) Benzoin, tolu
balsam, styrax, alcohol w/propellant.
Aerosol can 7 oz.
Use: Skin protectant.
BENZOL. Usually refers to benzene.

BENZO-MENTH TABLETS. (Vale) Benzocaine 2.2 mg/Tab. Bot. 1000s.
Use: Topical anesthetic.
• **BENZONATATE,** U.S.P. XXIII. Cap., U.S.P. XXIII. [go]-Meth-oxypoly-(ethyleneoxy)ethyl-p-butylaminobenzoate. 2,5,8,11,14,17,20,23,26-Nonaoxaoctacosan-28-yl p-(butylamino)benzoate. B.A.N.: 3,6,9,12,15,18,21,24,27-nonaoxaoctacosyl 4-N-butylaminobenzoate.
Use: Cough suppressant.
See: Tessalon, Perles (DuPont).
BENZONATATE SOFTGELS. (Various Mfr.) Benzonatate 100 mg. Cap. Bot. 100s, 1000s.
Use: Cough suppressant.
BENZOPHENONE.
See: Pan Ultra, Lot., Lipstick (Cummins).
W/Oxybenzone, dioxybenzone.
See: Solbar Lotion (Person & Covey).
BENZOPYRROLATE.
See: Benzopyrronium.
BENZOQUINOLIMINE.
See: Emete-Con (Pfizer).
BENZOQUINONIUM CHLORIDE.
Use: Skeletal muscle relaxant (No mfr. listed).
BENZOSULFIMIDE.
See: Saccharin, U.S.P. XXIII.
BENZOSULPHINIDE SODIUM. Name previously used for Saccharin Sodium.
• **BENZOXIQUINE.** USAN.
Use: Disinfectant.
BENZOYL p-AMINOSALICYLIC.
See: Benzapas, Pow., Tab. (Dorsey).
BENZOYLPAS CALCIUM. Benzoic acid, 4-(benzoylamino)-2-hydroxy-calcium salt (2:1), pentahydrate. Calcium 4-benzamidosalicylate (1:2) pentahydrate.
Use: Antitubercular.
See: Benzapas, Tab., Pow. (Dorsey).
• **BENZOYL PEROXIDE, HYDROUS,** U.S.P. XXIII. Gel., Lot., U.S.P. XXIII. Peroxide, dibenzoyl.
Use: Keratolytic.
See: Benzagel-5 & 10, Oint. (Dermik).
Benoxyl, Lot. (Stiefel)
Benzac AC, Gel, Liq. (Owen/Galderma).
Brevoxyl, Gel (Stiefel).
Clearasil Acne Treatment, Cream (Vicks).
Clearasil Antibacterial Acne Lotion (Vicks).
Dermoxyl, Gel (ICN).
Epi-Clear Antiseptic Lotion, Scrub (Squibb).
Exact, Cream (Premier).
Oxy-5 Acne Pimple Medication (SK-

Beecham).
Oxy-10 Maximum Strength Acne-Pimple Medication (SK-Beecham).
Oxy Wash Antibacterial Skin Wash (SK-Beecham).
Panoxyl, Bar (Stiefel).
Peroxin A5, A10, Gel (Dermol).
Persadox, Cream, Lot. (Ortho).
Persadox HP, Cream, Lot. (Owen/Galderma).
Persa-Gel, Gel (Ortho).
Theroxide, Liq., Lot. (Medicis).
Topex, Lot. (Vicks).
W/Chlorhydroxyquinoline, hydrocortisone.
See: Loroxide-HC, Lot. (Dermik).
Vanoxide-I IC, Lot. (Dermik).
W/Polyoxyethylene lauryl ether.
See: Benzac 5 & 10, Gel (Owen/Galderma).
Desquam-X, Gel (Westwood).
W/Sulfur.
See: Sulfoxyl Lotion (Stiefel).
N'-BENZOYLSULFANILAMIDE.
See: Sulfabenzamide.
W/Sulfacetamide, sulfathiazole, urea.
See: Sultrin, Tab, Cream (Ortho).
BENZPHETAMINE HYDROCHLORIDE.
N-Benzyl-N-α-dimethylphenethylamine HCl, dextro.
Use: Anorexiant.
See: Didrex, Tab. (Upjohn).
BENZPYRINIUM BROMIDE. 1-Benzyl-3-hydroxypyridinium bromide dimethylcarbamate.
• **BENZQUINAMIDE.** USAN. B.A.N. N,N-diethyl-1,3,4,6,7,11b-hexahydro-2-hydroxy-9,10-dimethoxy-2H-benzo[a]quinolizine-3-carboxamide acetate.
Use: Antiemetic agent.
See: Emete-Con, Vial (Roerig).
Quantril (Roerig).
BENZQUINAMIDE HYDROCHLORIDE.
See: Emete-Con. (Roerig).
BENZTHIANIDE. 3-Benzylthiomethyl-6-chloro-7-sulfamyl-2H-1,2,4-benzothiadiazine-1,1-di-oxide. Urease.
• **BENZTHIAZIDE,** U.S.P. XXIII. Tabs , U.S.P. XXIII. B.A.N. 3-Benzylthiomethyl-6-chloro-7-sulfamyl-1,2,4-benzothiadiazine 1,1-dioxide. 3-((benzylthio)-methyl)-6-chloro-2H-1,2,4,benzothiadiazine-7-sulfonamide 1,1-dioxide. 6-chloro-3[(phenylmethyl) thio] methyl - 2H-1,2,4, benzothiadiazine-7-sulfonamide 1,1-dioxide.
Use: Diuretic, antihypertensive.
See: Aquatag, Tab. (Solvay).
Exna, Tab. (Robins).
Hydrex, Tab. (Trimen).

Proaqua, Tab. (Solvay).
Urazide, Tab. (Hauck).
W/Reserpine.
See: Exna-R, Tab. (Robins).
BENZTROPINE. B.A.N. 3-Benzhydry-
loxytropane.
Use: Treatment of Parkinson's disease.
• **BENZTROPINE MESYLATE,** U.S.P. XXI-
II., Inj., Tab., U.S.P. XXIII., Methanesul-
fonate, 3α-(Diphenylmethoxy)-
1αH,5αH-tropane methanesulfonate.
Use: Parasympatholytic, antiparkinson-
ism.
W/sodium Cl.
See: Cogentin, Tab., Amp. (Merck &
Co.).
BENZTROPINE METHANESULFONATE.
See: Benztropine Mesylate.
BENZYDAMINE. B.A.N. 1-Benzyl-3-(3-di-
methyl-aminopropoxy)indazole.
Use: Anti-inflammatory, analgesic.
• **BENZYDAMINE HYDROCHLORIDE.**
USAN. 1-Benzyl-3- [3-(dimethylamino)-
propoxyl]-1H-indazole HCl. Tantum.
Use: Analgesic, anti-inflammatory, an-
tipyretic.
BENZYDROFLUMETHIAZIDE. 3-Benzyl-
3,4-dihydro-6-(trifluoromethyl)-1,2,4-
benzthiadiazine-7-sulfonamide, 1,1-
dioxide.
See: Bendroflumethiazide.
**BENZYHYDRYL-N-METHYLPIPER-
AZINE HCl.**
See: N- BENZYHYDRYL-N-
METHYLPIPERAZINE HCl.
• **BENZYL ALCOHOL,** N.F. XVIII. Phenyl-
carbinol.
Use: Antiseptic, local anesthetic.
See: Topic, Gel (Ingram).
Vicks Blue Mint, Regular & Wild Cher-
ry Medicated Cough Drops (Vicks).
• **BENZYL BENZOATE,** U.S.P. XXIII. Lot.,
U.S.P. XXIII. Benzoic acid, phenylmethyl
ester.
Use: 10% to 30% emulsion in scabies;
pharmaceutical necessity.
BENZYL BENZOATE SAPONATED. Tri-
ethanolamine 20 Gm, oleic acid 80 Gm,
benzyl benzoate q.s. 1000 ml.
BENZYL CARBINOL.
See: Phenylethyl Alcohol, U.S.P. XXIII.
**BENZYLPENICILLIN, BENZYLPENICIL-
LOIC, BENZYLPENILLOIC ACID.**
(Kremers-Urban)
Use: Assessment of penicillin sensitivi-
ty. [Orphan drug]
See: Pre-Pen/MDM.
BENZYL PENICILLIN-C-14. (Nuclear-
Chicago) Carbon-14 labelled penicillin;
prepared from phenyl-(acetic acid-1-C-

14), 6-aminopenicillanic acid as the
potassium salt. 23.4 mc/mM (62.9
mc/mg); radiochemical purity is 100%.
Vacuum-sealed glass vial 50 mi-
crocuries, 0.5 millicuries.
Use: Radioisotope.
BENZYL PENICILLIN G, POTASSIUM.
See: Penicillin G Potassium.
BENZYL PENICILLIN G, SODIUM.
See: Penicillin G Sodium.
• **BENZYLPENICILLOYL POLYLYSINE
CONCENTRATE,** U.S.P. XXIII. Inj.,
U.S.P. XXIII.
Use: Skin test antigen.
See: Pre-Pen (Kremers-Urban).
BEPANTHEN.
See: Panthenol.
BEPHEDIN. Benzyl ephedrine.
BEPHENIUM BROMIDE. N-Benzyl-N, N-
dimethyl-N-(2-phenoxyethyl)ammonium
bromide.
• **BEPHENIUM HYDROXYNAPHTHOATE,**
U.S.P. XXI. For Oral Susp., U.S.P. XXI.
Benzyldimethyl (2-phenoxy-ethyl)am-
monium-3-hydroxy-2-naphthoate. Ben-
zenemethanaminium,N,N-dimethyl-N-
(2-phenoxy-ethyl)-, salt with 3-hydroxy-
2-naphthalenecarboxylic acid (1:1).
Use: Anthelmintic (hookworms).
BEPHENIUM HYDROXYNAPHTHOATE.
B.A.N. Benzyldimethyl-2-phenoxyethy-
lammonium 3-hydroxy-2-naphthoate.
Use: Treatment of ancylostomiasis and
ascariasis.
• **BEPRIDIL HYDROCHLORIDE.** USAN.
Use: Vasodilator.
See: Vascor (McNeil).
• **BERACTANT.** USAN.
Use: Lung surfactant. [Orphan drug]
See: Survanta (Ross).
**BERACTANT INTRATHECAL SUSPEN-
SION.**
Use: Lung surfactant. [Orphan drug]
See: Survanta.
• **BERAPROST.** USAN.
Use: Improves ischemic syndromes.
• **BERAPROST SODIUM.** USAN.
Use: Improves ischemic action.
BERBERINE.
W/Hydrastine, glycerin.
See: Murine, Ophth. Soln.
BERBERINE HYDROCHLORIDE.
W/Borax, sodium Cl, boric acid, camphor
water, cherry laurel water, rose water,
thimerosol.
See: Lauro, eye irrigator and drops
(Otis Clapp).
• **BEREFRINE.** USAN.
Use. Mydriatic agent.

BER-EX. (Dolcin) Calcium succinate 2.8 gr, acetylsalicylic acid 3.7 gr/Tab. Bot. 100s, 500s.
Use: Anti-arthritic, antirheumatic.
BEROCCA PARENTERAL NUTRITION. (Roche) Vitamins B_1 3 mg, biotin 60 mcg, B_2 3.6 mg, niacinamide 40 mg, B_6 4 mg, d-panthenol 15 mg, C 100 mg, folic acid 0.4 mg/ml. Inj. **Amp.**: Duplex pkg. containing 1 ml Soln. 1 and 1 ml Soln. 2. Box 25s.; **Vial:** Duplex pkg. containing 20 ml vial (10 ml fill) of Soln 1 plus a 10 ml vial of Soln 2. Box 1s.
Use: Vitamin/mineral supplement.
BEROCCA PLUS TABLETS. (Roche) Vitamins A 5000 IU, E 30 IU, C 500 mg, B_1 20 mg, B_2 20 mg, niacinamide 100 mg, B_6 25 mg, biotin 0.15 mg, pantothenic acid 25 mg, folic acid 0.8 mg, B_{12} 50 mcg, iron 27 mg, cromium 0.1 mg, magnesium 50 mg, manganese 5 mg, copper 3 mg, zinc 22.5 mg/Tab. Bot. 100s.
Use: Vitamin/mineral supplement.
BEROCCA TABLETS. (Roche) Vitamins B_1 15 mg, B_2 15 mg, B_6 4 mg, niacinamide 100 mg, calcium pantothenate 18 mg, B_{12} 5 mcg, folic acid 0.5 mg, C 500 mg/Tab. Bot. 100s, 500s.
Use: Vitamin/mineral supplement.
BEROTEC. B_2 agonist.
See: Fenoterol HBr.
BERPLEX-C. (Alton) Vitamins B and C. Bot. 100s, 1000s.
Use: Vitamin supplement.
BERPLEX PLUS. (Schein) Iron 27 mg, vitamins A 5,000 IU, E 30 IU, C 500 mg, B_1 20 mg, B_2 20 mg, B_3 100 mg, B_5 25 mg, B_6 25 mg, B_{12} 50 mcg, biotin 0.15 mg, folic acid 0.8 mg, Cr, Mg, Mn, Cu and Zn. Tab. Bot. 100s.
Use: Vitamin/mineral supplement.
BERSOTRIN. (Kenyon) Vitamins B_1 15 mg, B_2 10 mg, C 300 mg, calcium pantothenate 10 mg, niacinamide 50 mg, B_6 5 mg/Cap. Bot. 100s.
Use: Vitamin supplement.
BERVITE. (Alton) Multiple vitamin. Bot. 100s, 1000s.
Use: Vitamin supplement.
• **BERYTHROMYCIN.** USAN. (1) 12-Deoxyery-thromycin; (2) Erythromycin B.
Use: Antiamebic, antibacterial.
BESAPRIN TABLETS. (Sanofi Winthrop) Aspirin, chlormezanone.
Use: Salicylate, analgesic, tranquilizer, muscle relaxant.
BESEROL TABLETS. (Sanofi Winthrop) Acetaminophen, chlormezanone.
Use: Analgesic, tranquilizer, muscle relaxant.

BESITEX B1. (Mills) Ephedrine ethylenediamine HCl 6 mg/Tab. Bot. 100s.
Use: Diet aid.
BESITEX B3. (Mills) Ephedrine ethylenediamine HCl 6 mg/Tab. Bot. 100s.
Use: Diet aid.
BESTA CAPSULES. (Hauck) Vitamins B_1 20 mg, B_2 15 mg, niacinamide 100 mg, calcium pantothenate 20 mg, E 50 IU, magnesium sulfate 70 mg, zinc 18.4 mg, B_{12} 4 mcg, B_6 25 mg, C 300 mg/Cap. Bot. 100s.
Use: Vitamin/mineral supplement.
BEST C CAPS. (Hauck) Ascorbic acid 500 mg/TR Cap. Bot. 100s.
Use: Vitamin C supplement.
BESTRONE INJECTION. (Bluco) Estrone in aqueous susp. 2 mg or 5 mg/ml. Vial 10 ml.
Use: Estrogen.
BETA-2. (Nephron) Isoetharine HCl 1% with glycerin, sodium bisulfite, parabens. Bot. 10 ml, 30 ml.
Use: Respiratory therapy, oral inhalant
BETA-ADRENERGIC BLOCKERS.
See: Brevibloc, Inj. (DuPont).
Blocadren, Tab. (Merck & Co..
Cartrol, Tab. (Abbott).
Corgard, Tab. (Princeton).
Inderal, Tab., Inj. (Wyeth-Ayerst).
Inderal LA, Sustained Release Cap. (Wyeth-Ayerst).
Kerlone, Tab. (Searle).
Levatol, Tab. (Reed-Carnrick).
Lopressor, Tab., Inj. (Geigy).
Nadolol, Tab. (Various Mfr.)
Propranolol HCl, Tab. (Various Mfr.).
Propranolol HCl, Inj. (SoloPak).
Sectral, Cap. (Wyeth-Ayerst).
Tenormin, Tab. (ICI Pharm.).
Timolol, Tab. (Various Mfr.).
Visken, Tab. (Sandoz).
BETA-ADRENERGIC BLOCKERS, OPHTHALMIC.
See: Betagan Liquifilm, Soln. (Allergan).
Betoptic, Soln. (Alcon).
Ocupress, Soln. (Otsuka).
OptiPranolol, Soln. (Bausch & Lomb).
Timoptic in Ocudose, Soln. (Merck & Co.).
Timoptic, Soln. (Merck & Co.).
• **BETA CAROTENE,** U.S.P. XXIII. Cap., U.S.P. XXIII. β,β-Carotene. All-trans-B-Carotene. (All-E)-1,1-(3,7,12,16-Tetramethyl-1,3,5,7,9,11,13,15,17-octadecanonaene-1,18-diyl) bis (2,6,6-trimethylcyclohexene).
Use: Ultraviolet screen.
See: Max-Caro (Marlyn).

Provatene (Solgar).
Solatene (Roche).
BETACETYLMETHADOL. B.A.N. β-4-Di-methylamino-1-ethyl-2,2-diphenylpentyl acetate.
Use: Narcotic analgesic.
BETACHRON E-R. (Inwood) Propranolol HCl 60 mg, 80 mg, 120 mg, 160 mg. ER Cap. 60 mg, 120mg, 160 mg: Bot. 100s. 80 mg: Bot. 100s, 250s.
Use: Beta-adrenergic blockers.
BETACREST. (Nutrition) **Kapule:** Vitamins B_1 15 mg, B_2 10 mg, B_6 5 mg, B_{12} 4 mcg, calcium pantothenate 20 mg, niacinamide 100 mg, C 600 mg, liver 125 mg. Bot. 60s. **Inj.:** Vitamins B_1 100 mg, B_2 2 mg, B_6 5 mg, B_{12} 30 mcg, niacinamide 125 mg, panthenol 10 mg, benzyl alcohol 1.5%/ml. Vial 30 ml.
Use: Vitamin supplement.
BETACREST KAPULE. (Nutrition) Vitamins B_1 30 mg, B_2 20 mg, B_6 10 mg, B_{12} 8 mcg, calcium pantothenate 40 mg, niacinamide 200 mg, C 600 mg, liver 250 mg/2 Cap. Bot. 60s.
Use: Vitamin/mineral supplement.
BETADINE. (Purdue Frederick) Povidone-iodine.
Aerosol Spray, Bot. 3 oz.
Antiseptic Gauze Pads 3" 9". Box 12s.
Antiseptic Lubricating Gel, Tube 5 Gm.
Disposable Medicated Douche, concentrated packette w/cannula and 6 oz water.
Douche, Bot. 1 oz, 4 oz, 8 oz.
Douche Packette, 0.5 oz (6 per carton).
Helafoam Solution Canister 250 Gm.
Mouthwash/Gargle, Bot. 6 oz.
Oint., Tube 1 oz, Jar 1 lb, 5 lb.
Oint., packette oz, oz.
Perineal Wash Conc. Kit, Bot. 8 oz w/dispenser.
Skin Cleanser, Bot. 1 oz, 4 oz.
Skin Cleanser Foam, Canister 6 oz.
Solution, 0.5 oz, 8 oz, 16 oz, 32 oz, gal.
Solution Packette, oz.
Solution Swab Aid, 100s.
Solution Swabsticks, 1s Box 200s; 3s Box 50s.
Surgical Scrub, Bot. pt, pt w/dispenser, qt, gal, packette 0.5 oz.
Surgi-prep Sponge-Brush 36s.
Vaginal Suppositories, Box 7s w/vaginal applicator.
Viscous Formula Antiseptic Gauze Pads: 3" 9", 5" 9". Box 12s.
Whirlpool Concentrate, Bot. gal.
Use: Antiseptic for uses indicated in product labeling.
BETADINE ANTISEPTIC. (Purdue Frederick) Povidone-iodine 10%. Vaginal gel. 18 g with applicator.
Use: Vaginal preparation.
BETADINE CREAM. (Purdue-Frederick) Povidone-iodine 5% mineral oil, polyoxyethylene stearate, polysorbate, sorbitan monostearate, white petrolatum. Cream Tube 14 Gm.
Use: Antiseptic/germicide.
BETADINE MEDICATED DISPOSABLE DOUCHE. (Purdue Frederick) Povidone-iodine 0.3% Soln. Vial 6 ml with 180 ml bot. Sanitized water.
Use: Vaginal preparation.
BETADINE MEDICATED DOUCHE. (Purdue Frederick) Povidone-iodine 10% (0.3% when diluted). Soln. In 15 and 240 ml packets.
Use: Vaginal preparation.
BETADINE MEDICATED PREMIXED DISPOSABLE DOUCHE. (Purdue-Frederick) Povidone-iodine 0.3% soln. Bot. 180 ml.
Use: Vaginal preparation.
BETADINE SHAMPOO. (Purdue-Frederick) Povidone-iodine 7.5%. Shampoo Bot. 118 ml.
Use: Antiseborrheic.
BETADINE VAGINAL GEL. (Purdue-Frederick) Povidone-iodine 10%, polyethylene glycols. Gel Tube w/appl. 18 Gm, 90 Gm.
Use: Antiseptic and germicide.
BETA-ESTRADIOL.
See: Estradiol, U.S.P. XXIII.
BETAEUCAINE HYDROCHLORIDE. Name previously used for Eucaine HCl.
BETAGAN. (Allergan) Levobunolol HCl 0.5% w/polyvinyl alcohol, benzalkonium Cl, sodium metabisulfite, EDTA. Bot. 5 ml, 10 ml, 15 ml.
Use: Beta-adrenergic blocking agent, ophthalmic.
BETAGEN. (Enzyme Process) Vitamins B_1 1 mg, B_2 1.2 mg, niacin 15 mg, B_6 18 mg, pantothenic acid 18 mg, choline 1.8 Gm, betaine 96 mg/6 Tab. Bot. 100s, 250s.
Use: Vitamin supplement.
BETAGEN OINTMENT. (Goldline) Povidone iodine. Oint. Tube oz. Jar lb.
Use: Antiseptic.
BETAGEN SOLUTION. (Goldline) Povidone iodine. Bot. pt, gal.
Use: Antiseptic.
BETAGEN SURGICAL SCRUB. (Goldline) Povidone iodine. Bot. pt, gal.
Use: Antiseptic.

BETA-GLUCOCEREBROSIDASE, RE-COMBINANT. (Genzyme)
Use: Treatment of Gaucher's disease.
[Orphan drug]
• **BETAHISTINE HYDROCHLORIDE.**
USAN. 2-(2-Methylaminoethyl) pyridine dihydrochloride.
Use: Meniere's disease. A diamine oxidase inhibitor. Increase microcirculation.
BETA-HYPOPHAMINE.
See: Vasopressin.
BETAINE. (Orphan Medical)
Use: Homocystinuria. [Orphan drug]
• **BETAINE HYDROCHLORIDE,** U.S.P. XXIII. Acidol HCl, lycine HCl.
Use: Replenisher adjunct (electrolyte).
W/Ferrous fumarate, docusate sodium, desiccated liver, vitamins, minerals.
See: Hemaferrin, Tab. (Western Research).
W/Pancreatin, pepsin, ammonium Cl.
See: Zypan, Tab. (Standard Process).
W/Pepsin.
See: Normacid, Tab. (Stuart).
BETALIN S. (Lilly) Thiamine HCl.
50 mg or 100 mg. Tab. Bot. 100s.
Use: Vitamin B₁ supplement.
BETAMEPRODINE. B.A.N. β 3 Ethyl 1 methyl-4-phenyl-4-propionyloxypiperidine.
Use: Narcotic analgesic.
BETAMETHADOL. B.A.N. β-6-Dimethylamino-4,4-diphenylheptan-3-ol.
Use: Narcotic analgesic.
• **BETAMETHASONE,** U.S.P. XXIII.
Cream, Syr., Tab., U.S.P. XXIII. 9-α-Fluoro-11β, 17,21-trihydroxy16β-methylpregna-1,4-diene-3,20-dione. 9α-Fluoro16β-methylprednisolone. Acetate and sodium phosphate.
Use: Glucocorticoid.
See: Celestone, Inj., Syr., Tab. (Schering).
• **BETAMETHASONE ACETATE,** U.S.P. XXIII. Pregna-1,4-diene-3,20-dione, 9-fluoro-11, 17-dihydroxy-16-methyl-21-(acetyloxy)-, (11β, 16β)-. 9-Fluoro-11β,17,21-trihydroxy-16β-methylpregna-1,4-diene-3,20-dione 21-acetate.
Use: Glucocorticoid.
BETAMETHASONE ACIBUTATE. B.A.N.
21-Acetoxy-9α-fluoro-11β-hydroxy-16β-methyl-17-(2-methylpropionyloxy)pregna-1,4-diene-3,20-dione.
Use: Corticosteroid.
• **BETAMETHASONE BENZOATE,** U.S.P. XXIII. Gel, U.S.P. XXIII. 9-Fluoro-11β 17,21-trihydroxy-16β-methylpregna-1,4-

diene-3,20-dione 17 benzoate.
Use: Glucocorticoid.
See: Benisone. (Warner-Chilcott).
Flurobate (Texas Pharmacal).
Uticort, Prods. (Parke-Davis).
• **BETAMETHASONE DIPROPIONATE,** U.S.P. XXIII. Topical Aerosol, Cream, Lot., Oint., U.S.P. XXIII.
Use: Glucocorticoid.
See: Alphatrex Prods. (Savage).
Diprolene Prods. (Schering).
Diprosone Prods. (Schering).
Psorion Cream (ICN).
• **BETAMETHASONE SODIUM PHOS-PHATE,** U.S.P. XXIII. Inj., U.S.P. XXIII.
Pregna-1,4-diene-3,20-dione, 9-fluoro-11,17-dihydroxy-16-methyl-21-(phosphonoxy)-, disodium salt, (11β, 16β). 9-Fluoro-11β,17,21-trihydroxy-16β-methylpregna-1,4-diene-3,20-dione 21-(disodium phosphate).
See: Celestone Phosphate Inj. (Schering).
• **BETAMETHASONE SODIUM PHOS-PHATE AND BETAMETHASONE AC-ETATE SUSPENSION, STERILE,** U.S.P. XXIII.
See: Celestone Soluspan (Schering).
• **BETAMETHASONE VALERATE,** U.S.P. XXIII. Cream, Lot., Oint., U.S.P. XXIII.
Topical Aerosol U.S.P. XXI. Pregna-1,4-diene-3,20-dione,9-fluoro-11,21-dihydroxy-16-methyl-17-[(1-oxopentyl)oxy]-,(11β,16β)-. 9-Fluoro-11β,17,21-trihydroxy-16β-methylpregna-1,4-diene-3,20-dione 17-valerate.
See: Betatrex Prods. (Savage).
Beta-Val Prods. (Lemmon).
Valisone Prods. (Schering).
Valnac Prods. (Schering).
• **BETAMICIN SULFATE.** USAN.
Use: Antibacterial.
BETANAPHTHOL. 2-Naphthol.
Use: Parasiticide.
BETAPACE. (Berlex) Sotalol HCl 80 mg, 160 mg, 240 mg/Tab. Bot. 100s, UD 100s.
Use: Beta-adrenergic blocking agent.
BETAPEN-VK. (Bristol) Penicillin V potassium. **Oral Soln.:** 125 mg/ml Bot. 100 ml. 250 mg/5 ml Bot. 100 ml, 200 ml. **Tab.:** 250 mg/Tab. Bot. 100s, 1000s; 500 mg/Tab. Bot. 100s.
Use: Antibacterial; penicillin.
beta-PHENYL-ETHYL-HYDRAZINE.
Phenelzine dihydrogen sulfate.
See: Nardil, Tab. (Parke-Davis).
BETAPRODINE. B.A.N. β-1,3-Dimethyl-4-phenyl-4-propionyloxypiperidine.
Use: Narcotic analgesic.

BETA-PROPIOLACTONE.
See: Betaprone, Vial (Forest).
BETA-PYRIDYL-CARBINOL. Nicotinyl alcohol. Alcohol corresponding to nicotinic acid.
See: Roniacol, Elix., Tab. (Roche Lab.).
BETASERON. (Berlex) Interferon beta 0.3 mg, albumin human 15 mg, dextrose 15 mg. Pow. for Inj. single-use vial 5 ml and 2 ml vial of diluent.
Use: Cytokine agent.
BETATREX. (Savage) Betamethasone valerate 0.1%. Cream, Oint. Tube 15 Gm, 45 Gm; Lot. Bot. 60 ml.
Use: Corticosteroid.
BETA-VAL CREAM. (Lemmon) Betamethasone valerate equivalent to 0.1% betamethasone base in cream base. Tube 15 Gm, 45 Gm.
Use: Corticosteroid.
• **BETAXOLOL HYDROCHLORIDE.** USAN.
Use: Antianginal, antihypertensive.
See: Betoptic, Ophth. (Alcon). Kerlone (Searle).
• **BETAXOLOL OPHTHALMIC SOLUTION,** U.S.P. XXIII.
• **BETHANECHOL CHLORIDE,** U.S.P. XXIII. Inj., Tab., U.S.P. XXIII. (2-Hydroxypropyl) trimethylammonium Cl Carbamate. Carbamylmethylcholine Cl.
Use: Parasympathomimetic.
See: Duvoid, Tab. (Norwich Eaton). Myotonachol, Tab., Amp. (Glenwood). Urabeth, Tab. (Major). Urecholine, Tab., Amp. (Merck & Co.). Vesicholine, Tab. (Star).
• **BETHANIDINE.** USAN. 2-Benzyl-1,3-dimethylguanidine.
Use: Hypotensive.
• **BETHANIDINE SULFATE.** USAN.
Use: Pulmonary surfactant. [Orphan drug]
BETHAPRIM. (Major) Trimethoprim 40 mg, sulfamethoxazole 200 mg/5 ml, alcohol 0.26%, saccharin and sorbitol. Susp.
Use: Anti-infective.
BETHAPRIM DS TABS. (Major) Trimethoprim 160 mg, sulfamethoxazole 800 mg/Tab. Bot. 100s, 500s, UD 100s.
Use: Anti-infective.
BETHAPRIM SS TABS. (Major) Trimethoprim 80 mg, sulfamethoxazole 400 mg/Tab. Bot. 100s, 500s.
Use: Anti-infective.
• **BETIATIDE.** USAN.
Use: Pharmaceutic aid.
BETOPTIC. (Alcon) Betaxolol HCl 0.5%. Bot. 2.5 ml, 10 ml, 15 ml.

Use: Beta-adrenergic blocking agent, ophthalmic.
BETOPTIC S. (Alcon) Betaxalol HCl 0.25%. Bot. 2.5 ml, 5 ml, 15 ml.
Use: Beta-adrenergic blocking agent, ophthalmic.
BETULINE. (Ferndale) Methyl salicylate, camphor, menthol, peppermint oil in a water soluble base. Lot. Bot. 60 ml, pt.
Use: External analgesic.
• **BEVANTOLOL HYDROCHLORIDE.** USAN.
Use: Antianginal, antihypertensive, cardiac depressant.
BEVONIUM METHYLSULFATE. B.A.N. 2-Benziloyloxy-methyl-1,1-dimethylpiperidinium methylsulfate.
Use: Antispasmodic.
BEXOMAL-C. (Hauck) Vitamins B_1 6 mg, B_2 7 mg, B_3 80 mg, B_5 10 mg, B_6 5 mg, B_{12} 6 mcg, C 250 mg/Tab. Bot. 50s.
Use: Vitamin supplement.
• **BEZAFIBRATE.** USAN.
Use: Antihyperlipoproteinemic.
See: Bezalip (Norwich Eaton).
BEZITRAMIDE. B.A.N. 4-[4-(2-Oxo-3-propionylbenzimidazolin-1-yl)piperidino]-2,2-diphenylbutyronitrile.
Use: Narcotic analgesic.
BEZON. (Whittier) Vitamins B_1 5 mg, B_2 3 mg, niacinamide 20 mg, pantothenic acid 3 mg, B_6 0.5 mg, C 50 mg, B_{12} 1 mcg/Cap. Bot. 30s, 100s.
Use: Vitamin supplement.
BEZON FORTE. (Whittier) Vitamins B_1 25 mg, B_2 12.5 mg, niacinamide 50 mg, pantothenic acid 10 mg, B_6 5 mg, C 250 mg/Cap. Bot. 30s, 100s.
Use: Vitamin supplement.
B-F-I POWDER. (Beecham Products) Bismuth-formic-iodide, zinc phenolsulfonate, bismuth subgallate, amol, potassium alum, boric acid, menthol, eucalyptol, thymol and inert diluents. Can 0.25 oz, 1.25 oz, 8 oz.
Use: Antiseptic.
B.G.O. (Calotabs) Iodoform, salicylic acid, sulfur, zinc oxide, phenol (liquefied) 1%, calamine, menthol, petrolatum, lanolin, mineral oil, undecylenic acid 1%. Jar 7/8 oz, Tube 1 oz.
Use: Antiseptic, antifungal.
BIALAMICOL. B.A.N. 3,3'-Diallyl-5,5-bis-diethyl-aminomethyl-4,4-dihydroxy-biphenyl. Biallylamicol.
Use: Treatment of amebiasis.
• **BIALAMICOL HCI.** USAN. 5,5'-Diallyl-α,α-bis-(diethylamino)-m,m-bitolyl-4,4-diol HCl.
Use: Antiamebic.

BIAMINE. (Forest) Thiamine HCl, 100 mg/ml, with 0.5% chlorobutanol. Vial 30 ml.
Use: Enzyme co-factor vitamin.
BIAPENEM.. USAN.
Use: Antibacterial.
BIAPHASIC INSULIN INJECTION. A suspension of insulin crystals in a solution of insulin buffered at pH 7. Insulin Novo Rapitard.
BIAVAX-II. (Merck & Co.) Rubella and mumps virus vaccine, live. See details under Meruvax-II and Mumpsvax. Single-dose vial w/diluent. Pkg. 1s, 10s.
Use: Agent for immunization.
BIAXIN. (Abbott) **Tab.:**Clarithromycin 250 mg, 500 mg. Bot. 60s, UD 100s. **Gran. for oral susp.:** 125mg/5ml Bot. 100ml, 200 ml; 250 mg/5ml Bot. 100 ml.
Use: Antibiotic.
BIBENZONIUM BROMIDE. B.A.N. 2-(1,2-Diphenylethoxy) ethyltrimethylammonium bromide.
Use: Cough suppressant.
BICIFADINE HYDROCHLORIDE. USAN.
Use: Analgesic.
BICILLIN. (Wyeth-Ayerst) Penicillin G benzathine 200,000 units/Tab. Bot. 36s.
Use: Antibacterial; penicillin.
BICILLIN C-R. (Wyeth-Ayerst) Penicillin G benzathine 150,000 units, penicillin G procaine 150,000 units/ml w/lecithin, povidone, methyl and propylparabens. Vial 10 ml. Bicillin 300,000 units, penicillin G procaine 300,000 units/1 ml w/lecithin, povidone, methyl and propylparaben. Tubex cartridge 1 ml. Pkg. 10s. Bicillin 600,000 units, penicillin G procaine 600,000 units with parabens, lecithin and povidone/2 ml Tubex cartridge. Pkg. 10s. Bicillin 1,200,000 units, penicillin G procaine 1,200,000 units with parabens, lecithin and povidone/4 single-dose disposable syringe, 10s, 4 ml.
Use: Antibacterial; penicillin.
BICILLIN C-R 900/300 INJECTION. (Wyeth-Ayerst) Penicillin G benzathine 900,000 units, penicillin G procaine 300,000 units with parabens, lecithin and povidone/2 ml. Tubex. Pkg. 10s.
Use: Antibacterial; penicillin.
BICILLIN LONG-ACTING. (Wyeth-Ayerst) Penicillin G benzathine 300,000 units/ml w/lecithin, povidone, methyl and propylparabens. 300,000 units/ml. Vial 10 ml 600,000 units/Tubex. 1,200,000 units/2 ml Tubex 10s. 2,400,000 units/4 ml single dose disposable syringe, 10s.
Use: Antibacterial; penicillin.

BICIROMAB.. USAN.
Use: Monoclonal antibody (antifibrin).
BICITRA. (Willen) Sodium citrate dihydrate 500 mg, citric acid monohydrate 334 mg, 5 mEq sodium ion/5 ml. Shohl's Solution. Bot. 4 oz, pt, gal, Unit-dose 15 ml, 30 ml.
Use: Systemic alkalinizer.
• **BICLODIL HYDROCHLORIDE.** USAN.
Use: Antihypertensive (vasodilator).
BiCNU. (Bristol-Myers/Bristol Oncology) Carmustine (BCNU) 100 mg, sterile diluent (dehydrated alcohol USP inj.) 3 ml/Vial.
Use: Antineoplastic agent.
BICOZENE CREAM. (Sandoz) Benzocaine 6%, resorcinol 1.66% in cream base. Tube oz.
Use: Local anesthetic.
BICYCLINE. (Knight) Tetracycline HCl 250 mg/Cap. Bot. 100s.
Use: Antibacterial; tetracycline.
BIDIMAZIUM IODIDE. B.A.N. 4-(Biphenyl-4-yl)- 2-(1-dimethylaminostyryl)-3-methylthiazolium iodide.
Use: Anthelmintic.
• **BIDISOMIDE.** USAN.
Use: Antiarrhythmic.
BIFE. (Jenkins) Thiamine HCl 1 mg, ferrous sulfate 3 gr/Tab. Bot. 1000s.
Use: Vitamin/iron supplement.
BIFLURANOL. B.A.N. erythro-4,4'-(1-Ethyl-2-methylethylene)di-(2-fluorophenol).
Use: Benign hypertrophy of the prostate.
• **BIFONAZOLE.** USAN.
Use: Antifungal.
BILAX. (Drug Industries) Dehydrocholic acid 50 mg, docusate sodium 100 mg/Cap. Bot. 100s, 500s.
Use: Laxative.
BILE ACIDS, OXIDIZED. Note also dehydrocholic acid.
W/Atropine methyl nitrate, ox and hog bile extract, phenobarbital.
See: G.B.S., Tab.(Forest).
W/Bile whole (desiccated), dessicated whole pancreas, homatropine methylbromide.
See: Pancobile, Tab. (Solvay).
W/Ox bile, steapsin, phenobarbital, homatropine methylbromide.
See: Oxacholin, Tab. (Roxane).
BILE ACID SUQUESTRANTS.
See: Cholybar (Parke-Davis)
Questran (Bristol Labs)
Questran Light (Bristol Labs)
Colestid (Upjohn)
BILE EXTRACT. (Various Mfr.) Pow. 0.25

lb, 1 lb.

W/Cascara sagrada, dandelion root, podophyllin, nux vomica.
See: Oxachol, Liq. (Roxane).

W/Dehydrocholic acid, homatropine methylbromide, phenobarbital.
See: Neocholan, Tab. (Merrell Dow).

W/Pancreatic substance, dl-methionine, choline bitartrate.
See: Licoplex, Tab. (Mills).

BILE EXTRACT, OX. Purified ox gall.
Lilly—Enseal 5 gr, Bot. 100s, 500s, 1000s.
C. D. Smith—Tab. 5 gr, Bot. 1000s.
Stoddard—Tab. 3 gr, Bot. 100s, 500s, 1000s.

W/Cellulase, pepsin, glutamic acid HCl, pancreatin.
See: Kanulase, Tab. (Dorsey).

W/Cellulase, pepsin, glutamic acid HCl, pancreatin, methscopolamine nitrate, pentobarbital.
See: Kanumodic, Tab. (Dorsey).

W/Colcynth compound extract, cascara sagrada extract, podophyllin, hyoscyamus extract.
See: Bileo-Secrin Compound Tablets (First Texas).

W/Dehydrocholic acid, homatropine methylbromide, phenobarbital.
See: Bilamide, Tab. (Norgine).

W/Dehydrocholic acid, pepsin, homatropine methylbromide.
See: Biloric, Cap. (Arcum).

W/Desoxycholic acid, oxidized bile acids, pancreatin.
See: Bilogen, Tab. (Organon).

W/Enzyme concentrate, pepsin, dehydrocholic acid, belladonna extract.
See: Ro-Bile, Tab. (Solvay).

W/Oxidized bile acids, steapsin, phenobarbital, homatropine methylbromide.
See: Oxacholin, Tab. (Philips).

W/Pepsin, pancreatic enzyme concentrate.
See: Konzyme, Tab. (Brunswick).
Nu'Leven, Tab. (Lemmon).
Nu'Leven Plus, Tab. (Lemmon).

W/Sodium salicylate, phenolphthalein, chionanthus extract, cascara sagrada extract, sodium glycocholate, sodium taurocholate.
See: Glycols, Tab. (Bowman).

BILEIN. Bile salts obtained from ox bile.

BILE-LIKE PRODUCTS.
See: Zanchol, Tab. (Searle).

BILE PRODUCTS.
See: Bile Salts.
Dehydrocholic Acid.
Desoxycholic Acid.

Ketocholanic Acid.

BILE SALTS. Sodium glycocholate and taurocholate. Note also Bile Extract, Ox and oxidized bile acids.
Lilly—Enseal 5 gr, Bot. 100s.
See: Bilein.
Bisol, Tab. (Paddock).
Ox Bile Extract.
Oxidized Bile Acids.

W/Belladonna, nux vomica compound Bile salts 60 mg, belladonna leaf extract 5 mg, nux vomica extract 2 mg, phenolphthalein 30 mg, sodium salicylate 15 mg, aloin 15 mg/Tab. Bot. 1000s.
Use: Laxative, antispasmodic.

W/Cascara extract, phenolphthalein, capsicum oleoresin.
See: Bilocomp, Tab. (Lannett).

W/Cascara sagrada, phenolphthalein, capsicum oleoresin, peppermint oil.
See: Torocol, Tab. (Plessner).

W/Cellulase, calcium carbonate, pancrelipase.
See: Accelerase, Cap. (Organon).

W/Cellulase, pancrelipase, calcium carbonate, belladonna alkaloids, phenobarbital.
See: Accelerase-PB, Cap. (Organon).

W/Dehydrocholic acid, pancreatic substance.
See: Depancol, Tab. (Parke-Davis).

W/Dehydrocholic acid, pepsin, pancreatin.
See: Progestive, Tab. (NCP).

W/Pancreatin, pepsin, dehydrocholic acid, desoxycholic acid.
See: Pepsatal, Tab. (Kenyon).

W/Pancrelipase, cellulase.
See: Cotazym-B, Tab. (Organon).

W/Papain, cascara sagrada extract, phenolphthalein, capsicum oleoresin.
See: Torocol Compound, Tab. (Plessner).

W/Pepsin, homatropine, methylbromide, amylase, lipase, protease.
See: Digesplen, Tab., Elix., Drops (Med. Prod.).

W/Phenolphthalein, chionanthus extract.
See: Bile Anthus Compound, Cap. (Scrip).

W/Sodium salicylate, phenolphthalein, chionanthus extract, bile extract, cascara sagrada extract.
See: Glycols, Tab. (Bowman).

BILE, WHOLE DESICCATED.
W/Pancreatin, mycozyme diastase, pepsin, nux vomica extract.
See: Enzobile, Tab. (Hauck).

BILEZYME. (Geriatric) Amylolytic enzyme 30 mg, proteolytic enzyme 6 mg, dehydrocholic acid 200 mg, desoxy-

cholic acid 50 mg/Tab. Bot. 42s, 100s, 500s.
Use: Digestive aid.

BILI-LABSTIX REAGENT STRIPS. (Miles Diagnostic) Reagent strips. Bot. 100s. Test for pH, protein, glucose, ketones, bilirubin and blood in urine.
Use: Diagnostic aid.

BILI-LABSTIX SG REAGENT STRIPS. (Miles Diagnostic) Bot. 100s. Urinalysis reagent strip test for specific gravity, pH, protein, glucose, ketone, bilirubin, and blood.
Use: Diagnostic aid.

BILIRUBIN REAGENT STRIPS. (Miles Diagnostic) Seralyzer reagent strip. Bot. 25s. Quantitative strip test for total bilirubin in serum or plasma.
Use: Diagnostic aid.

BILIRUBIN TEST.
See: Ictotest.(Miles Diagnostic).

BILIVIST. (Berlex) Ipodate sodium 500 mg/Cap. Bot. 120s.
Use: Radiopaque agent.

BILOCOMP TABLETS. (Lannett) Bile salts 1.5 gr, cascara extract 0.5 gr, phenolphthalein 0.5 gr, oleoresin capsicum 1/20 mln/Tab. Bot. 1000s.
Use: Laxative.

BILOGEST. (Mills) Mixed oxidized bile acids 65 mg, desoxycholic acid 60 mg, extract ox bile 40 mg, pepsin 100 mg, pancreatin 100 mg, inositol 40 mg, dimethionine 120 mg, betaine HCl 75 mg, choline bitartrate 100 mg, diazyme 10 mg/Tab. Bot. 100s.
Use: Gallbladder disorders, indigestion, cirrhosis, obesity.

BILOPAQUE. (Sanofi Winthrop) Tyropanoate sodium 750 mg/Cap. Catchcovers of 4 cap. Box 20s, Bot. 100s, 500s.
Use: Radiopaque agent.

BILORIC. (Arcum) Pepsin 9 mg, ox bile 160 mg/Cap. Bot. 100s, 1000s.
Use: Antispasmodic.

BILSTAN. (Standex) Bile salts 0.5 gr, cascara sagrada powder extract 0.5 gr, phenolphthalein 0.5 gr, aloin 1/8 gr, podophyllin gr/Tab. Bot. 100s.
Use: Laxative.

BILTRICIDE. (Miles) Praziquantel 600 mg/Tab. Bot. 6s.
Use: Anthelmintic.

BIMETHOXYCAINE LACTATE. Bis-[b-(o-methoxy-phenyl) isopropyl] amine lactate. Isocaine Lactate.

BINDARIT.. USAN.
Use: Antirheumatic.

BINDAZAC. B.A.N. 1-Benzylindazol-3-

yloxyacetic acid. Bendazac (I.N.N.).
Use: Anti-inflammatory.

BINEX-C.
See: C-BINEX.

• **BINIRAMYCIN.** USAN.
Use: Antibiotic.

• **BINOSPIRONE MESYLATE.** USAN.
Use: Anxiolytic.

BINTRON TABLETS. (Madland) Liver fraction 4.6 gr, ferrous sulfate 5 gr, vitamins B_1 3 mg, B_2 0.5 mg, B_6 0.15 mg, C 20 mg, calcium pantothenate 0.3 mg, niacinamide 10 mg/Tab. Bot. 100s, 1000s.
Use: Vitamin/mineral supplement.

BIO-ACEROLA C COMPLEX. (Solgar) Vitamin C 500 mg, citrus bioflavoids 10 mg, rutin 5 mg in a natural base of acerola, rose hips, buckwheat, black currant and green pepper concentrate powders, cherry flavored. Wafers. Bot. 50s, 100s.
Use: Vitamin supplement.

BIOBRANE. (Sanofi Winthrop) A temporary skin substitute available in various sizes.
Use: Temporary skin substitute.

BIOCAL 250. (Miles) Calcium 250 mg/Chew. Tab. Bot. 75s.
Use: Calcium supplement.

BIO-C.
See: C-BIO.

BIOCAL 500. (Miles) Calcium 500 mg/Tab. Bot. 75s.
Use: Calcium supplement.

BIOCEF. (Inter. Ethical Labs) **Cap.** Cephalexin 500 mg. Bot. 100s. **Pow. for Susp.:** Cephalexin 125 mg/5 ml, 250 mg/5 ml when reconstituted. 100 ml.
Use: Antibiotic.

BIO-CREST. (Nutrition) Citrus bioflavonoid complex 200 mg, vitamin C 250 mg, rutin 50 mg/Tabseal. Bot. 100s.
Use: Vitamin supplement.

BIOCULT-GC. (Medical Technology Corp.) Swab Test for gonorrhea. For endocervical, urethral, rectal and pharyngeal cultures. Box 1 test per kit.
Use: Diagnostic aid.

BIODEGRADABLE POLYMER IMPLANT CONTAINING CARMUSTINE.
Use: Treatment of recurrent malignant glioma. [Orphan drug]
See: Biodel Implant/BCNU.

BIODEL IMPLANT/BCNU. (Scios Nova) Biodegradable polymer implant containing carmustine.
Use: Treatment of recurrent malignant glioma.

BIODINE. (Major) Iodine 1%. Soln. Bot.

ㅔ, ㅔ
Use: Antiseptic, germicide.
BIO-FLAVONOID COMPOUNDS. Vitamins P.
BIO-FLAVONOID COMPOUND, CITRUS. W/Vitamins C.
See: C.V.P. Syr., Cap. (USV Pharm).
Mevanin-C, Cap. (Beutlich).
Mevatinic-C, Tab. (Beutlich).
Peridin-C, Tab. (Beutlich).
Pregent, Tab. (Beutlich).
BIOGASTRONE.
See: Carbenoxolone.
• **BIOLOGICAL INDICATOR FOR DRY-HEAT STERILIZATION, PAPER STRIP,** U.S.P. XXIII.
Use: Indicator.
• **BIOLOGICAL INDICATOR FOR ETHYL-ENE OXIDE STERILIZATION, PAPER STRIP,** U.S.P.XXII.
Use: Indicator.
• **BIOLOGICAL INDICATOR FOR STEAM STERILIZATION,** U.S.P. XXIII.
Use: Indicator.
BIO-MEDI-PEC. (Medi-Rx) Neomycin sulfate 300 mg, kaolin 6 Gm, pectin 0.13 Gm/fl oz. Bot. pt, gal.
Use: Antidiarrheal.
BIOMOX. (Inter. Ethical Labs) Amoxicillin 250 mg/Cap. Bot. 100s.
Use: Antibiotic.
BION TEARS. (Alcon) Dextran 70 0.1%, hydroxypropyl methylcellulose 2910 0.3%. Preservative free. Soln. In single-use 0.45 ml containers (28s).
Use: Artificial tears.
BIONATE 50-2. (Seatrace) Testosterone cypionate 50 mg, estradiol cypionate 2 mg/ml. Vial 10 ml.
Use: Androgen, estrogen combination.
BIOPHOSPHONATES.
See: Didronel (Norwich Eaton)
Didronel IV (MGI Pharma)
Aredia (Ciba)
BIORAL.
See: Carbenoxolone.
BIOS I.
See: Inositol.
BIO-TAB. (Inter. Ethical Labs) Doxycycline hyclate 100 mg, film coated. Tab. Bot. 50s, 100s, 500s.
Use: Antibiotic.
BIOTEL DIABETES. (Biotel) In vitro diagnostic test for diabetes and other metabolic disorders by screening for glucose in the urine. Test Kit 12s.
Use: In vitro diagnostic aid.
BIOTEL KIDNEY. (Biotel) In vitro diagnostic test for early detection of diseases of the kidneys, bladder and urinary tract

ㅔ, screening for hemoglobin, red blood cells and albumin in the urine. Test Kit 12s.
Use: In vitro diagnostic aid.
BIOTEL U.T.I. (Biotel) In vitro diagnostic home test to detect urinary tract infections by screening for nitrate in urine. Test Kit 12s.
Use: In vitro diagnostic aid.
BIOTEXIN.
See: Novobiocin.
BIOTHESIN. (Pal-Pak). Phosphorated carbohydrate solution cerium oxalate 120 mg, bismuth subnitrate 120 mg, benzocaine 15 mg, aromatics/Tab. 1000s.
Use: Antiemetic/antivertigo combination.
• **BIOTIN,** U.S.P. XXIII.
Use: Vitamin.
BIOTIN FORTE 3 MG. (Vitaline) B_1 10 mg, B_2 10 mg, B_3 40 mg, B_5 10 mg, B_6 25 mg, B_{12} 10 mg, C 200 mg, biotin 3 mg, FA 800 mcg, Zn 30 mg.
Use: Vitamin supplement.
BIOTIN FORTE 5 MG EXTRA STRENGTH. (Vitaline) B_1 10 mg, B_2 10 mg, B_3 40 mg, B_5 10 mg, B_6 25 mg, B_{12} 10 mcg, C 100 mg, biotin 5 mg, FA 800 mcg/Tab. Bot. 60s.
Use: Vitamin supplement.
BIO-TYTRA. (Approved) Neomycin sulfate 2.5 mg, gramicidin 0.25 mg, benzocaine 10 mg/Troche. Box 10s.
Use: Anti-infective.
BIPECTOL TABLETS. (Vale) Opium 1.2 mg, bismuth hydroxide 32.4 mg, kaolin colloidal 162 mg, pectin 32.4 mg/Tab. Bot. 1000s.
Use: Antidiarrheal.
• **BIPENAMOL HYDROCHLORIDE.** USAN.
Use: Antidepressant.
• **BIPERIDEN,** U.S.P. XXIII. 1-Piperidine-propanol,α-bicyclo[2.2.1]hept-5-en-2-yl-α-phenyl-α-5-Norbornen-2-yl-α-phenyl-1-piperidinepropanol.
Use: Anticholinergic.
• **BIPERIDEN HYDROCHLORIDE,** U.S.P. XXIII. Tab., U.S.P. XXIII. 1-Piperidine-propanol, -α-bicyclo[2.2.1]-hept-5-en-2-yl-α-phenyl-, hydrochloride. α-5-Norbornen-2-yl-α-phenyl-1-piperidinepropanol HCl.
Use: Anticholinergic, antiparkinson agent.
BIPERIDEN HYDROCHLORIDE and LACTATE. (Alpha-(Bicyclo[2,2,1] hept-5-en-2-yl)-alpha-phenyl-1-piperidine propanol.

Use: Anticholinergic, antiparkinson agent.
See: Akineton, Amp., Tab. (Knoll).
• **BIPERIDEN LACTATE INJECTION,** U.S.P. XXIII. 1- Piperidinepropanol, α-bicyclo[2.2.1]hept-5-en-2-yl-α-phenol, compound with 2-hydroxypropanoic acid (1:1). α-5-Norbornen-2-yl-α-phenyl-1-piperidine- propanol lactate (salt).
Use: Anticholinergic, antiparkinson agent.
BIPHASIC INSULIN INJECTION. B.A.N. A suspension of bovine and porcine insulin crystals in a solution of insulin buffered at pH 7.
Use: Hypoglycemic agent.
BIPHETAMINE 12.5. (Pennwalt) Dextroamphetamine (as resin complex) 6.25 mg, amphetamine (as resin complex) 6.25 mg/Cap. Bot. 100s.
Use: Diet aid.
BIPHETAMINE 20. (Pennwalt) Dextroamphetamine (as resin complex) 10 mg, amphetamine (as resin complex) 10 mg/Cap. Bot. 100s.
Use: Diet aid.
• **BIPHENAMINE HYDROCHLORIDE.** USAN. 2-Diethylaminoethyl-3-phenylsalicylate HCl.
Use: Topical anesthetic, antibacterial, antifungal.
BIPOLE-S. (Spanner) Testosterone 25 mg, estrone 2 mg/ml. Vial 10 ml.
Use: Androgen, estrogen combination.
BIRTH CONTROL.
See: Oral Contraceptive.
BIS (ACETOXYPHENYL) OXINDOL.
See: Oxyphenisatin.
• **BISACODYL,** U.S.P. XXIII. Supp., Tab., U.S.P. XXIII. Phenol, 4,4'-(2-pyridinylmethylene) bis-,diacetate (ester). Di-(p-acetoxyphenyl)-2-pyridylmethane. 4-4-(2-pyridylmethylene) diphenol diacetate (ester).
Use: Cathartic.
See: Bisacodyl Uniserts, Supp. (Upsher-Smith).
Bisco-Lax, Supp. (Raway).
Dacodyl, Tab., Supp. (Major).
Deficol, Tab., Supp. (Vangard).
Delco-Lax, Tab. (Delco).
Dulcagen, Tab., Supp. (Goldline).
Dulcolax, Tab., Supp. (Ciba Cons.).
Fleet Bisacodyl, Tab., Supp. (Fleet).
Theralax, Tab., Supp. (Beecham Labs).
• **BISACODYL TANNEX.** USAN. Water-soluble complex of bisacodyl and tannic acid.
Use: Contact laxative.

See: Clysodrast, packet (Barnes-Hind).
BISACODYL UNISERTS. (Upsher-Smith) Bisacodyl. Supp. **5 mg:** 12s. **10 mg:** 12s, 50s, 500s.
Use: Laxative.
BISALATE. (Allison) Sodium salicylate 5 gr, salicylamide 2.5 gr, sodium paraminobenzoate 5 gr, ascorbic acid 50 mg, butabarbital sodium 1/8 gr/Tab. Bot. 100s, 1000s.
Use: Antirheumatic.
• **BISANTRENE HYDROCHLORIDE.** USAN.
Use: Antineoplastic.
BISATIN.
See: Oxyphenisatin.
BISCOLAN HC SUPPOSITORIES. (Lannett) Same as Biscolan Supp. w/hydrocortisone acetate 10 mg/Supp. Box 12s.
BISCOLAN SUPPOSITORIES. (Lannett) Bismuth subgallate, benzocaine, resorcin, cod liver oil, lanolin, zinc oxide/Supp. Box 12s.
BISCO-LAX. (Raway) Bisacodyl 10 mg/Supp. Box of foil UD 12s, 50s, 100s, 500s, 1000s.
Use: Laxative.
BISHYDROXYCOUMARIN.
See: Dicumarol, U.S.P. XXIII.
BISMAPEC TABLETS. (Vale) Bismuth hydroxide 137.7 mg, colloidal kaolin 648 mg, citrus pectin 129.6 mg/Tab. Bot. 1000s.
Use: Antidiarrheal.
BISMU-KINO. (Denver) Bismuth oxycarbonate 10 gr, eucalyptus gum 6 gr, phenyl salicylate, camphor, menthol, carminative oils of nutmeg and clove in soothing, demulcent base w/alcohol 2%/fl oz. Bot. 4 oz, pt.
Use: Stomach and intestinal upset.
BISMUTH ALUMINATE. Magnesium trisilicate, aluminum hydroxide, magnesium carbonate coprecipitate.
See: Escot, Cap. (Solvay).
BISMUTH GLYCOLLYLARSANILATE. B.A.N. Bismuthyl N-glycoloylarsanilate. Glycobiarsol(I.N.N.).
Use: Treatment of amebiasis.
BISMUTH GLYCOLYLARSANILATE. Bismuthyl N-glycollylarsanilate.
Use: Antiamebic.
See: Glycobiarsol, N.F. XVIII.
BISMUTH HYDROXIDE.
See: Milk of Bismuth, U.S.P. XXIII.
BISMUTH, INSOLUBLE PRODUCTS.
See: Bismuth Subgallate (Various Mfr.). Bismuth Subsalicylate (Various Mfr.). Bismuth Tribromophenate (N.Y. Quinine).

BISMUTH, MAGMA. Name previously used for Milk of Bismuth.
• **BISMUTH, MILK OF,** N.F. XVIII.
Use: Astringent, antacid.
BISMUTH OXYCARBONATE.
See: Bismuth Subcarbonate.
BISMUTH POTASSIUM TARTRATE. Basic bismuth potassium bismuthotartrate.
Brewer—25 mg/ml Amp. 2 ml.
Miller—0.016 Gm/ml Amp. 2 ml, Box 12s, 100s; Bot. 30 ml, 60 ml.
Raymer—2.5% Amp. 2 ml, Box 12s, 100s.
Use: Agent for syphilis.
BISMUTH RESORCIN COMPOUND.
W/Bismuth subgallate, balsam Peru, benzocaine, zinc oxide, boric acid.
See: Bonate, Supp. (Suppositoria).
W/Bismuth subgallate, balsam Peru, zinc oxide, boric acid.
See: Versal, Supp. (Suppositoria).
W/Bismuth subgallate, zinc oxide, boric acid, balsam Peru.
See: Anulan, Supp. (Lannett).
BISMUTH SODIUM TARTRATE.
Use: I.M., syphilis.
BISMUTH SUBBENZOATE.
Use: Dusting powder for wounds.
BISMUTH SUBCARBONATE.
Use: Gastroenteritis, diarrhea.
W/Benzocaine, zinc oxide, boric acid.
See: Aracain Rectal Supp. (Commerce).
W/Calcium carbonate, magnesium carbonate.
See: Dimacid, Tab. (Otis Clapp).
W/Calcium carbonate, magnesium carbonate, aminoacetic acid, dried aluminum hydroxide gel.
See: Buffertabs, Tab. (Forest).
W/Charcoal and ginger.
See: Harv-a-carbs, Tab. (Forest).
W/Hydrocortisone acetate, belladonna extract, ephedrine sulfate, zinc oxide, boric acid, balsam Peru, cocoa butter.
See: Rectacort, Supp. (Century).
W/Kaolin, pectin.
See: K-C, Liq. (Century).
W/Paregoric, kaolin (colloidal), aluminum hydroxide, pectin.
See: Kapinal, Tab. (Jenkins).
W/Paregoric, phenyl salicylate, zinc phenolsulfonate, pepsin.
See: Bismuth, salol, zincand paregoric. (Bowman).
W/Pectin, kaolin, opium powder.
See: KBP/O, Cap. (Cole).
W/Phenyl salicylate, zinc phenolsulfonate, pepsin.
See: Bismuth, salol, zinc compound

(Bowman).
W/Phenyl salicylate, chloroform, eucalyptus gum, camphor.
See: Bismu-Kino, Liq. (Denver Chem.).
W/Ephedrine sulfate, belladonna extract, zinc oxide, boric acid, bismuth oxyiodide, balsam Peru.
See: Wyanoids, Preps. (Wyeth-Ayerst).
• **BISMUTH SUBGALLATE,** U.S.P. XXIII, (Various Mfr.) Dermatol.
Use: Topically for skin conditions; orally as an antidiarrheal.
W/Balsam Peru, zinc oxide, cod liver oil.
See: Pile-Gon, Oint. (E.J. Moore).
W/Benzocaine, resorcin, cod liver oil, lanolin, zinc oxide.
See: Biscolan, Supp. (Lannett).
W/Benzocaine, zinc oxide, boric acid, balsam Peru.
See: Anocaine, Supp. (Hauck).
W/Bismuth oxyiodide, bismuth resorcin compound, benzocaine, boric acid.
See: Bonate, Supp. (Suppositoria).
W/Bismuth resorcin compound, balsam Peru, benzocaine, zinc oxide, boric acid.
See: Bonate, Supp. (Suppositoria).
W/Bismuth resorcin compound, zinc oxide, boric acid, balsam Peru.
See: Anulan, Supp. (Lannett).
Versal, Supp. (Suppositoria).
W/Cod liver oil, benzocaine, lanolin, zinc oxide, resorcin, balsam Peru, hydrocortisone.
See: Doctient HC, Supp. (Suppositoria).
W/Hydrocortisone acetate, bismuth resorcin compound, zinc oxide, balsam Peru, benzyl benzoate.
See: Anusol-HC, Supp. (Parke-Davis).
W/Diethylaminoacet-2,6-xylidide, zinc oxide, aluminum subacetate, balsam Peru.
See: Xylocaine Suppositories (Astra).
W/Kaolin, colloidal.
See: Diastop, Liq. (Elder).
W/Kaolin colloidal, calcium carbonate, magnesium trisilicate, papain, atropine sulphate.
See: Kaocasil, Tab. (Jenkins).
W/Kaolin, opium, zinc phenolsulfonate, pectin.
See: Cholactabs, Tab. (Roxane).
W/Kaolin, pectin, zinc phenolsulfonate, opium powder.
See: Diastay, Tab. (Elder).
W/Opium powder, pectin, kaolin, zinc phenolsulfonate.
See: Bismuth, Pectin, Paregoric (Lemmon).
W/Zinc oxide, bismuth resorcin compound, balsam Peru, benzyl benzoate.
See: Anugesic, Supp., Oint. (Parke-

Davis).
Anusol, Supp., Oint. (Parke-Davis).
BISMUTH SUBIODIDE.
See: Bismuth oxyiodide.
• **BISMUTH SUBNITRATE,** U.S.P. XXIII.
Use: Gastroenteritis, amebic dysentery,
locally for wounds.
W/Calcium carbonate, magnesium car-
bonate.
See: Antacid No. 2, Tab. (Bowman).
Maygel, Tab. (Century).
W/Sodium bicarbonate, magnesium car-
bonate, diastase, papain.
Panacarb, Tab. (Lannett).
• **BISMUTH SUBSALICYLATE.** USAN. Ba-
sic bismuth salicylate.
Use: Agent for syphilis.
W/Calcium carbonate, glycocoll.
See: Pepto-Bismol, Tab. (Norwich).
W/Pectin, salol, kaolin, zinc sulfocarbolate,
aluminum hydroxide.
See: Wescola Antidiarrheal-Stomach
Upset (Western Research).
W/Phenylsalicylate, zinc phenolsulfonate,
methylcellulose, magnesium aluminum
silicate.
See: Pepto-Bismol, Liq. (Norwich).
BISMUTH TANNATE. (Various Mfr.) Tan-
bismuth.
Use: Astringent and protective in G.I.
disorders.
BISMUTH TRIBROMOPHENATE.
Use: Intestinal antiseptic.
BISMUTH VIOLET. (Table Rock) Bismuth
Violet. **Oint.** 1%. Jar oz, lb. **Soln.** 0.5%.
Bot. 0.5 oz, 6 oz, pt, gal. **Tr.** 0.5%. Bot. 6
oz, pt, also 1% w/benzoic and salicylic
acid. Bot. 0.5 oz, 6 oz, pt.
Use: Antibacterial, antifungal.
**BISMUTH, WATER-SOLUBLE PROD-
UCTS.**
See: Bismuth Potassium Tartrate (Vari-
ous Mfr.).
• **BISOBRIN LACTATE.** USAN. Meso-1,1'-
tetramethlenebis[1,2,3,4-tetrahydro-6,7-
dimethoxyisoquinoline]dilactate.
Use: Fibrinolytic.
• **BISOPROLOL.** USAN.
Use: Antihypertensive.
• **BISOPROLOL FUMARATE.** USAN.
Use: Antihypertensive.
See: Zebeta (Lederle).
Ziac, Tab. (Lederle).
BISOXATIN. B.A.N. 2,3-Dihydro-2,2-di(4-
hydroxy- phenyl)-1,4-benzoxazin-3-one.
Use: Laxative.
• **BISOXATIN ACETATE.** USAN.
Use: Cathartic.
BISPECIFIC ANTIBODY 520C9x22.
(Medarex)

Use: Serotherapy of ovarian cancer.
[Orphan drug]
• **BISPYRITHIONE MAGSULFEX.** USAN.
Use: Antibacterial, antidandruff.
BISQUADINE. (Sterwin) Alexidine.
BIS-TROPAMIDE. Tropicamide.
See: Mydriacyl, Soln. (Alcon).
BITE & ITCH LOTION. (Weeks & Leo)
Pramoxine HCl 1%, pyrilamine maleate
2%, pheniramine maleate 0.2%, chlor-
pheniramine maleate 0.2%. Bot. 4 oz.
Use: Minor skin irritations.
BITHIONOL. 2,2'-Thiobis(4,6-
dichlorophenol) B.A.N.
Use: Local anti-infective.
See: Actamer (Monsanto Chem.).
W/Allantoin, salicylic acid.
See: Domerine, Shampoo (Miles).
Bitin (No Mfr. currently listed).
Lorothidol (No Mfr. currently listed).
W/Resorcinol monoacetate, sulfur.
See: Acne-Dome, Preps. (Miles).
• **BITHIONOLATE SODIUM.** USAN. Dis-
odium 2,2'-thiobis-(4,6-dichlorophenox-
ide).
Use: Topical anti-infective.
BITIN. CDC Anti-infective agent.
See: Bithionol.
• **BITOLTEROL MESYLATE.** USAN.
Use: Bronchodilator.
See: Tornalate, Inhalation soln. (Dura).
BITRATE. (Arco) Phenobarbital 15 mg,
pentaerythritol tetranitrate 20 mg/Tab.
Bot. 100s.
Use: Sedative/hypnotic, antianginal.
• **BIZELESIN.** USAN.
Use: Antineoplastic.
B-JECT-100. (Hyrex) Vitamins B_1 100
mg, B_2 2 mg, B_3 100 mg, B_5 2 mg, B_6 2
mg/ml. Inj. Vial 10 ml, 30 ml.
Use: Vitamin B supplement.
**BLACK AND WHITE BLEACHING
CREAM.** (Schering-Plough) Hydro-
quinone 2%. Tube 0.75 oz, 1.5 oz.
Use: Skin bleaching agent.
BLACK AND WHITE OINTMENT.
(Schering-Plough) Resorcinol 3%. Tube
0.62 oz, 2.25 oz.
Use: Antiseptic, antipruritic.
BLACK DRAUGHT. (Chattem) Powdered
senna extract. **Tab.:** 600 mg. Bot. 30s.
Gran.: 1.65 Gm/0.5 tsp. Jar 22.5 Gm.
Use: Laxative.
BLACK DRAUGHT SYRUP. (Chattem)
Casanthranol 90 mg w/senna, rhubarb,
anise, methyl salicylate, ginger, pepper-
mint oil, spearmint oil, menthol, alcohol
5%, tartrazine/Tbsp. Bot. 2 oz, 5 oz.
Use: Laxative.
BLACK WIDOW SPIDER, ANTIVENIN.

See: Antivenin (Lactrodectus mactens), Inj. (Merck & Co.).

BLAIREX HARD CONTACT LENS CLEANER. (Blairex) Anionic detergent. Liq. Bot. 60 ml.
Use: Hard contact lens care.

BLAIREX LENS LUBRICANT. (Blairex) Isotonic. Sorbic acid 0.25%, EDTA 0.1%, borate buffer, NaCl, hydroxypropyl-methylcellulose, glycerin. Soln. Bot. 15 ml.
Use: Soft contact lens care.

BLAIREX STERILE SALINE SOLUTION. (Blairex) Normal saline 0.9%. Aerosol can 90 ml, 240 ml, 360 ml.
Use: Soft contact lens care.

BLAIREX SYSTEM. (Blairex Labs) Sodium Cl 135 mg/Tab. 200s, 365s w/15 ml bot.
Use: Soft contact lens care.

BLAIREX SYSTEM II. (Blairex Labs) Sodium Cl 250 mg/Tab. 90s, 180s w/27.7 ml bot.
Use: Soft contact lens care.

BLAUD STRUBEL. (Strubel) Ferrous sulfate 5 gr/Cap. Bot. 100s.
Use: Iron supplement.

BLEFCON. (Madland) Sodium sulfacetamide 30%. Oint. Tube 1/8 oz.
Use: Ophthalmic preparation.

BLENOXANE. (Bristol-Myers/Mead Johnson Oncology) Bleomycin sulfate 15 units/Vial. 1s, 10s.
Use: Antineoplastic agent.

• **BLEOMYCIN SULFATE, STERILE,** U.S.P. XXIII. Antibiotic obtained from cultures of Streptomyces verticillus.
Use: Antineoplastic. [Orphan drug]
See: Blenoxane, Inj. (Bristol).

BLEPH-10 LIQUIFILM. (Allergan) Sulfacetamide sodium 10%, polyvinyl alcohol 1.4%, thimerosal 0.005%, polysorbate 80, sodium thiosulfate, EDTA, purified water. Plastic dropper bot. 2.5 ml, 5 ml, 15 ml.
Use: Anti-infective, ophthalmic.

BLEPH-10 S.O.P. STERILE OPH-THALMIC OINTMENT. (Allergan) Sulfacetamide sodium 10%, phenylmercuric acetate 0.0008%, white petrolatum, mineral oil, nonionic lanolin derivatives. Tube 3.5 Gm.
Use: Anti-infective, ophthalmic.

BLEPHAMIDE LIQUIFILM. (Allergan) Sulfacetamide sodium 10%, prednisolone acetate 0.2%, polyvinyl alcohol 1.4%, EDTA, polysorbate 80, sodium thiosulfate, benzalkonium Cl. Dropper bot. 5 ml, 10 ml.
Use: Anti-inflammatory, anti-infective,

ophthalmic.

BLEPHAMIDE S.O.P. STERILE OPH-THALMIC OINTMENT. (Allergan) Prednisolone acetate 0.2%, sulfacetamide sodium 10%, phenylmercuric acetate 0.0008%, mineral oil, white petrolatum, nonionic lanolin derivatives. Tube 3.5 Gm.
Use: Anti-inflammatory, anti-infective, ophthalmic.

BLINX. (Pilkington Barnes-Hind) Sodium Cl, potassium Cl, sodium phosphate, benzalkonium Cl 0.005%, EDTA 0.02%. Soln. Bot. 120 ml.
Use: Extraocular irrigation solution.

BLIS. (Commerce) Boric acid 47.5%, salicylic acid 17%. Bot. 7 oz.
Use: Foot preparation.

BLISTERGARD. (Medtech) Alcohol 6.7%, pyroxylin solution, oil of cloves, B-hydroxyquinolone. Liq. Bot. 30 ml.
Use: Skin protectant.

BLISTEX. (Blistex) Padimate O 6.6%, oxybenzone 2.5%, dimethicone 2%, cocoa butter, lanolin, parabens, mineral oil, petrolatum. Tube 4.5 g.
Use: Lip balm.

BLISTEX ULTRA PROTECTION. (Blistex) Octyl methoxycinnamate, oxybenzone, octyl salicylate, menthyl anthranilate, homosalate, dimethicone. Tube 4.2 g.
Use: Lip balm.

BLISTIK. (Blistex) Padimate O 6.6%, oxybenzone 2.5%, dimethicone 2%. Lip balm stick 4.5 Gm.
Use: Lip protectant.

BLIS-TO-SOL. (Chattem) **Liq.:** Salicylic acid, undecylenic acid. Bot. 1 oz, 2 oz.
Pow.: Benzoic acid, salicylic acid. Bot. 2 oz.
Use: Antifungal, external.

BLM.
See: Bleomycin sulfate.

BLOCADREN. (Merck & Co.) Timolol maleate 5 mg, 10 mg or 20 mg/Tab. **5 mg:** Bot. 100s; **10 mg:** Bot. 100s, UD 100s; **20 mg:** Bot. 100s.
Use: Beta-adrenergic blocking agent.

BLOCK OUT BY SEA & SKI. (Carter) Padimate O, octyl methoxycinnamate, oxybenzone. Cream. Tube 120 Gm.
Use: Sunscreen.

BLOCK OUT CLEAR BY SEA & SKI. (Carter) Padimate O, octyl methoxycinnamate, octyl salicylate, SD alcohol 40. Lot. Bot. 120 ml.
Use: Sunscreen.

BLOOD, ANTICOAGULANTS.
See: Anticoagulants.

• **BLOOD CELLS, RED.** U.S.P. XXIII.
Use: Blood replenisher.
BLOOD COAGULATION.
See: Hemostatics.
BLOOD FRACTIONS.
See: Albumin (Human) Salt-Poor (Armour; Hyland).
BLOOD GLUCOSE CONCENTRATOR.
See: Glucagon (Lilly).
BLOOD GLUCOSE TEST.
See: Chemstrip bG Strips. (Boehringer Mannheim).
Dextrostix Reagent Strips. (Miles Diagnostic).
First Choice, Strips (Polymer Technology, Int.).
Glucostix Strips. (Miles Diagnostic).
Visidex II Reagent Strips. (Miles Diagnostic).
• **BLOOD GROUPING SERUM, ANTI-A.** U.S.P. XXIII.
Use: Diagnostic aid (in vitro, blood).
• **BLOOD GROUPING SERUM, ANTI B,** U.S.P. XXIII.
Use: Diagnostic aid (in vitro, blood).
• **BLOOD GROUPING SERUMS.** U.S.P. XXIII. Anti-Rh. (Anti-D) 85%-1ubes, 10 tests; Vial, with pipette, 5 ml Anti-Rh. (Anti C plus D) 17%-Tube, 10 tests; Vial, with pipette, 5 ml.
Use: Diagnostic aid in the determination of Rh. (D) and Rh. (C plus D) factors in red blood cells.
• **BLOOD GROUP SPECIFIC SUBSTANCES A, B AND AB,** U.S.P. XXIII.
Use: Blood neutralizer (isoagglutinins, group O blood).
BLOOD PLASMA.
See: Normal Human Plasma.
BLOOD PLASMA SUBSTITUTES.
See: Dextran (Cutter; Pharmachem).
BLOOD UREA NITROGEN TEST.
See: Azostix Strips. (Miles Diagnostic).
BLOOD VOLUME DETERMINATION.
See: Evans Blue, dye (City Chem).
• **BLOOD, WHOLE HUMAN,** U.S.P. XXIII.
Use: Blood replenisher.
BLU-6. (Bluco) Pyridoxine HCl 100 mg/ml. Vial 30 ml.
Use: Vitamin B supplement.
BLU-12 100. (Bluco) Cyanocobalamin 100 mcg /ml. Vial 30 ml.
Use: Vitamin B supplement.
BLU-12 1000. (Bluco) Cyanocobalamin 1000 mcg /ml. Vial 30 ml.
Use: Vitamin B supplement.
BLUBORO POWDER. (Herbert) Aluminum sulfate 53.9%, calcium acetate 43% w/boric acid, FD&C; Blue 1. Packet

1.9 Gm. Box 12s.
Use: Astringent.
BLUDEX. (Burlington) Methenamine 40.8 mg, methylene blue 5.4 mg, phenyl salicylate 18.1 mg, atropine sulfate 0.03 mg, hyoscyamine 0.03 mg, benzoic acid 4.5 mg/Tab. Bot. 100s, 1000s.
Use: Urinary antiseptic, antispasmodic.
BLUE. (Various Mfr.) Pyrethrins 0.3%, piperonyl butoxide 3%, petroleum distillate 1.2%. Gel Bot. 30 Gm, 480 Gm.
Use: Pediculicide.
BLUE GEL MUSCULAR PAIN RELIEVER. (Rugby) Menthol in a specially formulated base. Gel. Tube 240 g.
Use: Rubs & liniments.
BLUE STAR OINTMENT. (McCue Labs.) Salicylic acid, benzoic acid, methyl salicylate, camphor, lanolin, petrolatum. Jar 2 oz.
Use: Minor skin irritations, ringworm, corn or callus removal.
BLUTENE CHLORIDE. Tolonium chloride, Toluidine blue O chloride, 3-amino-7-dimethylamino-2-methyl-phenazathonium salt.
B-MAJOR. (Barth's) Vitamins B_1 7 mg, B_2 14 mg, niacin 2.35 mg, B_{12} 7.5 mcg, B_6 0.15 mg, pantothenic acid 0.37 mg, choline 85 mg, inositol 6 mg, biotin, folic acid, aminobenzoic acid/Cap. Bot. 1s, 3s, 6s, 12s.
Use: Vitamin/mineral supplement.
B.M.E. (Brothers) Aminophylline 32 mg, ephedrine sulfate 8 mg, phenobarbital 8 mg, chlorpheniramine maleate 2 mg, alcohol 15%/5 ml. Bot. pt.
Use: Bronchodilator, decongestant, sedative/hypnotic, antihistamine.
B-N. (Eric, Kirk & Gary). Bacitracin 500 units, neomycin sulfate 5 mg. Oint. Tube 0.5 oz.
Use: Anti-infective, external.
b-NAPHTHYL SALICYLATE. Betol, Naphthosalol, Salinaphthol.
Use: G.I. & G.U., antiseptic.
B-NUTRON TABLETS. (Nion) Vitamins B_1 2 mg, niacinamide 18 mg, B_2 3 mg, B_6 2.2 mg, cyanocobalamin 3 mcg, folic acid 0.4 mg, iron 6 mg, pantothenic acid 3.3 mg, B complex as provided by 150 mg Brewer's yeast/Tab. Bot. 100s, 500s.
Use: Vitamin/mineral supplement.
B and O SUPPRETTES NO. 15A & NO. 16A. (PolyMedica) Opium 30 mg or 60 mg, belladonna extract 15 mg/Supp. Jar 12s.
Use: Narcotic analgesic, antispasmodic.
BOBID. (Boyd) Phenylpropanolamine

HCl 50 mg, chlorpheniramine maleate 8 mg, methscopolamine bromide 2.5 mg/Cap. Bot. 100s.
Use: Decongestant, antihistamine, anticholinergic.
BO-CAL. (Fibertone) Calcium 250 mg, magnesium 125 mg, vitamin D_3 100 IU, boron 0.75 mg/Tab. Bot. 120s.
Use: Vitamin/mineral supplement.
BOILAID. (E.J. Moore) Benzocaine, tetracaine, ichthammol, resin cerate, thymol iodide. Jar oz.
Use: Anesthetic drawing salve.
BOIL-EASE ANESTHETIC DRAWING SALVE. (Commerce) Benzocaine 0.5%, ichthammol 1.86%, sulfur 0.44%, camphor 1.6%, juniper tar 0.11%, phenol 0.42%. Tube oz.
Use: Anesthetic drawing salve.
BOILnSOAK. (Alcon) Sodium Cl 0.7%, boric acid, sodium borate, thimerosal 0.001%, disodium edetate 0.1%. Bot. 8 oz, 12 oz.
Use: Soft contact lens care.
• **BOLANDIOL DIPROPIONATE.** USAN.
Use: Anabolic.
• **BOLASTERONE.** USAN.
Use: Anabolic.
BOLAX. (Boyd) Docusate sodium 240 mg, phenolphthalein 30 mg, dihydrocholic acid ¾ gr/Cap. Bot. 100s.
Use: Laxative.
BOLDENONE. B.A.N. 17β-Hydroxyandrosta-1,4-dien-3-one.
Use: Anabolic steroid.
• **BOLDENONE UNDECYLENATE.** USAN. 17β Hydroxyandrosta-1,4-dien-3-one 10 undecenoate. Parenabol. Under study.
Use: Anabolic.
• **BOLENOL.** USAN. 19-Nor-17-α-pregn-5-en-17-ol. 17α-ethyl-5-estren-17-ol. Under study.
Use: Anabolic.
• **BOLMANTALATE.** USAN. 17β-Hydroxyestr-4-en-3-one adamantane-1-carboxylate.
Use: Anabolic steroid.
BONACAL PLUS TABLETS. (Kenwood) Vitamins A 5000 IU, D 400 IU, C 100 mg, B_1 3 mg, B_2 3 mg, B_6 10 mg, B_{12} 4 mcg, niacinamide 20 mg, d-calcium pantothenate 3.3 mg, iron 42 mg, calcium 350 mg, manganese 0.33 mg, zinc 0.1 mg, magnesium 1.67 mg, potassium 1.67 mg/Tab. Bot. 100s.
Use: Vitamin/mineral supplement.
BONAL ITCH CREAM. (E.J. Moore) Benzocaine, dibucaine, tetracaine in water-washable base. Tube oz.
Use: Local anesthetic.

BONATE. (Suppositoria) Bismuth subgallate, balsam Peru, benzocaine, zinc oxide/Supp. Box 12s, 100s, 1000s.
Use: Anorectal preparation.
BONE MEAL W/VITAMIN D. (Natures Bounty) Calcium 220 mg, vitamin D 100 IU, phosphorus 100 mg, iron 0.45 mg, copper 0.05 mg, zinc 20 mcg, manganese 2.75 mcg, magnesium 0.925 mg. Tab. Bot. 100s, 250s.
Use: Vitamin/mineral supplement.
BONINE. (Pfipharmecs) Meclizine HCl 25 mg/Chew. tab. Pkg. 8s, 48s.
Use: Antiemetic/antivertigo.
BONTRIL PDM. (Carnrick) Phendimetrazine tartrate 35 mg/3 layer Tab. Bot. 100s, 1000s.
Use: Anorexiant.
BONTRIL SLOW RELEASE CAPSULES. (Carnrick) Phendimetrazine tartrate 105 mg/Cap. Bot. 100s.
Use: Anorexiant.
BOPEN-VK. (Boyd) Potassium phenoxymethyl penicillin 400,000 units/Tab. Bot. 100s.
Use: Antibacterial; penicillin.
BORAX. Sodium Borate, N.F. XVIII.
• **BORIC ACID,** N.F. XVIII. Cryst. or Pow.
Use: Mild antiseptic.
See: Borofax, Oint. (Burroughs Wellcome).
W/Combinations.
See: Saratoga Ointment (Blair).
BORIC ACID OINTMENT. (Various Mfr.) Topical ointment 5% or 10%. Tube, Jar 30 Gm, 52.5 Gm, 60 Gm, 120 Gm, 454 Gm. Ophth. oint. 0.5% or 10%. Tube, Jar. 3.5 Gm, 3.75 Gm, 30 Gm, 60 Gm, 480 Gm.
Use: Minor skin irritations.
2-BORNANONE. Camphor, U.S.P. XXIII.
BORNAPRINE. B.A.N. 3-Diethylaminopropyl 2-phenylbicyclo[2.2.1]-heptane-2-carboxylate.
Use: Spasmolytic.
See: Sormodren.
• **BORNELONE.** USAN.
Use: Ultraviolet screen.
• **BOROCAPTATE SODIUM B10.** USAN.
Use: Antineoplastic.
BOROFAIR. (Major) Acetic acid 2% in aluminum acetate soln. Bot. 60 ml.
Use: Otic preparation.
BOROFAX OINTMENT. (Burroughs Wellcome) Boric acid 5%. Tube 1.75 oz.
Use: Minor skin irritations.
BOROGLYCERIN. Glycerol borate. (Emerson) Bot. pt.
BOROGLYCERIN GLYCERITE. Boric acid 31 parts, glycerin 96 parts.

Use: Agent for dermatitis.

BOROPAK POWDER. (Glenwood) Aluminum sulfate and calcium acetate. One packet dissolved in a pint of water yields a 1:40 dilution. Pcks 2.4 Gm. 100s.
Use: Anti-inflammatory agent, topical.

BOROTANNIC COMPLEX. Boric acid 31 mg, tannic acid 50 mg.
W/salicylic acid, ethyl alcohol.
See: Onycho-Phytex, Liq. (Unimed).

BOSTON ADVANCE CLEANER. (Polymer Tech) Concentrated homogenous surfactant with friction-enhancing agents. Soln. Bot. 30 ml or with conditioner in convenience pack
Use: Hard contact lens care.

BOSTON ADVANCE CONDITIONING SOLUTION. (Polymer Tech) Sterile, buffered, slightly hypertonic. Polyaminopropyl biguanide 0.0015%, EDTA 0.05%. Bot. 120 ml or with cleaner in a convenience pack.
Use: Hard contact lens care.

BOSTON ADVANCE REWETTING DROPS. (Polymer Tech) Buffered, slightly hypertonic. Polyaminopropyl biguanide 0.0015%, EDTA 0.05%. Bot. 10 ml.
Use: Hard contact lens care.

BOSTON CLEANER. (Polymer Tech) Anionic sulfate surfactant with friction-enhancing agents, sodium Cl. Soln. Bot. 30 ml.
Use: Hard contact lens care.

BOSTON CONDITIONING SOLUTION. (Polymer Tech) Sterile, buffered, slightly hypertonic, low viscosity. EDTA 0.05%, chlorhexidine gluconate 0.006%. Bot. 120 ml.
Use: Hard contact lens care.

BOSTON RECONDITIONING DROPS. (Polymer Tech) Hydrophilic polyelectrolyte, polyvinyl alcohol, hydroxyethylcellulose, chlorhexidine gluconate, EDTA. Soln. Bot. 120 ml.
Use: Contact lens care.

BOTOX. (Allergan) Botulinum toxin type A 100 units, albumin 0.05 mg, sodium chloride 0.9mg. Pow. for inj. (lyophilized). Vials.
Use: Ophthalmic preparation.

BOTTOMBETTER. (Inno Visions) Petrolatum 49%, lanolin 15.5%, beeswax, sodium borate, lanolin alcohols, methylsalicylate, sorbitan sesquioleate, parabens, oxyquinolone, EDTA. Oint. Pkg. 18s.
Use: Diaper rash product.

BOTULINUM TOXIN TYPE A.
Use: Treatment of strabismus and ble-

pharospasm. [Orphan drug]
See: Botox (Allergan).
Occulinum (Allergan).

BOTULINUM TOXIN TYPE B.
Use: Cervical dystonia [Orphan drug]

BOTULINUM TOXIN TYPE F.
Use: Cervical dystonia; essential blepharospasm. [Orphan drug]

• **BOTULISM ANTITOXIN,** U.S.P. XXIII.
Use: Prophylaxis and treatment of the toxins of C. botulinum, Types A or B; passive immunizing agent.

BOUNTY BEARS. (Nature's Bounty) Vitamins A 2500 IU, D 400 IU, E 15 IU, C 60 mg, B_1 1.05 mg, B_2 1.2 mg, B_3 13.5 mg, B_6 1.05 mg, B_{12} 4.5 mcg, folic acid 0.3 mg/Tab. Bot. 100s.
Use: Vitamin/mineral supplement.

BOUNTY BEARS PLUS IRON. (Nature's Bounty) Vitamins A 2500 IU, D 400 IU, E 15 IU, C 60 mg, B_1 1.05 mg, B_2 1.2 mg, B_3 13.5 mg, B_6 1.05 mg, B_{12} 4.5 mcg, folic acid 0.3 mg, iron 15 mg/Tab. Bot. 100s.
Use: Vitamin/mineral supplement.

BOURBONAL.
See: Ethyl Vanillin, N.F. XVIII.

BOVINE COLOSTRUM.
Use: AIDS-related diarrhea. [Orphan drug]

BOVINE WHEY PROTEIN CONCENTRATE.
Use: Treatment of cryptosporidiosis. [Orphan drug]
See: Immuno-C.

BOWMAN COLD TABS. (Bowman) Acetaminophen 324 mg, phenylpropanolamine HCl 24.3 mg, caffeine 16.2 mg/Tab. Bot. 1000s, 5000s.
Use: Analgesic, decongestant.

BOWMAN'S POISON ANTIDOTE KIT. (Bowman) Syrup of ipecac 1 oz, 1 bottle; activated charcoal liquid 2 oz, 3 bottles.
Use: Antidote.

BOWSTERAL. (Bowman) Isopropanol 60%. Bot. pt, gal.
Use: Anti-rust disinfectant for surgical instruments.

• **BOXIDINE.** USAN. 1-[2-[[4'-(Trifluoromethyl)-4-biphenylyl]-oxy]ethyl]pyrrolidine.
Use: Adrenal steroid blocker.

BOYLEX. (Approved) Diperodon, hexachlorophene, rosin cerate, ichthammol, carbolic acid, thymol, camphor, juniper tar. Tube oz.
Use: Drawing salve.

BOYOL. (Pfeiffer) Ichthammol 10%, benzocaine, lanolin and petrolatum base. Salve Tube 30 Gm.

Use: Antiseptic, local anesthetic.
B-PAP. (Wren) Acetaminophen 120 mg, sodium butabarbital 15 mg/5 ml. Bot. pt, gal.
Use: Analgesic, sedative.
B-PAS.
See: Calcium Benzoylpas.
B-PLEX. (Goldline) Vitamins B₁ 15 mg, B₂ 15 mg, B₃ 100 mg, B₅ 18 mg, B₆ 4 mg, B₁₂ 5 mcg, C 500 mg, folic acid 0.5 mg/Tab. Bot. 100s.
Use: Vitamin/mineral supplement.
B-PLEX 100, INJECTABLE. (Jenkins) Vitamins B₁ 100 mg, B₂ 2 mg, B₆ 2 mg, panthenol 10 mg, niacinamide 125 mg, ethanolamide of gentisic acid 2.5%/ml. Vial 30 ml.
Use: Vitamin/mineral supplement.
B-PLEX 100 W/B₁₂. (Jenkins) Vitamins B₁ 100 mg, B₂ 2 mg, B₆ 5 mg, niacinamide 125 mg, panthenol 10 mg, B₁₂ 30 mcg, ethanolamide of gentisic acid 2.5%/ml. Vial 30 ml, 12s.
Use: Vitamin/mineral supplement.
B-P-M CREAM. (Durel) Burow's solution 5%, phenol 0.5%, menthol 0.5%, camphor 1% in Duromantel cream. Jar oz, 1 lb, 6 lb.
Use: Agent for eczema.
BP-PAPAVERINE. (Burlington) Papaverine HCl 150 mg/S.R. Cap. Bot. 50s.
Use: Vasodilator.
BQ COLD TABLETS. (Bristol-Myers) Acetaminophen 325 mg, phenylpropanolamine HCl 12.5 mg, chlorpheniramine maleate 2 mg/Tab. Card 16s, Bot. 16s, 30s, 50s.
Use: Analgesic, decongestant, antihistamine.
BRACE. (SK-Beecham) Denture adhesive. Tube 1.4 oz, 2.4 oz.
BRADOSOL BROMIDE. (Ciba) Domiphen bromide.
BRANCHAMIN 4%. (Travenol) Isoleucine 1.38 Gm, leucine 1.38 Gm, valine 1.25 Gm, phosphate 31.6 mOsm/100 ml. Bot. 500 ml.
Use: Adjunct to regular TPN therapy for highly stressed or traumatized patients.
BRANCHED CHAIN AMINO ACIDS.
Use: Amyotrophic lateral sclerosis. [Orphan drug]
BRASIVOL BASE. (Stiefel) Cleansing paste containing polyoxyethylene lauryl ether and a surfactant cleanser. Jar 4.1 oz.
Use: Degreasing skin cleanser.
BRASIVOL FINE, MEDIUM AND ROUGH. (Stiefel) Aluminum oxide scrub particles

in a surfactant cleansing base. **Fine:** Jar 5.1 oz. **Medium:** Jar 6 oz. **Rough:** Jar 6.5 oz.
Use: Scrub cleanser.
BREACOL DECONGESTANT COUGH MEDICATION. (Glenbrook) Dextromethorphan HBr 10 mg, phenylpropanolamine HCl 37.5 mg, alcohol 10%, chlorpheniramine maleate 4 mg/5 ml. Bot. 3 oz, 6 oz.
Use: Antitussive, decongestant, antihistamine.
BREATHEASY. (Pascal) Racemic epinephrine HCl soln. 2.2% inhaled by use of nebulizer. Bot. 0.25 oz, 0.5 oz, 1 oz.
Use: Bronchodilator.
BREEZEE MIST. (Pedinol) Aluminum chlorhydrate, undecylenic acid, menthol. Aerosol Bot. 4 oz.
Use: Antifungal, deodorant, antiperspirant, foot powder.
BREEZEE MIST ANTIFUNGAL. (Pedinol) Miconazole nitrate 2%, isobutane, talc, aluminum chlorhydrate, cyclomethicone, isopropyl myristate, propylene carbonate, menthol. Pow. Bot. 113 g.
Use: Antifungal.
BREONESIN. (Sanofi Winthrop-Breon) Guaifenesin 200 mg/Cap. Bot. 100s.
Use: Expectorant.
• **BREQUINAR SODIUM.** USAN.
Use: Antineoplastic.
• **BRETAZENIL.** USAN
Use: Antianxiety agent.
BRETHAIRE. (Geigy) Terbutaline sulfate inhaler 7.5 ml. (10.5 Gm) w/mouthpiece.
Use: Bronchodilator.
BRETHANCER. (Geigy) Inhaler (complete unit to be used with Brethaire).
BRETHINE. (Geigy) Terbutaline sulfate. **Tab.:** 2.5 mg. Bot. 100s, 1000s, UD 100s, Gy-Pak 90s, 100s. 5 mg. Bot. 100s, 1000s, UD 100s, Gy-Pak 90s, 100s. **Amp.:** 1 mg/ml. Box 10s, 100s.
Use: Bronchodilator.
• **BRETYLIUM TOSYLATE.** USAN. 2-Bromobenzyl-ethyldimethylammonium toluene-p-sulfonate.
Use: Hypotensive.
See: Bretylol, Inj. (American Critical Care).
BRETYLOL. (American Critical Care) Bretylium tosylate 50 mg/ml. Amp. 10 ml.
Use: Antiarrhythmic agent.
BREVIBLOC. (Anaquest) Esmolol HCl 10 mg/ml or 250 mg/ml, propylene glycol 25%. **10 mg/ml:** Vial 10 ml. **250 mg/ml:** Amp 10 ml.
Use: Beta-adrenergic blocking agent.

BREVICON. (Syntex) Norethindrone 0.5 mg, ethinyl estradiol 0.035 mg/Tab. 21 and 28 day (7 inert tabs) Wallette.
Use: Oral contraceptive.
BREVITAL SODIUM. (Lilly) Methohexital sodium. **Vial:** 500 mg/50 ml, 500 mg/50 ml w/diluent, 2.5 Gm/250 ml, 5 Gm/500 ml. **Amp.:** 2.5 Gm, 5 Gm.
Use: General anesthetic.
BREVOXYL. (Stiefel) Benzyol peroxide 4%, simethicone. Gel. Tube 42.5 Gm, 90 Gm.
Use: Anti-acne product.
BREWER'S YEAST. (Various Mfr.) Pow., Tab. 6 gr, 7.5 gr, 1 lb.
W/Docusate sodium.
See: Doss or Super Doss, Tab., Cap. (Ferndale).
W/Psyllium seed, plantago ovata, karaya gum.
See: Plantamucin Granule, (Elder).
BREXIN EX LIQUID. (Savage) Pseudoephedrine HCl 30 mg, guaifenesin 200 mg/5 ml.
Use: Decongestant, expectorant.
BREXIN EX TABLET. (Savage) Pseudoephedrine HCl 60 mg, guaifenesin 400 mg/Tab. Bot. 100s.
Use: Decongestant, expectorant.
BREXIN L.A. (Savage) Chlorpheniramine maleate 8 mg, pseudoephedrine HCl 120 mg/L.A. Tab. Bot. 100s.
Use: Antihistamine, decongestant.
BRICANYL INJECTION. (Lakeside) Terbutaline sulfate 1 mg/Amp. 1 ml. 10s.
Use: Bronchodilator.
BRICANYL TABLETS. (Lakeside) Terbutaline sulfate 2.5 mg or 5 mg/Tab. Bot. 100s, 1000s, UD 100s.
Use: Bronchodilator.
• BRIFENTANIL HYDROCHLORIDE. USAN.
Use: Analgesic.
BRIGEN-G. (Grafton) Chlordiazepoxide 5 mg, 10 mg or 25 mg/Tab. Bot. 500s.
Use: Antianxiety agent.
BRIJ 96 and 97. (ICI Americas) Polyoxyl 10 oleyl ether available as 96 and 97.
Use: Surface-active agent.
BRIJ-721. (ICI Americas) Polyoxyethylene 21 stearyl ether (100% active).
Use: Surface-active agent.
• BRIMONIDINE TARTRATE. USAN.
Use: Antihypertensive for treatment of glaucoma.
• BRINOLASE. USAN. Fibrinolytic enzyme produced by Aspergillus oryzae.
Use: Fibrinolytic.
BRIREL W/SUPERINONE. (Sanofi Winthrop) Hexahydropyrazine, hexahy-

drate.
Use: Anthelmintic.
BRISTOJECT. (Bristol) Prefilled disposable syringes w/needle.
  Aminophylline: 250 mg/10 ml.
  Atropine Sulfate: 5 mg/5 ml or 1 mg/ml. 10s.
  Calcium Cl: 10%. 10 ml. 10s.
  Dexamethasone: 20 mg/5 ml.
  Dextrose: 50%. 50 ml. 10s.
  Diphenhydramine: 50 mg/5 ml.
  Dopamine HCl: 200 mg/5 ml, 400 mg/10 ml.
  Ephedrine: 50 mg/10 ml.
  Epinephrine: 1:10,000. 10 ml. 10s.
  Lidocaine HCl.: 1%: 5 ml, 10 ml; 2%: 5 ml; 4%: 25 ml, 50 ml; 20%: 5 ml, 10 ml.
  Magnesium Sulfate: 5 Gm/10 ml. 10s.
  Metaraminol: 1%. 10 ml.
  Sodium Bicarbonate: 7.5%: 50 ml; 8.4%: 50 ml. 10s.
BRITISH ANTI-LEWISITE. Dimercaprol.
See: BAL.
BROBELLA-P.B. (Brothers) Atropine sulfate 0.0195 mg, hyoscine HBr 0.0065 mg, hyoscyamine sulfate 0.1040 mg, phenobarbital 0.25 gr/Tab. Bot. 100s, 1000s.
Use: Anticholinergic/antispasmodic, sedative/hypnotic.
BROCILLIN. (Brothers) Potassium penicillin G 400,000 units/Tab. or 5 ml. Bot. 100s. Bot. 80 ml.
Use: Antibacterial; penicillin.
• BROCRESINE. USAN. 0-(4-Bromo-3-hydroxybenzyl)hydroxylamine. Alpha(amino-oxy)-6-bromo-m-cresol.
Use: Histidine decarboxylase inhibitor.
See: Contramine phosphate.
• BROCRINAT. USAN.
Use: Diuretic.
BROCYCLINE. (Brothers) Tetracycline HCl 250 mg/Cap. Bot. 100s, 1000s.
Use: Antibacterial; tetracycline.
BROFED. (Marnel) Pseudoephedrine HCl 30 mg, brompheniramine maleate 4 mg/5 ml. Elix. Bot.
Use: Decongestant, antihistamine.
BROFEZIL. B.A.N. 2-(4-p-Bromophenylthiazol-2-yl)propionic acid.
Use: Anti-inflammatory.
• BROFOXINE. USAN.
Use: Antipsychotic.
BROLADE. (Brothers) Chlorpheniramine maleate 8 mg, phenylephrine HCl 20 mg, methscopolamine nitrate 2.5 mg/Cap. Bot. 50s, 500s.
Use: Antihistamine, decongestant, anticholinergic.

BROMACRYLIDE. N-(acrylamidomethyl)-3-bromopropionamide.
• **BROMADOLINE MALEATE.** USAN.
Use: Analgesic.
BROMALEATE. A mixture of 2-amino-2-methyl-1-propanol and 8-bromotheophylline.
See: Pamabrom.
BROMALINE ELIXIR. (Rugby) Phenylpropanolamine HCl 12.5 mg, brompheniramine maleate 2 mg, alcohol 2.3%. Elix. Bot. 118 ml, pt. and gal.
Use: Decongestant, antihistamine.
BROMALINE PLUS. (Rugby) Phenylpropanolamine HCl 12.5 mg, brompheniramine maleate 2 mg, acetaminophen 500 mg. Captabs. Bot. 24s.
Use: Decongestant, antihistamine, analgesic.
BROMALIX. (Century) Brompheniramine maleate 4 mg, phenylephrine HCl 5 mg, phenylpropanolamine HCl 5 mg, alcohol 2.3%/5 ml. Bot. 4 oz, pt, gal.
Use: Antihistamine, decongestant.
BROMANATE DC COUGH SYRUP. (Various Mfr.) Phenylpropanolamine HCl 12.5 mg, brompheniramine maleate 2 mg, codeine phosphate 10 mg, alcohol 0.95%. Syr. Bot. 120 ml, pt, gal.
Use: Decongestant, antihistamine, antitussive.
BROMANYL. (Various Mfr.) Bromodiphenhydramine HCl 12.5 mg, codeine phosphate 10 mg, alcohol 5%. Syr. Bot. pt, gal.
Use: Antihistamine, antitussive.
BROMAREST DX. (Warner Chilcott) Pseudoephedrine HCl 30 mg, brompheniramine maleate 2 mg, dextromethorphan HBr 10 mg, alcohol 0.95%. Butterscotch favor. Syr. Bot. 480 ml.
Use: Antitussive combination.
BROMATANE D.C. COUGH SYRUP. (Goldline) Brompheniramine maleate, phenylpropanolamine HCl, codeine phosphate. Bot. gal.
Use: Antihistamine, decongestant, antitussive.
BROMATANE DX COUGH SYRUP. (Goldline) Pseudoephedrine HCl 30 mg, brompheniramine maleate 2 mg, dextromethorphan HBr 10 mg. Bot. 480 ml.
Use: Decongestant, antihistamine, antitussive.
BROMATAPP ELIXIR. (Goldline) Brompheniramine maleate 2 mg, phenylephrine HCl 12.5 mg, alcohol 2.3%/5 ml. Bot. 4 oz, 8 oz, pt, gal.
Use: Antihistamine, decongestant.

BROMATAPP TABLETS. (Goldline) Brompheniramine maleate 12 mg, phenylpropanolamine HCl 75 mg/Tab. Bot. 100s, 1000s.
Use: Antihistamine, decongestant.
BROMAURIC ACID. Hydrogen tetrabromoaurate.
• **DROMAZEPAM.** USAN. 7-Bromo-1,3-dihydro-5-(2-Pyridyl)-2H-1,4-benzodiazepin-2-one.
Use: Antianxiety agent.
BROMAZINE.
See: Ambodryl HCl, Elix., Kapseal (Parke-Davis).
BROMBAY ELIXIR. (PBI) Brompheniramine maleate 2 mg/5 ml, alcohol 3%. Bot. 4 oz, pt, gal.
Use: Antihistamine.
• **BROMCHLORENONE.** USAN. 6-Bromo-5-chloro-2-benzoxazolinone. (Maumee) Vinyzene.
Use: Local anti-infective.
BROMEBRIC ACID. B.A.N. cis-3-Bromo-3-p-anisoylacrylic acid.
Use: Cytotoxic agent.
• **BROMELAINS.** USAN.
Use: Anti-inflammatory.
See: Dayto-Anase, Tab. (Dayton).
BROMENZYME. (Barth's) Bromelain 40 mg/Tab. Bot. 100s, 250s, 500s.
Use: Digestive aid.
BROMETHOL.
See: Avertin.
BROMEZYME. (Barth's) Bromelain 40 mg, papaya fruit, papain enzyme/Tab. Bot. 100s, 250s, 500s.
Use: Digestive aid.
BROMFED CAPSULES. (Muro) Brompheniramine maleate 12 mg, pseudoephedrine HCl 120 mg/TR Cap. Bot. 100s, 500s.
Use: Antihistamine, decongestant.
BROMFED-DM SYRUP. (Muro) Brompheniramine maleate 2 mg, pseudoephedrine HCl 30 mg, dextromethorphan HBr 10 mg/5 ml. Bot. 120 ml, 240 ml, 480 ml.
Use: Antihistamine, decongestant, antitussive.
BROMFED-PD CAPSULES. (Muro) Brompheniramine maleate 6 mg, pseudoephedrine HCl 60 mg/TR Cap. Bot. 100s, 500s.
Use: Antihistamine, decongestant.
BROMFED SYRUP. (Muro) Brompheniramine maleate 2 mg, pseudoephedrine HCl 30 mg/5 ml. Bot. 480 ml.
Use: Antihistamine, decongestant.
BROMFED TABLETS. (Muro) Brompheniramine maleate 4 mg, pseu-

doephedrine HCl 60 mg/Tab. Bot. 100s.
Use: Antihistamine, decongestant.
• **BROMFENAC SODIUM.** USAN.
Use: Analgesic.
BROMHEXINE. B.A.N. N-(2-Amino-3,5-
dibromobenzyl)-N-cyclohexylmethy-
lamine.
Use: Bronchial mucolytic.
• **BROMHEXINE HCl.** USAN. (1) 3,5-Dibro-
mo-Nα-cyclohexyl-Nα-methyltoluene-α,
2-diamine monohydrochloride. (2) N-cy-
clohexyl-N-methyl-(2-amino-3,-5-dibro-
mobenzyl) ammonium Cl.
Use: Expectorant, mucolytic.
See: Bisolvon (Boehringer Ingelheim).
BROMHEXINE.
Use: Mild/moderate keratoconjunctivitis
sicca. [Orphan drug]
BROMIDES.
See: Lanabrom, Elix. (Lannett).
Peacocks Bromides, Liq. (Natcon).
BROMIDE SALTS.
See: Calcium Bromide.
Ferrous Bromide.
Potassium Bromide.
Sodium Bromide.
Strontium Bromide.
BROMI-LOTION. (Gordon) Aluminum hy-
droxychloride 20%, emollient base. Bot.
1.5 oz, 4 oz.
Use: Antiperspirant.
• **BROMINDIONE.** USAN. 2-(4-Bro-
mophenyl)(2)2-(p-Bromophenyl)-1,3-in-
dandione.
Use: Anticoagulant.
Occ: Oircladin.
BROMI-TALC. (Gordon) Potassium alum,
bentonite, talc. Shaker can 3.5 oz, 1 lb, 5
lb.
Use: Bromidrosis, hyperhidrosis.
• **BROMOCRIPTINE.** USAN. 2-Bromo-
α-ergocryptine.
Use: Prolactin inhibitor.
• **BROMOCRIPTINE MESYLATE.** USAN
2-Bromo-α-ergocryptine mesylate.
Use: Prolactin inhibitor.
See: Parlodel, Tab. (Sandoz).
• **BROMOCRIPTINE MESYLATE,** U.S.P.
XXIII. Tab., U.S.P. XXIII.
Use: Prolactin inhibitor.
BROMODIETHYLACETYLUREA.
See: Carbromal.
**BROMODIPHENHYDRAMINE HY-
DROCHLORIDE.** B.A.N. U.S.P. XXIII.
N-2-(4-Bromobenzhydryloxy)ethyl-
dimethylamine. Bromazine (I.N.N.).
Use: Antihistamine.
**BROMODIPHENHYDRAMINE
HCL/CODEINE COUGH SYRUP.** (PBI)
Bromodiphenhydramine HCl 12.5 mg,

codeine phsophate 10 mg. Syr. Bot. 480
ml.
Use: Antitussive combination.
BROMOFROM. Tribromomethane.
BROMOISOVALERYL UREA. Alpha,
bromoisovaleryl urea.
See: Bromisovalum.
BROMOPHEN T.D. (Rugby) Phenyl-
propanolamine HCl 15 mg, phenyle-
phrine HCl 15 mg, brompheniramine
maleate 12 mg/Tab. Bot. 100s, 1000s.
Use: Decongestant, antihistamine.
BROMOPHIN.
See: Apomorphine HCl (Various Mfr.).
BROMO QUININE COLD TABLETS.
See: BQ Cold Tablets (Bristol-Myers).
BROMO-SELTZER. (Warner-Lambert)
Acetaminophen 325 mg, sodium bicar-
bonate 2.78 Gm, citric acid 2.22 Gm
(when dissolved, forms sodium citrate
2.85 Gm)/Dose. Large (2⅝ oz), King
(4.25 oz), Giant (9 oz), Foil pack, single
dose 48s.
Use: Antacid, analgesic.
**BROMO-SELTZER EFFERVESCENT
GRANULES.** (Warner-Lambert) Sodi-
um bicarbonate 2781 mg, aceta-
minophen 325 mg, citric acid 2224 mg,
sodium 761 mg, sugar. Bot. 127.5 g.
Use. Antacid, analgesic.
8-BROMOTHEOPHYLLINE. W/2-amino-
2-methyl-1-propanol.
See: Pamabrom.
**BROMOTHEOPHYLLINATE
AMINOISOBUTANOL.**
See: Pamabrom.
**BROMOTHEOPHYLLINATE
PYRANISAMINE.**
See: Pyrabrom.
**BROMOTHEOPHYLLINATE PYRIL-
AMINE.**
See: Pyrabrom.
BROMOTUSS W/CODEINE. (Rugby)
Bromodiphenhydramine HCl 12.5 mg,
codeine phosphate 10 mg, alcohol 5 %.
Syr. Bot. 120 ml, pt, gal.
Use: Antihistamine, antitussive.
• **BROMOXANIDE.** USAN.
Use: Anthelmintic.
• **BROMPERIDOL DECANOATE.** USAN.
Use: Antipsychotic.
**BROMPHEN DC W/CODEINE COUGH
SYRUP.** (Various Mfr.) Phenyl-
propanolamine HCl 12.5 mg,
brompheniramine maleate 2 mg,
codeine phosphate 10 mg, alcohol
0.95%. Syr. Bot. 120 ml, pt, gal.
Use: Decongestant, antihistamine, anti-
tussive.
BROMPHEN DX. (Rugby) Pseu-

doephedrine HCl 30 mg, brompheniramine maleate 2 mg, dextromethorphan HBr 10 mg, alcohol 0.95%. Syr. Bot. 480 ml.
Use: Decongestant, antihistamine, antitussive.

BROMPHEN EXPECTORANT. (Various Mfr.) Phenylpropanolamine HCl 5 mg, phenylephrine HCl 5 mg, brompheniramine maleate 2 mg, guaifenesin 100 mg, alcohol 3.5%. Liq. Bot. 120 ml, pt, gal.
Use: Decongestant, antihistamine, expectorant.

BROMPHENIRAMINE. B.A.N. 3-(4-Bromophenyl)-3-(2-pyridyl) propyldimethylamine.
Use: Antihistamine.

BROMPHENIRAMINE COUGH SYRUP. (Geneva) Pseudoephedrine HCl 30 mg, brompheniramine maleate 2 mg, dextromethorphan HBr 10 mg, alcohol 0.95%. Bot. 480 ml.
Use: Decongestant, antihistamine, antitussive.

BROMPHENIRAMINE DC. (Geneva) Phenylpropanolamine HCl 12.5 mg, brompheniramine maleate 2 mg, codeine phosphate 10 mg, alcohol 0.95%. Syr. Bot. 120 ml.
Use: Decongestant, antihistamine, antitussive.

• **BROMPHENIRAMINE MALEATE,** U.S.P. XXIII. Elix., Inj., Tab., U.S.P. XXIII. 2-[p-Bromo-α-[2-di- methylamino)ethyl]-benzyl]-pyridine maleate.
Use: Antihistamine.
See: Dimetane, Tab., Elix., Inj. (Robins). Symptom 3, Liq. (Parke-Davis). Veltane (Lannett).

BROMPHENIRAMINE MALEATE W/COMBINATIONS.
See: Bro-Expectorant W/Codeine, Liq. (Solvay).
Bromepaph, Preps. (Quality Generics).
Cortane, Preps. (Standex).
Cortapp, Elix. (Standex).
Dimetane Decongestant, Tab., Elix. (Robins).
Dimetane Expectorant, Liq. (Robins).
Dimetane Expectorant-DC, Liq. (Robins).
Dimetapp Extentabs, Elix. (Robins).
Eldatapp, Tab., Liq. (Elder).

BROMPTON'S COCKTAIL. Heroine or morphine 10 mg, cocaine 10 mg, alcohol, chloroform water, syrup.
Use: Narcotic agonist analgesic.

BROMTAPP. (Blue Cross) Brompheniramine maleate 4 mg, phenylephrine HCl 5 mg, phenylpropanolamine HCl 5 mg/5 ml. Bot. 16 oz, gal.
Use: Antihistamine, decongestant.

BRONCAJEN. (Jenkins) Pyrilamine maleate 10 mg, phenylephrine HCl 2 mg, potassium guaiacol sulfonate 2 gr, ammonium Cl 2 gr, ipecac ⅛ gr/Tab. Dot. 1000s.
Use: Antihistamine, decongestant, expectorant.

BRONCHIAL CAPSULES. (Various Mfr.) Theophylline 150 mg, guaifenesin 90 mg. Cap. Bot. 100s.
Use: Antiasthmatic, expectorant.

BRONCHOLATE CAPSULES. (Bock) Ephedrine HCl 12.5 mg, guaifenesin 200 mg/Cap. Bot. 100s, 1000s.
Use: Bronchodilator, expectorant.

BRONCHOLATE SOFTGELS. (Bock) Ephedrine HCl 12.5 mg, guaifenesin 200 mg. Cap. Bot. 100s.
Use: Bronchodilator, expectorant.

BRONCHOLATE SYRUP. (Bock) Ephedrine HCl 6.25 mg, guaifenesin 100 mg/5 ml. Bot. pt.
Use: Bronchodilator, expectorant.

BRONCHO SALINE. (Blairex) 0.9% sodium Cl for diluting bronchodilator solutions for inhalation. Soln. 90 ml, 240 ml w/metered dispensing valve.
Use: Inhalation diluent.

BRONCHOVENT. (Mills) Aminophylline 90 mg, guaifenesin 50 mg, amobarbital 16 mg/coated Tab. Bot. 100s.
Use: Bronchodilator, expectorant, sedative.

BRONDECON. (Parke-Davis) **Tab.:** Oxtriphylline 200 mg, guaifenesin 100 mg/Tab. Bot. 100s. **Elix.:** Oxtriphylline 100 mg, guaifenesin 50 mg/5 ml w/alcohol 20%. Bot. 8 oz, 16 oz.
Use: Bronchodilator, expectorant.

BRONDELATE. (Various Mfr.) Oxtriphylline 300 mg, guaifenesin 150 mg, alcohol 20%/5 ml. Elix. Bot. pt, gal.
Use: Bronchodilator, expectorant.

BRONICOF. (Jenkins) Ethylmorphine HCl 2.5 mg, syrup hydriodic acid 50%, potassium citrate 438 mg, sodium benzoate 10 mg, aromatics/5 ml. Bot. 3 oz, 4 oz, gal.
Use: Cough sedative, expectorant.

BRONITIN. (Whitehall) Theophylline hydrous 120 mg, guaifenesin 100 mg, ephedrine HCl 24.3 mg, pyrilamine maleate 16.6 mg/Tab. Bot. 24s, 60s.
Use: Bronchodilator.

BRONITIN MIST. (Whitehall) Epinephrine bitartrate in inhalation aerosol. Each

spray releases 0.3 mg epinephrine bitartrate equivalent to 0.16 mg epinephrine base. Bot 15 ml or 15 ml refills.
Use: Bronchodilator.
BRONKAID DUAL ACTION. (Sterling Health) Ephedrine sulfate 25 mg, guaifenesin 400 mg. Cap. Bot. 24s.
Use: Bronchodilator.
BRONKAID MIST. (Sanofi Winthrop) Epinephrine 0.5% in inhalation aerosol. Each spray releases 0.25 mg epinephrine. Aerosol 10 Gm or 16.7 Gm w/adapter; 15 Gm, 25 Gm refills.
Use: Bronchodilator.
BRONKAID MIST SUSPENSION. (Sanofi Winthrop) Epinephrine bitartrate 0.7%. Each spray releases 0.3 mg epinephrine bitartrate equivalent to 0.16 mg epinephrine base. Bot. 10 ml, 15 ml with and without adapter.
Use: Bronchodilator.
BRONKAID TABLETS. (Sanofi Winthrop) Ephedrine sulfate 24 mg, guaifenesin 100 mg, theophylline 100 mg/Tab. Box 24s, 60s.
Use: Bronchodilator, expectorant.
BRONKASMA TABLETS. (Sanofi Winthrop) Theophylline anhydrous, ephedrine sulphate, thenyldiamine.
Use: Bronchodilator.
BRONKEPHRINE. (Sanofi Winthrop) Ethylnorepinephrine HCl 2 mg/ml in a sterile isotonic solution of sodium chloride 0.7% w/sodium acetone bisulfite 0.2%, sodium hydroxide or HCl to adjust pH to 2.9-4.5. Amp. 1 ml. Box 25s.
Use: Bronchodilator.
BRONKODYL. (Sanofi Winthrop) Theophylline 100 mg or 200 mg/Cap. Bot. 100s. Theophylline 300 mg/SR Cap. Bot. 100s.
Use: Bronchodilator.
BRONKOLATE "G". (Parmed) Dyphylline 200 mg, guaifenesin 200 mg/Tab. Bot. 100s, 1000s.
Use: Bronchodilator, expectorant.
BRONKOLIXIR. (Sanofi Winthrop) Guaifenesin 50 mg, ephedrine sulfate 12 mg, theophylline 15 mg, phenobarbital 4 mg/5 ml. Bot. pt.
Use: Expectorant, bronchodilator, sedative/hypnotic.
BRONKOMETER. (Sanofi Winthrop) Isoetharine mesylate 0.61%, saccharin, menthol, alcohol 30%. Metered dose of 340 mcg isoetharine in fluoro hydrocarbon propellant. Bot. w/nebulizer 10 ml, 15 ml. Refill 10 ml, 15 ml.
Use: Bronchodilator.
BRONKOSOL. (Sanofi Winthrop)

Isoetharine HCl 1% w/glycerin, sodium bisulfite, parabens for oral inhalation. Bot. 10 ml, 30 ml.
Use: Bronchodilator.
BRONKOTABS. (Sanofi Winthrop) Ephedrine sulfate 24 mg, theophylline 100 mg, guaifenesin 100 mg, phenobarbital 8 mg/Tab. Bot. 100s, 1000s.
Use: Bronchodilator, expectorant, sedative/hypnotic.
BRONKOTUSS. (Hyrex) Chlorpheniramine maleate 4 mg, guaifenesin 100 mg, ephedrine sulfate 8.216 mg, hydriodic acid syrup 1.67 mg/5 ml w/alcohol 5%. Bot. pt, gal.
Use: Antihistamine, expectorant, decongestant.
BRONOPOL. B.A.N. 2-Bromo-2-nitropropane-1,3-diol.
Use: Antiseptic, preservative.
•**BROPERAMOLE.** USAN.
Use: Anti-inflammatory.
•**BROPIRIMINE.** USAN.
Use: Antineoplastic, antiviral.
BROSERPINE. (Brothers) Reserpine 0.25 mg/Tab. Bot. 250s, 1000s.
Use: Antihypertensive.
BROTANE ELIXIR. (Halsey) Bot. 16 oz, gal.
Use: Decongestant.
BROTANE EXPECTORANT. (Blue Cross) Guaifenesin 100 mg, brompheniramine maleate 2 mg, phenylephrine HCl 5 mg, phenylpropanolamine HCl 5 mg/5 ml, alcohol 3.5%. Bot. 16 oz.
Use: Expectorant, antihistamine, decongestant.
•**BROTIZOLAM.** USAN.
Use: Hypnotic.
BRO-T'S. (Brothers) Bromisovalum 0.12 Gm, carbromal 0.2 Gm/Tab. Bot. 100s, 1000s.
Use: Sedative, tranquilizer.
BRO-TUSS. (Brothers) Dextromethorphan HBr 15 mg, chlorpheniramine maleate 2 mg, phenylephrine HCl 5 mg, ammonium Cl 100 mg, sodium citrate 150 mg, vitamin C 30 mg/10 ml. Bot. 4 oz, pt, gal.
Use: Antitussive, antihistamine, decongestant, expectorant.
BRO-TUSS A.C. (Brothers) Acetaminophen 120 mg, codeine phosphate 10 mg, phenylephrine HCl 5 mg, chlorpheniramine maleate 2 mg, menthol 1 mg, alcohol 10%/5 ml. Bot. pt, gal.
Use: Analgesic, antitussive, decongestant, antihistamine.
BROWN MIXTURE. (Various Mfr.) Paregoric 12%, glycyrrhiza fluid extract, anti-

mony potassium tartrate, alcohol. Liq. Bot. 120 ml, pt, gal.
Use: Antidiarrheal.
BRUCELLA VACCINE. Undulant fever vaccine.
Use: I.M., S.C., undulant fever.
BRYREL SYRUP. (Sanofi Winthrop) Piperazine citrate anhydrous 110 mg/ml. Bot. oz
Use: Anthelmintic.
B-SCORBIC. (Pharmics) Vitamins C 300 mg, B_1 25 mg, B_2 10 mg, calcium pantothenate 10 mg, niacinamide 50 mg, lemon flavored complex 200 mg/Tab. Bot. 100s, 1000s.
Use: Vitamin supplement.
BSS.
See: Balanced Salt Solution.
BSS PLUS. (Alcon Surgical) Balanced salt solution with bicarbonate dextrose and glutathione. Two part solution reconstituted within 6 hrs. of surgery. Bot. 500 ml.
Use: Intraocular irrigating solution.
• **BUCAINIDE MALEATE.** USAN.
Use: Cardiac depressant.
BUCET. (UAD) Butalbital 50 mg, acetaminophen 650 mg. Cap. Bot. 100s.
Use: Analgesic.
BUCETIN. B.A.N. N-3-Hydroxybutyryl-p-phenetidine.
Use: Analgesic.
BUCHU.
See: Barosmin.
• **BUCINDOLOL HYDROCHLORIDE.** USAN. A Mead Johnson investigational drug.
Use: Investigative, antihypertensive.
BUCLADIN-S. (Stuart) Buclizine HCl 50 mg. Softab. Tab. Bot. 100s.
Use: Antiemetic/antivertigo.
BUCLIZINE. B.A.N. 1-(4-t-Butylbenzyl)-4-(4-chlor- obenzhydryl) piperazine.
Use: Antiemetic.
• **BUCLIZINE HYDROCHLORIDE.** USAN. 1-(p-tert Butylbenzyl)-4-(p-chloro-alpha-phenylbenzyl) piperazine dihydrochloride.
Use: Antiemetic, antinauseant.
See: Bucladin-S, Tab. (Stuart).
BUCLOSAMIDE. B.A.N. N-Butyl-4-chlorosalicyl-amide.
Use: Antimycotic.
• **BUCROMARONE.** USAN.
Use: Cardiac depressant (antiarrhythmic).
• **BUCRYLATE.** USAN.
Use: Surgical aid.
• **BUDESONIDE.** USAN.
Use: Anti-inflammatory.

BUFACET. (Jenkins) Acetylsalicylic acid 3.5 gr, acetophenetidin 2.5 gr, caffeine alkaloid 0.5 gr, aromatics, buffered w/aluminum hydroxide gel/Tab. Bot. 1000s.
Use: Analgesic.
BUF ACNE CLEANSING BAR. (3M Products) Salicylic acid 1%, sulfur 1% in detergent cleansing bar. 3.5 oz.
Use: Anti-acne.
BUF-BAR. (3M Personal Care) Sulpher 3% and titanium dioxide. Bar 105 Gm.
Use: Anti-acne.
BUF BODY SCRUB. (3M Products) Round cleansing sponge on plastic handles.
Use: Cleansing sponge.
BUFEXAMAC. B.A.N. 4-Butoxyphenylacetohydroxamic acid.
Use: Anti-inflammatory.
BUFF-A. (Mayrand) Aspirin acid 5 gr. buffered w/magnesium hydroxide, aluminum hydroxide dried gel. Tab. Bot. 100s, 1000s.
Use: Analgesic.
BUFF-A-COMP. (Mayrand) Aspirin 648 mg, caffeine 40 mg, butalbital 50 mg/Tab. Bot. 100s.
Use: Analgesic combination.
BUFF-A-COMP NO. 3. (Mayrand) Butalbital 50 mg, aspirin 325 mg, caffeine 40 mg, codeine phosphate 30 mg/Tab. Bot. 100s.
Use: Analgesic combination.
BUFFAPRIN. (Buffington) Aspirin 325 mg. buffered with magnesium oxide. Sugar, caffeine, lactose, salt free. Tab. Dispens-A-Kit 500s.
Use: Salicylate analgesic.
BUFFASAL. (Dover) Aspirin 325 mg/Tab. w/ magnesium oxide. Sugar, lactose, salt free. UD Box 500s.
Use: Salicylate analgesic.
BUFFASAL MAX. (Dover) Aspirin 500 mg/Tab w/magnesium oxide. Sugar, lactose, salt free.
Use: Salicylate analgesic.
BUFFERIN AF NITE TIME. (B-M Squibb) Acetaminophen 500 mg, diphenhydramine citrate 38 mg, simethicone. Cap shaped tab. Bot. 24s and 50s.
Use: Sleep aid, analgesic.
BUFFERED ASPIRIN. (Various Mfr.) Aspirin 325 mg with buffers. Tab. Bot. 100s, 500s, 1000s and UD 100s and 200s.
Use: Analgesic.
BUFFETS II. (JMI) Aspirin 226 mg, acetaminophen 162 mg, caffeine 32.4 mg, aluminum hydroxide 50 mg/Tab. Bot. 1000s.

Use: Analgesic combination.
BUFFEX. (Hauck) Aspirin 325 mg w/dihydroxyaluminum aminoacetate. Tab. Bot. 1000s, Sanipack 1000s.
Use: Salicylate analgesic.
BUFFINOL. (Otis Clapp) Aspirin 324 mg buffered w/magnesium oxide. Sugar, caffeine, lactose, salt free. Tab. Bot. 100s, 200s, 500s.
Use: Salicylate analgesic.
BUFFINOL EXTRA. (Otis Clapp) Aspirin 500 mg/Tab. Sugar, caffeine, lactose, salt free. Safety pack 500s.
Use: Salicylate analgesic.
BUF FOOT CARE KIT. (3M Products) Cleansing system for the feet.
Use: Foot preparation.
BUF FOOT CARE LOTION. (3M Products) Moisturizing lotion for feet.
Use: Foot preparation.
BUF FOOT CARE SOAP. (3M Products) Bar 3.5 oz.
Use: Foot preparation.
BUFILCON A. USAN.
Use: Contact lens material.
BUF KIT FOR ACNE. (3M Products) Cleansing sponge, cleansing bar. 3.5 oz w/booklet, holding tray.
Use: Anti-acne.
BUF LOTION. (3M Products) Moisturizing lotion.
Use: Emollient.
• **BUFORMIN.** USAN. 1-Butylbiguanide. Silubin.
Use: Oral hypoglycemic agent.
BUFOSAL. (Table Rock) Sodium salicylate 15 gr/dram w/calcium carbonate, sodium bicarbonate as granulated effervescent powder. Bot. 4 oz.
Use: Salicylate analgesic.
BUF-PED NON MEDICATED CLEANSING SPONGE. (3M Products) Abrasive cleansing sponge.
Use: Cleansing skin on feet.
BUF PUF BODYMATE. (3M Products) Oval two-sided cleansing sponge. Abrasive/gentle.
Use: Cleansing all areas of the body.
BUF-PUF MEDICATED. (3M Pharm) Water-activated. Salicylic acid 0.5% (reg. strength), alcohols benzoate, EDTA, triethanolamine and vitamin E acetate. Salicylic acid 2% (max. strength). Pads. Jar 30s.
Use: Anti-acne.
BUF-PUF NON-MEDICATED CLEANSING SPONGE. (3M Products) Abrasive cleansing sponge.
Use: Skin cleansing.
BUFROLIN. B.A.N. 6-Butyl-1,4,7,10-tetrahydro-4,10-dioxo-1,7-phenanthroline-2,8-dicarboxylic acid.
Use: Mast-cell stabilizer.
BUF-SUL TABLETS AND SUSPENSION. (Sheryl) Sulfacetamide 167 mg, sulfadiazine 167 mg, sulfamerazine 167 mg. Tab. 100s. Susp. pt.
Use: Antibacterial, sulfonamide.
BUF-TABS. (Blue Cross) Aspirin 5 gr/Tab. w/aluminum hydroxide, glycine magnesium carbonate. Bot. 100s.
Use: Salicylate analgesic.
BUFURALOL. B.A.N. 2-tert-Butylamino-1-(7-ethylbenzofuran-2-yl)ethanol.
Use: Beta adrenergic blocking agent.
BUFYLLINE. B.A.N. Theophylline compound with 2-amino-2-methylpropan-1-ol (1:1).
Use: Bronchodilator.
BUG-PRUF. (Scherer) n, n diethyl-m-toluamide (DEET) 94.525%, other isomers 4.975%, fragrance 0.5%. Bot. 2 oz.
Use: Insect repellent.
BUGS BUNNY. (Miles) Vitamins A 2500 IU, E 15 IU, C 60 mg, folic acid 0.3 mg, B_1 1.05 mg, B_2 1.2 mg, niacin 13.5 mg, B_6 1.05 mg, B_{12} 4.5 mcg, D 400 IU/Tab. Bot. 60s.
Use: Vitamin/mineral supplement.
BUGS BUNNY CHEWABLE VITAMINS AND MINERALS. (Miles) Vitamins A 5000 IU, D 400 IU, E 30 IU, C 60 mg, folic acid 0.4 mg, B_1 1.5 mg, B_2 1.7 mg, niacin 20 mg, B_6 2 mg, B_{12} 6 mcg, biotin 40 mcg, pantothenic acid 10 mg, iron 18 mg, calcium 100 mg, phosphorus 100 mg, iodine 150 mcg, magnesium 20 mg, copper 2 mg, zinc 15 mg/Tab. Bot 60s.
Use: Vitamin/mineral supplement.
BUGS BUNNY PLUS IRON. (Miles) Vitamins A 2500 IU, E 15 IU, C 60 mg, folic acid 0.3 mg, B_1 1.05 mg, B_2 1.2 mg, niacin 13.5 mg, B_6 1.05 mg, B_{12} 4.5 mcg, D 400 IU, iron 15 mg/Chew. tab. Bot. 60s.
Use: Vitamin/mineral supplement.
BUGS BUNNY WITH EXTRA C. (Miles) Vitamins A 2500 IU, D 400 IU, E 15 IU, C 250 mg, folic acid 0.3 mg, B_1 1.05 mg, B_2 1.2 mg, niacin 13.5 mg, B_6 1.05 mg, B_{12} 4.5 mcg/Tab. Bot. 60s.
Use: Vitamin/mineral supplement.
BULGARICUS-L.
See: L-BULGARICUS.
BULKOGEN. A mucin extracted from the seeds of *Cyanopsis tetragonaloba*.
BULLFROG. (Chattem) Benzophenone-3, octyl methoxycinnamate, isostearyl alcohol, aloe, hydrogenated vegetable oil, vitamin E. Waterproof. Stick 16.5 g.

Use: Sunscreen.
BULLFROG EXTRA MOISTURIZING GEL. (Chattem) Benzophenone-3, octocrylene, octyl methoxycinnamate, vitamin E, aloe. SPF 18. Tube 90 g.
Use: Sunscreen.
BULLFROG FOR KIDS. (Chattem). SPF 18. Octocrylene, octyl methoxycinnamate, octyl salicylate, vitamin E, aloe, alcohols benzoate. Gel Tube 60 Gm.
Use: Sunscreen.
BULLFROG SPORT LOTION. (Chattem) Benozophenone-3, octocrylene, octyl methoxycinnamate, octyl salicylate, titanium dioxide, diazolidinyl urea, EDTA, parabens, vitamin E, aloe. SPF 18. Bot. 120 ml.
Use: Sunscreen.
BULLFROG SUNBLOCK. (Chattem) SPF 18, 36. Benzophenone-3, octocrylene, octyl methoxycinnamate, aloe, vitamin E, isostearyl alcohol. PABA free. Waterproof. Gel Tube 120 g.
Use: Sunscreen.
• **BUMETANIDE.** U.S.P. XXIII, Tab., Inj., 3-Butylamino-4-phenoxy-5-sulfamoylbenzoic acid.
Use: Diuretic.
See: Bumex, Inj., Tab. (Roche).
• **BUMETRIZOLE.** USAN.
Use: Ultraviolet screen.
BUMEX. (Roche) Bumetanide 0.5 mg, 1 mg or 2 mg/Tab. 0.5 mg and 1 mg Bot. 100s, 500s, UD 100s. 2 mg Bot. 100s, UD 100s. Inj. Amp 2 ml, 0.25 mg/ml. Box 10s. Vial 2 ml, 4 ml or 10 ml, 0.25 mg/ml. Box 10s.
Use: Loop diuretic.
BUMINATE. (Hyland) Normal serum albumin (human) **25%** soln. in 20 ml w/o administration set; 50 ml and 100 ml w/administration set. **5%** soln. in 250 ml and 500 ml w/administration set.
Use: Albumin replacement.
• **BUNAMIDE HYDROCHLORIDE.** USAN.
Use: Anthelmintic.
BUNAMIODYL SODIUM. Sodium 3-butyramido-α-ethyl-2,4,6-triiodocinnamate.
Use: Diagnostic aid (radiopaque medium).
BUNAPROLAST. USAN.
Use: Anti-asthmatic.
BUNIODYL. B.A.N. 3-(3-Butyramido-2,4,6-triiodo- phenyl)-2-ethylacrylic acid. Bunamiodyl (I.N.N.).
Use: Radiopaque substance.
• **BUNOLOL HCl.** USAN. (±)-5-[3-(tert-butylamino)-2-hydroxypropoxy]-3,4-dihydro-1-(2H)-naphthalenone HCl.
Use: Antiadrenergic (β-receptors).

BUN REAGENT STRIPS. (Miles Diagnostic) Seralyzer reagent strips. A quantitative strip test for BUN in serum or plasma. Bot 25s.
Use: Diagnostic aid.
BUPHENINE. B.A.N. 1-(4-Hydroxyphenyl)-2-(1-methyl-3-phenylpropylamino)propan-1-ol.
Use: Peripheral vasodilator.
See: Perdilatal HCl.
• **BUPICOMIDE.** USAN.
Use: Antihypertensive.
BUPIVACAINE. B.A.N. USAN 1-Butyl-2-(2,6-xylylcarbamoyl)piperidide. 1-Butyl-2',6-pipecoloxylidide. (Abbott) **0.25%:** Amp. 20 ml, syr. 50 ml. **0.5%:** Amp. 20 ml, syr. 30 ml. **0.75%:** Amp. 20 ml, syr. 20 ml.
Use: Local anesthetic.
• **BUPIVACAINE IN DEXTROSE INJECTION,** U.S.P. XXIII.
Use: Local anesthetic.
• **BUPIVACAINE AND EPINEPHRINE INJECTION,** U.S.P. XXIII.
Use: Local anesthetic.
See: Marcaine w/Epinephrine, Inj. (Sanofi Winthrop).
• **BUPIVACAINE HYDROCHLORIDE,** U.S.P. XXIII. Inj. U.S.P. XXIII. 2-piperidinecarboxamide, 1-butyl-N-(2, 6-dimethylphenyl)-, monohydrochloride, monohydrate.
Use: Local anesthetic.
See: Marcaine, Injectable (Sanofi Winthrop).
Sensorcaine, Inj. (Astra).
BUPRENEX INJECTION. (Reckitt & Colman) Buprenorphine HCl 0.3 mg/ml w/50 mg anhydrous dextrose. Amp. 1 ml.
Use: Narcotic analgesic.
BUPRENORPHINE. B.A.N. N-Cyclopropylmethyl-7,8-dihydro-7α-(1-(S)-hydroxy-1,2,2-trimethylpropyl)-O[6]-methyl-6,14-endoethanonormorphine.
Use: Analgesic.
See: Buprenex, Inj. (Norwich Eaton).
• **BUPRENORPHINE HYDROCHLORIDE.** USAN.
Use: Analgesic.
• **BUPROPION HYDROCHLORIDE.** USAN.
Use: Antidepressant.
See: Wellbutrin (Burroughs Wellcome).
• **BURAMATE.** USAN. 2-Hydroxyethyl benzylcarbamate. Hyamate.
Use: Anticonvulsant, tranquilizer.
See: Hyamate (Xttrium).
BURDEO. (Hill) Aluminum subacetate 100 mg, boric acid 300 mg/oz. Bot. 3 oz.

Roll-on 8 oz.
Use: Deodorant.
BURN-A-LAY. (Ken-Gate) Chlorobutanol
0.75%, oxyquinoline benzoate 0.025%,
zinc oxide 2%, thymol 0.5%. Cream.
Tube oz.
Use: Burn remedy.
BURNATE. (Burlington) Vitamins A 4000
IU, D-2 400 IU, thiamine HCl 3 mg, ri-
boflavin 2 mg, niacinamide 10 mg, pyri-
dine HCl 2 mg, cyanocobalamin 5 mcg,
calcium pantothenate 0.5 mg, folic acid
0.4 mg, ascorbic acid 50 mg, ferrous fu-
marate 300 mg, calcium 200 mg, iodine
0.15 mg, copper 1 mg, magnesium 5
mg, zinc 1.5 mg/Tab. Bot. 100s.
Use: Vitamin/mineral supplement.
BURN GON. (E.J. Moore) Benzocaine,
cod liver oil, boric acid, lanolin. Tube
1.25 oz.
Use: Burn remedy.
BURN THERAPY.
See: Americaine, Preps. (American
Critical Care).
Amertan, Jelly (Lilly).
Burn-A-Lay, Cream (Ken-Gate).
Burnicin, Oint. (Quality Generics).
Burn-Quel, Aerosol (Halperin).
Butesin Picrate Oint. (Abbott).
Foille, Preps. (Carbisulphoil).
Kip, Preps. (Youngs Drug Prod.).
Nupercainal, Oint. (Ciba).
Silvadene, Cream (Marion).
Solarcaine, Preps. (Schering-Plough).
Sulfamylon, Cream (Sanofi Winthrop).
Unguentine, Preps. (Norwich).
BURN-QUEL. Halperin aerosol dis-
penser. 1 oz, 2 oz.
Use: Burn remedy.
BURNTAME SPRAY. (Otis Clapp) Benzo-
caine, in spray. Aerosol can 2.5 oz.
Use: Anesthetic/antiseptic burn remedy.
BUR-OIL-ZINC. (Durel) Zinc oxide, tal-
cum, lanolin, olive oil, Burow's solution.
Bot. 4 oz, pt, gal.
Use: Generalized and widespread
eczematous eruptions, acute and sub-
acute inflammatory processes, exfolia-
tive dermatitis.
BUR-OIL-ZINC LOTION PLUS. (Durel)
Menthol 0.25%, phenol 0.5% added to
Bur-oil-zinc compound. Bot. 4 oz, pt, gal.
Use: Antipruritic.
BURO-SOL ANTISEPTIC POWDER.
(Doak) Contents make a diluted Burow's
Solution. aluminum acetate topical soln.
plus benzethonium Cl. Pkg. (2.36 Gm)
12s, 100s. Bot. Pow. 4 oz, 1 lb, 5 lb.
Use: Astringent wet dressing.
BUROW'S SOLUTION. Aluminum Ac-

etate Topical Solution, U.S.P. XXIII.
See: Buro-Sol Pow. (Doak).
Domeboro, Pow., Tab. (Miles).
W/Boric acid, acetic acid.
See: Star-Otic, Drops (Star).
BURSUL. (Burlington) Sulfamethiazole
500 mg/Tab. Bot. 100s.
Use: Antibacterial; sulfonamide.
BUR-TUSS. (Burlington) Chlorpheni-
ramine maleate 2 mg, phenylephrine
HCl 5 mg, phenylpropanolamine HCl 5
mg, guaifenesin 100 mg, alcohol 2.5%/5
ml. Bot. pt, gal.
Use: Antihistamine, decongestant, ex-
pectorant.
BUR-ZIN. (Lamond) Aluminum acetate
solution 2%, zinc oxide 10%. Bot. 4 oz, 8
oz, pt, qt, gal. Also w/o lanolin.
Use: Antipruritic, counter-irritant.
• **BUSERELIN ACETATE.** USAN.
Use: Gonad-stimulating principle.
BUSPAR TABLETS. (Mead Johnson)
Buspirone HCl 5 mg or 10 mg/Tab.
Use: Antianxiety agent.
• **BUSPIRONE HYDROCHLORIDE.**
USAN.
Use: Antianxiety agent.
See: BuSpar, Tab. (Mead Johnson).
• **BUSULFAN.** U.S.P. XXIII. Tabs, U.S.P.
XXIII. Tetramethylene dimethanesul-
fonate. 1-4-Dimethanesulphonyloxybu-
tane. 1,4-Butanediol dimethanesul-
fonate.
Use: Chronic myeloid leukemia. [Or-
phan drug]
See: Myleran, Tab. (Burroughs Well-
come).
BUSULPHAN. B.A.N. Tetramethylene
di(methanesulphonate).
Use: Antineoplastic agent.
• **BUTABARBITAL,** U.S.P. XXIII 5-sec-
Butyl-5-ethylbarbituric acid.
Use: Sedative/hypnotic.
See: BBS, Tab. (Solvay).
Butisol, Prods. (Wallace).
Da-Sed, Tab. (Sheryl).
Expansatol, Cap. (Merit).
Medarsed, Elix., Tab. (Medar).
W/Acetaminophen.
See: G-3, Tab. (Hauck).
Sedapap, Elix. (Mayrand).
Sedapap-10, Tab. (Mayrand).
W/Acetaminophen, codeine phosphate.
See: G-3, Cap. (Hauck).
W/Acetaminophen, mephenesin.
See: T-Caps, Cap. (Burlington).
W/Acetaminophen, phenacetin, caffeine.
See: Windolor, Tab. (Winston).
W/Acetaminophen, salicylamide, phenyl-
toloxamine citrate.

See: Dengesic, Tab. (Scott-Alison).
Scotgesic, Cap., Elix. (Scott/Cord).
W/Ambutonium bromide, aluminum hydroxide, magnesium hydroxide.
See: Aludrox, Susp., Tab. (Wyeth-Ayerst).
W/Aminophylline, phenylpropanolamine HCl, chlorpheniramine maleate, aluminum hydroxide, magnesium trisilicate.
See: Asmacol, Tab. (Vale).
W/Carboxyphen.
See: Bontril Timed No. 2, Tab. (G. W. Carnrick).
W/Chlorpheniramine maleate, hyoscine HBr.
See: Pedo-Sol, Tab., Elix. (Warren Pharmacal).
W/Dihydroxypropyl theophylline, ephedrine HCl.
See: Airet R, Tab. (Baylor).
W/Ephedrine sulfate, theophylline.
See: Airet Y, Tab., Elix. (Baylor).
W/Ephedrine HCl, theophylline, guaifenesin.
See: Quibron Plus, Cap., Elix. (Bristol).
W/Ephedrine HCl, theophylline, isoproterenol.
W/Ephedrine sulfate, theophylline, guaifenesin.
See: Broncholate, Cap., Elix. (Bock).
W/l-Hyoscyamine.
See: Cystospaz-SR, Cap. (Webcon).
W/Hyoscyamine sulfate, atropine sulfate, hyoscine HBr, homatropine methylbromide.
See: Butabell HMB, Tab., Elix. (Saron).
W/Hyoscyamine sulfate, scopolamine methylnitrate, atropine sulfate.
See: Banatil, Cap., Elix. (Trimen).
W/Nitroglycerin.
See: Nitrodyl-B, Cap. (Bock).
W/Pentaerythritol tetranitrate.
See: Petn Plus (Saron).
W/Pentobarbital, phenobarbital.
See: Quiess, Tab. (Forest).
W/Phenazopyridine, hyoscyamine HBr.
See: Pyridium Plus, Tab. (Parke-Davis).
W/Phenazopyridine, scopolamine HBr, atropine sulfate, hyoscyamine sulfate.
See: Buren, Tab. (Ascher).
W/Phenobarbital, pentobarbital, hyoscyamine sulfate, hyoscine HBr, atropine sulfate.
See: Neoquess, Tab. (Forest).
W/Salicylamide.
See: Dapco, Tab. (Mericon).
W/Secobarbital.
See: Monosyl, Tab. (Arcum).
W/Secobarbital, pentobarbital, phenobarbital.

See: Quad-Set, Tab. (Kenyon).
W/Theophylline.
See: Theobid, Cap. (Meyer).
W/Theophylline, pseudoephedrine HCl.
See: Asmadil, Cap. (Solvay).
Ayr, Liq. (Ascher).
Ayrcap, Cap. (Ascher).
Az-Kap, Cap. (Keene).
B. A., Prods. (Federal).
Bronchobid, Duracap (Meyer).
• **BUTABARBITAL SODIUM.** U.S.P. XXIII.
Cap., Elix., Tab., U.S.P. XXIII. Sodium 5-sec-butyl-5-ethylbarbiturate. (Various Mfr.) **Tab.:** 15 mg. Bot. 1000s; 30 mg Bot. 100s, 1000s. **Elixir:** 30 mg/5ml Bot. pt.
Use: Sedative/hypnotic.
See: BBS, Tab. (Solvay).
Butalan, Elix. (Lannett).
Butisol Sodium, Elix., Tab. (Wallace).
Expansatol, Cap. (Merit).
Quiebar, Spantab, Tab (Nevin).
Renbu, Tab. (Wren).
Soduben Tab., Elix. (Arcum).
W/Acetaminophen.
See: Amino-Bar, Tab. (Bowman).
Minotal, Tab. (Carnrick).
W/Acetaminophen, aspirin, caffeine.
See: Dolor Plus, Tab. (Geriatric).
W/Acetaminophen, caffeine.
See: Dularin-TH, Tab. (Donner).
Phrenilin, Tab. (Carnrick).
W/Acetaminophen, mephenesin, codeine phosphate.
See: Bancaps-C, Cap. (Westerfield).
W/Acetaminophen, salicylamide.
See: Banesin Forte, Tab. (Westerfield).
Indogesic, Tab. (Century).
W/Acetaminophen, salicylamide, d-amphetamine sulfate, hexobarbital, secobarbital sodium, phenobarbital.
See: Sedragesic, Tab. (Lannett).
W/d-Amphetamine sulfate.
See: Bontril, Tab. (Carnrick).
W/Ascorbic acid, sodium p-aminobenzoate, salicylamide, sodium salicylate.
See: Bisalate, Tab. (Allison).
W/Atropine sulfate, hyoscyamine HBr, alcohol, hyoscine HBr.
See: Hyonatol Tab., Hyonatol B Elix., Hexett, Tab. (Bowman).
W/Belladonna extract
See: Butibel, Tab., Elix. (McNeil).
Quiebel, Elix., Cap. (Nevin).
W/Dehydrocholic acid, belladonna extract.
See: Decholin-BB, Tab. (Miles).
W/Methscopolamine bromide, aluminum hydroxide gel, dried, magnesium trisilicate.
See: Eulcin, Tab. (Leeds).

W/Pentobarbital sodium, phenobarbital sodium.
See: Trio-Bar, Tab. (Jenkins).
W/Salicylamide, mephenesin.
See: Metrogesic, Tab. (Metro).
W/Secobarbital sodium.
See: Monosyl, Tab. (Arcum).
W/Secobarbital sodium, pentobarbital sodium, phenobarbital.
See: Nidar, Tab. (Armour).
W/Secobarbital sodium, phenobarbital.
See: S.B.P., Tab. (Lemmon).
W/Simethicone, hyoscyamine sulfate, atropine sulfate, hyoscine HBr.
See: Sidonna, Tab. (Reed & Carnrick).
W/Theophylline, pseudoephedrine HCl.
See: Dilorbron, Cap. (Hauck).
BUTABELL HMB. (Saron) Butabarbital 15 mg, hyoscyamine sulfate 0.1037 mg, atropine sulfate 0.0194 mg, hyoscine HBr 0.0065 mg/Tab. Bot. 100s, 1000s.
Use: Sedative/hypnotic, anticholinergic/antispasmodic.
BUTACAINE.
Use: Local anesthetic.
See: Butyn Dental Oint. (Abbott).
• **BUTACETIN.** USAN. 4′-Tert-butoxyacetanilide.
Use: Analgesic.
• **BUTACLAMOL HYDROCHLORIDE.** USAN.
Use: Antipsychotic.
BUTAGEN CAPS. (Goldline) Phenylbutazone 100 mg/Cap. Bot. 100s, 500s.
Use: Antirheumatic.
BUTALAMINE. B.A.N. 5-(2-Dibutylaminoethyl)-amino-3-phenyl-1,2,4-oxadiazole.
Use: Vasodilator.
BUTALAN. (Lannett) Butabarbital sodium 33.3 mg/5 ml, alcohol 7%. Elix. Bot. pt, gal.
Use: Sedative/hypnotic.
• **BUTALBITAL,** U.S.P. XXIII. 5-Allyl-5-isobutyl-barbituric acid. Allylbarbituric Acid.
Use: Nonnarcotic analgesic.
See: Buff-A-Comp #3 (Mayrand).
Lotusate, Cap. (Sanofi Winthrop).
Sandoptal, Preps. (Sandoz).
W/Acetaminophen.
See: Phrenilin, Tab. (Carnrick).
Phrenilin Forte, Cap. (Carnrick).
W/Acetaminophen, codeine.
See: Phrenilin w/Codeine, Cap. (Carnrick).
W/Acetaminophen, caffeine.
See: Arbutal, Tab. (Arcum).
Buff-A-Comp, Tab., Cap. (Mayrand).
Esgic, Tab. (Gilbert).

Cefinal, Tab. (Alto).
Protension, Tab. (Blaine).
Repan, Tab. (Everett).
W/Aspirin, caffeine.
See: Duogesic, Cap. (Western Research).
Fiorinal, Cap., Tab. (Sandoz).
W/Aspirin, caffeine, codeine phosphate.
See: Buff-A-Comp, Tab w/Codeine. (Mayrand).
Fiorinal With Codeine, Cap. (Sandoz).
W/Caffeine, aspirin, acetaminophen.
See: Anaphen, Cap. (Hauck).
• **BUTALBITAL, ACETAMINOPHEN AND CAFFEINE TABLETS,** U.S.P. XXIII.
Use: Analgesic.
BUTALBITAL, ASPIRIN & CAFFEINE. (Various Mfr.) **Tab.:** Aspirin 325 mg, caffeine 40 mg, butalbital 50 mg. Bot. 20s, 100s, 1000s, UD 100s. **Cap.:** Aspirin 325 mg, caffeine 40 mg, butalbital 50 mg. Bot. 100s, 1000s.
Use: Nonnarcotic analgesic combination.
• **BUTALBITAL AND ASPIRIN TABLETS,** U.S.P. XXIII.
Use: Analgesic, sedative.
BUTALBITAL COMPOUND. (Various Mfr.) Tab., Cap. Bot. 100s, 500s, 1000s.
Use: Nonnarcotic analgesic.
W/Acetaminophen, butalbital.
See: Phrenilin (Carnrick).
Bancap (Forest).
Bucet, Cap. (UAD).
Tencon, Cap. (Inter. Ethical Labs).
Triaprin (Dunhall).
Sedapap-10 (Mayrand).
W/Acetaminophen, caffeine, butalbital.
See: Arcet, Tab. (EconoMed).
Esgic (Forest).
Fioricet (Sandoz).
Repan (Everett).
Amaphen (Trimen).
Butace (American Pharm.).
Endolor (Keene).
Esgic-Plus, Tab. (Forest).
G-1 (Hauck).
Isocet, Tab. (Rugby).
Margesic, Cap. (Marnel).
Medigesic Plus (U.S. Pharm. Corp.).
Phrenilin Forte (Carnrick).
Sedapap-10 (Mayrand).
Triad, Cap. (UAD).
W/Aspirin, butalbital.
See: Axotal (Adria).
W/Aspirin, caffeine, butalbital.
See: Fiorgen PF (Goldline).
Fiorinal (Sandoz).
Isollyl Improved (Rugby).
Lanorinal (Lannett).

Lorprn (Russ Pharm.).

B-A-C (Mayrand).

BUTALAN ELIXIR. (Lannett) Sodium butabarbital 0.2 Gm/30 ml. Bot. pt, gal.
Use: Sedative/hypnotic.

BUTALGIN.
See: Methadone HCl (Various Mfr.).

BUTALLYLONAL. 5-(2-Bromoallyl)-5-sec-butylbarbituric acid. (Pernocton).
Use: Hypnotic.

• **BUTAMBEN,** U.S.P. XXIII. Benzoic acid, 4-amino-,butyl ester. Butyl p-aminobenzoate.
Use: Local anesthetic.

• **BUTAMBEN PICRATE.** USAN.
Use: Topical anesthetic.
See: Butesin Picrate, Oint. (Abbott).

• **BUTAMIRATE CITRATE.** USAN.
Use: Antitussive.

• **BUTAMISOLE HYDROCHLORIDE.** USAN.
Use: Anthelmintic.

BUTAMYRATE. B.A.N. 2-(2-Diethylaminoethoxy)-ethyl 2-phenylbutyrate.
Use: Cough suppressant.

• **BUTANE,** N.F. XVIII.
Use: Aerosol propellant.

BUTANILICAINE. B.A.N. 2-Butylamino-6'-chloroacet-o-toluidide.
Use: Local anesthetic.

BUTANISAMIDE. 1-Butyl-1-(o-methoxyphenyl) urea.

• **BUTAPERAZINE MALEATE.** USAN.
Use: Antipsychotic.

BUTAPHYLLAMINE. Ambuphylline. Theophylline aminoisobutanol. Theophylline with 2-amino-2-methyl-1-propanol.

BUTAPRO ELIXIR. (Approved) Butabarbital sodium 0.2 Gm/30 ml. Bot. pt, gal.
Use: Sedative/hypnotic.

• **BUTAPROST.** USAN.
Use: Bronchodilator.

BUTAZONE. (Major) Phenylbutazone.
Cap.: 100 mg. Bot. 100s, 500s. **Tab.:** 100 mg. Bot. 500s.
Use: Antirheumatic.

• **BUTEDRONATE TETRASODIUM.** USAN.
Use: Diagnostic aid (bone imaging).

BUTELLINE.
See: Butacaine Sulfate (Various Mfr.).

• **BUTERIZINE.** USAN.
Use: Vasodilator.

BUTESIN PICRATE. n-Butyl-p-aminobenzoate. Butamben picrate.

BUTESIN PICRATE OINTMENT. (Abbott) Butamben picrate 1%. Tube oz.
Use: Local anesthetic.

BUTETHAL. (Various Mfr.) 5-Ethyl-5-

butylbarbituric acid.
Use: Sedative/hypnotic.

BUTETHAMATE. B.A.N. 2-Diethylaminoethyl 2-phenylbutyrate.
Use: Antispasmodic.

BUTETHAMINE FORMATE. 2-Isobutyl aminoethyl-p-aminobenzoate formate.

BUTETHAMINE HYDROCHLORIDE, 2-(Isobutylamino) ethyl-p-amino benzoate HCl.
See: Dentocaine (Amer. Chem. & Drug).

BUTETHANOL.
See: Tetracaine.

BUTHALITONE SODIUM. B.A.N. A mixture of 100 parts by weight of the monosodium derivative of 5-allyl-5-isobutyl-2-thiobarbituric acid and 6 parts by weight of dried sodium carbonate.
Use: Sedative/hypnotic.

• **BUTHIAZIDE.** USAN. 6-Chloro-3, 4-dihydro-3-isobutyl-2H-1,2,4-benzothiadiazine-7-sulfonamide 1,1-dioxide.
Use: Diuretic, antihypertensive.

BUTIBEL. (Wallace) Butabarbital sodium 15 mg, belladonna extract 15 mg/Tab or 5 ml. **Tab.** Bot. 100s. **Elix.:** (w/alcohol 7%) Bot. pt.
Use: Sedative/hypnotic, anticholinergic/antispasmodic.

• **BUTIKACIN.** USAN.
Use: Antibacterial.

• **BUTILFENIN.** USAN.
Use: Diagnostic aid.

• **BUTIROSIN SULFATE.** USAN. A mixture of the sulfates of the A and B forms of an antibiotic produced by Bacillus circularis.
Use: Antibacterial.

BUTISOL SODIUM. (Wallace) Butabarbital sodium. **Elix.:** 30 mg/5 ml. Bot pt, gal. **Tab.:** 15 mg, 30 mg. Bot. 100s, 1000s. 50 mg or 100 mg. Bot. 100s.
Use: Sedative/hypnotic.
See: Buticaps, Cap. (Wallace).
W/Belladonna extract.
See: Butibel, (Wallace).

• **BUTIXIRATE.** USAN.
Use: Analgesic, antirheumatic.

• **BUTOCONAZOLE NITRATE.** USAN.
Use: Antifungal.
See: Femstat, Cream (Syntex).

BUTOLAN. Benzylphenyl carbamate.

• **BUTONATE.** USAN.
Use: Anthelmintic.

• **BUTOPAMINE.** USAN.
Use: Cardiotonic.

• **BUTOPROZONE HYDROCHLORIDE.** USAN.

Use: Cardiac depressant (anti-arrhythmic).
BUTOPYRONOXYL. (Indalone) Butylmesityl oxide.
Use: Insect repellant.
• **BUTORPHANOL.** USAN.
Use: Analgesic, antitussive.
• **BUTORPHANOL TARTRATE,** U.S.P. XXIII. Inj., U.S.P. XXIII.
Use: Analgesic.
See: Stadol, Inj. (Bristol).
BUTOXAMINE. B.A.N. (±)-erythro-1-(2,5-Dimethoxyphenyl)-2-t-butylamino-propan-1-ol.
Use: Inhibitor of fatty acid mobilization.
• **BUTOXAMINE HYDROCHLORIDE.** USAN.α-[1-(Tertbutylamino)ethyl]-2,5-dimethoxybenzyl alcohol HCl.
Use: Oral hypoglycemic, antihpemic.
BUTRIPTYLINE. B.A.N. L(+)-3-(10,11-Di-hydro-5H-diben- zo[a,d]cycloheptene-5-yl)-2-methyl-propyldimethylamine.
Use: Antidepressant.
• **BUTRIPTYLINE HYDROCHLORIDE.** USAN. dl-10, 11-Dihydro-N, N, β-trimethyl-5H-dibenzo (a,d)cyclohep-tene-5-propylamine HCl.
Use: Antidepressant.
• **BUTYL ALCOHOL,** N.F. XVIII. Butyl alcohol is n-butyl alcohol.
Use: Pharmaceutic aid (solvent).
BUTYL AMINOBENZOATE. n-Butyl p-Aminobenzoate. Scuroforme.
Use: Local anesthetic.
W/Benzocaine, tetracaine HCl.
See: Cetacaine, Preps. (Cetylite).
W/Benzyl alcohol, phenylmercuric borate, benzocaine.
See: Dermathyn, Oint. (Davis & Sly).
W/Procaine, benzyl alcohol, in sweet almond oil.
See: Anucaine, Amp. (Calvin).
W/Tetracaine.
See: Pontocaine, Oint. (Sanofi Winthrop).
• **BUTYLATED HYDROXYANISOLE,** N.F. XVIII. tert-Butyl-4-methoxyphenol.
Use: Pharmaceutic aid (antioxidant).
• **BUTYLATED HYDROXYTOLUENE,** N.F. XVIII. B.A.N. 2,6-Di-tert-butyl-P-cresolution
Use: Pharmaceutic aid (antioxidant).
• **BUTYLPARABEN,** N.F. XVIII. Butyl p-Hydroxy-benzoate.
Use: Pharmaceutical aid (antifungal preservative).
BUTYLPHENAMIDE. N-n-butyl-3-phenyl-salicylamide.
BUTYLPHENYLSALICYLAMIDE.
See: Butylphenamide.

BUTYROPHENONE. Antipsychotic agent.
See: Haloperidol.
BUTYRYLCHOLINESTERASE.
Use: Treat cocaine overdose; post-surgical apnea. [Orphan drug]
B VITAMINS, PARENTERAL.
See: B-Ject-100 (Hyrex)
Becomject-100 (Mayrand)
B VITAMINS WITH VITAMIN C, PARENTERAL.
See: Key-Plex Injection (Hyrex)
Neurodep Injection (Medical Products)
Vicam Injection (Keene)
B-VITE INJECTION. (Bluco) Vitamins B_1 50 mg, B_2 5 mg, B_6 5 mg, niacinamide 125 mg, B_{12} 1000 mcg, dexpanthenol 6 mg, C 50 mg/10 ml. Mono vial w/benzyl alcohol 1% in water for injection.
Use: Vitamin supplement.
BVU.
See: Bromisovalum.
BW 12C.
Use: Sickle cell disease. [Orphan drug]
BYCLOMINE. (Major) Dicyclomine. **Cap.:** 10 mg. Bot. 100s, 250s, 1000s. **Tab.:** 20 mg. Bot. 100s, 250s, 1000s.
Use: Antispasmodic.
BYCLOMINE W/PHENOBARBITAL. (Major) **Cap.:** Dicyclomine HCl 10 mg, phenobarbital 15 mg. Bot. 250s, 1000s. **Tab.:** Dicyclomine HCl 20 mg, phenobarbital 15 mg. Bot. 100s, 250s, 1000s.
Use: Antispasmodic, sedative/hypnotic.
BYDRAMINE. (Major) Diphenhydramine HCl 12.5 mg/5 ml, alcohol 5%. Syr. Bot. 118 ml, pt, gal.
Use: Antihistamine.
BYDRAMINE COUGH. (Major) Diphenhydramine HCl 12.5 mg/5 ml, alcohol 5%. Syr. Bot. 118 ml, pt, gal.
Use: Antitussive.

C

C1-ESTERASE-INHIBITOR, HUMAN, PASTEURIZED.
Use: Prevention/treatment of angioedema. [Orphan drug]
C1 INHIBITOR.
Use: Treatment of angioedema. [Orphan drug]
C VITAMIN.
See: Ascorbic Acid, Prep.
• **CABUFOCON B.** USAN.
Use: Contact lens material.
CACHEXON. (Telluride Pharm)
See: L-GLUTATHIONE.
CACODYLIC ACID SALTS.

Ferric Salt.
Iron Salt.
Sodium Salt.
• **CACTINOMYCIN.** USAN. Dactinomycin 10%, actinomycin C_2 45%, actinomycin C_3 45%. Actinomycin C.
Use: Antineoplastic agent.
See: Sanamycin (FBA Pharm).
C-ACEROLA.
See: ACEROLA-C.
CADE OIL.
See: Juniper Tar.
CADE OIL CREAM NO. 26. (Durel) Cade oil 3%, ammoniated mercury 2%, in Duromantel cream. Jar 1 oz, 1 lb, 6 lb.
Use: Antipsoriatic.
CADE OIL CREAM NO. 27. (Durel) Cade oil 5%, sulfur 5%, salicylic acid 3% in Duromantel cream. Jar 1 oz, 1 lb, 6 lb.
Use: Antipsoriatic, keratolytic.
• **CADEXOMER IODINE.** USAN.
Use: Antiseptic, antiulcerative.
CAD-O-BATH. (Durel) Oil of cade 35%, polysorbate "20" 35%. Bot. 8 oz, pt, gal.
Use: Antipruritic, antipsoriatic.
C & E SOFTGELS. (Nature's Bounty) E 400 mg, C 500 mg/Cap. Bot. 50s.
Use: Vitamin supplement.
CAFATINE. (Major) Ergotamine tartrate 2 mg, caffeine 100 mg. Supp. Box 12s.
Use: Migraine combination.
CAFATINE PB. (Major) Ergotamine tartrate 2 mg, caffeine 100 mg, belladonna alkaloids 0.25 mg, pentobarbital 60 mg/Supp. Box foil 10s.
Use: Agent for migraine.
CAFEDRINE. B.A.N. L-7-[2-(β-Hydroxy-α-methylphenethylamino)ethyl]-theophylline.
Use: Analeptic.
CAFENOL. (Sanofi Winthrop) Aspirin, caffeine.
Use: Salicylate analgesic.
CAFERGOT P-B SUPPOSITORIES. (Sandoz) Ergotamine tartrate 2 mg, caffeine 100 mg, bellafoline 0.25 mg, pentobarbital 60 mg/Supp. Box 12s.
Use: Agent for migraine.
CAFERGOT P-B TABLETS. (Sandoz) Ergotamine tartrate 1 mg, caffeine 100 mg, bellafoline 0.125 mg, pentobarbital sodium 30 mg/Tab. SigPak dispensing pkg. of 90s, 250s.
Use: Agent for migraine.
CAFERGOT SUPPOSITORIES. (Sandoz) Ergotamine tartrate 2 mg, caffeine 100 mg in cocoa butter base. Supp. Box 12s.
Use: Agent for migraine.
CAFERGOT TABLETS. (Sandoz) Ergotamine tartrate 1 mg, caffeine 100 mg/S.C. Tab. Bot. 250s. SigPak dispensing pkg. of 90s.
Use: Agent for migraine.
CAFETRATE. (Schein) Ergotamine tartrate 2 mg, caffeined 100 mg/Supp. Box 12s.
Use: Agent for migraine.
OAFFEDRINE. (Thompson) Caffeine 200 mg/T.R. Cap. Bot. 20s.
Use: CNS stimulant.
• **CAFFEINE, U.S.P.** U.S.P. XXIII. 1H-purine-2,6-dione,3,-7-dihydro-1,3,7-trimethyl-xanthine. Guaranine; Methyltheobromine; Thein.
Use: CNS stimulant; apnea of prematurity [Orphan drug]
See: Enerjets, Loz. (Chilton).
Femicin, Tab. (SK-Beecham).
Nodoz, Tab. (Bristol-Myers).
Stim 250, Cap. (Scrip).
Tirend (SK-Beecham).
Vivarin, Tab. (J.B. Williams).
CAFFEINE CITRATED.
Use: CNS stimulant.
CAFFEINE SODIO-BENZOATE.
See: Caffeine sodium benzoate.
• **CAFFEINE SODIUM BENZOATE INJECTION, U.S.P.** U.S.P. XXIII. Approximately equal parts of caffeine and sodium benzoate. (Various Mfr.) Amp. (3¾ gr and 7.5 gr) 2 ml, Box 12s, 100s. Hypo Tab. (1 gr) Tube 20s, 100s and Pow.
Use: Orally, I.M. central nervous system stimulant.
CAFFEINE SODIUM SALICYLATE. (Various Mfr.) Bot. 1 oz; Pkg. 0.25 lb, 1 lb.
Use: See caffeine.
CAFFEINE-THEOPHYLLINE COMPOUND. w/Nux Vomica Ext.
See: Xanthinux, Tab. (Cole).
CAFFIN-T.D. (Kenyon) Caffeine 250 mg/Cap. Bot. 100s.
Use: CNS stimulant.
CAGOL. (Harvey) Guaiacol 0.1 Gm, eucalyptol 0.08 Gm, iodoform 0.2 Gm, camphor 0.05 Gm/2 ml in olive oil. Vial 30 ml.
Use: Expectorant.
CAINE-A.
See: A-CAINE.
CAINE-L.
See: L-CAINE.
CAINE-L E.
See: L-CAINE E.
CAINE-L VISCOUS.
See: L-CAINE VISCOUS.
CAINE-T.
See: T-CAINE.
CALADRYL. (Parke-Davis) Calamine

8%, pramoxine HCl 1%, alcohol 2.2%, camphor, diazolidinyl urea, parabens. Lot. Bot. 180 ml.
Use: Topical poison ivy treatment.
CALADRYL CLEAR. (Parke-Davis) Pramoxine HCl 1%, zinc acetate 0.1%, alcohol 2%, camphor, diazolidinyl urea, parabens. Lot. Bot. 180 ml.
Use: Topical poison ivy treatment.
CALADRYL FOR KIDS. (Parke-Davis) Calamine 8%, pramoxine HCl 1%, camphor, cetyl alcohol, diazolidinyl urea, parabens. Cream. Tube 45 g.
Use: Topical poison ivy treatment.
CALAFORMULA. (Eric, Kirk & Gary) Ferrous gluconate 130 mg, calcium lactate 130 mg, vitamins A 1000 IU, D 400 IU, B_1 2 mg, B_2 2 mg, niacinamide 5 mg, ascorbic acid 20 mg, folic acid 0.13 mg, magnesium 0.25 mg, copper 0.25 mg, zinc 0.25 mg, manganese 0.25 mg, potassium 0.075 mg/Cap. Bot. 50s, 100s, 500s, 1000s, 5000s.
Use: Vitamin/mineral supplement.
CALAFORMULA F. (Eric, Kirk & Gary) Calaformula plus fluorine 0.333 mg/Tab. Bot. 100s.
Use: Vitamin/mineral supplement, dental caries preventative.
CALA-GEN. (Goldline) Diphenhydramine HCl 1%, camphor, alcohol 2%. Lot. Bot. 178 ml.
Use: Minor skin irritations.
CALAHIST LOTION. (Walgreen) Diphenhydramine HCl 1%, calamine 8.1%, camphor 0.1%. Lot. Bot. 6 oz.
Use: Minor skin irritations.
CALAMATUM. (Blair) **Lot.:** Calamine, zinc oxide, phenol, camphor, benzocaine 3%, nongreasy base. Bot. 1125 ml. **Oint:** Calamine, zinc oxide, phenol, camphor, benzocaine. Tube 45 Gm.
Use: Minor skin irritations.
CALAMATUM AEROSOL SPRAY. (Blair) Benzocaine 3%, zinc oxide, calamine, phenol, camphor. Spray can 3 oz.
Use: Minor skin irritations.
• **CALAMINE, U.S.P.** U.S.P. XXIII. (Various Mfr.) : Calamine 8%, zinc oxide 8%, glycerin 2%, bentonite magma, calcium hydroxide soln. Lot. Bot. 120 ml, 240 ml, pt, gal.
Use: Astringent, mild antiseptic
CALAMINE, PHENOLATED. (Humco) Calamine 8%, zinc oxide 8%, glycerin 2%, bentonite magma, and phenol 1% in calcium hydroxide solution. Lot. Bot. 120, 240 ml.
Use: Astringent, mild antiseptic.
CALAMOX. (Hauck) Prepared calamine

0.17 Gm. Oint. Tube 60 Gm.
Use: Astringent, mild antiseptic.
CALAMYCIN. (Pfeiffer) Pyrilamine maleate, zinc oxide 10%, calamine 10%, benzocaine, chloroxylenol, zirconium oxide, isopropyl alcohol 10%. Lot. Bot. 120 ml.
Use: Minor skin irritations.
CALAN. (Searle) Verapamil HCl 40 mg, 80 mg or 120 mg/Tab. Bot. 100s, 500s, 1000s, UD 100s.
Use: Calcium channel blocking agent.
CALAN SR. (Searle) Verapamil HCl 180 mg or 240 mg/SR Capl. Bot. 60s, 100s, UD 100s.
Use: Calcium channel blocking agent.
CAL-BID. (Geriatric) Elemental calcium 250 mg, ascorbic acid 100 mg, vitamin D 125 IU/Tab. Bot. 100s.
Use: Vitamin/mineral supplement.
CAL CARB-HD. (Konsyl Pharm) Calcium 6.5 Gm per packet, simethicone. Pow. 7 Gm packets, Bot. 210 Gm.
Use: Nutritional supplement.
CALCET. (Mission) Elemental calcium 153 mg, vitamin D 100 units/Tab. Bot. 100s.
Use: Vitamin/mineral supplement.
CALCET PLUS. (Mission) Elemental calcium 152.8 mg, elemental iron 18 mg, vitamins A 5000 IU, D 400 IU, E 24.8 mg, B_1 2.25 mg, B_2 2.55 mg, B_3 30 mg, B_5 15 mg, B_6 3 mg, B_{12} 9 mcg, C 500 mg, folic acid 0.8 mg, zinc 15 mg/Tab. Bot. 100s.
Use: Vitamin/mineral supplement.
CALCIBIND. (Mission) Inorganic phosphate content 34%, sodium content 11%. Packets: Cellulose sodium phosphate 25 Gm. Single dose 90 packets, 300 Gm bulk pack.
Use: Urinary tract product.
CALCICAPS. (Nion) Calcium (dibasic calcium phosphate, calcium gluconate, calcium carbonate) 125 mg, vitamin D 67 IU, phosphorus 60 mg/Tab. Bot. 100s, 500s.
Use: Vitamin/mineral supplement.
CALCICAPS WITH IRON. (Nion) Calcium 125 mg, phosphorus 60 mg, vitamin D 67 IU, ferrous gluconate 7 mg, tartrazine/Tab. Bot. 100s, 500s.
Use: Vitamin/mineral supplement.
CALCICAPS M-Z. (Nion) Ca 400 mg, Mg 133 mg, Zn 5 mg, vitamin A 1667 mg, D 133 IU, Se. Tab. Bot. 90s.
Use: Vitamin combination.
CALCICAPS, SUPER. (Nion) Calcium 400 mg, phosphorus 41.7 mg, vitamin D 100 IU/Tab. Bot. 90s.

Use: Vitamin/mineral supplement.
CALCI-CHEW. (R & D) Calcium carbonate 1.25 Gm (500 mg calcium)/Chew. Tab. Bot. 100s.
Use: Antacid.
CALCIDAY-667. (Nature's Bounty) Calcium carbonate 667 mg (266.8 mg calcium)/Tab. Bot. 60s.
Use: Antacid.
CALCIDRINE SYRUP. (Abbott) Codeine 8.4 mg, calcium iodide anhydrous 152 mg, alcohol 6%/5 ml. Bot. 120 ml, 480 ml.
Use: Antitussive, expectorant.
• **CALCIFEDIOL, U.S.P.** U.S.P. XXIII. Cap., U.S.P. XXIII. 25-hydroxycholecalciferol; 25[OH]–D₃.
Use: Calcium regulator.
See: Calderol (Organon).
CALCIFEROL, U.S.P. U.S.P. XXIII. Ergosterol. (D₂) **Liq:** 8000 IU/ml. Bot. 60 ml. **Tab:** 50,000 IU. Bot. 100s. **Inj:** 500,000 IU/ml. Amp. 1 ml.
Use: Refractory rickets, familial hypophoshatemia, hypoparathyroidism.
CALCIJEX. (Abbott) Calcitriol injection 1 mcg or 2 mcg/ml. Amp. 1 ml.
Use: Hypocalcemia and hypoparathyroidism.
CALCIMAR INJECTION, SYNTHETIC. (Rhone-Poulenc Rorer) Calcitonin solution (Salmon origin) containing 200 IU/ml. Vial 2 ml.
Use: Treatment of Paget's disease.
CALCI-MIX. (R & D) Calcium carbonate 1250 mg. Cap. Bot. 100s.
Use: Nutritional supplement.
CALCIPARINE. (DuPont Critical Care) Heparin calcium in water for injection. **5000** units/0.2 ml prefilled syringe. **12,500** units/0.5 ml Amp. **20,000** units/0.8 ml Amp.
Use: Anticoagulant.
• **CALCIPOTRIENE.** USAN.
Use: Antipsoriatic.
See: Dovonex, Oint. (Westwood-Squibb).
CALCITONIN.
Use: Treatment of Paget's disease.
See: Calcimar (USV).
Cibacalcin (Ciba).
Miacalcin (Sandoz).
• **CALCITONIN HUMAN.** USAN. Hormone from thyroid gland.
Use: Plasma hypocalcemic hormone; symptomatic Paget's disease of bone [Orphan drug]
See: Cibacalcin (Ciba).
CALCITONIN SALMON.
See: Calcimar (USV).

Miacalcin (Sandoz).
Osteocalcin, Inj. (Arcola).
CALCITONIN SALMON NASAL SPRAY.
Use: Symptomatic Paget's disease of bone. [Orphan drug]
• **CALCITRIOL.** USAN. 9,10-seco(5Z,7E)-5,7,10(19)-cholestatriene-1a, 3b, 25-triol.
Use: Management of hypocalcemia in chronic renal dialysis patients.
See: Calcijex, Inj. (Abbott).
Rocaltrol, Cap. (Roche).
CALCIUM-600. (Schein) Calcium 600 mg. Tab. Bot. 60s.
Use: Nutritional supplement.
CALCIUM 600/VITAMIN D. (Schein) Ca 600 mg, D 125 IU. Tab. Bot. 60s.
Use: Vitamin supplement.
CALCIUM ACETATE.
Use: Hyperphosphatemia. [Orphan drug]
CALCIUM ACETATE MINERAL/ELECTROLYTES.
See: Phos-Ex 62.5 Mini-Tabs (Vitaline)
Phos-Ex 167 (Braintree)
PhosLo (Braintree)
Phos-Ex 250 (Vitaline)
Phos-Ex 125 (Vitaline)
CALCIUM ACETYLSALICYLATE. Kalmopyrin, kalsetal, soluble aspirin, tylcalsin.
Use: Salicylate analgesic.
CALCIUM ALUMINUM CARBONATE. W/Dl-Amino acetate complex.
See: Ancid Tab., Susp. (Sheryl).
CALCIUM AMINOSALICYLATE. Aminosalicylate calcium, N.F. XVIII.
CALCIUM AMPHOMYCIN.
See: Amphomycin.
• **CALCIUM AND MAGNESIUM CARBONATES TABLETS, U.S.P.** U.S.P. XXIII.
Use: Antacid.
CALCIUM ASCORBATE. (Freeda) **Tab.:** Calcium ascorbate 610 mg (equivalent to 500 mg ascorbic acid). Bot. 100s, 250s, 500s. **Pow.:** Calcium ascorbate 1 Gm (equivalent to 826 mg ascorbic acid) per ¼ tsp. Bot. 120 Gm, 448 Gm.
Use: Calcium supplement.
CALCIUM 4-BENZAMIDOSALICYLATE. Calcium Aminacyl B-PAS. Benzoylpas Calcium.
See: Benzapas, Pow., Tab. (Dorsey).
CALCIUM BENZAMIDOSALICYLATE. B.A.N. Calcium 4-benzamido-2-hydroxybenzoate.
Use: Treatment of tuberculosis.
CALCIUM BENZOYL-p-AMINOSALICYLATE.
See: Benzoylpas calcium.

CALCIUM BENZOYLPAS.
See: Benzoylpas calcium.
**CALCIUM BIS-DIOCTYL SULFOSUCCI-
NATE.**
See: Dioctyl Calcium
CALCIUM CARBIMIDE. Calcium
cyanamide. Sulfosuccinate.
CALCIUM CARBONATE.
Use: Hyperphosphatemia. [Orphan
drug]
CALCIUM CARBONATE 600/VITAMIN D.
(Major) Ca 600 mg, D 125 IU. Tab. Bot.
60s.
Use: Vitamin supplement.
CALCIUM CARBONATE, AROMATIC.
(Lilly) Calcium carbonate 10 gr/Tab. Bot.
100s, 1000s.
Use: Antacid.
**CALCIUM CARBONATE AND MAGNE-
SIA TABLETS, U.S.P.** U.S.P. XXIII.
Use: Antacid.
• **CALCIUM CARBONATE, MAGNESIA,
AND SIMETHICONE, U.S.P.** U.S.P.
XXIII. Tab
• **CALCIUM CARBONATE ORAL SUS-
PENSION, U.S.P.** U.S.P. XXIII.
Use: Antacid.
• **CALCIUM CARBONATE, PRECIPITAT-
ED, U.S.P.** U.S.P. XXIII. (Various Mfr.)
Precipitated chalk; carbonic acid, calci-
um salt (1:1).
Use: Antacid.
See: Alka Mints (Miles Labs).
Amitone, Tab. (Menley & James).
Antacid Tablets (Goldline).
Biocal Prods. (Miles).
Cal-Sup, Tab. (Riker).
Chooz (Schering-Plough).
Dicarbosil, Tab. (SK-Beecham).
Equilet (Mission).
Extra Strength Antacid (Various Mfr.).
Maalox Antacid (RPR).
Mallamint, Tab. (Mallard).
Mylanta (J & J-Merck).
Tums (SK-Beecham).
CALCIUM CARBONATE. (Various Mfr.)
500 mg/Tab. 100s, 120s, UD 100s; 600
mg/Tab. 60s, 72s, 150s, UD 100s; 650
mg/Tab. 100s, 1000s.
Use: Antacid.
CALCIUM CARBONATE. (Roxane) **Tab.:**
1250 mg. Bot. 100s, UD 100s. **Susp.:**
1250 mg/5 ml. Bot. 500 ml, UD 5 ml.
Use: Antacid.
**CALCIUM CARBONATE W/COMBINA-
TIONS.**
See: Accelerase, Cap. (Organon).
Alkets, Tab. (Upjohn).
Camalox, Tab., Susp. (Rhone-Poulenc
Rorer Consumer).

Ca-Plus, Tab. (Miller).
Co-Gel, Tab. (Arco).
Diatrol, Tab. (Otis Clapp).
Dimacid, Tab. (Otis Clapp).
Gas-Eze, Tab. (E.J. Moore).
Kanalka, Tab. (Lannett).
Kaocasil, Tab. (Jenkins).
Lactocal, Tab. (Laser).
Natabec, Prep. (Parke-Davis).
Titralac, Liq., Tab. (Riker).
CALCIUM CASEINATE.
See: Casec, Pow. (Mead Johnson).
CALCIUM CHANNEL BLOCKERS.
Use: Angina pectoris, vasospastic and
unstable angina.
See: Adalat, Cap. (Miles).
Calan, Inj., Tab, (Searle).
Calan SR, SR Cap. (Searle).
Cardene, Cap. (Syntex).
Cardene SR, SR Cap. (Syntex).
Cardene IV, Inj. (DuPont).
Cardizem, Tab. (Marion).
Diltiazem HCl, ER Cap. (Various Mfr.).
DynaCirc, Cap. (Sandoz).
Isoptin, Inj., Tab. (Knoll).
Isoptin SR, SR Cap. (Knoll).
Nimotop, Cap. (Miles).
Plendil, SR Tab. (Merck & Co.).
Procardia, Cap. (Pfizer).
Vascor, Tab. (McNeil).
Verapamil HCl, Inj., Tab. (Various Mfr.).
CALCIUM CHEL 330. (Geigy).
Use: Heavy metal antagonist.
See: Calcium Trisodium Pentetate.
• **CALCIUM CHLORIDE, U.S.P.** U.S.P.
XXIII. Inj., U.S.P. XXIII. 1 Gm (10 ml)
contains 272 mg (13.6 mEq) calcium.
Inj: 10% soln. Amp., vial, syringe 10 ml.
Use: Electrolyte.
• **CALCIUM CHLORIDE CA 45.** USAN.
Use: Radioactive agent.
• **CALCIUM CHLORIDE CA 47.** USAN.
Use: Radioactive agent.
• **CALCIUM CHLORIDE INJECTION,
U.S.P.** U.S.P. XXIII. (Upjohn) 1 Gm
Amp. 10 ml, 25s. (Torigian) 1 Gm Amp.
10 ml 12s, 25s, 100s. (Trent) 10% Amp.
10 ml (Cutter) 13.6 mEq./10 ml Vial.
Use: IV, hypocalcemic tetany.
• **CALCIUM CITRATE, U.S.P.** U.S.P. XXIII.
Use: Calcium supplement.
CALCIUM CYCLAMATE. Calcium cyclo-
hexanesulfamate.
CALCIUM CYCLOBARBITAL. Calcium
5-(l-cyclohexen-l-yl)-5-ethylbarbiturate.
Use: Central depressant.
**CALCIUM
CYCLOHEXANESULFAMATE.**
See: Calcium Cyclamate.
CALCIUM 600 + D. (Nature's Bounty)

Calcium 600 mg, vitamin D 125 IU. Film coat. Tab. Bot. 60s.
Use: Nutritional supplement.
CALCIUM DL -PANTOTHENATE. Calcium Pantothenate, Racemic, U.S.P. XXIII.
CALCIUM DIOCTYL SULFOSUCCINATE. Docusate Calcium, U.S.P. XXIII.
See: Surfak (Hoechst).
CALCIUM DISODIUM EDATHAMIL.
See: Edetate Calcium Disodium, U.S.P. XXIII.
CALCIUM DISODIUM EDETATE. Edetate Calcium Disodium, U.S.P. XXIII.
Use: Antidote for acute and chronic lead poisoning, lead encephalopathy.
See: Calcium Disodium Versenate (Riker).
CALCIUM DISODIUM VERSENATE. (Riker) Calcium Disodium Edetate U.S.P. Inj.: 200 mg/ml. Amp 5 ml.
Use: IV or IM for lead poisoning and/or lead encephalopathy.
CALCIUM EDETATE SODIUM. Edetate Calcium Disodium, U.S.P. XXIII.
Use: Antidote for acute and chronic lead poisoning or lead encephalopathy.
CALCIUM EDTA.
See: Calcium Disodium Versenate, Amp. (Riker).
CALCIUM FOLINATE. B.A.N. Calcium N-[4-(2-amino-5-formyl-5,6,7,8-tetrahydro-4-hydroxy-pteridinyl-6-methyl-aminobenzoyl]-L-glutamate.
Use: Antidote to folic acid antagonists.
See: Leucovorin Calcium.
•**CALCIUM GLUBIONATE.** USAN. 6.5% Calcium.
Use: Calcium replenisher.
See: Neo-Calglucon (Sandoz).
•**CALCIUM GLUCEPTATE, U.S.P.** U.S.P. XXIII. (Various Mfr.) 1.1 Gm (5 ml) contains 90 mg (4.5 mEq) calcium. Inj.: 1.1 Gm/5 ml. Amp. 5 ml. Vial 50 ml.
Use: Calcium electrolyte replacement.
See: Calcium Gluceptate (Abbott).
Calcium Gluceptate (I.M.S).
Calcium Gluceptate (Lilly).
CALCIUM GLUCOHEPTONATE. (Various Mfr.) Cal. D-glucoheptonate O.
Use: Calcium supplement.
•**CALCIUM GLUCONATE, U.S.P.** U.S.P. XXIII. 9% Calcium. Tab.: 500 mg (calcium 45 mg), 650 mg (calcium 58.5 mg), 975 mg (calcium 87.75 mg) or 1 Gm (calcium 90 mg). Bot. 100s, 200s, 500s, 1000s, UD 100s.
Use: Calcium replacement.
CALCIUM GLUCONATE GEL.

Use: Topical treatment of hydrogen fluoride burns. [Orphan drug]
CALCIUM GLYCEROPHOSPHATE. Neurosin. (Various Mfr.).
•**CALCIUM HYDROXIDE, U.S.P.** U.S.P. XXIII. Topical Soln. U.S.P. XXIII.
Use: Astringent; pharmaceutic necessity for calamine lotion.
CALCIUM HYDROXIDE POWDER. (Lilly) Powder 4 oz/Bot.
Use: Preparation of lime water solution.
CALCIUM HYPOPHOSPHITE. (N.Y. Quinine & Chem. Works).
CALCIUM IODIDE.
W/Codeine phosphate.
See: Calcidrine Syr. (Abbott).
W/Chloral hydrate, ephedrine HCl.
See: Iophed, Syr. (Marsh Labs).
CALCIUM IODIZED.
See: Cal-Lime-1, Tab. (Scrip).
W/Calcium creosotate.
See: Niocrese, Tab. (Noyes).
W/Ipecac, hyoscyamus extract, licorice extract.
See: Kaldifane, Tab. (Noyes).
CALCIUM IODOBEHENATE. Calioben. (Various Mfr.).
CALCIUM IPODATE. Ipodate Calcium, U.S.P. XXIII.
See: Oragrafin Calcium, Granules (Squibb).
CALCIUM KINATE GLUCONATE. Kinate is hexahydrotetrahydroxybenzoate. Calcium Quinate.
•**CALCIUM LACTATE, U.S.P.** U.S.P. XXIII. 13% Calcium. Tab.: 325 mg (42.25 mg Calcium) or 650 mg (84.5 mg Calcium). Bot. 100s, 1000s, UD 100s.
Use: Calcium deficiency and prophylaxis.
W/Calcium glycerophosphate.
See: Calphosan, Amp., Vial (Carlton).
W/Calcium glycerophosphate, phenol, sodium Cl solution.
See: Calpholan, Vial (Century).
Calphosan, Inj. (Brown).
W/Niacinamide, folic acid, ferrous gluconate, vitamins.
See: Pergrava No. 2, Cap. (Arcum).
W/Phenobarbital, extract hyoscyamus, terpin hydrate, guaifenesin.
See: Gylanphen, Tab. (Lannett).
W/Theobromine sodium salicylate, phenobarbital.
See: Theolaphen, Tab. (Elder).
W/Thiamine HCl.
See: Nycralan, Tab. (Lannett).
W/Zinc sulfate.
See: Zinc-220, Cap. (Alto).
•**CALCIUM LACTOBIONATE, U.S.P.**

U.S.P. XXIII.
Use: Calcium supplement.
CALCIUM LACTOPHOSPHATE. Lactic acid hydrogen phosphate calcium salt.
CALCIUM LEUCOVORIN. Leucovorin Calcium, U.S.P. XXIII. Inj., tab., powder for oral, powder for inj.
Use: For overdosage of folic acid antagonists; megalobastic anemias.
See: Leucovorin Calcium (Lederle). Wellcovorin (Burroughs Wellcome).
CALCIUM MANDELATE. Urisept (Grail).
Use: Urinary antiseptic, acidifier.
CALCIUM MAGNESIUM CHELATED. (Nature's Bounty) Ca 500 mg, Mg 250 mg/Tab. Bot. 50s, 100s.
Use: Vitamin supplement.
CALCIUM MAGNESIUM ZINC. (Nature's Bounty) Ca 333 mg, Mg 133 mg, Zn 8.3 mg/Tab. Bot. 100.
Use: Vitamin supplement.
CALCIUM NOVOBIOCIN. Calcium salt of an antibacterial substance produced by *Streptomyces niveus.*
Use: Anti-infective.
CALCIUM OROTATE.
See: Calora, Tab. (Miller).
CALCIUM OXYTETRACYCLINE. Oxytetracycline Calcium, N.F. XIV.
• **CALCIUM PANTOTHENATE, U.S.P.** U.S.P. XXIII. Tab., U.S.P. XXIII. β-Alanine, N-(2,4-dihydroxy-3,3-dimethyl-1-oxobutyl)-,calcium salt (2:1). vitamin B_5. D(+)-N-(alpha, gamma dihydroxy-beta,beta-dimethyl-butyryl)-beta aminopropionic acid, calcium salt, dextro form. Pantothenic Acid. Tab.
Use: Pantothenic acid (B_5) deficiency, coenzyme A precursor.
See: Calcium Pantothenate (Freeda). Calcium Pantothenate (Fibertone).
W/Ascorbic acid, niacinamide, vitamins B_1, B_2, B_6, B_{12}, A, D, E.
See: Tota-Vi-Caps Gelatin Capsule, Cap. (Elder).
W/Calcium carbonate.
See: Ilomel, Pow. (Warren-Teed).
W/Calcium carbonate, ferrous fumarate, niacinamide.
See: Prenatag, Tab. (Reid-Rowell).
W/Danthron.
See: Modane, Tab., Liq. (Warren-Teed). Parlax, Tab. (Parmed).
W/Docusate sodium.
See: Pantyl, Tab. (McGregor).
W/Docusate sodium, acetphenolisatin.
See: Android-Plus, Tab. (Brown). Peri-Pantyl, Tab. (McGregor).
W/Methoscopolamine nitrate, mephobarbital.

See: Ilocalm, Tabs. (Warren-Teed).
W/Niacinamide and vitamins.
See: Allbee C-800, Prods. (Robins). Allbee T, Cap. (Robins). Allbee with C, Cap. (Robins). Ferrovite, Tab. (Laser). Fumatinic, Tab. (Laser). Maintenance Vitamin Formula, Tab. (Burgin-Arden). Mulvidren, Tab. (Stuart). OB-Tabs, Tab. (Laser). Probec, Tab. (Stuart). Probec-T, Tab. (Stuart). Stuart Hematinic, Tab. (Stuart). Stuart Therapeutic Multivitamin, Tab. (Stuart).
W/Niacinamide, vitamins B_1, B_2, B_6.
See: Noviplex Capsules, Cap. (Elder).
W/Vitamins B_1, B_2, B_6, B_{12}, niacinamide, choline Cl, inositol, dl-methionine, testosterone, estrone, procaine.
See: Gerihorm, Inj. (Burgin-Arden).
W/Vitamin complex, ferrous fumarate, folic acid, calcium lactate, niacinamide.
See: Vitanate, Tab. (Century).
W/Vitamins A, D, B_1, B_2, C, niacinamide, calcium phosphorus, iron, B_6, B_{12}, E, magnesium, manganese, potassium, zinc, choline bitartrate, inositol.
See: Geriatric Vitamin Formula, Tab. (Burgin-Arden).
W/Vitamins A, E, C, zinc sulfate, magnesium sulfate, niacinamide, B_1, B_2, manganese Cl, B_6, folic acid, B_{12}.
See: Vicon Forte, Cap. (Glaxo).
W/Vitamin C, niacin, zinc sulfate, vitamins E, B_1, B_2, B_6, B_{12}.
See: Z-Bec, Tab. (Robins).
W/Vitamin complex, iron.
See: Vita-iron, Tab. (Century).
W/Vitamins,minerals, niacinamide.
See: Arcum-VM, Cap. (Arcum). Capre, Tab. (Marion). Orovimin, Tab. (Reid-Rowell). Os-Cal Forte, Tab. (Marion). Os-Vim, Tab. (Marion). Stuartinic, Tab. (Stuart). Theramin, Tab. (Arcum). Theron, Tab. (Stuart). Uplex, Cap. (Arcum).
W/Vitamins, minerals, methyl testosterone, ethinyl estradiol, niacinamide.
See: Geritag, Cap. (Reid-Rowell).
W/Vitamin C, niacinamide, zinc sulfate, magnesium sulfate, vitamins B_1, B_2, B_6.
See: Vicon-C, Cap. (Glaxo).
W/Zinc sulfate, niacinamide, magnesium sulfate, manganese sulfate, vitamin complex.
See: Vicon Plus, Cap. (Glaxo).

• **CALCIUM PANTOTHENATE, RACEMIC, U.S.P.** U.S.P. XXIII. β-Alanine, N-(2,4-dihydroxy-3,3-dimethyl-1-oxo- butyl)-, calcium salt (2:1), (±-Calcium DL-pantothenate (1:2).
Use: Vitamin B (enzyme cofactor).
See: Pantholin (Lilly).

• **CALCIUM PHOSPHATE, DIBASIC, U.S.P.** U.S.P. XXIII. Tab., U.S.P. XXIII.
Use: Calcium replenisher.
See: Dicalcium Phosphate.
Diostate D, Tab. (Upjohn).

CALCIUM PHOSPHATE, MONOCALCIUM.
See: Dicalcium Phosphate.

• **CALCIUM PHOSPHATE, TRIBASIC.** Tricalcium Phosphate, N.F. XVIII. 39% Calcium. Tab.
Use: Calcium replacement.
See: Posture (Wyeth-Ayerst).

CALCIUM-PHOSPHORUS-FREE.
See: Fosfree, Tab. (Mission).

• **CALCIUM POLYCARBOPHIL, U.S.P.** U.S.P. XXIII. Tab.
Use: Cathartic.
See: Fibercon, Tab. (Lederle).

CALCIUM POLYSULFIDE.
Use: Wet dressing, soak.
See: Vlemasque, Cream. (Permik).
Vleminckx, Soln. (Ulmer).

CALCIUM PROPIONATE.
See: Propionate-caprylate mixtures.

CALCIUM QUINATE.
See: Calcium Kinate Gluconate.

• **CALCIUM SACCHARATE, U.S.P.** U.S.P. XXIII.
Use: Sweetening agent.

CALCIUM SACCHARIN. Saccharin Calcium, U.S.P. XXIII.
Use: Sweetening agent.

CALCIUM SALICYLATE, THEO-BROMINE.
See: Theocalcin, Tab., Pow. (Knoll).

CALCIUM SALTS OF SENNOSIDES A & B.
Use: Laxative.
See: Gentle Nature, Tab. (Sandoz).
Nytilax, Tab. (Mentholatum).

• **CALCIUM SILICATE, U.S.P.** N.F. XVIII. A compound of calcium oxide and silicon dioxide.
Use: Pharmaceutic aid (tablet excipient).

• **CALCIUM STEARATE, U.S.P.** N.F. XVIII.
Use: Pharmaceutic aid (tablet lubricant).

CALCIUM SUCCINATE.
W/Aspirin.
See: Ber-Ex, Tab. (Dolcin).
Dolcin, Tab. (Dolcin).

W/Phenobarbital, salicylamide, vitamin C.
See: Calsuxaphen, Cap., Tab. (Lannett).

• **CALCIUM SULFATE, U.S.P.** N.F. XVIII.
Use: Pharmaceutic aid (tablet diluent).

CALCIUM THIOSULFATE.
Use: Wet dressing, soak.
See: Vlemasque Cream (Dermik).
Vleminckx, Soln. (Ulmer).

CALCIUM TRISODIUM PENTETATE.
Calcium trisodium (carboxymethylimino)-bis(ethyl-enenitrilo) tetra-acetic acid.
Use: Heavy metal antagonist.
See: Calcium Chel 330 (Geigy).

CALCIUM TRISODIUM PENTETATE.
B.A.N. Calcium chelate of the trisodium salt of diethylenetriamine-NNN′N″N″-penta-acetic acid.
Use: Chelating agent.

CALCIUM UNDECYLENATE. 10% calcium undecylenate Pow.
Use: Antifungal.
See: Caldesene, Pow. (Pharmacraft).
Cruex Squeeze Pow. (Pharmacraft).

CALCIUM WITH VITAMIN D. (Schein) Calcium 600 mg, vitamin D 125 IU Bot. 60s.
Use: Calcium supplement.

CALDECORT CREAM. (Pharmacraft) Hydrocortisone acetate equivalent to hydrocortisone 0.5% in lanolin, white petroleum, mineral oil base. Tube 15 Gm, 30 Gm.
Use: Corticosteroid, topical.

CALDECORT LIGHT CREAM. (Pharmacraft) Hydrocortisone acetate equivalent to hydrocortisone 0.5% w/aloe cream. Tube 15 Gm.
Use: Corticosteroid, topical.

CALDECORT SPRAY. (Pharmacraft) Hydrocortisone 0.5%. Aerosol can 1.5 oz
Use: Corticosteroid, topical.

CALDEE. (Jenkins) Ascorbic acid (sodium ascorbate equivalent to 10 mg vitamin C) 10 mg, vitamin D 200 IU, dicalcium phosphate 7.5 gr, irradiated yeast/Tab. Bot. 1000s.
Use: Vitamin/mineral supplement.

CALDEROL. (Organon) Calcifediol 20 mcg or 50 mcg/Tab. Bot. 60s.
Use: Metabolic bone disease or hypocalcemia in renal dialysis patients.

CALDESENE. (Pharmacraft) **Oint.:** Cod liver oil (vitamins A, D) zinc oxide 15%, lanolin, petroleum 54%, talc. Tube 37.5 Gm. **Pow.:** Calcium undecylenate 10%. Bot. 60 Gm, 120 Gm.
Use: Antifungal.

• **CALDIAMIDE SODIUM.** USAN.

Use: Pharmaceutic aid.

CAL-D-MINT. (Enzyme Process) Calcium 800 mg, magnesium 150 mg, iron 18 mg, iodine 0.1 mg, copper 2 mg, vitamin D 200 IU/2 Tab. Bot. 100s, 250s.
Use: Vitamin/mineral supplement.

CAL-D-PHOS. (Archer-Taylor) Dicalcium phosphate 4.5 gr, calcium gluconate 3 gr, vitamin D/Tab. Bot. 1000s.
Use: Vitamin/mineral supplement.

CALEL-D TABLETS. (Rhone-Poulenc Rorer) Calcium 500 mg, vitamin D 200 IU/Tab. Bot. 60s, 75s.
Use: Vitamin/mineral supplement.

CALFER-VITE. (Drug Industries) Iron (ferrous fumarate) 30 mg, vitamins A 5000 IU, D 400 IU, B_1 3 mg, B_2 3 mg, B_3 20 mg, B_5 5 mg, B_6 2 mg, B_{12} 2 mcg, C 75 mg, Cu, I, Mg, Zn, lemon bioflavonoid complex/Tab. Bot. 100s, 500s.
Use: Vitamin/mineral supplement.

CAL-GUARD. (Rugby) Calcium carbonate 50 mg. Softgol Cap. Bot. 60s.
Use: Nutritional supplement.

CALICARB. (Jenkins) Calcium carbonate 0.25 Gm, magnesium carbonate 0.15 Gm, bismuth subnitrate 60 mg, powdered ipecac 0.25 mg, aromatics/Tab. Bot. 1000s.
Use: Antacid.

CALICYLIC CREME. (Gordon) Salicylic acid 10%, mineral oil, cetyl alcohol, propylene glycol, white wax, sodium lauryl sulfate, oleic acid, methyl and propyl parabens, triethanolamine. 60 Gm.
Use: Keratolytic.

CAL-IM. (Standex; Kenyon) Calcium glycerophosphate 1%, calcium levulinate 1.5%. Vial 30 ml.
Use: Calcium supplement.

CALINATE-FA. (Reid-Rowell) Calcium 250 mg, vitamins A 4000 IU, D 400 IU, B_1 3 mg, B_2 3 mg, B_6 5 mg, B_{12} 1 mcg, folic acid 1 mg, C 50 mg, B_3 (niacinamide) 20 mg, B_5 (d panthenol 1 mg), iron 60 mg, iodine 0.02 mg, manganese 0.2 mg, magnesium 0.2 mg, zinc 0.1 mg, copper 0.15 mg/Tab. Bot. 100s.
Use: Vitamin/mineral supplement.

CALIOBEN.
See: Calcium Iodobehenate.

CALIVITE. (Apco) Calcium carbonate 885 mg, ferrous sulfate 199 mg, vitamins A 3600 IU, D 400 IU, C 75 mg, B_1 1.5 mg, B_2 1.95 mg, B_6 0.75 mg, nicotinic acid 15 mg, B_{12} activity 0.025 mcg, choline 1500 mcg, inositol 2500 mcg, pantothenic acid 75 mcg, folic acid 25 mcg, p-aminobenzoic acid 12 mcg, potassium 10 mg, magnesium 1 mg,

zinc 0.075 mg, manganese 0.02 mg, copper 0.01 mg, cobalt 0.02 mcg/Tab. Bot. 100s.
Use: Vitamin/mineral supplement.

CAL-LIME-1. (Scrip) Calcium iodized 1 gr/Tab. Bot. 1000s.

CALMOL 4. (Mentholatum) **Supp.:** Cocoa butter 80%, zinc oxide 10%, bismuth subgallate. Box 12s, 24s.
Use: Anorectal preparation.

CALMOSIN. (Spanner) Calcium gluconate, strontium bromide. Amp. 10 ml. 100s.

CALM-X. (Republic Drug) Dimehydrinate 50 mg. Tab. Pkg. 162.
Use: Antiemetic/antivertigo.

CAL-NOR. (Vortech) Calcium glycerophosphate 100 mg, calcium levulinate 150 mg/10 ml. Inj. Vial 100 ml.
Use: Calcium supplement.

CALOCARB TABLETS. (Vale) Calcium carbonate 648 mg/Tab. w/cinnamon flavor. Bot. 1000s.
Use: Antacid.

CALOMEL. Mercurous Cl.
Use: Cathartic.

CALOTABS. Reformulated. (Calotabs) Docusate sodium 100 mg, casanthranol 30 mg/Tab. Box 10s.
Use: Laxative.

CALOXIDINE (IODIZED CALCIUM).
See: Calcium Iodized.

CALPHOSAN. (Glenwood) Calcium glycerophosphate 50 mg, calcium lactate 50 mg/10 ml sodium Cl solution. Contains calcium 0.08 mEq/ml. Inj. Amp. 10 ml, Vial 60 ml.
Use: Calcium supplement.

CAL-PLUS. (Geriatric) Calcium carbonate 1500 mg/Tab. Bot. 100s.
Use: Calcium supplement.

CALSAN. (Burgin-Arden) Calcium glycerophosphate 10 mg, calcium levulinate 15 mg, chlorobutanol 0.5%/ml. Inj. Vial 100 ml.
Use: Calcium supplement.

CAL SUP INSTANT 1000. (3M Personal Care Products) Elemental calcium 1000 mg, vitamins D 400 IU, C 60 mg. Pow. Packet 12s.
Use: Vitamin/mineral supplement.

CAL SUP 600 PLUS. (3M Personal Care Products) Elemental calcium 600 mg, vitamins D 200 IU, C 30 mg/Tab. Bot. 60s.
Use: Vitamin/mineral supplement.

CALSUXAPHEN. (Lannett) Calcium succinate 2.5 gr, salicylamide 4 gr, phenobarbital 1/8 gr, vitamin C 30 mg/Cap., Tab. Bot. 250s, 500s, 1000s.
Use: Analgesic, sedative/hypnotic.

• **CALTERIDOL CALCIUM.** USAN.
Use: Pharmaceutic aid.
CALTRATE 600. (Lederle) Calcium carbonate 1.5 Gm (calcium 600 mg). Bot. 60s, 120s.
Use: Calcium supplement.
CALTRATE 600 + D. (Lederle) Calcium carbonate 1.5 Gm (elemental calcium 600 mg), vitamin D 125 IU/Tab. Bot. 60s.
Use: Vitamin/mineral supplement.
CALTRATE 600 + IRON. (Lederle) Calcium carbonate 600 mg, iron 18 mg, vitamin D 125 IU/Tab. Bot. 60s.
Use: Vitamin/mineral supplement.
CALTRATE JR. (Lederle) Calcium carbonate 750 mg (300 mg calcium)/Chew. Tab. Bot. 60s.
Use: Calcium supplement.
CALTRO. (Geneva Generics) Elemental calcium 250 mg, vitamin D 125 IU/Tab. Bot. 100s, 1000s.
Use: Vitamin/mineral supplement.
CAMA ARTHRITIS STRENGTH. (Sandoz Consumer) Aspirin 500 mg, magnesium oxide 150 mg, aluminum hydroxide gel 125 mg/Tab. Bot. 100s, 250s.
Use: Salicylate analgesic.
CAMALOX. (Rhone-Poulenc Rorer Consumer) **Liq.:** Aluminum hydroxide 225 mg, magnesium hydroxide 200 mg, calcium carbonate 250 mg/5 ml. Sodium content 1.2 mg/5 ml (0.05 mEq), vanilla-mint flavor. Bot. 360 ml.
Use: Antacid.
CAM-AP-ES. (Camall) Hydrochlorothiazide 15 mg, reserpine 0.1 mg, hydralazine HCl 25 mg/Tab. Bot. 100s.
Use: Antihypertensive.
CAMELLIA LOTION. (O'Leary) Moisturizer lotion for face, hands and body. For normal to oily skin. Bot. 4 oz.
Use: Emollient.
CAMEO OIL. (Medco Lab) Mineral oil, isopropyl myristate, lanolin oil, PEG-8-Dioleate. Plastic Bot. 8 oz, 16 oz, 32 oz.
Use: Emollient.
• **CAMIGLIBOSE.** USAN.
Use: Antidiabetic (Glucohydrolase inhibitor).
CAMOUFLAGE CRAYON. (O'Leary) Coverup for minor skin discolorations, under eye concealer, lipstick fixer. Available 6 shades. Crayon 0.05 oz.
Use: Skin coverup.
CAMPHO-PHENIQUE. (Sanofi Winthrop) Camphor 10.8%, phenol 4.7%. **Liq.:** 22.5 ml, 45 ml, 120 ml. **Gel:** 6.9 Gm, 15 Gm.
Use: External analgesic, antiseptic.

CAMPHO-PHENIQUE ANTIBIOTIC PLUS PAIN RELIEVER. (Sanofi Winthrop) Bacitracin 500 units, neomycin 3.5 mg, polymyxin B 5,000 units/Gm, lidocaine 40 mg. Oint.: Tube 5 Gm.
Use: Anti-infective, topical.
• **CAMPHOR, U.S.P.** U.S.P. XXIII. Spirit U.S.P. XXIII. Bicyclo- [2.2.1.]heptane-2-one, 1,7,7-trimethyl. 2-Bornanone.
Use: Topical antipruritic; anti-infective; pharmaceutic necessity for camphorated phenol, paregoric and flexible collodion, antitussive, expectorant, local counterirritant, nasal decongestant.
See: Vicks Inhaler (Vicks).
Vicks Regular and Wild Cherry Medicated Cough Drops (Vicks).
Vicks Medi-Trating Throat Lozenges (Vicks).
Vicks Sinex, Nasal Spray (Vicks).
Vicks Vaporub, Oint. (Vicks).
Vicks Vaposteam, Liq. (Vicks).
Vicks Va-Tro-Nol, Nose Drops (Vicks).
CAMPHOR, MONOBROMATED. 3-Bromo-2-bornanone.
• **CAMPHORATED, PARACHLOROPHENOL.** U.S.P. XXIII.
Use: Anti-infective (dental).
CAMPHORIC ACID. 1,2,2-Trimethyl-1,3-cyclopentanedicarboxylic acid.
CAMPHORIC ACID ESTER. Ester of p-Tolylmethylcarbinal as Diethanolamine Salt.
CAMPTROPIN. (Jenkins) Caffeine alkaloid 5 mg, camphor 12 mg, atropine sulfate 0.1 mg/Tab. Bot. 1000s.
Use: Expectorant, anticholinergic/antispasmodic.
• **CANDICIDIN, U.S.P.** U.S.P. XXIII. Oint., Vag. Tab., U.S.P. XXIII. An antifungal antibiotic derived from *Strep. griseus.*
Use: Local antifungal.
See: Candeptin, Vaginal Tab., Oint. (Julius Schmid).
Vanobid, Oint., Vaginal Tab. (Merrell Dow).
CANDIDA TEST. (SmithKline Diagnostics) Culture test for candida. 4s.
Use: Diagnostic aid.
• **CANDOXATRIL.** USAN.
Use: Antihypertensive.
• **CANDOXATRILAT.** USAN.
Use: Antihypertensive.
CANDYCON. (Allison) Chlorprophenpyridamine maleate 2 mg, phenylephrine HCl 5 mg/Tab. Bot. 50s.
Use: Antihistamine, decongestant.
CANNABINOIDS. Antiemetic/Antivertigo agent.
See: Dronabinol.

CANNABINOL. B.A.N. 6,6,9-Trimethyl-3-pentyl-ben-zo[c]chromen-l-ol.
CANNABIS. Antiemetic/Antivertigo agent.
See: Dronabinol.
CANOPAR. (Burroughs Wellcome).
See: Thenium closylate.
• **CANRENOATE POTASSIUM.** USAN.
Use: Aldosterone antagonist.
• **CANRENONE.** USAN.
Use: Aldosterone antagonist.
CANTHARIDIN.
Use: Keratolytic.
CANTIL. (Merrell Dow) Mepenzolate bromide 25 mg/Tab. Bot. 100s.
Use: Anticholinergic/antispasmodic.
CA-OROTATE. (Miller) Calcium (as calcium orotate) 50 mg/Tab. Bot. 100s.
Use: Calcium supplement.
C-A-P. (Eastman) Cellulose acetate phthalate.
CAP-A.
See: A-CAP.
CAPAHIST-DMH. (Freeport) Chlorpheniramine maleate 8 mg, phenylpropanolamine HCl 50 mg, atropine sulfate 1/100 gr, dextromethorphan HBr 20 mg/T.R. Cap.
Use: Antihistamine, decongestant, anticholinergic/antispasmodic, antitussive.
CAPASTAT SULFATE. (Lilly) Capreomycin sulfate 1 Gm/5 ml. Vial 5 ml.
Use: Antituberculous agent.
CAPITAL WITH CODEINE. (Carnrick)
Liq.: Acetaminophen 120 mg, codeine phosphate 12 mg/5 ml. Bot. pt. **Tab.:** Codeine phosphate 30 mg, acetaminophen 325 mg/Tab. scored. Bot. 100s.
Use: Narcotic analgesic combination.
CAPITROL CREAM SHAMPOO. (Westwood) 5,7-dichloro-8-hydroxyquinoline. Chloroxine 2% in a shampoo base, sodium octoxynol-3 sulfonate, PEG-6 lauramide, dextrin, stearyl alcohol/ceteareth-20, sodium lauryl sulfoacetate, docusate sodium, magnesium aluminum silicate, PEG-14M, EDTA, benzyl alcohol 1%, citric acid, water, color, fragrance. Tube 85 Gm.
Use: Antiseborrheic.
Ca-PLUS-PROTEIN. (Miller) Calcium (as contained in a calcium-protein complex made with specially isolated soy protein) 280 mg/Tab. Bot. 100s.
Use: Calcium supplement.
CAPNITRO. (Freeport) Nitroglycerin 6.5 mg/TR Cap. Bot. 100s.
Use: Antianginal agent.
• **CAPOBENATE SODIUM.** USAN. Sodium

6-(3,4,5-trimethoxybenzamido) Hexanoate.
Use: Cardiac depressant (antiarrhythmic).
• **CAPOBENIC ACID.** USAN. 6-(3,4,5-Trimethoxybenzamido)-hexanoic acid.
Use: Cardiac depressant (antiarrhythmic).
CAPOTEN. (Squibb) Captopril 12.5 mg, 25 mg, 37.5 mg, 50 mg or 100 mg/Tab. Bot 100s, UD 100s.
Use: Antihypertensive.
CAPOZIDE. (Squibb) Captopril/hydrochlorothiazide 25/15 mg, 25/25 mg, 50/15 mg or 50/25 mg/Tab. Bot. 100s.
Use: Antihypertensive.
CAPREOMYCIN. B.A.N.
Use: Antituberculosis agent.
See: Capastat sulfate (Lilly).
• **CAPREOMYCIN SULFATE STERILE, U.S.P.** U.S.P. XXIII. An antibiotic derived from *Streptomyces capreolus*. Caprocin.
Use: Antibiotic (tuberculostatic).
See: Capastat Sulfate, Amp. (Lilly).
CAPROCHLORONE. Levo-gamma-(o-chlorobenzyl) delta-oxo-gamma-phenyl-caproic acid.
• **CAPROMAB PENDETIDE.** USAN.
Use: Monoclonal antibody.
CAPROXAMINE. B.A.N. (E)-3'-Amino-4-methyl-hexanophenone O-(2-aminoethyl)oxime.
Use: Antidepressant.
CAPRYLATE-PROPIONATE MIXTURES.
See: Sopronol, Preps. (Wyeth-Ayerst).
CAPRYLATE, SALTS.
See: Sodium Caprylate.
Zinc Caprylate.
CAPRYLATE SODIUM, INJECTION. Ingram—Amp. 33%, 1 ml Pkg. 12s, 25s, 100s.
Use: Antifungal.
See: Sodium Caprylate Preps.
CAPSAICIN.
Use: External analgesic.
See: R-Gel (Healthline Labs).
Zostrix Cream (GenDerm).
CAPSICUM OLEORESIN.
W/Alcohol, benzocaine, oxyquinoline, thymol, capsicum oleoresin.
See: Dent's Dental Poultice (C. S. Dent).
W/Alcohol, chlorobutanol hydrous (chloroform derivative), phenol, eugenol, cresol.
See: Dent's Toothache Drops Treatment (C. S. Dent).
W/Benzocaine, phenol.
See: Dent's Toothache Gum (C. S. Dent).

W/Methyl salicylate, oil of camphor, oil of pine, turpentine oil.
See: Sloan's Liniment, Liq. (Warner-Lambert).
CAPSULES, EMPTY GELATIN. (Lilly) Lilly markets clear empty gelatin capsules in sizes 000,00,0,1,2,3,4,5.
• **CAPTAMINE HYDROCHLORIDE.** USAN. N-(2-mercaptoethyl)dimethylamine hydrochloride.
Use: Cutaneous depigmenting activity.
CAPTODIAME. B.A.N. 4-Butylthiobenzhydryl 2-dimethylaminoethyl sulfide.
Use: Tranquilizer.
See: Covatin hydrochloride.
CAPTODIAME HCl. 4-Butylthio-a-phenylbenzyl 2-dimethylaminoethyl sulfide. Covatin hydrochloride.
• **CAPTOPRIL, U.S.P.** U.S.P. XXIII. Tab., U.S.P. XXIII. Angiotensin I converting enzyme inhibitor.
Use: Antihypertensive agent.
See: Capoten, Tab. (Squibb).
• **CAPURIDE.** USAN.
Use: Hypnotic.
CAQUIN. (Forest) Hydrocortisone 1%, iodochlorhydroxyquin 3%, hydrophilic base. Cream. Tube 20 Gm.
Use: Corticosteroid, topical.
• **CARACEMIDE.** USAN.
Use: Antineoplastic.
CARAFATE. (Marion Merrell Dow) Sucralfate 1 Gm **Tab.:** Bot. 100s, 120s, 500s, UD 100s.**Susp.:** 1 Gm/10 ml. Bot. 420 ml.
Use: Anti-ulcer agent.
• **CARAMEL, U.S.P.** N.F. XVIII.
Use: Pharmaceutic aid (Color).
CARAMIPHEN. B.A.N. 2-Diethylaminoethyl 1-phenylcyclopentane-1-carboxylate.
Use: Treatment of the parkinsonian syndrome.
See: Parpanit hydrochloride.
Taoryi edisylate.
CARAMIPHEN EDISYLATE.
W/Phenylpropanolamine.
See: Tuss-Ornade, Prods. (SK-Beecham).
CARAMIPHEN ETHANEDISULFONATE.
W/Phenylephrine HCl, phenindamine tartrate.
See: Dondril, Tab. (Whitehall).
CARAMIPHEN HYDROCHLORIDE. 1-Phenylcyclo- pentanecarboxylic acid 2-diethyl-aminoethyl ester hydrochloride.
Use: Proposed antiparkinson agent.
• **CARAWAY, U.S.P.** N.F. XVIII. Oil, N.F. XVIII.
Use: Flavor.

CARBACHOL, U.S.P. U.S.P. XXI. Intraocular Soln., Ophth. Soln., U.S.P. XXI. Ethanaminium, 2-(aminocarbonyl)oxy-N,N,N-trimethyl-,Cl. CarbamycholineCl. CholineCl carbamate, Lentin, Carbolin.
Use: Parasympathomimetic agent; cholinergic.
See: Miostat Intraocular, Soln. (Alcon). Murocarb, Soln. (Muro).
W/Methylcellulose.
See: Isopto Carbachol, Soln. (Alcon).
CARBACRYLAMINE RESINS.
Use: Cation-exchange resin.
• **CARBADOX.** USAN. Methyl 3-quinoxalin-2-yl- methylenecarbazate
CARBAMATE.
See: Valmid, Tab. (Lilly).
• **CARBAMAZEPINE, U.S.P.** U.S.P. XXIII. Tab., U.S.P. XXIII. Oral Susp., U.S.P. XXIII. 5H-dibenz[b,f]azepine-5-carboxamide. (Various Mfr.) **Chew. Tab.:** 100 mg. Bot. 100s. **Tab.:** 200 mg. Bot. 100s, 500s, 1000s, UD 100s.
Use: Treatment of epilepsy and trigeminal neuralgia.
See: Carbamazepine (Rugby).
Epitol (Lemmon).
Tegretol, Tab. (Geigy).
CARBAMIDE. (Various Mfr.) Urea. Cream, Lot.
Use: Emollient.
See: Aquacare (Herbert).
Carmol 20 (Syntex).
Elaqua XX (Elder).
Nutraplus (Owen/Allercreme).
Rea-Lo (Whorton).
Ultra Mide Moisturizer (Baker/Cummins).
Ureacin-20 (Pedinol).
Ureacin-40 (Pedinol).
CARBAMIDE COMPOUNDS.
See: Acetylcarbromal (Various Mfr.).
Bromisovalum (Various Mfr.).
Bromural, Tab. (Knoll).
Carbrital, Elix., Kap. (Parke-Davis).
Carbromal (Various Mfr.).
Sedamyl, Tab. (Riker).
• **CARBAMIDE PEROXIDE TOPICAL SOLUTION, U.S.P.** U.S.P. XXIII. Urea compound w/hydrogen peroxide (1:1).
Use: Local anti-infective, anti-inflammatory, analgesic, dental discomfort.
See: Gly-Oxide (Marion).
Orajel Brace-aid Rinse (Commerce).
Orajel Perioseptic, Liq. (Del Pharm.).
Proxigel (Reed & Carnick).
CARBAMIDE PEROXIDE 6.5% IN GLYCERIN.
Use: Otic preparation.

See: Murine Ear Drops (Abbott).
Murine Ear Wax Removal System (Abbott).
CARBAMYLCHOLINE CHLORIDE.
See: Carbachol.
CARBAMYLMETHYLCHOLINE CHLORIDE.
See: Urecholine, Tab., Inj. (Merck & Co.).
• **CARBANTEL LAURYL SULFATE.**
USAN.
Use: Anthelmintic.
CARBAPENEM.
See: Imipenem-Cilastatin.
CARBARSONE, U.S.P. U.S.P. XXI.
Caps., U.S.P. XXI. (Various Mfr.) N-carbamoylarsanilic acid. Amabevan, ameban, amibiarson, arsambide, fenarsone, leucarsone, aminarsone, amebarsone.
p-Ureidobenzenearsonic acid.
Use: Acute and chronic amebiasis and trichomoniasis.
• **CARBASPIRIN CALCIUM.** USAN.
Use: Analgesic.
• **CARBAZERAN.** USAN.
Use: Cardiotonic.
• **CARBENICILLIN DISODIUM, STERILE,**
U.S.P. U.S.P. XXIII. Sterile, U.S.P. XXIII.
4-Thia-1-azabicyclo[3.2.0]-heptane-2-carboxylic acid, 6-[(carboxyphenylacetyl)-amino]-3,3-dimethyl-7-oxo-, disodium salt. N-(2-Carboxy-3,3-dimethyl-7-oxo-4-thia-1-azabicyclo-[3.2.0]-hept-6-yl)-2-phenylmalonamic acid disodium salt.
Use: Antibacterial.
See: Geopen, Vial (Roerig).
Pyopen, Inj. (Beecham Labs).
• **CARBENICILLIN INDANYL SODIUM,**
U.S.P. U.S.P. XXIII. Tabs., U.S.P. XXIII.
Use: Antibacterial.
See: Geocillin, Tab. (Roerig).
• **CARBENICILLIN PHENYL SODIUM.**
USAN.
Use: Antibacterial.
• **CARBENICILLIN POTASSIUM.** USAN.
Use: Antibacterial.
• **CARBENOXOLONE SODIUM.** USAN.
Use: Glucocorticoid.
CARBETAPENTANE CITRATE. 2-[2-(Diethylamino)ethoxy] ethyl 1-phenyl-cyclopentyl-1-carboxylate dihydrogen citrate.
Use: Antitussive.
W/Codeine phosphate, chlorpheniramine maleate, guaifenesin.
See: Tussar-2, Syr. (Rhone-Poulenc Rorer).
Tussar SF, Liq. (Rhone-Poulenc Rorer).

CARBETHOXYSYRINGOYL METHYL-RESERPATE.
See: Singoserp, Tab. (Ciba).
CARBETHYL SALICYLATE.
See: Sal-Ethyl Carbonate, Tab. (Parke-Davis).
• **CARBETIMER.** USAN.
Use: Antineoplastic.
• **CARBIDOPA, U.S.P.** U.S.P. XXIII. 2-(3,4-Dihydroxybenzyl)-2-hydrazinopropionic acid; (-)-Lα-hydrazino-α-methyl-β-(3,4-dihydroxybenzene) propanoic acid monohydrate.
Use: Decarboxylase inhibitor.
See: Lodosyn, Tab. (Merck & Co.).
W/Levodopa.
See: Sinemet, Tab. (Du Pont Pharma).
• **CARBIDOPA AND LEVODOPA**
TABLETS, U.S.P. U.S.P. XXIII.
Use: Treatment of parkinson's disease.
See: Sinemet, Tab. (Du Pont Pharma).
CARBIDOPA & LEVODOPA. (Lemmon)
Carbidopa 10 mg, levodopa 100 mg; carbidopa 25 mg, levodopa 100 mg; carbidopa 25 mg, levodopa 250 mg. Tab.
Bot. 100s, 1000s.
Use: Antiparkinson agent.
CARBIMAZOLE. B.A.N. Ethyl 3-methyl-2-thiolmidazoline-1-carboxylate.
Use: Antithyroid substance.
See: Bimazol.
Neo-Mercazole.
CARBIMAZOLE. 1-Ethoxycarbonyl-2:3-di-hydro-3- methyl-2-thioimidazole. Neo-Mercazole.
CARBINOXAMINE COMPOUND DROPS.
(PBI) Pseudoephedrine HCl 25 mg, carbinoxamine maleate 2 mg, dextromethorphan HBr 4 mg. Grape flavor.
Drop. Bot. 30 ml.
Use: Decongestant, antitussive, antihistamine.
CARBINOXAMINE COMPOUND SYRUP.
(PBI) Pseudoephedrine HCl 60 mg, dextromethorphan HBr 15 mg, carbinoxamine maleate 4 mg. Grape flavor. Syr. Bot. 120 ml, pt, gal.
Use: Decongestant, antitussive, antihistamine.
CARBIPHENE. B.A.N. α-Ethoxy-N-methyl-N [2-(N-methylphenethylamino)ethyl]diphenyl-acetamide.
Use: Analgesic.
• **CARBIPHENE HCl.** USAN. 2-Ethoxy-N-methyl-n-[2-(methylphenethylamino)ethyl]-2, 2-diphenyl-acetamide HCl.
Use: Analgesic.
CARBISET TABLETS. (Nutripharm)
Pseudoephedrine 60 mg, carbinoxam-

ine maleate 4 mg/Tab. Bot. 100s.
Use: Decongestant, antihistamine.
CARBISET-TR. (Nutripharm) Pseudoephedrine HCl 120 mg, carbinoxamine maleate 8 mg/Tab. Bot. 100s.
Use: Decongestant, antihistamine.
CARBOCAINE. (Cook-Waite) Mepivacaine I ICl 0%. Inj. Dental cartridge 1.8 ml.
Use: Local anesthetic.
CARBOCAINE. (Sanofi Winthrop) Mepivacaine HCl. **1%:** Vial 30 ml, 50 ml. **1.5%:** Vial 30 ml. **2%:** Vial 20 ml, 50 ml.
Use: Local anesthetic.
CARBOCAINE WITH NEO-COBEFRIN. (Cook-Waite) Mepivacaine HCl 2% with levonorefrin 1:20,000. Inj. Dental cartridge 1.8 ml.
Use: Local anesthetic.
• **CARBOCLORAL.** USAN. Ethyl (2,2,2,-trichloro-1-hydroxyethyl)carbamate.
Use: Hypnotic.
See: Chloralurethane.
  Prodorm (Parke-Davis).
• **CARBOCYSTEINE.** USAN.
Use: Mucolytic.
CARBODEC. (Rugby) Pseudoephedrine HCl 60 mg, carbinoxamine maleate 4 mg/5 ml. Syr. Bot. pt, gal.
Use: Decongestant, antihistamine.
CARBODEC DM PRODUCTS. (Rugby)
Syr.: Pseudoephedrine HCl 60 mg, carbinoxamine maleate 4 mg, dextromethorphan HBr 15 mg, alcohol <0.6%/5 ml. Bot. 30 ml, 120 ml, pt, gal.
Drops (Pediatric): Pseudoephedrine HCl 25 mg, carbinoxamine maleate 2 mg, dextromethorphan HBr 4 mg, alcohol 0.6%/ml. Bot. 30 ml.
Use: Decongestant, antihistamine, antitussive.
CARBODEC TR. (Rugby) Pseudoephedrine HCl 120 mg, carbinoxamine maleate 8 mg/Tab. Bot. 100s.
Use: Decongestant, antihistamine.
CARBOL-FUCHSIN PAINT. Original fuchsin formula known as Castellani's Paint. Basic Fuchsin 0.3%, phenol 4.5%, resorcinol 10%, acetone 5%, alcohol 10%. Bot. 30 ml, 120 ml, 480 ml.
Use: Local antifungal.
See: Carfusin, Soln. (Rhone-Poulenc Rorer).
  Castaderm, Lot. (Lannett).
  Castellani's Paint (Various Mfr.).
CARBOLONIUM BROMIDE. B.A.N. Hexamethylenedi(carbamoylcholine bromide). Hexcarbacholine Bromide (I.N.N.).

Use: Muscle relaxant.
• **CARBOMER, U.S.P.** N.F. XVIII. A polymer of acrylic acid, crosslinked with a polyfunctional agent.
Use: Pharmaceutic aid (suspending agent); emulsifying agent.
See: Carbopol 934 P (Goodrich).
CARBOMER. B.A.N. A polymer of acrylic acid crosslinked with allyl sucrose.
Use: Pharmaceutic aid.
See: Carbopol 934.
• **CARBOMER 910, U.S.P.** N.F. XVIII, USAN.
Use: Pharmaceutic aid.
• **CARBOMER 934.** N.F. XVIII, USAN.
Use: Pharmaceutic aid.
• **CARBOMER 934P, U.S.P.** USAN.
Use: Pharmaceutic aid.
• **CARBOMER 940, U.S.P.** N.F. XVIII, USAN.
Use: Pharmaceutic aid.
• **CARBOMER 941, U.S.P.** N.F. XVIII, USAN.
Use: Pharmaceutic aid.
• **CARBOMER 1342, U.S.P.** N.F. XVIII.
Use: Pharmaceutic aid.
CARBOMYCIN. An antibiotic from *Streptomyces halstedii.*
Use: Anti-infective.
• **CARBON DIOXIDE, U.S.P.** U.S.P. XXIII.
Use: Inhalation, respiratory stimulant.
See: Ceo-Two, Supp. (Beutlich).
• **CARBON MONOXIDE C 11,** U.S.P. 23.
Use: Diagnostic radiopharmaceutical.
CARBONIC ACID, DILITHIUM SALT. Lithium Carbonate, U.S.P. XXIII.
CARBONIC ACID, DISODIUM SALT. Sodium Carbonate, N.F. XVIII.
CARBONIC ACID, MONOSODIUM SALT. Sodium Bicarbonate, U.S.P. XXIII.
CARBONIC ANHYDRASE INHIBITORS.
See: Acetazolamide, Tab. (Various Mfr.).
  AK-ZOL, Tab. (Akorn).
  Daranide, Tab. (Merck & Co.).
  Dazamide, Tab. (Major).
  Diamox, Tab., Sequel, Vial (Lederle).
  Neptazane, Tab. (Lederle).
CARBONIS DETERGENS, LIQUOR.
See: Coal Tar Solution.
CARBONYL DIAMIDE.
See: Chap Cream (Ar-Ex).
• **CARBON TETRACHLORIDE, U.S.P.** N.F. XVII. Benzinoform. (Various Mfr.).
Use: Pharmaceutic aid (solvent).
• **CARBOPLATIN.** USAN.
Use: Antineoplastic.
• **CARBOPROST.** USAN.
Use: Oxytocic.

• **CARBOPROST TROMETHAMINE, U.S.P.** U.S.P. XXIII. Inj., U.S.P. XXIII.
Use: Oxytocic.
See: Prostin, Amp. (Upjohn).

CARBOSE D.
See: Carboxymethylcellulose sodium, Prep.

CARBOTABS. (Jenkins) Sodium bicarbonate 3¹/₃ gr, magnesium carbonate 1 gr, calcium carbonate gr, papain gr, pancreatin gr/Tab. Bot. 1000s.
Use: Antacid.

CARBOVIR.
Use: AIDS treatment. [Orphan drug]

CARBOWAX. 300, 400, 1540, 4000. Polyethylene glycol 300, 400, 1540, 4000.

CARBOXYMETHYLCELLULOSE SALT OF DEXTROAMPHETAMINE. Carboxyphen.
See: Bontril Timed Tab. (Carnrick).

• **CARBOXYMETHYLCELLULOSE SODIUM, U.S.P.** U.S.P. XXIII. Paste, Tab., U.S.P. XXIII. Cellulose, carboxymethyl ester, sodium salt. Carbose D, C.M.C. (Hercules Pow. Co.).
Use: Pharmaceutic aid (suspending agent, tablet excipient, viscosity-increasing agent); cathartic.
W/Acetphenolisatin, docusate sodium.
See: Scrip-Lax, Tab. (Scrip).
W/Alginic acid, sodium bicarbonate.
See: Pretts, Tabs. (Marion Merrel Dow).
W/Belladonna extract, kaolin, pectin, zinc phenosulfonate.
See: Gelcomul, Liq. (Commerce).
W/Digitoxin.
See: Foxalin, Cap. (Standex).
Thegitoxin (Standex).
W/Docusate sodium.
See: Dialose, Cap. (Stuart).
W/Docusate sodium, casanthranol.
See: Dialose Plus, Cap. (Stuart).
Disolan Forte, Cap. (Lannett).
Tri-Vac, Cap. (Rhode).
W/Docusate sodium, oxyphenisatin acetate.
See: Dialose Plus, Cap. (Stuart).
W/Methylcellulose.
See: Ex-Caloric, Wafer (Eastern Research).
W/Testosterone, estrone, sodium Cl.
See: Tostestro, Inj. (Bowman).

• **CARBOXYCELLULOSE SODIUM 12, U.S.P.** N.F. XVIII.
Use: Pharmaceutic aid (suspending agent, viscosity increasing agent).

CARBOXYMETHYLCYSTEINE. B.A.N. S-Carboxymethylcysteine.

Use: Mucolytic agent.

CARBOXYPHEN.
W/Butabarbital.
See: Bontril, Timed Tab. (Carnrick).

CARBROMAL. (Various Mfr.) Bromodiethylacetylurea, bromadel, nyctal, planadalin, uradal.
Use: Sedative/hypnotic.
W/Bromisovalum (Bromural).
See: Bro-T's, Tab. (Brothers).

CARBUTAMIDE. B.A.N. 1-Butyl-3-sulphanilylurea.
Use: Hypoglycemic agent.

CARBUTAMIDE. N-Butyl-N'-sulfanilylurea. BZ. 55; Invenol; Nadisan.
Use: Hypoglycemic agent.

• **CARBUTEROL HYDROCHLORIDE.** USAN.
Use: Bronchodilator.

CARDABID. (Saron) Nitroglycerine 2.5 mg/SR Tab. Bot. 60s, 100s.
Use: Antianginal agent.

• **CARDAMON, U.S.P.** N.F. XVIII. Oil, seed, Cpd. Tincture, N.F. XVIII.
Use: Flavor.

CARDEC DM DROPS. (Various Mfr.) Carbinoxamine maleate 2 mg, pseudoephedrine HCl 25 mg, dextromethorphan HBr 4 mg, alcohol <0.6%/ml. Drop. Bot. 30 ml.
Use: Antihistamine, decongestant, antitussive.

CARDEC DM PEDIATRIC SYRUP. (Schein) Pseudoephedrine HCl 60 mg, dextromethorphan HBr 15 mg, carbinoxamine maleate 4 mg, < 0.6% alcohol. Bot. pt.
Use: Decongestant, antitussive, antihistamine.

CARDEC DM SYRUP. (Various Mfr.) Carbinoxamine maleate 4 mg, pseudoephedrine HCl 60 mg, dextromethorphan HBr 15 mg, alcohol > 0.6%/5 ml. Bot. 30 ml, 120 ml, pt, gal.
Use: Antihistamine, decongestant, antitussive.

CARDEC-S. (Various Mfr.) Pseudoephedrine HCl 60 mg, carbinoxamine maleate 4 mg/5 ml. Syr. Bot. pt, gal.
Use: Decongestant, antihistamine.

CARDENE. (Syntex) Nicardipine 20 mg or 30 mg/Cap. Bot. 100s, 500s, UD 100s.
Use: Calcium channel blocking agent.

CARDENE IV. (Wyeth-Ayerst) Nicardipine HCl 2.5 ml, sorbitol 48 mg/ml. Inj. 10 ml amps.
Use: Calcium channel blocking agent.

CARDENE SR. (Syntex) Nicardipine HCl 30 mg, 45 mg, 60 mg/Cap. SR Bot. 60s,

200s, UD 100s.
Use: Calcium channel blocking agent.
CARDENZ. (Miller) Vitamins C 25 mg, E
5 mg, inositol 30 mg, p-aminobenzoic
acid 9 mg, A 2000 IU, B_6 1.5 mg, B_{12} 1
mcg, D 100 IU, niacinamide 20 mg,
magnesium 23 mg, iodine 0.05 mg,
potassium 8 mg/Tab. Bot. 100s.
Use: Vitamin/mineral supplement.
CARDIAMID.
See: Nikethamide. (Various Mfr.).
CARDIAZOL.
See: Metrazol, Preps. (Knoll).
CARDILATE. (Burroughs Wellcome) Ery-
thrityl tetranitrate 10 mg/Tab. Bot. 100s.
Use: Antianginal agent.
CARDIO-GREEN. (Becton-Dickinson) In-
docyanine Green. Inj. Vial 25 mg, 50
mg, with diluent. CG disposable units/10
mg, 40 mg.
Use: Diagnostic aid, ophthalmic.
CARDIO-GREEN DISPOSABLE UNIT.
(Hynson, Westcott & Dunning) Vial Car-
dio-Green, ampule aqueous solvent and
calibrated syringe. 10 mg.
Use: Diagnostic aid.
CARDI-OMEGA 3. (Thompson Medical)
EPA 180 mg, DHA 120 mg, cholesterol 5
mg, less than 2% RDA of vitamins A, B_1,
B_2, B_3, C, D, Fe, Ca/Cap. Bot. 60s.
Use: Vitamin/mineral supplement.
CARDIOPLEGIC SOLUTION.
Use: During open heart surgery.
See: Plegisol, Soln. (Abbott).
CARDIOQUIN TABLETS. (Purdue Fred-
erick) Quinidine polygalacturonate 275
mg equivalent to quinidine sulfate 200
mg/Tab. Bot. 100s, 500s.
Use: Antiarrhythmic agent.
CARDIOTROL-CK. (Roche Diagnostics)
Lyophilized human serum containing
three CK isoenzymes from human tis-
sue source. 10x2 ml.
Use: Suitable for use as a quality con-
trol for immunochemical or elec-
trophoretic assays.
CARDIOTROL-LD. (Roche Diagnostics)
Lyophilized human serum containing all
LD isoenzymes from human tissue
source. 10x1 ml.
Use: Suitable for use as a quality control for immunochemical or elec-
trophoretic assays.
CARDIZEM. (Marion Merrel Dow) Dilti-
azem HCl 30 mg, 60 mg, 90 mg or 120
mg/Tab. Bot. 100s, UD 100s.
Use: Calcium channel blocking agent.
CARDIZEM CD. (Marion Merrell Dow)
Diltiazem HCl 180 mg, 240 mg, 300
mg/Ext. Rel. Cap. Bot. 30s, 90s and UD

100s.
Use: Calcium channel blocking agent.
CARDIZEM SR. (Marion Merrel Dow) Dil-
tiazem 60 mg, 90 mg or 120 mg/S.R.
Cap. Bot. 100s, UD 100s.
Use: Calcium channel blocking agent.
CARDOPHYLLIN.
See: Aminophylline. (Various Mfr.).
CARDOXIN. (Vita Elixir) Digoxin 0.25
mg/Tab.
Use: Cardiotonic.
CARDURA. (Roerig) Doxazosin mesylate
1 mg, 2 mg, 4 mg, 8 mg/Tab. Bot. 100s.
Use: Antihypertensive.
CARENA.
See: Aminophylline (Various Mfr.).
CARFECILLIN. B.A.N. 6-(α-Phenoxycar-
bonyl- phenylacetamido) penicillanic
acid.
Use: Antibiotic.
• **CARFENTANIL CITRATE.** USAN.
Use: Narcotic analgesic.
CARFIN TABS. (Major) Warfarin sodium
2 mg, 2.5 mg, 5 mg, 7.5 mg or 10
mg/Tab. Bot. 100s, 200s (5 mg only).
Use: Anticoagulant.
CARGENTOS.
See: Silver Protein, Mild.
CARGESIC. (Rand) Bot. 2 oz
Use: Analgesic, counterirritant.
CARINDACILLIN. B.A.N. 6-(α-Indan-5-
yloxycarbonylphenylacetamido)penicil-
lanic acid.
Use: Antibiotic.
CARISOPRODOL, U.S.P. U.S.P. XXIII.
Tab., U.S.P. XXIII. N-isopropyl meproba-
mate. Isomeprobamate, N-isopropyl-2-
methyl-2-propyl-1, 3 propanediol dicar-
bamate. B.A.N. 2-Carbamoyloxymethyl-
2-N-isopropylcarbamoyloxymethylpenta
ne. (Various Mfr.) 350 mg. Tab. Bot. 30s,
60s, 100, 500s, 1000s, UD 100s.
Use: Skeletal muscle relaxant.
See: Rela, Tab. (Schering).
Soma, Tab. (Wallace).
• **CARISOPRODOL AND ASPIRIN
TABLETS, U.S.P.** U.S.P. XXIII.
Use: Analgesic, muscle relaxant.
See: Soma Compound Tab. (Wallace).
• **CARISOPRODOL, ASPIRIN, AND
CODEINE PHOSPHATE TABLETS,
U.S.P.** U.S.P. XXIII.
Use: Analgesic, muscle relaxant.
See: Soma Compound w/Codeine Tab.
(Wallace).
CARIA-PABA.
See: PABA-CARIA.
CARISOPRODOL COMPOUND. (Various
Mfr.) Carisoprodol 200 mg, aspirin 325
mg/Tab. Bot. 15s, 30s, 40s, 100s, 500s,

1000s.
Use: Skeletal muscle relaxant, salicylate analgesic.

CARI-TAB. (Jones Medical) Fluoride 0.5 mg, vitamins A 2000 IU, D 200 IU, C 75 mg/Softab. Bot. 100s.
Use: Vitamin supplement, dental caries preventative.

•**CARMANTADINE.** USAN.
Use: Treatment of parkinson's disease.

CARMOL 10. (Syntex) Urea (carbamide) 10% in hypoallergenic water-washable lotion base. Bot. 6 fl oz.
Use: Emollient.

CARMOL 20. (Syntex) Urea (carbamide) 20% in hypoallergenic vanishing cream base. Tube 3 oz, Jar lb.
Use: Emollient.

CARMOL-HC CREAM 1%. (Syntex) Micronized hydrocortisone acetate 1%, urea 10% in water-washable base. Tube 1 oz, Jar 4 oz.
Use: Corticosteroid.

•**CARMUSTINE.** USAN. 1,3bic-(2-chloroethyl)-1-nitrosourea.
Use: Antineoplastic.
See: Bicnu, Inj. (Bristol).

CARNATION FOLLOW-UP. (Carnation) Protein (from non-fat milk) 18 Gm, carbohydrate (from lactose and corn syrup) 89.2 Gm, fat 27.7 Gm, vitamins A, D, E, K, C, B_1, B_2, B_3, B_6, B_{12}, B_5, folic acid, biotin, choline, Ca, P, Cl, Mg, I, Mn, Cu, Zn, Fe 13 mg, inositol, cholesterol 11.4 mg, taurine, sodium 264 mg, potassium 913 mg. Pow. 360 Gm Con. 390 ml.
Use: Enteral nutritional therapy.

CARNATION GOODSTART. (Carnation) Protein 16 Gm, carbohydrate 74.4 Gm, fat 34.5 Gm, vitamins A, D, E, K, B_1, B_2, B_3, B_5, B_6, B_{12}, C, folic acid, biotin, choline, inositol, cholesterol 68 mg, taurine, Ca, P, Mg, Fe 10 mg, Zn, Mn, Cu, I, Cl, sodium 162 mg, potassium 663 mg. Pow 360 Gm Con. 390 ml.
Use: Enteral nutritional therapy.

CARNATION INSTANT BREAKFAST. (Carnation) Non-fat instant breakfast containing 280 K calories w/15 Gm protein and 8 oz whole milk. Pkt. 35 Gm, Ctn. 6s. Six flavors.
Use: Enteral nutritional supplement.

•**CARNIDAZOLE.** USAN. Methyl-nitro-imidazole.
Use: Antiparasitic, antiprotozoal.

CARNITINE-L.
See: L-CARNITINE.

CARNITOR. (Sigma-Tau) Levocarnitine. **Liq.:** 100 mg/ml. Bot. 10 ml. **Tab.:** 330 mg. Bot. 90s. **Inj.:** 1 Gm/5 ml. Single-dose amps 5 ml.
Use: Vitamin supplement.

•**CAROXAZONE.** USAN.
Use: Antidepressant.

CARPERIDINE. B.A.N. Ethyl 1-(2-carbamoylethyl)-4-phenylpiperidine-4-carboxylate.

CARPHENAZINE. B.A.N. 10-3-[4-(2-Hydroxyethyl)piperazin-1-yl]propyl-2-propionylphenothiazine.
Use: Tranquilizer.

CARPROFEN.
Use: Nonsteroidal anti-inflammatory drug; analgesic.
See: Rimadyl. (Roche).

•**CARRAGEENAN, U.S.P.** N.F. XVIII.
Use: Pharmaceutic aid (suspending agent, viscosity increasing agent).

CARRISYN. (Carrington Labs) Phase I AIDS, ARC.
Use: Antiviral, immunomodulator.

CARSALAM. B.A.N. 1,3-Benzoxazine-2,4-dione. O-Carbamoylsalicylic acid lactam.
Use: Analgesic.

•**CARSATRIN SUCCINATE.** USAN.
Use: Cardiotonic.

•**CARTAZOLATE.** USAN.
Use: Antidepressant.

•**CARTEOLOL HYDROCHLORIDE.** USAN.
Use: Anti-adrenergic.

CARTER'S LITTLE PILLS. (Carter Products) Bisacodyl 5 mg/Pill. Vial 30s, 85s.
Use: Laxative.

CARTICAINE. B.A.N. Methyl 4-methyl-3-(2-propylaminopropionamido)thiophene-2-carboxylate.
Use: Local anesthetic.

CARTROL. (Abbott) Carteolol 2.5 mg or 5 mg/Tab. Bot. 100s.
Use: Beta-adrenergic blocking agent.

CARTUCHO COOK WITH RAVOCAINE. (Sanofi Winthrop) Ravocaine, novocaine, levophed or neo-cobefrin.
Use: Dental anesthetic.

•**CARUBICIN.** USAN.
Use: Antineoplastic.

•**CARUMONAM SODIUM.** USAN.
Use: Antibacterial.

•**CARVEDILOL.** USAN.
Use: Antianginal, antihypertensive.

CAR-VIT. (Mericon) Ascorbic acid 60 mg, vitamins A acetate 4000 IU, D-2 400 IU, ferrous fumarate 90 mg (elemental iron 30 mg), oyster shell 600 mg (calcium 230 mg)/Cap. Bot. 90s, 1000s.
Use: Vitamin/mineral supplement.

•**CARVOTROLINE HYDROCHLORIDE.** USAN.

Use: Antipsychotic.
• **CARZELESIN.** USAN.
Use: Antineoplastic (site-selective DNA binding).
CARZENIDE. p-Sulfoamoylbenozoic acid.
Use: Carbonic anhydrase inhibitor.
CASA-DICOLE. (Blue Cross) Docusate sodium 100 mg, casanthrol 30 mg/Cap. Bot. 100s.
Use: Laxative.
• **CASANTHRANOL.** USAN. U.S.P. XXIII. A purified mixture of the anthranol glycosides derived from Cascara sagrada.
Use: Cathartic.
See: Black Draught, Prods. (Chattem Labs.).
W/Docusate sodium.
See: Bu-Lax-Plus, Cap. (Ulmer).
Calotabs, Tab. (Calotabs).
Comfolax-Plus, Cap. (Rhone-Poulenc Rorer).
Comfolax-Plus, Cap. (Searle).
Comfula-Plus (Searle).
Constiban, Cap. (Quality Generics).
Diolax, Cap. (Century).
Dio-Soft (Standex).
Disanthrol, Cap. (Lannett).
Disulans, Cap. (Noyes).
Easy-Lax Plus, Cap. (Walgreen).
Genericace, Cap. (Forest Pharm.).
Neo-Vardin D-S-S-C, Cap. (Scherer).
Nuvac, Cap. (LaCrosse).
Peri-Colace, Cap., Syr. (Mead Johnson).
Sodex, Cap. (Hauck).
Stimulax, Cap. (Geriatric).
Tonelax Plus, Cap. (A.V.P.).
W/Docusate sodium, sodium carboxymethylcellulose.
See: Dialose Plus, Cap. (Stuart).
Disolan Forte, Cap. (Lannett).
Tri-Vac, Cap. (Rhode).
W/Mineral oil, irish moss.
See: Neo-Kondremul, Liq. (Fisons).
CASCARA. (Lilly) Cascara 150 mg/Tab. Bot. 100s.
Use: Cathartic.
• **CASCARA FLUID EXTRACT, AROMATIC, U.S.P.** U.S.P. XXIII.
Use: Cathartic.
W/Psyllium husk powder, prune powder.
See: Casyllium, Pow. (Upjohn).
CASCARA GLYCOSIDES.
Use: Cathartic.
• **CASCARA SAGRADA, U.S.P.** U.S.P. XXIII. Extract, Fluidextract, U.S.P. XXIII. (Various Mfr.) 325 mg/Tab. Bot. 100s, 1000s.
Use: Cathartic.

• **CASCARA SAGRADA EXTRACT, U.S.P.** U.S.P. XXIII.
Use: Cathartic.
W/Bile salts, papain, phenolphthalein, capsicum oleoresin.
See: Torocol Compound, Tab. (Plessner).
W/Bile salts, phenolphthalein, capsicum oleoresin, peppermint oil.
See: Torocol, Tab. (Plessner).
W/Ox bile (desiccated), phenolphthalein, aloin, podophyllin.
See: Bilgon, Tab. (Reid-Rowell).
W/Oxgall, dandelion root, podophyllin, tincture nux vomica.
See: Oxachol, Liq. (Philips Roxane).
W/Pancreatin, pepsin, sodium salicylate.
See: Bocresin, Liq. (Scrip).
W/Phenolphthalein, sodium glycocholate, sodium taurocholate, aloin.
See: Bicholax, Tab. (Elder).
Oxiphen, Tab. (Webcon).
W/Sodium salicylate, phenolphthalein, chionanthus extract, bile extract, sodium glycocholate, sodium taurocholate.
See: Glycols, Tab. (Bowman).
• **CASCARA SAGRADA FLUID EXTRACT, U.S.P.** U.S.P. XXIII. (Parke-Davis) Alcohol 18%. Bot. pt, gal, UD 5 ml.
Use: Cathartic. [Orphan drug]
See: Cas-Evac, Liq. (Parke-Davis).
Bilstan (Standex).
CASCARA SAGRADA FLUID EXTRACT AROMATIC. Aromatic Cascara Fluid extract, U.S.P. XXIII. Liq. Alcohol $\simeq$ 18%/5 ml. Bot. 60 ml, 120 ml, pt, gal, UD 5 ml.
Use: Cathartic.
W/Psyllium husk powder, prune powder.
See: Casyllium, Granules (Upjohn).
CASCARIN.
See: Casanthranol (Various Mfr.).
CASEC. (Mead Johnson Nutrition) Calcium caseinate (derived from skim milk curd and calcium carbonate). Pow. Can 2.5 oz.
Use: Enteral nutritional supplement.
CASOATE-A. (Marcen) Hydrolyzed casein 100 mg, histidine monohydrochloride 4 mg, benzyl alcohol 5 mg, phenol 5 mg/ml. Vial 10 ml.
Use: Anti-ulcer agent.
CAST. (NMS) Color Allergy Screening Test: A visual ELISA test for quantitative determination of Human Immunoglobulin E in serum.
Use: Diagnostic aid.
CAST. (Biomerica) Reagent test for immunoglobulin E in serum. Tube Kit 25s.

Use: In vitro diagnostic aid.

CASTADERM. (Lannett) Resorcin, boric acid, acetone, fuchsin basic, phenol, alcohol 9%. Liq. Bot. 30 ml, 120 ml, 480 ml.
Use: Antifungal, external.

CASTEL MINUS. (Syosset) Resorcinol 10%, acetone, basic fuchsin, hydroxyethyl cellulose, alcohol 10%. Non-staining. Liq. Bot. 30 ml.
Use: Antifungal, external.

CASTEL PLUS. (Syosset) Resorcinol 10%, acetone, basic fuchsin, hydroxyethyl cellulose, alcohol 10%. Liq. Bot. 30 ml.
Use: Antifungal, external.

CASTELLANI PAINT. (Pedinol) Basic fuchsin, phenol resorcinol, acetone, alcohol. Bot. 30 ml, 120 ml, 480 ml. Also available as colorless solution without basic fuchsin. Bot. 30 ml, 120 ml, 480 ml.
Use: Antifungal, external.

CASTELLANI'S PAINT. (Arohor Taylor) Bot. 4 oz, 16 oz.
Use: Antifungal, external.

CASTELLANI'S PAINT. (Penta) Carbolfuchsin solution. Fuchsin 0.3%, phenol 4.5%, resorcinol 10%, acetone 1.5%, alcohol 13%. Bot. 1 oz, 4 oz, pt.
Use: Antifungal, external.

• **CASTOR OIL, U.S.P.** U.S.P. XXIII. Aromatic, Caps., U.S.P. XXIII. (Various Mfr.) Liq., emulsion. (Various Mfr.) Liq. Bot. 60 ml, 120 ml, pint.
Use: Cathartic; pharmaceutic aid (plasticizer).
See: Neoloid (Lederle).
   Purge (Fleming).

• **CASTOR OIL EMULSION, U.S.P.** U.S.P. XXIII.
Use: Cathartic.
See: Emulsoil (Paddock).
   Fleet Flavored (Fleet).

• **CASTOR OIL, HYDROGENATED, U.S.P.** N.F. XVIII.
Use: Cathartic.

CATAFLAM. (Geigy) Diclofenac 50 mg (as potassium) Tab. Bot. 100s, UD100s.
Use: Nonsteroidal antiinflammatory agent.

CATAPRES. (Boehringer Ingelheim) Clonidine HCl 0.1 mg, 0.2 mg or 0.3 mg/Tab. Bot. 100s. 0.1 mg, 0.2 mg: Bot. 1000s, UD 100s.
Use: Antihypertensive.

CATAPRES-TTS. (Boehringer Ingelheim) Clonidine 2.5 mg, 5 mg or 7.5 mg/Transdermal patch. Pkg. 4s, 12s.
Use: Antihypertensive.

CATARASE. (Iolab) Chymotrypsin 1:5,000 (300 units) in a 2-chamber vial with 2 ml sodium Cl.
Use: Ophthalmic enzyme.

CATARRHALIS, KILLED NEISSERIA. W/*Klebsiella pneumoniae, Diplococcus pneumoniae,* streptococci, staphylococci.
See: Combined Vaccine No. 4 W/Catarrhalis, Inj. (Lilly).

CATHOMYCIN CALCIUM. Calcium novobiocin.
Use: Anti-infective.

CATHOMYCIN SODIUM. Novobiocin sodium.
Use: Anti-infective.

CATIONIC RESINS.
See: Resins, Sodium Removing.

CATRIX. (Donell DerMedex) Octyl methoxycinnamate, menthyl anthranilate, benzophenone 3, titanium dioxide, sesame oil, cetearyl alcohol, urea, EDTA, imidazolidinyl urea, parabens. SPF 15. Cream Tube 30 g.
Use: Sunscreen.

CAV-X FLUORIDE TREATMENT. (Palisades) Stannous fluoride 0.4% gel. Bot. 121.9 Gm.
Use: Dental caries preventative.

C-BIO. (Barth's) Vitamin C 150 mg, citrus bioflavonoid complex 100 mg, rutin 50 mg/Tab. Bot. 100s, 500s, 1000s.
Use: Vitamin supplement.

C-B TIME. (Arco) Ascorbic acid 200 mg, vitamins B_1 10 mg, B_2 10 mg, B_6 5 mg, B_{12} 10 mcg, niacinamide 50 mg, calcium pantothenate 10 mg/Tab. Bot. 40s, 120s, 500s.
Use: Vitamin supplement.

C-B TIME 500. (Arco) Vitamins C 500 mg, B_1 10 mg, B_2 10 mg, B_6 5 mg, cyanocobalamin 10 mg, niacinamide 50 mg, calcium pantothenate 10 mg/Tab. Bot. 30s, 100s, 500s.
Use: Vitamin supplement.

C-B TIME LIQUID. (Arco) Vitamins C 300 mg, B_1 15 mg, B_2 10 mg, B_3 100 mg, B_5 20 mg, B_6 5 mg, B_{12} 5 mcg. Liq. Bot. 120 ml.
Use: Vitamin supplement.

C-BINNEX.
See: BINNEX-C.

C-CAPS 500. (Drug Industries) Vitamin C 500 mg/Cap. Bot. 100s.
Use: Vitamin C supplement.

CCD 1042. (Cocensys)
Use: Treatment of infantile spasms. [Orphan drug]

CCNU. Lomustine.
Use: Antineoplastic agent.

See: CeeNu, Tab. (Bristol).

C-CRYSTALS. (Nature's Bounty) Vitamin C 5,000 mg/tsp. Crystals. Bot. 180 Gm.
Use: Vitamin supplement.

CD4 HUMAN TRUNCATED 369 AA POLYPEPTIDE.
Use: AIDS treatment. [Orphan drug]

CD4 IMMUNOGLOBULIN G, RECOMBINANT HUMAN.
Use: AIDS treatment. [Orphan drug]

CD4, RECOMBINANT SOLUBLE HUMAN (rCD4).
Use: AIDS treatment. [Orphan drug]

CD5-T LYMPHOCYTE IMMUNOTOXIN.
Use: Rejection in bone marrow transplants. [Orphan drug]

CD-45 MONOCLONAL ANTIBODIES.
Use: Prevent graft rejection in organ transplants. [Orphan drug]

CDDP.
Use: Antineoplastic agent.
See: Cisplatin.

C.D.M. EXPECTORANT. (Lannett) Dextromethorphan HBr 10 mg, chlorpheniramine maleate 1 mg, phenylephrine HCl 5 mg, sodium citrate 15 mg, guaifenesin 25 mg/5 ml. Bot. pt, gal.
Use: Antitussive, antihistamine, decongestant, expectorant.

C.D.P. CAPS. (Goldline) Chlordiazepoxide HCl 5 mg, 10 mg or 25 mg/Cap. Bot. 100s, 500s, 1000s.
Use: Antianxiety agent.

CEA. (Abbott Diagnostics) Radioimmunoassay or enzyme immunoassay for quantitative measurement of carcinoembryonic antigen in human serum or plasma. Test kit 100s.
Use: Diagnostic aid.

CEA-ROCHE. (Roche Diagnostics) Radioimmunoassay capable of detecting and measuring plasma levels of CEA in the nanogram range. Sensitivity-0.5 ng./ml of CEA.
Use: Diagnostic aid.

CEA-ROCHE TEST KIT. (Roche Diagnostics) Carcinoembryonic antigen, a glycoprotein which is a constituent of the glycocalyx of embryonic entodermal epithelium. Test kit.
Use: Diagnostic aid.

CEBID TIME CELLES. (Hauck) Ascorbic acid 500 mg/Cap. Bot. 100s.
Use: Vitamin C supplement.

CEB NUGGETS. (Scott/Cord) Vitamins B_1 15 mg, B_2 15 mg, B_6 5 mg, B_{12} 5 mcg, C 600 mg, niacinamide 100 mg, E 40 IU, calcium pantothenate 20 mg, folic acid 0.1 mg/Nugget. Bot. 60s.
Use: Vitamin supplement.

CEBO-CAPS. (Forest) Placebo capsules.

CEBRALAN-M TABLETS. (Lannett) Vitamin B_1 10 mg, niacinamide 30 mg, B_{12} 3 mcg, C 100 mg, E 5 IU, A 10,000 IU, D 1000 IU, iron 15 mg, copper 1 mg, iodine 0.15 mg, manganese 1 mg, magnesium 5 mg, zinc 1.5 mg/Tab. Bot. 100s, 1000s.
Use: Vitamin/mineral supplement.

CEBRALAN M.T. TABLETS. (Lannett) Vitamins B_1 15 mg, B_2 10 mg, B_6 2 mg, pantothenic acid 10 mg, niacinamide 100 mg, B_{12} 7.5 mcg, C 150 mg, E 5 IU, A 25,000 IU, copper 1 mg, iron 15 mg, iodine 0.15 mg, manganese 1 mg, magnesium 5 mg, zinc 1.5 mg/Tab. Bot. 100s, 1000s.
Use: Vitamin/mineral supplement.

C & E CAPSULES. (Nature's Bounty) Vitamins C 500 mg, E 400 mg/Cap. Bot. 50s, 100s.
Use: Vitamin supplement.

CECLOR. (Lilly) **Pulv.:** Cefaclor 250 mg or 500 mg. Bot. 15s, 100s, UD 100s.
Oral Susp.: Cefaclor 125 mg, 250 mg/5ml. Bot. 75 ml, 150 ml; 187 mg, 375 mg/5 ml. Bot. 50 ml, 100 ml.
Use: Antibacterial, cephalosporin.

CECON SOLUTION. (Abbott) Ascorbic acid 10% in propylene glycol. Each drop from enclosed dropper supplies 2.5 mg ascorbic acid; each ml contains 100 mg Bot. w/dropper 50 ml.
Use: Vitamin C supplement.

• **CEDEFINGOL.** USAN.
Use: Antineoplastic adjunct; antipsoriatic.

CEEBEVIM. (Nature's Bounty) Vitamins B_1 15 mg, B_2 10.2 mg, B_3 50 mg, B_5 10 mg, B_6 5 mg, C 300 mg/Cap. Bot. 100s, 300s.
Use: Vitamin supplement.

CeeNU. (Bristol-Myers/Bristol Oncology) Lomustine (CCNU) 10 mg, 40 mg or 100 mg/Cap. Dose pk. of two cap. each of all three strengths.
Use: Antineoplastic agent.

CEEPA. (Geneva) Theophylline 130 mg, ephedrine HCl 24 mg, phenobarbital 8 mg/Tab. Bot. 100s, 1000s.
Use: Bronchodilator, decongestant, sedative/hypnotic.

CEEPRYN. Cetylpyridinium Cl.
Use: Antiseptic.
See: Cepacol Lozenges, Soln., Troches (Merrell Dow).

CEETOLAN CONCENTRATE. (Lannett) Cetyldimethylbenzyl ammonium Cl 1:5500/2 oz. Bot. diluted w/1 gal water. Bot. 2 oz.

Use: Mouthwash.

CEE WITH BEE. (Wesley) Vitamins B_1 15 mg, B_2 10.2 mg, B_3 50 mg, B_5 10 mg, B_6 5 mg, C 300 mg, tartrazine. Bot. 100s, 1000s.
Use: Vitamin supplement.

• **CEFACLOR, U.S.P.** U.S.P. XXIII. Capsules, For Oral Susp., For Oral Susp., U.S.P. XXIII.
Use: Antibacterial.
See: Ceclor, Cap. (Lilly).

• **CEFADROXIL, U.S.P.** U.S.P. XXIII. Caps., Tabs., Oral Susp., U.S.P. XXIII. 7-[[D-2-amino-2-(4 hydroxyphenyl) acetyl] amino]-3-methyl-8-oxo-5-thia-1-azabicyclo [4.2.0] Oct-2-ene-2-carboxylic acid monohydrate.
Use: Antibiotic.
See: Duricef, Cap., Tab., Susp. (Mead Johnson).

CEFADYL. (Apothecon) Cephapirin sodium 500 mg, 1 Gm or 2 Gm/Vial.; Piggyback vial 1 Gm, 2 Gm or 4 Gm; Bulk vial 20 Gm.
Use: Antibacterial, cephalosporin.

• **CEFAMANDOLE.** USAN.
Use: Antibacterial.

• **CEFAMANDOLE NAFATE, STERILE, U.S.P.** U.S.P. XXIII. For Inj. U.S.P. XXIII. 5-Thia-1-azabicyco(4.2.0)oct-2-ene-2-carboxylic acid, 7-(((formyloxy,)phenylacetyl)amino)-3-(((1-methyl-1H-tetrazol-5-yl)thio)methyl)-8-oxo-monosodium salt,(6R-(6a, 7 b (R))).
Use: Antibiotic.
See: Mandol, Amp. (Lilly).

• **CEFAMANDOLE SODIUM, U.S.P.** U.S.P. XXIII. For Inj., U.S.P., Sterile, U.S.P. XXIII.
Use: Antibiotic.

CEFANEX. (Apothecon) Cephalexin monohydrate 250 mg or 500 mg/Cap. Bot. 100s.
Use: Antibacterial, cephalosporin.

• **CEFAPAROLE.** USAN.
Use: Antibacterial.

CEFAPIRIN. B.A.N. 7-[α-(4-Pyridylthioacetamido)]- cephalosporanic acid.
Use: Antibiotic.

• **CEFATRIZINE.** USAN.
Use: Antibacterial.

• **CEFAZAFLUR SODIUM.** USAN.
Use: Antibacterial.

• **CEFAZOLIN, U.S.P.** U.S.P. XXIII.
Use: Antibiotic.

• **CEFAZOLIN SODIUM, STERILE, U.S.P.** U.S.P. XXIII. Inj., U.S.P. XXIII. Sodium salt of 3-[(5-methyl-1, 3, 4-thiadiazol-2-yl) thio]-methyl -8-oxo 7-[2-(1H-tetrazol-1-yl) acetanido]-5-thia-1-azabicyclo[4-2.0]oct-2-ene-2-carboxylic acid.
(Apothecon) **250 mg:** Vial; **500 mg, 1 g:** Vial, piggyback vial; **5 g, 10 g, 20 g:** bulk pkg.
Use: Antibiotic.
See: Ancef, Vial (SK-Beecham). Kefzol, Amp. (Lilly).

• **CEFBUPERAZONE.** USAN.
Use: Antibacterial.

• **CEFDINIR.** USAN.
Use: Antibacterial.

• **CEFEPIME HCl.** USAN.
Use: Antibacterial.

• **CEFETAMET.** USAN.
Use: Antibacterial.

• **CEFETECOL.** USAN.
Use: Antibacterial.

CEFINAL II. (Alto) Salicymide 150 mg, acetaminophen 250 mg, doxylamine succinate 25 mg/Tab. Bot. 100s.
Use: Analgesic combination.

• **CEFIXIME.** USAN. U.S.P. XXIII. Tab., Oral Susp., U.S.P. XXIII.
Use: Antibacterial, cephalosporin.
See: Suprax (Lederle).

CEFIZOX. (SK-Beecham) Semisynthetic cephalosporin equivalent to: **Vials: 1** Gm, 2 Gm, 10 Gm of ceftizoxime/Vial. **Piggyback Vials:** 1 Gm, 2 Gm/100 ml. **Minibags:** 1 Gm, 2 Gm/50 ml w/dextrose injection (D5W).
Use: Antibacterial, cephalosporin.

• **CEFMENOXINE HYDROCHLORIDE.** USAN. U.S.P. XXIII. Sterile, Inj. U.S.P. XXIII.
Use: Antibacterial.
See: Takeda (Abbott).

CEFMETAZOLE. USAN.
Use: Antibacterial.

• **CEFMETAZOLE SODIUM.** USAN.
Use: Antibacterial.
See: Zefazone (Upjohn).

• **CEFMETAZOLE SODIUM, STERILE, U.S.P.** U.S.P. XXIII.

CEFOBID. (Roerig) Cefoperazone sodium 1 Gm or 2 Gm/Vial. 1 Gm, 2 Gm PBU 10 pack.
Use: Antibacterial, cephalosporin.

CEFOL FILMTAB. (Abbott) Vitamins B_1 15 mg, B_2 10 mg, B_6 5 mg, B_{12} 6 mcg, C 750 mg, E 30 mg, calcium pantothenate 20 mg, niacinamide 100 mg, folic acid 500 mcg/Tab. Bot. 100s.
Use: Vitamin/mineral supplement.

• **CEFONICID MONOSODIUM.** USAN.
Use: Antibacterial.

• **CEFONICID SODIUM.** USAN.
Use: Antibacterial.

• **CEFONICID SODIUM, STERILE, U.S.P.** U.S.P. XXIII.

Use: Antibacterial.
• **CEFOPERAZONE SODIUM, STERILE, U.S.P.** U.S.P. XXIII.
Use: Antibacterial.
See: Cefobid, Inj. (Roerig).
• **CEFORANIDE FOR INJECTION, U.S.P.** U.S.P. XXIII.
Use: Antibacterial.
• **CEFORANIDE, STERILE, U.S.P.** U.S.P. XXIII.
Use: Antibacterial.
CEFOTAN. (Stuart) Cefotetan disodium 1 Gm/10 ml, 1 Gm/100 ml or 2 Gm/100 ml. Vial.
Use: Antibacterial, cephalosporin.
• **CEFOTETAN DISODIUM STERILE, U.S.P.** U.S.P. XXIII, USAN.
Use: Antibacterial.
See: Cefotan, Inj. (Stuart).
• **CEFOTAXIME SODIUM, U.S.P.** U.S.P XXII. Inj., U.S.P. XXIII.
Use: Antibacterial.
See: Claforan, Inj. (Hoechst).
CEFOTETAN DISODIUM. Cephalosporin
See: Cefotan (Stuart).
• **CEFOTETAN STERILE, U.S.P.** U.S.P. XXIII, USAN.
Use: Antibacterial.
• **CEFOTIAM FOR INJECTION, U.S.P.** U.S.P. XXIII.
Use: Antibacterial.
• **CEFOTIAM HYDROCHLORIDE.** USAN.
Use: Antibacterial.
• **CEFOTIAM HYDROCHLORIDE, STERILE, U.S.P.** U.S.P. XXIII.
Use: Antibacterial.
• **CEFOXITIN.** USAN.
Use: Antibacterial.
• **CEFOXITIN SODIUM, U.S.P.** U.S.P. XXII.
Use: Antibacterial.
• **CEFOXITIN SODIUM INJECTION, U.S.P.** U.S.P. XXIII.
Use: Antibacterial.
• **CEFOXITIN SODIUM, STERILE, U.S.P.** U.S.P. XXIII. 5-Thia-1-azabicyclo (4.2.0) oct-2-ene-2-carboxylic acid, 3-((aminocarbonyl) oxy) methyl)-7-methoxy-8-oxo-7-((2-thienylacetyl)-amino)-, sodium salt (6R-cis)-.
Use: Antibacterial.
See: Mefoxin, Inj. (Merck & Co.).
• **CEFPIMIZOLE.** USAN.
Use: Antibacterial.
• **CEFPIMIZOLE SODIUM.** USAN.
Use: Antibacterial.
• **CEFPIRAMIDE, U.S.P.** U.S.P. XXIII, Inj., USAN.
Use: Antibacterial.
• **CEFPIRAMIDE SODIUM.** USAN.

Use: Antibacterial.
• **CEFPIROME SULFATE.** USAN
Use: Antibacterial.
CEFPODOXIME PROXETIL.
Use: Antibiotic.
See: Vantin Tab. (Upjohn).
Vantin Gran. for Susp. (Upjohn).
• **CEFPROZIL.** USAN.
Use: Antibacterial.
See: Cefzil (Bristol Labs.)
• **CEFROXADINE.** USAN.
Use: Antibacterial.
• **CEFSULODIN SODIUM, STERILE, U.S.P.** U.S.P. XX1.
Use: Antibacterial.
• **CEFTAZIDIME, U.S.P.** U.S.P. XXIII, Inj., USAN.
Use: Antibacterial.
See: Ceptaz, Inj. (Glaxo).
Fortaz, Inj. (Glaxo).
Tazicef, Inj. (Abbott)
Tazidime, Inj. (Lilly).
CEFTIN. (Glaxo) Cefuroxime axetil 125 mg, 250 mg or 500 mg/Tab. Bot. 20s, 60s, UD 100s.
Use: Antibacterial, cephalosporin.
• **CEFTIZOXIME SODIUM, U.S.P.** U.S.P. XXIII.
Use: Antibacterial.
• **CEFTIZOXIME SODIUM INJECTION, U.S.P.** U.S.P. XXIII.
Use: Antibacterial.
• **CEFTRIAXONE SODIUM, STERILE, U.S.P.** U.S.P. XXIII.
Use: Antibacterial.
See: Rocephin, Inj. (Roche).
• **CEFUROXIME.** USAN. U.S.P. XXIII (6R, 7R)-3-Carbamoyloxymethyl-7-[(2Z)-2-(2-furyl)-2-methoxyiminoacetamido]-ceph-3-em-1-carboxylic acid.
Use: Antibiotic.
• **CEFUROXIME AXETIL.** USAN. U.S.P. XXIII. Tab.
Use: Antibiotic.
See: Ceftin, Tab. (Glaxo).
• **CEFUROXIME PIVOXETIL.** USAN
Use: Antibacterial.
• **CEFUROXIME SODIUM, U.S.P.** U.S.P. XXIII. Inj., U.S.P. XXIII.
• **CEFUROXIME SODIUM, STERILE, U.S.P.** U.S.P. XXIII.
Use: Antibiotic.
See: Kefurox, Inj. (Lilly).
Zinacef, Inj. (Glaxo).
CEFZIL. (Bristol Labs) Cefprozil. **Tab:** 250 mg, 500 mg. Bot. 100s and UD 100s. **Pow. Susp.:** 125 mg/5 ml, 250 mg/5 ml. Bubble gum flavor. Bot. 50 and 100 ml.
Use: Antibiotic.

CELESTONE. (Schering) **Tab.**: Betamethasone 0.6 mg. Bot. 100s, 500s, UD 21s. **Syr.**: Betamethasone 0.6 mg/5 ml, alcohol < 1%. Bot. 120 ml.
Use: Corticosteroid.
CELESTONE PHOSPHATE INJECTION. (Schering) Betamethasone sodium phosphate 4 mg/ml equivalent to betamethasone alcohol 3 mg/ml. Vial 5 ml.
Use: Corticosteroid.
CELESTONE SOLUSPAN. (Schering) Betamethasone sodium phosphate 3 mg, betamethasone acetate 3 mg, dibasic sodium phosphate 7.1 mg, monobasic sodium phosphate 3.4 mg, edetate disodium 0.1 mg, benzalkonium Cl 0.2 mg/ml. Vial 5 ml.
Use: Corticosteroid.
•**CELIPROLOL HYDROCHLORIDE.** USAN.
Use: Anti-adrenergic.
CELLABURATE. (Eastman) Cellulose acetate butyrate.
Use: Pharmaceutic aid (plastic filming agent).
CELLACEPHATE. B.A.N. A partial mixed acetate and hydrogen phthalate ester of cellulose.
Use: Enteric coating.
CELLASE W-100. W/Alpha-amylase W-100, proteinase W-300, lipase, estrone, testosterone, vitamins, minerals.
See: Geramine, Tab. (Brown).
CELLEPACBIN. (Arthrins) Vitamins A 1200 IU, B_1 1.5 mg, B_2 1.5 mg, B_6 0.75 mg, niacinamide 7.5 mg, panthenol 3 mg, C 20 mg, B_{12} 2 mcg, E 1 IU/Cap. Bot. 180s.
Use: Vitamin supplement.
CELLOTHYL. (Numark) Methylcellulose 0.5 Gm/Tab. Bot. 100s, 1000s.
Use: Laxative.
CELLUFRESH. (Allergan) Carboxymethylcellulose sodium 0.5%. In 0.3 ml single-use containers (4s).
Use: Ocular lubricant.
•**CELLULASE.** USAN. A concentrate of cellulose splitting enzyme derived from *Aspergillus niger* and other sources.
Use: Digestive aid.
W/Bile salts, mixed conjugated, pancrelipase.
See: Cotazym-B, Tab. (Organon).
W/Mylase, prolase, calcium carbonate, magnesium glycinate.
See: Zylase, Tab. (Vitarine).
W/Mylase, prolase, lipase.
See: Ku-Zyme, Cap. (Kremers-Urban).
W/Pepsin, glutamic acid, pancreatin, ox bile extract.

See: Kanulase, Tab. (Sandoz Consumer).
W/Pepsin, pancreatin, dehydrocholic acid.
See: Gastroenterase, Tab. (Wallace).
CELLULOSE. W/Hexachlorophene.
See: ZeaSorb, Pow. (Stiefel).
•**CELLULOSE ACETATE, U.S.P.** N.F. XVIII.
Use: Polymer membrane, insoluble.
•**CELLULOSE ACETATE PHTHALATE, U.S.P.** N.F. XVIII. Cellulose, acetate, 1,2-benzenedicarboxylate.
Use: Pharmaceutic aid (tablet-coating agent).
CELLULOSE, CARBOXYMETHYL, SODIUM SALT. Carboxymethylcellulose Sodium, U.S.P. XXIII.
CELLULOSE, HYDROXYPROPYL METHYL ETHER. Hydroxypropyl Methylcellulose, U.S.P. XXIII.
CELLULOSE METHYL ETHER.
See: Methylcellulose, Prep. (Various Mfr.).
•**CELLULOSE MICROCRYSTALLINE, U.S.P.** N.F. XVIII.
Use: Tablet diluent.
CELLULOSE, NITRATE. Pyroxylin, U.S.P. XXIII.
CELLULOSE, OXIDIZED. Oxidized Cellulose, U.S.P. XXIII.
Use: Local hemostatic.
CELLULOSE, OXIDIZED REGENERATED, U.S.P. U.S.P. XXIII.
•**CELLULOSE, POWDERED, U.S.P.** N.F. XVIII.
Use: Tablet and capsule diluent.
•**CELLULOSE SODIUM PHOSPHATE, U.S.P.** U.S.P. XXIII.
Use: Antiurolithic.
See: Calcibind (Mission).
CELLULOSIC ACID.
See: Oxidized Cellulose. (Various Mfr.).
CELLULOLYTIC. W/Amylolytic, proteolytic.
See: Trienzyme, Tab. (Forest Pharm.).
CELLULOLYTIC ENZYME.
See: Cellulase (Various Mfr.).
W/Amylolytic, proteolytic enzymes, lipase, phenobarbital, hyoscyamine sulfate, atropine sulfate.
See: Arco-Lipase Plus, Tab. (Arco).
W/Amylolytic enzyme, proteolytic enzyme, lipolytic enzyme, butisol sodium, belladonna.
See: Butibel-zyme, Tab. (McNeil).
W/Calcium carbonate, glycine, amylolytic and proteolytic enzymes.
See: Co-Gel, Tab. (Arco).
W/Proteolytic enzyme, amylolytic enzyme,

lipolytic enzyme.
See: Ku-Zyme, Cap. (Kremers-Urban).
Zymme, Cap. (Scrip).
W/Proteolytic, amylolytic, lipolytic enzymes, iron, ox bile.
See: Spaszyme, Tab. (Dooner).
CELLUVISC. (Allergan) Carboxymethylcellulose 1% ophthalmic soln. Single use containers 0.01 fl oz
Use: Artificial tear solution.
CELONTIN. (Parke-Davis) Methsuximide 150 mg or 300 mg/Kapseal. Bot. 100s.
Use: Anticonvulsant.
CEL-U-JEC. (Hauck) Betamethasone sodium phosphate 4 mg (equivalent to betamethasone alcohol 3 mg)/ml. Soln. Inj. Vial 5 ml.
Use: Corticosteroid.
CENAFED. (Century) **Tab.:** Pseudoephedrine HCl 30 mg or 60 mg. Bot. 100s, 1000s. **Syr.:** Pseudoephedrine HCl 30 mg/5 ml. Bot. 120 ml, pt, gal.
Use: Decongestant.
CENAFED PLUS. (Century Pharm.) Pseudoephedrine HCl 60 mg, triprolidine HCl 25 mg/Tab. Bot. 100s, 1000s.
Use: Decongestant, antihistamine.
CENA-K. (Century) Potassium and Cl 20 mEq/15 ml (10% KCl), saccharin. Bot. pt, gal.
Use: Potassium supplement.
CENALAX. (Century) Bisacodyl. **Tab.:** 5 mg. Bot. 100s, 1000s. **Supp.:** 10 mg. Pkg. 12s, 1000s.
Use: Laxative.
CENOLATE. (Abbott Hospital Prods) Sodium ascorbate 562.5 mg/ml (equivalent to 500 mg/ml ascorbic acid), sodium hydrosulfate 0.5%. Inj. Amp. 1 ml, 2 ml.
Use: Vitamin C supplement.
CENTER-AL. (Center) Allergenic extracts, alum precipitated 10,000 PNU/ml or 20,000 PNU/ml. Vial 10 ml, 30 ml.
Use: Treatment of allergy due to pollens or house dust.
CENTRAFREE. (Nature's Bounty) Iron 27 mg, vitamins A 5000 IU, D 400 IU, E 30 IU, B_1 2.25 mg, B_2 2.6 mg, B_3 20 mg, B_5 10 mg, B_6 3 mg, B_{12} 9 mcg, C 90 mg, folic acid 0.4 mg, biotin 45 mcg, Ca, Cl, Cr, Cu, I, K, Mg, Mn, Mo, P, Se, Zn/Tab. Bot. 100s.
Use: Vitamin/mineral supplement.
CENTRAL NERVOUS SYSTEM DEPRESSANTS.
See: Sedatives.
CENTRAL NERVOUS SYSTEM STIMULANTS.
See: Amphetamine (Various Mfr.).
D-Amphetamine (Various Mfr.).

Anorexigenic agents.
Caffeine (Various Mfr.).
Coramine, Liq., Inj. (Ciba).
Desoxyephedrine HCl, Tab. (Various Mfr.).
Desoxyn HCl, Tab. Gradumet. (Abbott).
Dexedrine, Preps. (SK-Beecham).
Methamphetamine HCl (Various Mfr.).
Ritalin HCl, Tab., Inj. (Ciba).
CENTRAX. (Parke-Davis) Prazepam. **Cap.:** 5 mg or 10 mg. Bot. 100s, 500s. 20 mg. Bot. 100s. **Tab.:** 10 mg. Bot. 100s, UD 100s.
Use: Antianxiety agent.
CENTROVITE ADVANCED FORMULA. (Rugby) Fe 18 mg, A 5000 IU, D 400 IU, E 30 IU, B_1 1.5 mg, B_2 1.7 mg, B_3 20 mg, B_5 10 mg, B_6 2 mg, B_{12} 6 mcg, C 60 mg, Fa 0.4 mg, biotin 30 mcg, Ca, Cl, Cr, Cu, i, vitamin K, Mg, Mn, Mo, Ni, P, Se, Si, Sn, V, Zn, K. Tab. Bot. 100s.
Use: Vitamin supplement.
CENTROVITE JR. (Rugby) Iron 18 mg, vitamins A 5000 IU, D 400 IU, E 15 IU, B_1 1.5 mg, B_2 1.7 mg, B_3 20 mg, B_5 10 mg, B_6 2 mg, B_{12} 6 mcg, C 60 mg, folic acid 0.4 mg, biotin 45 mcg, Cr, Cu, I, Mg, Mn, Mo, Zn/Chew. Tab. Bot. 60s.
Use: Vitamin/mineral supplement.
CENTRUM. (Lederle) Vitamins A 5000 IU, E 30 IU, C 90 mg, folic acid 400 mcg, B_1 2.25 mg, B_2 2.6 mg, B_6 3 mg, niacinamide 20 mg, B_{12} 9 mcg, D 400 IU, biotin 45 mcg, pantothenic acid 10 mg, calcium 162 mg, phosphorus 125 mg, iodine 150 mcg, iron 27 mg, magnesium 100 mg, potassium 30 mg, manganese 5 mg, chromium 25 mcg, selenium 25 mcg, molybdenum 25 mcg, zinc 15 mg, copper 2 mg, K 25 mcg, Cl 27.2 mg/Tab.
Use: Vitamin/mineral supplement.
CENTRUM ADVANCED FORMULA. (Lederle) Vitamins A 2500 IU, E 30 IU, C 60 mg, B_1 1.5 mg, B_2 1.7 mg, B_3 20 mg, B_5 10 mg, B_6 2 mg, B_{12} 6 mcg, D_2 400 IU, iron 9 mg, biotin 300 mcg per 15 ml. With I, Zn, Mn, Cr, Mo, alcohol. 6.6%. Liq. Bot. 236 ml.
Use: Vitamin/mineral supplement.
CENTRUM JR. (Lederle) Vitamins A 5000 IU, D 400 IU, E 30 IU, C 60 mg, folic acid 400 mcg, B_1 1.5 mg, B_6 2 mg, B_{12} 6 mcg, riboflavin 1.7 mg, niacinamide 20 mg, iron 18 mg, magnesium 20 mg, copper 2 mg, zinc 10 mg, biotin 45 mcg, panthothenic acid 10 mg, molybdenum 20 mcg, chromium 20 mcg, iodine 150 mcg, manganese 1 mg/Chew. Tab. Bot. 60s.

Use: Vitamin/mineral supplement.

CENTRUM JR. + EXTRA C. (Lederle) Vitamins A 5000 IU D 400 IU, E 30 IU, C 300 mg, folic acid 400 mcg, biotin 45 mcg, B_1 1.5 mg, pantothenic acid 10 mg, B_2 1.7 mg, nicacinamide 20 mg, B_6 2 mg, B_{12} 6 mcg, K-1 10 mcg, iron 18 mg, magnesium 40 mg, iodine 150 mcg, copper 2 mg, phosphorous 50 mg, calcium 108 mg, zinc 15 mg, manganese 1 mg, molybdenum 20 mcg, chromium 20 mcg/Chew. Tab. Cherry, orange, grape, lemon lime flavors. Bot. 15s.
Use: Vitamin/mineral supplement.

CENTRUM, JR. + EXTRA CALCIUM. (Lederle) Calcium 160 mg, iron 18 mg, vitamins A 5000 IU, D 400 IU, E 30 IU, B_1 1.5 mg, B_2 20 mg, B_3 20 mg, B_5 10 mg, B_6 2 mg, B_{12} 6 mcg, C 60 mg, folic acid 400 mcg, Cr, Cu, I, Mn, Mg, Mo, P, Zn, K 10 mcg, biotin 45 mcg/Chew. Tab. Bot. 15s.
Use: Vitamin/mineral supplement.

CENTRUM, JR. + IRON. (Lederle) Iron 18 mg, vitamins A 5000 IU, D 400 IU, E 30 IU, B_1 1.5 mg, B_2 20 mg, B_3 1.7 mg, B_5 10 mg, B_6 2 mg, B_{12} 6 mcg, C 60 mg, folic acid 0.4 mg, Ca, Cr, Cu, I, Mg, Mn, Mo, P, zinc 15 mg, biotin 45 mcg, K 10 mcg/Chew. Tab. Bot. 75s.
Use: Vitamin/mineral supplement.

CENTRUM SILVER GEL-TABS. (Lederle) Vitamins A 6,000 IU, D 400 IU, E 45 IU, B_1 1.5 mg, B_2 1.7 mg, B_3 20 mg, B_5 10 mg, B_6 3 mg, B_{12} 25 mcg, C 60 mg, K 10 mcg, biotin 30 mcg, folic acid 200 mcg, Fe 9 mg. With Ca 200 mg, Cu, I, Mg, P, Zn, Cl, Cr, Mn, Mo, Ni, K, Se, Si and V. Tab. Bot. 60s.
Use: Vitamin/mineral supplement.

CENTURION A-Z. (Mission) Fe 27 mg, A 5000 IU, D 400 IU, E 30 IU, B_1 2.25 mg, B_2 2.6 mg, B_3 20 mg, B_5 10 mg, B_6 3 mg, B_{12} 9 mcg, C 90 mg, Fa 0.4 mg, biotin 0.45 mg, Ca, Cl, Cr, Cu, I, K, Mg, Mn, Mo, P, Se, Zn, vitamin K. Tab. Bot. 130s.
Use: Vitamin supplement.

CEO-TWO. (Beutlich) Potassium bitartrate, sodium bicarbonate in polyethylene glycol base/Supp. 10s.
Use: Laxative.

CEPACOL. (Lakeside/SK-Beecham) Cetylpyridinium Cl 0.05%, alcohol 14%, tartrazine, saccharin. Liq. Bot. 360 ml, 540 ml, 720 ml, 960 ml.
Use: Antiseptic.

CEPACOL ANESTHETIC LOZENGES. (Lakeside/ SK-Beecham) Benzocaine 10 mg, cetylpyridinium Cl 0.07%, tar-

trazine, aromatics in citrus flavored hard candy base. Pkg. 18s, 324s.
Use: Anesthetic, antiseptic.

CEPACOL THROAT LOZENGES. (Lakeside/SK-Beecham) Cetylpyridinium Cl 0.07%, benzyl alcohol 0.3%, tartrazine, aromatics in mint flavored hard candy base. Pkg. 27s, 400s.
Use: Antiseptic.

CEPASTAT CHERRY FLAVOR LOZENGES. (Lakeside/SK-Beecham) Phenol 0.72%, menthol 0.12%, sorbitol saccharin. Box 18s.
Use: Anesthetic.

CEPASTAT LOZENGES. (Lakeside/ SK-Beecham) Phenol 1.45%, menthol 0.12%/Lozenge w/sorbitol, saccharin, eucalyptus oil. Pkg. 18s.
Use: Anesthetic.

CEPHACETRILE SODIUM. Sodium 7-(2-cyanoacetamido)-3-(hydroxy-methyl)-8-oxo-5-thia-1-aza-bicyclo [4.3.0]oct-2-ene-2-carboxylate acetate (ester).
Use: Antibacterial.

• **CEPHADRINE TABLETS, U.S.P.** U.S.P. XXIII.

• **CEPHALEXIN, U.S.P.** U.S.P. XXIII. Caps., Oral Susp., Tabs., U.S.P. XXIII. 7-(D-2-Amino-2-phenyl-acetamido) 3 methyl-8-oxo-5-thia-1-azabicyclo-[4.2.0]oct-2-3n3-2-carboxylic acid. 5-Thia-1-azabicyclo[4.2.0]oct-2-ene-2-carboxylic acid,7-[(aminophenylacetyl)amino]-3-methyl-8oxo-, monohydrate.
Use: Antibiotic.
See: Ceporex.
Keflex (Lilly).

• **CEPHALEXIN HYDROCHLORIDE.** USAN.
Use: Antibacterial.
See: Keftab (Lilly).

CEPHALEXIN MONOHYDRATE.
See: Biocef, Cap., Susp. (Inter. Ethical Labs).
Cefanex, Cap. (Apothecon).
Keflex, Pulvule, Susp. (Lilly).
Zartran, Cap. (Dartmouth).

CEPHALIN.
W/Lecithin with choline base, lipositol.
See: Alcolec, Cap., Granules (American Lecithin).

CEPHALORAM. B.A.N. 7-Phenylacetamidocephalosporanic acid.
Use: Antibiotic.

CEPHALORIDINE, STERILE. USAN 1-[[2-Carboxy-8-oxo-7-[2-(2-thienyl)acetamido]-5-thia-1-azabicyclo[4.2.0]oct-2-en-3-yl]methyl]pyridinium hydroxide inner salt.

Use: Antibacterial.
CEPHALOSPORIN C. B.A.N. 7-(5-Amino-5-carboxy-valeramido)cephalosporanic acid.
Use: Antibiotic.
•**CEPHALOTHIN SODIUM, U.S.P.** U.S.P. XXIII. Inj., Sterile, For Inj., U.S.P. XXIII. 7-(2-Thienyl acetamido) cephalosporanic acid sodium salt. 5-Thia-1-azabicy) clo[4.2.0]oct-2-ene-2-carboxylic acid,3-[(acetyloxy)methyl]-8-oxo-7-[(2-thienylacetyl)-amino]-,monosodium salt.
Use: Antibacterial, antibiotic.
See: Keflin, Vial (Lilly).
•**CEPHAPIRIN SODIUM, STERILE, U.S.P.** U.S.P. XXIII. Sodium 3-(hydroxymethyl)-8-oxo-7-[2-(4-pyridylthio) acetamido]-5-thia-1-azabicyclo[4.2.0]oct-2-ene-2-carboxylate acetate (ester).
Use: Antibiotic.
See: Cefadyl, Vial (Bristol).
CEPHAZOLIN SODIUM.
See: Ancef (SK-Beecham).
Kefzol (Lilly).
•**CEPHRADINE, U.S.P.** U.S.P. XXIII. Cap., Inj., Oral Susp., Sterile U.S.P. XXIII. 7-[D-2-Amino-2-(1,4-cyclohexadien-1-yl)-acetamido]-3-methyl-8-oxo-5-thia-1-azabicyclo[4.2.0]oct-2-ene-2-carboxylic acid monohydrate.
Use: Antibiotic.
See: Velosef, Cap., Inj., Susp. (Squibb).
CEPHULAC. (Marion Merrell Dow) Lactulose syrup 10 Gm/15 ml (less than galactose 2.2 Gm, lactose 1.2 Gm, other sugars 1.2 Gm). Bot. 473 ml, 1890 ml, UD 15 ml, 30 ml. Box 100s.
Use: Laxative.
CEPTAZ. (Glaxo) Ceftazidime pentahydrate with L-arginine at a concentration of 349 mg/Gm ceftazidime activity equivalent to anhydrous ceftazidime. Vial. 1 and 2 g, Infusion packs 1 and 2 g, Pharmacy bulk packages 10 Gm.
Use: Antibiotic, cephalosporin.
CERAMIDE TRIHEXOSIDEASE/ALPHA-GALACTOSIDASE A.
Use: Fabry's disease. [Orphan drug]
CERAPON. Triethanolamine Polypeptide Oleate-Condensate. (Purdue-Frederick).
See: Cerumenex, Drops (Purdue-Frederick).
CEREBID-150. (Saron) Papaverine HCl 150 mg/SR Cap. Bot. 100s, 1000s.
Use: Peripheral vasodilator.
CEREBID-200. (Saron) Papaverine HCl 200 mg/SR Tab. Bot. 100s, 1000s.
Use: Peripheral vasodilator.
CEREDASE. (Genzyme) Alglucerase. Inj.

10 U/ml or 80 U/ml. Bot. 5 ml.
Use: Enzyme replacement for Gaucher's disease.
CERELOSE.
See: Glucose (Various Mfr.).
CEREZYME. (Genzyme) Imiglucerase 212 units (equiv. to a withdrawal dose of 200 units). Pow. for Inj. Vials.
Use: Treatment for Gaucher's disease.
CERESPAN. (Rhone-Poulenc Rorer) Papaverine HCl 150 mg/SR Cap. Bot. 100s, 1000s.
Use: Peripheral vasodilator.
CERETEX. (Enzyme Process) Iron 15 mg, vitamins B_{12} 10 mcg, B_1 2 mg, B_6 1 mg, niacinamide 1 mg, pantothenic acid 0.15 mg, B_2 2 mg, iodine 15 mg/2 ml. Bot. 60 ml, 8 oz.
Use: Vitamin/mineral supplement.
CEREZYME. (Genzyme) Imiglucerase 20 ml vial containing 200 units lyophilized powder. Inj.
Use: Enzyme replacement therapy.
•**CERONAPRIL.** USAN.
Use: Antihypertensive.
CEROSE-DM. (Wyeth-Ayerst) Dextromethorphan HBr 15 mg, chlorpheniramine maleate 4 mg, phenylephrine HCl 10 mg/5 ml, alcohol 2.4%, saccharin. Sugar free. Liq. Bot. 120 ml, 480 ml.
Use: Antitussive, antihistamine, decongestant.
CERTAGEN. (Goldline) Iron 27 mg, vitamins A 5000 IU, D 400 IU, E 30 IU, B_1 2.25 mg, B_2 2.6 mg, B_3 20 mg, B_5 10 mg, B_6 3 mg, B_{12} 9 mcg, C 90 mg, folic acid 0.4 mg, biotin 45 mcg, Ca, Cl, Cr, Cu, I, K, Mg, Mn, Mo, P, Se, Zn, vitamin K. Bot. 30s, 100s, 130s, 1000s.
Use: Vitamin/mineral supplement.
CERTA-VITE. (Major) Vitamin A 5000 IU, D 400 IU, E 30 IU, K_1 25 mcg, C 60 mg, B_1 1.5 mg, B_2 1.7 mg, B_3 20 mg, B_6 2 mg, B_{12} 6 mcg, B_5 10 mg, folic acid 400 mcg, biotin 30 mcg, iron 18 mg, Ca, P, I, Mg, Cu, Zn, Mn, K, Cl, Cr, Mo, Se, Ni, Si, V, B. Tab. Bot. 130s.
Use: Vitamin-mineral supplement.
CERTA-VITE GOLDEN. (Major) Vitamin A 6000 IU, D 400 IU, E 45 IU, B_1 1.5 mg, B_2 1.7 mg, B_3 20 mg, B_5 10 mg, B_6 3 mg, B_{12} 25 mcg, C 60 mg, K 10 mcg, iron 9 mg, folic acid 200 mcg, calcium 200 mg, zinc 15 mg, biotin 30 mcg, Cl, Cr, Cu, I, K, Mg, Mn, Mo, Ni, P, Se, Si, V. Tab. Bot. 60s.
Use: Vitamin-mineral supplement.
CERUBIDINE. (Wyeth-Ayerst) Daunorubicin HCl 5 mg/ml once reconstituted w/4 ml water for injection. Vial 20 mg.

Use: Antineoplastic agent.
• **CERULETIDE.** USAN.
Use: Stimulant.
CERUMENEX DROPS. (Purdue Frederick) Triethanolamine polypeptide oleate-condensate 10%, chlorobutanol in propylene glycol 0.5%. Liq. Dropper bot. 6 ml, 12 ml.
Use: Otic preparation.
CERVICAL RIPENING AGENTS.
See: Prepidil (Upjohn).
CES. (I.C.N.) Conjugated estrogens 0.625 mg, 1.25 mg or 2.5 mg/Tab.
Use: Estrogen.
• **CESIUM CHLORIDE.** USAN.
Use: Myocardial scanning.
• **CETABEN SODIUM.** USAN.
Use: Antihyperlipoproteinemic.
CETACAINE. (Cetylite) Benzocaine 14%, butyl aminobenzoate 2%, tetracaine HCl 2%, benzalkonium Cl 0.5%, cetyl dimethyl ethyl ammonium bromide 0.005%. **Aerosol Spray:** 56 Gm. **Liq.:** 56 Gm. **Oint.:** Jar 37 Gm, flavored. **Hosp. Gel:** 29 Gm.
Use: Local anesthetic.
CETACIN. (Jenkins) Cetylpyridinium Cl 4 mg, sodium propionate 10 mg, benzocaine 6 mg/Tab. Bot. 1000s.
Use: Anesthetic, antiseptic.
CETACORT LOTION. (Owen) Hydrocortisone in concentrations of 0.25%, 0.5%, 1% w/cetyl alcohol, propylene glycol, stearyl alcohol, sodium lauryl sulfate, butylparaben, methylparaben, propylparaben, purified water. Bot. 120 ml (0.25% only), 60 ml (0.5%, 1%).
Use: Corticosteroid.
• **CETALKONIUM.** F.D.A. Benzylhexadecyldimethylammonium ion.
• **CETALKONIUM CHLORIDE.** USAN. Cetyldimethylbenzyl ammoniumCl.
Use: Antibacterial agent.
W/Phenylephrine, pyrilamine maleate, thimerosal.
See: Anti-B Mist (DePree).
CETAMIDE. (Alcon) Sulfacetamide sodium 10%, with parabens in white petrolatum, mineral oil, liquid lanolin. Sterile ophthalmic oint. Tube 3.5 Gm.
Use: Anti-infective, ophthalmic.
• **CETAMOLOL HYDROCHLORIDE.** USAN.
Use: Anti-adrenergic.
CETAPHIL. (Owen) Cetyl alcohol, stearyl alcohol, propylene glycol, sodium lauryl sulfate, methylparaben, propylparaben, butylparaben, purified water. Cream, Lot. Bot. 480 Gm (cream), 240 ml, 480 ml (lotion).

Use: Skin cleanser.
CETAPRED. (Alcon) Sulfacetamide sodium 10%, prednisolone acetate 0.25%, mineral oil, white petrolatum, liquid lanolin, parabens. Soln., Ophth. Oint. Tube 3.5 Gm.
Use: Anti-infective, ophthalmic.
CETAZOL. (Professional Pharmacal) Acetazolamide 250 mg/Tab. Bot. 100s.
Use: Anticonvulsant, diuretic.
• **CETIEDIL CITRATE.** USAN.
Use: Vasodilator.
• **CETIRIZINE HYDROCHLORIDE.** USAN.
Use: Antihistamine.
• **CETOCYCLINE HYDROCHLORIDE.** USAN.
Use: Antibacterial.
CETOMACROGOL 1000. B.A.N. Polyethylene glycol 1000 monocetyl ether. Polyoxyethylene glycol 1000 monocetyl ether.
Use: Pharmaceutical aid.
• **CETOPHENICOL.** USAN. D-threo-N-p-[acetyl-β-hydroxy-α-(hydroxymethyl)-phenethyl]-2,2-dichloroacetamide.
Use: Antibacterial agent.
• **CETOSTEARYL ALCOHOL, U.S.P. N.F.** XVIII.
Use: Pharmaceutic aid (emulsifying agent).
CETOXIME. B.A.N. N-Benzylanilinoacetamidoxime.
Use: Antihistamine.
• **CETRAXATE HYDROCHLORIDE.** USAN.
Use: Anti-ulcerative.
CETRIMONIUM CHLORIDE. B.A.N. HexadecyltrimethylammoniumCl.
Use: Antiseptic detergent.
• **CETYL ALCOHOL, U.S.P.** N.F. XVIII. 1-Hexadecanol.
Use: Emulsifying and stiffening agent.
CETYLCIDE SOLUTION. (Cetylite) Cetyldimethylethyl ammonium bromide 6.5%, benzalkonium Cl 6.5%, isopropyl alcohol 13%. Inert ingredients 74%, including sodium nitrite. Bot. 16 oz, 32 oz.
Use: Disinfectant.
CETYLDIMETHYL BENZYL AMMONIUM CHLORIDE.
See: Ceetolan Concentrate, Liq. (Lannett).
W/Benzocaine, ascorbic acid.
See: Locane, Troches (Reid-Rowell).
W/Phenylephrine HCl, pyrilamine maleate.
See: Dalihist, Nasal Spray (Dalin).
• **CETYL ESTERS WAX, U.S.P.** N.F. XVIII.
Use: Pharmaceutic aid (stiffening agent).
• **CETYLPYRIDINIUM CHLORIDE, U.S.P.**

U.S.P. XXIII. Topical Soln., Loz, U.S.P.
XXIII. 1-Hexadecyl-pyridiniumCl.
Use: Local anti-infective.
See: Bactalin (LaCrosse).
W/Benzocaine.
See: Axon Throat Loz. (McKesson).
Cpacol, Throat Loz., (Merrell Dow).
Coirex, Preps. (Reid-Rowell),
Lanazets, Loz. (Lannett).
Oradex-C, Troches (Commerce).
Semets, Troches (Beecham Labs).
Spec-T Sore Throat Loz. (Squibb).
Tyro-Loz (Kenyon).
Vicks Medi-Trating Throat Lozenges
(Vicks).
W/Benzocaine.
See: Cepacol Antiseptic Lozenges
(Merrell Dow).
W/Benzocaine, menthol, camphor, euca-
lyptus oil.
See: Vicks Medi-Trating Throat
Lozenges (Vicks).
W/Dextromethorphan HBr, benzocaine.
See: Thorzettes (Towne).
W/d-Methorphan HBr, phenyltoloxamine
dihydrogen citrate, sodium citrate.
See: Exo-Kol, Cough Syrup, Spray,
Tab. (Inwood).
W/Phenylephrine HCl, methapyrilene HCl,
menthol, eucalyptol, camphor, methyl
salicylate.
See: Vicks Sinex Nasal Spray (Vicks).
W/Phenylpropanolamide HCl, benzocaine,
terpin hydrate.
See: S.A.C. Throat Lozenges (Towne).
**CETYLTRIMETHYL AMMONIUM BRO-
MIDE.** (Bio Labs.) Cetrimide B.P.,
Cetavlon, CTAB.
Use: Antiseptic.
W/Lidocaine, hexachlorophene.
See: Aerosept, Aerosol (Dalin).
CEVALIN. (Lilly) Ascorbic acid 100 mg or
500 mg/ml. Inj. Amp. 10 ml (100 mg), 1
ml (500 mg).
Use: Vitamin C supplement.
CEVI-BID. (Geriatric) Ascorbic acid 500
mg/TR Caps. Bot. 30s, 100s, 500s.
Use: Vitamin C supplement.
CEVI-FER. (Geriatric) Ascorbic acid 300
mg, ferrous fumarate 20 mg, folic acid 1
mg/Cap. Bot. 30s, 100s.
Use: Vitamin/mineral supplement.
CE-VI-SOL. (Mead Johnson Nutrition)
Ascorbic acid 35 mg/0.6 ml, alcohol 5%.
Bot. w/dropper 50 ml.
Use: Vitamin C supplement.
CEVITAMIC ACID.
See: Ascorbic acid.
CEVITAN.
See: Ascorbic acid.

CEWIN TABLETS. (Sanofi Winthrop)
Ascorbic acid.
Use: Vitamin C supplement.
CEYLON GELATIN.
See: Agar.
CEZIN. (UAD) Vitamins B_1 20 mg, B_2 10
mg, B_3 100 mg, B_5 20 mg, B_6 5 mg, C
300 mg, magnesium sulfate 70 mg, zinc
sulfate 80 mg. Cap. Bot. 100s.
Use: Vitamin supplement.
CEZIN-S. (UAD) Vitamins A 10,000 IU, D
50 IU, E 50 IU, B_1 10 mg, B_2 5 mg, B_3 50
mg, B_5 10 mg, B_6 2 mg, C 200 mg, folic
acid 0.5 mg, zinc sulfate 80 mg, magne-
sium sulfate 70 mg, Mn Cl 4 mg/Cap.
Bot. 100s.
Use: Vitamin supplement.
C FACTORS "1000" PLUS. (Solgar) Vitamins C with rosehips 1000 mg, citrus
bioflavoinoids 250 mg, rutin 50 mg, hesperidin complex 25 mg. Tab. Bot. 50s,
100s, 250s.
Use: Vitamin supplement.
C.G. (Sig) Chorionic gonadotropin
(lyophilized) 10,000 units, mannitol 100
mg, supplied with diluent. Univial 10 ml.
Use: Chorionic gonadotropin.
CG DISPOSABLE UNIT.
See: Cardio Green, Vial (Hynson, West-
cott & Dunning).
CG RIA. (Abbott Diagnostics) Radioim-
munoassay for the quantitative measurement of total circulating serum
cholylglycine.
Use: Diagnostic aid.
CHAP CREAM. (Ar-Ex) Carbonyl diamide. Tube 1.5 oz, 3.25 oz. Jar 4 oz, 9
oz, 18 oz.
Use: Emollient.
CHAPOLINE CREAM LOTION. (Wade)
Glycerine, boric acid, chlorobutanol
0.5%, alcohol 10%. Bot. 4 oz, pt, gal.
Use: Emollient.
CHAPSTICK MEDICATED LIP BALM.
(Robins) **Jar:** Petrolatum 60%, camphor
1%, menthol 0.6%, phenol 0.5%, microcrystalline wax, mineral oil, cocoa butter,
lanolin, paraffin wax, parabens 7 Gm.
Squeezable tube: Petrolatum 67%,
camphor 1%, menthol 0.6%, phenol
0.5%, microcrystalline wax, mineral oil,
cocoa butter, lanolin, parabens 10 Gm.
Stick: Petrolatum 41%, camphor 1%,
menthol 0.6%, phenol 0.5%, paraffin
wax, mineral oil, cocoa butter, 2-octyl
dodecanol, arachidyl propionate,
polyphenyl methylsiloxane 556, white
wax, oleyl alcohol, isopropyl lanolate,
carnauba wax, isopropyl myristate, lanolin, cetyl alcohol, parabens 4.2 Gm.

Use: Mouth/throat product.
CHAPSTICK SUNBLOCK 15. (Robins Consumer) Padimate O 0.7%, oxybenzone 3%. Stick 4.25 Gm.
Use: Lip protectant, sunscreen.
CHAPSTICK SUNBLOCK 15 PETROLEUM JELLY PLUS. (Robins) White petrolatum 89%, padimate O 7%, oxybenzone 3%, aloe, lanolin. Stick 10 g.
Use: Lip protectant, sunscreen.
CHARCOAID. (Requa) Activated charcoal 30 Gm/150 ml in sorbitol. Bot. 150 ml.
Use: Antidote.
CHARCOAID 2000. (Requa) Activated charcoal 50 g in water. Bot. 240 ml.
Use: Antidote.
CHARCOAL. (Various Mfr.) Cap., Tab.
Use: Antiflatulent.
See: Charcoal (Paddock).
Charcoal (Rugby).
• **CHARCOAL, ACTIVATED, U.S.P.** U.S.P. XXIII.
Use: Antidote. Drug, chemical poisoning.
See: Actidose-Aqua (Paddock).
Charcoaid (Requa).
Liqui-Char (Jones Medical).
Superchar (Gulf-Bio Systems).
W/Nux vomica, bismuth subgallate, pepsin, berberis, diastase, pancreatin, hydrastis, papain.
See: Charcocaps, Cap. (Requa).
Charcotabs, Tab. (Requa).
CHARCOAL PLUS. (Kramer) Activated charcoal 200 mg, simethicone 40 mg. Tab. Bot. 120s.
Use: Antiflatulent.
CHARCOAL AND SIMETHICONE. Antiflatulent.
See: Charcoal Plus (Kramer).
Flatulex (Dayton).
CHARCOCAPS. (Requa) Activated charcoal 260 mg/Cap. Bot. 36s.
Use: Antiflatulent.
CHARDONNA-2. (Kremers-Urban) Belladonna extract 15 mg, phenobarbital 15 mg/Tab. Bot. 100s.
Use: Anticholinergic/antispasmodic, sedative/hypnotic.
CHARO SCATTER-PAKS. (Requa) Activated charcoal 5 Gm/Packet.
Use: Odor absorber.
CHAZ SCALP TREATMENT DANDRUFF SHAMPOO. (Revlon) Zinc pyrithione 1% in liquid shampoo.
Use: Antiseborrheic.
CHEALAMIDE INJECTION. (Vortech) Disodium edetate 150 mg/ml. Vial 20 ml.
Use: Chelating agent.

CHECKMATE. (Oral-B) Acidulated phosphate fluoride 1.23%. Bot. 2 oz, 16 oz.
Use: Dental caries preventative.
CHEK-STIX URINALYSIS CONTROL STRIPS. (Miles Diagnostic) Bot. 25s.
Use: Diagnostic aid.
CHELAFRIN.
See: Epinephrine.
CHELATED CALCIUM MAGNESIUM. (Nature's Bounty) Calcium^{++} 500 mg, magnesium 250 mg/Tab. Protein coated. Bot. 50s.
Use: Mineral supplement.
CHELATED CALCIUM MAGNESIUM ZINC. (Nature's Bounty) Calcium^{++} 333 mg, magnesium 133 mg, zinc 8.3 mg/Tab. Bot. 100s.
Use: Mineral supplement.
CHELATED MAGNESIUM. (Freeda) Magnesium amino acids chelate 500 mg (magnesium 100 mg)/Tab. Bot. 100s, 250s, 500s.
Use: Magnesium supplement.
CHELATED MANGANESE. (Freeda) Manganese 20 mg or 50 mg/Tab. Bot. 100s, 250s, 500s.
Use: Manganese supplement.
CHELATING AGENT.
See: BAL, Amp. (Hynson, Westcott & Dunning).
Calcium Disodium Versenate, Amp., Tab. (Riker).
Desferal, Amp. (Ciba).
Endrate Disodium, Amp. (Abbott).
Magora, Tab. (Miller).
CHELEN.
See: Ethyl Chloride.
CHEL-IRON. (Kinney) Iron choline citrate complex (ferrocholinate) 0.33 Gm equivalent to 40 mg of elemental iron/Tab. Bot. 100s.
Use: Iron supplement.
CHEL-IRON LIQUID. (Kinney) Ferrocholinate 0.417 Gm equivalent to 50 mg of elemental iron. Bot. 8 fl oz.
Use: Iron supplement.
CHEL-IRON PEDIATRIC DROPS. (Kinney) Ferrocholinate 0.208 Gm equivalent to 25 mg of elemental iron/ml. Bot. 60 ml with calibrated dropper.
Use: Iron supplement.
CHEL-IRON PLUS. (Kinney) Ferrocholinate 200 mg (equivalent to 24 mg elemental iron), vitamin B_{12} with intrinsic factor concentrate 1/3 units, vitamins C 50 mg, B_1 2 mg, B_2 2 mg, B_6 HCl 2 mg, niacin 25 mg/Tab. Bot. 100s.
Use: Vitamin/mineral supplement.
CHEMET. (McNeil-CPC) Succimer 100 mg. Cap. Bot. 100s.

Use: Chelating agent.

CHEMIPEN. Potassium phenethicillin.
Use: Antibacterial, penicillin.

CHEMOVAG SUPPS. (Forest Pharm.)
Sulfisoxazole 0.5 Gm/Supp. Bot. 12s
w/applicators.
Use: Antibacterial, sulfonamide.

CHEMOZINE. (Tennessee Pharm.) Sulfadiazine, 0.167 Gm, sulfamerazine 0.167
Gm, sulfamethazine 0.167 Gm/Tab. Bot.
100s, 1000s. Susp. Bot. pt, gal.
Use: Antibacterial, sulfonamide.

CHEMSTRIP 6. (Boehringer Mannheim)
Broad range test for glucose, protein,
pH, blood, ketones and leukocytes. Bot.
strip 100s.
Use: Diagnostic aid.

CHEMSTRIP 7. (Boehringer Mannheim)
Broad range test for glucose, protein,
pH, blood, ketones, bilirubin and leukocytes. Bot. strip 100s.
Use: Diagnostic aid.

CHEMSTRIP 8. (Boehringer Mannheim)
Broad range urine test for glucose, protein, pH, blood,ketones, bilirubin, urobilinogen and leukocytes. Bot. Strip
100s.
Use: Diagnostic aid.

CHEMSTRIP 9. (Boehringer Mannheim)
Broad range test for glucose, protein,
pH, blood, ketones, bilirubin, urobilinogen, nitrite and leukocytes in urine. Bot.
strip 100s.
Use: Diagnostic aid.

CHEMSTRIP 10 SG. (Boehringer
Mannheim) Broad range test for glucose, protein, pH, blood, ketones, bilirubin, urobilinogen, nitrite and leukocytes
in urine. Bot. Strip 100s.
Use: Diagnostic aid.

CHEMSTRIP 4 THE OB. (Boehringer
Mannheim) Broad range test for glucose, protein, blood and leukocytes in
urine. Bot. Strip 100s.
Use: Diagnostic aid.

CHEMSTRIP bG. (Boehringer
Mannheim) For measuring glucose in
blood. Bot. strip 25s, 50s.
Use: Diagnostic aid.

CHEMSTRIP 2 GP. (Boehringer
Mannheim) Broad range test for glucose
and protein. Bot. strip 100s.
Use: Diagnostic aid.

CHEMSTRIP-K. (Boehringer Mannheim)
Reagent papers for ketones in urine.
Bot. paper 25s, 100s.
Use: Diagnostic aid.

CHEMSTRIP 2 LN. (Boehringer
Mannheim) Broad range test for nitrite

and leukocytes. Bot. strip 100s.
Use: Diagnostic aid.

CHEMSTRIP MICRAL. (Boehringer
Mannheim) In vitro reagent strips to de-
tect albumin in urine. In 5s, 30s.
Use: Diagnostic aid.

CHEMSTRIP MINERAL. (Boehringer
Mannheim) In vitro reagent strips used
to detect albumin in urine. Strips. 5s,
30s.
Use: In vitro diagnostic aid.

CHEMSTRIP uG. (Boehringer
Mannheim) Use to test for glucose in
urine using the glucose oxidase method.
Bot. strip 100s.
Use: Diagnostic aid.

CHEMSTRIP uGK. (Boehringer
Mannheim) Broad range test for glucose
and ketones. Bot. strip 50s, 100s.
Use: Diagnostic aid.

CHENATAL. (Miller) Calcium 580 mg,
magnesium 200 mg, vitamins C 100 mg,
folic acid 0.4 mg, A 5000 IU, D 400 IU,
B_1 3 mg, B_2 3 mg, B_6 5 mg, B_{12} 9 mcg,
niacinamide 30 mg, pantothenic acid 5
mg, tocopherols (mixed) 10 mg, iron 20
mg, copper 1 mg, manganese 2 mg,
potassium 10 mg, zinc 25 mg, iodine 0.1
mg/2 Tabs. Bot. 100s.
Use: Vitamin/mineral supplement.

CHENODEOXYCHOLIC ACID.
Use: Gallstone solubilizing agent.
See: Chenodiol.

•**CHENODIOL.** USAN.
Use: Anticholelithogenic. [Orphan drug]
See: Chenix, Tab. (Reid-Rowell).

CHERACOL. (Roberts) Codeine phosphate 10 mg, guaifenesin 100 mg/5 ml,
alcohol 4.75%. Bot. 2 oz, 4 oz, pt.
Use: Antitussive, expectorant.

CHERACOL D. (Roberts) Dextromethorphan HBr 10 mg, guaifenesin 100 mg/5
ml, alcohol 4.75%. Bot. 2 oz, 4 oz, 6 oz.
Use: Antitussive, expectorant.

CHERACOL NASAL. (Roberts)
Oxymetazoline HCl 0.05%, phenylmercuric acetate 0.02 mg/ml, benzalkonium
chloride, glycine, sorbitol. Soln. Spray
30 ml.
Use: Decongestant.

CHERACOL PLUS. (Roberts) Phenylpropanolamine HCl 8.3 mg, dextromethorphan HBr 6.7 mg, chlorpheniramine maleate 1.3 mg/5 ml. Bot. 4 oz.
Use: Decongestant, antitussive, antihistamine.

CHERACOL SINUS. (Roberts) Pseudoephedrine sulfate 120 mg,

dexbrompheniramine 6 mg/Tab. SA. Pck 10s.
Use: Decongestant, antihistamine.
CHERACOL SORE THROAT. (Roberts) Phenol 1.4%, saccharin, sorbitol, alcohol 12.5%. Spray Bot. 177 ml.
Use: Mouth and throat product.
CHERALIN SYRUP. (Lannett) Potassium guaiacolsulfonate 88 mg, ammonium Cl 88 mg, antimony potassium tartrate 1 mg, codeine phosphate 10 mg/5 ml. Bot. pt, gal.
Use: Antitussive, expectorant.
CHERATUSSIN COUGH SYRUP. (Towne) Dextromethorphan HBr 45 mg, ammonium Cl 575 mg, citrate sodium 280 mg/Fl oz. Bot. 4 oz.
Use: Antitussive, expectorant.
CHERI-APRO. (Approved) Codeine phosphate 1 gr, potassium guaiacolsulfonate 8 gr, tartar emetic $\frac{1}{12}$ gr/Fl oz. Bot. 4 oz, gal.
Use: Antitussive, expectorant.
CHERO-TRISULFA-V. (Vita Elixir) Sulfadiazine 0.166 Gm, sulfacetamide 0.166 Gm, sulfamerazine 0.166 Gm, sodium citrate 0.5 Gm/5 ml. Susp. Bot. pt.
Use: Antibacterial, sulfonamide.
• **CHERRY JUICE, U.S.P.** N.F. XVIII.
Use: Flavor.
• **CHERRY SYRUP, U.S.P.** N.F. XVIII.
Use: Pharmaceutic aid (Vehicle).
CHESTAMINE. (Leeds) Chlorpheniramine maleate 8 mg or 12 mg/Cap. Bot. 50s.
Use: Antihistamine.
CHEST THROAT LOZENGES. (Lane) Eucalyptol, anise, horehound, tolu balsam, benzoin tincture, sugar, corn syrup. Pkg. 30s.
Use: Antiseptic.
CHEWABLE C. (Approved Pharm.) Vitamin C 100 mg, 250 mg, 300 mg and 500 mg/Tab. Bot. 100s.
Use: Vitamin supplement.
CHEW HIST. (Kenyon) Phenylephrine HCl 7.5 mg, chlorpheniramine maleate 2 mg, vitamin C 50 mg/Wafer. Bot. 100s.
Use: Decongestant, antihistamine.
CHEW-VIMS. (Barth's) Vitamins A 5000 IU, D 400 IU, B_1 3 mg, B_2 6 mg, niacin 1.71 mg, C 100 mg, B_{12} 5 mcg, E 5 IU/Tab. Bot. 30s, 90s, 180s, 360s.
Use: Vitamin supplement.
CHEW-VI-TAB. (Blue Cross) Vitamins A 2500 IU, D 400 IU, E 15 IU, C 60 mg, folic acid 0.3 mg, B_1 1.05 mg, B_2 1.2 mg, niacin 13.5 mg, B_6 1.05 mg, B_{12} 4.5 mcg/Tab. Bot. 100s.
Use: Vitamin supplement.

CHEW-VI-TAB WITH IRON. (Blue Cross) Vitamins A 5000 IU, C 60 mg, E 15 IU, folic acid 0.4 mg, B_1 1.5 mg, B_2 1.7 mg, niacin 20 mg, B_6 2 mg, B_{12} 6 mcg, D 400 IU, iron 18 mg/Tab. Bot. 100s.
Use: Vitamin/mineral supplement.
CHEW VITES. (Kenyon) Vitamins A 5000 IU, D 500 IU, B_1 2 mg, B_2 2 mg, B_6 1 mg, B_{12} 2 mcg, calcium pantothenate 2 mg, C 50 mg, niacinamide 10 mg, fluoride 0.05 mg/Tab. Bot. 100s.
Use: Vitamin/mineral supplement.
CHIBROXIN. (Merck & Co.) Norfloxacin 3 mg/ml. Soln. Drop. Bot. 5 ml.
Use: Ophthalmic antibiotic.
CHIGGEREX. (Scherer) Benzocaine 0.02%, camphor, menthol, peppermint oil, olive oil, clove oils, pegosperse, methylparaben, distilled water. Oint. Jar 50 Gm.
Use: Local anesthetic, counterirritant.
CHIGGERTOX. (Scherer) Benzocaine 2.1%, benzyl benzoate 21.4%, soft soap, isopropyl alcohol. Liq. Bot. oz.
Use: Local anesthetic.
CHILDREN'S ADVIL. (Wyeth-Ayerst) Ibuprofen 100 mg/5 ml. Bot. 119 ml, 473 ml.
Use: Nonsteroidal anti-inflammatory drug; analgesic.
CHILDREN'S ALLEREST. (Fisons) Phenylpropanolamine HCl 94 mg, chlorpheniramine maleate 6 mg. Chew. Tab. Bot. 24s.
Use: Pediatric decongestant, antihistamine.
CHILDREN'S FEVERALL. (Upsher-Smith) Acetaminophen 120 mg or 325 mg/Supp. Pkg. 6s.
Use: Analgesic.
CHILDREN'S FORMULA COUGH SYRUP. (Pharmakon) Guaifenesin 50 mg, dextromethorphan HBr 5 mg, sucrose, corn syrup. Alcohol free. Grape flavor. Syr. Bot. 118 ml, 236 ml.
Use: Expectorant, antitussive.
CHILDREN'S HOLD 4-HOUR COUGH SUPPRESSANT & DECONGESTANT. (Beecham Products) Dextromethorphan HBr 3.75 mg, phenylpropanolamine HCl 6.25 mg/Loz. Pkg. 10s.
Use: Antitussive, decongestant.
CHILDREN'S KAOPECTATE. (Upjohn) **Chew. Tab.:** Attapulgite 300 mg. Pck. 16s.
Liq.: Attapulgite 600 mg. Bot. 180 ml.
Use: Antidiarrheal.
CHILDREN'S MOTRIN. (McNeil-CPC) Ibuprofen 100 mg/5 ml, sucrose. Susp. Bot. 120 ml, 480 ml.

Use: Nonsteroidal anti-inflammatory agent, analgesic.
CHILDREN'S NO ASPIRIN ELIXIR. (Walgreen) Acetaminophen 80 mg/2.5 ml. Non-alcoholic. Bot. 4 oz.
Use: Analgesic.
CHILDREN'S NO-ASPIRIN TABLETS. (Walgreen) Acetaminophen 80 mg/Tab. Bot. 30s.
Use: Analgesic.
CHILDREN'S NYQUIL. (Vicks) Pseudoephedrine HCl 10 mg, chlorpheniramine maleate 0.6 mg, dextromethorphan HBr 5 mg/5 ml. Bot. 120 ml, 240 ml.
Use: Decongestant, antihistamine, antitussive.
CHILDREN NYQUIL NIGHTIME HEAD COLD, ALLERGY FORMULA. (Richardson-Vicks) Pseudoephedrine HCl 10 mg, chlorpheniramine maleate 0.67 mg/5 ml. Alcohol free. Sorbitol, sucrose. Grape flavor. Liq. Bot. 120 ml.
Use: Decongestant, antihistamine.
CHILDREN'S SUNKIST MULTIVITAMINS COMPLETE. (Ciba) Iron 18 mg, vitamin A 5000 IU, D_3 400 IU, E 30 IU, B_1 1.5 mg, B_2 1.7 mg, B_3 20 mg, B_5 10 mg, B_6 2 mg, B_{12} 6 mcg, C 60 mg, folic acid 400 mcg, Ca 100 mg, Cu, I, K, Mg, Mn, P, zinc 10 mg, biotin 40 mcg, K_1 10 mcg, sorbitol, aspartame, phenylalanine, tartrazine. Chew. Tab. Bot. 60s.
Use: Vitamin-mineral supplement.
CHILDREN'S SUNKIST MULTIVITAMINS + EXTRA C. (Ciba) Vitamin A 2500 IU, E 15 IU, D_3 400 IU, B_1 1.05 mg, B_2 1.2 mg, B_3 13.5 mg, B_6 1.05 mg, B_{12} 4.5 mcg, C 250 mg, folic acid 0.3 mg, vitamin K_1 5 mcg, sorbitol, aspartame, phenylalanine, tartrazine. Chew.Tab. Bot. 60s.
Use: Vitamin supplement.
CHILDREN'S SUNKIST MULTIVITAMININS + IRON. (Ciba) Iron 15 mg, vitamin A 2500 IU, E 15 IU, D_3 400 IU, B_1 1.05 mg, B_2 1.2 mg, B_3 13.5 mg, B_6 1.05 mg, B_{12} 4.5 mcg, C 60 mg, folic acid 0.3 mg, vitamin K_1 5 mcg, sorbitol, aspartame, phenylalanine, tartrazine. Chew. Tab. Bot. 60s.
Use: Vitamin with Iron supplement.
CHILDREN'S TYLENOL COLD TABLETS. (McNeil-CPC) Pseudoephedrine HCl 7.5 mg, chlorpheniramine maleate 0.5 mg, acetaminophen 80 mg, aspartame, sucrose, phenylalanine 4 mg. Chewable. Grape flavor. Tab. Bot. 24s.
Use: Decongestant, antihistamine, analgesic.

CHILDREN'S TYLENOL COLD LIQUID. (McNeil-CPC) Pseudoephedrine HCl 15 mg, chlorpheniramine maleate 1 mg, acetaminophen 160 mg, sorbitol, sucrose. Alcohol free. Grape flavor. Liq. Bot. 120 ml.
Use: Decongestant, antihistamine, analgesic.
CHILDREN'S TYLENOL COLD MULTI SYMPTOM PLUS COUGH. (McNeil-CPC) Acetaminophen 160 mg, dextromethorphan HBr 5 mg, chlorpheniramine maleate 1 mg, pseudoephedrine HCl 15 mg/5 ml. Liq. Bot. 120 ml.
Use: Decongestant, antihistamine, antitussive.
CHILDREN'S TYLENOL ELIXIR. (McNeil-CPC) Acetaminophen 160 mg/5 ml. Elix. Bot. 60 ml, 120 ml.
Use: Analgesic.
CHILDREN'S TY-TABS. (Major) Acetaminophen 80 mg. Tab. Bot. 100s, 1000s.
Use: Analgesic, antipyretic.
CHIMERIC M-T412 (HUMAN-MURINE) IgG MONOCLONAL ANTI-CD4.
Use: Multiple sclerosis. [Orphan drug]
CHIMERIC (MURINE VARIABLE, HUMAN CONSTANT) MAB TO CD20. (Idec Pharm)
Use: Treatment of non-Hodgkin's B-cell lymphoma. [Orphan drug]
CHINESE GELATIN.
See: Agar.
CHINESE ISINGLASS. 7-Iodo-8-hydroxyquinoline-5-sulfonic acid sodium salt. Yatren.
Use: Amebicide.
CHINIOFON. 7-Iodo-8-hydroxyquinoline-5-sulfonic acid, anayodin, yatren, quinoxyl.
Use: Amebicide.
CHINOSOL. (Vernon) 8-Hydroxyquinoline sulfate 7.5 gr/Tab. Vial 6s. Trit. Tab. ($^3/_5$ gr) Bot. 50s. Vial 110s. Pow. 1 oz.
Use: Antiseptic.
CHLAMYDIA TRACHOMATIS TEST.
Use: Diagnostic aid.
See: MicroTrak (Syva).
CHLAMYDIAZYME. (Abbott Diagnostics) Enzyme immunoassay for detection of *Chlamydia trachomatis* from urethral or urogenital swabs. Test kit 100s.
Use: Diagnostic aid.
CHLO-AMINE. (Hollister-Stier) Chlorpheniramine maleate 2 mg/Chew. Tab. Box 24x4 mg Tab. Packages.
Use: Antihistamine.
• **CHLOPHEDIANOL.** F.D.A. 2-Chloro-alpha-[2-(dimethylamino)ethyl] benzhydrol.

• **CHLOPHEDIANOL HCl.** USAN. a-(2-Di-methylaminoethyl)-o-chlorobenzyhydrol HCl.
Use: Antitussive.
CHLOR-4. (Mills) Chlorpheniramine maleate 4 mg/Tab. Bot. 100s.
Use: Antihistamine.
CHLOR, I 0.5%.
See: I-CHLOR 0.5%.
CHLORACOL 0.5%. (Horizon) Chloramphenicol 5 mg/ml with chlorobutanol, hydroxypropyl methylcellulose. Dropper bot. 7.5 ml.
Use: Anti-infective, ophthalmic.
CHLORAFED. (Hauck) Chlorpheniramine maleate 2 mg, pseudoephedrine HCl 30 mg/5 ml, alcohol, dye, sugar and corn free. Syr. Bot. 120 ml, 480 ml.
Use: Antihistamine, decongestant.
CHLORAFED H.S. TIMECELLES.
(Hauck) Chlorpheniramine maleate 4 mg, pseudoephedrine HCl 60 mg/SR Cap. Bot. 100s, 500s, UD 50s.
Use: Antihistamine, decongestant.
CHLORAFED TIMECELLES. (Hauck) Chlorpheniramine maleate 8 mg, pseudoephedrine HCl 120 mg/SA timecelles Bot. 100s, 500s. UD 50s.
Use: Antihistamine, decongestant.
CHLORAHIST. (Evron) Chlorpheniramine maleate **4 mg/Tab.:** Bot. 100s, 1000s. **8 mg or 12 mg/Cap.:** Bot. 250s, 1000s. **Syr. 2 mg/4 ml.:** Bot. qt.
Use: Antihistamine.
CHLORALFORMAMIDE. N-(2,2,2-trichloro-l-hydrox-yethyl) formamide.
• **CHLORAL HYDRATE, U.S.P.** U.S.P. XXIII. Caps., Syr. U.S.P. XXIII. 1,1-Ethanediol, 2,2,2-trichloro-ethanol. Chloral.
Use: Hypnotic and sedative.
See: Aquachloral Supprettes, Supp. (Webcon).
Noctec, Cap., Syr. (Squibb).
Generic Products:
Quality Generics (7.5 gr) Bot. 100s.
G.F. Harvey-Cap. (3 gr) Bot. 100s; (7.5 gr) Bot. 100s.
Lederle-Cap. (500 mg) 100s.
Pacific Pharm. Corp.-Cap. (7.5 gr) Bot. 100s, 1000s.
Parke, Davis-Cap. (500 mg) Bot. 100s, UD 100s.
Stayner-Cap. (250 mg or 500 mg) Bot. 100s,
(500 mg) Bot. 1000s, Crystals Bot. 1 lb. and 5 lbs.
West-Ward-Cap. (3 gr, 7.5 gr) Bot. 100s.
CHLORAL HYDRATE BETAINE (1:1) COMPOUND. Chloral Betaine.

CHLORALPYRINE DICHLORALPYRINE.
See: Dichloralantipyrine.
CHLORALURETHANE. Name used for Carbochloral.
CHLORAMAN. (Rasman) Chlorpheniramine maleate 12 mg/Tab. Bot. 100s, 500s, 1000s.
Use: Antihistamine.
• **CHLORAMBUCIL, U.S.P.** U.S.P. XXIII. Tab. U.S.P. XXIII. 4-[fb]p-[Bis(2-chlorethyl)-amino]-phenylbutyric acid. Benzenebutanoic acid. 4-[bis(2-chloroethyl)-amino]-.
Use: Antineoplastic.
See: Leukeran, Tab. (Burroughs Wellcome).
CHLORAMINE-T. Sodium paratoluenesulfan chloramide, chloramine, chlorozone.
Lilly-Tab. (0.3 Gm), Bot. 100s, 1000s.
Robinson, Pow., 1 oz.
Use: Antiseptic, deodorant.
See: Chlorazene (Badger).
• **CHLORAMPHENICOL, U.S.P.** U.S.P. XXIII. Caps., Cream, Oral Soln., Tab., Otic Soln., Sterile, Ophth. Soln., Ophth. Oint., for Ophth. Soln. Inj., U.S.P. XXIII. D(-)-threo-2, 2-Dichloro-N[Beta-hydroxy-alpha-(hy-droxymethyl)-p-nitrophenethyl]acetamide. (Various Mfr.)
Soln.: 5 mg/ml Bot. 7.5 ml, 15 ml; **Oint.:** 10 mg/g Tube 3.5 g; **Cap.:** 250 mg Bot. 100s.
Use: Antibacterial, antirickettsial.
See: AK-Chlor, Preps. (Akorn).
Chlorcetin.
Chloromycetin, Preps. (Parke-Davis).
Chloroptic Ophth. Oint. (Allergan).
Chloroptic S.O.P. Ophth. Oint. (Allergan).
Econochlor, Soln., Oint. (Alcon).
Kemicetine.
Mychel, Cap. (Rachelle).
Ophthochlor, Soln. (Parke-Davis).
Paraxin.
W/Polymixin B.
Use: Treatment of superficial ocular infections involving the conjunctiva and/or cornea caused by susceptible organisms.
See: Chloromyxin Ophthalmic Oint. (Parke-Davis).
W/Polymixin B, Hydrocortisone.
See: Ophthocort, Oint. (Parke-Davis).
• **CHLORAMPHENICOL AND HYDROCORTISONE ACETATE FOR OPHTHALMIC SUSPENSION, U.S.P.** U.S.P. XXIII.
Use: Antibiotic, anti-inflammatory.
See: Chloromycetin, Prods. (Parke-Davis).

• **CHLORAMPHENICOL, POLYMIXIN B SULFATE, AND HYDROCORTISONE ACETATE OPHTHALMIC OINTMENT,** U.S.P. U.S.P. XXIII.
Use: Antibiotic, anti-inflammatory.
See: Chloromycetin, Prods. (Parke-Davis).

• **CHLORAMPHENICOL AND POLYMYXIN B SULFATE OPHTHALMIC OINTMENT,** U.S.P. U.S.P. XXIII.
Use: Antibiotic.

• **CHLORAMPHENICOL PALMITATE,** U.S.P. U.S.P. XXIII. Oral Susp. U.S.P. XXIII.
Use: Antibacterial, antirickettsial.
See: Chloromycetin Palmitate, Oral Susp. (Parke-Davis).

• **CHLORAMPHENICOL PANTOTHENATE COMPLEX.** USAN. A complex consisting of 4 parts of chloramphenicol to one part of calcium pantothenate. Pantofenicol.
Use: Antibiotic.

• **CHLORAMPHENICOL AND PREDNISOLONE OPHTHALMIC OINTMENT,** U.S.P. U.S.P. XXIII.
Use: Antibiotic, steroid combination.
See: Chloromycetin, Prods. (Parke-Davis).

• **CHLORAMPHENICOL SODIUM SUCCINATE, STERILE, U.S.P.** U.S.P. XXIII. (Various Mfr.) 100 mg/ml Inj. Vial 1 g in 15 ml.
Use: Antibacterial, antirickettsial.
See: Chloromycetin Succinate, Inj., (Parke-Davis).
Mychel-S, IV. (Rachelle).

CHLORANIL. 2,3,5,6-Tetrachloro-1,4-benzoquinone.

CHLORASEPTIC CHILDREN'S LOZENGES. (Vicks) Benzocaine 5 mg/Loz. Pkg. 18s.
Use: Local anesthetic.

CHLORASEPTIC LIQUID. (Vicks) Total phenol 1.4% as phenol and sodium phenolate, saccharin. Menthol and cherry flavors. Bot. 180 ml, 360 ml (mouthwash/gargle); 45 ml, 240 ml, 360 ml (throat spray).
Use: Antiseptic, anesthetic.

CHLORASEPTIC LOZENGE. (Vicks) Total phenol 32.5 mg/lozenge as phenol and sodium phenolate. Menthol and cherry flavors. Pkg. 18s, 36s.
Use: Anesthetic, antiseptic.

CHLORATE. (Major) Chlorpheniramine maleate 4 mg/Tab. Bot. 24s, 100s, 1000s.
Use: Antihistamine.

CHLORAZANIL HCl. 2-Amino-4-(p-chloroanilino)-s-triazine HCl. Daquim.

CHLORAZENE. (Badger) Chloramine-T, sodium p-toluene-sulfonchloramide.
Pow.: UD Pkg. 20 Gm, 38 Gm, 50 Gm, 88 Gm, 200 Gm, 240 Gm, 320 Gm, Bot. 1 lb, 5 lb. **Aromatic Pow. (5%):** Bot. 1 lb, 5 lb. **Tab. (0.3 Gm):** Bot. 20s, 100s, 1000s, 5000s.
Use: Antiseptic, deodorant.

CHLORAZEPATE DIPOTASSIUM.
Use: Antianxiety agent, anticonvulsant.
See: Clorazepate dipotassium.

CHLORAZEPATE MONOPOTASSIUM.
See: Clorazepate monopotassium.

CHLORAZINE TABS. (Major) Prochlorperazine 5 mg or 10 mg/Tab. Bot. 100s.
Use: Antiemetic/antivertigo, antipsychotic.

CHLORAZONE.
See: Chloramine-T.

CHLOR BENZO MOR, A AND D OINTMENT. (Wade) Vitamins A and D fortified, chlorobutanol 3%, benzocaine 2%, benzyl alcohol 3%, actamer 1%, in lanolin and petrolatum base. Tube 1 oz, Jar 1 oz, lb.
Use: Antiseptic, local anesthetic.

CHLOR BENZO MOR SPRAY. (Wade) Vitamin A and D fortified, chlorobutanol 3%, benzocaine 2%, benzyl alcohol 3%, and actamer 1%, in lanolin and mineral oil base. Bot. 2 oz, 11 oz.
Use: Antiseptic, anesthetic.

CHLORBETAMIDE. B.A.N. Dichloro-N-(2,4-di- chlorobenzyl)-N-(2-hydroxyethyl)acetamide.
Use: Treatment of amebiasis.

CHLORBUTANOL.
See: Chlorobutanol, N.F. XVIII.

CHLORBUTOL.
See: Chlorobutanol, N.F. XVIII.

CHLORCYCLIZINE. B.A.N. 1-(4-Chlorobenzhydryl)-4-methylpiperazine.
Use: Antihistamine.

CHLORCYCLIZINE HYDROCHLORIDE, U.S.P. N.F. XVI. 1-(p-Chloro-α-phenylbenzyl)-4-methylpiperazine HCl. 1-(p-Chlorobenzhydryl)-4-methylpiperazine HCl. Histantin.
Use: Antihistamine.
W/Hydrocortisone acetate.
See: Mantadil, Cream (Burroughs Wellcome).
W/Pseudoephedrine HCl.
See: Fedrazil, Tab. (Burroughs Wellcome).

• **CHLORDANTOIN.** F.D.A. 5-(1-Ethylpentyl)-3-[(tri- chloromethyl) thio] hydantoin.

• **CHLORDANTOIN.** USAN. 5-(1-Ethyl-amyl)-3-trichloro- methyl thiohydantoin.
Use: Antifungal.
See: Sporostacin Cream (Ortho).
• **CHLORDIAZEPOXIDE, U.S.P.** U.S.P. XXIII. Tab., U.S.P. XXIII. 3H-1, 4-Benzo-diazepin-2-amine, 7-chloro-N-methyl-5-phenyl-, 4-oxide; 7-chloro-2-(methy-lamino)-5-phenyl-3H-1, 4-benzodi-azepine 4-oxide.
Use: Antianxiety agent.
See: A-poxide, Cap. (Abbott).
Brigen-G, Tab. (Grafton).
Libritabs, Tab. (Roche).
Menrium, Tab. (Roche).
W/Amitriptyline.
See: Limbitrol, Tab. (Roche).
• **CHLORDIAZEPOXIDE AND AMITRIPTY-LINE HCL TABLETS, U.S.P.** U.S.P. XXIII.
Use: Antianxiety agent.
See: Limbitrol, Tab. (Roche).
• **CHLORDIAZEPOXIDE HCl, U.S.P.** U.S.P. XXIII., Caps, Sterile U.S.P. XXIII. 7-Chloro-2-methylamino-5-phenyl-3H-1, 4-benzodiazepine-4-oxide HCl. Metha-minodiazopino HCl.
Use: Tranquilizer, sedative.
See: A-poxide, Cap. (Abbott).
Chlordiazachel, Cap. (Rachelle).
Librium, Cap., Inj. (Roche).
Screen, Cap. (Foy).
Zetran, Cap. (Hauck).
W/Clidinium bromide.
See: Librax, Cap. (Roche).
CHLORDIAZEPOXIDE W/CLINDINIUM BROMIDE. (Various Mfr.) Clindinium 2.5 mg, chlordiazepoxide HCl 5 mg/Cap. Bot. 30s, 100s, 500s, 1000s, UD 100s.
Use: Gastrointestinal anticholinergic combination. {CHLORDRINE S.R}. (Rugby) Pseudoephedrine HCl 120 mg, chlorpheniramine maleate 8 mg/Cap. Bot. 100s.
Use: Decongestant, antihistamine.
CHLOREN 4. (Wren) Chlorpheniramine maleate 4 mg/Tab. Bot. 100s, 1000s.
Use: Antihistamine.
CHLOREN 8 T.D. (Wren) Chlorpheni-ramine maleate 8 mg/Tab. Bot. 100s, 1000s.
Use: Antihistamine.
CHLOREN 12 T.D. (Wren) Chlorpheni-ramine maleate 12 mg/Tab. Bot. 100s, 1000s.
Use: Antihistamine.
CHLORESIUM. (Rystan) Oint.: Chloro-phyllin copper complex 0.5% in hy-drophilic base. Tube 1 oz, 4 oz, Jar lb.

Soln.: Chlorophyllin copper complex 0.2% in isotonic saline soln. Bot. 60 ml, 240 ml, qt.
Use: Healing agent, deodorizer.
CHLORESIUM TABLETS. (Rystan) Chlorophyllin copper complex 14 mg/Tab. Bot. 100s, 1000s.
Use: Oral deodorant.
CHLORESIUM TOOTH PASTE. (Rystan) Chlorophyllin copper complex. Tube 3.25 oz.
Use: Oral deodorant.
CHLORETHYL.
See: Ethyl Chloride.
CHLORGEST-HD. (Great Southern) Phenylephrine HCl 5 mg, chlorpheni-ramine maleate 4 mg, hydrocodone bitartrate 1.67 mg. Alcohol free. Liq. Bot. pt, gal.
Use: Decongestant, antihistamine, anti-tussive.
CHLORGUANIDE HYDROCHLORIDE.
See: Chloroguanide HCl (Various Mfr.).
CHLORHEXADOL. 2-Methyl-4-(2',2,2,-trichlor-1-hydroxyethoxy)-2-pentanol. Lora.
CHLORHEXADOL. B.A.N. 2-Methyl-4-(2,2,2-trichloro-1-hydroxyethoxy)pen-tan 2 ol.
Use: Hypnotic, sedative.
• **CHLORHEXIDINE.** F.D.A. 1,1'-Hexam-ethylenebis-[5-(-chlorophenyl) biguanide]
Use: Antiseptic.
See: BactoShield, Foam, Soln. (Am-sco).
BactoShield 2, Soln. (Amsco).
Hibiclens.
Hibiscrub.
Hibitane.
Lisium.
Rotersept.
• **CHLORHEXIDINE GLUCONATE.** USAN. 1,1'-Hex-amethylenebis [5-(-chlorophenyl)biguanide] dihydro-Cl. Oral rinse or topical skin cleanser.
Use: Antimicrobial. [Orphan drug] Bac-toShield, Foam, soln. (Amsco). Bac-toShield 2, soln. (Amsco).
See: Hibiclens, Liq. (Stuart).
Hibistat, Liq. (Stuart).
Peridex (Procter & Gamble).
• **CHLORHEXIDINE HYDROCHLORIDE.** USAN.
Use: Anti-infective, topical.
CHLORHYDROXYQUINOLIN.
See: Quinolor Compound, Oint. (Squibb).
CHLORINATED AND IODIZED PEANUT OIL. Chloriodized Oil.

• **CHLORINDANOL.** USAN. 7-Chloro-4-indanol.
Use: Antiseptic, spermaticide.

CHLORINE COMPOUND, ANTISEPTIC.
Antiseptics, Chlorine.

CHLORIODIZED OIL. Chlorinated and iodized peanut oil.

OI ILOΠIOONDAMINC OI ILOΠIDC.
4,5,6,7-Tetra-chloro-2-(2-dimethylaminoethyl)-isoindoline dimethoCl.

CHLORISONDAMINE CHLORIDE.
B.A.N. 4,5,6,7-Tetrachloro-2-(2-trimethylammonioethyl)-isoindolinium diCl.
Use: Hypotensive.

• **CHLORMADINONE ACETATE.** USAN. 6-Chloro-6-dehydro-17α-acetoxyprogesterone. 6-Chloro-17-hydroxypregna-4,6-diene-3,20 dione acetate.
Use: Progestin.

CHLOR MAL w/SAL + APAP S.C. (Richlyn) Chlorpheniramine maleate 2 mg, acetaminophen 150 mg, salicylamide 175 mg/Tab. Bot. 1000s.
Use: Antihistamine, analgesic.

CHLORMERODRIN. 3-Chloro-mercuri-2-methoxy-propylurea. Chloro (2-methoxy-3-ureidopropyl) mercury. Mercloran.
Use: Diuretic.

CHLORMERODRIN Hg 197 INJECTION.
Mercury-^{197}HG, [3-[(aminocarbonyl)amino]-2-methoxypropyl]-chloro-. Chloro(2-methoxy-3-ureido- propyl)mercury-^{197}Hg.
Use: Diagnostic aid (renal scanning).

CHLORMERODRIN Hg 203 INJECTION.
Mercury-^{203}Hg,[3-[(aminocarbonyl)amino]-(ureidopropyl)mercury-^{203}Hg.
Use: Diagnostic aid (tumor localization).

CHLORMETHIAZOLE. B.A.N. 5-(2-Chloroethyl)-4-methylthiazole.
Use: Hypnotic, sedative.

CHLORMEZANONE. Chlormethazanone. 2-(4-Chlorophenyl)-3-methyl-4-methathiazanone-1-2-dioxide.
Use: Antianxiety agent.
See: Trancopal, Cap. (Sanofi Winthrop).

CHLORMIDAZOLE. B.A.N. 1-(4-Chlorobenzyl)-2-methylbenzimidazole.
Use: Antifungal agent.

CHLOR-NIRAMINE ALLERGY TABS.
(Whiteworth) Chlorpheniramine maleate 4 mg/Tab. Bot. 24s, 100s.
Use: Antihistamine.

CHLOROAZODIN. Alpha, alpha, Azobis-(chloroformamidine).

• **CHLOROBUTANOL, U.S.P.** N.F. XVIII.
1,1,1-Trichloro-2-methyl-2-propanol.
Sedaform. (Various Mfr.).
Use: Anesthetic, antiseptic, hypnotic; pharmaceutic aid (antimicrobial preservative).
See: Cerumenex, Drops (Purdue-Fredorick).
Pre-Sert (Allergan).
W/Atropine sulfate, chlorpheniramine maleate, phenylpropanolamine HCl.
See: Decongestant, Inj. (Century).
W/Benzocaine, camphor.
See: Eardro, Liq. (Jenkins).
W/Calcium glycerophosphate, calcium levulinate.
See: Cal San, Inj. (Burgin-Arden).
W/Cetyltrimethylammonium Br, methapyrilene HCl, phenylephrine HCl, hydrocortisone.
See: T-Spray, Liq. (Saron).
W/Diphenhydramine HCl.
See: Ardeben, Inj. (Burgin-Arden).
W/Ephedrine HCl, sodium Cl.
See: Efedron HCl Nasal Jelly (Hart).
W/Estradiol cypionate, testosterone cypionate.
See: Depo-Testadiol, Vial (Upjohn).
Depotestogen, Vial (Hyrex).
W/Glycerin, anhydrous.
See: Ophthalgan, Liq. (Wyeth-Ayerst).
W/Liquifilm.
See: Liquifilm Tears (Allergan).
W/Methylcellulose.
See: Lacril (Allergan).
W/Myristyl-gamma-picolinium Cl.
See: Wet Tone, Soln. (Riker).
W/Nonionic lanolin derivative.
See: Lacri-Lube, Ophthalmic Ointment (Allergan).
W/Polyethylene glycol, polyoxyl 40 stearate.
See: Blink-N-Clean (Allergan).
W/Sodium Cl.
See: Ocean, Liq. (Fleming).
W/Tannic acid, isopropyl alcohol.
See: Outgro, Soln. (Whitehall).
W/Vitamins B_1, B_2, B_6, niacinamide, calcium pantothenate, benzyl alcohol.
See: Lanoplex, Inj. (Lannett).

• **CHLOROCRESOL, U.S.P.** U.S.P. XXIII.
Use: Antiseptic, disinfectant.

CHLORODRI. (Kenyon) Chlorpheniramine maleate 5 mg, phenylpropanolamine HCl 12.5 mg, atropine sulfate 0.2 mg/ml. Vial 10 ml.
Use: Antihistamine, decongestant,

CHLOROETHANE.
See: Ethyl Chloride. anticholinergic/

antispasmodic.
CHLOROFAIR. (Pharmafair) **Soln.:** Chloramphenicol 5 mg/ml. Bot. 7.5 ml **Oint.:** Chloramphenicol 10 mg/Gm in white petrolatum base with mineral oil, polysorbate 60. Tube 3.5 Gm.
Use: Anti-infective, ophthalmic.
• **CHLOROFORM, U.S.P.** N.F. XVII. Bot. 1 lb, 5 lb.
Use: Inhalation anesthetic; solvent.
CHLOROGUANIDE HYDROCHLORIDE. (Various Mfr.) (Proguanil HCl) 1-(p-Chlorophenyl)-5-isopropylbiguanidine HCl. Guanatol HCl.
Use: Antimalarial.
CHLOROHIST-LA. (Hauck) Xylometazoline HCl 0.1%. Soln. Spray 15 ml.
Use: Nasal decongestant.
CHLORO-IODOHYDROXYQUINOLINE.
See: Clioquinol, U.S.P. XXIII.
CHLOROMETAXYLENOL-p.
See: p-CHLOROMETAXYLENOL.
CHLOROMETHAPYRILENE CITRATE.
See: Chlorothen Citrate.
CHLOROMYCETIN. (Parke-Davis) Chloramphenicol.
Ophth. Oint.: (1%) in base of petrolatum, polyethylene. Tube 3.5 Gm.
Inj.: 100 mg/ml (as sodium succinate) when reconstituted. In 1 Gm in 15 ml vials
Ophth. Soln.: (25 mg) Bot. w/dropper 15 ml (dry). Soln. 5 mg/ml Plastic dropper Bot. 5 ml.
Oral: 150 mg/5 ml (palmitate), alcohol, sucrose, sodium benzoate 0.5%. Custard flavor. Bot. 60 ml.
Otic Drops: (0.5%) 5 mg/ml w/propylene glycol. Bot. 15 ml.
Use: Anti-infective.
CHLOROMYCETIN HYDROCORTISONE. (Parke-Davis) Hydrocortisone acetate 0.5% (2.5% as powder), chloramphenicol 0.25% (1.25% as powder), cholesterol, methylcellulose, benzethonium Cl 0.01%. Pow. Bot. with dropper 5 ml. Reconstitute with water.
Use: Anti-infective, ophthalmic.
CHLOROMYCETIN KAPSEALS. (Parke-Davis) Chloramphenicol 250 mg/Cap. Bot. 100s.
Use: Anti-infective.
CHLOROMYCETIN SODIUM SUCCINATE I.V. (Parke-Davis) Chloramphenicol sodium succinate dried powder which when reconstituted contains chloromycetin 100 mg/ml. Steri-vial 1 Gm, 10s.

Use: Anti-infective.
CHLOROPHENOL-p.
See: p-CHLOROPHENOL.
CHLOROPHENOTHANE. 1,1,1-Trichloro-2,2-bis(p-chlorophenyl) ethane. Gesarol, Neocid, Dicophane.
Use: Pediculocide.
CHLOROPHYLL. (Freeda Vitamins) Chlorophyll 20 mg/Tab. Bot. 100s, 250s, 500s.
Use: Deodorizer.
CHLOROPHYLL "A" OINTMENT.
See: Chloresium Oint. (Rystan).
CHLOROPHYLL "A" SOLUTION. (Chlorophyllin).
See: Chloresium Soln. (Rystan).
CHLOROPHYLL COMPLEX PERLES. (Standard Process) Natural chlorophyll extracted from alfalfa and tillandsia. Vitamin K 3.3 mg/6 Perles. Bot. 60s, 350s. Oint. Tube 1.5 oz, Jar 3 oz.
Use: Healing agent, deodorizer.
CHLOROPHYLL DERIVATIVES, SYSTEMIC.
See: chlorophyll (Freeda).
Derifil (Rystan).
Chlorosium (Rystan).
CHLOROPHYLL DERIVATIVES, TOPICAL.
See: Chloresium (Rystan).
CHLOROPHYLL TABLETS.
See: Derifil, Tab. (Rystan).
Nullo, Tab. (Depree).
CHLOROPHYLL, WATER-SOLUBLE. (Various Mfr.) Chlorophyllin.
See: Chloresium Prep. (Rystan).
Derifil, Pow. (Rystan).
CHLOROPHYLLIN.
Use: Healing agent, deodorizer.
• **CHLOROPHYLLIN COPPER COMPLEX.** USAN.
Use: Deodorant.
See: Nullo, Tab. (Chattem).
PALS, Tab. (Palisades).
• **CHLOROPROCAINE HCl, U.S.P.** U.S.P. XXIII. Inj., U.S.P. XXIII. beta, Diethylamino-ethyl 2-chloro-4-amino-benzoate HCl. 4-amino-2-chloro-, 2-(diethylamino) ethyl ester, HCl. 2-(Diethylamino) ethyl 4-amino-2-chlorobenzoate HCl. (Abbott) 2% or 3%. Concentration in Abboject Syringe, Ampule or Vial.
Use: Anesthetic (local).
See: Nesacaine, Vial (Pennwalt).
Nescaine-CE, Vial (Pennwalt).
CHLOROPTIC STERILE OPHTHALMIC SOLUTION. (Allergan) Chloramphenicol 0.5%, chlorobutanol 0.5%. **Soln.:** Dropper bot. 2.5 ml, 7.5 ml. **Oint.:** Chlo-

ramphenicol 10 mg/Gm in white petroleum base with mineral oil,polyoxyl 40 stearate, nonionic lanolin derivatives, PEG 300 and 0.5% chlorobutanol. Tube 3.5 Gm.
Use: Anti-infective, ophthalmic.

• **CHLOROQUINE, U.S.P.** U.S.P. XXIII. 7-Chloro-4-[[4-(die-thylamino)-1-methyl butyl]amino]quinoline.
Use: Pharmaceutic necessity for chloroquine HCl.
See: Aralen HCl Prods. (Sanofi Winthrop).

• **CHLOROQUINE HYDROCHLORIDE INJ., U.S.P.** U.S.P. XXIII.
Use: Antiamebic, antimalarial.
See: Aralen HCl (Sanofi Winthrop).

• **CHLOROQUINE PHOSPHATE, U.S.P.** U.S.P. XXIII. Tab. U.S.P. XXIII. Nivaquine.
Use: Febrile attacks of malaria; antiamebic; lupus erythematosus suppressant.
See: Aralen Phosphate, Tab. (Sanofi Winthrop).

CHLOROQUINE PHOSPHATE W/PRIMAQUIN PHOSPHATE.
See: Aralen Phosphate W/Primaquine Phosphate (Sanofi Winthrop.).

5-CHLORO-SALICYLANILIDE.

CHLOROSERPINE. (Various Mfr.) Chlorothiazide 250 mg or 500 mg, reserpine 0.125 mg/Tab. Bot. 100s, 1000s.
Use: Antihypertensive.

CHLOROTHEN. 2-[(5-Chloro-2-thenyl)(2-di- methylaminoethyl)amino]pyridine hydrochloride, citrate salts (Chlorothenylpyramine, chloromethapyrilene, pyrithen).
Use: Antihistamine.

CHLOROTHEN CITRATE. (Whittier) 2-[-(5-Chloro-2-thenyl)](2-dimethylamino)-ethyl]amino]pyridine dihydrogen citrate. Chloromethapyrilene, chlorothenylpyramine, pyrithen. Tab., Bot. 100s.
Use: Antihistamine.

W/Pyrilamine, thenylpyramine.
See: Derma-Pax, Liq. (Recsei).

CHLOROTHENYLPYRAMINE.
Chlorothen, Prep.

CHLOROTHEOPHYLLINATE W/BE-NADRYL.
See: Dramamine, Prep. (Searle).

• **CHLOROTHIAZIDE, U.S.P.** U.S.P. XXIII. Oral Susp., Tabs., U.S.P. XXIII. 6-Chloro-2H-1,2,4-benzothiadiazine-7-sulfonamide 1,1-dioxide.
Use: Diuretic.
See: Diuril, Tab., Susp. (Merck & Co.).
W/Methyldopa.

See: Aldoclor, Tab. (Merck & Co.).
W/Reserpine. Tab.: Chlorothiazide 250 mg or 500 mg, reserpine 0.125 mg. Bot. 100s, 1000s.
See: Diupres, Tab. (Merck & Co.).
Use: Diuretic.

• **CHLOROTHIAZIDE SODIUM FOR INJECTION, U.S.P.** U.S.P. XXIII.
Use: Diuretic.
See: Sodium Diuril, Vial (Merck & Co.).

CHLOROTHYMOL. 6-Chlorothymol.
Use: Antibacterial.

• **CHLOROTRIANISENE, U.S.P.** U.S.P. XXII. Cap., U.S.P. XXII. Chlorotris (p-methoxyphenyl)ethylene. Chlorotri-(4-methoxyphenyl)ethylene.
Use: Estrogen.
See: TACE, Cap. (Marion Merrell Dow).

β **CHLOROVINYL ETHYNYL CARBINOL.**
See: Placidyl, Cap. (Abbott).

• **CHLOROXINE, U.S.P.** USAN.
Use: Antiseborrheic.

• **CHLOROXYLENOL, U.S.P.** U.S.P. XXIII. 4-Chloro-3,5-xylenol. p-Chloro-m-xylenol; parachloro-metaxylenol; benzytol.
Use: Antiseptic.
W/Benzocaine, menthol, lanolin.
See: Unburn, Spray, Cream, Lot. (Leeming-Pacquin).
W/Hexachlorophene.
See: Desitin, Preps. (Leeming-Pacquin).
W/Methyl salicylate, menthol, camphor, thymol, eucalyptus oil, isopropyl alcohol.
See: Gordobalm, Balm (Gordon).

CHLORPAZINE. (Major) Prochlorperazine maleate 5 mg, 10 mg or 25 mg/Tab. Bot. 100s, UD 100s (5 mg, 10 mg only).
Use: Antipsychotic.

CHLORPHED INJECTION. (Hauck) Brompheniramine maleate 10 mg/ml. Vial 10 ml.
Use: Antihistamine.

CHLORPHED-LA. (Hauck) Oxymetazoline 0.05%. Soln. Spray 15 ml.
Use: Decongestant.

• **CHLORPHENESIN.** F.D.A. 3-(p-Chlorophenoxy)-1,2-propanediol.

CHLORPHENESIN. B.A.N. 3-(4-Chlorophenoxyl)-propane-1,2-diol.
Use: Antifungal agent.

• **CHLORPHENESIN CARBAMATE.** USAN. 3-(p-Chlorophenoxy)-2-hydroxypropyl carbamate.
Use: Muscle relaxant.
See: Maolate, Tab. (Upjohn).

• **CHLORPHENIRAMINE MALEATE,**

U.S.P. U.S.P. XXIII. Inj., Syr., Tab.,
U.S.P. XXIII. 2-[p-Chloro-alpha(2-dimethylaminoethyl)benzyl]pyridine maleate,
chlorprophenpyridamine maleate. 2-
Pyridinepropanamine, gamma-(4-
chlorophenyl)-N,N-dimethyl-,(Z)-2-
butenedioate(1:1).
Use: Antihistamine.
See: Alermine, Tab. (Reid-Rowell).
Chestamine, Cap. (Leeds).
Chlo-Amine, Tab. (Hollister-Stier).
Chloraman, Tab. (Rasman).
Chloren, Preps. (Wren).
Chlor-4, Tab. (Mills).
Chlor-Niramine, Tab. (Whiteworth).
Chlorophen, Vial (Medical Chem.).
Chlor-pen, Tab., Vial (American Chemical & Drug).
Chlor-Span, Cap. (Burlington).
Chlortab, Tab., Cap., Inj. (North American Pharmacal).
Chlor-Trimeton Maleate, Preps. (Schering).
Cosea, Preps. (Center).
Histacon, Tab., Syr. (Marsh Labs).
Histaspan, Cap. (Rhone-Poulenc Rorer).
Histex, Cap. (Hauck).
Nasahist (Keene).
Phenetron, Preps. (Lannett).
Polaramine, Tab., Syr. (Schering).
Pyranistan, Tab. (Standex).
Rhinihist, Elix. (Central).
Teldrin, Spansule (SK-Beecham).
Trymegen (Medco).
**CHLORPHENIRAMINE MALEATE
W/COMBINATIONS.**
See: Al-Ay, Preps. (Bowman).
Alka-Seltzer Plus, Tab. (Miles).
Allerdec, Cap. (Towne).
Allerest, Prods. (Pharmacraft).
Alumadrine, Tab. (Fleming).
A.R.M., Tab. (SK-Beecham).
Atussin-D.M. Expectorant, Liq. (Federal).
Bellafedrol A-H, Tab. (Lannett).
B.M.E., Liq. (Brothers).
Bobid, Cap. (Boyd)
Breacol Cough Medication, Liq. (Glenbrook).
Brolade, Cap. (Brothers).
Bur-Tuss Expectorant (Burlington).
CDM Expectorant (Lannett).
Cenahist, Cap. (Century).
Cenaid, Tab. (Century).
Centuss, Tab. (Century).
Chew-Hist, Wafer (Kenyon).
Chlorodri, Vial (Kenyon).
Chlorpel, Cap. (Santa).
Chlor-Trimeton, Preps. (Schering).

Codimal, Tab. (Central).
Col-Decon, Tab. (Quality Generics).
Colrex Compound, Preps. (Reid-Rowell).
Comtrex, Tab., Cap., Liq. (Bristol-Myers).
Conalsyn Croncap, Cap. (Cenci).
Contac, Cap. (SK-Beecham).
Cophene No. 2, Cap. (Dunhall).
Cophene-S, Syr. (Dunhall).
Coricidin, Preps. (Schering).
Corilin, Liq. (Schering).
Corizahist, Preps. (Mason).
Coryban-D, Cap. (Leeming).
Co-Tylenol, Preps. (McNeil).
Dallergy, Tab., Cap., Syr. (Laser).
Decobel, Cap. (Lannett).
Decojen, Tab., Vial (Jenkins).
Deconamine, Tab., Cap., Syr. (Berlex).
Dehist, Cap. (Forest).
Demazin, Tab., Syr. (Schering).
Derma-Pax, Lot. (Recsei).
Dezest, Cap. (Geneva Drugs).
Donatussin, Liq., Syr. (Laser).
Dristan, Preps. (Whitehall).
Drucon, Elix. (Standard Drug).
Efricon Expectorant (Lannett).
Extendryl, Tab., Cap., Syr. (Fleming).
F.C.A.H., Cap. (Scherer).
Fedahist, Prods. (Donner).
Fitacol (Standex).
Formadrin, Liq. (Kenyon).
Histabid, Cap. (Glaxo).
Histacon, Tab., Syr. (Marsh Labs).
Histapco, Tab. (Apco).
Histaspan-D, Cap. (Rhone-Poulenc Rorer).
Histaspan Plus, Cap. (Rhone-Poulenc Rorer).
Hista-Vadrin, Tab., Cap., Syr. (Scherer).
Histine Prods. (Freeport).
Histogesic, Tab. (Century).
Hycomine Compound, Tab. (DuPont).
Infantuss, Liq. (Scott/Cord).
Koryza, Tab. (Forest Pharm.).
Kronofed-A, Cap. (Ferndale).
Lanatuss Expectorant (Lannett).
Mapap CF, Tab. (Major).
Marhist (Marlop).
Neo-Pyranistan, Tab. (Standex).
Nilcol, Tab., Elix. (Parke-Davis).
Nolamine, Tab. (Carnrick).
Novafed A, Cap., Liq. (Marion Merrell Dow).
Novahistine, Preps. (Marion Merrell Dow).
Partuss, Liq. (Parmed).
Partuss T.D., Tab. (Parmed).
Phenahist, Preps. (Amid).

Phenchlor, Prods. (Freeport).
Phenetron Compound, Tab. (Lannett).
Polytuss-DM, Liq. (Rhode).
Pyma, Cap., Vial (Forest Pharm.).
Pyristan, Cap., Elix. (Arcum).
Pyranistan (Standex).
Quelidrine, Syr. (Abbott).
Rentuss, Cap., Syr. (Wren).
Rhinex D M, Tab., Syr. (Lemmon).
Rhinogesic, Tab. (Vale).
Rohist-D, Cap. (Rocky Mtn.).
Ryna, Liq. (Wallace).
Ryna-tussadine, Tab., Liq. (Wallace).
Salphenyl, Cap. (Hauck).
Scotcof, Liq. (Scott/Cord).
Scotnord (Scott/Cord).
Scotuss Liq. (Scott/Cord).
Shertus, Liq. (Sheryl).
Sialco, Tab. (Foy).
Sinarest, Tab. (Pharmacraft).
Sine-Off, Prods. (SK-Beecham).
Sino-Compound, Tab. (Bio-Factor).
Sinovan Timed, Cap. (Drug Ind.).
Sinucol, Cap., Vial (Tennessee).
Sinulin, Tab. (Carnrick).
Sinutab Extra Strength, Cap. (Warner-Lambert).
Spantuss, Tab., Liq. (Arco).
Statomin Maleate CC, Tab. (Bowman).
Sudafed Plus, Tab., Syr. (Burroughs Wellcome).
Symptrol, Cap. (Saron).
T.A.C., Cap. (Towne).
Tonecol, Tab., Syr. (A.V.P.).
Triamininc, Prods. (Sandoz Consumer).
Triamincin Chewables (Sandoz Consumer).
Trigelamine, Oint. (E.J. Moore).
Turbilixir, Liq. (Burlington).
Turbispan Leisurecaps, Cap. (Burlington).
Tusquelin, Syr. (Circle).
Tussar, Prods. (Rhone-Poulenc Rorer).
Valihist, Cap. (Otis Clapp).
d-CHLORPHENIRAMINE MALEATE.
See: Polarmine Expectorant, Tab., Syr. (Schering).
CHLORPHENIRAMINE MALEATE W/PSEUDOEPHEDRINE HCL. (Vitarine) Pseudoephedrine HCl 120 mg, chlorpheniramine maleate 8 mg/Cap. Bot. 100s, 1000s.
Use: Decongestant, antihistamine.
• **CHLORPHENIRAMINE POLISTIREX.** USAN.
Use: Antihistamine.
CHLORPHENIRAMINE RESIN W/COMBINATIONS.

See: Omni-Tuss, Liq. (Pennwalt).
CHLORPHENIRAMINE TANNATE. W/Carbetapentane tannate, ephedrine tannate, phenylephrine tannate.
See: Rynatuss Tab., Susp. (Wallace).
W/Phenylephrine tannate, pyrilamine tannate.
See: Rynatan, Tab., Susp. (Wallace).
CHLORPHENOCTIUM AMSONATE. B.A.N. 2,4-Di- chlorophenoxymethyl-dimethyloctylammonium 4,4'-diaminostilbene-2,2-disulfonate.
Use: Antifungal agent.
CHLORPHENOXAMINE. B.A.N. N-2-(4-Chloro-α-me-thylbenzhydryloxy)ethyl-dimethylamine.
Use: Antiparkinson agent.
CHLORPHTHALIDONE. 1-Oxo-3-(3'-sulfanyl-4-chlorophenyl)-3-hydroxy-isoindoline.
See: Chlorthalidone.
CHLOR-PRO 10. (Schein) Chlorpheniramine maleate 10 mg/ml, benzyl alcohol. Inj. Vial 30 ml.
Use: Antihistamine.
CHLORPROGUANIL. B.A.N. 1-(3,4-Dichlorophenyl)-5-isopropylbiguanide.
Use: Antimalarial.
• **CHLORPROMAZINE, U.S.P.** U.S.P. XXII. Supp. U.S.P. XXIII. 2-Chloro-10-[3-(dimethylamino)propyl]-phenothiazine. 10H-Phenothiazine-10-propanamine,2-chloro-N,N-dimethyl
Use: Antiemetic, tranquilizer.
See: Chloractil.
Largactil.
• **CHLORPROMAZINE HCI, U.S.P.** U.S.P. XXIII. Inj., Syr., Tab., Cap., Supp. U.S.P. XXIII.
Use: Antiemetic, tranquilizer.
See: Chlorzine, Inj. (Hauck).
Promachlor, Tab. (Geneva).
Promapar, Tab. (Parke-Davis).
Promaz, Inj. (Keene).
Sonazine, Tab. (Reid-Rowell).
Terpium, Tab. (Scrip).
Thorazine, Tab., Cap., Liq., Syr., Supp., Amp. (SK-Beecham).
CHLORPROMAZINE HCL INTENSOL ORAL SOLUTION. (Roxane) Chlorpromazine HCl concentrated oral soln. **30 mg/ml**: Bot. 120 ml. **100 mg/ml**: Bot. 240 ml.
Use: Antiemetic, antipsychotic.
• **CHLORPROPAMIDE, U.S.P.** U.S.P. XXII. Tabs. U.S.P. XXIII. 1-[(p-Chlorophenyl)-sulfonyl]-3-propylurea. Benzene-sulfonamide, 4-chloro-N-[(propylamino)carbonyl]-.
Use: Hypoglycemic agent.

See: Diabinese, Tab. (Pfizer Laboratories).
CHLORPROPHENPYRIDAMINE MALEATE.
See: Chlorpheniramine Maleate, U.S.P. XXIII.
•**CHLORPROTHIXENE, U.S.P.** U.S.P. XXIII. Inj., Oral Susp., Tab., U.S.P. XXIII. 1-Propanamine, 3-(2-chloro-9H-thioxanthene-9-ylidene)-N,N-dimethyl-,(Z)-; (Z)-2-Chloro-N,N-dimethylthioxanthene-D^9-propylamine.
Use: Tranquilizer; antiemetic.
See: Taractan, Tab., Conc., Inj. (Roche).
CHLORQUINALDOL. 5,7-Dichloro-8-hydroxyquinal-dine.
CHLORQUINALDOL. B.A.N. 5,7-Dichloro-8-hydroxy-2-methylquinoline.
Use: Antiseptic, fungicide.
CHLORQUINOL. A mixture of the chlorinated products of 8-hydroxyquinoline containing about 65% of 5,7-dichloro-8-hydroxyquinoline. Quixalin.
CHLOR-REST. (Rugby) Phenylpropanolamine HCl 18.7 mg, chlorpheniramine maleate 2 mg/Tab. Bot. 24s, 100s, 1000s.
Use: Decongestant, antihistamine.
CHLOR-SPAN. (Burlington) Chlorpheniramine maleate 8 mg/S.R. Cap. Bot. 60s.
Use: Antihistamine.
•**CHLORTETRACYCLINE AND SULFAMETHAZINE BISULFATES SOLUBLE POWDER, U.S.P.** U.S.P XXII.
Use: Antibiotic.
•**CHLORTETRACYCLINE BISULFATE, U.S.P.** U.S.P. XXIII.
Use: Antibiotic.
•**CHLORTETRACYCLINE HYDROCHLORIDE, U.S.P.** U.S.P. XXIII. Caps., Oint., Ophth. Oint., Soluble Powder, Sterile, Tab., U.S.P. XXIII. 7-Chlorotetracycline hydrochloride.
Use: Antibiotic.
See: Aureomycin, Oint. (Storz/Lederle)
•**CHLORTHALIDONE, U.S.P.** U.S.P. XXIII. Tabs. U.S.P. XXIII. 2-Chloro-5-(1-hydroxy-3-oxo-1-isoindolinyl)benzenesulfonamide. Benzenesulfonamide, 2-chloro-5-(2,3-dihydro-1-hydroxy-3-oxo-1H-isoindol-1-yl)-.
Use: Diuretic, antihypertensive.
See: Combipres, Tab. (Boehringer-Ingelheim).
    Hygroton, Tab. (Rhone-Poulenc Rorer).
    W/Reserpine.
    See: Demi-Regroton, Tab. (Rhone-

Poulenc Rorer).
    Regroton, Tab. (Rhone-Poulenc Rorer).
CHLORTHENOXAZIN. B.A.N. 2-(2-Chloroethyl)-2,3-dihydro-1,3-benzoxazin-4-one.
Use: Anti-inflammatory, analgesic.
CHLORTRIANISENE, U.S.P. U.S.P. XXI.
CHLOR-TRIMETON. (Schering) Chlorpheniramine maleate. **Inj.:** 10 mg/ml. Amp. 1 ml 100s. **Tab.:** 4 mg. Box 24s. Bot. 100s, 1000s. **Repetabs:** 8 mg. Box 24s, 48s. Bot. 100s, 1000s. 12 mg. Bot. 100s, 1000s. Blister packs 12s, 24s. **Syr.:** 2 mg/5 ml. Bot. 4 oz, pt, gal.
Use: Antihistamine.
CHLOR-TRIMETON 4-HOUR RELIEF TABLETS. (Schering) Chlorpheniramine maleate 4 mg, pseudoephedrine sulfate 60 mg/Tab. Box 24s, 48s.
Use: Antihistamine, decongestant.
CHLOR-TRIMETON 12 HOUR ALLERGY. (Schering-Plough) Chlorpheniramine maleate 8 mg, pseudoephedrine sulfate 120 mg/SR Tab. Box 24s, 48s. UD 96s.
Use: Antihistamine, decongestant.
CHLOR-TRIMETON 12-HOUR RELIEF TABLETS. (Schering) Chlorpheniramine maleate 8 mg, d-isophedrine sulfate 120 mg/Tab. Box 12s. Bot. 36s.
Use: Decongestant, antihistamine.
CHLOR-TRIMETON ALLERGY. (Schering-Plough) Chlorpheniramine maleate 4 mg. Tab. Pkg. 24s.
Use: Antihistamine.
CHLOR-TRIMETON W/COMBINATIONS. (Schering) Chlorpheniramine maleate.
    W/Acetaminophen.
    See: Coricidin, Tab. (Schering).
    W/Acetaminophen, phenylpropanolamine.
    See: Coricidin "D", Prods. (Schering).
    W/Phenylephrine HCl.
    See: Demazin, Prods. (Schering).
    W/Pseudoephedrine sulfate.
    See: Chlor-Trimeton Decongestant Tab. (Schering).
    Chlor-Trimeton 12 Hour Allergy (Schering-Plough).
    W/Salicylamide, phenacetin, caffeine, vitamin C.
    See: Coriforte, Cap. (Schering).
    W/Sodium salicylate, amino acetic acid.
    See: Corilin, Liq. (Schering).
CHLOR-TRIMETON SINUS. (Schering) Phenylpropanolamine HCl 12.5 mg, chlorpheniramine maleate 2 mg, acetaminophen 500 mg/Capl. Box 12s, 24s.
Use: Decongestant, antihistamine, analgesic.

CHLORTRON. (Pharmex) Chlorpheniramine maleate 10 mg/Vial. Vial 30 ml.
Use: Antihistamine.
CHLORZIDE. (Foy) Hydrochlorothiazide 50 mg/Tab. Bot. 1000s.
Use: Diuretic.
• **CHLORZOXAZONE, U.S.P.** U.S.P. XXIII. Tab., U.S.P. XXIII, 5-Chlorobenzoxazolin-2-one. 5-Chlorobenzoxazolinone. (Various Mfr.) **250 mg:** Tab. Bot. 100s, 1000s; **500 mg:** Tab. Bot. 100s, 500s, 1000s.
Use: Muscle relaxant.
See: Paraflex, Tab. (McNeil).
Parafon Forte DSC, Capl. (McNeil).
Remular-S (Inter. Ethical).
W/Acetaminophen.
See: Blanex, Cap. (Edwards).
• **CHLORZOXAZONE AND ACETA-MINOPHEN CAPSULES, U.S.P.** U.S.P. XXIII.
Use: Muscle relaxant, analgesic.
CHLORZOXAZONE AND ACETA-MINOPHEN TABLETS, U.S.P. U.S.P. XXI.
Use: Muscle relaxant, analgesic.
CHOICE 10. (Whiteworth) Potassium Cl 10% soln., unflavored. Bot. gal.
Use: Potassium supplement.
CHOICE 20. (Whiteworth) Potassium Cl 20% soln., unflavored. Bot. gal.
Use: Potassium supplement.
CHOLAC. (Alra) Lactulose 10 Gm/15 ml. Bot. 240 ml, pt, UD 30 ml.
Use: Laxative.
CHOLACRYLAMINE RESIN. An anion exchange resin consisting of a water soluble polymer having a molecular weight equivalent between 350 and 360 in which aliphatic quaternary amine groups are attached to an acrylic backbone by ester linkages.
CHOLAJEN. (Jenkins) Ox bile extract 3.5 gr, desoxycholic acid ⅛ gr, dehydrocholic acid gr, pancreatin 1 gr, betaine HCl 1 gr. Bot. 1000s.
Use: Laxative.
CHOLALIC ACID.
See: Cholic Acid.
CHOLAN-DH. (Pennwalt) Dehydrocholic acid 250 mg/Tab. Bot. 100s.
Use: Laxative.
CHOLAN-HMB. (Ciba Consumer) Dehydrocholic acid 250 mg/Tab. Bot. 100s.
Use: Laxative.
CHOLANIC ACID. Dehydrodesoxycholic acid.
CHOLEBRINE. (Mallinckrodt) Iocetamic acid (62% iodine) 750 mg/Tab. Bot. 100s, 150s.

Use: Radiopaque agent.
• **CHOLECALCIFEROL, U.S.P.** U.S.P. XXII. Vitamin D-3, activated 5,7-Cholestadien-3β-ol. 9,10-Secocholesta-5,7,-10(19)-trien-3-ol.
Use: Vitamin D deficiency.
See: Decavitamin Cap., Tab.
CHOLECYSTOGRAPHY AGENTS.
See: Bilopaque, Cap. (Sanofi Winthrop).
Iodized Oil (Various Mfr.).
Iophendylate Inj.
Pantopaque, Amp. (LaFayette).
Telepaque, Tab. (Sanofi Winthrop).
CHOLEDYL. (Parke-Davis) Oxtriphylline. **Tab.:** 100 mg. Bot. 100s; 200 mg. Bot. 100s, 1000s, UD 100s. **Elix.:** 100 mg/5 ml, alcohol 20%. Bot. pt. **Pediatric Syr.:** 50 mg/5 ml. Bot. pt.
Use: Bronchodilator.
CHOLEDYL SA. (Parke-Davis) Oxtriphylline 400 mg or 600 mg/Tab. Bot. 100s, UD 100s.
Use: Bronchodilator.
• **CHOLERA VACCINE, U.S.P.** U.S.P. XXII. (Lederle) India Strains, Vial 1.5 ml (Lilly) Vial 1.5 ml (Wyeth-Ayerst) Vial 1.5 ml, 20 ml.
Use: Active immunizing agent.
CHOLERETIC. Bile salts.
See: Bile Preps. and Forms.
Dehydrocholic Acid.
Desoxycholic Acid.
Tocamphyl, Tab. (Various Mfr.).
CHOLESTERIN.
See: Cholesterol.
• **CHOLESTEROL.** N.F. XVIII. Cholest-5-en-3β-ol. 5,6-Cholesten-3-Ol(Cholesterin). (Various Mfr.).
Use: Pharmaceutic aid (emulsifying agent).
CHOLESTEROL REAGENT STRIPS. (Miles Diagnostic) A quantitative strip test for cholesterol in serum. Seralyzer reagent strips. Bot. 25s.
Use: Diagnostic aid.
CHOLESTYRAMINE. An antihyperlipidemic agent used to lower cholesterol. Consists of anhydrous cholestyramine 4 Gm/dose.
See: Cholybar, Bar (Parke-Davis).
Questran, Pow. (Bristol Labs.).
Questran Light, Pow. (Bristol Labs.).
• **CHOLESTYRAMINE FOR ORAL SUS-PENSION, U.S.P.** U.S.P. XXIII.
Use: Ion-exchange resin (bile salts), antihyperlipoproteinemic.
• **CHOLESTYRAMINE RESIN, U.S.P.** U.S.P. XXIII. A styryl-divinyl-benzene copolymer (about 2% divinylbenzene)

containing quaternary ammonium groups.
Use: Resin producing insoluble bile acid complexes.
See: Questran, Pow. (Bristol).
CHOLIC ACID. 3,7,12-Trihydroxycholanic acid. Cholalic acid. Dehydrocholic Acid.
CHOLIDASE. (Freeda) Choline 185 mg, inositol 150 mg, vitamins B_6 2.5 mg, B_{12} 5 mcg, E 7.5 mg/Tab. Bot. 100s, 250s, 500s.
Use: Lipotropic/vitamin supplement.
CHOLINE. (Various Mfr.) Choline. Tab.: **250 mg:** Bot. 100s, 250s, 500s, 1000s. **500 mg:** Bot. 100s. **650 mg:** Bot. 90s, 100s, 250s, 500s.
Use: Lipotropic.
CHOLINE BITARTRATE.
W/Bile extract, pancreatic substance, dl-methionine.
See: Licoplex, Tab. (Mills).
W/Methionine, inositol, desiccated liver, vitamin B_{12}.
See: Limvic, Tab. (Briar).
W/Mucopolysaccharide, epinephrine neutralizing factor, pancreatic lipotropic fraction, dl-methionine, inositol, bile extract
See: Lipo-K, Cap. (Marcen).
W/d-Pantothenyl alcohol.
See: Ilopan-Choline, Tab. (Adria).
W/Safflower oil, whole liver, soybean, lecithin, inositol, methionine, natural to copherols, vitamins B_6, B_{12}, panthenol.
See: Nutricol, Cap., Vial (Nutrition Control).
CHOLINE CHLORIDE. (Various Mfr.).
Use: Liver supplement. [Orphan drug]
W/Inositol, methionine, vitamin B_{12}.
See: Cho-Meth, Vial (Kenyon).
Lychol-B, Inj. (Burgin-Arden).
W/Methionine, vitamins, niacinamide, panthenol.
See: Minoplex, Vial (Savage).
W/Panthenol, inositol, vitamins, minerals, estrone, testosterone.
See: Geramine, Inj. (Brown).
W/Panthenol, inositol, vitamins, minerals, estrone, testosterone, polydigestase.
See: Geramine, Tab. (Brown).
W/Vitamin B_1, niacinamide, B_2, B_6, calcium pantothenate, cyanocobalamin, B_{12}, inositol, dl-methionine, testosterone, estrone, procaine.
See: Gerihorm, Inj. (Burgin-Arden).
CHOLINE CHLORIDE, CARBAMATE.
Carbachol, U.S.P. XXIII.
CHOLINE CHLORIDE SUCCINATE.
See: Succinylcholine Chloride, U.S.P. XXIII.

CHOLINE CITRATE, TRICHOLINE CITRATE.
W/Inositol, methionine, vitamin B_{12}.
See: Cholimeth Tab. (Central).
CHOLINE DIHYDROGEN CITRATE. 2-Hydroxy-ethyl trimethylammonium citrate-U.S. vitamin 0.5 Gm. Bot. 100s, 500s.
Use: Lipotropic.
See: Cholinate, Liq. (Cenci).
CHOLINE MAGNESIUM TRISALICYLATE. (Sidmark) 500 mg, 750 mg or 1000 mg. Tab. Bot. 100s, 500s.
Use: Salicylate analgesic.
See: Trilisate, Tab. (Purdue Frederick).
CHOLINE SALICYLATE. B.A.N. Choline salt of salicylic acid.
Use: Analgesic, antipyretic.
CHOLINERGIC AGENTS.
(Parasympathomimetic Agents).
See: Mecholyl Cl, Inj. (Baker).
Mestinon, Tab., Syr., Amp. (Roche).
Mytelase, Cap. (Sanofi Winthrop).
Pilocarpine Nitrate (Various Mfr.).
Prostigmin Bromide, Tab. (Roche).
Prostigmin Methylsulfate, Inj. (Roche).
Tensilon, Inj. (Roche).
Urecholine, Inj., Tab. (Merck & Co.).
CHOLINERGIC BLOCKING AGENTS.
See: Parasympatholytic agents.
CHOLINESTERASE INHIBITORS.
Agents that inhibit the enzyme cholinesterase and enhance the effects of endogenous acetylcholine.
Use: Glaucoma therapy.
See: Eserine Sulfate, Oint., (Various, eg, Harber, Iolab, Pharmaderm).
Isopto Eserine, Soln., (Alcon).
Eserine Salicylate, Soln., (Alcon).
Use: Muscle stimulants.
See: Neostigmine Bromide, Tab., (Lannett).
Prostigmin, Tab., (Roche).
Neostigmine Methylsulfate, Inj., (Various Mfr.).
Prostigmin, Inj., (Roche).
CHOLINE THEOPHYLLINATE.
See: Oxtriphylline.
CHOLINE THEOPHYLLINATE. B.A.N. Choline salt of theophylline.
Use: Bronchodilator.
CHOLINOID. (Goldline) Choline 111 mg, inositol 111 mg, vitamins B_1 0.3 mg, B_2 0.3 mg, B_3 3.3 mg, B_5 1.7 mg, B_6 0.3 mg, B_{12} 1.7 mcg, C 100 mg, lemon bioflavonoid complex 100 mg/Cap. Bot. 100s.
Use: Lipotropic/vitamin supplement.
CHO-LIV-12. (Jenkins) Choline 100 mg,

cyanocobalamin 200 mcg, liver equal to vitamin B_{12} 10 mcg/ml. Vial 10 ml, 12s.
Use: Lipotropic/vitamin supplement.
CHOL METH IN B. (Esco) Choline bitartrate 235 mg, inositol 112 mg, methionine 70 mg, betaine anhydrous 50 mg, vitamins B_{12} 6 mcg, B_1 6 mg, B_6 3 mg, niacin 10 mg/Cap. Bot. 500s, 1000s.
Use: Vitamin supplement.
CHOLOGRAFIN MEGLUMINE. (Squibb) Iodipamide meglumine 10.3% (iodine 5.1%)/100 ml, Vial 100 ml. 52% (26% iodine)/20 ml, Vial 20 ml.
Use: Cholangiography, cholecystography.
CHOLOGRAFIN SODIUM. Disodium salt of N,N'-adipyl bis-(3-amino-2:4:6 triodobenzoic acid).
CHOLOXIN. (Flint) Sodium dextrothyroxine 1 mg, 2 mg or 4 mg/Tab. Tartrazine (2 mg, 4 mg only). Bot. 100s, Bot. 250s (2 mg, 4 mg only).
Use: Antihyperlipidemic.
CHOLYGLYCINE.
See: CG RIA, Kit (Abbott).
CHO-METH. (Kenyon) Methionine 30 mg, choline Cl 200 mg, inositol 100 mg, vitamin B_{12} 12 mcg/2 ml. Vial 30 ml.
Use: Nutritional supplement.
CHONDODENDRON TOMENTOSUM.
See: Curare.
CHONDROTIN SULFATE AND SODIUM HYALURONATE. A surgical aid in anterior segment procedures including cataract extraction and intraocular lens implantation.
See: Viscoat, Soln., (Cilco).
CHONDRUS. Irish Moss.
W/Petrolatum, Liq.
See: Kondremul, Liq. (Fisons).
CHOO E PLUS C. (Stayner) Vitamin E 100 IU, C 250 mg/Tab. Bot. 100s.
Use: Vitamin supplement.
CHOOZ. (Schering-Plough) Calcium carbonate 500 mg/Gum tab. Pkg. 16s.
Use: Antacid.
CHOREX 5. (Hyrex) Chorionic gonadotropin 5000 units, urea 100 mg, thimerosal 1 mg, sodium phosphate buffer/Vial 10 ml.
Use: Chorionic gonadotropin.
CHOREX 10. (Hyrex) Chorionic gonadotropin 10,000 units, urea 100 mg, thimerosal 1 mg, sodium phosphate buffer/Vial 10 ml.
Use: Chorionic gonadotropin.
CHORIGON. (Dunhall) Chorionic gonadotropin (dried) 1000 units/ml. Vial 10 ml.
Use: Chorionic gonadotropin.

• CHORIONIC GONADOTROPIN, U.S.P. U.S.P. XXIII. Inj., U.S.P. XXIII. 5000 IU/Vial w/diluent 10 ml, 10,000 IU/Vial w/diluent 10 ml (Serono) hCG 10,000 IU, mannitol 100 mg, benzyl alcohol 0.9%/10 ml Vial.
Use: Prepubertal cryptorchidism or induction of ovulation and pregnancy in anovulatory women.
See: Antuitrin-S (Parke-Davis).
A.P.L., Inj. (Wyeth-Ayerst).
C-G-10, Vial (Scrip).
Chorigon, Amp. (Dunhall).
Chorex 5, Vial (Hyrex).
Chorex 10, Vial (Hyrex).
Chorion-Plus, Vial (Pharmex).
Follutein, Vial (Squibb).
Gonadex (Continental Dist.).
Khorion (Hickam).
Neovital-Diluent, Inj. (Pasadena Research).
Rochoric, Inj. (Rocky Mtn.).
CHORION-PLUS. (Pharmex) Chorionic gonadotropin 10,000 units/Vial. Diluent: Glutamic acid 52 mcg, vitamin B_1 25 mg, procaine 1%/ml. Vial 10 ml.
Use: Chorionic gonadotropin.
CHORON 10. (Forest Pharm.) Chorionic gonadotropin 10,000 units/vial with diluent 10 ml. Also contains mannitol. Inj. Vial 10 ml.
Use: Chorionic gonadotropin.
CHROMAGEN. (Savage) Cap.: Ferrous fumarate 66 mg, vitamins C 250 mg, B_{12} activity 10 mcg, desiccated stomach substances 100 mg/soft gelatin cap. Bot. 100s, 500s. Inj.: Iron peptonized 100 mg, vitamin B_{12} 5 mcg, cyanocobalamin 25 mcg, lidocaine HCl 1%/2 ml. Vial 10 ml, 30 ml.
Use: Vitamin/mineral supplement.
CHROMALBIN. (Squibb) 100 uCi containing chromium CR 51 and human albumin.
CHROMA-PAK. (SoloPak) Chromium 4 mcg/ml: Vial 10 ml, 30 ml. 20 mcg/ml: Vial 5 ml. [Use]Use: Parenteral nutritional supplement.
CHROMARGYRE.
See: Merbromin (Various Mfr.).
• CHROMATE Cr-51, SODIUM FOR INJECTION, U.S.P. U.S.P. XXIII.
CHROMATED SOLUTION (^{51}Cr).
See: Chromitope sodium (Squibb).
CHROMELIN COMPLEXION BLENDER. (Summers) Dihydroxyacetone 5%, alcohol 50%. Bot. oz.
Use: Agent for vitiligo.
CHROMIC ACID, DISODIUM SALT. Sodi-

um Chromate Cr^{51} Inj., U.S.P. XXIII.
- **CHROMIC CHLORIDE, U.S.P.** U.S.P.
XXIII. Inj., U.S.P. XXIII. Chromium Cl
(CrCl3) hexahydrate. Chromium (3+) Cl
hexahydrate.
Use: Chromium deficiency treatment.
See: Chrometrace, Inj. (Armour).
- **CHROMIC CHLORIDE Cr^{51}.**
USAN.
Use: Radioactive agent.
See: Chromitope Cl (Squibb).
- **CHROMIC PHOSPHATE Cr^{51}.**
USAN.
Use: Radioactive agent.
- **CHROMIC PHOSPHATE P^{32}
SUSPENSION, U.S.P.** U.S.P. XXIII.
Use: Radioactive agent.
CHROMITOPE SODIUM. (Squibb) Chro-
mate Cr^{51}, Sodium for Inj. 0.25 mCi.
Use: Radioactive agent.
CHROMIUM. A trace metal used in IV nu-
tritional therapy that helps maintain nor-
mal glucose metabolism and peripheral
nerve function.
See: Chromium, Inj. (Various Mfr.).
Chromic Chloride, Inj. (Various Mfr.).
Chromium Chloride, Inj. (Various Mfr.).
Chroma-Pak, Inj. (Solopak)
Chromium Trace Metal Additive, Inj.
(IMS).
Concentrated Chrmic Chloride, Inj.
(American Regent).
- **CHROMONAR HCl.** USAN. Ethyl[[3-[2-
(di- ethylamino)-ethyl]-4-methyl-2-oxo-
2H-1-benzopyran-7-yl]oxy]acetate HCl.
Intensain.
Use: Coronary vasodilator.
CHRONULAC. (Marion Merrell Dow) Lac-
tulose 10 Gm/15 ml (< 2.2 Gm galac-
tose, 1.2 Gm lactose, 1.2 Gm other sug
ars). Bot. 473 ml, 1890 ml, UD 15 ml, 30
ml. Box 100s.
Use: Laxative.
CHRYSAZIN.
See: Danthron, N.F. XVIII.
CHUR-HIST. (Churchill) Chlorpheni-
ramine 4 mg/Kaptab. Bot. 100s.
Use: Antihistamine.
CHYMEX. (Adria) Bentiromide 500
mg/7.5 ml w/propylene glycol 40%.
Screening test for pancreatic exocrine
insufficiency.
Use: Diagnostic aid.
CHYMODIACTIN. (Smith) 4 nKat units,
1.4 mg sodium L-cysteinate HCl with
diluent. Pow. for Inj. Vial 2 ml.
Use: Proteolytic enzyme.
- **CHYMOPAPAIN.** USAN. Proteolytic en-
zyme isolated from papaya latex, differ

ing from papain in electrophoretic mobili-
ty, solubility and substrate specificity.
Use: Proteolytic enzyme.
- **CHYMOTRYPSIN, U.S.P.** U.S.P. XXIII.
Ophth. Soln. U.S.P. XXIII. An enzyme,
α-Chymotrypsin obtained in crystalline
form from mammalian pancreas by
aqueous acid extraction of its proen-
zyme, chymotrypsinogen, and subse-
quent conversion with trypsin to chy-
motrypsin.
Use: Proteolytic enzyme.
See: Catarase, Soln. (CooperVision).
W/Trypsin.
See: Orenzyme, Tab. (Marion Merrell
Dow).
W/Trypsin, neomycin palmitate.
See: Biozyme, Oint. (Armour).
C.I. BASIC VIOLET 3. Gentian Violet,
U.S.P. XXIII.
CIBA VISION CLEANER. (Ciba Vision)
Cocoamphocarboxyglycinate, sodium
lauryl sulfate, sorbic acid 0.1%, hexy-
lene glycol, EDTA 0.2%. Soln. 5 ml or 15
ml.
Use: Soft contact lens care.
CIBA VISION SALINE. (Ciba Vision)
Buffered, isotonic with NaCl, boric acid.
Soln. Bot. 90 ml, 240 ml, 360 ml.
Use: Solution for rinsing/storage of soft
contact lens.
CIBENZOLINE.
See: Cifenline Succinate. USAN.
- **CICLAFRINE HYDROCHLORIDE.**
USAN.
Use: Antihypotensive.
- **CICLAZINDOL.** USAN. 10-m-
Chlorophenyl-2,3,4,-10-tetrahydropyrlm-
ido[1,2-α]-indol-10-ol.
Use: Antidepressant.
- **CICLETANINE.**
Use: Antihypertensive.
CICLOPIROX. USAN.
Use: Antifungal.
- **CICLOPIROX OLAMINE, U.S.P.** U.S.P.
XXIII. Cream, U.S.P. XXIII.
Use: Antifungal.
See: Loprox, Cream (Hoechst).
- **CICLOPROFEN.** USAN. 2-(2-
Fluorenyl)propionic acid.
Use: Anti-inflammatory.
- **CICLOPROLOL HYDROCHLORIDE.**
USAN.
Use: Anti-adrenergic (beta receptor).
CICLOXOLONE. B.A.N. 3β-(cis-2-Car-
boxycyclo-hexylcarbonyloxy)-11-oxo-
olean-12-en-30-oic acid.
Use: Treatment of gastric ulcers.
CIDEX. (Surgikos) Activated dialdehyde
soln. Bot. qt, gal, 2.5 gal.

Use: Sterilizing, disinfecting agent.
CIDEX-7. (Surgikos) Glutaraldehyde 2% and vial of activator with aqueous potassium salt as buffer and sodium nitrite as a corrosive inhibitor. Soln. Bot. qt, 1 gal, 5 gal.
Use: Sterilizing, disinfecting agent.
CIDEX PLUS. (Surgikos) 3.2% glutaraldehyde. Soln. Gal. [Use]Use: Sterilizing, disinfecting agent.
C.I. DIRECT BLUE 53 TETRASODIUM SALT. Evans Blue, U.S.P. XXIII.
• **CIDOXIEPIN HCl.** USAN.
Use: Psychotherapeutic.
• **CIFENLINE SUCCINATE.** USAN. Formerly Cibenzoline.
Use: Cardiac depressant (antiarrhythmic).
• **CIGLITAZONE.** USAN.
Use: Antidiabetic.
CIGNOLIN.
See: Anthralin (Various Mfr.).
• **CILADOPA HYDROCHLORIDE.** USAN.
Use: Treatment of Parkinson's disease.
CILASTATIN-IMIPENEM. A formulation of imipenem, a thienamycin antibiotic, and cilastatin sodium, the inhibitor of the renal dipeptidase, dehydropeptidase-1.
Use: Antibiotic.
See: Primaxin I.V., Pow. (Merck & Co.). Primaxin I.M., Pow. (Merck & Co.)
• **CILASTATIN SODIUM.** USAN.
Use: Enzyme inhibitor.
W/Imipenem.
See: Primaxin, Inj. (Merck & Co.).
• **CILASTATIN SODIUM, STERILE, U.S.P.** U.S.P. XXIII.
Use: Enzyme inhibitor.
• **CILAZAPRIL.** USAN.
Use: Antihypertensive.
CILFOMIDE TABLETS. (Sanofi Winthrop) Inositol hexanicotinate.
Use: Hypolipidimic, peripheral vasodilator.
CILIARY NEUROTROPHIC FACTOR. (Regeneron Pharm)
Use: Treatment of amyotrophic lateral sclerosis. [Orphan drug]
CILIARY NEUROTROPHIC FACTOR (RECOMBINANT HUMAN).
Use: Treatment of motor neuron disease. [Orphan drug]
CILLIUM. (Whiteworth) Psyllium seed husk pow. 4.94 Gm, 14 calories/rounded tsp. Bot. 420 Gm, 630 Gm.
Use: Laxative.
CILOXAN. (Alcon) Ciprofloxacin HCl/ml 3.5 mg (equivalent to 3 mg base). Soln., Drop-Tainer dispensers. 2.5 ml, 5 ml.
Use: Antibiotic.

• **CIMATEROL.** USAN.
Use: Repartitioning agent.
• **CIMETIDINE, U.S.P.** U.S.P. XXIII. Tab., U.S.P. XXIII. 1-Methyl-3-[2-(5-methylimidazol-4-ylmethylthio)ethyl]guanidine-2-carbonitrile.
Use: H$_2$ receptor histamine antagonist.
See: Tagamot, Tab., Inj. (SK Boooham).
• **CIMETIDINE HYDROCHLORIDE.** USAN.
Use: H$_2$ receptor histamine antagonist.
CIMETIDINE HCl. (Endo) Cimetidine HCl 150 mg, phenol 5 mg/ml. Inj. In 2 ml vials and 8 ml multiple dose vials.
Use: Histamine H$_2$ antagonist.
CINACORT SPAN. (Foy) Triamcinolone acetonide 40 mg/ml. Vial 5 ml.
Use: Corticosteroid.
• **CINALUKAST.** USAN.
Use: Antiasthmatic.
• **CINANSERIN HYDROCHLORIDE.** USAN. 2'-[[3-(Dimethylamino)propyl]thio]cinnamanilide HCl.
Use: Serotonin antagonist.
CINCHONA BARK. (Various Mfr.).
Use: Antimalarial, tonic.
W/Anhydrous quinine, cinchonidine, cinchonine, quinidine, quinine.
See: Totaquine, Pow. (Various Mfr.).
W/Iron oxide, nux vomica, vitamin B$_1$, alcohol.
See: Briatonic, Liq. (Briar).
CINCHONIDINE SULFATE.
CINCHONINE SALTS. (Various Mfr.).
Use: Quinine dihydrochloride.
CINCHOPHEN. 2-Phenylcinchoninic acid.
Use: Analgesic.
CINEPAZATE. B.A.N. Ethyl 4-(3,4,5-trimethoxy-cinnamoyl)piperazin-1-ylacetate.
Use: Treatment of angina.
• **CINEPAZET MALEATE.** USAN.
Use: Antianginal.
CINEPAZIDE. B.A.N. 1-Pyrrolidin-1-ylcarbonyl-methyl-4-(3,4,5-trimethoxycinnamoyl)-piperazine.
Use: Peripheral vasodilator.
• **CINFLUMIDE.** USAN.
Use: Muscle relaxant.
• **CINGESTOL.** USAN. 19-Nor-17α-pregn-5-en-20-yn-17-ol.
Use: Progestogen.
CINNAMALDEHYDE.
• **CINNAMEDRINE.** USAN. a-[1-(Cinnamyl-methylamine)-ethyl] benzyl alcohol.
Use: Uterine antispasmodic.
See: Midol, Tab. (Glenbrook).
CINNAMIC ALDEHYDE. Name previous-

ly used for Cinnamaldehyde.
• **CINNAMON, U.S.P.** N.F. XVIII.
Use: Flavoring agent.
• **CINNAMON OIL, U.S.P.** N.F. XVIII. (Various Mfr.).
Use: Pharmaceutic aid.
CINNAMYL EPHEDRINE HCl.
W/Acetaminophen, homatropine methylbromide.
See: Periodic, Cap. (Towne).
• **CINNARIZINE.** USAN. 1-Diphenylmethyl-4-trans-cinnamylpiperazine; 1-Benzhydryl-4-cinnamylpiperazine; F.D.A. 1-Cinnamyl-4-diphenyl-methylpiperazine.
Use: Antihistamine.
CINNOPENTAZONE. INN for Cintazone.
CINOBAC. (Oclassen) Cinoxacin **250 mg/Pulv.:** Bot. 40s. **500 mg/Pulv.:** Bot. 50s.
Use: Urinary anti-infective.
• **CINODINE HYDROCHLORIDE.** USAN.
Use: Antibacterial.
• **CINOXACIN, U.S.P.** U.S.P. XXIII. Cap., U.S.P. XXIII 1-Ethyl-4-oxo[1,3]dioxolo-[4,5-g]cinnoline-3-carboxylic acid.
Use: Antibacterial.
See: Cinobac, Cap. (Dista).
CINOXACIN. (Biocraft) **250 mg:** Cap. Bot. 40s, 100s; **500 mg:** Cap. Bot. 50s, 100s.
Use: Antibacterial.
• **CINOXATE, U.S.P.** U.S.P. XXIII. Lot., U.S.P. XXIII. 2-Ethoxyethyl p-methoxycinnamate.
Use: Ultraviolet screen.
See: Sundare Prods. (Cooper).
W/Methyl anthranilate.
See: Maxafil Cream (Cooper).
CINOXOLONE. B.A.N. Cinnamyl 3β-acetoxy-11-oxo-olean-12-en-30-oate.
Use: Treatment of gastric ulcer.
• **CINPERENE.** USAN. 1-Cinnamyl-4-(2,6-dioxo-3-phenyl-3-piperidyl)piperidine.
Use: Tranquilizer.
CIN-QUIN. (Reid-Rowell) Quinidine sulfate. (Contains 83% anhydrous quinidine alkaloid.) **Tab.:** 100 mg, 200 mg or 300 mg. Bot. 100s, 1000s, UD 100s. **Cap.:** 200 mg. Bot. 100s. 300 mg. Bot. 100s, 1000s, UD 100s.
Use: Antiarrhythmic.
• **CINROMIDE.** USAN.
Use: Anticonvulsant.
• **CINTAZONE.** USAN. 2-Pentyl-6-phenyl-1H-pyrazolo [1,2-a] cinnoline-1,3(2H)-dione.
Use: Anti-inflammatory.
• **CINTRIAMIDE.** USAN.
Use: Antipsychotic.
• **CIOTERONEL.** USAN.

Use: Treatment of acne, adrogenic alopecia and keloid (antiandrogen).
CIPRALAN. (Hoffman-LaRoche) Cifenline succinate, formerly cibenzoline.
Use: Antiarrhythmic agent.
• **CIPREFADOL SUCCINATE.** USAN.
Use: Analgesic.
CIPRO. (Miles Pharm.) Ciprofloxacin HCl 250 mg, 500 mg or 750 mg/Tab. Bot. 50s, UD 100s.
Use: Antibacterial, fluoroquinolone.
CIPRO I.V. (Miles Pharm.) Ciprofloxacin 200 mg and 400 mg (with lactic acid). Inj. Vial: 20 ml (1%), 40 ml (1%). Flex Bot.: 100 ml (in 5% dextrose) and 200 ml (in 5% dextrose).
Use: Antibacterial, fluoroquinolone.
• **CIPROCINONIDE.** USAN.
Use: Adrenocortical steroid.
• **CIPROFIBRATE.** USAN.
Use: Antihyperlipoproteinemic.
• **CIPROFLOXACIN.** USAN. U.S.P. XXIII
Use: Antibacterial.
• **CIPROFLOXACIN HYDROCHLORIDE.** USAN. U.S.P. XXIII
Use: Antibacterial.
See: Ciloxan, Soln. (Alcon).
Cipro (Miles).
• **CIPROSTENE CALCIUM.** USAN.
Use: Platelet anti-aggregatory agent.
• **CIRAMADOL.** USAN.
Use: Analgesic.
• **CIRAMADOL HYDROCHLORIDE.** USAN.
Use: Analgesic.
CIRBED. (Boyd) Papaverine HCl 150 mg/Cap. Bot. 100s.
Use: Antispasmodic.
CIRCAVITE-T. (Circle) Iron 12 mg, vitamins A 10,000 IU, D 400 IU, E 15 mg, B_1 10.3 mg, B_2 10 mg, B_3 100 mg, B_5 18.4 mg, B_6 4.1 mg, B_{12} 5 mcg, C 200 mg, Cu, Mg, Mn, zinc 1.5 mg. Bot. 100s.
Use: Vitamin/mineral supplement.
• **CIROLEMYCIN.** USAN.
Use: Antibacterial, antineoplastic.
• **CISAPRIDE.** USAN.
Use: Peristaltic stimulant.
• **CISPLATIN, U.S.P.** U.S.P. XXIII.
Use: Antineoplastic agent.
See: Platinol, Inj. (Bristol).
CIS-RETINOIC ACID. (13-cis-Retinoic Acid).
Use: Anti-acne.
See: Isotretinoin.
Accutane (Roche).
CITANEST HCl. (Astra) **Plain:** Prilocaine HCl 4%/1.8 ml dental cartridge.
Use: Local anesthetic.
CITANEST HCl FORTE. (Astra) Prilo-

caine HCl 4% with epinephrine 1:
200,000. Contains sodium metabisulfite.
Dental cartridge 1.8 ml. Inj.
Use: Local anesthetic.
• **CITENAMIDE.** USAN.
Use: Anticonvulsant.
CITHAL CAPSULES. (Table Rock) Watermelon seed extract 2 gr, theobromine 4 gr, phenobarbital 0.25 gr/Cap. Bot. 100s, 500s.
Use: Antihypertensive.
CITRACAL. (Mission) Calcium citrate 950 mg/Tab. Bot. 100s.
Use: Calcium supplement.
CITRACAL 1500 + D. (Mission) Calcium citrate 1500 mg, vitamin D 200 IU/Tab. Bot. 60s.
Use: Vitamin/calcium supplement.
CITRACAL LIQUITAB. (Mission) Calcium citrate 2376 mg/Effervescent tab. Box. 30s.
Use: Calcium supplement.
CITRA FORTE. (Boyle) Hydrocodone bitartrate 5 mg, ascorbic acid 30 mg, pheniramine maleate 2.5 mg, pyrilamine maleate 3.33 mg, potassium citrate 150 mg/5 ml. Bot. pt, gal.
Use: Antitussive, vitamin C supplement, antihistamine.
CITRAMIN-500. (Thurston) Vitamin C 500 mg, rose hips, acerola with mixed bioflavonoids/Loz. Bot. 100s, 250s, 1000s.
Use: Vitamin/mineral supplement.
CITRANOX. (Alconox)
Use: Liquid acid detergent for manual and ultrasonic washers.
CITRA pH. (Val Med) Sodium citrate dihydrate 450 mg/30 ml. Soln. 30 ml.
Use: Antacid.
CITRASAN B. (Sandia) Lemon bioflavonoid complex 300 mg, vitamins C 300 mg, B_1 30 mg, B_2 10 mg, B_6 5 mg, B_{12} 4 mcg, calcium pantothenate 10 mg, niacinamide 50 mg/Tab. Bot. 100s, 1000s.
Use: Vitamin supplement.
CITRASAN K-250. (Sandia) Vitamins C 250 mg, K 1 mg, lemon bioflavonoid 250 mg/Tab. Bot. 100s, 1000s.
Use: Vitamin supplement.
CITRASAN K LIQUID. (Sandia) Vitamins C 125 mg, K 0.66 mg, lemon bioflavonoid complex 125 mg/5 ml. Bot. pt, gal.
Use: Vitamin supplement.
CITRATE ACID.
See: Bicitra Soln. (Willen).
CITRATE AND CITRIC ACID SOLUTION.
Use: Alkalinizer.

See: Polycitra (Willen).
Polycitra-LC (Willen).
Polycitra-K (Willen).
Oracit (Carolina Medical Products.).
Bicitra (Willen).
CITRATE OF MAGNESIA. (Various Mfr.) Magnesium citrate. Soln. Bot. 300 ml.
Use: Laxative.
CITRATED NORMAL HUMAN PLASMA.
See: Plasma, Normal Human.
CITRESCO-K. (Esco) Vitamins C 100 mg, K 0.7 mg, citrus bioflavonoid complex 100 mg/Cap. Bot. 100s, 500s, 1000s.
Use: Vitamin supplement.
• **CITRIC ACID, U.S.P.** U.S.P. XXIII. 1,2,3-Propanetricarboxylic acid, 2-hydroxy-.
Use: Component of anticoagulant solutions and drug products.
CITRIC ACID AND D-GLUCONIC ACID IRRIGANT.
Use: Genitourinary irrigant. [Orphan drug]
See: Renacidin (Guardian).
• **CITRIC ACID, MAGNESIUM OXIDE, AND SODIUM CARBONATE IRRIGATION, U.S.P.** U.S.P. XXIII.
Use: Irrigating solution.
CITRIN.
See: Vitamin P.
CITRIN CAPSULES. (Table Rock) Watermelon seed extract 4 gr/Cap. Bot. 100s, 500s.
Use: Antihypertensive.
CITROCARBONATE. (Upjohn) Sodium bicarbonate 0.78 Gm, sodium citrate anhydrous 1.82 Gm/3.9 Gm. Bot. 4 oz, 8 oz.
Use: Antacid.
CITROCARBONATE EFFERVESCENT GRANULES. (Roberts-Hauck) Sodium bicarbonate 780 mg, sodium citrate anhydrous 1820 mg, sodium 700.6 mg/5 ml. Bot. 150 g.
Use: Antacid, analgesic.
CITRO CEE, SUPER. (Marlyn) Bioflavonoids 500 mg, rutin 50 mg, vitamin C 500 mg, rose hips powder 500 mg/Tab. Bot. 50s, 100s.
Use: Vitamin supplement.
CITRO-FLAV 200. (Goldline) Citrus bioflavonoid compound 200 mg/Cap. Bot. 100s, 1000s.
Use: Vitamin supplement.
CITROLEUM SUNBURN CREME. (Citroleum) Bot. 4 oz.
CITROLITH. (Beach) Potassium citrate 50 mg, sodium citrate 950 mg/Tab. Bot. 100s, 500s.
Use: Urinary alkalinizer.

CITROMA. (Century) Magnesium citrate. Oral soln. Bot. 10 oz.
Use: Laxative.

CITROMA LOW SODIUM. (National Magnesia) Magnesium citrate. Oral soln w/lemon or cherry flavor in sugar-free vehicle. Bot. l0 oz.
Use: Laxative.

CITROPAM. (Jenkins) No. 1 Ammonium Cl 0.5 Gm, citric acid 0.5 Gm, potassium guaiacolsulfonate 0.5 Gm/fl oz. Bot. 3 oz, 4 oz, gal. Also Citropam No. 2 w/codeine phosphate 30 mg/fl oz. Bot. 3 oz, 4 oz, gal.
Use: Expectorant.

CITROTEIN. (Sandoz Nutrition) Sucrose, pasteurized egg white solids, amino acids, maltodextrin, citric acid, natural and artificial flavors, mono and diglyc erides, partially hydrogenated soybean oil, 0.66 cal/ml, protein 40.7 Gm, carbohydrate 120.7 Gm, fat 1.55 Gm, sodium 698 mg, potassium 698 mg/L. Tartrazine (orange flavor only). Pow. 1.57 oz/packet, Can 14.16 oz. Orange, grape and punch flavors.
Use: Enteral nutritional supplement.

CITROVORUM FACTOR. Leucovorin Calcium, U.S.P. XXIII.
See: Leucovorin Calcium (Lederle) Folinic Acid.

CITRUCEL. (SK-Beecham) Methylcellulose 2 Gm/heaping tbsp. dose w/citric acid. Bot. 16 oz, 30 oz.
Use: Laxative.

CITRUCEL SUGAR FREE. (SK-Beecham) Methylcellulose 2 Gm, aspartame, phenylalanine 52 mg. Pow. Can. 479 Gm.
Use: Laxative.

CITRUS BIOFLAVONOID COMPOUND.
See: Bioflavonoid Compounds (Various Mfr.).
C.V.P., Syr. (USV Pharm.).
Vitamin P.
W/Ascorbic acid, phenyltoloxamine dihydrogen citrate, salicylamide, acetyl p-aminophenol, caffeine, racemic amphetamine sulfate.
See: Euphenex, Tab. (Westerfield).

CITRUS-FLAV C 500. (Fibertone) Citrus bioflavonoids complex 200 mg, vitamin C 200 mg, hesperidin complex 40 mg, acerola 50 mg, rutin 10 mg, in citrus base of orange and lemon powder, grapefruit concentrate powder and citrus pectin. Tabs. Bot. 100s, 250s.

C-JECT. (Lincoln) Ascorbic acid 2000 mg, sodium bisulfite 0.1%, disodium sequestrene 0.01%/10 ml. Amp. 10 ml,

"Score-Break" Box 25s.

C-JECT WITH B. (Lincoln) When mixed with 10 ml of diluent, each vial contains: Vitamins C 2000 mg, B_1 50 mg, B_2 5 mg, B_6 10 mg, nicotinamide 100 mg, methylparaben 0.89 mg, propylparaben 0.22 mg, sodium bisulfite 10 mg, disodium sequestrene 1 mg. Box of 6 lyophilized plugs and 6 10 ml vials of Sterile Diluent.

CKA CANKER AID. (Pannett Prod.) Benzocaine, aluminum hydrate, magnesium trisilicate, sodium acid carbonate. Pow.
Use: Cold-canker sore.

CK(CPK) REAGENT STRIPS. (Miles Diagnostic) Seralyzer reagent strips for creatnine phosphokinase in serum or plasma. Bot. 25s.
Use: Diagnostic aid.

•**CLADRIBINE.** USAN.
Use: Antineoplastic. [Orphan drug]
See: Leustatin (Ortho Biotech).

CLAFORAN. (Hoechst) Cefotaxime sodium 1 Gm, 2 Gm or 10 Gm/Vial. Infusion Bot.: 1 Gm, 2 Gm. Viaflex (pre-mixed frozen) Bag: 1 Gm, 2 Gm. Add-Vantage System: Vial 1 Gm, 2 Gm.
Use: Antibacterial, cephalosporin.

CLAMIDOXIC ACID. B.A.N. [2-(3,4-Dichlorobenz-amido)phenoxy]acetic acid.
Use: Antirheumatic.

•**CLAMOXYQUIN HYDROCHLORIDE.** USAN. 5-Chloro-7-(((3-(diethylamino)propyl)-amino)methyl)-8-quinolinol dihydrochloride.
Use: Amebicide.

CLARETIN-12.
See: Vitamin B_{12}.

CLARITHROMYCIN. A semi-synthetic macrolide antibiotic.
See: Biaxin Filmtabs, Tabs., Oral Susp. (Abbott).

CLARITIN. (Schering) Loratadine.
Use: Antihistamine.

•**CLAVULANATE POTASSIUM, U.S.P.** U.S.P. XXIII.
Use: Inhibitor (β-lactamase).

•**CLAVULANATE POTASSIUM, STERILE, U.S.P.** U.S.P. XXIII.
Use: Inhibitor (β-lactamase).

CLAVULANATE POTASSIUM AND TICARCILLIN.
Use: Antibacterial, pencillin.
See: Timentin, Pow. for Inj. (SK-Beecham).
Timentin, Soln. (SK-Beecham).

CLAVULANIC ACID/AMOXICILLIN.
Use: Antibacterial, penicillin.
See: Augmentin Tab. (Beecham Labs).

CLAVULANIC ACID/TICARCILLIN.

Use: Antibacterial, penicillin.
See: Timentin Pow. for Inj. (Beecham Labs).
•**CLAZOLAM.** USAN.
Use: Tranquilizer.
•**CLAZOLIMINE.** USAN.
Use: Diuretic.
•**CLAZURIL.** USAN.
Use: Coccidiostat.
CLEAN-N-SOAK. (Allergan) Cleaning agent with phenylmercuric nitrate 0.004%. Bot. 4 oz.
Use: Hard contact lens care.
CLEARASIL 10%. (Vicks Prods) Benzoyl peroxide 10%. Bot. oz.
Use: Anti-acne.
CLEARASIL ADULT CARE MEDICATED BLEMISH STICK. (Vicks Prods) Sulfur 8%, resorcinol 1%, bentonite 4%, laureth-4, titanium dioxide. Stick 1/8 oz.
Use: Anti-acne.
CLEARASIL ANTIBACTERIAL SOAP. (Vicks Prods) Triclosan 0.75%, glycerin, bentonite, titanium dioxide. 3.25 oz.
Use: Skin cleanser.
CLEARASIL CLEARSTICK. (Procter & Gamble) Salicylic acid 1.25%, alcohol 39%, aloe vera gel, menthol, EDTA. Liq. 35 ml.
Use: Anti-acne.
CLEARASIL CLEARSTICK, MAXIMUM STRENGTH. (Procter & Gamble) Salicylic acid 2%, alcohol 39%, aloe vera gel, menthol, EDTA. Liq. 35 ml.
Use: Anti-acne.
CLEARASIL CLEARSTICK FOR SENSITIVE SKIN, MAXIMUM STRENGTH. (Procter & Gamble) Salicylic acid 2%, alcohol 39%, aloe vera gel, menthol, EDTA. Liq. 35 ml.
Use: Anti-acne.
CLEARASIL DAILY FACE WASH. (Procter & Gamble) Triclosan 0.3%, glycerin, aloe vera gel, EDTA. Liq. Bot. 135 ml.
Use: Antiseptic and germicide.
CLEARASIL DOUBLE CLEAR. (Richardson-Vicks) **Regular strength:** Salicylic acid 1.25%, alcohol 40% in pads. Bot. 32s. **Maximum strength:** Salicylic acid 2%, alcohol 40% in pads. Bot. 32s.
Use: Anti-acne.
CLEARASIL DOUBLE TEXTURED PADS. (Procter & Gamble) **Pads, regular strength:** Salicylic acid 2%, alcohol 40%, glycerin, aloe vera gel, EDTA. In 40s. **Pads, maximum strength:** Salicylic acid 2%, alcohol 40%, menthol, aloe vera gel, EDTA. In 40s.
Use: Anti-acne.
CLEARASIL MAXIMUM STRENGTH.

(Richardson-Vicks) Pads, maximum strength: Salicylic acid 2%, alcohol 40%, witch hazel distillate, quaternium-22l aloe vera gel, menthol, Jar 32s. Pads, regular strength: Salicylic acid 1.25%, alcohol 40%, witch hazel distillate, quaternium-22, aloe vera gel, menthol. Jar 32s.
Use: Anti-acne.
CLEARASIL MAXIMUM STRENGTH ACNE TREATMENT CREAM. (Vicks Prods) Benzoyl peroxide 10% in tinted or vanishing base. Tube 19.5 Gm, 30 Gm.
Use: Anti-acne.
CLEARASIL MEDICATED ASTRINGENT. (Vicks Prods) Salicylic acid 0.5%, alcohol 43%. Bot. 4 oz.
Use: Anti-acne.
CLEAR AWAY. (Schering-Plough) Salicyclic acid 40%. Disc Pck. 18s.
Use: Keratolytic.
CLEAR AWAY PLANTAR. (Schering-Plough) Salicyclic acid 40%. Disc (for feet) Pck. 24s.
Use: Keratolytic.
CLEARBLUE EASY. (Whitehall) Dip stick for in-home pregnancy test. Kit 1,2s.
Use: Diagnostic aid.
CLEARBLUE PREGNANCY TEST. (VLI) Dip stick for pregnancy test. Kit 2s.
Use: Diagnostic aid.
CLEAR BY DESIGN. (SK-Beecham) Benzoyl peroxide 2.5% in an invisible, greaseless gel base. Tube 1.5 oz, 3 oz.
Use: Anti-acne.
CLEAREX ACNE CREAM. (Approved) Allantoin, sulfur, resorcinol, d-panthenol, isopropanol. Tube 1.5 oz.
Use: Anti-acne.
CLEAR EYES ACR EYE DROPS. (Ross) Naphazoline HCl 0.012%, glycerin 0.2%, zinc sulfate 0.25%, benzalkonium Cl, boric acid, EDTA. Bot. 15 ml, 30 ml.
Use: Ophthalmic decongestant.
CLEAR EYES EYE DROPS. (Ross) Naphazoline HCl 0.012%, benzalkonium Cl 0.01%, disodium edetate 0.1%, glycerin 0.2%, boric acid, sodium borate. Bot. 0.5 oz, 1 oz.
Use: Ophthalmic vasoconstrictor, lubricant.
CLEARLY CALA-GEL. (TecLabs) Diphenhydramine HCl, zinc acetate, menthol, EDTA. Gel In 180 g.
Use: Antihistamine, topical.
CLEARPLAN. (VLI) Ovulation prediction test. Box 10s.
Use: Diagnostic aid.
•**CLEBOPRIDE.** USAN.

Use: Antiemetic.

CLEFAMIDE. B.A.N. αα-Dichloro-N-(2-hydroxy-ethyl)-N-[4-(4-nitrophenoxy)benzyl]acetamide.
Use: Treatment of amebiasis.

• **CLEMASTINE.** USAN. (+)-2-[2-(4-Chloro-α-methyl- benzhydryloxy)ethyl]-1-methylpyrrolidine. Tavegil hydrogen fumarate.
Use: Antihistamine.
See: Tavist, Tab., Syr. (Sandoz).

• **CLEMASTINE FUMARATE.** USAN.
Use: Antihistamine.

• **CLEMASTINE FUMARATE TABLETS, U.S.P.** U.S.P. XXIII.
Use: Antihistamine.

CLEMIZOLE. B.A.N. 1-(4-chlorobenzyl)-2-pyrrolidin-1-ylmethylbenzimidazole.
Use: Antipruritic.

CLEMIZOLE HCl. 1-p-Chlorobenzyl-2-pyrrolidyl-methyl benzimidazole. Reactrol.

CLEMIZOLE PENICILLIN. B.A.N. Benzylpenicillin combined with 1-(4-chlorobenzyl)-2-pyrrolidin-1-ylmethyl-benzimidazole. Neopenyl.
Use: Antibiotic.

CLENS. (Alcon) Cleansing agent with benzalkonium Cl 0.02%, EDTA 0.1%. Soln. Bot. 60 ml.
Use: Hard contact lens care.

• **CLENTIAZEM MALEATE.** USAN.
Use: Antianginal, antihypertensive.

CLEOCIN HCl. (Upjohn) Clindamycin HCl 75 mg, 150 mg or 300 mg/Cap. Tartrazine. Bot. 100s. (75 mg); 16s, 100s, UD 100s (150 mg, 300 mg).
Use: Anti-infective.

CLEOCIN PEDIATRIC. (Upjohn) Clindamycin palmitate HCl equivalent to clindamycin 75 mg/5 ml when reconstituted as directed. Bot. 100 ml.
Use: Anti-infective.

CLEOCIN PHOSPHATE. (Upjohn) Clindamycin phosphate equivalent to clindamycin 150 mg/ml. **300 mg:** Vial 2 ml w/disodium edetate 1 mg, benzyl alcohol 18.9 mg. Pack 25s, 100s. **600 mg:** Vial 4 ml w/disodium edetate 2 mg, benzyl alcohol 37.8 mg. Pack 25s, 100s. **900 mg:** Vial 6 ml. Pack 25s, 100s. **9000 mg:** Bulk Vial 60 ml. Pack 5s.
Use: Anti-infective.

CLEOCIN T. (Upjohn) Clindamycin phosphate 10 mg/ml. Topical soln., gel. Bot. 30 ml, 60 ml, pt. (topical soln.). Bot. 7.5 Gm, 30 Gm (gel). Lot. Bot. 60 ml.
Use: Anti-infective.

CLEOCIN VAGINAL. (Upjohn) Clindamycin phosphate 2%, mineral oil, benzyl alcohol, propylene glycol, polysorbate 60, sorbitan, monostearate. Cream. Tube with 7 disposable applicators 40 Gm.
Use: Anti-infective.

CLERZ DROPS FOR HARD LENSES. (Ciba Vision) Hypertonic solution with hydroxyethyl cellulose, sorbic acid, poloxamer 407, EDTA 0.1%, thimerosal 0.001%. Soln. Bot. 25 ml.
Use: Hard contact lens care.

CLERZ DROPS FOR SOFT LENSES. (Ciba Vision) Hypertonic solution with hydroxyethyl cellulose, sodium borate, poloxamer 407, sorbic acid, thimerosal 0.001%, EDTA 0.1%. Soln. Bot. 25 ml.
Use: Soft contact lens care.

CLERZ 2 FOR HARD LENSES. (Alcon) Isotonic solution with hydroxyethyl cellulose, poloxamer 407, sodium Cl, potassium Cl, sodium borate, boric acid, sorbic acid, EDTA. Soln. Bot. 5 ml, 15 ml.
Use: Hard contact lens care.

CLERZ 2 FOR SOFT LENSES. (Ciba Vision) Isotonic solution with sodium Cl, potassium Cl, hydroxyethyl cellulose, poloxamer 407, sodium borate, boric acid, sorbic acid, EDTA. Soln. Bot. 5 ml, 15 ml.
Use: Soft contact lens care.

CLETOQUINE. B.A.N. 7-Chloro-4-[4-(2-hydroxy- ethylamino)-1-methylbutyl]aminoquinoline.
Use: Anti-inflammatory.

• **CLIDINIUM BROMIDE, U.S.P.** U.S.P. XXIII. Cap., U.S.P. XXIII. 1-Methyl-3-benzil-oyloxy-quinuclidinium bromide. 3-Hydroxy-1-methyl-quinuclidinium bromide benzilate.
Use: Anticholinergic.
See: Quarzan, Cap. (Roche).
W/Chlordiazepoxide.
See: Librax, Cap. (Roche).

CLINAFLOXACIN HCl. USAN.
Use: Antibacterial.

CLINDA-DERM. (Paddock) Clindamycin phosphate 1%, isopropyl alcohol 51.5%, propylene glycol. Soln. Bot. 50 ml.
Use: Anti-acne.

• **CLINDAMYCIN.** USAN. Methyl 7-chloro-6,7,8-tri-deoxy-6-(trans-1-methyl-4-propyl-L-2-pyrrolidine-carboxamido)-1-thio-L-threo-α-D-galactooctopy-ranoside.
Use: Topical antibiotic for acne. Oral as antibiotic. Vaginal as anti-infective. AIDS associated pneumonia [Orphan drug]
See: Cleocin T (Upjohn).
Cleocin (Upjohn).

Cleocin Vaginal Cream (Upjohn).
• **CLINDAMYCIN HYDROCHLORIDE,
U.S.P.** U.S.P. XXIII. Cap. U.S.P. XXIII.
Use: Antibacterial.
See: Cleocin HCl A.D.T., Cap. (Upjohn).
• **CLINDAMYCIN PALMITATE HY-
DROCHLORIDE, U.S.P.** U.S.P. XXIII.
Oral Soln. U.S.P. XXIII.
Use: Antibacterial.
See: Cleocin Pediatric (Upjohn).
Cleocin T, Liq. (Upjohn).
• **CLINDAMYCIN PHOSPHATE, U.S.P.**
U.S.P. XXIII. Inj., Topical Soln., Sterile,
Topical Susp., Gel, U.S.P. XXIII.
Use: Antibacterial.
See: Cleocin phosphate, Inj. (Upjohn).
Clinda-Derm, Soln. (Paddock).
CLINDAMYCIN PHOSPHATE. (Various
Mfr.) Clindamycin phosphate 1%. Topi-
cal Soln. Bot. 30 ml, 60 ml, 60 ml appli-
cator bottle.
Use: Antibacterial.
CLINDEX. (Rugby) Clidinium bromide 2.5
mg, chlordiazepoxide HCl 5 mg/Cap.
Bot. 100s, 500s, 1000s.
Use: Anticholinergic/antispasmodic.
CLINISTIX REAGENT STRIPS. (Miles Di-
agnostic) Glucose oxidase, peroxidase
and orthotolidine. Diagnostic test for glu-
cose in urine. Bot. 50s.
Use: Diagnostic aid.
CLINITEST. (Miles Diagnostic) 2-drop
and 5-drop combination packages w/col-
or charts for both 2-drop and 5-drop use.
Reagent tablets containing copper sul-
fate, sodium hydroxide, heat-producing
agents. Patient's plastic set; Tab. refills.
Box: 100s, 500s, sealed in foil. **Child-re-
sistant bot.:** 36s, 100s.
Use: Diagnostic aid.
CLINOCAINE HCl.
See: Procaine HCl.
CLINORIL. (Merck & Co.) Sulindac 150
mg or 200 mg/Tab. Bot. 100s, UD 100s.
Unit-of-use 60s, 100s.
Use: Nonsteroidal anti-inflammatory
drug; analgesic.
CLINOXIDE CAPSULES. (Geneva
Generics) Clidinium 2.5 mg, chlor-
diazepoxide HCl, 5 mg. Cap. Bot. 100s,
500s.
Use: Gastrointestinal anticholinergic
combination.
• **CLIOQUINOL, U.S.P.** U.S.P. XXIII.
Comp. Pow., Cream, Oint., U.S.P. XXIII.
5-Chloro-7-iodo-8-quinolinol. Quinambi-
cide, Rometin. Iodohydroxyquin.
Use: Topical antifungal.
See: HCV Creame (Saron).
Quin III, Cream (Lemmon).

Quinoform, Oint., Cream, Lot. (C & M
Pharmacal).
Torofor, Cream, Oint. (Torch).
Vioform, Prep. (Ciba).
W/Aluminum acetate solution, hydrocorti-
sone.
See: Hydrelt, Cream, Oint. (Elder).
W/Hydrocortisone acetate,
See: Viotag Cream (Reid-Rowell).
W/Hydrocortisone acetate, lidocaine.
See: Lidaform-HC, Creme, Lot. (Miles
Pharm).
W/Hydrocortisone, coal tar solution.
See: Tar-Quin-HC, Oint. (Jenkins).
W/Hydrocortisone, lidocaine.
See: Bafil Lotion (Scruggs).
HIL-20 Lotion (Reid-Rowell).
W/Hydrocortisone, chlorobutanol.
See: Hc-Form, Jelly (Recsei).
W/Hydrocortisone, coal tar extract.
See: Racet LCD, Cream (Lemmon).
W/Hydrocortisone and pramoxine HCl.
See: Dermarex Cream (Hyrex).
Sherform-HC, Oint. (Sheryl).
Stera-Form Creme (Mayrand).
V-Cort, Cream (Scrip).
W/Methylcellulose, aluminum hydroxide,
atropine sulfate, hyoscine HBr,
hyoscyamine sulfate.
See: Enterex, Tab. (Person & Covey).
W/Nystatin.
See: Nystaform, Oint. (Miles Pharm).
• **CLIOQUINOL AND HYDROCORTISONE
CREAM, U.S.P.** U.S.P. XXIII.
Use: Topical antifungal.
See: Bafil, Cream (Skruggs).
Caquin Cream (Forest).
Coidocort Cream (Coast).
Corticoid, Cream (Jenkins).
Domeform-HC, Cream (Miles Pharm).
Hi-Form Cream (Blaine).
Hydrelt, Cream (Elder).
Hysone, Cream (Hauck).
Ido-Cortistan Oint. (Standex).
Iodocort, Cream (Ulmer).
Iohydro, Cream (Freeport).
Kencort, Cream (Kenyon).
Lanvisone, Cream (Lannett).
Maso-Form, Cream (Mason).
Mity-Quin Cream (Reid-Rowell).
Racet, Cream (Lemmon).
Racet Forte, Cream (Lemmon).
Vioform-Hydrocortisone, Cream, Oint.,
Lot. (Ciba).
Vio-Hydrocort, Cream, Oint. (Quality
Generics).
• **CLIOQUINOL AND HYDROCORTISONE
OINTMENT, U.S.P.** U.S.P. XXIII.
Use: Topical antifungal.
See: Hysone, Cream (Hauck).

Vioform-Hydrocortisone, Cream, Oint., Lot. (Ciba).

Vio-Hydrocort, Cream, Oint. (Quality Generics).

CLINOXIDE. (Geneva G) Clidinium bromide 2.5 mg, chlordiazepoxide HCl 5 mg/Cap. Bot. 100s, 500s.
Use: Anticholinergic/antispasmodic.

CLIPOXIDE. (Schein) Clidinium bromide 2.5 mg, chlordiazepoxide HCl 5 mg/Cap. Bot. 100s, 500s.
Use: Anticholinergic/antispasmodic.

•**CLIPROFEN.** USAN.
Use: Anti-inflammatory.

•**CLOBAMINE MESYLATE.** USAN.
Use: Antidepressant.

•**CLOBAZAM.** USAN. 7-Chloro-1-methyl-5-phenyl-1,5-benzodiazepine-2,4-dione.
Use: Tranquilizer.

CLOBENZTROPINE. 3-(p-Chloro-a-phenylbenzyl-oxy)tropane.

•**CLOBETASOL PROPIONATE.** USAN.
Use: Corticosteroid.
See: Temovate, Cream, Oint., Scalp application (Glaxo Dermatology).

CLOBETASONE. B.A.N. 21-Chloro-9α-fluoro-17α-hydroxy-16β-methylpregna-1,4-diene-3,11,20-trione.
Use: Corticosteroid.

•**CLOBETASONE BUTYRATE.** USAN.
Use: Corticosteroid.

CLOCIGUANIL. B.A.N. 4,6-Diamino-1-(3,4-dichlorobenzyloxy)-1,2-dihydro-2,2-dimethyl-1,3,5-triazine.
Use: Antimalarial.

•**CLOCORTOLONE ACETATE.** USAN.
Use: Glucocorticoid.

•**CLOCORTOLONE PIVALATE, U.S.P.** U.S.P. XXIII. Cream, U.S.P. XXIII.
Use: Glucocorticoid.

CLOCREAM. (Upjohn) Vitamins A and D in vanishing base. Tube oz.
Use: Emollient.

•**CLODANOLENE.** USAN.
Use: Relaxant (skeletal muscle).

•**CLODAZON HYDROCHLORIDE.** USAN.
Use: Antidepressant.

CLODERM. (Hermal) Clocortolone pivalate cream 0.1%. Tube 15 Gm, 45 Gm.
Use: Corticosteroid.

•**CLODRONIC ACID.** USAN.
Use: Regulator.

•**CLOFAZIMINE, U.S.P.** U.S.P. XXIII. Cap., U.S.P. XXIII. USAN. 3-(p-Chloroanilino) 10-(p-chlorophenyl)-2,10-dihydro-2-(isopropylimino)-phena-zine.
Use: Tuberculostatic, leprostatic. [Orphan drug]
See: Lamprene, Cap. (Geigy).

•**CLOFIBRATE, U.S.P.** U.S.P. XXIII. Cap., U.S.P. XXIII. Ethyl 2-(p-chlorophenoxy) 2-methyl-propionate. Propanoic acid, 2-(4-chlorophenoxy)-2-methyl-, methyl ester.
Use: Antihyperlipidemic.
See: Atromid S, Cap. (Wyeth-Ayerst).

•**CLOFILIUM PHOSPHATE.** USAN.
Use: Cardiac depressant.

•**CLOFLUCARBAN.** USAN. 4,4'-Dichloro-3-(trifluoro-methyl)-carbanilide. Irgasan, CF3.
Use: Antiseptic.

CLOFLUPEROL. B.A.N. 4-(4-Chloro-3-trifluoro-methylphenyl)-1-[3-(4-fluorobenzoyl)propyl]piperidin-4-ol.
Use: Neuroleptic.

•**CLOGESTONE ACETATE.** USAN. 6-Chloro-3β, 17-dihydroxypregna-4,6-dien-20-one diacetate. Under study.
Use: Progesterone.

CLOGUANAMILE. B.A.N. 1-Amidino-3-(3-chloro-4- cyanophenyl)urea.
Use: Antimalarial.

CLOMACRAN. B.A.N. NN-Dimethyl-3-(2-chloro-9, 10-dihydroacridin-9-yl)propylamine.
Use: Tranquilizer.

•**CLOMACRAN PHOSPHATE.** USAN. 2-Chloro-9-[3-(dimethyl-amino)propyl] acridan phosphate (1:1). Under study.
Use: Tranquilizer.

•**CLOMEGESTONE ACETATE.** USAN. 6-Chloro- 17-acetoxy-1,6α-methyl-4,6-pregnadiene-3,20- dione. Under study.
Use: Progestin.

•**CLOMETHERONE.** USAN. 6α-Chloro-16α-methyl-pregn-4-ene-3,20-dione.
Use: Anti-estrogen.

CLOMID. (Marion Merrell Dow) Clomiphene citrate 50 mg/Tab. Carton 30s.
Use: Ovulation stimulant.

•**CLOMINOREX.** USAN.
Use: Anorexic.

•**CLOMIPHENE CITRATE, U.S.P.** U.S.P. XXIII. Tab., U.S.P. XXIII. 2-[p-(2-Chloro-1,2-diphenyl-vinyl)phenoxy]triethylamine dihydrogen citrate. Ethanamine, 2-[4-(2-chloro-1,2-diphenylethenyl)-phenoxy]-N,N-diethyl-,2-hydroxy-1,2,3-propanetricarboxylate(1:1). (Lemmon) 50 mg/Tab. Pkg. 10s, 30s.
Use: Ovulation stimulant.
See: Clomid, Tab. (Marion Merrell Dow).
Milophene, Tab. (Milex).
Serophene, Tab. (Serono).

CLOMIPRAMINE HCl. USAN. 3-Chloro-

5-[3-(dimethyl-amino)propyl]-10, 11-di-hydro-5H-dibenz-[b,f] azepine monohydrochloride.
Use: Antidepressant.
See: Anafranil (Ciba).
CLOMOCYCLINE. B.A.N. N^2-(Hydroxymethyl)-chlortetracycline.
Use: Antibiotic.
• **CLONAZEPAM, U.S.P.** U.S.P. XXIII. Tab., U.S.P. XXIII. 5-(o-Chlorophenyl)-1,3-di-hydro-7-nitro-2H-1,4-benzodiazepin-2-one. B.A.N. 5-(2-Chlorophenyl)-1,3-di-hydro-7-nitro-2H-1,4-benzodiazepin-2-one. Rivotril.
Use: Anticonvulsant.
See: Klonopin, Tab. (Roche).
• **CLONIDINE.** USAN. 2-(2,6-Dichloroanilino)-2-imida-zoline.
Use: Antihypertensive.
See: Catapres (Boehringer Ingelheim).
• **CLONIDINE HYDROCHLORIDE, U.S.P.** U.S.P. XXIII. Tabs., U.S.P. XXIII. Benzamine, 2,6-dichloro-N-2-imidazolidinylidene-, monoCl. (1)2-(2,6-Dichloranilino)-2-imidazoline monohydrochloride. (2)2-(2,6-Dichloro-phenylamino)-2-imidazoline HCl.
Use: Hypotensive. Epidural use for pain in cancer patients [Orphan drug]
See: Catapres, Tab. (Boehringer Ingelheim).
• **CLONIDINE HYDROCHLORIDE AND CHLORTHALIDONE TABLETS, U.S.P.** U.S.P. XXIII.
Use: Antihypertensive, diuretic.
See: Combipres, Tab. (Boehringer Ingelheim).
CLONITAZENE. B.A.N. 2-(4-Chlorobenzyl)-1-(2-diethylaminoethyl)-5-nitrobenzimidazole.
Use: Narcotic analgesic.
• **CLONITRATE.** USAN. 3-Chloro-1,2-propanediol dinitrate. Dylate.
Use: Coronary vasodilator.
• **CLONIXERIL.** USAN.
Use: Analgesic.
• **CLONIXIN.** USAN.
Use: Analgesic.
• **CLOPAMIDE.** USAN. **(1)** 4-Chloro-N-(2,6-dimethylpiperidino)-3-sulfamoylbenzamide; **(2)** 4-chloro-3-sulfamoylbenzoic acid 1,5-dimethylpentamethylenehydrazide.
Use: Antihypertensive, diuretic.
See: Aquex, Tab. (Lannett).
• **CLOPENTHIXOL.** USAN. BAN. 4-[3-(2-Chlorothioxanthen-9-ylidene)propyl]-1-piperazine-ethanol.
Use: Antipsychotic.

See: Sordinol (Wyeth-Ayerst).
• **CLOPERIDONE HYDROCHLORIDE.** USAN. 3-[3-[4-(m-Chlorophenyl)-1-piperazinyl] propyl]-2,-4-(IH, 3H)-quinazolinedione HCl.
Use: Sedative, tranquilizer.
CLOPHEDIANOL HCl.
See: Acutuss, Tab., Expect, (Philips Roxane).
CLOPHENOXATE HCl. 2-Dimethyllamino-ethyl p-chlorphenoxyacetate HCl.
Use: Cerebral stimulant.
• **CLOPIMOZIDE.** USAN.
Use: Antipsychotic.
• **CLOPIPAZAN MESYLATE.** USAN.
Use: Antipsychotic.
CLOPIRAC. USAN. 1-p-Chlorophenyl-2,5-dimethylpyrrol-3-ylacetic acid.
Use: Anti-inflammatory.
CLOPONONE. B.A.N. β,4-Dichloro-α-dichloro-acetamidopropiophenone.
Use: Antiseptic.
CLOPRA. (Quantum) Metoclopramide 10 mg (as monohydrochloride monohydrate)/Tab. Bot. 100s, 500s, 1000s.
Use: Antiemetic, gastrointestinal stimulant.
• **CLOPREDNOL.** USAN.
Use: Glucocorticoid.
• **CLOPROSTENOL SODIUM.** USAN.
Use: Prostaglandin.
CLOQUINATE. B.A.N. Chloroquine di-(8-hydroxy-7-iodoquinoline-5-sulfonate).
Use: Treatment of amebiasis.
• **CLORAZEPATE DIPOTASSIUM.** USAN. 7-Chloro-2,3-dihydro-2,2-dihydroxy-5-phenyl-IH-1,4-benzodiazepine-3-carboxylic acid dipotassium salt.
Use: Antianxiety, minor tranquilizer, anticonvulsant.
See: Tranxene, Cap. (Abbott).
• **CLORAZEPATE MONOPOTASSIUM.** USAN.
Use: Minor tranquilizer.
CLORAZEPIC ACID. B.A.N. 7-Chloro-2,3-dihydro-2,2-dihydroxy-5-phenyl-1H-1,4-benzodiazepine-3-carboxylic acid.
Use: Sedative.
• **CLORETHATE.** USAN.
Use: Sedative/hypnotic.
• **CLOREXOLONE.** USAN. 5-Chloro-2-cyclohexyl-6-sulfamoylisoindolin-1-one.
Use: Diuretic.
See: Nefrolan.
CLORFED II. (Stewart-Jackson) Chlorpheniramine 4 mg, pseudoephedrine 60 mg/Tab. Bot. 100s.
Use: Antihistamine, decongestant.

CLORFED CAPSULES. (Stewart-Jackson) Chlorpheniramine 8 mg, pseudoephedrine 120 mg/Cap. 100s.
Use: Antihistamine, decongestant.
CLORFED EXPECTORANT. (Stewart-Jackson) Pseudoephedrine 30 mg, guaifensen 100 mg, codeine 10 mg. Bot. pt.
Use: Decongestant, expectorant, antitussive.
CLORGYLINE. B.A.N. N-3-(2,4-Dichlorophenoxy) propyl-N-methylprop-2-ynylamine.
Use: Monoamine oxidase inhibitor, antidepressant.
CLORINDIONE. B.A.N. 2-(4-Chlorophenyl)indane-1,3-dione.
Use: Anticoagulant.
• **CLOROPERONE HYDROCHLORIDE.** USAN.
Use: Antipsychotic.
• **CLOROPHENE.** USAN. 4-Chloro-alpha-phenyl-o-cresol.
Use: Disinfectant.
See: Santophen 1 (Monsanto).
CLORPACTIN WCS-90. (Guardian) Sodium oxychlorosene. Bot. 2 Gm, 5s.
Use: Antiseptic.
• **CLORPRENALINE HYDROCHLORIDE.** USAN. (formerly Isoprophenamine HCl) 1-(α-Chlorophenyl)-2-isopropyl-aminoethanol hydrochloride hydrate. Vortel.
Use: Bronchodilator.
• **CLORSULON.** USAN.
Use: Antiparasitic, fasciolicide.
• **CLORTERMINE HCl.** USAN. o-Chloro-α,α-dimethylphenethylamine HCl.
Use: Anorexic.
• **CLOSANTEL.** USAN.
Use: Anthelmintic.
• **CLOSIRAMINE ACETURATE.** USAN.
Use: Antihistamine.
CLOSTEBOL ACETATE. B.A.N. 17β-Acetoxy-4-chloroandrost-4-en-3-one.
Use: Anabolic steroid.
• **CLOTHIAPINE.** USAN. 2-Chloro-11-(4-methyl-piperazin-1-yl)dibenzo[b,f][1,4]thiazepine.
Use: Tranquilizer.
• **CLOTHIXAMIDE MALEATE.** USAN. 4-[3-(2-Chlorothioxanthen-9-ylidene)propyl]-N-methyl-1-piperazinepropionamide dimaleate.
Use: Tranquilizer.
• **CLOTICASONE PROPIONATE.** USAN.
Use: Anti-inflammatory.
• **CLOTRIMAZOLE, U.S.P.** U.S.P. XXIII. Cream, Lot., Topical Soln., Vaginal Tab.,

U.S.P. XXIII. l-(o-Chloro-α,α-diphenylbenzyl)-imidazole. (Various Mfr.) **Vaginal Tab.:** 100 mg, in 7s with applicator. **Vaginal cream:** 1% Tube 45 g with applicator.
Use: Antifungal, candida infections.
See: FemCare,Vaginal Ta., Cream. (Schering-Plough).
Gyne-Lotrimin, Cream, Vaginal Tab. (Schering-Plough).
Lotrimin, Cream, Soln. (Schering).
Mycelex, Cream, Soln., Tab. (Miles Pharm).
Mycelex-7, Vaginal Cream, Tab. (Miles).
Mycelex-G, Vaginal Supp. (Miles Pharm).
CLOTRIMAZOLE. (NMC) Clotrimazole 1%, benzyl alcohol. Vaginal cream. In 45 g with 7 disposable applicators.
Use: Antifungal agent.
CLOTRIMAZOLE. (Taro) Clotrimazole 1% in a vanishing cream base, benzyl alcohol 1%, cetostearyl alcohol. Cream. Tube 15 g, 30 g, 45 g, 2 x 45 g.
Use: Antifungal agent.
• **CLOTRIMAZOLE AND BETAMETHASONE DIPROPIONATE CREAM, U.S.P.** U.S.P. XXIII.
Use: Antifungal, anti-inflammatory.
• **CLOVE OIL, U.S.P.** N.F. XVIII.
Use: Pharmaceutic aid (flavor).
CLOVERINE. (Medtech) White salve. Tin oz.
Use: Minor skin irritations.
CLOVOCAIN. (Vita Elixir) Benzocaine, oil of cloves.
Use: Local anesthetic.
• **CLOXACILLIN BENZATHINE, U.S.P.** U.S.P. XXIII. Intramammary Soln., Sterile, U.S.P. XXIII.
Use: Antibiotic.
• **CLOXACILLIN SODIUM, U.S.P.** U.S.P. XXIII., Cap., Intramammary Soln., Sterile, For Oral Soln., U.S.P. XXIII. 4-Thia-1-azabicyclo[3.2.0]heptane-2-carboxylic acid,6-[[[3-(2-chlorophenyl)-5-methyl-isoxazoly]carbonyl]amino]-3,3-dimethyl-7-oxo-,monosodium salt, monohydrate. Monosodium 6-[3-(o-chlorophenyl)-5-methyl-4-isoxazolecarboxamido]-3,3-dimethyl-7-oxo-4-thia-1-azabicyclo[3.2.0]heptane-2-carboxylate monohydrate.
Use: Antibiotic for resistant staph infections.
See: Cloxapen, Cap. (Beecham Labs). Tegopen, Cap., Granules (Bristol).
CLOXAPEN. (Beecham Labs) Cloxacillin sodium 250 mg or 500 mg/Cap. Bot.

100s.
Use: Antibacterial, penicillin.
• **CLOXYQUIN.** USAN.
Use: Antibacterial.
• **CLOZAPINE.** USAN. 8-Chloro-11-(4-methylpiperazin-1-yl)-5H-dibenzo[b,e][1,4]-diazepine.
Use: Antipsychotic.
See: Clozaril (Sandoz).
CLOZARIL. (Sandoz) Clozapine 25 mg or 100 mg/Tab. UD 100s, total daily dose packages of 150 mg, 200 mg, 250 mg, 300 mg, 400 mg, 500 mg, 600 mg/day.
Use: Antipsychotic.
CLUSIVOL SYRUP. (Whitehall) Vitamins A 2500 U.S.P. units, D-2 400 U.S.P. units, C 15 mg, B_{12} 2 mcg, B_1 1 mg, B_2 1 mg, niacinamide 5 mg, d-panthenol 3 mg, B_6 0.6 mg, manganese, 0.5 mg, zinc 0.5 mg, magnesium 3 mg/5 ml. Bot. 8 fl oz, 16 fl oz.
Use: Vitamin/mineral supplement.
CLYSODRAST. (Rhone-Poulenc Rhone-Poulenc Rorer) Tannic acid, 2.5 Gm, bisacodyl 1.5 mg per packet. Pow. Box 25s, 50s.
Use: Laxative.
C-MAX. (Bio-Tech) Vitamin C 1000 mg, magnesium 40 mg, zinc 5 mg, potassium 10 mg, manganese 1 mg, pectin in a base of rose hips 10 mg. Tabs. Bot. 100s.
Use: Vitamin/mineral supplement.
C.M.C. CELLULOSE GUM.
See: Carboxymethylcellulose Sodium, Preps.
CMV. (Wampole-Zeus) Cytomegalovirus antibody test system for the qualitative and semi-quantitative detection of CMV antibody in human serum. Test 100s.
Use: Diagnostic aid.
CMV-IGIV.
Use: Immune serum.
See: Cytomegalovirus Immune Globulin Intravenous, (Human).
Pow. for Inj. (Massachusetts Public Health Biologic Laboratories)
COADVIL. (Whitehall) Ibuprofen 200 mg, pseudoephedrine HCl 30 mg/Tab. Bot. 100s.
Use: Analgesic, decongestant.
COAGULATION FACTOR IX.
Use: Treatment of hemophilia B. [Orphan drug]
See: Mononine.
COAGULATION FACTOR IX (HUMAN).
Use: Treatment of hemophilia B. [Orphan drug]
See: AlphaNine.
COAGULANTS.

See: Hemostatics.
• **COAL TAR.** U.S.P. XXIII. Oint., Soln., U.S.P. XXIII.
Use: Topical antieczematic; antipsoriatic.
See: Balnetar, Liq. (Westwood).
Estar, Gel (Westwood).
L.C.D. Compound, Oint., Soln. (Al may).
Polytar Bath, Liq. (Stiefel).
Protar Protein, Shampoo (Dermol).
Tarbonis, Cream (Reed & Carnrick).
Zetar, Preps. (Dermik).
W/Allantoin, hydrocortisone.
See: Alphosyl-HC, Lot., Cream (Reed & Carnrick).
W/Hydrocortisone.
See: Doak Oil Forte, Liq. (Doak).
Tarcortin, Cream (Reed & Carnrick).
W/Iodoquinol, hydrocortisone.
See: ZeTar-Quin, Cream (Dermik).
W/Mercury oleate, salicylic acid, phenol, p-nitrophenol.
See: Prosol, Emulsion (Torch).
W/Zinc oxide.
See: Tarpaste, Paste (Doak).
COAL TAR BATH. (Durel) Coal tar solution 20%, polysorbate "20" 5%, isopropanol 75%. Bot. 8 oz, pt, gal.
Use: Tar-containing preparation, topical.
COAL TAR CREAM COTASOL. (Durel) Coal tar solution 5% in Duromantel cream. Jar 1 oz, 1 lb, 6 lb.
Use: Tar-containing preparation, topical.
COAL TAR, DISTILLATE.
Use: Tar-containing preparation, topical.
See: Lavatar, Liq. (Doak).
Syntar, Cream (Elder).
W/Sulfur, salicylic acid.
See: Pragmatar, Oint. (Menley & James).
COAL TAR EXTRACT.
Use: Tar-containing preparation, topical.
W/Allantoin, hexachlorophene.
See: Sebical Cream (Reed & Carnrick).
W/Allantoin, hexachlorophene, glycerin, lanolin.
See: Pso-Rite, Cream (DePree).
W/Allantoin, salicylic acid, perhydrosqualine.
See: Skaylos Cream (Ambix).
Skaylos Lotion (Ambix).
W/Salicylic acid, resorcinol, benzoic acid.
See: Mazon Cream (SK-Beecham).
COAL TAR PASTE.
Use: Tar-containing preparation, topical.
W/Zinc paste.
See: Tarpaste, Paste (Doak).
• **COAL TAR TOPICAL SOLUTION, U.S.P.** U.S.P. XXIII. Liquor Carbonis Deter-

gens. L.C.D.
Use: Anti-eczematic, topical.
See: Advanced Formula Tegrin, Shampoo (Block).
Balnetar, Liq. (Westwood).
Estar, Gel (Westwood).
L.C.D. Compound Oint., Soln. (Almay).
MG217 Medicated, Shampoo, Cond. (Triton).
Psorigel, Gel (Owen).
PsoriNail, Liq. (Summers).
Wright's Soln. (Fougera).
Zetar, Emulsion, Shampoo (Dermik).
W/Allantoin, psorilan, myristate.
See: Iocon, Shampoo (Owen).
Psorelief, Cream (Quality Generics).
W/Hydrocortisone, iodoquinol.
See: Cor-Tar-Quin, Cream, Lot. (Miles Pharm).
W/Hydrocortisone alcohol, clioquinololine, diperodon HCl, vitamins A, D.
See: Pentarcort, Cream (Dalin).
W/Robane (perhydrosqualene).
See: Skaylos Shampoo (Ambix).
W/Salicylic acid.
See: Epidol, Soln. (Spirt).
Ionil T, Shampoo (Owen).
W/Salicylic acid, sulfur, protein.
See: Vanseb-T Tar Shampoo (Herbert).
CO-APAP. (Various Mfr.) Pseudoephedrine HCl 30 mg, chlorpheniramine maleate 2 mg, dextromethorphan HBr 15 mg, acetaminophen 325 mg/Tab. Bot. 24s, 50s, 100s, 1000s.
Use: Decongestant, antihistamine, antitussive, analgesic.
COBALAMINE CONCENTRATE, U.S.P. U.S.P. XXI.
Use: Hematopoietic vitamin.
See: Vitamin B_{12} (Various Mfr.).
COBALT CHLORIDE.
W/Ferrous gluconate, vitamin B_{12}, duodenum whole desiccated.
See: Bitrinsic-E, Cap. (Elder).
COBALT GLUCONATE.
W/Ferrous gluconate, vitamin B_{12} activity, desiccated stomach substance, folic acid.
See: Chromagen, Cap., Inj. (Savage).
COBALT-LABELED VITAMIN B_{12}.
See: Rubratope-57 (Squibb).
COBALT STANDARDS FOR VITAMIN B_{12}.
See: Cobatope-57, and Cobatope-60 (Squibb).
• **COBALTOUS CHLORIDE Co 57.** USAN.
Use: Radioactive agent.
• **COBALTOUS CHLORIDE Co 60.** USAN.
Use: Radioactive agent.

COBATOPE-57. (Squibb) Cobaltous Cl Co 57.
COBEX 1000. (Standex) Vitamin B_{12} 1000 mcg/10 ml. Vial 30 ml.
Use: Vitamin B_{12} supplement.
CO-BILE. (Western Research) Hog bile 64.8 mg, pancreas substance 64.8 mg, papain-pepsin complex 97.2 mg, diatase malt 16.2 mg, papain 48.6 mg, pepsin 48.6 mg/Tab. Bot. 1000s.
Use: Digestive enzyme.
COBIRON. (Pharmex) Cyanocobalamin 100 mcg, hydroxycobalamine 50 mcg, ferrous gluconate 60 mg, liver inj. 5 mcg/2 ml, procaine HCl 2%, phenol 0.5%. Vial 30 ml.
Use: Vitamin/mineral supplement.
• **COCAINE, U.S.P.** U.S.P. XXIII. Methyl 3β-Hydroxy-1αH,-5αH-tropane-2β-carboxylate Benzoate (Ester) Alkaloid.
Use: Anesthetic (topical).
• **COCAINE HYDROCHLORIDE, U.S.P.** U.S.P. XXIII. Tab., for Topical Soln., U.S.P. XXIII. 8-Azabicyclo[3.2.1]octane-2-carboxylic acid, 3-(benzoyloxy)-8-methyl-, methyl ester, hydrochloride. Methyl 3β-hydroxy-1αH,5αH-tropan-2β-carboxylate, benzoate (ester) HCl.
Use: Mucosal anesthetic (topical).
COCAINE VISCOUS. (Roxane) Cocaine viscous 4%, 10%. Soln. Top. Bot. 4 ml, 10 ml.
Use: Local anesthetic.
CO-CARBOXYLASE. B.A.N. Pyrophosphoric ester of aneurine.
Use: Co-enzyme.
COCCIDIOIDIN.
See: Spherulin (Berkeley Biologicals).
COCCULIN.
See: Picrotoxin, Inj. (Various Mfr.).
COCILAN SYRUP. (Approved) Euphorbia, wild lettuce, cocillana, squill, senega, cascarin (bitterless). Bot. gal. Available w/codeine. Bot. gal.
COCILLANA.
W/Euphorbia pilulifera, squill, antimony potassium tartrate, senega.
See: Cylana Syr. (Bowman)
• **COCOA, U.S.P.** N.F. XVIII. Syr., N.F. XVI-II.
Use: Pharmaceutic aid (flavor; flavored vehicle).
• **COCOA BUTTER, U.S.P.** N.F. XVIII.
Use: Pharmaceutic aid (suppository base).
CODACTIDE. B.A.N. D-Ser[1]-Lys[17,18]-β[1]-[18]-corticotrophin amide.
Use: Corticotrophic peptide.
CODALAN NO. 1. (Lannett) Codeine phosphate 8 mg, acetaminophen 500

mg, caffeine 30 mg/Tab. Bot. 100s, 500s, 1000s.
Use: Narcotic analgesic combination.
CODALAN NO. 2. (Lannett) Codeine phosphate 15 mg/Tab. Bot. 100s, 500s, 1000s.
Use: Narcotic analgesic combination.
CODALAN NO. 3. (Lannett) Codeine phosphate 30 mg/Tab. Bot. 100s, 500s, 1000s.
Use: Narcotic analgesic combination.
CODAMINE PEDIATRIC SYRUP. (Barre-National) Hydrocodone bitartrate 2.5 mg, phenylpropanolamine HCl 12.5 mg. Bot. pt.
Use: Antitussive, decongestant.
CODAMINE SYRUP. (Goldline) Hydrocodone bitartrate 5 mg, phenylpropanolamine HCl 25 mg/5 ml. Bot. pt, gal.
Use: Antitussive, decongestant.
CODANOL OINTMENT. (A.P.C.) Vitamins A, D, hexachlorophene, zinc oxide. Tube 1.5 oz, 4 oz, Jar lb.
Use: Minor skin irritations.
CODAP. (Reid-Rowell) Codeine phosphate 32 mg, acetaminophen 325 mg/Tab. Bot. 250s.
Use: Narcotic analgesic combination.
CODASA I. (Stayner) Codeine phosphate 0.25 gr, aspirin 5 gr/Cap. Bot. 100s, 500s.
Use: Narcotic analgesic combination.
CODASA II. (Stayner) Codeine phosphate 0.5 gr, aspirin 5 gr/Cap. Bot. 100s, 500s.
Use: Narcotic analgesic combination.
CODASA FORTE. (Stayner) Codeine phosphate 0.5 gr, aspirin 10 gr/Cap. Bot. 100s, 500s.
Use: Narcotic analgesic combination.
CODASA TABS. (Stayner) Codeine phosphate 0.25 gr or 0.5 gr, aspirin 5 gr/Tab. Bot. 100s, 1000s.
Use: Narcotic analgesic combination.
CODEGEST EXPECTORANT. (Great Southern) Guaifenesin 100 mg, phenylpropanolamine HCl 12.5 mg, codeine phosphate 10 mg. Alcohol, dye free. Liq. Bot. pt, gal.
Use: Antitussive, decongestant, expectorant.
CODEHIST DH ELIXIR. (Geneva Generics) Pseudoephedrine 30 mg, chlorpheniramine maleate 2 mg, codeine phosphate 10 mg, alcohol 5.7%. Bot. 120 ml, 480 ml.
Use: Decongestant, antihistamine, antitussive.
•**CODEINE, U.S.P.** U.S.P.-XXIII. 7,8-Dide-

hydro-4,5α-epoxy-3-methoxy-17-methylmorphinan-6α-ol monohydrate. Crystal or Pow. Bot. ⅛ oz, 1 oz.
Use: Analgesic (narcotic); antitussive.
CODEINE COMBINATIONS.
See: Actifed-C, Expectorant, Syr. (Burroughs-Wellcome).
Anexsia w/Codeine, Tab. (Boooham Labs).
APAP w/Codeine, Tab. (Central).
A.P.C. w/Codeine, Tab. (Various Mfr.).
Ascriptin W/Codeine No. 2, Tab. (Rhone-Poulenc Rorer).
Ascriptin W/Codeine No. 3, Tab. (Rhone-Poulenc Rorer).
Buff-A-Compound, Tab. (Mayrand).
Calcidrine Syr. (Abbott).
Capital w/Codeine, Susp. (Carnrick).
Cheracol, Syr. (Upjohn).
Chlor-Trimeton Expectorant (Schering).
Codalan, Tab. (Lannett).
Codasa I and II, Cap. (Stayner).
Colrex Compound, Cap., Elix. (Reid-Rowell).
Cosanyl Cough Syrup (Health Care Ind.).
Drucon w/Codeine, Liq. (Standard Drug).
Empirin No. 1, No. 2, No. 3, No. 4, Tab. (Burroughs-Wellcome).
Fiorinal w/Codeine, Cap. (Sandoz).
G-3, Cap. (Hauck).
Golacol, Syr. (Arcum).
Novahistine, Expectorant (Marion Merrell Dow).
Nucofed, Liq. (Beecham).
Partuss AC (Parmed).
Pediacof, Syr. (Sanofi Winthrop).
Phenaphen #2, #3, #4, Cap. (Robins).
Phenaphen-650, Cap. (Robins).
Phenatuss, Liq. (Dalin).
Phenergan Expectorant w/Codeine, Troches (Wyeth-Ayerst).
Proval No. 3, Tab. (Reid-Rowell).
Prunicodeine, Syr. (Lilly).
Robitussin A-C, DAC (Robins).
Tega-Code, Cap. (Ortega).
Tolu-Sed, Elix. (Scherer).
Tussar-2, Syr. (Rhone-Poulenc Rorer).
Tussar SF, Liq. (Rhone-Poulenc Rorer).
Tussi-Organidin, Liq. (Wallace).
Tylenol w/Codeine No. 1, No. 2, No. 3, No. 4 Tab. (McNeil).
Tylenol w/Codeine, Elix. (McNeil).
Vasotus, Liq. (Sheryl).
CODEINE METHYLBROMIDE. Eucodin.
Use: Antitussive.
•**CODEINE PHOSPHATE, U.S.P.** U.S.P.

XXIII. Inj., Tab., U.S.P. XXIII. (Various Mfr.) Pow. Bot. ⅛ oz, 0.25 oz, 0.5 oz, 1 oz.
Use: Narcotic analgesic, antitussive.
•**CODEINE POLISTIREX.** USAN.
Use: Antitussive.
CODEINE RESIN COMPLEX COMBINATIONS.
See: Omni-Tuss, Liq. (Pennwalt).
•**CODEINE SULFATE, U.S.P.** U.S.P. XXIII.
Tab., U.S.P. XXIII. 7,8-Didehydro-4,5α-epoxy-3-methoxy-17-methyl-morphinan-6α-ol sulfate.
Use: Narcotic analgesic, antitussive.
CODELCORTONE.
See: Prednisolone.
CODICLEAR DH SYRUP. (Central) Hydrocodone bitartrate 5 mg, guaifenesin 100 mg/5 ml. Bot. 4 oz, pt.
Use: Antitussive, expectorant.
CODIMAL. (Central) Chlorpheniramine maleate 2 mg, pseudoephedrine HCl 30 mg, acetaminophen 325 mg/Cap. Bot. 24s, 100s, 1000s.
Use: Antihistamine, decongestant, analgesic.
CODIMAL DH SYRUP. (Central) Hydrocodone bitartrate 1.66 mg, phenylephrine HCl 5 mg, pyrilamine maleate 8.33 mg/5 ml. Bot. 4 oz, pt, gal.
Use: Antitussive, decongestant, antihistamine.
CODIMAL DM. (Central) Dextromethorphan HBr 10 mg, phenylephrine HCl 5 mg, pyrilamine maleate 8.33 mg/5 ml, alcohol 4%, saccharin, sorbitol. Sugar free. Bot. 4 oz, pt, gal.
Use: Antitussive, decongestant, antihistamine.
CODIMAL EXPECTORANT. (Central) Phenylpropanolamine HCl 25 mg, guaifenesin 100 mg/5 ml. Menthol. Bot. 4 oz, pt.
Use: Decongestant, expectorant.
CODIMAL-L.A. (Central) Chlorpheniramine maleate 8 mg, pseudoephedrine HCl 120 mg/SR Cap. Bot. 100s, 1000s.
Use: Antihistamine, decongestant.
CODIMAL-L.A. HALF CAPSULES. (Central) Pseudoephedrine HCl 60 mg, chlorpheniramine maleate 4 mg, sucrose. Cap. Bot. 100s.
Use: Decongestant, antihistamine.
CODIMAL PH SYRUP. (Central) Codeine phosphate 10 mg, phenylephrine HCl 5 mg, pyrilamine maleate 8.33 mg/5 ml. Bot. 4 oz, pt, gal.
Use: Antitussive, decongestant, antihistamine.
CODIMAL TABLETS. (Central) Chlor-

pheniramine maleate 2 mg, pseudoephedrine HCl 30 mg, acetaminophen 325 mg/Tab. Bot. 24s, 100s, 1000s.
Use: Antihistamine, decongestant, analgesic.
•**COD LIVER OIL, U.S.P.** U.S.P. XXIII.
Emulsion.
Use: Vitamin A and D therapy.
See: Cod Liver Oil Concentrate Cap. (Schering).
W/Anesthesin, zinc oxide, hydroxyquinoline.
See: Medicone Dressing. (Medicone).
W/Benzocaine.
See: Morusan, Oint. (Beecham Labs).
W/Creosote. (Bryant) Cod liver oil 9 min, creosote 1 min/Cap. Bot. 100s.
W/Malt extract (Burroughs Wellcome) Vitamins A 6450 IU, D 645 IU. Bot. 10 fl oz, 20 fl oz.
W/Methylbenzethonium Cl.
See: Benephen, Prods. (Halsted).
W/Viosterol.
(Abbott) Vitamins A 2800 IU, D 255 IU/Gm. Bot. 12 fl oz.
(Squibb) Vitamins A 2000 IU, D 440 IU/Gm. Bot. 4 fl oz, 12 fl oz.
W/Zinc oxide.
See: Desitin, Preps. (Leeming).
COD LIVER OIL CONCENTRATE.
(Schering) Concentrate of cod liver oil with vitamins A and D added. **Cap.:** Bot. 40s, 100s. **Tab.:** Bot. 100s, 240s. Also W/Vitamin C. Bot. 100s.
Use: Vitamin supplement.
COD LIVER OIL OINTMENT.
See: Moruguent, Oint. (Beecham Labs).
•**CODORPHONE HYDROCHLORIDE.**
USAN.
Use: Analgesic.
•**CODOXIME.** USAN.
Use: Antitussive.
•**CODOXY.** (Halsey) Oxycodone HCl 4.5 mg, oxycodone terephthalate 0.38 mg, aspirin 325 mg/Tab. Bot. 100s.
Use: Narcotic analgesic combination.
COGENTIN. (Merck & Co.) Benztropine Mesylate **Tab.:** 0.5 mg Bot. 100s; 1 mg Bot. 100s, UD 100s; 2 mg Bot. 100s, 1000s, UD 100s. **Inj.:** Benztropine mesylate 1 mg/ml w/sodium Cl 9 mg and water for injection q.s. to 1 ml Amp. 2 ml, Box 6s.
Use: Antiparkinson agent.
CO-GESIC. (Central) Hydrocodone bitartrate 5 mg, acetaminophen 500 mg/Tab. Bot. 100s, 500s.
Use: Narcotic analgesic combination.
COGNEX. (Parke-Davis) Tacrine HCl 10

mg, 20 mg, 30 mg, 40 mg. Cap. Bot. 120s, UD 100s.
Use: Psychotherapeutic agent.
CO-HEP-TRAL. (Davis & Sly) Folic acid 10 mg, vitamin B_{12} 100 mcg, liver injection q.s./ml. Vial 10 ml.
Use: Vitamin/mineral supplement.
COLABID TABS. (Major) Probenecid 500 mg, colchicine 0.5 mg/Tab. Bot. 100s, 1000s.
Use: Agent for gout.
COLACE. (Bristol-Myers) Docusate sodium. **Cap.:** 50 mg or 100 mg. Bot. 30s, 60s, 250s, 1000s, UD 100s. **Syr.:** 60 mg/15 ml with alcohol < 1%. Bot. 240 ml, 480 ml. **Liq.:** 150 mg/15 ml. Bot. 30 ml, 480 ml with calibrated droppers.
Use: Laxative.
COLAGYN. (Smith) Zinc sulfocarbolate, potassium, oxyquinoline sulfate, lactic acid, boric acid. Jelly. Tube w/applicator and refill 6 oz. Douche Pow. 3 oz, 7 oz, 14 oz.
COLANA SYRUP. (Hance) Euphorbia pilulifera tincture 8 ml, wild lettuce syrup 8 ml, cocillana tincture 2.5 ml, squill compound syrup 1.5 ml, cascara 0.25 Gm, menthol 4.8 mg/fl oz. Bot. 4 fl oz, gal. Also w/Dionin 15 mg/fl oz. Bot. gal.
COLASPASE. B.A.N. L-Asparagine amidohydrolase obtained from cultures of *Escherichia coli.*
See: Crasnitin.
CO-LAV. (Copley) Polyethylene glycol 3350 Gm, sodium chloride 1.46 Gm, potassium chloride 0.745 Gm, sodium bicarbonate 1.68 Gm, sodium sulfate 5.68 Gm per L. Liq. Jug 4 L.
Use: Bowel evacuant.
COLAX. (Rugby) Docusate sodium 100 mg, phenolphthalein 65 mg/Tab. Bot. 30s.
Use: Laxative.
COLBENEMID. (Merck & Co.) Probenecid 0.5 Gm, colchicine 0.5 mg/Tab. Bot. 100s.
Use: Agent for gout.
•**COLCHICINE, U.S.P.** U.S.P. XXIII. Tab., Inj. U.S.P. XXIII. Acetamide, N-(5,6,7,9-tetrahydro-1,2,3,10-tetrame-thoxy-9-oxobenzo[a]heptalen-7-yl)-.(Various Mfr.).
Use: Gout suppressant. Treat multiple sclerosis [Orphan drug]
W/Benemid.
See: Colbenemid, Tab. (Merck & Co.).
W/Methyl salicylate. (Parke-Davis) Colchicine gr, methyl salicylate 3 min/Cap. Bot. 100s, 500s, 1000s.
Use: Orally, gout therapy.

W/Probenecid.
See: Benn-C, Tab. (Scrip).
Colbenemid, Tab. (Merck & Co.).
Robenecid with colchicine, Tab. (Robinson).
W/Sodium salicylate.
See: Salcoce, Tab. (Cole).
W/Sodium salicylate, calcium carbonate, dried aluminum hydroxide gel, phenobarbital.
See: Apcogesic, Tabs. (Apco).
W/Sodium salicylate, potassium iodide.
See: Bricolide, Tab. (Briar).
COLCHICINE SALICYLATE.
W/Phenobarbital, sodium p-aminobenzoate, vitamin B_1, aspirin.
See: Doloral, Tab. (Alamed).
COLD CREAM, U.S.P. U.S.P. XXI.
Use: Emollient; water in oil emulsion ointment base.
COLDONYL. (Dover) Acetaminophen, phenylephrine HCl/Tab. Sugar, lactose and salt free. UD Box 500s.
Use: Analgesic, decongestant.
COLDRAN. (Blue Cross) Phenylephrine HCl 5 mg, chlorpheniramine maleate 2 mg, salicylamide 1.5 gr, acetaminophen 0.5 gr, caffeine/Tab. Bot. 30s.
Use: Decongestant, antihistamine, analgesic.
COLD RELIEF. (Rugby) Phenylpropanolamine HCl, chlorpheniramine maleate 2 mg, dextromethorphan HBr 10 mg, acetaminophen 325 mg/Tab. Bot. 50s.
Use: Decongestant, antihistamine, antitussive, analgesic.
COLDRINE. (Hauck) Acetaminophen 200 mg, pseudoephedrine HCl 30 mg/Tab. Bot. 1000s.
Use: Analgesic, decongestant.
COLD SORE LOTION. (McKesson) Bot. 0.25 oz.
Use: Cold sores.
COLD SORE LOTION. (Purepac) Camphor, benzoin, aluminum Cl. Bot. 0.5 oz.
Use: Cold sores.
COLD TABLETS. (Walgreen) Phenylphrine HCl 5 mg, chlorpheniramine maleate 2 mg, acetaminophen 325 mg/Tab. Bot. 50s.
Use: Decongestant, antihistamine, analgesic.
COLD TABLETS MULTIPLE SYMPTOM. (Walgreen) Acetaminophen 500 mg, pseudoephedrine HCl 30 mg, chlorpheniramine maleate 2 mg, dextromethorphan HBr 10 mg/Tab. Bot. 50s.
Use: Analgesic, decongestant, antihistamine, antitussive.

COLD VACCINES, ORAL. (Sherman) Oral Tabs.
See: Entoral, Pulvule (Lilly).
COLESTID. (Upjohn) Colestipol HCl 5 Gm/pkt. Box 30s, Bot. 500 Gm.
Use: Antihyperlipidemic.
• **COLESTIPOL HYDROCHLORIDE, U.S.P.** U.S.P. XXIII. For Oral Susp., U.S.P. XXIII.
Use: Antihyperlipoproteinemic.
See: Colestid (Upjohn).
COL-EVAC. (Forest) Potassium bitartrate, bicarbonate of soda and a blended base of polyethylene glycols. Supp. 2s, 12s.
COLEXUSS. (Jenkins) White pine 56.7 mg, wild cherry 56.7 mg, American spikenard 6 mg, poplar bud 6 mg, sanguinaria 5 mg, menthol 0.5 mg/fldr. Bot. 3 oz, 4 oz, gal.
Use: Cough syrup.
COLFANT. (Jenkins) Paregoric 2 min (pow. opium $^1/_{125}$ gr), sodium bicarbonate 1 gr, magnesium trisilicate gr, catnip extract gr, chamomile extract gr (Matricaria), oil fennel q.s./Tab. Bot. 1000s.
Use: Narcotic analgesic, antacid.
COLFED-A CAPSULES. (Parmed) Pseudoephedrine HCl 120 mg, chlorphenlramine maleate 8 mg. Bot 100s.
• **COLFORSIN.** USAN.
Use: Antiglaucoma agent.
• **COLFOSCERIL PALMITATE.** Synthetic pulmonary surfactant.
Use: Prevention/treatment of hyaline membrane disease. [Orphan drug]
See: Exosurf (Burroughs Wellcome).
• **COLFOSCERIL PALMITATE.** USAN.
Use: Antiatelectic.
COLIMYCIN SODIUM METHANESULFONATE.(Parke-Davis).
See: Colistimethate Sodium.
COLIMYCIN SULFATE. (Parke-Davis).
See: Coly-Mycin, Preps. (Parke-Davis).
• **COLISTIMETHATE SODIUM, STERILE, U.S.P.** U.S.P. XXIII. Sodium Colistin Methanesulfonate. Colistin methane sulfonic acid, pentasodium salt. Pentasodium colistin methanesulfonate.
Use: Antibiotic.
See: Coly-Mycin-M, Injectable (Parke-Davis).
COLISTIN. B.A.N. A mixture of polypeptides produced by strains of *Bacillus polymyxa var. colistinus.*
Use: Antibiotic.
COLISTIN BASE.
W/Neomycin base, hydrocortisone acetate, thonzonium bromide, polysorbate 80, acetic acid, sodium acetate.

See: Coly-Mycin Otic W/Neomycin and Hydrocortisone, Liq. (Parke-Davis).
COLISTIN METHANESULFONATE.
See: Colistimethate Sodium.
COLISTIN AND NEOMYCIN SULFATES AND HYDROCORTISONE ACETATE OTIC SUSPENSION, U.S.P. U.S.P. XXIII.
Use: Antibiotic, anti-inflammatory.
• **COLISTIN SULFATE, U.S.P.** U.S.P. XXIII. Oral Susp., U.S.P. XXIII. The sulfate salt of an antibiotic substance elaborated by *Aerobacillus colistinus.*
Use: Antibacterial.
See: Colymycin-S Ophthalmic (Parke-Davis).
Coly-Mycin S Susp. (Parke-Davis).
COLISTIN SULFOMETHATE. B.A.N. An antibiotic obtained from colistin sulfate by sulfomethylation with formaldehyde and sodium bisulfite.
Use: Anti-infective.
CO-LIVER. (Standex) Folic acid 1 mg, vitamin B_{12} 100 mcg, liver 10 mcg/ml. Vial 10 ml.
Use: Vitamin/mineral supplement.
COLLADERM. (C & M Pharmacal) Purified water, glycerin, soluble collagen, hydrolysed elastin, allantoin, ethylhydroxy cellulose, sorbic, octoxynol-9. Bot. 2.3 oz.
Use: Emollient.
COLLAGENASE.
See: Santyl (Knoll).
COLLAGENASE ABC OINTMENT. (Advance Biofactures) Collagenase 250 units/Gm in white petrolatum. 25 Gm, 50 Gm.
Use: Topical enzyme preparation.
COLLAGEN IMPLANT. (Lacrimedics) In 0.2 mm, 0.3 mm, 0.4 mm, 0.5 mm. 0.6 mm. Box 12s.
use: Collagen implant, ophthalmic.
COLLAGEN IMPLANT.
See: Zyderm I. (Collagen Corp.).
Zyderm II. (Collagen Corp.).
COLLASTIN OIL FREE MOISTURIZER. (Dermol) Soluble collagen, hydrolyzed elastin. Lot. Bot. 60 ml.
Use: Emollient.
• **COLLODION, U.S.P.** U.S.P. XXIII. Flexible, U.S.P. XXIII.
Use: Topical protectant.
COLLOIDAL ALUMINUM HYDROXIDE.
See: Aluminum Hydroxide Gel, U.S.P. XXIII.
COLLOIDAL GOLD.
See: Aureotope (Squibb).
COLLOIDAL SILVER IODIDE.
See: Neo-Silvol, Soln. (Parke-Davis).

COLLYRIUM FOR FRESH EYES. (Wyeth-Ayerst) Neutral borate solution with boric acid, sodium borate, thimerosal ≤ 0.002%. Bot. 120 ml.
Use: Extraocular irrigating solution.

COLLYRIUM FRESH EYE DROPS. Tetrahydrozoline HCl 0.05%, benzalkonium chlorido 0.01%, EDTA 0.1%, glycerin 1%. Bot. 15 ml.
Use: Ophthalmic vasoconstrictor/mydriatic.

COLOCARE. (Helena Labs) In-home fecal test. Kit. 3s.
Use: Diagnostic aid.

COLOCTYL. (Vitarine) Docusate sodium 100 mg/Cap. Bot. 100s, 1000s, UD 1000s.
Use: Laxative.

COLOGEL. (Lilly) Methylcellulose 450 mg/5 ml, alcohol 5%, saccharin. Bot. 16 fl oz.
Use: Laxative.

COLONY STIMULATING FACTOR.
Use: Adjunct during antineoplastic therapy.
See: Leukine (Immunex)
Neupogen (Amgen).
Prokine (Hoechst-Roussel).

COLOR ALLERGY SCREENING TEST.
See: CAST (Biomerica).

COLOR OVULATION TEST. (Biomerica) Monoclonal antibody-based enzyme immunoassay test for hLH in urine. Kit. 9-day test kit.
Use: To predict ovulation.

COLOSCREEN. (Helena Labs) Occult blood screening test. Kit 12s, 25s, 50s. 3 tests per kit.
Use: Diagnostic aid.

COLOSCREEN/VPI. (Helena Labs) Occult blood screening test. Box 100s, 1000s.
Use: Diagnostic aid.

COLOVAGE. (Dyna Pharm) Powder for reconstitution to produce 1 gal soln. Containing sodium Cl 5.53 Gm, potassium Cl 2.82 Gm, sodium bicarbonate 6.36 Gm, sodium sulfate anhydrous 21.5 Gm, polyethylene glycol 3350. Pkg. 1s.
Use: Laxative.

COL-PROBENECID. (Various Mfr.) Probenecid 500 mg, colchicine 0.5 mg/Tab. Bot. 100s, 1000s, UD 100s.
Use: Agent for gout.

COLTAB CHILDREN'S. (Hauck) Phenylephrine HCl 2.5 mg, chlorpheniramine maleate 1 mg/Chew. tab. Bot. 30s.

Use: Decongestant, antihistamine.

• **COLTEROL MESYLATE.** USAN.
Use: Bronchodilator.

COLY-MYCIN M PARENTERAL. (Parke-Davis) Colistimethate sodium equivalent 150 mg colistin base per vial.
Use: Anti-infective.

COLY-MYCIN S ORAL SUSPENSION. (Parke-Davis) Colistin sulfate 300 mg/60 ml. For oral susp. Bot. 300 mg.
Use: Anti-infective.

COLY-MYCIN S OTIC DROPS W/NEOMYCIN AND HYDROCORTISONE. (Parke-Davis) Colistin base as the sulfate 3 mg, neomycin base as the sulfate 3.3 mg, hydrocortisone acetate 10 mg, thonzonium bromide 0.5 mg/ml, polysorbate 80, acetic acid, sodium acetate, thimerosal. Dropper bot. 5 ml, 10 ml.
Use: Anti-infective.

COLYTE. (Reed & Carnrick) **2L:** PEG (Polyethylene glycol-electrolyte solution) 3350 120 Gm, sodium sulfate 11.36 Gm, sodium bicarbonate 3.36 Gm, sodium Cl 2.92 Gm, potassium Cl 1.49 Gm. **1 gal:** PEG 3350 227.1 Gm, sodium sulfate 21.5 Gm, sodium bicarbonate 6.36 Gm, sodium Cl 5.53 Gm, potassium Cl 2.82 Gm. **6 L:** PEG 3350 360 Gm, sodium sulfate 34.08 Gm, sodium bicarbonate 10.08 Gm, sodium Cl 8.76 Gm, potassium Cl 4.47 Gm. Pack 5.
Bot. 2 L, gal, 4L, 6L.
Use: Bowel evacuant for GI exams.

COMBICAL D. (Mills) Calcium 375 mg, vitamin D 400 IU, phosphorus 180 mg, magnesium 144 mg/3 Tab. Bot. 1000s.
Use: Vitamin/mineral supplement.

COMBICHOLE. (Trout) Dehydrocholic acid 2 gr, desoxycholic acid 1 gr/Tab. Bot. 100s, 1000s.
Use: Hydrocholeretic.

COMBIPRES TABLETS. (Boehringer Ingelheim) **0.1 mg:** Clonidine HCl 0.1 mg, chlorthalidone 15 mg/Tab. Bot. 100s, 1000s. **0.2 mg:** Clonidine HCl 0.2 mg, chlorthalidone 15 mg/Tab. Bot. 100s, 1000s. **0.3 mg:** Clonidine HCl 0.3 mg, chlorthalidone 15 mg/Tab. Bot. 100s.
Use: Antihypertensive.

COMBISTIX REAGENT STRIPS. (Miles Diagnostic) Protein test-tetrabromphenol blue, citrate buffer, protein-absorbing agent; glucose test area-glucose oxidase, orthotolidin and a catalyst; pH test area methyl red and bromthymol blue. Box, strips, 100s.
Use: Diagnostic aid.

COMFORTCARE GP WETTING & SOAK-ING. (Pilkington Barnes Hind) Buffered, isotonic. Chlorhexidine gluconate 0.005%, EDTA 0.02%, octyl phenoxy (oxyethylene) ethanol, povidone, polyvinyl alcohol, propylene glycol, hydroxyethyl cellulose, NaCl. Soln. Bot. 120 ml or 240 ml.
Use: Contact lens care.

COMFORT DROPS. (Barnes-Hind) Isotonic solution containing naphazoline 0.03%, benzalkonium Cl 0.005%, edetate disodium 0.02%. Bot. 15 ml.
Use: Hard contact lens care.

COMFORT EYE DROPS. (Pilkington Barnes-Hind) Naphazoline HCl 0.03%, disodium edetate 0.02%, benzalkonium Cl 0.005%. Plastic dropper bot. 15 ml.
Use: Ophthalmic decongestant.

COMFORT GEL LIQUID. (Walgreen) Aluminum hydroxide compressed gel 200 mg, magnesium hydroxide 200 mg, simethicone 20 mg/5 ml. Bot. 12 oz.
Use: Antacid, antiflatulent.

COMFORT GEL TABLETS. (Walgreen) Magnesium hydroxide 85 mg, simethicone 25 mg, aluminum hydroxide-magnesium carbonate codried gel 282 mg/Tab. Bot. 100s.
Use: Antacid, antiflatulent.

COMFORTINE. (Dermik) Zinc oxide 12%, vitamins A and D, lanolin in protective base. Oint. Tube 1.5 oz, 4 oz.
Use: Emollient.

COMFORT TEARS. (Pilkington Barnes-Hind) Hydroxyethyl cellulose, benzalkonium Cl 0.005%, edetate disodium 0.02%. Bot. 15 ml.
Use: Soft contact lens care.

COMHIST L.A. CAPSULES. (Norwich Eaton) Phenylephrine HCl 20 mg, chlorpheniramine maleate 4 mg, phenyltoloxamine citrate 50 mg/Cap. Bot. 100s.
Use: Decongestant, antihistamine.

COMHIST TABLETS. (Norwich Eaton) Phenylephrine HCl 10 mg, chlorpheniramine maleate 2 mg, phenyltoloxamine citrate 25 mg/Tab. Bot. 100s.
Use: Decongestant, antihistamine.

COMPAL. (Reid-Rowell) Dihydrocodeine 16 mg, acetaminophen 356.4 mg, caffeine 30 mg/Cap. Bot. 100s.
Use: Analgesic combination.

COMPAT NUTRITION ENTERAL DELIVERY SYSTEM. (Sandoz Nutrition) Top fill feeding containers 600 ml, 1400 ml. Gravity delivery set. Pump delivery set. Compat enteral feeding pump.
Use: Enteral nutritional supplement.

COMPAZINE. (SK-Beecham) Prochlorperazine as the maleate. **Tab.:** 5 mg, 10 mg or 25 mg. Bot. 100s, 1000s, UD 100s (except for 25 mg). **Inj.:** Edisylate salt 5 mg/ml. Amp. 2 ml, vial 10 ml, disposable syringe 2 ml. **SR Spansule:** Maleate salt 10 mg, 15 mg or 30 mg. Bot. 50s, 500s, UD 100s. **Supp.:** 2.5 mg, 5 mg or 25 mg. Box 12s. **Syr.:** Edisylate salt 5 mg/5 ml. Bot. 4 fl oz.
Use: Antiemetic, antipsychotic.

COMPETE. (Mission) Iron 27 mg, vitamins A 5000 IU, D 400 IU, E 45 IU, B_1 2.25 mg, B_2 2.6 mg, B_3 30 mg, B_6 25 mg, B_{12} 9 mcg, C 90 mg, folic acid 0.4 mg, Zn/Tab. Bot. 100s.
Use: Vitamin/mineral supplement.

COMPLEAT-B MEAT BASE FORMULA. (Sandoz Nutrition) Beef, nonfat milk, hydrolyzed cereal solids, maltodextrin, pureed fruits and vegetables, corn oil, mono and diglycerides. Bot. 250 ml, Can 250 ml.
Use: Enteral nutritional supplement.

COMPLEAT-MODIFIED FORMULA MEAT BASE. (Sandoz Nutrition) Hydrolyzed cereal solids, calcium caseinate, pureed fruits and vegetables, corn oil, beef puree, mono and diglycerides. Can 250 ml.
Use: Enteral nutritional supplement.

COMPLEAT-REGULAR FORMULA. (Sandoz Nutrition) Deionized water, beef puree, hydrolyzed cereal solids, green bean puree, pea puree, nonfat milk, corn oil, maltodextrin, peach puree, orange juice, mono and diglycerides, carrageenan, vitamins, minerals. Bot. 250 ml, Can 250 ml.
Use: Enteral nutritional supplement.

COMPLETE. (Mission) Vitamins A 5000 IU, D 400 IU, E 45 IU, C 90 mg, B_1 2.25 mg, folic acid 0.4 mg, B_2 2.6 mg, B_3 30 mg, B_6 25 mg, B_{12} 9 mcg, ferrous gluconate 233 mg, zinc 22.5 mg/Tab. Bot. 100s, 1000s.
Use: Vitamin/mineral supplement.

COMPLETONE ELIXIR FORT. (Sanofi Winthrop) Ferrous gluconate.
Use: Iron supplement.

COMPLEX 15 CREAM. (Baker/Cummins) Jar 4 oz.
Use: Emollient.

COMPLEX 15 LOTION. (Baker/Cummins) Bot. 8 oz.
Use: Emollient.

COMPLEX ZINC CARBONATES. *See:* Zinc (Sublingual Products).

COMPLY LIQUID. (Sherwood) Sodium caseinate, calcium caseinate, hydrolyzed cornstarch, sucrose, corn oil,

soy lecithin, vitamins A, B_1, B_2, B_3, B_5, B_6, B_{12}, C, D, E, K, folic acid, biotin, choline, Ca, Cl, Cu, Fe, I, Mg, Mn, P, Zn. Can 250 ml, Bot. 200 ml.
Use: Enteral nutritional supplement.
COMPOUND 42.
See: Warfarin (Various Mfr.).
COMPOUND B.
See: Corticosterone (Various Mfr.).
COMPOUND CB3025.
See: Alkeran, Tab. (Burroughs Wellcome).
COMPOUND E. (Kendall).
See: Cortisone Acetate. (Various Mfr.).
COMPOUND F.
See: Hydrocortisone (Various Mfr.).
COMPOUND Q.
Use: Antiviral.
See: Trichosanthine (Genelabs).
COMPOUND S.
Use: Antiviral.
See: Retrovir (Burroughs).
Zidovudine.
COMPOUND W. (Whitehall) Salicylic acid 17% w/w in flexible collodion vehicle w/ether 63.5%. Bot. 0.31 oz.
Use: Keratolytic.
COMPOZ. (Medtech) **Tab.**: Diphenhydramine HCl 50 mg Pkg. 12s, 24s. **Cap.**: Diphenhydramine HCl 25 mg Pkg. 16s.
Use: OTC sleep aid.
COMPRECIN.
See: Penetrex (Warner-Lambert).
COMTREX. (Bristol-Myers) Acetaminophen 325 mg, pseudoephedrine HCl 30 mg, chlorpheniramine maleate 2 mg, dextromethorphan HBr 10 mg/Tab. Bot. 24s, 50s.
Use: Analgesic, decongestant, antihistamine, antitussive.
COMTREX A/S. (Bristol-Myers) **Tab.**: Pseudoephedrine HCl 30 mg, chlorpheniramine maleate 2 mg, acetaminophen 500 mg. Bot. 24s, 50s. **Capl.**: Pseudoephedrine HCl 30 mg, chlorpheniramine maleate 2 mg, acetaminophen 500 mg. Bot. 50s, UD 24s.
Use: Decongestant, antihistamine, analgesic.
COMTREX CAPLETS. (Bristol-Myers) Acetaminophen 325 mg, pseudoephedrine HCl 30 mg, chlorpheniramine maleate 2 mg, dextromethorphan HBr 10 mg/Capl. Bot. 24s, 50s.
Use: Analgesic, decongestant, antihistamine, antitussive.
COMTREX COUGH FORMULA. (Bristol-Myers) Pseudoephedrine HCl 15 mg, dextromethorphan 7.5 mg, guaifenesin 50 mg, acetaminophen 125 mg/5 ml, al-

cohol 20%. Bot. 120 ml, 240 ml.
Use: Decongestant, antitussive, expectorant, analgesic.
COMTREX DAY-NIGHT. (Bristol-Myers) **Night:** Pseudoephedrine HCl 30 mg, chlorpheniramine maleate 2 mg, dextromethorphan HBr 10 mg, acetaminophen 325 mg/Tab. Pkg. 6s. **Day:** Pseudoephedrine HCl 30 mg, dextromethrophan HBr 10 mg, acetaminophen 500 mg/Tab. Pkg. 18s.
Use: Antitussive, decongestant, antihistamine.
COMTREX LIQUID. (Bristol Myers) Pseudoephedrine HCl 10 mg, dextromethorphan HBr 3.3 mg, chlorpheniramine maleate 0.67 mg, acetaminophen 108.3 mg, alcohol 20%, sucrose. Bot. 180 ml.
Use: Decongestant, antitussive, antihistamine.
COMTREX, MAXIMUM STRENGTH. (Bristol-Myers) Pseudoephedrine HCl 30 mg, dextromethorphan HBr 15 mg, chlorpheniramine maleate 2 mg, acetaminophen 500 mg. Cap. 24s, 50s.
Use: Decongestant, antihistamine, antitussive.
COMTREX LIQUID MULTI-SYMPTOM COLD RELIEVER. (Bristol-Myers) Acetaminophen 650 mg, phenylpropanolamine HCl 25 mg, chlorpheniramine maleate 4 mg, dextromethorphan HBr 20 mg/30 ml, alcohol 20%. Bot. 6 oz, 10 oz.
Use: Analgesic, decongestant, antihistamine, antitussive.
COMTREX LIQUI-GELS. (Bristol-Myers) Acetaminophen 325 mg, phenylpropanolamine HCl 12.5 mg, chlorpheniramine maleate 2 mg, dextromethorphan HBr 10 mg/Tab. Blister pkg. 24s, 50s.
Use: Analgesic, decongestant, antihistamine, antitussive.
CONAR. (Beecham Labs) Dextromethorphan HBr 15 mg, phenylephrine HCl 10 mg/5 ml. Bot. pt.
Use: Antitussive, decongestant.
CONAR-A TAB. (Beecham Labs) Dextromethorphan HBr 15 mg, phenylephrine HCl 10 mg, acetaminophen 300 mg, guaifenesin 100 mg/Tab. Bot. 100s. UD 20s.
Use: Antitussive, decongestant, analgesic, expectorant.
CONAR EXPECTORANT. (Beecham Labs) Dextromethorphan HBr 15 mg, phenylephrine HCl 10 mg, guaifenesin 100 mg/5 ml. Bot. 4 oz, pt.
Use: Antitussive, decongestant,

expectorant.

CONCEIVE OVULATION PREDICTOR. (Quidel) In vitro diagnostic test for luteinizing hormone in urine.
Use: Pregnancy test.

CONCENTRAID. (Ferring Labs) Desmopressin acetate 0.1 mg/ml (0.1 mg equals 400 IU arginine vasopressin). Soln. Disposable intranasal pipettes containing 20 mcg/2 ml.
Use: Posterior pituitary hormones.

CONCENTRATED CLEANER. (Bausch & Lomb) Anionic sulfate surfactant with friction-enhancing agents and sodium chlorine. Soln. Bot. 30 ml.
Use: Contact lens care.

CONCENTRATED MILK OF MAGNESIA-CASCARA. (Roxane) Magnesium hydroxide 2.34 g, aromatic cascara fluid extract 5 ml, alcohol 7%. Liq. 15 ml.
Use: Laxative.

CONCENTRATED MULTIPLE TRACE ELEMENT. (American Regent) Zinc (as sulfate) 5 mg, copper (as sulfate) 1 mg, manganese (as sulfate) 0.5 mg, chromium (as chloride) 10 mcg. Vial. 10 ml.
Use: Therapeutic supplement.

CONCENTRATED OLEOVITAMIN A & D. *See:* Oleovitamin A & D, Concentrated, Cap. (Various Mfr.).

CONCENTRATED PHILLIPS' MILK OF MAGNESIA. (Phillips) Magnesium hydroxide 800 mg/5 ml, sorbitol and sugar. Strawberry and orange vanilla creme flavors. Liq. 8 fl. oz.
Use: Antacid, laxative.

CONCENTRATED TUBERCULIN.

CONCENTRIN CAPS. (Parke-Davis) Dextromethorphan HBr 15 mg, pseudoephedrine HCl 30 mg, guaifenesin 100 mg/Cap. Bot. 12s.
Use: Antitussive, decongestant, expectorant.

CONDOL SUSPENSION. (Sanofi Winthrop) Dipyrone, chlormezanone.
Use: Analgesic, muscle relaxant.

CONDOL TABLETS. (Sanofi Winthrop) Dipyrone, chlormezanone.
Use: Analgesic, muscle relaxant.

CONDRIN-LA. (Hauck) Phenylpropanolamine HCl 75 mg, chlorpheniramine maleate 12 mg. Bot. 1000s.
Use: Decongestant, antihistamine.

CONDYLOX. (Oclassen) Podofilox 0.5%, alcohol 95%. Soln. Bot. 3.5 ml.
Use: Keratolytic.

CONEST. (Grafton) Conjugated estrogens 0.625 mg, 1.25 mg or 2.5 mg/Tab. Bot. 100s, 1000s.
Use: Estrogen.

CONEX-DA. (Forest) Phenylpropanolamine HCl 37.5 mg, chlorpheniramine maleate 4 mg/Tab. Bot. 100s, 1000s.
Use: Decongestant, antihistamine.

CONEX PLUS. (Forest) Phenylpropanolamine HCl 25 mg, chlorpheniramine maleate 4 mg, acetaminophen 325 mg/Tab. Bot. 1000s.
Use: Decongestant, antihistamine, analgesic.

CONEX SYRUP. (Forest) Phenylpropanolamine HCl 12.5 mg, guaifenesin 100 mg/5 ml. Bot. 4 oz.
Use: Decongestant, expectorant.

CONEX WITH CODEINE. (Forest) Codeine phosphate 10 mg, guaifenesin 100 mg, phenylpropanolamine HCl 12.5 mg/5 ml. Bot. 4 oz.
Use: Antitussive, expectorant, decongestant.

CONFIDENT. (Block) Carboxymethylcellulose gum, ethylene oxide polymer, petrolatum/mineral oil base. Tube 0.7 oz, 1.4 oz, 2.4 oz.
Use: Denture adhesive.

CONGESPIRIN FOR CHILDREN ASPIRIN-FREE CHEWABLE COLD TABLETS. (Bristol-Myers) Acetaminophen 81 mg, phenylephrine HCl 1.25 mg, saccharin/Chew. Tab. Bot. 24s.
Use: Analgesic, decongestant, antipyretic.

CONGESPIRIN FOR CHILDREN, ASPIRIN-FREE LIQUID COLD MEDICINE. (Bristol-Myers) Acetaminophen 130 mg, phenylpropanolamine HCl 6.25 mg/15 ml, alcohol 10%. Bot. 3 oz.
Use: Analgesic, decongestant.

CONGESPIRIN FOR CHILDREN, COUGH SYRUP. (Bristol-Myers) Dextromethorphan hydrobromide 5 mg/5 ml. Bot. 3 oz.
Use: Antitussive.

CONGESS. (Fleming) *Sr.:* Guaifenesin 250 mg, pseudoephedrine HCl 120 mg/SR Cap. *Jr.:* Guaifenesin 125 mg, pseudoephedrine HCl 60 mg/TR Cap. Bot. 100s, 1000s.
Use: Expectorant, decongestant.

CONGESS JR. (Fleming) Pseudoephedrine HCl 60 mg, guaifenesin 125 mg/Cap. Bot. 100s, 1000s.
Use: Decongestant, expectorant.

CONGESS SR. (Fleming) Pseudoephedrine HCl 120 mg, guaifenesin 250 mg/Cap. Bot. 100s, 1000s.
Use: Decongestant, expectorant.

CONGESTAC. (Menley & James) Pseudoephedrine HCl 60 mg, guaifenesin

400 mg/Tab. Bot. 24s.
Use: Decongestant, expectorant.
CONGESTANT D. (Rugby) Phenyl-propanolamine HCl 12.5 mg, chlorpheni-ramine maleate, acetaminophen 325 mg, sucrose. Tab. Bot. 100s, 1000s.
Use: Decongestant, antihistamine.
CONGESTERONE. (Kenyon) Conjugated estrogens 0.625 mg, 1.25 mg or 2.5 mg/Tab. Bot. 100s.
Use: Estrogen.
CONGO RED. Injection.
Use: Hemostatic in hemorrhagic disorders.
CONJUGATED ESTROGENS.
See: Estrogens, Conjugated (Various Mfr.).
Use: Estrogen.
CONJUNCTAMIDE. (Horizon) Pred-nisolone acetate 0.5%, sodium sulfac-etamide 10%, hydroxypropyl methylcel-lulose, polysorbate 80, sodium thiosul-fate, benzalkonium Cl 0.01%. Susp. Dropper bot. 5 ml, 15 ml.
Use: Corticosteroid, anti-infective, oph-thalmic.
CONJUTABS. (Rand) **Conjutabs 62:** Es-trogens 0.625 mg/Tab. **Conjutabs 125:** Estrogens 1.25 mg/Tab. **Conjutabs 250:** Estrogens 2.5 mg/Tab. (Enteric coated) Bot. 100s, 500s.
Use: Estrogen.
CONRAY. (Mallinckrodt) Iothalamate meglumine 60% (28.2% iodine), EDTA. Inj. Vial 20 ml, 30 ml, 50 ml, 100 ml, 150 ml.
Use: Radiopaque agent.
CONRAY-30. (Mallinckrodt) Iothalamate meglumine 30% (14.1% iodine), EDTA. Inj. Vial 300 ml.
Use: Radiopaque agent.
CONRAY-43. (Mallinckrodt) Iothalamate meglumine 43% (20.2% iodine), EDTA. Inj. Vial 50 ml, 100 ml, 250 ml.
Use: Radiopaque agent.
CONRAY-325. (Mallinckrodt) Iothalamate sodium 54.3% (32.5% iodine), EDTA. Inj. Vial 30 ml, 50 ml.
Use: Radiopaque agent.
CONRAY-400. (Mallinckrodt) Iothalamate sodium 66.8% (40% iodine), EDTA. Inj. Vial 25 ml, 50 ml.
Use: Radiopaque agent.
CONSIN COUMOUND SALVE. (Wiscon-sin) Carbolic acid ointment. Jar 2 oz, lb.
Use: Minor skin irritations.
CONSTAB 100. (Kenyon) Docusate sodi-um 100 mg/Tab. Bot. 100s, 1000s.
Use: Laxative.
CONSTILAC. (Alra) Lactulose syrup 10

Gm/15 ml. Bot. 8 oz, 16 oz, UD 30 ml.
Use: Laxative.
CONSTONATE 60. Docusate sodium 100 mg, 250 mg/Cap. Bot. 100s, 1000s.
Use: Laxative.
CONSTULOSE. (Barre-National) Lactu-lose 10 Gm, galactose < 2.2 Gm, lac-tose 1.2 Gm, other sugars < 1.2 Gm/15 ml. Syr. Bot. 237 ml, 946 ml.
Use: Laxative. analgesic.
CONTAC-12 HOUR CAPLETS. (SK-Beecham) Phenylpropanolamine HCl 75 mg, chlorpheniramine maleate 12 mg/Capl. Bot. 10s, 20s.
Use: Decongestant, antihistamine.
CONTAC-12 HOUR CAPSULES. (SK-Beecham) Phenylpropanolamine HCl 75 mg, chlorpheniramine maleate 8 mg/CA Cap. Pkg. 10s, 20s.
Use: Decongestant, antihistamine.
CONTAC COUGH & CHEST COLD LIQ-UID. (SK-Beecham) Pseudoephedrine HCl 15 mg, dextromethorpan HBr 5 mg, guaifenesin 50 mg, acetaminophen 125 mg, alcohol 10%, saccharin, sorbitol. Liq. Bot. 4 fl. oz.
Use: Decongestant, antitussive, expec-torant, analgesic.
CONTAC COUGH AND SORE THROAT FORMULA. (SK-Beecham) Dex-tromethorphan HBr 5 mg, aceta-minophen 125 mg, alcohol 10%. Bot. 120 ml.
Use: Antitussive, analgesic.
CONTACT DAY & NIGHT COLD & FLU CAPLETS. (SK-Beecham) **Night:** Pseudoephedrine HCl 60 mg, diphenhy-dramine HCl 50 mg, dextromethorphan HBr 30 mg, acetaminophen 650 mg/Cap. Pkg. 5s. **Day:** Pseu-doephedrine HCl 60 mg, dextromethor-phan HRr 30 mg, acetaminophen 650 mg/Cap. Pkg. 15s.
Use: Decongestant, antihistamine, anti-tussive, analgesic.
CONTAC JR. (SK-Beecham) Pseu-doephedrine HCl 15 mg, aceta-minophen 160 mg, dextromethorphan HBr 5 mg, saccharin, sorbitol/5 ml. Bot. 4 oz.
Use: Decongestant, analgesic, antitus-sive.
CONTAC MAXIMUM STRENGTH 12-HOUR CAPLETS. (SK-Beecham) Phenylpropanolamine HCl 75 mg, chlor-pheniramine maleate 12 mg/Capl. Pkg. 20s.
Use: Decongestant, antihistamine.
CONTAC NIGHTTIME COLD. (SK-Beecham) Acetaminophen 167 mg, dex-

tromethorphan HBr 5 mg, pseu-
doephedrine HCl 10 mg, doxylamine
succinate 1.25 mg/5 ml, alcohol 25%.
Bot. 177 ml.
Use: Analgesic, antitussive, deconges-
tant, antihistamine.
**CONTAC NON-DROWSY FORMULA SI-
NUS.** (SK-Beecham) Pseudoephedrine
HCl 30 mg, acetaminophen 500
mg/Cap. Pkg. 24s.
Use: Decongestant, analgesic.
CONTAC SEVERE COLD FORMULA.
(SK-Beecham) Phenylpropanolamine
HCl 12.5 mg, acetaminophen 500 mg,
chlorpheniramine maleate 2 mg, dextromethorphan HBr 15 mg/Capl. Pkg.
10s, 20s.
Use: Decongestant, analgesic, antihistamine, antitussive.
**CONTAC SEVERE COLD & FLU HOT
MEDICINE.** (SK-Beecham) Pseudoephedrine HCl 60 mg, chlorpheni-
ramine maleate 4 mg, dextromethor-
phan HBr 20 mg, acetaminophen 650
mg/Pow. Pkg. 6 packs.
Use: Decongestant, antihistamine, anti-
tussive.
**CONTAC SEVERE COLD & FLU NIGHT-
TIME LIQUID.** (SK-Beecham) Pseu-
doephedrine HCl 10 mg, chlorpheni-
ramine maleate 0.67 mg, dextromethor-
phan HBr 5 mg, acetaminophen 167 mg,
alcohol 18.5%, saccharin, sorbitol, glu-
cose. Liq. Bot. 180 ml.
Use: Decongestant, antihistamine, anti-
tussive.
CONTACT LENS PRODUCTS, SOFT.
(Hydrogel).
Use: Rinsing/storage solutions.
See: Allergan Hydrocare Preserved
Saline (Allergan).
Boil n Soak (Alcon).
Lensrins (Allergan).
Opti-Soft (Alcon).
ReNu Saline (Bausch & Lomb).
Saline Solution, Sterile Preserved
(Bausch & Lomb).
Murine Preserved All-Purpose Saline
Solution (Ross).
Sensitive Eyes Plus (Bausch & Lomb).
Sensitive Eyes Saline (Bausch &
Lomb).
Soft Mate Saline for Sensitive Eyes
(Sola/Barnes-Hind).
Allergan Sorbi-Care Saline (Allergan).
Sterile Saline (Bausch & Lomb).
Blairex Sterile Saline (Blairex).
Hypo-Clear (Bausch & Lomb).
Lens Plus Preservative Free (Aller-
gan).

Ciba Vision Saline (Ciba Vision).
Hypo-Clear (Bausch & Lomb).
Purisol 4 (Amcon).
Unisol (Wesley-Jessen).
Unisol 4 (Wesley-Jessen).
Soft Mate Saline Preservative-Free
(Sola/Barnes-Hind).
Use: Salt tablets for normal saline.
See: Soft Rinse 135 (Professional Sup-
plies).
Amcon 250 (Amcon).
Easy Eyes (Eaton Medicals).
Marlin Salt System II (Marlin).
Soft Rinse 250 (Professional Sup-
plies).
Use: Surfactant cleaning solutions.
See: Ciba Vision Cleaner (Ciba Vision).
Daily Cleaner (Bausch & Lomb).
Preflex for Sensitive Eyes (Alcon).
DURAcare II (Blairex).
LC-65 (Allergan).
Lens Clear (Allergan).
Lens Plus Daily Cleaner (Allergan).
Mira Flow Extra Strength (Ciba Vi-
sion).
Murine Contact Lens Cleaner (Ross).
Opti-Clean II (Alcon).
Pliagel (Wesley-Jessen).
Sensitive Eyes Saline/Cleaning Solu-
tion (Bausch & Lomb).
Sof/Pro-Clean (Sherman).
Sof/Pro-Clean (s.a.) (Sherman).
Soft Mate Hands Off Daily Cleaner
(Sola/Barnes-Hind).
Soft Mate Protein Remover
(Sola/Barnes-Hind).
Soft Mate Daily Cleaning for Sensitive
Eyes (Sola/Barnes-Hind).
Use: Enzymatic cleaners.
See: Allergan Enzymatic (Allergan).
Extenzyme Protein Cleaner (Allergan).
Opti-zyme Enzymatic Cleaner (Alcon).
ReNu Effervescent Enzymatic Cleaner
(Bausch & Lomb).
ReNu Thermal Enzymatic Cleaner
(Bausch & Lomb).
Ultrazyme Enzymatic Cleaner (Aller-
gan).
Use: Re-wetting solutions.
See: Adapettes for Sensitive Eyes (Al-
con).
Clerz Drops (Wesley-Jessen).
Clerz 2 (Wesley-Jessen).
Comfort Tears (Sola/Barnes-Hind).
Lens Drops (Ciba Vision).
Lens Fresh (Allergan).
Lens Lubricant (Bausch & Lomb).
Lens Plus Rewetting Drops (Allergan).
Lens-Wet (Allergan).
Murine Sterile Lubricating and Rewet-

ting Drops (Ross).
Opti-Tears (Alcon).
Sensitive Eye Drops (Bausch & Lomb).
Soft Mate Comfort Drops (Sola/Barnes-Hind).
Soft Mate Lens Drops (Sola/Barnes-Hind)
Sterile Lens Lubricant (Blairex).
Use: Chemical disinfection systems.
See: Allergan Hydrocare Cleaning and Disinfecting (Allergan).
Aosept (Ciba Vision).
Disinfecting Solution (Bausch & Lomb).
Flex-Care (Alcon).
Lens Plus Oxysept System (Allergan).
Lensept (Ciba Vision).
MiraSept System (Wesley-Jessen).
Opti-Free (Alcon).
Pure Sept (Ross).
Quik-Sept System (Bausch & Lomb).
ReNu Multi-Action (Bausch & Lomb).
Soft Mate (Sola/Barnes-Hind).
Soft Mate Consept (Sola/Barnes-Hind).
CONTE-PAK-4. (SoloPak) Zinc 5 mg, copper 1 mg, manganese 0.5 mg, chromium 10 mcg. Vial 1 ml, 10 ml, 30 ml.
Use: Parenteral nutritional supplement.
CONTRACEPTIVES.
See: Oral Contraceptives (Various Mfr.).
Foams, Vaginal.
See: Delfen, Vaginal Foam (Ortho Pharm.).
Emko, Vaginal Foam (Emko).
Intrauterine System.
See: Progestasert, (Alza)
Jellies & Creams, Vaginal.
See: Colagyn, Jel (Smith).
Colagyn, Jel (Smith).
Conceptrol, Cream, Gel (Ortho).
Gynol II, Gel (Ortho).
Immolin, Cream-Jel (Schmid).
Koromex-A, Jelly (Holland-Rantos).
Koromex, Cream or Jelly (Holland-Rantos).
Ortho-Creme (Ortho).
Ortho-Gynol, Jelly (Ortho).
Miscellaneous.
See: Norplant (Wyeth-Ayerst).
VCF, Film (Apothecus).
Suppositories, Vaginal.
See: Intercept, Inserts (Ortho).
Lorophyn, Supp., Jelly (Eaton).
CONTRIN. (Geneva) Iron (from ferrous fumarate) 110 mg, B$_{12}$ 15 mcg, IFC (intrinisic factor as concentrate or from stomach preparations) 240 mg, C 75

mg, folic acid 0.5 mg/Cap. Bot. 100s.
CONTROL. (Thompson) Phenylpropanolamine HCl 75 mg/TR Cap. Bot. 14s, 28s, 56s.
Use: OTC diet aid.
CONTROL-I. (Schein) Pyrethrins 0.3%, piperonyl butoxide technical 3%. Lig. Bot. 118 ml.
Use: Pediculicide.
CONTUSS LIQUID. (Parmed) Phenylpropanolamine HCl 20 mg, phenylephrine HCl 5 mg, guaifenesin 100 mg, alcohol 5%, saccharin, sorbitol, sucrose. Liq. Bot. 16 fl. oz.
Use: Antihistamine, decongestant, antitussive.
CONVATEC PRODUCTS. (Conva-Tec) A series of health care products for the convalescent patient including:
Accuseal Bedside Drainage Bag w/Washport or Filter;
Accuseal Leg Bag;
Active Life Ostomy Pouch, Closed Open;
Duoderm Hydroactive Dressing w/Adhesive Border, Burnpak, Granules or Ulcerpak;
Durahesive Wafer w/low profile flange;
Stomahesive, Paste, Powder, Wafers, Wafer w/Sure Fit Accordian Flange;
Sur-Fit, Closed Pouch, Disposable Convex Inserts, Drainable Pouch, Flexible, Irrigation Sleeve, O.R. Set, System, Pouch Covers, Urostomy Pouch w/Covers;
Urihesive, System, System w/Accuseal Connection;
Wound Manager Drainage Pouch;
Visi-Flow Irrigation Starter Set.
CONVERSPAZ. (Ascher) Cellulase 5 mg, protease 10 mg, amylase 30 mg, lipase 13 mg, l-hyoscyamine sulfate 0.0625 mg/Cap. Bot. 100s.
Use: Digestive enzymes.
COOL-MINT LISTERINE. (Warner-Lambert) Thymol, eucalyptol, methyl salicylate, menthol, alcohol 21.6%. Liq. Bot. 90 ml, 180 ml, 360 ml, 540 ml, 720 ml, 960 ml.
Use: Mouthwash.
COOPERVISION BALANCED SALT SOLUTION. (CooperVision) Sterile intraocular irrigation soln. Bot. 15 ml, 500 ml.
Use: Intraocular irrigating solution.
COPAVIN PULVULES. (Lilly) Codeine sulfate 15 mg, papaverine HCl 15 mg/Cap. Bot. 100s.
Use: Antitussive.
COPE. (Mentholatum) Aspirin 421.2 mg, magnesium hydroxide 50 mg, aluminum

hydroxide 25 mg, caffeine 32 mg/Tab. Bot. 36s, 60s.
Use: Salicylate analgesic, antacid.
COPHENE-B. (Dunhall) Brompheniramine maleate 10 mg/ml/Inj. Vial 10 ml with methyl and propyl parabens.
Use: Antihistamine.
COPHENE #2. (Dunhall) Chlorpheniramine maleate 12 mg, pseudoephedrine HCl 120 mg/Time Cap. Bot. 100s, 500s.
Use: Antihistamine, decongestant.
COPHENE INJECTABLE. (Dunhall) Atropine sulfate 0.2 mg, phenylpropanolamine HCl 12.5 mg, chlorpheniramine maleate 5 mg/ml. Pkg. 10 ml.
Use: Anticholinergic/antispasmodic, decongestant, antihistamine.
COPHENE-PL. (Dunhall) Phenylephrine HCl 20 mg, phenylpropanolamine HCl 20 mg, chlorpheniramine maleate 5 mg/5 ml. Bot. 16 oz.
Use: Decongestant, antihistamine.
COPHENE-S. (Dunhall) Dihydrocodone bitartrate 3 mg, phenylephrine HCl 20 mg, phenylpropanolamine HCl 20 mg, chlorpheniramine maleate 5 mg/5 ml Bot. pt.
Use: Antitussive, decongestant, antihistamine.
COPHENE-X. (Dunhall) Carbetapentane citrate 20 mg, phenylephrine HCl 10 mg, phenylpropanolamine HCl 10 mg, chlorpheniramine maleate 2.5 mg, potassium guaiacolsulfonate 45 mg/Cap. Bot. 100s.
Use: Antitussive, decongestant, antihistamine, expectorant.
COPHENE-XP SYRUP. (Dunhall) Carbetapentane citrate 20 mg, phenylephrine HCl 10 mg, phenylpropanolamine HCl 20 mg, chlorpheniramine maleate 2.5 mg, potassium guaiacolsulfonate 45 mg/5 ml. Bot. pt.
Use: Antitussive, decongestant, antihistamine, expectorant.
COPOLYMER 1, (COP 1).
Use: Treat multiple sclerosis. [Orphan drug]
COPPER. (Abbott) Copper 0.4 mg/ml (as 0.85 mg cupric Cl.) Inj. Vial 10 ml, 30 ml.
Use: Parenteral nutritional supplement.
•**COPPER GLUCONATE, U.S.P.** U.S.P. XXIII.
Use: Copper supplement.
COPPERHEAD BITE THERAPY.
See: Antivenin, Snake Polyvalent Inj. (Wyeth-Ayerst).
COPPERIN. (Vernon) Iron ammonium citrate, copper (6 gr). "A" adult dose, " B"

children dose. Bot. 30s, 100s, 500s.
Use: Mineral supplement.
COPPERTONE. (Schering-Plough) A series of sun-care products marketed under the Coppertone name including Waterproof Lotions SPF 4, 6, 8, 15 and 25. Bot. 4 fl oz, 8 fl oz. Oil SPF 2: Bot. 4 fl oz, 8 fl oz; Lite Formula Oil SPF 2: Bot. 4 fl oz; Lite Lotion SPF 4: Bot. 4 fl oz; Dark Tanning Body Mousse SPF 4: Tube 4 oz; Suntanning Gel SPF 4: Tube 3 oz; Noskote SPF 8: Tube 0.44 oz, Jar 1 oz; Noskote SPF-15: Jar 1 oz. Contain one or more of the following ingredients: Padimate O, oxybenzone, homosalate, ethylhexyl p-methocinnamate.
Use: Sunscreen.
COPPERTONE DARK TANNING SPRAY. (Schering-Plough) Padimate 0 in spray base (SPF 2). Bot. 8 fl oz.
Use: Sunscreen.
COPPERTONE FACE. (Schering-Plough) A series of sunscreen lotions with SPF 2, 4, 6 and 15 in a non-greasy base with Padimate O, oxybenzone (SPF 15 only).
Use: Sunscreen.
COPPERTONE KIDS SUNBLOCK. (Schering Plough) **SPF 15:** Ethylhexyl p-methoxycinnamate, oxybenzone, 2-ethylhexyl salicylate, homosalate. Lot. Bot. 120 ml, 240 ml. **SPF 30:** Octocrylene, ethylhexyl p-methoxycinnamate, oxybenzone, 2-ethylhexyl salicylate. Lot. Bot. 120 ml, 240 ml.
Use: sunscreen.
COPPERTONE LIPKOTE. (Schering-Plough) Ethylhexyl p-methoxycinnamate, oxybenzone. SPF 15. Stick 4.5 g.
Use: Sunscreen.
COPPERTONE MOISTURIZING SUNBLOCK. (Schering-Plough) **SPF 45:** Ethylhexyl p-methoxycinnamate, 2-ethylhexyl salicylate, octocrylene, oxybenzone. Lot. Bot. 120 ml, 300 ml. **SPF 30, 25:** Ethylhexyl p-methoxycinnamate, oxybenzone, 2-ethylhexyl salicylate, homosalate. Lot. Bot. SPF 30: 120 ml, 240 ml; SPF 25: 120 ml. **SPF 15:** Ethylhexyl p-methoxycinnamate, oxybenzone. Lot. Bot. 120 ml, 240 ml, 300 ml.
Use: Sunscreen.
COPPERTONE MOISTURIZING SUNSCREEN. (Schering-Plough) Ethylhexyl p-methoxycinnamate, oxybenzone, benzyl alcohol, vitamin E, aloe. PABA free. SPF 6, 8. Waterproof. Lot. Bot. 120 ml, 240 ml.
Use: Sunscreen.
COPPERTONE MOISTURIZING SUNTAN. (Schering-Plough) **SPF 4:**

ethylhexyl p-methoxycinnamate, oxybenzone, benzyl alcohol, vitamin E, aloe. PABA free. Waterproof. Lot. Bot. 120 ml, 240 ml. **SPF 2:** homosalate, vitamin E, aloe. PABA free. Waterproof. Oil. Bot. 120 ml.
Use: Sunscreen.
COPPERTONE NOSKOTE. (Schering Plough) Homosalate 8%, oxybenzone 3%. (SPF 8) Oint. Jar 13.2 Gm, 30 Gm.
Use: Sunscreen.
COPPERTONE SPF-25 SUNBLOCK LOTION. (Schering-Plough) Ethylhexyl p-methoxycinnamate, oxybenzone, padimate 0 in lotion base (SPF-25). Bot. 4 fl oz.
Use: Sunscreen.
COPPERTONE SPORT. (Schering-Plough) Ethylhexyl p-methoxycinnamate, oxybenzone. SPF 4, 8, 15, 30. Lot. Bot. 120 ml.
Use: Sunscreen.
COPPERTONE TAN MAGNIFIER SUN-TAN. (Schering-Plough). **SPF 2:** Triethanolamine salicylate. Oil Bot. 120 ml. **SPF 4: Lotion:** Ethylhexyl p-methoxycinnamate. Bot. 120 ml. **Gel:** 2-phenylbenzimidazole-5-sulfonic acid. Tube 120 g.
Use: Sunscreen
COPPER TRACE METAL ADDITIVE. (IMS) Copper 1 mg. Inj. Vial 10 ml.
COPPER UNDECYLENATE.
W/Sodium propionate, sodium caprylate, propionic acid, undecylenic acid, salicylic acid.
CO-PYRONIL 2. (Dista) Chlorpheniramine maleate 4 mg, pseudoephedrine HCl 60 mg/Pulvule. Bot. 100s, 1000s.
Use: Antihistamine, decongestant.
CORAB. (Abbott Diagnostics) Radioimmunoassay for detection of antibody to hepatitis B core antigen. Test kit 100s.
Use: Diagnostic aid.
CORAB-M. (Abbott Diagnostics) Radioimmunoassay for the qualitative determination of specific IgM antibody to hepatitis B virus core antigen (Anti-HBc IgM) in human serum or plasma and may be used as an aid in the diagnosis of acute or recent hepatitis B infection.
Use: Diagnostic aid.
CORACE INJECTION. (Forest Pharm.) Cortisone acetate 50 mg/ml. Vial 10 ml.
Use: Glucocorticoid.
CORACIN. (Roberts Hauck) Hydrocortisone acetate 1%, neomycin sulfate 0.5%, bacitracin zinc 400 units, polymyxin B sulfate 10,000 units/Gm in white petrolatum and mineral oil base.

Oint. Tube 3.5 Gm.
Use: Corticosteroid, anti-infective, ophthalmic.
CORAL. (Lorvic) Fluoride ion 1.23%, 0.1 molar phosphate. Jar 250 Gm, Coral II: 180 disposable cup units//carton.
Use: Phosphate/fluoride prophylaxis paste.
CORAL/PLUS. (Lorvic) Free fluoride ion 2.2%, recrystallized kaolinite. Tube 250 Gm.
CORAL SNAKE (NORTH AMERICAN) ANTIVENIN.
See: Antivenin (Micrurus fulvius). (Wyeth-Ayerst).
CORANE CAPSULES. (Forest Pharm.) Pyrilamine maleate 25 mg, pheniramine maleate 10 mg, phenylpropanolamine HCl 25 mg, phenylephrine HCl 10 mg/Cap. Bot. 100s, 500s, 1000s.
Use: Antihistamine, decongestant.
CORBICIN-125. (Arthrins) Vitamin C 125 mg/Cap. Bot. 100s.
Use: Vitamin C supplement.
CORDARONE. (Wyeth-Ayerst) Amiodarone HCl 200 mg/Tab. Bot. 60s.
Use: Antiarrhythmic.
CORDRAN. (Dista) Flurandrenolide 0.025%, 0.05% in emulsified petrolatum base/Gm. **0.025%:** Tube 30 Gm, 60 Gm, Jar 225 Gm. **0.05%:** Tube 15 Gm, 30 Gm, 60 Gm, Jar 225 Gm.
Use: Corticosteroid.
CORDRAN LOTION. (Dista) Flurandrenolide 0.05%, cetyl alcohol, benzyl alcohol, stearic acid, glyceryl monostearate, polyoxyl 40 stearate, glycerin, mineral oil, menthol, purified water. Squeeze bot. 15 ml, 60 ml.
Use: Corticosteroid.
CORDRAN-N CREAM & OINTMENT. (Dista) Flurandrenolide 0.5 mg, neomycin sulfate 5 mg/Gm. Tube 15 Gm, 30 Gm, 60 Gm.
Use: Corticosteroid.
CORDRAN SP. (Dista) Flurandrenolide 0.025%, 0.05% in emulsified base w/cetyl alcohol, stearic acid, polyoxyl 40 stearate, mineral oil, propylene glycol, sodium citrate, citric acid, purified water. **0.025%:** Tube 30 Gm, 60 Gm, Jar 225 Gm. **0.05%:** Tube 15 Gm, 30 Gm, 60 Gm, Jar 225 Gm.
Use: Corticosteroid.
CORDRAN TAPE. (Dista) Flurandrenolide 4 mcg/sq. cm. Roll 7.5 cm × 60 cm, 7.5 cm 200 cm.
Use: Corticosteroid.
CORDROL. (Vita Elixir) Prednisolone 5 mg, 10 mg or 20 mg/Tab. Bot. 100s.

Use: Corticosteroid.
COREGA POWDER. (Block) Denture adhesive containing polyethyleneoxide polymer w/peppermint oil, karaya gum. Pkg.: pocket 0.7 oz; medium 1.15 oz; economy 3.55 oz.
Use: Denture adhesive.
CORGARD. (Bristol Myers Squibb) Nadolol 20 mg, 40 mg, 80 mg, 120 mg or 160 mg/Tab. Bot 100s, 1000s, UD 100s.
Use: Beta-adrenergic blocker.
• **CORIANDER OIL, U.S.P.** N.F. XVIII.
Use: Pharmaceutic aid (flavor).
CORICIDIN. (Schering) Chlorpheniramine maleate 2 mg, acetaminophen 325 mg/Tab. Bot. 12s, 24s, 48s, 100s, 1000s.
Use: Antihistamine, analgesic.
CORICIDIN "D" DECONGESTANT TABLETS. (Schering) Chlorpheniramine maleate 2 mg, acetaminophen 325 mg, phenylpropanolamine HCl 12.5 mg/Tab. Bot. 12s, 24s, 48s, 100s. Dispensary pack 200s.
Use: Antihistamine, analgesic, decongestant,
CORICIDIN DEMILETS. (Schering-Plough) Phenylpropanolamine HCl 6.25 mg, chlorpheniramine maleate 1 mg, acetaminophen 80 mg, saccharin, lactose. Tab. Bot. 24s, 36s.
Use: Pediatric decongestant, antihistamine, analgesic.
CORICIDIN EXTRA STRENGTH SINUS HEADACHE TABLETS. (Schering) Acetaminophen 500 mg, phenylpropanolamine HCl 12.5 mg, chlorpheniramine maleate 2 mg/Tab. Box 24s.
Use: Analgesic, decongestant, antihistamine.
CORICIDIN MAX STRENGTH SINUS HEADACHE. (Schering-Plough) Phenylpropanolamine HCl 12.5 mg, chlorpheniramine maleate 2 mg, acetaminophen 500 mg/Tab. Box 24s.
Use: Decongestant, antihistamine, analgesic.
CORILIN INFANT LIQUID. (Schering) Chlorpheniramine maleate 0.75 mg, sodium salicylate 80 mg/ml, alcohol <1%. Bot. 30 ml.
Use: Antihistamine, salicylate analgesic.
CORMED.
See: Nikethamide (Various Mfr.).
• **CORMETHASONE ACETATE.** USAN.
Use: Anti-infammatory.
CORN FIX. (Last) Turpentine oil 2.4%, liquefied phenol 2.25%. Bot. 0.3 oz.

Use: Cauterizing agent.
CORN HUSKERS LOTION. (Warner-Lambert Prods.) Glycerin 6.7%, SD alcohol, algin, TEA-oleoyl sarcosinate, guar gum, methylparaben, calcium sulfate, calcium Cl, TEA-fumarate, TEA-borate. Bot. 4 oz, 7 oz.
Use: Emollient.
• **CORN OIL, U.S.P.** N.F. XVIII.
Use: Pharmaceutic aid (solvent, oleaginous vehicle).
See: G. B. Prep Emulsion (Gray). Lipomul-Oral, Liq. (Upjohn).
CORNS-O-POPPIN. (Ries-Hamly) Salicylic acid 6.5%, benzoic acid 12%.
Use: Cauterizing agent.
COROTROPE. (Winthop Pharm.) Milrinone for IV use.
Use: Cardiotonic agent.
CORPUS LUTEUM, EXTRACT (WATER SOLUBLE).
See: Progesterone, Preps. (Various Mfr.).
CONQUE. (Geneva Generics) I lydrocortisone 1%, iodochlorhydroxyquin 3%. Cream. Tube 20 Gm.
Use: Corticosteroid.
CORRECTIVE MIXTURE W/PAREGORIC. (Beecham Labs) Zinc sulfocarbolate 10 mg, phenyl salicylate 22 mg, bismuth subsalicylate 85 mg, pepsin 45 mg, paregoric 0.6 ml/5 ml, alcohol 2%. Bot. Gal.
Use: Antidiarrheal.
CORRECTOL EXTRA GENTLE. (Schering-Plough) Docusate sodium 100 mg. Cap. Bot. 30s.
Use: Laxative.
CORRECTOL TABLETS. (Plough) Docusate sodium 100 mg, yellow phenolphthalein 65 mg/Tab. Box 15s, 30s, 60s, 90s.
Use: Laxative.
CORT-T.
See: T-CORT.
CORTAGEL. (Inter-Hermes) Hydrocortisone acetate 0.5%. Gel. Tube. 15 Gm, 30 Gm.
Use: Corticosteroid.
CORTAID. (Upjohn) Hydrocortisone acetate 0.5%. **Spray:** 1.5 fl oz, alcohol 46%. Bot. 45 ml.
Use: Corticosteroid.
CORTAID, MAXIMUM STRENGTH. (Upjohn) **Cream:** Hydrocortisone in parabens 1%, cetyl and stearyl alcohols, glycerin and white petrolatum. Tube 15 Gm, 30 Gm.
Use: Corticosteroids.
CORTAID MAXIMUM STRENGTH

ƐΠΠAY. (Upjohn) I lydrocortisone 1%, alcohol 55%, glycerin, methylparaben. Pump spray. Bot. 45 ml.
Use: Topical corticosteroid.

CORTAN. (Blue Cross) Prednisone 5 mg/Tab. Bot. 1000s.
Use: Corticosteroid.

CORTANE D.C. EXPECTORANT. (Standex) Brompheniramine maleate 2 mg, guaifenesin 100 mg, phenylephrine HCl 5 mg, phenylpropanolamine HCl 5 mg, codeine phosphate 10 mg, alcohol 3.5%/5 ml. Bot. pt.
Use: Antihistamine, expectorant, decongestant, antitussive.

CORTANE EXPECTORANT. (Standex) Brompheniramine maleate 2 mg, guaifenesin 100 mg, phenylephrine 5 mg, phenylpropanolamine HCl 5 mg, alcohol 3.5%/5 ml. Bot. pt.
Use: Antihistamine, expectorant, decongestant.

CORTAPP ELIXIR. (Standex) Brompheniramine maleate 5 mg, phenylephrine HCl 5 mg, phenylpropanolamine HCl 5 mg, alcohol 2.3%/5 ml. Bot. pt.
Use: Antihistamine, decongestant.

CORTATRIGEN EAR SUSPENSION. (Goldline) Hydrocortisone 1%, neomycin sulfate 5 mg, polymyxin B sulfate 10,000 units/ml. Bot. 10 ml.
Use: Corticosteroid, anti-infective, otic.

CORTATRIGEN MODIFIED EAR DROPS. (Goldline) Bot. 10 ml.
Use: Corticosteroid, anti-infective, otic.

CORT-DOME. (Miles Pharm) Hydrocortisone alcohol. **Cream:** 0.25%: 1 oz, 4 oz; 0.5%: 1 oz; 1%: 1 oz. **Lot.:** 0.25%: 4 oz; 0.5%: 4 oz; 1%: 1 oz.
Use: Corticosteroid.

CORT-DOME HIGH POTENCY. (Miles Pharm.) Hydrocortisone acetate 25 mg in a monoglyceride base. Supp. Box foil 12s.
Use: Corticosteroid.

CORTEF ACETATE OINTMENT. (Upjohn) Hydrocortisone acetate 10 mg/Gm, lanolin (anhydrous), white petrolatum, mineral oil. Tube 20 Gm (10 mg/Gm).
Use: Corticosteroid.

CORTEF FEMININE ITCH CREAM. (Upjohn) Hydrocortisone acetate equivalent to hydrocortisone 5 mg/Gm. Tube 0.5 oz.
Use: Corticosteroid.

CORTEF ORAL SUSPENSION. (Upjohn) Hydrocortisone 10 mg/5 ml (as 13.4 mg hydrocortisone cypionate). Oral susp.

Bot. 4 oz.
Use: Corticosteroid.

CORTEF TABLETS. (Upjohn) Hydrocortisone. **5 mg/Tab.:** Bot. 50s; **10 mg or 20 mg/Tab.:** Bot. 100s.
Use: Corticosteroid.

CORTENEMA. (Solvay) Hydrocortisone 100 mg in aqueous solution w/carboxypolymethylene, polysorbate 80, methylparaben 0.18%/60 ml. Bot. w/applicator. UD 1s.
Use: Corticosteroid.

CORTENIL.
See: Desoxycorticosterone Acetate, Preps. (Various Mfr.).

CORT-H.
See: H-CORT.

CORTICAL HORMONE PRODUCTS.
See: Adrenal Cortex Extract (Various Mfr.).
Aristocort, Preps. (Lederle).
Corticotropin, Preps. (Various Mfr.).
Hydrocortisone, Preps. (Various Mfr.).
Cortisone Acetate, Preps. (Various Mfr.).
Decadron LA, Inj. (Merck & Co.).
Decadron, Tab., Elix., Inj. (Merck & Co.).
Desoxycorticosterone Acetate, Preps. (Various Mfr.).
Dexamethasone, Tab. (Various Mfr.).
Fludrocortisone (Various Mfr.).
Hydeltrasol, Inj. (Merck & Co.).
Hydrocortone Acetate, Inj. (Merck & Co.).
Hydrocortone Phosphate, Inj. (Merck & Co.).
Kenacort, Prep. (Squibb).
Lipo-Adrenal Cortex, Inj. (Upjohn).
Medrol, Preps. (Upjohn).
Methylprednisolone, Tab. (Various Mfr.).
Prednisolone, Tab. (Various Mfr.).
Prednisone, Tab. (Various Mfr.).
Triamcinolone, Tab. (Various Mfr.).

CORTICOID. (Jenkins) Hydrocortisone alcohol 10 mg, clioquinol 30 mg, methylparaben 0.5 mg, propylparaben 0.5 mg/Gm. Tube 20 Gm.
Use: Corticosteroid, antifungal, anti-infective.

•**CORTICORELIN OVINE TRIFLUTATE.** USAN.
Use: Diagnostic aid for adrenal cortical function and Cushings syndrome. [Orphan drug]

CORTICOSTEROID/MYDRIATIC COMBO, OPHTHALMICS. Prednisolone acetate 0.25%, atropine sulfate 1%.
Use: Treatment of anterior uveitis.

See: Mydrapred, Susp. (Alcon).
CORTICOTROPIN HIGHLY PURIFIED.
See: H. P. Acthar Gel. Vial. (Armour).
• **CORTICOTROPIN INJECTION, U.S.P.**
U.S.P. XXIII. ACTH, Adrenocorticotropic
hormone or adrenocorticotrop(h)in or
corticotropin.
Use: Adrenal corticotropic hormone;
adrenocortical steroid (anti-inflamma-
tory); diagnostic aid (adrenocortical in-
sufficiency).
See: Cortrophin Gel, Vial, Amp.
(Organon).
• **CORTICOTROPIN FOR INJECTION,**
U.S.P. U.S.P. XXIII.
Use: Adrenal corticotropic hormone;
adrenocortical steroid (anti-inflamma-
tory); diagnostic aid (adrenocortical in-
sufficiency).
See: ACTH.
Acthar (Armour).
• **CORTICOTROPIN INJECTION, REPOSI-**
TORY, U.S.P. U.S.P. XXIII. (Various
Mfr.).
Use: IM anterior pituitary hormone ther-
apy; adrenocortical steroid (anti-in-
flammatory); diagnostic aid (adreno-
cortical insufficiency).
See: Acthar Gel Vial (Armour).
ACTH Gel Purified (Various Mfr.).
Cortrophin Gel Amp., Vial (Organon).
H.P. Acthar Gel, Vial (Armour).
CORTIFOAM. (Reed & Carnrick) Hydro-
cortisone acetate 10% in an aerosol
foam w/propylene glycol, emulsifying
wax, steareth 10, cetyl alcohol, methyl-
paraben, propylparaben, trolamine, wa-
ter, inert propellants. Container 20 Gm
w/rectal applicator for 14 applicatorfuls.
Use: Corticosteroid.
CORTIN 1% CREAM. (C & M Pharmacal)
Hydrocortisone 1%, clioquinol 3%. Tube
20 Gm.
Use: Corticosteroid, antifungal, anti-in-
fective.
CORTINAL. (Kenyon) Micronized hydro-
cortisone alcohol in a nonallergenic wa-
ter washable base 5 mg/Gm. Tube 1 oz.
Use: Corticosteroid.
CORTISOL.
See: Hydrocortisone, U.S.P. XXIII.
Note: Cortisol was the official published
name for hydrocortisone in U.S.P. XXI-
II. The name was changed back to Hy-
drocortisone, U.S.P. in Supplement 1
to the U.S.P. XXIII.
CORTISOL CYCLOPENTYLPROPI-
ONATE.
See: Cortef Fluid, Susp., Tab. (Upjohn).
• **CORTISONE ACETATE, U.S.P.** U.S.P.

XXIII. Sterile Susp., Tab., U.S.P. XXIII.
17,21-Dihydroxypregn-4-ene 3,11,20-tri-
one 21 acetate. (Kendall's Compound E)
(Upjohn) 5 mg, 10 mg, 25 mg/Tab. Bot.
50s, 100s, 500s.
Use: Adrenocortical steroid (anti-inflam-
matory).
See: Cortistan (Standex).
Cortone Acetate, Tab. (Merck & Co.).
CORTISPORIN CREAM. (Burroughs
Wellcome) Polymyxin B sulfate 10,000
units, neomycin sulfate 5 mg, hydrocorti-
sone acetate 5 mg/Gm, methylparaben
0.25%. Tube 7.5 Gm.
Use: Anti-infective, corticosteroid.
CORTISPORIN OINTMENT. (Burroughs
Wellcome) Polymyxin B sulfate 5000
units, bacitracin zinc 400 units,
neomycin sulfate 5 mg, hydrocortisone
(1%) 10 mg/Gm in petrolatum base.
Tube 30 Gm.
Use: Anti-infective, corticosteroid.
CORTISPORIN OPHTHALMIC OINT-
MENT. (Burroughs Wellcome)
Polymyxin B sulfate 10,000 units, bacitracin 400 units, neomycin sulfate 3.5
mg, hydrocortisone (1%) 10 mg/Gm in
petrolatum base. Tube 3.5 Gm.
Use: Anti-infective, corticosteroid, oph-
thalmic.
CORTISPORIN OPHTHALMIC SUSPEN-
SION. (Burroughs Wellcome) Polymyxin B sulfate 10,000 units, neomycin sulfate 3.5 mg, hydrocortisone (1%) 10 mg,
in sterile, isotonic saline, thimerosal,
cetyl alcohol, glyceryl monostearate, liquid petrolatum, polyoxyl 40 stearate,
propylene glycol/ml. Dropper bot. 7.5 ml
Sterile.
Use: Anti-infective, corticosteroid, ophthalmic.
CORTISPORIN OTIC SOLUTION STER-
ILE. (Burroughs Wellcome) Polymyxin
B sulfate 10,000 units, neomycin sulfate
5 mg, hydrocortisone 10 mg/ml, glycerin,
propylene glycol, vitamin K metabisulfite
0.1%. Dropper bot. 10 ml Sterile.
Use: Anti-infective, corticosteroid,
otic.
CORTISPORIN OTIC SUSPENSION.
(Burroughs Wellcome) Polymyxin B sulfate 10,000 units, neomycin sulfate 5
mg, hydrocortisone free alcohol 10
mg/ml, cetyl alcohol, propylene glycol,
polysorbate 80, thimerosal. Dropper bot.
10 ml Sterile.
Use: Anti-infective, corticosteroid,
otic.
CORTISTAN. (Standex) Cortisone 25
mg/10 ml.

Use: Corticosteroid.
• **CORTIVAZOL.** USAN. 11B,17,21-trihy-
droxy-6, 16α-dimethyl-2′-phenyl-2H-
pregna-2,4,6-trieno[3,2-c]-pyrazol-20-
one 21-acetate.
Use: Anti-inflammatory.
CORTIZONE-5. (Thompson Med.) Hydro-
cortisone 0.5%, glycerin, mineral oil,
white petrolatum. Tube 30 Gm.
Use: Corticosteroid.
CORTIZONE-S, MAXIMUM STRENGTH.
(Thompson Medical) Hydrocortisone
0.5%. Tube.
Use: Corticosteroid.
• **CORTODOXONE.** USAN. 17,21-Dihy-
droxy-pregn-4-ene-3,20-dione. Cortex-
olone.
Use: Anti-inflammatory.
CORTOGEN ACETATE. Cortisone acetate.
CORTONE ACETATE. (Merck & Co.)
Cortisone acetate. **5 mg/Tab.:** Bot. 50s.
10 mg/Tab.: Bot. 100s. **25 mg/Tab.:** Bot.
100s, 500s, 1000s, UD 100s. **Inj.:** 50
mg/ml. Vial 10 ml.
Use: Corticosteroid.
CORTOXIDE GEL. (Syosset) Hydrocorti-
sone 0.5% or 1% in gel base. Bot. 1.5
oz.
Use: Corticosteroid.
CORTRIL TOPICAL OINTMENT 1%.
(Pfizer Laboratories) Hydrocortisone
1%, cetyl and stearyl alcohol, propylene
glycol, sodium lauryl sulfate, petrolatum,
cholesterol, mineral oil, methyl and
propyl parabens in ointment base. Tube
0.5 oz.
Use: Corticosteroid.
CORTROSYN INJECTION. (Organon)
Cosyntropin 0.25 mg, mannitol 10 mg,
lyophilized powder/ml. Vial. Pkg. w/1 ml
amp. diluent. Box 10s. Vial.
Use: Corticosteroid.
CORT-T.
See: T-CORT.
CORT-TOP OINTMENT. (Standex) Topi-
cal hydrocortisone 1%. Tube 20 Gm.
Use: Corticosteroid.
CORUBEEN. (Spanner) Vitamin B_{12}
crystalline 1000 mcg/ml. Vial 10 ml.
Use: Vitamin B_{12} supplement.
CORYZA BRENGLE. (Hauck) Pseu-
doephedrine HCl 30 mg, aceta-
minophen 200 mg/Cap. Bot. 1000s.
Use: Decongestant, analgesic.
CORZIDE. (Bristol Myers Squibb) Nadolol
40 mg, bendroflumethiazide 5 mg/Tab or
Nadolol 80 mg, bendroflumethiazide 5
mg/Tab. Bot. 100s.
Use: Antihypertensive.

CORZYME. (Abbott Diagnostics) Enzyme
immunoassay for detection of antibody
to hepatitis B core antigen in serum or
plasma. Test kit 100s.
Use: Diagnostic aid.
CORZYME-M. (Abbott Diagnostics) En-
zyme immunoassay for the detection of
IgM antibody to hepatitis B core antigen
(Anti-HBc IgM) in human serum or plas-
ma. Test kit 100s.
Use: Diagnostic aid.
COSANYL. (Health Care Industries)
Codeine sulfate 10 mg, d-pseu-
doephedrine HCl 30 mg/5 ml, alcohol
6% in peach flavored base. Bot. 4 oz, pt,
gal.
Use: Antitussive, decongestant.
COSANYL-DM. (Health Care Industries)
Dextromethorphan HBr 15 mg, d-pseu-
doephedrine HCl 30 mg/5 ml, alcohol
6% in a peach flavor. Bot. 4 oz, gal.
Use: Antitussive, decongestant.
COSMEGEN. (Merck & Co.) Actinomycin
D (dactinomycin) 0.5 mg (lyophilized
powder)/3 ml.
Use: Antineoplastic agent.
COSMOLINE.
See: Petrolatum.
COSULID. (Ciba) Sulfachloropyridazine.
• **COSYNTROPIN.** USAN.
Use: Adrenal corticotropic hormone.
See: Cortrosyn, Vial (Organon).
COTAPHYLLINE TABS. (Major) Oxtri-
phylline 100 mg or 200 mg/Tab. Bot.
100s, 500s.
Use: Bronchodilator.
COTARNINE CHLORIDE. Cotarnine hy-
drochloride.
COTARNINE HYDROCHLORIDE.
See: Cotarnine Chloride.
COTAZYM. (Organon) Pancrelipase, li-
pase 8000 units, protease 30,000 units,
amylase 30,000 units, calcium carbon-
ate 25 mg/Cap. Bot. 100s, 500s.
Use: Digestive enzymes.
COTAZYM-S. (Organon) Pancrelipase
spheres, lipase 5,000 units, protease
20,000 units, amylase 20,000 units/Cap.
Bot. 100s, 500s.
Use: Digestive enzymes.
COTININE FUMARATE. (-)-1-Methyl-5-
(3-pyridyl)-2 pyrrolidinone compound
(2:1) with fumaric acid.
Use: Psychomotor stimulant.
COTOLATE TABS. (Major) Benztropine 1
mg or 2 mg/Tab. Bot. 100s, 1000s.
Use: Antiparkinson agent.
COTRIM. (Lemmon) Sulfamethoxazole
400 mg, trimethoprim 80 mg/Tab. Bot.
100s, 500s.

Use: Anti-infective.
COTRIM D.S. (Lemmon) Sulfamethoxazole 800 mg, trimethoprim 160 mg/Tab. Bot. 100s, 500s, UD 100s.
Use: Anti-infective.
COTRIM PEDIATRIC. (Lemmon) Sulfamethoxazole 200 mg, trimethoprim 40 mg/5 ml. Bot. 480 ml.
Use: Anti-infective.
COTRIM S.S. (Lemmon) Sulfamethoxazole 400 mg, trimethoprim 800 mg/Tab. Bot. 100s.
Use: Anti-infective.
CO-TRIMOXAZOLE. B.A.N. Compounded preparations of trimethoprim and sulfamethoxazole in the proportions of 1 part to 5 parts.
Use: Antibacterial.
• **COTTON, PURIFIED, U.S.P.** U.S.P. XXIII.
Use: Surgical aid.
• **COTTONSEED OIL, U.S.P.** N.F. XVIII.
Use: Pharmaceutic aid, solvent, oleaginous vehicle.
CO TUSS V LIQUID. (Rugby) Hydrocodone bitartrate 5 mg, guaifenesin 100 mg. Bot. 480 ml.
Use: Antitussive, expectorant.
COTYLENOL CHEWABLE COLD TABLET. (McNeil Prods.) Acetaminophen 80 mg, phenylpropanolamine HCl 3.125 mg, chlorpheniramine maleate 0.5 mg/Tab. Bot. 24s.
Use: Analgesic, decongestant, antihistamine.
COTYLENOL CHILDREN'S CHEWABLE COLD TABLET. (McNeil Prods.) Acetaminophen 80 mg, chlorpheniramine maleate 0.5 mg, pseudoephedrine HCl 7.5 mg/Tab. Bot. 24s.
Use: Analgesic, antihistamine, decongestant.
COTYLENOL CHILDREN'S LIQUID COLD FORMULA. (McNeil Prods.) Acetaminophen 160 mg, chlorpheniramine maleate 1 mg, pseudoephedrine HCl 15 mg, sorbitol/5 ml. Bot. 4 oz.
Use: Analgesic, antihistamine, decongestant.
COTYLENOL COLD FORMULA. (McNeil Prods.) Chlorpheniramine maleate 2 mg, dextromethorphan HBr 15 mg, pseudoephedrine HCl 30 mg, acetaminophen 325 mg/Tab. or Capl. **Tab.:** Box 24s, Bot. 50s, 100s. **Capl.:** Bot. 24s, 50s.
Use: Antihistamine, antitussive, decongestant, analgesic.
COTYLENOL LIQUID COLD FORMULA. (McNeil Prods.) Acetaminophen 650 mg, chlorpheniramine maleate 4 mg,

pseudoephedrine HCl 60 mg, dextromethorphan HCl 30 mg/30 ml, alcohol 7.5%, sorbitol. Bot. 5 oz.
Use: Analgesic, antihistamine, decongestant, antitussive.
COUGH FORMULA COMTREX. (Bristol-Myers) Pseudoephedrine HCl 15 mg, dextromethorphan HBr 7.5 mg, guaifenesin, saccharin, sucrose. Liq. Bot. 120 ml, 240 ml.
Use: Antitussive, expectorant.
COUGH SYRUP. (Goldline) Phenylephrine HCl 5 mg, dextromethorphan HBr 10 mg, guaifenesin 100 mg, alcohol free. Bot. 120 ml.
Use: Decongestant, antitussive, expectorant.
COUGH-X. (Ascher) Dextromethorphan 5 mg, benzocaine 2 mg. Loz. Pkg. 9s.
Use: Local anesthetic, antitussive.
COUMADIN. (DuPont) Warfarin sodium crystalline. **Tab.:** 1 mg, 2 mg, 2.5 mg, 5 mg, 7.5 mg or 10 mg/Tab. Bot. 100s, 1000s, UD 100s. **Inj.:** 50 mg/Vial w/diluent sodium Cl, thimerosal, sodium hydroxide to adjust pH. Vial 50 mg with 2 ml amp. diluent. Box 6s.
Use: Anticoagulant.
COUMARIN.
Use: Anticoagulant.
COUMARIN AND INDANDIONE DERIVATIVES.
Use: Anticoagulant.
See: Coumadin, Tab. (DuPont).
Warfarin Sodium, Tab. (Various Mfr.)
Panwarfin, Tab. (Abbott)
Sofarin, Tab. (Lemmon)
Miradon, Tab. (Schering)
• **COUMERMYCIN.** USAN. Antibiotic derived from *Streptomyces rishiriensis*.
Use: Antibiotic.
• **COUMERMYCIN SODIUM.** USAN.
Use: Antibiotic.
COUNTERPAIN RUB. (Squibb Mark) Methyl salicylate, eugenol, menthol. Oint. Tube 1 oz.
Use: External analgesic.
COVANGESIC. (Wallace) Phenylpropanolamine HCl 12.5 mg, phenylephrine HCl 7.5 mg, chlorpheniramine maleate 2 mg, pyrilamine maleate 12.5 mg, acetaminophen 275 mg, tartrazine/Tab. Bot. 24s.
Use: Decongestant, antihistamine, analgesic.
COVERMARK. (O'Leary) Neutral cream, hypoallergenic, opaque, greaseless. Jars 1 oz, 3 oz, available in eleven shades.
Use: Conceals birthmarks and skin dis-

colorations.

COVERMARK STICK. (O'Leary) For normal to oily skin, available in 7 shades.
Use: Conceals birthmarks and skin discolorations.

CO-XAN SYRUP. (Central) Theophylline anhydrous 150 mg, ephedrine HCl 25 mg, guaifenesin 100 mg, codeine phosphate 15 mg, alcohol 10%/15 ml. Bot. 1 pt.
Use: Bronchodilator, decongestant, expectorant, antitussive.

CPA TR. (Schein) Phenylpropanolamine HCl 75 mg, chlorpheniramine maleate 12 mg/Cap. Bot. 100s, 1000s.
Use: Decongestant, antihistamine.

CPLEX. (Arcum) Vitamins B_1 10 mg, B_2 10 mg, B_6 5 mg, B_{12} 10 mcg, niacinamide 100 mg, calcium pantothenate 25 mg, C 150 mg, liver 50 mg, dried yeast 50 mg/Cap. Bot. 100s, 1000s.
Use: Vitamin/mineral supplement.

C.P.M. TABLETS. (Goldline) Chlorpheniramine 4 mg/Tab. Bot. 1000s.
Use: Antihistamine.

C-REACTIVE PROTEIN TEST.
See: LA test-CRP kit. (Fisher).

CREAM CAMELLIA. (O'Leary) Jar 2 oz.
Use: Emollient.

CREATININE REAGENT STRIPS. (Miles Diagnostic) Seralyzer reagent strips. A quantitative strip test for creatinine in serum or plasma. Bot. 25s.
Use: Diagnostic aid.

CREMAGOL. (Cremagol) Emulsion of liquid petrolatum, agar agar, acacia, glycerin. Bot. 14 oz. W/cascara 11 gr/oz, Bot. 14 oz. W/phenolphthalein 2 gr/oz, Bot. 14 oz.
Use: Laxative.

CREMESONE. (Dalin) Hydrocortisone alcohol 5 mg/Gm. Tube 1 oz.
Use: Corticosteroid.

CREOMULSION COUGH MEDICINE. (Creomulsion) Beechwood creosote, cascara, ipecac, menthol, white pine, wild cherry w/alcohol. For Adults. Bot. 4 fl oz, 8 fl oz.
Use: Coughs and bronchial irritations due to colds.

CREOMULSION FOR CHILDREN. (Creomulsion) Beechwood creosote, cascara, ipecac, menthol, white pine, wild cherry w/alcohol. For Children. Bot. 4 fl oz, 8 fl oz.
Use: Coughs and bronchial irritations due to colds.

CREON 10. (Solvay) Lipase 10,000 USP units, amylase 33,200 USP units, protease 37,500 USP units. DR Cap. Bot.

100s, 250s.
Use: Digestive enzyme.

CREON 20. (Solvay) Lipase 20,000 USP units, amylase 66,400 USP units, protease 75,000 USP units. DR Cap. Bot. 100s, 250s.
Use: Digestive enzyme.

CREON 25. (Solvay) Lipase 25,000 units, amylase 74,700 units, protease 62,500 units, pancreatin 300 mg. Cap. Bot. 100s.
Use: Digestive enzyme.

CREOSOTE. Wood creosote, creosote, beechwood creosote.
W/Ipecac, menthol, licorice, white pine, wild cherry, cascara, vitamin C.
See: Creozets, Loz. (Creomulsion).

CREOTERP. (Jenkins) Terpin hydrate 2 gr, potassium iodide ⅛ gr, creosote min, eucalyptol min/Tab. Bot. 1000s.
Use: Antitussive.

CREO-TERPIN. (Lee) Dextromethorphan HBr 10 mg/15 ml, tartrazine, alcohol 25%, terpin hydrate, creosote. Liq. Bot. 120 ml.
Use: Antitussive.

CRESCORMON. (KabiVitrum) Somatotropin 4 IU/Vial. IM administration.
Use: Growth hormone.
Note: Crescormon will be available only for patients who qualify for treatment; full documentation for prospective patients to be submitted to Kabi Group Inc. for approval.

• **CRESOL, U.S.P.** N.F. XVIII. Mixture of 3 isomeric cresols. Phenol, methyl cresol.
Use: Antiseptic, disinfectant.

CRESOL PREPARATIONS.
Use: Antiseptic, disinfectant.
See: Cresol, Soln. (Various Mfr.).
Cresylone, Liq. (Parke-Davis).
Saponated Cresol Soln.

CRESTABOLIC. (Nutrition) Protein anabolic steroid, methandriol dipropionate 50 mg/ml, benzyl alcohol 5% in sesame oil. Vial 10 ml.
Use: Anabolic steroid.

m-CRESYL-ACETATE.
See: Cresylate, Liq. (Recsei).

CRESYLATE. (Recsei) M-cresyl-acetate 25%, isopropanol 25%, chlorobutanol 1%, benzyl alcohol 1%, castor oil 5%, propylene glycol/15 ml. Bot. 15 ml, pt.
Use: Otic preparation.

CRESYLIC ACID. Same as Cresol.

• **CRISNATOL MESYLATE.** USAN.
Use: Antineoplastic.

• **CRILVASTATIN.** USAN.
Use: Antihyperlipidemic.

CRITICARE HN. (Mead Johnson Nutri-

tion) High nitrogen elemental diet. Protein 14%, fat 4.3%, carbohydrate 81.5%. Bot. 8 oz.
Use: Enteral nutritional supplement.
CROFERRIN. (Forest Pharm.) Iron peptonate 50 mg, liver injection 2.5 mcg, vitamin B_{12} 12.5 mcg, lidocaine HCl 1%, phenol 0.5%, sodium citrate 0.125%, sodium bisulfite 0.009%/ml. Vial 10 ml, 30 ml.
Use: Vitamin/mineral supplement.
•**CROFILCON A.** USAN.
Use: Contact lens material.
•**CROMITRILE SODIUM.** USAN.
Use: Antihistamine.
CROMOGLYCIC ACID. B.A.N. 1,3-Di-(2-car-boxy-4-oxochromen-5-yloxy)propan-2-ol.
Use: Treatment of allergic airway obstruction.
CROMOLYN SODIUM.
Use: Treatment of mastocytosis. [Orphan drug]
See: Gastrocrom
CROMOLYN SODIUM. (Dey) 20 mg/2 ml. Inhalation. In unit-dose vials.
Use: Respiratory inhalant.
CROMOLYN SODIUM 4% OPHTHALMIC SOLUTION.
Use: Vernal keratoconjunctivitis. [Orphan drug]
CRONETAL.
See: Disulfiram.
CROPROPAMIDE. B.A.N. NN-Dimethyl-2-(N-propyl- crotonamido)butyramide.
Use: Respiratory stimulant.
•**CROSCARMELLOSE SODIUM, N.F.** N.F. XVIII.
Use: Tablet disintegrant.
•**CROSPOVIDONE, U.S.P.** N.F. XVIII.
Use: Pharmaceutic aid (tablet excipient).
CROSS ASPIRIN. (Cross) Aspirin 325 mg/Tab. Sugar, salt and lactose free. Bot. 100s, 1000s.
Use: Salicylate analgesic.
CROTAB. (Therapeutic Antibodies) *See:* ANTIVENIN, POLYVALENT CROTALID (OVINE) FAB.
CROTALIDAE ANTIVENIN POLYVALENT. (Wyeth) 1 vial of lyophilized serum, 1 vial of bacteriostatic water 10 ml, USP, 1 vial normal horse serum. Inj. Vials combination Pkg.
Use: Antivenin.
CROTALINE ANTIVENIN, POLYVALENT. Antivenin Crotalidae Polyvalent, U.S.P. XXIII. North and South American Antisnakebite serum.
Use: Passive immunizing agent.

•**CROTAMITON, U.S.P.** U.S.P. XXIII. Cream, U.S.P. XXIII. N-Crotonyl-N-ethyl-o-toluidine.
Use: Antipruritic.
See: Eurax, Cream, Lot. (Geigy).
CROTETHAMIDE. B.A.N. 2-(N-Ethylcrotonamido)-NN-dimethylbutyramide.
Use: Respiratory stimulant.
CRPA, CRPA LATEX TEST. (Laboratory Diagnostics) Rapid latex agglutination test for the qualitative determination of C reactive protein. CRPA, 1 ml—CRP Positest Control, 0.5 ml CRPA Latex Test Kit.
Use: Diagnostic aid.
CRUDE TUBERCULIN.
See: Tuberculin, Old, Vial (Parke-Davis).
CRUEX CREAM. (Ciba Consumer) Total undecylenate 20% as undecylenic acid and zinc undecylenate. Tube 0.5 oz.
Use: Antifungal, external.
CRUEX SPRAY POWDER. (Pharmacraft) Undecylenic acid 2% and zinc undecylenate 20%. Aerosol can 1.8 oz, 3.5 oz, 5.5 oz.
Use: Antifungal, external.
CRUEX SQUEEZE POWDER. (Pharmacraft) Calcium undecylenate 10%. Plastic squeeze bot. 1.5 oz.
Use: Antifungal, external.
CRYPTOLIN. (Hoechst) Gonadorelin in nasal spray.
Use: Cryptorchism treatment.
CRYPTOSPORIDIUM HYPERIMMUNE BOVINE COLOSTRUM IgG CONCENTRATE.
Use: Treat diarrhea in AIDS patients. [Orphan drug]
CRYPTOSPORIDIUM PARVUM BOVINE IMMUNOGLOBULIN CONCENTRATE.
Use: Treat infection of GI tract in immunocompromised patients. [Orphan drug]
CRYSPEN-400. (Knight) Buffered penicillin G potassium 400,000 units/Tab. Bot. 100s.
Use: Antibacterial, penicillin.
CRYSTALLINE TRYPSIN. Highly purified preparation of enzyme as derived from mammalian pancreas glands.
See: Tryptar, Inj. (Armour).
CRYSTALS-C.
See: C-CRYSTALS.
CRYSTAL VIOLET.
See: Methylrosaniline Chloride, U.S.P.
CRYSTAMINE. (Dunhall) Cyanocobalamin 100 mcg or 1000 mcg/ml, benzyl alcohol. Vial 10 ml, 30 ml.

Use: Vitamin B$_{12}$ supplement.
CRYSTI-1000. (Roberts Hauck) Cyanocobalamine crystalline 1000 mcg/ml. Inj. Vial 10 ml, 30 ml.
Use: Vitamin B$_{12}$.
CRYSTICILLIN 300 A.S. (Apothecon) Sterile procaine penicillin G suspension U.S.P. 300,000 units/ml, lecithin, povidone, sodium citrate, sodium formaldehyde sulfoxylate, sodium carboxymethylcellulose, methylparaben, propylparaben. Vial 10 ml.
Use: Antibacterial, penicillin.
CRYSTICILLIN 600 A.S. (Apothecon) Sterile procaine penicillin G suspension 600,000 units/1.2 ml, lecithin, phenol, povidone, sodium citrate, sodium carboxymethylcellulose, sodium formaldehyde sulfoxylate, methylparaben, propylparaben. Vial 12 ml.
Use: Antibacterial, penicillin.
CRYSTI-LIVER. (Hauck) Liver injection (equivalent to B$_{12}$ 10 mcg), crystalline B$_{12}$ 100 mcg, folic acid 0.4 mg. Vial 10 ml.
Use: Vitamin/mineral supplement.
CRYSTOGRAFIN. Meglumine diatrizoate.
Use: Contrast medium.
C-SOLVE. (Syosset) Alcohol 36%, glycerin, polysorbate 20, laureth-4, water soluble cellulose gum, PVA, collagen, gelatin hydrolysate, midazolidinyl urea, sorbic acid. Lot. Bot. 50 ml.
Use: Lotion base.
C SPERIDIN. (Marlyn) Hesperidin 100 mg, lemon bioflavonoids 100 mg, vitamin C 500 mg/SR Tab. Bot. 100s.
Use: Vitamin supplement.
C-SYRUP-500. (Ortega) Ascorbic acid 500 mg/5 ml. Bot. pt, gal.
Use: Vitamin C supplement.
CTAB.
See: Cetyl Trimethyl Ammonium Bromide.
C-TUSSIN. (Century) Codeine phosphate 10 mg, pseudoephedrine HCl 30 mg, guaifenesin 100 mg/5 ml, alcohol 7.5%. Bot. 120 ml, gal.
Use: Antitussive, decongestant, expectorant.
CULMINAL. (Culminal) Benzocaine 3% in water miscible cream base. Tube oz.
Use: Local anesthetic.
CULTURETTE 10 MINUTE GROUP A STEP ID. (Marion Merrel Dow) Latex slide agglutination test for group A streptococcal antigen on throat swabs. Kit 55 determinations.
Use: Diagnostic aid.

CUMETHAROL. B.A.N. 4,4′-Dihydroxy-3,3-(2-methoxy-ethylidene)dicoumarin.
Use: Anticoagulant.
• **CUPRIC ACETATE Cu 64.** USAN.
Use: Radioactive agent.
• **CUPRIC CHLORIDE, U.S.P.** U.S.P. XXII., Inj., U.S.P. XXIII.
Use: Copper deficiency treatment.
See: Copperace, Inj. (Armour).
• **CUPRIC SULFATE, U.S.P.** U.S.P. XXIII. Inj., U.S.P. XXIII.
Use: Antidote to phosphorus.
W/Zinc sulfate, camphor.
See: Dalibour, Pow. (Doak).
CUPRID. (Merck & Co.) Trientine HCl 250 mg/Cap. Bot. 100s.
Use: Chelating agent.
CUPRIMINE. (Merck & Co.) Penicillamine 125 mg or 250 mg/Cap. Bot. 100s.
Use: Penicillamine.
• **CUPRIMYXIN.** USAN.
Use: Antibacterial.
CUPRI-PAK. (SoloPak) Copper **0.4 mg/ml:** Vial 10 ml, 30 ml. **2 mg/ml:** Vial 5 ml.
Use: Parenteral nutritional supplement.
CURARE.
Use: Muscle relaxant.
See: d-Tubocurarine Salts (Various Mfr.).
CURARE ANTAGONIST.
See: Neostigmine Methylsulfate Inj. (Various Mfr.).
Tensilon, Amp. (Roche).
CURITY INCONTINENT CARE PRODUCTS. (Kendall).
Use: Management of adult bladder control problems.
CUROSURF. (Chiesi Pharm)
See: PULMONARY SURFACTANT REPLACEMENT.
CURRAL.
See: Diallyl Barbituric Acid, Tab. (Various Mfr.).
CURRETAB. (Solvay) Medroxyprogesterone acetate 10 mg/Tab. Bot. 50s.
Use: Progestin.
CUTAR BATH OIL. (Summers) Liquor carbonis detergens 7.5% in liquid petrolatum, isopropyl myristate, acetylated lanolin, lanolin alcohols extract. Bot. 180 ml.
Use: Emollient.
CUTEMOL EMOLLIENT CREAM. (Summers) Allantoin 0.2%, liquid petrolatum, acetylated lanolin, lanolin alcohols extract, isopropyl myristate, water. Jar 2 oz.
Use: Emollient.
CUTICURA ACNE CREAM. (DEP Corp.)

MADE 2 MISTAKES TODAY

1. COMING IN TO WORK
2. TALKING TO THIS GREG YAHOO

WILL BE IN TUES. AM

Form 180
Revised 10/90

RITE AID PRESCRIPTION

Name _____ R̥ No. _____

Address _____ Phone _____

Third Party Cardholder
I.D. No. _____ Date _____

Plan _____

Plan No. _____ Group No. _____ Price _____

R̥

Call (Josh)

614-262-9184

Dr. _____ Dr. _____
      Dispense As Written   Substitution Permissible

Address _____ Phone _____

Refill _____ Times   DEA No. _____

OVER →

Benzoyl peroxide 5%. Bot. 30 Gm.
Use: Anti-acne.
CUTICURA MEDICATED SHAMPOO.
(Jeffrey Martin) Sodium lauryl sulfate,
sodium stearate, salicylic acid, protein,
sulfur. Tube 3 oz.
Use: Antidandruff shampoo.
CUTICURA MEDICATED SOAP. (DEP
Corp.) Triclocarban 1%, petrolatum,
sodium tallowate, sodium cocoate, glyc-
erin, mineral oil, sodium Cl, tetrasodium
EDTA, sodium bicarbonate, magnesium
silicate, iron oxides. Bar 3.5 oz, 5.5 oz.
Use: Antibacterial skin care.
CUTICURA OINTMENT. (DEP Corp.)
Precipitated sulfur 0.5%, phenol 0.1%,
oxyquinoline 0.05%. Tube 52.5 Gm.
Use: Anti-acne.
CUTIVATE. (Glaxo) Fluticasone propi-
onate. **Cream:** 0.05%. Jar 15,30,60 Gm.
Oint.: 0.005%. Jar 15, 30, 60 Gm.
Use: Corticosteroid, topical.
CUTTER INSECT REPELLENT. (Milos)
N,N-Diethyl-meta-toluamide 28.5%, oth-
er isomers 1.5%. Vial 1 oz; Foam, Can 2
oz; Spray 7 oz, 14 oz aerosol can; As-
sortment Pack; First Aid Kits, Trial Pack,
6s; Marine Pack 3s; Camp Pack 4s;
Pocket Pack, Travel Pack.
Use: Insect repellent.
CY 1503. (Cytel)
Use: Anti-thromboembolic. [Orphan
drug]
CY 1899. (Cytel)
Use: Treatment of hepatitis B. [Orphan
drug]
CYADE-GEL. (Kenyon) Adenosine-5-
monophosphate 100 mg, vitamin B_{12}
100 mcg/ml. Vial 10 ml.
Use: Adenosine phosphate.
CYANIDE ANTIDOTE PACKAGE. (Lilly)
2 Amp. (300 mg/10 ml) sodium nitrite; 2
Amp. (12.5 Gm/50 ml) w/sodium thiosul-
fate; 12 aspirols amyl nitrite 5 min/Pkg.
Check exact dosage before administra-
tion.
Use: Antidote.
CYANOCOB. (Paddock) Vitamin B_{12}
1000 mcg/ml. Bot. 1000 ml, Vial 10 ml.
Use: Vitamin B_{12} supplement.
• **CYANOCOBALAMIN, U.S.P.** U.S.P. XXI-
II. Inj. U.S.P. XXIII.α-(5,6-Dimethyl-benz-
imidazol-1-yl)cobamide cyanide. Vitamin
B_{12}.
Use: Vitamin B_{12} supplement.
See: Redisol, Inj., Tab. (Merck & Co.).
• **CYANOCOBALAMIN CO 57, U.S.P.** USP
XXII. Cap., Oral Soln., U.S.P. XXIII.
Use: Diagnostic aid (pernicious ane-
mia).

• **CYANOCOBALAMIN CO 60, U.S.P.**
U.S.P. XXII. Cap., Oral Soln., U.S.P.
XXII.
Use: Diagnostic aid (pernicious ane-
mia).
CYANOCOBALAMIN CRYSTALLINE.
Use: Vitamin B_{12} supplement.
See: Vitamin B_{12}, Inj., Tab. (Various
Mfr.).
Cobex, Inj. (Pasadena).
Crystamine, Inj. (Dunhall).
Rubcamin PC, Inj. (Apothecon).
Berubigen, Inj. (Upjohn).
Betalin 12, Inj. (Lilly).
Crysti-12, Inj. (Hauck).
Crysti 1000, Inj. (Roberts Hauck).
Cyanoject, Inj. (Mayrand).
Cyomin, Inj. (Forest).
Kaybovite-1000, Inj. (Kay).
Redisol, Inj. (Merck & Co.).
Rubesol-1000, Inj. (Central).
Sytobex, Inj. (Park-Davis).
CYANOJECT. (Mayrand) Vitamin B_{12}
1000 mcg/ml, benzyl alcohol. Vial 10 ml,
30 ml.
Use: Vitamin B_{12} supplement.
CYANOVER. (Research Supplies)
Cyanocobalamin 100 mcg, liver injection
10 mcg, folic acid 10 mg/ml. Lyo-layer
vial 10 ml with vial of diluent 10 ml.
Use: Vitamin/mineral supplement.
CYCLAMATE SODIUM. Cyclohexane-
sulfamate dihydrate salt.
• **CYCLAMIC ACID.** USAN. N-Cyclohexyl-
sulfamic acid. Hexamic Acid. Cyclohexa-
nesulfamic acid. Currently banned in
U.S.
Use: Sweetening agent.
CYCLAN CAPS. (Major) Cyclandelate
200 mg or 400 mg/Tab. Bot. 100s,
1000s, UD 100s. 400 mg: Bot. 250s
also.
Use: Vasodilator.
CYCLANDELATE. 3,3,5-Trimethylcyclo-
hexyl mandelate.
Use: Vasodilator.
See: Cyclan, Cap. (Major).
Cyclospasmol, Tab., Cap. (Wyeth-Ay-
erst).
CYCLARBAMATE. B.A.N. 1,1-Di(phenyl-
carbamoyl-oxymethyl)cyclopentane.
Use: Muscle relaxant; tranquilizer.
• **CYCLAZOCINE.** USAN. 3-(Cyclopropyl-
methyl)-1,2,3,4,5,6-hexahydro-6, 11-di-
methyl-2,6-methano-3-benzazocin-8-ol.
This product is under study.
Use: Analgesic.
• **CYCLINDOLE.** USAN.
Use: Antidepressant.

CYCLINEX-1. (Ross) Protein 7.5 g (from carnitine, cystine, histidine, isoleucine, leucine, lysine, methionine, phenylalanine, taurine, threonine, tryptophan, tyrosine, valine), fat 27 g (from palm oil, hydrogenated coconut oil, soy oil), carbohydrate 52 g (from hydrolyzed corn starch), linoleic acid 2000 mg, Fe 10 mg, Na 215 mg, K 760 mg, Ca, vitamins A, B_1, B_2, B_3, B_5, B_6, B_{12}, C, D, E, K, biotin, choline, folic acid, inositol, Cl, Cu, I, Mg, Mn, P, Se, Zn and 515 Cal per 100 g. Nonessential amino acid free. Pow. Can 350 g.
Use: Enteral nutritional supplement.

CYCLINEX-2. (Ross) Protein 15 g (from carnitine, cystine, histidine, isoleucine, leucine, lysine, methionine, phenylalanine, taurine, threonine, tryptophan, tyrosine, valine), fat 20.7 g (from palm oil, hydrogenated coconut oil, soy oil), carbohydrate 40 g (from hydrolyzed cornstarch), Fe 17 mg, Na 1175 mg, K 1830 mg, Ca, vitamins A, B_1, B_2, B_3, B_5, B_6, B_{12}, C, D, E, K, biotin, choline, folic acid, inositol, Cl, Cu, I, Mg, Mn, P, Se, Zn and 480 Cal per 100 g. Nonessential amino acid free. Pow. Can 325 g.
Use: Enteral nutritional supplement.
• **CYCLIRAMINE MALEATE.** USAN.
Use: Antihistamine.
• **CYCLIZINE.** U.S.P. XXIII. Piperazine, 1-(diphenylmethyl)-4-methyl-1-(Diphenylmethyl)-4-methyl piperazine.
Use: Anticholinergic.
See: Marzine (hydrochloride).
Valoid (hydrochloride or lactate).
• **CYCLIZINE HYDROCHLORIDE, U.S.P.** U.S.P. XXIII. Tab. U.S.P. XXIII. 1-Diphenylmethyl-4-methylpiperazine. N-Benzhydryl-N-methyl piperazine. Piperazine, 1-(diphenylmethyl)-4-methyl-,monohydrochloride.
Use: Antiemetic.
See: Marezine HCl and lactate, Preps. (Burroughs Wellcome).
W/Ergotamine tartrate, caffeine.
See: Migral, Tab. (Burroughs Wellcome).
• **CYCLIZINE LACTATE INJECTION, U.S.P.** U.S.P. XXIII. A sterile soln. of cyclizine lactate in water for injection.
Use: Antihistamine, antiemetic.
CYCLOBARBITAL. 5-(1-Cyclohexen-1-yl)-5-ethylbarbituric acid.
Use: Central depressant.
CYCLOBARBITAL CALCIUM. Cyclobarbitone, namuron, palinum, cyclobarbital Cal. 5-(1-Cyclohexenyl)-5-Ethylbarbituric Acid.

Use: Sedative/hypnotic.
CYCLOBARBITONE. B.A.N. 5-(Cyclohex-1-enyl)-5-ethylbarbituric acid.
Use: Hypnotic; sedative.
• **CYCLOBENDAZOLE.** USAN.
Use: Anthelmintic.
CYCLOBENZAPRINE HCl, U.S.P. U.S.P. XXIII. Tab., U.S.P. XXIII. 5-(3-Dimethylamino-propylidene)-dibenzo(a.e.)cycloheptatriene HCl. (Various Mfr.) 10 mg. Tab. Bot. 30s, 100s, 1000s.
Use: Musculoskeletal relaxant.
See: Flexeril, Tab. (Merck & Co.).
CYCLOCORT CREAM. (Lederle) Amcinonide 0.1% in Aquatain hydrophilic base. Tubes 15 Gm, 30 Gm, 60 Gm.
Use: Corticosteroid.
CYCLOCORT OINTMENT. (Lederle) Amcinonide 0.1% in ointment base. Tube 15 Gm, 30 Gm, 60 Gm.
Use: Corticosteroid.
CYCLOCUMAROL. 3,4-Dihydro-2-methoxy-2-methyl-4-phenyl-2H,5H-pyrano[3,2c][1]benzopyran-5-one.
Use: Anticoagulant.
CYCLOFENIL. B.A.N. 4,4'-Diacetoxybenz-hydrylidenecyclohexane.
Use: Treatment of infertility.
• **CYCLOFILCON A.** USAN.
Use: Contact lens material.
CYCLOGEN. (Central) Dicyclomine HCl 10 mg, sodium Cl 0.9%, chlorobutanol hydrate 0.5%. Vial 10 ml, Box 12s.
Use: Antispasmodic.
CYCLOGUANIL EMBONATE. B.A.N. 4,6-Diamino-1-(4-chlorophenyl)-1,2-dihydro-2,2-dimethyl-1,3,5-triazine compound with 4,4'-methylenedi-(3-hydroxy-2-naphthoic acid) (2:1).
Use: Antimalarial.
• **CYCLOGUANIL PAMOATE.** USAN. 4,6-Diamino-1-(p-chlorophenyl)-1,2-dihydro-2,2-dimethyl-s-triazine compound (2:1) with 4,4'-methylenebis- [3-hydroxy-2-naphthoic acid].
Use: Antimalarial.
CYCLOGYL. (Alcon) Cyclopentolate HCl Soln. 0.5%, 1% or 2%. Droptainer 2 ml, 5 ml, 15 ml.
Use: Cycloplegic, mydriatic.
• **CYCLOHEXIMIDE.** USAN.
Use: Antipsoriatic.
• **CYCLOMETHICONE, U.S.P.** N.F. XVIII.
Use: Pharmaceutic aid (wetting agent).
CYCLOMETHYCAINE. B.A.N. 3-(2-Methylpiperidino)propyl 4-cyclohexyloxybenzoate.
Use: Local anesthetic.
CYCLOMETHYCAINE AND METHAPYRILENE.

Use: Topical anesthetic.
See: Surfadil Cream, Lot. (Lilly).
CYCLOMETHYCAINE SULFATE, U.S.P.
U.S.P. XXI. Creme, Jelly, Oint., Supp.,
U.S.P. XXI. 3-(2-Methylpiperidino)
propyl p-(cyclohexyloxy) benzoate sul-
fate.
Use: Topical anesthetic.
See: Surfacaine, Prep. (Lilly).
W/Methapyrilene.
See: Surfadil, Cream, Lot. (Lilly).
CYCLOMETHYCAINE AND
THENYLPYRAMINE.
See: Surfadil Cream, Lot. (Lilly).
CYCLOMYDRIL. (Alcon) Phenylophrino
HCl 1%, cyclopentolate HCl 0.2%, ben-
zalkonium Cl 0.01%, EDTA. Droptainer
2 ml, 5 ml.
Use: Mydriatic.
CYCLONIL. (Seatrace) Dicyclomine HCl
10 mg/ml. Vial 10 ml.
Use: Anticholinergic/antispasmodic.
CYCLOPAL. 5-Allyl-5(2-cyclopenten-1-
yl)-barbituric acid. Cyclopentenyl allyl-
barbituric acid.
CYCLOPAR. (Parke-Davis) Tetracycline
HCl 250 mg or 500 mg/Cap. 250 mg:
Bot. 100s, 1000s. 500 mg: Bot. 100s,
UD 100s.
Use: Antibacterial, tetracycline.
CYCLOPENTAMINE HYDROCHLORIDE,
U.S.P. U.S.P. XXI. Nasal Soln., U.S.P.
XXI. N-a-Dimethylcyclopentaneethy-
lamine HCl.
Use: Adrenergic (vasoconstrictor).
See: Clopane Hydrochloride, Nasal
Soln. (Dista).
W/Aludrine.
See: Aerolone Compound, Soln. (Lilly).
W/Chlorpheniramine.
See: Hista-Clopane, Pulvule (Lilly).
CYCLOPENTENYL - ALLYL - BARBI-
TURIC ACID.
See: Cyclopal.
• CYCLOPENTHIAZIDE. USAN. 6-Chloro-
3-(cyclo-pentylmethyl)-3,4-dihydro-2H-
1,2,4-benzothiadiazine-7-sulfonamide
1,1-dioxide.
Use: Diuretic, anti-hypertensive.
See: Navidrex.
• CYCLOPENTOLATE HYDROCHLORIDE,
U.S.P. U.S.P. XXIII. Ophth. Soln., U.S.P.
XXIII. β-Di-methyl-aminoethyl (1-hydrox-
ycyclopentyl) phenylacetate HCl. 2-(Di-
methylamino)ethyl 1-Hydroxy-α-phenyl-
cyclopentane- acetate HCl. Benze-
neacetic acid, α-(1-hydroxy-
cyclopentyl)-,2-(dimethylamino)ethyl ester, hydrochloride. (Various Mfr.) 1%
Soln. Bot. 2 ml, 5 ml, 15 ml.

Use: Anticholinergic (ophthalmic).
See: AK-Pentolate, Soln. (Akorn).
Cyclogyl, Soln. (Alcon).
W/Phenylephrine HCl.
See: Cyclomydril, Soln. (Alcon).
CYCLOPENTYLPROPIONATE.
See: Depo-Testosterone, Vial (Upjohn).
• CYCLOPHENAZINE HYDROCHLORIDE.
USAN.
Use: Antipsychotic.
• CYCLOPHOSPHAMIDE, U.S.P. U.S.P.
XXIII. Inj., Tabs., U.S.P. XXIII. N,N-bis(2-
Chloroethyl)-tetrahydro-,2- oxide, mon-
odydrate. 2 H-1,3,2-Oxazaphosphorin-
2-amine. phordiamidic acid cyclic ester
monohydrate. 2-[bis(2-Chloroethyl)
amino] tetrahydro-2H-1,3,2-oxazaphos-
phorine-2-Oxide.
Use: Antineoplastic, immunosuppres-
sive.
See: Cytoxan, Tab., Vial (Bristol Oncol-
ogy).
• CYCLOPROPANE, U.S.P. U.S.P. XXIII.
Trimethylene.
Use: Inhalation anesthetic.
• CYCLOSERINE, U.S.P. U.S.P. XXIII.
Caps., U.S.P. XXIII. D-(+)-4-Amino-3-
isoxazolidinone. 3-Isoxazolidinone, 4-
amino-, (R)-. An antibiotic produced by
Streptomycin orchidaceus. Oxamycin.
Use: Antibacterial (tuberculostatic).
See: Seromycin, Cap. (Lilly).
L-CYCLOSERINE.
Use: Treat Gaucher's disease. [Orphan
drug]
CYCLOSPASMOL CAPSULES. (Wyeth-
Ayerst) Cyclandelate 200 mg or 400
mg/Cap. Bot. 100s.
Use: Vasodilator.
CYCLOSPASMOL TABLETS. (Wyeth-
Ayerst) Cyclandelate 100 mg/Tab. Bot.
100s, 500s.
Use: Vasodilator.
CYCLOSPORIN A.
Use: Immunosuppressant.
See: Cyclosporine, U.S.P. XXIII.
• CYCLOSPORINE, U.S.P. U.S.P. XXIII.
Use: Immunosuppressive.
See: Sandimmune, Inj., Oral Soln.
(Sandoz).
CYCLOSPORINE OPHTHALMIC.
Use: Severe keratoconjunctivitis sicca;
graft rejection following keratoplasty.
[Orphan drug]
CYCLO-TAB. (Jenkins) Butabarbital sodi-
um 5.4 mg, pentobarbital sodium 5.4
mg, phenobarbital sodium 5.4 mg,
hyoscyamine HBr 0.1037 mg, scopo-
lamine HBr 0.0065 mg, atropine sulfate
0.0194 mg/Tab. Bot. 1000s.

Use: Sedative/hypnotic, anticholinergic/antispasmodic.

CYCRIMINE. B.A.N. 1-Cyclopentyl-1-phenyl-3- piperidinopropan-1-ol.
Use: Treatment of the parkinsonian syndrome.

CYCRIN. (ESI Pharma) Medroxyprogesterone acetate 2.5 mg, 5 mg. Tab. Bot. 100s.
Use: Progestin.

CYDONOL MASSAGE LOTION. (Gordon) Isopropyl alcohol 14%, methyl salicylate, benzalkonium Cl. Bot. 4 oz, gal.
Use: Counterirritant.

•**CYHEPTAMIDE.** USAN.
Use: Anticonvulsant.

CYKLOKAPRON. (KabiVitrum) **Tab.**: Tranexamic acid 500 mg. Bot. 100s. **Inj.**: 100 mg/ml. Amp. 10 ml.
Use: Hemostatic.

CYLERT CHEWABLE TABLETS. (Abbott) Pemoline 37.5 mg/Tab. Bot. 100s.
Use: Psychotherapeutic agent.

CYLERT TABLETS. (Abbott) Pemoline 18.75, 37.5 or 75 mg/Tab. Bot. 100s.
Use: Psychotherapeutic agent.

CYLEX SUGAR FREE. (Pharmacon) Benzocaine 15 mg, cetylpyridinium Cl 5 mg, sorbitol. Loz. Pkg. 12s.
Use: Antiseptic, analgesic.

CYLEX THROAT. (Pharmacon) Benzocaine 15 mg, cetylpyridinium Cl 5 mg, sorbitol. Loz. Pkg. 12s.
Use: Antiseptic, analgesic.

CYNOBAL. (Arcum) Cyanocobalamin 100 mcg or 1000 mcg/ml. Inj. **100 mcg:** Vial 30 ml. **1000/mcg/ml.:** Inj. Vial 10 ml, 30 ml.
Use: Vitamin B$_{12}$ supplement.

CYOMIN. (Forest) Cyanocobalamin 1000 mcg/ml. Vial 10 ml, 30 ml.
Use: Vitamin B$_{12}$ supplement.

•**CYPENAMINE HCl.** USAN. 2-Phenylcyclopentylamine HydroCl.
Use: Antidepressant.

•**CYPOTHRIN.** USAN.
Use: Insecticide.

•**CYPRAZEPAM.** USAN.
Use: Sedative.

CYPRENORPHINE. B.A.N. N-Cyclopropylmethyl-7,8-dihydro-7α-(1-hydroxy-1-methylethyl)-O^6-methyl-6, 14-endoethenonormorphine.
Use: Narcotic antagonist.

•**CYPROHEPTADINE HYDROCHLORIDE, U.S.P.** U.S.P. XXIII. Syrup, Tabs., U.S.P. XXIII. 4-(5H-Dibenzo-[a,d]cyclohepten-5-ylidene)-1-methylpiperidene HydroCl. 1-Methyl-4-(5-dibenzo-[a,e]cyclohepta-trienylidene) piperidine HCl monohydrate.
Use: Antihistamine, antipruritic.
See: Periactin, Tab., Syr. (Merck & Co.).

•**CYPROLIDOL HYDROCHLORIDE.** USAN. Diphenyl (2-(4-pyridyl)cyclopropyl)-methanol hydrochloride.
Use: Psychotherapeutic agent.

•**CYPROTERONE ACETATE.** USAN. 6-Chloro-17-hydroxy-1α-2α-methylenepregna-4,6-diene-3, 20-dione acetate.
Use: Anti-androgen. [Orphan drug]

•**CYPROXIMIDE.** USAN.
Use: Antidepressant.

CYREN A.
See: Diethylstilbestrol Prep. (Various Mfr.).

CYRIMINE HCl. 1-Phenyl-1-cyclopentyl-3-piperidino-1-propanol HCl.
Use: Antispasmodic.
See: Pagitane HCl, Tab. (Lilly).

CYRONINE. (Major) Liothyronine sodium 25 mcg/Tab. Bot. 100s.
Use: Thyroid hormone.

CYSTAGON. (Mylan) Cysteamine bitartrate 50 mg, 150 mg/Cap. Bot. 500s.
Use: Treatment of nephropathic cystinosis.

CYSTAMIN.
See: Methenamine, Tab. (Various Mfr.).

CYSTAMINE. (Tennessee) Methenamine 2 gr, phenyl salicylate 0.5 gr, phenazopyridine HCl 10 mg, benzoic acid ⅛ gr, hyoscyamine sulfate gr, atropine sulfate gr/SC Tab. Bot. 100s, 1000s.
Use: Urinary anti-infective.

•**CYSTEAMINE.** USAN.
Use: Antiurolithic, cysteine calculi, nephropathic cystinosis. [Orphan drug]

•**CYSTEAMINE HYDROCHLORIDE.** USAN.
Use: Treatment of nephropathic cystinosis.
See: Cystagon.

•**CYSTEINE HCl, U.S.P.** U.S.P. XXIII. Lotion, U.S.P. XXIII. L-Cysteine hydrochloride monohydrate.
Use: Amino acid for replacement therapy, treatment of photosensitivity in erythropoietic protoporphyria. [Orphan drug]
See: Cysteine HCl (Abbott).

CYSTEX. (Numark) Methenamine 162 mg, sodium salicylate 162.5 mg, benzoic acid 32 mg/Tab. Bot. 40s.
Use: Urinary anti-infective.

CYSTIC FIBROSIS GENE THERAPY.
Use: Cystic fibrosis. [Orphan drug]
CYSTIC FIBROSIS TRANSMEMBRANE CONDUCTANCE REGULATOR GENE.
(Genetic Therapy)
Use: Treatment of cystic fibrosis. [Orphan drug]
• **CYSTINE.** USAN. An essential amino acid. Delta—Bot. 100 Gm; Mann—Bot. 25 Gm; Abbott—50 mg/ml HCl salt solution.
Use: Amino acid replacement therapy, an additive for infants on TPN.
CYSTO. (Freeport) Methenamine 40.8 mg, methylene blue 5.4 mg, phenyl salicylate 18.1 mg, atropine sulfate 0.03 mg, hyoscyamine 0.03 mg, benzoic acid 4.5 mg/Tab. Bot. 1000s.
Use: Urinary anti-infective.
CYSTO-CONRAY. (Mallinckrodt) Iothalamate meglumine 43% (iodine 20.2%) with EDTA. Soln. Vial 50 ml, 100 ml. Bot. 250 ml.
Use: Radiopaque agent.
CYSTO-CONRAY II. (Mallinckrodt) Iothalamate meglumine 17.2% (iodine 8.1%) with EDTA. Soln. Bot. 250 ml, 500 ml.
Use: Radiopaque agent.
CYSTOGRAFIN. (Squibb) Meglumine diatrizoate 30% (bound iodine 14%), EDTA 0.04%. Bot. 100 ml, 300 ml.
Use: Radiopaque agent.
CYSTOGRAFIN-DILUTE. (Squibb) Diatrizoate meglumine 18% (organically-bound iodine 85 mg)/ml. Vial 300 ml, 500 ml.
Use: Radiopaque agent.
CYSTO-SPAZ. (Polymedica) l-Hyoscyamine 0.15 mg/Tab. Bot. 100s.
Use: Anticholinergic/antispasmodic.
CYSTO-SPAZ-M. (Polymedica) Hyoscyamine sulfate 375 mcg/Cap. Bot. 100s.
Use: Anticholinergic/antispasmodic.
CYSTREA. (Moore Kirk) Methenamine 2 gr, phenyl salicylate 0.5 gr, methylene blue 1/5 gr, benzoic acid gr, hyoscyamine alkaloid gr, atropine sulfate gr/Tab. Bot. 100s, 1000s.
Use: Urinary anti-infective.
CYTADREN. (Ciba) Aminoglutethimide 250 mg/Tab. Bot. 100s.
Use: Adrenal steroid inhibitor.
• **CYTARABINE, U.S.P.** U.S.P. XXIII. Sterile, U.S.P. XXIII. 2(1H)-Pyrimidihone, 4-amino-1-β- -arabinofuranosyl-. 1-β- -Arabinofuranosylcytosine. (Various Mfr.) 100 mg or 500 mg. Pow. for inj. Vials.

Use: Antineoplastic agent.
See: Cytosar, Inj. (Upjohn).
CYTARABINE, DEPOFOAM ENCAPSULATED.
Use: Neoplastic meningitis. [Orphan drug]
• **CYTARABINE HYDROCHLORIDE.** USAN. 1-Arabinoluranosylcytosine hydrochloride.
Use: Management of acute leukemias.
See: Cytosar-U, Vial (Upjohn).
CYTOGAM. (Connaught) Cytomegalovirus immune globulin intravenous (human).
Use: Cytomegalovirus disease associated with kidney transplantation.
CYTOMEGALOVIRUS IMMUNE GLOBULIN (HUMAN).
Use: Cytomegalovirus disease associated with organ transplant. [Orphan drug]
CYTOMEGALOVIRUS IMMUNE GLOBULIN (HUMAN) IV.
Use: CMV pneumonia in bone marrow transplants. [Orphan drug]
CYTOMEL. (SK-Beecham) Liothyronine sodium 5 mcg, 25 mcg or 50 mcg/Tab. Bot. 100s. 25 mcg: Bot. 1000s.
Use: Thyroid hormone.
CYTOSAR-U. (Upjohn) Cytarabine 20 mg/ml in powder, 50 mg/ml reconstituted. Vial 100 mg, 500 mg.
Use: Antineoplastic agent.
CYTOSINE ARABINOSIDE HCl. Cytarabine HCl.
See: Cytosar-U (Upjohn).
CYTOTEC. (Searle) Misoprostol 200 mcg/Tab. Bot. 100s, UD 100s.
Use: Prostaglandins.
CYTOVENE. (Syntex) Ganciclovir (as sodium) 500 mg/Pow. Vial. 10 ml.
Use: Antiviral agents.
CYTOX. (MPL) Cyanocobalamin 500 mcg, vitamins B_6 20 mg, B_1 100 mg, benzyl alcohol 2% in isotonic solution of sodium Cl/ml. Inj. Vial 10 ml.
Use: Vitamin supplement.
CYTOXAN LYOPHILIZED. (Bristol-Myers/Mead Johnson Oncology) Cyclophosphamide. Vial 500 mg.
Use: Antineoplastic agent.
CYTOXAN POWDER. (Bristol-Myers/Mead Johnson Oncology) Cyclophosphamide powder 100 mg, 200 mg, 500 mg, 1 Gm or 2 Gm/Vial.
Use: Antineoplastic agent.
CYTOXAN TABLETS. (Bristol-Myers/Mead Johnson Oncology) Cyclophosphamide 25 mg or 50 mg/Tab.

25 mg/Tab.: Bot. 100s; **50 mg/Tab.**: Bot. 100s, 1000s, UD 100s.
Use: Antineoplastic agent.

D

D₂. One of the D vitamins.
See: Ergocalciferol.
D₃. One of the D vitamins.
See: Cholecalciferol.
DAA.
See: Dihydroxy Aluminum Aminoacetate.
• **DACARBAZINE,** U.S.P. XXIII. Inj., U.S.P. XXIII. 5-(3,3-Dimethyltriazeno) imidazole-4-carboxamide.
Use: Antineoplastic.
See: Dtic-Dome, Inj. (Miles Pharm).
D.A. CHEWABLE TABLETS. (Dura) Phenylephrine HCl 10 mg, chlorpheniramine 2 mg, methscopolamine nitrate 1.25 mg/Tab. Bot. 100s.
Use: Decongestant, antihistamine, anticholinergic.
DACODYL. (Major) **Tab.**: Bisacodyl 5 mg /Tab. Bot. 100s, 250s, 1000s. UD 100s. **Supp.**: Bisacodyl 10 mg. Box 12s, 100s.
Use: Laxative.
DACRIOSE. (Iolab) Isotonic, buffered solution of purified water, sodium Cl, potassium Cl, sodium hydroxide, sodium phosphate, benzalkonium CL 0.01%, edetate disodium 0.03%. Bot. 0.5 oz, 1 oz, 4 oz.
Use: Irrigating solution, ophthalmic.
• **DACTINOMYCIN,** U.S.P. XXIII. Inj., U.S.P. XXIII. Actinomycin D.
Use: Antineoplastic.
See: Cosmegen, Vial (Merck & Co.).
DACURONIUM BROMIDE. B.A.N. 3α-Acetoxy-17β-hydroxy-5α-androstan-2β,16β-di-(1-methyl-1-piperidinium) dibromide.
Use: Neuromuscular blocking agent.
DAILY CARE. (Pfizer) Zinc oxide 10%, mineral oil, white petrolatum, parabens. Oint. Tube 57 g.
Use: Diaper rash product.
DAILY CLEANER. (Bausch & Lomb) Isotonic solution with sodium Cl, sodium phosphate, tyloxapol, hydroxyethyl cellulose, polyvinyl alcohol with thimerosal 0.004%, EDTA 0.2%. Soln. Bot. 45 ml.
Use: Soft contact lens care.
DAILY CONDITIONING TREATMENT. (Blistex) Padimate O 7.5%, oxybenzone 3.5%, petrolatum. Stick 11.4 Gm. SPF 15.
Use: Lip protectant, sunscreen.

DAILY LIP PROTECTOR. (Retsews Corp.) Padimate O 7.5%, oxybenzone 3.5%, cetyl alcohol, aloe, cocoa butter, lanolin, vitamins A and E, petrolatum. SPF 15. Lip balm 7.5 g.
Use: Lip protectant, sunscreen.
DAILY VITAMIN LIQUID. (PBI) Vitamins A 2500 IU, D 400 IU, E 15 IU, C 60 mg, B₁ 1.2 mg, B₂ 1.2 mg, B₆ 1.05 mg, B₁₂ 4.5 mcg, niacinamide 13.5 mg/5 ml. Bot. 8 oz, pt, gal.
Use: Vitamin supplement.
DAILY VITAMINS. (Kirkman) Vitamins A 5000 IU, D 400 IU, C 50 mg, B₁ 3 mg, B₂ 2.5 mg, B₆ 1 mg, B₁₂ 1 mcg, niacinamide 20 mg, d-calcium pantothenate 1 mg/Tab. Bot. 100s.
Use: Vitamin supplement.
DAILY VITAMINS W/IRON. (Kirkman) Vitamins A 5000 IU, D 400 IU, B₁ 2 mg, B₂ 2.5 mg, B₆ 1 mg, B₁₂ 1 mcg, niacinamide 20 mg, d-calcium pantothenate 1 mg, iron 18 mg/Tab. Bot. 100s.
Use: Vitamin/mineral supplement.
DAILY-VITE W/IRON & MINERALS. (Rugby) Elemental iron 18 mg, vitamins A 5000 IU, D 400 IU, E 30 mg, B₁ 1.5 mg, B₂ 1.7 mg, B₃ 20 mg, B₅ 10 mg, B₆ 2 mg, B₁₂ 6 mcg, C 60 mg, folic acid 0.4 mg, Ca, Cl, Cr, Cu, I, K, Mg, Mn, Mo, P, Se, zinc 15 mg, biotin 30 mcg, vitamin K 50 mcg/Tab. Bot. 100s, 365s, 1000s.
Use: Vitamin/mineral supplement.
DAIRY EASE. (Sanofi Winthrop) Lactase 3300 FCC units, mannitol. Tab. Bot. 60s.
Use: Lactase enzyme.
DAISY 2 PREGNANCY TEST. (Advanced Care) Home pregnancy test. Test kit 2s.
Use: Diagnostic aid.
DAKIN'S SOLUTION.
See: Sodium Hypochlorite Solution Diluted.
DAKIN'S SOLUTION-FULL STRENGTH. (Century) Sodium hypochlorite 0.5%. Soln. Bot. pt, gal.
Use: Anti-infective, external.
DAKIN'S SOLUTION-HALF STRENGTH. (Century) Sodium hypochlorite 0.25%. Soln. Bot. pt.
Use: Anti-infective, external.
DAKRINA. (Dakryon) Polyvinyl alcohol 0.6%, povidone 5%, vitamin C, polymer solubilized vitamin A palmitate 350 IU, EDTA 0.05%. Drop. Bot. 15 ml.
Use: Ophthalmic.
DALALONE. (Forest) Dexamethasone sodium phosphate 4 mg/ml, methyl and propyl parabens, sodium bisulfite. Vial 5 ml.
Use: Corticosteroid.

DALALONE D.P. (Forest) Dexamethasone acetate 16 mg/ml, polysorbate 80, carboxymethylcellulose, sodium bisulfite, EDTA, benzyl alcohol. Vial 1 ml, 5 ml.
Use: Corticosteroid.

DALALONE L.A. (Forest) Dexamethasone 8 mg/ml, polysorbate 80, carboxymethylcellulose, sodium bisulfite, EDTA, benzyl alcohol. Vial 5 ml.
Use: Corticosteroid.

D-ALA-PEPTIDE T.
Use: Antiviral.
See: Peptide T (Carl Biotech/National Institute of Mental Health).

DALEDALIN TOSYLATE. USAN. 3-Methyl-3-[3-(methylamino) ropyl]-1-phenylindoline mono-p-toluene sulfonate.
Use: Antidepressant.

DALEX. (Dalin) Dextromethorphan HBr 45 mg, phenylephrine HCl 15 mg, chlorpheniramine maleate 6 mg, guaifenesin 180 mg, ammonium Cl 600 mg/fl oz.
Syr.: Bot. 4 oz, pt. **Loz.:** 10s, 18s. **Cap.:** 20s. **Pediatric:** Bot. 4 oz. **TR:** 15s.
Use: Antitussive, decongestant, antihistamine, expectorant.

• **DALFOPRISTIN.** USAN.
Use: Antibacterial agent.

DALGAN. (Wyeth-Ayerst) Dezocine 5 mg, 10 mg or 15 mg/ml. **5 mg/ml:** Vial (SD) 1 ml. **10 mg/ml:** Vial (SD) 1 ml, Vial (MD) 10 ml, syringes (prefilled) 1 ml. **15 mg/ml:** Vial (SD) 1 ml, syringes (prefilled) 1 ml.
Use: Narcotic analgesic.

DALICOTE. (Dalin) Hexachlorophene, pyrilamine maleate, diperodon HCl 0.25%, dimethyl polysiloxane, silicone, zinc oxide, camphor. Lot. Bot. 4 fl oz.
Use: Antihistamine, antipruritic, anesthetic.

DALIDERM LIQUID. (Dalin) Ethyl alcohol 66%, quaternium ammonium compound, carbolic acid, benzoic acid, salicylic acid, resorcin, camphor, tannic acid, coal tar solution, chlorothymol. Bot. 0.5 oz, 1 oz.
Use: Antipruritic, antifungal, keratolytic.

DALIDERM POWDER. (Dalin) Zinc undecylenate, sodium propionate, quaternium ammonium compound, salicylic acid, boric acid, aluminum acetate, alum. Can 2 oz, 3.5 oz.
Use: Antipruritic, antifungal, keratolytic.

DALIDYNE. (Dalin) Methylbenzethonium Cl, tannic acid, benzocaine, ethyl alcohol, benzyl alcohol, camphor, menthol, chlorothymol. Lot. Bot. 0.25 oz, 0.5 oz, 1 oz.
Use: Counterirritant for mouth.

DALIDYNE JEL. (Dalin) Benzocaine, cherry-flavored base. Tube 10 Gm.
Use: Local anesthetic, topical.

DALIDYNE THROAT SPRAY. (Dalin) Lidocaine, cetyldimethylbenzyl ammonium Cl, ethyl alcohol. Aerosol ⅓ oz.
Use: Anesthetic, antiseptic.

DALIFORT. (Dalin) Vitamins A 25,000 IU, D 400 IU, C 500 mg, B_1 10 mg, B_2 5 mg, B_6 5 mg, B_{12} 5 mcg, niacinamide 100 mg, d-calcium pantothenate 20 mg, iron 10 mg, magnesium oxide 5 mg, zinc sulfate 1.5 mg, copper sulfate 1 mg/Tab. Bot. 30s, 100s.
Use: Vitamin/mineral supplement.

DALIHIST. (Dalin) Phenylephrine HCl 0.5%, pyrilamine maleate 0.15%, cetyl benzyldimethyl ammonium Cl 0.04% in aqueous isotonic solution. Spray 20 ml.
Use: Decongestant, antihistamine.

DALIMYCIN. (Dalin) Oxytetracycline HCl 250 mg/Cap. Bot. 24s, 100s.
Use: Antibacterial, tetracycline.

DALISEPT. (Dalin) Vitamins A 750 IU, D 75 IU, diperodon HCl 1%, methylbenzethonium Cl 0.1%. Tube 2 oz, 4 oz. Jar 16 oz.
Use: Anesthetic, topical w/vitamins.

DALIVIM FORTE. (Dalin) Iron ammonium citrate 18 gr, liver fraction 3 gr, vitamins B_{12} 60 mcg, A palmitate 10,000 IU, D 1000 IU, B_1 12 mg, B_2 4 mg, niacinamide 20 mg, B_6 2 mg, calcium pantothenate 12 mg, mixed tocopherols 30 mg, calcium glycerophosphate 65 mg, manganese glycerophosphate 17.5 mg/oz. Bot. 4 oz, 8 oz, 16 oz.
Use: Vitamin/mineral supplement.

DALIVIM FORTE TABLETS. (Dalin) Iron 100 mg, desiccated liver 150 mg, vitamins B_{12} 10 mcg, A palmitate 1667, D 167 IU, C 50 mg, B_1 3 mg, B_2 3 mg, niacinamide 10 mg, B_6 0.5 mg, calcium pantothenate 2 mg, calcium glycerophosphate 11 mg, manganese glycerophosphate 3 mg/Tab. Bot. 50s, 100s.
Use: Vitamin/mineral supplement.

DALLERGY. (Laser) Chlorpheniramine maleate 8 mg, phenylephrine HCl 20 mg, methscopolamine nitrate 2.5 mg/ER Capl. Bot. 100s.
Use: Antihistamine, decongestant, anticholinergic.

DALLERGY-D SYRUP. (Laser) Chlorpheniramine maleate 2 mg, phenylephrine HCl 5 mg/5ml. Bot. 4oz.
Use: Antihistamine, decongestant.

DALLERGY-JR CAPSULES. (Laser) Brompheniramine maleate 6 mg, pseudoephedrine HCl 60 mg/Cap. Bot. 100s, 1000s.
Use: Antihistamine, decongestant.
DALLERGY SYRUP. (Laser) Chlorpheniramine maleate 2 mg, phenylephrine HCl 10 mg, methscopolamine nitrate 0.625 mg/5 ml. Bot. pt, gal.
Use: Antihistamine, decongestant, anticholinergic/antispasmodic.
DALLERGY TABLETS. (Laser) Chlorpheniramine maleate 4 mg, phenylephrine HCl 10 mg, methscopolamine nitrate 1.25 mg/Tab. Bot. 100s, 1000s.
Use: Antihistamine, decongestant, anticholinergic/antispasmodic.
DALMANE. (Roche) Flurazepam HCl 15 mg or 30 mg/Cap. Bot. 100s, 500s, Prescription Pak 300s. RNP (Reverse Numbered Packages) 4 rolls × 25 cap. or 4 cards 25 cap. UD 100s.
Use: Sedative/hypnotic.
• **DALTEPARIN SODIUM.** USAN.
Use: Anticoagulant; antithrombotic.
• **DALTROBAN.** USAN.
Use: Platelet aggregation inhibitor.
• **DALVASTATIN.** USAN.
Use: Antihyperlipidemic.
DAMACET-P. (Mason) Hydrocodone bitartrate 5 mg, acetaminophen 500 mg/Tab. Bot. 100s, 500s.
Use: Narcotic analgesic combination.
DAMASON-P. (Mason) Hydrocodone bitartrate 5 mg, aspirin 224 mg, caffeine 32 mg/Tab. Bot. 100s, 500s.
Use: Narcotic analgesic combination.
DAMBOSE.
See: Inositol, Tabs.
D-AMP. (Dunhall) Ampicillin trihydrate 500 mg/Cap. Bot. 100s.
Use: Antibacterial, penicillin.
• **DANAPAROID SODIUM.** USAN.
Use: Antithrombotic.
DANATROL CAPSULES. (Sanofi Winthrop) Danazol.
Use: Gonadotropin inhibitor.
• **DANAZOL,** U.S.P. XXIII. Cap., U.S.P. XXIII. 17α-Pregna-2,4-dien-20-yno-[2,3-d]isoxazol-17-ol.
Use: Pituitary gonadotropin suppressant.
See: Danocrine, Cap. (Sanofi Winthrop).
DANDRUFF SHAMPOO. (Walgreen) Zinc pyrithione 2 Gm/100 ml. Bot. 11 oz. Tube 7 oz.
Use: Antiseborrheic.
DANOCRINE. (Sanofi Winthrop) Danazol 50 mg, 100 mg or 200 mg/Cap. Bot.

100s.
Use: Gonadotropin inhibitor.
DANOGAR TABLETS. (Sanofi Winthrop) Danazol.
Use: Gonadotropin inhibitor.
DANOL CAPSULES. (Sanofi Winthrop) Danazol.
Use: Gonadotropin inhibitor.
DANTRIUM. (Procter & Gamble) Dantrolene sodium. **25 mg/Cap.**: Bot. 100s, 500s, UD 100s; **50 mg/Cap.**: Bot. 100s; **100 mg/Cap.**: Bot. 100s, UD 100s.
Use: Skeletal muscle relaxant.
DANTRIUM I.V. (Procter & Gamble) Dantrolene sodium 20 mg/Vial. Vial 70 ml.
Use: Skeletal muscle relaxant.
• **DANTROLENE.** USAN. 1(((5-(4-nitrophenyl)-2-furanyl) methylene) amino) 2,4-nidazolidinedione.
Use: Skeletal muscle relaxant.
• **DANTROLENE SODIUM.** USAN.
Use: Skeletal muscle relaxant.
See: Dantrium, Cap. (Norwich Eaton).
DAPACIN COLD CAPSULES. (Ferndale) Phenylpropanolamine 12.5 mg, chlorpheniramine maleate 2 mg, acetaminophen 325 mg. Bot. 100s.
Use: Decongestant, antihistamine, analgesic.
DAPA EXTRA STRENGTH TABLETS. (Ferndale) Acetaminophen 500 mg/Cap. Bot. 50s, 100s, 1000s, UD 100s.
Use: Analgesic.
DAPA TABLETS. (Ferndale) Acetaminophen 324 mg/Tab. Bot. 100s, 1000s, UD 100s.
Use: Analgesic.
DAPCO. (Schlicksup) Salicylamide 300 mg, butabarbital 15 mg/Tab. Bot. 100s, 1000s.
Use: Salicylate analgesic, sedative/hypnotic.
DAPIRAZOLE HCL.
Use: Ophthalmic alpha adrenergic blocking agent.
See: Rev-Eyes, Pow. (Storz/Lederle).
• **DAPSONE,** U.S.P. XXIII. Tab., U.S.P. XXIII. Benzenamine, 4,4'-sulfonyl-bis-. Diaminodiphenylsulfone. 4,4-Sulfonyldianiline.
Use: Treatment of leprosy; dermitis herpetiformis suppressant; prevention/treatment of **Pneumocystis carinii** pneumonia. [Orphan drug]
DARAGEN. (Owen/Golderma) Collagen polypeptide, benzalkonium Cl in a mild amphoteric base. Shampoo. Bot. 8 oz.
Use: Shampoo.
DARA SOAPLESS SHAMPOO.

(Owen/Golderma) Purified water, potassium coco hydrolyzed protein, sulfated castor oil, pentasodium triphosphate, sodium benzoate, sodium lauryl sulfate, fragrance. Shampoo. Bot. 8 oz, 16 oz.
Use: Scalp protectant.

DARANIDE. (Merck & Co.) Dichlorphenamide 50 mg/Tab. Bot. 100s.
Use: Agent for glaucoma.

DARAPRIM. (Burroughs Wellcome) Pyrimethamine 25 mg/Tab. Bot. 100s.
Use: Antimalarial.

DARBID. (SK-Beecham) Isopropamide iodide 5 mg/Tab. Bot. 50s.
Use: Anticholinergic/antispasmodic.

DARCO G-60. (ICI Americas) Activated carbon from lignite.
Use: Purifier.

•**DARGLITAZONE SODIUM.** USAN.
Use: Oral hypoglycemic.

DARICON. (Beecham Labs) Oxyphencyclimine HCl 10 mg/Tab. Bot. 60s, 500s.
Use: Antispasmodic.

•**DARODIPINE.** USAN.
Use: Antihypertensive, bronchodilator, vasodilator.

DARVOCET-N 50. (Lilly) Propoxyphene napsylate 50 mg, acetaminophen 325 mg/Tab. Bot. 100s (Rx Pak) 500s; Blister pkg. 10 × 10s.
Use: Narcotic analgesic combination.

DARVOCET-N 100. (Lilly) Propoxyphene napsylate 100 mg, acetaminophen 650 mg/Tab. Bot. 100s (Rx Pak) 500s; Blister pkg. 10 × 10s; 500 single cut blisters; UD rolls 20 × 25s.
Use: Narcotic analgesic combination.

DARVON. (Lilly) Propoxyphene HCl 65 mg/Pulv. Bot. 100s. Rx Pak 500s; Blister pkg. 10 × 10s; UD rolls 20 × 25s.
Use: Narcotic analgesic.

DARVON COMPOUND-65. (Lilly) Propoxyphene HCl 65 mg, aspirin 389 mg, caffeine 32.4 mg/Pulv. Bot. 100s (Rx Pak) 500s; Blister pkg. 10 × 10s.
Use: Narcotic analgesic combination.

DARVON-N. (Lilly) Propoxyphene napsylate. Tab.: 100 mg. Bot. 100s (Rx Pak), 500s; Blister pkg. 10 × 10s; Rx Pak 20 × 50s.
Use: Narcotic analgesic.

DA-SED TABLET. (Sheryl) Butabarbital 0.5 gr/Tab. Bot. 100s.
Use: Sedative/hypnotic.

DASIN. (SK-Beecham) Ipecac 3 mg, acetylsalicylic acid 130 mg, camphor 15 mg, caffeine 8 mg, atropine sulfate 0.13 mg/Cap. Bot. 100s, 500s.
Use: Analgesic, anticholinergic/antispasmodic.

DATURINE HBr.
See: Hyoscyamine Salts (Various Mfr.).

•**DAUNORUBICIN HCL,** U.S.P. XXIII. For Inj., U.S.P. XXIII. An antibiotic produced by *Streptomyces ceruleorubidus.* 3-Acetyl-1,2,3,-4,6,11-hexahydro-3,5, 12-trihydroxy-10-methoxy-6,11-dioxonaphthacen-1-yl-3-amino-2,3,6-trideoxy-β-D-galactopyranoside.
Use: Antineoplastic.
See: Cerubidine, Inj. (Wyeth-Ayerst).

•**DAUNORUBICIN HYDROCHLORIDE.** USAN.
Use: Antineoplastic.

DAVITAMON K.
See: Menadione Inj., Tab. (Various Mfr.).

DAVOSIL. (Hoyt) Silicon carbide in glycerin base. Jar 8 oz, 10 oz.
Use: Agent for oral hygiene.

DAYALETS. (Abbott) Vitamins B_1 1.5 mg, B_2 1.7 mg, A 5000 IU, C 60 mg, D 400 IU, niacinamide 20 mg, B_6 2 mg, B_{12} 6 mcg, E 30 IU, folic acid 0.4 mg/Filmtab. Bot. 100s.
Use: Vitamin supplement.

DAYALETS PLUS IRON. (Abbott) Vitamins B_1 1.5 mg, B_2 1.7 mg, niacinamide 20 mg, B_6 2 mg, C 60 mg, A 5000 IU, D 400 IU, E 30 IU, B_{12} 6 mcg, iron 18 mg, folic acid 0.4 mg/Filmtab. Bot. 100s.
Use: Vitamin/mineral supplement.

DAY CAPS. (Towne) Vitamins A 5500 IU, D 400 IU, B_1 3 mg, B_2 3 mg, B_6 0.5 mg, B_{12} 4 mcg, C 50 mg, calcium pantothenate 5 mg, niacinamide 20 mg/Cap. Bot. 120s, 300s.
Use: Vitamin supplement.

DAY CAP TABS-M. (Towne) Vitamins A 5500 IU, D 400 IU, B_1 3 mg, B_2 3 mg, B_6 0.5 mg, B_{12} 4 mcg, C 50 mg, niacinamide 20 mg, calcium pantothenate 5 mg, l-Lysine HCl 15 mg, iron 10 mg, zinc 1.5 mg, manganese 1 mg, iodine 0.1 mg, copper 1 mg, potassium 5 mg, magnesium 6 mg/Cap. or tab. Bot. 100s, 250s.
Use: Vitamin/mineral supplement.

DAYCARE. (Vicks Health Care) **Expectorant Liq.:** Pseudoephedrine HCl 10 mg, dextromethorphan HBr 3.3 mg, guaifenesin 33.3 mg, acetaminophen 108 mg, alcohol 10% and saccharin. Bot. 180 ml, 300 ml.
Use: Decongestant, antitussive, expectorant, analgesic.

DAY-NIGHT COMTREX. (Bristol-Myers) Pseudoephedrine HCl 30 mg, chlorpheniramine maleate 2 mg, dextromethorphan HBr 10 mg, aceta-

minophen 325 mg/Tab. Pkg. 6s.
Use: Decongestant, antihistamine, anti-
tussive, analgesic.
DAYPRO. (Searle) Oxaprozin 600
mg/Tab. Bot. 100s, UD 100s.
Use: Nonsteroidal anti-inflammatory.
DAY TAB. (Towne) Vitamins A 5000 IU, D
400 IU, B_1 15 mg, B_2 10 mg, C 600 mg,
niacinamide 20 mg, B_6 5 mg, folic acid
400 mcg, pantothenic acid 10 mg, zinc
15 mg, copper 2 mg, B_{12} 5 mcg/Tab.
Bot. 100s, 200s.
Use: Vitamin/mineral supplement.
DAY TAB ESSENTIAL. (Towne) Vitamins
A 5000 IU, D 400 IU, E 15 IU, C 60 mg,
folic acid 0.4 mg, B_1 1.5 mg, B_2 1.7 mg,
niacin 20 mg, B_6 2 mg, B_{12} 6 mcg/Tab.
Bot. 200s.
Use: Vitamin supplement.
DAY TABS, NEW. (Towne) Vitamins A
5000 IU, E 15 IU, D 400 IU, C 60 mg,
folic acid 0.4 mg, B_1 1.5 mg, B_2 1.7 mg,
niacin 20 mg, B_6 20 mg, B_{12} 6 mcg/Tab.
Bot 100s, 250s.
Use: Vitamin supplement.
DAY TAB PLUS IRON. (Towne) Iron 18
mg, vitamins A 5000 IU, D 400 IU, B_1 1.5
mg, B_2 1.7 mg, niacinamide 20 mg, C 60
mg, B_6 2 mg, pantothenic acid 10 mg,
B_{12} 6 mcg, folic acid 0.1 mg/Tab. Bot.
100s.
Use: Vitamin/mineral supplement.
DAY TABS PLUS IRON, NEW. (Towne)
Vitamins A 5000 IU, E 15 IU, D 400 IU, C
60 mg, folic acid 0.4 mg, B_1 1.5 mg, B_2
1.7 mg, niacin 20 mg, B_6 20 mg, B_{12} 6
mcg, iron 18 mcg/Tab. Bot. 250s.
Use: Vitamin/mineral supplement.
DAY TAB STRESS COMPLEX. (Towne)
Vitamins A 5000 IU, C 600 mg, B_1 15
mg, B_2 10 mg, niacin 100 mg, D 400 IU,
E 30 IU, B_6 5 mg, folic acid 400 mcg, B_{12}
6 mcg, pantothenic acid 20 mg, iron 18
mg, zinc 15 mg, copper 2 mg/Tab. Bot.
60s.
Use: Vitamin/mineral supplement.
DAY TAB WITH IRON. (Towne) Vitamins
A 5000 IU, D 400 IU, E 15 IU, C 60 mg,
folic acid 1.5 mg, B_1 15 mg, B_2 1.7 mg,
niacin 20 mg, B_6 2 mg, B_{12} 6 mcg, iron
18 mg/Tab. Bot. 200s.
Use: Vitamin/mineral supplement.
DAYTO-ANASE. (Dayton) Bromelains
50,000 IU (protease activity). Tab. Bot.
60s.
Use: Enzyme.
DAYTO HIMBIN. (Dayton) Yohimbine 5.4
mg/Tab. Bot. 60s.
Use: Alpha adrenergic blocker.
DAYTO SULF. (Dayton) Sulfathiazole

3.42%, sulfacetamide 2.86%, sulfabenzamide 3.7%, urea 0.64%. Cream. Tube
78 Gm with 8 disposable applicators.
Use: Anti-infective, vaginal.
DAY-VITE. (Drug Industries) Vitamins A
10,000 IU, D-3 1000 IU, E 6.7 mg, C 100
mg, B_1 5 mg, B_2 5 mg, B_6 2 mg, B_{12} 2
mcg, niacinamide 25 mg, calcium pan-
tothenate 10 mg/Tab. Bot. 100s, 500s.
Use: Vitamin supplement.
DAZAMIDE TABS. (Major) Acetazo-
lamide 250 mg/Tab. Bot. 100s, 250s,
1000s, UD 100s.
Use: Diuretic.
•**DAZANDROL MALEATE.** USAN.
Use: Antidepressant.
•**DAZEPINIL HYDROCHLORIDE.** USAN.
Use: Antidepressant.
•**DAZMEGREL.** USAN.
Use: Inhibitor (thromboxane syn-
thetase).
•**DAZOPRIDE FUMARATE.** USAN.
Use: Peristaltic stimulant.
•**DAZOXIBEN HYDROCHLORIDE.**
USAN.
Use: Antithrombotic.
DB ELECTRODE PASTE. (Day-Baldwin)
Tube 5%.
DBED. Dibenzylethylenediamine dipeni-
cillin G.
Use: Antibacterial, penicillin.
See: Benzathine penicillin G Susp.
DCA.
See: Desoxycorticosterone acetate
preps. (Various Mfr.).
DCF. Pentostatin (2'-deoxycoformycin).
Use: Antibiotic.
See: Nipent, Pow. (Parke-Davis).
DCP. (Towne) Calcium 180 mg, phospho-
rus 105 mg, vitamins D 66.7 IU/Tab. Bot.
100s.
Use: Vitamin/mineral supplement.
DC SOFTGELS. (Goldline) Docusate cal-
cium 240 mg/Cap. Bot. 100s, 500s.
Use: Laxative.
DC 240. (Goldline) Docusate calcium 240
mg/Cap. Bot. 100s, 500s.
Use: Laxative.
DDAVP. (Rhone-Poulenc Rhone-Poulenc
Rorer) Desmopressin acetate 0.1 mg,
chlorobutanol 5 mg, sodium Cl 9 mg/ml.
Vial 2.5 ml w/applicator tubes for nasal
administration.
Use: Antidiuretic.
DDAVP INJECTION. (Rhone-Poulenc
Rorer).
Desmopressin acetate 4 mcg, chlorobu-
tanol 5 mg, sodium Cl 9 mg/ml. Amp. 1
ml.
Use: Antidiuretic.

ddC. Dideoxycytidine.
Use: Antiviral.
See: HIVID (Roche).
ddI. Didanosine.
Use: Antiviral agent.
See: Videx, Tab., Pow. (Bristol-Myers Squibb).
D-DIOL. (Burgin-Arden) Testosterone cypionate 50 mg, estradiol cypionate 2 mg/ml. Vial 10 ml.
Use: Androgen, estrogen.
DDS.
See: Dapsone Tab., U.S.P. XXIII.
DDT.
See: Chlorophenothane.
DEACETYLLANATOSIDE C.
See: Deslanoside, U.S.P. XXIII.
DEADLY NIGHTSHADE LEAF, U.S.P.
See: Belladonna Leaf, U.S.P. XXIII.
1-DEAMINO-8-D-ARGININE VASO-PRESSIN. Desmopressin acetate.
Use: Posterior pituitary hormone.
See: Concentraid, Soln. (Ferring Labs.). DDAVP, Inj., Soln. (Rhone-Poulenc Rorer).
DEBA.
See: Barbital (Various Mfr.).
DEBRISAN. (Johnson & Johnson) Dextranomer **Beads:** Spherical hydrophilic 0.1-0.3 mm diameter. Bot. 25 Gm, 60 Gm, 120 Gm. Pk. 7 × 4 Gm, 14 × 14 Gm. U.S. distributor Johnson & Johnson Products. **Paste:** 10 Gm. Foil packets 6s.
Use: Wound and ulcer cleansing.
• **DEBRISOQUIN SULFATE.** USAN. 3,4-Dihydro-2(IH) isoquinolinecarboxamidine sulfate. Formerly Isocaramidine Sulfate.
Use: Hypotensive agent.
DEBROX. (Marion) Carbamide peroxide 6.5% in anhydrous glycerol. Plastic squeeze bot. 0.5 oz, 1 oz.
Use: Otic preparation.
DECABID. (Lilly) Indecainide HCl 50 mg, 75 mg or 100 mg/SR tab. Bot. 100s, UD 100s. [Approved but not marketed].
Use: Antiarrhythmic.
DECA-BON. (Barrows) Vitamins A 3000 IU, D 400 IU, C 60 mg, B_1 1 mg, B_2 1.2 mg, niacinamide 8 mg, B_6 1 mg, panthenol 3 mg, B_{12} 1 mcg, biotin 30 mcg/0.6 ml. Drops Bot. 50 ml.
Use: Vitamin supplement.
DECADERM. (Merck & Co.) Dexamethasone 0.1% w/isopropyl myristate gel, wood alcohols, refined lanolin alcohol, microcrystalline wax, anhydrous citric acid, anhydrous sodium phosphate dibasic. Tube 30 Gm.

Use: Corticosteroid.
DECADROL. (Paddock) Dexamethasone sodium phosphate 4 mg/ml. Vial 5 ml.
Use: Corticosteroid.
DECADRON. (Merck & Co.) Dexamethasone. **Tab.:** 0.25 mg: Bot. 100s; 0.5 mg: Bot. 100s, UD 100s; 0.75 mg: 100s, UD 100s; 1.5 mg: Bot. 50s, UD 100s; 4 mg: Bot. 50s, UD 100s; 6 mg: Bot. 50s, UD 100s. **Elix.:** 0.5 mg/5 ml, benzoic acid 0.1%, alcohol 5% Bot. w/dropper 100 ml, Bot. w/out dropper 237 ml.
Use: Corticosteroid.
W/Neomycin sulfate.
See: NeoDecadron, Ophth. Soln., Ophth. Oint., Topical, Cream (Merck & Co.).
DECADRON-LA SUSPENSION. (Merck Sharp & Dohme) Dexamethasone acetate equivalent to 8 mg dexamethasone/ml w/sodium Cl 6.67 mg, creatinine 5 mg, disodium edetate 0.5 mg, sodium carboxymethylcellulose 5 mg, polysorbate 80 0.75 mg, sodium hydroxide to adjust pH, benzyl alcohol 9 mg, sodium bisulfite 1 mg, water for injection q.s. 1 ml. Vial 1 ml, 5 ml.
Use: Corticosteroid.
DECADRON PHOSPHATE. (Merck & Co.) Dexamethasone sodium phosphate equivalent in various forms:
Ophth. Soln.: 0.1% w/creatinine, sodium citrate, sodium borate, polysorbate 80, hydrochloric acid to adjust pH, disodium edetate, sodium bisulfite 0.1%, water for injection, phenylethanol 0.25%, benzalkonium Cl 0.02%. Ocumeter dispenser 5 ml.
Use: Ophthalmic and otic anti-inflammatory agent.
Ophth. Oint.: 0.05% w/white petrolatum and mineral oil. Tube 3.5 Gm.
Use: Ophthalmic and otic corticosteroid.
Cream: 0.1% w/stearyl alcohol, cetyl alcohol, mineral oil, polyoxyl 40 stearate, sorbitol solution, methyl polysilicone emulsion, creatinine, purified water, sodium citrate, disodium edetate, sodium hydroxide to adjust pH, methylparaben 0.15%, sorbic acid 0.1%. Tube 15 Gm, 30 Gm.
Use: Topical corticosteroid.
Turbinaire: Dexamethasone sodium phosphate 0.1 mg equivalent to dexamethasone 0.084 mg w/fluorochlorohydrocarbons as propellants and alcohol 2%. Aerosol w/nasal applicator. Container 170 sprays; refill package without nasal applicator.
Use: Nasal corticosteroid.

W/Neomycin.
Use: Corticosteroid, anti-infective.
See: NeoDecadron, Ophth. Soln., Ophth. Oint., Topical Cream (Merck & Co.)
W/Xylocaine **Inj.:** Dexamethasone sodium phosphate equivalent to dexamethasone phosphate 4 mg, lidocaine HCl 10 mg, citric acid 10 mg, creatinine 8 mg, sodium bisulfite 0.5 mg, disodium edetate 0.5 mg, sodium hydroxide to adjust pH, water for injection, methylparaben 1.5 mg, propylparaben 0.2 mg/ml. Vial 5 ml.
Use: Corticosteroid.

DECADRON PHOSPHATE INJECTION. (Merck & Co.) Dexamethasone sodium phosphate 4 mg or 24 mg/ml, creatinine 8 mg, sodium citrate 10 mg, disodium edetate 0.5 mg (24 mg/ml only), sodium hydroxide to adjust pH, sodium bisulfite 1 mg, methylparaben 1.5 mg, propylparaben 0.2 mg/ml. **4 mg/ml:** Vial 1 ml, 5 ml, 25 ml. **24 mg/ml** (for I.V. use only): Vial 5 ml, 10 ml.
Use: Corticosteroid.

DECADRON PHOSPHATE RESPI-HALER. (Merck & Co.) Dexamethasone sodium phosphate equivalent to 0.1 mg dexamethasone phosphate (approximately 0.084 mg dexamethasone) w/fluorochlorohydrocarbons as propellants, alcohol 2%. Aerosol for oral inhalation, 170 sprays in 12.6 Gm pressurized container.
Use: Bronchodilator.

DECADRON W/XYLOCAINE. (Merck & Co.) Dexamethasone sodium phosphate 4 mg, lidocaine HCl 10 mg/ml/ml. Soln. Vial 15 ml.
Use: Adrenal cortical steroid.

DECA-DURABOLIN. (Organon) Nandrolone decanoate injection w/benzyl alcohol 10%. **50 mg/ml:** Multidose vial 2 ml. **100 mg/ml:** Multidose vial 2 ml, syringe 1 ml. **200 mg/ml:** Multidose vial 1 ml, syringe 1 ml.
Use: Anabolic steroid.

DECA-DURABOLIN REDIJECT SYRINGES. (Organon) Nandrolone decanoate 50 mg, 100 mg or 200 mg/ml. Syringe 1 ml Box 25s.
Use: Anabolic steroid.

DECAGEN. (Goldline) Elemental iron 30 mg, vitamins A 9000 IU, D 400 IU, E 30 mg, B_1 10 mg, B_2 10 mg, B_3 20 mg, B_5 20 mg, B_6 5 mg, B_{12} 10 mcg, C 90 mg, folic acid 0.4 mg, Ca, Cr, Cu, I, K, Mg, Mn, Mo, P, Se, zinc 15 mg, vitamin K 25 mcg, biotin 45 mcg/Tab. Bot. 130s, 1000s.
Use: Vitamin/mineral supplement.

DECAJECT. (Mayrand) Dexamethasone sodium phosphate 4 mg/ml. Vial 5 ml, 10 ml.
Use: Corticosteroid.

DECAJECT-L.A. (Mayrand) Dexamethasone acetate 8 mg/ml suspension, polysorbate 80, carboxymethylcellulose, sodium bisulfite, EDTA, benzyl alcohol. Inj vial 5 ml
Use: Corticosteroid.

DECAJEST LA. (Mayrand) Dexamethasone acetate 8 mg/ml. Vial 5 ml.
Use: Corticosteroid.

DECALIX. (Pharmed) Dexamethasone 0.5 mg/5 ml Bot. 100 ml.
Use: Corticosteroid.

DECAMETH. (Foy) Dexamethasone sodium phosphate injection 4 mg/5 cc vial.
Use: Corticosteroid.

DECAMETH L.A. (Foy) Dexamethasone sodium phosphate injection. 8 mg/ml. Vial/5 ml.
Use: Corticosteroid.

DECAMETH TABLETS. (Foy) Dexamethasone 0.75 mg/Tab. Bot. 1000s.
Use: Corticosteroid.

DECAMETHONIUM IODIDE. B.A.N. Decamethylenedi(trimethylammonium iodide)
Use: Muscle relaxant.

DECAPRYN. (Marion Merrell Dow) Doxylamine succinate 12.5 mg/Tab. Bot. 100s.
Use: Antihistamine.
W/Pyridoxine HCl.
See: Bendectin, Tab. (Marion Merrell Dow).

DECASONE INJECTION. (Forest Pharm.) Dexamethasone sodium phosphate equivalent to dexamethasone phosphate 4 mg/ml. Vial 5 ml.
Use: Corticosteroid.

DECASPRAY. (Merck & Co.) Topical dexamethasone aerosol. Every second of spray dispenses approximately 0.075 mg of dexamethasone. Dexamethasone 10 mg, isopropyl myristate, isobutane in pressurized container 25 Gm.
Use: Corticosteroid, topical.

DECAVITAMIN CAPSULES AND TABLETS, U.S.P. XXI. Vitamins A 4000 IU, D 400 IU, C 70 mg, calcium pantothenate 10 mg, B_{12} 5 mcg, folic acid 100 mcg, nicotinamide 20 mg, B_6 2 mg, B_2 2 mg, B_1 2 mg/Cap. or Tab.
Use: Vitamin therapy.

DECCASOL-T. (Kenyon) Vitamins B_1 10 mg, B_2 5 mg, B_6 2 mg, pantothenic acid 10 mg, niacinamide 30 mg, B_{12} 3 mcg, C

100 mg, E 5 IU, A 10,000 IU, D 1000 IU, iron 15 mg, copper 1 mg, manganese 1 mg, magnesium 5 mg, zinc 1.5 mg/Tab. Bot. 100s.
Use: Vitamin/mineral supplement.

DECHLORISON ACETATE. 9-alpha, 11-beta, di-chloro-1,4-pregnadiene-17-alpha, 21-diol-3,20-dione-21 acetate. Diloderm.

DECHOLIN. (Miles Pharm) Dehydrocholic acid 250 mg/Tab. Bot. 100s, 500s.
Use: Hydrocholeric.

DECICAIN. Tetracaine HCl.

•**DECITABINE.** USAN.
Use: Antineoplastic.

•**DECLABEN.** USAN.
Use: Antiarthritic, emphysema therapy adjunct.

•**DECLENPERONE.** USAN.
Use: Sedative.

DECLOMYCIN HCl. (Lederle) Demeclocycline HCl. **Cap.:** 150 mg Bot. 100s. **Tab.:** 150 mg Bot. 100s; 300 mg Bot. 48s.
Use: Antibacterial, tetracycline.

DECOBEL LANACAPS. (Lannett) Belladonna alkaloids 0.128 mg, phenylpropanolamine HCl 50 mg, chlorpheniramine maleate 1 mg, pheniramine maleate 12.5 mg/Cap. Bot. 100s, 1000s.
Use: Decongestant, antihistamine.

DECOFED. (Various Mfr.) Pseudoephedrine HCl 30 mg/5 ml. Syr. Bot. 120 ml, 240 ml, pt, gal.
Use: Decongestant.

DECOHIST CAPSULES. (Towne) Chlorpheniramine maleate 1 mg, phenylpropanolamine HCl 12.5 mg, salicylamide 180 mg, caffeine 15 mg/Cap. Bot. 18s.
Use: Antihistamine, decongestant, analgesic.

DECOHISTINE DH LIQUID. (Pennex) Pseudoephedrine HCl 30 mg, chlorpheniramine maleate 2 mg, codeine phosphate 10 mg, alcohol. Liq. Bot. 120 ml, pt and gal.
Use: Decongestant, antihistamine, antitussive.

DECOHISTINE ELIXIR. (PBI) Phenylephrine HCl 5 mg, chlorpheniramine maleate 2 mg, alcohol 5%. Elix. Bot. 120 ml, pt. and gal.
Use: Decongestant, antihistamine.

DECOJEN INJECTION. (Jenkins) Atropine sulfate 0.2 mg, phenylpropanolamine HCl 12.5 mg, chlorpheniramine maleate 5 mg, water for injection q.s./ml. Vial 10 ml, 12s.

Use: Anticholinergic/antispasmodic, decongestant, antihistamine.

DECONADE. (H.L. Moore) Phenylpropanolamine HCl 75 mg, chlorpheniramine maleate 12 mg/Cap. Bot. 100s, 1000s.
Use: Decongestant, antihistamine.

DECONAMINE SR CAPSULES. (Berlex) Chlorpheniramine maleate 8 mg, d-pseudoephedrine HCl 120 mg/Cap. Bot. 100s, 500s.
Use: Antihistamine, decongestant.

DECONAMINE SYRUP, DYE FREE. (Berlex) Chlorpheniramine maleate 2 mg, d-pseudoephedrine HCl 30 mg/5 ml, sorbitol. Bot. 473 ml.
Use: Antihistamine, decongestant.

DECONAMINE TABLETS, DYE-FREE. (Berlex) Chlorpheniramine maleate 4 mg, d-pseudoephedrine HCl 60 mg/Tab. Bot. 100s.
Use: Antihistamine, decongestant.

DECONGESTABS. (Various Mfr.) Phenylpropanolamine HCl 40 mg, phenylephrine HCl 10 mg, chlorpheniramine maleate 5 mg, phenyltoloxamine citrate 15 mg/Tab. Bot. 100s, 500s, 1000s.
Use: Decongestant, antihistamine.

DECONGESTANT EXPECTORANT LIQUID. (Schein) Pseudoephedrine HCl 30 mg, codeine phosphate 10 mg, guaifenesin 100 mg, alcohol 7.5%. Bot. 480 ml.
Use: Decongestant, antitussive, expectorant.

DECONGESTANT FORMULA MEDIQUELL. (Parke-Davis Prods) Dextromethorphan HBr 30 mg, pseudoephedrine HCl 60 mg/Square.
Use: Antitussive, decongestant.

DECONGESTANT TABLETS. (Various Mfr.) Phenylpropanolamine HCl 40 mg, phenylephrine HCl, chlorpheniramine maleate 5 mg, phenyltoloxamine citrate 15 mg/Tab. Bot. 100s, 1000s.
Use: Decongestant, antihistamine.

DECONSAL II CAPSULES. (Adams) Pseudoephedrine 60 mg, guaifenesin 600 mg/Cap. Bot. 100s.
Use: Decongestant, expectorant.

DECONSAL PEDIATRIC. (Adams) Codeine phosphate 10 mg, pseudoephedrine HCl 30 mg, guaifenesin 100 mg/5 ml, alcohol 6%. Syr. Bot. 480 ml.
Use: Decongestant, expectorant.

DECONSAL SPRINKLE CAPSULE. (Adams) Phenylephrine HCl 10 mg, guaifenesin 300 mg/S.R. Cap. Bot. 100s.

Use: Decongestant, expectorant.

•DECTAFLUR. USAN.
Use: Dental caries prophylactic.

DECUBITEX. (I.C.P) **Oint.:** Biebrich scarlet red sulfonated 0.1%, balsam Peru, castor oil, zinc oxide, starch, sodium propionate, parabens. Jar 15 Gm, 60 Gm, 120 Gm, lb. **Pow.:** Biebrich scarlet red sulfonated 0.1%, starch, zinc oxide, sodium propionate, parabens. Bot. 30 Gm, UD 1 Gm.
Use: Wound-healing agent, emollient, antipruritic.

DECYLENES. (Rugby) Undecylenic acid, zinc undecylenate. Oint. Tube 30 Gm, lb.
Use: Antifungal, external.

DEEP DOWN PAIN RELIEF RUB. (Beecham Products) Methyl salicylate 15%, menthol 5%, camphor 0.5%. Tube 1.25 oz, 3 oz.
Use: External analgesic.

DEEP STRENGTH MUSTEROLE. (Schering-Plough) Methyl salicylate 30%, menthol 3%, methyl nicotinate 0.5% Tube 1.25 oz, 3 oz.
Use: External analgesic.

DEFED-60. (Ferndale) Pseudoephedrine 60 mg/Tab. Bot 1000s.
Use: Decongestant.

DEFEN-LA. (Horizon) Pseudoephedrine HCl 60 mg, guaifenesin 600 mg. SR Tab. Bot. 100s.
Use: Decongestant, expectorant.

•DEFEROXAMINE. USAN.
Use: Chelating agent for iron.

•DEFEROXAMINE HYDROCHLORIDE. USAN.
Use: Chelating agent for iron.

•DEFEROXAMINE MESYLATE, U.S.P. XXIII. Sterile, U.S.P. XXIII. N-[5-[3-[(5-aminopentyl) hydroxycar- bamoyl]propionamido]-pentyl]-3-[[5-(N-hydroxyacetamido) entyl]-carbamoyl]-propionohydroxamic acid.
Use: Iron depleter.
See: Desferal, Amp. (Ciba).

DEFIBROTIDE.
Use: Thrombotic thrombocytopenic purpura. [Orphan drug]

DEFICOL. (Vangard) Bisacodyl 5 mg/Tab. Bot. 100s, 1000s.
Use: Laxative.

•DEFLAZACORT. USAN.
Use: Anti-inflammatory.

d4T.
Use: Antiviral.
See: Stavudine (B-M Squibb).

DEGEST-2. (Pilkington Barnes-Hind) Naphazoline HCl 0.012%, benzalkonium Cl 0.0067%, disodium edetate 0.02%. Bot. 15 ml.
Use: Ophthalmic decongestant.

DEHYDREX.
Use: Recurrent corneal erosion. [Orphan drug]

•DEHYDROACETIC ACID, N.F. XVII.
Use: Pharmaceutic aid (preservative).

DEHYDROCHOLATE SODIUM INJ., U.S.P. XXI. Sodium 3,7,12-trioxo-5β-Cholan-24-oate.
Use: Relief of liver congestion; diagnosis of cardiac failure.
See: Decholine Sodium, Inj. (Miles Pharm).

7-DEHYDROCHOLESTEROL, ACTIVATED. (Various Mfr.) Vitamin D-3.

•DEHYDROCHOLIC ACID, U.S.P. XXIII. Tab., U.S.P. XXIII. 3,7,12-Trioxo-5β-cholan-24-oic acid. Ketocholanic acid, oxidized cholic acid, bile acids oxidized.
Use: Orally, hydrocholeretic and choleretic.
See: Atrocholin,Tab. (Glaxo).
  Cholan-DH, Tab. (Pennwalt).
  Ketocholanic acid.
  Neocholan, Tab. (Merrell Dow).
W/Amyloytic and proteolytic enzymes, desoxycholic acid.
See: Bilezyme, Tab. (Geriatric).
W/Bile, homatropine methylbromide, pepsin.
See: Biloric, Caps. (Arcum).
W/Bile, homatropine methylbromide, phenobarbital.
See: Bilamide, Tab. (Norgine).
W/Bile extract, pepsin, pancreatin.
See: Progestive, Tab. (NCP).
W/Desoxycholic acid.
See: Combichole, Tab. (F. Trout).
  Ketosox, Tab. (Ascher).
W/Docusate sodium.
See: Dubbalax-B, Cap. (Redford).
  Dubbalax-N, Cap. (Redford).
  Neolax, Tab. (Central).
W/Docusate sodium, phenolphthalein.
See: Bolax, Cap. (Boyd).
  Sarolax (Saron).
  Tripalax, Cap. (Redford).
W/Homatropine methylbromide.
See: Cholan V, Tab. (Pennwalt).
  Dranochol, Tab. (Marin).
W/Homatropine methylbromide, sodium pentobarbital.
See: Homachol, Tab. (Lemmon).
W/Methscopolamine, ox bile, amobarbital.
See: Hydrochol Plus, Tab. (Elder).
W/Ox bile, homatropine methylbromide, phenobarbital.

See: Bilamide, Tab. (Norgine).
W/Pancreatin, pepsin, bile salts, desoxycholic acid.
See: Pepsatal, Tab. (Kenyon).
W/Pancreatin, pepsin, ox bile, belladonna extract.
See: Ro-Bile, Tab. (Solvay).
W/Pepsin, pancreatin, ox bile extract, papain.
See: Canz, Tab. (Cole).
W/Pepsin, pancreatin enzyme concentrate, cellulase.
See: Gastroenterase, Tab (Wallace).
W/Phenobarbital, homatropine methylbromide.
See: Cholan-HMB, Tab. (Pennwalt).
W/Phenobarbital, homatropine methylbro mide, gerilase, geriprotase, desoxycholic acid.
See: Bilezyme Plus, Tabs. (Geriatric).
W/Phenolphthalein, docusate sodium.
See: Sarolax, Cap. (Saron).
DEHYDROCHOLIN.
Use: Hydrocholeretic.
See: Dehydrocholic acid.
DEHYDRODESOXYCHOLIC ACID.
See: Cholanic acid.
DEHYDROEMETINE. B.A.N. 3-Ethyl-1,6,7,11b-tetrahydro-9,10-dimethoxy-2-(1,2,3,4-tetrahydro-6,7-dimethoxy-1-iso-quinolylmethyl)-4H-benzo[a]-quinolizine. 2,3-Dehydroemetine.
Use: Treatment of amebiasis.
DEKASOL. (Seatrace) Dexamethasone phosphate 4 mg/ml. Vial 5 ml, 10 ml.
Use: Corticosteroid.
DEKASOL L.A. (Seatrace) Dexamethasone acetate 8 mg/ml. Vial 5 ml.
Use: Corticosteroid.
DE-KOFF. (Whiteworth) Terpin hydrate w/dextromethorphan. Elix. Bot. 4 oz.
Use: Antitussive, expectorant.
DELACORT LOTION. (Mericon) Hydrocortisone 0.5%. Bot. 4 oz.
Use: Corticosteroid, topical.
DELADIOL-40. (Steris) Estradiol valerate 40 mg/ml, castor oil, benzyl benzoate, benzyl alcohol. Vial 10 ml.
Use: Estrogen.
DELADUMONE. (Bristol Myers Squibb) Testosterone enanthate 90 mg, estradiol valerate 4 mg in sesame oil/ml, chlorobutanol 0.5%. Vial 5 ml, 1 dose (1 ml).
Use: Androgen, estrogen combination.
• **DELAPRIL HYDROCHLORIDE.** USAN.
Use: Antihypertensive, enzyme inhibitor.
DEL-AQUA-5. (Del-Ray) Benzoyl peroxide 5%. Tube 1.5 oz.

Use: Anti-acne.
DEL-AQUA-10. (Del-Ray) Benzoyl peroxide 10%. Tube 1.5 oz.
Use: Anti-acne.
DELAQUIN LOTION. (Schlicksup) Hydrocortisone 0.5%, iodoquin 3%. Bot. 3 oz.
Use: Corticosteroid, anti-fungal.
DELATEST. (Dunhall) Testosterone enanthate 100 mg/ml, chlorobutanol in sesame oil. Amp. 10 ml.
Use: Androgen.
DELATESTADIOL. (Dunhall) Testosterone enanthate 90 mg, estradiol valerate 4 mg/ml, chlorobutanol in sesame oil. Amp. 10 ml.
Use: Androgen, estrogen combination.
DELATESTRYL. (Gynex) Testosterone enanthate 200 mg/ml in sesame oil, chlorobutanol 0.5%. Vial 5 ml.
Use: Androgen.
• **DELAVIRDINE MESYLATE.** USAN.
Use: Antiviral.
DELCID. (Lakeside) Aluminum hydroxide 600 mg, magnesium hydroxide 665 mg/5 ml, alcohol 0.3%, saccharin. Bot. 8 oz.
Use: Antacid.
DEL-CLENS. (Del-Ray) Soapless cleanser. Bot. 8 oz.
Use: Skin cleanser.
DELCORT. (Hauck) Hydrocortisone 0.5%, paraben base. Cream. Pack. 1 gm.
Use: Corticosteroid.
DELCORT. (Hauck) Hydrocortisone 1%. Cream. Tube 20 gm, Jar 1 lb.
Use: Corticosteroid.
DELCO-LAX. (Delco) Bisacodyl 5 mg/Tab. Bot. 1000s.
Use: Laxative.
DELCOZINE. (Delco) Phendimentrazine tartrate 70 mg/Tab. Bot. 1000s, 5000s.
Use: Anorexiant.
DELESTREC. Estradiol 17-undecanoate.
Use: Estrogen.
DELESTROGEN. (Mead Johnson) Estradiol valerate **10 mg/ml:** In sesame oil, chlorobutanol 0.5%. Vial 5 ml. **20 mg/ml:** In castor oil, benzyl benzoate 20%, benzyl alcohol 2%. Vial 5 ml or 1 ml unimatic single dose syringe. **40 mg/ml:** In castor oil, benzyl benzoate 40%, benzyl alcohol 2%. Vial 5 ml.
Use: Estrogen.
DELFEN CONTRACEPTIVE FOAM. (Ortho) Nonoxynol-9 12.5% in an oil-in-water emulsion at pH 4.5 to 5.0. Starter can with applicator 20 Gm. Refill 20 Gm, 50 Gm.
Use: Spermicide.

DELINAL. Propenzolate HydroCl.

• **DELMADINONE ACETATE.** USAN. 6-Chloro-17-hydroxypregna-1, 4, 6-triene-3, 20-dione acetate.
Use: Progestin.
See: Delmate (Syntex).

DEL-MYCIN. (Del-Ray) Erythromycin 2%, ethyl alcohol 66%.Topical soln. Bot. 60 ml.
Use: Anti-acne.

DELSYM COUGH SUPPRESSANT LIQUID. (McNeil Prods) Dextromethorphan HBr 30 mg/5 ml. Bot. 3 oz.
Use: Antitussive.

DELTA-1-CORTISONE.
Use: Corticosteroid.
See: Deltasone, Tab. (Upjohn).

DELTA-1-HYDROCORTISONE.
Use: Corticosteroid.
See: Prednisolone (Various Mfr.).

DELTA-CORTEF. (Upjohn) Prednisolone 5 mg/Tab. Bot. 100s, 500s.
Use: Corticosteroid.

DELTACORTONE. Prednisone.
Use: Corticosteroid.

DELTA-CORTRIL. Prednisolone.
Use: Corticosteroid.

DELTA-D. (Freeda) Vitamin D_3 400 IU/Tab. Bot. 250s, 500s.
Use: Vitamin D supplement.

• **DELTAFILCON A.** USAN.
Use: Contact lens material.

• **DELTAFILCON B.** USAN.
Use: Contact lens material.

DELTAPEN. (Trimen) Potassium penicillin G (U.S.P.) 400,000 units/5 ml. Oral Susp. Bot. "16 dose." Tab. Bot. 100s.
Use: Antibacterial, penicillin.

DELTASONE. (Upjohn) Prednisone. **2.5 mg:** Tab. Bot. 100s. **5 mg:** Tab. Bot. 100s, 500s, UD 100s, Dosepak 21s. **10 mg, 20 mg:** Tab. Bot. 100s, 500s, UD 100s. **50 mg:** Tab. Bot. 100s, UD 100s.
Use: Corticosteroid.

DELTA-TRITEX. (Dermol) Triamcinolone acetonide. **Cream:** 0.1% Tube 30 and 80 gm. **Oint.:** 0.1% Tube 30 gm.
Use: Corticosteroid, topical.

DELTAVAC. (Trimen) Sulfanilamide 15%, aminacrine HCl 0.2%, allantoin 2%. Vaginal cream: Tube with applicator 113.4 Gm.
Use: Vaginal anti-infective, antiseptic.

DEL-TRAC. (Del-Ray) Acne lotion. Bot. 2 oz.
Use: Anti-acne.

DELTRA-STAB.
Use: Corticosteroid.
See: Prednisolone (Various Mfr.).

DEL-STAT. (Del-Ray) Abradent cleaner.

Jar 2 oz.
Use: Anti-acne.

DEL-VI-A. (Del-Ray) Vitamin A 50,000 IU/Cap. Bot. 100s.
Use: Vitamin A supplement.

DELYSID. Lysergic acid diethylamide.
Use: Potent psychotogenic.

DEMADEX. (Boehringer Mannheim) **Tab.:** Torsemide 5 mg, 10 mg, 20 mg, 100 mg. Bot. UD 100s. **Inj.:** Torsemide 10 mg/ml. Amps. 2 ml or 5 ml.
Use: Diuretics, loop.

DEMAZIN. (Schering-Plough) **Syr.:** Chlorpheniramine maleate 2 mg, phenylpropanolamine HCl 12.5 mg/5 ml, alcohol 7.5%, menthol. Bot. 4 oz. **Tab.:** Chlorpheniramine maleate 4 mg, phenylpropanolamine HCl 25 mg. Box 24s. Bot. 100s, 1000s.
Use: Antihistamine, decongestant.

• **DEMECARIUM BROMIDE,** U.S.P. XXIII. Ophth. Soln. U.S.P. XXIII.
Use: Cholinergic, (ophthalmic).
See: Humorsol, Soln. (Merck & Co.).

• **DEMECLOCYCLINE,** U.S.P. XXIII. Oral susp., U.S.P. XXII. 7-Chloro-4-(dimethylamino)-1,4,4α,5,5α,6,11,12α-octahydro-3,6,10,-12,12α-pentahydroxy-1,11-dioxo-2-naphthacene-carboxamide.
Use: Antibacterial.
See: Declomycin Prods. (Lederle). Ledermycin Prods. (Lederle).

• **DEMECLOCYCLINE HYDROCHLORIDE,** U.S.P. XXIII. Cap., Tab., U.S.P. XXIII.
Use: Antibacterial.
See: Declomycin HCl, Preps. (Lederle).

• **DEMECLOCYCLINE HYDROCHLORIDE AND NYSTATIN CAPSULES,** U.S.P. XXIII.
Use: Antibacterial.
See: Declostatin, Cap. (Lederle).

• **DEMECLOCYCLINE HYDROCHLORIDE AND NYSTATIN TABLETS,** U.S.P. XXII.
Use: Antibacterial.
See: Declostatin, Tab. (Lederle).

DEMECOLCINE. B.A.N. N-Methyl-N-deacetyl-colchicine.
Use: Antimitotic, leukemia therapy.

• **DEMECYCLINE.** USAN.
Use: Antibacterial.

DEMEROL APAP. (Sanofi Winthrop) Meperidine HCl 50 mg, acetaminophen 300 mg/Tab. Bot. 100s.
Use: Narcotic analgesic combination.

DEMEROL HYDROCHLORIDE. (Sanofi Winthrop) Meperidine HCl. **Syr.:** 50 mg/5 ml, saccharin. Bot. 16 fl oz. **Inj.:** Detecto-Seal, Carpuject, Sterile Cartridge-Needle Unit. **2.5%** (25 mg/ml), **5%**

(50 mg/ml), **7.5%** (75 mg/ml), **10%** (100 mg/ml), Box 10s. **Uni-Amp 5%:** 0.5 ml (25 mg)/Amp., 1 ml (50 mg)/Amp., 1.5 ml (75 mg)/Amp., 2 ml (100 mg)/Amp. Box 25s; **10%:** 1 ml (100 mg)/Amp. Box 25s. **Uni-Nest 5%:** 0.5 ml (25 mg)/Amp., 1 ml (50 mg)/Amp., 1.5 ml (75 mg)/Amp., 2 ml (100 mg)/Amp. Box 25s; **10%:** 1 ml/Amp. Box 25s. **Vial: 5%** multiple-dose vial/30 ml Box 1s. **Tab.:** 50 mg or 100 mg. Bot. 100s, 500s.
Use: Narcotic analgesic.

DEMETHYLCHLORTETRACYCLINE HCl.
Use: Antibacterial, tetracycline.
See: Demeclocycline HCl, U.S.P. XXIII.

DEMI-REGROTON. (Rhone-Poulenc Rhone-Poulenc Rorer) Chlorthalidone 25 mg, reserpine 0.125 mg/Tab. Bot. 100s, 1000s.
Use: Antihypertensive, diuretic.

•**DEMOXEPAM.** USAN. 7-Chloro-1, 3-dihydro-5-phenyl-2H-1, 4-benzodiazepin-2-one-4-oxide.
Use: Minor tranquilizer.

DEMSER. (Merck & Co.) Metyrosine 250 mg/Cap. Bot. 100s.
Use: Antihypertensive.

DEMULEN 1/35-21. (Searle) Ethynodiol diacetate 1 mg, ethinyl estradiol 35 mcg/Tab. Compack disp. 21s, 6×21, 2421. Refill 21s, 1221.
Use: Oral contraceptive.

DEMULEN 1/35-28. (Searle) Ethynodiol diacetate 1 mg, ethinyl estradiol 35 mcg/Tab.Compack 28s: 21 active tabs, 7 placebo tabs. Compack 6×28, 2428. Refill 28s, 1228.
Use: Oral contraceptive.

DEMULEN 1/50-21. (Searle) Ethynodiol diacetate 1 mg, ethinyl estradiol 50 mcg/Tab. Compack Disp. 21s, 6×21, 2421. Refill 21s, 1221.
Use: Oral contraceptive.

DEMULEN 1/50. (Searle) Ethynodiol diacetate 1 mg, ethinyl estradiol 50 mcg/Tab. Compack 28s: 21 active tabs, 7 placebo tabs. Compack Disp. of 28, 6 ×28, 2428. Refill 28s, 1228.
Use: Oral contraceptive.

DENALAN DENTURE CLEANSER. (Whitehall) Sodium percarbonate 30%. Bot. 7 oz., 13 oz.
Use: Agent for oral hygiene.

•**DENATONIUM BENZOATE,** N.F. XVIII. Bitrex (MacFarlan Smith, Ltd. Scotland) Benzyldiethyl [(2, 6-xylylcarbamoyl) methyl] ammonium benzoate.
Use: Denaturant for ethyl alcohol.
See: Bitrex.

DENCORUB. (Last) Methyl salicylate 20%, menthol 0.75%, camphor 1%, eucalyptus oil 0.5%. Tube 1.25 oz, 2.75 oz.
Use: External analgesic.

DENCORUB ANALGESIC LIQUID. (Last) Oleoresin capsicum suspension in aqueous vehicle. Bot. 6 oz.
Use: External analgesic.

DENGESIC. (Scott-Alison) Salicylamide 100 mg, acetaminophen 240 mg, phenyltoloxamine dihydrogen citrate 30 mg, butabarbital ⅛ gr/Tab. Bot. 60s, 500s.
Use: Analgesic, sedative/hypnotic.

•**DENOFUNGIN.** USAN.
Use: Antifungal, antibacterial.

DENOREX. (Whitehall) Coal tar solution 9%, menthol 1.5%. Shampoo Bot. 4 oz, 8 oz.
Use: Antiseborrheic.

DENOREX EXTRA STRENGTH. (Whitehall) Coal tar solution 12.5%, menthol 1.5%, alcohol 10.4%. Shampoo. Bot. 120, 240, 360 ml.
Use: Antiseborrheic.

DENOREX MOUNTAIN FRESH. (Whitehall) Coal tar solution 9%, menthol 1.5%. Bot. 4 oz, 8 oz.
Use: Antiseborrheic.

DENOREX WITH CONDITIONERS. (Whitehall) Coal tar solution 9%, menthol 1.5%. Bot. 4 oz, 8 oz.
Use: Antiseborrheic.

DENQUEL. (Procter & Gamble) Potassium nitrate 5%, calcium carbonate, glycerin, flavors. Tube 1.6 oz, 3 oz, 4.5 oz.
Use: Agent for oral hygiene, preparation for sensitive teeth.

DENTAL CARIES PREVENTIVE. (Hoyt) Fluoride ion 1.2%, alumina abrasive. 2 Gm Box 200s, Jar 9 oz.
Use: Dental caries preventative.

•**DENTAL TYPE SILICA,** U.S.P. XXIII.

DENTROL. (Block) Carboxymethylcellulose, polyethelyne oxide homopolymer, peppermint and spearmint in mineral oil base. Bot. 0.9 oz, 1.8 oz.
Use: Denture adhesive.

DENT'S DENTAL POULTICE. (C.S. Dent) Glycerin mineral oil, polyoxyethylene sorbitan monooleate. Bot. 0.125 oz, 0.25 oz.
Use: Dental poultice.

DENT'S EAR WAX DROPS. (C.S. Dent) Glycerin, mineral oil, polyoxyethylene sorbitan monooleate. Bot. 0.125 oz, 0.25 oz.
Use: Otic preparation.

DENT'S LOTION-JEL. (C.S. Dent) Benzocaine in special base. Tube 0-2 oz.

Use: Local anesthetic, oral.

DENT'S TOOTHACHE DROPS TREAT-MENT. (C.S. Dent) Alcohol 60%, chlorobutanol anhydrous (chloroform derivative) 0.09%, propylene glycol, eugenol. Bot. 0.125 oz.
Use: Local anesthetic, oral.

DENT'S TOOTHACHE GUM. (C.S. Dent) Benzocaine, eugenol, petrolatum in base of cotton and wax. Box 0.035 oz.
Use: Local anesthetic, oral.

DENT-ZEL-ITE. (Last) **Oral Mucosal Analgesic:** Benzocaine 5%, alcohol, glycerin. Bot. $^1/_{16}$ oz,. **Temporary Dental Filling:** Sandarac gum, alcohol. Bot. oz,. **Toothache Drops:** Eugenol 85% in alcohol. Bot. oz.
Use: Local anesthetic, oral.

DENYL SODIUM.
Use: Anticonvulsant.
See: Diphenylhydantoin Sodium, Cap. (Various Mfr.).

DEODORIZERS, SYSTEMIC. Chlorophyll derivatives (chlorophyllin).
Use: **Oral:** Control of fecal and urinary odors in colostomy, ileostomy or incontinence. **Topical:** Reduce pain and inflammation (wounds, burns, surface ulcers, skin irritation).
See: Chlorophyll, Tab. (Freeda). Derifil, Tab. (Rystan). Chloresium, Tab., Soln., Oint. (Rystan).

DEOXYADENOSINE, 2-CHLORO-2¹. (St. Jude Children's Hospital)
Use: Antineoplastic. [Orphan drug]

DEOXYCHOLIC ACID.
See: Desoxycholic Acid, Tab. (Various Mfr.).

2'DEOXYCOFOMYCIN. Pentostatin.
Use: Antibiotic.
See: Nipent, Pow. (Parke-Davis).

DEOXYCYTIDINE, 5-AZA-2'. (Pharmachemie U.S.A.)
Use: Antineoplastic. [Orphan drug]

DEOXYNOJIRMYCIN. (Searle) Butyl-DNJ.
Use: Antiviral.

DEPAKENE. (Abbott) Valproic acid. **Cap.:** 250 mg. Bot. 100s, UD 100s. **Syr.:** 250 mg/5 ml, sorbitol. Bot. 480 ml.
Use: Anticonvulsant.

DEPAKOTE. (Abbott) Divalproex sodium 125 mg, 250 mg or 500 mg/enteric coated tab and 125 mg/sprinkle cap. **125 mg:** Bot. 100s. **250 mg:** Bot. 100s, UD 100s. **500 mg:** Bot. 100s, UD 100s. **125 mg sprinkle:** Bot. 100s, UD 100s.
Use: Anticonvulsant.

dep ANDRO 100. (Forest) Testosterone cypionate in cottonseed oil 100 mg/ml, benzyl alcohol. Vial 10 ml.
Use: Androgen.

dep ANDRO 200. (Forest) Testosterone cypionate in cottonseed oil 200 mg/ml, benzyl benzoate, benzyl alcohol. Vial 10 ml.
Use: Androgen.

dep ANDROGYN. (Forest) Testosterone cypionate 50 mg, estradiol cypionate 2 mg/ml, chlorobutanol, cottonseed oil. Vial 10 ml.
Use: Androgen, estrogen combination.

DEPA-SYRUP. (Alra) Valproic acid syrup 250 mg/5 ml. Bot. 4 oz, 16 oz.
Use: Anticonvulsant.

DEPEN TABLETS. (Wallace) Penicillamine 250 mg/Tab. Bot. 100s.
Use: Penicillamine.

DEPEPSEN. Amylosulfate sodium.
Use: Digestive aid.

dep GYNOGEN. (Forest) Estradiol cypionate in cottonseed oil 5 mg/ml, cottonseed oil, chlorobutanol. Vial 10 ml.
Use: Estrogen.

dep MEDALONE 40. (Forest) Methylprednisolone acetate in aqueous suspension 40 mg/ml, polyethylene glycol, myristyl-gamma-picolinium Cl. Vial 5 ml.
Use: Corticosteroid.

dep MEDALONE 80. (Forest) Methylprednisolone acetate 80 mg/ml, polyethylene glycol, myristyl-gamma-picolinium Cl. Vial 5 ml.
Use: Corticosteroid.

DEPOESTRA. (Tennessee Pharm.) Estradiol cypionate 5 mg/ml. Vial 10 ml.
Use: Estrogen.

DEPO-ESTRADIOL. (Upjohn) Estradiol cypionate 1 mg or 5 mg/ml, chlorobutanol anhydrous 5.4 mg/ml, cottonseed oil. **1 mg/ml:** Vial 10 ml. **5 mg/ml:** Vial 5 ml.
Use: Estrogen.

DEPOGEN. (Sig) Estradiol valerate 10 mg or 20 mg/ml in oil. Vial 10 ml.
Use: Estrogen.

DEPOGEN. (Hyrex) Estradiol cypionate 5 mg/ml, cottonseed oil, chlorobutanol. Vial 10 ml.
Use: Estrogen.

DEPOJECT. (Mayrand) Methylprednisolone acetate 40 mg or 80 mg/ml suspension with polyethylene glycol and myristyl-gamma-picolinium Cl. Inj. Vial 5 ml.
Use: Corticosteroid.

DEPO-MEDROL. (Upjohn) Methylprednisolone acetate, 20 mg/Inj. Vial. 5 ml, 10 ml. Methylprednisolone acetate, 40

mg/Inj. Vial. 5 ml, 10 ml. Methylprednisolone acetate 80 mg/Inj. Vial. 1 ml, 5 ml.
Use: Glucocorticoid.
DEPONIT. (Wyeth-Ayerst) Nitroglycerin transdermal delivery system containing 5 mg or 10 mg/24 Hrs. Box 30s.
Use: Vasodilator, antianginal.
DEPOPRED 40. (Hyrex) Methylprednisolone acetate suspension 40 mg/ml, polyethylene glycol, myristyl-gamma-picolinum Cl. Vial 5 ml, 10 ml.
Use: Corticosteroid.
DEPOPRED 80. (Forest) Methylprednisolone acetate 80 mg/Inj. Vial. 5 ml.
Use: Glucocorticoid.
DEPO-PROVERA. (Upjohn) Medroxyprogesterone acetate 100 mg or 400 mg/ml. **100 mg/ml:** Suspended in polyethylene glycol 3350 27.6 mg, polysorbate 80 1.84 mg, sodium Cl 8.3 mg, methylparaben 1.75 mg, propylparaben 0.194 mg/ml. Vial 5 ml. **400 mg/ml:** Suspended in polyethylene glycol 3350 20.3 mg, sodium sulfate (anhydrous) 11 mg, myristyl-gamma-picolinium Cl 1.69 mg/ml. Vial 2.5 ml, 10 ml, 1 ml U-Ject.
Use: Progestin.
DEPOTEST. (Hyrex) Testosterone cypionate. **100 mg:** With cottonseed oil, benzyl alcohol. **200 mg:** With cottonseed oil, benzyl benzoate, benzyl alcohol. Vial 10 ml.
Use: Androgen.
DEPO-TESTADIOL. (Upjohn) Testosterone cypionate 50 mg, estradiol cypionate 2 mg, chlorobutanol 5.4 mg, cottonseed oil 874 mg/ml. Vial 1 ml, 10 ml.
Use: Androgen estrogen combination.
DEPOTESTOGEN. (Hyrex) Testosterone cypionate 50 mg, estradiol cypionate 2 mg, chlorobutanol 5 mg/ml in cottonseed oil/ml. Vial 10 ml.
Use: Androgen, estrogen combination.
DEPO-TESTOSTERONE. (Upjohn) Testosterone cypionate. **100 mg/ml:** In benzyl alcohol 9.45 mg, cottonseed oil 736 mg/ml. Vial 1 ml, 10 ml. **200 mg/ml:** In benzyl benzoate 0.2 ml, benzyl alcohol 9.45 mg, cottonseed oil 560 mg/ml. Vial 1 ml, 10 ml.
Use: Androgen.
DEPRENYL. Selegiline HCl.
See: Eldepryl (Somerset).
DEPRODONE. B.A.N. 11 β 17α-Dihydroxypregna-1, 4-diene-3,20-dione.
Use: Corticosteroid.
DEPROIST EXPECTORANT WITH CODEINE. (Geneva Marsam) Pseudoephedrine HCl 30 mg, codeine phosphate 10 mg, guaifenesin 100 mg/5 ml. Bot. 120 ml, 480 ml.
Use: Decongestant, antitussive, expectorant.
DEPROL TABLETS. (Wallace) Meprobamate 400 mg, benactyzine HCl 1 mg/Tab. Bot. 100s, 500s.
Use: Antidepressant.
• **DEPROSTIL.** USAN.
Use: Antisecretory.
DEP-TEST. (Sig) Testosterone cypionate 100 mg/ml. Vial 10 ml.
Use: Androgen.
DEPTROPINE. B.A.N. 3-(10, 11-Dihydrodibenzo-[a, d]cycloheptadien-5-yloxy)tropane.
Use: Bronchodilator.
DEQUALINIUM CHLORIDE. B.A.N. Decamethylenedi-(4-aminoquinaldinium Cl).
Use: Antiseptic.
DEQUASINE. (Miller) L-lysine 20 mg, l-cysteine 100 mg, dl-methionine 50 mg, vitamin C 200 mg, iron 5 mg, Cu, I, Mg, Mn, Zn. Tab. Bot. 100s.
Use: Vitamin/mineral supplement.
DERIFIL. (Rystan) Chlorophyllin copper complex 100 mg/Tab. Bot. 30s, 100s, 1000s.
Use: Internal deodorant.
DERMABASE. (Paddock) Mineral oil, petrolatum, cetostearyl alcohol, propylene glycol, sodium lauryl sulfate, isopropyl palmitate, imidazolidinyl urea, methyl and propylparabens. Cream. Jar 1 lb.
Use: Emollient.
DERMACARE. (Jenkins) Hexachlorophene, camphor, menthol, lanolin. Lot. Bot. 2 oz, 6 oz, pt, gal.
Use: Antiseptic.
DERMACOAT AEROSOL SPRAY. (Century) Benzocaine 4.5%. Bot. 7 oz.
Use: Local anesthetic, topical.
DERMACORT CREAM. (Solvay) Hydrocortisone 0.5% or 1% in a water soluble cream of stearyl alcohol, cetyl alcohol, isopropyl palmitate, citric acid, polyoxyethylene 40 stearate, sodium phosphate, propylene glycol, water, benzyl alcohol, buffered to pH 5.0. 0.5% in 30 Gm, 1% in 1 lb.
Use: Corticosteroid, topical.
DERMACORT LOTION. (Solvay) Hydrocortisone 1% in lotion base, buffered to pH 5.0. Paraben free. Bot. 120 ml.
Use: Corticosteroid, topical.
DERMA-COVER. (Scrip) Sulfur, salicylic acid, hyamine 10x, isopropyl alcohol 22%, in powder film forming base. Bot. 2

oz.
Use: Keratolytic.

DERMAFLEX. (Zila) Lidocaine 2.5%, alcohol 79%. Gel. Tube 15 g.
Use: Local anesthetic, topical.

DERMA-GUARD. (Greer) Protective adhesive pow. Can w/sifter top, 4 oz. Spray top Bot. 4 oz, pkg. 1 lb. Rings. Pkg. 5s, 10s.
Use: Skin protectant.

DERMAL-RUB BALM. (Hauck) Menthol racemic 7%, camphor 1%, methyl salicylate 1%, cajuput oil 1%. Cream. Jar 1 oz, 1 lb.
Use: External analgesic.

DERMA-MEDICONE. (Medicone) Benzocaine 20 mg, oxyquinoline sulfate 10.5 mg, menthol 4.8 mg, ichthammol 10 mg, zinc oxide 137 mg/Gm w/petrolatum, lanolin, perfume, certified color. Oint. Tube 1 oz, Jar lb.
Use: Local anesthetic, antipruritic, vasoconstrictor.

DERMA MEDICONE-HC. (Medicone) Hydrocortisone acetate 10 mg, benzocaine 20 mg, oxyquinoline sulfate 10.5 mg, ephedrine HCl 1.1 mg, menthol 4.8 mg, ichthammol 10 mg, zinc oxide 137 mg/Gm, petrolatum, lanolin, perfume. Oint. Tube 7 Gm, 20 Gm.
Use: Corticosteroid, local anesthetic, antipruritic.

DERMAMYCIN. (Pfeiffer) Diphenhydramine HCl 2% in a base of parabens, polyethylene glycol monostearate and propylene glycol. Cream 28.35 g.
Use: Topical antihistamine.

DERMANEED. (Hanlon) Zirconium oxide 4.5%, calamine 6%, zinc oxide 4%, actamer 0.1% in bland lotionized base. Bot. 4 oz.
Use: Antipruritic.

DERMA-PAX. (Recsei) Methapyrilene HCl 0.22%, chlorothenylpyramine maleate 0.06%, pyrilamine maleate 0.22%, benzyl alcohol 1%, chlorobutanol 1%, isopropyl alcohol 40%. Liq. 4 oz, pt.
Use: Topical antipruritic, antihistamine.

DERMA-PAX HC. (Recsei) Hydrocortisone 0.5%, pyrilamine maleate 0.2%, pheniramine maleate 0.2%, chlorpheniramine 0.06%, benzyl alcohol 1%. Liq. Bot. 60 ml, 120 ml, 480 ml.
Use: Topical corticosteroid, antihistamine.

DERMAREST. (Del) Diphenhydramine HCl 2%, resorcinol 2%, aloe vera gel, benzalkonium chloride, EDTA, menthol, methylparaben, propylene glycol. Gel Tube 29.25 Gm, 56.25 Gm.
Use: Antihistamine.

DERMAREST DRICORT. (Del) Hydrocortisone 1%, white petrolatum cream. Bot. 14 Gm.
Use: Topical corticosteroid.

DERMAREST PLUS. (Del) **Gel:** Diphenhydramine HCl 2%, menthol 1%, aloe vera gel, benzalkonium chloride, isopropyl alcohol, methylparaben; propylene glycol. Tube 15 Gm, 30 Gm. **Spray:** Diphenhydramine HCl 2%, menthol 1%, aloe vera gel, benzalkonium chloride, methylparaben propylene glycol, SDA 40 alcohol, EDTA. Bot. 60 ml.
Use: Antihistamine.

DERMA-pH SKIN LOTION. (Day-Baldwin) pH 4.6 to 4.9. Mentholated or plain. Plastic squeeze bot. 4 oz, 8 oz. Plastic bot. gal.

DERMASEPT ANTIFUNGAL. (PharmaKon) Tannic acid 6.098%, zinc Cl 5.081%, benzocaine 2.032%, methylbenzethonium HCl, tolnaftate 1.017%, undecylenic acid 5.081%, ethanol 38B 58.539%, phenol, benzyl alcohol, benzoic acid, coal tar, camphor, menthol. Liq. Bot. 30 ml.
Use: Antifungal (topical).

DERMASIL. (Chesebrough-Ponds) Glycerin and dimethicone in a base containing cyclomethicone, sunflower seed oil, petrolatum, borage seed oil, lecithin, vitamin E acetate, vitamin A palmitate, vitamin D_3, corn oil, EDTA, methylparaben, DMDM hydantoin. Lot. Bot. 120 ml, 240 ml.
Use: Emollient.

DERMA-SMOOTHE/FS OIL. (Hill) Fluocinolone acetonide 0.01%. Oil. Bot. 4 oz.
Use: Antipsoriatic, antiseborrheic.

DERMA-SMOOTHE OIL. (Hill) Refined peanut oil, mineral oil in lipophilic base.
Use: Antipruritic, skin protectant.

DERMA SOAP. (Ferndale) Dowicil 0.1%. 4 oz w/dispenser.
Use: Antiseptic.

DERMA-SOFT. (Vogarell) Medicated cream. Salicylic acid, castor oil, triethanolamine. Tube ¾ oz.
Use: Keratolytic.

DERMA-SONE 1%. (Hill) Hydrocortisone 1%, pramoxine HCl 1%, cetyl alcohol, glyceryl monosterate, isopropyl myristate, potassium sorbate, furcelleran.
Use: Corticosteroid, topical.

DERMASORCIN. (Lamond) Resorcin 2%, sulfur 5%. Bot. 1 oz, 2 oz, 4 oz, 8 oz, pt, 32 oz, 0.5 gal.
Use: Anti-acne, antiseborrheic.

DERMASTRINGE. (Lamond) Bot. 4 oz, 6 oz, 8 oz, pt, 32 oz, gal.
Use: Skin cleanser.

DERMASUL. (Lamond) Sulfur 5%. Bot. 1 oz, 2 oz, 4 oz, 8 oz, pt, 32 oz, 0.5 gal, gal.
Use: Anti-acne, antiseborrheic.

DERMATHYN. (Davis & Sly) Benzyl alcohol 3%, benzocaine 3.5%, butyl-p-aminobenzoate 1%, phenylmercuric borate. Tube 1 oz.
Use: Local anesthetic.

DERMATIC BASE. (Whorton) Compounding cream base. Bot. 16 oz.
Use: Cream and lotion base.

DERMATOL.
See: Bismuth subgallate, Preps. (Various Mfr.).

DERMATOP. (Hoechst-Roussel) Prednicarbate 0.1%, white petrolatum, lanolin alcohols, mineral oil, cetostearyl alcohol, EDTA, lactic acid. Cream 15 g, 60 g.
Use: Corticosteroids, topical.

DERMATOPHYTIN (Trichophytin). (Hollister-Stier) Prepared from the filtrates of mixtures of 21-day maltose broth cultures of Trichophyton mentagrophytes, *T rubrum* and *T tonsurans*. Vial 5 ml (undiluted) and 5 ml (diluted 1:30).
Use: Diagnostic aid.

DERMATOPHYTIN "O" (Oidiomycin). (Hollister-Stier) Prepared from the filtrate of a 21-day maltose broth culture of *Candida albicans* (Monillia). Vials 5 ml (undiluted) and 5 ml (diluted 1:100).
Use: Diagnostic aid.

DERMA VIVA. (Rugby) Mineral oil, glyceryl stearate, laureth-4, lanolin oil, PEG-100 stearate, PEG-40 stearate, PEG-4 dilaurate, trolamine, diocetyl sodium sulfosuccinate, parabens. Lot. Bot. 237 ml.
Use: Emollient.

DERMAX. (Dermco) Methphenoxydiol 100 mg, (3-(2-methosyphenoxy)-1, 2-propanediol). Bot. 100s, 1000s.
Use: Tension states.

DERMED. (Holloway) Vitamins A and D with hydrogenated vegetable oil. Cream. Tube 60 Gm, 120 Gm.
Use: Emollient.

DERMEZE. (Premo) Thenylpyramine HCl 2%, benzocaine 2%, tyrothricin 0.25 mg/Gm. Massage Lot. Bot. 5³/₄ oz.
Use: Topical antihistamine, antibiotic, anesthetic.

DERMICORT. (Republic Drug) **Cream:** Hydrocortisone 0.5%. Tube 30 Gm.
Lot.: Hydrocortisone 0.5%. Bot. 60 ml.
Use: Corticosteroid.

DERMOL HC. (Dermol) **Cream:** Hydro-

cortisone 1%. Tube 30 g. **Oint.:** Hydrocortisone 1%. Tube 30 g.
Use: Anorectal preparation.

DERMOLATE ANTI-ITCH. (Schering-Plough) Hydrocortisone 0.5% petrolatum, mineral oil, chlorocresol. Cream Tube 15 Gm, 30 Gm.
Use: Topical corticosteroid.

DERMOLIN. (Hauck) Menthol racemic, methyl salicylate, camphor, mustard oil, isopropyl alcohol 8%. Bot. 3 oz, pt, gal.
Use: Liniment, topical.

DERMOPLAST AEROSOL SPRAY. (Wyeth-Ayerst) Benzocaine 20%, menthol 0.5%, in water-dispersible base of Tween 85, PEG 400 monolaurate, methylparaben as preservative, propellants. Spray 2.75 oz, 6 oz.
Use: Topical anesthetic, antipruritic.

DERMOVAN. (Owen/Galderma) Glyceryl stearate, spermaceti, mineral oil, glycerin, cetyl alcohol, butylparaben, methylparaben, propylparaben, purified water. Vanishing-type base, Jar 1 lb.
Use: Skin protectant.

DERMOXYL. (ICN) Benzoyl peroxide 2.5%, 5%, 10%. Gel. Tube 30 g.
Use: Anti-acne.

DERM/T TAR EMOLLLIENT.
See: T/DERM TAR EMOLLIENT.

DERMTEX HC. (Pfeiffer) Hydrocortisone 0.5% in a glycerin base. Tube 15 Gm.
Use: Corticosteroid, topical.

DERMUSPRAY. (Warner-Chilcott) Trypsin 0.1 mg, Balsam Peru 72.5 mg, castor oil 650 mg/0.82 ml. Aer. Bot. 120 Gm.
Use: Topical enzyme combination.

DERM-VI SOAP.
See: VI-DERM SOAP.

D.E.S.
See: Diethylstilbestrol.

DESACCHROMIN. A nonprotein bacterial colloidal dispersion of polysaccharide.

•**DESCICLOVIR.** USAN.
Use: Antiviral.

•**DESCINOLONE ACETONIDE.** USAN.
Use: Glucocorticoid.

DESENEX. (Ciba) **Cream:** Undecylenic acid, zinc undecylenate 25%. Tube 0.5 oz, 1 oz. **Oint.:** Undecylenic acid 5%, zinc undecylenate 20%. Tube 0.9 oz, 1.8 oz, Can 1 lb. **Pow.:** Undecylenic acid 5%, zinc undecylenate 20%. Can 1.5 oz, 3 oz, Carton 1 lb. **Liq.:** Undecylenic acid 10%, isopropyl alcohol 47.1%. Pump spray bot. 1.5 oz. **Spray Pow.:** Undecylenic acid 5%, zinc undecylenate 20%. Aerosol can 2.7 oz, 5.5 oz. **Penetrating Foam:** Undecylenic acid 10%,

isopropyl alcohol 29.2%. Can 1.5 oz.
Use: Antifungal, external.
DESENEX FOOT & SNEAKER SPRAY.
(Pharmacraft) Aluminum chlorhydrex
w/alcohol 89.3%. Aerosol can 2.7 oz.
Use: Foot deodorant, antiperspirant.
DESENEX MAXIMUM STRENGTH.
(Fisons) Total undecylenate 25%, lano-
lin, parabono, whito potrolatum. Oint.
Tube 15 Gm.
Use: Topical anti-inflammatory.
DE SERPA. (de Leon) Reserpine 0.25 mg
or 0.5 mg/Tab. Bot. 100s, 500s, 1000s
(0.25 mg only).
Use: Antihypertensive.
DESERPIDINE. An alkaloid derived from
Rauwolfia canescens. 11-
Desmethoxyreserpine (Raunormine).
Use: Antihypertensive.
See: Harmonyl, Tab. (Abbott).
W/Hydrochlorothiazide.
See: Oreticyl, Tab. (Abbott).
W/Methyclothiazide.
See: Enduronyl and Enduronyl Forte,
Tab. (Abbott).
DESERT PURE CALCIUM. (Cal•White
Mineral Co.) Calcium (from calcium car-
bonate) 500 mg, vitamin D 125 IU. Tab.
Bot. 200s.
Use: Minerals and electrolytes.
DESFERAL. (Ciba) Deferoxamine mesy-
late 500 mg/5 ml. Amp. 4s.
Use: Antidote.
DESFERRIOXAMINE. B.A.N. 30-Amino-
3,14,25-tri- hydroxy-3,9,14,20,25-penta-
azatriacontane-2,10,- 13,21,24-pen-
taone. Deferoxamine (I.N.N.).
Use: Chelating agent.
• **DESFLURANE.** USAN.
Use: General anesthetic.
See: Suprane (Anaquest).
• **DESIPRAMINE HYDROCHLORIDE,**
U.S.P. XXIII. Cap., Tab., U.S.P. XXIII.
Use: Antidepressant.
See: Norpramin, Tab. (Marion Merrell
Dow).
Pertofrane, Cap. (USV).
DESITIN. (Leeming) **Pow.:** Talc. Can 3
oz, 7 oz, 10 oz. **Oint.:** Cod liver oil, zinc
oxide 40%, talc, petrolatum, lanolin.
Tube 1 oz, 2 oz, 4 oz, 8 oz, Jar 1 lb.
Use: Topical astringent, skin protectant.
DESITIN WITH ZINC OXIDE. (Pfizer)
Cornstarch 88.2%, zinc oxide 10%.
Pow. 28 g, 397 g.
Use: Diaper rash product.
• **DESLORELIN.** USAN
Use: Gonadotropin inhibitor. [Orphan
drug]

DESMA. (Tablicaps) Diethylstilbesterol 25
mg/Tab. Patient dispenser 10s.
Use: Estrogen.
• **DESMOPRESSIN ACETATE.** USAN.
Use: Treatment of diabetes insipidus.
Mild hemophilia A and von Wille-
brand's disease [Orphan drug]
See: Stimate (Armour).
DDAVP, Liq. (Rhone Poulone Rorer).
DESOGEN. (Organon) Desogestrel 0.15
mg, ethinyl estradiol 0.03 mg/Tab. Pck.
28s.
Use: Oral contraceptive.
• **DESOGESTREL.** USAN.
Use: Progestin.
W/ Ethinyl estradiol.
See: Desogen, Tab. (Organon).
Ortho-Cept, Tab.(Ortho).
DESOMORPHINE. B.A.N. 7,8-Dihydro-6-
deoxy- morphine.
Use: Narcotic analgesic.
• **DESONIDE.** USAN. 16-alpha-Hydrox-
yprednisolone-16, 17 acetonide. B.A.N.
11 β,21-Dihydroxy-16α, 17 α-isopropy-
lidenedioxypregna-1,4-diene-3,20-
dione.
Use: Anti-inflammatory, corticosteroid.
See: Tridesilon, Cream (Miles Pharm).
DESONIDE CREAM. (Owen/Galderma)
Desonide 0.05% in cream base. Tube
15 Gm, 60 Gm.
Use: Corticosteroid, topical.
DESOWEN. (Owen/Galderma) Desonide
0.05%. Cream. Tube 15 Gm, 60 Gm.
Use: Corticosteroid, topical.
• **DESOXIMETASONE,** U.S.P. XXIII.
Cream, Gel, Oint., U.S.P. XXIII.
Use: Adrenocortical steroid.
• **DESOXYCORTICOSTERONE
TRIMETHYLACETATE.** 11-Deoxycorti-
costerone pivalate.
Use: Adrenocortical steroid (salt-regu-
lating).
**DESOXYEPHEDRINE HYDROCHLO-
RIDE.** (Various Mfr.) Dextro-l-phenyl-2-
methylaminopropane, d-phenyliso-
propylmethylamine, d-N-methylamphet-
amine.
Use: CNS stimulant.
See: Methamphetamine HCl, Prep.
**dl-DESOXYEPHEDRINE HYDROCHLO-
RIDE.**
See: dl-Methamphetamine HCl.
dl-NOREPHEDRINE HYDROCHLORIDE.
alpha-Hydroxy-beta-aminopropylben-
zene HCl.
See: Phenylpropanolamine Hydrochloride (Various Mfr.).
DESOXYMETHASONE. B.A.N. 9α-Fluo-

ro-11β,-21-dihydroxy-16α-methylpregna-1,4-diene-3,20-dione.
Use: Topical corticosteroid.
DESOXYN. (Abbott) Methamphetamine HCl. **Tab.:** 5 mg. Bot. 100s. **Gradumets:** 5 mg. Bot. 100s; 10 mg. Bot. 100s; 15 mg. Bot. 100s, 500s.
Use: CNS stimulant.
DESOXY NOREPHEDRINE.
Use: CNS stimulant.
See: Amphetamine HCl, Preps. (Various Mfr.).
DESOXYRIBONUCLEASE.
W/Fibrinolysin.
Use: Topical enzyme preparation.
See: Elase, prep. (Parke-Davis).
DESPEC LIQUID. (Inter. Ethical Labs.) Phenylpropanolamine HCl 20 mg, phenylephrine HCl 5 mg, guaifenesin 100 mg, alcohol 5%. Liq. Bot. 118 ml.
Use: Decongestant, expectorant.
DESQUAM-E. (Westwood) Benzoyl peroxide 2.5%, 5% or 10%. Gel. Tube 42.5 Gm.
Use: Anti-acne.
DESQUAM-X 2.5%, 5% or 10% GEL. (Westwood) Benzoyl peroxide 2.5%, 5% or 10%, water base with laureth-4 6%. Tube 1.5 oz.
Use: Anti-acne.
DESQUAM-X 5% or 10% WASH. (Westwood) Benzoyl peroxide 5% or 10% in a lathering base of sodium oxtoxynol-3 sulfonate, docusate sodium, magnesium aluminum silicate, methylcellulose, EDTA. Bot. 5 oz.
Use: Anti-acne.
D-EST. (Burgin-Arden) Estradiol cypionate 5 mg/ml. Vial 10 ml.
Use: Estrogen.
DE-STAT. (Sherman) Surfactant cleaner, benzalkonium Cl 0.01%, EDTA 0.25%. Soln. Bot. 118 ml.
Use: Hard contact lens care.
DE-STAT 3. (Sherman) Octylphenoxy-polyethoxyethanol, benzyl alcohol 0.1%, trisodium edetate 0.5%. Soln. Bot. 118 ml.
Use: Hard contact lens care.
DESYREL. (Mead Johnson) Trazodone HCl 50 mg or 100 mg. **50 mg:** Bot. 100s, 1000s, UD 100s. **100 mg:** Bot. 500s.
Use: Antidepressant.
DESYREL DIVIDOSE. (Mead Johnson) Trazodone HCl 150 mg or 300 mg/Dividose tab. Dividose design breakable into fragments for dosing convenience. Bot. 100s, 500s (150 mg).
Use: Antidepressant.
DETACHOL. (Ferndale) Bland, nonirritat-

ing liquid for removing adhesive tape. Pkg. 4 oz.
Use: Adhesive remover.
DE TAL. (de Leon) Phenobarbital 0.25 gr, hyoscyamine sulfate 0.1037 mg, atropine sulfate 0.0194 mg, hyoscine HBr 0.0065 mg/Tab. or 5 ml. **Tab.:** Bot. 100s. **Elix.:** With alcohol 20%. Bot. pt.
Use: Sedative/hypnotic, anticholinergic/antispasmodic.
DETANE. (Del Pharmaceuticals) Benzocaine 7.5%. Tube 0.5 oz.
Use: Local anesthetic.
• **DETERENOL HYDROCHLORIDE.** USAN.
Use: Adrenergic.
DETERGENTS, Surface-Active.
See: pHisoDerm, Liq. (Sanofi Winthrop).
pHisoHex, Liq. (Sanofi Winthrop).
Zephiran, Prods. (Sanofi Winthrop).
DETIGON HYDROCHLORIDE.
See: Chlophedianol HCl (Various Mfr.).
• **DETIRELIX ACETATE.** USAN.
Use: Antagonist.
DET-O-JET. (Alconox).
Use: Liquid detergent for mechanical, instrument and cage washers.
DETUSS. (Various Mfr.) Phenylpropanolamine HCl 75 mg and caramiphen edisylate 40 mg/TR Cap. Bot. 100s, 500s, 1000s.
Use: Decongestant, antitussive.
DETUSSIN EXPECTORANT LIQUID. (Various Mfr.) Pseudoephedrine HCl 60 mg, hydrocodone bitartrate 5 mg, guaifenesin 200 mg, alcohol. Liq. Bot. 480 ml.
Use: Decongestant, antitussive, expectorant.
DETUSSIN LIQUID. (Various Mfr.) Pseudoephedrine HCl 60 mg, hydrocodone bitartrate 5 mg, alcohol. Liq. Bot. 480 ml.
Use: Decongestant, antitussive.
• **DEUTIERIUM OXIDE.** USAN.
Use: Radioactive agent.
• **DEVAZEPIDE.** USAN.
Use: Antispasmodic, gastrointestinal.
DEWITT'S PILLS. (DeWitt) Blister Pack 20s, 40s, 80s.
Use: Analgesic, diuretic.
DEXACIDIN OINTMENT. (Iolab) Neomycin sulfate 3.5 mg, dexamethasone 1 mg, polymyxin B sulfate 10,000 units/Gm. Tube 3.5 Gm.
Use: Anti-infective, corticosteroid, ophthalmic.
DEXACIDIN OPHTHALMIC SUSPENSION. (Iolab) Neomycin 3.5 mg, polymyxin B sulfate 10,000 units, dex-

amethasone 1 mg/ml. Bot. 5 ml.
Use: Anti-infective, corticosteroid, ophthalmic.

DEX-A-DIET CAFFEINE FREE. (O'Connor) Phenylpropanolamine HCl 75 mg/Cap. or Capl. Pkg. 3s, 6s, 20s, 40s. *Use:* Diet aid.

DEX-A-DIET ORIGINAL FORMULA. (O'Connor) Phenylpropanolamine HCl 75 mg, ascorbic acid 200 mg/Cap. Pkg. 3s, 6s, 10s, 24s, 48s. *Use:* Diet aid.

DEXAFED. (Mallard) Phenylephrine HCl 5 mg, dextromethorphan HBr 10 mg, guaifenesin 100 mg/5 ml. Syr. Bot. 120 ml. *Use:* Decongestant, antitussive, expectorant.

DEXAMETH. (Major) **Tab.**: Dexamethasone 0.25 mg, 0.5 mg, 0.75 mg, 1.5 mg or 4 mg. Bot. 100s (0.25 mg, 0.5 mg, 1.5 mg); Bot. 100s, 1000s, Unipak 12s (0.75 mg); Bot. 50s, 100s (4 mg). **Elix.**: 0.5 mg/5 ml, alcohol 5%. Bot. 100 ml, 240 ml. *Use:* Corticosteroid.

• **DEXAMETHASONE,** U.S.P. XXIII. Tab., Elix., Gel, Ophth. Susp., Topical Aerosol, U.S.P. XXIII. Pregna-1,4-diene-3,20-dione,9-fluoro-11,17,21-trihydroxy-16-methyl-, (11β,16α). 9-fluoro-11β, 17,21-trihydroxy-16α-methyl-, pregna-1,4-diene-3,20-dione.
Use: Adrenal corticosteroid (anti-inflammatory). Dose: Individualized according to disease, 0.75 mg is equivalent to 4 mg triamcinolone, 5 mg prednisone/prednisolone, 20 mg hydrocortisone or 25 mg cortisone.
See: Aeroseb-Dex, Aerosol (Herbert).
Decaderm in Estergel (Merck & Co.).
Decadron, Tab., Elix. (Merck & Co.).
Decameth, Inj. (Foy).
Decameth L.A., Inj. (Foy).
Decaspray, Aerosol (Merck & Co.).
Dexaport, Tab. (Freeport).
Dexone TM, Tab. (Solvay).
Dezone, Tab. (Solvay).
Hexadrol, Tab., Elix., Cream (Organon).
Maxidex Ophth. Liq. (Alcon).
W/Neomycin sulfate.
See: NeoDecadron, Prep. (Merck & Co.)
NeoDecaspray, Aerosol (Merck & Co.).
W/Neomycin sulfate, polymyxin B sulfate.
See: Maxitrol Ophth. Susp., Oint. (Alcon).

DEXAMETHASONE. (Steris) 0.1%.

Susp. Bot. 5 ml.
Use: Corticosteroid, ophthalmic.

• **DEXAMETHASONE ACEFURATE.** USAN.
Use: Anti-inflammatory, topical steroid.

• **DEXAMETHASONE ACETATE,** U.S.P. XXIII. Sterile Susp., U.S.P. XXIII.
Use: Adrenocortical steroid (anti-inflammatory).
See: Dexone LA, Ind. (Kay).

• **DEXAMETHASONE DIPROPIONATE.** USAN.
Use: Anti-inflammatory.

DEXAMETHASONE INTENSOL ORAL SOLUTION. (Roxane) Dexamethasone 1 mg/ml concentrated oral soln. Bot. 30 ml w/calibrated dropper.
Use: Corticosteroid.

DEXAMETHASONE OPHTHALMIC. (Various Mfr.) Dexamethasone 0.1%. Susp. Bot. 5 ml.
Use: Ophthalmic.

• **DEXAMETHASONE SODIUM PHOSPHATE,** U.S.P. XXIII. Inhalation Aerosol, Cream, Ophth. Oint., Ophth. Soln., Inj., U.S.P. XXIII. Pregn-4-ene-3,20-dione, 9-fluoro-11, 17-dihydroxy-16-methyl-21-(phosphonooxy)-disodium salt, (11β, 16α)-9-Fluoro-11β, 17,21-trihydroxy-16α-methylpregna-1,4-diene-3,20-dione-21-(dihydrogen phosphate) disodium salt. (Various Mfr.) **Soln.**: 0.1%. Bot. 5 ml; **Oint.**: 0.05%. Tube 3.5g.
Use: Adrenocortical steroid (anti-inflammatory).
See: AK-Dex, Soln., Oint. (Akorn).
Decadron Phosphate, Preps. (Merck & Co.).
Decadron Phosphate Respihaler (Merck & Co.).
Decaject, Vial (Mayrand).
Decameth, Inj. (Foy).
Dexone, Inj. (Keene, Hauck).
Dezone, Inj. (Solvay).
Hexadrol Phosphate, Inj. (Organon).
Maxidex, Oint. (Alcon).
Savacort D, Inj. (Savage).
Solurex, Inj. (Hyrex).
W/Lidocaine (Xylocaine).
See: Decadron Phosphate w/Xylocaine, Inj. (Merck & Co.).
W/Neomycin sulfate.
See: NeoDecadron, Prods. (Merck & Co.).
W/Neomycin and polymixin B sulfates.
See: Dexacidin, Prods. (CooperVision).

• **DEXAMISOLE.** USAN.
Use: Antidepressant.

DEXAMPHETAMINE.

See: Dextroamphetamine (Various Mfr.).

DEXAPHEN SA TABLETS. (Major) Pseudoephedrine sulfate 120 mg, dexbrompheniramine maleate 6 mg. In 10s, 20s, 40s, 100s, 500s.
Use: Decongestant, antihistamine.

DEXAPORT. (Freeport) Dexamethasone 0.75 mg/Tab. Bot. 1000s.
Use: Corticosteroid.

DEXASONE. (Various Mfr.) Dexamethasone sodium phosphate 4 mg/ml, methyl and propyl parabens, sodium bisulfite. Vial 5 ml, 10 ml, 30 ml.
Use: Corticosteroid.

DEXASONE INJECTION. (Hauck) Dexamethasone sodium phosphate 4 mg/ml. Vial 5 ml, 30 ml.
Use: Corticosteroid.

DEXASONE-L.A. INJECTION. (Hauck) Dexamethasone acetate 8 mg/ml. Vial 5 ml.
Use: Corticosteroid.

DEXASPORIN OINTMENT. (Various Mfr.) Dexamethasone 0.1%, neomycin sulfate equivalent to 0.35% neomycin base and 10,000 units polymyxin B sulfate/Gm, white petrolatum, lanolin, mineral oil, parabens. Oint. Tube 3.5, 5 Gm.
Use: Steroid, antibiotic (ophthalmic).

DEXASPORIN SUSPENSION. (Various Mfr.) Dexamethasone 0.1%, neomycin sulfate equivalent to 0.35%, neomycin base and 10,000 units polymyxin B sulfate/ml, hydroxypropyl methylcellulose, polysorbate 20, banzalkonium chloride. Drops. Bot. 5 ml.
Use: Steroid antibiotic (ophthalmic).

DEXATRIM-15. (Thompson) Phenylpropanolamine HCl 75 mg/TR Cap. Bot. 20s, 40s.
Use: Diet aid.

DEXATRIM-15 W/VITAMIN C. (O'Connor) Phenylpropanolamine HCl 75 mg, vitamin C 180 mg/TR Cap. Bot. 20s.
Use: Diet aid.

DEXATRIM MAXIMUM STRENGTH. (Thompson) Phenylpropanolamine HCl 75 mg/Tab. ER Bot. 20s.
Use: Diet aid.

DEXATRIM PLUS VITAMINS. (O'Connor) Phenylpropanolamine HCl 75 mg, vitamins B_1 1.5 mg, B_2 1.7 mg, B_3 20 mg, B_5 10 mg, B_6 2 mg, B_{12} 6 mcg, C 60 mg, biotin 30 mcg, folic acid 0.4 mg, cromium 50 mcg, copper 2 mg, iron 7.5 mg, iodine 150 mg, manganese 3 mg, zinc 15 mg/TR Cap. Bot. 16s.
Use: Diet aid, vitamin/mineral supplement.

DEXATRIM PRE-MEAL. (Thompson) Phenylpropanolamine HCl 25 mg/TR Cap. Bot. 30s.
Use: Diet aid.

• **DEXBROMPHENIRAMINE MALEATE,** U.S.P. XXIII. (+)-2-[p-Bromo-α-[2-(dimethylamino) ethyl]-benzyl]pyridine maleate. Dextro form of brompheniramine. Dextroparabromdylamine 1-(p-bromophenyl-1-(2- pyridyl)-3-dimethylamino propane maleate. (+)-2-(p-Bromo-α-2-(dimethylamithenzyl)-pyridine-M aleate (1:1).
Use: Antihistamine.
W/Pseudoephedrine sulfate.
See: Disophrol Chronotab, Tab. (Schering-Plough).
Drixoral S.A., Tab. (Schering-Plough).

DEXCHLOR. (Schein) Dexchlorpheniramine maleate 4 mg/RA Tab. Bot. 100s.
Use: Antihistamine.

• **DEXCHLORPHENIRAMINE MALEATE,** U.S.P. XXIII. Syr., Tab., U.S.P. XXIII. d-2-[p-Chloroalpha(2-di- methyl-amino-ethLL) Lenzyl] pyridine bimaleate. (+)-2-[p-Chloro-α-[2-(dimethylamino)-ethyl]benzyl]pyridine Maleate (1:1) Dextro-Chlorpheniramine Maleate.
Use: Antihistamine.
See: Polaramine, Repetabs Tab., Tab., Syr. (Schering-Plough).
W/Pseudoephedrine sulfate, guaifenesin, alcohol.
See: Polaramine Expectorant (Schering-Plough).

• **DEXCLAMOL HYDROCHLORIDE.** USAN.
Use: Sedative.

DEXEDRINE. (SK-Beecham) Dextroamphetamine sulfate. **Tab.:** 5 mg Bot. 100s, 1000s. **Spansule:** 5 mg Bot. 50s; 10 mg, 15 mg Bot. 50s, 500s.
Use: CNS stimulant.

• **DEXETIMIDE.** USAN. (+)-3-(1-Benzyl-4-piperidyl)-3-phenylpiperidine-2,6-dione.
Use: Treatment of Parkinson's disease.

• **DEXFENFLURAMINE HYDROCHLORIDE.** USAN.
Use: Antiobesity.

• **DEXIBUPROFEN LYSINE.** USAN.
Use: Nonsteroidal anti-inflammatory; analgesic.

• **DEXIMAFEN.** USAN.
Use: Antidepressant.

• **DEXIVACAINE.** USAN.
Use: Anesthetic.

• **DEXMEDETOMIDINE.** USAN.
Use: Sedative/hypnotic.

DEXONE. (Solvay) Dexamethasone 0.5 mg, 0.75 mg, 1.5 mg or 4 mg/Tab. Bot.

100s, UD 100s. Box 1s, 10s, 150s.
Use: Corticosteroid.
DEXONE. (Hauck) Dexamethasone sodium phosphate 4 mg/ml. Amp. 5 ml.
Use: Corticosteroid.
DEXONE. (Keene) Dexamethasone sodium phosphate 4 mg/ml, methyl and propyl parabens, sodium bisulfite. Vial 5 ml, 10 ml.
Use: Corticosteroid.
DEXONE L.A. (Keene) Dexamethasone acetate suspension equivalent to dexamethasone 8 mg, polysorbate 80, carboxymethylcellulose, sodium bisulfite, EDTA, benzyl alcohol. Vial 5 ml.
Use: Corticosteroid.
• **DEXORMAPLATIN.** USAN.
Use: Antineoplastic.
• **DEXOXADROL HYDROCHLORIDE.** USAN. d-2-(2,2-Diphenyl-1,3-dioxolan-4-yl) piperidine HCl. Dextro form of dioxadrol HCl.
Use: Antidepressant.
• **DEXPANTHENOL,** U.S.P. XXIII. Preparation, U.S.P. XXIII. (+)-2,4-Dihydroxy-N-(3-hydroxypropyl)-3,3-di-methylbutyramide.
Use: Treatment of paralytic ileus and postoperative distention.
See: Ilopan, Inj. (Adria).
Panthoderm (USV).
DEXPANTHENOL WITH CHOLINE BITARTRATE.
See: Ilopan-choline (Adria).
• **DEXPEMEDOLAC.** USAN.
Use: Analgesic
• **DEXPROPANOLOL HCl.** USAN. (±)-I-(Iso- propylamino)-3-(I-naphthyloxy)-2-propanol HCl.
Use: Cardiac depressant (Antiarrhythmic).
• **DEXRAZOXANE.** USAN.
Use: Cardioprotectant. [Orphan drug]
DEXTRAN. B.A.N. Polyanhydroglucose.
Use: Blood volume expander.
See: LMWD-Dextran 40 (Pharmchem).
Macrodex, Soln. (Pharmacia).
DEXTRAN 6%. (Abbott)
See: Dextran 75, I.V. (Abbott).
• **DEXTRAN 40.** USAN. Polysaccharide (m.w. 40,000) produced by the action of Leuconostoc mesenteroides on saccharose.
Use: Blood suspension stabilizer.
DEXTRAN 45, 75. Polysaccharide (m.w. 45,000, 75,000) produced by the action of Leuconostoc mesenteroides on saccharose. Rheotran (45).
Use: Blood volume expander, antithrombogenic agent.

• **DEXTRAN 70.** USAN. A polysaccharide. Macrodex, Soln. (Pharmacia).
Use: Blood volume expander.
• **DEXTRAN 75.** USAN. Dextran 75 6% in 0.9% saline. Flask 500 ml; Dextran 75 6% in 5% dextrose. Flask 500 ml.
Use: Blood plasma expander.
DEXTRAN ADJUNCT.
Use: Plasma expander.
See: Promit (Pharmacia) Inj.
DEXTRAN AND DEFEROXAMINE.
Use: Acute iron poisoning. [Orphan drug]
DEXTRANOMER. B.A.N. Dextran cross-linked with epichlorohydrin.
Use: Promoter of wound healing.
DEXTRAN SULFATE.
Use: Antiviral. [Orphan drug]
See: Uendex (Ueno Fine Chem Industry Ltd.)
• **DEXTRATES,** N.F. XVIII. Mixture of sugars (approximately 92% dextrose monohydrate and 8% higher saccharides; dextrose equivalent is 95 to 97%) resulting from the controlled enzymatic hydrolysis of starch.
Use: Pharmaceutic aid (tablet binder and diluent).
DEXTRIFERRON. B.A.N. A colloidal solution of ferric hydroxide in complex with partially hydrolyzed dextrin.
Use: Treatment of iron-deficiency anemias.
See: Imferon, Amp. (Merrell Dow).
• **DEXTRIN,** N.F. XVIII.
Use: Pharmaceutic aid (tablet and capsule diluent).
• **DEXTROAMPHETAMINE.** USAN.
Use: Stimulant (central).
DEXTROAMPHETAMINE WITH AMPHETAMINE AS RESIN COMPLEX.
See: Biphetamine 12.5, 20, Cap. (Pennwalt).
DEXTROAMPHETAMINE PHOSPHATE. Monobasic d-a-methylphenethlyamine phosphate. (+)-α-Methylphenethylamine phosphate.
Use: CNS stimulant.
See: d-Amphetamine Phosphate combinations.
• **DEXTROAMPHETAMINE SULFATE,** U.S.P. XXIII. Cap., Elix., Tab., U.S.P. XXIII. Benzeneethanamine, α-methyl-, sulfate (2:1). (+)-α-Methylphenethylamine sulfate (2:1). d-Amphetamine sulfate, d-Methyl-phenylamine sulfate.
Use: Central stimulant.
See: Dexampex, Cap., Tab. (Lemmon).
Dexedrine, Preps. (SK-Beecham).

Diphylets, Granucaps (Solvay).
Tidex Tab. (Allison).
DEXTROAMPHETAMINE SULFATE W/COMBINATIONS.
Use: CNS stimulant.
See: Amphodex, Cap. (Jamieson-McK-ames).
Delcobese (Delco).
Min-Gera, Tab. (Scrip).
Trimex, Trimex #2, Cap. (Mills).
DEXTRO-CHECK NORMAL CONTROL.
(Miles Diagnostic) Clear liquid containing measured amount of glucose 0.10% w/v.
Use: Perform check of Glucometer refluctance photometer or Dextrometer refluctance photometer using Dextrostix and Glucometer II Blood Glucose Meter using Glucostix.
DEXTRO-CHEK CALIBRATORS. (Miles Diagnostic) Clear liquid soln. containing measured amounts of glucose. Low calibrator contains 0.05% w/v glucose. High calibrator contains 0.30% w/v glucose.
Use: Dextrostix to perform calibration procedure for Glucometer reflectance photometer.
DEXTRO-CHLORPHENIRAMINE MALEATE.
Use: Antihistamine.
See: Polaramine, Repetab, Tab., Expect., Syr. (Schering-Plough).
• **DEXTROMETHORPHAN, U.S.P. XXIII.**
(+)-3-Methoxy-N-methylmorphinan.
Use: Cough suppressant.
See: Benylin DM Cough Syrup(Parke-Davis).
Delsym, Liq. (Pennwalt).
W/Benzocaine, menthol, peppermint oil.
See: Vicks Formula 44 Cough Control Discs, Loz. (Vicks).
• **DEXTROMETHORPHAN HYDROBRO-MIDE, U.S.P. XXIII.** Syr., U.S.P. XXIII. d-3-Methoxy-N-methylmorphinan. (+)-3-Methoxy-17-methyl-9α, 13α,-14α-morphinan HBr. Dormethan. d-Methorphan.
Use: Antitussive.
See: Benylin DM Cough Syr. (Parke-Davis).
Dicodethal, Elix. (Lannett).
Mediquell, Tab. (Warner-Lambert).
St. Joseph Cough Syr. (Schering-Plough).
Symptom 1, Liq. (Parke-Davis).
Tus-F, Liq. (Orbit).
Tussade Tab. (Westerfield).
DEXTROMETHORPHAN HBr W/ BEN-ZOCAINE.
Use: Nonnarcotic antitussives.
See: Spec-T, Loz. (Apothecon).

Vicks Formula 44 Cough Control Discs, Loz. (Richardon Vicks)
Vicks Cough Silencers, Loz. (Richardson-Vicks)
DEXTROMETHORPHAN HBr W/COMBI-NATIONS.
See: Ambenyl-D, Liq. (Marion).
Anatuss DM, Syr., Tab. (Mayrand).
Anti-Tuss D.M., Liq. (Century).
Anti-Tussive, Tab. (Canright).
Bayer Prods. (Glenbrook).
Breacol Cough Medication, Liq. (Glenbrook).
Capahist-DMH, Cap. (Freeport).
C.D.M., Expectorant (Lannett).
Centuss, MLT, Tab. (Century).
Cerose-DM, Liq. (Wyeth-Ayerst).
Cheracol-D, Cough Syr. (Upjohn).
Cheratussin, Cough Syr. (Towne).
Chexit, Tab. (Sandoz Consumer).
Children's Hold 4-Hour Cough Suppressant & Decongestant, Loz. (Calgon).
Codimal DM, Liq. (Central).
Colrex, Syr. (Solvay).
Comtrex, Cap., Liq. Tab. (Bristol-Myers).
Congespirin Cough Syrup (Bristol-Myers).
Contac Jr., Liq. (SK-Beecham).
Coricidin Children's Cough Syrup (Schering-Plough).
Dimacol, Cap. (Robins).
Donatussin, Syr. (Laser).
Dorcol Ped. Cough Syr. (Sandoz Consumer).
Dristan Cough Formula, Syr. (Whitehall).
End-A-Koff, Jr. Syr. (Quality Generics).
Formula 44 Prods. (Vicks).
Halls Mentho-Lyptus Decongestant Cough Formula, Liq. (Warner-Lambert).
Histalets, DM, Syr. (Reid Provident).
Infantuss, Liq. (Scott/Cord).
Mapap CF, Tab. (Major).
Maximum Strength Tylenol Flu, Tab. (McNeil-CPC).
Niltuss, Syr. (Minn. Pharm.).
Nyquil, Liq. (Vicks).
Orthoxicol, Syr. (Upjohn).
Partuss, Liq. (Parmed).
Phenergan, Pediatric, Liq. (Wyeth-Ayerst).
Polytuss-DM, Liq. (Rhode).
Rentuss, Tab., Syr. (Wren).
Rentuss, Tab. (Wren).
Robitussin-DM, Syr., Loz. (Robins).
Robitussin Cold & Cough, Cap. (Robins).

Robitussin-CF (Robins).
Rondec DM, Drops, Syr. (Ross).
Scotcof Liq. (Scott/Cord).
Scotuss, Pediatric Cough Syr.
   (Scott/Cord).
Shertus, Liq. (Sheryl).
Silexin, Syr. (Clapp).
Sorbase Cough Syr. (Fort David).
Spec-T Sore Throat-Cough Suppres-
   sant Loz. (Squibb).
Sudafed Cough Syr. (Burroughs Well-
   come).
Synatuss-One, Liq. (Freeport).
Thor, Cough Syr. (Towne).
Tolu-Sed DM, Liq. (Scherer).
Tonecol, Syr., Tab. (A.V.P.).
Triaminic-DM Cough Formula (San-
   doz, Consumer).
Triaminicol, Syr. (Sandoz, Consumer).
Trind-DM, Syr. (Mead Johnson).
Tusquelin, Syr. (Circle).
Tussagesic, Tab., Susp. (Sandoz,
   Consumer).
Unproco, Cap. (Solvay).
Vicks Cough Prods. (Vicks).
Vicks Daycare, Liq. (Vicks).
Vicks Formula 44 Prods. (Vicks).
Vicks Nyquil, Liq. (Vicks).
Wal-Tussin DM, Syr. (Walgreen).
• **DEXTROMETHORPHAN POLISTIREX.**
   USAN.
   Use: Antitussive.
DEXTROMORAMIDE. B.A.N. (+)-1-(3-
   Methyl-4-morpholino-2, 2-diphenylbu-
   tyryl) pyrrolidine.
   Use: Narcotic analgesic.
DEXTROMORAMIDE TARTRATE. dl-(3-
   Methyl-4-morpholino-2, 2-d-phenyl-bu-
   tyryl) pyrrolidine.
   Use: Narcotic analgesic.
DEXTRO-PANTOTHENYL ALCOHOL.
   See: Panthenol (Various Mfr.).
   Ilopan (Adria).
DEXTROPROPOXYPHENE. B.A.N.
   α-(+)-4-Di-methylamino-3-methyl-1,2-
   diphenyl-2-propionyl-oxy-butane. α-(+)-
   1-Benzyl-3-dimethylamino-2-methyl-1-
   phenylpropyl propionate.
DEXTROPROPOXYPHENE HCl.
   Use: Analgesic.
   See: Propoxyphene HCl, Cap. (Various
   Mfr.).
DEXTRORPHAN. B.A.N. (+)-3-Hydroxy-
   N-methylmorphinan.
   Use: Narcotic analgesic.
• **DEXTROSE,** U.S.P. XXIII. Inj., U.S.P.
   XXIII. d-Glucose. -Glucose, monohy-
   drate.
   Use: Fluid and nutrient replenisher.
   W/Calcium ascorbate and benzyl alcohol

injection
   See: Calscorbate, Amp. (Cole).
   W/Psyllium mucilloid.
   See: V-lax, Pow. (Century).
**DEXTROSE 5% AND ELECTROLYTE
   #48.** (Travenol) Dextrose 50 Gm, calories 180/L with Na$^+$ 25, K$^+$ 20, Mg^{++} 3,
   Cl$^-$ 24, phosphate 3, acetate 23 with os-
   molarity 348 mOsm/L. Soln. Bot. 250 ml,
   500 ml, 1000 ml.
   Use: Parenteral nutritional supplement.
**DEXTROSE 5% AND ELECTROLYTE
   #75.** (Travenol) Dextrose 50 Gm, calo-
   ries 180/L with Na$^+$ 40, K$^+$ 35, Cl$^-$ 48,
   phosphate 15 and lactate 20 with osmo-
   larity 402 mOsm/L. Soln. Bot. 250 ml,
   500 ml, 1000 ml.
   Use: Parenteral nutritional supplement.
DEXTROSE-ALCOHOL INJECTION.
   Use: Parenteral nutritional supplement.
   See: 5% alcohol and 5% dextrose in
   water (Abbott, Baxter, Kendall Mc-
   Gaw)
DEXTROSE-ELECTROLYTE SOLUTION.
   Dextrose 2.5% w/0.45% sodium chlo-
   ride (Various Mfr.). Soln. 250, 500,
   1000 ml.
   Dextrose 5% w/0.11% sodium chloride
   (Kendal McGaw). Soln. 500, 1000
   ml.
   Dextrose 5% w/0.2% sodium chloride
   (Various Mfr.). Soln. 250, 500, 1000
   ml.
   Dextrose 5% w/0.33% sodium chloride
   (Various Mfr.). Soln. 250, 500, 1000
   ml.
   Dextrose 5% w/0.45% sodium chloride
   (Various Mfr.). Soln. 250, 500, 1000
   ml.
   Dextrose 5% w/0.9% sodium chloride
   (Various Mfr.). Soln. 250, 500, 1000
   ml.
   Dextrose 10% w/0.45% sodium chloride
   (Kendall McGaw). Soln. 1000 ml.
   Dextrose 10% w/0.9% sodium chloride
   (Various Mfr.). Soln. 500, 1000 ml.
   Potassium chloride 0.075% in D-5-W
   (Baxter). Soln. 1000 ml.
   Potassium chloride 0.15% in D-5-W
   (Various Mfr.). Soln. 1000 ml.
   Potassium chloride 0.224% in D-5-W
   (Various Mfr.). Soln. 1000 ml.
   Potassium chloride 0.3% in D-5-W (Vari-
   ous Mfr.). Soln. 500, 1000 ml.
   0.075% potassium chloride in 5% dex-
   trose and 0.2% sodium chloride (Vari-
   ous Mfr.). Soln. 1000 ml.
   0.15% potassium chloride in 5% dex-
   trose and 0.2% sodium chloride (Various Mfr.). Soln. 250, 500, 1000 ml.

0.224% potassium chloride in 5% dextrose and 0.2% sodium chloride (Various Mfr.). Soln. 1000 ml.

0.3% potassium chloride in 5% dextrose and 0.2% sodium chloride (Various Mfr.). Soln. 1000 ml.

0.15% potassium chloride in 5% dextrose and 0.33% sodium chloride (Baxter). Soln. 500, 1000 ml.

0.224% potassium chloride in 5% dextrose and 0.33% sodium chloride (Baxter). Soln. 1000 ml.

0.3% potassium chloride in 5% dextrose and 0.33% sodium chloride (Various Mfr.). Soln. 1000 ml.

0.075% potassium chloride in 5% dextrose and 0.45% sodium chloride (Various Mfr.). Soln. 1000 ml.

0.15% potassium chloride in 5% dextrose and 0.45% sodium chloride (Various Mfr.). Soln. 500, 1000 ml.

0.224% potassium chloride in 5% dextrose and 0.45% sodium chloride (Various Mfr.). Soln. 1000 ml.

0.3% potassium chloride in 5% dextrose and 0.45% sodium chloride (Various Mfr.). Soln. 1000 ml.

0.15% potassium chloride in 5% dextrose and 0.9% sodium chloride (Baxter). Soln. 1000 ml.

0.3% potassium chloride in 5% dextrose and 0.9% sodium chloride (Baxter). Soln. 1000 ml.

Isolyte G with 5% dextrose (Kendall McGaw) 70 mEq NH$_4$$^+$. Soln. 1000 ml.

Isolyte G with 10% dextrose (Kendall McGaw) 70 mEq NH$_4$$^+$. Soln. 1000 ml.

5% dextrose and electrolyte #75 (Baxter). Soln. 250, 500, 1000 ml.

Ionosol T and 5% dextrose (Abbott). Soln. 250, 500, 1000 ml.

Isolyte M and 5% dextrose (Kendall McGaw). Soln. 1000 ml.

Dextrose 5% in Ringer's (Various Mfr.). Soln. 500, 1000 ml.

Dextrose 2.5% in half-strength lactated Ringer's (Various Mfr.). Soln. 250, 500, 1000 ml.

Dextrose 5% in lactated Ringer's (Various Mfr.). Soln. 250, 500, 1000 ml.

5% dextrose and electrolyte #48 (Baxter). Soln. 250, 500, 1000 ml.

Ionosol MB and 5% dextrose (Abbott). Soln. 250, 500, 1000 ml.

Ionosol B and 5% dextrose (Abbott). Soln. 500, 1000.

Isolyte H with 5% dextrose (Kendall McGaw). Soln. 1000 ml.

Normosol-M and 5% dextrose (Abbott). Soln. 500, 1000.

Plasma-Lyte 56 and 5% dextrose (Baxter). Soln. 500, 1000.

Isolyte P with 5% dextrose (Kendall McGaw). Soln. 250, 500, 1000.

Isolyte S with 5% dextrose (Kendall McGaw). 23 mEq gluconate. Soln. 1000 ml.

Normosol-R and 5% dextrose (Abbott). 23 mEq gluconate. Soln. 500, 1000 ml.

Plasma-Lyte 148 and 5% dextrose (Baxter). 23 mEq gluconate. Soln. 500, 1000 ml.

Ionosol MB and 10% dextrose (Abbott). Soln. 500 ml.

10% dextrose with electrolytes (Abbott). Soln. 21 mEq gluconate. Soln. 500 ml in 1000 ml partial fill container.

10% dextrose and electrolyte no. 48 injection (Baxter). Soln. 250 ml.

Isolyte R with 5% dextrose (Kendall McGaw). Soln. 1000 ml.

Plasma-Lyte M and 5% dextrose (Baxter). Soln. 500, 1000 ml.

Plasma-Lyte R and 5% dextrose (Baxter). Soln. 1000 ml.

Isolyte E with 5% dextrose (Kendall McGaw). 8 mEq citrate. Soln. 1000 ml.
Use: Parenteral nutritional supplement.

• **DEXTROSE EXCIPIENT,** N.F. XVIII.
Use: Pharmaceutic aid (tablet excipient).

50% DEXTROSE WITH ELECTROLYTE PATTERN A. (McGaw) Dextrose 500 Gm/L, calories 1,700 cal/L, Na$^+$ 84 mEq, K$^+$ 40 mEq, CA^{++} 10 mEq, Mg^{++} 16 mEq, Cl$^-$ 115 mEq, osmolarity 2,800 mOsm/L, sulfate 16 mEq, gluconate 13 mEq. Soln. 500 ml in 1000 ml partial fill container.
Use: Parenteral nutritional supplement.

50% DEXTROSE WITH ELECTROLYTE PATTERN B. (Kendall McGaw) Dextrose 500 Gm/L, calories 1,700 cal/L, Na$^+$ 32 mEq, CA^{++} 9 mEq, Mg $^{++}$ 16 mEq, Cl$^-$ 32 mEq, osmolarity 2,615 mOsm/L, sulfate 16 mEq, gluconate 4.2 mEq. Soln. 500 ml in 1000 ml partial fill container.
Use: Parenteral nutritional supplement.

50% DEXTROSE WITH ELECTROLYTE PATTERN N. (McGaw) Dextrose 500 Gm/L, calories 1,700 cal/L, Na$^+$ 90 mEq, K$^+$ 80 mEq, Mg $^{++}$ 16 mEq, Cl$^-$ 150 mEq, phosphate 28 mEq, osmolarity 2,875 mOsm/L, sulfate 16 mEq. 500 ml in 1000 ml partial fill container.
Use: Parenteral nutritional supplement.

DEXTROSE LARGE VOLUME PARENTERALS. (Abbott Hospital Prods). Dextrose 2 0.5% in Water-1000 ml.

Dextrose 2 0.5% in 0.5 Sterile Lactose Ringer's or in 0.5 Sterile Saline-1000 ml.

Dextrose 5% in Water-150 ml, 250 ml, 500 ml, 1000 ml in Abbo-Vac glass or LifeCare flexible plastic container; partial-fill glass; 50 in 200 ml, 50 in 300 ml, 100 in 300 ml, 400 in 500 ml; partial-fill plastic: 50 in 150 ml, 100 in 150 ml.

Dextrose 5% in Lactose Ringer's-250 ml, 500 ml, 1000 ml glass; 500 ml, 1000 ml plastic container.

Dextrose 5% in Ringer's-500 ml, 1000 ml.

Dextrose 5% in Saline 0.9% or in 0.25, 0.33 or 0.5 Sterile Saline-250, 500, 1000 ml glass or plastic container.

Dextrose 10% in Water-250 ml, 500 ml, 1000 ml containers.

Dextrose 20% in Water-500 ml.

Dextrose 50% in Water-500 ml. Dextrose 20%, 30%, 40%, 50%, 60%, 70% Injections, U.S.P. in partial-fill container, 500 ml in 1000 ml.

Dextrose Injection 50%. Bot. 1000 ml.

Dextrose 50% and Injection w/Electrolytes in partial-fill container, 500 ml in 1000 ml.

Dextrose Injection 70%. Bot. 1000 ml.
Use: Parenteral nutritional supplement.

DEXTROSE SMALL VOLUME PARENTERALS. (Abbott Hospital Prods) **Dextrose 5%:** 50 ml, 100 ml pressurized pintop vial. **Dextrose 10%:** 5 ml amp.; **Dextrose 25%:** 10 ml syringe. **Dextrose 50%:** 50 ml Abboject syringe (18 G X 1.5[dp]), 50 ml Fliptop vial. **Dextrose 70%:** 70 ml pressurized pintop vial.
Use: Parenteral nutritional supplement.

• **DEXTROSE & SODIUM CHLORIDE INJECTION,** U.S.P. XXIII. (Abbott) 10% Dextrose and 0.225% Sodium Cl. Inj. Single dose container 500 ml.
Use: Parenteral nutritional supplement.

DEXTROSTIX. (Miles Diagnostic) A cellulose strip containing glucose oxidase and indicator system. Bot. 25s, 100s. Box 10s.
Use: Blood-glucose test.

DEXTROTHYROXINE SODIUM, U.S.P. XXI. Tab., U.S.P. XXI. D-Tyrosine, 0-(4-hydroxy-3, 5-diiodophenyl)- 3, 5-diiod-, monosodium salt hydrate.
Use: Anticholesteremic.
See: Choloxin, Tab. (Flint).

DEXULE. (Approved) Vitamins A 1333 IU, D 133 IU, B_1 0.33 mg, B_2 0.4 mg, C 10 mg, niacinamide 3.3 mg, iron 3.3 mg, calcium 29 mg, phosphorous 15 mg,

methylcellulose 100 mg, benzocaine 3 mg/Cap. Bot. 21s, 90s.
Use: Vitamin/mineral supplement.

DEXYL. (Pinex) Dextromethorphan HBr 15 mg, vitamin C 20 mg/Tab. Box 20s.
Use: Antitussive, vitamin C supplement.

DEY-DOSE EPINEPHRINE. (Dev Labs) Racemic epinephrine (as HCl) equal to 2.25% epinephrine base, chlorobutanol, sodium metabisulfite. Soln. for nebulization. Vial 0.25 ml.
Use: Bronchodilator.

DEY-DOSE ISOETHARINE HCl. (Dey Labs) Isoetharine HCl 1% with glycerin, sodium metabisulfite and parabens. Soln. for nebulization. Vial 0.25 ml, 0.5 ml.
Use: Brochodilator.

DEY-DOSE ISOPROTERENOL HCl. (Dey Labs) Isoproterenol HCl 0.5% (1:200). Soln. for nebulization. Vial 0.5 ml.
Use: Bronchodilator.

DEY-DOSE METAPROTERENOL SULFATE. (Dey Labs) Metaproterenol sulfate 0.5%. Inhaler 0.3 ml.
Use: Bronchodilator.

DEY-LUTE. (Dey Labs) Isoetharine HCl with sodium metabisulfite, glycerin. Soln. **0.08%:** UD 3 ml; **0.1%:** UD 5 ml; **0.17%:** UD 3 ml; **0.25%:** UD 2 ml.
Use: Bronchodilator.

DEY-LUTE METAPROTERENOL SULFATE. (Dey Labs) Metaproterenol sulfate 0.6%. Soln. for inhalation 2.5 ml.
Use: Bronchodilator.

DEY PAK SODIUM CHLORIDE 3%. (Dey) Sodium chloride 3%. Soln. Vial 3 ml, 5 ml, 100s and 10 ml, 15 ml, 50s.
Use: To induce sputum production for specimen collection.

DEY-PAK SODIUM CHLORIDE 10%. (Dey) Sodium chloride 10%. Soln. Vial 10 ml, 15 ml, 50s.
Use: To induce sputum production for specimen collection.

• **DEZAQUANINE.** USAN.
Use: Antineoplastic.

• **DEZAQUANINE MESYLATE.** USAN.
Use: Antineoplastic.

DEZEST. (Geneva Marsam) Atropine sulfate, phenylpropanolamine HCl, chlorpheniramine maleate. Bot. 100s.
Use: Anticholinergic/antispasmodic, decongestant, antihistamine.

• **DEZINAMIDE.** USAN.
Use: Anticonvulsant.

• **DEZOCINE.** USAN.
Use: Analgesic.
See: Dalgan (Wyeth-Ayerst).

D-FILM. (Ciba Vision) Poloxamer 407, EDTA 0.25%, benzalkonium Cl 0.025%. Gel Tube 25 Gm.
Use: Hard contact lens care.
DFMO. Eflornithine HCl.
Use: Anti-infective.
See: Ornidyl, Inj. (Marion Merrell Dow).
DFP. Disopropyl fluorophosphate (Various Mfr.).
d-GLUCOSE. Dextrose.
Use: Parenteral nutritional supplement.
See: D-2½-W, Soln. (Various Mfr.).
D-5-W, Soln. (Various Mfr.).
D-7.7-W, Soln. (Kendall McGaw).
D-10-W, Soln. (Various Mfr.).
D-20-W, Soln. (Various Mfr.).
D-25-W, Soln. (Various Mfr.).
D-30-W, Soln. (Various Mfr.).
D-38-W, Soln. (Kendall McGaw).
D-38.5-W, Soln. (Abbott).
D-40-W, Soln. (Various Mfr.).
D-50-W, Soln. (Various Mfr.).
D-60-W, Soln. (Various Mfr.).
D-70-W, Soln. (Various Mfr.).
DHC PLUS. (Purdue Frederick) Dihydrocodeine bitartrate 16 mg, acetaminophen 356.4 mg, caffeine 30 mg. Cap.Bot. 100s.
Use: Narcotic analgesic combination.
DHEA. (Elan Corp) EL10.
Use: Antiviral, immunomodulator.
D.H.E. 45. (Sandoz) Dihydroergotamine mesylate 1 mg/ml, methanesulfonic acid, alcohol 6.1%, glycerin 15%. Inj. in 1 ml amps.
Use: Agent for migraine.
DHPG. Ganciclovir sodium.
Use: Antiviral agent.
See: Cytovene, Pow. (Syntex).
BW B759U (Burroughs Wellcome).
DHS CONDITIONING RINSE. (Person & Covey) Conditioning ingredients. Bot. 8 oz.
Use: Dermatological hair conditioner.
DHS SHAMPOO. (Person & Covey) Blend of cleansing surfactants and emulsifiers. Plastic bot. w/dispenser 8 oz, 16 oz.
Use: Dermatological hair and scalp shampoo.
DHS TAR GEL SHAMPOO. (Person & Covey) Coal Tar, U.S.P. 0.5% Bot. 8 oz.
Use: Antiseborrheic, antipsoriatic.
DHS TAR SHAMPOO. (Person & Covey) Coal tar 0.5% in DHS shampoo. Bot. 4 oz, 8 oz, 16 oz.
Use: Antiseborrheic, antipsoriatic.
DHS ZINC SHAMPOO. (Person & Covey) Zinc pyrithione 2% in DHS shampoo. Bot. 6 oz, 12 oz.

Use: Antiseborrheic.
DHT. (Roxane) Dihydrotachysterol. **Tab.:** 0.125 mg, 0.2 mg or 0.4 mg/Tab. Bot. 50s, UD 100s (0.125 mg). 100s, UD 100s (0.2 mg). 50s (0.4 mg). **Intensol:** Dihydrotachysterol 0.2 mg/ml, alcohol 20%. Bot. 30 ml w/dropper.
Use: For postoperative tetany; idiopathic tetany; hypoparathyroidism.
DIABETA TABLETS. (Hoechst) Glyburide. **1.25 mg:** Bot. 50s. **2.5 mg:** Bot. 100s, UD 100s. **5 mg:** Bot. 100s.
Use: Antidiabetic agent.
DIABETIC TUSSIN DM. (Health Care Products) Dextromethorphan HBr 10 mg, guaifenesin 100 mg, saccharin, methylparaben, menthol, alcohol & dye free. Liq. Bot. 118 ml.
Use: Antitussive, expectorant.
DIABETIC TUSSIN EX. (Health Care Products) Guaifenesin 100 mg/5 ml, saccharin, menthol, methylparaben. Liq. Bot. 118 ml.
Use: Expectorant.
DIABINESE. (Pfizer Laboratories) Chlorpropamide. **100 mg/Tab.:** Bot. 100s, UD 100s; **250 mg/Tab.:** Bot. 100s, 1000s.
Use: Antidiabetic agent.
DIABISMUL LIQUID. (Forest) Opium 7 mg, pectin 80 mg, kaolin 2500 mg/ 15 ml. Bot. 8 oz.
Use: Antidiarrheal.
DIABISMUL TABLETS. (Forest) Bismuth subcarbonate 125 mg, powdered opium 1.23 mg, calcium carbonate 125 mg/Tab. Bot. 1000s.
Use: Antidiarrheal.
DIACETAMATE. B.A.N. 4-Acetamidophenyl acetate.
Use: Analgesic.
DIACETIC ACID TEST.
See: Acetest, Tab. (Miles Diagnostic).
DIACETO. (Archer-Taylor) Aspirin 3.5 gr, acetophenetidin 2.5 gr, caffeine 0.5 gr/Tab. Bot. 100s, 1000s.
Use: Analgesic.
DIACETO W/CODEINE. (Archer-Taylor) Codeine 0.25 gr, 0.5 gr/Tab. or Cap. Bot. 500s, 1000s.
Use: Narcotic analgesic.
DIACETO W/GELSEMIUM. (Archer-Taylor) Phenobarbital 0.5 gr, gelsemium 3 min./Tab. Bot. 1000s.
Use: Sedative/hypnotic.
• **DIACETOLOL HYDROCHLORIDE.** USAN.
Use: Anti-adrenergic.
DIACETRIZOATE, SODIUM.
See: Diatrizoate (Various Mfr.).
• **DIACETYLATED MONOGLYCERIDES,**

N.F. XVIII. Glycerin esterfied with edible fatty acids and acetic acid.
Use: Plasticizer.
DIACETYLCHOLINE CHLORIDE. Succinylcholine Cl.
See: Anectine Chloride, Inj., Pow. (Burroughs-Wellcome).
DIACETYL-DIHYDROXY-DIPHENYLISATIN.
See: Oxyphenisatin acetate (Various Mfr.).
DIACETYLDIOXYPHENYLISATIN.
See: Oxyphenisatin acetate (Various Mfr.).
DIACETYLMORPHINE SALTS. Heroin. Illegal in U.S.A. by Federal statute because of its addiction-causing nature.
DIACETYLNALORPHINE. B.A.N. O^3O^6-Diacetyl-N-allylnormorphine.
Use: Narcotic analgesic.
DI-ADEMIL.
See: Hydroflumethiazide, Tab. (Various Mfr.).
DIAGNIOL.
See: Sodium Acetrizoate.
DIAGNOSTIC AGENTS.
See: Acholest, Kit (Fougera).
Baroflave, Pow. (Lannett).
Cardio-Green, Vial (Hynson Westcott & Dunning).
Cardiografin, Vial (Squibb).
Cea-Roche, Kit (Roche).
Cholografin, Prep. (Squibb).
Coccidioidin, Vial (Cutter).
Dextrostix, Strip (Miles Diagnostic).
Dey-Pak Sodium Chloride (Dey).
Diptheria Toxin for Schick Test (Various Mfr.).
Evans Blue Dye, Inj. (New World Trading Corp.).
EZ Detect Strep-A Test (Biomerica).
Fertility Tape (Weston Labs.).
First Choice (Polymer Technology Int.).
Fluorescein Sodium Ophth. Soln. (Various Mfr.).
Fluor-I-Strip (Wyeth-Ayerst).
Fluor-I-Strip A.T. (Wyeth-Ayerst).
Fluress, Ophth. Soln. (Barnes-Hind).
Glucola, Soln. (Miles Diagnostic).
Hema-Combistix Strips (Miles Diagnostic).
Hemastix Strips (Miles Diagnostic).
Histalog, Amp. (Lilly).
Histoplasmin, Vial (Parke-Davis).
Indigo Carmine (Various Mfr.).
HIVAB HIV-1/HIV-2 (rDNA) EIA (Abbot).
Immunex CRP (Wampole).
Mannitol Soln., Inj. (Merck & Co.).

Mono-Latex (Wampole).
Mono-Plus (Wampole).
Phenolsulfonphthalein (Various Mfr.).
Phentolamine Methanesulfonate, Inj. (Various Mfr.).
Regitine, Amp., Tab. (Ciba).
Rheumanosticon Slide Test (Organon).
Rheumatex (Wampole).
Rheumaton (Wampole).
Rocky Mountain Spotted Fever Antigen, Vial (Lederle).
SureCell Chlamydia Test (Kodak).
SureCell Herpes (HSV) Test (Kodak).
SureCell Strep A Test (Kodak).
Sodium Dehydrocholate, Inj. (Various Mfr.).
Tes-Tape (Lilly).
See also: Cholecystography Agents.
Kidney Function Agents.
Liver Function Agents.
Urography Agents.
DIAGNOSTIC AGENTS.
See: Persantine IV (DuPont-Merck).
DIAGNOSTIC AGENTS FOR URINE.
See: Acetest, Tab. (Miles Diagnostic).
Albustix, Strip (Miles Diagnostic).
Biotel Diabetes (Biotel).
Biotel Kidney (Biotel).
Biotel U.T.I. (Biotel).
Bumintest, Tab. (Miles Diagnostic).
Chemstrip Micral, Strips (Boehringer Mannheim).
Clinistix, Strip (Miles Diagnostic).
Clinitest, Tab. (Miles Diagnostic).
Fortel Midstream (Biomerica).
Fortel Plus (Biomerica).
Hema-Combistix, Strip (Miles Diagnostic).
HCG-nostick (Organon Teknika).
Hemastix, Strip (Miles Diagnostic).
Hematest, Tab. (Miles Diagnostic).
Icotest, Tab. (Miles Diagnostic).
Ketostix, Strip (Miles Diagnostic).
Pheniplate, Preps.(Miles Diagnostic).
Phenistix, Strip (Miles Diagnostic).
SureCell hCG-Urine Test (Kodak).
Uristix, Strip (Miles Diagnostic).
Wampole One-Step hCG (Wampole).
DIALLYBARBITURIC ACID. Allobarbital, Allobarbitone, Curral.
W/Acetaminophen, aluminum aspirin, aspirin.
See: Allylgesic, Tab. (Elder).
DIALLYLAMICOL. Diallyl-diethylaminoethyl phenol di HCl.
DIALLYLNORTOXIFERINE.
See: Alloferin (Roche).
DIALMINATE. Mixture of magnesium carbonate and (alminate) dihydroxyalu-

minum glycinate.
W/Aspirin.
See: Bufferin, Preps. (Bristol-Myers).
DIALONE TABS. (Major)
Methandrostenolone 5 mg/Tab. Bot.
100s.
Use: Anabolic steroid.
DIALOSE. (Stuart) Docusate potassium
100 mg/Cap. Bot. 36s, 100s, UD 100s.
Use: Laxative.
DIALOSE. (J & J-Merck) Docusate sodi-
um 100 mg. Tab. Bot. 36s.
Use: Laxative.
DIALOSE PLUS. (Stuart) Docusate
potassium 100 mg, casanthranol 30
mg/Cap. Bot. 36s, 100s, 500s, UD 100s.
Use: Laxative.
DIALOSE PLUS. (J & J-Merck) Docusate
sodium 100 mg, yellow phenolphthalein
65 mg. Tab. Bot. 100s.
Use: Laxative.
DIALUME. (RPR) Aluminum hydroxide
gel 500 mg/Cap. Bot. 500s.
Use: Antacid.
**DIALYTE PATTERN LM W/1.5% DEX-
TROSE.** (Gambro) Dextrose 15 g/L,
Na^+ 131, Ca^{++} 3.5, Mg^{++} 0.5, Cl^- 94 and
lactate 40 with osmolarity 345 mOsm/L.
Soln. Bot. 1000 ml, 2000 ml.
Use: Peritoneal dialysis solution.
**DIALYTE PATTERN LM W/2.5% DEX-
TROSE.** (Gambro) Dextrose 25 g/L,
Na^+ 131.5, Ca^{++} 3.5, Mg^{++} 0.5, Cl^- 94
and lactate 40 with osmolarity 395
mOsm/L. Soln. Bot. 2000 ml.
Use: Peritoneal dialysis solution.
**DIALYTE PATTERN LM W/4.25% DEX-
TROSE.** (Gambro) Dextrose 42.5 g/L,
Na^+ 131.5, Ca^{++} 3.5, Mg^{++} 0.5, Cl^- 94
and lactate 40 with osmolarity 485
mOsm/L. Soln. Bot. 2000 ml.
Use: Peritoneal dialysis solution.
DIAMETHINE.
See: Dimethyl tubocurarine (Various
Mfr.).
DIAMINEDIPENICILLIN G.
See: Benzethacil (Various Mfr.).
DIAMINE T.D. (Major) Brompheniramine
maleate 8 mg or 12 mg/TR tab. Bot.
100s, 250s, 1000s.
Use: Antihistamine.
**DI-AMINO ACETATE COMPLEX W/CAL-
CIUM ALUMINUM CARBONATE.**
Cap. IU.
See: Ancid Tab., Susp. (Sheryl).
DIAMINODIPHENYLSULFONE. Dap-
sone, U.S.P. XXIII.
Use: Treatment of malaria.
See: Avlosulfon, Tab. (Wyeth-Ayerst).
Diasone Sodium, Tab. (Abbott).

Glucosulfone Sodium, Inj. (Various
Mfr.).
DIAMINOPROPYL TETRAMETHYLENE.
See: Spermine.
3,4-DIAMINOPYRIDINE.
Use: Lambert-Eaton myasthenic syndrome. [Orphan drug]
• **DIAMOCAINE CYCLAMATE.** USAN. (1)
1-(2-Anilinoethyl)-4-[2-(diethylamino)-
ethoxy]-4-phenylpiperidine bis(cyclohexanesulfamate); (2) Cyclohexanesul-
famic acid compound with 1-(2-anili-
noethyl)-4-[2-(diethylamino)ethoxy]-4-ph
enylpiperidine (2:1).
Use: Local anesthetic.
DIAMOX. (Lederle) Acetazolamide. **Tab.:**
125 mg Bot. 100s. 250 mg Bot. 100s,
1000s, UD 10 × 10s. **Inj. Vial:** Sterile
sodium salt 500 mg (sodium hydroxide
to adjust pH).
Use: Diuretic, anticonvulsant.
DIAMOX SEQUELS. (Lederle) Acetazolamide 500 mg/Cap. Bot. 30s, 100s.
Use: Diuretic, anticonvulsant.
DIAMPROMIDE. B.A.N. N-[2-(N-
Methylphen-ethylamino)propyl]propio-
nanilide.
Use: Analgesic.
DIAMTHAZOLE. B.A.N. 6-(2-Diethy-
laminoethoxy)-2-dimethylaminobenzoth-
iazole.
Dimazole (I.N.N.).
Use: Antifungal.
DIAMTHAZOLE DIHYDROCHLORIDE.
Asterol.
DIANEAL W/1.5% DEXTROSE. (Travenol) Dextrose 15 Gm/L, Na^+ 141,
Ca^{++} 3.5, Mg^{++} 1.5, Cl^- 101, lactate 45
with osmolarity 364 mOsm/L. Soln. Bot.
1000 ml, 2000 ml.
Use: Peritoneal dialysis solution.
DIANEAL 137 W/1.5% DEXTROSE. (Travenol) Dextrose 15 Gm/L, Na^+ 132,
Ca^{++} 3.5, Mg^{++} 1.5, Cl^- 102, lactate 35
with osmolarity 347 mOsm/L. Soln. Bot.
2000 ml.
Use: Peritoneal dialysis solution.
DIANEAL W/4.25% DEXTROSE. (Travenol) Dextrose 42.5 Gm/L, Na^+ 141,
Ca^{++} 3.5, Mg^{++} 1.5, Cl^- 101, lactate 45
with osmolarity 503 mOsm/L. Soln. Bot.
2000 ml.
Use: Peritoneal dialysis solution.
DIANEAL 137 W/4.25% DEXTROSE.
(Travenol) Dextrose 42.5 Gm/L, Na^+
132, Ca^{++} 3.5, Mg^{++} 1.5, Cl^- 102, lactate
35 with osmolarity 486 mOsm/L. Soln.
Bot. 2000 ml.
Use: Peritoneal dialysis solution.
DIANEAL PD-2 PERITONEAL DIALYSIS

SOLN WITH 1.1% AMINO ACID. *Use:* Nutritional supplement for dialysis patients. [Orphan drug]

• **DIAPAMIDE.** USAN. *Use:* Diuretic, antihypertensive.

DIAPANTIN. (Janssen) Isoprofamide bromide. *Use:* Anticholinergic.

DIAPARENE. (Glenbrook) Methylbenzethonium Cl. Pow. Bot. 4 oz, 9 oz, 12.5 oz, 14 oz. *Use:* Surface-active disinfectant.

DIAPARENE MEDICATED. (Lehn & Fink) Methylbenzethonium Cl with white petrolatum 0.1%, glycerin, mineral oil, stearyl alcohol. Cream. Tube 30, 60, 120 Gm. *Use:* Antimicrobial.

DIAPARENE OINTMENT. (Glenbrook) Methylbenzethonium Cl 0.1% w/petrolatum, glycerin. Tube 1 oz, 2 oz, 4 oz. *Use:* Antimicrobial.

DIAPARENE PERI-ANAL CREAM. (Glenbrook) Methylbenzethonium Cl 1:1000, zinc oxide, starch, cod liver oil, white petrolatum, lanolin, calcium caseinate. Cream Tube 1 oz, 2 oz, 4 oz. *Use:* Antimicrobial, astringent.

DIAPARESS. (Jenkins) Cod liver oil, diperodon HCl 0.25%, zinc oxide, starch, aluminum acetate, balsam Peru. Tube 1.5 oz. *Use:* Skin protectant.

DIAPER GUARD. (Del) Dimethicone 1%, white petrolatum 66%, cocoa butter, parabens, vitamins A, D_3, E, zinc oxide. Oint. Tube 49.6 Gm, 99.2 Gm. *Use:* Diaper rash product.

DIAPER RASH. (Various Mfr.) Zinc oxide, cod liver oil, lanolin, methylparaben, petrolatum, talc. Oint. Tube 113 Gm. *Use:* Diaper rash product.

DIAPHENYLSULFONE. Dapsone, U.S.P. XXIII. *Use:* Leprostatic.

DIAPID. (Sandoz,) Lypressin synthetic lysine-8-vasopressin. Equiv. to 50 U.S.P. units posterior pituitary/ml (0.185 mg/ml). Nasal spray. Bot. 8 ml. *Use:* Pituitary hormone.

DI-AP-TROL. (Foy) Phendimetrazine tartrate 35 mg/Tab. Bot. 100s, 1000s. *Use:* Anorexiant.

DIA-QUEL. (MiLance) Opium 18 mg (equivalent to 4.5 ml paregoric), homatropine MBr 0.9 mg, pectin 144 mg/ml with alcohol 10%. Liq. Bot. 120 ml. *Use:* Antidiarrheal.

DIARREST. (Dover) Calcium carbonate, pectin/Tab. Sugar, lactose and salt free. UD box 500s. *Use:* Antidiarrheal.

DIARRHEA RELIEF WITH PAREGORIC. (Weeks & Leo) Bismuth subsalicylate 63 mg, kaolin 675 mg, pectin 27 mg, paregoric 0.6 mg/5 ml Bot. 4 oz. *Use:* Antidiarrheal.

DIARRHEA THERAPY. *See:* Antidiarrheals.

DIASERP TABS. (Major) Chlorothiazide 250 mg or 500 mg/Tab. w/reserpine. Bot. 100s. *Use:* Antihypertensive.

DIASORB. (Columbia) Activated nonfibrous attapulgite. **Liq.:** 750 mg per 5 ml. Bot. 120 ml. **Tab.:** 750 mg. Pkg. 24s. *Use:* Antidiarrheal.

DIASPORAL CREAM. (Doak) Formerly Sulfur Salicyl Diasporal. Sulfur 3%, salicylic acid 2%, isopropyl alcohol in diasporal base. Cream Jar 3³/₄ oz. *Use:* Antiseptic, topical.

DIASTASE. *See:* Aspergillus oryzae enzyme. W/Bismuth subnitrate, sodium bicarbonate, magnesium carbonate, papain. *See:* Panacarb, Tab. (Lannett). W/Carica papaya enzyme. *See:* Caripeptic, Liq. (Upjohn).

DIASTIX REAGENT STRIPS. (Miles Diagnostic) Broad range test for glucose in urine. Containing glucose oxidase, peroxidase, potassium iodide/w blue background dye. Tab. Pkg. 50s, 100s. *Use:* Diagnostic aid.

DIATRIZOATE. 3,5-diacetamido-2,4,6-triiodobenzoic acid.

• **DIATRIZOATE MEGLUMINE,** U.S.P. XXII. Inj., U.S.P. XXIII. Benzoic acid, 3,5-bis(acetylamino)-2,4,6-triiodo compound with 1-deoxy-1-(methylamino)-glucitol (1:1). *Use:* Diagnostic aid (radiopaque medium). *See:* Angiovist 282, Inj. (Berlex). Cardiografin, Vial (Squibb). Cystographin, Inj. (Squibb). Gastrografin, Liq. (Squibb). Hypaque-Cysto, Liq. (Sanofi Winthrop). Hypaque Meglumine (Sanofi Winthrop). Renografin, Inj. (Squibb). Reno-M-DIP, Inj. (Squibb). Reno-M-30, Inj. (Squibb). Reno-M-60, Inj. (Squibb). Urovist, Prods. (Berlex). W/Iodipamide methylglucamine. *See:* Sinografin, Vial (Squibb). W/Sodium Diatrizoate.

See: Renovist, Inj. (Squibb).
• **DIATRIZOATE MEGLUMINE AND DIA-
TRIZOATE SODIUM INJECTION,**
U.S.P. XXIII.
Use: Diagnostic aid (radiopaque medium).
See: Angiorist 292, Inj. (Berlex).
Angiovist 370, Inj. (Berlex).
Gastrovist, Soln. (Berlex).
Hypaque-M Prods. (Sanofi Winthrop).
• **DIATRIZOATE MEGLUMINE AND DIA-
TRIZOATE SODIUM SOLUTION,**
U.S.P. XXIII.
Use: Diagnostic aid (radiopaque medium).
See: Gastrografini Soln. (Squibb).
Renografin-60, Soln. (Squibb).
Renografin-76, Soln. (Squibb).
Renovist, Soln. (Squibb).
**DIATRIZOATE MEGLUMINE 52.7% AND
IODIPAMIDE MEGLUMINE 25.8% (38%
IODINE).**
Use: Diagnostic aid, radiopaque agent.
See: Sinografin, Inj. (Squibb Diagnostics).
DIATRIZOATE METHYLGLUCAMINE.
Use: Diagnostic aid (radiopaque medium).
See: Diatrizoate Meglumine, U.S.P.
XXIII.
**DIATRIZOATE METHYLGLUCAMINE
SODIUM.** Sodium salt of N-methylglucamine salt of 3,5-diacetamido-2,4,6-triiodobenzoate.
Use: Diagnostic aid (radiopaque medium).
• **DIATRIZOATE SODIUM,** U.S.P. XXIII.
Inj., Soln., U.S.P. XXIII. Benzoic acid,
3,5-bis(acetylamino)-2,4,6-triiodo-,
monosodium salt.
Use: Diagnostic aid (radiopaque medium).
See: Hypaque Prods. (Sanofi
Winthrop).
Urovist Sodium, Inj. (Berlex).
W/Meglumine diatrizoate.
See: Gastrografin, Liq.(Squibb).
Renografin-60, -76, Vial (Squibb).
Renovist II, Vial (Squibb).
W/Methylglucamine diatrizoate, sodium
citrate, disodium ethylenediamine
tetra-acetate dihydrate, methylparaben, propylparaben.
See: Renovist, Vial (Squibb).
**DIATRIZOATE SODIUM 41.66% (24.9%
IODINE).**
Use: Diagnostic aid, radiopaque agent.
See: Hypaque sodium, Soln. (Sanofi
Winthrop.).
DIATRIZOATE SODIUM (59.87%

IODINE).
Use: Diagnostic aid, radiopaque agent.
See: Hypaque Sodium, Soln. (Sanofi
Winthrop.).
• **DIATRIZOATE SODIUM I-125.** USAN.
Use: Radioactive agent.
• **DIATRIZOATE SODIUM I-131.** USAN.
Use: Radioactive agent.
• **DIATRIZOIC ACID.** USAN. 3,5-Diacetamido-2,4,6-tri-iodobenzoic acid.
Use: Radiopaque substance.
See: Amidotrizoic Acid.
Hypaque sodium salt.
• **DIATRIZOIC ACID,** U.S.P. XXIII. Benzoic
acid, 3,5-bis(acetylamino)-2,4,6-triiodo-.
3,5-Diacetamido-2,4,6-triiodobenzoic
acid.
Use: Radiopaque medium (urographic).
DIATROL. (Otis Clapp) Calcium carbonate 261 mg, pectin 65 mg. In 100s, 200s,
500s.
Use: Antacid.
• **DIAZEPAM,** U.S.P. XXIII. Cap., Extended-Release Cap., Inj., Tab: U.S.P. XXIII.
2H-1,4-Benzodiazepan-2-one, 7-chloro-
1,3-dihydro-1-methyl-5-phenyl-. 7-
Chloro-1,3-dihydro-1-methyl-5-phenyl-
2H-1,4-benzodiazepin-2-one. B.A.N. 7-
Chloro-1,3-dihydro-1-methyl-5-phenyl-2
H-1,4-benzodiazepin-2-one. (Various
Mfr.) **Tab.:** 2 mg Bot. 100s, 500s, 1000s,
5000s; 5 mg or 10 mg Bot. 100s, 500s,
1000s, 2500s, 5000s; **Inj.:** 5 mg/ml
Amps 2 ml; vial 1, 2, 5, 10 ml; syringe 1,
2 ml.
Use: Agent for control of emotional disturbances; sedative; tranquilizer.
Oral Soln. (Roxane): 5 mg/5 ml. In UD 5
ml, 10 ml patient cups.
Concentrated Oral Soln. (Roxane): 5
mg/ml In 30 ml w/dropper.
See: Valium, Tab. (Roche).
Valrelease, S.R. Cap. (Roche).
Zetran (Hauck).
DIAZEPAM INTENSOL. (Roxane) Diazepam 5 mg/ml. Oral Soln. In 30 ml
with dropper.
Use: Antianxiety agent.
DIAZEPAM VISCOUS RECTAL SOLUTION.
Use: To treat acute repetitive seizures.
[Orphan drug]
• **DIAZIQUONE.** USAN.
Use: Antineoplastic.
DIAZMA. (Pharmex) Diphylline 250
mg/ml. Vial 10 ml.
Use: Antiasthmatic.
DIAZOMYCINS A, B, & C. Antibiotic obtained from *Streptomyces ambofaciens.*
Under study.

• **DIAZOXIDE,** U.S.P. XXIII. Cap., Oral Susp., Inj., U.S.P. XXIII. 7-Chloro-3-methyl-2H-1,-2, 4-benzothiadiazine-1, 1-dioxide.
Use: Glucose elevating agent.
See: Proglycem Capsules (Medical Market Specialists).
Proglycem Suspension (Medical Market Specialists).
DIAZOXIDE, PARENTERAL.
Use: Antihypertensive.
See: Diazoxide Injection USP, Inj. (Various Mfr.).
Hyperstat IV, Inj. (Schering).
• **DIBASIC CALCIUM PHOSPHATE DIHYDRATE,** U.S.P. XXIII.
Use: Replenisher (calcium); pharmaceutic aid (tablet base).
See: D.C.P. 340, Tab. (Parke-Davis).
Diostate D, Tab. (Upjohn).
DIBATROL. (Metro Med) Chlorpropamide 100 mg or 250 mg/Tab. Bot. 100s, 1000s.
Use: Antidiabetic agent.
DIBENCIL.
See: Benzathine Penicillin G. (Various Mfr.).
DIBENT. (Hauck) Dicyclomine 10 mg/ml with chlorobutanol. Inj. Vial 10 ml.
Use: GI anticholinergic/antispasmodic.
DIBENZEPIN. B.A.N. 10-(2-Dimethylaminoethyl)-5-methyldibenzo[b,e][1,4]diazepin-11-one.
Use: Antidepressant.
• **DIBENZEPIN HCl.** USAN. 10-[2-(Dimethylamino)ethyl]-5,10-dihydro-5-methyl-IIH-dibenzo-[b,e][1,4]diazepin-11-one monohydroCl.
Use: Antidepressant.
• **DIBENZOTHIOPHENE.** USAN.
Use: Keratolytic.
DIBENZYLETHYLENEDIAMINE DIPENICILLIN G, U.S.P.
See: Benzethacil.
DIBENZYLINE. (SK-Beecham) Phenoxybenzamine HCl 10 mg/Cap. Bot. 100s.
Use: Antihypertensive.
DIBROMODULCITOL.
Use: Antineoplastic. [Orphan drug]
• **DIBROMSALAN.** USAN. 4′, 5-Dibromosalicylanilide. Diaphene.
Use: Germicide.
• **DIBUCAINE,** U.S.P. XXIII. Cream, Oint., U.S.P. XXIII. 2-Butoxy-N-[2-(diethylamino)ethyl]-cinchoninamide.
Use: Local anesthetic.
See: D-caine, Oint. (Century).
Dulzit, Cream (Del).
Nupercainal, Oint. (Ciba).

W/Benzocaine.
See: Extend, Tab. (E.J. Moore).
W/Benzocaine, tetracaine.
See: Bonal Itch Cream, (E.J. Moore).
W/Dextrose.
See: Nupercaine Heavy Soln. (Ciba).
W/Sodium bisulfite.
See: Nupercainal, Cream, Oint. (Ciba).
W/Zinc oxide, bismuth subgallate, acetone sodium bisulfite.
See: Nupercainal, Oint., Supp. (Ciba).
• **DIBUCAINE HYDROCHLORIDE,** U.S.P. XXIII. Inj., U.S.P. XXIII. 2-Butoxy-N-(2-diethylamino-ethyl) cinchoninamide HCl. (Cinchocaine, Percaine).
Use: Surface and spinal anesthesia.
See: Nupercaine HCl, soln., (Ciba).
W/Antipyrine, hydrocortisone, polymyxin B sulfate, neomycin sulfate.
See: Otocort, Liq. (Lemmon).
W/Colistin sodium methanesulfonate, citric acid, sodium citrate.
See: Coly-Mycin M, Injectable (Warner-Chilcott).
DIBUPYRONE. B.A.N. Sodium N-(2,3-dimethyl-1-phenyl-5-oxopyrazolin-4-yl)-N-isobutylamino-methanesulphonate.
Use: Analgesic.
DIBUTOLINE SULFATE. Ethyl(2-hydroxy-ethyl)-dimethylammonium sulfate (2:1) bis(dibutyl-carbamate).
Use: Anticholinergic/antispasmodic.
DI-CAL CAPTABS. (Rugby) Calcium 116 mg, vitamin D 133 IU, phosphorus 90 mg. Bot. 1000s.
Use: Calcium, vitamin D supplement.
DICALCIUM PHOSPHATE. Dibasic Calcium Phosphate, U.S.P., Anhydrous Monocalcium Phosphate. (Various Mfr.) **Cap.:** 7.5 gr or 10 gr. **Tab.:** 7.5 gr, 10 gr or 15 gr. **Wafer:** 15 gr.
Use: Calcium supplement.
See: Irophos-D, Cap. (Lannett).
W/Calcium gluconate and Vitamin D. (Various Mfr.) Cap., Tab., Wafer.
See: Calcicaps, Tab. (Nion).
Di-Cal, Cap. (Kenyon).
W/Iron and Vitamin D. (Various Mfr.).
Lilly—Pulv., Bot. 100s.
W/Vitamin D. (Squibb) Calcium 85 mg, phosphorus 60 mg, vitamin D 41 IU.
DI-CAL D. (Abbott) Calcium 117 mg, vitamin D 133 IU, phosphorus 90 mg. Tab. Bot. 100s, 500s.
Use: Calcium, phosphorus, vitamin D supplement.
DICAL-D WITH VITAMIN C. (Abbott) Dibasic calcium phosphate containing calcium 116.7 mg, phosphorus 90 mg, vitamin D 133 IU, ascorbic acid 15

mg/Cap. Bot. 100s.
Use: Calcium, phosphorus and Vitamin C supplement.
DICAL-DEE. (Barre) Vitamins D 350 IU, dibasic calcium phosphate 4.5 gr, calcium gluconate 3 gr/Cap. Bot. 100s, 1000s.
Use: Calcium supplement.
DICALDEL. (Faraday) Dibasic calcium phosphate 300 mg, calcium gluconate 200 mg, vitamin D 33 IU/Cap. Bot. 100s, 250s, 500s, 1000s.
Use: Calcium supplement.
DICAL-D WAFERS. (Abbott) Dibasic calcium phosphate containing calcium 232 mg, phosphorus 180 mg, vitamin D 200 IU/Wafer. Box 51s.
Use: Calcium, phosphorus supplement.
DICALTABS. (Faraday) Dibasic calcium phosphate 108 mg, calcium gluconate 140 mg, vitamin D 35 IU/Tab. Bot. 100s, 250s, 1000s.
DICARBOSIL. (SK-Beecham) Calcium carbonate 500 mg/Chew. Tab. Roll 12s.
Use: Antacid.
DI-CET. (Sanford & Son) Methylbenzethonium Cl 24.4 Gm, sodium carbonate monohydrate 48.8 Gm, sodium nitrite 24.4 Gm, trisodium ethylenediamine tetra-acetate monohydrate 2.4 Gm. Pow. Pkg. 2.4 Gm, Box 24s.
Use: Dental instrument disinfectant.
DICHLORALANTIPYRINE. Dichloralphenazone. Chloralpyrine. A complex of 2 mol. chloral hydrate with 1 mol. antipyrine. Sominat.
W/Isometheptene mucate, N-acetyl-p-amino-phenol.
See: Midrin, Cap. (Carnrick).
DICHLORALPHENAZONE. B.A.N. A complex of chloral hydrate and phenazone. Dichloralantipyrine (Various Mfr.).
Use: Hypnotic.
DICHLORAMINE T. (Various Mfr.) (1% to 5% in chlorinated paraffin). P-Toluenesulfone-dichloramine.
Use: Antiseptic
DICHLOREN.
See: Mechlorethamine HCl, Sterile Inj. (Various Mfr.).
DICHLORISONE ACETATE. 9a, 11b-dichloro-dl,-4-pregnadiene-17a,21-diol-3,20-dione-21-acetate.
DICHLORMETHAZANONE. 2-(3,4-dichlorophenyl)-3-methyl-4-metathiazanone-1-dioxide.
DICHLOROACETATE SODIUM.
Use: Lactic acidosis; hypercholesterolemia. [Orphan drug]

DICHLOROACETIC ACID.
Use: Cauterizing agent.
See: Bichloracetic Acid, Liq. (Glenwood).
• **DICHLORODIFLUOROMETHANE,** N.F. XVII.
Use: Aerosol propellant.
DICHLORODIPHENYL TRICHLOROETHANE.
See: Chlorophenothane (Various Mfr.).
DICHLOROPHEN. B.A.N. Di(5-chloro-2-hydroxy-phenyl) methane.
Use: Anthelmintic.
DICHLOROPHENARSINE. B.A.N. 3-Amino-4-hydroxyphenyldichloroarsine.
Use: Antifungal.
DICHLOROPHENARSINE HYDROCHLORIDE. (Chlorarsen, Clorarsen, Fontarsol, Halarsol).
DICHLOROPHENE. Didroxane. G-4, bis(5-Chloro-2-hydroxyphenyl) methane. Related to hexachlorophene.
W/Parachlorometaxylenol, propyl-paraaminobenzoate, hexachlorophene, benzocaine.
See: Triguent, Oint. (Commerce).
W/Undecylenic acid.
See: Fungicidal Talc. (Gordon).
Onychomycetin, Liq. (Gordon).
W/Undecylenic acid, salicylicacid, hexachlorophene.
See: Podiaspray, aerosol pow. (Dalin).
• **DICHLOROTETRAFLUOROETHANE,** N.F. XVII. 1, 2-Dichlorotetrafluoroethane.
Use: Aerosol propellant.
DICHLOROXYLENOL. B.A.N. 2,4-Dichloro-3,5-xylenol.
Use: Bactericide.
DICHLORPHENAMIDE, U.S.P. XXI. Tab. U.S.P. XXI. 1,3-Benzenedisulfonamide, 4,5-di- chloro-. 1,3-Disulfamyl-4-5-dichloro-benzene. B.A.N. 4,5-Dichlorobenzene-1,3-disulfonamide.
Use: Agent for glaucoma.
DICHOLIN. (Kenyon) Ox bile extract 3/8 gr, iron lactate gr, calumba gr, chamomile flowers 1 gr, rhubarb 1 gr/Cap. Bot. 100s, 1000s.
DICHROMIUM TRIOXIDE. B.A.N. Chromium sesquioxide.
Use: Diagnostic aid.
• **DICIRENONE.** USAN.
Use: Hypotensive.
DICKEY'S OLD RELIABLE EYE WASH. (Dickey Drug) Berberine sulfate, boric acid, propyl parasept, methyl parasept. Plastic dropper bot. 8 ml, 12 ml, 1 oz.
Use: Counter-irritant, ophthalmic.
• **DICLOFENAC POTASSIUM.** USAN.

Use: Anti-inflammatory.
See: Cataflam, Tab. (Geigy).
• **DICLOFENAC SODIUM.** USAN.
Use: Anti-inflammatory.
See: Voltaren (Geigy).
• **DICLORALUREA.** USAN.
Use: Food additive.
DICLOXACIL. (Goldline) Dicloxacillin
sodium 250 mg or 500 mg/Cap. Bot.
100s.
Use: Antibacterial, penicillin.
• **DICLOXACILLIN.** USAN.6-[3-(2,6-
Dichlorophenyl)-5-methyl-4-isoxazole-
carboxamido]-3,3-dimethyl-7-oxo-4-thia-
1-azabicyclo[3.2.0]-heptane-2-car-
boxylic acid.
Use: Antibiotic.
See: Dynapen, Cap., Susp. (Bristol).
Pathocil, Cap., Susp. (Wyeth-Ayerst).
• **DICLOXACILLIN SODIUM,** U.S.P. XXII.
Cap., Sterile, For Oral Susp. U.S.P. XXII.
Use: Penicillinase-resistant penicillin.
See: Dycill, Cap. (Beecham).
Dynapen, Cap., Soln. (Bristol).
DICODETHAL ELIXIR. (Lannett) Dex-
tromethorphan HBr 10 mg/5 ml in el. ter-
pin hydrate. Bot. pt, gal.
Use: Antitussive, expectorant.
DICOLE. (Blue Cross) Docusate sodium
100 mg/Cap. Bot. 100s.
Use: Laxative.
DICOPHANE.
See: Chlorophenothane (Various Mfr.),
DDT.
DICOUMARIN.
See: Dicumarol, Preps. (Various Mfr.).
DICOUMAROL.
See: Dicumarol, U.S.P. XXIII.
• **DICUMAROL,** U.S.P. XXII. Tab., U.S.P.
XXII. Cap., U.S.P. XXI. 2H-1-Benzopy-
ran-2-one 3,3'-methylenebis 4-hy-
droxy-3,3-methylenebis(4-hydroxy-
coumarin). Dicoumarol. Dicoumarin.
Bishydroxycoumarin. Melitoxin. (Abbott)
Tab. 25 mg or 50 mg Bot. 100s, 1000s;
100 mg Bot. 1000s.
Use: Anticoagulant.
• **DICYCLOMINE HYDROCHLORIDE,**
U.S.P. XXIII. Cap., Inj., Syr., Tab., U.S.P.
XXIII. Bicyclohexyl-1-carboxylic acid, 2-
(diethylamino) ethyl 3w534 HCl. 2-(Di-
ethylamino)ethyl (Bicyclohexyl)-1-car-
boxylate hydroCl.
Use: Antispasmodic.
See: Antispas, Inj. (Keene).
Bentyl, Amp. Syringe, Cap., Tab., Syr.
(Merrell Dow).
Dysaps, Tab., Liq., Inj. (Savage).
Nospaz, Vial (Solvay).
Stannitol (Standex).

W/Aluminum hydroxide, magnesium hy-
droxide, methylcellulose.
See: Triactin Liq., Tab. (Norwich Eaton).
W/Phenobarbital.
See: Bentyl with Phenobarbital, Prods.
(Merrell Dow).
DICYCLON-M. (Kenyon) Dicyclomine
HCl 10 mg, pyrilamine maleate 10 mg,
pyridoxine HCl 10 mg/Tab. Bot. 100s,
1000s.
Use: Anticholinergic/antispasmodic.
DICYCLON NO.1. (Kenyon) Dicyclomine
HCl 10 mg/Tab. Bot. 100s, 1000s.
Use: Anticholinergic/antispasmodic.
DICYCLON NO. 2. (Kenyon) Dicyclomine
HCl 10 mg, phenobarbital 15 mg/Tab.
Bot. 100s, 1000s.
Use: Anticholinergic/antispasmodic,
sedative/hypnotic.
DICYCLON NO. 3. (Kenyon) Dicyclomine
HCl 20 mg, phenobarbital 15 mg/Tab.
Bot. 100s, 1000s.
Use: Anticholinergic/antispasmodic,
sedative/hypnotic.
DICYNENE. (Baxter)
Use: Hemostatic agent.
See: Ethamsylate.
DICYSTEINE.
See: Cystine, Pow. (Various Mfr.)
• **DIDANOSINE.** USAN.
Use: Antiviral, systemic.
See: Videx, Tab., Pow. (Bristol Myers
Squibb).
DIDEHYDRODIDEOXYTHYMIDINE.
Use: Antiviral.
See: Stavudine (B-M Squibb).
DI-DELAMINE GEL. (Commerce) Tripe-
lennamine HCl 0.5%, diphenhydramine
HCl 1%, benzalkonium Cl 0.12% in clear
gel. Tube 1.25 oz.
Use: Antipruritic.
DI-DELAMINE SPRAY. (Commerce)
Tripelennamine HCl 0.5%, diphenhy-
dramine HCl 1%, benzalkonium Cl
0.12%. Spray pump 4 oz.
Use: Antipruritic.
DIDEOXYCYTIDINE. (Roche).
Use: Antiviral.
See: HIVID.
2,3 DIDEOXYCYTIDINE. (Hoffman
LaRoche; NCI; Bristol-Myers).
Use: Antiviral (AIDS).
DIDEOXYINISINE.
Use: Antiviral.
See: Videx, Tab., Pow. (Bristol-Myers
Squibb).
DIDREX. (Upjohn) Benzphetamine HCl.
25 mg/Tab.: Bot. 100s; **50 mg/Tab.:** Bot.
100s, 500s.
Use: Anorexiant.

DIDRONEL. (Procter & Gamble) Etidronate disodium 200 mg or 400 mg/Tab. Bot. 60s. **IV Infusion:** Etidronate disodium 300 mg/6 ml amp.
Use: Hypercalcemia of malignancy.
• **DIENESTROL,** U.S.P. XXIII. Cream, U.S.P. XXIII. Non-steroid, synthetic estrogen. Dienoestrol. 4,4'-(Diethylideneethylene)diphenol. (Ortho) Dienestrol 0.01%. Tube 78 Gm w/applicator.
Use: Estrogen therapy, atrophic vaginitis.
See: D V, Cream (Merrell Dow).
D V, Supp. (Merrell Dow).
Ortho Dienestrol Cream (Ortho).
W/Sulfanilamide, aminacrine HCl, allantoin.
See: AVC/Dienestrol Cream, Supp. (Merrell Dow).
DIET-AID, MAXIMUM STRENGTH. (O'-Connor) Phenylpropanolamine HCl 75 mg/Cap. Pkg. 20s.
Use: Diet aid.
DIET-AID PLUS VITAMIN C, MAXIMUM STRENGTH. (O'Connor) Phenylpropanolamine HCl 75 mg, vitamin C 180 mg/Cap. Pkg. 20c.
Use: Diet aid.
DIET AIDS, NONPRESCRIPTION.
Use: Diet aid.
See: Appedrine, Tab. (Thompson).
Dex-A-Diet Plus Vitamin C, Cap. (O'-Connor).
Diet Ayds, Candy (DEP Corp.).
Dieutrim T.D., Cap. (Legere).
Extra Strength Grapefruit Diet Plan w/Diadax, Cap. (O'Connor).
Grapefruit Diet Plan w/Diadax, Cap., Tab. (O'Connor).
Maximum Strength Dexatrim Plus Vitamin C, Cap. (Thompsom).
Slim-Mint, Gum (Thompson).
DIET AYDS. (DEP) Benzocaine 6 mg/square. Bot. 48s.
Use: Diet aid.
DIETHADIONE. B.A.N. 5,5-Diethyloxazine-2,4-dione.
Use: Analeptic agent.
• **DIETHANOLAMINE,** N.F. XVIII.
Use: Pharmaceutic acid (alkalizing agent).
DIETHAZINE. B.A.N. 10-(2-Diethylaminoethyl)-Phenothiazine.
Use: Treatment of Parkinsonian syndrome.
DIETHANOLAMINE.
See: Diolamine.
DIETHAZINE HCl. 10-(β-Diethylaminoethyl)-pheno-thiazine HCl. Diparcol.

DIETHOXIN. Intracaine HCl.
DIETHYLDITHIOCARBAMATE.
Use: Trial drug for AIDS. [Orphan drug]
See: Imuthiol.
DIETHYLENEDIAMINE CITRATE. Piperazine Citrate, Piperazine Hexahydrate.
See: Antepar, Syr., Tab., Wafer (Burroughs Wellcome).
DIETHYLMALONYLUREA.
See: Barbital, Tab. (Various Mfr.).
• **DIETHYL PHTHALATE,** N.F. XVIII.
Use: Plasticizer.
DIETHYL-N META TOLUAMIDE.
See: N-DIETHYL META TOLUAMIDE.
• **DIETHYLPROPION HCl,** U.S.P. XXIII.
Tab., U.S.P. XXIII. 1-Phenyl-2-diethylaminopropanone-1 HCl. 2-(Di- ethylamino)proplophenone HCl.
Use: Anorexiant.
See: D.E.P.-75
Tenuate, Tab. (Merrell Dow).
Tepanil, Tab. (Riker).
Tepanil Ten-Tab. Tab. (Riker).
• **DIETHYLSTILBESTROL,** U.S.P. XXIII.
Inj., Tab., U.S.P. XXIII. Supp. U.S.P. XXI. Phenol 4,4'-(1,2-diethyl-1,2-othonediyl)bis . (Cyron A, Domestrol, Estrobene, Fonatol, New-Oestranol I, Oestrogenine, Oestromie-nin, Palestrol, Synthoestrin, Stiboestroform, Stilbestrol, Synestrin) alpha, alpha-Diethyl-4,4-stilbenediol.
Use: Estrogen.
See: Acnestrol, Lot. (Dermik).
Mase-Bestrol, Tab. (Mason).
W/Clioquinol, sulfanilamide.
See: D.I.T.I. Creme (Dunhall).
W/Nitrofurazone, diperodon HCl.
See: Furacin-E Urethral Inserts (Eaton).
• **DIETHYLSTILBESTROL DIPHOSPHATE,** U.S.P. XXIII. Inj., U.S.P. XXIII.
Use: Estrogen.
See: Stilphostrol, Inj., Tab. (Miles Pharm).
DIETHYLSTILBESTROL DIPROPIONATE, a,a'-Diethyl-4, 4 stilbenediol dipropionate. Cyren B, Estilben, Estroben DP, New-Oestranol 11, Orestol, Pabestrol D, Stilbestronate, Stilboestrol DP, Stilronate, Synestrin Amp. (Various Mfr.) Amp. in oil, 0.5 mg, 1 mg or 5 mg/ml. Tab. 0.5 mg, 1 mg or 5 mg.
Use: Estrogen.
DIETHYLTHIAMBUTENE. B.A.N. 3-Diethyl-amino-1, 1-di(2-thienyl)but-1-ene.
Use: Narcotic analgesic.
• **DIETHYLTOLUAMIDE,** U.S.P. XXIII. Topical Soln., U.S.P. XXIII. Benzamide, N, N-diethyl-3-methyl-N, N-Diethyl-m-tolu-

amide.
Use: Repellent (arthropod).
See: RV Pellent, Oint. (Elder).
N, N-DIETHYLVANILLAMIDE.
See: Ethamivan, Inj. (Various Mfr.).
DIET-TRIM. (Pharmex) Phenylpropanolamine, carboxymethylcellulose,
benzocaine/Tab. Bot. 21s, 90s.
Use: Diet aid.
DIET-TUSS. (Approved) Dextromethor-
phan 30 mg, thenylpyramine HCl, pyril-
amine maleate 80 mg, sodium salicylate
200 mg, sodium citrate 600 mg, ammo-
nium Cl 100 mg/fl oz. Sugar free. Bot. 4
oz.
Use: Antitussive, antihistamine, anal-
gesic, expectorant.
DIEUTRIM T.D. (Legere) Phenyl-
propanolamine 75 mg, benzocaine 9
mg, sodium carboxymethylcellulose 75
mg/SR Cap. Bot. 100s, 1000s.
Use: Diet aid.
• **DIFENOXIMIDE HYDROCHLORIDE.**
USAN.
Use: Antiperistaltic.
• **DIFENOXIN.** USAN. 1-(3-Cyano-3, 3-
diphenyl-propyl)-4-phenylpiperidine-4-
carboxylic acid.
Use: Antidiarrheal.
W/Atropine sulfate.
See: Motofen (Carnrick).
DIFETARSONE. B.A.N. NN'-Ethylene-1,
2-diarsanilic acid.
Use: Arsenicalcium.
• **DIFLORASONE DIACETATE,** U.S.P.
XXIII. Cream, Oint., U.S.P. XXIII. 6α,
9α-difluoro 11β, 17, 21trihydroxy-16β
methyl-pregna-1, 4-diene-3, 20-dione
17, 21 diacetate.
Use: Anti-inflammatory, antipruritic.
See: Florone, Cream, Oint. (Upjohn).
Maxiflor, Cream, Oint. (Herbert).
Psorcon, Cream, Oint. (Dermik).
• **DIFLOXACIN HYDROCHLORIDE.**
USAN.
Use: Anti-infective (DNA gyrase in-
hibitor).
• **DIFLUANINE HCl.** USAN. (McNeil) 1-(2-
Anilinoethyl)-4-[4, 4-bis(p-
fluorophenyl)butyl]-piperazine trihydro-
Cl.
Use: CNS stimulant.
DIFLUCAN. (Roerig) Fluconazole. **Tab.:**
50 mg, 100 mg or 200 mg. Bot. 30s, UD
100s. **Inj.:** 200 mg or 400 mg Vial 100
ml, 200 ml. **Pow. for Oral Susp.:** 10
mg/ml in 350 mg or 40 mg/ml in 1400
mg.
Use: Antifungal.
• **DIFLUCORTOLONE.** USAN. 6α,9-Difluo-

ro-11β, 21-dihydroxy-16α-methylpreg-
na-1, 4-diene-3, 20-dione.
Use: Glucocorticoid.
• **DIFLUCORTOLONE PIVALATE.** USAN.
Use: Glucocorticoid.
• **DIFLUMIDONE SODIUM.** USAN.
Use: Anti-inflammatory agent.
• **DIFLUNISAL,** U.S.P. XXIII. Tab., U.S.P.
XXIII.
Use: Analgesic, anti-inflammatory
agent.
See: Dolobid, Tab. (Merck & Co.).
• **DIFTALONE.** USAN.
Use: Anti-inflammatory agent.
• **DIFLUPREDNATE.** USAN. 6α, 9-difluoro-
11β, 17, 21-trihydroxypregna-1, 4-diene-
3, 20-dione 21-acetate-17-butyrate.
Use: Anti-inflammatory agent.
DI-GEL ADVANCED FORMULA. (Scher-
ing-Plough) Magnesium hydroxide 128
mg, calcium carbonate 280 mg, sime-
thicone 20 mg/Tab. Bot. 30s, 60s, 90s.
Use: Antacid, antiflatulent.
DI-GEL LIQUID. (Schering-Plough) Aluminum hydroxide (equivalent to dried
gel) 200 mg, magnesium hydroxide 200
mg, simethicone 20 mg/5 ml, saccharin,
sorbitol. Bot. 180 ml, 360 ml.
Use: Antacid, antiflatulent.
DIGESTAMIC. (Metro Med) Pancreali-
pase 300 mg, pepsin 100 mg/Tab. Bot.
50s.
Use: Digestive aid.
DIGESTAMIC LIQUID. (Metro Med) Bel-
ladonna leaf fluid extract 0.64 min./5 ml.
Bot. 8 oz.
Use: Anticholinergic/antispasmodic.
DIGESTANT. (Canright) Pancreatin 5.25
gr, ox bile extract 2 gr, pepsin 5 gr, be-
taine HCl 1 gr/Tab. Bot. 100s, 1000s.
Use: Digestive aid.
DIGESTIVE COMPOUND. (Thurston) Be-
taine HCl 3.25 gr, pepsin 1 gr, papain 2
gr, mycozyme 2 gr, ox bile 2 gr/2 Tab.
Bot. 100s, 500s.
Use: Digestive aid.
DIGESTIVE ENZYMES.
See: Cotazym Capsules (Organon).
Cotazym-S Capsules (Organon).
Creon Capsules (Solvay).
Dizmeys Tablets (Recsei Labs.).
Festal II Tablets (Hoechst-Roussel).
Hi-Vegi-Lip Tablets (Freeda).
Ilozyme Tablets (Adria).
Ku-Zyme HP Capsules (Kremers-Ur-
ban).
Pancrease Capsules (McNeil Pharm.)
Pancreatin Enseals Tablets (Lilly).
Pancreatin Tablets (Lilly).
VioKase Pow., Tab. (Robins).

**DIGESTIVE PRODUCTS, MISCELLA-
NEOUS.**
Use: Digestive enzyme supplement.
See: Ku-Zyme, Cap. (Kremers-Urban).
Arco-Lase, Tabs. (Arco).
Converzyme, Cap. (Ascher).
Digestozyme, Tab. (Various Mfr.).
Nu'Leven, Tab. (Lemmon).
Enzobile Improved (Hauck).
Sto-Zyme (Misemer).
DIGESTOZYME TABS. (Goldline) Pan-
creatin, pepsin, bile salts. Bot. 1000s.
Use: Digestive aid.
DIGIBIND. (Burroughs Wellcome) Digox-
in Immune Fab (ovine) fragments 40
mg, sorbitol 75 mg/Vial. Box 1s.
Use: Antidote.
DIGITALIS GLYCOSIDES.
Use: Cardiotonic.
See: Acylanid, Tab. (Sandoz).
Cedilanid, Tab. (Sandoz).
Cedilanid-D, Amp. (Sandoz).
Crystodigin, Tab. Amp., Vial (Lilly).
Deslanoside, Inj. (Various Mfr.).
Digiglusin, Tab. (Lilly).
Digitaline Nativelle, Soln., Tab., Elix.
(Savage).
Digitoxin, Preps. (Various Mfr.)
Digoxin, Preps. (Various Mfr.).
Gitaligin, Tab. (Schering).
Gitalin, Tab. (Various Mfr.).
Lanatoside C, Inj., Tab. (Various Mfr.).
Lanoxin, Tab., Inj., Elix. (Burroughs
Wellcome).
Purodigin, Tab. (Wyeth-Ayerst).
DIGITALIS LEAF, POWDERED.
Use: Cardiotonic.
See: Pil-Digis, Pill (Key).
DIGITALIS TINCTURE.
Use: Cardiotonic.
• **DIGITOXIN,** U.S.P. XXIII. Inj., Tab., U.S.P.
XXIII. (Various Mfr.) Amp. (0.2 mg/ml) 1
ml, Cap. in oil, 0.1 mg or 0.2 mg. Tab.
0.1 mg, 0.2 mg.
Use: Digitalis therapy, cardiotonic.
See: Crystodigin, Tab. (Lilly).
De-Tone 0.1, 0.2, Tab. (Scrip).
Digitaline Nativelle, Preps. (Savage).
Maso-Toxin, Tab. (Mason).
W/Carboxymethylcellulose and sodium.
See: Foxalin, Cap. (Standex).
DIGITOXIN, ACETYL.
Use: Cardiotonic.
See: Acylanid, Tab. (Sandoz).
α-**DIGITOXIN MONOACETATE.**
Use: Cardiotonic.
See: Acetyldigitoxin, Tab. (Various Mfr.).
• **DIGOXIN,** U.S.P. XXIII. Elix., Inj., Tab.
U.S.P. XXIII. Crystalline glycoside isolat-

ed from lvs. of digitalis lanata. 0.25
mg/Tab. Bot. 1000s, UD 100s.
Use: Cardiotonic.
See: Lanoxin, Preps. (Burroughs Well-
come).
Masoxin, Tab. (Mason).
DIGOXIN ANTIBODY.
See: Digidote.
DIGOXIN I-125 IMUSAY. (Abbott Diag-
nostics) Digoxin diagnostic kit for the
quantitative determination of serum
digoxin. 100s, 300s.
Use: Diagnostic aid.
**DIGOXIN IMMUNE FAB (OVINE) FRAG-
MENTS.**
Use: Antidote. [Orphan drug]
See: Digibind, Inj. (Burroughs Well-
come).
DIGOXIN RIABEAD. (Abbott Diagnos-
tics) Solid-phase radioimmunoassay for
quantitative measurement of serum
digoxin. Test kit 100s, 300s.
Use: Diagnostic aid.
DIHEMATOPORPHYRIN ETHERS.
Use: Antineoplastic. [Orphan drug]
• **DIHEXYVERINE HYDROCHLORIDE.**
USAN.
Use: Anticholinergic.
DIHISTINE D.H. (Goldline) Pseu-
doephedrine HCl 30 mg, chlorpheni-
ramine maleate 2 mg, codeine phos-
phate 10 mg. Elix. Bot. 4 oz, pt, gal.
Use: Decongestant, antihistamine, anti-
tussive.
DIHISTINE ELIXIR. (Various Mfr.)
Phenylephrine HCl 5 mg, chlorpheni-
ramine maleate 2 mg/5 ml. Bot. pt, gal.
Use: Decongestant, antihistamine.
DIHISTINE EXPECTORANT. (Goldline)
Pseudoephedrine HCl 30 mg, codeine
phosphate 10 mg, guaifenesin 100 mg,
alcohol 7.5%. Bot. 4 oz, pt, gal.
Use: Decongestant, antitussive, expec-
torant.
DIHYDAN SOLUBLE.
See: Phenytoin Sodium (Various Mfr.).
DIHYDRALLAZINE. B.A.N. 1,4-Dihy-
drazinophthalazine.
Use: Hypotensive.
DIHYDROCODEINE. Paracodin.
Drocode.
Use: Antitussive, analgesic.
DIHYDROCODEINE COMPOUND. (Vari-
ous Mfr.) Dihydrocodeine bitartrate 16
mg, aspirin 356.4 mg, caffeine 30 mg.
Cap. Bot. 100s, 500s.
Use: Narcotic analgesic.
• **DIHYDROCODEINONE BITARTRATE.**
U.S.P. XXIII.

Use: Narcotic.
See: Hydrocodone Bitartrate, U.S.P.
XXIII.
W/Caffeine, phenacetin, aspirin.
See: Drocogesic #3, Tab. (Rand).
Duradyne DHC, Liq. (Forest).
W/Caffeine, aspirin.
See: Synalgos-DC, Cap. (Wyeth-Ay-
erst).
W/Caffeine, acetaminophen.
See: DHC Plus, Cap. (Purdue Freder-
ick).
**DIHYDROCODEINONE RESIN COM-
PLEX.**
W/Phenyltoloxamine resin complex.
See: Tussionex, Preps. (Pennwalt).
DIHYDRO-DIETHYLSTILBESTROL.
See: Hexestrol, Tab., Vial (Various Mfr.).
DIHYDROERGOCORNINE. Ergot alka-
line component of hydergine.
See: Circanol, Tab. (Riker).
Deapril-ST, Tab. (Mead Johnson).
DIHYDROERGOCRISTINE. Ergot alka-
loid component of hydergine.
See: Circanol, Tab. (Riker).
Deapril-ST, Tab. (Mead Johnson).
DIHYDROERGOCRYPTINE. Ergot alka-
loid component of hydergine.
See: Circanol, Tab. (Riker).
Deapril-ST, Tab. (Mead Johnson).
DIHYDROERGOTAMINE. (D.H.E. 45)
(Sandoz) Dihydroergotamine mesylate.
Amp.
• **DIHYDROERGOTAMINE MESYLATE,**
U.S.P. XXIII. Inj., U.S.P. XXIII. Dihy-
droergotamine methanesulfonate.
Use: Agent for migraine, antiadrenergic.
See: DHE 45, Amp. (Sandoz).
W/Scopolamine HBr, phenobarbital sodi-
um, barbital sodium, Sandoptal.
See: Plexonal, Tab. (Sandoz).
• **DIHYDROERGOTAMINE MESYLATE,
HEPARIN SODIUM, and LIDOCAINE
HYDROCHLORIDE INJECTION,** U.S.P.
XXII. Inj.
DIHYDROERGOTOXINE. Ergoloid mesy-
late.
Use: Psychotherapeutic agent.
See: Gerimal, Tab. (Rugby).
Hydergine, Tab. (Sandoz).
Ergoloid Mesylates, Tab. (Various
Mfr.).
Ergoloid Mesylates, Tab. (Various
Mfr.).
Hydergine, Tab. (Sandoz).
Niloric, Tab. (Ascher).
Hydergine LC, Cap. (Sandoz).
Hydergine, Liq. (Sandoz).
DIHYDROFOLLICULAR HORMONE.
See: Estradiol (Various Mfr.).

DIHYDROFOLLICULINE.
See: Estradiol (Various Mfr.).
DIHYDROHYDROXYCODEINONE. Oxy-
codone. (Ducodal, Eukodal, Eucodal).
Use: Narcotic analgesic.
**DIHYDROHYDROXYCODEINONE HCl or
BITARTRATE.** Oxycodone HCl or Bitar-
trate.
W/Combinations.
See: Cophene-S, Syr. (Dunhall).
Corizahist-D, Syr. (Mason).
Damason-P, Tab. (Mason).
Percobarb, Cap. (DuPont).
Percodan, Tab. (DuPont).
Triaprin-DC, Cap. (Dunhall).
DIHYDROMORPHINONE HCl.
See: Dilaudid, Preps. (Knoll).
• **DIHYDROSTREPTOMYCIN SULFATE,**
U.S.P. XXIII. Boluses, Inj., Sterile, U.S.P.
XXIII.
Use: Antibiotic.
• **DIHYDROTACHYSTEROL,** U.S.P. XXIII.
Cap., Oral Soln., Tab., U.S.P. XXIII.
9,10-Seco-5,7,22-ergostartien-3-β-ol.
(Roxane) 0.2 mg/Tab. Bot. 100s, UD
100s.
Use: For postoperative tetany; idiopath-
ic tetany; hypoparathyroidism.
See: Hytakerol, Cap., Soln. (Sanofi
Winthrop).
DIHYDROTESTOSTERONE. An-
drostane-17-beta-ol-3-one.
See: Stanolone.
DIHYDROTHEELIN.
See: Estradiol (Various Mfr.).
DIHYDROXYACETONE.
See: Chromelin, Liq. (Summers).
QT, Liq. (Schering-Plough).
Sudden Tan, Liq. (Schering-Plough).
• **DIHYDROXYALUMINUM AMINOAC-
ETATE,** U.S.P. XXIII. Cap., Magma,
Tab., U.S.P. XXIII. Aluminum, (glycinato-
N,O) dihydroxy-hydrate. (Glycinato)-di-
hydroxyaluminum hydrate. Aluminum di-
hydroxyaminoacetate; basic aluminum
aminoacetate. (Glycinato) dihydroxyalu-
minum.
Use: Antacid.
W/Methscopolamine bromide, sodium lau-
ryl sulfate, magnesium hydroxide.
See: Alu-Scop, Cap., Susp. (Wester-
field).
W/Phenobarbital and atropine methyl ni-
trate.
See: Harvatrate A, Tab. (O'Neal).
W/Salicylsalicylic acid, aspirin.
See: Salsprin, Tab. (Seatrace).
DIHYDROXYCHOLECALCIFEROL.
See: Rocaltrol. (Roche).
24, 25 DIHYDROXYCHOLECALCIFER-

OL. (Lemmon/Tag)
Use: Uremic osteodystrophy. [Orphan drug]
DIHYDROXYESTRIN.
See: Estradiol (Various Mfr.).
DIHYDROXYFLUORANE. Fluorescein.
DIHYDROXYPHENYLISATIN.
See: Oxyphenisatin (Various Mfr.).
DIHYDROXYPHENYLOXINDOL.
See: Oxyphenisatin (Various Mfr.).
DIHYDROXYPROPYLTHEOPHYLLINE.
Dyphylline.
See: Neothylline, Tab., Elix., Inj. (Lemmon).
DIHYDROXY(STEARATO)ALUMINUM.
Aluminum Monostearate, N.F. XVIII.
DIIODOHYDROXYQUIN.
Use: Amebicide.
See: Iodoquinol, U.S.P. XXIII.
DI-IODOHYDROXYQUINOLINE. B.A.N.
8-Hydroxy-5,7-di-iodoquinoline.
Use: Treatment of amebiasis.
DIIODOHYDROXYQUINOLINE.
See: Iodoquinol, U.S.P. XXIII.
DIISOPROMINE HCl. N,N-diisopropyl-3,3-diphenylpropylamine HCl. (Lab. for Pharmaceutical Development, Inc.).
See: Desquam-X (Westwood).
• **DIISOPROPANOLAMINE,** N.F. XVII.
Use: Pharmaceutic aid (alkalinizing agent).
DIISOPROPYL PHOSPHOROFLUORI-DATE.
See: Isofluorophate, U.S.P. XXIII.
Floropryl, Oint. (Merck & Co.).
DIISOPROPYL SEBACATE.
See: Delavan, Cream (Miles Pharm).
DILACOR XR. (Rhone-Poulenc Rorer)
Diltiazem HCl **120 mg:** Cap. SR 100s.
240 mg: Cap. SR 100s, UD 100s.
Use: Calcium channel blocking agent.
DILAMINATE. Mixture of magnesium carbide and dihydroxy aluminum glycinate.
Use: Antacid.
DILANTIN. (Parke-Davis) Phenytoin. **30′**
Susp.: 30 mg/5 ml. Bot. 8 oz, UD 5 ml.
125 Susp.: 125 mg/5 ml. Bot. 8 oz, UD 5 ml. **Infatab:** 50 mg/Tab. Bot. 100s, UD 100s.
Use: Anticonvulsant.
DILANTIN SODIUM. (Parke-Davis) Extended phenytoin sodium. **Kapseal:** 30 mg, 100 mg. Bot. 100s, 1000s, UD 100s. **Amp.:** (w/propylene glycol 40%, alcohol 10%, sodium hydroxide) 100 mg/2 ml. UD 10s; 250 mg/5 ml. Amp. 10s, UD 10s.
Use: Anticonvulsant.
DILANTIN SODIUM W/PHENOBARBI-TAL KAPSEAL. (Parke-Davis) Pheny-

toin sodium 100 mg, phenobarbital 16 mg or 32 mg/Cap. Bot. 100s, 1000s, UD 100s (32 mg only).
Use: Anticonvulsant, sedative/hypnotic.
DILANTIN-30 PEDIATRIC. (Parke-Davis)
Phenytoin 30 mg/5 ml, alcohol 0.6%.
Susp. Bot. 240 ml, 5 ml.
Use: Anti-convulsant.
DILATRATE SR. (Reed & Carnrick)
Isosorbide dinitrate 40 mg/SR Cap. Bot. 100s.
Use: Antianginal.
DILAUDID COUGH SYRUP. (Knoll) Hydromorphone HCl 1 mg, guaifenesin 100 mg/ 5ml. Alcohol 5%. Bot. pt.
Use: Narcotic analgesic, expectorant.
DILAUDID HP AMPULE. (Knoll) Hydromorphone 10 mg/ml. Box 10s; 50 mg/5 ml. Box 1s.
Use: Narcotic analgesic.
DILAUDID HYDROCHLORIDE. (Knoll)
Hydromorphone HCl. **Amp.** (w/sodium citrate 0.2%, citric acid soln. 0.2%): 1 mg, 2 mg or 4 mg/ml. Box 10s. 2 mg, Box 25s. **Multiple Dose Vial:** 2 mg/ml. Bot. 20 ml. **Tab.:** 1 mg. Bot. 100s. 2 mg Bot. 100s, 500s. Strip pack 4 × 25s. 3 mg Bot. 100s. 4 mg 100s, 500s. Strip pack 4 × 25s. **Pow:** Vial, 15 gr Multiple dose vial 10 ml, 20 ml. 2 mg/ml. **Rectal Supp.:** (in cocoa butter base, w/colloidal silica 1%): 3 mg/Supp. Box 6s.
Use: Narcotic analgesic.
W/Guaifenesin.
See: Dilaudid Cough Syrup. (Knoll).
• **DILEVALOL HYDROCHLORIDE.** USAN.
Use: Antihypertensive, anti-adrenergic.
DILITHIUM CARBONATE. Lithium Carbonate, U.S.P. XXIII.
Use: Antipsychotic.
DILOCAINE. (Hauck) Lidocaine HCl 1% or 2%. Bot. 50 ml.
Use: Local anesthetic.
DILOR. (Savage) Dyphylline. **Tab.:** 200 mg. Bot. 100s, 1000s, UD 100s. **Elix.:** 160 mg/15 ml. Bot. pt.
Use: Bronchodilator.
DILOR 400. (Savage) Dyphylline 400 mg. Bot. 100s, 1000s, UD 100s.
Use: Bronchodilator.
DILOR G LIQUID. (Savage) Dyphylline 300 mg, guaifenesin 300 mg/15 ml. Bot. pt, gal.
Use: Bronchodilator, expectorant.
DILOR G TABLETS. (Savage) Dyphylline 200 mg, guaifenesin 200 mg/Tab. Bot. 100s, 1000s, UD 100s.
Use: Bronchodilator, expectorant.
DILOXANIDE. B.A.N. 4-(N-Methyldichloroacetamido) phenol.

Use: Treatment of amebiasis.
• **DILTIAZEM EXTENDED-RELEASE CAP-SULES,** U.S.P. XXIII.
Use: Vasodilator.
• **DILTIAZEM HYDROCHLORIDE.** USAN.
Use: Vasodilator.
DILTIAZEM HCl EXTENDED-RELEASE CAPSULES. (Various Mfr.) Diltiazem HCl 00 mg, 90 mg or 120 mg. Bot. 100s, 500s, 1000s.
Use: Vasodilator.
• **DILTIAZEM MALATE.** USAN.
Use: Vasodilator.
DIMACOL. (Robins) Pseudoephedrine HCl 30 mg, dextromethorphan HBr 10 mg, guaifenesin 100 mg/Cap. or 5 ml. **Cap.** Bot. 100s, 500s, Pre-Pack 12s, 24s. **Liq.** (w/alcohol 4.75%) Bot. pt.
Use: Decongestant, nonnarcotic antitussive, expectorant.
DIMAPHEN ELIXIR. (Major) Phenylpropanolamine HCl 12.5 mg, brompheniramine maleate 2 mg, alcohol 2.5%, saccharin, sorbitol. Elix. Bot. 120 ml, 240 ml, pt. gal.
Use: Decongestant, antihistamine.
DIMAPHEN OTC TABS. (Major) Phenylpropanolamine HCl 25 mg, brompheniramine maleate 4 mg. Tab. Bot. 24s.
Use: Decongestant, antihistamine.
DIMAPHEN TIME-TABS. (Major) Phenylpropanolamine HCl 75 mg, brompheniramine maleate 12 mg/Tab. Bot. 12s, 24s.
Use: Decongestant, antihistamine.
DIMAZOLE (I.N.N.). Diamthazole, B.A.N.
• **DIMEFADANE.** USAN. N, N-Dimethyl-3-phenyl-1-indanamine.
Use: Nonnarcotic analgesic.
• **DIMEFLINE HYDROCHLORIDE.** USAN.
Use: Respiratory stimulant.
• **DIMEFOLCON A.** USAN.
Use: Contact lens material.
DIMENEST. (Forest Pharm.) Dimenhydrinate 50 mg/ml. Vial 10 ml.
Use: Antiemetic/antivertigo.
• **DIMENHYDRINATE,** U.S.P. XXIII. Syr., Tab., Inj., U.S.P. XXIII. Beta-dimethylaminoethyl benzohydryl ether-8-chlorotheophyllinate. 8-Chlorotheophylline 2-(Diphenylmethoxy)-N, N-dimethylethylamine compound (1:1). IH-Purine-2,6-dione,8-chloro-3,7-dihydro-1,3-dimethyl-, compound with 2-(diphenylmethoxy)-N,N-dimethylethanamine (1:1). Gravol.
Use: Antiemetic, antihistamine.
See: Dimenest, Inj. (Forest Pharm.).
Dimentabs, Tab. (Bowman).
Dipendrate, Tab. (Kenyon).

Dramamine, Preps. (Upjohn).
Dramocen, Inj. (Central).
Dymenate, Inj. (Keene).
Eldadryl, Preps. (Elder).
Eldodram, Tab. (Elder).
Hydrate, Vial (Hyrex).
Reidamine, Inj. (Solvay).
Signate, Inj. (Sig).
Trav-Arex, Cap. (Quality Generics).
Traveltabs, Tab. (Geneva Marsam).
Vertab, Cap. (UAD).
DIMENOXADOLE. B.A.N. 2-Dimethylaminoethyl2-ethoxy-2, 2-diphenylacetate.
Use: Narcotic analgesic.
DIMENTABS. (Bowman) Dimenhydrinate 50 mg/Tab. Bot. 100s.
Use: Antiemetic/antivertigo.
DIMEPHEPTANOL. B.A.N. 6-Dimethylamino-4, 4-diphenylheptan-3-ol.
Use: Narcotic analgesic.
• **DIMEPRANOL ACEDOBEN.** USAN.
Use: Immunomodulator.
DIMEPREGNEN. B.A.N. 3β-Hydroxy-6α, 16α-dimethylpregn-4-en-20-one.
Use: Anti-estrogen.
DIMEPROPION. B.A.N. α-Dimethylaminopropio- phenone. Metamfepramone (I.N.N.).
Use: Anorexigenic.
• **DIMERCAPROL,** U.S.P. XXIII. Inj. U.S.P. XXIII. 2, 3-Dimercaptol-1-propanol.
Use: Antidote to gold, arsenic and mercury poisoning; metal complexing agent.
See: BAL Amp. (Hynson, Wescott & Dunning).
DIMESONE. B.A.N. 9α-Fluoro- 11β, 21-dihydroxy-16α, 17-dimethylpregna-1, 4-diene-3, 20-dione.
Use: Anti-inflammatory steroid.
DIMETANE. (Robins) Brompheniramine maleate. **Tab.:** 4 mg Bot. 100s, 500s, Pre-Pack 24s. **Extentab:** 8 mg or 12 mg Bot. 100s, 500s. **Elix.:** 2 mg/5 ml Bot. 4 oz, pt, gal. **Amp.:** 10 mg/ml, pH adjusted with sodium hydroxide. 1 ml Box 25s.
Use: Antihistamine.
W/Phenylephrine HCl, phenylpropanolamine HCl.
See: Dimetapp Elix., Extentab (Robins).
DIMETANE-DC COUGH SYRUP. (Robins) Brompheniramine maleate 2 mg, phenylpropanolamine HCl 12.5 mg, codeine phosphate 10 mg/5 ml w/alcohol 0.95%. Bot. pt, gal.
Use: Antihistamine, decongestant, antitussive.
DIMETANE DECONGESTANT CAPLETS. (Robins) Brompheniramine

maleate 4 mg, phenylephrine HCl 10 mg/Capl. Bot. 24s, 48s.
Use: Antihistamine, decongestant.
DIMETANE DECONGESTANT ELIXIR. (Robins) Brompheniramine maleate 2 mg, phenylephrine HCl 5 mg/5 ml, alcohol 2.3%, saccharin. Bot. 4 oz.
Use: Antihistamine, decongestant.
DIMETANE-DX COUGH SYRUP. (Robins) Pseudoephedrine HCl 30 mg, brompheniramine maleate 2 mg, dextromethorphan HBr 10 mg, alcohol 0.95%, saccharin, sorbitol. Bot. pt.
Use: Decongestant, antihistamine, antitussive.
DIMETANE EXTABS. (Robins) Brompheniramine maleate 8 mg/Tab. Pkg. 12s. Bot. 100s, 500s.
Use: Antihistamine.
DIMETAPP COLD & ALLERGY. (Robins) Brompheniramine maleate 1 mg, phenylpropanolamine HCl 6.25 mg, aspartame, phenylalanine 8 mg, sorbitol. Tab. Chew. Bot. Pck.
Use: Pediatric decongestant and antihistamine.
DIMETAPP COLD & FLU CAPLET. (Robins) Phenylpropanolamine HCl 12.5 mg, brompheniramine maleate 2 mg, acetaminophen 500 mg/Capl. Bot. 24s, 48s.
Use: Decongestant, antihistamine, analgesic.
DIMETAPP DM ELIXIR. (Robins) Phenylpropanolamine HCl 12.5 mg, brompheniramine maleate 2 mg, dextromethorphan HBr 10 mg, 2.3% alcohol, saccharin, sorbitol. Elix. Bot. 120 ml, 240 ml.
Use: Decongestant, antihistamine, antitussive.
DIMETAPP ELIXIR. (Robins) Brompheniramine maleate 2 mg, phenylpropanolamine HCl 12.5 mg/5 ml alcohol 2.3%, saccharin, sorbitol. Bot, 4 oz, 8 oz, pt, gal, Dis-Co Pack 5 ml 10 × 10s.
Use: Antihistamine, decongestant.
DIMETAPP EXTENTABS. (Robins) Brompheniramine maleate 12 mg, phenylpropanolamine HCl 75 mg/Tab. Bot. 100s, 500s, Dis-Co Pack 100s. Blister pack 12s, 24s.
Use: Antihistamine, decongestant.
DIMETAPP 4-HOUR LIQUI-GELS. (Robins) Brompheniramine maleate 4 mg, phenylpropanolamine HCl 25 mg, sorbitol. Cap. Pck. 12s.
Use: Decongestant and antihistamine.
DIMETAPP SINUS. (Robins) Pseudoephedrine HCl 30 mg, ibuprofen 200

mg/Cap. Bot. 20s, 40s.
Use: Decongestant and analgesic.
DIMETAPP TABLETS. (Robins) Brompheniramine maleate 4 mg, phenylpropanolamine HCl 12.5 mg/Tab. Blisterpak 24s.
Use: Antihistamine, decongestant.
• **DIMETHADIONE.** USAN. 5, 5-Dimethyl-2, 4-oxazolidine-dione. Eupractone (Travenol).
Use: Anticonvulsant.
DIMETHAZAN. 1, 3-Dimethyl-7-(2-dimethylamino-ethyl) xanthine.
• **DIMETHICONE.** N.F. XVIII. Dimethylsiloxane polymers, dimethyl polysiloxane.
Use: Prosthetic aid, component of barrier creams.
See: Covicone, Cream (Abbott).
Silicone, Oint. (Various Mfr.).
• **DIMETHICONE 350.** USAN.
Use: Prosthetic aid for soft tissue.
DIMETHINDENE. B.A.N. 2- 1-[2-(2-Dimethylaminoethyl) inden-3-yl]ethyl pyridine.
Use: Antihistamine.
DIMETHISOQUIN. B.A.N. 3-Butyl-1-(2-dimethyla-minoethoxy)isoquinoline. Quinisocaine (I.N.N.).
Use: Antipruritic.
• **DIMETHISTERONE.** USAN.
Use: Progesterone.
DIMETHOLIZINE PHOSPHATE. 1-(2-Methoxy phenyl) 4 (3-methoxypropyl)piperazine phosphate. Ansiv.
DIMETHOTHIAZINE. B.A.N. 10-(2-Dimethylamino- propyl)-2-dimethysulfamoylphenothiazine.
Use: Agent for migraine.
DIMETHOXANATE. B.A.N. 2-(2-Dimethylamino-ethoxy) ethyl phenothiazine-10-carboxylate.
Use: Cough suppressant.
DIMETHOXYPHENYL PENICILLIN SODIUM.
See: Methicillin sodium (Various Mfr.).
DIMETHPYRIDENE MALEATE. Dimethindene Maleate, U.S.P. XXIII.
See: Dimethindene Maleate, U.S.P. XXIII.
DIMETHYLAMINOPHENAZONE.
See: Aminopyrine (Various Mfr.).
DIMETHYLAMINO PYRAZINE SULFATE.
See: Ampyzine Sulfate.
DIMETHYLCARBAMATE. of 3-Hydroxy-1-Methylpyridinium Bromide.
See: Mestinon, Tab. (Roche).
DIMETHYLHEXESTROL DIPROPIONATE. Promethestrol Dipropionate.
See: Meprane Dipropionate, Tab. (Reed

& Carnrick).

DIMETHYL POLYSILOXANE.
See: Dimethicone (Various Mfr.).
W/Benzocaine, bismuth subcarbonate, carbamide, hexachlorophene, phenylephrine HCl, pyrilamine maleate, zinc oxide.
W/Hexachlorophene, zinc oxide, pyrilamine maleate, tetracaine HCl, methyl salicylate, zirconium oxide.
• **DIMETHYL SULFOXIDE,** U.S.P. XXIII. Irrigation, U.S.P. XXIII. Methyl sulfoxide. DMSO.
Use: Anti-inflammatory agent, topical.
See: Rimso-50 (Research Ind.).
DIMETHYLTHIAMBUTENE. B.A.N. 3-Dimethylamino-1, 1-di-(2-thienyl)but-1-ene.
Use: Narcotic analgesic.
DIMETHYLTUBOCURARINE. B.A.N. Dimethyl ether of (+)-tubocurarine.
Use: Neuromuscular blocking agent.
DIMETHYL-TUBOCURARINE IODIDE.
Use: Skeletal muscle relaxant.
See: Metocurine Iodide, U.S.P. XXIII.
DIMETHYLURETHIMINE.
See: Meturedepa (Armour).
• **DIMOXAMINE HYDROCHLORIDE.** USAN.
Use: Memory adjuvant.
DIMYCOR. (Standard Drug) Pentaerythritol tetranitrate 10 mg, phenobarbital 15 mg/Tab. Bot. 1000s.
Use: Antianginal, sedative/hypnotic.
DINACRIN. (Sanofi Winthrop) Isonicotinic acid, hydrazide.
Use: Antituberculous agent.
DINATE. (Blaine) Dimenhydrinate 50 mg/ml. Vial 10 ml.
Use: Antiemetic/antivertigo.
• **DINOPROSTONE.** USAN. 7-[3α-Hydroxy-2β-[(3S)-hydroxy-trans-oct-1-enyl]-5-oxocyclopent-1-yl]-cis-hept-5-enoic acid.
Use: Smooth muscle activator; agent for cervical ripening.
See: Prostaglandin E-2.
Prepidil (Upjohn).
• **DINSED.** USAN. N,N'-Ethylenebis (3-nitrobenzenesulfonamide).
Use: Coccidiostat.
DIOCTIN. (Janssen) Difenoxin HCl.
Use: Antidiarrheal.
DIOCTO. (Purepac) Docusate sodium 100 mg or 200 mg/Cap. Bot. 100s.
Use: Laxative.
DIOCTO-C. (Various Mfr.) Docusate sodium 60 mg, casanthranol 30 mg/15 ml. Syr. Bot. 240 ml, pt, gal.

Use: Laxative.
DIOCTO-K. (Rugby) Docusate potassium 100 mg/Cap. Bot. 100s, 1000s.
Use: Laxative.
DIOCTO-K PLUS. (Rugby) Docusate sodium 100 mg, casanthranol 30 mg. Cap. Bot. 100s, 1000s.
Use: Laxative.
DIOCTOLOSE. (Goldline) Docusate potassium 100 mg/Cap. Bot. 100s, 1000s.
Use: Laxative.
DIOCTOLOSE PLUS CAPSULES. (Goldline) Docusate 100 mg, casanthranol 30 mg/Cap. Bot. 100s, 1000s.
Use: Laxative.
DIOCTYL CALCIUM SULFOSUCCINATE. Docusate Calcium, U.S.P. XXIII.
Use: Laxative.
DIOCTYL POTASSIUM SULFOSUCCINATE.
W/Glycerin, potassium oleate and stearate.
See: Rectalad, Liq. (Wallace).
DIOCTYL SODIUM SULFOSUCCINATE. B.A.N. Docusate Sodium, U.S.P. XXIII.
Use: Non-laxative fecal softener.
DIODONE INJECTION.
See: Iodopyracet injection.
DIOEZE. (Century) Dioctyl sodium sulfosuccinate 250 mg/Cap. Bot. 100s, 1000s.
Use: Laxative.
• **DIOHIPPURIC ACID I-125.** USAN.
Use: Radioactive agent.
• **DIOHIPPURIC ACID I-131.** USAN.
Use: Radioactive agent.
DIO-HIST. (Approved) Dextromethorphan 30 mg, thenylpyramine HCl 80 mg, phenylephrine HCl 20 mg, potassium tartrate 1/24 gr/oz. Bot. 4 oz.
Use: Antihistamine.
D-DIOL. (Burgin-Arden) Testosterone cypionate 50 mg, estradiol cypionate 2 mg/ml. Vial 10 ml.
Use: Androgen, estrogen.
DIOLAMINE. Diethanolamine.
DIOLOSTENE.
See: Methandriol.
DIONEX. (Interstate) Docusate sodium 100 mg or 250 mg/Cap. Bot. 100s, 250s, 1000s.
Use: Laxative.
DIONIN. Ethylmorphine HCl.
Use: Orally; cough depressant, ocular lymphagogue.
DIONOSIL OILY. (Glaxo) Propyliodone 60% in peanut oil. Inj. Vial 20 ml.
Use: Bronchographic contrast medium.

DIOPHYLLIN.
See: Aminophylline, Preps. (Various Mfr.).

DIOPTERIN. Pteroyldiglutamic acid, PDGA, Pteroyl-alpha-glutamylglutamic acid.
Use: Antineoplastic agent.

DIORAPIN. (Standex) Estrogenic conjugate 0.625 mg, methyltestosterone 5 mg/Tab. Bot. 100s. Estrone 2 mg, testosterone 25 mg/ml. Inj. Vial 10 ml.
Use: Estrogen, androgen combination.

DIOSATE D. (Towne) Docusate sodium. Cap. 100 mg or 250 mg/Tab. Bot. 100s.
Use: Laxative.

DIOSMIN. Buchu resin obtained from lvs. of barosma serratifolia and alliedrutaceae.

DIO-SOFT. (Standex) Docusate sodium 100 mg, casanthranol 30 mg/Cap. Bot. 100s.
Use: Laxative.

DIOSTATE D. (Upjohn) Vitamin D 400 IU, calcium 343 mg, phosphorus 265 mg/3 Tab. Bot. 100s.
Use: Vitamin/mineral supplement.

• **DIOTYROSINE I-125.** USAN.
Use: Radioactive agent.

DIOVAL XX. (Keene) Estradiol valerate 20 mg/ml. Vial 10 ml.
Use: Estrogen.

DIOVAL 40. (Keene) Estradiol valerate 40 mg/ml. Vial 10 ml.
Use: Estrogen.

DIOVOCYLIN. (Ciba)
See: Estradiol, Preps. (Various Mfr.).

• **DIOXADROL HYDROCHLORIDE.** USAN.
Use: Antidepressant.

DIOXAMATE. B.A.N. 4-Carbamoyloxymethyl-2-methyl-2-nonyl-1,3-dioxolan.
Use: Treatment of Parkinsonian syndrome.

DIOXAPHETYL BUTYRATE. B.A.N. Ethyl 4-morpholino-2,2-diphenylbutyrate.
Use: Narcotic analgesic.

DIOXINDOL. Diacetylhydroxyphenylisatin.

DIOXYANTHRANOL.
See: Anthralin, N.F. (Various Mfr.).

DIOXYANTHRAQUINONE. 1,8-Dihydroxy-anthra- quinone.
See: Danthron, U.S.P. XXIII.

• **DIOXYBENZONE,** U.S.P. XXII. Dioxybenzone and Oxybenzone Cream, U.S.P. XXII. Methanone, (2-hydroxy-4-methoxyphenyl)(2-hydroxyphenyl)1.
Use: Sunscreen agent.
W/Oxybenzone, benzophene.

See: Solbar, Lot. (Person & Covey).

DIPALMITOYLPHOSPHATIDYL-CHOLINE. Colfosceril palmitate.
Use: Synthetic lung surfactant.
See: Exosurf Neonatal, Pow. (Burroughs Wellcome).

DIPALMITOYLPHOSPHATIDYL-CHOLINE/PHOSPHATIDYLGLYCEROL.
Use: Neonatal respiratory distress syndrome. [Orphan drug]

DIPARCOL HYDROCHLORIDE. Diethazine.

DIPEGYL.
See: Nicotinamide, Preps. (Various Mfr.).

DIPENICILLIN G.
See: Benzethacil.

DIPENINE BROMIDE. B.A.N. 2-Dicyclopentyl-acetoxy-ethyltriethylammonium bromide.
Use: Antispasmodic.
See: Diponium Bromide (I.N.N.).

DIPENTUM. (Pharmacia) Osalazine sodium 250 mg/Cap. Bot. 100s, 500s.
Use: Ulcerative colitis.

DIPERODON. B.A.N. 3-Piperidinopropane-1,2-diol di(phenylcarbamate).
Use: Local anesthetic.

DIPERODON, U.S.P. XXII. Oint., U.S.P. XXII. 3-Piperidino-1,2-propanediol dicarbanilate (ester) monohydrate.
Use: Local anesthetic.

DIPERODON HYDROCHLORIDE.
Use: Anesthetic.
See: Diothane Oint. (Merrell Dow). Proctodon, Cream (Solvay).
W/Bacitracin, neomycin sulfate, polymyxin.
See: Epimycin A, Oint. (Delta).
W/Benzalkonium Cl, ichthammol, thymol, camphor, juniper tar.
See: Boro Oint. (Scrip).
W/Furacin (nitrofurazone).
See: Furacin E Urethral Inserts (Eaton). Furacin H.C. Urethral Inserts (Eaton).
W/Furacin (nitorfurazone) and Microfur (nituroxime).
See: Furacin Otic, Drops. (Eaton).
W/Hydrocortisone, polymyxin B sulfate, neomycin.
See: My Cort Otic #1, Ear Drops (Scrip).
W/Hydroxyquinoline Benzoate.
See: Diothane, Oint. (Merrell Dow).
W/Methapyrilene HCl, pyrilamine maleate, allantoin, benzocaine, menthol.
See: Antihistamine Cream (Towne).
W/Thimerosal, isopropyl alcohol.
See: Earobex, Ear Drops (Hauck).

DIPHEMANIL METHYLSULFATE. B.A.N.

4-Benzhydrylidene-1, 1-dimethylpiperi-
dinium methyl-sulfate.
Use: Parasympatholytic.
DIPHENADIONE. 2-(Diphenylacetyl)-1-3,
indandione.
Use: Anticoagulant.
See: Dipaxin, Tab. (Upjohn).
DIPHENATIL.
See: Diphemanil methylsulfate.
DIPHENATOL. (Rugby) Diphenoxylate
HCl 2.5 mg, atropine sulfate 0.025 mg.
Tab. Bot. 100s, 500s, 1000s.
Use: Antidiarrheal.
DIPHEN COUGH. (PBI) Diphenhy-
dramine HCl 12.5 mg/5 ml. Syr. Bot. 118
ml, pt, gal.
Use: Antitussive.
DIPHENHIST. (Rugby) Diphenhy-
dramine. **Captabs:** 25 mg Bot. 100s, UD
24s. **Elix.:** 12.5 mg/5 ml. Bot. 120 ml, pt,
gal.
Use: Antihistamine.
• **DIPHENHYDRAMINE AND PSEU-
DOEPHEDRINE CAPSULES.** U.S.P.
XXIII.
Use: Antihistamine, decongestant.
• **DIPHENHYDRAMINE CITRATE,** U.S.P.
XXIII.
Use: Antihistamine.
• **DIPHENHYDRAMINE HYDROCHLO-
RIDE.** U.S.P. XXIII. Cap., Elix., Inj.,
U.S.P. XXIII. Ethanamine, 2-(diphenyl-
methoxy)-N,N-dimethyl-,HCl. 2-
(Diphenyl- methoxy)-N,N-dimethylethy-
lamine HCl.
Use: Antihistamine.
See: Bax, Cap., Elix., Expectorant
(McKesson).
Benachior, Syr. (Jenkins).
Benadryl Hydrochloride, Preps.
(Parke-Davis).
Benahist, Preps. (Keene).
Bentrac, Cap. (Kenyon).
Benylin Cough Syrup (Warner-Lam-
bert).
Clearly Cala-gel (Tec Labs).
Diphen-Ex, Syr. (Quality Generics).
Diphenhydramine HCl (Weeks & Leo).
Fenylhist, Cap. (Hauck).
Histine Prods. (Freeport).
Hyrexin, Inj. (Hyrex).
Mouthkote P/R, Oint., Spray (Parnell).
Span-Lanin, Cap. (Scrip).
Tusstat, Expectorant (Century).
W/Ammonium Cl, menthol.
See: Bentrac Expectorant, Liq. (Keny-
on).
Eldadryl Expectorant, Liq. (Elder).
Fenylex, Expectorant (Hauck).
Tusstat Expectorant (Century).

W/Antihistamines.
See: Symptrol, Syr., Cap., Inj. (Saron).
W/Benzethonium Cl.
See: Bendylate, Inj. (Solvay).
W/Chlorobutanol.
See: Ardeben, Inj. (Burgin-Arden).
W/Pheniramine maleate pyrilamine
maleate, phenylephrine HCl, phenyl-
propanolamine HCl.
See: Symptrol, Syr. (Saron).
W/Zinc oxide.
See: Ziradryl, Lot. (Parke-Davis).
• **DIPHENIDOL.** USAN. α,α-Diphenyl-1-
piperidinebutanol.
Use: Antiemetic.
See: Vontrol, Preps. (SK-Beecham).
• **DIPHENIDOL HCl.** USAN. αα-Diphenyl-
1- piperidinebutanol HCl.
Use: Antiemetic.
• **DIPHENIDOL PAMOATE.** USAN.
α,α-Diphenyl-1-piperidinebutanol com-
pound with 4,4′-methylenebis [3-hy-
droxy-2-naphthoic acid](2:1).
Use: Antiemetic.
DIPHENMETHANIL METHYLSULFATE.
4-Diphenylmethylene-1,1-di-
methylpiperidinium methylsulfate.
See: Diphemanil Methylsulfate (Various
Mfr.).
• **DIPHENOXYLATE HCl,** U.S.P. XXIII. 4-
Piperidinecarboxylic acid, 1-(3-cyano-
3,3-diphenylpropyl-4-phenyl-, ethyl es-
ter, HCl, 2,2-Diphenyl-4-(4-carbethoxy-
4-phenyl-1-pyeridino)butyronitrite ethyl
ester HCl. Ethyl 1-(3-Cyano-3,3
diphenyl-propyl)-4-phenylisonipecotate
Hydrochloride.
Use: Antiperistaltic to treat diarrhea.
W/Atropine.
See: Diaction, Tab. (Boots Pharm.).
Lomotil, Tab., Liq. (Searle).
• **DIPHENOXYLATE HYDROCHLORIDE
AND ATROPINE SULFATE,** U.S.P. XXI-
II. Oral Soln., Tab., U.S.P. XXIII.
Use: Antiperistaltic.
DIPHENYLAN SODIUM. (Lannett)
Phenytoin sodium, prompt 30 mg (27.6
mg phenytoin) or 100 mg (92 mg pheny-
toin)/Cap. Bot. 500s, 1000s.
Use: Anticonvulsant.
DIPHENYLHYDROXYCARBINOL. Ben-
zhydrol HCl.
DIPHENYLHYDANTOIN. Phenytoin,
U.S.P. XXIII.
Use: Anticonvulsant.
DIPHENYLHYDANTOIN SODIUM.
Phenytoin Sodium, U.S.P. XXIII.
Use: Anticonvulsant.
DIPHENYLISATIN.
See: Oxyphenisatin (Various Mfr.).

DIPHOSPHONIC ACID.
See: Etidronic acid.
DIPHOSPHOPYRIDINE (DPN). Antialcoholic. Under study.
DIPHOSPHOTHIAMIN. Cocarboxylase.
See: Coenzyme-B, Cap., and Inj. (Inwood).
DIPHOXAZIDE. N¹-(b-hydroxy-b,b-diphenylpropionyl)-N²-acetylhdrazine. Inductin.
• **DIPHTHERIA ANTITOXIN,** U.S.P. XXIII. (Squibb/Connaught) 20,000 units/Vial. (not < 500 units/ml).
Use: I.M., slow I.V. infusion; protection, treatment of diphtheria.
• **DIPHTHERIA & TETANUS TOXOIDS,** U.S.P. XXIII.
Use: Agent for immunization.
• **DIPHTHERIA & TETANUS TOXOIDS ABSORBED,** U.S.P. XXIII. (Dow, Lilly, Squibb/Connaught) Vial 5 ml.
Use: Agent for immunization.
DIPHTHERIA & TETANUS TOXOIDS ADSORBED, ALUMINUM PHOSPHATE ADSORBED. (Wyeth-Ayerst) Tubex 0.5 ml. Vial 5 ml. Pkg. 10s. Available in pediatric and adult strengths. 10 Lf units diphtheria and 5 Lf units tetanus per 0.5 ml dose. 1.5 Lf units diphtheria, 5 Lf units tetanus per 0.5 ml dose.
Use: Agent for immunization.
DIPHTHERIA/TETANUS TOXOIDS, ADSORBED. (Lederle).
Pediatric: 12.5 Lf units diphtheria, 5 Lf units tetanus per 0.5 ml dose. Vial 5 ml.
Adult: 2 Lf units diphtheria, and 5 Lf units tetanus per 0.5 ml dose. Vial 5 ml Disp. syringe 0.5 ml.
Use: Agent for immunization.
• **DIPHTHERIA & TETANUS TOXOIDS & PERTUSSIS VACCINE,** U.S.P. XXIII.
Use: Prevention against diphtheria, tetanus and pertussis.
See: Acel-Imune, Vial (Lederle).
Tri-immunol, Vial (Lederle).
Tripedia, Vial (Connaught).
DIPHTHERIA & TETANUS TOXOIDS & PERTUSSIS VACCINE ADSORBED. (Lederle) Vaccine Vial 7.5 ml.
Use: Agent for immunization.
DIPHTHERIA & TETANUS TOXOIDS & PERTUSSIS VACCINE COMBINED, ALUMINUM HYDROXIDE ADSORBED.
See: Triogen, Vial (Parke-Davis).
DIPHTHERIA & TETANUS TOXOIDS & PERTUSSIS VACCINE COMBINED, ALUMINUM PHOSPHATE-ADSORBED.

See: Tri-Immunol, Vial (Lederle)-Ramon, Diphtheria Anatoxin).
Use: Agent for immunization.
DIPHYLLINE.
See: Diazma, Vial (Pharmex).
DIPIMOL. (Everett) Dipyridamole 25 mg, 50 mg or 75 mg/Tab. Bot. 100s, 500s, 1000s.
Use: Antianginal.
DIPIPANONE. B.A.N. 4,4-Diphenyl-6-piperidino-heptan-3-one.
Use: Narcotic analgesic.
DIPIVALYL EPINEPHRINE.
See: Propine (Allergan).
• **DIPIVEFRIN.** USAN.
Use: Adrenergic.
DIPIVEFRIN HCl. (Schein) 0.1% Soln. 5 ml, 10 ml, 15 ml.
Use: Agent for glaucoma.
• **DIPIVEFRIN HYDROCHLORIDE,** U.S.P. XXIII. Ophth. Soln., U.S.P. XXIII.(+)-3,4-dihydroxy-a-(methylamino) methyl benzyl alcohol 3,4-dipivalate HCl.
Use: Treatment of chronic open-angle glaucoma.
See: Propine, Soln. (Allergan).
DIPONIUM BROMIDE (I.N.N.). Dipenine Bromide, B A N
DIPRENORPHINE. B.A.N. N-Cyclopropylmethyl-7,8-dlhydro-7 α-(1-hydroxy-1-methylethyl)-0⁶-methyl-6,14 endoethanonormorphine.
Use: Narcotic antagonist.
DIPRIDAMOLE. (Foy) Dipyridamole 25 mg/Tab. Bot. 1000s.
Use: Antianginal.
DIPRIVAN. (Zeneca) Propofol 10 mg/ml. Inj. Amp. 20 ml, 50 ml or 100 ml infusion vials.
Use: General anesthetic.
DIPROLENE AF CREAM. (Schering) Betamethasone dipropionate cream equivalent to 0.05% betamethasone. 15 Gm, 45 Gm.
DIPROLENE CREAM 0.05%. (Schering) Betamethasone dipropionate 0.05% in cream base. Tube 15 Gm.
Use: Anti-inflammatory, antipruritic (topical).
DIPROLENE OINTMENT 0.05%. (Schering) Betamethasone dipropionate 0.05%, in ointment base. Tube 15 Gm, 45 Gm.
Use: Anti-inflammatory, antipruritic (topical).
DIPROPHYLLINE. B.A.N. 7-(2,3-Dihydroxypropyl)- theophylline.
Use: Bronchodilator.
DIPROPYLACETIC ACID.
See: Valproic Acid.

DIPROSONE AEROSOL 0.1%. (Schering) Betamethasone dipropionate 6.4 mg (equiv. to 5 mg bethamethasone) in vehicle of mineral oil, caprylic-capric triglyceride w/isopropyl alcohol 10%, inert hydrocarbon propellants. (propane and isobutane). Can 85 Gm.
Use: Anti-inflammatory agent, topical.
DIPROSONE CREAM 0.05%. (Schering) Betamethasone dipropionate 0.64 mg (equiv. to 0.5 mg betamethasone) w/mineral oil, white petrolatum, polyethylene glycol 1000 monocetyl ether, cetostearyl alcohol, phosphoric acid, monobasic sodium phosphate with 4-chloro-m-cresol as preservative. Tube 15 Gm, 45 Gm.
Use: Anti-inflammatory agent, topical.
DIPROSONE LOTION 0.05%. (Schering) Betamethasone dipropionate 0.64 mg (equivalent to 0.5 mg betamethasone) w/isopropyl alcohol (46.8%), purified water. Bot. 20 ml, 60 ml.
Use: Anti-inflammatory agent, topical.
DIPROSONE OINTMENT 0.05%. (Schering) Betamethasone dipropionate 0.64 mg (equivalent to 0.5 mg betamethasone) in white petrolatum and mineral oil base. Tube 15 Gm, 45 Gm.
Use: Anti-inflammatory agent, topical.
DIPTHERIA EQUINE ANTITOXIN.
Use: Prophylaxis and treatment of diptheria.
• **DIPYRIDAMOLE,** U.S.P. XXIII. Tab., U.S.P. XXIII. 2,6-Di[di(2-hydroxy-ethyl)-amino]-4,8-dipiperidinopyrimido-[5,4-d]-pyrimidine.
Use: Coronary vasodilator.
See: Persantine.
• **DIPYRIDAMOLE.** USAN. 2,2′,2″-2,-(4,8-Dipiperidinopyrimido[5,4-d]pyrimidine-2,6-diyl)-dinitrilo]tetraethanol.
Use: Coronary vasodilator.
See: Dipimol, Tab. (Everett).
Dipridamole, Tab. (Foy).
Persantine, Tab. (Boehringer-Ingelheim).
Persantine IV (DuPont-Merck).
• **DIPYRITHIONE.** USAN.
Use: Antibacterial, antifungal.
• **DIPYRONE.** USAN, FDA. Sodium N-(2,3-dimethyl-1-phenyl-5-oxopyrazolin-4-yl)-N-methylamino-methanesulfonate. Sodium noramidopyrine methanesulfonate. Sodium phenyldimethylpyrazolon-me-thylamino-methane sulfonate, sodium (anti-pyrinylmethylamino)-methane sulfonate hydrate; methylmelubrin, methampyrone,4-Sod. methanesulfonate methylamine-antipyrine.

Use: Analgesic, antipyretic.
DIROX TABLETS. (Sanofi Winthrop) Paracetamol.
Use: Analgesic.
DISACCHARIDE TRIPEPTIDE GLYCEROL DIPALMITOYL.
Use: Antineoplastic. [Orphan drug]
DISALCID. (Riker) Salsalate. **Tab.:** 500 mg or 750 mg. Bot. 100s, 500s, UD 100s. **Cap.:** 500 mg. Bot. 100s.
Use: Salicylate analgesic.
DISANTHROL CAPSULES. (Lannett) Docusate sodium 100 mg, casanthranol 30 mg/Cap. Bot. 100s, 1000s.
Use: Laxative.
DISCASE. (Omnis Surgical) Chymopapain 5 units/2 ml. Vial 5 ml.
Use: Intradiscal injection for herniated lumbar intervertebral discs.
DISINFECTING SOLUTION. (Bausch & Lomb) Sodium Cl, sodium borate, boric acid, chlorhexidine gluconate 0.005%, EDTA 0.1%, thimerosal 0.001%. Bot. 355 ml.
Use: Soft contact lens care.
• **DISIQUONIUM CHLORIDE.** USAN.
Use: Antiseptic.
DISMISS DOUCHE. (Schering) Sodium Cl, sodium citrate, citric acid, cetaryl octoate, ceteareth-27, fragrance. Pow. for dilution. Pkg. 2s.
Use: Vaginal preparation.
DISOBROM. (Various Mfr.) Pseudoephedrine sulfate 120 mg, dexbrompheniramine maleate 6 mg Tab. Bot. 30s, 100s, 1000s.
Use: Decongestant, antihistamine.
• **DISOBUTAMIDE.** USAN.
Use: Cardiac depressant.
DISODIUM CARBONATE. Sodium Carbonate, N.F. XVIII.
DISODIUM CHROMATE. Sodium Chromate Cr 51 Injection, U.S.P. XXIII.
DISODIUM CHROMOGLYCATE.
See: Intal (Fisons).
Nasalcrom (Fisons).
DISODIUM CLODRONATE.
Use: Treatment of hypercalcemia of malignancy. [Orphan drug]
DISODIUM CLODRONATE TETRAHYDRATE.
Use: Increased bone resorption due to malignancy. [Orphan drug]
DISODIUM EDATHAMIL.
See: Edathamil Disodium (Various Mfr.).
DISODIUM EDETATE. Disodium ethylenediaminetetra acetate.
See: Edetate Disodium, U.S.P. XXIII.
DISODIUM PHOSPHATE.

See: Sodium Phosphate, U.S.P. XXIII.
**DISODIUM PHOSPHATE HEPTAHY-
DRATE.** Sodium Phosphate, U.S.P.
XXIII.
**DISODIUM SILIBININ DIHEMISUCCI-
NATE.**
Use: Antidote for mushroom poisoning.
[Orphan drug]
**DISODIUM THIOSULFATE PENTAHY-
DRATE.** Sodium Thiosulfate, U.S.P.
XXIII.
DI-SODIUM VERSENATE.
See: Edathamil Disodium (Various
Mfr.).
• **DISOFENIN.** USAN.
Use: Diagnostic aid.
DISOLAN. (Lannett) Docusate sodium
100 mg, phenolphthalein 65 mg/Cap.
Bot. 100s, 500s, 1000s.
Use: Laxative.
DISOLAN FORTE CAPSULES. (Lannett)
Casanthranol 30 mg, sodium car-
boxymethylcellulose 400 mg, docusate
sodium 100 mg/Cap. Bot. 100s, 500s,
1000s.
Use: Laxative.
DISONATE. (Lannett) Docusate sodium.
Cap.: 60 mg, 100 mg or 240 mg. Bot.
100s, 500s, 1000s. **Liq.:** 10 mg/ml Bot.
pt. **Syr.:** 20 mg/5 ml Bot. pt, gal.
Use: Laxative.
DISOPHROL. (Schering) Pseu-
doephedrine sulfate 60 mg,
dexbrompheniramine maleate 2 mg.
Tab. Bot. 100s.
Use: Decongestant, antihistamine.
DISOPHROL CHRONOTABS. (Schering)
Dexbrompheniramine maleate 6 mg,
pseudoephedrine sulfate 120 mg/SA
Tab. Bot. 100s.
Use: Antihistamine, decongestant.
DISOPLEX. (Lannett) Docusate sodium
100 mg, sodium carboxymethylcellulose
400 mg. Cap. Bot. 100s, 500s, 1000s.
Use: Laxative.
• **DISOPYRAMIDE.** USAN. 4-Di-isopropy-
lamino-2-phenyl-2-(2-pyridyl)butyra-
mide.
Use: Antiarrhythmic.
See: Rythmodan.
• **DISOPYRAMIDE PHOSPHATE,** U.S.P.
XXIII. Cap., U.S.P. XXIII.
Use: Antiarrhythmic.
• **DISOPYRAMIDE PHOSPHATE EXTEND-
ED-RELEASE CAPSULES,** U.S.P.
XXIII.
Use: Antiarrhythmic.
DI-SOSUL. (Drug Industries) Docusate
sodium 50 mg/Tab. Bot. 100s, 500s.
Use: Laxative.

DI-SOSUL FORTE. (Drug Industries) Do-
cusate sodium 100 mg, casanthranol 30
mg/Tab. Bot. 100s, 500s.
Use: Laxative.
DISOTATE. (Forest) Disodium edetate
150 mg/ml. Vial 20 ml.
Use: Treatment of hypercalcemia.
• **DISOXARIL.** USAN.
Use: Antiviral.
DI-SPAZ. (Vortech) Dicyclomine HCl.
Cap.: 10 mg. Bot. 1000s. **Inj.:** 10 mg.
Vial 10 ml.
Use: Gastrointestinal antispasmodic.
DISPOS-A-MED. (Parke-Davis)
Isoetharine HCl 0.5% or 1%, isopro-
terenol HCl 0.25% or 0.5%. Can of pre-
filled sterile tubes 0.5 ml, 50s.
Use: Bronchodilator.
DISPOS-A-MED ISOPROTERENOL HCL.
(Parke-Davis) Isoproterenol 0.25% or
0.5%, glycerin, sodium bisulfate. Soln.
Vial 0.5 ml. (Use only with Dispos-a-vial
solutions.)
Use: Bronchodilator.
DISPOS-A-VIAL. (Parke-Davis) Sodium
Cl 0.45% or 0.9%. Container 3 ml, 5 ml.
Box 100s.
Use: Oral inhalation.
DISTAQUAINE.
See: Penicillin V.
DISTIGMINE BROMIDE. B.A.N. NN'-
Hexamethyl- enedi-[1-methyl-3-(methyl-
carbamoyloxy)-pyridinium bromide].
Use: Anticholinesterase.
DISTIGMINE BROMIDE. Hexamarium
bromide.
DISULFAMIDE. B.A.N. 5-Chlorotoluene-
2,4-disulfonamide.
Use: Diuretic.
• **DISULFIRAM,** U.S.P. XXIII. Tab., U.S.P.
XXIII. Bis-(diethylthiocarbamoyl)disul-
fide. Tetraethylthiuram Disulfide.
Use: Treatment of alcoholism.
See: Antabuse, Tab. (Wyeth-Ayerst).
DISULFONAMIDE.
See: Dia-Mer-Sulfonamides (Various
Mfr.).
DITATE D.S. (Savage) Testosterone
enanthate 360 mg, estradiol valerate 16
mg, benzyl alcohol 2% in sesame oil.
Syringe 2 ml Box 10s. Vial 2 ml.
Use: Androgen, estrogen combination.
• **DITEKIREN.** USAN.
Use: Antihypertensive (renin inhibitor).
DITHIAZANINE. B.A.N. 3-Ethyl-2-[5-(3-
ethyl-benzothiazolin-2-ylidene)penta-
1,3-dienyl]benzothiazolium.
Use: Anthelmintic.
DITHRANOL.
See: Anthralin, U.S.P. XXIII. (Various

Mfr.).

D.I.T.I. CREME. (Dunhall) Iodoquinol 100 mg, sulfanilamide 500 mg, diethylstilbestrol 0.1 mg/Gm Jar. 4 oz.
Use: Anti-infective, vaginal.

D.I.T.I.-2 CREME. (Dunhall) Sulfanilamide 15%, aminacrine HCl 0.2%, allantoin 2%. Tube 142 Gm.
Use: Anti infective, vaginal.

DITOPHAL. B.A.N. SS'-Diethyl dithioisophthalate.
Use: Antileprotic.

DITROPAN. (Marion Merrell Dow) Oxybutynin Cl 5 mg/Tab. Bot. 100s, 1000s, UD identification pak 100s.
Use: Urinary tract agent.

DITROPAN SYRUP. (Marion Merrell Dow) Oxybutynin Cl. 5 mg/5 ml Bot. 473 ml.
Use: Urinary tract agent.

DIUCARDIN. (Wyeth-Ayerst) Hydroflumethiazide 50 mg/Tab. Bot. 100s.
Use: Diuretic, antihypertensive.

DIULO. (Searle) Metolazone. 2.5 mg, 5 mg or 10 mg/Tab. Bot. 100s.
Use: Diuretic, antihypertensive.

DIUPRES. (Merck & Co.) Chlorothiazide 250 mg or 500 mg, reserpine 0.125 mg/Tab. Bot. 100s, 1000s.
Use: Antihypertensive.

DIURESE. (American Urologicals) Trichlormethiazide 4 mg/Tab. Bot. 100s, 1000s.
Use: Diuretic.

DIURETIC COMBINATIONS.
See: Moduretic, Tab. (Merck & Co.).
Spironolactone w/Hydrochlorothiazide, Tab. (Various Mfr.).
Alazide, Tab. (Major).
Aldactazide, Tab. (Searle).
Dyazide, Cap. (SKB).
Maxzide, Tab. (Lederle).
Maxzide-25 MG, Tab. (Lederle).
Spironazide, Tab. (Schein).
Spirozide, Tab. (Rugby).
Triamterene w/Hydrochlorthiazide, Cap. (Various Mfr.).
Triamterene w/Hydrochlorothiazide, Tab. (Various Mfr.).

DIURETICS, LOOP.
See: Bumex, Inj., Tab. (Roche).
Edecrin, Tab. (Merck & Co.).
Edecrin Sodium, Inj. (Merck & Co.).
Fumide, Tab. (Everett).
Furomide M.D., Inj. (Hyrex).
Furosemide, Inj., Tab. (Various Mfr.).
Furosemide, Oral Soln. (Roxane).
Lasix, Inj., Oral Soln., Tab. (Hoechst-Roussel).
Luramide, Tab. (Major).

DIURETICS, OSMOTIC.
See: Glyrol, Soln. (Iolab).
Ismotic, Soln. (Alcon).
Mannitol, Inj. (Various Mfr.).
Osmitrol, Inj. (Baxter).
Osmoglyn, Soln. (Alcon).
Ureaphil, Inj. (Abbott).

DIURETICS, POTASSIUM-SPARING.
See: Alatone, Tab. (Major).
Aldactone, Tab. (Searle).
Amiloride HCl, Tab. (Various Mfr.).
Dyrenium, Cap. (SK-Beecham).
Midamor, Tab. (Merck & Co.).
Spironolactone, Tab. (Various Mfr.).

DIURETICS, THIAZIDES.
See: Anhydron, Tab. (Lilly).
Aquatag, Tab. (Solvay).
Aquatensen, Tab. (Wallace).
Chlorothiazide, Tab. (Various Mfr.).
Chlorthalidone, Tab. (Various Mfr.).
Diachlor, Tab. (Major).
Diaqua, Tab. (Hauck).
Diucardin, Tab. (Wyeth-Ayerst).
Diulo, Tab. (Searle).
Diurese, Tab. (American Urologicals).
Diurigen, Tab. (Goldline).
Diuril, Oral Susp., Tab. (Merck & Co.).
Diuril Sodium, Inj. (Merck & Co.).
Enduron, Tab. (Abbott).
Esidrix, Tab. (Ciba).
Ethon, Tab. (Major).
Exna, Tab. (Robins).
Hydrex, Tab. (Trimen).
Hydrochlorothiazide, Tab. (Various Mfr.).
Hydrochlorothiazide, Oral Soln. (Roxane).
HydroDIURIL, Tab. (Merck & Co.).
Hydroflumethiazide, Tab. (Various Mfr.).
Hydromal, Tab. (Hauck).
Hydromox, Tab. (Lederle).
Hydro-T, Tab. (Major).
Hydro-Z-50, Tab. (Mayrand).
Hydrozide-50, Tab. (T.E. Williams).
Hygroton, Tab. (Rhone-Poulenc Rhone-Poulenc Rorer).
Hylidone, Tab. (Major).
Lozol, Tab. (Rhone-Poulenc Rhone-Poulenc Rorer).
Metahydrin, Tab. (Merrell Dow).
Methyclothiazide, Tab. (Various Mfr.).
Mictrin, Tab. (Econo Med).
MyKrox (Pennwalt).
Naqua, Tab. (Schering).
Naturetin, Tab. (Princeton).
Niazide, Tab. (Major).
Oretic, Tab. (Abbott).
Proaqua, Tab. (Solvay).
Renese, Tab. (Pfizer).

Saluron, Tab. (Bristol Labs.).
Thalitone, Tab. (Boehringer-I).
Thiuretic, Tab. (Warner-Chilcott).
Trichlorex, Tab. (Lannett).
Trichlormethiazide, Tab. (Various Mfr.).
Zaroxolyn, Tab. (Pennwalt).
DIURETIC TABLETS. (Faraday) Buchu
leaves 150 mg, uva ursi leaves 150 mg,
juniper berries 120 mg, bone meal, pars-
ley, asparagus/Tab. Bot. 100s.
Use: Diuretic.
DIURIGEN TABLETS. (Goldline)
Chlorothiazide 500 mg/Tab Bot. 100s,
1000s.
Use: Diuretic.
**DIURIGEN W/RESERPINE 250
TABLETS.** (Goldline). Chlorothiazide
250 mg, reserpine 0.125 mg. Tab. Bot.
100s, 1000s.
Use: Antihypertensive combination.
**DIURIGEN W/RESERPINE 500
TABLETS.** (Goldline). Chlorothiazide
500 mg, reserpine 0.125 mg. Tab. Bot.
100s, 1000s.
Use: Antihypertensive combination.
DIURIL. (Merck & Co.) Chlorothiazide,
U.S.P. **Tab.:** 250 mg Bot. 100s, 1000s;
500 mg Bot. 100s, 1000s, UD 100s.
Oral Susp.: 250 mg/5 ml w/methyl-
paraben 0.12%, propylparaben 0.02%,
benzoic acid 0.1%, alcohol 0.5%. Bot.
237 ml.
Use: Diuretic, antihypertensive.
W/Methyldopa.
See Aldoclor, Tab. (Merck & Co.).
W/Reserpine.
See: Diupres, Tab. (Merck & Co.).
DIURIL SODIUM INTRAVENOUS. (Mer-
ck & Co.) Chlorothiazide sodium equiva-
lent to 0.5 Gm chlorothiazide w/mannitol
0.25 Gm sodium hydroxide, thimerosal
0.4 mg. Vial 20 ml.
Use: Diuretic, antihypertensive.
DIUTENSEN-R. (Wallace) Methycloth-
iazide 2.5 mg, reserpine 0.1 mg/Tab.
Bot. 100s, 500s.
Use: Antihypertensive combination.
• **DIVALPROEX SODIUM.** USAN.
Use: Anticonvulsant.
DIVINYL OXIDE. Vinyl ether, divinyl ether.
Use: Inhalation anesthetic.
DIZMISS. (Bowman) Meclizine HCl 25
mg/Tab. Bot. 100s, 1000s.
Use: Antiemetic/antivertigo.
dl-METHAMPHETAMINE HCl. dl-Des-
oxyephedrine HCl.
See: Oxydess, Tab. (North American).
W/Pyrilamine maleate, phenyltoloxamine
dihydrogen citrate, didesoxyephedrine
HCl, codeine phosphate, ammonium Cl,

potassium guaiacolsulfonate, chloro-
form, phenylpropanolamine tartar emet-
ic.
See: Meditussin-X Liquid (Hauck).
DM COUGH. (PBI) Dextromethorphan
HBr 10 mg/5 ml, alcohol 5%. Syr. Bot.
120 ml, pt, gal.
Use: Antitussive.
DMCT. (Lederle) Demethylchlortetracy-
cline.
Use: Anti-infective, tetracycline.
See: Declomycin HCl, Preps. (Lederle).
D-MED 800. (Ortega) Methylprednisolone
acetate 80 mg/ml suspension, polyethyl-
ene glycol, myristyl-gamma-picolinium
chloride. Inj. Vial. 5 ml.
Use: Glucocorticosteroid.
d-METHORPHAN HBr.
See: Dextromethorphan HBr (Various
Mfr.).
d-METHYLPHENYLAMINE SULFATE.
See: Dextroamphetamine Sulfate,
U.S.P. XXIII. (Various Mfr.).
**DML DERMATOLOGICAL MOISTURIZ-
ING LOTION.** (Person & Covey) Purified water, petrolatum, glycerin, methyl
glucose sesquisterate, dimethicone,
methyl gluceth-20 sesquisterate, benzyl
alcohol, volatile silicone, glyceryl
stearate, stearic acid, palmitic acid, cetyl
alcohol, xanthan gum, magnesium aluminum silicate carbomer 941, sodium
hydroxide. Bot. 8 oz.
Use: Emollient.
DML FACIAL MOISTURIZER. (Person &
Covey) Octyl methoxycinnamate 8%,
oxybenzone 4%, benzyl alcohol, petrolatum, EDTA. SPF 15. Cream 45 g.
Use: Sunscreen.
DML FORTE. (Person & Covey) Petrolatum, PPG-2 myristyl ether propionate,
glyceryl stearate, glycerin, stearic acid,
d-panthenol, DEA-cetyl phosphate,
simethicone, PVP eicosene copolymer,
benzyl alcohol, cetyl alcohol, silica, dis-
odium EDTA, BHA, magnesium alu-
minum silicate, sodium carbomer 1342.
Tube 113 Gm.
Use: Emollient.
DMSO.
See: Dimethyl sulfoxide.
DNR.
See: Cerubidine (Wyeth-Ayerst).
DOAK-OIL. (Doak) Tar distillate 2%, in a
lanolin, mineral oil suspension. Pl. Bot. 8
oz.
Use: Antiseborrheic.
DOAK OIL FORTE. (Doak) Tar distillate
5%. Bot. 4 oz.
Use: Antiseborrheic.

DOAK TAR LOTION. (Doak) Tar distillate 5%. Bot. 4 oz.
Use: Antiseborrheic.
DOAK TAR SHAMPOO. (Doak) Tar distillate 3% in shampoo base. Bot. 4 oz.
Use: Antiseborrheic.
DOAK TERSASEPTIC. (Doak) Liquid cleanser, pH 6.8. Bot. 4 oz, pt, gal.
Use: Liquid detergent.
DOAN'S BACKACHE SPRAY. (DEP Corp.) Methyl salicylate 15%, menthol 8.4%, methyl nicotinate 0.6%. Aerosol can 4 oz.
Use: External analgesic.
DOAN'S PILLS. (DEP Corp.) Magnesium salicylate 325 mg/Tab. Ctn. 24s, 48s.
Use: Analgesic.
• **DOBUTAMINE.**
Use: Cardiac stimulant.
• **DOBUTAMINE HYDROCHLORIDE.** U.S.P. XXIII. For Inj., U.S.P. XXIII.
Use: Cardiac stimulant.
See: Dobutrex, Inj. (Lilly).
• **DOBUTAMINE LACTOBIONATE.** USAN.
Use: Cardiac stimulant.
• **DOBUTAMINE TARTRATE.** USAN.
Use: Cardiac stimulant.
DOBUTREX SOLUTION. (Lilly) Dobutamine HCl 250 mg. Inj. Vial 20 ml.
Use: Inotropic agent.
• **DOCEBENONE.** USAN.
Use: Inhibitor (5-lipoxygenase).
See: Antiallergic; antiasthmatic.
• **DOCETAXEL.** USAN.
Use: Antineoplastic.
• **DOCONAZOLE.** USAN.
Use: Antifungal.
DOCTAR. (Savage) Coal tar 0.5%, conditioner. Shampoo. Bot. 100 ml.
Use: Antiseborrheic.
DOCTASE. (Purepac) Docusate sodium 100 mg, casanthranol 30 mg/Cap. Bot. 100s.
Use: Laxative.
DOCTOR BERRY'S SKIN TONER.
See: DR. BERRY'S SKIN TONER.
DOCTOR CALDWELL SENNA LAXATIVE.
See: DR. CALDWELL SENNA LAXATIVE.
DOCTOR DERMI-HEAL.
See: DR. DERMI-HEAL.
DOCTOR DRAKE'S COUGH MEDICINE.
See: DR. DRAKE'S COUGH MEDICINE.
DOCTOR SCHOLL'S.
See: DR. SCHOLL'S.
DOCTYL. (Approved) Docusate sodium 100 mg/Tab. Bot. 40s, 100s, 1000s.
Use: Laxative.

DOCTYLAX. (Approved) Docusate sodium 100 mg, acetophenolisatin 2 mg, prune conc. ¾ mg/Tab. Bot. 40s, 100s, 1000s.
Use: Laxative.
DOCUCAL-P SOFTGELS. (Parmed) Docusate (as calcium) 60 mg, phenolphthalein 65 mg/Cap. Bot. 100s, 1000s.
Use: Laxatives.
• **DOCUSATE CALCIUM,** U.S.P. XXIII. Cap., U.S.P. XXIII. 1, 4-Bis(2-ethylhexyl)sulfosuccinate, calcium salt. Calcium bis-dioctyl-sulfosuccinate.
Use: Fecal softener.
See: Surfak, Cap. (Hoechst).
Doxidan, Cap. (Hoechst).
Danthron, Tab. (Goldline).
DOCUSATE WITH CASANTHRANOL. (Various Mfr.) Docusate (as sodium) 100 mg, casanthranol 30 mg/Cap. Bot. 100s, 1000s, UD 100s.
Use: Laxative.
• **DOCUSATE POTASSIUM,** U.S.P. XXIII. Cap., U.S.P. XXIII.
Use: Stool softener.
See: Dialose, Cap. (Stuart).
Dialose Plus, Cap. (Stuart).
Kasof, Cap. (Stuart).
• **DOCUSATE SODIUM,** U.S.P. XXIII. Cap., Soln., Syr., Tab., U.S.P. XXIII. Aerosol OT. (Am. Cyanamid). Bis-(2-ethoxy)-S-sodium sulfosuccinate. Sodium 1, 4-Bis (2-ethylhexyl) Sulfosuccinate.
Use: Pharmaceutical aid (surfactant), stool softener.
See: Colace, Cap., Liq., Syr. (Mead Johnson).
Coloctyl, Cap. (Vitarine).
Comfolax, Cap. (Searle).
Consta B100, Tab. (Kenyon).
Correctol Extra Gentle, Cap. (Schering-Plough).
Dialose, Tab. (J & J-Merck).
Diomedicone, Tab (Medicone).
Diosate Caps. (Towne).
Diosux, Cap. (Jenkins).
Disonate, Cap., Tab. Syr., Liq. (Lannett).
Doss, Super Doss, Tab. (Ferndale).
Doxinate, Cap., Liq. (Hoechst).
DSS (Parke-Davis).
Duosol, Cap. (Kirkman Sales).
Dynoctol, Cap. (Solvay).
Easy-Lax, Cap. (Walgreen).
Konsto, Cap. (Freeport).
Laxatab, Tab. (Freeport).
Liqui-Doss, Liq. (Ferndale).
Modane Soft, Cap. (Adria).
Peri-Doss, Cap. (Ferndale).
Regul-Aid, Syr. (Quality Generics).

Regutol, Tab. (Schering-Plough).
Revac Supprettes, Supp. (Webcon).
Stulex, Tab. (Bowman).
Surfak, Cap. (Hoechst).
W/Ascorbic acid, ferrous fumarate.
See: Hemaspan Cap. (Bock).
W/Betaine HCl, zinc, manganese, molybdenum.
See: Hemaferrin (Western Research).
W/Bisacodyl.
See: Laxadan, Supp. (Lemmon).
W/Brewer's yeast.
See: Doss or Super Doss, Tab. (Ferndale).
W/Casanthranol.
See: Calotabs, Tab. (Calotabs).
Constiban (Quality Generics).
Diolax, Cap. (Century).
Dio Soft (Standex).
Disanthrol, Cap. (Lannett).
Di-Sosul Forte, Tab. (Drug).
Easy-Lax Plus, Cap. (Walgreen).
Genericace, Cap. (Forest Pharm.).
Neo-Vadrin D-D-S, Cap. (Scherer).
Nuvac, Cap. (LaCrosse).
Peri-Colace, Cap., Syr. (Mead Johnson).
W/Casanthranol, sodium carboxymethylcellulose.
See: Dialose Plus, Cap. (Stuart).
Disolan Forte, Cap. (Lannett).
Tri-Vac, Cap. (Rhode).
W/Dehydrocholic acid.
See: Dubbalax-B, Cap. (Redford).
Dubbalax-N, Cap. (Redford).
Neolax, Tab. (Central).
W/D-calcium pantothenate and acetphenolisatin.
See: Peri-Pantyl, Tab. (McGregor).
W/Ferrous fumarate, Vitamin C.
See: Hemaspan, Cap. (Bock).
Recoup, Tab. (Lederle).
W/Ferrous fumarate, vitamins.
See: Bevitone, Tab. (Lemmon).
W/Ferrous fumarate, betaine HCl, desiccated liver, vitamins, minerals.
See: Hemaferrin, Tab. (Western Research).
W/Glycerin.
See: Rectalad Enema, Liq. (Wampole).
W/Isobornyl thiocyanoacetate.
See: Barc, Cream, Liq. (Commerce).
W/Petrolatum.
See: Milkinol, Liq., Emulsion (Kremers-Urban).
W/Phenolphthalein.
See: Correctol, Tab. (Schering-Plough).
Disolan, Cap. (Lannett).
Ex-Lax Prods. (Sandoz Consumer).
Feen-A-Mint, Pills (Schering-Plough).

W/Phenolphthalein, dehydrocholic acid.
See: Bolax, Cap. (Boyd).
Sarolax, Cap. (Saron).
Tripalax, Cap. (Redford).
W/Polyoxyethylene nonyl phenol, sodium edetate, and 9-aminoacridine HCl.
See: Vagisec Plus Supp. (Schmid).
W/Senna concentrate.
See: Gentlax S, Tab. (Blair).
Sarolax (Saron).
Senokap-DDS, Cap. (Purdue Frederick).
Senokot S, Tab. (Purdue Frederick).
W/Sodium propionate, propionic acid, salicylic acid.
See: Prosal, Liq. (Gordon).
W/Vitamin-mineral combination.
See: Geriplex-FS, Kapseal (Parke-Davis).
Materna 1.60, Tab. (Lederle).
DODERLEIN BACILLI.
See: Redoderlein, Vial (Forest Pharm.).
DODICIN. B.A.N. 3,6,9-Triazaheneicosanoic acid.
Dodecyldi(aminoethyl)glycine.
Use: Surface active agent.
DOFAMIUM CHLORIDE. B.A.N. 2-(N-Dodecanoyl-N-methylamino)ethyldimethyl-(phenylcarbamoyl- methyl)ammonium Cl.
Use: Antiseptic.
• **DOFETILIDE.** USAN.
Use: Antiarrhythmic.
DOFUS. (Miller) Freeze dried *Lactobacillus acidophilus* minimum of 100,000,000 organisms/Cap. w/*Lactobacillus bifidus* organisms added. Bot. 60s.
Use: To restore intestinal flora.
DOK. (Major) Docusate sodium. **Caps.:** 250 mg. Bot. 100s, 1000s. **Liq.:** 150 mg/15 ml. Bot. pt. **Syrup:** 60 mg/15 ml. Bot. pt, gal.
Use: Laxative.
DOK-250. (Major) Docusate sodium 250 mg. Cap. Bot. 100s.
Use: Laxative.
DOKTORS SPRAY. (Scherer) Phenylephrine HCl 0.25%, chlorobutanol, sodium bisulfite, benzalkonium chloride. Soln. Bot. 30 ml.
Use: Nasal decongestant.
DOLACET C-3. (Hauck) Hydrocodone bitartrate 5 mg, acetaminophen 500 mg/Cap. Bot. 50s, 100s, 500s.
Use: Narcotic analgesic.
DOLAMIDE TABS. (Major) Chlorpropamide 100 mg or 250 mg/Tab. Bot. 100s, 500s, 1000s.
Use: Antidiabetic agent.

DOLAMIN. (Harvey) Ammonium sulfate 0.75% with sodium Cl, benzyl alcohol. Amp. 10 ml. In 12s, 25s, 100s.
Use: Antineuralgic.

DOLANEX ELIXIR. (Lannett) Acetaminophen 325 mg/5 ml, alcohol 23%. Bot. pt, gal.
Use: Analgesic.

DOLANTIN.
See: Meperidine HCl, U.S.P. XXIII.

DOLCIN. (Dolcin) Aspirin 3.7 gr, calcium succinate 2.8 gr/Tab. Bot. 100s, 200s.
Use: Analgesic.

DOLDRAM. (Dram) Salicylamide 7.5 gr/Tab. Bot. 100s.
Use: Salicylate analgesic.

DOLEAR. (Eastwood) Bot. 0.5 oz.
Use: Otic preparation.

DOLENE AP-65. (Lederle) Propoxyphene HCl 65 mg, acetaminophen 650 mg/Tab. Bot. 100s, 500s.
Use: Narcotic analgesic.

DOLENE COMPOUND-65. (Lederle) Propoxyphene HCl 65 mg, aspirin 389 mg, caffeine 32.4 mg/Cap. Bot. 100s, 500s.
Use: Narcotic analgesic.

DOLENE PLAIN. (Lederle) Propoxyphene HCl 65 mg/Cap. Bot. 100s, 500s.
Use: Narcotic analgesic.

DOLOBID. (Merck & Co.) Diflunisal 250 mg or 500 mg/Tab. Unit-of-use 60s, UD 100s.
Use: Salicylate analgesic.

DOLOMITE. (Nature's Bounty) Magnesium 78 mg, calcium 130 mg/Tab. Bot. 100s, 250s.
Use: Mineral supplement.

DOLOMITE. (Blue Cross) Calcium 426 mg, magnesium 246 mg/3 Tab. w/guar and acacia gum. Bot. 250s.
Use: Mineral supplement.

DOLOMITE PLUS CAPSULES. (Barth's) Magnesium 37 mg, calcium 187 mg, phosphorous 50 mg, iodine 0.25 mg/Cap. Bot. 100s, 500s, 1000s.
Use: Mineral supplement.

DOLOMITE TABLETS. (Faraday) Calcium 150 mg, magnesium 90 mg/Tab. Bot. 250s.
Use: Mineral supplement.

DOLONIL. (Parke-Davis)
See: Pyridium Plus, Tab. (Parke-Davis).

DOLOPHINE HYDROCHLORIDE. (Lilly) Methadone HCl. **Amp.:** (10 mg/ml; sodium Cl 0.9%) 1 ml 12s, 100s. **Vial:** (10 mg/ml) 20 ml (sodium Cl 0.9%, chlorobutanol 0.5%). 1s, 25s. **Tab.:** 5 mg, Bot. 100s. 10 mg, Bot. 100s.

Use: Narcotic analgesic.

DOLOPIRONA TABLETS. (Sanofi Winthrop) Dipyrone with chlormezanone.
Use: Analgesic, muscle relaxant, antianxiety agent.

DOLORAL. (Progressive Enterprises) Colchicine salicylate 0.1 mg, phenobarbital 8 mg, sodium p-amino-benzoate 15 mg, vitamins B₁ 25 mg, aspirin 325 mg/Tab. Bot. 100s, 1000s.
Use: Agent for gout, antiarthritic.

DOLORGON. (Kenyon) Mephenesin 200 mg, salicylamide 75 mg, acetyl-p-aminophenol 75 mg, ascorbic acid 50 mg/Tab. Bot. 100s, 1000s.
Use: Analgesic.

DOLOSAL.
See: Meperidine HCl.

DOLSED. (American Urologicals) Methenamine 40.8 mg, phenylsalicylate 18.1 mg, atropine sulfate 0.03 mg, hyoscyamine 0.03 mg, benzoic acid 4.5 mg, methylene blue 5.4 mg. Tab. Bot. 100s, 1000s.
Use: Urinary anti-infective.

DOLVANOL.
Use: Narcotic analgesic.
See: Meperidine HCl.

• **DOMAZOLINE FUMARATE.** USAN.
Use: Anticholinergic.

DOMEBORO. (Miles Pharm) Aluminum sulfate and calcium acetate when added to water gives therapeutic effect of Burow's. One pkg. or Tab./pt. water approximately equivalent to 1:40 dilution. **Pkg.:** 2.2 Gm, 12s, 100s. **Effervescent Tab.:** Box 12s, 100s, 1000s.
Use: Anti-inflammatory agent, topical.

DOMEBORO OTIC. (Miles Pharm) Acetic acid 2% (in aluminum acetate solution). Soln. Bot. 60 ml with dropper.
Use: Otic preparation.

DOME-PASTE BANDAGE. (Miles Pharm) Zinc oxide, calamine and gelatin bandage. Pkg. 4′ × 10 yd. and 3′ 10 yd. impregnated gauze bandage.
Use: Treatment of conditions of the extremities.

DOMESTROL.
See: Diethylstilbestrol, Preps. (Various Mfr.).

D.O.M.F.
Use: Germicide.
See: Merbromin (Mercurochrome) (City Chem.).

• **DOMIODOL.** USAN.
Use: Mucolytic.

• **DOMIPHEN BROMIDE.** USAN. Dodecyl-dimethyl-2-phenoxyethylammonium

bromide. Phenododecinium Bromide (I.N.N.).
Use: Antiseptic.
See: Bradosol.
Domibrom.
DOMOL BATH AND SHOWER OIL. (Miles Pharm.) D_1-isopropyl sebacate, isopropyl myristate with mineral oil. Bot. 240 ml.
Use: Emollient.
• **DOMPERIDONE.** USAN.
Use: Antiemetic.
DONATUSSIN DC SYRUP. (Laser) Hydrocodone bitartrate 2.5 mg, phenylephrine HCl 7.5 mg, guaifenesin 50 mg/5 ml. Bot. 120 ml, 480 ml.
Use: Antitussive, decongestant, expectorant.
DONATUSSIN PEDIATRIC DROPS. (Laser) Guaifenesin 20 mg, chlorpheniramine maleate 1 mg, phenylephrine HCl 2 mg/ml. Drop. bot. 30 ml.
Use: Expectorant, antihistamine, decongestant.
DONATUSSIN SYRUP. (Laser) Phenylephrine 10 mg, chlorpheniramine maleate 2 mg, dextromethorphan HBr 7.5 mg, guaifenesin 100 mg. Bot. pt, gal.
Use: Decongestant, antihistamine, antitussive, expectorant.
DONDRIL. (Whitehall) Dextromethorphan HBr 10 mg, phenylephrine HCl 5 mg, chlorpheniramine maleate 1 mg/Tab. Bot. 24s.
Use: Antitussive, decongestant, antihistamine.
• **DONETIDINE.** USAN.
Use: Antagonist (to Histamine H_2 receptors).
DONNA. (Arcum) Menthol, thymol, eucalyptol, exsiccated alum, boric acid. 4 oz, 14 oz.
Use: Vaginal preparation.
DONNACIN. (Pharmex) Phenobarbital 16.2 mg, hyoscyamine sulfate 0.1037 mg, atropine sulfate 0.194 mg, hyoscine HBr 0.0065 mg/5 ml or Tab. **Elix.:** Bot. pt, gal. **Tab.:** Bot. 1000s.
Use: Anticholinergic/antispasmodic.
DONNAFED Jr. (Jenkins) Ephedrine HCl ¹/₁₆ gr, belladonna extract gr (total alkaloids, 0.0006 gr), salicylamide 1.25 gr/Tab. Bot. 1000s.
Use: Decongestant, anticholinergic, analgesic.
DONNAGEL. (Wyeth-Ayerst) Attapulgite 600 mg **Chew. Tab.:** Pkg. 18s; **Liq.:** Bot. 120 ml, 240 ml.
Use: Antidiarrheal.
DONNAMAR. (H.L. Moore) Atropine sul-

fate 0.0194 mg, scopolamine HBr 0.0065 mg, hyoscyamine HBr or SO_4 0.1037 mg, phenobarbital 16.2 mg/5 ml, alcohol 23%. Elix. Bot. 120 ml, pt, gal.
Use: Anticholinergic/antispasmodic.
DONNAMAR. (Marnel) Hyoscyamine sulfate 0.125 mg. Tab. Bot. 100s.
Use: Anticholinergic/antispasmodic.
DONNAPHEN ELIXIR. (Approved) Phenobarbital 16.2 mg, hyoscyamine sulfate 0.1037 mg, atropine sulfate 0.0194 mg, hyoscine HBr 0.0065 mg/5 ml. Bot. pt, gal.
Use: Anticholinergic/antispasmodic.
DONNAPINE TABS. (Major) Belladonna alkaloids, phenobarbital. Bot. 100s, 1000s, UD 100s.
Use: Sedative, anticholinergic/antispasmodic.
DONNA-SED ELIXIR. (Vortech) Atropine sulfate 0.0194 mg, scopolamine HBr 0.0065, hyoscyamine HBr or SO_4 0.1037 mg, phenobarbital 16.2 mg, alcohol 23%. Liq. Bot. 118 ml, gal.
Use: Gastrointestinal anticholinergic.
DONNATAL. (Robins) Hyoscyamine sulfate 0.1037 mg, atropine sulfate 0.0194 mg, scopolamine HBr 0.0065 mg, phenobarbital 16.2 mg. **Cap. & Tab.:** Bot. 100s, 1000s. **Elix.:** w/alcohol 23%. Bot. 4 oz, pt, gal, Dis-Co pack 5 ml, 100s.
Use: Sedative, anticholinergic/antispasmodic.
DONNATAL DIS-CO UD PACK. (Robins) Hyoscyamine sulfate 0.1037 mg, atropine sulfate 0.0194 mg, hyoscine HBr 0.0065 mg, phenobarbital 16.2 mg (0.25 gr)/Tab. or 5 ml. **Tab.:** UD 100s. **Elix.:** UD (5 ml) 25s.
Use: Sedative, anticholinergic/antispasmodic.
DONNATAL EXTENTABS. (Robins) Hyoscyamine sulfate 0.3111 mg, atropine sulfate 0.0582 mg, scopolamine HBr 0.0195 mg, phenobarbital 48.6 mg (³/₄ gr)/Tab. Bot. 100s, 500s, Dis-Co pack 100s.
Use: Sedative, anticholinergic/antispasmodic.
DONNATAL #2. (Robins) Phenobarbital 32.4 mg (0.5 gr), hyoscyamine sulfate 0.1037 mg, atropine sulfate 0.0194 mg, scopolamine HBr 0.0065 mg/Tab. Bot. 100s, 1000s.
Use: Sedative, anticholinergic/antispasmodic.
DONNAZYME. (Robins) Hyoscyamine sulfate 0.0518 mg, atropine sulfate 0.0097 mg, scopolamine HBr 0.0033 mg, phenobarbital 8.1 mg (¹/₈ gr), pepsin

150 mg/Tab. in outer layer, pancreatin 300 mg, bile salts 150 mg/Tab. in core. Bot. 100s, 500s.
Use: Anticholinergic/antispasmodic, digestive aid.
DON'T. (Commerce) Sucrose octa acetate 5%, isopropyl alcohol 54%. Bot. 0.45 oz.
Use: Used to discourage nail biting and thumb sucking.
• **DOPAMANTINE.** USAN.
Use: Antiparkinsonian.
DOPAMINE. (Astra) Dopamine. **Amp.:** 200 mg/5 ml Amp. Box 10s; 400 mg/10 ml Amp. Box 5s. **Additive Syringe:** 200 mg/5 ml Syr. Box 1s; 400 mg/10 ml Syr. Box 1s.
Use: Inotropic agent.
• **DOPAMINE HYDROCHLORIDE,** U.S.P. XXIII. Inj., U.S.P. XXIII. 4-(2-Aminoethyl)pyrocatechol HCl.
Use: Adrenergic
Intropin, Amp. (American Critical Care).
• **DOPAMINE HYDROCHLORIDE AND DEXTROSE INJECTION,** U.S.P. XXIII.
Use: Adrenergic, emergency treatment of low blood pressure.
DOPAR. (Procter & Gamble) Levodopa 100 mg or 250 mg/Cap. Bot. 100s. 500 mg/Cap. Bot. 100s, 1000s.
Use: Anti-parkinson agent.
• **DOPEXAMINE.** USAN.
Use: Cardiovascular agent.
• **DOPEXAMINE HYDROCHLORIDE.** USAN.
Use: Cardiovascular agent.
DOPRAM. (Robins) Doxapram HCl 20 mg/ml, 0.9% benzyl alcohol. Vial 20 ml.
Use: Respiratory stimulant.
DORAL. (Wallace) Quazepam 7.5 mg or 15 mg/Tab. Bot. 100s, UD 100s.
Use: Sedative/hypnotic.
DORCOL CHILDREN'S COUGH SYRUP. (Sandoz Consumer) Dextromethorphan HBr 5 mg, pseudoephedrine HCl 15 mg, guaifenesin 50 mg/5 ml. Bot. 120 ml, 240 ml.
Use: Antitussive, decongestant, expectorant.
DORCOL CHILDREN'S DECONGESTANT LIQUID. (Sandoz Consumer) Pseudoephedrine HCl 15 mg/5 ml. Bot. 4 oz.
Use: Decongestant.
DORCOL CHILDREN'S LIQUID COLD FORMULA. (Sandoz Consumer) Pseudoephedrine HCl 15 mg, chlorpheniramine maleate 1 mg/5 ml. Bot. 4 oz.

Use: Decongestant, antihistamine.
DORCOL FEVER AND PAIN REDUCER. (Dorsey) Acetaminophen 160 mg/5 ml. Bot. 4 oz.
Use: Analgesic.
DORICO DROPS. (Sanofi Winthrop) Paracetamol.
Use: Analgesic.
DORICO TABLETS. (Sanofi Winthrop) Paracetamol.
Use: Analgesic.
DORIGLUTE TABS DEA. (Major) Glutethimide 0.5 Gm/Tab. Bot. 100s, 250s, 1000s.
Use: Nonbarbiturate hypnotic.
DORMAREX. (Republic) Pyrilamide maleate 25 mg/Cap. Pkg. 20s. Bot. 40s, 100s.
Use: Nonprescription sleep aid.
DORMAREX 2. (Republic) Diphenhydramine HCl 50 mg/Tab. Pkg. 16s. Bot. 32s.
Use: Nonprescription sleep aid.
DORME. (A.V.P.) Promethazine HCl 12.5 mg, 25 mg or 50 mg/Cap. Bot. 100s.
Use: Antihistamine.
DORMEER. (Pasadena Research) Scopolamine aminoxide HBr 0.2 mg/Cap. Bot. 100s, 1000s.
Use: Sedative/hypnotic.
DORMETHAN.
See: Dextromethorphan HBr. (Various Mfr.).
DORMIN. (Randob) Diphenhydramine HCl 25 mg, lactose. Cap. Bot. 32s, 72s.
Use: Sleep aid.
DORMIN SLEEPING CAPLETS. (Randob) Diphenhydramine HCl 25 mg/Cap. Bot. 32s.
Use: Sleep aid.
DORMIRAL.
See: Phenobarbital, Preps. (Various Mfr.).
DORMONAL.
See: Barbital, Preps. (Various Mfr.).
DORMUTOL. (Approved) Scopolamine aminoxide HBr 0.2 mg/Cap. Bot. 24s, 60s.
Use: Sedative/hypnotic.
DORNASE.
Use: Treatment of cystic fibrosis. [Orphan drug]
DORNASE ALFA.
See: Pulmozyme, Soln. (Genentech).
• **DORSATINE HYDROCHLORIDE.** USAN.
Use: Antihistamine.
DORYX PELLETS. (Parke-Davis) Doxycycline hyclate 100 mg/Cap. Bot. 50s.
Use: Anti-infective, tetracycline.
• **DORZOLAMIDE HYDROCHLORIDE.**

USAN.
Use: Treatment of glaucoma and ocular hypertension (carbonic anhydrase inhibitor).

D.O.S. CAPS. (Goldline) Dioctyl sodium sulfosuccinate SG 100 mg or 250 mg/Cap. Bot. 100s, 1000s.
Use: Laxative.

DOSS SYRUP. (PBI) Docusate sodium 20 mg/5 ml. Bot. pt, gal.
Use: Laxative.

•**DOTHIEPIN HCL.** USAN. 11-(3-Dimethylaminopropylidene)-6H-dibenzo[b,e]thiepin hydrochloride. Dosulepin (I.N.N.).
Use: Antidepressant.
See: Prothiaden (hydrochloride).

DOTIROL. (Sanofi Winthrop) Ampicillin trihydrate available in Cap, Susp., Inj. (IV, IM.).
Use: Antibacterial, penicillin.

DOUBLE ACTION TOOTHACHE RELIEF KIT. (C.S. Dent) Toothache drops, acetaminophen 325 mg/Tab. Box 8s.
Use: Treatment of toothache.

DOUBLE SAL TABLETS. (Vale) Sodium salicylate 640 mg/EC Tab. Dot. 1000s.
Use: Salicylate analgesic.

DOUBLE STRENGTH GAVISCON-2. (SK-Beecham) Aluminum hydroxide 160 mg, magnesium trisilicate 40 mg, alginic acid, calcium stearate, sodium bicarbonate, sucrose. Tab. Bot. 48s.
Use: Antacid.

DOUCHE. (Jenkins) Boric acid, borax, tannic acid, sodium salicylate, zinc sulfate, alum, hydrastine HCl, thymol, sodium bicarbonate and tartaric acid/Tab. Bot. 1000s.
Use: Vaginal preparation.

DOVACET CAPSULES. (Vale) Dover's powder 24.3 mg, aspirin 324 mg, caffeine 32.4 mg/Tab. Bot. 1000s.
Use: Analgesic.

DOVAPHEN CAP. (Jenkins) Dover's powder 16.2 mg (opium 1.62 mg), ipecac 1.62 mg, aspirin 2.5 gr, phenacetin 1.5 gr, caffeine $^1/_8$ gr, camphor 0.25 gr, atropine sulfate gr/Cap. Bot. 1000s.
Use: Analgesic.

DOVAPHEN JR. (Jenkins) Dover's powder 8.1 mg, acetophenetidin 0.5 gr, atropine sulfate $^1/_{4000}$ gr, salicylamide 0.5 gr, caffeine gr/Tab. Bot. 1000s.
Use: Analgesic.

DOVER'S POWDER. Ipecac 1 part, opium 1 part, lactose 8 parts.
Use: Analgesic, sedative, diaphoretic.
W/Acetophenetidin, atropine sulfate, aspirin, camphor, caffeine, sodium sulfate, dried.
See: Dovium, Cap. (Hance).
W/Acetophenetidin, atropine sulfate, salicylamide, caffeine.
See: Dovaphen Jr., Tab. (Jenkins).
W/Acetophenetidin, camphor, aspirin, caffeine, atropine sulfate.
See: Analgestine, Cap. (Hauck).
W/Acetophenetidin, sodium citrate, potassium guaiacolsulfonate.
See: Doverlyn, Cap., Tab. (Davis & Sly).
W/A.P.C. camphor monobromated.
See: Coldate, Tab. (Elder).
W/Aspirin, phenacetin, camphor monobromated, caffeine.
See: Coldate, Tab. (Elder).
W/Atropine sulfate, A.P.C., camphor.
See: Dasin, Cap. (Beecham-Massengill).

DOVIUM. (Hance) Dover's powder 0.5 gr, acetophenetidin 1.5 gr, atropine sulfate 1/500 gr, aspirin 2 gr, camphor 0.25 gr, caffeine $^1/_8$ gr, sodium sulfate, dried, 7.5 gr/Cap. Bot. 100s, 1000s.
Use: Analgesic, antipyretic.

DOVONEX. (Westwood-Squibb) Calcipotriene 0.005%. Oint. Tube 30, 60 or 100 g.
Use: Antipsoriatic.

DOWICIL 200.
See: Derma Soap (Ferndale).

DOW-ISONIAZID. (Merrell Dow) Isoniazid 300 mg/Tab. Bot. 30s.
Use: Antituberculous agent.

•**DOXACURIUM CHLORIDE.** USAN.
Use: Neuromuscular blocking agent.
See: Nuromax (Burroughs Wellcome).

DOXAMIN. (Forest) Thiamine HCl 100 mg, vitamin B_6 100 mg/ml. Vial 10 ml.
Use: Vitamin supplement.

DOXAPAP-N TABS. (Major) Propoxyphene napsylate 100 mg, acetaminophen 650 mg Bot. 100s, 500s.
Use: Narcotic analgesic.

DOXAPHENE CAPSULES. (Major) Propoxyphene HCl 65 mg/Cap. Bot. 1000s.
Use: Narcotic analgesic.

DOXAPHENE COMPOUND 65 CAPS. (Major) Propoxyphene HCl, acetaminophen. Bot. 1000s.
Use: Narcotic analgesic.

•**DOXAPRAM HYDROCHLORIDE,** U.S.P. XXIII. Inj., U.S.P. XXIII. 1-Ethyl-4-(2-morpholinoethyl)-3,3- diphenyl-2-pyrrolidinone HCl.
Use: Respiratory and CNS stimulant.
See: Dopram, Vial (Robins).

•**DOXAPROST.** USAN.

Use: Bronchodilator.
DOXATE. Docusate sodium.
Use: Laxative.
•**DOXAZOSIN MESYLATE.** USAN.
Use: Antihypertensive.
See: Cardura, Tab. (Roerig).
•**DOXEPIN HYDROCHLORIDE,** U.S.P.
XXIII. Cap., Oral Soln., U.S.P. XXIII.
Use: Psychotherapeutic drug.
See: Adapin, Cap. (Lotus).
Sinequan, Cap. (Roerig).
DOXIDAN. (Hoechst) Yellow phenolph-
thalein 65 mg, docusate calcium 60
mg/Cap. Bot. 30s, 100s, 1000s, UD
100s, Display Pack 10s.
Use: Laxative.
DOXINATE. (Hoechst) Docusate sodium.
Cap.: 240 mg/Cap. Bot. 100s. **Soln:** 50
mg/ml 5% alcohol. Bot. 60 ml, gal.
Use: Laxative.
•**DOXOFYLLINE.** USAN.
Use: Bronchodilator.
•**DOXORUBICIN.** USAN.
Use: Antineoplastic agent.
•**DOXORUBICIN HYDROCHLORIDE,**
U.S.P. XXIII. Inj., U.S.P. XXIII. 14-Hy-
droxydaunorubicin. An antibiotic pro-
duced by *Streptomyces peuceticus* var.
caesius.
Use: Antineoplastic agent.
See: Adriamycin (Adria).
•**DOXPICOMINE HYDROCHLORIDE.**
USAN.
Use: Analgesic.
DOXY 100. (Lyphomed) Doxycycline hy-
clate for injection. Pow. 100 mg/Vial.
Use: Anti-infective, tetracycline.
DOXY 200. (Lyphomed) Doxycycline hy-
clate. Pow. 200 mg/Vial.
Use: Anti-infective, tetracycline.
DOXYBETASOL. B.A.N. 9α-Fluoro-11β,
17α-dihydroxy-16β-methylpregna-1,4-
diene-3,20-dione.
Use: Corticosteroid.
DOXY-CAPS. (Edwards) Doxycycline hy-
clate 100 mg/Cap. Bot. 50s.
Use: Anti-infective, tetracycline.
DOXYCHEL CAPSULES. (Rachelle)
Doxycycline hyclate 50 mg or 100
mg/Cap. Bot. 50s, 500s, UD 100s.
Use: Anti-infective, tetracycline.
DOXYCHEL INJECTABLE. (Rachelle)
Doxycycline hyclate 100 mg or 200
mg/Vial.
Use: Anti-infective, tetracycline.
DOXYCHEL TABLETS. (Rachelle) Doxy-
cycline hyclate 50 mg or 100 mg/Tab.
Bot. 50s, 500s.
Use: Anti-infective, tetracycline.
•**DOXYCYCLINE,** U.S.P. XXIII. For Oral

Susp. U.S.P. XXIII. 4-(Dimethylamino)-
1,4,4a,5,5a,6,11,12a-octahydro-
3,5,10,12,12a-pentahydroxy-6-methyl-
1,11-dioxo-2-naphthacenecarboxamide.
Use: Antibiotic.
See: Vibramycin for Oral Susp. (Pfizer
Laboratories).
Vibramycin IV. (Roerig).
•**DOXYCYCLINE CALCIUM ORAL SUS-
PENSION,** U.S.P. XXIII.
Use: Antibiotic.
•**DOXYCYCLINE FOSFATEX.** USAN.
Use: Antibacterial.
•**DOXYCYCLINE HYCLATE,** U.S.P. XXIII.
Cap., Inj., Sterile, Tab., Delayed Release
Tab., U.S.P. XXIII. 2-Naphthacenecar-
boxamide, 4-(dimethyl-amino)-
1,4,4a,5,5a,6,11,12a-octahydro-
3,5,10,12-12a-pentahydroxy-6-methyl-
1,11-dioxo-, HCl compound with ethanol
monohydrate.
Use: Antibacterial.
See: Bio-Tab, Tab. (Inter. Ethical Labs).
Doxy-Caps, Cap. (Edwards).
Vibra-Tabs, Tab. (Pfizer Laboratories).
Vibramycin, Cap., Tab., Vial (Pfizer
Laboratories).
Vivox, Cap., Tab. (Squibb Mark).
•**DOXYLAMINE SUCCINATE,** U.S.P. XXI-
II. Syr., Tab., U.S.P. XXIII. 2-[α-(2-Di-
methylamino-ethoxy)-α-methyl-
benzyl]pyridine bisuccinate.
Use: Antihistamine.
See: Decapryn, Prep. (Merrell Dow).
Unisom, Tab. (Pfizer).
W/Acetaminophen, ephedrine sulfate, dex-
tromethorphan HBr, alcohol.
See: Nyquil, Liq. (Vick).
W/Dextromethorphan HBr, alcohol.
See: Consotuss Antitussive, Syr. (Mer-
rell Dow).
W/Dextromethorphan HBr, sodium citrate,
alcohol.
See: Vicks Formula 44 Cough Mixture,
Syr. (Vicks).
W/Mercodol.
See: Mercodol w/Decapryn, Syr. (Mer-
rell Dow).
DOXY-LEMMON CAPSULES. (Lemmon)
Doxycycline hyclate equivalent to 100
mg of doxycycline base/Cap. Bot. 50s,
500s, UD 100s.
Use: Anti-infective, tetracycline.
DOXY-LEMMON TABLETS. (Lemmon)
Doxycycline hyclate equivalent to 100
mg of doxycycline base/Tab. Bot. 50s,
500s, UD 100s.
Use: Anti-infective, tetracycline.
DOXY-TABS. (Rachelle) Doxycycline hy-
clate 100 mg/FC Tab. Bot. 50s, 500s.

Use: Anti-infective, tetracycline.
DOXY-TABS-50. (Rachelle) 50 mg/Tab.
Bot. 50s.
Use: Anti-infective, tetracycline.
DPPC. Colfosceril palmitate.
Use: Lung surfactant.
See: Exosurf Neonatal (Burroughs Wellcome).
•**DRAFLAZINE.** USAN.
Use: Cardioprotectant.
DRAMAJECT. (Mayrand) Dimenhydrinate 50 mg/ml. Vial 10 ml.
Use: Antiemetic/antivertigo.
DRAMAMINE II. (Upjohn) Meclizine HCl 25 mg/Tab. Pck. 8s.
Use: Antiemetic/antivertigo agent.
DRAMAMINE CHILDREN'S. (Upjohn) Dimenhydrinate 12.5 mg/5 ml, alcohol 5%, sucrose. liq. Bot. 120 ml.
Use: Antiemetic/antivertigo agent.
DRAMAMINE LIQUID. (Upjohn) Dimenhydrinate 12.5 mg/4 ml Bot. 90 ml, pt.
Use: Antiemetic/antivertigo.
DRAMAMINE TABLETS. (Upjohn) Dimenhydrinate 50 mg/Tab. Bot. 36s, 100s, 1000s, Blister pkg. 12s, UD 100s.
Use: Antiemetic/antivertigo.
DRAMANATE. (Pasadena) Dimenhydrinate 50 mg/ml. Inj. Vial 10 ml.
Use: Antiemetic/antivertigo.
DRAMARIN.
See: Dramamine, Preps. (Searle).
DRAMOJECT. (Mayrand) Dimenhydrinate 50 mg/ml, benzyl alcohol, propylene glycol. Inj. Vial 10 ml.
Use: Antiemetic/antivertigo.
DRAMYL.
See: Dramamine, Preps. (Searle).
DRANOCHOL. (Marin) Dehydrocholic acid 200 mg, homatropine methylbromide 5 mg/Tab. Bot. 60s, 500s, 1000s.
Use: Hydrocholeretic, antispasmodic.
DRAWING SALVE. (Whiteworth) Tube oz.
Use: Healing agent, topical.
DRAWING SALVE with TRIQUINODIN. (Towne) Tube 2 oz.
Use: Healing agent, topical.
DR. BERRY'S SKIN TONER. (Last) Hydroquinone 2%. Jar oz.
Use: Skin bleaching agent.
DR. CALDWELL SENNA LAXATIVE. (Mentholatum) Senna 7%, alcohol 4.5%. Bot. 130 ml, 360 ml.
Use: Laxative.
DRC PERI-ANAL CREAM. (Xttrium) Lassar's paste 37.5%, anhydrous lanolin, U.S.P. 37.5%, cold cream 25%. Tube 5 oz.
Use: Skin protectant, perianal.

DR. DERMI-HEAL. (Quality Formulations) Zinc oxide 25%, allantoin 1%, peruvian balsam, castor oil, white petrolatum. Oint. Tube 75 Gm.
Use: Astringent.
DR. DRAKE'S COUGH MEDICINE. (Last) Dextromethorphan HBr 10 mg/5 ml Bot. 2 oz.
Use: Antitussive.
•**DRIBENDAZOLE.** USAN.
Use: Anthelmintic.
DRI-A CAPS. (Barth's) Vitamin A 10,000 IU/Cap. Bot. 100s, 500s.
Use: Vitamin A supplement.
DRI A&D CAPS. (Barth's) Vitamins A 10,000 IU, D 400 IU/Cap. Bot. 100s, 500s.
Use: Vitamin A and D supplement.
DRI-E. (Barth's) Vitamin E. **100 IU/Cap.:** Bot. 100s, 500s, 1000s. **200 IU/Cap.:** Bot. 100s, 250s, 500s. **400 IU/Cap.:** Bot. 100s, 250s.
Use: Vitamin E supplement.
DRI/EAR. (Pfeiffer) Boric acid 2.75% in isopropyl alcohol. Soln. Dropper bot. 30 ml.
Use: Otic preparation.
•**DRIED ALUMINUM HYDROXIDE GEL,** U.S.P. XXIII.
Use: Antacid.
See: Aluminum Hydroxide Gel, dried.
DRIED YEAST.
See: Yeast, dried.
DRIMINATE TABS. (Major) Dimenhydrinate 50 mg/Tab. Bot. 100s, 1000s.
Use: Antiemetic/antivertigo.
DRINOPHEN CAPSULES. (Lannett) Phenylpropanolamine HCl 15 mg, acetylsalicylic acid 230 mg, acetaminophen 200 mg, caffeine 15 mg/Cap. Bot. 1000s.
Use: Decongestant, analgesic.
DRISDOL. (Sanofi Winthrop) Ergocalciferol (Vitamin D) 8000 IU/ml in propylene glycol. Bot. 60 ml.
Use: Refractory rickets; hypophosphatemia; hypoparathyroidism.
DRISDOL 50,000 UNIT CAPSULES. (Sanofi Winthrop) Vitamin D-2, 50,000 IU/Cap. Bot. 50s.
Use: Refractory rickets; hypophosphatemia; hypoparathyroidism.
DRISTAN 12 HOUR. (Whitehall) Chlorpheniramine maleate 4 mg, phenylephrine HCl 20 mg/Cap. Bot. 6s, 10s, 15s.
Use: Antihistamine, decongestant.
DRISTAN ALLERGY. (Whitehall) Pseudoephedrine HCl 60 mg, brompheniramine maleate 4 mg/Cap. Bot. 20s.

Use: Decongestant and antihistamine.
DRISTAN CAPSULES. (Whitehall)
Phenylephrine HCl 5 mg, chlorpheniramine maleate 2 mg, acetaminophen
325 mg/Cap. Bot. 16s, 36s, 75s.
Use: Decongestant, antihistamine,
analgesic.
DRISTAN COLD. (Whitehall) Phenylephrine HCl 5 mg, chlorpheniramine
maleate 2 mg, acetaminophen 325
mg/Tab. Bot. 24s, 50s, 100s.
Use: Decongestant, antihistamine,
analgesic.
DRISTAN COLD & FLU. (Whitehall) Ac-
etaminophen 500 mg, pseudoephedrine
HCl 60 mg, chlorpheniramine maleate 4
mg, dextromethorphan HBr 20 mg/Pow.
Pkts. 6s.
Use: Analgesic, decongestant, antihist-
amine, antitussive.
DRISTAN JUICE MIX-IN. (Whitehall) Ac-
etaminophen 500 mg, pseudoephedrine
HCl 60 mg, dextromethorphan 20
mg/Pow. Pkts. 5s.
Use: Analgesic, decongestant, antitus-
sive.
DRISTAN 12-HR NASAL. (Whitehall)
Oxymetazoline HCl 0.05%. Bot. 15 ml,
30 ml. Spray (menthol): 15 ml.
Use: Nasal decongestant.
**DRISTAN MAXIMUM STRENGTH
CAPLETS.** (Whitehall) Pseu-
doephedrine HCl 30 mg, aceta-
minophen 500 mg/Capl. Bot. 24s.
Use: Decongestant, analgesic.
DRISTAN MENTHOL NASAL MIST.
(Whitehall) Phenylephrine HCl 0.5%,
pheniramine maleate 0.2%. Bot. 0.5 oz,
1 oz.
Use: Decongestant, antihistamine.
DRISTAN NASAL MIST. (Whitehall)
Phenylephrine HCl 0.5%, pheniramine
maleate 0.2%. Regular: 15 ml, 30 ml.
Menthol: 15 ml.
Use: Decongestant, antihistamine.
DRISTAN NO DROWSINESS COLD.
(Whitehall) Pseudoephedrine HCl 30
mg, acetaminophen 500 mg/Cap. Bot.
20s.
Use: Decongestant, analgesic.
DRISTAN SALINE SPARY. (Whitehall)
Sodium chloride. Soln. Bot. 15 ml.
Use: Nasal product. {DRISTAN SINUS}.
(Whitehall) Pseudoephedrine HCl 30
mg, ibuprofen 200 mg/Cap. Pkg. 20s.
Bot. 40s.
Use: Decongestant; analgesic.
DRITHO-CREME. (Dermik) Anthralin
0.1%, 0.25% or 0.5%. Tube 50 Gm.
Use: Antipsoriatic.

DRITHO-CREME HP 1.0%. (Dermik) An-
thralin 1%. Tube 50 Gm.
Use: Antipsoriatic.
DRITHO-SCALP. (Dermik) Anthralin
0.25% or 0.5%. Tube 50 Gm.
Use: Antipsoriatic.
DRIXORAL. (Schering) Dexbrompheniramine maleate 6 mg, pseudoephedrine
sulfate 120 mg. SA Tab. Box 10s, 20s,
40s. Bot. 48s, 100s.
Use: Antihistamine, decongestant.
DRIXORAL. (Schering-Plough) Pseu-
doephedrine sulfate 30 mg, brompheni-
ramine maleate 2 mg, sorbitol, sugar.
Syrup. Bot. 118 ml.
Use: Decongestant, antihistamine.
DRIXORAL ALLERGY SINUS. (Scher-
ing-Plough) Pseudoephedrine sulfate 60
mg, dexbrompheniramine maleate 3
mg, acetaminophen 500 mg/Tab. Bot.
24s.
Use: Decongestant, antihistamine.
**DRIXORAL COUGH & CONGESTION
LIQUID CAPS.** (Schering-Plough)
Pseudoephedrine HCl 60 mg, dex-
tromethorphan HBr 30 mg, sorbitol.
Cap. Pkg. 10s.
Use: Decongestant, antihistamine.
**DRIXORAL COUGH & SORE THROAT
LIQUID CAPS.** (Schering-Plough) Dex-
tromethorphan HBr 15 mg, aceta-
minophen 325 mg, sorbitol. Cap. Pkg.
10s.
Use: Decongestant, antihistamine.
DRIXORAL COUGH LIQUID CAPS.
(Schering-Plough) Dextromethorphan
HBr 30 mg. Cap. Pkg. 10s.
Use: Antitussive.
DRIXORAL NON-DROWSY FORMULA.
(Schering-Plough) Pseudoephedrine
sulfate 120 mg, sugar. Tab. Pkg. 10s,
20s.
Use: Decongestant.
DRIXORAL PLUS. (Schering) Pseu-
doephedrine sulfate 60 mg,
dexbrompheniramine maleate 3 mg, ac-
etaminophen 500 mg/TR Tab. Bot. 24s.
Use: Decongestant, antihistamine,
analgesic.
**DRIXORAL SUSTAINED-ACTION
TABLETS.** (Schering-Plough) Psue-
doephedrine sulfate 120 mg,
dexbrompheniramine maleate 6 mg,
sugar, lactose. Tab. Pkg. 10s. Bots. 20s,
40s.
Use: Decongestant, antihistamine.
DRIZE. (Ascher) Phenylpropanolamine
HCl 75 mg, chlorpheniramine maleate
12 mg/SR Cap. Bot. 100s.
Use: Decongestant, antihistamine.

• **DROBULINE.** USAN.
Use: Cardiac depressant.
• **DROCINONIDE.** USAN.
Use: Anti-inflammatory.
DROCODE.
See: Dihydrocodeine.
DROMORAN, LEVO. Levorphanol, Levorphan.
See: Levo-Dromoran, Vial, Amp., Tab. (Roche).
• **DRONABINOL,** U.S.P. XXIII. Cap, U.S.P. XXIII. USAN.
Use: Antiemetic. [Orphan drug]
See: Marinol, Gel Cap. (Roxane).
DROP CHALK. (Various Mfr.) Calcium carbonate, prepared. Prepared chalk.
• **DROPERIDOL,** U.S.P. XXIII. Inj., U.S.P. XXIII. 1-[fb]1-[3-(p-Fluorobenzoyl)propyl-1,2,3,6-tetrahydro-4-pyridyl]-2-benzimidazolinone.
Use: Tranquilizer.
See: Inapsine, Inj. (Janssen).
W/Fentanyl citrate.
Use: Tranquilizer.
See: Innovar, Inj. (Janssen).
• **DROPRENILAMINE.** USAN.
Use: Vasodilator.
DROPROPIZINE. B.A.N. 1-(2,3-Dihydroxypropyl)-4-phenylpiperazine.
Use: Antitussive.
DROSTANOLONE. B.A.N. 17β-Hydroxy-2α-methyl-5α-androstan-3-one.
Use: Anabolic steroid.
DROTEBANOL. B.A.N. 3,4-Dimethoxy-17-methyl-morphinan-6β, 14-diol.
Use: Analgesic, antitussive.
DROTIC STERILE OTIC SOLUTION. (Ascher) Hydrocortisone 10 mg (1%), polymyxin B sulfate 10,000 units, neomycin 5 mg/ml, preservatives. Dropper bot. 10 ml.
Use: Otic preparation.
• **DROXACIN SODIUM.** USAN.
Use: Antibacterial
• **DROXIFILCON A.** USAN.
Use: Contact lens material.
DROXYPROPINE. B.A.N. 1-[2-(2-Hydroxyethoxy)- ethyl]-4-phenyl-4-propionylpiperidine.
Use: Cough suppressant.
DR. SCHOLL'S ADVANCED PAIN RELIEF CORN REMOVERS. (Schering-Plough) Salicylic acid 40% in a rubber-based vehicle. Disc. 6s.
Use: Keratolytic.
DR. SCHOLL'S ATHLETE'S FOOT. (Schering-Plough) **Pow.:** Tolnaftate 1%. Talc. 63 g. **Spray Liq.:** Tolnaftate 1%, alcohol 36%. 113 ml. **Spray Pow.:** Tolnaf-

tate 1%, SD alcohol 40 14%. 99 g.
Use: Antifungal, external.
DR. SCHOLL'S ATHLETE'S FOOT CREAM. (Schering-Plough) Tolnaftate 1%. Tube 0.5 oz.
Use: Antifungal, external.
DR. SCHOLL'S CALLOUS REMOVERS. (Schering-Plough) Salicylic acid 40% in a rubber-based vehicle. 6 pads, 4 discs. Extra thick in 4 discs.
Use: Keratolytic.
DR. SCHOLL'S CLEAR AWAY. (Schering-Plough) Salicylic acid 40% in a rubber-based vehicle. Disc 18s.
Use: Keratolytic.
DR. SCHOLL'S CLEAR AWAY ONESTEP. (Schering-Plough) Salicylic acid 40% in a rubber-based vehicle. Strip 14s.
Use: Keratolytic.
DR. SCHOLL'S CLEAR AWAY PLANTAR. (Schering Plough) Salicylic acid 40% in a rubber-based vehicle. Disc 24s.
Use: Keratolytic.
DR. SCHOLL'S CORN/CALLOUS REMOVER. (Schering-Plough) Salicylic acid 12.6% in a flexible collodion, alcohol 18%, ether 55%, hydrogenated vegetable oil. Liq. 10 ml with 3 cushions.
Use: Keratolytic.
DR. SCHOLL'S CORN/CALLOUS SALVE. (Schering-Plough) Salicylic acid 15%. Tube 0.4 oz.
Use: Keratolytic.
DR. SCHOLL'S CORN REMOVER. (Schering-Plough) Salicylic acid 40% in a rubber-based vehicle. Discs: 6s as wrap-arounds, 9s as ultra thin, small, waterproof, regular, soft and extra-thick.
Use: Keratolytic.
DR. SCHOLL'S CORN SALVE. (Schering-Plough) Salicylic acid 15%. Jar 0.4 oz.
Use: Keratolytic.
DR. SCHOLL'S CRACKED HEEL RELIEF, (Schering-Plough) Lidocaine 2%, benzalkonium Cl 0.13%. Cream 5.6 g.
Use: Local anesthetic, topical.
DR. SCHOLL'S INGROWN TOENAIL RELIEVER. (Schering-Plough) Sodium sulfide 1%. Bot. 0.33 oz.
Use: Foot preparation.
DR. SCHOLL'S MAXIMUM STRENGTH TRITIN. (Schering-Plough) **Pow.:** Tolnaftate 1% 56 g. **Spray Pow.:** Tolnaftate 1%, SD alcohol 40 14%, 85 g.
Use: Antifungal, external.
DR. SCHOLL'S MOISTURIZING CORN REMOVER KIT. (Schering-Plough) Sal-

icylic acid 40% in a rubber-based vehicle, moisturizing cream, pain relief cushions. Disc 6s.
Use: Keratolytic.
DR. SCHOLL'S ONESTEP CORN REMOVERS. (Schering-Plough) Salicylic acid 40% in a rubber-based vehicle. Strips 6s.
Use: Keratolytic.
DR. SCHOLL'S PRO COMFORT JOCK ITCH SPRAY. (Schering-Plough) Tolnaftate 1%. Aerosol can 3.5 oz.
Use: Antifungal, external.
DR. SCHOLL'S WART REMOVER KIT. (Schering-Plough) Salicylic acid 17% in a flexible collodion, alcohol 17%, ether 52%. Liq. 10 ml with brush and 6 adhesive pads.
Use: Keratolytic.
DR. SCHOLL'S ZINO PADS/WITH MEDICATED DISKS. (Schering-Plough) Salicylic acid 20% or 40%. Protective pads designed for use with and without salicylic acid-impregnated disks.
Use: Keratolytic.
DRUCON. (Standard Drug) Phenylephrine HCl 5 mg, chlorpheniramine maleate 2 mg, menthol 1 mg, alcohol 5%/5 ml Elix. Bot. pt, gal.
Use: Decongestant, antihistamine.
DRUCON C R. (Standard Drug) Phenylephrine HCl 25 mg, chlorpheniramine maleate 4 mg/Tab. Bot. 100s.
Use: Decongestant, antihistamine.
DRUCON WITH CODEINE. (Standard Drug) Codeine phosphate 10 mg, phenylephrine HCl 10 mg, chlorpheniramine maleate 2 mg, menthol 1 mg, alcohol 5%/5 ml. Bot. pt.
Use: Antitussive, decongestant, antihistamine.
DRY EYES. (Bausch & Lomb) White petrolatum, mineral oil, lanolin. Oint. Tube 0.7 g, 3.5 g, UD 24s.
Use: Ocular lubricant.
DRY EYE THERAPY. (Bausch & Lomb) Glycerin 0.3%, calcium Cl, magnesium Cl, potassium Cl, sodium Cl, sodium citrate, sodium phosphate, zinc Cl. Drop. Single-use Bot. 0.3 ml.
Use: Ophthalmic.
DRY SKIN CREME. (Gordon) Cetyl alcohol, lubricating oils in a water soluble base. Jar 2 oz, 1 lb, 5 lb.
Use: Emollient.
DRYSOL. (Person & Covey) Aluminum Cl hexahydrate 20% in 93% SD alcohol 40. Bot. 37.5 ml.
Use: Astringent.
DRYSUM SHAMPOO. (Summers) Alcohol 15%, acetone 6%. Plastic bot. 4 oz.
Use: Drying agent for oily hair.
DRY-T.
See: T-DRY.
DRY-T, JR.
See: T-DRY, JR.
DRYTERGENT. (C & M Pharmacal) TEA-dodecylbenzenesulfonate, boric acid, lauramide DEA, propylene glycol, purified water, color, fragrance. Bot. 8 oz, 16 oz, 1 gal.
Use: Anti-acne.
DRYTEX. (C & M Pharmacal) Salicylic acid 2%, benzalkonium Cl 0.1%, nonionic wetting agent, acetone 10%, isopropyl alcohol 40%, purified water, color, perfume. Lot. Bot. 240 ml.
Use: Anti-acne.
DSMC PLUS. (Geneva Marsam) Docusate potassium 100 mg. Cap. Bot. 100s.
Use: Laxative.
DSS. (Dioctyle sodium sulfosuccinate) Docusate sodium.
Use: Laxative.
See: Regutol, Tab. (Schering-Plough).
    Docusate Sodium, Cap. (Roxane).
    Colace, Cap. (Mead Johnson).
    Docusate Sodium, Cap. (Various, eg, Geneva, Marsam, Lederle, Major, Purepac, Rugby, Schein, URL).
    Disonate, Cap. (Lannett).
    DOK, Cap. (Major).
    DOS, Softgel, Cap. (Goldline).
    D-S-S, Cap. (Warner Chilcott).
    Modane Soft, Cap. (Adria).
    Pro-Sof, Cap. (Vangard).
    Regulax SS, Cap. (Republic).
D-S-S. (Warner Chilcott) Docusate sodium 100 mg/Cap. Bot. 100s, 1000s and UD 100s.
Use: Laxative.
D-S-S PLUS CAPSULES. (Warner-Chilcott) Docusate sodium 100 mg, casanthranol 30 mg/Cap. Bot. 100s, 1000s, UD 100s.
Use: Laxative.
DST. Dihydrostreptomycin.
See: Dihydrostreptomycin, Preps. (Various Mfr.).
D-TEST 100. (Burgin-Arden) Testosterone cypionate 100 mg/ml. Vial 10 ml.
Use: Androgen.
D-TEST 200. (Burgin-Arden) Testosterone cypionate 200 mg/ml. Vial 10 ml.
Use: Androgen.
DTIC. Dacarbazine.
Use: Antineoplastic.
See: Decarbazine, Inj. (Various Mfr.).
    DTIC-Dome, Inj,; (Miles Pharm).

DTIC-DOME. (Miles Pharm) Dacarbazine 100 mg or 200 mg. Vial 10 ml, 20 ml.
Use: Antineoplastic agent.

DTP. Diptheria and tetanus toxoids and pertussis vaccine, adsorbed.
Use: Toxoid.
See: Diptheria and Tetanus Toxoids and Pertussis Vaccine, Inj. (Connaught). Tri-Immunol, Inj. (Lederle).

DUADACIN. (Hoechst) Phenylpropanolamine HCl 12.5 mg, chlorpheniramine maleate 2 mg, acetaminophen 325 mg/Cap. Bot. 100s, 1000s.
Use: Decongestant, antihistamine, analgesic.

DUAL-WET. (Alcon Lenscare) Polyvinyl alcohol, duasorb water soluble polymetric system, benzalkonium Cl 0.01%, disodium edetate 0.05%. Bot. 2 oz.
Use: Hard contact lens care.

• **DUAZOMYCIN.** USAN. Antibiotic isolated from broth filtrates of *Streptomyces ambofaciens.*
Use: Antineoplastic agent.

DUAZOMYCIN A. Name used for Duazomycin.

DUAZOMYCIN B. Name used for Azotomycin.

DUAZOMYCIN C. Name used for Ambomycin.

DUBILE. (Kenyon) Ox bile extract 1.5 gr, mixed oxidized bile acids 1.5 gr, homatropine MBr $^1/_{120}$ gr/Tab. Bot. 100s, 1000s.

DULCAGEN SUPPOSITORIES. (Goldline) Bisacodyl 10 mg/Supp. Box 12s, 100s.
Use: Laxative.

DULCAGEN TABLETS. (Goldline) Bisacodyl 5 mg/Tab. Bot. 100s.
Use: Laxative.

DULCOLAX. (Ciba Consumer) Bisacodyl. **EC Tab.:** 5 mg. Box 10s, 25s, 50s, 100s. Bot. 1000s, UD 100s.
Supp.: 10 mg. Box 2s, 4s, 8s, 50s, 500s.
Bowel Prep Kit: 4 tab., 1 supp./Kit. 5s/box.
Use: Laxative.

DULL-C. (Freeda) Ascorbic acid 4 Gm/tsp. Pow. Bot. 100 Gm, 500 Gm, 1000 Gm.
Use: Vitamin supplement.

• **DULOXETINE HYDROCHLORIDE.** USAN.
Use: Antidepressant.

DULPHALAC. (Solvay) Lactulose 10 Gm/5 ml. Syr. Bot. 240 ml, 480 ml, 960 ml, UD 30 ml.
Use: Laxative.

DUO. (Norcliff Thayer) Surgical adhesive.

Tube 0.5 oz.

DUO-CET. (Mason) Hydrocodone bitartrate 5 mg, acetaminophen 500 mg/Tab. Bot. 100s.
Use: Narcotic analgesic.

DUO-CYP. (Keene) Testosterone cypionate 50 mg, estradiol cypionate 2 mg/ml. Vial 10 ml.
Use: Androgen, estrogen combination.

DUODENAL SUBSTANCE. W/Ox bile extract, pancreatin, papain.
See: Digenzyme, Tab. (Burgin-Arden).

DUODENUM WHOLE, DESICCATED & DEFATTED. W/Ferrous gluconate, Vitamin B_{12}, cobalt Cl.
See: Bitrinsic-E, Cap. (Elder).

DUODERM. (Conva Tec) **Sterile dressing:** 10 cm × 10 cm. Pack 5s. 20 cm 20 cm. Pack 3s. **Sterile gran:** Packet 4 Gm. Pack 5s.
Use: Wound-healing agent.

DUODERM EXTRA THIN. (ConvaTec) Flexible hydroactive sterile dressings. 4" x 4", 6" x 6". Pck. 10s.
Use: Topical drug

DUOFILM. (Stiefel) Salicylic acid 16.7%, lactic acid 16.7% in flexible collodion. Bot. 15 ml w/applicator.
Use: Keratolytic.

DUO-FLOW. (CooperVision) Poloxamer 188, benzalkonium Cl 0.013%, EDTA 0.25%. Soln. Bot. 120 ml.
Use: Hard contact lens care.

DUO-K. (Various Mfr.) Potassium 20 mEq, chloride 3.4 mEq/15 ml (from potassium gluconate and potassium Cl). Bot. pt, gal.
Use: Mineral supplement.

DUOLUBE. (Bausch & Lomb) White petrolatum, mineral oil. Sterile, preservative and lanolin free. Oint. Tube 3.5 Gm.
Use: Lubricant, ophthalmic.

DUO-MEDIHALER. (Riker) Isoproterenol HCl 0.16 mg, phenylephrine bitartrate 0.24 mg. In 15 ml (300 metered doses) or 22.5 ml (450 metered doses) medihaler. Refill vial 15 ml, 22.5 ml.
Use: Bronchodilator.

DUOMINE. (Kenyon) Dextromethorphan HBr 7.5 mg, chlorpheniramine maleate 10 mg, ammonium Cl 80 mg, potassium guaiacolate 90 mg, tartar emetic 0.8 mg/5 ml. Bot. 4 oz, pt, gal.
Use: Antitussive, antihistamine, expectorant.

DUOMYCIN. *See:* Aureomycin, Preps. (Lederle).

• **DUOPERONE FUMARATE.** USAN.

Use: Neuroleptic.

DUOPLANT. (Stiefel). Salicylic acid 27%, alcohol 50%, flexible collodion, hydroxypropylcellulose, lactic acid. Liq. Bot. 14 Gm.
Use: Ketatolytic (wart removal).

DUOSOL. (Kirkman Sales) Docusate sodium 100 mg or 250 mg/Cap. Bot. 100s, 1000s.
Use: Laxative.

DUOTAL. (Approved) 1.5 gr: Secobarbital sodium ³/₄ gr, amobarbital gr/Cap. 3 gr: Secobarbital sodium 1.5 gr, amobarbital 1.5 gr/Cap. Bot. 100s, 500s, 1000s.
Use: Sedative/hypnotic.

DUOTAL.
See: Guaiacol Carbonate (Various Mfr.).

DUO-TRACH KIT. (Astra) Lidocaine HCl 4%. Inj. 5 ml disp. syringe with laryngotracheal cannula.
Use: Local anesthetic.

DUOTRATE 30. (Jones Medical) Pentaerythritol tetranitrate 30 mg/SR Cap. Bot. 100s.
Use: Antianginal.

DUOTRATE 45. (Jones Medical) Pentaerythritol tetranitrate 45 mg/SR Cap. Bot. 100s.
Use: Antianginal.

DUOVIN-S. (Spanner) Estrone 2.5 mg, progesterone 25 mg/ml. Vial 10 ml.
Use: Estrogen, progestin combination.

DUO-WR, No. 1 & No. 2. (Whorton) **No. 1:** Salicylic acid, compound tincture benzoin. **No. 2:** Compound tincture benzoin, formaldehyde. Bot. 0.25 oz.
Use: Keratolytic.

DUPHALAC. (Solvay) Lactulose 10 Gm/15 ml (< 2.2 Gm galactose, 1.2 Gm lactose, 1.2 Gm or less of other sugars). Syr. Bot. 240 ml, pt, qt, UD 30 ml.
Use: Laxative.

DUPLAST. (Beiersdorf) Adhesive coated elastic cloth. 8"×4" Strip. Box 10s. 10'5" Strip. Box 8s, 10s.

DUPLEX SHAMPOO. (C & M Pharmacal) Sodium lauryl sulfate, lauramide DEA, purified water. Bot. pt, gal.
Use: Shampoo.

DUPLEX T SHAMPOO. (C & M Pharmacal) Sodium lauryl sulfate, purified water, lauramide DEA, solution of coal tar, alcohol 8.3%. Bot. pt, gal.
Use: Antiseborrheic.

DUPONOL.
See: Gardinol-type detergents (Sodium Lauryl Sulfate) (Various Mfr.).

DURABOLIN. (Organon) Nandrolone phenpropionate 25 mg/ml in sesame oil,

benzyl alcohol 5%. Inj. Vial 5 ml.
Use: Anabolic steroid.
See: Deca-Durabolin, Inj. (Organon).

DURABOLIN. (Organon) Nandrolone phenpropionate 50 mg/ml in sterile sesame oil, benzyl alcohol 10%. Inj. Vial 2 ml.
Use: Anabolic steroid.

DURACARE. (Blairex) Buffered hypertonic salt solution, non-ionic detergents with thimerosal 0.004%, EDTA 0.1%. Soln. Bot. 30 ml.
Use: Soft contact lens care.

DURACARE II. (Blairex Lab.) Buffered hypertonic salt solution, ethylene and propylene oxide, octylphenoxypolyethoxyethanol, lauryl sulfate salt of imidazoline, sodium bisulfite 0.1%, sorbic acid 0.1%, trisodium EDTA 0.25%. Soln. Bot. 30 ml.
Use: Contact lens care.

DURA-CHORION PLUS. (Pharmex) Estradiol valerate 10 mg/ml. Vial 10 ml.
Use: Estrogen.

DURACID. (Fielding) Calcium carbonate 325 mg, aluminum hydroxide-magnesium carbonate 175 mg. Chew. Tab. Bot. 100s.
Use: Antacid.

DURA-ESTRIN. (Hauck) Estradiol cypionate in oil 5 mg/ml. Inj. Vial 10 ml.
Use: Estrogen.

DURAGEN. (Hauck) Estradiol valerate in oil 20 mg or 40 mg/ml. Inj. Vial 10 ml.
Use: Estrogen.

• **DURAGESIC.** (Janssen) Fentanyl 2.5 mg, 5 mg, 7.5 mg or 10 mg/transdermal patch. Carton 5s.
Use: Narcotic analgesic.

DURA-GEST. (Dura) Phenylpropanolamine HCl 45 mg, phenylephrine HCl 5 mg, guaifenesin 200 mg/Cap. Bot. 100s, 500s.
Use: Decongestant, expectorant.

DURA-KELLIN. (Pharmex) Estrone 2 mg, potassium estrone sulfate 1 mg, sodium phosphate buffer, sodium carboxymethylcellulose 0.2%, thimerosal 1:20,000, benzyl alcohol 1.5%/ml. Vial 10 ml.
Use: Estrogen combination.

DURALEX. (American Urologicals) Pseudoephedrine HCl 120 mg, chlorpheniramine maleate 8 mg/SR Cap. Bot. 100s, 1000s.
Use: Decongestant, antihistamine.

DURALONE INJECTION. (Hauck) Methylprednisolone acetate 40 mg or 80 mg/ml Susp. for Inj. **40 mg:** Vial 10 ml.

80 mg: Vial 5 ml.
Use: Corticosteroid.
DURALUTIN INJECTION. (Roberts Hauck) Hydroxyprogesterone caproate in oil 250 mg/ml. Vial 5 ml.
Use: Progesterone.
DURA-METH. (Foy) Methylprednisolone 40 mg/ml. Vial 5 ml, 10 ml.
Use: Corticosteroid.
DURAMIST PLUS. (Pfeiffer) Oxymetazoline HCl 0.05%. Spray. 15 ml.
Use: Nasal decongestant.
DURAMORPH. (Elkins-Sinn) Morphine sulfate. Inj. 0.5 mg/ml or 1 mg/ml. Amp. 10 ml Box 10s. Preservative free.
Use: Narcotic analgesic.
DURANDROL. (Pharmex) Methandriol dipropionate 50 mg/ml. Vial 10 ml.
DURANEST HCl. (Astra) Etidocaine. **1%:** Vial 30 ml. **1% w/epinephrine 1:200,000:** Vial 30 ml. **1.5% w/epinephrine 1:200,000:** Amp. 20 ml.
Use: Local anesthetic.
DURAPAM. (Major) Flurazepam HCl 15 mg or 30 mg/Cap. Bot. 100s, 500s.
Use: Sedative/hypnotic.
•**DURAPATITE.** USAN.
Use: Prosthetic aid.
DURAQUIN. (Parke Davis) Quinidine gluconate 330 mg/SR Tab. Bot. 100s, UD 100s.
Use: Cardiac depressant.
DURASCREEN. (Reed & Carnrick) SPF 15. Ethylhexyl p-methoxycinnamate, 2-ethylhexyl salicylate, oxybenzone, parabens, titanium dioxide. Waterproof. Lot. Bot. 105 ml.
Use: Sunscreen.
DURA-TAP/PD. (Dura) Pseudoephedrine HCl 60 mg, chlorpheniramine maleate 4 mg. Cap. Bot. 100s.
Use: Decongestant, antihistamine.
DURATEARS NATURALE. (Alcon) White petroleum, anhydrous liquid lanolin, mineral oil. Oint. Tube 3.5 Gm.
Use: Lubricant, ophthalmic.
DURATEST-200/DURATEST-100. (Hauck) Testosterone cypionate in oil 100 mg or 200 mg/ml. Inj. Vial 10 ml.
Use: Androgen.
DURA-TESTOSTERONE. (Pharmex) Testosterone enthanate 200 mg/ml. Vial 10 ml.
Use: Androgen.
DURATESTRIN. (Hauck) Estradiol cypionate 2 mg, testosterone cypionate 50 mg/ml with chlorobutanol in cottonseed oil. Vial 10 ml.
Use: Estrogen, androgen combination.
DURA-TESTRONE. (Pharmex) Testos-

terone enthanate 90 mg, estradiol valerate 4 mg/ml.
Use: Androgen, estrogen combination.
DURA-TESTERONE FORTE. (Pharmex) Testosterone enthanate 180 mg, estradiol valerate 8 mg/ml. Vial 10 ml.
Use: Androgen, estrogen combination.
DURATHATE-200 INJECTION. (Hauck) Testosterone enanthate in oil 200 mg/ml. Vial 10 ml.
Use: Androgen.
DURATION MENTHOLATED VAPOR SPRAY. (Schering-Plough) Oxymetazoline HCl 0.05%, aromatics. Squeeze bot. 15 ml.
Use: Nasal decongestant.
DURATION MILD NASAL SPRAY. (Schering-Plough) Phenylephrine HCl 0.5%. Bot. 15 ml.
Use: Decongestant.
DURATION NASAL SPRAY. (Schering-Plough) Oxymetazoline HCl 0.05%. Aqueous soln. Squeeze bot. 15 ml, 30 ml.
Use: Nasal decongestant.
DURATESTRIN. (Hauck) Testosterone cypionate 50 mg, estradiol cypionate 2 mg/ml. Vial 10 ml.
Use: Androgen, estrogen combination.
DURATUSS. (Whitby) Pseudoephedrine HCl 120 mg, guaifenesin 600 mg. LA Tab. Bot. 100s.
Use: Decongestant, expectorant.
DURATUSS HD. (Whitby) Hydrocodone bitartrate 2.5 mg, pseudoephedrine HCl 30 mg, guaifenesin 100 mg, alcohol 5%. Elixir Bot. 473 ml.
Use: Antitussive, expectorant, decongestant.
DURA-VENT. (Dura) Phenylpropanolamine HCl 75 mg, guaifenesin 600 mg. SR Tab. Bot. 100s.
Use: Decongestant, expectorant.
DURA-VENT/A. (Dura) Phenylpropanolamine HCl 75 mg, chlorpheniramine maleate 10 mg. SR Cap. Bot. 100s.
Use: Decongestant, antihistamine.
DURA-VENT/DA. (Dura) Phenylephrine HCl 20 mg, chlorpheniramine maleate 8 mg, methscopolamine nitrate 2.5 mg. SR Tab. Bot. 100s.
Use: Decongestant, antihistamine, anticholinergic.
DURAZYME. (Blairex) Nonionic detergent preserved w/thimerosal 0.004%, EDTA 0.1% in sterile buffered hypertonic salt soln. Bot. 30 ml.
Use: Contact lens care.
DURICEF. (Mead Johnson) Cefadroxil.

Tab.: 1 Gm. Bot. 100s. **Cap.:** 500 mg. Bot. 100s, 500s. **Susp.:** 125 mg/5 ml, 250 mg/5 ml or 500 mg/5 ml Bot. 50 ml, 100 ml.
Use: Antibacterial, cephalosporin.
DUROLENE OINTMENT. (Durel) Glyceryl monostearate, petrolatum, cholesterol, polyoxyethyl sorbitol monolaurate. Jar 1 lb, 6 lb.
Use: Ointment base.
DUROMANTEL CREAM. (Durel) Spermaceti, cetyl alcohol, stearyl alcohol, glycerine, alcohol sulfates, aluminum acetate solution, purified water, methyl and propyl parasepts. Jar 1 lb, 6 lb.
DUROSHAM. (Durel) Soapless shampoo concentrate. Bot. 6 oz, gal.
Use: Shampoo.
DUSOTAL. (Harvey) Sodium amobarbital ¾ gr, sodium secobarbital gr/Cap. Bot. 1000s. (3 gr) Bot. 1000s.
Use: Sedative/hypnotic.
• **DUSTING POWDER, ABSORBABLE,** U.S.P. XXIII. Starch-derivative dusting pow.
Use: Surgical aid (glove lubricant).
DUSTING POWDER, SURGICAL.
See: B-F-I Powder (Calgon).
DUTCH DROPS. Oil of turpentine, sulfurated.
DUTCH OIL. Oil of turpentine, sulfurated.
DUVOID. (Norwich Eaton) Bethanechol Cl 10 mg, 25 mg or 50 mg/Tab. Bot. 100s, UD ctn. 100s.
Use: Urinary tract product.
D V CREAM. (Merrell Dow) Dienestrol 0.01% w/lactose, propylene glycol, stearic acid, diglycol stearate, TEA, benzoic acid, butylated hydroxytoluene, disodium edetate, buffered w/lactic acid to an acid pH. Tube 3 oz, w/applicator.
Use: Estrogen, vaginal.
D-VASO-S. (Dunhall) Pentylenetetrazole 50 mg, niacin 50 mg, dimenhydrinate 25 mg, alcohol 18%, sherry wine vehicle. Bot. pt.
D-10-W. (Various Mfr.) Dextrose in water injection 10% (amps 3 ml); vials 250 ml, 500 ml, 1000 ml; 17 ml fill in 20 ml, 500 ml fill in 1000 ml, 1000 ml fill in 2000 ml vials.
Use: Carbohydrate.
DWELLE. (DaKryon) Potassium sorbate 0.2%, polyvinyl alcohol, poly (N-glucose) EDTA 0.05% . Drop. Bot. 15 ml.
Use: Artificial tear solution.
DWIATOL. (Kenyon) Hyoscyamine HBr 0.256 mg, hyoscine HBr 0.0144 mg, atropine sulfate 0.048 mg, phenobarbital 0.5 gr/Tab. Bot. 100s, 1000s.

Use: Anticholinergic/antispasmodic.
D-XYLOSE.
See: Xylo-Pfan. (Adria).
DYANTOIN CAPS. (Major) Phenytoin sodium 100 mg/Cap. Bot. 100s, 1000s.
Use: Anticonvulsant.
DX 114 FOOT POWDER. (Amlab) Zinc undecylenate 1%, salicylic acid 1%, benzoic acid 1%, ammonium alum 5%, boric acid 10.5% w/zinc stearate, chlorophyll, talc, kaolin, starch, calcium silicate, oil of wormwood. Cont. 2 oz.
Use: Antifungal, external.
DYAZIDE. (SK-Beecham) Triamterene 37.5 mg, hydrochlorothiazide 25 mg/Cap. Bot. 1000s, UD 100s, Patient Pack 100s.
Use: Diuretic, antihypertensive.
DYCILL. (Beecham Labs) Dicloxacillin sodium 250 mg or 500 mg/Cap. Bot. 100s.
Use: Antibacterial, penicillin.
DYCLONE. (Astra) Dyclonine HCl 0.5% or 1%. Soln. Bot. 30 ml.
Use: Local anesthetic, topical.
• **DYCLONINE HCl,** U.S.P. XXIII. Gel, Topical Soln., U.S.P. XXIII. 4'-Butoxy-3-piperidinopropiophenone. HCl.
Use: Topical anesthetic.
See: Dyclone, Soln. (Astra).
W/Benzethonium chloride
See: Skin Shield, Liq. (Del).
W/Neomycinsulfate, polymyxin B sulfate, hydrocortisone acetate.
See: Neo-polycin HC, Oint. (Merrell Dow).
DYCOMENE. (Hance) Hydrocodone bitartrate ⅙ gr, pyrilamine maleate 1 gr/fl. oz. Bot. 3 oz, gal.
Use: Antitussive, sleep aid.
DYES.
See: Antiseptic, Dyes.
DYFLEX-200 TABLETS. (Econo Med) Dyphylline 200 mg/Tab. Bot. 100s, 1000s.
Use: Bronchodilator.
DYFLEX-G TABLETS. (Econo Med) Dyphylline 200 mg, guaifenesin 200 mg/Tab. Bot. 100s, 1000s.
Use: Bronchodilator, expectorant.
DYFLOS. B.A.N. Di-isopropyl phosphorofluoridate. Di-isopropyl fluorophosphonate.
Use: Agent for glaucoma.
DYLATE. Clonitrate.
Use: Coronary vasodilator.
DYLINE-GG LIQUID. (Seatrace) Dyphylline 100 mg, guaifenesin 100 mg/5 ml. Bot. pt, gal.

Use: Bronchodilator, expectorant.
DYLINE-GG TABLETS. (Seatrace) Dyphylline 200 mg, guaifenesin 200 mg/Tab. Bot. 100s, 1000s.
Use: Bronchodilator, expectorant.
•**DYMANTHINE HYDROCHLORIDE.** USAN. N,N- dimethyloctadecylamine hydrochloride.
Use: Anthelmintic.
DYMELOR. (Lilly) Acetohexamide 250 mg or 500 mg/Tab. Bot. 50s, 200s, 500s, Blister Pkg. 10 × 10s.
Use: Antidiabetic agent.
DYMENATE. (Keene) Dimenhydrinate 50 mg/ml. Vial 10 ml.
Use: Antiemetic/antivertigo.
DYNACIN. (Medicis Dermatologics) Minocycline HCl 50 mg, 100 mg. Cap. **50 mg:** Bot. 100s; **100 mg:** Bot. 50s.
Use: Tetracycline.
DYNACIRC. (Sandoz) Isradipine.
Use: Calcium channel blocker.
DYNACORYL.
See: Nikethamide, Preps. (Various Mfr.).
DYNA-HEX SKIN CLEANSER. (Western Medical) Chlorhexidine gluconate 4%, isopropyl alcohol 4%. Liq. Bot. 120 ml, 240 ml, 480 ml, 1 gal.
Use: Antiseptic/germicide.
DYNA-HEX 2 SKIN CLEANSER. (Western Medical) Chlorhexidine gluconate 2%, isopropyl alcohol 4%. Liq. Bot. 120 ml, 2409 ml, 480 ml, 1 gal.
Use: Antiseptic/germicide.
DYNAMINE.
Use: Antispasmodic. [Orphan drug]
DYNAPEN. (Bristol) Sodium dicloxacillin. **Cap.:** 125 mg, 250 mg or 500 mg. Bot. 24s, 50s, 100s. **Susp.:** 62.5 mg/5 ml. Bot. 80 ml, 100 ml, 200 ml.
Use: Antibacterial, penicillin.
DYNAPLEX. (Alton) Vitamin B complex. Bot. 100s, 1000s.
Use: Vitamin B supplement.
DYNARSAN.
See: Acetarsone, Tab.
DY-O-DERM. (Owen) Purified water, isopropyl alcohol, acetone, dihydroxyacetone, FD&C yellow No. 6, FD&C blue No. 1, FD&C red No. 33. Bot. 4 oz.
Use: Water-soluble vitiligo stain.
DY-PHYL-LIN. (Foy) Dyphylline 250 mg/ml with benzyl alcohol. Inj. Vial 10 ml.
Use: Bronchodilator.
•**DYPHYLLINE,** U.S.P. XXIII. Elixir, Inj., Tab., U.S.P. XXIII. 7-(2,3-Dihydroxypropyl) Theophylline, Hyphylline.
Use: Vasodilator, bronchodilator.

See: Brophylline, Inj., Granucaps (Solvay).
Dilor, Preps. (Savage).
Emfabid TD, Tab. (Saron).
Lardet, Inj. (Standex).
Neothylline, Tab. (Lemmon).
Prophyllin, Oint., Pow. (Rystan).
W/Chlorpheniramine maleate, guaifenesin, dextromethorphan HBr, phenylephrine HCl.
See: Hycoff-A, Syr. (Saron).
W/Guaifenesin.
See: Bronkolate-G, Tab. (Parmed).
Dilor-G, Liq., Tab. (Savage).
Embron, Syr., Cap. (Amid).
Neothylline GG, Liq. (Lemmon).
DYPHYLLINE GG ELIXIR. (Goldline) Bot. pt.
Use: Bronchodilator.
DYPROTEX. (Blistex) Micronized zinc oxide 40%, petrolatum 37.6%, dimethicone 2.5%, cod liver oil, aloe extract, zinc stearate. Pads. Pkgs. 3s (9 applications).
Use: Astringent (diaper rash).
DYRENIUM. (SK-Beecham) Triamterene. **50 mg/Cap.:** Bot. 100s, UD 100s, **100 mg/Cap.:** Bot. 100s, 1000s, UD 100s.
Use: Diuretic.
DYRETIC. (Keene) Furosemide 10 mg/ml. Vial 10 ml.
Use: Diuretic.
DYREXAN-OD. (Trimen) Phendimetrazine tartrate 105 mg. SR Cap. Bot. 100s.
Use: Anorexiant.
DYSENAID JR. (Jenkins) Paregoric 5 min., bismuth subgallate 1 gr, kaolin 1 gr, pectin 1/8 gr/Tab. Bot. 1000s.
Use: Antidiarrheal.
DYSPEL. (Dover) Acetaminophen, ephedrine sulfate, atropine sulfate. Sugar, lactose and salt free. Tab. UD Box 500s.
Use: Analgesic.

E

EAASE. (Neuro Genesis/Matrix) D, L-phenylalanine 500 mg, L-glutamine 15 mg, L-tyrosine 25 mg, L-carnitine 10 mg, L-arginine pyroglutamate 10 mg, L-ornithine/L-aspartate 10 mg, Cr 0.033 mg, Se 0.012 mg, B_1 0.33 mg, B_2 5 mg, B_3 3.3 mg, B_5 0.33 mg, B_6 0.33 mg, B_{12} 1 mcg, E 5 IU, biotin 0.05 mg, FA 0.066 mg, Fe 1 mg, Zn 2.5 mg, Ca 35 mg, I 0.25 mg, Cu 0.33 mg, Mg 25 mg/Cap. Bot.42s

Use: Oral nutritional supplement.

EACA. (Lederle) Epsilon aminocaproic acid.
Use: Antifibrinolytic agent.
See: Amicar (Lederle).

EARDRO. (Jenkins) Benzocaine 15 Gm, antipyrine 0.7 Gm, glycerol q.s./0.5 oz. Liq. Dropper Bot. 0.5 oz.
Use: Otic preparation.

EAR DROPS. (Weeks & Leo) Carbamide peroxide 6.5% in an anhydrous glycerin base. Bot. oz.
Use: Otic preparation.

EAR-DRY. (Scherer) Isopropyl alcohol, boric acid 2.75%. Dropper bot. 30 ml.
Use: Otic preparation.

EAREX EAR DROPS. (Approved) Benzocaine 0.15 Gm, antipyrine 0.7 Gm/0.5 oz. Bot. 0.5 oz.
Use: Otic prepartion.

EAR-EZE. (Hyrex) Hydrocortisone 1%, chloroxylenol 0.1%, pramoxine HCl 1%. Dropper bot. 15 ml.
Use: Corticosteroid, antibacterial, local anesthetic (otic).

EAROCOL EAR DROPS. (Hauck) Benzocaine 1.4%, antipyrine 5.4%, glycerin, oxyquinoline sulfate. Soln. Dropper bot. 15 ml.
Use: Otic preparation.

EARTHNUT OIL. Peanut Oil.

EASPRIN. (Parke-Davis) Aspirin 15 gr/EC Tab. Bot. 100s.
Use: Salicylate analgesic.

EAST-A. (Eastwood) Therapeutic lotion. Bot. 16 oz.
Use: Emollient.

EAST-GESIC. (Eastwood) Tab. Bot. 100s.

EASY-LAX. (Walgreen) Docusate sodium 100 mg/Cap. Bot. 60s.
Use: Laxative.

EASY-LAX PLUS. (Walgreen) Docusate sodium 100 mg, casanthranol 30 mg/Cap. Bot. 60s.
Use: Laxative.
Use: Anti-infective.

EAZOL. (Hauck) Fructose, dextrose, orthophosphoric acid with controlled hydrogen ion concentration. Bot. 473 ml.
Use: Antinauseant.

E-BASE. (Barr) Erythromycin. **Cap.:** 333 mg. Bot. 100s, 500s, 1000s. **Tab.:** 500 mg. Bot. 100s, 500s.

• **EBASTINE.** USAN.
Use: Antihistamine.

EBV-VCA. (Wampole-Zeus) Epstein-Barr virus, viral capsid antigen antibody test. Qualitative and semi-quantitative detection of EBV antibody in human serum. Test 100s.

Use: Diagnostic aid.

EBV-VCA Ig. (Wampole-Zeus) Epstein-Barr virus, viral capsid antigen Ig antibody. Qualitative and semiqualitative detection of EBV-VCA Ig antibody in human serum. Test 50s.
Use: Diagnostic aid.

ECBOLINE. Ergotoxine.

ECEE PLUS. (Edwards) Vitamin E 165 mg, ascorbic acid 100 mg, magnesium sulfate 70 mg, zinc sulfate 80 mg/Tab. Bot. 100s.
Use: Vitamin/mineral supplement.

• **ECHOTHIOPHATE IODIDE,** U.S.P. XXIII. Ophth. Soln. U.S.P. XXIII. Ethanaminium, 2-[(diethoxyphosphinyl)-thio]-N,N,N-trimethyl-, iodide. (2-Mercaptoethyl)-trimethylammonium iodide S-ester with O,O-diethyl phosphorothioate. Bot. 100s.
Use: Glaucoma; cholinergic.
See: Echodide, Ophth. Soln. (Alcon). Phospholine Iodide, Pow. (Wyeth-Ayerst).

• **ECLANAMINE MALEATE.** USAN.
Use: Antidepressant.

• **ECLAZOLAST.** USAN.
Use: Antiallergic, inhibitor.

ECLIPSE AFTER SUN. (Dorsey) Petrolatum, glycerin, oleth-3 phosphate, carbomer-934, imidazolidinyl urea, benzyl alcohol, cetyl esters wax. Lot. Bot. 180 ml.
Use: Emollient.

ECLIPSE LIP AND FACE PROTECTANT. (Dorsey) Padimate O, oxybenzone. Stick 4.5 Gm.
Use: Sunscreen for lips.

ECLIPSE ORIGINAL SUNSCREEN. (Dorsey) Padimate O, glyceryl PABA. Lot. Bot. 120 ml.
Use: Sunscreen.

ECLIPSE SUNTAN, PARTIAL. (Dorsey) Padimate O. Lot. Bot. 120 ml.
Use: Sunscreen.

• **ECONAZOLE.** USAN.
Use: Antifungal.

• **ECONAZOLE NITRATE.** USAN. U.S.P. XXIII
Use: Antifungal.

ECONO B & C. (Vanguard) Vitamins B_1 15 mg, B_2 10.2 mg, B_3 50 mg, B_5 10 mg, B_6 5 mg, C 300 mg/Capl. Bot. 100s, 1000s, UD 100s.
Use: Vitamin B supplement.

ECONOPRED OPHTHALMIC. (Alcon) Prednisolone acetate 0.125%, benzalkonium Cl 0.01% w/hydroxymethyl cellulose. Susp. Droptainer 5 ml, 10 ml.
Use: Anti-inflammatory, ophthalmic.

ECONOPRED PLUS. (Alcon) Prednisolone acetate 1%, benzalkonium Cl 0.01%, w/ hydroxymethyl cellulose. Susp. Droptainer 5 ml, 10 ml.
Use: Corticosteroid, ophthalmic.
ECOSONE CREAM. (Star) Hydrocortisone 0.5% in a water-soluble cream base. Tube oz.
Use: Corticosteroid.
ECOTHIOPATE IODIDE. B.A.N. S-2-Dimethylaminoethyl diethyl phosphorothioate methiodide.
Use: Agent for glaucoma.
ECOTRIN MAXIMUM STRENGTH. (SK Beecham) Acetylsalicylic acid 500 mg. **Tab.:** Bot. 60s, 150s. **Cap.:** Bot. 60s.
Use: Analgesic.
ECOTRIN REGULAR STRENGTH TABLETS. (SK-Beecham) Aspirin 325 mg/EC Tab. Bot. 100s, 250s, 1000s.
Use: Salicylate analgesic.
ECTOL. (Approved) Chlorpheniramine maleate, pyrilamine maleate, diperodon, hexachlorphene, benzalkonium, menthol, camphor. Tube oz.
Use: Antihistamine, antipruritic.
ECTYLUREA. B.A.N. (2-Ethylcrotonoyl) urea.
Use: Sedative.
ED A-HIST. (Edwards) Phenylephrine HCl 10 mg, chlorpheniramine maleate 4 mg/5 ml, alcohol 5%. Liq. Bot. 400 ml.
Use: Decongestant, antihistamine.
EDATHAMIL. Edetate ethylenediaminetetraacetic acid.
See: Nullapons (General Aniline).
EDATHAMIL CALCIUM-DISODIUM. Calcium disodium ethylenediamine tetraacetate.
See: Calcium Disodium Versenate, Amp. & Tab. (Riker).
EDATHAMIL DISODIUM. Disodium salt of ethylene diamine tetraacetic acid.
See: Endrate, Amp. (Abbott).
• **EDATREXATE.** USAN.
Use: Antineoplastic.
EDECRIN. (Merck & Co.) Ethacrynic acid 25 mg or 50 mg/Tab. Bot. 100s.
Use: Diuretic.
EDECRIN SODIUM INTRAVENOUS. (Merck & Co.) Ethacrynate sodium equivalent to 50 mg ethacrynic acid w/mannitol 62.5 mg, thimerosal 0.1 mg/Vial. Vial 50 ml for reconstitution.
Use: Diuretic.
• **EDETATE CALCIUM DISODIUM,** U.S.P. XXIII. Inj., U.S.P. XXIII. Calciate (2-), [[N,N-1,2-ethanediylbis[N-(carboxymethyl)-glycinato]](4-)-N,N,O,O,-O'',O']-, disodium, hydrate, (OC-6-21)-.

Disodium (ethylenedinitrilo)tetraceto calciate (2-) hydrate.
Use: Pharmaceutic aid (Chelating agent).
See: Calcium Disodium Versenate, Amp., Tab. (Riker).
• **EDETATE DIPOTASSIUM.** USAN.
Use: Chelating agent.
• **EDETATE DISODIUM,** U.S.P. XXIII. Inj., U.S.P. XXIII. Glycine, N,N'-1,2-ethanediylbis[N-(carboxymethyl)]-, disodium salt, dihydrate. Disodium (ethylenedinitrilo)tetraacetate dihydrate.
Use: Chelating agent.
See: Endrate, Amp. (Abbott).
Sodium Versenate (Riker).
W/Benzalkonium Cl, boric acid, potassium Cl, sodium carbonate anhydrous.
See: Swim-Eye Drops (Savage).
W/Phenylephrine HCl, methapyrilene HCl, benzalkonium Cl, sodium bisulfite.
See: Allerest Nasal Spray (Pharmacraft).
W/Phenylephrine HCl, benzalkonium Cl, sodium bisulfate.
See: Sinarest, Aerosol (Pharmacraft).
W/Potassium Cl, benzalkonium Cl, isotonic boric acid.
See: Dacriose (Smith, Miller & Patch).
W/Prednisolone sodium phosphate, niacinamide, sodium bisulfite, phenol.
See: P.S.P. IV. Inj. (Solvay).
Solu-Pred, Vial (Kenyon).
W/Sodium thiosulfate, salicylic acid, isopropyl alcohol, propylene glycol, menthol, colloidal alumina.
See: Tinver Lotion (Barnes-Hind).
• **EDETATE SODIUM.** USAN. Tetrasodium (ethylenedinitrilo)-tetraacetate, or tetrasodium ethylenediaminetetraacetate.
Use: Chelating agent.
See: Disodium Versenate (Riker).
Vagisec, Liq. (Julius Schmid).
• **EDETATE TRISODIUM.** USAN. Trisodium hydrogen (ethylenedinitrilo) tetraacetate, or trisodium hydrogen ethylenediaminetetraacetate.
Use: Chelating agent.
• **EDETIC ACID,** N.F. XVIII. (Ethylenedinitrilo) tetraacetic acid.
Use: Pharmaceutic (Metal-complexing agent).
• **EDETOL.** USAN.
Use: Alkalinizing agent.
• **EDIFOLONE ACETATE.** USAN.
Use: Cardiac depressant (antiarrhythmic).
EDITHAMIL.
See: Edathamil.

• **EDOBACOMAB.** USAN.
Use: Anti-endotoxin monoclonal anti-
body.
EDOGESTRONE. B.A.N. 17-Acetoxy-
3,3-ethylene-dioxy-6-methylpregn-5-en-
20-one.
Use: Progestational steroid.
• **EDOXUDINE.** USAN.
Use: Antiviral.
EDROFURADENE. Name used for Nifur-
dazil.
• **EDROPHONIUM CHLORIDE,** U.S.P.
XXIII. Inj. U.S.P. XXIII. Dimethylethyl (3-
hydroxyphenyl) ammonium chloride.
Ethyl (m-hydroxyphenyl)di-methyl- am-
monium chloride. Benzenaminium, N-
ethyl-3-hydroxy-N,N-dimethyl-chloride.
Use: Antidote to curare principles; di-
anogsitc aid (myathenia gravis).
See: Enlon, Inj. (Anaquest).
Tensilon Chloride, Vial (Roche).
ED-SPAZ. (Edwards) Hyoscyamine sul-
fate 0.125 mg/Tab. Bot. 100s.
Use: Anticholinergic/antispasmodic.
EDTA.
See: Edathamil (Various Mfr.).
ED-TLC. (Edwards) Phenylephrine HCl 5
mg, chlorpheniramine maleate 2 mg, hy-
drocodone bitartrate 1.67 mg/5 ml. Liq.
Bot. 473 ml.
Use: Decongestant, antihistamine, anti-
tussive.
ED-TUSS HC. (Edwards) Phenylephrine
HCl 10 mg, chlorpheniramine maleate 4
mg, hydrocodone bitartrate 2.5 mg, alco-
hol 5%/5 ml. Liq. Bot. 480 ml.
Use: Decongestant, antihistamine, antitussive.
E.E.S. 400 FILMTAB. (Abbott) Ery-
thromycin ethylsuccinate representing
400 mg erythromycin activity/Tab. Pkg.
100s, 500s, UD 100s.
Use: Anti-infective.
E.E.S. DROPS.(Abbott) Erythromycin ethylsuccinate representing erythromycin
activity 100 mg/2.5 ml when reconstituted w/water. Dropper Bot. 50 ml.
Use: Anti-infective.
E.E.S. GRANULES. (Abbott) Erythromycin ethylsuccinate representing
erythromycin activity 200 mg/5 ml oral
susp. Gran. Bot. 60 ml, 100 ml, 200 ml,
UD 5 ml.
Use: Anti-infective.
E.E.S. LIQUID-200 & 400. (Abbott) Erythromycin ethylsuccinate representing
erythromycin activity 200 mg/5 ml. Bot.
100 ml, 480 ml; erythromycin activity
400 mg/5 ml. Bot. 100 ml, 480 ml.

Use: Anti-infective.
EFED-II. (Alto) Ephedrine sulfate 25
mg/Cap. Box 24s.
Use: Decongestant.
EFEDRON NASAL. (Hyrex) Ephedrine
HCl 0.6%, chlorobutanol 0.5% w/sodium
Cl, menthol and cinnamon oil in a water-
soluble jelly base. Tube 20 Gm
Use: Decongestant.
• **EFEGATRAN SULFATE.** USAN.
Use: Antithrombotic.
E-FEROL SPRAY. (Forest Pharm.) Alpha
tocopherol equivalent to 30 IU Vitamin
E/ml. Can 6 oz.
E-FEROL SUCCINATE. (Forest Pharm.)
d-alpha Tocopherol acid succinate,
equivalent to Vitamin E. **100 or 400
IU/Cap.**: Bot. 100s, 500s, 1000s. **200
IU/Cap.**: Bot. 50s, 100s, 500s, 1000s. **50
IU/Tab.**: Bot. 100s, 500s, 1000s.
Use: Vitamin E supplement.
E-FEROL VANISHING CREAM. (Forest
Pharm.) Alpha tocopherol. Jar 2 oz.
Use: Emollient.
EFFECTIN TABLETS. (Sanofi Winthrop)
Bitolterol mesylate.
Use: Bronchodilator.
**EFFECTIVE STRENGTH COUGH FOR-
MULA.** (Barre-National) Chlorpheni-
ramine maleate 2 mg, dextromethor-
phan HBr 15 mg, alcohol 10%. Liq. Bot.
240 ml.
Use: Antihistamine, antitussive.
**EFFECTIVE STRENGTH COUGH FOR-
MULA WITH DECONGESTANT.**
(Barre-National) Pseudoephedrine HCl
20 mg, dextromethorhan HBr 10 mg, ,
alcohol 10%. Liq. Bot. 240 ml.
Use: Decongestant, antitussive.
EFFER-K. (Nomax) Potassium 25 mEq.
(as bicarbonate and citrate), saccharin.
Effervescent tab. Box foil 30s, 250s.
Use: Mineral supplement.
EFFEXOR. (Wyeth-Ayerst) Venlafaxine
25 mg, 37.5 mg, 50 mg, 75 mg or 100
mg / Tab. Bot. 100s, Redipak 100s.
Use: Antidepressant.
**EFFICOL COUGH WHIP, SUPPRES-
SANT, DECONGESTANT.** (Block)
Phenylpropanolamine HCl 6.25 mg,
dextromethorphan HBr 2.5 mg/5 ml Bot.
8 oz.
Use: Decongestant, antitussive.
**EFFICOL COUGH WHIP, SUPPRES-
SANT, DECONGESTANT, ANTIHISTA-
MINE.** (Block) Dextromethorphan HBr
2.5 mg, phenylpropanolamine HCl 6.25
mg, chlorpheniramine maleate 1 mg/5
ml Bot. 8 oz.
Use: Antitussive, decongestant, antihis-

tamine.
EFIDAC/24. (Ciba) Pseudoephedrine HCl 240 mg / Tab. Pkg. 6s, 12s.
Use: Decongestant.
• **EFLORNITHINE HYDROCHLORIDE.** USAN.
Use: Antineoplastic, antiprotozoal. [Orphan drug]
See: Ornidyl (Marion Merrell Dow).
EFO-DINE OINTMENT. (Fougera) Povidone-iodine oint. Foilpac oz, Tube oz. Jar lb.
EFRICON EXPECTORANT LIQUID.
(Lannett) Phenylephrine HCl 5 mg, chlorpheniramine maleate 2 mg, codeine phosphate 11 mg, ammonium chloride 90 mg, potassium guaiacolsulfonate 90 mg, sodium citrate 60 mg/5 ml. Bot. pt, gal.
Use: Decongestant, antihistamine, antitussive, expectorant.
EFUDEX. (Roche) Fluorouracil. **Soln:** Fluorouracil 2% or 5%, w/propylene glycol, hydroxypropyl cellulose, parabens, disodium edetate. Drop Dispenser 10 ml. **Cream:** Fluorouracil 5%, in vanishing cream base w/white petrolatum, stearyl alcohol, propylene glycol, polysorbate 60, parabens. Tube 25 Gm.
Use: Antineoplastic agent.
EGRAINE. A protein binder from oats.
• **EGTAZIC ACID.** USAN.
Use: Pharmaceutic aid.
EHDP.
See: Etidronate Disodium.
EHRLICH 594.
See: Acetarsone, Tab.
EHRLICH 606.
See: Arspheramine (Various Mfr.).
EL 10. (Elan Corporation)
Use: Antiviral, immunomodulator.
• **ELANTRINE.** USAN.
Use: Anticholinergic.
ELASE-CHLOROMYCETIN OINTMENT.
(Parke-Davis) Fibrinolysin 10 units, desoxyribonuclease 6666 units, chloramphenicol 100 mg. Tube 10 Gm. Fibrinolysin 30 units, desoxyribonuclease 20,000 units, chloramphenicol 300 mg and thimerosal. In 30 Gm.
Use: Topical enzyme preparation.
ELASE OINT. & PWD. FOR SOL. (Parke-Davis) **Pow.:** Fibrinolysin 25 units, desoxyribonuclease 15,000 units, thimerosal 0.1 mg/Vial as lyophilized powder. May be reconstituted with 10 ml of isotonic sodium Cl Soln. **Oint.:** Fibrinolysin 30 units, desoxyribonuclease 20,000 units, thimerosal 0.12 mg/30 Gm Tube. Fibrinolysin 10 units, desoxyribonucle-

ase 6,666 units/10 Gm w/thimerosal 0.04 mg as preservative. Ointment base of liquid petrolatum, polyethylene w/sucrose, sodium Cl. Tube 10 Gm, 30 Gm.
Use: Enzyme preparation, topical.
• **ELASTOFILCON A.** USAN.
Use: Contact lens material.
ELAVIL. (Merck & Co.) Amitriptyline HCl. **Tab.: 10 mg:** Bot. 100s, 1000s; **25 mg:** Bot. 100s, 1000s; **50 mg:** Bot. 100s, 1000s; **75 mg, 100 mg:** Bot. 100s; **150 mg:** Bot. 30s, 100s. All strengths in UD 100s. **Inj.:** Vial 10 mg/ml w/dextrose 44 mg, methylparaben 1.5 mg, propylparaben 0.2 mg/ml w/water for injection. q.s. Vial 1 ml, 10 ml.
Use: Antidepressant.
ELDEC KAPSEALS. (Parke-Davis) Elemental iron 3.3 mg, Vitamins A 1667 IU, E 10 mg, B_1 10 mg, B_2 0.9 mg, B_3 17 mg, B_5 10 mg, B_6 0.7 mg, B_{12} 2 mcg, C 67 mg, folic acid 0.3 mg, calcium iodine/Cap. Bot. 100s.
Use: Vitamin/mineral supplement.
ELDECORT. (ICN) Hydrocortisone 2.5%, light mineral oil, propylene glycol, allantoin / Cream. Tube 15 g, 30 g.
Use: Topical corticosteroid.
ELDEPRYL. (Somerset) Selegiline 5 mg. Tab. Bot. 60s.
Use: Antiparkinson agent.
ELDERCAPS. (Mayrand) Vitamins A 4000 IU, D-2 400 IU, E 25 mg, ascorbic acid 200 mg, thiamine mononitrate 10 mg, riboflavin 5 mg, pyridoxine HCl 2 mg, niacinamide 25 mg, d-calcium pantothenate 10 mg, zinc sulfate 25.3 mg, magnesium sulfate 70 mg, manganese sulfate 5 mg, folic acid 1 mg/Cap. Bot. 100s.
Use: Vitamin/mineral supplement.
ELDER'S RVP. Red Vet. Petrolatum.
Use: Dermatoses.
ELDERTONIC ELIXIR. (Mayrand) Vitamins B_1 0.17 mg, B_2 0.19 mg, B_3 2.22 mg, B_5 1.11 mg, B_6 0.22 mg, B_{12} 0.67 mcg, alcohol 13.5%, Mg, Mn, zinc 1.67 mg/5 ml. Bot. pt, gal, 240 ml.
Use: Vitamin/mineral supplement.
ELDISINE.
See: Vindesine sulfate.
ELDO-B & C. (Canright) Vitamins C 250 mg, B_1 25 mg, B_2 10 mg, niacinamide 150 mg, B_6 5 mg, d-calcium pantothenate 20 mg/Tab. Bot. 100s, 1000s.
Use: Vitamin supplement.
ELDOFE. (Canright) Ferrous fumarate 225 mg/Chew. tab. Bot. 100s, 1000s.
Use: Iron supplement.
ELDOFE-C. (Canright) Ferrous fumarate

225 mg, ascorbic acid 50 mg/Tab. Bot. 100s.
Use: Vitamin/mineral supplement.
ELDONAL. (Canright) Pentobarbital sodium 0.25 gr, hyoscyamine sulfate 0.1075 mg, atropine sulfate 0.0195 mg, hyoscine HBr 0.007 mg/Tab. or 5 ml. Tab. Bot. 100s, 1000s. Elix, Bot, pt,
Use: Sedative/hypnotic, anticholinergic/antispasmodic.
ELDONAL-L.A. (Canright) Hyoscyamine sulfate 0.3225 mg, atropine sulfate 0.0585 mg, hyoscine HBr 0.021 mg, pentobarbital sodium gr/Cap. Bot. 50s.
Use: Anticholinergic/antispasmodic, sedative/hypnotic.
ELDONAL-S. (Canright) Hyoscyamine sulfate 0.1075 mg, atropine sulfate 0.0195 mg, hyoscine HBr 0.007 mg, pentobarbital sodium 32.5 mg/Tab. Bot. 100s, 1000s.
Use: Anticholinergic/antispasmodic, sedative/hypnotic.
ELDOPAQUE. (Elder) Hydroquinone 2% in a tinted sunblocking cream base. Tube 15 Gm, 30 Gm.
Use: Skin bleaching agent.
ELDOPAQUE FORTE. (Elder) Hydroquinone 4% in a tinted sunblocking cream base. Tube 15 Gm, 30 Gm.
Use: Skin bleaching agent.
ELDOQUIN. (Elder) Hydroquinone 2% in a vanishing cream base. Tube 15 Gm, 30 Gm.
Use: Skin bleaching agent.
ELDOQUIN FORTE. (Elder) Hydroquinone 4% in vanishing cream base. Tube 15 Gm, 30 Gm.
Use: Skin bleaching agent.
ELDOVITE. (Canright) Vitamin/mineral formula. Bot. 100s.
Use: Vitamin/mineral supplement.
ELECAL. (Western Research) Calcium 250 mg, magnesium 15 mg/Tab. Bot. 1000s.
Use: Mineral supplement.
ELECTROLYTE #48 INJECTION. Pediatric maintenance electrolyte solution. Dextrose 5% in electrolyte #48 w/sodium 25 mEq, potassium 20 mEq, magnesium 3 mEq, chloride 22 mEq, lactate 23 mEq, phosphate 3 mEq/L.
Use: Water, caloric, electrolyte supplement.
ELECTROLYTE #75 and 5% DEXTROSE.
See: 5% Dextrose and Electrolyte #75.
ELECTROLYTE THERAPY.
See: K.M.C., Amp. (Ingram).
Lytren, Ready-to-Use, Liq. (Mead Johnson).

ELEGEN-G. (Grafton) Amitriptyline 10 mg, 25 mg or 50 mg/Tab. Bot. 100s, 1000s.
Use: Antidepressant.
ELEVITES. (Barth's) Vitamins A 6000 IU, D 400 IU, B_1 1.5 mg, B_2 3 mg, C 60 mg, B_{12} 10 mcg, niacin 1 mg, E 10 IU, malt diastase 15 mq, iron 15 mq, calcium 381 mg, phosphorus 0.172 mg, citrus bioflavonoid complex 15 mg, rutin 15 mg, nucleic acid 3 mg, redbone marrow 30 mg, peppermint leaves 10 mg, wheat germ 30 mg/Tab. or Cap. Bot. 100s, 500s, 1000s.
Use: Vitamin/mineral supplement.
•**ELFAZEPAM.** USAN.
Use: Appetite stimulant.
ELIMITE. (Herbert) Permethrin 5%. Cream. Tube 60 Gm.
Use: Scabicide/pediculicide.
ELIXICON. (Berlex) Theophylline 100 mg/5 ml with methyl and propyl parabens. Susp. Bot. 237 ml.
Use: Bronchodilator.
ELIXIRAL. (Vita Elixir) Phenobarbital 16.2 mg, hyoscyamine sulfate 0.1037 mg, atropine sulfate 0.194 mg, hyoscine HBr 0.0065 mg/5 ml. Liq. pt, gal.
Use: Sedative/hypnotic, anticholinergic/antispasmodic.
ELIXOPHYLLIN CAPSULES, DYE-FREE. (Forest) Anhydrous theophylline 100 mg or 200 mg/Cap. **100 mg:** Bot. 100s; 200 mg: Bot. 100s, 500s, UD 100s.
Use: Bronchodilator.
ELIXOPHYLLIN ELIXIR. (Forest) Anhydrous theophylline 80 mg, alcohol 20%/15 ml. Bot. pt, qt, gal.
Use: Bronchodilator.
ELIXOPHYLLIN-GG ORAL LIQUID. (Forest) Theophylline 100 mg, guaifenesin 100 mg/15 ml. Alcohol free. Bot. 240, 480 ml.
Use: Antiasthmatic combination.
ELIXOPHYLLIN-KI ELIXIR. (Forest) Anhydrous theophylline 80 mg, potassium iodide 130 mg, alcohol 10%/15 ml. Bot. 237 ml.
Use: Antiasthmatic combination.
ELLESDINE. (Janssen) Pipenperone.
Use: Tranquilizer.
ELMIRON. (Baker Norton)
See: PENTOSAN SODIUM POLYSULPHATE.
ELOCON CREAM. (Schering) Mometasone furoate 0.1%, hexylene glycol, phosphoric acid, propylene glycol stearate, stearyl alcohol, ceteareth-20, titanium dioxide, aluminum starch octenyl succinate, white wax, white

petrolatum. 15 Gm, 45 Gm.
Use: Corticosteroid, topical.
ELOCON LOTION.(Schering) Mometasone furoate 0.1%. Bot. 30 ml, 60 ml.
Use: Corticosteroid, topical.
ELOCON OINTMENT. (Schering) Mometasone furoate 0.1%, hexylene glycol, propylene glycol stearate, white wax, white petrolatum. 15 Gm, 45 Gm.
Use: Corticosteroid, topical.
E-LOR. (UAD) Propoxyphene HCl 65 mg, acetaminophen 650 mg/Tab. Bot. 100s.
Use: Narcotic analgesic.
ELPHEMET. (Canright) Phendimetrazine tartrate 35 mg/Tab. Bot. 100s, 1000s.
Use: Anorexiant.
ELPRECAL. (Canright) Vitamins A 5000 IU, D 400 IU, B_1 3 mg, B_2 2 mg, B_6 0.1 mg, B_{12} 1 mcg, C 50 mg, E 2 IU, calcium pantothenate 2.5 mg, niacinamide 15 mg, inositol 5 mg, choline 5 mg, calcium lactate 500 mg, ferrous sulfate 50 mg, copper 1 mg, manganese 1 mg, magnesium 2 mg, potassium 2 mg, zinc 0.5 mg, sulfur 1 mg/Cap. Bot. 100s.
Use: Vitamin/mineral supplement.
• **ELSAMITRUCIN.** USAN.
Use: Antineoplastic.
ELSERPINE. (Canright) Reserpine 0.25 mg/Tab. Bot. 100s, 1000s.
Use: Antihypertensive.
ELSPAR. (Merck & Co.) Asparaginase 10,000 IU, mannitol 80 mg/Vial 10 ml.
Use: Antineoplastic agent.
• **ELUCAINE.** USAN.
Use: Anticholinergic.
ELVANOL. (DuPont) Polyvinyl alcohol.
EMAGRIN. (Otis Clapp) Salicylamide, caffeine, aspirin/Tab. Sugar, lactose and salt free. Bot. 100s.
Use: Salicylate analgesic.
EMAGRIN FORTE TABLETS. (Clapp) Phenylephrine 5 mg, acetaminophen 261 mg, guaifenesin 101 mg, caffeine 32 mg. Bot. 100s, 200s, 500s.
Use: Decongestant, analgesic, expectorant.
EMAGRIN PROFESSIONAL STRENGTH. (Otis Clapp) Aspirin, salicylamide, caffeine. Sugar, lactose and salt free. Safety pack 500s, Medipak 200s, Aidpak 100s, Unit box 10s, 20s. Bot. 1000s.
Use: Salicylate analgesic.
EMBECHINE. Aliphatic chloroethylamine.
Use: Antineoplastic.
EMBRAMINE. B.A.N. N-2-(4-Bromo-α-methylbenzhydryloxy)ethyldimethylamine.
Use: Antihistamine.

EMBUTRAMIDE. B.A.N. N-[2-Ethyl-2-(3-methoxy-phenyl)butyl]-4-hydroxybutyramide.
Use: Narcotic analgesic.
EMCODEINE TABS. (Major) Aspirin with codeine as #2, #3 or #4. Bot. 100s, 500s.
Use: Narcotic analgesic combination.
EMCYT. (Kabi Pharmacia) Estramustine phosphate sodium equivalent to 140 mg estramustine phosphate/Cap. Bot. 100s.
Use: Antineoplastic agent.
EMDOL. (Approved) Salicylamide, para-aminobenzoic acid, sodium calcium succinate, vitamin D-1250. Bot. 100s, 1000s.
Use: Analgesic combination.
EMECHECK. (Savage) Phosphoric acid 21.5 mg, glucose, fructose/5 ml, methylparaben, cherry flavor. Liq. Bot. 120 ml.
Use: Antiemetic.
EMEPRONIUM BROMIDE. B.A.N. Ethyldimethyl-1-methyl-3,3-diphenylpropylammonium bromide.
Use: Anticholinergic.
EMERGENCY KITS
See: Ana-Kit (Hollister-Stier).
AtroPen Auto-Injector (Survival Technology).
Cyanide Antidote Package (Lilly).
Emergent-Ez Kit (Healthfirst Corp).
EpiPen Auto-Injector (Center Labs).
EpiPen Jr. Auto-Injector (Center Labs).
LidoPen Auto-Injector (Survival Technology).
Poison Antidote Kit (Bowman).
EMERGENT-EZ. (Healthfirst Corp.) Adrenalin 2 amp., aminophylline 1 amp., ammonia inhalants (3), amyl nitrite inhalants (2), atropine 2 amp., Benadryl 2 amp., nitroglycerin 1 bottle, Solu-Cortef 1 mix-o-vial, Talwin 1 amp., Tigan 1 amp., Valium 2 amp., Wyamine 2 amp., plastic air way (1), disposable syringes, tracheotomy needle (1) and tourniquet (1)/kit.
Use: Emergency kit.
EMEROID. (Delta) Zinc oxide 5%, diperodon HCl 0.25%, bismuth subcarbonate 0.2%, pyrilamine maleate 0.1%, phenylephrine HCl 0.25%, in a petrolatum base containing cod liver oil. Tube 1.25 oz.
Use: Anorectal preparation.
EMERSAL. (Medco Lab) Ammoniated mercury 5%, salicylic acid 2.5%, castor oil 23%, liquid petrolatum, polyoxyl 40 stearate, polysorbate 80, water. Lot. Plastic bot. 120 ml.
Use: Antipsoriatic.

EMESIS. (Kenyon) Levulose and dextrose 57.6 Gm, orthophosphoric acid 0.5 Gm/100 ml. Bot. 4 oz, pt, gal.
Use: Antiemetic.
EMERSON 1% SODIUM FLUORIDE DENTAL GEL. (Emerson) Red and plain. Bot. 2 oz.
Use: Dental caries preventative.
EMETICS.
See: Apomorphine HCl. Cupric Sulfate. Ipecac Syr.
• **EMETINE HYDROCHLORIDE,** U.S.P. XXIII. Inj., U.S.P. XXIII. Emetan, 6, 7, 10,11-tetramethoxy-,diHCl. (Lilly) Amp. 65 mg/1 ml.
Use: Antiamebic.
EMETROL. (Bock) Oral soln. containing balanced amounts of levulose (fructose) and dextrose (glucose) with orthophosphoric acid, stabilized at an optimal pH. Bot. 120 ml, 480 ml.
Use: Antiemetic.
EMFASEEM. (Saron) **Liq.:** Dyphylline 100 mg, guaifenesin 50 mg/15 ml w/alcohol 5%. Bot. pt. **Cap.:** Dyphylline 200 mg, guaifenesin 100 mg/Cap. Bot. 100s, 1000s. Unident 100s. **Inj.:** Vial 10 ml.
Use: Antiasthmatic combination.
EMGEL. (Glaxo) Erythromycin 2%. Gel. Tube 27 Gm.
Use: Anti-infective.
EM-GG. (Econo Med) Guaifenesin 100 mg/5 ml. Bot. pt.
Use: Expectorant.
• **EMILIUM TOSYLATE.** USAN.
Use: Cardiac depressant.
EMINASE. (Beecham) Anistreplase 30 units/vial.
Use: Thrombolytic enzyme.
EMITRIP TABS. (Major) Amitriptyline **10 mg or 25 mg/Tab.:** Bot. 100s, 250s, 1000s, UD 100s. **50 mg/Tab.:** Bot. 100s, 250s, 1000s, UD 100s. **75 mg/Tab.:** Bot. 100s, 250s, UD 100s. **100 mg/Tab.:** Bot. 100s, 250s, 1000s, UD 100s. **150 mg/Tab.:** Bot. 100s, 250s.
Use: Antidepressant.
EMKO BECAUSE CONTRACEPTOR. (Emko-Schering) Nonoxynol-9 (8% concentration). Contraceptor container w/applicator. Tube 10 Gm.
Use: Vaginal contraceptive.
EMKO PRE-FIL. (Schering) Nonoxynol-9 (8% concentration). Aerosol Can 30 Gm, Refill 60 Gm.
Use: Vaginal contraceptive.
EMKO VAGINAL FOAM. (Schering) Nonoxynol-9 (8% concentration). Kit Aerosol w/applicator 40 Gm, Refill 40 Gm, 90 Gm.

Use: Vaginal contraceptive.
EMLA. (Astra) Lidocaine 2.5%, prilocaine 2.5% / Cream. Tube 5 g, 30 g.
Use: Local anesthetic, topical.
EMOLLIA-CREME. (Gordon) Cetyl alcohol, lubricating oils in water-soluble base. Jar 4 oz, 5 lb.
Use: Emollient.
EMOLLIA-LOTION. (Gordon) Water-dispersable waxes, lubricating bland oils in a water-soluble lotion base. Bot. 1 oz, 4 oz, gal.
Use: Emollient.
EMPIRIN ASPIRIN TABLETS. (Burroughs Wellcome) Aspirin 325 mg/Tab. Bot. 50s, 100s, 250s.
Use: Analgesic.
EMPIRIN WITH CODEINE. (Burroughs Wellcome) Aspirin 325 mg with codeine phosphate 15 mg, 30 mg or 60 mg/Tab. **No. 2:** Codeine phosphate 15 mg (0.25 gr). Bot. 100s. **No. 3:** Codeine phosphate 30 mg (0.5 gr). Bot. 100s, 500s, 1000s, Dispenserpak 25s. **No. 4:** Codeine phosphate 60 mg (1 gr). Bot. 100s, 500s, 1000s, Dispenserpak 25s.
Use: Narcotic analgesic combination.
EMULAVE. (CooperCare)
See: Aveenobar Oilated (CooperCare).
EMUL-O-BALM. (Pennwalt) Menthol, camphor, methyl salicylate. Bot. 2 oz, 8 oz, gal.
Use: External analgesic.
EMULSOIL. (Paddock) Castor oil 95%. Bot. 60 ml.
Use: Laxative.
E-MYCIN. (Upjohn) Erythromycin. **250 mg**/EC Tab.: Bot. 100s, 500s, UD 100s, Unit-of-Use 40s. 333 mg/EC Tab.: Bot. 100s, 500s, UD 100s.
Use: Anti-infective.
EMYLCAMATE. B.A.N. 1-Ethyl-1-methylpropyl carbamate.
Use: Tranquilizer, muscle relaxant.
• **ENADOLINE HYDROCHLORIDE.** USAN.
Use: Analgesic.
• **ENALAPRIL MALEATE.** USAN.
Use: Antihypertensive.
See: Vasotec, Tab. (Merck & Co.).
W/Hydrochlorothiazide.
See: Vaseretic, Tab. (Merck & Co.).
• **ENALAPRILAT.** USAN.
Use: Antihypertensive.
• **ENALKIREN.** USAN.
Use: Antihypertensive.
• **ENAZADREM PHOSPHATE.** USAN.
Use: Antipsoriatic.
ENBUCRILATE. B.A.N. Butyl 2-cyanoacrylate.

Use: Surgical tissue adhesive.

•**ENCAINIDE HYDROCHLORIDE.** USAN.
Use: Cardiac depressant.
See: Enkaid, Cap. (Bristol).

ENCARE. (Thompson Medical)
Nonoxynol-9 (2.27%). Supp. 12s, 24s.
Use: Vaginal contraceptive.

•**ENCLOMIPHENE.** USAN. Cisclomiphene
is name previously used.

•**ENCYPRATE.** USAN. Ethyl N-benzylcy-
clopropane-carbamate.
Use: Antidepressant.

ENDAFED. (UAD Labs) Pseudoephedrine HCl 120 mg, brompheniramine maleate 12 mg/Cap. Bot. 100s.
Use: Decongestant, antihistamine.

ENDAGEN-HD. (Abana) Phenylephrine
HCl 5 mg, chlorpheniramine maleate 2
mg, hydrocodone bitartrate 1.67 mg.
Bot. 473 ml.
Use: Decongestant, antihistamine, anti-
tussive.

ENDAL. (UAD Labs) Phenylephrine HCl
20 mg, guaifenesin 300 mg/TR tab., dye
free. Bot. 100s.
Use: Decongestant, expectorant.

ENDAL EXPECTORANT. (UAD Labs)
Codeine phosphate 10 mg, phenylpropanolamine HCl 12.5 mg, guaifen
esin 100 mg/5 ml w/alcohol 5%. Bot. pt.
Use: Antitussive, decongestant, expectorant.

ENDAL-HD. (UAD Labs) Phenylephrine
HCl 5 mg, chlorpheniramine maleate 2
mg, hydrocodone bitartrate 1.67 mg
w/menthol, sucrose. Liq. Bot. 480 ml.
Use: Decongestant, antihistamine, antitussive.

ENDAL-HD PLUS. (UAD) Hydrocodone
bitartrate 2 mg, phenylephrine HCl 5 mg,
chlorpheniramine maleate 2 mg/5 ml.
Liq. Bot. 473 ml.
Use: Antitussive, decongestant, antihistamine.

ENDECON. (DuPont) Phenylpropanolamine HCl 25 mg, acetaminophen 325 mg/Tab. Bot. 60s.
Use: Decongestant, analgesic.

ENDEP. (Roche) Amitriptyline HCl 10 mg,
25 mg, 50 mg, 75 mg, 100 mg or 150
mg/Tab. **10 mg:** Bot. 100s, Tel-E-Dose
100s. **25 mg:** Bot. 100s, 500s, Tel-E-
Dose 100s. **50 mg:** Bot. 100s, 500s, Tel-
E-Dose 100s. **75 mg:** Bot. 100s, Tel-E-
Dose 100s. **100 mg:** Bot. 100s, Tel-E-
Dose 100s. **150 mg:** Bot 100s.
Use: Antidepressant.

END LICE. (Thompson) Pyrethrins 0.3%,
piperonyl butoxide techical 3%. Liq. Bot.
177 ml.

Use: Pediculicide.

ENDOBENZILINE BROMIDE. N,N-(dimethyl)-aminoethyl-α-(bicyclo[2.2.1]-5-
neptenyl) mandelate methyl bromide.
Use: Anticholinergic.

ENDOCAINE. Pyrrocaine.
Use: Local anesthetic.

ENDOJODIN.
See: Entodon.

ENDOLOR. (Keene) Butalbital 50 mg,
caffeine 40 mg, acetaminophen 325
mg/Cap. Bot. 100s.
Use: Sedative/hypnotic, analgesic.

ENDOMYCIN. A new antibiotic obtained
from cultures of Streptomyces endus.
Under study.

ENDOPHENOLPHTHALEIN. (Roche) Di-
acetyldioxphenylisatin-isacen-bisatin.
Use: Laxative.
See: Diacetylhydroxphenylisatin, Prep.
(Various Mfr.)

•**ENDRALAZINE MESYLATE.** USAN.
Use: Antihypertensive.

ENDRATE. (Abbott Hospital Prods) Edetate disodium 150 mg/ml. Amp. 20 ml.
Use: Treatment of hypercalcemia, control of ventricular arrhythmias associated with digitalis toxicity.

•**ENDRYSONE.** USAN.
Use: Anti-inflammatory.

ENDURON. (Abbott) Methyclothiazide
2.5 mg or 5 mg/Tab. **2.5 mg:** Bot. 100s,
1000s. **5 mg:** Bot. 100s, 1000s, UD
100s.
Use: Diuretic.

ENDURONYL. (Abbott) Methyclothiazide
5 mg, deserpidine 0.25 mg/Tab. Bot.
100s, 1000s, UD 100s.
Use: Antihypertensive, diuretic.

ENDURONYL FORTE. (Abbott) Methyclothiazide 5 mg, deserpidine 0.5
mg/Tab. Bot. 100s, 1000s.
Use: Antihypertensive, diuretic.

ENEBAG 2. (Lafayette) Air contrast barium enema bag. Case 24s.
Use: Radiopaque agent.

ENEBAG XL. (Lafayette) Air contrast barium enema bag 3000 ml w/lumen tubing,
enema tip and side clamp. Case 24s.
Use: Radiopaque agent.

ENECAT. (Lafayette) Barium sulfate suspension CT colon exam kit. Case 12s.
Use: Radiopaque agent.

ENEMARK. (Lafayette) Rectal marker.
85% w/v liquid barium. Case of 12 kits.
Use: Rectal marker during radiation
therapy.

ENER-B. (Nature's Bounty) Vitamin B_{12}
400 mcg/unit. Nasal gel. Unit 12s.
Use: Vitamin supplement.

ENERJETS. (Chilton) Caffeine 65 mg/Loz. pkg. 10s.
Use: Analeptic.

ENESET 1. (Lafayette) Barium sulfate suspension 300 ml/air contrast examination kit. Unit-of-use kit. Case 12s.
Use: Radiopaque agent.

ENESET 2. (Lafayette) Barium sulfate suspension 450 ml/contrast examination kit. Unit-of-use kit. Case 12s.
Use: Radiopaque agent.

ENESET 600. (Lafayette) Barium sulfate suspension 600 ml/air contrast examination kit. Unit-of-use kit. Case 12s.
Use: Radiopaque agent.

ENFAMIL. (Mead Johnson Nutrition) Vitamins A 2000 IU, D 400 IU, E 20 IU, C 52 mg, B_1 0.5 mg, B_2 1 mg, B_6 0.4 mg, B_{12} 1.5 mcg, niacin 8 mg, calcium 440 mg, phosphorus 300 mg, folic acid 100 mcg, pantothenic acid 3 mg, inositol 30 mg, biotin 15 mcg, K-1 55 mcg, choline 100 mg, iron 1.4 mg, potassium 650 mg, chloride 400 mg, copper 0.6 mg, iodine 65 mcg, sodium 175 mg, magnesium 50 mg, zinc 5 mg, manganese 100 mg/Qt. Concentrated Liq. 13 fl oz, Instant Pow. lb.
Use: Enteral nutritional supplement.

ENFAMIL HUMAN MILK FORTIFIER. (Mead Johnson) Whey protein, casein, corn syrup solids, lactose, protein 0.7 Gm, carbohydrate 2.7 Gm, fat 0.04 Gm, calories 14. Pow. Packet 0.95 Gm, Box 100s.
Use: Enteral nutritional supplement.

ENFAMIL WITH IRON. (Mead Johnson Nutrition) Iron 12 mg/Qt. Pkg. Con. Liq. 13 fl oz. 24s. Pow. 1 lb. 6s.
Use: Enteral nutritional supplement.

ENFAMIL WITH IRON READY TO USE. (Mead Johnson Nutrition) Ready-to-use Enfamil with Iron infant formula 20 kcal/fl oz. Can 8 fl oz, 6-can pack; 32 fl oz, 6 cans per case.
Use: Enteral nutritional supplement.

ENFAMIL NEXT STEP. (Mead Johnson Nutritionals) Protein 17.3 g, carbohydrates 74 g, fat 33.3 g/liter, with appropriate vitamins and minerals. **Liq.:** 390 ml concentrate, 1 qt ready-to-use. **Pow.:** 360 g, 720 g.
Use: Complete, concentrated oral nutrition.

ENFAMIL NURSETTE. (Mead Johnson Nutrition) Ready-to-feed Enfamil 20 kcal/fl oz, 4 fl oz, 6 fl oz and 8 fl oz. 4 bottles/sealed carton. W/Iron. Ready to use. Bot. 6 fl oz 4s, 24s.
Use: Enteral nutritional supplement.

ENFAMIL PREMATURE FORMULA. (Mead Johnson) Nonfat milk, whey protein concentrate, corn syrup solids, lactose, coconut oil, corn oil, medium chain triglycerides, soy lecithin. Protein 2.8 Gm, carbohydrate 10.7 Gm, fat 4.9 Gm, calories 96. Pow. Nursettes 120 ml.
Use: Enteral nutritional supplement.

ENFAMIL READY TO USE. (Mead Johnson Nutrition) Ready-to-use Enfamil infant formula 20 kcal/fl oz. Can 8 fl oz, 6-can pack; 32 fl oz, 6 cans per case.
Use: Enteral nutritional supplement.

•**ENFLURANE,** U.S.P. XXIII. 2-Chloro-1,1,2-trifluoroethyl difluoromethyl ether. Ethrane (Ohio Medical).
Use: Anesthetic (inhalation).

ENGERIX-B. (SKF) Hepatitis B vaccine (recombinant). **Inj.:** 20 mcg hepatitis B surface antigen/ml. Single dose vial. **Pediatric Inj.:** 10 mcg hepatitis B surface antigen/ml. Single dose vial.
Use: Vaccine.

•**ENGLITAZONE SODIUM.** USAN.
Use: Antidiabetic agent.

•**ENILCONAZOLE.** USAN.
Use: Antifungal.

•**ENISOPROST.** USAN.
Use: Antiulcerative. Reduce transplant rejection [Orphan drug]

ENISYL. (Person & Covey) L-Lysine monohydrochloride 334 mg or 500 mg/Tab. Bot. 100s, 250s.
Use: Dietary supplement.

ENKAID. (Bristol) Encainide HCl 25 mg, 35 mg or 50 mg/Cap. Bot. 100s, UD 100s.
Use: Antiarrhythmic.

•**ENLIMOMAB.** USAN.
Use: Monoclonal antibody.

ENLON INJECTION. (Anaquest) Edrophonium Cl 10 mg/ml, phenol 0.45%, sodium sulfite 0.2%. Vial 15 ml.
Use: Cholinergic muscle stimulant.

ENLON-PLUS. (Anaquest) Edrophonium chloride 10 mg, atropine sulfate 0.14 mg. Inj. Amp. 5 ml, Multi-dose Vial 15 ml.
Use: Cholinergic muscle stimulant.

•**ENLOPLATIN.** USAN.
Use: Antineoplastic.

ENNEX OINTMENT. (Ennex) Aloe vera extract 37.5%. **Skin Oint.:** Zinc oxide 12.5%, coal tar 1.5%, alcohol 4.5%. Tube oz. **Hemorrhoidal Oint.:** Tube oz.
Use: Anti-inflammatory, astringent, antipruritic.

•**ENOFELAST.** USAN.
Use: Anti-asthmatic.

•**ENOLICAM SODIUM.** USAN.
Use: Anti-inflammatory, antirheumatic.

ENOMINE CAPSULES. (Major) Phenyl-

propanolamine 45 mg, phenylephrine 5 mg, guaifenesin 200 mg/Cap. Bot. 100s, 500s.
Use: Decongestant, expectorant.
ENOVID. (Searle) Norethynodrel, mestranol 5 mg or 10 mg/Tab. **5 mg:** Norethynodrel 5 mg, mestranol 75 mcg. Bot. 100s, 6 × 20s calendar-pak. **10 mg:** Norethynodrel 9.85 mg, mestranol 0.15 mg. Bot. 50s.
Use: Estrogen, progestin combination.
ENOVID-E 21. (Searle) Norethynodrel 2.5 mg, mestranol 0.1 mg/Tab. Compack disp. 21s, 6 × 21. Refill 21s, 12 × 21.
Use: Estrogen, progestin combination.
ENOVIL. (Hauck) Amtriptyline HCl 10 mg/ml. Vial 10 ml.
Use: Antidepressant.
• **ENOXACIN.** USAN.
Use: Antibacterial.
See: Penetrex.
ENOXAPARIN.
See: Lovenox (Rhone-Poulenc Rorer).
• **ENOXIMONE.** USAN.
Use: Cardiotonic.
ENOXOLONE. B.A.N. 3β-Hydroxy-11-oxo-olean-12-en-30-oic acid.
Use: Treatment of skin diseases.
ENPIPRAZOLE. B.A.N. 1-(2-Chlorophenyl)-4-[2-(1-methylpyrazol-4-yl)ethyl]piperazine.
Use: Psychotropic drug.
• **ENPIROLINE PHOSPHATE.** USAN.
Use: Antimalarial.
• **ENPROFYLLINE.** USAN.
Use: Bronchodilator.
• **ENPROMATE.** USAN.
Use: Antineoplastic.
• **ENPROSTIL.** USAN.
Use: Antisecretory, antiulcerative.
ENRICH. (Ross) Liquid food with fiber providing complete, balanced nutrition as a full liquid diet, liquid supplement, or tube feeding. One serving provides 5 Gm dietary fiber. 1100 calories/L. 1530 calories provides 100% US RDA for vitamins and minerals. Can Ready-to-Use 8 fl oz (vanilla, chocolate).
Use: Enteral nutritional supplement.
ENSIDON. (Geigy) Opipramol HCl.
ENSURE. (Ross) Liquid food providing 1.06 calories/ml. Can be used as a full liquid diet, liquid supplement or tube feeding. Two quarts (2000 calories) provides 100% US RDA for vitamins and minerals for adults and children over 4 yrs. **Ready-to-Use:** Bot. 8 fl oz (vanilla). Can 8 fl oz (chocolate, black walnut, coffee, strawberry, eggnog, vanilla), 32 fl oz (vanilla, chocolate). **Pow.:** Can 14 oz

(400 Gm) (vanilla).
Use: Enteral nutritional supplement.
ENSURE HN. (Ross) High nitrogen low residue liquid food providing complete, balanced nutrition as tube feeding or oral supplement with 1.06 calories/ml. Provides 100% US RDA for vitamins and minerals for adults and children over 4 yrs. 1400 calories (1321 ml). Ready-to-Use: Can 8 fl oz (vanilla).
Use: Enteral nutritional supplement.
ENSURE OSMOLITE. (Ross).
See: Osmolite (Ross).
ENSURE PLUS. (Ross) High calorie liquid food w/caloric density of 1500 calories/L. Six servings (8 oz and 2130 calories each) provides 100% US RDA for vitamins and minerals for adults and children. Ready-to-Use: Bot. 8 fl oz (vanilla). Can 8 fl oz (chocolate, vanilla, eggnog, coffee, strawberry).
Use: Enteral nutritional supplement.
ENSURE PLUS HN. (Ross) High-calorie, high-nitrogen liquid food providing 1.5 calories/ml; 1420 calories provides 100% US RDA for vitamins and minerals for adults and children. Calorie/nitrogen ratio is 150:1. Can 8 fl oz (vanilla).
Use: Enteral nutritional supplement.
ENSURE PUDDING. (Ross) 17% US RDA vitamins and minerals for adults and children/5 oz. serving. Can 4s (chocolate, vanilla, tapioca, butterscotch).
Use: Nutritional supplement.
ENTAB 650. (Mayrand) Aspirin 650 mg/EC tab. Bot. 100s.
Use: Salicylate analgesic.
ENTERO-TEST. (HDC Corp.) Cap. To identify duodenal parasites; to diagnose and locate upper GI bleeding, pH disorders, achlorhydria and esophageal reflux. Bot. 10s, 25s.
Use: Diagnostic aid.
ENTERO-TEST PEDIATRIC. (HDC Corp.) To identify duodenal parasites; to diagnose and locate upper GI bleeding, pH disorders, achlorhydria and esophageal reflux. Cap. Bot. 10s, 25s.
Use: Diagnostic aid.
ENTEROTUBE. (Roche Diagnostics) Culture-identification method for enterobacteriaceae ACA. Test kit 25s.
Use: Diagnostic aid.
ENTERTAINER'S SECRET THROAT RELIEF SPRAY. (KLI Corp.) Sodium carboxymethylcellulose, potassium Cl, dibasic sodium phosphate, methyl and propyl parabens. Soln. 60 ml with pump spray.

Uses Saliva substitute.
ENTEX. (Procter & Gamble) Phenyle-
phrine HCl 5 mg, phenylpropanolamine
HCl 45 mg, guaifenesin 200 mg/Cap.
Bot. 100s, 500s.
Use: Decongestant, expectorant.
ENTEX LA. (Procter & Gamble) Phenyl-
propanolamine HCl 75 mg, guaifenesin
400 mg/T.R. Tab. Bot. 100s, 500s.
Use: Decongestant, expectorant.
ENTEX LIQUID. (Procter & Gamble)
Phenylephrine HCl 5 mg, phenyl-
propanolamine HCl 20 mg, guaifenesin
100 mg/5 ml, alcohol 5%. Elix. Bot. 480
ml.
Use: Decongestant, expectorant.
ENTEX PSE. (Procter & Gamble) Pseu-
doephedrine 120 mg, guaifenesin 600
mg. Prolonged action. Tab. Bot. 100s.
Use: Decongestant, expectorant.
ENTIRE B W/C. (Pharmex) Vitamin B
complex with vitamin C. Cap. Bot. 100s,
1000s.
Use: Vitamin supplement.
ENTODON. Propiodal, Entoidoin, Endo-
jodin, 2-Hydroxytrimethylene-bis-
(trimethylammonium iodide).
ENTOIDOIN.
See: Entodon.
ENTOLASE HP. (Robins) Lipase 8,000
units, protease 50,000 units, amylase
40,000 units/Cap. (enteric coated mi-
crobeads). Bot. 100s, 250s.
Use: Digestive enzymes.
ENTOZYME. (Robins) Pepsin 250 mg in
outer core, pancreatin 300 mg, bile salts
150 mg in enteric coated inner core/Tab.
Bot. 100s, 500s.
Use: Digestive enzymes.
ENTRITION HALF STRENGTH.
(Biosearch) Calcium and sodium ca-
seinates, maltodextrin, corn oil, soy
lecithin, mono- and diglycerides, protein
17.5 Gm, carbohydrate 68 Gm, fat 17.5
Gm, sodium 350 mg, potassium 600 mg,
calories 0.5/ml, osmolarity 120
mOsm/kg, water, vitamins A, B_1, B_2, B_3,
B_5, B_6, B_{12}, C, D, E, K, Ca, P, Mg, I, Fe,
Zn, Mn, Cu, Cl, biotin, choline, folic acid.
Pouch 1 L.
Use: Enteral nutritional supplement.
ENTRITION HN ENTRI-PAK.
(Biosearch). Sodium and calcium ca-
seinates, soy protein isolate, maltodex-
trin, corn oil, soy lecithin, mono and
diglycerides, vitamins A, B_1, B_2, B_3, B_5,
B_6, B_{12}, C, D, E, K, folic acid, biotin,
choline, Ca, Cl, Cu, Fe, I, Mg, Mn, P, Zn.
Pouch 1 L.
Use: Enteral nutritional supplement.

ENTROBAG SET. (Lafayette) Entero
clysis set. Case 6 sets.
Use: Enteroclysis of the small intestine.
ENTROBAR. (Lafayette) Barium sulfate
50%w/v susp. Bot. 500 ml, case 12 Bot.
Use: Radiopaque agent.
ENTROKIT. (Lafayette) Barium sulfate
susp. (Entrobar), methylcellulose (En-
trolcel). Case 4 kits.
Use: Radiopaque agent.
ENTROLCEL. (Lafayette) Methylcellu-
lose 1.8% w/w concentrate for dilution at
time of use. Bot. 500 ml, case 24 Bot.
Use: Diagnostic aid.
•**ENTSUFFEN SODIUM.** USAN.
Use: Detergent.
E.N.T. SYRUP. (Springbok) Brompheni-
ramine maleate 4 mg, phenylephrine
HCl 5 mg, phenylpropanolamine HCl 5
mg/5 ml. Bot. 16 oz.
Use: Antihistamine, decongestant.
E.N.T. TABLETS. (Springbok) Phenyle-
phrine HCl 25 mg, phenylpropanolamine
HCl 50 mg, chlorpheniramine maleate 8
mg/SA Tab. Bot. 100s, 500s.
Use: Decongestant, antihistamine.
ENTUSS. (Roberts/Hauck) **Tab.:** Hy-
drocodone bitartrate 5 mg, guaifenesin
300 mg/Tab. Bot. 100s. **Syr.:** 5 mg hydrocodone bitartate, 300 mg potassium
guaiacolsulfonate/5 ml. Alcohol free.
Bot. 120 ml, 480 ml.
Use: Antitussive, expectorant.
ENTUSS-D JUNIOR. (Roberts/Hauck)
Pseudoepherine HCl 30 mg, hydrocodone bitartrate 2.5 mg, guaifenesin
100 mg w/alcohol 5%, saccharin, sorbitol, sucrose. Liq. Bot.120 ml, pt.
Use: Antitussive, expectorant combination.
ENTUSS-D LIQUID. (Roberts/Hauck) Hydrocodone bitartrate 5 mg, pseu-
doephedrine 30 mg/5 ml. Sugar, alcohol,
corn and dye free. Bot. 16 oz.
Use: Antitussive, decongestant.
ENTUSS-D TABLETS. (Roberts/Hauck)
Pseudoephedrine 30 mg, hydrocodone
bitartrate 5 mg, guaifenesin 300 mg/Tab.
Bot. 100s.
Use: Decongestant, antitussive, expec-
torant.
ENUCLENE. (Alcon Surgical) Tyloxapol
0.25%, benzalkonium Cl 0.02%, hydrox-
ypropyl methylcellulose 0.85%. Soln.
Drop-tainer 15 ml.
Use: Artificial eye care.
ENULOSE. (Barre-National) Lactulose 10
Gm, galactose 2.2 Gm, lactose 1.2 Gm,
other sugars $\leq$ 1.2 Gm. Syr. pt, 2 qt.
Use: Laxative.

• **ENVIRADENE.** USAN.
  Use: Antiviral.
ENVIRO-STRESS. (Vitaline) Vitamins B$_1$
  50 mg, B$_2$ 50 mg, B$_3$ 100 mg, B$_5$ 50 mg,
  B$_6$ 50 mg, B$_{12}$ 25 mcg, C 600 mg, E 30
  IU, folic acid 0.4 mg, zinc 30 mg, Mg, Se,
  PABA. Tab. Bot. 90s, 1000s.
  Use: Vitamin/mineral supplement.
• **ENVIROXIME.** USAN.
  Use: Antiviral.
ENVISAN TREATMENT MULTIPACK.
  (Marion) Dextranomer with PEG 3000
  and PEG 600. Paste 10 Gm packets
  with nylon net and semi-occlusive film.
  Use: Wound debridement.
ENZEST. (Barth's) Seven natural en-
  zymes, calcium carbonate 250 mg/Tab.
  Bot. 100s, 250s, 500s.
  Use: Digestive enzymes, antacid.
ENZOBILE IMPROVED. (Hauck) Pancre-
  atic enzyme concentrate 100 mg, ox bile
  extract 100 mg, cellulase 10 mg in inner
  core and pepsin 150 mg in outer layer.
  EC tab. Bot. 100s.
  Use: Digestive enzymes.
ENZONE. (UAD) Hydrocortisone acetate
  1%, pramoxine HCl 1% in hydrophilic
  base w/stearic acid, aquaphor, isopropyl
  palmitate, polyoxyl-40, stearate, tri-
  ethanolamine lauryl sulfate. Cream.
  Tube 30 Gm w/rectal applicator.
  Use: Corticosteroid combination.
**ENZYMATIC CLEANER FOR EXTEND-
  ED WEAR.** (Alcon) Highly purified pork
  pancreatin to dilute in saline solution.
  Tab. Pkg. 12s.
  Use: Soft contact lens care.
ENZYME FORMULA #E-2. (Barth's) Amy-
  lase 30 mg, lipase 25 mg, bile salts 1 gr,
  wilzyme 10 mg, pepsin 2 gr, pancreatin
  0.5 gr, calcium carbonate 4 gr/Tab. Bot.
  100s, 250s.
  Use: Digestive aid.
ENZYMES.
  See: Alpha Chymar, Vial (Armour).
    Ananase, Tab. (Rhone-Poulenc Ror-
    er).
    Cholinesterase (Various Mfr.).
    Chymotrypsin.
    Cotazym, Cap. (Organon).
    Creon (Solvay).
    Diastase (Various Mfr.).
    Dornavac, Vial (Merck & Co.).
    Fibrinolysin. Hyaluronidase (Various
    Mfr.).
    Neutrapen, Vial (Riker).
    Pancreatin (Various Mfr.).
    Papain (Various Mfr.).
    Papase, Tab. (Warner-Chilcott).

    Penicillinase (Various Mfr.).
    Pepsin (Various Mfr.).
    Plasmin. Rennin (Various Mfr.).
    Taka-Diastase, Prep. (Parke-Davis).
    Travase, Oint. (Flint).
    Thrombolysin, I.V. Inj. (Merck & Co.).
    Varidase, Prep. (Lederle).
EPA CAPSULES. (Nature's Bounty) N-3
  fat content (mg) EPA 180 mg, DHA 120
  mg, vitamin E 1 IU. Bot. 50s, 100s.
  Use: Nutritional supplement.
• **EPHEDRINE,** U.S.P. XXIII. l-α-[1-(Methy-
  lamino)-ethyl]benzyl alcohol. (Various
  Mfr.) ()-erythro-α-[1-(Methylamino)eth-
  yl]benzyl Alcohol.
  Use: Adrenergic (bronchodilator).
  See: Bofedrol Inhalant (Bowman).
    Racephedrine HCl (Various Mfr.).
  W/Procaine.
  See: Ephedrine and Procaine, Rx "A",
    Amp. (Lilly).
  W/Pyrilamine maleate, guaifenesin, theo-
  phylline.
  W/Theophylline, guaifenesin, phenobarbi
  tal.
  See: Duovent, Tab. (Riker).
EPHEDRINE & AMYTAL. (Lilly)
  Ephedrine sulfate 25 mg, amobarbital
  50 mg/Pulv. Bot. 100s.
  Use: Decongestant, sedative/hypnotic.
EPHEDRINE HYDROCHLORIDE, U.S.P.
  XXIII. l-a-[1-(Methylamino) ethyl]benzyl
  alcohol hydrochloride. ()-erythro-α-[1-
  (Methylamino)ethyl]-benzyl Alcohol hy-
  drochloride. (Various Mfr.); Cryst. Box
  oz, 0.25 oz, 4 oz.
  Use: Adrenergic (bronchodilator).
EPHEDRINE HCl W/COMBINATIONS.
  See: Asma-lief, Tab., Susp. (Quality
    Generics).
    Ceepa, Tab. (Geneva).
    Co-Xan, Elix. (Central).
    Derma Medicone (Medicone).
    Derma Medicone HC, Oint.
    (Medicone).
    Ectasule, Ectasule Minus, Cap. (Flem-
    ing).
    Golacal, Syr. (Arcum).
    Kie, Tab., Syr. (Laser).
    Lardet Expectorant, Tab. (Standex).
    Lardet, Tab. (Standex).
    Mudrane GG, Tab. (Poythress).
    Mudrane, Tab. (Poythress).
    Pyrralan DM, Expectorant (Lannett).
    Quadrinal, Tab., Susp. (Knoll).
    Quelidrine, Syr. (Abbott).
    Quibron Plus (Bristol).
    Tedral-25, Tab. (Parke-Davis).
    T-E-P Compound, Tab. (Stanlabs).
    Theofedral, Tab. (Redford).

Theofenal, Susp., Tab. (Spencer-Mead).

EPHEDRINE HYDROCHLORIDE NASAL JELLY.
See: Efedron Nasal (Hyrex).

EPHEDRINE and PHENOBARBITAL. (Jenkins) Phenobarbital 0.25 gr, ephedrine HCl gr/Tab. Bot. 1000s. Use: Sedative/hypnotic, decongestant.

EPHEDRINE-RELATED COMPOUNDS.
See: Sympathomimetic Agents.

• **EPHEDRINE SULFATE,** U.S.P. XXIII. Cap., Inj., Nasal Soln., Syr., Tab., U.S.P. XXIII. ()-erythro-α-[1-(Methylamino)ethyl]-benzyl Alcohol. Benzenemethanol, α-[1-(methylamino)ethyl]-, sulfate (2:1) (salt). (Various Mfr). (Abbott) Inj. 50 mg/1 ml amp.
Use: Adrenergic (bronchodilator, nasal decongestant).
See: Ectasule Minus Jr. and Sr., Cap. (Fleming).
Slo-Fedrin, Cap. (Dooner).

EPHEDRINE SULFATE W/COMBINATIONS
See: B.M.E., Elix. (Brothers).
Bronkaid, Tab. (Sanofi Winthrop Products).
Bronkolixir, Elix. (Sanofi Winthrop).
Bronkotabs (Sanofi Winthrop).
Ectasule, Cap. (Fleming).
Ectasule Minus, Cap. (Fleming).
Eponal, Prep. (Cenci).
Marax DF, Syr. (Roerig).
Marax, Tab., Syr. (Roerig).
Neogen, Supp. (Premo).
Pazo, Oint., Supp. (Bristol-Myers).
Rectacort, Supp. (Century).
Va-Tro-Nol, Nose Drops (Vicks).
Wyanoids, Preps. (Wyeth-Ayerst).

• **EPHEDRINE SULFATE AND PHENOBARBITAL CAPSULES,** U.S.P. XXIII.
Use: Adrenergic (Bronchodilator).

1-EPHENAMINE PENICILLIN G. Compenamine.

EPHENYLLIN. (CMC) Theophylline 130 mg, ephedrine HCl 24 mg, phenobarbital 8 mg/Tab. Bot. 100s, 500s, 1000s.
Use: Bronchodilator, decongestant, sedative/hypnotic.

EPHRINE NASAL SPRAY. (Walgreen) Phenylephrine HCl 0.5%. Bot. 20 ml.
Use: Decongestant.

EPHRINITE NO. 1. (Kenyon) Phenylephrine HCl 5 mg, prophenpyridamine 12.5 mg/Tab. Bot. 100s.
Use: Decongestant.

EPI-C. (Lafayette Pharm.) Barium sulfate 150%. Susp. Bot. 450 ml.
Use: Diagnostic aid.

• **EPICILLIN.** USAN. 6-(D-α-Aminocyclohexa-1,4-dien-1-ylacetamido)penicillanic acid.
Use: Antibiotic.
See: Dexacillin.

EPIDERMAL GROWTH FACTOR (HUMAN).
Use: Acoolorato oornoal hoaling. [Orphan drug]

EPI-DERM BALM. (Pedinol) Methyl salicylate, menthol, propylene glycol, alcohol. Bot. gal.
Use: External analgesic.

EPIFOAM. (Reed & Carnrick) Hydrocortisone acetate 1%, pramoxine HCl 1% in base of propylene glycol, cetyl alcohol, PEG-100 stearate, glyceryl stearate, laureth-23, polyoxyl-40 stearate, methylparaben, propylparaben, trolamine, or hydrochloric acid to adjust pH, purified water, butane, propane inert propellant. Aerosol container 10 Gm.
Use: Corticosteroid, topical.

EPIFORM-HC. (Delta) Hydrocortisone 1%, iodohydroxyquin 3% in cream base. Tube 20 Gm.
Use: Corticosteroid, antifungal, topical.

EPIFRIN STERILE OPHTHALMIC SOLUTION. (Allergan) Levo-epinephrine HCl 0.25%, 0.5%, 1% or 2%, benzalkonium Cl, sodium metabisulfite, edetate disodium, purified water. 0.25% also contains sodium Cl. Bot. w/dropper 15 ml.
Use: Agent for glaucoma.

EPILEPSY.
See: Anticonvulsants.

E-PILO. (Iolab Pharm.) Pilocarpine HCl 1%, 2%, 3%, 4% or 6%, epinephrinebitartrate 1%, benzalkonium Cl 0.01%, edetate disodium 0.01%. Bot. 10 ml w/dropper-tip plastic vial.
Use: Agent for glaucoma.

EPILYT. (Stiefel) Propylene glycol, glycerin, oleic acid, quaternium-26, lactic acid, BHT. Lotion. Bot. 118 ml.
Use: Emollient.

• **EPIMESTROL.** USAN. 3-Methoxy-estra-1,3,5(10)-triene-16α, 17α-diol. Stimovul (Organon).
Use: Anterior pituitary activator.

EPIMYCIN A. (Delta) Polymyxin B sulfate 5000 units, bacitracin 400 units, neomycin sulfate 3.5 mg, diperodon HCl 10 mg/Gm. Oint. Tube 0.5 oz.
Use: Anti-infective, external.

EPINAL. (Alcon) Epinephrine 0.5%, 1% as borate complex, benzalkonium Cl 0.01%, ascorbic acid, acetylcysteine, boric acid, sodium carbonate. Dropper

Bot. 7.5 ml
Use: Agent for glaucoma.
EPINEPHRAN.
See: Epinephrine, Preps. (Various Mfr.).
• **EPINEPHRINE,** U.S.P. XXIII. Inh., Soln., Aerosol, Inj., Nasal Soln., Ophth. Soln., Sterile Oil Susp., U.S.P. XXIII. ()-3,4-Dihydroxy-alpha-[(methylamino) methyl]benzyl Alcohol. 1,2-Benzenediol,4-[1-hydroxy-2-(methylamino)ethyl]- Inhalation. Adnephrine, adrenal, adrenamine, adrenine, epinephran, eptreman, hemisine, hemostatin, nephridine, levorenine, paranephrin, renaglandin, renalina, supra-capsulin, suprarenaline, suprarenin, renoform, renostypticin, renostyptin, styptirenal, supradin, supranephrane, surrenine, takamina, vasoconstrictine, vasotonin, hypernephrin, renaleptine, scurenaline, nieraline. **Pediatric Inj.:** (Abbott) Soln. 0.01 mg/ml; 5 ml single-dose Abboject Syringe.
Use: Asthma, hayfever, acute allergic states, cardiac arrest, acute hypersensitivity reactions.
See: Asthma Meter, Aerosol (Rexall).
Asmolin, Vial (Lincoln).
Emergency Ana-Kit (Hollister-Stier)
W/Chlorobutanol, sodium bisulfite.
See: Ana-Guard Epinephrine, Inj. (Hollister Stier/Miles).
W/Lidocaine HCl.
See: Ardecaine 1%, 2%, Inj. (Burgin-Arden).
EPINEPHRINE BORATE.
Use: Adrenergic (ophthalmic).
See: Epinal Ophth. Soln. (Alcon).
Eppy/N Ophth. Soln. (Sola/Barnes-Hind).
EPINEPHRINE HYDROCHLORIDE.
Use: Adrenergic, ophthalmic.
See: Adrenalin Cl, Soln. (Parke-Davis).
Epifrin, Ophth. Soln. (Allergan).
Epinal, Ophth. Soln. (Alcon).
Sus-Phrine, Amp., Vial (Berlex).
Vaponefrin Solution & Nebulizer, Vial (Fisons).
W/Benzalkonium Cl, sodium Cl, sodium metabisulfite.
See: Glaucon, Soln. (Alcon).
W/Pilocarpine HCl.
See: Epicar, Soln. (Barnes-Hind).
EPINEPHRINE, RACEMIC.
See: Asthmanefrin Solution (SK-Beecham).
EPINEPHRINE-RELATED COMPOUNDS.
See: Sympathomimetic Agents.
• **EPINEPHRYL BORATE.** F.D.A. Cyclic (-)- 4-[l-hydroxy-2-(methylamino)ethyl]-o-phenylene borate.
• **EPINEPHRYL BORATE OPHTHALMIC SOLUTION,** U.S.P. XXIII. ()-3,4-Dihydroxy-α-[(methyl-amino)methyl]benzyl alcohol, cyclic 3,4-ester w/boric acid.
Use: Adrenergic (ophthalmic).
See: Epinal (Alcon).
Eppy (Barnes-Hind).
EPIOSTRIOL. B.A.N. Estra-1,3,5(10)-triene-3,16β,17β-triol. 16-epiestriol.
Use: Estrogen.
EPIPEN AUTO-INJECTOR. (Center) Epinephrine injection 1:1000. Delivers dose of 0.3 mg. Pkg. 1s, 2s, 2 ml injectors.
Use: Emergency kit.
EPIPEN JR. AUTO-INJECTOR. (Center) Epinephrine injection 1:2000. Delivers dose of 0.15 mg. Pkg. 1s, 2s, 2 ml injectors.
Use: Emergency kit.
EPIPHENETHICILLIN. L-(a-phenoxy-propionamido) penicillanic acid.
• **EPIPROPIDINE.** USAN. 1,1-Bic(2,3-epoxypropyl)-4,4bipiperidine. Eponate.
Use: Antineoplastic.
EPIRENAN.
See: Epinephrine (Various Mfr.).
• **EPIRIZOLE.** USAN.
Use: Analgesic, anti-inflammatory.
• **EPIRUBICIN HYDROCHLORIDE.** USAN.
Use: Antineoplastic.
EPISONE. (Delta) Hydrocortisone 10 mg in a base containing steryl alcohol, white petrolatum, mineral oil, propylene glycol, polyoxyl 40 stearate, purified water, methyl and propyl parabens. Tube oz.
Use: Corticosteroid.
• **EPITETRACYCLINE HYDROCHLORIDE,** U.S.P.XXII.
Use: Antibiotic.
• **EPITHIAZIDE.** USAN. 3-[(2,2,2-Trifluoroethylthio)methyl]-6-chloro-3,4-dihydro-2H-1,2,4-benzothiadiazine-7-sulfonamide 1,1-dioxide.
Use: Hypotensive and diuretic.
EPITOL. (Lemmon) Carbamazepine 200 mg/Tab. Bot. 500s, 1000s, UD 100s.
Use: Anticonvulsant.
E-PLUS. (Drug Industries) Vitamins E 73.5 mg, niacin 20 mg, lemon bioflavonoid complex 25 mg, C 50 mg, B_6 2 mg, B_1 5 mg/Tab. Bot. 100s, 500s.
Use: Vitamin supplement.
EPO.
See: Epogen (Amgen).
Procrit (Ortho Biotech).
• **EPOETIN ALFA.** USAN.
Use: Recombinant human erythropoietin, antianemic. [Orphan drug]

See: Epogen (Amgen).
Procrit (Ortho Biotech).
• **EPOETIN BETA.** USAN.
Use: Recombinant human erythropoi-
etin, antianemic. [Orphan drug]
EPOGEN. (Amgen) Epoetin Alfa (Erythro-
poietin; EPO) 2,000 units, 3,000 units,
4,000 units, 10,000 units, Preservative
free. Vial 1 ml.
Use: Recombinant human erythropoi-
etin.
• **EPOPROSTENOL.** USAN.
Use: Inhibitor (platelet). [Orphan drug]
• **EPOPROSTENOL SODIUM.** USAN.
Use: Inhibitor (platelet).
• **EPOSTANE.** USAN.
Use: Interceptive agent.
**EPOXYTROPINE TROPATE METHYL-
BROMIDE.**
See: Methscopolamine Bromide (Vari-
ous Mfr.).
EPPY/N. (Barnes-Hind) Epinephryl bo-
rate ophthalmic soln. 0.5%, 1% or 2%.
Bot. 7.5 ml.
Use: Agent for glaucoma.
• **EPRISTERIDE.** USAN.
Use: Treatment of benign prostate hy-
pertrophy.
EPROMATE. (Major) Aspirin 325 mg,
meprobamate 200 mg Tab. Bot. 100s,
500s.
Use: Salicylate analgesic, antianxiety
agent.
• **EPROSARTAN.** USAN.
Use: Antihypertensive.
EPSAL. (Press) Saturated soln. of epsom
salts 80% in ointment form. Jar 0.5 oz, 2
oz.
Use: Drawing ointment.
EPSIVITE 100. (Standex) Vitamin E 100
IU/Cap. Bot. 100s.
Use: Vitamin E supplement.
EPSIVITE 200. (Standex) Vitamin E 200
IU/Cap. Bot. 100s.
Use: Vitamin E supplement.
EPSIVITE 400. (Standex) Vitamin E 400
IU/Cap. Bot. 100s.
Use: Vitamin E supplement.
EPSIVITE FORTE. (Standex) Vitamin E
1000 IU/Cap. Bot. 100s.
Use: Vitamin E supplement.
EPSOM SALT.
See: Magnesium Sulfate.
EPT. (Parke-Davis Prods) In-home preg-
nancy test.
Use: Diagnostic aid.
E.P.T. PLUS. (Warner-Lambert) Reagent
in-home kit for urine testing. Pregnancy
test. Kit 1s.
Use: Diagnostic aid.

E.P.T. STICK TEST. (Warner-Lambert)
Reagent in-home kit for urine testing.
Pregnancy test. Kit 1s.
Use: Diagnostic aid.
EPTOIN.
See: Phenytoin Sodium (Various Mfr.).
EQUAGESIC. (Wyeth-Ayerst) Meproba-
mate 200 mg, aspirin 325 mg/Tab. Bot.
100s, Redi-pak 100s.
Use: Antianxiety agent, salicylate anal-
gesic.
EQUAL. (Nutrasweet) Aspartame. **Pack-
et:** 0.035 oz. (1 Gm). Box 50s, 100s,
200s. **Tab.:** Bot. 100s.
Use: Artificial sweetener.
EQUALACTIN. (Numark) Polycarbophil
500 mg (as calcium
polycarbophil)/Chew. tab.
Use: Antidiarrheal or laxative.
EQUANIL. (Wyeth-Ayerst) Meprobamate
200 mg or 400 mg/Tab. **200 mg:** Bot.
100s. **400 mg:** Bot. 100s, 500s, Redipak
25s.
Use: Antianxiety agent.
EQUAZINE M. (Rugby) Aspirin 325 mg,
meprobamate 200 mg, tartrazine tab.
Bot. 100s, 500s.
Use: Salicylate analgesic, antianxiety
agent.
EQUILET. (Mission) Calcium carbonate
500 mg/Chew. tab. Strip packed in 100s.
Use: Antacid.
• **EQUILIN,** U.S.P. XXIII. Estra-1, 3-5 (10),
7-tetraen-17 one, 3 hydroxy-3-Hydrox-
estra-1,3,5 (10), 7-tetraen-17-one.
Use: Estrogen.
EQUIPERTINE CAPSULES. (Sanofi
Winthrop) Oxypertine.
Use: Antianxiety agent, tranquilizer.
ERADACIL CAPSULES. (Sanofi
Winthrop) Rosoxacin.
Use: Antigonococcal agent.
ERAMYCIN. (Wesley) Erythromycin 250
mg (as stearate)/FC tab. Bot. 100s,
500s.
Use: Anti-infective.
• **ERBULOZOLE.** USAN.
Use: Radiosensitizer; antineoplastic.
ERCAF. (Geneva Marsam) Ergotamine
tartrate 1 mg, caffeine 100 mg/Tab. Bot.
100s, 1000s.
Use: Agent for migraine.
ERGAMISOL. (Janssen) Levamisole
(base) 50 mg/Tab. Blister pack 36s.
Use: Antineoplastic agent.
ERGO CAFF. (Rugby) Ergotamine tar-
trate 1 mg, caffeine 100 mg/Tab. Bot.
100s.
Use: Agent for migraine.
• **ERGOCALCIFEROL,** U.S.P. XXIII. Cap.,

Tab., Oral Soln. U.S.P. XXIII. 9, 10-Sec-oergosta-5,7,10(19),22-tetraen-3-ol, (3β-. Irradiated Ergosta-5,7,22-trien-3-beta-ol).
Use: Treatment of refractory rickets; familial hypophosphatemia; hypoparathyroidism.
See: Calciferol.
Drisdol, Liq., Cap. (Sanofi Winthrop).
Geltabs, Cap. (Upjohn).
ERGOCORNINE. (Various Mfr.) Ergot alkaloid.
Use: Peripheral vascular disorders.
ERGOCRISTINE. (Various Mfr.) Ergot alkaloid.
Use: Vascular disorders.
ERGOCRYPTINE. (Various Mfr.) Ergot alkaloid.
Use: Peripheral vascular disorders.
•**ERGOLOID MESYLATES,** U.S.P. XXIII. Oral Soln., Tab., U.S.P.XXII. (Lederle)
0.5 mg: Dihydroergocornine 0.167 mg, dihydroergocristine 0.167 mg, dihydroergocryptine 0.167 mg/0.5 mg Sublingual Tab. **1 mg:** Dihydroergocornine 0.333 mg, dihydroergocristine 0.333 mg, dihydro-ergocryptine 0.333 mg/1 mg Tab. Bot. 100s, 1000s.
Use: Psychotherapeutic agent.
See: Hydergine Prods. (Sandoz).
ERGOMAR. (Fisons) Ergotamine tartrate 2 mg/Sublingual Tab. Pkg. 20s.
Use: Agent for migraine.
ERGOMETRINE MALEATE.
See: Ergonovine (Various Mfr.).
ERGONAL. (Vita Elixir) Ergot powder 259.2 mg, aloin 8.1 mg, apiol fluid green 290 mg, oil pennyroyal 28 mg/Cap. Bot. 24s.
Use: Oxytocic.
ERGONOVINE. (Various Mfr.) Ergobasine, erolklinine, ergometrine, ergostetrine, ergotocine.
Use: Oxytocic.
See: Ergonovine Maleate.
•**ERGONOVINE MALEATE,** U.S.P. XXIII. Inj., Tab., U.S.P. XXIII. 9,10-Didehydro-N-[(S)-2-hydroxy-1-methylethyl]-6-methylergoline-8β-carboxamide maleate.
Use: IV, IM, orally, oxytocic.
See: Ergotrate Maleate, Preps. (Lilly).
ERGOSTAT. (Parke-Davis) Ergotamine tartrate 2 mg/Sublingual Tab. Vial UD 24s.
Use: Agent for migraine.
ERGOSTEROL, ACTIVATED OR IRRADIATED.
See: Ergocalciferol, U.S.P. XXIII.

ERGOSTETRINE.
See: Ergonovine (Various Mfr.).
•**ERGOTAMINE TARTRATE,** U.S.P. XXIII. Inj., Inhalation Aerosol, Tab., U.S.P. XXIII. Ergotaman-3,6,18-trione, 12-hydroxy-2-methyl-5-(phenylmethyl)-2,3-dihydroxybutanedioate (2:1) (salt). Femergin.
Use: Analgesic (specific in migraine).
See: Ergomar, Tab. (Fisons).
Ergostat, Tab. (Parke-Davis).
Gynergen, Amp., Tab. (Sandoz).
Medihaler-Ergotamine, Vial (Riker).
W/Belladonna alkaloids, acetophenetidin, caffeine.
See: Wigraine, Tab., Supp. (Organon).
W/Belladonna alkaloids, pentobarbital.
See: Cafergot P-B, Supp., Tab. (Sandoz).
W/Belladonna alkaloids, phenobarbital.
See: Bellergal, Tab. (Dorsey).
W/Caffeine.
See: Cafergot, Tab., Supp. (Sandoz).
W/Caffeine, homatropine methylbromide.
See: Ergotatropin, Tab. (Cole).
W/Cyclizine HCl, caffeine.
See: Migral Tab. (Burroughs Wellcome).
W/1-Hyoscyamine sulfate, phenobarbital.
See: Ergkatal, Tab. (Gilbert).
•**ERGOTAMINE TARTRATE AND CAFFEINE SUPPOSITORIES,** U.S.P. XXIII.
Use: Vascular headache.
See: Cafergot, Supp. (Sandoz).
•**ERGOTAMINE TARTRATE AND CAFFEINE TABLETS,** U.S.P. XXIII.
Use: Vascular headache.
See: Cafergot, Tab. (Sandoz).
Ergocaf, Tab. (Robinson).
Lanatrate, Tab. (Lannett).
ERGOT, FLUID EXTRACT. (Various Mfr.) Ergot 1 Gm/ml Bot. 4 oz, pt.
ERGOTIDINE.
See: Histamine (Various Mfr.).
ERGOTOCINE.
See: Ergonovine (Various Mfr.).
ERGOTRATE.
See: Ergonovine (Various Mfr.).
ERGOTRATE-H.
See: Ergonovine (Various Mfr.).
ERGOT-RELATED PRODUCTS.
See: Cafergot, Supp., Tab. (Sandoz).
Cafergot P-B, Supp., Tab. (Sandoz).
DHE-45, Amp. (Sandoz).
Ergonovine (Various Mfr.).
Ergotamine (Various Mfr.).
Ergotrate (Various Mfr.).
Gynergen, Amp., Tab. (Sandoz).
Hydergine, Sub. Tab. (Sandoz).

Hydro-Ergot, Tab. (Interstate).
Methergine, Amp., Tab. (Sandoz).
Trigot, Sublingual Tab. (Squibb).
Wigraine, Supp., Tab. (Organon).
ERGOZIDE. (Jenkins) Carbolic acid
2.25%, ergot extract 2.5%, zinc oxide
10%, balsam Peru 1.25%, oil cade
0.3%, Pkg. lh.
ERIDIUM. (Hauck) Phenazopyridine HCl
100 mg/Tab. Bot. 32s, 1000s.
Use: Urinary analgesic.
ERIODICTIN.
See: Vitamin P & Rutin.
•**ERIODICTYON,** N.F. XVIII. Flext., Aromatic Syrup, N.F. XVIII.
Use: Pharmaceutic aid (flavor).
See: Vitamin P & Rutin.
E-R-O. (Scherer) Propylene glycol, glycerol. Bot. w/dropper tip 15 ml.
Use: Otic preparation.
•**ERSOFERMIN.** USAN.
Use: Wound healing agent.
ERTINE. (Approved) Hexachlorophene,
benzocaine, cod liver oil, allantoin, boric
acid, lanolin. Tube 1.5 oz.
Use: Burn and first aid remedy.
ERWINIA ASPARAGINASE.
Use: Antineoplastic agent. [Orphan
drug]
ERYC. (Parke-Davis) Erythromycin enteric coated 250 mg/Tab. Bot. 40s, 100s,
500s, UD 100s.
Use: Anti-infective.
ERYCETTE. (Ortho Derm) Erythromycin
2% 20 mg/ml. Pkg. 60 pledgets.
Use: Anti-acne.
ERYDERM 2%. (Abbott) Erythromycin
topical soln. 2%. Bot. 60 ml.
Use: Anti-acne.
ERYGEL. (Herbert) Erythromycin 2%.
Gel Tube 30 Gm.
Use: Anti-infective, external.
ERYMAX TOPICAL SOLUTION. (Herbert) Erythromycin 2% Soln. 60 ml, 120
ml.
Use: Anti-acne.
ERYPAR. (Parke-Davis) Erythromycin
stearate 250 mg or 500 mg/Filmseal.
250 mg: Bot. 100s, 500s. **500 mg:** Bot.
100s.
Use: Anti-infective.
ERYPED. (Abbott) Erythromycin ethylsuccinate granules for oral susp. representing erythromycin activity of 400
mg/5 ml. Bot. 60 ml, 100 ml, 200 ml, UD
5 ml, 100s.
Use: Anti-infective.
ERY-SOL. (Dermol) Erythromycin 2% /
Soln. Bot. 66 ml.
Use: Anti-acne.

ERY-TAB. (Abbott) Erythromycin enteric
coated 250 mg, 333 mg or 500 mg/Tab.
250 mg: Bot. 30s, 40s, 100s, 500s, UD
100s. **333 mg:** Bot. 100s, 500s, UD
100s. **500 mg:** Bot. 100s, UD 100s.
Use: Anti-infective.
•**ERYTHRITYL TETRANITRATE, DILUTED,** U.S.P. XXIII.
Use: Coronary vasodilator.
•**ERYTHRITYL TETRANITRATE
TABLETS,** U.S.P. XXIII. (Various Mfr.)
Erythritol, erythrol tetranitrate, nitroerythrite, tetranitrin, tetranitrol.
Use: Coronary vasodilator.
See: Anginar, Tab. (Pasadena Research Labs.). Cardilate, Tab. (Burroughs Wellcome).
W/Phenobarbital.
See: Cardilate-P, Tab. (Burroughs Wellcome).
ERYTHROCIN LACTOBIONATE, I.V.
(Abbott Hospital Prods) Erythromycin
lactobionate. Pow. 500 mg/vial w/benzyl
alcohol 90 mg; 1 Gm/vial w/benzyl alcohol 180 mg. Pkg. Vial 5s.
Use: Anti-infective.
ERYTHROCIN LACTOBIONATE PIGGYBACK. (Abbott Hospital Prods) Erythromycin lactobionate for injection, 500
mg/dispensing vial. 5 mg/ml of erythromycin after reconstitution w/90 mg
benzyl alcohol. Pow. Pkg. 5 100 ml dispensing vials.
Use: Anti-infective.
ERYTHROCIN STEARATE. (Abbott) Erythromycin stearate 250 mg or 500
mg/Tab. **250 mg:** Bot. 40s, 100s, 500s,
UD 100s; **500 mg:** Bot. 100s.
Use: Anti-infective.
•**ERYTHROMYCIN,** U.S.P. XXIII. Delayed-release Cap., Oint., Ophth. Oint., Delayed-release Tab., Tab., Topical Soln.,
Topical Gel, U.S.P. XXIII. An antibiotic
from Streptomyces erythreus. (Upjohn)
Tab. 100 mg. Bot. 100s; 250 mg. Bot.
25s, 100s. (Various Mfr.) 5 mg/g Oint.
Tube 3.5 g, 3.75 g, UD 1 g.
Use: Antibiotic.
See: AK-Mycin, Oint. (Akorn).
A/T/S, Gel (Hoechst-Roussel).
Del-Mycin, Soln. (Del Ray).
Emgel, Gel (Glaxo).
E-Mycin, Tab. (Upjohn).
Erymax, Soln. (Herbert).
EryDerm, Soln. (Abbott).
Ery-sol, Soln. (Dermol).
Erythrocin, Prep. (Abbott).
Erythromycin, Gel (Glades).
Erythromycin Base, Filmtab (Abbott).
Ilotycin, Prep. (Dista).

PCE, Tab. (Abbott).
Robimycin, Tab. (Robins).
Romycin, Topical Soln. (Roberts).
RP-Mycin, Tab. (Solvay).
T-Stat, Pads (Westwood-Squibb).
Theramycin Z, Soln. (Medicis).
ERYTHROMYCIN. (Glades) Erythromycin 2%, alcohol 95% / Gel. Tube 30 g, 60 g.
Use: Anti-acne.
•**ERYTHROMYCIN ACISTRATE.** USAN.
Use: Antibiotic.
•**ERYTHROMYCIN AND BENZOYL PEROXIDE TOPICAL GEL,** U.S.P. XXIII.
Use: Antibiotic, keratolytic.
ERYTHROMYCIN BASE FILMTAB. (Abbott) Erythromycin base 250 mg or 500 mg/Tab. **250 mg:** Bot. 100s, 500s, UD 100s. **500 mg:** Bot 100s.
Use: Anti-infective.
•**ERYTHROMYCIN ESTOLATE,** U.S.P. XXIII. Cap., Oral Susp., for Oral Susp., Tab., U.S.P. XXIII. Supp., Erythromycin 2-propionate dodecyl sulfate. Lauryl sulfate salt of the propionic acid ester of erythromycin.
Use: Antibiotic.
See: Ilosone, Preps. (Dista).
•**ERYTHROMYCIN ETHYLSUCCINATE,** U.S.P. XXIII. Inj., Tab., for Oral Susp., Oral Susp., Sterile, U.S.P. XXIII. Erythromycin 2-(Ethylsuccinate).
Use: Antibiotic.
See: E.E.S. Prods. (Abbott). E-mycin E, Liq. (Upjohn). Pediamycin Prods. (Ross). Pediazole, Liq. (Ross). Wyamycin-E, Liq. (Wyeth-Ayerst).
•**ERYTHROMYCIN ETHYLSUCCINATE AND SULFISOXAZOLE ACETYL FOR ORAL SUSPENSION,** U.S.P. XXIII.
Use: Antibiotic, anti-infective.
See: Pediazole, Susp. (Ross).
•**ERYTHROMYCIN GLUCEPTATE, STERILE,** U.S.P. XXIII.
Use: Antibacterial.
See: Ilotycin Gluceptate, Amp. (Dista).
ERYTHROMYCIN GLUCOHEPTONATE.
See: Erythromycin Gluceptate, U.S.P. XXIII. Ilotycin Glucoheptonate, Amp. (Dista).
•**ERYTHROMYCIN LACTOBIONATE FOR INJECTION,** U.S.P. XXIII.
Use: Antibacterial.
See: Erythrocin Lactobionate, Vial (Abbott).
ERYTHROMYCIN 2-PROPIONATE DODECYL SULFATE. Erythromycin Estolate, U.S.P. XXIII.
Use: Antibacterial.
•**ERYTHROMYCIN PLEDGETS,** U.S.P.

XXIII.
Use: Antibiotic.
ERYTHROMYCIN PROPIONATE LAURYL SULFATE.
Use: Anti-infective.
See: Erthromycin Estolate. Ilosone, Preps. (Dista).
•**ERYTHROMYCIN STEARATE,** U.S.P. XXIII. Tab., for Oral Susp., U.S.P. XXII.
Use: Antibacterial.
See: Erythrocin Stearate Prods. (Abbott).
Erypar Filmseal, Tab. (Parke-Davis).
Wyamycin-S, Tab. (Wyeth-Ayerst).
ERYTHROMYCIN SULFATE.
Use: Anti-infective.
ERYTHROMYCIN TOPICAL. (Various Mfr.) 2% Gel. Tube 30 g, 60 g.
Use: Anti-acne agent, anti-infective.
See: Benzamycin (Dermik).
Emgel (Glaxo).
Erygel (Herbert).
ERYTHROPOLETIN (RECOMBINANT HUMAN).
Use: Antianemic. [Orphan drug]
•**ERYTHROSINE SODIUM,** U.S.P. XXII. Topical Soln., Soluble Tab., U.S.P. XXII.
Use: Diagnostic aid (dental disclosing agent).
ERYZOLE. (Alra) Erythromycin ethylsuccinate 200 mg, acetyl sulfisoxazole 600 mg/5 ml when reconstituted. Gran for Susp. 100 ml, 150 ml, 200 ml.
Use: Anti-infective.
ESCLABRON. Guaithylline.
Use: Antiasthmatic.
ESERDINE FORTE TABS. (Major) Methyclothiazide, reserpine 0.5 mg/Tab. Bot. 100s.
Use: Diuretic, antihypertensive.
ESERDINE TABS. (Major) Methyclothiazide, reserpine 0.25 mg/Tab. Bot. 100s, 250s.
Use: Diuretic, antihypertensive.
ESERINE. Physostigmine as alkaloid, salicylate or sulfate salt.
Use: Agent for glaucoma.
ESERINE SALICYLATE. (Alcon) Physostigmine 0.5%. Soln. 2 ml.
Use: Agent for glaucoma.
ESERINE SULFATE STERILE OPHTHALMIC OINTMENT. (CooperVision) Physostigmine sulfate 0.25%. Tube 3.5 Gm.
Use: Agent for glaucoma.
ESERINE SULFATE. (Robinson) Physostigmine sulfate 0.25%. Oint. Tube oz.
Use: Agent for glaucoma.
ESGIC CAPSULES. (Forest) Butalbital

50 mg, caffeine 40 mg, acetaminophen 325 mg/Cap. Bot. 100s.
Use: Sedative/hypnotic, analgesic.

ESGIC TABLETS. (Forest) Butalbital 50 mg, caffeine 40 mg, acetaminophen 325 mg/Tab. Bot. 100s.
Use: Sedative/hypnotic, analgesic.

ESGIC-PLUS. (Forest) Acetaminophen 500 mg, butalbital 50 mg, caffeine 40 mg/Tab. Bot. 100s, 500s.
Use: Analgesic, sedative/hypnotic.

ESIDRIX. (Ciba) Hydrochlorothiazide 25 mg, 50 mg/Tab. **25 mg:** Bot. 100s, 1000s, UD 100s. **50 mg:** Bot. 100s, 360s, 720s, 1000s, UD 100s. **100 mg:** Bot. 100s.
Use: Diuretic, antihypertensive.
W/Apresoline.
See: Apresoline-Esidrix, Tab. (Ciba).

ESIMIL. (Ciba) Hydrochlorothiazide 25 mg, guanethidine monosulfate 10 mg/Tab. Bot. 100s, Consumer Pack 100s.
Use: Diuretic, antihypertensive.

ESKALITH. (SKF) Lithium carbonate. **Cap.:** 300 mg. Bot. 100s, 500s; **Tab.:** 300 mg. Bot. 100s.
Use: Antipsychotic agent.

ESKALITH CR. (SKF) Lithium carbonate 450 mg/CR tab. Bot. 100s.
Use: Antipsychotic agent.

• **ESMOLOL HYDROCHLORIDE.** USAN. (1) Benzenepropanoic acid, 4-[2-hydroxy-3-[(1-methylethyl)amino]propoxy]-, methyl ester, hydrochloride, (±)-; (2) (±)-Methyl p.[2-hydroxy-3-(isopropyl-amino)propoxy]hydro cinnamate hydrochloride.
Use: Short acting beta-adrenergic blocking agent.
See: Brevibloc, Inj. (DuPont).

E-SOLVE. (Syosset) Alcohol 75%, propylene glycol, diethanolamide, polysorbate 80, talc, titanium dioxide, iron oxides, povidone, water soluble cellulose gum. Lot. Bot. 50 ml.
Use: Lotion base.

E-SOLVE-2. (Syosset) Erythromycin 2%, alcohol 80%, propylene glycol, lauramide DEA, zinc acetate, hydroxypropyl cellulose, iron oxides. Topical soln. Bot. 60 ml.
Use: Anti-acne.

E-SON. (Eastwood) Bot. 100s.
• **ESORUBICIN HYDROCHLORIDE.** USAN.
Use: Antineoplastic.

ESOTERICA DRY SKIN TREATMENT LOTION. (Norcliff Thayer) Bot. 13 fl oz.
Use: Emollient.

ESOTERICA FACIAL. (Medicis) Hydroquinone 2%, padimate O 3.3%, oxybenzone 2.5%, sodium bisulfites, parabens, EDTA. Cream, Tube 85 Gm.
Use: Topical drug.

ESOTERICA MEDICATED FADE CREAM, (Norcliff Thayer) Hydroquinone 2%, padimate O 3.3%, oxybenzone 2.5%. Cream. Jar 90 Gm.
Use: Skin bleaching agent.

ESOTERICA MEDICATED FADE CREAM, FACIAL. (Norcliff Thayer) Hydroquinone 2%, padimate O 3.3%, oxybenzone 2.5% in cream base. Jar 90 Gm, scented or unscented.
Use: Skin bleaching agent.

ESOTERICA MEDICATED FADE CREAM, REGULAR. (Norcliff Thayer) Hydroquinone 2%. Cream. Jar 90 Gm.
Use: Skin bleaching agent.

ESOTERICA SENSITIVE SKIN FORMULA. (SK-Beecham) Hydroquinone 1.5% with mineral oil, sodium bisulfite, parabens, EDTA. Cream. Jar 85 Gm.
Use: Skin bleaching agent.

ESPOTABS. (Combe) Yellow phenolphthalein 97.2 mg/Tab. Bot. 12s, 30s, 60s.
Use: Laxative.

• **ESPROQUIN HYDROCHLORIDE.** USAN.
Use: Adrenergic.

ESSENTIAL-8. Liquid amino acid protein supplement.
Use: Protein supplement.
See: Vivonex Diets, Liq. (Norwich Eaton).

ESTAR. (Westwood) Tar equivalent to 5% coal tar, U.S.P. in a hydro-alcoholic gel w/alcohol 13.8%. Tube 3 oz.
Use: Antipsoriatic, antipruritic.

• **ESTAZOLAM.** USAN.
Use: Sedative/Hypnotic.
See: ProSom (Abbott).

ESTER-C PLUS. (Solgar) Vitamin C 500 mg, citrus bioflavonoid complex 25 mg, acerola 10 mg, rutin 5 mg, rose hips 10 mg, calcium 62 mg/Cap. Bot. 50s.
Use: Vitamin supplement.

EST-D.
See: D-EST.

ESTER-C PLUS, EXTRA POTENCY. (Solgar) Vitamin C 1000 mg, citrus bioflavonoid complex 200 mg, acerola 25 mg, rutin 25 mg, rose hips 25 mg, calcium 125 mg/Tab. Bot. 30s.
Use: Vitamin supplement.

• **ESTERIFILCON A.** USAN.
Use: Contact lens material.

ESTILBEN.
See: Diethylstilbestrol Dipropionate

(Various Mfr.).
ESTINYL. (Schering) Ethinyl estradiol. **0.02 mg, 0.05 mg/Tab., coated:** Bot. 100s, 250s; **0.5 mg/Tab.:** Bot. 100s.
Use: Estrogen.
ESTOLATE. Erythromycin.
See: Erythromycin Propionate Lauryl Sulfate.
ESTOPEN.
See: Benzylpenicillin 2-diethylaminoethyl ester Hl.
ESTRACE. (Mead Johnson Labs) Estradiol micronized 0.5 mg, 1 mg or 2 mg/Tab. Bot. 100s.
Use: Estrogen.
ESTRACE VAGINAL CREAM. (Mead Johnson) 17β Estradiol 0.1 mg/Gm. Tube 42.5 Gm.
Use: Estrogen.
ESTRACON. (Freeport) Conjugated estrogens 1.25 mg/Tab. Bot. 1000s.
Use: Estrogen.
ESTRA-D. (Seatrace) Estradiol cypionate in oil 5 mg/ml Inj. Vial 10 ml.
Use: Estrogen.
ESTRADERM TRANSDERMAL. (Ciba) Estradiol. **0.05:** Each 10 × 10 cm. system contains 4 mg of estradiol for nominal delivery of 0.05 mg estradiol/day. Patient calendar packs of 8 and 24 systems. Ctn 6s. **0.1:** Each 20 × 20 cm. system contains 8 mg estradiol for nominal delivery of 0.1 mg estradiol/day. Patient calendar packs of 8 and 24 systems. Ctn. 6s.
Use: Estrogen.
• **ESTRADIOL,** U.S.P. XXIII. Pellets, Sterile Susp., Tab., U.S.P. XXIII. Estra-1,3,5(10)-triene-3,17-β-diol. Beta-estradiol, agofollin, dihydroxyestrin, dihydrotheelin, gynergon, gynoestryl. The form now known to be physiologically active is the "beta" form rather than the "alpha" form.
Use: Estrogen-replacement therapy.
See: Aquagen, Vial, Aq. (Remsen).
  Estrace, Tab., Vaginal Creme (Mead Johnson).
  Estraderm, Transdermal (Ciba).
  Femogen, Susp., Tab. (Fellows-Testagar).
  Progynon, Pellets (Schering).
W/Estriol, estrone. Hormonin No. 1 and 2, Tab. (Carnrick).
W/Estrone, estriol.
See: Sanestro, Tab. (Sandia).
W/Estrone, potassium estrone sulfate.
See: Tri-Estrin, Inj. (Keene).
W/Progesterone, testosterone, procaine HCl, procaine base.

See: Horm-Triad, Vial (Bell).
W/Testerone.
W/Testosterone and chlorobutanol in cottonseed oil.
See: Depo-Testadiol, Vial (Upjohn).
Transdermal.
See: Estraderm, Patch (Ciba).
ESTRADIOL CYCLOPENTYLPROPIONATE, Estradiol 17-beta(3-cyclopentyl)propionate. Estradiol Cypionate, U.S.P. XXIII. W/Testosterone cypionate.
See: Depo-Testadiol, Vial (Upjohn).
• **ESTRADIOL CYPIONATE,** U.S.P. XXIII. Inj. U.S.P. XXIII. Estradiol 17-β-(3-Cyclopentyl)propionate Estradiol 17-cyclopentanepropionate. Estra-1,3,5-(10)-triene-3,17-diol,(17 beta)-, 17-cyclopentane-propanoate.
Use: Estrogen.
See: Estradiol cyclopentylpropionate.
  Depo-Estradiol Cypionate, Inj. (Upjohn).
  Depogen, Inj. (Hyrex).
  D-Est, Inj. (Burgin-Arden).
  Estro-Cyp, Vial (Keene).
  Estroject-L.A., Vial (Mayrand).
  Hormogen Depot, Inj. (Hauck).
  Span-F, Inj. (Scrip).
W/Testosterone cypionate.
See: D-Diol, Inj. (Burgin-Arden).
  Dep-Tesestro, Inj. (ICN).
  Duo-Cyp, Vial (Keene).
  Duracrine, Inj. (Ascher).
  Menoject, L.A., Vial (Mayrand).
  T.E. Ionate P.A., Inj. (Solvay).
W/Testosterone cypionate, chlorobutanol.
See: Depo-Testadiol (Upjohn).
  Span F.M., Inj. (Scrip).
  T.E. Ionate P.A., Inj. (Solvay).
ESTRADIOL DIPROPIONATE. Estra-1,3,5(10)-triene-3,17 β-diol dipropionate. Ovocyclin Dipropionate.
Use: Estrogen.
• **ESTRADIOL ENANTHATE.** USAN. Estradiol 17-enanthate.
Use: Estrogen.
ESTRADIOL, ETHINYL.
See: Ethinyl Estradiol.
ESTRADIOL MONOBENZONATE.
See: Estradiol Benzoate.
ESTRADIOL PHOSPHATE.
See: Estradurin, Secule (Wyeth-Ayerst).
• **ESTRADIOL UNDECYLATE.** USAN. Estradiol 17-undecanoate.
Use: Estrogen.
See: Delestrec.
• **ESTRADIOL VAGINAL CREAM,** U.S.P.

XXIII.
Use: Estrogen.
• **ESTRADIOL VALERATE,** U.S.P. XXIII.
Inj., U.S.P. XXIII. Estra-1,3,5(10)-triene-
3,17-diol (17β)-,17-pentano-ate. Estra-
diol 17-valerate. (Various Mfr.) Inj. **10
mg/ml:** Vial 5 or 10 ml; **20 mg/ml:** Vial
10 ml; **40 mg/ml·** Vial 10 ml
Use: ogen.
See: Ardefem 10, 20, Inj. (Burgin-Ar-
den).
Deladiol, Inj. (Steris).
Delestrogen, Vial (Mead Johnson).
Depogen, Inj. (Sig).
Dioval, Preps. (Keene).
Duragen, Inj. (Roberts Hauck).
Duratrad, Inj. (Ascher).
Estate, Inj. (Savage).
Estra-L, Inj. (Pasadena Research).
Gynogen L.A., Inj. (Forest).
Span-Est, Inj. (Scrip).
Valergen, Inj. (Hyrex).
W/Benzyl alcohol.
See: Estate, Vial (Savage).
Reposo E-40, Vial (Paddock).
W/Hydroxyprogesterone caproate.
See: Hy-Gestradol, Inj. (Pasadena-Re-
search).
Hylutin-Est, Inj. (Hyrex).
W/Testosterone cypionate.
See: Depo-Testadiol, Inj. (Upjohn).
W/Testosterone enanthate.
See: Ardiol 90/4, 180/8, Inj. (Burgin-Ar-
den).
Deladumone, Vial (Squibb Mark).
Delatestadiol, Vial (Dunhall).
Duoval-P.A., I.M. (Solvay).
Estra-Testrin, Inj. (Pasadena Re-
search).
Span-Est-Test 4, Inj. (Scrip).
Teev, Inj. (Keene).
Tesogen L.A., Inj. (Sig).
Testanate, Vial (Kenyon).
Valertest, Inj. (Hyrex).
W/Testosterone enanthate, benzyl al-
cohol, sesame oil.
See: Repose-TE (Paddock).
ESTRADOL. (Kenyon) Ethinyl estradiol.
No. 1: 0.02 mg/Tab. **No. 2:** 0.05 mg/Tab.
Bot.
Use: Estrogen.
ESTRA-L. (Pasadena Research) Estradi-
ol valerate in castor oil. **20 mg/ml:** Vial
10 ml. 40 mg/ml: Vial 10 ml.
Use: Estrogen.
ESTRALUTIN.
See: Relutin (Solvay).
• **ESTRAMUSTINE.** USAN. Estradiol 3-bis
(2-chloroethyl) carbamate 17-(dihydro-
gen phosphate), disodium salt.

Use: Antineoplastic agent.
• **ESTRAMUSTINE PHOSPHATE SODIUM.**
USAN.
Use: Antineoplastic agent.
See: Emcyt, Cap. (Pharmacia).
ESTRATAB. (Solvay) **Tab.:** Esterified es-
trogens, principally sodium estrone sul-
fate 0.3 mg, 0.625 mg, 1.25 mg or 2.5
mg/Tab. Bot. 100s, 1000s.
Use: Estrogen.
ESTRATEST. (Solvay) Esterified estro-
gens 1.25 mg, methyltestosterone 2.5
mg/Tab. Bot. 100s, 1000s.
Use: Estrogen, androgen combination.
ESTRATEST H.S. (Solvay) Esterified es-
trogens 0.625 mg, methyltestosterone
1.25 mg/Tab. Bot. 100s.
Use: Estrogen, androgen combination.
ESTRA-TESTRIN. (Pasadena Research)
Testosterone enanthate 90 mg, estradiol
valerate 4 mg in oil/ml. Inj. Vial 10 ml.
Use: Androgen, estrogen combination.
• **ESTRAZINOL HYDROBROMIDE.** USAN.
dl-trans-3-Methoxy-8-aza-19-nor-17a-
pregna-1,3,5-trien-20-yn-17-ol hydro-
bromide.
Use: Estrogen.
ESTRIN.
See: Estrone.
ESTRINEX. (Adria)
See: TOREMIFENE.
• **ESTRIOL,** U.S.P. XXIII.
Use: Estrogen.
ESTRITONE NO. 1. (Kenyon) Conjugated
estrogens equine 0.625 mg, methyl-
testosterone 5 mg/Tab. Bot. 100s,
1000s.
Use: Estrogen, androgen combination.
ESTRITONE NO. 2. (Kenyon) Conjugated
estrogens equine 1.25 mg, methyl-
testosterone 10 mg/Tab. Bot. 100s,
1000s.
Use: Estrogen, androgen combination.
ESTROBENE DP.
See: Diethylstilbestrol Dipropionate
(Various Mfr.).
ESTRO-CYP. (Keene) Estradiol cypi-
onate 5 mg/ml in oil. Inj. Vial 10 ml.
Use: Estrogen.
ESTROFEM. (Pasadena Research)
Estradiol cypionate 5 mg/ml in oil. Inj.
Vial 10 ml.
Use: Estrogen.
• **ESTROFURATE.** USAN. (1)21, 23-
Epoxy-19-24-dinor-17α-chola-
1,3,5(10),7,20,22-hexaene-3,17-diol-3-
acetate; (2) 17-(3-furyl) estra-1,3,5-
(10),7-tetraene-3,17β-diol-3-acetate.
Use: Estrogen.
ESTROGENIC SUBSTANCES, CONJU-

GATED. (Water-soluble) A mixture containing the sodium salts of the sulfate esters of the estrogenic substances, principally estrone and equilin that are of the type excreted by pregnant mares. **Cream.**
See: Premarin Vaginal Cream (Wyeth-Ayerst). **Intravenous.**
See: Estroject, Vial (Mayrand).
Premarin (Wyeth-Ayerst).
Tab.
See: Aquagen, Inj. (Remsen).
Ces (ICN).
Estroquin, Tab. (Sheryl).
Estrosan, Tab. (Recsei).
Evestrone, Tab. (Delta).
Genisis, Tab. (Organon).
Menotabs, Tab. (Fleming).
Orapin (Standex).
Prelestrin, Tab. (Pasadena Research).
Premarin, Tab. (Wyeth-Ayerst).
Tag-39 H, Tab. (Solvay).
W/Ethinyl estradiol.
See: Demulen, Tab. (Searle).
W/Meprobamate.
See: Milprem, Tab. (Wallace).
PMB 200, Tab. (Wyeth-Ayerst).
PMB 400, Tab. (Wyeth-Ayerst).
W/Methyltestosterone.
See: Menotab-M #1 and 2, Tab. (Fleming).
Premarin with Methyltestosterone, Tab. (Wyeth-Ayerst).
ESTROGENIC SUBSTANCES IN AQUE-OUS SUSPENSION. (Wyeth-Ayerst) Sterile estrone suspension 2 mg/ml. Vial 10 ml.
Use: Estrogen.
ESTROGENIC SUBSTANCES MIXED.
May be a crystalline or an amorphous mixture of the naturally occurring estrogens obtained from the urine of pregnant mares. **Aqueous Susp.**
See: Gravigen Inj. (Bluco).
Lanestrin, Vial (Lannett).
Cap.
See: Urestrin, Cap. (Upjohn).
W/Androgen therapy, vitamins, iron, d-des-oxyephedrine HCl.
See: Mediatric, Preps. (Wyeth-Ayerst).
W/Methyltestosterone.
See: Premarin w/methyltestosterone, Tab. (Wyeth-Ayerst).
W/Testosterone.
See: Andrestraq, Vial (Central).
ESTROGEN-ANDROGEN THERAPY.
See: Androgen-Estrogen Therapy.
• **ESTROGENS, CONJUGATED,** U.S.P. XXIII. Inj. U.S.P. XXIII.
Use: Estrogen.

See: Conest, Tab. (Century).
Congens, Tab. (Blaine).
Congesterone, Tab. (Kenyon).
Estrocon, Tab. (Savage).
Ganeake, Tab. (Geneva).
Menotab, Tab. (Fleming).
PMB, Tab. (Wyeth-Ayerst).
Premarin, Tab., I.V. (Wyeth-Ayerst).
Premarin Vaginal Cream (Wyeth-Ayerst).
Premarin with Methyltestosterone, Tab. (Wyeth-Ayerst).
Sodestrin and Sodestrin-H, Tab. (Solvay).
Tag-39, Tab. (Solvay).
Zeste, Tab. (Ascher).
ESTROGENS EQUINE.
See: Estrogen. PMB, Tab. (Wyeth-Ayerst).
Premarin, Tab., I.V. (Wyeth-Ayerst).
Premarin Vaginal Cream (Wyeth-Ayerst).
Premarin with Methyltestosterone, Tab. (Wyeth-Ayerst).
• **ESTROGENS, ESTERIFIED,** U.S.P. XXIII. Tab., U.S.P. XXIII.
Use: Estrogen.
See: Amnestrogen, Tab. (Squibb).
Estratab (Solvay).
Evex, Tab. (Syntex).
Menest, Tab. (SK-Beecham).
Ms-Med, Tab. (Dunhall).
• **ESTROGENS, ESTERIFIED & ANDRO-GENS.**
Use: Estrogen & Androgen supplementation.
See: Estratest.
ESTROGENS, NATURAL.
Use: Estrogen.
See: Depogen, Vial (Hyrex).
Estradiol, Preps. (Various Mfr.).
Estrone, Preps. (Various Mfr.).
Estrogenic Substance (Various Mfr.).
PMB, Tab. (Wyeth-Ayerst).
Premarin, Tab., I.V. (Wyeth-Ayerst).
Premarin Vaginal Cream (Wyeth-Ayerst).
Premarin with Methyltestosterone, Tab. (Wyeth-Ayerst).
ESTROGENS, SYNTHETIC.
See: Dienestrol, Preps. (Various Mfr.).
Diethylstilbestrol, Preps. (Various Mfr.).
Hexestrol, Preps. (Various Mfr.).
Meprane, Tab. (Reed & Carnrick).
TACE, Cap. (Merrell Dow).
Vallestril, Tab. (Searle).
ESTROGESTIN A. (Harvey) Estrogenic substance 1 mg, progesterone 10 mg/ml in peanut oil. Vial 10 ml.

Use: Estrogen, progestin combination.
ESTROGESTIN C. (Harvey) Estrogenic substance 1 mg, progesterone 12.5 mg/ml in peanut oil. Vial 10 ml.
Use: Estrogen, progestin combination.
ESTROJECT. (Mayrand) Estrogenic substance. **2 mg/ml:** Vial 10 ml, 30 ml. **5 mg/ml:** Vial 10 ml.
Use: Estrogen.
ESTROJECT-LA. (Mayrand) Estradiol cypionate in oil 5 mg/ml. Inj. Vial 10 ml.
Use: Estrogen.
ESTROLAN. (Lannett) Estrogenic substance natural in oil 10,000 IU/ml. Vial 30 ml.
Use: Estrogen.
•**ESTRONE,** U.S.P. XXIII. Inj., Sterile susp., U.S.P. XXIII. 3-Hydroxy-estra-1,3,5(10)-trien-17-one. Oil Inj., Femidyn, follicular hormone, folliculin, follicunodis, cristallovar, glandubolin, hiestrone, ketohydroxy-estratriene, ketohydroxyestrin. 1 mg equals 10,000 IU.
Use: Estrogen.
See: Aquest, Inj. (Dunhall).
  Bestrone Suspension, Inj. (Bluco).
  Estrogenic Substances in Aqueous Susp. (Wyeth-Ayerst).
  Foygen, Vial (Foy).
  Menagen, Cap. (Parke-Davis).
  Menformon (A), Vial (Organon).
  Par-Supp, Vag. Supp. (Parmed).
  Propagon-S, Inj. (Spanner).
  Theelin, Vial, Aqueous and Oil (Parke-Davis).
W/Hydrocortisone acetate.
See: Estro-V HC, Supp. (Webcon).
W/Estradiol, potassium estrone sulfate.
  Tri-Orapin (Standex).
W/Estradiol, vitamin B_{12}.
See: Ovest, Tab. (Trimen).
  Ovulin, Inj. (Sig).
W/Estriol, estradiol. Hormonin, Tab. (Carnrick).
W/Estrogens.
See: Estrogenic Mixtures, Preps. (Various Mfr.).
  Estrogenic Substances, Preps. (Various Mfr.).
W/Lactose.
See: Estrovag, Supp. (Fellows-Testagar).
W/Potassium estrone sulfate.
See: Dura-Keelin, Vial (Pharmex).
  Mer-Estrone, Inj. (Keene).
  Sodestrin, Inj. (Solvay).
  Spanestrin-P, Vial (Savage).
W/Progesterone.
See: Duovin-S, Inj. (Spanner).
W/Testosterone.

See: Andesterone, Vial (Lincoln).
  Anestro, Inj. (Hauck).
  Di-Hormone, Susp. (Paddock).
  Di-Met Susp. (Organon).
  Diorapin (Standex).
  Dl-Steroid, Vial (Kremers-Urban).
  Estratest, Tab. (Solvay).
W/Testosterone, progesterone.
See: Tripole-F, Inj. (Spanner).
W/Testosterone, sodium carboxymethylcellulose, sodium Cl.
See: Tostestro, Inj. (Bowman).
W/Testosterone, vitamins.
See: Android-G, Vial (Brown).
  Geratic Forte, Inj. (Keene Pharm.).
  Geriamic, Tab. (Vortech).
  Geritag, Inj., Cap. (Solvay).
W/Testosterone, vitamin and mineral formula, amino acids.
See: Geramine, Tab., Inj. (Brown).
W/Testosterone propionate.
ESTRONE "5". (Keene) Estrone 5 mg/ml, sodium carboxymethyl- cellulose, povidone, benzyl alcohol, methyl and propyl parabens. Inj. Vial 10 ml.
Use: Estrogen.
ESTRONE SULFATE, PIPERAZINE.
See: Ogen, Tab., Vaginal Cream (Abbott).
ESTRONE SULFATE, POTASSIUM.
See: Estrogen, Vial (Med. Chem.).
  Kaytron, Inj. (Pasadena Research).
ESTRONE SULFATE POTASSIUM W/ESTRONE.
See: Dura-Keelin, Vial (Pharmex).
ESTRONOL AQUEOUS. (Central) Estrone 2 mg/ml w/preservatives and stabilizers. Inj. Vial 10 ml, 30 ml.
Use: Estrogen.
ESTRONOL-LA. (Central) Estradiol cypionate in oil 5 mg/ml w/chlorobutanol 0.5%. Inj. Vial 10 ml, Box 6s.
Use: Estrogen.
•**ESTROPIATE,** U.S.P. XXIII. Vaginal Cream, Tab., U.S.P. XXIII. Estrone hydrogen sulfate compound with piperazine (1:1). Piperazine estrone sulfate.
Use: Estrogen.
See: Ogen, Tab., Vaginal Cream (Abbott).
ESTROPIPATE. (Various Mfr.) Sodium estrone sulfate 0.625 mg (equiv. to 0.75 mg estropipate). Tab. Bot. 100s.
Use: Estrogen.
ESTROQUIN TABLET. (Sheryl) Purified conjugated estrogens 1.25 mg/Tab. Bot. 100s.
Use: Estrogen.
ESTROVIS. (Parke-Davis) Quinestrol 100 mcg/Tab. Bot. 100s.

Use: Estrogen.
• **ETAFEDRINE HCL.** USAN.
Use: Bronchodilator.
See: Mercodol w/Decapryn, Liq. (Merrell Dow).
Nethamine (Merrell Dow).
• **ETAFILCON A.** USAN.
Use: Contact lens material.
ETALENT. (Roger) Ethaverine HCl 100 mg/Cap. Bot. 50s, 500s.
Use: Peripheral vasodilator.
ETAMIPHYLLINE. B.A.N. 7-(2-Diethylaminoethyl)- theophylline.
Use: Smooth muscle relaxant.
• **ETANIDAZOLE.** USAN.
Use: Antineoplastic (hypoxic cell radiosensitizer).
E-TAPP ELIXIR. (Edwards) Brompheniramine maleate 4 mg, phenylephrine HCl 5 mg, phenylpropanolamine HCl 5 mg/5 ml, alcohol 2.3%. Bot. gal.
Use: Antihistamine, decongestant.
• **ETAROTENE.** USAN.
Use: Keratolytic, topical.
• **ETAZOLATE HYDROCHLORIDE.** USAN.
Use: Antipsychotic.
ETENZAMIDE. B.A.N. 2-Ethoxybenzamide.
Use: Analgesic.
ETERNA 27 CREAM. (Revlon) Pregnenolone acetate 0.5% in cream base.
Use: Emollient.
• **ETEROBARB.** USAN.
Use: Anticonvulsant.
• **ETHACRYNATE SODIUM FOR INJECTION,** U.S.P. XXIII. Sodium [2,3-dichloro-4-(2-methylenebutyryl)-phenoxy]acetate.
Use: Diuretic.
See: Edecrin Sodium I.V., Inj. (Merck & Co.).
• **ETHACRYNIC ACID,** U.S.P. XXIII. Tab., U.S.P. XXIII. Acetic acid, [2,3-dichloro-4-(2-methylene-1-oxobutyl)phenoxy].
Use: Diuretic.
See: Edecrin, Tab. (Merck & Co.).
• **ETHAMBUTOL HCl,** U.S.P. XXIII. Tab., U.S.P. XXIII. (+)-2,2-(Ethylenediimino)-di-1-butanol Di HCl.
Use: Antitubercular.
See: Myambutol HCl (Lederle).
ETHAMICORT.
See: Hydrocortamate.
ETHAMIVAN. B.A.N. NN-Diethylvanillamide.
Use: Central nervous system stimulant.
ETHAMOLIN. (Reed & Carnrick) Ethanolamine oleate 5%. Inj. Amp. 2 ml.
Use: Sclerosing agent.
• **ETHAMSYLATE.** USAN. Diethylammonium 2,5-dihydroxybenzenesulfonate. Dicynene.
Use: Hemostatic.
ETHANOL. (Various Mfr.) Alcohol, anhydrous. Alcohol, U.S.P. XXIII.
ETHANOLAMINE. Olamine.
• **ETHANOLAMINE OLEATE.** USAN.
Use: Sclerosing agent. [Orphan drug]
See: Ethamolin (Reed & Carnrick).
ETHAQUIN. (Ascher) Ethaverine HCl 100 mg/Tab. Bot. 100s, 500s, 1000s.
Use: Peripheral vasodilator.
ETHASULFATE SODIUM. Sodium 2-Ethyl-1-hexanol sulfate.
ETHATAB. (Glaxo) Ethaverine HCl 100 mg/Tab. Bot. 100s, 500s. UD 100s.
Use: Peripheral vasodilator.
ETHATAB. (Whitby) Ethaverine HCl 10 mg/Tab. Bot. 100s, UD 100s.
Use: Peripheral vasodilator.
ETHAVERINE HYDROCHLORIDE. The ethyl analog of papaverine HCl, 6,7-diethoxy-1-(3,4-diethoxybenzyl) isoquinoline HCl. Diquinol HCl, Preparin HCl, Perperine HCl. The tetraethyl homolog of papaverine is 2 to 4 times more active and less than half as toxic as the parent drug.
Use: Antispasmodic.
See: Etalent, Cap. (Roger).
Ethaquin, Tab. (Ascher).
Neopavrin, Tab., Elix, (Savage).
Spasodil, Tab. (Rand).
ETHAVEROL "75." (Pharmex) Ethaverine HCl 75 mg/ml. Vial 10 ml.
Use: Peripheral vasodilator.
ETHAVEX-100 TABLETS. (Econo Med) Ethaverine HCl 100 mg/Tab. Bot. 100s, 1000s.
Use: Peripheral vasodilator.
• **ETHCHLORVYNOL,** U.S.P. XXIII. Cap., U.S.P. XXIII. 1-Chloro-3-ethyl-1-penten-4-yn-3-ol.
Use: Hypnotic, sedative.
See: Placidyl, Cap. (Abbott).
Serensil, Prods. (Ciba).
ETHEBENECID. B.A.N. 4-Diethylsulamoyl benzoic acid.
Use: Uricosuric.
ETHENOL, HOMOPOLYMER. Polyvinyl Alcohol, U.S.P. XXIII.
ETHENZAMIDE. o-Ethoxybenzamide.
• **ETHER,** U.S.P. XXIII. Ethyl ether.
Use: General anesthetic.
ETHIAZIDE. B.A.N. 6-Chloro-3-ethyl-3,4-dihydro-1,2,4-benzothiadiazine-7-sulfonamide 1,1-dioxide.
Use: Diuretic.
• **ETHINYL ESTRADIOL,** U.S.P. XXIII. Tab., U.S.P. XXIII. 17-Ethinyl-3,17-estra-

diol. 19-Norpregna-1,3,5(10)-trien-20-yne-3,17-diol,(17α)-. 19-Nor-17α-pregna-1, 3,5-(10)-trien-20-yne-3,17-diol.
Use: Estrogen. Turner's syndrome [Orphan drug]
See: Estinyl, Tab. (Schering).
Feminone, Tab. (Upjohn).
Lynoral, Tab. (Organon)
Menolyn, Tab. (Arcum).
Ovogyn, Tab. (Pasadena Research).
ETHINYL ESTRADIOL W/COMBINATIONS
See: Ardiatric, Tab. (Burgin-Arden).
Brevicon, Tab. (Syntex).
Demulen, Tab. (Searle).
Desogen, Tab. (Organon).
GenCept, Tab. (Gencon).
Halodrin, Tab. (Upjohn).
Jenest-28, Tab. (Organon).
Loestrin, Tab. (Parke-Davis).
Loestrin 1.5/30, Tab. (Parke-Davis).
Lo/Ovral, Tab. (Wyeth-Ayerst).
Modicon 21 and 28, Tab. (Ortho).
Nelulen, Tab. (Watson Labs).
Nordette, Tab. (Wyeth-Ayerst).
Norinyl, Prods. (Syntex).
Norlestrin, Tab. (Parke-Davis).
Norlestrin Fe, Tab. (Parke-Davis).
Ortho-Cept, Tab. (Ortho).
Ortho-Cyclen, Tab. (Ortho).
Ortho-Novum 1/35, 21 and 28 (Ortho).
Ortho Tri-Cyclen, Tab. (Ortho).
Os-Cal-Mone, Tab. (Marion).
Ovcon-35, Tab. (Mead Johnson).
Ovcon-50, Tab. (Mead Johnson).
Ovlin, Vial (ICN).
Ovral, Tab. (Wyeth-Ayerst).
Triphasil, Tab. (Wyeth-Ayerst).
ETHINYL ESTRADIOL AND DIMETHIS-TERONE TABLETS.
Use: Estrogen, progestin combination.
ETHINYL ESTRENOL.
See: Lynestrenol (Organon).
•**ETHIODIZED OIL INJECTION,** U.S.P. XXIII.
Use: Diagnostic aid (radiopaque medium).
See: Ethiodol, Inj. (Savage).
•**ETHIODIZED OIL I-131.** USAN. Radioactive iodine addition to ethyl ester of poppyseed oil. Ethiodal-131.
Use: Antineoplastic, radioactive agent.
ETHIODOL. (Savage) Ethiodized oil. Fatty acid ethyl ester of poppy-seed oil, iodine 37%. Inj. Amp. 10 ml, Box 2s.
Use: Diagnostic aid.
•**ETHIOFOS.** USAN. Formerly gammaphos.
Use: Radioprotector. [Orphan drug]
•**ETHIONAMIDE,** U.S.P. XXIII. Tab., U.S.P.

XXIII. 2-Ethylthioisonicotinamide. 4-Pyridinecarbothioamide, 2-ethyl.
Use: Tuberculostatic.
See: Trecator S.C., Tab. (Wyeth-Ayerst).
ETHISTERONE. 17-Hydroxy-17a-pregn-4-en-20-yn-3-one.
See: Anhydrohydroxyprogesterone (Various Mfr.).
ETHMOZINE. (Roberts) Moricizine HCl 200 mg, 250 mg or 300 mg/Tab. Bot. 21s, 100s, UD 100s.
Use: Antiarrhythmic.
ETHOCAINE.
See: Procaine HCl (Various Mfr.).
ETHOCYLORVYNOL. β-Chlorovinyl ethyl ethynyl carbinol. Ethchlorvynol, U.S.P. XXIII.
ETHODRYL.
See: Diethylcarbamazine Citrate.
ETHOGLUCID. B.A.N. 1,2:15,16-Diepoxy-4,7,10,-13-tetraoxahexadecane.
Use: Antineoplastic agent.
ETHOHEPTAZINE. B.A.N. Ethyl hexahydro-1-methyl-4-phenylazepine-4-carboxylate.
Use: Analgesic.
ETHOHEPTAZINE CITRATE. Ethyl Hexahydro-1-methyl-4-phenylazepine-4-carboxylate Dihydrogen citrate. Ethyl Hexahydro-1-methyl-4-phenyl-1H-azepine-4-carboxylate Citrate (1:1).
ETHOHEXADIOL. Ethyl hexanediol, 2-ethylhexane-1,3-diol, Rutgers 612. Used in Comp. Dimethyl Phthalate.
Use: Insect repellent.
ETHOMOXANE. B.A.N. 2-Butylaminomethyl-8-ethoxy-1,4-benzodioxan.
Use: Adrenaline antagonist.
•**ETHONAM NITRATE.** USAN. Ethyl 1-(1,2,3-4-tetrahydro-1-naphthyl)imidazole-5-carboxylate nitrate.
Use: Fungicide.
•**ETHOPROPAZINE HYDROCHLORIDE,** U.S.P. XXIII. Tab. U.S.P. XXIII. 10H-Phenothiazine-10-ethanamine, N,N-diethyl-α-methyl-,monohydrochloride. 10-[2-(Diethylamino)propyl]-phenothiazine monohydrochloride. Lysivane.
Use: Antiparkinsonian.
See: Parsidol HCl, Tab. (Warner-Chilcott).
ETHOSALAMIDE. B.A.N. 2-(2-Ethoxyethoxy) benzamide.
Use: Analgesic; antipyretic.
•**ETHOSUXIMIDE,** U.S.P. XXIII. Cap., U.S.P. XXIII. 2-Ethyl-2-methyl-succinimide.

Use: Anticonvulsant.
See: Zarontin, Cap., Syr. (Parke-Davis).
ETHOSUXIMIDE. (Copley) Ethosuximide
250 mg/5 ml / Syrup. Bot. 483 ml.
Use: Anticonvulsant.
ETHOTOIN. B.A.N. 3-Ethyl-5-phenylimi-
dazoline-2,4-dione.
Use: Anticonvulsant.
See: Peganone, Tab. (Abbott).
ETHOVAN. Ethyl Vanillin.
ETHOXZOLAMIDE. 6-Ethoxy-2-benzoth-
iazolesulfonamide.
Use: Carbonic anhydrase inhibitor.
ETHRANE. (Anaquest) Enflurane.
Volatile Liq. Bot. 125 ml, 250 ml.
Use: General anesthetic.
• **ETHYBENZTROPINE.** USAN. 3-
(diphenylmethoxy)-8-ethylnortropane.
Panolid. Methylbenztropine.
Use: Anticholinergic.
• **ETHYL ACETATE,** N.F. XVIII.
Use: Flavor.
ETHYL AMINOBENZOATE. Anesthesin,
anesthrone, benzocaine, parathesin.
Use: Local anesthetic.
See: Benzocaine (Various Mfr.).
ETHYL BISCOUMACETATE. B.A.N. Eth-
yl di(4-hydroxycoumarin-3-yl)acetate.
Use: Anticoagulant.
ETHYL BISCOUMACETATE. 3,3-(Car-
boxymethylene) bis (4-hydroxy-
coumarin) ethyl ester. Ethyl Bis (4-hy-
droxy-2-oxo-2H-1-benzopyran-3-yl) ac-
etate.
ETHYL BROMIDE. (Various Mfr.) Bro-
moethane.
Use: General anesthetic.
ETHYL CARBAMATE.
See: Urethan (Various Mfr.).
• **ETHYLCELLULOSE,** N.F. XVIII.
Use: Tablet binder.
• **ETHYLCELLULOSE AQUEOUS DIS-
PERSION,** N.F. XVIII.
Use: Tablet binder.
ETHYL CHAULMOOGRATE.
Use: Hansen's disease, sarcoidosis.
• **ETHYL CHLORIDE,** U.S.P. XXIII.
Chloroethane.
Use: Local anesthetic.
See: Gebauer-Spra-Pak. Stratford-
Cook-Spray, 100 Gm.
• **ETHYL DIBUNATE.** USAN. Ethyl 2,7-di-t-
butyl-naphthalene-1-sulfonate.
Use: Cough suppressant.
ETHYL DIIODOBRASSIDATE. Iodobras-
sid. Lipoiodine.
**ETHYLDIMETHYLAMMONIUM BRO-
MIDE.**
See: Ambutonium Bromide.
ETHYLENE. (Various Mfr.) Ethene.

Use: General anesthetic.
• **ETHYLENEDIAMINE,** U.S.P. XXIII.
Use: Component of aminophylline.
ETHYLENEDIAMINE SOLUTION. (67%
w/v).
Use: Solvent (Aminophylline Inj.).
**ETHYLENEDIAMINETETRAACETIC
ACID.**
See: Edathamil, EDTA (Various Mfr.).
**ETHYLENEDIAMINE TETRAACETIC
ACID DISODIUM SALT.**
See: Endrate Disodium, Amp. (Abbott).
ETHYLESTRENOL. B.A.N. 17α-Eth-
ylestr-4-en-17β-ol.
Use: Anabolic steroid.
ETHYLHYDROCUPREINE HCl. 6 Ethyl-
hydrocupreine monohydrochloride.
Use: Antiseptic.
ETHYLMETHYLTHIAMBUTENE. B.A.N.
3-Ethyl-methylamino-1,1-di-(2-
thienyl)but-1-ene.
Use: Narcotic analgesic.
ETHYLMORPHINE HYDROCHLORIDE.
7,8-Didehydro-4,5α-epoxy-3-ethoxy-17-
methyl-morphinan-6α-ol Hydrochloride.
Dionin.
Use: Narcotic.
ETHYL NITRITE SPIRIT. Ethyl nitrite.
Sweet Spirit of Niter. Spirit of Nitrous
Ether.
• **ETHYLNOREPINEPHRINE HCl,** U.S.P.
XXIII. Inj., U.S.P. XXIII.
Use: Bronchodilator.
See: Bronkephrine, Amp. (Sanofi
Winthrop).
• **ETHYL OLEATE,** N.F. XVIII.
Use: Pharmaceutic aid (vehicle).
ETHYL OXIDE; ETHYL ETHER,
Use: Solvent.
ETHYLPAPAVERINE HCl.
See: Ethaverine HCl (Various Mfr.).
• **ETHYLPARABEN,** N.F. XVIII. Ethyl p-Hy-
droxybenzoate.
Use: Pharmaceutic aid (antifungal
preservative).
ETHYL PYROPHOSPHATE. B.A.N.
Tetraethyl pyrophosphate.
Use: Treatment of myasthenia gravis.
ETHYLSTIBAMINE. Astaril, neostibosan.
Use: Antimony therapy.
ETHYL VANILLATE. Ethyl-hydroxy-
methoxy-benzoate.
• **ETHYL VANILLIN,** N.F. XVIII. 3-Ethoxy-4-
hydroxybenzaldehyde.
Use: Flavor.
• **ETHYNERONE.** USAN.
Use: Progestin.
• **ETHYNODIOL DIACETATE,** U.S.P. XXIII.
19-Nor-17α-pregn-4-en-20-yne-3B,17-
diol diacetate; 17α-ethynyl-4-estrene-

3β,17β-diol diacetate.
Use: As progesterone, progestin.
See: Ovulen, Tab. (Searle).
W/Ethinyl estradiol.
Demulen, Preps. (Searle).
Nelulen, Tab. (Watson Labs).
W/Mestranol.
See: Ovulen, Tab. (Searle).
• **ETHYNODIOL DIACETATE AND ETHINYL ESTRADIOL TABLETS,** U.S.P. XXIII.
Use: Oral contraceptive.
• **ETHYNODIOL DIACETATE AND MESTRANOL TABLETS,** U.S.P. XXIII.
Use: Oral contraceptive.
ETHYNYLESTRADIOL.
See: Ethinyl Estradiol, U.S.P. (Various Mfr.)
Mestranol (Various Mfr.).
ETHYNYLESTRADIOL 3-METHYL ETHER.
See: Enovid, Tab. (Searle).
• **ETIBENDAZOLE.** USAN.
Use: Anthelmintic.
ETICYLOL. (Ciba) Ethinyl estradiol.
Use: Estrogen.
• **ETIDOCAINE.** USAN. (±)-2-(N-Ethyl-propylamino)-butyro-2,6-xylidide.
Use: Local anesthetic.
See: Duranest (base and hydrochloride).
• **ETIDRONATE DISODIUM,** U.S.P. XXIII.
Tab., U.S.P. XXIII. The disodium salt of (1-Hydroxyethylidene) diphosphonic acid.
Use: Treatment of symptomatic Paget's disease of bone (osteitis deformans). Degenerative metabolic bone disease [Orphan drug]
See: Didronel, Tab. (Procter & Gamble).
• **ETIDRONIC ACID.** USAN. (1-Hydroxy-ethylidene) diphosphonic acid.
Use: Bone calcium regulator.
• **ETIFENIN.** USAN.
Use: Diagnostic aid.
ETIFOXINE. B.A.N. 6-Chloro-2-ethyl-amino-4-methyl-4-phenyl-4H-3,1-ben-zoxazine.
Use: Tranquilizer.
• **ETINTIDINE HYDROCHLORIDE.** USAN.
Use: Antagonist.
ETISAZOLE. V.B.A.N. 3-Ethylamino-1,2-benzisothiazole.
Use: Fungicide, veterinary medicine.
• **ETOCRYLENE.** USAN.
Use: Ultraviolet screen.
• **ETODOLAC.** USAN.
Use: Anti-inflammatory.
See: Lodine (Wyeth-Ayerst).
• **ETOFENAMATE.** USAN.

Use: Analgesic, anti-inflammatory.
• **ETOFORMIN HYDROCHLORIDE.** USAN.
Use: Antidiabetic.
• **ETOMIDATE.** USAN.
Use: Hypnotic.
ETOMIDE HYDROCHLORIDE. Bandol. Carbiphene HCl.
ETONITAZENE. B.A.N. 1-(2-Diethyl-laminoethyl)-2-(4-ethoxybenzyl)-5-ni-trobenzimidazole.
Use: Narcotic analgesic.
• **ETONOGESTREL.** USAN.
Use: Progestin.
• **ETOPOSIDE,** U.S.P. 23, Cap., U.S.P. 23.
Use: Antineoplastic.
See: Vepesid, Inj., Cap. (Bristol).
ETOPOSIDE. (Gensia) Etoposide 20 mg/ml, alcohol 30.5%, benzyl alcohol 30 mg, polysorbate 80 mg, PEG 300 650 mg, citric acid 2 mg/ml. Inj. Vials 5 ml, 25 ml.
Use: Antineoplastic.
• **ETOPOSIDE PHOSPHATE.** USAN.
Use: Antineoplastic.
• **ETOPRINE.** USAN.
Use: Antineoplastic.
ETOQUINOL SODIUM. Name used for Actinoquinol sodium.
ETORPHINE. B.A.N. 7,8-Dihydro-7α-[1(R)-hydroxy-1-methylbutyl]-0⁶-methyl-6,14-endoethenomorphine.
Use: Narcotic analgesic.
ETOVAL.
See: Butethal, N.F. (Various Mfr.).
• **ETOXADROL HYDROCHLORIDE.** USAN.
Use: Anesthetic.
ETOXERIDINE. B.A.N. Ethyl 1-[2-(2-hy-droxyethoxy)ethyl]-4-phenylpiperidine-4-carboxylate.
Use: Narcotic analgesic.
• **ETOZOLIN.** USAN.
Use: Diuretic.
ETRAFON (2-10). (Schering) Perphenazine 2 mg, amitriptyline HCl 10 mg/Tab. Bot. 100s, 500s, UD 100s.
Use: Psychotherapeutic combination.
ETRAFON (2-25). (Schering) Perphenazine 2 mg, amitriptyline HCl 25 mg/Tab. Bot. 100s, 500s, UD 100s.
Use: Psychotherapeutic combination.
ETRAFON-A (4-10). (Schering) Perphenazine 4 mg, amitriptyline HCl 10 mg/Tab. Bot. 100s, UD 100s.
Use: Psychotherapeutic combination.
ETRAFON FORTE TABLETS (4-25). (Schering) Perphenazine 4 mg, amitriptyline HCl 25 mg/Tab. Bot. 100s, 500s, UD 100s.

Use: Psychotherapeutic combination.
• **ETRETINATE.** USAN.
Use: Antipsoriatic.
See: Tegison, Cap. (Roche).
ETRYNIT. Propatyl nitrate.
Use: Coronary agent.
• **ETRYPTAMINE ACETATE.** USAN. 3-(2-Aminobutyl)-indole Acetate.
Use: Central stimulant.
See: Monase (Upjohn).
ETS-2%. (Paddock) Erythromycin topical 2%. Soln. Bot. 60 ml.
Use: Anti-acne.
ETTRIOL TRINITRATE.
See: Propatyl nitrate.
ETYBENZATROPINE. Ethybenztropine.
ETYNODIOL ACETATE. Ethynodiol Diacetate.
EUBASIN.
See: Sulfapyridine (Various Mfr.).
EUCAINE HCl. 2,2,6-Trimethyl-4-piperidinol benzoate HCl.
EUCALYPTAMINT. (Ciba) Menthol 8%, eucalyptus oil, SD 3A alcohol. Gel. Tube 60 g.
Use: Rubs and liniments.
EUCALYPTAMINT MAXIMUM STRENGTH. (Ciba) Menthol 16%, lanolin, eucalyptus oil. Oint. Tube 60 ml
Use: Rubs and liniments.
EUCALYPTOL. 1,8-Epoxy-p-menthane.
Use: Pharmaceutic aid (flavor), antitussive, nasal decongestant.
See: Vicks Sinex, Nasal Spray (Vicks).
Vicks Va-Tro-Nol, Nose Drops (Vicks).
Vicks Prods. (Vicks).
• **EUCALYPTUS OIL,** N.F. XVIII.
Use: Flavor, antitussive, nasal decongestant, expectorant, topical analgesic.
See: Vicks Prods. (Vicks).
Victors Regular, Cherry Loz. (Vicks).
EUCAPINE SYRUP. (Lannett) Ammonium Cl 10 gr, potassium guaiacol-sulfonate 8 gr. White pine and wild cherry syrup. Bot. pt, gal.
Use: Expectorant.
• **EUCATROPINE HYDROCHLORIDE,** U.S.P. XXIII. Ophth. Soln., U.S.P. XXIII. 1,2,2,6-Tetramethyl-4-piperidyl mandelate HCl. Benzeneacetic acid, alpha-hydroxy-, 1,2,2,6-tetramethyl-4-piperidinyl ester hydrochloride. (Glogau) Crystal, Bot. Gm.
Use: Pharmaceutical necessity for ophthalmic dosage form.
EUCERIN. (Beiersdorf) Unscented moisturizing formula. **Creme:** Jar 120 Gm, lb. **Lot.:** Bot. 240 ml, 480 ml.
Use: Emollient.

EUCERIN CLEANSING. (Beiersdorf) Sodium laureth sulfate, cocoamphocarboxyglycinate, cocamidopropyl betaine, cocamide MEA, PEG-7 glyceryl cocoate, PEG-5 lanolate, PEG-120 methyl glucose dioleate, lanolin alcohol, imidazolidinyl urea. Soap free. Lot. Bot. 240 ml.
Use: Skin cleanser.
EUCERIN DRY SKIN CARE DAILY FACIAL. (Beiersdorf) Ethylhexyl p-methoxycinnamate, titanium dioxide, 2-phenylbenzimidazole-5- sulfonic acid, 2-ethylhexyl salicylate, mineral oil, cetearyl alcohol, castor oil, lanolin alcohol, EDTA. SPF 20. Lot. Bot. 120 ml.
Use: Sunscreen.
EUCERIN PLUS. (Beiersdorf) Mineral oil, hydrogenated castor oil, 5% sodium lactate, 5% urea, glycerin, lanolin alcohol. Lot. Bot. 177 ml.
Use: Emollient.
EUCODAL.
See: Oxycodone (No Mfr. currently lists).
EUCORAN.
See: Nikethamide (Various Mfr.).
EUCUPIN DIHYDROCHLORIDE.
Isoamylhydrocupreine dihydrochloride.
EUDAL-SR. (UAD) Pseudoephedrine 120 mg, guaifenesin 400 mg/SR Tab. Bot. 100s.
Use: Decongestant, expectorant.
EUFLAVINE.
See: Acriflavine (Various Mfr.).
• **EUGENOL,** U.S.P. XXIII. (Various Mfr.) 4-Allyl-2-methoxy-phenol. Phenol, 2-methoxy-4-(2-propenyl)-.
Use: Dental analgesic, oral anesthetic.
See: Benzodent, Oint. (Vicks).
EUKADOL.
See: Dihydrohydroxycodeinone, Preps. (No Mfr. currently lists).
EULCIN. (Leeds) Methscopolamine bromide 2.5 mg, butabarbital sodium 10 mg, aluminum hydroxide gel, dried, 250 mg, magnesium trisilicate 250 mg/Tab. Bot. 100s.
Use: Anticholinergic/antispasmodic, sedative/hypnotic, antacid.
EULEXIN. (Schering) Flutamide 125 mg/Cap. 100s, 500s, UD 100s.
Use: Antineoplastic agent.
EUMYDRIN DROPS. (Sanofi Winthrop) Atropine methonitrate.
Use: Anticholinergic/antispasmodic.
EUNERYL.
See: Phenobarbital (Various Mfr.).
EUPHORBIA COMPOUND. (Sherwood) Euphorbia pilulifera fluidextract 1.5 ml,

iobelia tincture 2.2 ml, nitroglycerin spirit 0.29 ml, sodium iodide 1.04 Gm, sodium bromide 1.04 Gm, alcohol 24%/30 ml. Bot. pt, gal.
Use: Sedative/hypnotic, expectorant.
EUPHORBIA PILULIFERA. W/Cocillana, squill, antimony potassium tartrate, senega.
See: Cylana, Syr. (Bowman).
W/Phenyl salicylate and various oils.
See: Rayderm, Oint. (Velvet Pharmacal).
EUPRACTONE. (Travenol) Dimethadione.
EUPRAX. Albution.
•**EUPROCIN HCl.** USAN. O^6-Isopentylhydrocupreine dihydrochloride.
Use: Topical anesthetic.
See: Eucupin HCl.
EUQUININE. Quinine ethyl carbonate.
Use: Antimalarial, antipyretic.
EURAX CREAM. (Westwood) Crotamiton 10% in vanishing-cream base of glyceryl monostearate, anhydrous lanolin, PEG 6-32, glycerin, polysorbate 80, water, benzyl alcohol, mineral oil, white wax, quaternium-15, fragrance. Tube 60 Gm.
Use: Scabicide/pediculicide.
EURAX LOTION. (Westwood) Crotamiton 10% in emollient-lotion base of glyceryl monostearate, anhydrous lanolin, PEG 6-32, glycerin, polysorbate 80, water, benzyl alcohol, light mineral oil, carboxymethylcellulose, simethicone, quaternium-15, fragrance. Bot. 60 Gm, 454 Gm.
Use: Scabicide/pediculicide.
EVAC-Q-KIT. (Adria) Each kit contains: **Evac-Q-Mag:** Magnesium citrate 300 ml, citric acid, potassium citrate. **Evac-Q-Tabs:** 2 tab. phenolphthalein 130 mg/Tab. **Evac-Q-Sert:** 2 supp. containing potassium bitartrate, sodium bicarbonate/supp. in polyethylene glycol base. Patient instruction sheet.
Use: Bowel evacuant.
EVAC-Q-KWIK. (Adria) Each kit contains: **Evac-Q-Mag:** magnesium citrate **300 ml,** citric acid, potassium citrate in cherry-flavored base. **Evac-Q-Tabs:** 2 tab. phenolphthalein 130 mg. **Evac-Q-Kwik Supp.:** bisacodyl 10 mg.
Use: Bowel evacuant.
EVAC SUPPOSITORIES. (Burgin-Arden) Sodium bicarbonate, sodium biphosphate, dioctyl sodium sulfosuccinate 50 mg/Supp.
Use: Laxative.
EVAC TABLETS. (Burgin-Arden) Guar gum 300 mg, danthron 50 mg, sodium

100 mg/Tab.
Use: Laxative.
EVACTOL. (Delta) Docusate sodium 100 mg, sodium carboxymethyl cellulose 200 mg/Cap. Pkg. 10s, Bot. 10s, 30s, 100s.
Use: Laxative.
EVAC-U-GEN. (Walker) Yellow phenolphthalein 97.2 mg w/corn syrup, lactose, saccharin/Chew. Tab. Bot. 35s, 100s.
Use: Laxative.
EVAC-U-LAX. (Hauck) Yellow phenolphthalein 80 mg/Chew. tab. Bot. 100s.
Use: Laxative.
EVALOSE. (Copley) Lactulose 10 g/15 ml, galactose < 1.6 g, lactose < 1.2 g, other sugars ≤ 1.2 g / Syrup. Bot. 240 ml, 960 ml.
Use: Laxative.
•**EVANS BLUE,** U.S.P. XXIII. Inj., U.S.P. XXIII. 1,3-Naphthalenedisulfonic acid, 6,6-[(3,3-dimethyl[1,1-biphenyl]-4,4-diyl)bis(azo)]bis[4-amino-5-hydroxy]-, tetrasodium salt. Azovan Blue, B.A.N. Pure diazo dye. Amp. (0.5%) 5 ml 12s, 25s, 100s. (New World Trading Corp.) Inj. 5 ml amps.
Use: Diagnostic aid (blood volume determination).
EVERONE. (Hyrex) Testosterone enanthate in oil 100 mg or 200 mg/ml. Vial 10 ml.
Use: Androgen.
EVICYL TABLETS. (Sanofi Winthrop) Inositol hexanicotinate.
Use: Hypolipidemic, peripheral vasodilator.
EVIRON. (Delta) Ferrous fumarate 160 mg, copper 1 mg, ascorbic acid 75 mg/Tab.
Use: Mineral supplement.
E-VISTA. (Seatrace) Hydroxyzine HCl 50 mg/ml Inj. Vial 10 ml.
Use: Antianxiety agent.
E-VITAL CREME. (Pasadena Research) Vitamins E 100 IU, A 250 IU, D 100 IU, d-panthenol 0.2%, allantoin 0.1%/Gm. Jar 2 oz, lb.
Use: Emollient.
E-VITAMIN OINTMENT. (Forest) d-alpha tocopherol acetate 30 IU/Gm. Tube 1.5 oz. Jar 2 oz, lb.
Use: Emollient.
EWIN NINOS TABLETS. (Sanofi Winthrop) Aspirin.
Use: Salicylate analgesic.
EXACT. (Premier) Benzoyl peroxide 5%, parabens. Cream Jar 19.5 Gm.
Use: Anti-acne.
•**EXAMETAZINE.** USAN.

Use: Diagnostic aid, cerebrovascular disease.
• **EXAPROLOL HYDROCHLORIDE.** USAN.
Use: Antiadrenergic.
EX-AQUA. (E.J. Moore) Extract of buchu, extract of uva ursi, extract of corn silk, extract of juniper, caffeine/Tab. Bot. 80s.
Use: Diuretic.
EX-CALORIC WAFERS. (Eastern Research) Carboxymethylcellulose 181 mg, methylcellulose 272 mg/Wafer. Bot. 100s, 500s, 5000s.
Use: Diet aid.
EXCEDRIN ASPIRIN FREE. (Bristol-Myers) Acetaminophen 500 mg, caffeine 65 mg/Cap. Bot. 24s, 50s, 100s.
Use: Nonnarcotic analgesic combination.
EXCEDRIN EXTRA STRENGTH. (Bristo-Myers USP) Acetaminophen 250 mg, aspirin 250 mg, caffeine 65 mg. **Capl.:** Bot. 24s, 50s, 80s. **Tab.:** Bot. 12s, 30s, 60s, 100s, 165s, 225s.
Use: Analgesic combination.
EXCEDRIN P.M. ASPIRIN FREE. (Bristol-Myers) Acetaminophen 500 mg, diphenhydramine citrate 38 mg/ **Tab.:** Bot. 10s, 30s, 50s, 80s. **Capl.:** Bot. 30s, 50s. **Liq.:** Acetaminophen 167 mg or 1000 mg, diphenhydramine HCl 8.3 mg/5 ml or 50 mg/30 ml, alcohol 10%, sucrose. Bot. 180 ml.
Use: Analgesic, sleep aid.
EXCEDRIN SINUS. (Bristol-Myers) Pseudoephedrine HCl 30 mg, acetaminophen 500 mg/Tab. Bot. 24s.
Use: Decongestant, analgesic.
EXCEDRIN SINUS CAPLET. (Bristol-Myers) Acetaminophen 500 mg, pseudoephedrine HCl 30 mg/Tab. Bot. 24s.
Use: Analgesic, decongestant.
EXCITA EXTRA. (Schmid) Nonoxynol 9 5.6% (Ribbed). Condom. Box 12s.
Use: Condom with spermicide.
EXGEST LA TABLETS. (Carnrick) Phenylpropanolamine HCl 75 mg, guaifenesin 400 mg. Bot. 100s or 500s.
Use: Decongestant, expectorant.
EXIDINE-2 SCRUB. (Baxter) Chlorhexidine gluconate 2%, isopropyl alcohol 4%. Soln. Bot. 120 ml.
Use: Antiseptic, germicide.
EXIDINE-4 SCRUB. (Baxter) Chlorhexidine gluconate 4%, isopropyl alcohol 4%. Soln. Bot. 120 ml, 240 ml, 480 ml, 887 ml, 1 gal.
Use: Antiseptic, germicide.
EXIDINE SKIN CLEANSER. (Xttrium) Chlorhexidine gluconate 4%, isopropyl

alcohol 4%. Bot. 120 ml, 240 ml, 16 oz, 32 oz, gal.
Use: Antiseptic, germicide.
EX-LAX. (Sandoz) Yellow phenolphthalein 90 mg/chocolate Chew. Tab. or unflavored pill. Chocolate Tab. 6s, 18s, 48s, 72s. Unflavored pill 8s, 30s, 60s.
Use: Laxative.
EX-LAX CHOCOLATED. (Sandoz) Yellow phenolphthalein 90 mg/Chew. Tab. In 6s, 18s, 48s, 72s.
Use: Laxative.
EX-LAX EXTRA GENTLE. (Sandoz) Phenolphthalein 65 mg, docusate sodium 75 mg/Tab. Pkg. 24s, 48s.
Use: Laxative.
EX-LAX GENTLE NATURE. (Sandoz) Calcium salts of sennosides A&B. Tab. 16s.
Use: Laxative.
EX-LAX MAXIMUM RELIEF. (Sandoz) Yellow phenolphthalein 135 mg. Tab. Pkg. 24s.
Use: Laxative.
EX-LAX UNFLAVORED. (Sandoz) Yellow phenolphthalein 90 mg/Tab. 8s, 30s, 60s.
Use: Laxative.
EXNA. (Robins) Benzthiazide 50 mg/Tab. Bot. 100s.
Use: Diuretic, antihypertensive.
EXOCAINE. (Commerce) Methyl salicylate 25%. Tube 1.3 oz.
Use: External analgesic.
EXOCAINE PLUS. (Commerce) Methyl salicylate 30%. Jar 4 oz, Tube 1.3 oz.
Use: External analgesic.
EXOL. Di-isobutyl ethoxy ethyl dimethyl benzyl ammonium Cl.
EXONIC OT. Dioctyl Sodium Sulphosuccinate.
Use: Laxative.
EXORBIN. (Various Mfr.) Polyaminomethylene resin.
EXOSURF (Burroughs Wellcome) Dipalmitoylphosphatidylcholine (DPPC). Lyophilized pow. Vial 10 ml.
Use: Synthetic lung surfactant.
EXPECTORANT DM COUGH SYRUP. (Weeks & Leo) Dextromethorphan HBr 15 mg, guaifenesin 100 mg/5 ml, alcohol 7.125%. Bot. 6 oz.
Use: Antitussive, expectorant.
EXPENDABLE BLOOD COLLECTION UNIT—ACD. (Travenol) Citric acid 540 mg, sodium citrate 1.49 Gm, dextrose 1.65 Gm/67.5 ml.
Use: Anticoagulant.
EXSEL. (Herbert) Selenium sulfide 2.5% in shampoo/lotion base. Bot. 4 oz.

Use: Antiseborrheic.
EXTEN STRONE 10. (Schlicksup) Estradiol valerate 10 mg/ml. Vial 10 ml.
Use: Estrogen.
EXTEND. (E.J. Moore) Benzocaine, dibucaine. Tube oz.
Use: Local anesthetic.
EXTENDRYL CHEWABLE TABLETS, (Fleming) Chlorpheniramine maleate 2 mg, phenylephrine HCl 10 mg, methscopolamine nitrate 1.25 mg/Chew. tab. Bot. 100s, 1000s.
Use: Antihistamine, decongestant, anticholinergic/antispasmodic.
EXTENDRYL JUNIOR. (Fleming) Chlorpheniramine maleate 4 mg, phenylephrine HCl 10 mg, methscopolamine nitrate 1.25 mg/TD Cap. 100s, 1000s.
Use: Antihistamine, decongestant, anticholinergic/antispasmodic.
EXTENDRYL SENIOR. (Fleming) Chlorpheniramine maleate 8 mg, phenylephrine HCl 20 mg, methscopolamine nitrate 2.5 mg/TD Cap. Bot. 100s, 1000s.
Use: Antihistamine, decongestant, anticholinergic/antispasmodic.
EXTENDRYL SYRUP. (Fleming) Chlorpheniramine maleate 2 mg, phenylephrine HCl 10 mg, methscopolamine nitrate 1.25 mg/5 ml. Bot. pt, gal.
Use: Antihistamine, decongestant, anticholinergic/antispasmodic.
EXTENZYME SOFLENS PROTEIN CLEANER. (Allergan) Papain, sodium Cl, sodium carbonate, sodium borate, edetate disodium. Vial w/Tab. 24s. Refill 36s.
Use: Soft contact lens care.
EXTRA ACTION COUGH. (Rugby) Dextromethorphan HBr 15 mg, guaifenesin 100 mg w/alcohol 1.4%, corn syrup, saccharin. Syr. Bot. 118 ml.
Use: Antitussive, expectorant.
EXTRA STRENGTH ASPIRIN CAPSULES. (Walgreen) Aspirin 500 mg/Cap. Bot. 80s.
Use: Salicylate analgesic.
EXTRA STRENGTH BAYER PLUS. (Sterling Health) Aspirin buffered with calcium carbonate, magnesium carbonate, magnesium oxide 500 mg / Capl. Bot. 30s, 60s.
Use: Salicylate analgesic.
EXTRA STRENGTH BAYER ENTERIC 500 ASPIRIN. (Sterling Health) 500 mg. Tab. Enteric coated. Bot. 60s.
Use: Analgesic.
EXTRA STRENGTH DOAN'S PM. (Ciba) Magnesium salicylate 500 mg, diphenhydramine HCl 25 mg / Capl. Pkg. 20s.

Use: Sleep aid.
EXTRA STRENGTH GAS-X. (Sandoz Consumer) Simethicone 125 mg/Tab. Pkg. 18s.
Use: Antiflatulent.
EXTRA STRENGTH TYLENOL HEADACHE PLUS. (McNeil-CPC) Acetaminophen 500 mg, calcium carbonate 250 mg / Capl. Bot. 100s.
Use: Nonnarcotic analgesic combination.
EXTRA STRENGTH TYLENOL PM. (McNeil-CPC) Diphenhydramine 25 mg, acetaminophen 500 mg / **Tab.**: 24s, 50s; **Capl.**: 24s, 50s; **Gelcap:** 20s, 40s.
Use: Sleep aid.
EXTRA STRENGTH VICKS COUGH DROPS. (Richardson-Vicks) Menthol 8.4 mg (menthol flavor) or menthol 10 mg (cherry and honey lemon flavors), corn syrup, sucrose / Loz. Pkg. 9s, 30s.
Use: Mouth and throat product.
EXTREME COLD FORMULA. (Major) Pseudoephedrine HCl 30 mg, chlorpheniramine maleate 1 mg, dextromethorphan HBr 15 mg, acetaminophen 500 mg/Cap. Bot. 10s.
Use: Decongestant, antihistamine, antitussive, analgesic.
EYE FACE AND BODY WASH STATION. (Lavoptik) Sodium Cl 0.49 Gm, sodium biphosphate 0.4 Gm, sodium phosphate 0.45 Gm/100 ml, benzalkonium Cl 0.005%. Bot. 32 oz.
Use: Emergency wash.
EYE IRRIGATING SOLUTION. (Rugby) Sodium Cl, sodium phosphate mono- and dibasic, benzalkonium Cl, EDTA. Soln. Bot. 118 ml.
Use: Extraocular irrigating solution.
EYE IRRIGATING WASH. (Roberts Hauck) Boric acid 1.2%, potassium Cl 0.38%, sodium carbonate anhydrous, EDTA, benzalkonium Cl. Soln. Bot. 120 ml.
Use: Ophthalmic irrigation solution.
EYE-LUBE-A. (Optopics) Glycerin 0.25%, EDTA, NaCl, benzalkonium chloride. Soln. Bot. 15 ml.
Use: Ocular lubricant.
EYE MO. (Sanofi Winthrop) Boric acid, benzalkonium Cl, phenylephrine HCl, zinc sulfate.
Use: Astringent, ophthalmic.
EYE-SED OPHTHALMIC SOLUTION. (Scherer) Boric acid 2.17%, zinc sulfate 0.217%, benzalkonium Cl 0.01% in purified water. Bot. 15 ml.
Use: Astringent, ophthalmic.
EYESINE. (Akorn) Tetrahydrozoline HCl

0.05%, boric acid, sodium borate, sodium chloride, benzalkonium chloride 0.1%, EDTA. Drops. Bot. 15 ml.
Use: Vasoconstrictor/mydriatic (ophthalmic).
EYE-STREAM. (Alcon) Sodium Cl, potassium Cl, calcium Cl, magnesium Cl, benzalkonium Cl 0.013%, sodium citrate, sodium acetate. Bot. 30 ml, 120 ml.
Use: Irrigating agent, ophthalmic.
EYE WASH. (Bausch & Lomb) Sodium Cl Soln. Bot. 4 oz. w/eye cup.
Use: Irrigating agent, ophthalmic.
EYE WASH. (Goldline) Boric acid, potassium Cl, EDTA, anhydrous sodium carbonate, benzalkonium Cl. Soln. Bot. 118 ml.
Use: Ophthalmic irrigation solution.
EYE WASH. (Lavoptik) Sodium Cl 0.49%, sodium biphosphate 0.4%, sodium phosphate 0.45%, benzalkonium Cl. Soln. Bot. 180 ml with eye cup.
Use: Ophthalmic irrigation solution.
EZ-DETECT. (Biomerica) Occult blood screening test. Kit 3s.
Use: Diagnostic aid.
EZ DETECT STREP-A TEST. (Biomerica) Coated stick test for detection of group A streptococci taken directly from a throat swab.
Use: Diagnostic aid.
EZE PAIN. (Halsey) Acetaminophen 2.5 gr, salicylamide, caffeine/Cap. Bot. 21s.
Use: Analgesic.
EZIDE. (Econo Med) Hydrochlorothiazide 50 mg/Tab. Bot. 100s, 1000s.
Use: Diuretic.
EZOL. (Stewart-Jackson) Butalbital 50 mg, caffeine 40 mg, acetaminophen 325 mg. Bot. 100s.
Use: Sedative/hypnotic, analgesic.
EZOL #3. (Stewart Jackson) Aceta minophen 650 mg, codeine 30 mg. Bot. 100s.
Use: Narcotic analgesic combination.

F

FACES ONLY CLEAR SUNSCREEN BY COPPERTONE. (Schering-Plough) Ethylhexyl p-methoxycinnamate, oxybenzone. SPF 6. Gel 55.5 g.
Use: Sunscreen.
FACES ONLY MOISTURIZING SUN-BLOCK BY COPPERTONE. (Schering-Plough) Ethylhexyl p-methoxycinnamate, oxybenzone. SPF 15. Lot. Bot. 55.5 ml.
Use: Sunscreen.

FACT HOME PREGNANCY TEST. (Advanced Care) Accurate test for pregnancy in 45 minutes, for use as early as 3 days after a missed period. 1 Test kit 1s.
Use: Diagnostic aid.
FACTOR VII-a RECOMBINANT, DNA ORIGIN.
Use: Antihemophilic, von Willebrand's disease. [Orphan drug]
FACTOR VIII.
See: Antihemophilic Factor.
• **FACTOR IX COMPLEX,** U.S.P. XXIII.
Use: Hemostatic.
FACTOR XIII.
Use: Congenital Factor XIII deficiency. [Orphan drug]
See: Fibrogammin.
FACTREL. (Wyeth-Ayerst) Gonadorelin HCl 100 mcg or 500 mcg/Vial w/Amp. of 2 ml sterile diluent.
Use: Diagnostic aid.
FACTS PLUS. (Advanced Care Products) Reagent in-home kit for urine testing. Pregnancy test. Kit 1s, 2s.
Use: Diagnostic aid.
• **FADROZOLE HYDROCHLORIDE.** USAN.
Use: Antineoplastic.
FALGOS TABLETS. (Sanofi Winthrop) Acetylsalicylic acid.
Use: Salicylate analgesic.
• **FAMCICLOVIR.** USAN.
Use: Antiviral.
See: Famvir, Tab. (SK-Beecham).
FALMONOX. (Sanofi Winthrop) Teclozan. Susp., Tab..
Use: Amebicide.
• **FAMOTIDINE.** USAN.
Use: Antagonist (to histamine hydrogen receptors).
See: Pepcid, Tab., Susp., Inj. (Merck & Co.).
• **FAMOTIN HCl.** USAN. 1-[(p-Chlorophenoxy)-methyl] -3, 4-dihydroisoquinoline HCl.
Use: Antiviral.
FAMPROFAZONE. B.A.N. 4-Isopropyl-2-methyl-3-[N-methyl-N-(α-methyl-phenethyl)aminomethyl]-1-phenyl-5-pyrazolone.
Use: Analgesic; antipyretic.
FAMVIR. (SK-Beecham) Famciclovir 500 mg. Tab. 30s, UD50s.
Use: Management of acute herpes zoster (shingles).
• **FANETIZOLE MESYLATE.** USAN.
Use: Immunoregulator.
FANSIDAR. (Roche) Sulfadoxine 500 mg, pyrimethamine 25 mg/Tab. Box 25s.
Use: Antimalarial.

• **FANTRIDONE HCl.** USAN. 5-[3-(Di-methylamino)-propyl]-6(5H)-phenan-thridinone monohydrochloride monohydrate.
Use: Antidepressant.

FARA-GEL ANTACID TABLETS. (Faraday) Tab. Bot. 100s.
Use: Antacid.

FARAMALS. (Faraday) Vitamins A 10,000 IU, D 2000 IU, B_1 6 mg, B_2 4 mg, B_6 0.5 mg, folic acid 0.1 mg, C 100 mg, calcium pantothenate 5 mg, niacinamide 30 mg, E 5 IU, B_{12} 3 mcg/Tab. Bot. 100s, 250s, 500s, 1000s.
Use: Vitamin/mineral supplement.

FARAMALS-M. (Faraday) Faramals plus calcium 103 mg, cobalt 0.1 mg, copper 1 mg, iodine 0.15 mg, iron 10 mg, magnesium 6 mg, molybdenum 0.2 mg, phosphorus 80 mg, potassium 5 mg, zinc 1.2 mg/Tab. Bot. 100s, 250s, 500s, 1000s.
Use: Vitamin/mineral supplement.

FARAMINS. (Faraday) Vitamins B_1 20 mg, B_2 6 mg, C 40 mg, niacinamide 20 mg, calcium pantothenate 3 mg, B_6 0.5 mg, powdered whole dried liver 125 mg, dried debittered yeast 125 mg, choline dihydrogen citrate 20 mg, inositol 20 mg, dl-methionine 20 mg, folic acid 0.1 mg, B_{12} 10 mcg, ferrous gluconate 30 mg, dicalcium phosphate 250 mg, copper sulfate 5 mg, magnesium sulfate 10 mg, manganese sulfate 5 mg, cobalt sulfate 0.2 mg, potassium Cl 2 mg, potassium iodide 0.15 mg/Tab. Bot. 100s, 250s, 500s, 1000s.
Use: Vitamin/mineral supplement.

FARATOL. (Faraday) Vitamins A 12,500 IU, D 1000 IU, B_1 20 mg, B_2 6 mg, B_6 0.5 mg, B_{12} 15 mcg, folic acid 0.1 mg, niacinamide 10 mg, calcium pantothenate 3 mg, C 60 mg, E 5 IU, choline dihydrogen citrate 20 mg, inositol 20 mg, dl-methionine 20 mg, whole dried liver 100 mg, dried debittered yeast 100 mg, dicalcium phosphate 200 mg, ferrous gluconate 30 mg, potassium iodide 0.2 mg, magnesium sulfate 7.2 mg, copper sulfate 5 mg, manganese sulfate 3.4 mg, cobalt sulfate 0.2 mg, potassium Cl 1.3 mg, zinc sulfate 2 mg, molybdenum 0.2 mg in a base of alfalfa/Tab. Bot. 100s, 250s, 500s, 1000s.
Use: Vitamin/mineral supplement.

FARBITAL COMPOUND CAPSULES. (Major) Butalbital, caffeine, aspirin. Bot. 100s.
Use: Sedative/hypnotic, salicylate analgesic.

FARBITAL COMPOUND WITH CODEINE #3. (Major) Butalbital, caffeine, aspirin, codeine 30 mg. Bot. 1000s.
Use: Sedative/hypnotic, salicylate analgesic.

FARBITAL TABS. (Major) Butalbital. Bot. 100s.
Use: Sedative/hypnotic.

FARNOQUINONE. 2-Difarnesyl-3-methyl-1, 4-naphthoquinone.

FASTIN. (Beecham Labs) Phentermine HCl 30 mg/Cap. Bot. 100s, 450s. Pack 150s. (5 × 30s).
Use: Anorexiant.

FAT EMULSION, INTRAVENOUS.
See: Liposyn 10% (Abbott).
Liposyn 20% (Abbott).
Travamulsion 10% (Travenol).
Travamulsion 20% (Travenol).
Intralipid 10% (Kabi Vitrum).
Intralipid 20% (Kabi Vitrum).
Soyacal 10% (Alpha Therapeutic).
Soyacal 20% (Alpha Therapeutic).
Liposyn II 10% (Abbott).
Liposyn II 20% (Abbott).

FATHER JOHN'S MEDICINE PLUS. (Oakhurst) Phenylephrine HCl 2.5 mg, chlorpheniramine maleate 1 mg, dextromethorphan HBr 7.5 mg, guaifenesin 30 mg, ammonium Cl 100 mg, sodium citrate/5 ml. Bot. 120 ml, 240 ml.
Use: Decongestant, antihistamine, antitussive, expectorant.

FATTIBASE. (Paddock) Preblended fatty acid suppository base composed of triglycerides of coconut oil and palm kernel oil. Jar 1 lb, 5 lb.
Use: Fatty acid suppository base.

FATTY ACIDS, UNSATURATED.
See: Fats, Unsaturated.
Undecylenic Acid (Various Mfr.).

FAT, UNSATURATED.
See: Arcofac, Emul. (Armour).
Lufa, Cap. (USV Pharm.).

FAZADINIUM BROMIDE. 1,1'-Azobis(3-methyl-2- phenylimidazo[1,2-α]pyridinium bromide).
Use: Neuromuscular blocking agent.

• **FAZARABINE.** USAN.
Use: Antineoplastic.

F.C.A.H. CAPSULES. (Scherer) Chlorpheniramine maleate 4 mg, acetaminophen 162 mg, salicylamide 162 mg/Cap. Bot. 100s, 500s.
Use: Antihistaminic, analgesic.

• **FEBANTEL.** USAN.
Use: Anthelmintic.

FEBERIN. (Arcum) Ferrous gluconate 3 gr, vitamins C 25 mg, B_1 2 mg, B_6 1 mg, B_2 1 mg, niacinamide 5 mg/Tab. Bot.

100s, 1000s.
Use: Vitamin/mineral supplement.
FEBRILE ANTIGENS. (Laboratory Diagnostics) Group O antigens (somatic) are dyed blue and group H antigens (flagellars) are dyed red for clear identification for detection of bacterial agglutinins, bacterial infections. Vial 5 ml.
Use: Diagnostic aid.
FEBRIN. (Jenkins) Acetophenetidin 0.1 Gm, acetylsalicylic acid 0.12 Gm, caffeine 15 mg, camphor monobromated 60 mg/Tab. Bot. 1000s.
Use: Analgesic combination.
FEBRINOL. (Vitarine) Acetaminophen 325 mg/Tab. Bot. 100s, 1000s.
Use: Analgesic.
FE-BRONE. (Forest Pharm.) Vitamins B_{12} 1 IU, folic acid 1 mg, ferrous sulfate exsiccated (powdered) 200 mg, ferrous sulfate exsiccated (timed) 200 mg, C acid 100 mg, B_6 0.5 mg, B_1 2 mg, B_2 1 mg, copper 0.9 mg, zinc 0.5 mg, manganese 0.3 mg/Cap. Bot. 30s, 100s, 1000s.
Use: Vitamin/mineral supplement.
FEDAHIST GYROCAPS. (Kremers-Urban) Pseudoephedrine HCl 65 mg, chlorpheniramine maleate 10 mg/SR Cap. Bot. 100s.
Use: Decongestant, antihistamine.
FEDAHIST TIMECAPS. (Kremers-Urban) Pseudoephedrine HCl 120 mg, chlorpheniramine maleate 8 mg/SR Cap. Bot. 100s.
Use: Decongestant, antihistamine.
FEDRAZIL. (Burroughs Wellcome) Pseudoephedrine HCl 30 mg, chlorcyclizine HCl 25 mg/Tab. Box 24s. Bot. 100s.
Use: Decongestant, antihistamine.
FEDRINAL. (H.L. Moore) Ephedrine HCl 12 mg, phenobarbital 12 mg, potassium iodide 160 mg, theophylline anhydrous 31.2 mg/5 ml. Bot. pt, gal.
Use: Decongestant, sedative/hypnotic, expectorant, bronchodilator.
FEEN-A-MINT DUAL FORMULA. (Plough) Docusate sodium 100 mg, yellow phenolphthalein 65 mg/Tab. Box 15s, 30s, 60s.
Use: Laxative.
FEEN-A-MINT GUM. (Plough) Yellow phenolphthalein 97.2 mg/Chewing gum Tab. Box 5s, 16s, 40s.
Use: Laxative.
FEEN-A-MINT MINT. (Plough) Yellow phenolphthalein 97.2 mg/Chewable mint tab. Box 20s.
Use: Laxative.
FEEN-A-MINT PILLS. (Plough) Docusate

sodium 100 mg, yellow phenolphthalein 65 mg/Tab. Box 15s, 30s, 60s.
Use: Laxative.
FEG-L. (Western Research) Ferrous gluconate 300 mg/Tab. Handicount 28s (36 bags of 28 tab.).
Use: Iron supplement.
FEIBA VH IMMUNO. (Immuno-U.S.) Freeze-dried anti-inhibitor coagulant complex. Heparin free. Vapor heated. Inj. Vial with diluent and needle.
Use: Antihemophilic.
FELBAMATE. USAN.
Use: Treatment of Lennox-Gastaut Syndrome. [Orphan drug]
FELBATOL. (Wallace Labs) Felbamate, lactose 400 mg or 600 mg/tab., Felbamate, 600 mg/5 ml/susp. **Tab.:** Bot. 100s and UD 100s. **Susp.:** 240 ml and 960 ml.
Use: Antiepileptic. Due to 10 cases of aplastic anemia associated with felbamate use (including 2 deaths), the FDA and Carter-Wallace recommend that use of the drug be suspended unless use of the physician decides that withdrawal would pose an even greater risk to the patient. Patients should not discontinue the drug on their own. There has been no product recall at this time (8/94).
• **FELBINAC.** USAN.
Use: Anti-inflammatory.
FELDENE. (Pfizer Laboratories) Piroxicam 10 mg or 20 mg/Cap. **10 mg:** Bot 100s. **20 mg:** Bot. 100s, 500s, UD 100s.
Use: Nonsteroidal anti-inflammatory drug; analgesic.
FELLOBOLIC INJECTION. (Forest Pharm.) Methandriol dipropionate 50 mg/ml. Vial 10 ml.
• **FELODIPINE.** USAN.
Use: Vasodilator.
See: Plendil, Tab. (Merck & Co.).
• **FELYPRESSIN.** USAN. 2-(Phenylalanine)-8-lysine vasopressin.
Use: Vasoconstrictor.
FEMAGENE. (Tennessee) Boric acid, sodium borate, lactic acid, menthol, methylbenzethonium Cl, parachlorometaxylenol, lactose, surface-active agents. Pow. 6 oz.
Use: Feminine hygiene.
FEMAZOLE TABS. (Major) Metronidazole 250 mg or 500 mg/Tab. **250 mg:** Bot. 100s, 250s, 500s. **500 mg:** Bot. 50s, 100s.
Use: Anti-infective.
FEMCAPS. (Buffington) Acetaminophen, caffeine, ephedrine sulfate, atropine sul-

fate/Tab. Sugar, lactose and salt free Dispens-a-Kit 500s, Aidpaks 100s.
Use: Analgesic, bronchodilator, anticholinergic/antispasmodic.

FEMCARE. (Schering-Plough) **Vaginal Cream:** Clotrimazole 1%, benzyl alcohol, cetearyl alcohol, cetyl esters wax, octyldodecanol, polysorbate 60, sorbitan monostearate. Tube. 45 Gm. **Vaginal Tab.:** Clotrimazole 100 mg, in 7s with applicator.
Use: Vaginal yeast infection.

FEMCET. (Russ) Acetaminophen 325 mg, butalbital 50 mg, caffeine 40 mg/Cap. Bot. 100s.
Use: Analgesic, sedative/hypnotic.

FEMERGIN.
See: Ergotamine Tartrate (Various Mfr.).

FEMIDINE. (A.V.P.) Povidone-iodine. Bot. 240 ml.
Use: Cleansing douche.

FEMIDYN.
See: Estrone (Various Mfr.).

FEMILAX. (G & W Labs) Docusate sodium 100 mg, phenolphthalein 65 mg/Tab. Bot. 30s, 60s, 90s.
Use: Laxative.

FEMINIQUE DISPOSABLE DOUCHE. (Schmid) Sodium benzoate, sorbic acid, lactic acid, octoxynol-9. Twin-pack Bot. 150 ml.
Use: Douche.

FEMINIQUE DISPOSABLE DOUCHE. (Schmid) Vinegar and water. Soln. Twin-packs. Bot. 150 ml.
Use: Douche.

FEMINONE. (Upjohn) Ethinyl estradiol 0.05 mg/Tab. Bot. 100s.
Use: Estrogen.

FEMIRON. (Beecham Products) Iron 20 mg/Tab. Bot 40s, 120s.
Use: Iron supplement.

FEMIRON MULTI-VITAMINS AND IRON. (Beecham Products) Iron 20 mg, vitamins A 5,000 IU, D 400 IU, B_1 1.5 mg, riboflavin 1.7 mg, niacinamide 20 mg, C 60 mg, B_6 2 mg, B_{12} 6 mcg, calcium pantothenate 10 mg, folic acid 0.4 mg, E 15 mg/Tab. Bot. 40s, 120s.
Use: Vitamin/mineral supplement.

FEMOTRONE. (Bluco) Progesterone in oil 50 mg/ml. Vial 10 ml.
Use: Progestin.

FEMSTAT VAGINAL CREAM. (Syntex) Butoconazole nitrate 2% in water-washable emollient cream. Tube 28 Gm w/applicators.
Use: Antifungal, vaginal.

•**FENALAMIDE.** USAN. (1) Ethyl N-[2-(diethylamino)-ethyl]-2-ethyl-2-phenyl-

malonamate; (2) Phenylethylmalonic acid monoethyl ester diethylaminoethylamide.
Use: Smooth muscle relaxant.

FENAMISAL. Phenyl aminosalicylate.

•**FENAMOLE.** USAN. 5-Amino-1-phenyl-1H-tetrazol.
Use: Anti-inflammatory agent

FENAPRIN TABLETS. (Sanofi Winthrop) Aspirin, chlormezanone.
Use: Salicylate analgesic, antianxiety agent.

FENAROL. (Sanofi Winthrop) Chlormezanone 100 mg or 200 mg/Tab. Bot. 100s.
Use: Antianxiety agent.

FENARSONE.
See: Carbarsone (Various Mfr.).

•**FENBENDAZOLE.** USAN.
Use: Anthelmintic.

•**FENBUFEN.** USAN.
Use: Anti-inflammatory.

FENCAMFAMIN. B.A.N. N-Ethyl-3-phenylbicyclo-[2.2.1]hept-2-ylamine.
Use: Central nervous system stimulant; appetite suppressant.

•**FENCILBUTIROL.** USAN.
Use: Choleretic.

•**FENCLOFENAC.** USAN. 2-(2,4-Dichlorophenoxy)-phenylacetic acid.
Use: Anti-inflammatory.

•**FENCLONINE.** USAN. dl-3-(p-Chlorophenyl)-alanine. Under study by Pfizer.
Use: Serotonin biosynthesis inhibitor.

•**FENCLORAC.** USAN.
Use: Anti-inflammatory.

FENCLOZIC ACID. B.A.N. 2-(4-Chlorophenyl)-thiazol-4-ylacetic acid.
Use: Anti-inflammatory.

FEND. (Mine Safety Appliances).
A-2—Water soluble cream which forms a physical barrier to water insoluble irritants. Tube 3 oz, Jar lb.
E-2—This cream combines the functions of the water soluble Fend A-2 and water insoluble Fend I-2 creams. Tube 3 oz, Jar lb.
I-2—Water insoluble cream which forms a physical barrier to water soluble irritants. Tube 3 oz, Jar lb.
S-2—A silicone cream which forms a barrier against a combination of water soluble and water insoluble irritants. Tube 3 oz, Jar lb.
X—Industrial cold cream which rubs well into the skin and serves as a skin conditioner. Tube 3 oz, Jar lb.
Use: Skin protectant.

FENDOL. (Buffington) Salicylamide, caf-

feine, acetaminophen, phenylephrine HCl/Tab. Sugar, lactose and salt free. Dispens-A-Kit 500s. Bot. 100s.
Use: Analgesic combination.
•**FENDOSAL.** USAN.
Use: Anti-inflammatory.
FENESIN. (Dura) Guaifenesin 600 mg/SR Tab. Bot. 100s, 600s.
Use: Expectorant.
•**FENESTREL.** USAN. 5-Ethyl-6-methyl-4-phenyl-3-cyclohexene-1-carboxylic acid. Under study.
Use: Nonsteroid estrogen.
•**FENETHYLLINE HYDROCHLORIDE.** USAN. 7-[2-[(α-Methylphenethyl)-amino]-ethyl]theophylline hydrochloride.
Use: Stimulant center.
•**FENFLURAMINE HYDROCHLORIDE.** USAN. N-ethyl-α-methyl-m-(trifluoromethyl)-phenethylamine hydrochloride.
Use: Sympathomimetic (anorexiant).
See: Pondimin, Tab. (Robins).
•**FENGABINE.** USAN.
Use: Mood regulator.
•**FENIMIDE.** USAN. 3-Ethyl-2-methyl-2-phenylsuccinimide.
Use: Tranquilizer.
•**FENISOREX.** USAN. (±)-cis-7-Fluoro-1-phenylisochroman-3-ylmethylamine.
Use: Anorexigenic.
•**FENMETOZOLE HYDROCHLORIDE.** USAN.
Use: Antidepressant antagonist.
•**FENMETRAMIDE.** USAN.
Use: Antidepressant.
•**FENNEL OIL,** N.F. XVIII.
Use: Pharmaceutic aid (flavor).
•**FENOBAM.** USAN.
Use: Sedative.
•**FENOCTIMINE SULFATE.** USAN.
Use: Gastric antisecretory.
FENOFIBRATE.
Use: Antihyperlipidemic.
See: Lipidil, Cap. (Fournier).
•**FENOLDOPAM MESYLATE.** USAN.
Use: Antihypertensive.
•**FENOPROFEN.** USAN. 2-(3-phenoxyphonyl) propionic acid. (±)-m-Phenoxyhydratropic acid; (2) dl-2-(3-phenoxyphenyl)-propionic acid.
Use: Anti-inflammatory, analgesic.
•**FENOPROFEN CALCIUM,** U.S.P. XXIII. Cap., Tab., U.S.P. XXIII.
Use: Anti-inflammatory, analgesic.
See: Nalfon, Cap., Tab. (Dista).
•**FENOTEROL.** USAN. (1)3,5-Dihydroxy-α-[[(p-hydroxy-α-methylphenethyl) amino] methyl]-benzyl alcohol; (2) 1-(3,5-Dihydroxyphenyl)-2-[[1-(4-hydroxybenzyl)ethyl]amino] ethanol.

Use: Bronchodilator.
•**FENPIPALONE.** USAN.
Use: Anti-inflammatory.
FENPIPRAMIDE. B.A.N. 2,2-Diphenyl-4-piperidonobutyramide.
Use: Spasmolytic.
FENPIPRANE. B.A.N. 1-(3,3-Diphenylpropyl)-piperidine.
Use: Spasmolytic.
•**FENPRINAST HYDROCHLORIDE.** USAN.
Use: Anti-allergic, bronchodilator.
•**FENPROSTALENE.** USAN.
Use: Luteolysin.
•**FENQUIZONE.** USAN.
Use: Diuretic.
•**FENRETINIDE.** USAN.
Use: Antineoplastic.
•**FENSPIRIDE HYDROCHLORIDE.** USAN.
Use: Bronchodilator, anti-adrenergic.
•**FENTANYL.**
Use: Narcotic analgesic.
See: Duragesic, Transdermal (Janssen).
•**FENTANYL CITRATE,** U.S.P. XXIII. Inj. U.S.P. XXIII. N-(1-phenethyl-4-piperidyl) propionanilide citrate. Propanamide, N-phenyl N [1 (2 phenyl-ethyl)-4-piperidinyl]-,2-hydroxy-1,2,3-propanetricarboxylate (1:1).
Use: Narcotic analgesic.
See: Sublimaze, Inj. (Janssen).
FENTANYL CITRATE AND DROPERIDOL. (Astra) Fentanyl 0.05 mg, droperidol 2.5 mg/ml. Inj. Amp and Vial 2 ml, 5 ml.
Use: General anesthetic.
See: Innovar, Inj. (Janssen).
FENTANYL TRANSDERMAL SYSTEM.
See: Duragesic-25 (Janssen). Duragesic-50 (Janssen). Duragesic-75 (Janssen). Duragesic-100 (Janssen).
•**FENTIAZAC.** USAN.
Use: Anti-inflammatory.
•**FENTICLOR.** USAN. Di-(5-chloro-2-hydroxyphenyl)-sulfide.
Use: Antiseptic, fungicide.
•**FENTICONAZOLE NITRATE.** USAN.
Use: Antifungal.
FENTON ELIXIR. (Sanofi Winthrop) Ferrous gluconate.
Use: Iron supplement.
FENYLHIST. (Hauck) Diphenhydramine HCl 25 mg or 50 mg/Cap. Bot. 1000s.
Use: Antihistamine.
FENYRAMIDOL HCl. Phenyramidol HCl.
•**FENYRIPOL HYDROCHLORIDE.** USAN. α-(2-pyrimidinylaminomethyl) benzyl al-

cohol hydrochloride.
Use: Skeletal muscle relaxant.
FEOCYTE. (Dunhall) Iron 110 mg, vitamins C 100 mg, B$_6$ 2 mg, B$_{12}$ 50 mcg, copper sulfate 2 mg, folic acid 0.8 mg, desiccated liver/Prolonged Action Tab. Bot. 100s.
Use: Vitamin/mineral supplement
FEOCYTE INJECTABLE. (Dunhall) Peptonized iron 15 mg, vitamin B$_{12}$ 200 mcg, liver injection N.F. beef 10 units, sodium citrate 10 mg, benzyl alcohol 2%/ml. Vial 10 ml.
Use: Vitamin/mineral supplement.
FE-O.D. (Trimen) Iron 100 mg, ascorbic acid 500 mg/Tab. Bot. 100s.
Use: Vitamin/mineral supplement.
FEOSOL CAPSULES. (SK-Beecham) Dried ferrous sulfate 159 mg (50 mg iron)/SR Cap. Bot. 30s, 100s, 500s, UD 100s.
Use: Iron supplement.
FEOSOL ELIXIR. (SK-Beecham) Ferrous sulfate (44 mg iron) 220 mg/5 ml, alcohol 5%. Bot. 16 oz.
Use: Iron supplement.
FEOSOL TABLETS. (SK-Beecham) Dried ferrous sulfate 200 mg (65 mg iron)/Tab. Bot. 100s, 1000s, UD 100s.
Use: Iron supplement.
FEOSTAT. (Forest) **Tab.:** Ferrous fumarate 100 mg (33 mg iron)/Chew. tab. Bot. 100s, 1000s. **Drops:** Ferrous fumarate 45 mg (15 mg iron)/0.6 ml. Bot. 60 ml.
Use: Iron supplement.
FEOSTAT SUSPENSION. (Forest) Ferrous fumarate 100 mg (33 mg iron)/5 ml. Bot. 240 ml.
Use: Iron supplement.
FE-PLUS PROTEIN. (Miller) Iron (as an iron-protein complex) 50 mg/Tab. Bot. 100s.
Use: Iron supplement.
FEPRAZONE. B.A.N. 4-(3-Methylbut-2-enyl)-1,2-diphenylpyrazolidine-3,5-dione.
Use: Analgesic; anti-inflammatory.
FERANCEE. (J & J-Merck) Elemental iron 67 mg (from 200 mg ferrous fumarate), vitamin C 150 mg Tab. Bot. 100s.
Use: Vitamin/mineral supplement.
FERANCEE-HP. (Stuart) Elemental iron 110 mg (from 330 mg ferrous fumarate), ascorbic acid 350 mg, sodium ascorbate 281 mg/Tab. Bot. 60s.
Use: Vitamin/mineral supplement.
FERATAB. (Upsher-Smith) Ferrous sulfate 300 mg (60 mg iron)/Tab. Bot. 100s.

Use: Iron supplement.
FERATE-C. (Vale) Ferrous fumarate 150 mg, ascorbic acid 200 mg, docusate sodium 25 mg/Tab. Bot. 100s, 1000s.
Use: Vitamin/mineral supplement.
FER-GEN-SOL DROPS. (Goldline) Ferrous sulfate drops. Bot. 50 ml.
Use: Iron supplement.
FERGON. (Sanofi Winthrop) Pure ferrous gluconate. **Tab.:** 320 mg equal to approximately 37 mg ferrous iron/Tab. Bot. 100s, 500s, 1000s. **Elix.:** 300 mg = 35 mg iron/5 ml. Bot. 16 fl. oz.
Use: Iron supplement.
FERGON PLUS. (Sanofi Winthrop) Iron 58 mg (from ferrous gluconate) vitamin B$_{12}$ w/intrinsic factor concentrate 0.5 units, ascorbic acid 75 mg/Capl. Bot. 100s.
Use: Vitamin/mineral supplement.
FER-IN-SOL. (Mead Johnson Nutrition) **Drops:** Elemental iron 15 mg/0.6 ml, alcohol 0.02%. Bot. w/dropper 50 ml. **Syr.:** 18 mg/5 ml. Alcohol 5%. Bot. 16 fl oz. **Cap.:** 60 mg. Bot. 100s.
Use: Iron supplement.
FER-IRON. (Rugby) Ferrous sulfate 75 mg (iron 15 mg)/0.6 ml. Drops. Bot. 50 ml.
Use: Iron supplement.
FERMETONE COMPOUND CAPSULES. (Sanofi Winthrop) Pancreatin.
Use: Digestive enzyme.
FERNCORT LOTION. (Ferndale) Hydrocortisone acetate 0.5% in lotion base. Bot. 120 ml.
Use: Corticosteroid.
FEROCYL. (Hudson) Ferrous fumarate 150 mg (iron 50 mg), docusate sodium 100 mg/TR Cap. Bot. 100s.
Use: Iron supplement.
FERO-FOLIC 500. (Abbott) Ferrous sulfate controlled-release (equivalent to 105 mg iron), vitamin C 500 mg, folic acid 800 mcg/Filmtab. Bot. 100s, 500s.
Use: Vitamin/mineral supplement.
FERO-GRAD 500 FILMTAB. (Abbott) Sodium ascorbate 500 mg, ferrous sulfate equivalent to 105 mg iron/CR Filmtab. Bot. 30s, 100s, 500s, UD 100s.
Use: Iron supplement.
FERO-GRADUMET FILMTAB. (Abbott) Ferrous sulfate 525 mg controlled-release equivalent to 105 mg iron/Filmtab. Bot. 100s.
Use: Iron supplement.
FEROLIX. (Century) Ferrous sulfate 5 gr, alcohol 5%/10 ml Elix. Bot. 8 oz, pt, gal.
Use: Iron supplement.
FEROSAN FORTE. (Sandia) Ferrous fu-

marate 300 mg, liver-stomach concentrate 150 mg, vitamin B_{12} w/intrinsic factor concentrate 7.5 mcg, intrinsic factor concentrate 150 mg, B_{12} 7.5 mcg, ascorbic acid 75 mg, folic acid 1 mg, sorbitol 50 mg/Tab. Bot. 100s.
Use: Vitamin/mineral supplement.

FEROSAN SYRUP. (Sandia) Ferrous fumarate 91.2 mg, B_1 10 mg, B_6 3 mg, B_{12} 25 mcg/5 ml 16 oz, gal.
Use: Iron supplement.

FEROSPACE. (Hudson) Ferrous sulfate 250 mg (iron 50 mg)/TR Cap. Bot. 100s.
Use: Iron supplement.

FEROTRINSIC. (Rugby) Iron 36.3 mg (from ferrous fumarate), vitamins B_{12} 15 mcg, C 75 mg, intrinsic factor (as concentrate or from stomach preparations) 240 mg, folic acid 0.5 mg/Cap. 100s, 1000s.
Use: Vitamin/mineral supplement.

FEROWEET. (Barth's) Vitamins B_1 6 mg, B_2 12 mg, niacin 4 mg, iron 30 mg, B_{12} 10 mcg, B_6 95 mcg, pantothenic acid 50 mcg/3 Cap. Bot. 100s, 500s, 1000s.
Use: Vitamin/mineral supplement.

FERRACOMP. (Hauck) Liver 2 mcg, vitamins B_{12} 15 mcg, B_1 10 mg, B_2 5 mg, B_6 1 mg, calcium pantothenate 1 mg, niacinamide 10 mg, iron 31.3 mg/ml. Vial 30 ml.
Use: Vitamin/mineral supplement.

FERRALET. (Mission) Ferrous gluconate 320 mg (37 mg iron)/Tab. Bot. 100s.
Use: Iron supplement.

FERRALET PLUS. (Mission) Ferrous gluconate equivalent to 46 mg iron, ascorbic acid 400 mg, folic acid 0.8 mg, vitamin B_{12} 25 mcg/Tab. Bot. 100s.
Use: Vitamin/mineral supplement.

FERRALET S.R.. (Mission) Ferrous gluconate 320 mg (iron 37 mg)/SR Tab. Bot. 30s.
Use: Iron supplement.

FERRALYN LANACAPS. (Lannett) Ferrous sulfate 250 mg (iron 50 mg)/TR Cap. Bot. 100s, 500s, 1000s.
Use: Iron supplement.

FERRANOL. (Robinson) Ferrous fumarate 3 gr or 5 gr/Tab. Bot. 100s, 1000s.
Use: Iron supplement.

FERRA-TD. (Goldline) Ferrous sulfate 250 mg (iron 50 mg)/TR Cap. Bot. 100s, 1000s.
Use: Iron supplement.

FERRETS. (Pharmics) Ferrous fumarate 325 mg, iron 106 mg/Tab. Bot. 100s.
Use: Iron supplement.

FERRIC AMMONIUM CITRATE. Ammonium iron (Fe^{+++}) citrate.

Use: Iron supplement.
FERRIC AMMONIUM SULFATE. (Various Mfr.).
Use: Astringent.
FERRIC AMMONIUM TARTRATE. (Various Mfr.).
Use: Iron supplement.
FERRIC CACODYLATE. (Various Mfr.).
Use: Leukemias & iron deficiency.
FERRIC CHLORIDE. (Various Mfr.).
Use: Astringent.
•**FERRIC CHLORIDE Fe 59.** USAN.
Use: Radioactive agent.
FERRIC CITROCHLORIDE TINCTURE. Iron (3+) chloride citrate.
Use: Hematinic.
•**FERRIC FRUCTOSE.** USAN. Fructose iron complex with potassium (2:1).
Use: Hematinic.
FERRIC GLYCEROPHOSPHATE. Glycerol phosphate iron (3+) salt.
Use: Pharmaceutic necessity.
FERRIC HYPOPHOSPHITE. Iron (3+) phosphinate.
Use: Pharmaceutic necessity.
•**FERRICLATE CALCIUM SODIUM.** USAN.
Use: Hematinic.
•**FERRIC OXIDE, RED,** N.F. XVIII.
Use: Pharmaceutic aid (color).
•**FERRIC OXIDE, YELLOW,** N.F. XVIII.
Use: Pharmaceutic aid (color).
FERRIC "PEPTONATE." (Various Mfr.).
See: Iron Peptonized.
FERRIC PYROPHOSPHATE, SOLUBLE. Iron (3+) citrate pyrophosphate.
FERRIC QUININE CITRATE, "GREEN." (Various Mfr.).
Use: Iron supplement.
FERRIC SUBSULFATE SOLUTION. (Various Mfr.).
Use: Local use on the skin.
FERRIZYME. (Abbott Diagnostics) Enzyme immunoassay for qualitative determination of ferritin in human serum or plasma. Test kit 100s.
Use: Diagnostic aid.
FERROCHOLATE.
See: Ferrocholinate.
FERROCHOLINATE. Ferrocholate. Ferrocholine. A chelate prepared by reacting equimolar quantities of freshly precipitated ferric hydroxide with choline dihydrogen citrate.
Use: Iron supplement.
See: Chel-Iron, Preps. (Kinney).
FERROCHOLINE.
See: Ferrocholinate.
Kelex, Tabseal. (Nutrition).
FERRO-CYTE. (Spanner) Iron peptonate

20 mg, liver injection (20 mg/ml) 0.25 ml, vitamins B_1 22 mg, B_2 0.5 mg, B_6 2.5 mg, B_{12} 30 mcg, niacinamide 25 mg, panthenol 1 mg/ml. Inj. Multiple dose vial 10 ml.
Use: Vitamin/mineral supplement.
FERRO-DOCUSATE T.R. (Parmed) Ferrous fumarate 150 mg (iron 50 mg), docusate sodium 100 mg/TR Cap. Bot. 100s.
Use: Iron supplement.
FERRO-DOK TR. (Major) Ferrous fumarate 150 mg (iron 50 mg), docusate sodium 100 mg/TR Cap. Bot. 100s.
Use: Iron supplement.
FERRO-DSS. (Geneva Marsam) Ferrous fumarate 150 mg (iron 50 mg), docusate sodium 100 mg/TR Cap. Bot. 100s.
Use: Iron supplement.
FERRODYL CHEWABLE TABLETS. (Arcum) Ferrous fumarate 320 mg, vitamin C 200 mg/Tab. Bot. 100s, 1000s.
Use: Vitamin/mineral supplement.
FERROMAR. (Marnel) Ferrous fumarate 201.5 mg (iron 65 mg), vitamin C 200 mg/SR Capl. Bot. 100s.
Use: Iron Supplement.
FERROMAX (INTRAMUSCULAR IRON). (Kenyon) Iron peptonized 100 mg, copper gluconate 0.2 mg, cobalt Cl 4 mg, pectin 10 mg/ml. Vial 10 ml.
Use: Mineral supplement.
FERRONEED. (Hanlon) Ferrous gluconate 300 mg, ascorbic acid 60 mg/Cap. Bot. 100s.
Use: Vitamin/mineral supplement.
FERRONEED T-CAPS. (Hanlon) Ferrous fumarate 250 mg, thiamine HCl 5 mg, ascorbic acid 50 mg/TD Cap. Bot. 100s.
Use: Vitamin/mineral supplement.
FERRONEX. (Pasadena Research) Iron from ferrous gluconate 2.9 mg, Vitamins B_{12} equivalent 1 mcg, B_2 0.75 mg, B_3 50 mg, B_5 1.25 mg, B_{12} 15 mcg, procaine 2%/ml. Inj. Vial 30 ml.
Use: Vitamin/mineral supplement.
FERRO-SEQUELS. (Lederle) Ferrous fumarate 150 mg (equivalent to 50 mg elemental iron), dioctyl sodium sulfosuccinate 100 mg/TD Cap. Bot. 30s, 100s, 1000s, UD 10×10s.
Use: Iron supplement.
FERROSPAN CAPSULES. (Imperial Lab.) Ferrous fumarate 200 mg, ascorbic acid 100 mg/Tab. Bot. 100s, 1000s.
Use: Vitamin/mineral supplement.
FERROSYN INJECTION. (Standex) Cyanocobalamin 30 mcg, liver 2 mcg, ferrous gluconate 100 mg, riboflavin 1.5 mg, panthenol 2.5 mg, niacinamide 100

mg, procaine 2%. Vial 30 ml.
Use: Vitamin/mineral supplement.
FERROSYN S.C. (Standex) Iron 60 mg, vitamin B_{12} 5 mcg, magnesium 0.6 mg, copper 0.3 mg, manganese 0.1 mg, potassium 0.5 mg, zinc 0.15 mg/Tab. Bot. 100s, 1000s.
Use: Vitamin/mineral supplement.
FERROSYN SEE TABS. (Standex) Iron 34 mg, ascorbic acid 60 mg/Tab. Bot. 100s, 1000s.
Use: Vitamin/mineral supplement.
FERROSYN TAB. (Standex) Iron 60 mg, vitamin B_{12} 5 mcg, magnesium 0.6 mg, copper 0.3 mg, manganese 0.1 mg, potassium 0.5 mg, zinc 0.15 mg/Tab. Bot. 100s.
Use: Vitamin/mineral supplement.
FERROUS BROMIDE. (Various Mfr.).
Use: In chorea & tuberculous cervical adenitis.
FERROUS CARBONATE MASS. Vallet's mass. (Various Mfr.).
Use: Iron supplement.
FERROUS CARBONATE, SACCHARATED. (Various Mfr.).
Use: Iron supplement.
•**FERROUS CITRATE Fe-59 INJECTION,** U.S.P. XXIII.
Use: Radioactive agent.
•**FERROUS FUMARATE,** U.S.P. XXIII. Tab., U.S.P. XXIII.
Use: Hematinic.
See: Childron, Susp. (Fleming).
  Eldofe, Tab. (Canright).
  El-Ped-Ron, Liq. (Elder).
  Farbegen, Cap. (Hickam).
  Feco-T, Cap. (Blaine).
  Ferretts, Tab. (Pharmics).
  Fumasorb, Tab. (Marion).
  Fumerin, Tab. (Laser).
  Ircon, Tab. (Key).
  Laud-Iron, Tab., Susp. (Amfre-Grant).
  Maniron, Meltab. (Bowman).
W/Ascorbic Acid.
See: C-Ron, Preps. (Solvay).
  Cytoferin, Tab. (Wyeth-Ayerst).
  Eldofe-C, Tab. (Canright).
  Ferancee, Tab. (J & J-Merck).
  Ferancee-HP, Tab. (Stuart).
  Ferrodyl Chewable Tab. (Arcum).
  Ferromar, SR Cap. (Marnel).
  Min-Hema Chewable, Tab. (Scrip).
W/Ascorbic acid and folic acid.
See: Fer-Regules, Cap. (Quality Generics).
  Ferro-Docusate T.R., Cap. (Parmed)
  Ferro Dok TR, Cap. (Major)
  Ferro-DSS S.R., Cap. (Geneva Marsam)

Ferro-Sequels, Cap. (Lederle).
W/Norethindrone, mestranol.
See: Ortho Novum Fe-28, Fe-28, 1 mg
Fe-28, Tab. (Ortho).
W/Vitamins and minerals.
See: Stuart Formula, Tab. (Stuart).
Stuart Prenatal, Tab. (Stuart).
Stuartnatal 1 + 1, Tab. (Stuart).
Theron, Tab. (Stuart).
Vitanate, Tab. (Century).
• **FERROUS FUMARATE AND DOCUSATE
SODIUM EXTENDED-RELEASE
TABLETS, U.S.P..** U.S.P. XXIII.
Use: Iron supplement.
• **FERROUS GLUCONATE,** U.S.P. XXIII.
Cap., Elixir, Tab., U.S.P. XXIII. Iron (2+)
Gluconate.
Use: Iron deficiency.
See: Entron, Cap., Tab. (LaCrosse).
Fergon Prods. (Sanofi Winthrop Prod-
ucts).
W/Ascorbic acid, desiccated liver, vitamin
B complex.
See: I.L.X. w/B$_{12}$, Tab. (Kenwood).
Stuart Hematinic, Liq. (Stuart).
W/Polyoxyethylene glucitan monolaurate.
See: Simron, Cap. (Morroll Dow).
FERROUS IODIDE. (Various Mfr.).
Use: In chronic tuberculosis.
FERROUS IODIDE SYRUP. (Various
Mfr.).
Use: In chronic tuberculosis.
FERROUS LACTATE. (Various Mfr.).
Use: Iron deficiency.
• **FERROUS SULFATE,** U.S.P. XXIII. Tab.,
Dried, Syr., Oral Soln., U.S.P. XXIII.
Use: Iron deficiency.
See: Feosol, Spansule, Tab., Elix. (SK-
Beecham).
Fer-iron, Drops (Rugby).
Ferralyn, Cap. (Lannett).
Fero-Gradumet, Tab. (Abbott).
Ferolix, Elix. (Century).
Ferrous Sulfate Filmseals, Tab.
(Parke Davis).
Fesotyme SR, Cap. (Elder).
Irospan, Cap., Tab. (Fielding).
Mol-Iron, Prods. (Schering).
Telefon, Cap. (Kenyon).
W/Ascorbic acid.
See: Fero-Grad-500, Tab. (Abbott).
Mol-Iron W/Vitamin C, Tab., Chrono-
sules (Schering).
W/Ascorbic acid, folic acid.
See: Fero-Folic-500, Tab. (Abbott).
W/Cyanocobalamin, ascorbic acid, folic
acid.
See: Intrin, Cap. (Merit).
W/Folic acid.

See: Folvron, Cap. (Lederle).
W/Maalox.
See: Fermalox, Tab. (Rhone-Poulenc
Rorer Consumer).
FERROUS SULFATE FILMSEALS.
(Parke-Davis) Ferrous sulfate 5 gr/DR
Tab. Bot. 1000s, UD 100s.
Use: Iron supplement.
• **FERROUS SULFATE Fe 59.** USAN.
Use: Radioisotope.
FERTILITY TAPE. (Weston Labs.) Regu-
lar, extrasensitive, less-sensitive. W/Fer-
tility Testor, cervical glucose test. Pkg.
test 60s.
Use: Diagnostic aid.
• **FERTIRELIN ACETATE.** USAN.
Use: Hormone (gonadotropin-releas-
ing).
• **FERUMOXIDES.** USAN.
Use: Superparamagnetic diagnostic.
• **FERUMOXSIL.** USAN.
Use: Superparamagnetic diagnostic.
FERUSAL. (Vitarine) Ferrous sulfate 325
mg/Tab.
Use: Iron supplement.
FESTAL II. (Hoechst) Lipase 6000 units,
amylase 30,000 units, protease 20,000
units/Tab. Bot. 100s, 500s.
Use: Digestive enzyme.
FESTALAN. (Hoechst) Lipase 6000 units,
amylase 30,000 units, protease 20,000
units, atropine methylnitrate 1 mg/EC
Tab. Bot. 100s, 1000s.
Use: Digestive enzyme.
FETINIC. (Hauck) Iron 3.6 mg, vitamins
B$_{12}$ equivalent 2 mcg, B$_1$ 10 mg, B$_2$ 0.5
mg, B$_3$ 10 mg, B$_5$ 1 mg, B$_6$ 1 mg, B$_{12}$ 15
mcg, chlorobutanol 0.5%, benzyl alcohol
2%/ml. Vial 30 ml.
Use: Vitamin/mineral supplement.
FETINIC-MW. (Hauck) Iron 66 mg (from
ferrous fumarate), vitamins B$_{12}$ 5 mcg, C
60 mg/SR Cap. Bot. 100s.
Use: Vitamin/mineral supplement.
• **FETOXYLATE HYDROCHLORIDE.**
USAN.
Use: Relaxant.
FEVERALL, CHILDREN'S. (Upsher-
Smith) Acetaminophen 120 mg/Supp.
Pkg. 6s.
Use: Analgesic.
FEVERALL, INFANTS'. (Upsher-Smith)
Acetaminophen 80 mg. Supp. Pkg. 6s.
Use: Analgesic.
FEVERALL, JUNIOR STRENGTH. (Up-
sher-Smith) Acetaminophen 325
mg/Supp. Pkg. 6s.
Use: Analgesic.
FEVERALL SPRINKLE. (Upsher-Smith)
Acetaminophen 80 mg or 160 mg/Cap.

Bot. 20s.
Use: Analgesic.
• **FEZOLAMINE FUMARATE.** USAN.
Use: Antidepressant.
FGN-1. (Cell Pathways)
Use: Treatment of adenomatous polyposis coli. [Orphan drug]
• **FIACITABINE (FIAC).** USAN.
Use: Antiviral.
• **FIALURIDINE (FIAU).** USAN.
Use: Antiviral.
FIAU. (Oclassen)
Use: Treatment of hepatitis B. [Orphan drug]
FIBERALL. (Ciba Consumer) Calcium carbophil 1250 mg (equiv. to 1000 mg polycarbophil). Chew. Tab. Lemon-flavor. Pkg. 18s.
Use: Laxative.
FIBERALL NATURAL FLAVOR. (Ciba Consumer) **Pow.:** Psyllium hydrophilic mucilloid 3.4 Gm, wheat bran, sodium < 10 mg, potassium 60 mg, calories 6/5.9 Gm, saccharin. Can 150 Gm, 300 Gm, 450 Gm. **Wafer:** Psyllium hydrophilic mucilloid 3.4 Gm, wheat bran, oats, sucrose. Box 14s.
Use: Laxative.
FIBERALL ORANGE FLAVOR. (Ciba Consumer) Psyllium hydrophilic mucilloid 3.4 Gm, wheat bran, sodium < 10 mg, potassium 60 mg, calories 6/5.9 Gm Pow. Can 150 Gm, 300 Gm, 450 Gm.
Use: Laxative.
FIBERCON. (Lederle) Calcium polycarbophil 500 mg/Tab. Bot. 36s, 60s.
Use: Laxative.
FIBER GUARD. (Wyeth-Ayerst) All natural high fiber supplement 530 mg/Tab. Bot. 100s, 200s.
Use: Fiber supplement.
FIBERLAN. (Elan) Protein 50 Gm, fat 40 Gm, carbohydrates 160 Gm, Na 920 mg, K 1.56 Gm, fiber 14 g/per L. With vitamins A, C, B, B_2, B_3, D, E, B_5, B_6, B_{12}, K, Ca, Fe, folic acid, P, I, Mg, Zn, Cu, biotin, Mn, choline, Cl, Se, Cr, Mo. Liq. Bot. 237 ml.
Use: Enteral nutritional therapy.
FIBER-LAX. (Rugby) Calcium polycarbophil 625 mg (equiv. to 500 mg polycarbophil)/Tab. Bot. 60s.
Use: Laxative.
FIBERMED HIGH-FIBER SNACKS. (Purdue Frederick) One serving (15 snacks) contains 5 Gm dietary fiber. Box 8 oz. Packs of 24 × 1.3 oz.
Use: Fiber supplement.
FIBERMED HIGH-FIBER SUPPLEMENT. (Purdue Frederick) Each supplement

contains 5 Gm dietary fiber. Box 14s. Institutional pack, Box 144s of two supplements.
Use: Fiber supplement.
FIBERNORM. (G & W) Calcium polycarbophil 625 mg/Tab. Bot. 60s.
Use: Laxative.
FIBER RICH (O'Connor) Phenylpropanolamine HCl 75 mg/Tab. Bot. 24s.
Use: Diet aid.
FIBRAD. (Ross) Fiber 7 Gm, sodium < 15 mg, potassium < 25 mg. Pow. Bot. 414 Gm.
Use: Nongelling dietary fiber source for enteral use.
FIBRE TRIM TABLETS. (Schering) Grain and citrus fruit concentrated dietary fiber. Bot. 100s, 250s.
Use: Diet aid.
FIBRE TRIM w/CALCIUM TABLETS. (Schering) Grain and citrus fruit concentrated dietary fiber w/calcium. Bot. 90s, 225s.
Use: Diet aid.
FIBRIN HYDROLYSATE.
See: Aminosol, Soln. (Abbott).
• **FIBRINOGEN I-125.** USAN.
Use: Diagnostic aid.
FIBRINOGEN (HUMAN). Partially purified fibrinogen prepared by fractionation from normal human plasma.
Use: Coagulant (clotting factor).
FIBRINOLYSIN (HUMAN) WITH DESOXYRIBONUCLEASE. Plasmin. An enzyme prepared by activating a human blood plasma fraction with streptokinase.
Use: Topical enzyme preparation.
See: Elase, Oint., Pow. (Parke-Davis).
FIBRINOLYSIS INHIBITOR.
See: Amicar Syr., Tab., Vial (Lederle).
FIBRONECTIN. USAN.
Use: Treatment of nonhealing corneal ulcers or epithelial defects. [Orphan drug]
FILAXIS. (Amlab) Vitamins A 25,000 IU, D 1250 IU, C 150 mg, E 5 IU, B_1 12 mg, B_2 5 mg, B_6 0.5 mg, B_{12} 5 mcg, calcium pantothenate 5 mg, niacinamide 100 mg, iron 15 mg, iodine 0.15 mg, magnesium 10 mg, potassium 5 mg, calcium 75 mg, phosphorous 60 mg/Tab. Bot. 30s, 100s. Available w/B_{12}. Bot. 30s, 60s, 100s.
Use: Vitamin/mineral supplement.
• **FILGRASTIM (G-CSF).** USAN.
Use: Biological response modifier; antineoplastic adjunct. [Orphan drug]
See: Neupogen (Amgen).

FILIBON. (Lederle) Vitamins A 5000 IU, D 400 IU, B_1 1.5 mg, B_6 2 mg, niacinamide 20 mg, B_2 1.7 mg, B_{12} 6 mcg, E 30 mg, C 60 mg, folic acid 0.4 mg, elemental iron 18 mg, iodine 150 mcg, magnesium 100 mg, elemental calcium 125 mg/Tab. Bot 100s.
Use: Vitamin/mineral supplement.

FILIBON F.A. (Lederle) Elemental calcium 250 mg, elemental iron 45 mg, vitamins A 8000 IU, D 400 IU, E 30 mg, B_1 1.7 mg, B_2 2 mg, B_3 20 mg, B_6 4 mg, B_{12} 8 mcg, C 60 mg, folic acid 1 mg, I, Mg/Tab. Bot. 100s.
Use: Vitamin/mineral supplement.

FILIBON FORTE. (Lederle) Vitamins A 8000 IU, D 400 IU, E 45 mg, C 90 mg, niacinamide 30 mg, B_6 3 mg, B_1 2 mg, B_2 2.5 mg, folic acid 1 mg, B_{12} 12 mcg, calcium 300 mg, iron 45 mg, magnesium 100 mg, iodine 200 mcg/Tab. Bot. 100s.
Use: Vitamin/mineral supplement.

• **FILIPIN.** USAN.
Use: Antifungal.

FINAC. (C & M Pharmacal) Sulfur 2% in tinted lotion base. Bot. 60 ml.
Use: Anti-acne.

• **FINASTERIDE.** USAN.
Use: Benign prostatic hypertrophy therapy; antineoplastic.
See: Proscar, Tab. (Merck & Co.).

FIOGESIC. (Sandoz) Phenylpropanolamine HCl 25 mg, pyrilamine maleate 12.5 mg, pheniramine maleate 12.5 mg, calcium carbaspirin 382 mg (equiv. to 300 mg ASA)/Tab. Bot. 100s.
Use: Decongestant, antihistamine, analgesic.

FIORGEN TABS PF. (Goldline) Butabarbital 50 mg, aspirin 325 mg, caffeine 40 mg/Tab. Bot. 100s, 1000s.
Use: Sedative/hypnotic, salicylate/analgesic.

FIORICET. (Sandoz) Acetaminophen 325 mg, butalbital 50 mg, caffeine 40 mg/Tab. Bot. 100s, 500s. SandoPak 100s.
Use: Analgesic, sedative/hypnotic.

FIORINAL. (Sandoz) Butalbital (Sandoptal) 50 mg, caffeine 40 mg, aspirin 325 mg/Tab. or Cap. **Tab.:** Bot. 100s, 1000s. Sandopak 100s. **Cap.:** Bot. 100s, 500s. Control Pak 25s.
Use: Sedative/hypnotic, salicylate analgesic.

FIORINAL WITH CODEINE NO. 3 CAPSULES. (Sandoz) Butalbital (Sandoptal) 50 mg, caffeine 40 mg, aspirin 325 mg, codeine phosphate 30 mg/Cap. Bot. 100s. Control Pak 25s.

Use: Sedative/hypnotic, analgesic combination.

FIRE ANT VENOM, ALLERGENIC EXTRACT, IMPORTED.
Use: Skin test, immunotherapy. [Orphan drug]

FIRMDENT. (Moyco) Formerly Moy. Karaya gum 94.6%, sodium borate 5.36% Pkg. 3 oz.
Use: Denture adhesive.

FIRST AID CREAM. (Johnson & Johnson) Cetyl alcohol, glyceryl stearate, isopropyl palmitate, stearyl alcohol, synthetic beeswax. Tube 0.8 oz, 1.5 oz, 2.5 oz.
Use: Antiseptic, skin protectant.

FIRST AID CREAM. (Walgreen) Benzocaine 3%, allantoin 0.2%, benzyl alcohol 4%, phenol 0.25%. Tube 1.5 oz.
Use: Anesthetic, antiseptic.

FIRST CHOICE. (Polymer Technology International) 50s.
Use: In vitro reagent test strips for blood glucose monitoring.

FIRST RESPONSE OVULATION PREDICTOR. (Tambrands) Monoclonal antibody-based enzyme immunoassay test for hLH in urine. Test kit 1s.
Use: Diagnostic aid.

FIRST RESPONSE PREGNANCY TEST. (Tambrands) Reagent in-home kit for urine testing. Test kit 1s.
Use: Diagnostic aid.

FISH OIL CONCENTRATE, NATURAL. Natural fish oil concentrate containing EPA (Eicosapentaenoicacid) and DHA (Docosahexaenoic acid).
Use: Fish oil.
See: Comega, Cap. (Upsher-Smith).

FITACOL. (Standex) Atropine sulfate 0.2 mg, phenylpropanolamine 12.5 mg, chlorpheniramine maleate 0.5 mg, chlorobutanol 0.5 mg, water q.s./ml. Bot. pt.
Use: Anticholinergic/antispasmodic, decongestant, antihistamine.

FITACOL STANKAPS. (Standex) Belladonna alkaloidal salts 0.16 mg (atropine sulfate 0.024 mg, scopolamine HBr 0.014 mg, hyoscyamine sulfate 0.122 mg), phenylpropanolamine HCl 50 mg, chlorpheniramine maleate 1 mg, pheniramine maleate 12.5 mg/Cap. Bot. 100s.
Use: Anticholinergic/antispasmodic, decongestant, antihistamine.

5-FC.
See: Flucytosine.

5-FU.
See: Fluorouracil.

523 TABLETS. (Enzyme Process) Pancreatin 200 mg 4x/Tab. Tryspin, chymotrypsin, amylase, lipase enzymes from pancreatin, raw beef pancreas. Bot. 100s, 250s.
Use: Digestive enzyme.

FIXODENT. (Vicks Prods) Calcium sodium poly (vinyl methyl ether-maleate), carboxymethylcellulose sodium in a petrolatum base. Tube 0.75 oz, 1.5 oz, 2.5 oz.
Use: Denture adhesive cream.

•**FK-565.** USAN.
Use: Immunomodultor.

FLAGYL. (Searle) Metronidazole 250 mg or 500 mg/Tab. **250 mg:** Bot. 50s, 100s, 250s, 1000s, 2500s, UD 100s; **500 mg:** Bot. 50s, 100s, 500s, UD 100s.
Use: Anti-infective.

FLAGYL I.V. (Searle) Metronidazole HCl sterile lyophilized powder in single-dose vials equivalent to 500 mg metronidazole. Carton 10s.
Use: Anti-infective.

FLAGYL I.V. RTU. (Searle) Metronidazole ready-to-use, premixed, 500 mg/100 ml Soln. Vial (glass), Box 6s; Container, (plastic), Box 24s.
Use: Anti-infective.

FLANDERS BUTTOCKS OINTMENT. (Flanders) Zinc oxide, castor oil, balsam peru, boric acid in an emollient base. 60 Gm.
Use: Minor skin irritations.

FLAREX. (Alcon) Fluorometholone acetate 0.1%, benzalkonium chloride, 0.01% EDTA. Susp. Bot. 2.5 ml, 5 ml, 10 ml.
Use: Corticosteroid (Ophthalmic).

FLATULENCE TABLETS. (Vale) Nux vomica 16.2 mg, cascara sagrada extract 64.8 mg, ginger 48.6 mg, capsicum 16.2 mg/Tab. w/asafetida.
Use: Laxative, antiflatulent.

FLATULEX. (Dayton) **Tab.:** Simethicone 80 mg, activated charcoal 250 mg/Tab. Bot. 100s. **Drops:** Simethicone 40 mg/0.6 ml. Bot. 30 ml with calibrated dropper.
Use: Antiflatulent.

FLATUS. (Foy) Nux vomica extract 0.25 gr, cascara extract 1 gr, ginger ¾ gr, capsicum gr/Tab. w/asfetida qs. Bot. 1000s.
Use: Antiflatulent, laxative.

FLAV-A-D. (Kirkman) Vitamins A 5000 IU, D 1000 IU, C 100 mg/Tab. Bot. 100s, 1000s. Also w/fluoride. Bot. 100s, 1000s.
Use: Vitamin supplement.

FLAVINE.
See: Acriflavine Hydrochloride (Various Mfr.).

FLAVINOID-C. (Barth's) **Tab.:** Vitamin C 150 mg, hesperidin complex 10 mg, citrus bioflavonoid 50 mg, rutin 20 mg/Tab. Bot. 100s, 500s, 1000s. **Liq.:** Vitamin C 100 mg, bioflavonoid complex 100 mg/5 ml. Bot. 4 oz.
Use: Vitamin supplement.

•**FLAVODILOL MALEATE.** USAN.
Use: Antihypertensive.

FLAVOLUTAN.
See: Progesterone (Various Mfr.).

FLAVONOID COMPOUNDS.
See: Bio-Flavonoid Compounds Vitamin P.

FLAVONS-500. (Freeda) Citrus bioflavonoids complex 500 mg, hesperidin complex/Tab. Bot. 100s, 250s, 500s.
Use: Vitamin supplement.

FLAVORCEE. (Nature's Bounty) Ascorbic acid 100 mg or 250 mg/Chew. Tab. **100 mg:** Bot. 100s; **250 mg:** Bot. 250s.
Use: Vitamin C supplement.

FLAVORED DILUENT. (Roxane) Flavored vehicle for the immediate administration of crushed tablet or capsule product. Bot. 500 ml, UD 15 ml × 100.
Use: Flavored vehicle.

•**FLAVOXATE HCl.** USAN. 2-Piperidinoethyl-3-methyl-4-oxo-2-phenyl-4H-1-benzopyran-8-carboxylate HCl.
Use: Urinary antispasmodic.
See: Urispas, Tab. (SK-Beecham).

FLAVUROL. Merbromin.
Use: Antiseptic.

FLAXEDIL TRIETHIODIDE. Gallamine triethiodide soln.
Use: Skeletal muscle relaxant.

•**FLAZALONE.** USAN. p-Fluoro-phenyl 4-(p-fluorophenyl)-4-hydroxy-1-methyl-3-piperidyl ketone. 3-(4-Fluorobenzoyl)-4-(4-fluorophenyl)-1-methylpiperidin-4-ol.
Use: Anti-inflammatory.

•**FLECAINIDE ACETATE.** USAN.
Use: Cardiac depressant.

FLEET BABYLAX. (Fleet) Glycerin 4 ml in disposable pre-lubricated rectal applicator. Liq. pkg. 6s.
Use: Laxative.

FLEET BAGENEMA. (Fleet) Castile soap or Fleets bisacodyl prep.
Use: Laxative.

FLEET BISACODYL PREP PACKETS. (Fleet) Bisacodyl 10 mg/10 ml packet. 36 packets/box.
Use: Laxative.

FLEET ENEMA. (Fleet) Sodium biphos-

phate 19 Gm, sodium phosphate 7 Gm/118 ml. Bot. w/rectal tube 4.5 oz. Pediatric size 67.5 ml, 135 ml.
Use: Laxative.
FLEET FLAVORED CASTOR OIL EMULSION. (Fleet) 1 oz delivers 30 ml castor oil. Bot. 1.5 oz, 3 oz.
Use: Laxative.
FLEET GLYCERIN SUPPOSITORIES. (Fleet) Adult: Jar 12s, 24s, 50s. Child Size: Jar 12s.
Use: Laxative.
FLEET LAXATIVE. (Fleet) Bisacodyl. EC Tab.: 5 mg/Tab. Bot. 24s. Supp.: 10 mg. Box 4s.
Use: Laxative.
FLEET MINERAL OIL ENEMA. (Fleet) Mineral oil 4.5 fl oz in an unbreakable vinyl squeeze bottle.
Use: Laxative.
FLEET PHOSPHO-SODA. (Fleet) Sodium phosphate 18 Gm, sodium biphosphate 48 Gm/100 ml (96.4 mEq sodium/20 ml). Bot. 45 ml, 90 ml, 240 ml.
Use: Laxative.
FLEET PREP KITS. (Fleet) A series of different laxative kits for use prior to barium enema, bowel surgery, proctoscopy, colonoscopy, etc. w/complete patient instruction form:
Prep Kit #1: Fleet Phospho-Soda 45 ml, Fleet Bisacodyl Tablets 45 mg, Fleet Bisacodyl Suppository 110 mg.
Prep Kit #2: Fleet Phospho-Soda 45 ml, Fleet Bisacodyl Tablets 45 mg, 1 Fleet Bagenema set for large volume enema, including optional Castile Soap Packet. 20 ml.
Prep Kit #3: Fleet Phospho-Soda 45 ml, Fleet Bisacodyl Tablets 45 mg, Fleet Bisacodyl Enema 130 ml. 10 mg.
Prep Kit #4: Fleet Flavored Castor Oil Emulsion 45 ml, Fleet Bisacodyl Tablets 45 mg, Fleet Bisacodyl Suppository 110 mg.
Prep Kit #5: Fleet Flavored Castor Oil Emulsion 45 ml, Fleet Bisacodyl Tablets 45 mg, 1 Fleet Bagenema set for large volume enema, including optional Castile Soap Packet. 20 ml.
Prep Kit #6: Fleet Flavored Castor Oil Emulsion 45 ml, Fleet Bisacodyl Tablets 45 mg, Fleet Bisacodyl Enema 130 ml. 10 mg.
Use: Laxative.
FLEET RELIEF ANESTHETIC HEMORRHOIDAL OINTMENT. (Fleet) Pramoxine HCl 1%. Six disposable pre-filled applicators. Tube 30 Gm.
Use: Anorectal preparation.

• **FLEROXACIN.** USAN.
Use: Antibacterial.
• **FLESTOLOL SULFATE.** USAN.
Use: Anti-adrenergic.
• **FLETAZEPAM.** USAN.
Use: Relaxant.
FLETCHER'S CASTORIA for CHILDREN. (Mentholatum) Senna 6.5%, alcohol 3.5%. Liq. Bot. 75 ml, 150 ml.
Use: Laxative.
FLEX-ALL 454. (Chattem) Menthol 7%, alcohol, allantoin, aloe vera gel, boric acid, carbomer 940, diazolidinyl urea, eucalyptus oil, glycerin, iodine, parabens, methyl salicylate, peppermint oil, polysorbate 60, potassium iodide, propylene glycol, thyme oil, triethanolamine. Gel Tube. 240 Gm.
Use: External analgesic.
FLEX ANTI-DANDRUFF SHAMPOO. (Revlon) Zinc pyrithione 1% in liquid shampoo.
Use: Antiseborrheic.
FLEX ANTI-DANDRUFF STYLING MOUSSE. (Revlon) Zinc pyrithione 0.1%. Aerosol foam.
Use: Antiseborrheic.
FLEXAPHEN. (Trimen) Chlorzoxazone 250 mg, acetaminophen 300 mg/Cap. Bot. 100s.
Use: Skeletal muscle relaxant combination.
FLEX-CARE FOR SENSITIVE EYES. (Alcon Lenscare) Sterile solution of chlorhexidine 0.005%, edetate disodium 0.1%. Bot. 120 ml, 237 ml, 355 ml.
Use: Contact lens care.
FLEXERIL. (Merck) Cyclobenzaprine HCl 10 mg/Tab. Bot. 100s, UD 100s.
Use: Muscle relaxant.
FLEXIBLE HYDROACTIVE DRESSINGS/GRANULES.
See: Intra Site (Smith & Nephew).
    Shur-Clens (Calgon Vestal).
    DuoDerm (ConvaTec).
    Sorbsan (Dow B. Hickam).
FLEX-O.
See: O-FLEX.
FLEXOJECT. (Mayrand) Orphenadrine citrate 30 mg/ml. Inj. Vial 10 ml, amps 2 ml.
Use: Muscle relaxant.
FLEXON. (Keene) Orphenadrine citrate 30 mg/ml. Inj. Vial 10 ml.
Use: Muscle relaxant.
FLEXSOL. (Alcon Lenscare) Sterile, buffered, isotonic aqueous soln. of sodium Cl, sodium borate, boric acid, adsor-

bobase. Bot. 6 oz.
Use: Soft contact lens care.
FLINTSTONES. (Miles) Vitamin A 2500
IU, E 15 mg, C 60 mg, folic acid 0.3 mg,
B_1 1.05 mg, B_2 1.2 mg, niacin 13.5 mg,
B_6 1.05 mg, B_{12} 4.5 mcg, D 400
IU/Chew. Tab. Bot. 60s, 100s.
Use: Vitamin supplement.
FLINTSTONES COMPLETE. (Miles) Ele-
mental iron 18 mg, vitamins A 5000 IU, D
400 IU, E 30 mg, B_1 1.5 mg, B_2 1.7 mg,
B_3 20 mg, B_5 10 mg, B_6 2 mg, B_{12} 6
mcg, C 60 mg, folic acid 0.4 mg, biotin
40 mcg, Ca, Cu, I, Mg, P, zinc 15
mg/Chew. Tab. Bot. 60s, 100s.
Use: Vitamin/mineral supplement.
FLINTSTONES WITH EXTRA C. (Miles)
Vitamins A 2500 IU, D 400 IU, E 15 mg,
C 250 mg, folic acid 0.3 mg, B_1 1.05 mg,
B_2 1.2 mg, niacin 13.5 mg, B_6 1.05 mg,
B_{12} 4.5 mcg/Tab. Bot. 60s, 100s.
Use: Vitamin supplement.
FLINTSTONES WITH IRON. (Miles) Vitamins A 2500 IU, E 15 mg, C 60 mg, folic
acid 0.3 mg, B_1 1.05 mg, B_2 1.2 mg,
niacin 13.5 mg, B_6 1.05 mg, B_{12} 4.5
mcg, D 400 IU, iron 15 mg/Chew. Tab.
Bot. 60s.
Use: Vitamin/mineral supplement.
FLO-COAT. (Lafayette Pharm.) Barium
sulfate 100%. Susp. Bot. 1850 ml.
Use: Radiopaque agent.
• **FLOCTAFENINE.** USAN.
Use: Analgesic.
FLORAJEN. (Jenkins) Fluoride 0.5 mg,
vitamins A 4000 IU, D 400 IU, ascorbic
acid 75 mg, B_1 2 mg, B_2 2 mg, niaci-
namide 18 mg, B_6 1 mg, calcium pan-
tothenate dextro 5 mg, cyanocobalamin
2 mcg/Tab. Bot. 100s, 500s, 1000s.
Use: Vitamin/mineral supplement.
FLORANTYRONE. B.A.N. 4-(Fluoran-
then-8-yl)-4-oxobutyric acid.
Use: Stimulation of bile acid secretion.
FLOR-D CHEWABLE TAB. (Derm
Pharm.) Fluoride 1 mg, vitamins A 4000
IU, D 400 IU, C 75 mg, B_1 1.5 mg, B_2 1.8
mg, niacinamide 15 mg, B_6 1 mg, B_{12} 3
mcg, calcium pantothenate 10 mg/Tab.
Bot. 100s.
Use: Vitamin/mineral supplement.
FLOR-D DROPS. (Derm Pharm.) Fluo-
ride 0.5 mg, vitamins A 3000 IU, D 400
IU, C 60 mg, B_1 1 mg, B_2 1.2 mg, niaci-
namide 8 mg/0.6 ml. Bot. 60 ml.
Use: Vitamin/mineral supplement.
• **FLORDIPINE.** USAN.
Use: Antihypertensive.
FLORICAL. (Mericon) Sodium fluoride
8.3 mg, calcium carbonate 364 mg

(equivalent to 145.6 mg calcium)/Cap.
Bot. 100s, 500s.
Use: Mineral supplement.
FLORIDA FOAM. (Hill) Benzalkonium Cl,
aluminum subacetate, boric acid 2%.
Bot. 8 oz.
Use: Soap substitute, antiseborrheic,
antifungal, anti-acne.
FLORIDA SUNBURN RELIEF. (Pharma-
cel) Benzyl alcohol 3%, phenol 0.4%,
camphor 0.2%, menthol 0.15%. Lot. Bot.
60 ml.
Use: Topical.
FLORINEF ACETATE TABLETS.
(Apothecon) Fludrocortisone acetate,
0.1 mg/Tab. Bot. 100s.
Use: Mineralocorticoid.
FLORONE CREAM. (Dermik) Diflorasone
diacetate 0.5 mg/Gm (0.05%) w/stearic
acid, sorbitan mono-oleate, polysorbate
60, sorbic acid, citric acid, propylene gly-
col, purified water. Tube 15 Gm, 30 Gm,
60 Gm.
Use: Corticosteroid.
FLORONE E. (Dermik) Diflorasone diac-
etate 0.5 mg. Tube 15 Gm, 30 Gm, 60
Gm.
Use: Corticosteroid.
FLORONE OINTMENT. (Dermik) Diflo-
rasone diacetate 0.5 mg/Gm (0.05%)
W/polyoxypropylene 15-stearyl ether,
stearic acid, lanolin alcohol and white
petrolatum. Tube 15 Gm, 30 Gm, 60
Gm.
Use: Corticosteroid.
FLOROPRYL. (Merck & Co.)
Isoflurophate 0.025% in sterile oph-
thalmic ointment in polyethylene-mineral
oil gel. Tube 3.5 Gm.
Use: Agent for glaucoma.
FLORVITE CHEWABLE TABLETS.
(Everett) Vitamins, fluoride 0.5
mg/Chew. tab. Bot 100s.
Use: Dental caries preventative.
FLORVITE HALF STRENGTH. (Everett)
Elemental fluoride 0.5 mg, vitamins A
2500 IU, D 400 IU, E 15 mg, B_1 1.05 mg,
B_2 1.2 mg, B_3 13.5 mg, B_6 1.05 mg, B_{12}
4.5 mcg, C 60 mg, folic acid 0.3
mg/Chew. Tab. Bot. 100s.
Use: Vitamin/mineral supplement, dental caries preventative.
FLORVITE & IRON DROPS. (Everett) Elemental fluorine. **0.25 mg:** Vitamins A
1500 IU, D 400 IU, E 5 mg, B_1 0.5 mg,
B_2 0.6 mg, B_3 8 mg, B_6 0.4 mg, C 35 mg,
iron 10 mg/ml. **0.5 mg:** Vitamins A 1500
IU, D 400 IU, E 5 mg, B_1 0.5 mg, B_2 0.6
mg, B_3 8 mg, B_6 0.4 mg, C 35 mg, iron
10 mg/ml. Bot. 50 ml.

Use: Vitamin/mineral supplement, dental caries preventative.

FLORVITE & IRON CHEWABLE.
(Everett) Fluoride 1 mg, iron 12 mg, vitamins A 2500 IU, D 400 IU, E 15 mg, B$_1$ 1.05 mg, B$_2$ 1.2 mg, B$_3$ 13.5 mg, B$_6$ 1.05 mg, B$_{12}$ 4.5 mcg, C 60 mg, folic acid 0.3 mg/Chew. tab. Bot. 100s.
Use: Vitamin/mineral supplement, dental caries preventative.

FLORVITE PEDIATRIC DROPS.
(Everett) Elemental fluorine. **0.25 mg/ml:** vitamins A 1500 IU, D 400 IU, E 5 mg, B$_1$ 0.5 mg, B$_2$ 0.6 mg, B$_3$ 8 mg, B$_6$ 0.4 mg, B$_{12}$ 2 mcg, C 35 mg/ml. **0.5 mg/ml:** vitamins A 1500 IU, D 400 IU, E 5 mg, B$_1$ 0.5 mg, B$_2$ 0.6 mg, B$_3$ 8 mg, B$_6$ 0.4 mg, B$_{12}$ 2 mcg, C 35 mg, iron 10 mg/ml Bot. 50 ml.
Use: Vitamin/mineral supplement, dental caries preventative.

FLORVITE TABLETS-1 mg. (Everett) Elemental fluorine 1 mg, vitamins A 2500 IU, D 400 IU, E 15 mg, B$_1$ 1.05 mg, D$_2$ 1.2 mg, B$_3$ 13.5 mg, B$_6$ 1.05 mg, B$_{12}$ 4.5 mcg, C 60 mg, folic acid 0.3 mg/Chew. tab. Bot. 100s, 1000s.
Use: Vitamin/mineral supplement, dental caries preventative.

FLOSEQUINAN.
See: Manoplax (Boots).
• **FLOXACILLIN.** USAN.
Use: Antibacterial.
• **FLOXIN.** (Ortho) **Tab.:** Ofloxacin, 200 mg, 300 mg or 400 mg. Bot. 50s, 100s. **Inj.:** 200 mg flexible container; 400 mg Vial 10 ml, 20 ml; Bot. 100 ml; flexible container.
Use: Antibacterial, fluoroquinolone.

FLOXURIDINE, U.S.P. XXI. Sterile, U.S.P. XXI. 2′-Deoxy-5-fluorouridine.
Use: Antiviral agent.
See: FUDR, Vial (Roche).

FLUANISONE. B.A.N. 4 Fluoro-a-[4-(2-methoxy-phenyl)piperazin-1-yl]butyrophenone.
Use: Neuroleptic.
• **FLUAZACORT.** USAN.
Use: Anti-inflammatory.
• **FLUBANILATE HYDROCHLORIDE.** USAN. Ethyl N-[2(dimethylamino)ethyl]-m-(trifluoromethyl) carbanilate HCl.
Use: Antidepressant.
• **FLUBENDAZOLE.** USAN.
Use: Antiprotozoal.
FLUCARBRIL. 1-Methyl-6-(trifluromethyl)carbostyril.
Use: Muscle relaxant, analgesic.
• **FLUCINDOLE.** USAN.
Use: Antipsychotic.

FLUCLOROLONE ACETONIDE. B.A.N. 9α,-11β-Dichloro-6α-fluoro-21-hydroxy-16α,17α-isopropylidenedioxypregna-1,4-diene-3,20-dione.
Use: Corticosteroid.
• **FLUCLORONIDE.** USAN. 9, 11β-Dichloro-6α-fluoro-16α, 17, 21-trihydroxypregna-1, 4-diene-3, 20-dione cyclic 16, 17-acetal with acetone.
Use: Glucocorticoid.
FLUCLOXACILLIN. B.A.N. 6-[3-(2-Chloro-6-fluorophenyl)-5-methylisoxazole-4-carboxamido]-penicillanic acid.
Use: Antibiotic.
FLU, COLD & COUGH MEDICINE. (Major) Pseudoephedrine HCl 60 mg, chlorpheniramine 4 mg, dextromethorphan HBr 20 mg, acetaminophen 500 mg. Pow. Pck. 6s.
Use: Decongestant, antihistamine, antitussive, analgesic.
• **FLUCONAZOLE.** USAN.
Use: Antifungal.
See: Diflucan (Rocrig).
• **FLUCRYLATE.** USAN. 2,2,2-Trifluoro-1-methylethyl-2-cyanoacrylate.
Use: Surgical aid (tissue adhesive).
• **FLUCYTOSINE,** U.S.P. XXIII. Cap. U.S.P. XXIII. 5-Fluorocytosine.
Use: Antifungal.
See: Ancobon, Cap. (Roche).
• **FLUCYTOSINE.** USAN. 4-Amino-5-fluoro-1,2-dihydropyrimidin-2-one. 5-Fluorocytosine.
Use: Antifungal.
See: Alcobon.
• **FLUDALANINE.** USAN.
Use: Antibacterial.
FLUDARA. Fludarabine 50 mg. Pow. for recon. Vial. 6 ml.
Use: Antineoplastic.
• **FLUDARABINE PHOSPHATE.** USAN.
Use: Antineoplastic. [Orphan drug]
See: Fludara, Pow. (Berlex).
• **FLUDAZONIUM CHLORIDE.** USAN.
Use: Anti-infective, topical.
• **FLUDEOXYGLUCOSE F 18 INJECTION,** U.S.P. XXIII. USAN.
Use: Diagnostic aid. For brain disorders, thyroid disorders, liver disorders, cardiac disease and neoplastic disease.
• **FLUDOREX.** USAN.
Use: Anorexic, anti-emetic.
• **FLUDROCORTISONE ACETATE,** U.S.P. XXIII. Tab. U.S.P. XXIII. 9-alpha-Fluorohydrocortisone. Pregn-4-ene-3,20-dione,21-(acetyloxy)-9-fluoro-11,-17-dihydroxy-, (11 beta)-.9-Fluoro-11 beta, 17,21-trihydroxypregn-4-ene-3,20-dione

21-acetate.
Use: Adrenocortical steroid (salt-regulation).
See: Florinef Acetate, Tab. (Squibb).
•**FLUFENAMIC ACID.** USAN. N-(α, α, α-Trifluoro-m-tolyl) anthranilic acid.
Use: Anti-inflammatory agent.
•**FLUFENSIAL.** USAN.
Use: Analgesic.
FLUGESTONE. B.A.N. 9α-Fluoro-11β,17-dihydroxy-pregn-4-ene-3,20-dione.
Use: Progesterone steroid.
FLUIDEX. (O'Connor) Natural botanical ingredients. Tab. Bot. 36s, 72s.
Use: Diuretic.
FLU-IMUNE. (Lederle) Influenza virus vaccine. Vial 5 ml (10 doses). (Purified surface antigen).
Use: Vaccine, viral.
FLUITRAN. Trichlormethiazide.
FLUMADINE. (Forest) **Tab.:** Rimantadine HCl 100 mg. Bot. 20s, 100s, 500s, 1000s. **Syr.:** Rimantadine HCl 50 mg/5ml. Bot. 60 ml, 240 ml, 480 ml.
Use: Antiviral.
•**FLUMAZENIL.** USAN.
Use: Antagonist (to benzodiazepine).
See: Mazicon (Roche).
Romazicon, Inj. (Hoffman-La Roche).
FLUMECINOL.
Use: Hyperbilirubinemia in newborns. [Orphan drug]
See: Zixoryn.
FLUMEDROXONE. B.A.N. 17α-Hydroxy-6α-trifluoromethylpregn-4-ene-3,20-dione.
Use: Agent for migraine.
•**FLUMEQUINE.** USAN.
Use: Antibacterial.
•**FLUMERIDONE.** USAN.
Use: Anti-emetic.
•**FLUMETHASONE.** USAN. 6α,9α-Difluoro-11β, 17α,21-trihydroxy-16α-methyl-pregna-1,4-diene-3,20- dione. 6α,9α-Difluoro-16α-methylprednisolone.
Use: Corticosteroid.
See: Locorten [21-pivalate] (Ciba).
FLUMETHIAZIDE. 6-Trifluoromethyl-7-sulfamyl-1,2,4-benzothiadiazine-1,1-dioxide.
Use: Diuretic.
See: Rautrax, Tab. (Squibb).
FLUMETHIAZIDE. B.A.N. 6-Trifluoromethyl-1,2,4-benzothiadiazine-7-sulphonamide 1,1-dioxide.
Use: Diuretic.
•**FLUMETRAMIDE.** USAN.
Use: Relaxant.
•**FLUMEZAPINE.** USAN.

Use: Antipsychotic, neuroleptic.
•**FLUMINOREX.** USAN.
Use: Anorexic.
•**FLUMIZOLE.** USAN.
Use: Anti-inflammatory.
FLUNARIZINE.
Use: Alternating hemiplegia. [Orphan drug]
See: Sibelium.
•**FLUNARIZINE HCl.** USAN. (E)-1-[Bis-(p-fluorophenyl) methyl]-4-cinnamyl-piperazine dihydrochloride.
Use: Vasodilator.
•**FLUNIDAZOLE.** USAN.
Use: Antiprotozoal.
•**FLUNISOLIDE.**
See: AcroBid (Key Pharm.).
Nasalide (Syntex).
•**FLUNISOLIDE ACETATE.** USAN. Fluoxolonate.
Use: Anti-inflammatory.
•**FLUNITRAZEPAM.** USAN. 5-Fluorophenyl-1,3-dihydro-1-methyl-7-nitro-2H-1,4-benzodiazepin-2-one.
Use: Hypnotic.
•**FLUNIXIN.** USAN.
Use: Anti-inflammatory, analgesic.
FLUOCET. (NMC Labs) Fluocinolone acetonide cream 0.025% or 0.01%. Tube 15 Gm, 60 Gm.
Use: Corticosteroid.
FLUOCINOLIDE. Fluocinonide, U.S.P. XXIII.
•**FLUOCINOLONE ACETONIDE,** U.S.P. XXIII. Cream, Oint., Topical Soln. U.S.P. XXIII. Pregna-1,4-diene-3,20-dione,6,9-difluoro-11,21-dihydroxy-16,17-[(1-methylethylidene)bis(oxy)], (6α,11β,-16α)-. 9a-Difluoro-16a-hydroxyprednisolone-16, 17-acetonide. 6α,9α-Difluoro-11β,16α,17,21-tetrahydroxypregna-1,4-diene-3,20-dione. Cyclic 16,-17-Acetal with Acetone.
Use: Adrenocortical steroid (topical anti-inflammatory).
See: Fluonid, Cream, Oint., Soln. (Herbert).
Synalar, Cream, Oint., Soln. (Syntex). W/Neomycin sulfate.
See: Neo-Synalar (Syntex).
•**FLUOCINONIDE,** U.S.P. XXIII. Cream, Gel, Oint., U.S.P. XXIII. F.D.A. 6α, 9α-Difluoro-11β-16α, 17α-21-tetrahydroxypregna-1,4-diene-3,20-dione, cyclic 16, 17-acetal with acetone, 21-acetate. B.A.N. 21-Acetoxy-6α,9α-difluoro-11β-hydroxy-16α, 17α-iso- propylidenedioxypregna-1,4-diene-3,20-dione. Fluocinolone 16α, 17α-acetonide 21 acetate.

Use: Corticosteroid.
See: Lidex, Cream, Oint., Soln. (Syntex).
   Lidex-E, Cream (Syntex).
   Metosyn.
   Topsyn, Gel (Syntex).
• **FLUOCINONIDE TOPICAL SOLUTION,** U.S.P. XXIII.
   Use: Corticosteroid.
• **FLUOCORTIN BUTYL.** USAN. Butyl-6α-fluoro-11β-hydroxy-16α-methyl-3,20-dioxopregna-1,4-dien-21oate.
   Use: Anti-inflammatory.
• **FLUOCORTOLONE.** USAN. 6α-Fluoro-11β,21-dihy- droxy-16α-methylpregna-1,4-diene-20-dione. (Berlin) 6α-Fluoro-11β, 21-dihydroxy-16α-methylpregna-1, 4-diene-3, 20-dione.
   Use: Corticosteroid.
   See: Ultralanum [21-hexanoate]
• **FLUOCORTOLONE CAPROATE.** USAN.
   Use: Glucocorticoid.
FLUOGEN. (Parke-Davis) Influenza virus vaccine, trivalent—Immunizing antigen, ether extracted. Vial 5 ml, UD syringe 0.5 ml. The 5 ml vial contains sufficient product to deliver ten 0.5 ml doses.
   Use: Vaccine, viral.
FLUONEX. (ICN) Fluocinonide 0.05%. Cream. Tube. 15 Gm, 30 Gm.
   Use: Topical corticosteroid.
FLUONID. (Herbert) Fluocinolone Acetonide. **Soln.:** 0.01%. Bot. 20 ml, 60 ml.
   Use: Corticosteroid.
FLUOPROMAZINE. B.A.N. 10-(3-Dimethylaminopropyl)-2-trifluoromethylpiamothiazine. Triflupromazine (I.N.N.).
   Use: Tranquilizer.
FLUORACAINE. (Akorn) Proparacaine HCl 0.5%, fluorescein sodium 0.25%, glycerin, povidone, thimerosal 0.01%. Dropper Bot. 5 ml.
   Use: Local anesthetic, ophthalmic.
• **FLUORESCEIN,** U.S.P. XXIII. Inj. U.S.P. XXIII.
   Use: Diagnostic aid (corneal trauma indicator).
• **FLUORESCEIN SODIUM,** U.S.P. XXIII. Ophth. Strip, U.S.P. XXIII. Spiro[isobenzofuran-1(3H), 9-[9H]xanthene]-3-one, 3′6-dihydroxy, disodium salt. (Various Mfr.) Soluble fluorescein. Bot. 1 oz.
   Use: 2% soln. in diagnosis of eye conditions. (circulation time).
   See: AK-Fluor, Amp., Vial (Akorn).
   Fluor-I-Strip. (Wyeth-Ayerst).
   Fluorets, Strips (Akorn).
   Ful-Glo, Strips (Sola/Barnes-Hind).
   Funduscein, Amp. (Iolab).
   Ophthifluor, Amp. (Deklerht).
   Plak-Lite Soln. (Internat. Pharm.).

FLUORESCEIN SODIUM I.V.
   See: Fluorescite, Amp. (Alcon).
FLUORESCEIN SODIUM 2% SOLUTION. (Alcon) Drop-Tainer 15 ml, Steri-Unit 2 ml 12s.
   Use: Diagnostic aid, ophthalmic.
FLUORESCEIN SODIUM 2%. (Iolab) A sterile aqueous solution containing fluorescein sodium 2%. Dropperette 1 ml, Box 12s.
   Use: Diagnostic aid, ophthalmic.
FLUORESCEIN SODIUM W/ PROPARACAINE HCl. (Pasadena) Proparacaine HCl 0.5%, fluorescein sodium 0.25%, thimerosal 0.01%, povidone, glycerin, EDTA. Ophthalmic soln. Dropper Bot. 5 ml.
   Use: Local anesthetic, diagnostic aid, ophthalmic.
FLUORESCITE. (Alcon) Fluorescein as sodium salt. Inj. Soln. **10%:** Amp. 5 ml, Box 12s, Disposable Syringe 5 ml, 12s; **25%:** Amp 2 ml. Box 12s.
   Use: Diagnostic aid, ophthalmic.
FLUORESOFT. (Various Mfr.) Fluorexon 0.35%. Soln. Pipette 0.5 ml, Box 12s.
   Use: Diagnostic aid, ophthalmic.
FLUORETS. (Akorn) Fluorescein sodium 1 mg. Strip. Box 100s.
   Use: Diagnostic aid, ophthalmic.
FLUOREXON.
   See: Fluoresoft (Holles).
FLUORIDE. (Kirkman) Fluoride 1 mg (sodium fluoride 2.21 mg). Tab. Bot. 1000s.
   Use: Dental caries preventative.
FLUORIDE LOZ. (Kirkman) Fluoride 1 mg (sodium fluoride 2.21 mg). Loz. Bot. 1000s.
   Use: Dental caries preventative.
FLUORIDE SODIUM.
   See: Dentafluor Chewable, Tab. (Western Pharm.).
   Karidium, Top. Soln., Tab. (Lorvic).
   Karigel, Gel (Lorvic).
FLUORIDE-T.
   See: T-FLUORIDE.
FLUORIDE THERAPY.
   See: Adeflor Preps. (Upjohn).
   Cari-Tab, Softab Tab. (Stuart).
   Coral Prods. (Lorvic).
   Fluorineed, Chew. Tab. (Hanlon).
   Fluorinse, Liq. (Pacemaker).
   Fluora, Loz. (Kirkman).
   Gal-Kam, Preps. (Scherer).
   Luride Preps. (Hoyt).
   Mulvidren-F, Softab Tab. (Stuart).
   Point Two, Rinse (Hoyt).
   Poly-Vi-Flor, Drops, Tab. (Mead Johnson).

Soluvite-F, Drops (Pharmics).
Tri-Vi-Flor, Drops, Tab. (Mead Johnson).
FLUORIGARD. (Colgate-Palmolive) Fluoride 0.02% (from sodium fluoride 0.05%), alcohol 6%, tartrazine. Bot. 180 ml, 300 ml, 480 ml.
Use: Dental caries preventative
FLUORI-METHANE SPRAY. (Gebauer) Dichlorodifluoromethane 15%, trichloromonofluoromethane 85%. Bot. 4 oz.
Use: "Painful motion" syndromes.
FLUORINEED. (Hanlon) Fluoride 1 mg/Chew. Tab. Bot. 100s, 1000s.
Use: Dental caries preventative.
FLUORINSE. (Oral-B) Fluoride 0.09% from sodium fluoride 0.2%. Bot. 480 ml.
Use: Dental caries preventative.
FLUORINSE. (Pacemaker) Fluoride mouthwash. Pack. Fluoride ion level 0.05% or 0.2%. UD Bot. 32 oz. Concentrate 1 oz, 4 oz, gal.
Use: Dental caries preventative.
FLUOR-I-STRIP. (Wyeth-Ayerst) Fluorescein sodium 9 mg/ophthalmic strip. Box. 300s.
Use: Diagnostic aid, ophthalmic.
FLUOR-I-STRIP-A.T. (Wyeth-Ayerst) Fluorescein sodium 1 mg/ophthalmic strip. Box 300s (150 × 2).
Use: Diagnostic aid, ophthalmic.
FLUORITAB. (Fluoritab) Sodium fluoride 2.2 mg equivalent to 1 mg of fluorine (as fluoride ion) w/inert organic filler 75.8 mg/Tab. Bot. 100s; Liq. dropper bot. (fluorine 0.25 mg from 0.55 mg sodium fluoride/Drop) 19 ml.
Use: Dental caries preventative.
5-FLUOROCYTOSINE.
See: Ancobon, Cap. (Roche).
• **FLUORODOPA f 18.** U.S.P. XXIII, Inj. USAN.
Use: Diagnostic radiopharmaceutical.
FLUOROGESTONE ACETATE. 9-Fluoro-11β, 17-dihydroxypregn-4-ene-3, 20-dione, 17-acetate.
Use: Progestin.
FLUOROHYDROCORTISONE ACETATE. 9-α- Fluorohydrocortisone.
See: Fludrocortisone Acetate (Various Mfr.).
• **FLUOROMETHOLONE,** U.S.P. XXIII. Cream, Ophth. Susp., U.S.P. XXIII. Pregna-1,4-diene-3,20-diene, 9-fluoro-11,17-dihydroxy-6-methyl-,(6α,11β)-. 6α-Methyl-9α-fluoro-21-desoxyprednisolone. 9-Fluoro-11β, 17-dihydroxy-6α-methylpregna-1, 4-diene-3, 20-dione. B.A.N. 9α-Fluoro-11β-17α-dihy-

droxy-6α-methylpregna-1,4-diene-3,20-dione.
Use: Glucocorticoid.
See: Fluor-Op, Susp. (Iolab).
FML, Liquifilm, Ophth. Susp., Oint. (Allergan).
Oxylone, Cream Ophth. Susp. (Upjohn).
W/Neomycin sulfate.
See: Neo-Oxylone, Oint. (Upjohn).
• **FLUOROMETHOLONE ACETATE.** USAN.
Use: Glucocorticoid, anti-inflammatory.
FLUOR-OP. (Iolab Pharm.) Fluorometholone 0.1% (1 mg/ml) susp. Bot. 5 ml, 10 ml, 15 ml w/dropper.
Use: Corticosteroid.
FLUOROPHENE.
Use: Antiseptic.
FLUOROPLEX TOPICAL. (Herbert)
Soln.: Fluorouracil 1% in a propylene glycol base. Plastic bot. w/dropper 30 ml. **Cream:** Fluorouracil 1% in emulsion base w/benzyl alcohol 0.5%, emulsifying wax, mineral oil, isopropyl myristate, sodium hydroxide, purified water. Tube 30 Gm.
Use: Topical treatment of multiple actinic (solar) keratoses.
FLUOROQUINOLONES.
Use: Anti-infective.
See: Ciloxan (Alcon).
Cipro (Miles).
Cipro I.V. (Miles).
Floxin (Ortho).
Maxaquin (Searle).
Noroxin (Merck Sharp and Dohme).
Penetrex (Rhone-Poulenc Rhone-Poulenc Rorer).
• **FLUOROSALAN.** USAN. 3, 5-dibromo-3′-trifluoromethyl salicylanilide. Fluorophene.
Use: Antiseptic.
FLUOR-O-SOL. (Hoyt) Fluoride 1.2% with silicon dioxide abrasive. Jar 50 Gm, Carton 6s.
Use: Dental caries preventative.
FLUOROTHYL. Bis (2, 2, 2-trifluoroethyl) ether.
See: Flurothyl.
• **FLUOROURACIL,** U.S.P. XXIII. Cream, Inj., Topical Soln., U.S.P. XXIII. 5-Fluorouracil. (Roche) Amp. 10 ml, 500 mg, Box 10s.
Use: Malignancies, antineoplastic. [Orphan drug]
See: Adrucil, Inj. (Adria).
Efudex, Soln., Cream (Roche).
Fluoroplex, Soln., Cream (Herbert Labs.).

FLUOSOL. (Alpha Therapeutic) Perfluorochemicals 20%. Emulsion in 400 ml flexible plastic bag. Additive solutions 1 and 2 supplied in a separate continuous oxygenation kit.
Use: Perfluorochemical emulsion.
FLUOTHANE. (Wyeth-Ayerst) Halothane.
Bot. 125 ml, 250 ml.
Use: Inhalation anesthetic.
• **FLUOTRACEN HYDROCHLORIDE.** USAN.
Use: Antipsychotic, antidepressant.
• **FLUOXETINE HCl.** USAN.
Use: Antidepressant.
See: Prozac, Pulv., Liq. (Dista).
FLU-OXINATE. (Pasadena) Benoxinate HCl 0.4%, fluorescein sodium 0.25%, chlorobutanol 1%, povidone, glycerin, EDTA. Ophthalmic soln. Dropper bot. 5 ml.
Use: Local anesthetic, diagnostic aid, ophthalmic.
• **FLUOXYMESTERONE,** U.S.P. XXIII.
Tab., U.S.P. XXIII. 9-α-Fluoro-11-β-hydroxy-17-α-methyltestosterone. 9-Fluoro-11β, 17β-dihydroxy-17-methylandrost-4-en-3-one. (Various Mfr.) 10 mg Tab. Bot. 100s.
Use: Androgen.
See: Android-F, Tab. (Brown).
   Halotestin, Tab. (Upjohn).
   Ora-Testryl, Tab. (Squibb Mark).
W/Ethinyl estradiol.
See: Halodrin, Tab. (Upjohn).
FLUOXYMESTERONE. B.A.N. 9α-Fluoro-11β, 17 β-dihy 17α-methylandrost-4-en-3-one. 9α-Fluoro-11 β-hydroxymethyltestosterone.
Use: Androgen, anabolic steroid.
FLUPENTHIXOL. B.A.N. 9-3-[4-(2-Hydroxyethel)-piperazin-1-yl]propylidene-2-trifluoromethylthioxanthene.
Use: Tranquilizer.
• **FLUPERAMIDE.** USAN.
Use: Antiperistaltic.
• **FLUPEROLONE ACETATE.** USAN.
9α-Fluoro-21-methylprednisolone, 9α-Fluoro-11β,17α,21-trihy-droxy-21-methylpregna-1:4-diene-3:20-dione acetate. Methral.
Use: Corticosteroid.
FLUPHENAZINE DECANOATE.
See: Prolixin Decanoate, Soln. (Princeton).
Use: Antipsychotic.
• **FLUPHENAZINE ENANTHATE,** U.S.P. XXIII. Inj., U.S.P. XXIII. 4-(3-(2-(Trifluoromethyl)phenothiazine-10-yl)-propyl)-1-piperazine-ethanol.
Use: Tranquilizer.

See: Prolixin Enanthate Prods. (Princeton).
• **FLUPHENAZINE HYDROCHLORIDE,** U.S.P. XXIII. Elixir, Inj., Oral Soln., Tab., U.S.P. XXIII. 1-(2-Hydroxyethyl)-4-[3-(2-trifluoromethyl)-10H-Phenothiazinyl-propyl]-piperazine diHCl. 4-(3-(2-(Trifluoromethyl) phenothiazine-10-yl) propyl)-1-piperazine-ethanol Dihydrochloride.
Use: Tranquilizer.
See: Permitil, Preps. (Schering).
   Prolixin, Tab., Elix., Vial (Princeton).
• **FLUPIRTINE MALEATE.** USAN.
Use: Analgesic.
FLUPREDNIDENE. B.A.N. 9α-Fluoro-11β-17 α,21-trihydroxy-16-methylenepregna-1,4-diene-3, 20-dione.
Use: Glucocorticosteroid.
• **FLUPREDNISOLONE VALERATE.** USAN.
6-Fluoro-11β, 17, 21-trihydroxypregna-1, 4-diene-3,20-dione 17-valerate.
Use: Glucocorticoid.
FLUPROFEN. B.A.N. 2-(2'-Fluoro-biphenyl-4-yl)-propionic acid.
Use: Anti-inflammatory, analgesic.
• **FLUPROQUAZONE.** USAN.
Use: Analgesic.
• **FLUPROSTENOL SODIUM.** USAN.
Use: Prostaglandin.
• **FLUQUAZONE.** USAN.
Use: Anti-inflammatory.
• **FLURADOLINE HYDROCHLORIDE.** USAN.
Use: Analgesic.
FLURA DROPS. (Kirkman) Fluoride.
Drops: 0.25 mg (from 0.55 mg sodium fluoride). Bot. 24 ml. **Rinse:** 0.02% (from 0.05% sodium fluoride). Bot. 480 ml.
Use: Dental caries preventative.
FLURA-LOZ. (Kirkman) Sodium fluoride 2.2 mg providing 1 mg fluoride/ Loz. Bot. 100s, 1000s.
Use: Dental caries preventative.
• **FLURANDRENOLIDE,** U.S.P. XXIII.
Cream, Oint., Lotion, Tape, U.S.P. XXIII.
Use: Adrenocortical steroid (topical anti-inflammatory).
See: Cordran, Preps.(Dista).
FLURANDRENOLONE. 6α-Fluoro-16α-hydroxyhydrocortisone 16, 17-acetonide.
Use: Corticosteroid.
FLURANDRENOLONE. B.A.N. 6α-Fluoro-11β,-21-dihydroxy-16α, 17α-isopropylidenedioxypregn-4-ene-3,20-dione. 6α-Fluoro-16α, 17α-isopropylidenedioxyhydrocortisone. Fludroxycortide (I.N.N.).
Use: Corticosteroid.
FLURA-DROPS. (Kirkman) Fluoride 0.25

mg (from sodium fluoride 0.55 mg) per drop. Bot. 30 ml.
Use: Dental caries preventative.
FLURA-TABLETS. (Kirkman) Sodium fluoride 2.21 mg, equivalent to 1 mg fluoride ion/Tab. Bot. 100s, 1000s.
Use: Dental caries preventative.
•**FLURAZEPAM HYDROCHLORIDE,** U.S.P. XXIII. Cap., U.S.P. XXIII. 7-Chloro-1-[2-(diethylamino)ethyl]-5-(o-fluorophenyl)-3,-dihydro-2H-1,4-benzo-diazepin-2-one dihydrochloride. B.A.N. 7-Chloro-1-(2-diethylamino-ethyl)-5-(2-fluorophenyl)-1,3-dihydro-2H-1,4-ben-zodiazepin-2-one.
Use: Hypnotic.
See: Dalmane, Cap. (Roche).
•**FLURBIPROFEN, U.S.P.** U.S.P. XXIII.
Use: Anti-inflamatory; analgesic.
FLURBIPROFEN. (Various Mfr.) Flurbiprofen 50 mg or 100 mg. Tab. 100s, 500s.
Use: Anti-inflammatory; analgesic.
•**FLURBIPROFEN SODIUM,** U.S.P. XXIII, Ophth., USAN. 2-(2-Fluorobiphenyl-4-yl)propionic acid.
Use: Anti-inflammatory; analgesic.
See: Ocufen, Drops (Allergan).
FLURESS. (Pilkington Barnes-Hind) Fluorescein sodium 0.25%, benoxinate HCl 0.4% in isotonic boric acid soln., chlorobutanol 1%. Bot. 5 ml.
Use: Local anesthetic, diagnostic aid.
•**FLURETOFEN.** USAN.
Use: Anti-inflammatory, antithrombotic.
•**FLURFAMIDE.** USAN.
Use: Enzyme inhibitor.
•**FLUROCITABINE.** USAN.
Use: Antineoplastic.
FLURO-ETHYL. (Gebauer) Ethyl Cl 25%, dichlorotetrafluoroethane 75%. Aerosol can 255 Gm.
Use: Topical anesthetic.
•**FLUROGESTONE ACETATE.** USAN.
Use: Progestin.
FLUROSYN. (Rugby) **Cream:** Fluocinolone acetonide 0.01% or 0.025%. Tube 15 Gm, 60 Gm, 425 Gm. **Oint:** Fluocinolone acetonide 0.025% in a white petrolatum base. Tube 15 Gm, 60 Gm.
Use: Corticosteroid topical.
FLUROTHYL, U.S.P. XXI. Bis (2,2,2-trifluoroethyl) ether. Hexafluorodiethyl ether. B.A.N. Di-(2,2,2-trifluoroethyl) ether. Bis(2,2,2-trifluoroethyl)ether.
Use: Central nervous system stimulant, shock inducing agent (convulsant).
See: Indoklon.
•**FLUROXENE.** USAN. 2,2,2-Trifluoroethyl vinyl ether. Fluoromar.

Use: General inhalation anesthetic.
FLU-SHIELD. (Wyeth-Ayerst) Influenza virus vaccine, trivalent—Immunizing antigen, ether extracted. Vial 5 ml, UD syringe 0.5 ml. The 5 ml vial contains sufficient product to deliver ten 0.5 ml doses.
Use: Vaccine, viral.
•**FLUSPIPERONE.** USAN.
Use: Antipsychotic.
•**FLUSPIRILENE.** USAN. 8-[4, 4-bis(p-Fluorophenyl)butyl]-1-phenyl-1,3,8-triaza-spiro-[4.5] decan-4-one.
Use: Tranquilizer, antipsychotic.
See: Imap (McNeil).
•**FLUTAMIDE.** USAN.
Use: Antiandrogen.
See: Eulexin Cap. (Schering).
FLUTEX. (Syosset) Triamcinolone acetonide. **Cream:** 0.025%, 0.1%, 0.5% Tube 15 Gm, 30 Gm, 60 Gm, 120 Gm, 240 Gm. **Oint.:** 0.025%, 0.1%, 0.5% Tube 30 Gm, 60 Gm, 120 Gm.
Use: Corticosteroid, topical.
•**FLUTIAZIN.** USAN.
Use: Anti-inflammatory.
•**FLUTICASONE PROPIONATE.** USAN.
Use: Anti-inflammatory.
See: Cutivate (Glaxo).
FLUTRA. Trichlormethiazide.
Use: Diuretic.
•**FLUTROLINE.** USAN.
Use: Antipsychotic.
•**FLUVASTATIN SODIUM.** USAN
Use: Antihyperlipidemic.
See: Lescol, Cap. (Sandoz).
FLUVIRIN. (Adams) Influenza virus vaccine. Vial 5 ml (Purified Surface Antigens).
Use: Agent for immunization.
•**FLUZINAMIDE.** USAN.
Use: Anticonvulsant.
FLUZONE. (Connaught) Influenza virus vaccine. Vial 5 ml (10 doses) (Whole-virus); Vial 5 ml, UD syringes 0.5 ml (Split-virus).
Use: Agent for immunization.
FML S.O.P. (Allergan) Fluorometholone 0.1% Oint. Tube 3.5 Gm.
Use: Corticosteroid, ophthalmic.
FML FORTE. (Allergan) Fluorometholone 0.25%, benzalkonium Cl 0.005%, EDTA, polysorbate 80, polyvinyl alcohol 1.4%. Susp. Dropper bot. 2 ml, 5 ml, 10 ml, 15 ml.
Use: Corticosteroid, ophthalmic.
FML LIQUIFILM. (Allergan) Fluorometholone 0.1%, polyvinyl alcohol 1.4%, benzalkonium Cl, edetate disodium, sodium Cl, sodium phosphate

monobasic, monohydrate, sodium phosphate dibasic (anhydrous), polysorbate 80, purified water, sodium hydroxide to adjust pH. Dropper bot. 1 ml, 5 ml, 10 ml, 15 ml.
Use: Corticosteroid, ophthalmic.
FML-S. (Allergan) Fluorometholone 0.1%, sulfacetomide sodium 10%. Susp. Dropper Bot. 5 ml, 10 ml.
Use: Corticosteroid, ophthalmic.
FOAMICON. (Invamed) Aluminum hydroxide 80 mg, magnesium trisilicate 20 mg, alginic acid, clacium stearate, compressible sugar, sodium bicarbonate, sucrose. Chew. Tab. Bot. 100s.
Use: Antacid.
•**FOCOFILCON A.** USAN.
Use: Contact lens material.
FOILLE. (Blistex) Benzocaine 2%, benzyl alcohol 4% in a bland vegetable oil base. Oint. Tube 30 Gm.
Use: Local anesthetic.
FOILLECORT. (Blistex) Hydrocortisone acetate 0.5%. Cream. Tube 3.5 Gm.
Use: Corticosteroid, topical.
FOILLE MEDICATED FIRST AID. (Blistex) **Aerosol:** Benzocaine 5% with chloroxylenol 0.1% in a bland vegetable oil base with benzyl alcohol. Spray 92 Gm. **Oint.:** Benzocaine 5%, chloroxylenol 0.1% in a bland vegetable oil base. Tube 30 Gm. **Lot.:** Benzocaine 5%, chloroxylenol 0.1% in a bland vegetable oil base with benzyl alcohol 30 ml.
Use: Local anesthetic.
FOILLE PLUS. (Blistex) **Cream:** Benzocaine 5%, benzyl alcohol 4% in a nonstaining washable base. Tube 3.5 Gm. **Soln.:** Benzocaine 5%, benzyl alcohol, alcohol 77.8%. Aerosol spray 105 Gm.
Use: Local anesthetic.
FOLABEE. (Vortech) Liver inj. B_{12} equivalent to 10 mcg, crystalline B_{12} 100 mcg, folic acid 0.4 mg. Inj. Vial 10 ml.
Use: Anemia.
FOLACIN.
See: Folic acid.
FOLACINE.
See: Folic acid. (Various Mfr.).
FOLATE, SODIUM.
See: Folvite, Soln. (Lederle).
FOLEX PFS INJECTION. (Adria) Methotrexate sodium 25 mg/ml. Preservative free. Inj. Vial. 2 ml, 4 ml, 8 ml.
Use: Antineoplastic agent.
•**FOLIC ACID,** U.S.P. XXIII. Inj., Tab. U.S.P. XXIII. Pteroylglutamic acid. N-[p-[[[(2-Amino-4-hydroxy-6-pteridinyl)-methyl]-amino] benzoyl]-L-glutamic

acid. L-Glutamic acid, N-[4-[[(2-amino-1,4-dihydro-4-oxo-6-pteridinyl)methyl]-amino]benzoyl]-. Vitamin Bc.
Use: Anemia.
See: Folvite, Tab., Soln. (Lederle).
FOLIC ACID. (Various Mfr.) Tab. **0.4 mg:** Bot. 100s. **0.8 mg:** Bot. 100s. **1 mg:** Bot. 30s, 100s, 1000s, UD 100s.
Use: Treatment of folic acid deficiency.
FOLIC ACID. (LyphoMed) 5 mg/ml w/ benzyl alcohol 1.5%, EDTA. Inj. Vials 10 ml.
Use: Treatment of folic acid deficiency.
FOLIC ACID ANTAGONISTS.
See: Methotrexate Inj., Tab. (Lederle).
FOLIC ACID SALTS.
See: Folvite, Tab., Soln. (Lederle).
FOLINIC ACID. Leucovorin Calcium, U.S.P. XXIII. (Various Mfr.)
FOLIVER "12." (Pharmex) Vitamin B_{12} activity from liver inj. equivalent to cyanocobalamin 10 mcg, folic acid 1 mg, B_{12} 100 mcg/ml. Vial 10 ml, Univial 10 ml.
Use: Anemia.
FOL-LI-BEE. (Foy) Liver inj. equivalent to cyanocobalamin 10 mcg, folic acid 1 mg, cyanocobalamin 100 mcg/ml, phenol 0.5% pl l adjusted w/sodium hydroxide and/or HCl. Vial 10 ml multi-dose, Monovials.
Use: Anemia.
FOLLICLE STIMULATING HORMONE, HUMAN. Menotropins, Pergonal.
FOLLICORMON.
See: Estradiol Benzoate. (Various Mfr.).
FOLLICULAR HORMONES.
See: Estrone (Various Mfr.).
FOLLICULIN.
See: Estrone (Various Mfr.).
FOLLUTEIN. (Squibb Mark) Chorionic gonadotropin (HCG). Pow. with 10 ml diluent. 10,000 units (W/Sodium Cl 83 mg, sodium hydroxide, phenol 0.5%). Pow. for inj.
Use: Chorionic gonadotropin.
FOLTRIN. (Vitarine) Liver and stomach concentrate 240 mg, B_{12} 15 mcg, iron 110 mg, C 75 mg, folic acid 0.5 mg/Cap. Bot. 100s, 1000s.
Use: Vitamin/mineral supplement.
•**FOMEPIZOLE.** USAN.
Use: Antidote (alcohol dehydrogenase inhibitor).
FOMOCAINE. B.A.N. 4-(3-Morpholinopropyl)-benzyl phenyl ether.
Use: Local anesthetic.
FONATOL.
See: Diethylstilbestrol (Various Mfr.).
FONAZINE MESYLATE. 10-[2-(Dimethy-

lamino)propyl]-N, N-dimethylphenoth-iazine-2-sulfonamide methanesulfonate.
Use: Serotonin inhibitor.

FONTARSOL.
See: Dichlorophenarsine Hydrochloride.

FORALICON PLUS ELIXIR. (Forbes) Vitamins B_{12} 16.7 mcg, B_0 4 mg, iron 200 mg (equivalent to elemental iron 24 mg), niacinamide 40 mg, folic acid 0.8 mg, sorbitol soln. q.s./15 ml. Bot. 8 oz, 16 oz.
Use: Vitamin/mineral supplement.

FORANE. (Anaquest) Isoflurane. Gas. Volume 100 ml.
Use: General anesthetic.

FORDUSTIN. (Sween) Cornstarch based powder with deodorizing action. Bot. 3 oz, 8 oz.
Use: Baby powder.

FORMADON SOLUTION.(Gordon) Formalin solution 3.7% to 4% (10% of U.S.P. strength) in an aqueous perfumed base. Bot. 1 oz, 4 oz, 0.5 gal, gal.
Use: Bromhidrosis, hyperhidrosis.

FORMADRIN. (Kenyon) Chlorpheniramine maleate 12 mg, potassium guaiacol sulfonate 8 gr, ammonium Cl 8 gr, tartar emetic $1/12$ gr, dl-desoxyephedrine HCl 2 mg/oz. Bot. 4 oz.
Use: Antihistamine, expectorant.

• **FORMALDEHYDE SOLUTION,** U.S.P. XXIII. A 37% aqueous solution.
Use: For poison ivy, fungus infections of the skin, hyperhidrosis and as an astringent disinfectant.

FORMALIN.
See: Formaldehyde Solution (Various Mfr.).

FORMALYDE-10. (Pedinol) Formaldehyde 10%, FDA-40 alcohol. Spray Bot. 60 ml.
Use: Bromhidrosis, hyperhidrosis.

FORMA-RAY SOLUTION. (Gordon) Formalin 7.4% to 8% (20% of USP strength) in aqueous, scented, tinted solution. Bot. 1.5 oz, 4 oz.
Use: Drying agent following laser treatment for verrucae, excessive perspiration and odor.

FORMEBOLONE. B.A.N. 2-Formyl-11α, 17β-dihydroxy-17α-methylandrosta-1,4-dien-3-one.
Use: Anabolic steroid.

FORMIC ACID.
W/Silicic acid.
See: Nyloxin, Inj. (Hynson, Westcott & Dunning).

FORMINITRAZOLE. B.A.N. 2-Formamido-5-nitrothiazole.
Use: Treatment of trichomoniasis.

• **FORMOCORTAL.** USAN. 3-(2-Chloroethoxy)-9-fluoro-11β, 16α, 17, 21-tetrahydroxy-20-oxopregna-3, 5-diene-6-carboxaldehyde, cyclic 16, 17-acetal with acetone, 21-acetate.
Use: Glucocorticoid.

FORMULA 44 COUGH CONTROL DISCS. (Vicks)
See: Vicks Formula 44 Cough Discs (Vicks).

FORMULA 44 COUGH MIXTURE. (Vicks) Chlorpheniramine maleate 2 mg, dextromethorphan HBr 15 mg, alcohol 10%/5 ml. Liq. Bot. 120 ml, 240 ml.
Use: Antihistamine, antitussive.

FORMULA 44D DECONGESTANT COUGH MIXTURE. (Vicks) Pseudoephedrine HCl 20 mg, dextromethorphan HBr 10 mg, guaifenesin 67 mg, alcohol 10%/5 ml. Liq. Bot. 120 ml, 240 ml.
Use: Decongestant, antitussive, expectorant.

FORMULA "K". (Pharmex) Calcium gluconate 1.5 Gm, potassium Cl 4.47 Gm, magnesium sulfate 60 mg/ml. Vial 30 ml.
Use: Mineral supplement.

FORMULA 44M COUGH AND COLD. (Vicks) Pseudoephedrine HCl 15 mg, dextromethorphan HBr 7.5 mg, chlorpheniramine maleate 1 mg, acetaminophen 125 mg/5 ml, alcohol 20%, saccharin, sucrose. Liq. Bot. 120 ml, 240 ml.
Use: Decongestant, antitussive, antihistamine, analgesic.

FORMULA NO. 81. (Fellows) Liver (beef) for inj. 1 mcg, ferrous gluconate 100 mg, niacinamide 100 mg, B_2 1.5 mg, panthenol 2.5 mg, B_{12} 3 mcg, procaine HCl 25 mg/2 ml. Vial 30 ml.
Use: Vitamin/mineral supplement.

FORMULA 1207. (Thurston) Iodine, liver fraction No. 2, caseinates/Tab. Bot. 100s, 250s.
Use: Mineral supplement.

FORMULA B. (Major) Vitamins B_1 15 mg, B_2 15 mg, B_3 100 mg, B_5 18 mg, B_6 18 mg, B_{12} 5 mcg, C 500 mg, folic acid 0.5 mg/Tab. Bot 250 g.
Use: Vitamin supplement.

FORMULA-Q. (Major) Quinine sulfate 65 mg, vitamin E 400 IU (as dl-alpha tocopheryl acetate. Cap. Bot. 50s.
Use: For treatment of nocturnal leg cramps.

FORMYL TETRAHYDROPTEROYLGLUTAMIC ACID. Leucovorin Calcium, U.S.P. XXIII.

FORMULA VM-2000 TABLETS. (Solgar) Vitamins A 5000 IU, D 200 IU, E 67.1 mg, B_1 50 mg, B_2 50 mg, B_3 50 mg, B_5 50 mg, B_6 50 mg, B_{12} 50 mcg, C 150 mg, folic acid 0.4 mg, zinc 15 mg, iron 5 mg, boron, Ca, Cr, Cu, I, K, Mg, Mn, Mo, Se, Beta carotene 7500 IU, Betaine, biotin 50 mcg, choline, bioflavonoids, amino acids, glutamic acid, hesperidin, inositol, l-glutethione, PABA, rutin. Tab. Bot. 30s, 60s, 90s, 180s.
Use: Vitamin/mineral supplement.

FORTA DRINK POWDER. (Ross) Whey protein concentrate, sucrose, vitamins A, B_1, B_2, B_3, B_5, B_6, B_{12}, C, D, E, folic acid, biotin, Ca, Cu, Fe, I, Mg, Mn, P, Zn. Can. 482 gm.
Use: Enteral nutritional supplement.

FORTA-FLORA. (Barth's) Whey-lactose 90%, pectin. **Pow.:** Jar lb. **Wafer:** Bot. 100s.

FORTAGESIC TABLETS. (Sanofi Winthrop) Paracetamol, pentazocine.
Use: Narcotic analgesic.

FORTA INSTANT CEREAL. (Ross) Lactose-free oat or bran cereal provides 6.25 Gm dietary fiber/serving. Can 1 lb 1 oz.
Use: Enteral nutritional supplement.

FORTA INSTANT PUDDING. (Ross) Lactose-free in pudding base. Can 1 lb 12 oz. Vanilla, chocolate, butterscotch flavors.
Use: Enteral nutritional supplement.

FORTA PUDDING MIX. (Ross) Milk protein isolate, sucrose, hydrolyzed cornstarch, modified tapioca starch, partially hydrogenated soybean oil, vitamins A, B_1, B_2, B_3, B_5, B_6, B_{12}, C, D, E, folic acid, biotin, Ca, Fe, P, I, Mg, Zn, Cu, Mn, tartrazine. Can 794 Gm.
Use: Enteral nutritional supplement.

FORTA SHAKE POWDER. (Ross) Nonfat dry milk, sucrose, vitamins A, B_1, B_2, B_3, B_5, B_6, B_{12}, C, D, E, folic acid, biotin, Ca, Cu, Fe, I, Mg, Mn, P, Zn, tartrazine. Can lb, pkt. 1.4 oz. Can 1 lb 2.7 oz, pkt. 1.6 oz.
Use: Enteral nutritional supplement.

FORTA SOUP MIX. (Ross) Milk protein isolate, sodium and calcium caseinate, hydrolyzed cornstarch, modified tapioca starch, powdered shortening (partially hydrogenated coconut oil), vitamins A, B_1, B_2, B_3, B_5, B_6, B_{12}, C, D, E, folic acid, biotin, Ca, Cu, Fe, I, Mg, Mn, P, Zn. Chicken flavor. Can. 454 Gm.
Use: Enteral nutritional supplement.

FORTAZ. (Glaxo Pharmaceuticals) Ceftazidime powder for parenteral administration 500 mg, 1 Gm, 2 Gm, or 6 Gm Vial. **Pow. 500 mg:** Tray 25s. **1 Gm:** Tray 25s, Infusion Pack Tray 10s. **2 Gm:** Tray 10s, Infusion Pack Tray 10s. **6 Gm:** Pharmacy Bulk Pkg. Tray 6s. **Inj.:** 1 g, 2 g Vial 50 ml, premixed, frozen.
Use: Antibacterial, cephalosporin.

FORTE L.I.V. (Foy) Cyanocobalamin 15 mcg liver injection equivalent to vitamin B_{12} activity 1 mcg, ferrous gluconate 50 mg, B_2 0.75 mg, panthenol 1.25 mg, niacinamide 50 mg, citric acid 8.2 mg, sodium citrate 118 mg/ml, procaine HCl 2%. Bot. 30 ml.
Use: Vitamin supplement.

FORTEL MIDSTREAM. (Biomerica) Reagent in home urine test for pregnancy. 1 test stick per kit.
Use: Pregnancy test.

FORTEL OVULATION. (NMS) Monoclonal antibody-based home test to predict ovulation. Kit 1s.
Use: Diagnostic aid.

FORTEL PLUS. (Biomerica) Reagent in home urine pregnancy test. Kit contains urine collection cup, dropper, test device.
Use: Pregnancy test.

FORTRAL. (Sanofi Winthrop) Pentazocine as solution and tablets.
Use: Narcotic analgesic.

FORTRAMIN. (Thurston) Vitamins E 200 IU, A 6000 IU, D 600 IU, B_1 4.5 mg, B_2 4.5 mg, B_6 4.5 mg, B_{12} 5 mcg, C 2.75 mg, rutin 8 mg, hesperidin complex 10 mg, lemon bioflavonoids 15 mg, d-calcium pantothenate 50 mg, para-aminobenzoic acid 7.5 mg, biotin 10 mg, folic acid 24 mcg, niacinamide 20 mg, desiccated liver 25 mg, iron 3 mg, calcium 75 mg, phosphorous 34 mg, manganese 10 mg, copper 0.5 mg, zinc 0.5 mg, iodine 0.375 mg, potassium 500 mg, magnesium 5 mg/Tab. Bot. 100s, 250s.
Use: Vitamin/mineral supplement.

• **FOSARILATE.** USAN.
Use: Antiviral.

• **FOSAZEPAM.** USAN. 7-Chloro-1-dimethylphosphinylmethyl-1,3-dihydro-5-phenyl-2H-1,4-benzodiazepin-2-one.
Use: Hypnotic.

• **FOSCARNET SODIUM.** USAN.
Use: Antiviral.
See: Foscavir, Inj. (Astra).

FOSCAVIR. (Astra) foscarnet Sodium 24 mg/ml. Inj. Bot. 250 ml, 500 ml.
Use: Antiviral.

FOSFESTROL. B.A.N. trans-$\alpha\alpha'$ Diethylstilbene-4,4-diol bis(dihydrogen phosphate).

Use: Treatment of carcinoma of the prostate.

• **FOSFOMYCIN.** USAN.
Use: Antibacterial.

• **FOSFOMYCIN TROMETHAMINE.** USAN.
Use: Antibacterial.

• **FOSFONET SODIUM.** USAN.
Use: Antiviral.

FOSFREE. (Mission) Calcium lactate 250 mg, calcium gluconate 250 mg, calcium carbonate 300 mg, calcium 175.7 mg, ferrous gluconate 125 mg (iron 14.5 mg), vitamins A 1500 IU, B_1 5 mg, B_2 2 mg, B_3 10 mg, B_5 1 mg, B_6 3 mg, B_{12} 2 mcg, C 50 mg, D 150 IU/Tab. Bot. 100s.
Use: Vitamin/mineral supplement.

• **FOSINOPRIL.**
Use: Angiotensin converting enzyme inhibitor, antihypertensive.
See: Monopril (Mead Johnson).

• **FOSINOPRIL SODIUM.** USAN.
Use: Antihypertensive, enzyme inhibitor.
See: Monopril (Mead Johnson).

• **FOSINOPRILAT.** USAN.
Use: Antihypertensive.

• **FOSPHENYTOIN SODIUM.** USAN.
Use: Anticonvulsant. [Orphan drug]

• **FOSPIRATE.** USAN.
Use: Anthelmintic.

• **FOSQUIDONE.** USAN.
Use: Antineoplastic.

• **FOSTEDIL.** USAN.
Use: Vasodilator.

FOSTEX 5% BPO. (Westwood) Benzyl peroxide 5% in Laureth-4 base. Gel 45 Gm.
Use: Anti-acne.

FOSTEX 10% BPO CLEANSING BAR. (Westwood) Benzoyl peroxide 10%. Bar 3.75 oz.
Use: Anti-acne.

FOSTEX 10% BPO WASH. (Westwood) Benzoyl peroxide 10% with water base. Liq. Bot. 150 ml.
Use: Anti-acne.

FOSTEX ACNE MEDICATION CLEASING. (Bristol-Myers) Salicylic acid 2%, EDTA, stearyl alcohol. Cream. 118 g.
Use: Anti-acne.

FOSTEX MEDICATED COVER-UP. (Westwood) Sulfur 2% in a flesh-tinted greasless base. Cream Tube 30 Gm.
Use: Anti-acne.

• **FOSTRIECIN SODIUM.** USAN.
Use: Antineoplastic.

FOSTRIL. (Westwood) Sulfur 2% in greaseless base. Lot. Tube 30 ml.
Use: Anti-acne.

FOTOTAR CREAM. (Elder) Coal tar 1.6% (from 2% coal tar extract) in emollient moisturizing cream base. Tube 90 Gm, 480 Gm.
Use: Chronic skin disorders.

FOURSALCO. (Jenkins) Salicylic acid 0.5 gr, sodium bicarbonate 3 gr, magnesium salicylate 2 gr, strontium salicylate 2 gr, acetophenetidin 0.25 gr, methyl salicylate, pancreatin 1/40 gr, diastase gr/Tab. Bot. 1000s.
Use: Analgesic.

4-WAY COLD TABLETS. (Bristol-Myers) Aspirin 324 mg, phenylpropanolamine HCl 12.5 mg, chlorpheniramine maleate 2 mg/Tab. Bot. 36s, 60s, Card 15s.
Use: Analgesic, decongestant, antihistamine.

4-WAY FAST ACTING NASAL SPRAY. (Bristol-Myers) Phenylephrine HCl 0.5%, naphazoline HCl 0.05%, pyrilamine maleate 0.2%, buffered isotonic aqueous soln., thimerosal. Atomizer 15 ml, 30 ml.
Use: Decongestant, antihistamine.

4-WAY LONG ACTING NASAL SPRAY. (Bristol-Myers) Oxymetazoline HCl 0.05% in isotonic buffered soln. Spray Bot. 15 ml.
Use: Nasal decongestant.

FOWLER'S SOLUTION. Potassium Arsenite Solution (Various Mfr.).

FOXALIN. (Standex) Digitoxin 0.1 mg, sodium carboxymethylcellulose/Cap. Bot. 100s.
Use: Cardiac glycoside.

FOXGLOVE.
See: Digitalis (Various Mfr.).

FOYGEN AQUEOUS. (Foy) Estrogenic substance or estrogens 2 mg/ml with sodium carboxymethylcellulose, povidone, benzyl alcohol, methyl and propyl parabens. Inj. Vial 10 ml.
Use: Estrogen.

FOYPLEX INJECTION. (Foy) Sterile injectable soln. of nine water-soluble vitamins. Packaged as 2 separate solutions for extemporaneous combination.
Use: Parenteral nutritional supplement.

FRAMYCETIN. B.A.N. An antibiotic produced by *Streptomyces decaris.*
Use: Antibiotic.

FRANODIL. (Sanofi Winthrop) Ephedrine sulfate, theophylline, anhydrous, chlormezanone.
Use: Bronchodilator.

FRANOL. (Sanofi Winthrop) Theophylline anhydrous, ephedrine sulfate, phenobarbital, thenyldiamine HCl.
Use: Bronchodilator.

FREAMINE III. (Kendall McGaw) Amino acid 8.5% or 10%. Bot. 500 ml, 1000 ml.
Use: Parenteral nutritional supplement.
FREAMINE III W/ELECTROLYTES. (Kendall McGaw) Amino acid 3% with electrolytes. Bot. 1000 ml.
Use: Parenteral nutritional supplement.
FREAMINE 8.5% III W/ELECTROLYTES. (Kendall McGraw) Sodium 60 mEq/L, potassium 60 mEq/L, magnesium 10 mEq/L, Cl 60 mEq/L, phosphate 40 mEq/L, acetate 125 mEq/L. Soln. Bot. 500 ml, 1000 ml.
Use: Parenteral nutritional supplement.
FREAMINE HBC. (American McGaw) High branched 6.9% amino acid formulation for hypercatabolic patients. Bot. 1000 ml.
Use: Parenteral nutritional supplement.
FREEDAVITE. (Freeda) Iron 30 mg (from ferrous fumarate), vitamins A 5000 IU, D 400 IU, E 3 IU, B_1 5 mg, B_2 3 mg, B_3 25 mg, B_5 5 mg, B_6 0.5 mg, B_{12} 2 mcg, C 60 mg, choline, inositol, Ca, Cu, K, Mg, Mn, Zn. Bot. 100s, 250s, 500s.
Use: Vitamin/mineral supplement.
FREEZONE. (Whitehall) Salicylic acid 13.6%, alcohol 20.5%, ether 64.8% in flexible collodion base. Bot. 9.3 ml 13 oz.
Use: Keratolytic.
• **FRENTIZOLE.** USAN.
Use: Immunoregulator.
FRESH n' FEMININE. (Walgreen) Benzethonium Cl 0.2% Bot. 8 oz.
Use: Vaginal preparation.
• **FRUCTOSE,** U.S.P. XXIII. Inj., U.S.P. XXIII. (Abbott) (Cutter) Soln. 10%. Bot. 1000 ml.
Use: Nutrient.
See: Frutabs, Tab. (Pfanstiehl).
• **FRUCTOSE AND SODIUM CHLORIDE INJECTION,** U.S.P. XXIII.
Use: Fluid, nutrient and electrolyte replenisher.
FRUITY CHEWS. (Goldline) Vitamins A 2500 IU, D 400 IU, E 15 mg, B_1 1.05 mg, B_2 1.2 mg, B_3 13.5 mg, B_6 1.05 mg, B_{12} 4.5 mcg, C (as sodium ascorbate and ascorbic acid) 60 mg, folic acid 0.3 mg/Chew. Tab. Bot. 100s.
Use: Vitamin/mineral supplement.
FRUITY CHEWS WITH IRON. (Goldline) Elemental iron 12 mg, vitamins A 2500 IU, D 400 IU, E 15 mg, B_1 1.05 mg, B_2 1.2 mg, B_3 13.5 mg, B_6 1.05 mg, B_{12} 4.5 mg, C (as sodium ascorbate and ascorbic acid) 60 mg, folic acid 0.3 mg, zinc 8 mg/Chew. Tab. Bot. 100s.
Use: Vitamin/mineral supplement.

FRUSEMIDE. 4-Chloro-N-furfuryl-5-sulfamoylanthranilic acid. Lasix.
FRUSEMIDE. B.A.N. 4-Chloro-N-furfuryl-5-sulphamoylanthranilic acid. Furosemide (I.N.N.).
Use: Diuretic.
FRUTABS. (Pfanstiehl) Fructose 2 Gm. Tab. Bot. 100s.
Use: Carbohydrate.
FTA-ABS. (Wampole-Zeus) Fluorescent treponemal antibody-absorbed test in vitro for confirming a positive reagin test for syphillis. Test 100s.
Use: Diagnostic aid.
FTA-ABS/DS. (Wampole-Zeus) Fluorescent treponemal antibody-absorbed test in vitro for confirming a positive reagin test for syphilis. Test 100s.
Use: Diagnostic aid.
• **FUCHSIN, BASIC,** U.S.P. XXIII. Basic Fuchsin is a mixture of rosaniline and pararosaniline HCl. Basic Magenta.
Use: Ingredient in Carbo-Fuchsin Solution anti-infective (topical).
FUDR. (Roche) Floxuridine 500 mg sterile pow. for inj. Vial 5 ml.
Use: Antineoplastic agent.
FUL-GLO. (Sola/Barnes-Hind) Fluorescein sodium 0.6 mg/Strip. Box 300s.
Use: Diagnostic aid, ophthalmic.
FULLER. (Birchwood) Pkg. 1 shield.
Use: Anorectal protective garment.
FULVICIN P/G. (Schering) Griseofulvin ultramicrosize 125 mg, 165 mg, 250 mg or 330 mg/Tab. Bot. 100s.
Use: Antifungal.
FULVICIN-U/F. (Schering) Griseofulvin microsize 250 mg or 500 mg/Tab. Bot. 60s, 250s.
Use: Antifungal.
FUMAGILLIN. B.A.N. A crystalline antibiotic produced during the growth of a strain of *Aspergillus fumigatus*.
• **FUMARIC ACID.** N.F. XVIII. 2-Butenedioic acid.
Use: Acidifier.
FUMASORB. (Milance) Ferrous fumarate 200 mg (iron 66 mg)/Tab. Bot. 30s, 60s.
Use: Iron supplement.
FUMATINIC CAPSULES. (Laser) Iron 90 mg (from ferrous fumarate), vitamins C 100 mg, B_{12} 15 mcg, folic acid 1 mg/SR Cap. Bot. 100s, 1000s.
Use: Vitamin/mineral supplement.
FUMERIN. (Laser) Ferrous fumarate 195 mg equivalent to iron 64 mg/Tab. Bot. 100s, 1000s.
Use: Iron supplement.
FUMERON. (Vitarine) Ferrous fumarate 330 mg, vitamin B_1 5 mg/TR Cap.

Use: Vitamin/mineral supplement.
- **FUMOXICILLIN.** USAN.
Use: Antibacterial.
FUNDUSCEIN. (Iolab) Fluorescein sodium. Inj. **10%:** Amp. 5 ml. 12s. **25%:** Amp. 3 ml. 12s.
Use: Diagnostic aid, ophthalmic.
FUNGACETIN OINTMENT. (Blair) Triacetin (glyceryl triacetate) 25% in a water-miscible ointment base. Tube 30 Gm.
Use: Antifungal, external.
FUNGATIN. (Major) Tolnaftate 1%. Cream Tube 15 Gm.
Use: Antifungal, external.
FUNGICIDES.
See: Aftate, Prods. (Plough).
Arcum, Preps. (Arcum).
Asterol.
Basic Fuchsin (Various Mfr.).
Desenex, Prods. (Pharmacraft).
Dichlorophene.
Miconazole Nitrate (Various Mfr.).
Nifuroxime (Various Mfr.).
Nitrofurfuryl Methyl Ether (Various Mfr.).
Phenylmercuric Preps. (Various Mfr.).
Propionate, Sodium (Various Mfr.).
Propionic Acid (Various Mfr.).
Sporanox, Cap. (Janssen).
Undecylenic Acid (Various Mfr.).
- **FUNGIMYCIN.** USAN.
Use: Antifungal.
FUNGINAIL. (Kramer) Resorcinol 1%, salicyclic acid 2%, parachlorometaxylenol 2%, benzocaine 0.5%, acetic acid 2.5%, propylene glycol, hydroxypropyl methylcellulose, alcohol 0.5%. Bot. 30 ml.
Use: Antifungal, external.
FUNGIZONE. (Squibb) Amphotericin B 3%, thimerosal, titanium dioxide. **Lot.:** Plastic bot. 30 ml. **Cream, Oint:** Tube 20 Gm.
Use: Antifungal, external.
FUNGIZONE INTRAVENOUS. (Squibb) Amphotericin B 50 mg, sodium desoxycholate 41 mg, sodium phosphate 25.2 mg/Vial (lyophilized).
Use: Antifungal.
FUNGIZONE FOR LABORATORY USE IN TISSUE CULTURE. (Squibb) Amphotericin B 50 mg, sodium desoxycholate 41 mg/Vial 20 ml.
Use: Laboratory.
FUNGOID. (Pedinol) Undecylenic acid 25%. Soln. Bot. 29.57 ml.
Use: Antifungal, external.
FUNGOID CREME. (Pedinol) Miconazole nitrate 2%, mineral oil. Tube 56.7 g.

Use: Antifungal, external.
FUNGOID HC CREME. (Pedinol) Miconazole nitrate 2%, hydrocortisone 1%. In 56.7 g, 1 g dual packets.
Use: Antifungal, external.
FUNGOID TINCTURE. (Pedinol) Miconazole nitrate 2%, alcohol. Soln. Bot. with brush applicator 7.39 ml, 29.57 ml.
Use: Antifungal, external.
FURACIN SOLUBLE DRESSING. (Roberts) Nitrofurazone 0.2% in a water-soluble, non-drying, ointment-like base of polyethylene glycols. Jar 454 Gm, Tube 28 Gm, 56 Gm.
Use: Burn preparation.
FURACIN TOPICAL CREAM. (Roberts) Furacin 0.2% in a water miscible, self-emulsifying cream w/glycerin, cetyl alcohol, mineral oil, ethoxylated fatty alcohol, methylparaben, propylparaben, water. Tube 28 Gm.
Use: Burn preparation.
FURACIN TOPICAL SOLUTION. (Roberts) Nitrofurazone 0.2%. Bot. 480 ml.
Use: Burn preparation.
FURADANTIN ORAL SUSPENSION. (Procter & Gamble) Nitrofurantoin 5 mg/ml. Bot. 60 ml, 470 ml.
Use: Urinary anti-infective.
FURALAZINE HYDROCHLORIDE. 3-Amino-6-[2-(5-nitro-2-furyl)vinyl]-as-triazine HCl.
Use: Antimicrobial compound.
FURALTADONE. (±)-5-Morpholinomethyl-3-[(5-nitrofurfurylidene)amino]-2-oxazolidinone.
FURANITE TABS. (Major) Nitrofurantoin 50 mg or 100 mg/Tab. Bot. 100s.
Use: Urinary anti-infective.
- **FURAPROFEN.** USAN.
Use: Anti-inflammatory.
- **FURAZOLIDONE,** U.S.P. XXIII. Oral Susp., Tab., U.S.P. XXIII. 2-Oxazolidone, 3-(((5-nitro-2 furanyl) methylene)amino). 3[(5-Nitrofurfurylidene)-amino]-2-oxazolidinone.
Use: Antimicrobial agent.
See: Furoxone Tab., Susp. (Norwich Eaton).
- **FURAZOLIUM CHLORIDE.** USAN.
Use: Antibacterial.
- **FURAZOLIUM TARTRATE.** USAN.
Use: Antibacterial.
FURAZOSIN HCl. 1-(4-Amino-6, 7-dimethoxy-2-quin-azolinyl)-4-(2-furoyl)piperazine monohydrochloride. Under study.
Use: Antihypertensive.
- **FUREGRELATE SODIUM.** USAN.

Use: Inhibitor (thromboxene synthetase).

FURETHIDINE. 1-(2-Tetrahydrofurfuryloxyethyl)-4-phenylpiperidine-4-carboxylic acid ethyl ester.

FURETHIDINE. B.A.N. Ethyl 4-phenyl-1-[2-(tetrahydrofurfuryloxy)ethyl]piperidine-4-carboxylate.
Use: Narcotic analgesic.

•**FURODAZOLE.** USAN.
Use: Anthelmintic.

FURONATAL FA. (Metro Med) Vitamins A 8000 IU, D 400 IU, E 30 IU, C 60 mg, folic acid 1 mg, B_1 2 mg, B_2 2.8 mg, B_6 2.5 mg, B_{12} 8 mcg, niacinamide 20 mg, iron 65 mg, calcium 125 mg/Tab. Bot. 100s, 1000s.
Use: Vitamin/mineral supplement.

•**FUROSEMIDE,** U.S.P. XXIII. Inj., Tab., U.S.P. XXIII. 4-Chloro-N-(furfuryl-)-5-sulfamoylanthranilic acid. Benzoic acid, 5-(aminosulfonyl)-4-chloro-2[(2-furanylmethyl)amino]. (Abbott) 10 mg/ml. Inj. Single dose syringe 2 ml, 5 ml, 10 ml, single dose vial 2 ml, 10 ml, partial fill single dose vial 4 ml.
Use: Diuretic.
See: Furnide, Tab. (Everett).
Furomide, Vial (Hyrex).
Lasix, Tab., Inj., Soln. (Hoechst-Roussel).

FUROSEMIDE. (Roxane) Furosemide. **10 mg/ml:** Soln. Dropper bot. 60 ml. **40 mg/5 ml:** Soln. Bot. 5 ml, 10 ml, 500 ml.
Use: Diuretic.

FUROSEMIDE. (Various Mfr.) **Tab.: 20 mg or 80 mg:** Bot. 100s, 500s, 1000s, UD 100s; **40 mg:** Bot. 60s, 100s, 500s, 1000s, UD 100s. **Oral Soln.:** 10 mg/ml Bot. 60 ml, 120 ml. **Inj.:** 10 mg/ml Vial 10 ml, single dose vial 2 ml, 4 ml, 10 ml.
Use: Diuretic.

FUROXONE. (Procter & Gamble) Furazolidone. **Tab.:** 100 mg. Bot. 20s, 100s. **Liq.:** 50 mg/15 ml. Bot. 60 ml, 473 ml.
Use: Antibacterial.

•**FURSALAN.** USAN. 3, 5-Dibromo-N-(tetrahydrofurfuryl)- salicylamide. Under study.
Use: Germicide.

FUSAFUNGINE. B.A.N. An antibiotic produced by *Fusarium lateritium.*

•**FUSIDATE SODIUM.** USAN. (I) Sodium 3α, 11α, 16β-trihydroxy-29-nor-8α,9β,13α,14β-dammara-17(20),24-dien-21-oate 16-acetate. Fucidine (Squibb).
Use: Antibacterial.
See: Fucidine (Squibb).

•**FUSIDIC ACID.** USAN. An antibiotic produced by a strain of Fusidium. cis-16β-Acetoxy-3α,-11 α-dihydroxy-4α,8, 14-trimethyl-18-nor-5α,-8α,9β,13α,14β-cholesta-17(20),24-dien-21-oic acid.
Use: Antibacterial.

G

G-4.
See: Dichlorophene.

G-11. (Givaudan) Hexachlorophene Pow. for mfg.
See: Hexachlorophene, U.S.P. XXIII.

GABAPENTIN.
Use: Anticonvulsant.
See: Neurontin, Cap. (Parke-Davis).

GABBROMICINA.
See: AMINOSIDINE.

GACID TAB. (Arcum) Magnesium trisilicate 500 mg, aluminum hydroxide 250 mg/Tab. Bot. 100s, 1000s.
Uco: Antacid.

•**GADOBENATE DIMEGLUMINE.** USAN.
Use: Diagnostic imaging aid.

•**GADODIAMIDE.** USAN.
Use: Diagnostic aid, paramagnetic.
See: Omniscan, Vial (Sanofi Winthrop).

GADOPENTETATE DIMEGLUMINE.
Use: Radiopaque agent.
See: Magnevist (Berlex).

•**GADOTERIDOL.** USAN.
Use: Diagnostic aid, paramagnetic.
See: ProHance, Inj. (Squibb Diagnostics).

•**GALLAMINE TRIETHIODIDE,** U.S.P. XXIII. Inj. U.S.P. XXIII. [v-Phenenyltris(oxyethylene)] tris[triethylam-monium] Triiodide. Ethanaminium, 2,2′,2″-[1,2,3-benzenetriyltris(oxy)]tris-[N,N,N-triethyl]-,triiodide.
Use: Skeletal muscle relaxant.
See: Flaxedil (Davis & Geck).

•**GALLIUM CITRATE Ga-67 INJECTION,** U.S.P. XXIII.
Use: Diagnostic aid (radiopaque medium).

•**GALLIUM NITRATE.**
Use: Treatment of cancer-related hypercalcemia. [Orphan drug]
See: Ganite (Fujisawa).

GALLOCHROME.
See: Merbromin (Various Mfr.).

GALLOTANNIC ACID.
See: Tannic Acid, Preps. (Various Mfr.).

GALLSTONE SOLUBILIZING AGENTS.
See: Actigall, Cap. (Ciba).
Chenix, Tab. (Reid-Rowell).
Moctanin. (Ethitek).

GAMASTAN. (Cutter) Immune serum globulin (human) U.S.P. Vial 2 ml, 10 ml.
Use: Immune serum.

GAMAZOLE TABS. (Major) Sulfamethoxazole 500 mg/Tab. Bot. 100s, 500s, 1000s.
Use: Antibacterial, sulfonamide.

• **GAMFEXINE.** USAN. N,N-Dimethyl-a-phenyl-cyclo-hexanepropylamine.
Use: Antidepressant.

GAMIMUNE N. (Cutter Biologicals) Immune globulin IV (human) 5% in maltose 10%. Inj. Vial 10 ml, 50 ml, 100 ml.
Use: Immune serum.

GAMIMUNE N 10%. (Miles) Immune globulin IV (human) 10%. Inj. Vial 50 ml, 100 ml, 200 ml.
Use: Immune serum.

GAMMA BENZENE HEXACHLORIDE. B.A.N. a-1,2,3,4,5,6-Hexachlorocyclohexane. Lindane, U.S.P. XXIII.
Use: Antiparaasitic.

GAMMAGARD. (Hyland) Immune globulin intravenous (human) 2.5 Gm or 5 Gm/Vial. Inj. Dried concentrate w/diluent.
Use: Immune serum.

GAMMA GLOBULIN.
See: Immune Globulin Intramuscular.

GAMMA INTERFERON, 1-B.
See: Actimmune (Genentech).

GAMMAR. (Armour) Immune globulin, (human) U.S.P. Vial 2 ml, 10 ml.

GAMMAR-IV. (Armour) Immune globulin (human). Sucrose 5%, albumin 3% (1 Gm or 5 Gm). In 1 Gm single-dose vial with 20 ml sterile water for inj.; 2.5 Gm single-dose vial with 50 ml sterile water for inj.; 5 Gm single-dose vial with 100 ml sterile water for inj.; 5 Gm pharmacy bulk pack.
Use: Immune serum.

GAMOLENIC ACID. B.A.N. cis, cis, cis-Octadeca-6,9,12-trienoic acid.
Use: Treatment of hypercholesterolemia.

GAMULIN Rh. (Armour) Rho (D) Immune globulin (Human). Vial, syringe 1 dose.
Use: Rh-negative mothers after delivery of an Rh-positive infant.

• **GANCICLOVIR.** USAN.
Use: Antiviral.
See: Cytovene (Syntex).

• **GANCICLOVIR SODIUM.** USAN.
Use: Antiviral.
See: Cytovene (Syntex).

G AND W PRODUCTS. (G & W) G and W markets the following products under the G & W brand name:
Aminophylline Rectal Supp., 250 mg,

500 mg.
Aspirin Rectal Supp., 125 mg, 300 mg, 600 mg.
Bisacodyl Supp., 10 mg.
Glycerin Supp., Adult and Infant Sizes.
Hemorrhoidal Rectal Ointment.
Hemorrhoidal Rectal Supp., Formula C-116 and Formula C-119.
Hemorrhoidal Rectal Supp. w/Hydrocortisone Acetate 10 mg or 25 mg/Supp.
Vaginal Sulfa Cream.

GANEAKE. (Geneva) Conjugated Estrogens, 0.625 mg, 1.25 mg or 2.5 mg/Tab. Bot. 100s, 1000s.
Use: Estrogen.

GANGLIONIC BLOCKING AGENTS.
See: Arfonad, Amp. (Roche).
Dibenzyline HCl, Cap. (SK-Beecham).
Hexamethonium Cl and Bromide (Various Mfr.).
Hydergine, Amp., Tab. (Sandoz).
Inversine, Tab. (Merck & Co.).
Priscoline HCl, Tab., Vial (Ciba).
Regitine, Amp., Tab. (Ciba).

GANGLIOSIDES AS SODIUM SALTS.
Use: Retinitis pigmentosa. [Orphan drug]

• **GANIRELIX ACETATE.** USAN.
Use: Treatment of gonadal steroid dependent diseases (LHRH antagonist).

GANITE. (Fujisawa). Gallium nitrate. 25 mg/ml. Vial. 20 ml.
Use: Treatment of cancer-related hypercalcemia.

GANTANOL. (Roche) Sulfamethoxazole. **Tab.:** 0.5 Gm/Tab. Bot. 100s, 500s, Tel-E-Dose 100s. **Susp:** 0.5 Gm/5 ml (cherry flavor) Bot. 1 pt.
Use: Antibacterial, sulfonamide.

GANTANOL DS. (Roche) Sulfamethoxazole 1 Gm/Tab. Bot. 100s.
Use: Antibacterial, sulfonamide.

GANTRISIN, AZO. (Roche)
See: Azo Gantrisin, Tab. (Roche).

GANTRISIN INJECTABLE. (Roche) Sulfisoxazole diolamine 4 mg/ml. W/sodium metabisulfite 2 mg. Pkg. 10s.
Use: Antibacterial, sulfonamide.

GANTRISIN, LIPO. (Roche) Acetyl Sulfisoxazole.
Use: Antibacterial, sulfonamide.
See: Lipo Gantrisin, Susp. (Roche).

GANTRISIN PEDIATRIC SUSPENSION. (Roche) Acetyl sulfisoxazole 0.5 Gm/5 ml. Bot. 120 ml, 480 ml.
Use: Antibacterial, sulfonamide.

GANTRISIN TABLETS. (Roche) Sulfisoxazole 0.5 Gm/Tab. Tel-E-Dose Pkg. 100s (10 strips of 10), Bot. 100s, 500s.
Use: Antibacterial, sulfonamide.

W/Phenylazo-diamino-pyridine HCl.
See: Azo Gantrisin, Tab. (Roche).
GARAMYCIN. (Schering) **Cream:** Gentamicin sulfate 1.7 mg (equivalent to gentamicin base 1 mg). Methylparaben 1 mg, butylparaben 4 mg as preservatives, stearic acid, propylene glycol monostearate, isopropyl myristate, propylene glycol, polysorbate 40, sorbitol soln., water/Gm. Tube 15 Gm. **Oint.:** Gentamicin sulfate 1.7 mg (equivalent to gentamicin base 1 mg), methylparaben 0.5 mg, propylparaben 0.1 mg in petrolatum base/Gm. Tube 15 Gm.
Use: Anti-infective, external.
GARAMYCIN INJECTABLE. (Schering) Gentamicin sulfate. Inj. equivalent to 40 mg gentamicin base, methylparaben 1.8 mg, propylparaben 0.2 mg, as preservatives, sodium bisulfite 3.2 mg, disodium edetate 0.1 mg/ml Vial 2 ml (80 mg), 20 ml (800 mg); Syringe 1.5 ml (60 mg), 2 ml (80 mg); **Pediatric Inj.:** 10 mg/ml w/methylparaben 1.3 mg, propylparaben 0.2 mg, sodium bisulfite 3.2 mg, edetate disodium 0.1 mg/ml. Vial 2 ml (20 mg).
Use: Antibacterial, aminoglycoside.
GARAMYCIN INTRATHECAL INJECTION. (Schering) Gentamicin sulfate equivalent to 2 mg/ml gentamicin base, 8.5 mg sodium Cl/ml. Amp. 2 ml.
Use: Antibacterial, aminoglycoside.
GARAMYCIN I.V. PIGGYBACK. (Schering) Gentamicin sulfate equivalent to 1 mg gentamicin base, 8.9 mg sodium Cl, (no preservatives). Inj. Bot. 60 ml (60 mg), 80 ml (80 mg).
Use: Antibacterial, aminoglycoside.
GARAMYCIN OPHTHALMIC OINTMENT-STERILE. (Schering) Gentamicin sulfate equivalent to 3 mg, gentamicin, methylparaben and propylparaben as preservatives/Gm in petrolatum base. Tube 3.5 Gm
Use: Anti-infective, ophthalmic.
GARAMYCIN OPHTHALMIC SOLUTION, STERILE. (Schering) Gentamicin sulfate equivalent to 3 mg gentamicin, disodium phosphate, monosodium phosphate, sodium Cl, benzalkonium Cl/ml. Plastic dropper bot. 5 ml.
Use: Anti-infective, ophthalmic.
GARAMYCIN PEDIATRIC INJECTION. (Schering) Gentamicin sulfate equivalent to 10 mg per ml as sulfate. Vials 2 ml.
Use: Aminoglycoside.
GARDAN. (Sanofi Winthrop) Dipyrone.
Use: Analgesic, antipyretic, anti-inflammatory.

GARDENAL.
See: Phenobarbital. (Various Mfr.).
GARDINOL TYPE DETERGENTS. Aurinol, Cyclopon, Dreft, Drene, Duponol, Lissapol, Maprofix, Modinal, Orvus, Sandopan, Sadipan.
Use: Detergents.
GARDOL. Sodium Lauryl Sarcosinate.
GARFIELD. (Menley & James) Vitamin A 2500 IU, Vitamin D 400 IU, Vitamin E 15 IU, Vitamin C 60 mg, folic acid 0.3 mg, Vitamin B_1 1.05 mg, Vitamin B_2 1.2 mg, Vitamin B_3 13.5 mg, Vitamin B_6 1.05 mg, Vitamin B_{12} 4.5 mcg, sucrose, lactose. Chew. Tab. Bot. 60s.
Use: Vitamin supplement.
GARFIELD COMPLETE W/ MINERALS. (Menley & James) Vitamin A 5000 IU, Vitamin D 400 IU, Vitamin E 30 IU, Vitamin C 60 mg, folic acid 0.4 mg, Vitamin B_1 1.5 mg, Vitamin B_2 1.7 mg, Vitamin B_3 20 mg, Vitamin B_6 2 mg, Vitamin B_{12} 6 mcg, biotin 40 mcg, Vitamin B_5 10 mg, iron 18 mg, calcium 100 mg, Cu 2 mg, P 100 mg, I 150 mcg, Mg 20 mg, zinc 15 mg, aspartame, phenylalanine, sorbital. Chew. Tab. Bot. 60s
Use: Vitamin-mineral supplement.
GARFIELD PLUS EXTRA C. (Menley & James) Vitamin A 2500 IU, Vitamin D 400 IU, Vitamin E 15 IU, Vitamin C 250 mg, folic acid 0.3 mg, Vitamin B_1 1.05 mg, Vitamin B_2 1.2 mg, Vitamin B_3 13.5 mg, Vitamin B_6 1.05 mg, Vitamin B_{12} 4.5 mcg, sucrose, lactose. Chew. Tab. Bot. 60s.
Use: Vitamin supplement.
GARFIELD PLUS IRON. (Menley & James) Vitamin A 2500 IU, Vitamin D 400 IU, Vitamin E 15 IU, Vitamin C 60 mg, folic acid 0.3 mg, Vitamin B_1 1.05 mg, Vitamin B_2 1.2 mg, Vitamin B_3 13.5 mg, Vitamin B_6 1.05 mg, Vitamin B_{12} 4.5 mcg, iron 15 mcg, sucrose, lactose. Chew. Tab. Bot. 60s.
Use: Vitamins with iron.
GARFIELDS TEA. (Last) Senna leaf powder 68.3%. Bot. 2 oz.
Use: Laxative.
GARITABS. (Blue Cross) Iron 50 mg, vitamins B_1 5 mg, B_2 5 mg, C 75 mg, niacinamide 30 mg, B_5 2 mg, B_6 0.5 mg, B_{12} 3 mcg Bot. 1000s.
Use: Vitamin/mineral supplement.
GARITONE. (Halsey) Bot. 16 oz.
Use: Dietary supplement.
GARI-TONIC HEMATINIC. (Blue Cross) Vitamins B_1 5 mg, niacinamide 100 mg, B_2 5 mg, pantothenic acid 4 mg, B_6 1 mg, B_{12} 6 mcg, choline bitartrate 100

mg, iron 100 mg/30 ml Bot. 16 oz.
Use: Vitamin/mineral supplement.
GARLIC. Allium.
Use: Intestinal antispasmodic.
See: Allimin, Tab. (Mosso).
GARLIC CAPSULES. (Miller) Garlic 166
mg/Cap. Bot. 100s.
Use: Intestinal antispasmodic.
GARLIC CONCENTRATE.
W/Parsley Concentrate.
See: Allimin, Tab. (Mosso).
GARLIC OIL.
See: Natural Garlic Oil, Cap. (Spirt).
GARLIC OIL CAPSULES. (Kirkman) Bot.
100s.
GAS-EZE. (E.J. Moore) Aluminum hy-
droxide, magnesium hydroxide, calcium
carbonate, glycine, mannitol, oil pepper-
mint/Tab. Bot. 50s, Pak 36s.
Use: Antacid.
GAS PERMEABLE DAILY CLEANER.
(Pilkington Barnes-Hind) Nonionic aque-
ous solution cleaning agents in alkaline
buffered medium w/edetate disodium
2%, thimerosal 0.004%. Bot. 30 ml.
Use: Gas permeable contact lens care.
**GAS PERMEABLE LENS STARTER
SYSTEM.** (Barnes-Hind) Daily cleanser,
Bot. 3 ml, Wetting and soaking soln.,
Bot. 60 ml, Hydra-Mat II spin cleansing
unit. Kit.
Use: Gas permeable contact lens care.
**GAS PERMEABLE WETTING & SOAK-
ING SOLUTION.** (Barnes-Hind) Sterile
aqueous, isotonic soln. of low viscosity,
buffered to physiological pH. Bot. 60 ml,
120 ml.
Use: Gas permeable contact lens care.
GASTRIC ACIDIFIERS.
See: Acidulin, Pulv. (Lilly)
Glutamic Acid HCl (Various Mfr.).
GASTRIC MUCIN.
(Wilson) Granules 8 oz., 1 lb.
Use: Anti-ulcer.
W/Magnesium glycinate, aluminum hy-
droxide gel.
See: Mucogel, Tab. (Inwood).
GASTROCCULT. (SmithKline Diagnos-
tics) Occult blood screening test. In 40s.
Use: Diagnostic aid.
GASTROCROM. (Fisons) Cromolyn sodi-
um 100 mg/Cap. Bot. 100s.
Use: Respiratory inhalant.
See: Cromolyn Sodium.
GASTROGRAFIN. (Squibb) Diatrizoate
methyl-glucamine 66%, sodium diatri-
zoate 10%. Soln. Bot. 120 ml.
Use: Radiopaque agent.
GASTROINTESTINAL TESTS.
See: Entero-test, Cap. (HDC)

Entero-Test, Ped. Cap. (HDC).
Gastro-Test (HDC).
GASTRON. (Sanofi Winthrop) Pancre-
atin.
Use: Digestive enzyme.
GASTROSED. (Hauck) Hyoscyamine
sulfate. **Soln.:** 0.125 mg/ml. Dropper
Bot. 5 ml. Alcohol free. **Tab.:** 0.125 mg
Bot. 100s.
Use: Anticholinergic/antispasmodic.
GASTRO-TEST. (HDC Corp.) To deter-
mine stomach pH and to diagnose and
locate gastric bleeding. Test 25s.
Use: Diagnostic aid.
GAS-X. (Sandoz Consumer) Simethicone
80 mg/Chew. Tab. Pkg. 12s, 30s.
Use: Antiflatulent.
GAS-X, EXTRA STRENGTH. (Sandoz
Consumer) Simethicone 125 mg/Chew.
Tab. Box 18s.
Use: Antiflatulent.
•**GAUZE, ABSORBENT,** U.S.P. XXIII.
Use: Surgical aid.
•**GAUZE, PETROLATUM,** U.S.P. XXIII.
Use: Surgical aid.
GAVISCON. (SK-Beecham) Aluminum
hydroxide 80 mg, magnesium trisilicate
20 mg, alginic acid, sodium bicarbonate,
sucrose, calcium stearate. Chew. Tab.
Bot. 30s, 100s.
Use: Antacid.
**GAVISCON-2 DOUBLE STRENGTH
TABLETS.** (SK-Beecham) Aluminum
hydroxide 160 mg, magnesium trisilicate
40 mg, alginic acid, sodium bicarbonate,
sucrose, Chew. Tab. Bot. 48s.
Use: Antacid.
**GAVISCON EXTRA STRENGTH RELIEF
FORMULA LIQUID.** (SK-Beecham) Aluminum hydroxide 254 mg, magnesium
carbonate 237.5 mg, parabens, EDTA,
saccharin, sorbitol, simethicone, sodium
alginate/5 ml. Bot. 355 ml.
Use: Antacid.
**GAVISCON EXTRA STRENGTH RELIEF
FORMULA TABLETS.** (SK-Beecham)
Aluminum hydroxide 160 mg, magnesium carbonate 105 mg, alginic acid,
sodium bicarbonate, sucrose, calcium
stearate. Chew. Tab. Bot. 30s, 100s.
Use: Antacid.
GAVISCON LIQUID. (SK-Beecham) Alu-
minum hydroxide 31.7 mg, magnesium
carbonate 119.3 mg/5 ml Bot. 177 ml,
355 ml.
Use: Antacid.
GBA.
See: Gamma hydroxybutyrate.
G.B.H. LOTION. (Century) Gamma ben-
zene hexachloride 1%. Bot. 2 oz, pt, gal.

Use: Scabicide/pediculicide.
G.B.S. (Forest) Dehydrocholic acid 125 mg, phenobarbital 8 mg, homatropine methylbromide 2.5 mg/Tab. 100s, 1000s.
Use: Hydrocholeretic.
G-CSF.
See: Neupogen (Amgen).
GEBAUER'S 114. (Gebauer) Dichlorotetrafluoroethane 100%. Can 8 oz.
Use: Local anesthetic.
GEBAUER ETHYL CHLORIDE. (Gebauer) Ethyl Cl. Bot. 4 oz, metal tube 100 Gm.
Use: Local anesthetic.
GEE-GEE. (Bowman) Guaifenesin 200 mg/Tab. Bot. 1000s.
Use: Expectorant.
GEFARNATE. B.A.N. A mixture of steroisomers of 3,7-dimethylocta-2,6-dienyl 5,9,13-trimethyl-tet-radeca-4,8,12-trienoate. Geranyl farnesylacetate. Gefarnil.
Use: Treatment of peptic ulcer.
GEL II. (Oral-B) Fluoride 0.5% (from sodium flouride 1.1%). Tube 60 Gm.
Use: Dental caries preventative.
GEL II TOPICAL GEL. (Oral-B) Fluoride ion 1.23% from sodium fluoride and hydrofluoric acid (acidulated phosphate fluoride). Bot. 480 Gm.
Use: Dental caries preventative.
GEL-A-CAP. (Kenyon) Gelatin 10 gr/Cap. Bot. 100s, 1000s.
GELADINE. (Barth's) Gelatin, protein, vitamin D/Cap. Bot. 100s, 500s.
GELAMAL. (Halsey) Magnesium-aluminum hydroxide gel. Bot. 12 oz.
Use: Antacid.
• **GELATIN,** N.F. XVIII.
Use: Pharmaceutic aid.
• **GELATIN FILM, ABSORBABLE,** U.S.P. XXIII.
Use: Local hemostatic.
See: Gelfilm (Upjohn).
GELATIN FILM, STERILE.
See: Neupogen (Amgen).
GELATIN POWDER, STERILE.
See: Gelfoam Powder (Upjohn).
GELATIN SPONGE.
See: Gelfilm (Upjohn).
• **GELATIN SPONGE, ABSORBABLE,** U.S.P. XXIII.
Use: Local hemostatic.
See: Gelfoam, Paks (Upjohn).
GELATIN, ZINC.
See: Zinc gelatin. (Various Mfr.).
GEL-CLEAN. (Barnes-Hind) Gel formulated with nonionic surfactant. Tube 30 Gm.

Use: Hard contact lens care.
GEL-DI.
See: DI-GEL.
GELFILM. (Upjohn) Sterile, absorbable gelatin film. Envelope 1s. 100 mm × 125 mm. Also available as Ophth. Sterile 25 50 mm. Box 6s.
Use: Hemostatic.
GELFOAM. (Upjohn)
STERILE SPONGES:
Size 12-3mm 20 × 60 mm (12 sq. cm) 3 mm. Box 4 sponges in individual envelopes.
Size 12-7mm. 20 × 60 mm (12 sq. cm.) 7 mm. Box 12 sponges in individual envelopes, jar 4 sponges.
Size 50-10mm. 62.5 × 80 mm (50 sq. cm.) 10 mm. Box 4 sponges in individual envelopes.
Size 100-10mm. 80 × 125 mm (100 sq. cm.) 10 mm. Box 6 sponges in individual envelopes.
Size 200-10mm. 80 × 250 mm (200 sq. cm.) 10 mm. Box 6 sponges in individual envelopes.
Compressed size 100 (intended primarily for application in the dry state). 80 × 125 mm. Boxoo of 6 sponges in individual envelopes.
PACKS:
Packs size 2 cm. (Designed particularly for nasal packing). 2 × 40 cm. Single jar. (Packing cavities).
Size 6 cm. 6 × 40 cm. Box 6 sponges in individual envelopes.
Use: Hemostatic, topical.
GELFOAM COMPRESSED. (Upjohn) Size 100 (80 × 125 mm.) Box 6s.
Use: Hemostatic, topical.
GELFOAM DENTAL PACK. (Upjohn) Size 4, 20 mm × 20 mm 7 mm. Jar 15 sponges. Size 2, 10 mm 20 mm (2 sq. cm.) 7 mm. Jar 15 sponges.
Use: Hemostatic, topical.
GELFOAM POWDER. (Upjohn) Sterile Jar 1 Gm.
Use: Hemostatic.
GELFOAM PROSTATECTOMY CONES. (Upjohn) Prostatectomy cones (for use with Foley catheter). 13 cm, 18 cm in diameter. Box 6s.
Use: Hemostatic.
GEL JET GELATIN CAPSULES. (Kirkman) Bot. 100s, 250s.
GEL-KAM. (Scherer) Fluoride 0.1% (stannous fluoride 0.4%). Cinnamon fla-

vor. Gel. Bot. w/applicator tip 69 Gm, 105 Gm, 129 Gm.
Use: Dental caries preventative.

GELOCAST. (Beiersdorf) Unna's Boot medicated bandage: Semi-rigid cast impregnated with zinc oxide mixtures. Box 4 inches × 10 yd, 3 inches 10 yd.
Use: Unna's cast dressing

GELPIRIN. Acetaminophen 125 mg, aspirin 240 mg, caffeine 32 mg. Tab. Bot. 100s, 1000s.
Use: Analgesic.

GELPIRIN CCF. (Atra) Acetaminophen 325 mg, guaifenesin 25 mg, phenylpropanolamine maleate 12.5 mg/Tab. Bot. 50s, 200s, 500s.
Use: Analgesic, expectorant, decongestant.

GELSAF SUPER. (Robinson) Safflower oil 750 mg/Cap. Bot. 100s, 1000s, Pkg. 30s, Bulk pkg. 5000s.
Use: Enteral nutritional supplement.

GELSAF SUPER W/B₆. (Robinson) Safflower oil 912 mg, vitamin B_6 0.5 mg/Cap. or Safflower oil 1150 mg, B_6 3 mg/Cap. Bot. 100s, 250s, 1000s.
Use: Enteral nutritional supplement.

GELSEMIUM. (Various Mfr.) Pkg. oz.
Use: For neuralgia.
W/APC.
See: APC Combinations.

GELSEMIUM W/COMBINATIONS.
See: Briacel, Tab. (Briar).
   Bricor, Tab. (Briar).
   Cystitol, Tab. (Briar).
   Lanased, Tab. (Lannett).
   Ricor, Tab. (Vortech).
   Sodadide, Tab. (Scrip).
   UB, Tab. (Scrip).
   Urisan-P, Tab. (Sandia).
   Uriseptic w/Gelsemium, Tab. (Spencer-Mead).
   Uritol, Tab. (Kenyon).
   Urothyn Improved, Tab. (Solvay).
   Urseptic, Tab. (Century).
   U-Tract, Tab. (Bowman).

GELSOLIN, RECOMBINANT HUMAN. (Biogen)
Use: Treatment of cystic fibrosis. [Orphan drug]

GEL-TIN. (Young Dental) Fluoride 0.1% (from stannous flouride 0.4%) Gel Bot. 57 Gm, 623 Gm.
Use: Dental caries preventative.

GELUSIL. (Parke-Davis) Magnesium hydroxide 200 mg, aluminum hydroxide 200 mg, simethicone 25 mg/5 ml **Liq.:** Bot. 355 ml. **Susp.:** Bot. 180 ml, 360 ml. **Chew. Tab.:** Bot. 100s.
Use: Antacid.

•**GEMCADIOL.** USAN.
Use: Antihyperlipoproteinemic.
•**GEMCITABINE.** USAN.
Use: Antineoplastic.
•**GEMCITABINE HYDROCHLORIDE.** USAN.
Use: Antineoplastic.
•**GEMEPROST.** USAN.
Use: Prostaglandin.
•**GEMFIBROZIL,** U.S.P. XXIII. Cap. U.S.P. XXIII. 2,2-Dimethyl-5-(2,5-xyly-loxy) valeric acid.
Use: Treatment of hypercholesterolemia.
See: Lopid, Cap. (Parke-Davis).

GENABID. (Goldline) Papaverine HCl 150 mg/TR Cap. Bot. 100s, 1000s.
Use: Peripheral vasodilator.

GENAC TABLETS. (Goldline) Triprolidine HCl 2.5 mg, pseudoephedrine HCl 60 mg/Tab. Bot. 24s, 100s.
Use: Antihistamine, decongestant.

GENAGESIC TABS. (Goldline) Propoxyphene HCl 165 mg, acetaminophen 650 mg/Tab. Bot. 100s, 500s.
Use: Narcotic analgesic combination.

GENAHIST. (Goldline) Diphenhydramine HCl 25 mg/Cap or Tab. Bot. 24s.
Use: Antihistamine.

GENAHIST LIQUID. (Goldline) Diphenhydramine 12.5 mg/5 ml. Elix. 120 ml.
Use: Antihistamine.

GENALLERATE TABLETS. (Goldline) Chlorpheniramine maleate 4 mg/Tab. Bot. 24s.
Use: Antihistamine.

GENAMIN COLD SYRUP. (Goldline) Phenylpropanolamine HCl 12.5 mg, chlorpheniramine maleate 2 mg. Alcohol free. In 120 ml.
Use: Decongestant, antihistamine.

GENAMIN EXPECTORANT. (Goldline) Phenylpropanolamine 12.5 mg, guaifenesin 100 mg, alcohol 5%. In 120 ml.
Use: Decongestant, expectorant.

GENAPAP CHILDREN'S CHEWABLE TABS. (Goldline) Acetaminophen 80 mg/Tab. Bot. 30s.
Use: Analgesic.

GENAPAP CHILDREN'S ELIXIR. (Goldline) Acetaminophen 160 mg/5 ml. Cherry flavor. Bot. 120 ml.
Use: Analgesic.

GENAPAP EXTRA STRENGTH CAPLETS. (Goldline) Acetaminophen 500 mg/Cap. Bot. 50s, 100s.
Use: Analgesic.

GENAPAP INFANTS' DROPS. (Goldline) Acetaminophen 100 mg/ml, alcohol 7%.

Soln. Dropper bot. 15 ml.
Use: Analgesic.
GENAPAP TABLETS. (Goldline) Aceta-
minophen 325 mg/Tab. Bot. 100s.
Use: Analgesic.
GENAPAX. (Key) Gentian violet 5
mg/tampon. Box 12s.
Use: Antifungal, vaginal.
GENAPHED TABLETS. (Goldline) Pseu-
doephedrine HCl 30 mg/Tab. Bot. 24s,
100s.
Use: Decongestant.
GENASAL. (Goldline) Oxymetazoline
0.05%. Soln. 15 ml, 30 ml.
Use: Decongestant.
GENASOFT CAPSULES. (Goldline) Do-
cusate sodium 100 mg/Cap. Bot. 60s.
Use: Laxative.
GENASOFT PLUS CAPSULES. (Gold-
line) Docusate sodium 100 mg, casan-
thranol 30 mg/Cap. Bot. 60s.
Use: Laxative.
GENASPOR ANTIFUNGAL CREAM.
(Goldline) Tolnaftate 1%. Bot. 15 Gm.
Use: Antifungal, external.
GENASYME TABLETS. (Goldline) Sime-
thicone 80 mg/Tab. Bot. 100s.
Use: Antiflatulent.
GENATAP ELIXIR. (Goldline) Brompheni-
ramine maleate 2 mg, phenyl-
propanolamine HCl 12.5 mg, alcohol
2.3%/5 ml. Bot. 120 ml.
Use: Antihistamine, decongestant.
GENATON. (Goldline) Aluminum hydroxide 80 mg, magnesium trisilicate 20 mg,
alginic acid, sodium bicarbonate, sodi-
um 18.4 mg, sucrose, sugar. Chew. Tab.
Bot. 100s.
Use: Antacid.
**GENATON EXTRA STRENGTH
TABLETS.** (Goldline) Aluminum hydrox-
ide 160 mg, magnesium carbonate 105
mg, alginic acid, sodium bicarbonate,
sodium 29.9 mg, sucrose, calcium
stearate. Chew. Tab. Bot. 100s.
Use: Antacid.
GENATON LIQUID. (Goldline) Aluminum
hydroxide 31.7 mg, magnesium carbon-
ate 137.3 mg, sodium alginate, sodium
13 mg, EDTA, saccharin, sorbitol/5 ml.
Bot. 355 ml.
Use: Antacid.
GENATROPINE HCl. Atropine-N-oxide
HCl. Aminoxytropine Tropate HCl.
See: X-tro, Cap. (Xttrium).
GENATUSS DM SYRUP. (Goldline) Dex-
tromethorphan HBr 10 mg, guaifenesin
100 mg. Bot. 120 ml.
Use: Antitussive, expectorant.
GENATUSS SYRUP. (Goldline) Guaifen-

esin 100 mg/5 ml, alcohol 3.5%. Bot.
120 ml.
Use: Expectorant.
GEN-BEE WITH C. (Goldline) Vitamins
B$_1$ 15 mg, B$_2$ 10.2 mg, B$_3$ 50 mg, B$_5$ 10
mg, B$_6$ 5 mg, C 300 mg, tartrazine. Cap.
Bot. 130s, 1000s.
Use: Vitamin supplement.
GENCALC 600 TABLETS. (Goldline)
Calcium 600 mg (from calcium carbon-
ate 1.5 Gm)/Tab. Bot. 60s.
Use: Calcium supplement.
GENCEPT. (Gencon) **0.5/35:** Norethin-
drone 0.5 mg, ethinyl estradiol, 35
mcg/Tab (with 7 inert tabs) Pkgs 21s and
28s; **1/35:** norethindrone 1 mg, ethinyl
estradiol 35 mcg/Tab (with 7 inert tabs)
Pkgs 21s and 28s; **10/11:** norethindrone
0.5 mg and 1 mg, ethinyl estradiol 35
mcg/Tab (with 7 inert tabs). Pkg 21s and
28s.
Use: Oral contraceptives.
GENCOLD CAPSULES. (Goldline)
Phenylpropanolamine HCl 75 mg, chlor-
pheniramine maleate 8 mg/SR Tab. Bot.
10s.
Use: Decongestant, antihistamine.
GENEBS EXTRA STRENGTH CAPLETS.
(Goldline) Acetaminophen 500 mg/Cap.
Bot. 100s, 1000s.
Use: Analgesic.
GENEBS EXTRA STRENGTH TABLETS.
(Goldline) Acetaminophen 500 mg/Tab.
Bot. 100s, 1000s.
Use: Analgesic.
GENEBS TABLETS. (Goldline) Aceta-
minophen 325 mg/Tab. Bot. 100s,
1000s.
Use: Analgesic.
GENERET-500. (Goldline) Iron 105 mg,
Vitamins B$_1$ 6mg, B$_2$ 6 mg, B$_3$ 30 mg, B$_5$
10 mg, B$_6$ 5 mg, B$_{12}$ 25 mcg, C (as sodi-
um ascorbate) 500 mg. TR Tab. Bot.
60s.
Use: Vitamin/mineral supplement.
GENERIX-T. (Goldline) Elemental iron 15
mg, vitamins A 10,000 IU, D 400 IU, E
5.5 mg, D$_1$ 15 mg, B$_2$ 10 mg, B$_3$ 100 mg,
B$_5$ 10 mg, B$_6$ 2 mg, B$_{12}$ 7.5 mcg, C 150
mg, Cu, I, Mg, Mn, zinc 1.5 mg. Tab. Bot.
100s, 1000s.
Use: Vitamin/mineral supplement.
GENEX CAPS. (Goldline) Phenylpropanolamine HCl 18 mg, acetaminophen 325 mg/Cap. Bot. 100s,
1000s.
Use: Decongestant, analgesic.
GENITAL HERPES TREATMENT.
See: Acyclovir.
Zovirax Cap., Oint. (Burroughs Well-

come).

GENITE. (Goldline) Pseudoephedrine HCl 10 mg, doxylamine succinate 1.25 mg, dextromethorphan HBr 5 mg, acetaminophen 167 mg, alcohol 25%/5 ml. Bot. 177 ml.
Use: Decongestant, antihistamine, antitussive, analgesic.

GENITOURINARY IRRIGANTS.
See: Acetic acid for Irrigation (Various Mfr.).
Glycine (Aminoacetic Acid) For Irrigation (Various Mfr.).
Neosporin G.U. Irrigant, Soln. (Burroughs-Wellcome).
Renacidin, Pow., Soln. (Guardian).
Resectisol, Soln. (Kendall McGaw).
Sorbitol (Various Mfr.)
Sorbitol-Mannitol (Abbott)
Sodium Chloride for Irrigation (Various Mfr.)
Sterile Water for Irrigation (Various Mfr.)
Suby's Solution G (Various Mfr.)

GEN-K POWDER. (Goldline) Potassium Cl. Pow. 20 mEq/packet. Box 30s.
Use: Potassium supplement.

GEN-K TABS. (Goldline) Effervescent potassium. Bot. 30s.
Use: Potassium supplement.

GENNA TABLETS. (Goldline) Senna concentrate 217 mg/Tab. Bot. 100s, 1000s.
Use: Laxative.

GENNIN TABLETS. (Goldline) Buffered aspirin 5 gr. Bot. 100s.
Use: Salicylate analgesic.

GENOPHYLLIN.
See: Aminophylline (Various Mfr.).

GENOPTIC LIQUIFILM STERILE OPHTHALMIC SOLUTION. (Allergan) Gentamicin sulfate equivalent to 3 mg gentamicin/ml w/polyvinyl alcohol 1.4%, edetate disodium, HCl, benzalkonium Cl. Bot. 1 ml, 5 ml.
Use: Anti-infective, ophthalmic.

GENOPTIC S.O.P. STERILE OPHTHALMIC OINTMENT. (Allergan) Gentamicin sulfate equivalent to 3 mg gentamicin/Gm w/white petrolatum, methylparaben, propylparaben. Oint. Tube 3.5 Gm.
Use: Anti-infective, ophthalmic.

GENORA 0.5/35 TABLETS. (Rugby) Norethindrone 0.5 mg, ethinyl estradiol 0.035 mg/Tab. Pkg. 21s; 28s (7 inert tab.)
Use: Oral contraceptive.

GENORA 1/35-21 TABLETS. (Rugby) Norethindrone 1 mg, ethinylestradiol 0.035 mg/Tab. Pkg. 126s (6-pak).
Use: Oral contraceptive.

GENORA 1/35-28 TABLETS. (Rugby) Norethindrone 1 mg, ethinylestradiol 0.035 mg/Tab., 7 inert tab. Pkg. 168s (6-pak).
Use: Oral contraceptive.

GENORA 1/50-21 TABLETS. (Rugby) Norethindrone 1 mg, mestranol 0.05 mg/Tab. Pkg. 126s (6-pak).
Use: Oral contraceptive.

GENORA 1/50-28 TABLETS. (Rugby) Norethindrone 1 mg, mestranol 0.05 mg/Tab., 7 inert tab. Pkg. 168s (6-pak).
Use: Oral contraceptive.

GENPREP OINTMENT. (Goldline) Live yeast cell derivative supplying 2000 units skin respiratory factor/oz of ointment w/shark liver oil 3%, phenylmercuric nitrate 1:10,000. Tube 2 oz.
Use: Anorectal preparation.

GENPRIL. (Goldline) Ibuprofen 200 mg. Tab. 50s, 100s.
Use: Nonsteroidal anti-inflammatory agent.

GENPRIN. (Goldline) Aspirin 325 mg. Tab. 100s.
Use: Salicylate analgesic.

GENSALATE SODIUM. Sodium gentisate. (Sodium salt of 2,5-dihydroxybenzoic acid).
Use: Analgesic.

GENSAN TABLETS. (Goldline) Aspirin 400 mg, caffeine 32 mg/Tab. Bot. 100s.
Use: Analgesic combination.

GEN/T SUPPOSITORIES.
See: T/GEN SUPPOSITORIES.

GENTAB-LA CAPLETS. (Genetco) Guaifenesin 400 mg, phenylpropanolamine HCl 75 mg/Capl. 100s, 500s.
Use: Expectorant, decongestant.

GENTACIDIN OPHTHALMIC OINTMENT. (Iolab) Gentamicin 3 mg/Gm. Oint. Tube 3.5 Gm.
Use: Anti-infective, ophthalmic.

GENTACIDIN OPHTHALMIC SOLUTION. (Iolab) Gentamicin sulfate 3 mg/ml. Soln. Bot. 5 ml.
Use: Anti-infective, ophthalmic.

GENTAFAIR. (Pharmafair) **Oint.:** Gentamicin 3 mg/Gm with liquid lanolin, white petrolatum, mineral oil, parabens. Tube 3.75 Gm, 15 Gm. **Soln.:** Gentamicin 3 mg/ml, polyoxyl 40 stearate, polyethylene glycol. Dropper bot. 5 ml, 15 ml.
Use: Anti-infective, ophthalmic.

GENT-AK. (Akorn) **Oint.:** Gentamicin 3 mg/Gm with liquid lanolin, white petrola-

tum, mineral oil, parabens. Tube 3.5 Gm, 5 Gm, 15 Gm. **Soln.:** Gentamicin 3 mg/ml with polyoxyl 40 stearate, polyethylene glycol. Bot. 5 ml, 15 ml.
Use: Anti-infective, ophthalmic.
GENTAMICIN IMPREGNATED PMMA BEADS ON SURGICAL WIRE.
Use: Chronic osteomyelitis. [Orphan drug]
GENTAMICIN LIPOSOME INJECTION.
Use: **Mycobacterium avium** -intracellulare infection. [Orphan drug]
• **GENTAMICIN SULFATE,** U.S.P. XXIII. Cream, Oint., Inj., Ophth. Oint., Ophth. Soln., Sterile, U.S.P. XXIII. (Schering) Produced by *Micromonospora purpurea.* (Various Mfr.) **Ophthalmic Oint.:** 3 mg/g Tube 3.5 g; **Ophthalmic Soln.:** 3 mg/ml Bot. 5 ml, 15 ml.
Use: Antibacterial.
See: Apogen, Inj. (Beecham Labs).
Garamycin, Preps. (Schering).
Genoptic, Preps. (Allergan).
Gentaciden, Preps. (Iolab).
Gentak, Preps. (Akorn).
• **GENTAMICIN AND PREDNISOLONE ACETATE OPHTHALMIC SUSPENSION,** U.S.P. XXIII.
Use: Antibiotic, anti-inflammatory.
• **GENTIAN VIOLET,** U.S.P. XXIII. Topical Soln., Cream, U.S.P. XXIII. Methylrosaniline Cl. Bismuth Violet.
Use: Topical anti-infective.
See: Genapax, tampon. (Key).
GVS, Vaginal cream and inserts. (Savage).
W\Surfactants.
See: Hyva, Vaginal Tab. (Holland-Rantos).
GENTISATE SODIUM. 5-Hydroxysalicylate sodium, 2,5-Dihydroxy benzoate sodium.
• **GENTISIC ACID ETHANOLAMIDE,** N.F. XVIII.
Use: Pharmaceutic aid.
GENTLAX. (Blair) Standardized senna concentrate 326 mg, malt extract, sucrose/Gran. 180 Gm.
Use: Laxative.
GENTLAX S TABLETS. (Blair) Standardized senna concentrate 187 mg, docusate sodium 50 mg. Tab. Bot. 30s, 60s.
Use: Laxative.
GENTLE NATURE NATURAL VEGETABLE LAXATIVE.(Sandoz Consumer) Sennosides A and B as calcium salts. 20 mg/Tab. Box 16s, 32s.
Use: Laxative.

GENTLE SHAMPOO. (Ulmer) Bot. 4 oz, gal.
Use: Mild, neutral shampoo.
GENTRAN 40. (Baxter) Dextran 40 10% w/sodium Cl 0.9% or Dextran 40 10% w/dextrose 5%. Inj. Plastic Bot. 500 ml.
Use: Plasma expander.
GENTRAN 70. (Baxter) Dextran 70 6% w/sodium Cl 0.9%. Inj. Plastic Bot. 500 ml.
Use: Plasma expander.
GENTRAN 75. (Baxter) Dextran 75 6% in sodium Cl 0.9%. Inj. Bot. 500 ml.
Use: Plasma expander.
GENTRASUL. (Bausch & Lomb) Gentamicin 3 mg. **Oint.:** 3.5 Gm. **Soln.:** Dropper bot. 5 ml.
Use: Anti-infective, ophthalmic.
GENTZ RECTAL WIPES. (Roxane) Pramoxine HCl 1%, alcloxa 0.2%, witch hazel 50%, propylene glycol 10%. Box 100s, 120s (individually wrapped disposable wipes).
Use: Anorectal preparation.
GENUINE BAYER ASPIRIN. (Glenbrook) Aspirin 325 mg/FC Tab. Bot. 12s, 24s, 50s, 200s, 300s.
Use: Salicylate analgesic.
GEN-XENE. (Alra) Clorazepate dipotassium 3.75 mg, 7.5 mg or 15 mg/Tab. Bot. 30s, 100s, 500s, UD 100s.
Use: Antianxiety agent, anticonvulsant.
GEOCILLIN. (Roerig) Carbenicillin indanyl sodium 382 mg/Tab. Bot. 100s, UD 100s.
Use: Antibacterial, penicillin.
GEOPEN. (Roerig) Carbenicillin Disodium. Inj. **Vial:** 1 Gm, 2 Gm, 5 Gm. Pkg. 10s. **Piggyback Vial:** 2 Gm, 5 Gm, 10 Gm. **Bulk Pharmacy Pack:** 30 Gm.
Use: Antibacterial, penicillin.
• **GEPIRONE HYDROCHLORIDE.** USAN. Marketed by Mead Johnson.
Use: Antianxiety, antidepressant.
GERA PLUS. (Towne) Iron 50 mg, vitamine B_1 5 mg, B_2 5 mg, C 75 mg, niacinamide 30 mg, calcium pantothenate 2 mg, B_6 0.5 mg, B_{12} 3 mcg/Tab. Bot. 100s.
Use: Vitamin/mineral supplement.
GERAVITE ELIXIR. (Hauck) Lysine monohydrochloride 150 mg, vitamins B_1 1 mg, B_2 1.2 mg, niacinamide 100 mg, B_{12} 10 mcg/15 ml w/alcohol 15%. Bot. 16 oz, gal.
Use: Vitamin/mineral supplement.
GERBER BABY FORMULA LOW IRON. (Mead Johnson) Protein (from non-fat

milk) 14.7 Gm, carbohydrate (from lactose) 71.3 Gm, fat (from palm olein, soy, coconut and high oleic sunflower oils) 36 Gm, linoleic acid 5.9 Gm, vitamins A, D, E, K, C, B_1, B_2, B_3, B_5, B_6, B_{12}, folic acid, biotin, choline, inositol, Ca, P, Mg, Fe 3.4 mg, Zn, Mn, Cu, I, Na 220 mg, K 720 mg, Cl, taurine, calories per L 666.7 **Ready to use liq.**: Bot. 943 ml. **Concentrated liq.**: Bot. 433 ml. **Pow.**: Can 457 Gm and 914 Gm.
Use: Enteral nutritional therapy.
GERBER BABY FORMULA WITH IRON. (Mead Johnson) Protein (from non-fat milk) 14.7 Gm, carbohydrate (from lactose) 71.3 Gm, fat (from palm olein, soy, coconut and high oleic sunflower oils) 36 Gm, with linoleic acid 5.9 Gm, vitamins A, D, E, K, C, B_1, B_2, B_6, B_{12}, B_3, folic acid, B_5, biotin, choline, inositol, Ca, P, Mg, Fe 12 mg, Zn, Mn, Cu, I, Na 220 mg, K 720 mg, Cl, taurine, calories per L 666.7. **Ready to use liq.**: Bot. 943 ml. **Concentrated liq.**: Bot. 433 ml. **Pow.**: Can 457 Gm.
Use: Enteral nutritional therapy.
GERBER SOY BABY FORMULA. (Mead Johnson) Protein (from soy protein isolate) 20 Gm, carbohydrate (from corn syrup solids and sugar) 66.7 Gm, fat (from palm olein, soy, coconut and high oleic sunflower oils) 35.3 Gm, linoleic acid 5.7 Gm, vitamins A, D, E, K, C, B_1, B_2, B_3, B_5, B_6, B_{12}, folic acid, biotin, choline, inositol, Ca, P, Mg, Fe 12 mg, Zn, Mn, Cu, I, Na 313.3 mg, K 766.7 mg, Cl, L-methionine, L-carnitine, taurine, calories per L 666.7. **Pow.**: Can 400 Gm.
Use: Enteral nutritional therapy.
GEREF. (Serono) Sermorelin acetate 50 mcg (lyophilized). Pow. for Inj. Amp. 2 ml w/sodium Cl. 0.9%.
Use: Diagnostic aid.
GERI-ALL-D. (Barth's) Vitamins A 10,000 IU, D 400 IU, B_1 7 mg, B_2 14 mg, C 200 mg, niacin 4.17 mg, B_{12} 25 mcg, E 50 IU, B_6 0.35 mg, pantothenic acid 0.63 mg, trace minerals and other factors. 2 Cap. Bot. 1 mo., 3 mo. and 6 mo. supply of Geri-All regular and Geri-All-D.
Use: Vitamin/mineral supplement.
GERIATRAZOLE. (Kenyon) Vitamins B_{12} 50 mg, B_2 2 mg, liver-painless 2 mcg, dl-methionine 10 mg, inositol 20 mg, d-panthenol 20 mg, B_1 20 mg, B_6 5 mg, niacinamide 75 mg, pentylenetetrazole 10 mg/ml. Vial 30 ml.
Use: Vitamin/mineral supplement.

GERIATRIC SUPPLEMENTS W/MULTI-VITAMINS/MINERALS.
See: Geravite, Elix. (Hauck).
Gerimed, Tab. (Fielding).
Geriplex FS, Caps. (Parke-Davis).
Hep-Forte, Cap. (Marlyn).
Megadose, Tab. (Arco).
Mega VM-80, Tab. (Nature's Bounty)
Optivite P.M.T., Tab. (Optimox).
Strovite Plus, Tab. (Everett).
Ultra-Freeda, Tab. (Freeda)
Ultra-Freeda Iron Free, Tab. (Freeda).
Vigortol, Liq. (Rugby).
Viminate, Elix. (Various Mfr.).
Viopan-T, Tab. (Trimen).
Vita-Plus G Softgels (Scot-Tussin).
GERIATROPLEX. (Morton) Cyanocobalamin 30 mcg, liver inj. 0.1 ml vitamins B_{12} activity 2 mcg, ferrous gluconate 50 mg, B_2 1.5 mg, calcium pantothenate 2.5 mg, niacinamide 100 mg, citric acid 16.4 mg, sodium citrate 23.6 mg/2 ml. Vial 30 ml.
Use: Vitamin/mineral supplement.
GERIDEN. (Kenyon) Methyltestosterone 2 mg, ethinyl estradiol 0.01 mg, rutin 10 mg, vitamins C 30 mg, B_{12} 2 mcg, A 5000 IU, D 500 IU, E 2 IU, calcium pantothenate 3 mg, B_1 2.5 mg, B_6 0.5 mg, niacinamide 15 mg, iron 5 mg, copper 0.2 mg, manganese 1 mg, magnesium 5 mg, potassium 2 mg, choline bitartrate 40 mg, PABA 10 mg, inositol 20 mg/Cap. Bot. 100s, 1000s.
Use: Vitamin/mineral hormone supplement.
GERI-DERM. (Barth's) Vitamins A 400,000 IU, D 40,000 IU, E 200 IU, panthenol 800 mg/4 oz. Jar 4 oz.
Use: Skin supplement.
GERIDIUM TABLETS. (Goldline) Phenazopyridine HCl 100 mg or 200 mg/Tab. Bot. 100s, 1000s.
Use: Urinary analgesic, anti-infective.
GERIFORT PLUS. (A.P.C.) Vitamins A 10,000 IU, B_1 5 mg, B_2 6 mg, B_6 2 mg, C 75 mg, D-2 1000 IU, niacinamide 60 mg, iron 10 mg, calcium 115 mg, phosphorous 83 mg, iodine 0.1 mg, calcium pantothenate 10 mg, d-alpha tocopheryl acid succinate 3 IU, cobalamin concentrate 3 mcg, choline bitartrate 70 mg, inositol 35 mg, biotin 15 mcg, Zn 0.2 mg, magnesium 2 mg, manganese 0.5 mg, potassium 0.15 mg/Amcap. Bot. 100s.
Use: Vitamin/mineral supplement.
GERIJEN IMPROVED. (Jenkins) Testosterone 10 mg, estrone 1 mg, cyanocobalamin 50 mcg, niacinamide 50 mg, inositol 5 mg, methionine 5 mg,

choline Cl 5 mg/ml, pectin 0.25%. Vial 10 ml.

GERILETS. (Abbott) Vitamins A 5000 IU, D 400 IU, E 45 IU, C 90 mg (from sodium ascorbate), folic acid 0.4 mg, B_1 2.25 mg, B_2 2.6 mg, niacin 30 mg, B_6 3 mg, B_{12} 9 mcg, biotin 0.45 mg, pantothenic acid 15 mg, iron 27 mg (from ferrous sulfate)/Tab. Bot. 100s.
Use: Vitamin/mineral supplement.

GERIMAL. (Rugby) Ergoloid Mesylates 0.5 mg or 1 mg/**Sublingual Tab.**: Bot. 100s, 500s, 1000s; 1 mg/**Oral Tab.**: Bot. 100s, 500s, 1000s.
Use: Psychotherapeutic agent.

GERIMED. (Fielding) Vitamins A 5000 IU, D 400 IU, E 30 mg, B_1 3 mg, B_2 3 mg, B_3 25 mg, B_6 2 mg, B_{12} 6 mcg, C 120 mg, calcium 370 mg, zinc 15 mg, Mg, phosphorous 130 mg/Tab. Bot. 60s.
Use: Vitamin/mineral supplement.

GERINEED. (Hanlon) Vitamins A 5000 IU, B_1 20 mg, B_2 5 mg, niacinamide 20 mg, D_6 0.5 mg, calcium pantothenate 5 mg, B_{12} 5 mcg, rutin 25 mg, C 50 mg, E 10 IU, choline 50 mg, inositol 50 mg, calcium lactate 1.64 mg, iron sulfate 10 mg, copper 1 mg, iodine 0.5 mg, manganese 1 mg, magnesium sulfate 1 mg, potassium sulfate 5 mg, zinc sulfate 0.5 mg/Cap. Bot. 100s.
Use: Vitamin/mineral supplement.

GERIOT. (Goldline) Iron 50 mg (from ferrous sulfate), vitamins B_1 5 mg, B_2 5 mg, B_3 30 mg, B_5 2 mg, B_6 0.5 mg, B_{12} 3 mcg, C 75 mg Tab. Bot. 100s.
Use: Vitamin/mineral supplement.

GERIPLEX-FS. (Parke-Davis) Vitamins A 5000 IU, B_1 5 mg, B_2 5 mg, B_{12} 2 mcg, nicotinamide 15 mg, C 50 mg, choline dihydrogen citrate 20 mg, E 5 mg, iron 6 mg, copper sulfate 4 mg, manganese sulfate 4 mg, zinc sulfate 0.5 mg, calcium 59 mg, docusate sodium 100 mg, aspergillus oryzea enzymes 162.5 mg/Kapseal Bot. 100s.
Use: Vitamin/mineral supplement.

GERI-PLUS. (Approved) Vitamins A 12,500 IU, D 1200 IU, B_1 15 mg, B_2 10 mg, C 75 mg, niacinamide 30 mg, calcium pantothenate 2 mg, B_6 0.5 mg, E 5 IU, Brewer's yeast 10 mg, B_{12} 15 mcg, iron 11.58 mg, desiccated liver 15 mg, choline bitartrate 30 mg, inositol 30 mg, calcium 59 mg, phosphorous 45 mg, zinc 0.68 mg, francium dicalcium phosphate 200 mg, Mn, enzymatic factors, amino acids/Cap. Bot. 50s, 100s, 1000s.
Use: Vitamin/mineral supplement.

GERI-PLUS ELIXIR. (Approved) Vitamins

B_1 25 mg, B_2 10 mg, B_6 1 mg, niacinamide 100 mg, calcium pantothenate 5 mg, B_{12} 20 mcg, iron ammonium citrate 100 mg, choline 200 mg, inositol 100 mg, magnesium Cl 2 mg, manganese citrate 2 mg, zinc acetate 2 mg, amino acids/fl oz. Bot. pt.
Use: Vitamin/mineral supplement.

GERISPAN. (Robinson) Vitamins A 12,500 IU, D 1000 IU, B_1 5 mg, B_2 2.5 mg, niacinamide 40 mg, B_6 1 mg, calcium pantothenate 4 mg, B_{12} 2 mcg, C 75 mg, E 2 IU, choline bitartrate 31.4 mg, inositol 15 mg, calcium 75 mg, phosphorus 58 mg, iron 30 mg, magnesium 3 mg, manganese 0.5 mg, potassium 2 mg, zinc 0.5 mg/Cap. Bot. 100s, 1000s, Bulk Pack 5000s.
Use: Vitamin/mineral supplement.

GERITOL COMPLETE TABLETS. (Beecham Products) Vitamins A 5000 IU, E 30 IU, C 60 mg, folic acid 400 mcg, B_1 1.5 mg, B_2 1.7 mg, niacinamide 20 mg, D_6 2 mg, D_{12} 6 mcg, D 400 IU, K 50 mcg, biotin 300 mcg, pantothenic acid 10 mg, calcium 162 mg, phosphorous 125 mg, iodine 150 mcg, iron (as ferrous fumarate) 50 mg, magnesium 100 mg, copper 2 mg, manganese 7.5 mg, potassium 37.5 mg, chloride 34.1 mg, cromium 15 mcg, molybdenum 15 mcg, selenium 15 mcg, zinc 15 mg, nickel 5 mcg, silicon 80 mcg, Sn. V/Tab. Bot. 14s, 40s, 100s, 180s, 300s.
Use: Vitamin/mineral supplement.

GERITOL TONIC LIQUID. (Beecham Products) Iron 50 mg (from iron ammonium citrate), Vitamins B_1 2.5 mg, B_2 2.5 mg, niacinamide 50 mg, panthenol 2 mg, pyridoxine 0.5 mg, B_{12} 0.75 mcg, methionine 25 mg, choline bitartrate 50 mg/15 ml. Alcohol 12%. Bot. 120 ml, 360 ml, 720 ml.
Use: Vitamin/mineral supplement.

GERIVITES. (Various Mfr.) Iron (from ferrous sulfate) 50 mg, vitamins D_1 5 mg, B_2 5 mg, B_3 30 mg, B_5 2 mg, B_6 0.5 mg, B_{12} 3 mcg, C 75 mg/Tab. Bot. 40s, 100s, 1000s.
Use: Vitamin/mineral supplement.

GERIX ELIXIR. (Abbott) Vitamins B_1 6 mg, B_2 6 mg, niacin 100 mg, iron 15 mg, B_6 1.6 mg, cyanocobalamin 6 mcg, alcohol 20%/30 ml. Bot. 480 ml.
Use: Vitamin/mineral supplement.

GERLIPO. (Kenyon) Choline bitartrate 250 mg, methionine 150 mg, inositol 100 mg, desiccated whole liver 100 mg, B-cotrate 100 mg, vitamins B_1 1.5 mg, B_2 1 mg, B_6 0.1 mg, d-calcium pantothenate

2 mg, niacinamide 15 mg/3 Tab. Bot. 100s, 1000s.
Use: Vitamin/mineral supplement.
GERMANIN. (CDC)
Use: Anti-infective.
See: Suramin sodium (Naphuride sodium).
GERMICIN. (CMC) Benzlakonium Cl 50%. Bot. pt., gal.
Use: Antiseptic, germicide.
GER-O-FOAM. (Geriatric) Methylsalicylate 30%, benzocaine 3%, volatile oils. Aerosol can 4 oz.
Use: Analgesic, anesthetic.
GERTEROL DEPO. (Fellows) Medroxyprogesterone acetate 50 mg or 100 mg/ml. Vial 5 ml.
Use: Progestin.
GESIC. (Lexalabs) Aspirin 226.8 mg, caffeine 32.4 mg, codeine 32.4 mg/Tab. Bot. 100s.
Use: Narcotic analgesic combination.
•**GESTACLONE.** USAN. (1) 17β-Acetyl-6-chloro-1β, 1a,2β,8β,9α,10,11,12,13,14α-,15,16β,1 6a,17-tetradecahydro-10β,13β-dimethyl-3H-dicyclopropa[1,2:16,17]cyclopenta-[a]-phenanthren-3-one.
Use: Progestin.
GESTIN. (Dalin) Formerly G.I. 8. Bot. 4 oz, 8 oz.
•**GESTODENE.** USAN.
Use: Progestin.
GESTONEED. (Hanlon) Calcium lactate 1069 mg, vitamins C 100 mg, nicotinic acid 18 mg, B_2 2.4 mg, B_1 1.8 mg, B_6 9 mg, D 500 IU, A 6000 IU/Cap. Bot. 100s.
Use: Vitamin/mineral supplement.
•**GESTONORONE CAPROATE.** USAN. 17-Hydroxy-19-norpregn-4-ene-3,20-dione hexanoate.
Use: Progestin.
•**GESTRINONE.** USAN.
Use: Progestin.
GESTRONOL, B.A.N. 17-Hydroxy-19-norpregn-4-ene-3,20-dione.
Use: Progesterone steroid.
GETS-IT. (Oakhurst) Salicyclic acid, zinc Cl, collodion in ether ≃ 35%, alcohol ≃ 28%. Liq. Bot. 12 ml.
Use: Keratolytic.
•**GEVOTROLINE HYDROCHLORIDE.** USAN.
Use: Antipsychotic.
GEVRABON. (Lederle) Vitamins B_1 5 mg, B_2 2.5 mg, B_{12} 1 mcg, niacinamide 50 mg, B_6 1 mg, pantothenic acid 10 mg, choline 100 mg, zinc 2 mg, iodine 100 mg, magnesium 2 mg, manganese 2 mg, iron 15 mg/30 ml w/alcohol 18%.

Bot. 480 ml.
Use: Vitamin/mineral supplement.
GEVRAL. (Lederle) Vitamins A 5000 IU, B_1 1.5 mg, B_2 1.7 mg, B_6 2 mg, B_{12} 6 mcg, folic acid 0.4 mg, C 60 mg, E 30 mg, niacinamide 20 mg, calcium 162 mg, phosphorous 125 mg, elemental iron 18 mg, magnesium 100 mg, iodine 150 mcg/Tab. Bot. 100s.
Use: Vitamin/mineral supplement.
GEVRAL PROTEIN. (Lederle) Calcium caseinate, sucrose, protein 15.6 Gm, carbohydrate 7.05 Gm, fat 0.52 Gm, sodium 50 mg, potassium 13 mg, calories 95.3/26 Gm. Pow. Can. 8 oz, 5 lb.
Use: Enteral nutritional supplement.
GEVRAL T. (Lederle) Vitamins A 5000 IU, D 400 IU, B_1 2.25 mg, B_2 2.6 mg, B_6 3 mg, B_{12} 9 mcg, C 90 mg, E 45 IU, niacinamide 30 mg, calcium 162 mg, folic acid 0.4 mg, phosphorous 125 mg, elemental iron (from ferrous fumarate) 27 mg, magnesium 100 mg, iodine 225 mcg, copper 1.5 mg, zinc 22.5 mg/Tab. Bot. 100s.
Use: Vitamin/mineral supplement.
GG-CEN CAPSULES. (Central) Guaifenesin 200 mg/Cap. Bot. 24s, 100s.
Use: Expectorant.
GI STIMULANTS.
See: Clopra, Tab. (Quantum).
Maxolon, Tab. (Beecham).
Metoclopramide, Tab. (Various Mfr.).
Metoclopramide HCl, Inj. (Quad).
Octamide, Tab. (Adria).
Reclomide, Tab. (Major).
Reglan, Inj., Syr., Tab. (Robins).
GL-2 SKIN ADHERENT. (Gordon) Ready to use. Bot. pt, qt, gal.
G L-7 SKIN ADHERENT. (Gordon) Plastic material which may be used full strength or diluted with 3 to 10 parts 99% isopropyl alcohol, acetone or naphtha. Pkg. pt, qt, gal.
GLANDUBOLIN.
See: Estrone (Various Mfr.).
GLAUBER'S SALT.
See: Sodium Sulfate (Various Mfr.).
GLAUCON SOLUTION. (Alcon) Epinephrine HCl 1% or 2% w/benzalkonium Cl, sodium Cl 0.01%, sodium metabisulfite, EDTA. Dropper bot. 10 ml.
Use: Agent for glaucoma.
GLAUCTABS. (Akorn) Methazolamide 25 mg, 50 mg. Tab. Bot. 100s.
Use: Diuretics.
•**GLAZE, PHARMACEUTICAL,** N.F. XVIII.
Use: Pharmaceutic aid (tablet coating).
•**GLEMANSERIN.** USAN.
Use: Anti-anxiety agent.

- **GLEPTOFERRON.** USAN.
  Use: Hematinic.
- **GLIAMILIDE.** USAN.
  Use: Antidiabetic.
  GLIBENCLAMIDE. B.A.N. 1- 4-[2-(5-Chloro-2-methoxybenzamido)ethyl]benzenesulphonyl-3-cyclohexylurea glyburide.
  Use: Oral hypoglycemic agent.
- **GLIBORNURIDE.** USAN. endo-1-[(IR)-(2-Hydroxy-3-bornyl)]-3-(p-tolysulfonyl)urea. Glutril.
  Use: Oral hypoglycemic agent.
- **GLICETANILE SODIUM.** USAN.
  Use: Antidiabetic.
- **GLIFLUMIDE.** USAN.
  Use: Antidiabetic.
  GLIM.
  See: Gardinol Type Detergents (Various Mfr.).
- **GLIMEPIRIDE.** USAN.
  Use: Hypoglycemic.
- **GLIPIZIDE.** USAN.
  Use: Antidiabetic.
  See: Glucotrol, Tab. (Pfizer).
  GLIQUIDONE. B.A.N. 1-Cyclohexyl-3-p-[2-(3,4-dihydro-7-methoxy-4,4-dimethyl-1,3-dioxo-2(1H)-isoquinolyl)ethyl]phenylsulfonylurea.
  Use: Oral hypoglycemic agent.
  GLISOXEPIDE. B.A.N. 3-[4-(Perhydroazepin-1-ylureidosulfonyl)phenethylcarbamoyl]-5-methylis-oxazole.
  Use: Oral hypoglycemic agent.
  GLOBULIN, GAMMA.
  See: Gamma Globulin (Various Mfr.). Poliomyelitis Immune Globulin, Human, Vial. (Various Mfr.).
  GLOBULIN, HEPATITIS B IMMUNE.
  See: H-BIG, Vial (Abbott).
- **GLOBULIN, IMMUNE,** U.S.P. XXIII.
  Use: I.M., measles prophylactic and polio; passive immunizing agent.
  See: Gammagee, Vial (Merck, Sharp & Dohme).
- **GLOBULIN, Rho(D) IMMUNE,** U.S.P. XXIII.
  Use: Immunosuppressive.
  GLOBULIN, POLIOMYELITIS IMMUNE. Human.
  See: Poliomyelitis Immune Globulin (Various Mfr.).
- **GLOXIMONAM.** USAN.
  Use: Antibacterial.
  GLUBIONATE CALCIUM.
  See: Neo-Calglucon, Syrup (Dorsey).
- **GLUCAGON,** U.S.P. XXIII. Inj., U.S.P. XXIII. (Lilly) 1 unit/ml w/diluent. 10 units

w/10 ml diluent. Glucagon HCl 1 mg or 10 mg w/diluent; soln. contains lactose, glycerin 1.6% w/phenol 0.2% as a preservative. Vial.
  Use: Hypoglycemic shock.
  GLUCAGON EMERGENCY KIT. (Lilly) Glucagon 1 mg, lactose 49 mg w/diluent. Inj. 1 ml Hyporet.
  Use: Emergency treatment of hypoglycemia.
  GLUCAMIDE. (Lemmon) Chlorpropamide 100 mg or 250 mg/Tab. Bot. 100s, 250s, 500s, 1000s, UD 100s.
  Use: Antidiabetic.
  GLUCEANA LIQUID. (Ross) Calcium and sodium caseinate, amino acids, hydrolyzed cornstarch, fructose, soy fiber, safflower oil, soy oil, soy lecithin, vitamins A, B_1, B_2, B_3, B_5, B_6, B_{12}, C, D, E, K, folic acid, Cl, Ca, P, Mg, I, Mn, Cu, Zn, Fe, Se, Cr, Mo, biotin, choline. Can 8 oz. Ready-to-use.
  Use: Enteral nutritional supplement.
- **GLUCEPTATE SODIUM.** USAN.
  Use: Pharmaceutic aid.
  d-GLUCITOL (d-Sorbitol)/Homatropine methylbromide.
  See: ProBilagol, Liq. (Purdue Frederick).
  GLUCOCEREBROSIDASE-BETA-GLUCOSIDASE.
  Use: Treatment of Gaucher's disease.
  See: Ceredase, Inj. (Genzyme).
  GLUCOCEREBROSIDASE, RECOMBINANT RETROVIRAL VECTOR. (Genetic Therapy)
  Use: Treatment for Gaucher's disease. [Orphan drug]
  GLUCOCORTICOIDS.
  See: Cortical Hormone Products.
  GLUCOLET AUTOMATIC LANCING DEVICE. (Miles Diagnostic) To obtain sample for blood glucose testing. Automatic spring loaded lancing device.
  Use: Diagnostic aid.
  GLUCOLET ENDCAPS. (Miles Diagnostic) To obtain sample for blood glucose testing. Controls depth of lancet penetration. Regular or super puncture.
  Use: Diagnostic aid.
  GLUCOMETER II BLOOD GLUCOSE METER. (Miles Diagnostic) Electronic meter for blood glucose testing.
  Use: Diagnostic aid.
  D-GLUCONIC ACID, CALCIUM SALT. Calcium Gluconate, U.S.P. XXIII.
  GLUCONIC ACID SALTS.
  See: Calcium Gluconate. Ferrous Gluconate. Magnesium Gluconate.

Potassium Gluconate.
• **GLUCOSAMINE.** USAN. 2-Amino-2-de-
oxy-β-D-glucopyranose.
Use: Pharmaceutic aid.
W/Nystatin, oxytetracycline.
See: Terrastatin, Cap., Soln. (Pfizer).
W/Tetracycline HCl, nystatin.
See: Tetrastatin Cap., Susp. (Pfizer).
W/Tetracycline.
See: Tetracyn, Cap., Syr. (Roerig).
W/Oxytetracycline.
See: Terramycin, Prep (Pfizer).
GLUCOSE.
See: Pal-A-Dex, Pow. (Baker).
**GLUCOSE-40 OPHTHALMIC
OINTMENT.** (Iolab) Liquid glucose 40%
in white petrolatum, anhydrous lanolin
with parabens. Tube 3.5 Gm.
Use: Hyperosmolar preparation.
GLUCOSE ELEVATING AGENTS.
See: B-D Glucose, Chew. Tab. (Becton
Dickinson).
Glucagon, Pow. for Inj. (Lilly).
Glutose, Gel. (Paddock).
Insta-Glucose, Gel. (ICN).
Insulin Reaction, Gel. (Sherwood).
Proglycem, Cap., Oral. Susp. (Medical
Market).
• **GLUCOSE ENZYMATIC TEST STRIP,**
U.S.P. XXIII.
Use: Diagnostic aid (in vitro, reducing
sugars in urine).
GLUCOSE (HK) REAGENT STRIPS.
Reagent strip test for detection of glu-
cose in serum or plasma. Bot. 50s.
Use: Diagnostic aid.
GLUCOSE & KETONE URINE TEST.
(Major) Reagent test for glucose and ke-
tones in urine. Bot. 100s.
Use: Diagnostic aid.
• **GLUCOSE, LIQUID,** N.F. XVIII. (Various
Mfr.) Cerelose, Dextrose.
Use: As a 5% to 50% solution as nutri-
ent; for acute hepatitis and dehydra-
tion; to increase blood volume; phar-
maceutic aid (tablet binder, coating
agent).
D-GLUCOSE, MONOHYDRATE. Dex-
trose, U.S.P. XXIII.
GLUCOSE OXIDASE. W/peroxidase,
potassium iodide.
See: Diastix, Vial, Tab. (Miles Diagnos-
tic).
GLUCOSE POLYMERS.
See: Polycose, Pow., Liq. (Ross).
GLUCOSE REAGENT STRIPS. (Miles
Diagnostic) A quantitative strip test for
glucose in serum or plasma. Seralyzer
reagent strips. Bot. 50s.
Use: Diagnostic aid.

GLUCOSE TEST.
See: Combistix (Miles Diagnostic).
First Choice, Strips (Polymer Technol-
ogy Int.).
Glucose Reagent Strips (Miles Diag-
nostic).
**GLUCOSE TOLERANCE TEST PREPA-
RATION.**
See: Glucola (Miles Diagnostic).
GLUCOSTIX REAGENT STRIPS. (Miles
Diagnostic) Cellulose strip containing
glucose oxidase and indicator system.
Bot. 50s, 100s, UD 25s.
Use: Diagnostic aid.
GLUCOSULFONE SODIUM, INJ..
See: Sodium Glucosulfone Injection.
GLUCO SYSTEM LANCETS. (Miles Di-
agnostic) Disposable lancets for use in
Miles Diagnostic Autolet or Glucolet.
Use: Diagnostic aid.
GLUCOTROL. (Roerig) Glipizide 5 mg or
10 mg/Tab. Bot. 100s, UD 100s.
Use: Antidiabetic.
GLUCOTROL-XL. (Pfizer) Glipizide 5 mg
or 10 mg. ER Tab. Bot. 100s, 500s.
Use: Antidiabetic.
GLUCOVITE. (Vale) Ferrous gluconate
260 mg, vitamins B_1 1 mg, B_2 0.5 mg, C
10 mg/Tab. Bot. 1000s, 5000s.
Use: Vitamin/mineral supplement.
GLUCUROLACTONE. Gamma lactone
of glucofuranuronic acid.
See: Preltron-Oral, Tab. (Pasadena Re-
search).
GLUCURONATE SODIUM.
See: Preltron, Inj. (Pasadena Re-
search).
GLU-K. (Western Research) Potassium
gluconate 486 mg/Tab. Bot. 1000s.
Use: Potassium supplement.
GLUKOR. (Hyrex) Chorionic go-
nadotropin 200 IU/ml when reconstitut-
ed. Pow. for inj. Vial 10 ml, 25 ml w/dilu-
ent.
Use: Chorionic gonadotropin.
GLUSIDE.
See: Saccharin (Various Mfr.).
GLUTAMATE SODIUM.
W/Niacin, vitamins, minerals.
See: L-Glutavite, Cap. (Cooper).
GLUTAMIC ACID HYDROCHLORIDE.
Acidogen, aciglumin, glutasin.
Use: Gastric acidifier.
See: Acidulin, Pulv. (Lilly).
W/Cellulase, pepsin, pancreatin, ox bile
extract.
See: Kanulase, Tab. (Dorsey).
GLUTAMIC ACID SALTS.
See: Calcium Glutamate (Various Mfr.).
• **GLUTARAL CONCENTRATE,** U.S.P.

XXIII.
Use: Disinfectant.
See: Cidex (Surgikos).
GLUTARALDEHYDE. (City Chem.) Glutaraldehyde 25% in water. Pkg. 3 kg; (Wyeth-Ayerst) Sonacide Soln., Gal, 5 Gal.
Use: Germicide.
GLUTAREX-1. (Ross) Protein 15 g, fat 23.9 g, carbohydrates 46.3 g, linoleic acid 1800 mg, Fe 9 mg, Na 190 mg, K 675 mg, Ca, vitamins A, B_1, B_2, B_3, B_5, B_6, B_{12}, C, D, E, K, biotin, choline, folic acid, inositol, Cl, Cu, I, Mg, Mn, P, Se, Zn and 480 Cal per 100 g. Lysine and tryptophan free. Pow. Can 350 g.
Use: Enteral nutritional supplement.
GLUTAREX-2. (Ross) Protein 30 g, fat 15.5 g, carbohydrates 30 g, Fe 13 mg, Na 880 mg, K 1370 mg, Ca, vitamins A, B_1, B_2, B_3, B_5, B_6, B_{12}, C, D, E, K, biotin, choline, folic acid, inositol, Cl, Cu, I, Mg, Mn, P, Se, Zn and 410 Cal per 100 g. Lysine and tryptophan free. Pow. Can 325 g.
Use: Enteral nutritional supplement.
L-GLUTATHIONE.
Use: Treatment of AIDS-associated cachexia. [Orphan drug]
See: Cachexon.
GLUTETHIMIDE. B.A.N. 2-Ethyl-2-phenylglutatimide.
Use: Non-barbiturate hypnotic.
• **GLUTETHIMIDE,** U.S.P. XXIII. Cap., Tab., U.S.P. XXIII. Alpha-ethyl-alpha-phenyl-glutarimide. 2-Ethyl-2-phenylglutarimide.
Use: Non-barbiturate hypnotic.
See: Doriden, Cap. (Rhone-Poulenc Rorer).
GLUTOFAC. (Kenwood) Vitamins C 300 mg, B_1 15 mg, B_2 10 mg, niacinamide 50 mg, B_6 50 mg, calcium pantothenate 20 mg, magnesium 133 mg, selenium 25 mcg, GTF chromium complex 25 mcg/Tab. Trace amounts of Mg, K, Fe, Cu, P. Bot. 90s.
Use: Vitamin/mineral supplement.
GLUTOL. (Paddock) Dextrose 100 Gm/180 ml. Bot. 180 ml.
Use: Diagnostic aid.
GLUTOSE. (Paddock) Liquid glucose (40% dextrose). Concentrated glucose for insulin reactions. Gel. Bot. 60 Gm.
Use: Glucose elevating agent.
GLYATE. (Geneva Marsam) Guaifenesin 100 mg/5 ml, alcohol 3.5%. Syr. Bot. 118 ml, 480 ml.
Use: Expectorant.
• **GLYBURIDE.** USAN.

Use: Antidiabetic.
See: Diabeta (Hoechst).
Glynase, Tab. (Upjohn).
Micronase, Tab. (Upjohn).
GLYCALOX. B.A.N. A polymerized complex of glycerol and aluminum hydroxide. Glucalox (I.N.N.).
Use: Treatment of gastric hyperacidity.
GLYCARNINE IRON.
See: Ferronord, Tab. (Cooper).
GLYCATE CHEWABLES. (Forest) Glycine 150 mg, calcium carbonate 300 mg/Tab. Bot. 1000s.
Use: Antacid.
• **GLYCERIN,** U.S.P. XXIII. Ophth. Soln., Oral Soln., U.S.P. XXIII. 1,2,3-Propanetriol.
Use: Pharmaceutic aid (humectant, solvent).
See: Corn Huskers Lot. (Warner-Lambert).
Ophthalgan Ophthalmic, Soln. (Wyeth-Ayerst).
Osmoglyn (Alcon).
W/ Dimethicone.
See: Dermasil, Lot. (Chesebrough-Ponds).
W/Urea.
See: Kerid Ear Drops (Blair).
• **GLYCERIN SUPPOSITORIES,** U.S.P. XXIII. (Various Mfr.) Glycerin, sodium stearate.
Use: Rectal evacuant, cathartic.
• **GLYCEROL, IODINATED.** USAN.
Use: Expectorant.
• **GLYCERYL BEHENATE,** N.F. XVIII.
Use: Pharmaceutic aid.
GLYCERYL GUAIACOLATE.
Use: Expectorant.
See: Guaifenesin, U.S.P. XXIII.
GLYCERYL GUAIACOLATE CARBAMATE. Methocarbamol.
See: Robaxin, Tab., Inj. (Robins).
Robaxin 750, Tab. (Robins).
GLYCERYL GUAIACOLETHER.
See: Guaifenesin.
• **GLYCERYL MONOSTEARATE,** N.F. XVIII. (Various Mfr.) Monostearin.
Use: Pharmaceutic aid (emulsifying agent).
GLYCERYL-T. (Rugby) Theophylline 150 mg, guaifenesin 90 mg/Cap. Bot. 100s, 1000s.
Use: Bronchodilator, expectorant.
GLYCERYL TRIACETATE.
See: Triacetin.
GLYCERYL TRIACETIN. (Various Mfr.) Triacetin.
See: Enzactin, Aerosal, Pow., Cream (Wyeth-Ayerst).

Fungacetin, Oint, Liq. (Blair Labs.).
GLYCERYL TRINITRATE OINTMENT.
See: Nitrol, Oint. (Kremers-Urban).
GLYCERYL TRINITRATE TABLETS.
See: Nitroglycerin (Various Mfr.).
Nitroglyn, Tab. (Key Corp.).
GLYCETS-ANTACID TABLETS. (Weeks
& Leo) Calcium carbonate 350 mg,
simethicone 25 mg/Chew. Tab. Bot.
100s.
Use: Antacid/antiflatulent.
**GLYCINATO DIHYDROXYALUMINUM
HYDRATE.**
See: Dihydroxyaluminum Aminoac-
etate, U.S.P. XXIII.
• **GLYCINE,** U.S.P. XXIII. Irrigation, U.S.P.
XXI. Aminoacetic Acid.
Use: Myasthenia gravis treatment, irri-
gating solution.
W/Aluminum hydroxide-magnesium car-
bonate coprecipitated gel.
See: Glycogel, Tab., Susp. (Central).
W/Aluminum, magnesium hydroxide, mag-
nesium trisilicate, belladonna extract,
mannitol, peppermint oil.
See: Gas-Eze, Tab. (E.J. Moore).
W/Calcium Carbonate.
See: Antacid No. 6, Tab. (Bowman).
Glycate Chewables, Tab. (O'Neal).
P.H. Tab. (Scrip).
Titralac, Liq., Tab. (Riker).
W/Calcium carbonate, amylolytic, prote-
olytic cellulolytic enzymes.
See: Co-gel, Tab. (Arco).
W/Chlortrimeton, sodium salicylate.
See: Corilin, Liq. (Schering).
W/Glutamic acid, alanine.
See: Prostall, Cap. (Metabolic Prods.).
W/Magnesium trisilicate, calcium carbon-
ate.
See: P.H. Tab., Chewable, Mix (Scrip).
GLYCINE, ALUMINUM SALT.
See: Dihydroxyaluminum Aminoac-
etate, U.S.P. XXIII.
GLYCINE HYDROCHLORIDE. (Various
Mfr.).
Use: Gastric acidifier.
GLYCOBIARSOL, U.S.P. XXI. Tab.,
U.S.P. XXI. Bismuthyl-N-Glycolylarsani-
late, Chemo Puro, Pow. for Mfr. (Hydro-
gen N-glycoloylarsanilato) oxobismuth.
Use: Amebiasis, Trichomonas vaginalis,
Monilia albicans.
GLYCOBIARSOL. (I.N.N.) Bismuth Gly-
collylarsanilate, B.A.N.
GLYCOCOLL. Glycine.
See: Aminoacetic Acid (Various Mfr.).
GLYCOCYAMINE. Guanidoacetic acid.
GLYCOFED TABLETS. (Pal-Pak) Pseu-
doephedrine 30 mg, guaifenesin 100

mg. Bot. 1000s.
Use: Decongestant, expectorant.
GLYCO IOPHEN SOLUTION. (Wade)
Tincture of iodine, phenol 2%, glycerine
q.s., peppermint oil. Bot. 2 oz, 4 oz, pt,
gal.
Use: Antiseptic.
• **GLYCOL DISTERATE.** USAN.
Use: Pharmaceutic aid.
GLYCOL MONOSALICYLATE.
W/Oil of mustard, camphor, menthol,
methyl salicylate.
See: Musterole, Oint., Cream (Plough).
GLYCOPHENYLATE BROMIDE.
See: Mepenzolate Methylbromide.
• **GLYCOPYRROLATE,** U.S.P. XXIII. Inj.,
Tab., U.S.P. XXIII. 1-Methyl-3-pyrrolidyl
a-phenylcyclopentaneglycolate metho-
bromide. 3-Hydroxy-1,1-dimethylpyrroli-
dinium bromideα-cyclopentylmandelate.
Use: Anticholinergic.
See: Robinul, Tab., Inj. (Robins).
Robinul Forte, Tab. (Robins).
GLYCOPYRRONIUM BROMIDE. B.A.N.
3-α-Cyclo-pentylmandeloyloxy-1,1-di-
methylpyrrolidinium bromide.
Use: Anticholinergic.
GLYCOTUSS. (Vale) Guaifenesin 100
mg/Tab. Bot. 100s, 1000s.
Use: Expectorant.
GLYCOTUSS-dM. (Pal-Pak) Guaifenesin
100 mg, dextromethorphan HBr 10
mg/Tab. Bot. 100s, 1000s.
Use: Expectorant, antitussive.
• **GLYCYRRHIZA,** U.S.P. XXIII. Pure ex-
tract, Fluidextract, U.S.P. XXIII. Licorice
root.
Use: Flavoring agent.
• **GLYCYRRHIZA EXTRACT, PURE, U.S.P.**
U.S.P. XXIII.
Use: Flavoring agent.
• **GLYCYRRHIZA FLUIDEXTRACT, N.F.**
N.F. XVIII.
Use: Flavoring agent.
W/Camphorated opium tincture, tartar
emetic, glycerin.
See: Brown Mixture. (Bowman).
W/Pepsin-papain complex, pancreas, malt
diastase, charcoal, ox bile.
See: Pepsocoll, Tab. (Western Re-
search Labs.).
GLYDANILE SODIUM. (1)5'-Chloro-2-[p-
[(5-isobutyl-2-pyrimidinyl)sulfamoyl]-
phenyl]-o-acetanilidide monosodium
salt; (2) 4-[N-(5-isobutyl-2-pyrimidinyl)-
sulfamoyl] phenylacetic acid-5-chloro-2-
methoxyanilide sodium salt.
Use: Antidiabetic.
• **GLYHEXAMIDE.** USAN.
Use: Antidiabetic.

GLYLORIN. (Cellergy Pharm)
See: MONOLAURIN.
• **GLYMIDINE SODIUM.** USAN. [N-[5-(2-Methoxyethoxy)-2-idinyl] benzene-sulfonamido]-sodium.
Use: Oral hypoglycemic agent.
GLYMOL.
See: Petrolatum Liquid (Various Mfr.).
GLYNASE. (Upjohn) Glyburide **1.5 mg or 3 mg:** Tab. (Micronized). Bot. 30s, 60s, 90s, 100s, 500s, 1000s, UD 100. **6 mg:** Tab. Bot. 100s, 500s.
Use: Antidiabetic.
GLYNAZAN EXPECTORANT. (Scherer) Theophylline sodium glycinate 60 mg (equivalent to theophylline 30 mg), guaifenesin 50 mg, sodium citrate 100 mg/5 ml. Bot. pt.
Use: Bronchodilator, expectorant.
• **GLYOCTAMIDE.** USAN. 1-Cyclooctyl-3(p-tolylsulfonyl) urea.
Use: Hypoglycemic agent.
GLY-OXIDE. (SK-Beecham) Carbamide peroxide 10% in flavored anhydrous glycerol. Liq. bot. 15 ml, 60 ml w/applicator.
Use: Mouth and throat product.
GLYOXYLDIUREIDE.
See: Allantoin (Various Mfr.).
• **GLYPARAMIDE.** USAN. 1-(p-Chlorophenylsulfonyl)-3-(p-dimethylaminophenyl) urea.
Use: Oral hypoglycemic agent.
GLYPRESSIN. (Ferring)
See: TERLIPRESSIN.
GLYTUSS. (Mayrand) Guaifenesin 200 mg/Tab. Bot. 100s.
Use: Expectorant
GLYVENOL. (Ciba) Tribenoside. Not available in U.S.
Use: Venoprotective agent.
GM-CSF. Granulocyte macrophage colony stimulating factor.
See: Leukine (Immunex).
Prokine (Hoechst-Roussel).
G-MYTICIN CREME AND OINTMENT. (Pedinol) Gentamicin sulfate equivalent to gentamicin base 1 mg. Tube 15 Gm.
Use: Anti-infective.
• **GODODIAMIDE.** USAN.
Use: Diagnostic aid.
GO-EVAC. (Copley) Polyethylene glycol 3350 59 g, sodium sulfate 5.685 g, sodium bicarbonate 1.685 g, sodium chloride 1.465 g, potassium chloride 0.743 g/L. Pow. Jug 4 L.
Use: Bowel evacuants.
GOLACOL. (Arcum) Codeine sulfate 30 mg, papaverine HCl 30 mg, emetine HCl 2 mg, ephedrine HCl 15 mg, q.s./30 ml.

Alcohol 6.25%. Syr. Bot. 4 oz, 16 oz, gal. Orange flavor.
Use: Antitussive.
GOLD (Au^{198}). Colloid Radio.
Use: Antineoplastic agent.
See: Radio Gold (Au^{198}).
GOLD Au 198 INJECTION.
Use: Antineoplastic; diagnostic for liver scanning.
GOLD COMPOUNDS.
See: Gold Sodium Thiosulfate (Various Mfr.).
Myochrysine, Amp. (Merck, Sharp & Dohme).
Ridaura, Cap. (SKF).
Solganal, Vial (Schering).
GOLD SODIUM THIOMALATE, U.S.P. XXI. Inj., U.S.P. XXI. Gold, mercaptobutanedioato(1-)-, disodium salt, monohydrate. (Disodium mercaptosuccinato) gold monohydrate.
Use: Rheumatoid arthritis.
See: Aurolate, Inj. (Pasadena).
Myochrysine, Amp. (Merck, Sharp & Dohme).
GOLD SODIUM THIOSULFATE. Sterile, Auricidine, Aurocidin, Aurolin, Auropin, Aurocan, Novaorycin, Solfooricol and Thiochrysine.
Use: Antirheumatic agent.
GOLD THIOGLUCOSE.
See: Aurothioglucose, U.S.P. XXIII.
GOLDEN BALM. (Jenkins) Methyl salicylate, menthol, camphor/fl oz. Bot. 3 oz, pt, gal.
Use: External analgesic.
GOLDEN-WEST COMPOUND. (Golden-West) Gentian root, licorice root, cascara sagrada, damiana leaves, senna leaves, psyllium seed, buchu leaves, crude pepsin. Box 1.5 oz.
Use: Laxative.
GOLDICIDE CONCENTRATE. (Pedinol) N-Alkyl-dimethylbenzylammonium chloride, cetyl dimethyl ammonium Cl. Bot. (Conc.) oz. Ctn. 10s.
Use: Chemical disinfection of surgical and podiatry instruments.
GOLD SEAL CALCIUM 600. (Walgreen) Calcium 1200 mg/Tab. Bot. 60s.
Use: Calcium supplement.
GOLD SEAL CALCIUM 600 WITH VITAMIN D. (Walgreen) Calcium 1200 mg, vitamin D/Tab. Bot. 60s.
Use: Calcium supplement.
GOLD SEAL CHEWABLE VITAMIN C. (Walgreen) Ascorbic acid 250 mg or 500 mg/Tab. Bot. 100s.
Use: Vitamin C supplement.
GOLD SEAL FERROUS GLUCONATE.

(Walgreen) Iron 37 mg/Tab. Bot. 100s.
Use: Iron supplement.
GOLD SEAL FERROUS SULFATE TABLETS. (Walgreen) Ferrous sulfate 325 mg/Tab. Bot. 100s, 1000s.
Use: Iron supplement.
GOLD SEAL TIME RELEASE FERROUS SULFATE. (Walgreen) Iron 50 mg/Tab. Bot. 100s.
Use: Iron supplement.
GOLYTELY. (Braintree) Pow. for oral soln. after reconstitution containing PEG-3350 236 Gm, sodium sulfate 22.74 Gm, sodium bicarbonate 6.74 Gm, sodium Cl 5.86 Gm, potassium Cl 2.97 Gm when made up to 4 L. Disposable container 4800 ml.
Use: Laxative.
GONACRINE.
See: Acriflavine (Various Mfr.).
• **GONADORELIN ACETATE.** USAN.
Use: Gonad-stimulating principle. [Orphan drug]
See: Cryptolin Prods. (Hoechst).
• **GONADORELIN HYDROCHLORIDE.** USAN.
Use: Gonad-stimulating principle.
GONADOTROPIC SUBSTANCE.
See: Gonadotropin Chorionic.
GONADOTROPINS.
See: Pergonal, Pow. for Inj. (Serona).
• **GONADOTROPIN, CHORIONIC,** U.S.P. XXIII. For Inj., U.S.P. XXIII. Human Pregnancy Urine.
Use: In the female: Chronic cystic mastitis, functional sterility, dysmenorrhea, premenstrual tension, threatened abortion. In the male: Cryptorchidism, hypogenitalism, dwarfism, impotency, enuresis.
See: Android HCG, Inj. (Brown).
Antuitrin "S", Vial (Parke-Davis).
A.P.L., Secules (Wyeth-Ayerst).
Chopion-Plus, Vial (Pharmex).
Corgonject, Vial (Mayrand).
Dura-Chroion Plus, Vial (Pharmex).
Follutein Pow. (Squibb).
Libigen, Vial (Savage).
Pregnyl, Amp. (Organon).
W/Vitamin B$_1$, glutamic acid, procaine HCl.
See: Glukor, Vial (Brown).
GONADOTROPIN, PITUITARY ANT. LOBE. Extracted from anterior lobe of equine pituitaries (not pregnant mare urine) (rat unit = 1 Fevold-Hisaw unit).
GONADOTROPIN RELEASING HORMONE ANALOG.
See: Lupron, Inj. Susp. (TAP Pharm.)
Zoladex, Implant (ICI Pharma.)

GONADOTROPIN RELEASING HORMONES.
See: Lutrepulse, Pow. for Inj. (Ortho).
Supprelin, Inj. (Ortho).
Synarel, Soln. (Syntex).
GONADOTROPIN SERUM. Pregnant mare's serum.
GONADOTROPIN SPECIAL DILUENT. (Kenyon) Sodium succinate 0.5%, sodium nicotinate 1%, glutamic acid 52.5 ppm, propylparaben 0.02%, chlorobutanol 0.5%. Vial 10 ml.
GONAK. (Akorn) Hydroxypropyl methylcellulose 2.5%, boric acid, EDTA, benzalkonium Cl 0.01%, sodium borate. Soln. Bot. 15 ml.
Use: Ophthalmic preparation.
GONIC. (Hauck) Chorionic gonadotropin 10,000 units/vial. Pow. for inj. Vial 10 ml w/diluent.
Use: Chorionic gonadotropin.
GONIOSCOPIC HYDROXYPROPYL METHYLCELLULOSE.
See: Goniosol Lacrivial, Soln. (Smith, Miller & Patch).
GONIOSCOPIC PRISM SOLUTION. (Alcon) Hydroxyethyl cellulose preserved with thimerosal 0.004%, edetate sodium 0.1%. Soln. Plastic dispenser 15 ml.
Use: Ophthalmic preparation.
GONIOSOL. (Iolab) Gonioscopic hydroxypropylmethylcellulose 2.5%. Bot. 15 ml.
Use: Ophthalmic preparation.
GONODECTEN TEST KIT. (United States Packaging) Tube test for urethral dischrge from males, for detection of neisseria gonorrhoeae. Test kit 10s, 25s.
Use: Diagnostic aid.
GONORRHEA TESTS.
See: Biocult-GC (Medical Tech.).
Gonodecten Test Kit (United States Packaging).
Gonozyme Diagnostic Kit (Abbott).
Isocult for Neisseria gonorrhoeae (SmithKline Diagnostics).
MicroTrak Neisseria gonorrhoeae Culture Test (Syva).
GONOZYME. (Abbott Diagnostics) Enzyme immunoassay for detection of *neisseria gonorrhoeae* in urogenital swab specimens. Test kit 100s.
Use: Diagnostic aid.
GOOD SAMARITAN OINTMENT. (Good Samaritan) Tube 1.25 oz.
Use: Counter-irritant.
GOODY'S HEADACHE POWDERS. (Goody) Aspirin 520 mg, acetaminophen 250 mg, caffeine 32.5 mg/dose. Pow. Pkg. 2s, 6s, 24s.
Use: Analgesic.

GO PAIN. (DePree) **Cream:** Methyl salicylate, chlorobutanol, menthol, camphor, thymol. Tube 1.5 oz, 4 oz. **Oral Gel:** Benzocaine, eugenol. Tube ³⁄₈ oz. **Throat spray:** 4 oz.
Use: External analgesic.

GO PAIN EXTRA STRENGTH BALM. (DePree) Methyl salicylate. Jar 3³⁄₄ oz.
Use: External analgesic.

GORDOBALM. (Gordon) Chloroxylenol, methyl salicylate, menthol, camphor, thymol, eucalyptus oil, isopropyl alcohol 16%, fast-drying gum base. Bot. 4 oz, gal.
Use: External analgesic.

GORDOCHOM. (Gordon) Undecylenic acid 25%, chloroxylenol 3%, penetrating oil base. Liq. Bot. 15 ml, 30 ml w/applicator.
Use: Antifungal, external.

GORDOFILM. (Gordon) Salicylic acid 16.7%, lactic acid 16.7% in flexible collodian. Bot. 15 ml.
Use: Keratolytic.

GORDOGESIC CREAM. (Gordon) Methyl salicylate 10% in absorption base. Jar 2.5 oz, 1 lb.
Use: External analgesic.

GORDOMATIC CRYSTALS. (Gordon) Sodium borate, sodium bicarbonate, sodium Cl, thymol, menthol, eucalyptus oil. Jar 8 oz, 7 lb.
Use: Counter irritant.

GORDOMATIC LOTION. (Gordon) Menthol, camphor, propylene glycol, isopropyl alcohol. Bot. 1 oz, 4 oz, gal.
Use: Counter-irritant.

GORDOMATIC POWDER. (Gordon) Menthol, thymol camphor, eucalyptus oil, salicylic acid, alum bentonite, talc. Shaker can 3.5 oz. Can 1 lb, 5 lb.
Use: Counter-irritant.

GORDOPHENE. (Gordon) Neutral coconut oil soap 15%, glycerin with Septi-Chlor (trichlorohydroxy diphenyl ether) broad spectrum antimicrobial and bacteriostatic agent. Bot. 4 oz, gal.
Use: Surgical soap.

GORDO-POOL WHIRLPOOL CONCENTRATE. (Gordon) Bot. pt.
Use: Water softener, cleanser.

GORDO-VITE A CREME. (Gordon) Vitamin A 100,000 IU/oz. in water soluble base. Jar 0.5 oz, 2.5 oz, 4 oz, lb, 5 lb.
Use: Emollient.

GORDO-VITE A LOTION. (Gordon) Vitamin A 100,000 IU/oz. Plastic bot. 4 oz, gal.
Use: Emollient.

GORDO-VITE E CREME. (Gordon) Vitamin E 1500 IU/oz in water soluble base. Jar 2.5 oz, lb.
Use: Emollient.

GORD-UREA. (Gordon) Urea 22% or 40% in petrolatum base. Jar oz.
Use: Emollient.

GORMEL CREAM. (Gordon) Urea 20% in emollient base. Jar 0.5 oz, 2.5 oz, 4 oz, 1 lb, 5 lb.
Use: Emollient.

• **GOSERELIN.** USAN.
Use: LHRH agonist.
See: Zoladex (Stuart).

GOSERELIN ACETATE.
Use: Gonadotropin-releasing hormone analog.
See: Zoladex (ICI Pharma.).

GOSSYPOL.
Use: Antineoplastic. [Orphan drug]

GOTAMINE. (Vita Elixir) Ergotamine tartrate 1 mg, caffeine 100 mg/Tab.
Use: Agent for migraine.

GOUT, AGENTS FOR.
See: Allopurinol, Tab. (Various Mfr.).
Anturane, Tab., Cap. (Ciba).
Benemid, Tab. (Merck & Co.).
ColBenemid, Tab. (Merck & Co.).
Colchicine, Inj. (Lilly).
Colchicine, Tab. (Various Mfr.).
Col-Probenecid, Tab. (Various Mfr.).
Probalan, Tab. (Lannett).
Proben-C, Tab. (Various Mfr.).
Probenecid, Tab. (Various Mfr.).
Probenecid w/Colchicine, Tab. (Various Mfr.).
Sulfinpyrazone, Tab., Cap. (Various Mfr.).
Zyloprim, Tab. (Burroughs Wellcome).

• **GOVAFILCON A.** USAN.
Use: Contact lens material (hydrophilic).

GP-500. (Marnel) Pseudoephedrine HCl 120 mg, guaifenesin 500 mg. Tab. Bot. 100s.
Use: Decongestant, expectorant.

• **GRAMICIDIN,** U.S.P. XXIII.
Use: Antibacterial.
W/Neomycin.
See: Spectrocin Oint. (Squibb).
W/Neomycin sulfate, polymyxin B sulfate, thimerosal.
See: Neo-Polycin Ophthalmic Soln. (Merrell Dow).
W/Neomycin sulfate, polymyxin B sulfate, benzocaine.
See: Tricidin, Oint. (Amlab).
W/Neomycin sulfate, triamcinolone, nystatin.
See: Mycolog Cream, Oint. (Squibb).
W/Polymyxin B sulfate, neomycin sulfate.
See: AK-Spore Ophth. Soln. (Akorn).

Neosporin, Ophthalmic Soln. (Burroughs Wellcome).

Neosporin-G Cream (Burroughs Wellcome).

Ocutricin Ophth. Soln. (Bausch & Lomb).

W/Polymyxin B sulfate, neomycin sulfate, hydrocortisone acetate.

See. Cortisporin, Cream (Burroughs Wellcome).

GRAMINEAE POLLENS.
See: Allergenic Extracts, Timothy and Related Pollens (Parke-Davis).

• **GRANISETRON.** USAN.
Use: Antiemetics.
See: Kytril, Vial (SmithKine-Beecham).

GRANULDERM. (Copley) Trypsin 0.1 mg, balsam Peru 72.5 mg, castor oil 650 mg/0.82 ml. Aerosol Spray 113.4 Gm.
Use: Topical enzyme preparation.

GRANULEX. (Hickam) Trypsin 0.1 mg, balsam Peru 72.5 mg, castor oil 650 mg w/emulsifier/0.82 ml. Spray can 2 oz, 4 oz.
Use: Wound-healing agent.

GRANULOCYTE-COLONY STIMULATING FACTOR.
See: Neupogen (Amgen).

GRANULOCYTE MACROPHAGE-COLONY STIMULATING FACTOR.
AIDS-related neutropenia. [Orphan drug]
See: Leukine (Immunex).
Prokine (Hoechst-Roussel).

GRAPEFRUIT DIET PLAN with DIADEX, MAXIMUM STRENGTH CAPSULES.
(O'Conner) Phenylpropanolamine HCl 37.5 mg, grapefruit extract, sugar/S.R. Cap. Bot. 20s.
Use: Diet aid.

GRAPEFRUIT DIET PLAN with DIADAX TABLETS. (O'Connor) Natural grapefruit extract, phenylpropanolamine HCl 12.5 mg/Chew. tab. Bot. 42s, 90s.
Use: Diet aid.

GRATUS STROPHANTHIN. Quabain.

GRAVINEED. (Hanlon) Vitamins C 100 mg, E 10 IU, B_1 3 mg, B_2 2 mg, B_6 10 mg, B_{12} 5 mcg, A 4000 IU, D 400 IU, niacin 10 mg, folic acid 0.1 mg, iron fumarate 40 mg, calcium 67 mg/Cap. Bot. 100s.
Use: Vitamin/mineral supplement.

GREEN MINT. (Block) Urea, glycine, polysorbate 60, sorbitol, alcohol 12.2%, peppermint oil, menthol, chlorophyllin-copper complex. Bot. 7 oz, 12 oz.
Use: Mouth and throat product.

GREEN SOAP, U.S.P. XXIII.
Use: Detergent.

GRIFULVIN V. (Ortho Derm) Griseofulvin microsize. **Tab:** 250 mg. Bot. 100s; 500 mg. Bot. 100s, 500s. **Susp:** 125 mg/5 ml. Bot. 120 ml.
Use: Antifungal.

GRILLODYNE TABLETS. (Forest Pharm.) Aspirin 3.5 gr, phenacetin 2.5 gr, caffeine alkaloid 0.5 gr, phenobarbital 0.25 gr/Tab. Bot. 1000s.
Use: Salicylate analgesic, sedative/hypnotic.

GRISACTIN. (Wyeth-Ayerst) Griseofulvin microsize. **Cap.: 125 mg:** Bot. 100s; **250 mg:** Bot. 100s, 500s. **Tab.: 500 mg:** Bot. 60s.
Use: Antifungal.

GRISACTIN ULTRA. (Wyeth-Ayerst) Griseofulvin ultramicrosize 125 mg, 250 mg or 330 mg/Tab. Bot. 100s.
Use: Antifungal.

• **GRISEOFULVIN,** U.S.P. XXIII. Cap., Oral Susp., Tab., Ultramicrosized Tab., U.S.P. XXIII. An antibiotic. 7-Chloro-4,6-dimethoxy-coumaran-3-one-2-spiro-1'-(2-methoxy-6-methylcyclohex-2-en-4-one). 7-Chloro-2,4,6-trimethoxy-6-methylspiro[benzofuran-2(3H), 1[2]-cyclohexene]-3,4-dione. Spiro[benzofuran-2(3H)-1-[2]cyclohexene]-3,4-dione,7-chloro-2,4,6-trimethoxy-6-methyl-, (1s-trans)-. Fulcin, Grisovin. (Various Mfr.) 165 mg or 330 mg. Tab. Bot. 100s.
Use: Antifungal (antibiotic).
See: Fulvicin P/G, Tab. (Schering).
Fulvicin-U/F, Tab. (Schering).
Grifulvin V, Tab., Susp. (Ortho).
Grisactin, Cap., Tab. (Wyeth-Ayerst).
Grisactin Ultra, Tab. (Wyeth-Ayerst).

GRISEOFULVIN MICROCRYSTALLINE.
Use: Antifungal.
See: Fulvicin U/F, Tab. (Schering).
Grifulvin V, Tab., Susp. (Ortho).
Grisactin, Cap., Tab. (Wyeth-Ayerst).

GRISEOFULVIN ULTRAMICROSIZE.
Use: Antifungal.
See: Fulvicin P/G, Tab.(Schering).
Gris-Peg, Tab. (Dorsey).

GRIS-PEG TABLETS. (Herbert) Griseofulvin ultramicrosize 125 mg or 250 mg/Tab. **125 mg:** Bot. 100s, 500s. **250 mg:** Bot. 100s, 250s, 500s.
Use: Antifungal.

GROWTH HORMONE. Extract of human pituitaries containing predominantly growth hormone.
See: Crescormon.

GROWTH HORMONE RELEASING FACTOR.
Use: Long-term treatment of growth fail-

ure. [Orphan drug]

G-STROPHANTHIN. Ouabain.

GUAIACOHIST. (Pharmex) Potassium guaiacolsulfonate 40 mg, sodium iodide 50 mg, chlorpheniramine maleate 5 mg/ml. Vial 30 ml.
Use: Expectorant, antihistamine.

GUAIACOL. (Various Mfr.) Methylcatechol.
Use: Expectorant.

GUAIACOL. (Jenkins) Guaiacol 0.1 Gm, eucalyptol 0.08 Gm, iodoform 0.02 Gm, camphor 0.05 Gm, sesame oil q.s./2 ml. Vial 10 ml.
Use: Expectorant.
W/Methyl salicylate, menthol.
See: Guaiamen, Cream (Lannett).

GUAIACOL CARBONATE. (Various Mfr.) (Duotal).
Use: Expectorant.

GUAIACOL GLYCERYL ETHER.
See: Guaifenesin.

GUAIACOL POTASSIUM SULFONATE.
See: Bronchial, Syr. (DePree)
W/Ammonium Cl, sodium citrate, benzyl alcohol, carbinoxamine maleate.
See: Clistin Expectorant, Syr. (McNeil).
W/Dextromethorphan I IDr.
Bronchial DM, Syr. (DePree).
W/Dextromethorphan HBr, chlorpheniramine maleate, ammonium Cl, tartar emetic.
See: Duomine, Syr. (Kenyon).
W/Pheniramine maleate, pyrilamine maleate, codeine phosphate.
See: Tritussin, Syr. (Towne).

GUAIADOL. (Medwick) Aqueous. Vial 30 ml.

GUAIADOL COMPOUND. (Medical Chem.) Naiouli oil 100 mg, eucalyptol 80 mg, guaiacol 100 mg, iodoform 20 mg, camphor 50 mg/2 ml. Aqueous or in oil. Vial 30 ml.

GUAIADOL COMPOUND. (Medwick) Oil. Vial 30 ml.

GUAIAMEN. (Lannett) Methyl salicylate, guaiacol, menthol in greaseless base. 4 oz, 1 lb.
Use: Analgesic, expectorant.

GUAIANESIN.
See: Guaifenesin.
Use: Expectorant.

•**GUAIAPATE.** USAN.
Use: Antitussive.

GUAIFED CAPSULES. (Muro) Guaifenesin 250 mg, pseudoephedrine HCl 120 mg/TR Cap. Bot. 100s, 500s.
Use: Expectorant, decongestant.

GUAIFED PD CAPSULES. (Muro) Pseudoephedrine HCl 60 mg, guaifenesin

300 mg/TR Cap. Bot. 100s, 500s.
Use: Decogestant, expectorant.

GUAIFED SYRUP. (Muro) Pseudoephedrine HCl 30 mg, guaifenesin 200 mg. Bot. 118 ml, 473 ml.
Use: Decongestant, expectorant.

•**GUAIFENESIN,** U.S.P. XXIII. Cap., Syr., Tab., U.S.P. XXIII. Methphenoxydiol. 3-(o-methoxyphenoxy)-1,2-propanediol.
Synonyms:
Glyceryl Guaiacolate.
Glyceryl Guaiacol Ether.
Guaianesin.
Guaifylline.
Guayanesin.
Use: Expectorant.
See: Anti-tuss, Liq. (Century).
Consin-GG, Syr. (Wisconsin).
Diabetic Tussin Ex, Liq. (Health Care Products).
Dilyn, Liq., Tab. (Elder).
2/G, Liq. (Merrell Dow).
G-100, Syr. (Bock).
GG-Cen, Syr (Central)
Glycotuss, Tab., Syr. (Vale).
Glytuss, Tab. (Mayrand).
G-Tussin, Syr. (Quality Generics).
Humibid L.A., Tab. (Adams).
Hytuss, Tab., Cap. (Hyrex).
Robitussin, Syr. (Robins).
Tursen, Tab. (Wren).
Wal-Tussin, Syr. (Walgreen).
W/Combinations.
See: Actifed C Expectorant, Liq. (Burroughs Wellcome).
Actol Exp., Syr., Tab. (Beecham Labs).
Airet G.G., Cap., Elix. (Baylor Labs).
Ambenyl-D, Liq. (Marion).
Anatuss DM, Syr., Tab. (Mayrand).
Anti-tuss D.M., Liq. (Century).
Antitussive Guaiacolate, Syr. (Med. Chem.).
Asbron G, Tab., Elix. (Dorsey).
Bur-Tuss Expectorant (Burlington).
Brexin, Cap., Liq. (Savage).
Bri-stan, Liq. (Briar)
Broncholate, Cap., Elix. (Bock).
Bronchovent, Tab. (Mills).
Bronkolate-G, Tab. (Parmed).
Bronkolixir, Elix. (Sanofi Winthrop).
Bronkotabs, Tab. (Sanofi Winthrop).
Bro-Tane, Expectorant (Scrip).
C.D.M., Expectorant (Lannett).
Cerylin, Liq. (Spencer-Mead).
Cheracol-D, Syr. (Upjohn).
Chlor-Trimeton, Expectorant (Schering).
Colrex, Expectorant (Solvay).
Conar-A, Susp., Tab. (Beecham Labs).

Conar Expectorant, Liq. (Beecham Labs).
Congestac, Tab. (SK-Beecham).
Consin-DM, Syr. (Wisconsin).
Coricidin Children's Cough Syr. (Schering).
Cortane D.C., Exp. (Standex).
Dextro-Tuss GG, Liq. (Ulmer).
Dilaudid, Syr. (Knoll).
Dilor-G, Tab., Liq. (Savage).
Dilyn, Liq. (Elder).
Dimacol, Cap. (Robins).
Dimetane Expectorant, Liq. (Robins).
Dimetane Expectorant-DC, Liq. (Robins).
DM Plus, Liq. (West-Ward).
Donatussin, Syr. (Laser).
Duovent, Tab. (Riker).
Emfaseem, Liq., Tab. (Saron).
Entex, Cap., Liq. (Norwich Eaton).
Formula 44D Decongestant Cough Mixture, Syr. (Vicks).
G-100/DM, Syr. (Bock).
G-Bron Elix. (Laser).
2G/DM, Liq. (Merrell Dow).
Glycotuss-DM, Tab. (Vale).
Guiatussin w/Codeine, Liq. (Spencer-Mead).
Guistrey Fortis, Tab. (Bowman).
Gylanphen, Tab. (Lannett).
Histussinol, Syr. (Bock).
Hycoff-A, Syr. (Saron).
Hycotuss Expectorant, Liq. (DuPont).
Hylate, Tab., Syr. (Hyrex).
Isoclor Expectorant (American Critical Care).
Lanatuss, Expectorant (Lannett).
Lardet Expectorant, Tab. (Standex).
Mudrane GG, Tab., Elix. (Poythress).
Neospect, Tab. (Lemmon).
Novahistine Cough Formula, Liq. (Merrell Dow).
Novahistine DMX, Liq. (Merrell Dow).
Novahistine, Expectorant (Merrell Dow).
Panaphyllin, Susp. (Panamerican).
Partuss-A, Tab. (Parmed).
Partuss AC (Parmed).
Phenatuss, Liq. (Dalin).
PMP, Expectorant, Syr. (Schlicksup).
Polaramine Expectorant (Schering).
Poly-Histine Expectorant (Bock).
Polytuss-DM, Liq. (Rhode).
P.R. Syrup, Liq. (Fleming).
Queltuss, Syr., Tab. (Westerfield).
Quibron, Cap., Liq. (Bristol).
Quibron-300, Cap. (Bristol).
Quibron Plus, Cap., Elix. (Bristol).
Rentuss, Cap., Syr. (Wren).
Rhinex DM (Lemmon).

Robitussin AC, CF, DAC, DM, PE (Robins).
Robitussin-DM Cough Calmers, Loz. (Robins).
Robitussin Cold & Cough, Cap. (Robins).
Robitussin Severe Congestion, Cap. (Robins).
Hondec-DM, Syr. (Ross).
Rymed, Prods. (Edwards).
Santussin, Cap. (Sandia).
Scotcof, Liq. (Scott/Cord).
Silexin, Cough Syr. (Clapp).
Slo-Phyllin GG, Cap., Syr. (Dooner).
Sorbase Cough Syr. (Fort David).
Sorbase II Cough Syr. (Fort David).
Spen-Histine Expectorant (Spencer-Mead).
Sudafed Cough Syr. (Burroughs Wellcome).
Tolu-Sed, Liq. (Scherer).
Tolu-Sed DM, Liq. (Scherer).
Triaminic Expectorant (Sandoz Consumer).
Trihista-Phen, Liq. (Recsei).
Tri-Histin Expectorant (Recsei).
Tri-Mine, Expectorant (Spencer-Mead).
Trind-DM, Liq. (Mead Johnson).
Trind, Liq. (Mead Johnson).
Tussafed, Expectorant (Calvital).
Tussar-2, Syr. (Rhone-Poulenc Rorer).
Tussar SF, Liq. (Rhone-Poulenc Rorer).
Tussend, Liq. (Merrell Dow).
Verequad, Tab., Susp. (Knoll).
Vicks Cough Syr. (Vicks).
Vicks Formula 44D Decongestant Cough Mixture, Syr. (Vicks).
Wal-Tussin DM, Syr. (Walgreen).

• **GUAIFENESIN AND CODEINE PHOS-PHATE SYRUP,** U.S.P. XXIII.
Use: Expectorant, antitussive.

GUAIFENESIN & PSEUDOEPHEDRINE HCL & CODEINE PHOSPHATE SYRUP. (Schein) Pseudoephedrine HCl 30 mg, codeine phosphate 10 mg, guaifenesin 100 mg, alcohol 1.4 %. Bot. 473 ml.
Use: Decongestant, antitussive, expectorant.

GUAIMAX-D. (Central) Pseudoephedrine HCl 120 mg, guaifenesin 600 mg. ER Tab. Bot. 100s.
Use: Decongestant, expectorant.

GUAIODOL AQUEOUS. (Kenyon) Potassium guaiacolsulfonate 40 mg, sodium iodide 50 mg in saturated aqueous naiouli, guaiacol, eucalyptol, menthol/ml. Vial 30 ml.

Use: Expectorant.
GUAIODOL COMPOUND. (Kenyon)
Naiouli oil 0.1 Gm, eucalyptol 0.08 Gm,
guaiacol 0.1 Gm, iodoform 0.02 Gm,
camphor 0.05 Gm/2 ml. Vial 30 ml.
Use: Expectorant.
GUAIPAX TABLETS. (Vitarine) Phenyl-
propanolamine HCl 75 mg, guaifenesin
400 mg/Tab. Bot. 100s, 500s, 1000s.
Use: Decongestant, expectorant.
GUAIPHENESIN. B.A.N. 3- -
Methoxyphenoxy-propane-1:2-diol.
Guaiacol glycerol ether.
Use: Cough suppressant.
GUAIPHOTOL. (Foy) Iodine 1/30 gr, calci-
um cresoate 4 gr/Tab. Bot. 1000s.
Use: Expectorant.
GUAITAB TABLETS. (Muro) Pseu-
doephedrine HCl 60 mg, guaifenesin
400 mg, lactose/Tab. Bot. 100s.
Use: Decongestant, expectorant.
• **GUAITHYLLINE.** USAN. 3-(o-Methoxy-
phenoxy)-1,2- propanediol w/theo-
phylline
Use: Antiasthmatic.
GUAMECYCLINE. B.A.N. N-(4-Guanidi-
noformi-midoylpiperazin-1-
ylmethyl)tetracycline.
Use: Antibiotic.
GUAMIDE.
See: Sulfaguanidine (Various Mfr.).
• **GUANABENZ.** USAN.[(2,6-Dichloroben-
zylidene)-amino] guanidine.
Use: Antihypertensive.
See: Wytensin, Tab. (Wyeth-Ayerst).
• **GUANABENZ ACETATE,** U.S.P. XXIII.
Tab., U.S.P. XXIII.
Use: Antihypertensive.
GUANACLINE. B.A.N. 1-(2-Guanidi-
noethyl)-1,-2,3,6-tetrahydro-4-picoline.
Use: Hypotensive.
• **GUANADREL SULFATE,** U.S.P. XXIII.
Tab., U.S.P. XXIII. (1,4-Dioxaspiro[4.5]
dec-2-ylmethyl)guanidine sulfate (2:1).
Use: Antihypertensive.
See: Hylorel, Tab. (Fisons).
• **GUANCYDINE.** USAN.
Use: Antihypertensive.
• **GUANETHIDINE MONOSULFATE,**
U.S.P. XXIII. Tab., U.S.P. XXIII. [2-(Hex-
ahydro-1(2H)-azocinyl)-ethyl]guanidine
sulfate (2:1), or [2-(hexahydro-1(2H)-
azocinyl)-ethyl] guanidine hydrogen sul-
fate.
Use: Antihypertensive. Reflex sympa-
thetic dystrophy and causalgia [Or-
phan drug]
W/Hydrochlorothiazide.
See: Esimil, Tab. (Ciba).
GUANETHIDINE SULFATE, U.S.P. XXI.

Tab. U.S.P. XXI. Guanidine, 2-(hexahy-
dro-1(2H)-azocinyl)ethyl-, sulfate (2:1).
[2-(Hexahydro-1-(2H)-azocinyl)ethyl]
guanidine sulfate.
Use: Antihypertensive.
See: Ismelin, Tab. (Ciba).
W/Hydrochlorothiazide.
See: Esimil, Tab. (Ciba).
• **GUANFACINE HYDROCHLORIDE.**
USAN.
Use: Antihypertensive.
See: Tenex, Tab. (Robins).
GUANIDINE HCl. (Key) Guanidine HCl
125 mg/Tab. Bot. 100s.
Use: Cholinergic muscle stimulant.
GUANISOQUIN. 7-Bromo- 3,4-dihydro-2-
(1H)-iso-quinoline carboxamidine sul-
fate (2:1).
Use: Antihypertensive.
• **GUANISOQUIN SULFATE.** USAN.
Use: Antihypertensive.
• **GUANOCLOR SULFATE.** USAN.[[2-(2,6-
Di-chlorophenoxy)-ethyl]amino] guani-
dine sulfate.
Use: Antihypertensive.
• **GUANOCTINE HYDROCHLORIDE.**
USAN.
Use: Antihypertensive.
• **GUANOXABENZ.** USAN.
Use: Antihypertensive.
GUANOXAN. B.A.N. 2-Guanidinomethyl-
1,4 benzodioxan.
Use: Hypotensive.
• **GUANOXAN SULFATE.** USAN. (1,4-
Benzodioxan-2-ylmethyl)-guanidine-
sulfate. Envacar.
Use: Antihypertensive.
• **GUANOXYFEN SULFATE.** USAN. (3-
Phenoxypropyl) guanidine sulfate.
Use: Antihypertensive, antidepressant.
GUARDAL. (Morton) Vitamins A 10,000
IU, B₁ 20 mg, B₂ 8 mg, C 50 mg, niaci-
namide 10 mg, calcium d-pantothenate
5 mg, iron 10 mg, dried whole liver 100
mg, yeast 100 mg, choline bitartrate 30
mg, B₆ 0.5 mg, B₁₂ 8 mcg, mixed toco-
pherols 5 mg, dicalcium phosphate an-
hydrous 150 mg, magnesium sulfate
dried 7.2 mg, sodium 1 mg, potassium
Cl 1.3 mg/Tab. Bot. 100s.
Use: Vitamin/mineral supplement.
GUARDEX. (Archer-Taylor) Tube 4 oz, 1
lb, 4.5 lb.
Use: Emollient.
• **GUAR GUM,** N.F. XVIII.
Use: Pharmaceutic aid (tablet binder;
tablet disintegrant).
W/Danthron, docusate sodium.
See: Guarsol, Tab. (Western Research).

W/Standardized senna concentrate.
See: Gentlax B, Granules, Tab. (Blair).
GUAYANESIN.
Use: Expectorant.
See: Guaifenesin (Various Mfr.).
GUIACOUGH CF LIQUID. (Schein)
Phenylpropanolamine HCl 12.5 mg,
dextromethorphan HBr 10 mg, guaifen-
esin 100 mg. Bot. 118 ml.
Use: Decongestant, antitussive, expec-
torant.
GUIACOUGH PE LIQUID. (Schein) Pseu-
doephedrine HCl 30 mg, guaifenesin
100 mg, alcohol 1.4%. Bot. 118 ml.
Use: Decongestant, expectorant.
GUIAMID EXPECTORANT. (Vangard)
Guaifenesin 100 mg/5 ml, alcohol 3.5%.
Bot. pt, gal.
Use: Expectorant.
GUIAPHED ELIXIR. (Various Mfr.) Theo-
phylline 45 mg, ephedrine sulfate 36 mg,
guaifenesin 150 mg, phenobarbital 12
mg, alcohol 19%/15 ml Liq. Bot. 480 ml.
Use: Antiasthmatic combination.
GUIATUSS A.C. SYRUP. (Various Mfr.)
Codeine phosphate 10 mg, guaifenesin
100 mg, alcohol 3.5%/5 ml. Syr. Bot. 120
ml, pt, gal.
Use: Antitussive, expectorant.
GUIATUSS BERTUSS COUGH SYRUP.
(Alton) Bot. 4 oz, 8 oz, 16 oz, gal.
Use: Cough preparation.
GUIATUSS CF SYRUP. (Barre National)
Phenylpropanolamine HCl 12.5 mg,
dextromethorphan HBr 10 mg, guaifen-
esin 100 mg/Syr. Bot. 120 ml.
Use: Antitussive, expectorant.
GUIATUSS DAC LIQUID. (Various Mfr.)
Pseudoephedrine HCl 30 mg, codeine
phosphate 10 mg, guaifenesin 100 mg,
alcohol. Liq. Bot. 120 ml, 480 ml.
Use: Decongestant, antitussive, expec-
torant.
**GUIATUSS DM BERTUSS COUGH
SYRUP.** (Alton) Bot. 4 oz, 8 oz, 16 oz,
gal.
Use: Cough preparation.
GUIATUSS D.M. LIQUID. (Various Mfr.)
Dextromethorphan HBr 10 mg, guaifen-
esin 100 mg. Bot. 120 ml, 240 ml, pt, gal.
Use: Antitussive, expectorant.
GUIATUSS SYRUP. (Various Mfr.)
Guaifenesin 100 mg/5 ml. Syr. Bot. 120
ml, 240 ml, pt, gal.
Use: Expectorant.
GUIATUSS PE. (Barre-National) Pseu-
doephedrine HCl 30 mg, guaifenesin
100 mg, alcohol 1.4%. Liq. Bot. In 120
ml.
Use: Decongestant, expectorant.

**GUIATUSSIN W/CODEINE EXPECTO-
RANT.** (Rugby) Codeine phosphate 10
mg, guaifenesin 100 mg/5 ml, alcohol
3.5%. Syr. Bot. 120 ml, pt, gal.
Use: Antitussive, expectorant.
**GUIATUSSIN W/DEXTROMETHOR-
PHAN.** (Rugby) Dextromethorphan HBr
15 mg, guaifenesin 100 mg, alcohol
1.4%. Liq. Bot. 480 ml.
Use: Antitussive, expectorant.
GUISTREY FORTIS. (Bowman) Guaifen-
esin 100 mg, phenylephrine HCl 10 mg,
chlorpheniramine maleate 1 mg/Tab.
Bot. 1000s.
Use: Expectorant, decongestant, anti-
histamine.
GULFASIN TABS. (Major) Sulfisoxazole
500 mg/Tab. Bot. 100s, 250s, 1000s.
Use: Antibacterial, sulfonamide.
GUNCOTTON, SOLUBLE. Pyroxylin.
• **GUSPERIMUS TRIHYDROCHLORIDE.**
USAN.
Use: Immunosuppresant
GUSTALAC. (Geriatric) Calcium carbon-
ate 300 mg, defatted skim milk pow. 200
mg/Tab. Bot. 100s, 250s, 1000s.
Use: Antacid/calcium supplement.
GUSTASE. (Geriatric) Gerilase (standard
amylolytic enzyme) 30 Gm, geriprotase
(standard proteolytic enzyme) 6 mg,
gericellulase (standard cellulolytic enzyme) 2 mg/Tab. Bot. 42s, 100s, 500s.
Use: Digestive aid.
GUSTASE PLUS. (Geriatric) Phenobarbi-
tal 8 mg, homatropine methylbromide
2.5 mg, gerilase 30 mg, geriprotase 6
mg, gericellulase 2 mg/Tab. Bot. 42s,
100s, 500s.
Use: Sedative/hypnotic, anticholiner-
gic/antispasmodic, digestive aid.
• **GUTTA PERCHA,** U.S.P. XXIII.
Use: Dental restoration agent.
GLYNAPHEN TABLETS. (Lannett) Phe-
nobarbital ⅛ gr, hyoscyamus extract gr,
terpin hydrate 2 gr, guaifenesin 1 gr, cal-
cium lactate 1 gr/Tab. Bot. 1000s.
G-VITAMIN.
See: Riboflavin (Various Mfr.).
G-WELL LOTION. (Goldline) Bot. 2 oz,
pt.
Use: Scabicide.
G-WELL SHAMPOO. (Goldline) Bot. 2
oz, pt, gal.
Use: Pediculicide.
GYNECORT. (Combe) Hydrocortisone
acetate 0.5%. Cream. Tube 15 Gm.
Use: Corticosteroid, topical.
GYNECORT 10, EXTRA STRENGTH.
(Combe) Hydrocortisone acetate 1%,
parabens, zinc pyrithione. Cream. Tube

15 Gm.
Use: Corticosteroid.
GYNE-LOTRIMIN COMBINATION PACK.
(Schering-Plough) **Vaginal Tab.**: Clotrimazole 500 mg. Pkg. 7s; **Topical Cream:** Clotrimazole 1%. Tube 7 g.
Use: Antifungal, vaginal.
GYNE-LOTRIMIN VAGINAL CREAM 1%.
(Schering) Clotrimazole ≃ 5 Gm/applicatorful. Tube 45 Gm, 45 Gm twin-packs w/applicator.
Use: Antifungal, vaginal.
GYNE-LOTRIMIN VAGINAL TABLETS.
(Schering) Clotrimazole 100 mg/Tab. Box 7 Tab. w/applicator, Box 6s.
Use: Antifungal, vaginal.
GYNE-MOISTRIN. (Schering-Plough) Polyglyceryl methacrylate, propylene glycol, parabens. Gel. Tube 45 g.
Use: Vaginal preparation.
GYNERGON.
See: Estradiol (Various Mfr.).
GYNE-SULF. (G & W) Sulfathiazole 3.42%, sulfacetamide 2.86%, sulfabenzamide 3.7%, urea 0.64%. Cream. Tube with applicator 82.5 Gm.
Use: Anti-infective, vaginal.
dep GYNOGEN. (Forest) Estradiol cyplonate in cottonseed oil 5 mg/ml, cottonseed oil, chlorobutanol. Vial 10 ml.
Use: Estrogen.
GYNOGEN L.A. 10. (Forest) Estradiol valerate in sesame oil 10 mg/ml. Vial 10 ml.
Use: Estrogen.
GYNOGEN L.A. 20. (Forest) Estradiol valerate in castor oil 20 mg/ml. Vial 10 ml.
Use: Estrogen.
GYNOGEN L.A. 40. (Forest) Estradiol valerate in castor oil 40 mg/ml. Inj. Vial 10 ml.
Use: Estrogen.
GYNOL II CONTRACEPTIVE VAGINAL JELLY. (Ortho) Nonoxynol-9 in 2% concentration. Starter 75 Gm tube w/applicator. Refill 75 Gm, 114 Gm/Tube.
Use: Contraceptive.
GYNO-PETRARYL. (Janssen) Econazole nitrate.
Use: Antifungal, vaginal.
GYNOVITE PLUS. (Optimox) Vitamins A 833 IU, D 67 IU, E 55 mg (as d-alpha tocopheryl acid succinate), B_1 1.7 mg, B_2 1.7 mg, B_3 3.3 mg, B_5 1.7 mg, B_6 3.3 mg, B_{12} 21 mcg, C 30 mg, calcium 83 mg, iron 3 mg, folic acid 0.067 mg, boron, betaine, biotin, Cr, Cu, hesperidin, I, inositol, Mg, Mn, PABA, pancreatin, rutin, Se, Zinc 2.5 mg. Tab. Bot.

180s.
Use: Multivitamin with calcium and iron.

H

HABITROL. (Basel Pharm) Nicotine transdermal system. Dose absorbed in 24 hours, 21 mg, 14 mg, 7; total nicotine content (respectively) 52.5 mg, 35 mg, 17.5. Patch. Box 30 systems.
Use: Smoking deterrent.
HACHIMYCIN. B.A.N. An antibiotic produced by Streptomyces hachijoensis.
Use: Antibiotic used in the treatment of trichomoniasis.
See: Trichomycin.
HAIR BOOSTER VITAMIN. (Nature's Bounty) Vitamin B_3 35 mg, B_5 100 mg, B_{12} 6 mcg, folic acid 0.4 mg, zinc 15 mg, Cu, iron 18 mg, I, Mn, choline, inositol, PABA, protein, tartrazine. Tab. Bot. 60s.
Use: Vitamin/mineral supplement.
•HALAZEPAM, U.S.P. XXII.
Use: Sedative.
See: Paxipam, Tab. (Schering).
•HALCINONIDE, U.S.P. XXIII. Cream, Oint., Topical Soln., U.S.P. XXIII. Corticosteroid halcinonide. 21-Chloro-9-fluoro-11,16,17-trihydroxy-pregna-4-ene-3,20-dione, cyclic 16,17 acetal.
Use: Anti-inflammatory.
See: Halog Cream, Oint., Soln. (Princeton).
HALCION. (Upjohn) Triazolam 0.125 mg or 0.25 mg/Tab. **0.125 mg:** Bot. 100s, Visipak 100s. (4 × 25s). **0.25 mg:** Bot. 100s, UD 100s, Visipak 100s. (4 × 25s).
Use: Sedative/hypnotic.
HALDOL. (McNeil Pharm) Haloperidol. **Tab.:** 0.5 mg, 1 mg, 2 mg, 5 mg or 10 mg/Tab. Bot. 100s, 1000s, UD blisterpacks 10 × 10s. 20 mg/Tab. Bot. 100s, UD blisterpacks 10 × 10s. **Conc. Soln.:** 2 mg/ml. Bot. 15 ml, 120 ml, 240 ml. **Inj.:** (w/methylparaben 1.8 mg, propylparaben 0.2 mg, lactic acid) amp. 5 mg/ml. Box 10 1 ml, multidose vial of 10 ml Prefilled Syringe 10 1 ml.
Use: Antipsychotic.
HALDOL CONCENTRATE. (McNeil-CPC) Haloperidol 2 mg/ml. Bot. 15, 120, 240 ml.
Use: Antipsychotic agent.
HALDOL DECANOATE. (McNeil Pharm) Haloperidol 70.5 mg/ml to provide Haldol 50 mg/ml. Inj. Amp. 1 ml. Box 3s, 10s.
Use: Antipsychotic.
HALDRONE. (Lilly) Paramethasone ac-

etate 1 mg or 2 mg/Tab. Bot. 100s.
Use: Corticosteroid.
HALENOL, CHILDREN'S. (Halsey) Acetaminophen 160 mg/5 ml. Elix. Bot. 120 ml, 240 ml, pt, gal.
Use: Analgesic.
HALENOL ELIXIR. (Blue Cross) Acetaminophen 120 mg/5 ml, alcohol 7%. Bot. 4 oz.
Use: Analgesic.
HALERCOL. (Mallard) Vitamins A 5000 IU, D 400 IU, E 1.36 mg, B_1 1.5 mg, B_2 2 mg, B_3 20 mg, B_5 1 mg, B_6 0.1 mg, B_{12} 1 mcg, C 37.5 mg/Cap. Bot. 100s.
Use: Vitamin supplement.
HALETHAZOLE. B.A.N. 5-Chloro-2-[4-(2-diethyl-aminoethoxy)phenyl]benzothiazole.
Use: Antifungal agent.
HALEY'S M-O. (Sterling Health) Mineral oil 25%, milk of magnesia in emulsion base. Flavored or regular. Bot. 240 ml, 480 ml, 960 ml.
Use: Laxative.
HALFORT-T. (Blue Cross) Vitamins C 300 mg, B_1 15 mg, B_2 10 mg, niacin 100 mg, B_6 5 mg, B_{12} 4 mcg, pantothenic acid 20 mg/Tab. Bot. 100s.
Use: Vitamin supplement.
HALFPRIN 81. (Kramer) Aspirin 81 mg. EC Tab. Bot. 90s.
Use: Salicylate analgesic.
HALF STRENGTH ENTRITION ENTRI-PAK. (Biosearch) Protein 17.5 Gm (Na and Ca caseinates), carbohydrate 68 Gm (maltodextrin), fat 17.5 Gm (corn oil, soy lecithin, mono- and diglycerides), sodium 350 mg, potassium 600 mg, m Osm/120 kg H_2O, calories 0.5/ml, vitamins A, B_1, B_2, B_3, B_5, B_6, B_{12}, C, D, E, K, P, Ca, Mg, I, Fe, Zn, Mn, Cu, Cl, biotin, choline, folic acid. Liq. Pouch 1 L.
Use: Enteral nutritional therapy.
HALF STRENGTH INTROLAN. (Elan) Protein 22.5 g, fat 18 g, carbohydrates 70 g, Na 345 mg, K 585 mg/L. Vitamins A, C, B_1, B_2, B_3, D, E, B_6, B_{12}, B_5, K, Ca, Fe, folic acid, P, I, Mg, Zn, Cu, biotin, Mn, choline, Cl, Se, Cr, Mo. Liq. In 1000 ml New Pak closed systems with and without color check.
Use: Enteral nutritional supplement.
HALI-BEST. (Barth's) Vitamins A 10,000 IU, D 400 IU/Cap. Bot. 100s, 500s.
Use: Vitamin supplement.
HALIBUT LIVER OIL.
Use: Vitamin supplement.
HALIVER OIL.
See: Halibut Liver Oil (Various Mfr.).
HALLS MENTHO-LYPTUS DECONGES-

TANT LIQUID. (Warner-Lambert Prods) Dextromethorphan HBr 15 mg, phenylpropanolamine HCl 37.5 mg, menthol 14 mg, eucalyptus oil 12.7 mg/10 ml, alcohol 22%. Bot. 90 ml.
Use: Antitussive, decongestant.
HALL'S MENTHO-LYPTUS COUGH LOZENGES. (Warner-Lambert Prods) Menthol and eucalyptus oil in varying amounts and flavors. Stick-Pack 9s. Bag 30s.
Use: Mouth and throat product.
HALLS-PLUS MAXIMUM STRENGTH. (Warner-Lambert) Menthol 10 mg, corn syrup, sugar. Cherry, honey-lemon and regular flavors. Tab. Pkg. 10s, 25s.
Use: Mouth and throat product.
• **HALOBETASOL PROPIONATE.**
Use: Corticosteroid, topical.
See: Ultravate (Westwood Squibb).
HALOBEX T. (Halsey) Dietary supplement.
• **HALOFANTRINE HYDROCHLORIDE.** USAN.
Use: Antimalarial. [Orphan drug]
HALOFED. (Halsey) **Tab.:** Pseudoephedrine HCl 30 mg or 60 mg. Bot. 100s, 1000s. **Syr.:** Pseudoephedrine HCl 30 mg/5 ml. Bot. 120 ml, 240 ml, pt, gal.
Use: Decongestant.
• **HALOFENATE.** USAN. 2-Acetamidoethyl (4-chlorophenyl) (3-trifluoromethylphenoxy)-acetate.
Use: Hypolipemic agent.
See: Livipas (Merck, Sharp & Dohme).
HALOGAN. (Blue Cross) Chloroxylenol, acetic acid, glycerin, benzalkonium Cl. Bot. 0.5 oz.
Use: Otic preparation.
HALOG CREAM. (Westwood Squibb) Halcinonide 0.025% or 0.1%, in specially formulated cream base consisting of glyceryl monostearate, cetyl alcohol, myristyl stearate, isopropyl palmitate, polysorbate 60, propylene glycol, purified water. **0.1%:** Tube 15 Gm, 30 Gm, 60 Gm, Jar 240 Gm. **0.025%:** Tube 15 Gm, 60 Gm.
Use: Corticosteroid, topical.
HALOG E CREAM. (Westwood Squibb) Halcinonide 0.1% in hydrophilic vanishing cream base consisting of propylene glycol dimethicone 350, castor oil, cetearyl alcohol, ceteareth-20, propylene glycol stearate, white petrolatum, water. Tube 15 Gm, 30 Gm, 60 Gm.
Use: Corticosteroid, topical.
HALOG OINTMENT. (Westwood Squibb) Halcinonide 0.1%, in Plastibase (plasti-

cized hydrocarbon gel), PEG 400, PEG 6000 distearate, PEG 300, PEG 1540, butylated hydroxy toluene. Tube 15 Gm, 30 Gm, 60 Gm, Jar 240 Gm.
Use: Corticosteroid, topical.

HALOG SOLUTION. (Westwood Squibb) Halcinonide 0.1%, edetate disodium, PEG 300, purified water, butylated hydroxy toluene as preservative. Bot. 20 ml, 60 ml.
Use: Corticosteroid, topical.

• **HALOPEMIDE.** USAN.
Use: Antipsychotic.

HALOPENIUM CHLORIDE. B.A.N. 4-Bromo-benzyl-3-(4-chloro-2-isopropyl-5-methyl-phenoxy)-propyldimethylammonium chloride.
Use: Antiseptic.

• **HALOPERIDOL,** U.S.P. XXIII. Tab., Inj., Oral Soln. U.S.P. XXIII. 4[-4-p-Chlorophenyl-4-hydroxy-piperidino]-4′-fluorobutyrophenone. Serenace Soln.
Use: Antipsychotic, tranquilizer.
See. Haldol, Tab., Conc., Inj. (McNeil).

• **HALOPERIDOL DECANOATE.** USAN.
Use: Antipsychotic.

• **HALOPREDONE ACETATE.** USAN.
Use: Anti-inflammatory

• **HALOPROGESTERONE.** USAN. 6α-Fluoro-17α-bromo-progesterone.
Use: Progestin.

• **HALOPROGIN,** U.S.P. XXIII. Cream, Top. Soln., U.S.P. XXIII. 3-Iodo-2-propynyl-2, 4, 5-trichlorophenyl ether.
Use: Antimicrobic.
See: Halotex, Cream, Soln. (Westwood).

HALOPYRAMINE. B.A.N. 2-(4-Chloro-N-2-pyridylbenzylamino)ethyldimethylamine. Chloropyramine (I.N.N.).
Use: Antihistamine.

HALOTESTIN. (Upjohn) Fluoxymesterone 2 mg, 5 mg or 10 mg. **2 mg:** Bot. 100s; **5 mg:** Bot. 100s; **10 mg:** Bot. 30s, 100s.
Use: Androgen.
W/Ethinyl estradiol.
See: Halodrin, Tab. (Upjohn).

HALOTEX CREAM. (Westwood) Haloprogin 1% in water dispersible base composed of PEG-400, PEG-4000, diethyl sebacate, polyvinylpyrrolidone. Tube 15 Gm, 30 Gm.
Use: Antifungal, topical.

HALOTEX SOLUTION. (Westwood) Haloprogin 1% in a clear colorless vehicle of diethyl sebacate w/alcohol 75%. Bot. 10 ml, 30 ml.
Use: Antifungal, topical.

• **HALOTHANE,** U.S.P. XXIII. 2-Bromo-2-chloro-1-1,1-trifluoroethane. Fluothane.
Use: General anesthetic (inhalation).
See: Fluothane, Liq. (Wyeth-Ayerst). Halothane, 250 ml Liq. (Abbott).

HALOTUSSIN. (Halsey) Guaifenesin 100 mg/5 ml. Bot. 4 oz, 8 oz, pt, gal.
Use: Expectorant.

HALOTUSSIN-DM. (Halsey) Dextromethorphan HBr 10 mg, guaifenesin 100 mg. In 120 ml, 240 ml, pt, gal.
Use: Antitussive, expectorant.

HALOTUSSIN-DM SUGAR-FREE LIQUID. (Halsey) Dextromethorphan HBr 10 mg, guaifenesin 100 mg. In 120 ml, 240 ml, 480 ml, gal.
Use: Antitussive, expectorant.

HALQUINOL. B.A.N. A mixture of the chlorinated products of 8-hydroxyquinoline containing about 65% of 5,7-dichloro-8-hydroxyquinoline.
Use: Anti-infective.

• **HALQUINOLS.** USAN. 5, 7-Dichloro-8-quinolinol; 5-chloro-8-quinolinol and 7-chloro-8-quinolinol In proportions resulting naturally from chlorination of 8-quinolinol.
Use: Antimicrobial, topical.
See: Quinolor (Squibb). Tarquinor (Squibb).

HALTRAN TABLETS. (Upjohn) Ibuprofen 200 mg/ Tab. Bot. 30s, 50s. Blister pkg. 12s.
Use: Nonsteroidal anti-inflammatory drug analgesic.

HAMA. Hydroxy-aluminum magnesium aminoacetate.

HAMAMELIS WATER.
See: Succus Cineraria Maritima, Soln. (Walker Pharm).
Witch hazel (Various Mfr.).
Tucks (Parke-Davis).

• **HAMYCIN.** USAN.
Use: Antifungal.

HANG-OVER-CURE. (Silvers) Calcium carbonate, glycine, thiamine HCl, pyridoxine HCl, aspirin. Cont. Tab. 6 Gm.
Use: Antacid, analgesic combination.

HANIFORM. (Hanlon) Vitamins A 25,000 IU, D 1,000 IU, B_1 10 mg, B_2 5 mg, C 150 mg, niacinamide 150 mg/Cap. Bot. 100s.
Use: Vitamin supplement.

HANIPLEX. (Hanlon) Vitamins B_1 20 mg, B_2 10 mg, B_6 1 mg, calcium pantothenate 10 mg, B_{12} 5 mcg, niacin 20 mg, liver concentrate 50 mg, C 150 mg/Cap. Bot. 100s.
Use: Vitamin supplement.

HANSEN'S DISEASE. Leprosy.
See: Diasone, Sodium, Tab. (Abbott).

Ethyl Chaulmoograte (Various Mfr.).
Isoniazid (Various Mfr.).
HAPONAL. (Kenyon) Atropine sulfate
0.0195 mg, hyoscine HBr 0.0065 mg,
hyoscyamine sulfate 0.1040 mg, pheno-
barbital 0.25 gr./Tab. Bot. 100s, 1000s.
Use: Anticholinergic/antispasmodic,
codative/hypnotic.
HARBOLIN. (Arcum) Hydralazine HCl 25
mg, hydrochlorothiazide 15 mg, reser-
pine 0.1 mg/Tab. Bot. 100s, 1000s.
Use: Antihypertensive combination.
• **HARD FAT,** N.F. XVIII.
Use: Pharmaceutic necessity.
HARTSHORN. Ammonium Carbonate.
HAUGASE. (Madland) Trypsin, chy-
motrypsin. Bot. 50s, 250s.
Use: Enzyme preparation.
HAUTOSONE. (Forest Pharm.) Hydro-
cortisone 0.5% in Triusol (three polyols)
15 Gm. Box 6s.
Use: Corticosteroid, topical.
HAVAB. (Abbott Diagnostics) Radioim-
munoassay or enzyme immunoassay
for detection of antibody to hepatitis A
virus. Test kit 100s.
Use: Diagnostic aid.
HAVAB EIA. (Abbott Diagnostics) En-
zyme immunoassay for the detection of
antibody to hepatitis A virus.
Use: Diagnostic aid.
HAVAB-M. (Abbott Diagnostics) Radioim-
munoassay for the detection of specific
IgM antibody to hepatitis A virus. Test kit
100s.
Use: Diagnostic aid.
HAVAB-M EIA. (Abbott Diagnostics) En-
zyme immunoassay for the detection of
IgM antibody to hepatitis A virus.
Use: Diagnostic aid.
**HAWAIIAN TROPIC ALOE PABA SUN-
SCREEN.** (Tanning Research) Padi-
mate 0, oxybenzone. Cream Bot. 120
Gm.
Use: Sunscreen.
HAWAIIAN TROPIC BABY FACES. (Tan-
ning Research) SPF 20. Octyl
methoxycinnamate, octocrylene, ben-
zophenone-3, menthyl anthranilate,
PABA free, waterproof. Gel Tube 120 g.
Use: Sunscreen.
**HAWAIIAN TROPIC BABY FACES SUN-
BLOCK.** (Tanning Research) Octyl
methoxycinnamate, benzophenone-3,
octyl salicylate, titanium dioxide, oc-
tocrylene, PABA free, waterproof. **SPF
35:** Lot. Bot. 60 ml, 120 ml, 300 ml. **SPF
50:** Lot. Bot. 120 ml.
Use: Sunscreen.
HAWAIIAN TROPIC COOL ALOE WITH

I.C.E. (Tanning Research) Lidocaine,
menthol, aloe, SD alcohol 40, diazolidinyl urea, EDTA, vitamins A and E, tartrazine. Gel. Jar 360 g.
Use: Emollient.
HAWAIIAN TROPIC DARK TANNING.
(Tanning Research) **Gel:** Phenylbenzimidazole sulfonic acid. SPF 2. Bot. 240
ml. **Oil:** 2-ethylhexyl methoxycinnamate,
octyl dimethyl PABA, waterproof. Bot.
240 ml.
Use: Sunscreen.
**HAWAIIAN TROPIC DARK TANNING
WITH SUNSCREEN.** (Tanning Research) **Oil:** Ethylhexyl p-methoxycinnamate, octyl dimethyl PABA. Waterproof.
SPF 4. Bot. 240 ml. **Gel:** Phenylbenzimi-
dazole, sulfonic acid. PABA free. SPF 4.
Tube 240 g.
Use: Sunscreen.
**HAWAIIAN TROPIC JUST FOR KIDS
SUNBLOCK.** (Tanning Research) **SPF
30:** Homosalate, octyl methoxycinna-
mate, benzophenone-3, menthyl an-
thranilate, octyl salicylate. PABA free.
Waterproof. Lot. Bot. 88.7 ml. **SPF 45:**
Octyl methoxycinnamate, benzophe-
none-3, octyl salicylate, octocrylene, ti-
tanium dioxide. PABA free. Waterproof.
Lot. Bot. 88.7 ml.
Use: Sunscreen.
**HAWAIIAN TROPIC LIP BALM SUN-
BLOCK.** (Tanning Research) Padimate
0, oxybenzone. Stick 4 Gm.
Use: Sunscreen.
HAWAIIAN TROPIC 8 PLUS. (Tanning
Research) Octyl methoxycinnamate,
benzophenone-3, menthyl anthranilate.
PABA free. Waterproof. SPF 8+.
Gel 120 g.
Use: Sunscreen.
HAWAIIAN TROPIC 10 PLUS. (Tanning
Research) Octyl methoxycinnamate,
benzophenone-3, menthyl anthranilate.
PABA free. Waterproof. SPR 10+. Gel
120 g.
Use: Sunscreen.
HAWAIIAN TROPIC 15 PLUS. (Tanning
Research) Octyl methoxycinnamate, oc-
tocrylene, benzophenone-3, menthyl an-
thranilate, PABA free, waterproof. Gel
Tube 120 g.
Use: Sunscreen.
**HAWAIIAN TROPIC 15 PLUS SUN-
BLOCK.** (Tanning Research) Menthyl
anthranilate, octyl methoxycinnamate,
benzophenone-3. PABA free. Water-
proof. Lot. Bot. 7.5 ml, 15 ml, 60 ml, 120
ml, 240 ml, 300 ml.
Use: Sunscreen.

HAWAIIAN TROPIC 15 PLUS SUN-BLOCK LIP BALM. (Tanning Research) Padimate O, oxybenzone. SPF 15, waterproof. Stick 4.2 Gm.
Use: Sunscreen.
HAWAIIAN TROPIC 45 PLUS SUN-BLOCK LIP BALM. (Tanning Research) Octyl methoxycinnamate, benzophenone-3, octyl salicylate, titanium dioxide, menthyl anthranilate. PABA free. Waterproof. SPF 45+. Lip balm 4.2 g.
Use: Sunscreen.
HAWAIIAN TROPIC PROTECTIVE TANNING. (Tanning Research) Titanium dioxide. PABA free. Waterproof. SPF 6. Lot. Bot. 240 ml
Use: Sunscreen.
HAWAIIAN TROPIC PROTECTIVE TANNING DRY. (Tanning Research) SPF 6. **Oil:** 2-ethylhexyl p-methoxycinnamate, homosalate, menthyl anthranilate. Waterproof. Bot. 180 ml. **Gel:** Phenylbenzimidazole, sulfonic acid, benzophenone-4. Tube 180 g.
Use: Sunscreen.
HAWAIIAN TROPIC SELF TANNING SUNBLOCK. (Tanning Research) Octyl methoxycinnamate, benzophenone-3, aloe, cetyl alcohol, stearyl alcohol, cocoa butter, parabens, vitamin E. PABA free. SPF 15. Cream 93.75 ml.
Use: Sunscreen.
HAWAIIAN TROPIC SPORT SUNBLOCK. (Tanning Research) SPF 15, SPF 30. Methoxycinnamate, octocrylene, benzophenone-3, octyl salicylate, titanium dioxide. PABA free. Waterproof. Lot. Bot. 88.7 ml.
Use: Sunscreen.
HAWAIIAN TROPIC SUNBLOCK. (Tanning Research) Titanium dioxide, octyl methoxycinnamate, benzophenone-3, octyl salicylate, octocrylene. PABA free. Waterproof. **SPF 30+:** Lot. Bot. 120 ml. **SPF 45+:** Lot. Bot. 120 ml, 300 ml.
Use: Sunscreen.
HAWAIIAN TROPIC SWIM 'N' SUN. (Tanning Research) Padimate O, oxybenzone. Lot. Bot. 120 ml.
Use: Sunscreen.
HAYFEBROL LIQUID. (Scot-Tussin) Pseudoephedrine HCl 30 mg, chlorpheniramine 2 mg/Syr. Bot. 118 ml.
Use: Decongestant, antihistamine.
HAZOGEL BODY AND FOOT RUB. (Nortech) Witch hazel 70%, isopropanol 20% in a neutralized resin vehicle. Bot. 4 oz.
Use: Astringent, antipruritic.
H-BIG HEPATITIS B IMMUNE GLOBULIN (HUMAN). (Abbott Diagnostics) Hepatitis B immune globulin (human). Vial 4 ml, 5 ml.
Use: Immune serum.
HC, 1%. (C&M Pharm.) Hydrocortisone 1%, petrolatum base. Oint. Tube 15, 20, 30, 60, 120, 240 Gm, lb.
Use: Corticosteroids.
HC DERMA-PAX. (Recsei) Hydrocortisone 0.5% in liquid base. Dropper Bot. 2 oz.
Use: Corticosteroid, topical.
HCG.
See: Chorionic Gonadotropin.
HCG-nostick. (Organon Teknika) Sol Particle Immunoassay (SPIA) for detection of hCG in urine. Stick 30s.
Use: Pregnancy test.
H-CORT. (Torch) Hydrocortisone micronized pow. Bot. 5 Gm, 10 Gm, 100 Gm.
Use: Extemporaneous prescription compounding.
HCV CREME. (Saron) Hydrocortisone alcohol 1%, clioquinol 3%. Tube 15 Gm, 45 Gm.
Use: Corticosteroid, antifungal (topical)
HD 85. (Lafayette) High density barium suspension 85% w/v. Bot. 4 x 2000 ml.
Use: Radiopaque agent.
HD 200 PLUS. (Lafayette Pharm) Barium sulfate 98%. Pow. Bot. 312 Gm.
Use: Radiopaque agent.
HEAD & SHOULDERS CONDITIONER. (Procter & Gamble) Pyrithione zinc 0.3%. Bot. 4 oz, 11 oz.
Use: Antiseborrheic.
HEAD & SHOULDERS DRY SCALP. (Procter & Gamble) Pyrithione zinc 1%, regular and conditioning formulas. Shampoo. Bot. 210 ml, 330 ml, 450 ml.
Use: Antiseborrheic.
HEAD & SHOULDERS INTENSIVE TREATMENT DANDRUFF SHAMPOO. (Procter & Gamble) Selenium sulfide 1%, regular and conditioning forumlas. Shampoo. Bot. 120 ml, 210 ml, 330 ml.
Use: Antiseborrheic.
HEAD & SHOULDERS SHAMPOO. (Procter & Gamble) Pyrithione zinc 1%. **Cream:** Tube 51 Gm, 75 Gm, 120 Gm, 210 Gm. **Lot:** 120 ml, 210 ml, 330 ml, 450 ml.
Use: Antiseborrheic.
HEALON. (Kabi Pharmacia) Sodium hyaluronate 10 mg/ml. Inj. Syringe 0.4 ml, 0.55 ml, 0.85 ml, 2 ml.
Use: Surgical aid, ophthalmic.
HEALON GV. (Kabi Pharmacia) Sodium hyaluronate 14 mg/ml Inj. Syringe 0.55

ml, 0.85 ml.
Use: Surgical aid, ophthalmic.
HEALON YELLOW. (Kabi Pharmacia)
Sodium hyaluronate 10 mg, fluorescein
sodium 0.005 mg/ml Inj. Syringe 0.55
ml, 0.85 ml.
Use: Surgical and dignostic aid, oph-
thalmic.
HEALTHBREAK. (Lemar Labs) Silver ac-
etate 6 mg. Chewing gum. Pack 24s.
Use: Smoking deterrent.
HEARTBURN ANTACID. (Walgreen) Alu-
minum hydroxide dried gel 80 mg, mag-
nesium trisilicate 60 mg/ Tab. Bot. 100s.
Use: Antacid.
HEART MUSCLE DEPRESSANT.
See: Pronestyl HCl, Cap., Vial (Squibb).
HEART MUSCLE EXTRACTS. Adeno-
sine-5-Mono-phosphate sodium.
HEATROL. (Otis Clapp) **Tab.:** Sodium Cl
635 mg, potassium Cl 40.6 mg, calcium
phosphate 31.5 mg, magnesium car-
bonate 9.1 mg/Tab. Safety pk. 1000s,
Medipak 200s, Aidpak 100s, Dispenser
350s.
Use: Fluid/electrolyte replacement.
HEAVY METAL POISONING, ANTIDOTE.
See: BAL., Amp. (Hynson, Westcott &
Dunning).
Calcium Disodium Versenate, Amp.,
Tab. (Riker).
HEB CREAM BASE. (Barnes-Hind)
Washable, hypoallergenic, odorless
base. Jar lb.
Use: Extemporaneous prescription
compounding.
HEDAQUINIUM CHLORIDE. B.A.N.
Hexadecamethylenedi-(2-isoquinolinium
chloride).
Use: Antifungal.
HEDEX CAPLETS. (Winthrop Products)
Paracetamol.
Use: Analgesic.
HEET LINIMENT. (Whitehall) Methyl sali-
cylate 15%, camphor 3.6%, oloeoresin
capsicum 0.025%, alcohol 70%. Bot. 2¹/₃
oz, 5 oz.
Use: External analgesic.
• **HEFILCON A.** USAN.
Use: Contact lens material.
• **HELFILCON B.** USAN.
Use: Contact lens material.
HELISTAT. (Marion Merrell Dow) Ab-
sorbable collagen hemostatic sponge.
Pkg. 5s.
Use: Collagen hemostat.
• **HELIUM,** U.S.P. XXIII.
Use: Diluent for gases.
HEMABATE. (Upjohn) Carboprost
tromethamine equivalent to 250 mcg

carboprost, tromethamine 83 mcg/ml.
Inj. Amp 1 ml.
Use: Abortifacient.
HEMA-CHEK SLIDES. (Ames) Fecal oc-
cult blood test containing slide tests, de-
veloper and applicators. Pkg. 100s,
300s, 1000s.
Use: Diagnostic aid.
HEMA-COMBISTIX REAGENT STRIPS.
(Ames) Four-way strip test for urinary
pH, glucose, protein and occult blood.
Strip. Bot. 100s.
Use: Diagnostic aid.
HEMAFATE T.D. CAPSULES. (Knight)
Bot. 60s.
Use: Hematinic.
HEMAFERRIN TABLETS. (Western Re-
search) Ferrous fumarate 150 mg, des-
iccated liver 50 mg, docusate sodium 25
mg, betaine HCl 100 mg, folic acid 0.4
mg, vitamins C 50 mg, B_6 2 mg, manganese 2 mg, B_{12} 5 mcg, copper 1 mg,
zinc 2 mg, molybdenum 0.4 mg/Tab. 28
Pack 1000s.
Use: Vitamin/mineral supplement.
HEMAFOLATE. (Canright) Ferrous gluconate 293 mg, liver fraction II 250 mg,
gastric substance 100 mg, vitamins C 50
mg, B_{12} 10 mcg/Tab. Bot. 100s, 1000s.
Use: Vitamin/mineral supplement.
HEMA-FORTE. (Stayner) Vitamins B_1 5
mg, B_2 5 mg, B_6 1 mg, calcium pantothenate 2 mg, niacinamide 25 mg,
desiccated liver 300 mg, iron 25 mg, inositol 25 mg, choline bitartrate 25 mg,
B_{12} 5 mcg, C 50 mg/Tab. Bot. 100s,
1000s.
Use: Vitamin/mineral supplement.
HEMALIVE LIQUID. (Barth's) Vitamins B_1
3.15 mg, B_2 3.33 mg, niacin 22.5 mg, B_6
0.81 mg, B_{12} 6 mcg, biotin 3.6 mcg, iron
60 mg, choline, inositol, liver fraction No.
1, pantothenic acid/15 ml. Bot. 8 oz, 24
oz.
Use: Vitamin/mineral supplement.
HEMALIVE TABLETS. (Barth's) Vitamins
B_{12} 25 mcg, iron 75 mg, B_1 2.5 mg, B_2 5
mg, niacin 1.4 mg, C 30 mg, liver 240
mg, B_6, pantothenic acid, aminobenzoic
acid, choline, inositol, Mg, Mn,
Cu/3 Tab. Bot. 100s, 500s, 1000s.
Use: Vitamin/mineral supplement.
HEMANEED. (Hanlon) Hematinic B_{12}, in-
trinsic factor, Fe/Cap. Bot. 100s.
Use: Vitamin/mineral supplement.
HEMAPOIETIC AGENTS.
See: Iron products.
Lipotropic Preparations.
Liver Products.
Vitamins.

HEMASPAN TABLETS. (Bock) Iron 110 mg (from ferrous fumarate), ascorbic acid 200 mg, docusate sodium 20 mg/Tab. Bot. 100s, 1000s.
Use: Iron supplement.

HEMASTIX REAGENT STRIPS. (Ames) Cellulose strip, impregnated with a peroxide and orthotolidine for detection of hematuria and hemoglobinuria. Strip Bot. 50s.
Use: Diagnostic aid.

HEMAT. (Kenyon) Iron 57.4 mg, vitamins B_1 3 mg, B_2 2 mg, B_{12} 1 mcg, niacinamide 5 mg, desiccated liver 2 gr, stomach substance 50 mg/Tab. Bot. 100s, 1000s.
Use: Vitamin/mineral supplement.

HEMATEST REAGENT TABLETS. (Ames) Reagent Tab. for blood in the feces. Bot. 100s.
Use: Diagnostic aid.

HEMATINIC. (Canright) Ferrous gluconate 180 mg, desiccated liver 200 mg, vitamins B_{12} 1 mcg, C 25 mg, B_1 3.3 mg, copper gluconate 0.3 mg/Tab. Bot. 100s, 1000s.
Use: Vitamin/mineral supplement.

HEMATINIC CAPSULES. (Robinson) Vitamins B_1 1 mg, B_2 2 mg, B_{12} 1 mcg, iron 40 mg, desiccated liver 200 mg/Cap. Bot. 100s, 1000s.
Use: Vitamin/mineral supplement.

HEMATINICS.
See: Iron Products.
  Ferric Compounds.
  Ferrous Compounds.
  Liver Products.
  Vitamin B_{12}.
  Vitamin Products.

HEMATRIN. (Towne) Iron 50 mg, vitamins B_{12} 10 mcg, B_1 10 mg, B_2 10 mg, B_6 2 mg, C 150 mg, copper 2 mg, niacinamide 50 mg, calcium pantothenate 5 mg, desiccated liver 200 mg/Captab. Bot. 60s, 100s.
Use: Vitamin/mineral supplement.

HEMATRIN NO. 1. (Kenyon) Ferrous sulfate extract 200 mg, desiccated liver N.F. 200 mg, stomach substance 100 mg, vitamin C 50 mg, folic acid 1 mg, B_{12} w/intrinsic factor concentrate 0.25 IU, B_{12} N.F. (from cobalamin concentrate) 6.26 mcg/Tab. Bot. 1000s.
Use: Vitamin/mineral supplement.

HEMATRIN NO. 2. (Kenyon) Intrinsic factor w/vitamin B_{12} 0.5 IU, liver stomach concentrate 175 mg, vitamins B_{12} concentrate 10 mcg, folic acid 0.2 mg, ferrous sulfate exsiccate 400 mg, C 75 mg/Cap. Bot. 100s, 1000s.

Use: Vitamin/mineral supplement.
HEME ARGINATE.
Use: Acute porphyria; myelodysplastic syndromes. [Orphan drug]
HEMESELECT. (SmithKline Diagnostics) Occult blood screening test. Box 40 test kits.
Use: Fecal testing.
HEMIACIDRIN. Citric acid, glucono-delta-lactone, magnesium carbonate.
Use: Genitourinary irrigant.
See: Renacidin, Pow. (Guardian).
  Renacidin, Soln. (Guardian).
HEMEX. (Vogarell) Oint. Tube 1.25 oz. Supp. Box 12s.
Use: Anorectal preparation.
HEMIN.
Use: Acute intermittent porphyria. [Orphan drug]
See: Panhematin, Inj. (Abbott).
HEMIN AND ZINC MESOPORPHYRIN.
Use: Acute porphyric syndromes. [Orphan drug]
HEMISINE.
See: Epinephrine (Various Mfr.).
HEMISUCCINOXYPREGNENOLONE, DELTA-5 - Panzalone.
HEMOCAINE OINTMENT. (Mallard) Diperodon HCl 0.25%, pyrilamine maleate 0.1%, phenylephrine HCl 0.25%, bismuth subcarbonate 0.2%, zinc oxide 5% in a cod liver oil and petrolatum base. Oint. 37.5 Gm.
Use: Local anesthetic, anorectal.
HEMOCCULT SENSA. (SmithKline Diagnostics) Occult blood screening tests.
Use: Fecal testing.
HEMOCCULT SLIDES. (SmithKline Diagnostics) Occult blood detection (fecal). In 100s, 1000s and tape dispensers (test 100s).
Use: Diagnostic aid.
HEMOCCULT II. (SmithKline Diagnostics) Occult blood detection (fecal). In 102s, kit 100s.
Use: Diagnostic aid.
HEMOCYTE. (U.S. Pharm) Ferrous fumarate 324 mg (FE 106 mg)/Tab. Bot. 100s.
Use: Iron supplement.
HEMOCYTE-F. (U.S. Pharm) Iron 106 mg (from ferrous fumarate), folic acid 1 mg/Tab. 100s.
Use: Iron supplement.
HEMOCYTE PLUS. (U.S. Pharm) Iron 106 mg (from ferrous fumarate), sodium ascorbate 200 mg, vitamins B_1 10 mg, B_2 6 mg, B_6 5 mg, B_{12} 15 mcg, folic acid 1 mg, niacinamide 30 mg, calcium pantothenate 10 mg, zinc sulfate 80 mg,

magnesium sulfate 70 mg, manganese sulfate 4 mg, copper sulfate 2 mg/Tabule. Bot. 100s.
Use: Vitamin/mineral supplement.
HEMOCYTE PLUS ELIXIR. (US Pharm) Polysaccharide iron complex 36 mg, vitamin B_3 13.3 mg, B_5 3.3 mg, B_6 1.3 mg, B_{12} 1 mcg, folic acid 0.33 mg, zinc 5 mg, Mn 1.3 mg/15 ml, alcohol 13%, sucrose. Bot. 473 ml.
Use: Vitamin/mineral supplement.
HEMOCYTE-V. (U.S. Pharm) Liver injection 2 mcg, vitamin B_{12} 15 mcg, B_1 10 mg, B_2 0.5 mg, B_3 10 mg, B_6 1 mg, B_5 1 mg, iron (ferrous gluconate) 3.63 mg, d-glucose 1%, chlorobutanol 0.5%, benzyl alcohol 2% per ml. Inj. Vial 10 ml multiple dose.
Use: Iron and liver combination.
HEMOFIL M. (Hyland Therapeutic) Stable dried preparation of Antihemophilic Factor in concentrated form. Alubm (human) 12.5 mg/ml when reconstituted. Bot. 10 ml, 20 ml, 30 ml with diluent.
Use: Antihemophilic product.
HEMOFIL T. (Hyland) Antihemophilia Factor (Human), method four, dried, heat-treated 225-375 IU/10 ml; 450-650 IU/20 ml; 675-999 IU/30ml; 1000-1600 IU/30 ml.
Use: Treatment of Hemophilia A, for prevention and control of hemorrhagic episodes.
HEMOGEST. (Mills) Betaine HCl 50 mg, ferrous fumarate 100 mg, folic acid 0.05 mg, zinc gluconate 5 mg, copper gluconate 10 mg, manganese gluconate 5 mg, vitamins B_1 1 mg, B_2 1 mg, B_6 0.5 mg, B_{12} 1 mcg, niacinamide 10 mg/Tab. Bot. 100s.
Use: Vitamin/mineral supplement.
HEMOGLOBIN REAGENT STRIPS. (Ames) Seralyzer reagent strips. Bot. 50s. Quantitive strip test for hemoglobin in whole blood.
Use: Diagnostic aid.
HEMOPHILUS b CONJUGATE VACCINE.
Use: Vaccine, bacterial.
See: HibTITER, Inj. (Lederle/Praxis Biologicals).
Pedvax HIB, Pow. (MSD).
ProHIBIT, Inj. (Connaught).
HEMORHEOLOGIC AGENT. Pentoxifylline.
See: Trental, Tab. (Hoechst-Roussel).
HEMORRHOIDAL HC. (Various Mfr.) Hydrocortisone acetate 10 mg, bismuth subgallate 2.25%, bismuth resorcin compound 1.75%, benzyl benzoate

1.2%, balsam Peru 1.8%, zinc oxide 11%/Supp. Bot. 12s, 50s, 100s, UD 12s.
Use: Anorectal preparation.
HEMORRHOIDAL OINTMENT. (Goldline) Live yeast cell derivative supplying skin respiratory factor 2000 units/oz of ointment w/shark liver oil 3%, phenyl mercuric nitrate 1[ratio]10,000
Use: Anorectal preparation.
HEMORRHOIDAL SUPPOSITORIES. (Goldline) Bismuth subgallate 2.25%, bismuth resorcin compound 1.75%, benzyl benzoate 1.2%, balsam Peru 1.8%, zinc oxide 11%/Supp. Box 12s.
Use: Anorectal preparation.
HEMORRHOIDAL UNISERTS. (Upsher-Smith) Bismuth subgallate 2.25%, bismuth resorcin compound 1.75%, benzyl benzoate 1.2%, balsam Peru 1.8%, zinc oxide 11%/Supp. Carton 12s, 50s.
Use: Anorectal preparation.
HEMOSTATICS, LOCAL.
See: Absorbable Gelatin Sponge (Upjohn).
Gelfilm (Upjohn).
Gelfoam, Preps.(Upjohn).
Helistat (Marion Merrell Dow).
Hemotene (Astra).
Oxidized Cellulose.
Thrombin (Various Mfr.).
HEMOSTATICS, SYSTEMIC.
See: Adrenosem Salicylate, Preps. (Beecham-Massengill).
Aquamephyton, Inj. (Merck, Sharp & Dohme).
Carbazochrome Salicylate.
Mephyton, Tab. (Merck, Sharp & Dohme).
HEMOSTATIC TROPICAL. Thrombin.
See: Thrombinar, Pow. (Armour).
Thrombostat, Pow. (Parke-Davis).
HEMOSTATIN.
See: Epinephrine (Various Mfr.).
HEMOTENE. (Astra) Absorbable collagen hemostat/1 Gm. Pkg. 5s.
Use: Hemostatic, topical.
HEMO-VITE. (Drug Industries) Ferrous fumarate to equal iron 79 mg, copper sulfate 1 mg, vitamins C 150 mg, B_1 5 mg, B_2 5 mg, B_6 1 mg, calcium pantothenate 10 mg, niacinamide 50 mg, folic acid 2 mg, intrinsic factor, B_{12} 0.5 NF unit/Tab. Bot. 100s, 500s.
Use: Vitamin/mineral supplement.
HEMOVITE LIQUID. (Drug Industries) Vitamin B_{12} crystallin 8.34 mcg, B_6 2 mg, ferric pyrophosphate soluble to equal iron 100 mg, folic acid 0.25 mg, niacinamide 13.3 mg/5 ml. Bot. 473 ml.
Use: Vitamin/mineral supplement.

HEMOZYME ELIXIR. (Barrows) Vitamins B_1 5 mg, B_2 5 mg, B_6 1 mg, panthenol 4 mg, niacinamide 1 mg, B_{12} 3 mcg, iron 100 mg, choline bitartrate 100 mg, dl-methionine 100 mg, yeast extract, alcohol 12%/fl oz. Bot. 12 oz.
Use: Vitamin/mineral supplement.

HEM-PREP. (G & W) Shark liver oil, phenylmercuric nitrate 1:10,000, bismuth subgallate, zinc oxide, benzocaine/Supp. Bot. 12s, 24s.
Use: Anorectal preparation.

HEMRIL-HC UNISERTS. (Upsher-Smith) Hydrocortisone acetate 25 mg/Supp. 12s.
Use: Anorectal preparation.

HEMRIL UNISERTS. (Upsher-Smith) Bismuth subgallate 2.25%, bismuth resorcin compound 1.75%, benzyl benzoate 1.2%, balsam Peru 1.8%, zinc oxide 11%/Supp. 12s, 50s.
Use: Anorectal preparation.

HENBANE.
See: Hyoscyamus (Various Mfr.).

HENYDIN-M. (Arcum) Thyroid desiccated pow. 0.5 gr, vitamins B_1 1 mg, B_2 0.5 mg, B_6 0.5 mg, niacinamide 2.5 mg/Tab. Bot. 100s, 1000s.
Use: Vitamin supplement.

HENYDIN-R. (Arcum) Thyroid desiccated pow. 1 gr, vitamins B_1 2 mg, B_2 1 mg, B_6 1 mg, niacinamide 5 mg/Tab. Bot. 100s, 1000s.
Use: Vitamin supplement.

HEPANE-LS EXTRA. (Kenyon) Vitamin B_{12} activity 40 mcg/ml. Vial 10 ml.
Use: Vitamin supplement.

HEPARIN, 2-0-DESULFATED.
Use: Treatment of cystic fibrosis. [Orphan drug]
See: Aeropin.

HEPARIN ANTAGONIST.
See: Protamine Sulfate (Various Mfr.).

HEPARIN CALCIUM.
Use: Anticoagulant.
See: Calciparine, Inj. (American Critical Care).

• **HEPARIN CALCIUM,** U.S.P. XXIII. Inj., U.S.P. XXIII.
Use: Anticoagulant.

HEPARIN LOCK FLUSH SOLUTION. (Winthrop Pharm) **10 USP units/1 ml:** Cartridge 2 ml HEP-PAK containing 1 cartridge heparin lock flush Soln. (1 ml) and 2 cartridges sodium Cl Inj. HEP-PAK-2 containing 1 cartridge heparin lock flush soln. (1 ml) and 1 cartridge sodium Cl Inj. **10 USP units/2 ml:** Cartridge 2 ml. **100 USP units/1 ml:** Cartridge 2 ml HEP-PAK containing 1 car-

tridge heparin lock flush soln (1 ml) and 2 cartridges sodium Cl Inj. HEP-PAK-2 containing 1 cartridge of heparin lock flush soln (1 ml) and 1 cartridge sodium Cl Inj. **100 USP units/2 ml:** Cartridge 2 ml.
Use: Maintaining patency of indwelling IV catheter.

HEPARIN LOCK FLUSH SOLUTION. (Wyeth-Ayerst) Heparin sodium 10 units or 100 units/1 ml vial. Pkg. 50 Tubex 1 ml, 2 ml.
Use: Clearing intermittent infusion sets.

• **HEPARIN SODIUM.** U.S.P. XXIII. Inj., Lock Flush Soln., U.S.P. XXIII. (Upjohn) 1000 units/ml. Vial 10 ml, 30 ml 5000 units/ml. Vial 1 ml, 10 ml 10,000 units/ml. Vial 1 ml, 4 ml (Winthrop Pharm) 5000 USP units/1 ml. Carpuject 1 ml fill in 2 ml cartridge.
Use: I.M., I.V. or S.C., anticoagulant in prevention and treatment of thrombosis or embolism. Note: Protamine sulfate is antidote.
See: Hepathrom, Amp., Vial (Fellows-Testagar).
Heprinar, Inj. (Armour).
Lipo-Hepin, Amp., Vial (Riker).
Lipo-Hepin/BL, Amp., Vial (Riker).
Liquaemin, Vial (Organon).
W/Choline Cl, Vitamin B_{12}, folic acid, niacinamide.
Hep-Plex, Vial (Kenyon).
W/Vit. B_{12}, folic acid, niacinamide, choline Cl.
See: Heparin-B, Vial (Medical Chem.).

HEPARIN SODIUM AND 0.45% SODIUM CHLORIDE. (Abbott) 12,500, 25,000 units in 250 ml Inj.
Use: Anticoagulant.

HEPARIN SODIUM AND 0.9% SODIUM CHLORIDE. (Travenol) Inj.: 1000 units in 500 ml Viaflex. 2000, 5000 units in 1000 ml Viaflex.
Use: Anticoagulant.

HEPARIN SODIUM LOCK FLUSH SOLUTION.
Use: Anticoagulant.
See: Heparin Lock Flush, Inj. (Various).
Hep-Lock, Inj. (Elkins-Sinn).
Hep-Lock U/P, Inj. (Elkins-Sinn).

HEPATAMINE. (Kendall McGaw) Amino acid 8%. Inj. Bot. 500 ml.
Use: Parenteral nutritional supplement.

HEPATIC-AID II INSTANT DRINK POWDER. (Kendall McGaw) Amino acids (high BCAA, low AAA), maltodextrin, sucrose, partially hydrogenated soybean oil, lecithin, mono and diglycerides. In 3 oz packet of 12s.

Use: Enteral nutritional supplement.

• **HEPATITIS B IMMUNE GLOBULIN,** U.S.P. XXIII.
Use: Passive immunizing agent.
See: Hep-B-Gammagee, Inj. (Merck, Sharp & Dohme).

HEPATITIS B VACCINE, RECOMBINANT.
Use: Agent for immunization.
See: Recombivax-HB, Inj. (Merck, Sharp & Dohme).

• **HEPATITIS B VIRUS VACCINE INACTIVATED,** U.S.P. XXIII.
Use: Active immunizing agent.
See: Heptavax-B (Merck, Sharp & Dohme).

HEP-B-GAMMAGEE. (Merck, Sharp & Dohme) Hepatitis B Immune Globulin. Vial 5 ml.
Use: Agent for immunization.

HEPFOMIN R INJECTION. (Keene) Liver inj. equivalent to cyanocobalamin 10 mcg, folic acid 0.4 mg, cyanocobalamin 100 mcg. Vial 10 ml.
Use: Parenteral nutritional supplement.

HEP-FORTE.(Marlyn) Vitamins A 1200 IU, E 6.7 mg, B_1 1 mg, B_2 1 mg, B_3 10 mg, B_5 2 mg, B_6 0.5 mg, B_{12} 1 mcg, C 10 mg, folic acid 0.06 mg, zinc 2 mg, choline 21 mg, inositol 10 mg, biotin 3.3 mg, dl-methionine 10 mg, dried yeast 64.8 mg, desiccated liver 194.4 mg, liver concentrate 64.8 mg, liver fraction number 2 64.8 mg, lecithin/Cap. Bot. 100s, 300s, 500s.
Use: Vitamin/liver supplement.

HEP-LOCK. (Elkins-Sinn) Sterile heparin sodium soln. in saline 10 units or 100 units/ml. Dosette 1 ml, 2 ml, multiple dose vial 10 ml, 30 ml.
Use: Maintenance of patency of heparin lock catheters.

HEP-LOCK PF. (Elkins-Sinn) Preservative-free heparin flush soln. 10 units/ml or 100 units/ml. Vial 1 ml.
Use: Maintenance of patency of heparin lock catheters.

HEP-PLEX. (Kenyon) Heparin sodium 2500 units, vitamin B_{12} 50 mcg, choline Cl 100 mg, folic acid 2 mg, niacinamide 50 mg in isotonic saline/ml. Vial 10 ml.
Use:

HEPROFAX.
See: Mucoplex (Stuart).

HEPTABARBITONE. B.A.N. 5-(Cyclohept-1-enyl)-5-ethylbarbituric acid.
Use: Sedative/hypnotic.

HEPTALAC. (Copley) Lactulose 10 g/15 ml, galactose < 1.6 g, lactose < 1.2 g, other sugars ≤ 1.2 g/ Syrup. Bot. 473 ml,

1920 ml.
Use: Laxative.

HEPTAMINOL. B.A.N. 6-Amino-2-methylheptan-2-ol.
Use: Coronary vasodilator.

HEPTAVAX-B. (Merck, Sharp & Dohme) Hepatitis B surface antigen. **Adult:** 20 mcg/ml. Vial 3 ml. **Pediatric:** 10 mcg/0.5 ml. Vial 0.5 ml.
Use: Agent for immunization.

HEPTUNA PLUS. (Roerig) Vitamins B_1 3.1 mg, B_2 2 mg, B_6 1.6 mg, niacinamide 15 mg, calcium pantothenate 0.9 mg, B_{12} 5 mcg, with intrinsic factor concentrate 25 mg, C 150 mg from sodium ascorbate, desiccated liver 50 mg, iron 100 mg (from ferrous sulfate), copper 1 mg, molybdenum 0.2 mg, calcium 37.4 mg, iodine 0.05 mg, manganese 0.033 mg, magnesium 2 mg, phosphorus 29 mg, potassium 1.7 mg/Cap. Bot. 100s.
Use: Vitamin/mineral supplement.

HERBAL CELLULEX. (Nature's Bounty) Vitamin C 83 mg, K 33 mg, iron 9 mg/Tab. Bot. 90s.
Use: Vitamin supplement.

HERBAL LAXATIVE. (Nature's Bounty) Senna concentrate 125 mg, cascara sagrada 20 mg, buckthorn bark PDR. Tab. Bot. 100s.
Use: Laxative.

HERMAL BATH OIL. (Hermal) Soybean oil-based bath oil. Bot. 8 oz, 32 oz.
Use: Emollient.

HEROIN. Forbidden in U.S.A. by Federal statute because of its addiction-causing nature.
See: Diacetylmorphine.

HERPECIN-L. (Campbell) Allantoin, octylp-(dimethylamino)-benzoate (Padimate O), titanium dioxide, pyridoxine HCl in a balanced, acidic lipid system. Lip balm. Tube 2.5 Gm.
Use: Cold sore treatment.

HERPES SIMPLEX VIRUS GENE. (Genetic Therapy)
Use: Treatment of brain tumors. [Orphan drug]

HERPETROL. (Alva) L-lysine, vitamin A, E, B_2, ascorbic acid, Zn/Tab. Bot. 42s, 84s.
Use: Nutritional supplement.

HERPLEX LIQUIFILM. (Allergan) Idoxuridine 0.1%, polyvinyl alcohol 1.4%. Soln. Bot. w/dropper 15 ml.
Use: Antiviral.

HERRICK LACRIMAL PLUG. (Lacrimedics) Silicone plug 0.3 mm or 0.5 mm Pkg. 2 plugs.
Use: Punctal plug.

HES. Hetastarch.
Use: Plasma expander.
See: Hespan, Inj. (DuPont Critical Care).
HESACORB. (Jenkins) Citrus bioflavonoids compound 100 mg, vitamin C 100 mg/Cap. Bot. 1000s.
Use: Vitamin supplement.
HES-BIC. (Kenyon) **Cap.:** Purified hesperidin 100 mg, ascorbic acid 100 mg. **Tab.:** Purified hesperidin 200 mg, ascorbic acid 200 mg. Bot. 100s, 1000s.
Use: Vitamin supplement.
HESPAN INJECTION. (DuPont Critical Care) Hetastarch 6 Gm, sodium Cl 0.9%/100 ml. Bot. 500 ml.
Use: Plasma volume expander.
HESPERIDIN.
Use: Capillary fragility and permeability, hemorrhage.
See: Vitamin P; also Rutin.
W/Combinations.
See: A.C.N., Tab. (Person & Covey).
Ceebec, Tab. (Person & Covey).
HesBic, Cap., Tab. (Kenyon).
Hesper Bitabs, Tab. (Merrell Dow).
Nialcx, Tab. (Mallard).
Norlmex-Plus, Cap. (Vortech).
Pregent, Tab. (Beutlich).
Vita Cebus, Tab. (Cenci).
HESPERIDIN W/C. (Various Mfr.).
Use: Vitamin supplement.
See: Min-Hest, Cap. (Scrip).
HESPERIDIN METHYL CHALCONE.
Use: Vitamin P supplement.
• **HETACILLIN POTASSIUM,** U.S.P. XXII. Cap., Intramammary Inf., Oral Susp., Tab., Sterile, U.S.P. XXII.
Use: Antibacterial.
• **HETAFLUR.** USAN.
Use: Dental caries prophylactic.
• **HETASTARCH.** USAN.
Use: Plasma volume extender.
See: Hespan, Inj. (American Critical Care).
• **HETERONIUM BROMIDE.** USAN. (±)-3-Hydroxy-1, 1-dimethypyrrolidinium bromide, α-phenyl-2-thiopheneglycolate. Hetrum Cl.
Use: Anticholinergic.
HEXABAMATE #1. (Rugby) Tridihexethyl Cl 25 mg, meprobamate 200 mg/Tab. Bot. 100s, 500s.
Use: Anticholinergic combination.
HEXABAMATE #2. (Rugby) Tridihexethyl Cl 25 mg, meprobamate 400 mg/Tab. Bot. 100s, 500s.
Use: Anticholinergic combination.
HEXABAX. (Kirkman) Skin cleanser. Bot. pt.

Use: Antibacterial, topical.
HEXA-BETALIN. (Lilly) Pyridoxine HCl. Inj. Vial 100 mg/ml. Ctn. 10s, vial 10 ml.
Use: Vitamin B_6 supplement.
HEXABRIX SOLUTION. (Mallinckrodt) Ioxaglate meglumine 39.3%, ioxaglate sodium 19.6% (32% iodine). Vial 20 ml, 30 ml, 50 ml, 100 ml fill in bot. 150 ml, 200 ml fill in bot. 250 ml, bot. 150 ml.
Use: Radiopaque agent.
HEXACHLORCYCLOHEXANE.
See: Benzene Hexachloride, Gamma.
• **HEXACHLOROPHENE,** U.S.P. XXIII. 2,2'-methylenebis[3,4,6-trichlorophenol]. Di-(3,5,6-trichloro-2-hydroxy-phenyl)]methane. Hexachlorophene (I.N.N.).
Use: Antiseptic.
See: Derl.
Gamophen, Leaves, Bar (Arbrook).
pHisoHex Prods. (Winthrop Pharm).
W/Soya protein complex.
See: Soy-Dome Cleanser, Liq. (Miles Pharm).
• **HEXACHLOROPHENE CLEANSING EMULSION,** U.S.P. XXIII.
Use: Anti-infective, topical detergent.
• **HEXACHLOROPHENE LIQUID SOAP, DETERGENT LIQUID,** U.S.P. XXIII.
See: pHisoHex Liq. Prods. (Winthrop Pharm).
Use: Anti-infective, topical detergent.
HEXACOSE. Mixture of C-6 alcohols derived from oxidation of tetracosane— $C_{24}H_{50}$.
See: Hexathricin, Aerospra (Lincoln).
HEXACREST. (Nutrition) Vitamin B_6 100 mg/ml, benzyl alcohol 1.5%. Vial 10 ml.
Use: Vitamin B_6 supplement.
HEXADECADROL.
See: Dexamethasone.
HEXADIENOL. Hexacose.
HEXADIMETHRINE BROMIDE. B.A.N. Poly-(NNN'N-tetra-methyl-N-trimethyl-enehexamethylenediammonium dibromide). Polybrene.
Use: Heparin antagonist.
HEXADROL. (Organon) Dexamethasone. **Tab.:** 4 mg. Bot. 100s, UD 100s, Strip 10 X 10s. **Elix.:** 0.5 mg/5 ml, alcohol 5%. Bot. 120 ml.
Use: Corticosteroid.
HEXADROL PHOSPHATE. (Organon) Dexamethasone sodium phosphate 4 mg/ml, 10 mg/ml or 20 mg/ml, benzyl alcohol. **4 mg/ml:** Vial 1 ml, 5 ml, disposable syringe 1 ml. **10 mg/ml:** Vial 10 ml, disposable syringe 1 ml. **20 mg/ml:** Vial 5 ml, disposable syringe 5 ml.
Use: Corticosteroid.

• **HEXAFLUORENIUM.** F.D.A. Hexamethylene bis-[9-fluorenyldimethylammonium ion]
Use: Muscle relaxant.
HEXAFLUORODIETHYL ETHER. Name used for Flurothyl.
HEXAHYDROXYCYCLOHEXANE.
See: Inositol, Preps. (Various Mfr.).
HEXAKOSE. Mixture of tetracosanes and oxidation products.
See: Hexathricin, Aerospra (Lincoln).
W/Benzethonium Cl, p-chloro-m-xylenol, ethyl p-aminobenzoate and tyrothricin.
See: Hexathricin, Aeropak (Lincoln).
HEXALEN. (US Bioscience) Altretamine.
Use: Antineoplastic.
HEXAMARIUM BROMIDE. (Hexamethylene bis(3-pyridyl N-methylcarbamate) dimethyl bromide.
HEXAMETHONIUM.
W/Rauwiloid.
See: Rauwiloid w/hexamethonium, Tab. (Riker).
HEXAMETHONIUM BROMIDE. B.A.N. Vegolysen. Hexamethylene (bistrimethyl ammonium) bromide.
Use: Hypotensive.
HEXAMETHONIUM CHLORIDE. (Various Mfr.) Hexamethylene (bistrimethylammonium) Cl.
HEXAMETHONIUM IODIDE. B.A.N. Hexamethylenedi(trimethylammonium iodide).
Use: Hypotensive.
HEXAMETHONIUM TARTRATE. B.A.N. Hexamethylenedi(trimethylammonium hydrogen tartrate).
Use:
HEXAMETHYLAMINE.
See: Hexastat. Hypotensive.
HEXAMETHYLENAMINE.
See: Methenamine (Various Mfr.).
HEXAMETHYLENETETRAMINE.
See: Methenamine, U.S.P. XXIII. Hexamethylenetetramine Mandelate.
HEXAMETHYLMELAMINE. Altretamine.
Use: Antineoplastic.
See: Hexalen.
HEXAMETHYLPARAROSANILINE CHLORIDE.
See: Bismuth Violet, Soln. (Table Rock).
HEXAMETHYLROSANILINE CHLORIDE.
See: Gentian Violet.
HEXAMINE.
See: Methenamine (Various Mfr.).
HEXAMINE HIPPURATE. B.A.N. A 1:1 complex of hexamine and hippuric acid.
Use: Antiseptic.
HEXAPRADOL HCl. a-(1-

Aminohexyl)benzhydrol HCl.
Use: CNS stimulant.
HEXAPROFEN. B.A.N. 2-(4-Cychlohexylphenyl)-propionic acid.
Use: Anti-inflammatory, antipyretic, analgesic.
HEXAPROPYMATE. B.A.N. 1-(2-Propynyl)cyclohexanol carbamate. Merinax.
Use: Sedative/hypnotic.
HEXATE. (Davis & Sly) Atropine sulfate $1/2000$ gr, extract of hyoscyamus 0.25 gr, methylene blue gr, methanamine 0.5 gr, benzoic acid 0.5 gr, salol 0.5 gr./Tab. Bot. 1000s.
Use: Urinary anti-infective.
HEXATHRICIN AEROSPRA. (Lincoln) Hexadienol 8 Gm, benzethonium Cl 80 mg, p-chloro m-xylenol 800 mg, tyrothricin 40 mg, ethyl-p-aminobenzoate 1.6 Gm/6 oz. Aeropak 3 oz.
Use: Counterirritant, antifungal (topical).
HEXATHRICIN EPISIOTOMY AEROSPRA. (Lincoln) Hexakose (hexadienol) 4.2 Gm, p-chloro-m-xylenol 420 mg, benzethonium Cl 55 mg, ethyl-p-aminobenzoate 2.77 Gm/3 oz. can. Aerospra can 3 oz.
HEXAVITAMIN. (A.V.P.) Vitamins A 5000 IU, D 400 IU, C 75 mg, B_1 2 mg, B_2 3 mg, niacin 20 mg/Tab. Bot. 500s.
Use: Vitamin supplement.
HEXAVITAMIN. (Upsher-Smith) Tab. Bot. 100s, 1000s, UD 100s.
Use: Vitamin supplement.
HEXAVITAMIN CAPSULES and TABLETS, U.S.P. XXI. Vitamins A 5000 IU, B_1 2 mg, B_2 3 mg, C 75 mg, D 400 IU, nicotinamide 20 mg/Tab. or Cap. Bot. 100s, 500s, 1000s, UD 100s. (Various Mfr.).
Use: Multivitamin.
See: Hepicebrin, Tab. (Lilly).
HEXAVITAMINS SC. (Halsey).
Use: Vitamin supplement.
HEXAVITAMIN TABLETS. (A.V.P.) Vitamins A 5000 IU, D 400 IU, C 75 mg, B_1 2 mg, B_2 3 mg, niacin 20 mg/Tab. Bot. 500s.
Use: Vitamin supplement.
HEXAVITAMIN TABLETS, N.F. (Forest Pharm.) Vitamin A 1.5 mg, D 10 mcg, C 75 mg, B_1 2 mg, B_2 3 mg, nicotinamide 20 mg/SC Tab. Bot. 1000s.
Use: Vitamin supplement.
HEXAZOLE. B.A.N. 4-Cyclohexyl-3-ethyl-1,2,4-triazole.
Use: Central nervous system stimulant.
HEXCARBACHOLINE BROMIDE (I.N.N.). Carbolinium Bromide. B.A.N.

HEXCARBACHOLINE BROMIDE. 1,6-Hexame-thylenebiscarbaminoylcholine bromide.
• **HEXEDINE.** USAN. 2,6-bis(2-Ethylhexyl)hexahydro-7a-methyl-1H imidasol[1,5c]imidazole.
Use: Antibacterial.
HEXENE-OL. Hexacose.
HEXENOL. Hexacose.
HEXETHAL SODIUM. (Hebaral) Sodium ethylhexylbarbiturate.
Use: Sedative/hypnotic.
HEXETIDINE. B.A.N. 5-Amino-1,3-bis(beta-ethylhexyl)-5-methylhexahydropyrimide. Triocil.
Use: Bactericide, fungicide.
HEXITOL IRRIGANTS.
Use: Genitourinary irrigants.
See: Resectisol, Soln. (Kendall McGaw).
Sorbitol, Soln. (Kendall McGaw).
Sorbitol, Soln. (Travenol).
Sorbitol Mannitol, Soln. (Abbott).
HEXOBARBITAL, U.S.P. XXI.
See: Sombulex, Tab. (Riker).
W/Acetaminophen, salicylamide, d-amphetamine sulfate, secobarbital sodium, butabarbital sodium, phenobarbital.
See: Sedragesic, Tab. (Lannett).
W/Dihydrohydroxycodeinone HCl, dihydrohydroxy-codeinone terephthalate, homatropine terephthalate, aspirin, phenacetin, caffeine.
See: Percobarb, Cap. (Du Pont).
W/Dihydrohydroxycodeinone terephthalate, dihydrohydroxycodeinone HCl, homatropine terephthalate, aspirin, phenacetin, caffeine.
See: Percobarb-Demi, Cap. (Du Pont).
• **HEXOBENDINE.** USAN. Hexobendine HCl. 1,2-Di-[N-methyl-3-(3,4,5-trimethoxybenzoyloxy)propylamino]ethane.
Use: Coronary vasodilator.
HEXOESTROL.
See: Hexestrol (Various Mfr.).
HEXOPAL. (Winthrop Products) Inositol hexanicotinate.
Use: Hypolipidemic, peripheral vasodilator.
HEXOPRENALINE. B.A.N. NN'-Di-[2-(3,4-dihydroxyphenyl)-2-hydroxyethyl]hexamethylenediamine.
Use: Bronchodilator.
• **HEXOPRENALINE SULFATE.** USAN.
Use: Bronchodilator; tocolytic.
• **HEXYLENE GLYCOL,** N.F. XVIII.
Use: Pharmaceutic aid (humectant, solvent).
HEXYLRESORCINOL, U.S.P. XXIII. Pil,

U.S.P. XXI. Loz., U.S.P. XXIII. 4-Hexylresorcinol. (Various Mfr.).
Use: Anthelmintic (intestinal roundworms and trematodes), minor throat irritations.
See: Listerine Antiseptic Throat Loz. (Warner-Lambert).
Sucrets Sore Throat Loz. (Calgon).
HEXYPHEN-2. (Robinson) Trihexyphenidyl HCl 2 mg/Tab. Bot. 100s.
Use: Antiparkinson agent.
HEXYPHEN-5. (Robinson) Trihexyphenidyl HCl 5 mg/Tab. Bot. 100s, 1000s.
Use: Antiparkinson agent.
H.H.R. (Geneva Generics) Hydralazine HCl 25 mg, hydrochlorothiazide 15 mg, reserpine 0.1 mg/Tab. Bot. 100s, 1000s.
Use: Antihypertensive.
HIBICLENS. (Stuart) Chlorhexidine gluconate 4%, isopropyl alcohol 4%, in a non-alkaline base. Bot. 4 oz, 8 oz, 16 oz, 32 oz, gal. Packette 15 ml.
Use: Antiseptic, germicide.
HIBICLENS SPONGE BRUSH. (Stuart) Chlorhexidine gluconate impregnated sponge brush. Unit-of-use 22 ml sponge brushes.
Use: Antiseptic, germicide.
HIBISCRUB. Chlorhexidine gluconate. B.A.N.
Use: Surgical hand scrub.
HIBISTAT. (Stuart) Chlorhexidine gluconate 0.5%. **Liq.:** Isopropyl alcohol 70%, emollients. Bot. 4 oz, 8 oz. **Towelettes:** Unit-of-use pocket-size towelette impregnated with 5 ml Hibistat.
Use: Antiseptic, germicide.
HIBPLEX. (Standex) Vitamins B_1 100 mg, B_2 2 mg, B_3 100 mg, panthenol 2 mg/ml. Vial 30 ml.
Use: Vitamin supplement.
HibTITER VACCINE. (Lederle/Praxis Biologics) Purified Hemophilus b saccharide 10 mcg, diphtheria CRM_{197} protein 25 mcg. Inj. single-dose vials.
Use: Agent for immunization.
HI B WITH C. (Towne) Vitamin C 300 mg, B_1 15 mg, B_2 10.2 mg, niacin 50 mg, B_6 5 mg, pantothenic acid 10 mg/Cap. Bot. 100s.
Use: Vitamin supplement.
HI-COR 1.0. (C & M Pharmacal) Hydrocortisone 1% in a nonionic, ester-free, salt-free, paraben-free washable base. Tube 30 Gm, Jar 60 Gm, lb.
Use: Corticosteroid, topical.
HI-COR 2.5. (C & M Pharmacal) Hydrocortisone 2.5% in a nonionic, ester-free, salt-free, paraben-free washable base.

Tube 30 Gm. Jar 60 Gm.
Use: Corticosteroid, topical.
HIESTRONE.
See: Estrone (Various Mfr.).
HIGH B12. (Barth's) Vitamin B_{12}, desiccated liver. Cap. Bot. 100s, 500s.
Use: Vitamin/liver supplement.
HIGH POTENCY COLD CAP. (Weeks & Leo) Salicylamide 325 mg, chlorpheniramine maleate 4 mg, dextromethorphan HBr 15 mg, caffeine 16.2 mg/Tab. Bot. 18s.
Use: Salicylate analgesic, antihistamine, antitussive.
HIGH POTENCY PAIN RELIEVERS. (Weeks & Leo) Acetaminophen 300 mg, salicylamide 300 mg/Cap. Bot. 20s, 40s.
Use: Analgesic.
HIGH POTENCY VITAMINS AND MINERALS. (Burgin-Arden) Vitamins A 25,000 IU, D 400 IU, B_1 10 mg, B_2 5 mg, C 150 mg, niacinamide 100 mg, calcium 103 mg, phosphorous 80 mg, iron 10 mg, B_6 1 mg, B_{12} 5 mcg, magnesium 5.5 mg, manganese 1 mg, potassium 5 mg, zinc 1.4 mg/Tab. Bot. 100s.
Use: Vitamin/mineral supplement.
HILL-SHADE LOTION. (Hill) Para-aminobenzoic acid, alcohol 65%. SPF 22.
Use: Sunscreen.
HI-POTENCY B-COMPLEX. (Kenyon) Vitamins B_1 20 mg, B_2 12 mg, B_6 2 mg, B_{12} 3 mcg, C 50 mg, calcium pantothenate 5 mg, folic acid 0.1 mg, niacinamide 25 mg, liver fraction II 30 mg, yeast 175 mg, iron gluconate 30 mg, iron reduced 10 mg, choline bitartrate 20 mg, inositol 20 mg, dl-methionine 20 mg/Tab. Bot. 100s, 1000s.
Use: Vitamin/mineral supplement.
HI-PO-VITES TABLETS. (Nature's Bounty) Iron 5.8 mg, vitamins A 25,000 IU, D 400 IU, E 15 mg, B_1 25 mg, B_2 25 mg, B_3 50 mg, B_5 12.5 mg, B_6 15 mg, B_{12} 50 mcg, C 150 mg, folic acid 0.4 mg, Ca, Cu, I, K, Mg, Mn, P, Zn, biotin 1 mcg, PABA, choline bitartrate, betaine, rutin, inositol, citrus bioflavanoids, desiccated liver, bone meal, lecithin. Tab. Bot. 100s.
Use: Vitamin/mineral supplement.
HIPPRAMINE.
See: Methenamine hippurate.
HIPPUTOPE. (Squibb) Radio-iodinated sodium iodohippurate (^{131}I) Inj. Bot. 1 m Ci, 2 m Ci.
Use: Diagnostic aid.
HIPREX. (Merrell Dow) Methenamine hippurate 1 Gm/Tab. Bot. 100s.
Use: Urinary anti-infective.

HI-PRO WAFERS. (Mills) Casein-lactalbumin fusion 13.3 gr, dl-methionine 5 mg, l-lysine mono-hydrochloride 16.7 mg, l-cystine 5 mg/Tab. Bot. 336s.
HI-RIBO. (Kenyon) Vitamin B_2 riboflavin-5-phos, 50 mg/ml. Vial 10 ml.
Use: Vitamin supplement.
HISMANAL. (Janssen) Astemizole 10 mg/Tab. 100s, UD 100s.
Use: Antihistamine.
HISTACHLOR. (Kenyon) Chlorpheniramine maleate 4 mg/Tab. Bot. 100s, 1000s.
Use: Antihistamine.
HISTACHLOR D-8, D-12. (Kenyon) Chlorpheniramine maleate 8 mg, 12 mg/DA Tab. Bot. 1000s.
Use: Antihistamine.
HISTACHLOR T-8, T-12. (Kenyon) Chlorpheniramine maleate 8 mg or 12 mg/TR Cap. Bot. 100s, 1000s.
Use: Antihistamine.
HISTACHLOR W/A.P.C. (Kenyon) Chlorpheniramine maleate 2 mg, salicylamide 3.5 gr, phenacetin 2.5 gr, caffeine 0.5 gr./Tab. Bot. 100s, 1000s.
Use: Antihistamine, analgesic.
HISTACOMP SYRUP. (Approved) Thenylpyramine HCl 80 mg, ammonium Cl 10 gr, sodium citrate 5 gr, antimony potassium tartrate $^1/_{24}$ gr, menthol, aromatics q.s./fl oz. Syr. Bot. 4 oz, 8 oz. Also available w/dextromethorphan. Bot. 4 oz.
Use: Cough preparation.
HISTACOMP TABLETS. (Approved) Pyrilamine maleate 25 mg, aspirin 3.5 gr, phenacetin 2.5 gr, caffeine 0.5 gr./Tab. Bot. 30s, 100s, 1000s.
Use: Antihistamine, analgesic.
HISTACON. (Marsh Labs) Chlorpheniramine maleate 12 mg, ephedrine HCl 15 mg/SR Tab. Bot. 100s, 1000s.
Use: Antihistamine, decongestant.
HISTACON SYRUP. (Marsh Labs) Chlorpheniramine maleate 3 mg, ephedrine HCl 4 mg/5 ml, alcohol 5%. Bot. pt.
Use: Antihistamine, decongestant.
HISTA-DERFULE. (Forest) Chlorpheniramine maleate 4 mg, acetaminophen 325 mg, phenylpropanolamine HCl 25 mg, powdered opium 2 mg/Cap. Bot. 100s, 1000s.
Use: Antihistamine, analgesic, decongestant.
HISTAFED C COUGH SYRUP. (Life Labs) Pseudoephedrine 30 mg, triprolidine 1.25 mg, codeine phosphate 10 mg, alcohol 4.3%. In 120 ml, pt, gal.
Use: Decongestant, antihistamine, antitussive.

HISTAGESIC D.M. (Bowman) Phenylpropanolamine HCl 25 mg, chlorpheniramine maleate 4 mg, dextromethorphan HBr 10 mg, acetaminophen 324
mg/Tab. Bot. 100s, 1000s.
Use: Decongestant, antihistamine, antitussive, analgesic.
HISTAGESIC MODIFIED. (Bowman) Acetaminophen 324 mg, phenylephrine
HCl 10 mg, chlorpheniramine maleate 4
mg/Tab.
Use: Analgesic, decongestant, antihistamine.
HISTAGESIC MODIFIED TABLETS.
(Jones Medical) Phenylephrine HCl 10
mg, chlorpheniramine maleate 4 mg, acetaminophen 324 mg/Tab. Bot. 1000s.
Use: Decongestant, antihistamine,
analgesic.
HISTAJECT. (Mayrand) Brompheniramine maleate 10 mg/ml, methyl and
propyl parabens. Inj. Vial 10 ml.
Use: Antihistamine.
HISTAJEN. (Jenkins) Codeine phosphate
10 mg, pyrilamine maleate 12 mg, ammonium Cl 175 mg, potassium citrate
131 mg, alcohol 2%/5 ml. Syr. Bot. 3 oz,
4 oz, gal.
Use: Antitussive, antihistamine, expectorant.
HISTAJEN JR. (Jenkins) Chlorpheniramine maleate 1 mg, acetophenetidin
75 mg, caffeine 15 mg, salicylamide 105
mg/Tab. Bot. 1000s.
Use: Antihistamine, analgesic.
HISTALET. (Solvay) **Syr.:** Pseudoephedrine HCl 45 mg, chlorpheniramine maleate 3 mg/5 ml. Bot. 480 ml.
Forte: Phenylephrine HCl 10 mg, pyrilamine maleate 25 mg, chlorpheniramine
maleate 4 mg, phenylpropanolamine
HCl 50 mg/SR Tab. Bot. 100s, 250s.
Use: Decongestant, antihistamine.
HISTALET FORTE. (Major) Phenylpropanolamine HCl 50 mg, phenylephrine HCl 10 mg, chlorpheniramine
maleate 4 mg, pyrilamine maleate 25
mg, lactose, sugar. Tab. Bot. 100s, 500s.
Use: Decongestant, antihistamine.
HISTALET X. (Solvay) **Syr.:** Pseudoephedrine HCl 45 mg, guaifenesin
200 mg/5 ml, alcohol 15%. Bot. 480 ml.
Tab.: Pseudoephedrine HCl 120 mg,
guaifenesin 400 mg/Tab. Bot. 100s.
Use: Decongestant, expectorant.
HISTAMIC CAPSULES. (Metro Med)
Phenylpropanolamine HCl 50 mg,
phenylephrine HCl 25 mg, phenyltoloxamine citrate 30 mg, chlorpheniramine
maleate 12 mg/SR Cap. Bot. 100s,

1000s.
Use: Decongestant, antihistamine.
HISTAMIC TABLETS. (Metro Med)
Phenylpropanolamine HCl 40 mg,
phenylephrine HCl 10 mg, phenyltolox-
amine citrate 15 mg, chlorpheniramine
maleate 5 mg/Tab. Bot. 100s, 1000s.
Use: Decongestant, antihistamine.
HISTAMINE. 2-(4-Imidazolyl) ethylamine.
Use: Diagnostic aid.
HISTAMINE ACID PHOSPHATE.
See: Histamine Phosphate, U.S.P. XXI-
II.
HISTAMINE DIHYDROCHLORIDE.
W/Methyl nicotinate, oleoresincapicum,
glycomonosalicylate.
Use: External analgesic.
See: Akes-N-Pain Rub, Oint. (E.J.
Moore).
W/Menthol, thymol, methyl salicylate.
See: Imahist Unction (Gordon).
HISTAMINE H₂ ANTAGONISTS.
See: Axid Pulvules, Cap. (Lilly).
Cimetidine HCl, Inj. (Endo).
Pepcid, Tab., Pow. (MSD).
Pepcid IV, Inj. (MSD).
Tagamet, Tab., Liq., Inj. (SK-
Beecham).
Zantac, Tab. Syr. Inj. (Glaxo and
Roche).
HISTAPCO. (Apco) Chlorpheniramine
maleate 4 mg, ipecac and opium pow.
0.25 gr, (contains opium 0.025 gr), cam-
phor monobromated ⅛ gr, salicylamide
2 gr, phenacetin 1.5 gr, caffeine alkaloid
gr, atropine sulfate gr/Tab.
Use: Antihistamine, analgesic, anti-
cholinergic combination.
HISTAQUAD. (Richlyn) Phenyl-
propanolamine HCl 25 mg, pyrilamine
maleate 12.5 mg, pheniramine maleate
12.5 mg, phenylephrine HCl 2.5
mg/Cap. Bot. 1000s.
Use: Decongestant, antihistamine.
HISTAQUAD. (Richlyn) Pyrilamine
maleate 6.25 mg, phenyltoloxamine dihydrogen citrate 6.25 mg, prophenpyridamine maleate 6.25 mg/Tab. Bot.
1000s.
Use: Antihistamine.
HISTARON-4. (Approved) Chloro-
prophenpyridamine maleate 4 mg/Tab.
Bot. 100s, 500s, 1000s.
Use: Antihistamine.
HISTARON-12. (Approved) Chloro-
prophenpyridamine maleate 12 mg/Cap.
Bot. 100s, 500s, 1000s.
Use: Antihistamine.
HISTASPAN-D. (USV) Chlorpheniramine
maleate 8 mg, phenylephrine HCl 20

mg, methscopolamine nitrate 2.5
mg/Cap. in sustained-release micro-
dialysis cells. Bot. 100s, 1000s.
Use: Antihistamine, decongestant, anticholinergic.
HISTATAB PLUS. (Century) Chlorpheni-
ramine maleate 2 mg, phenylephrine
HCl 5 mg/ Iab. Bot. 100s, 1000s.
Use: Antihistamine, decongestant.
HISTATIME FORTE. (Major) Phenylpropanolamine HCl 50 mg, phenylephrine HCl 10 mg, chlorpheniramine
maleate 4 mg, pyrilamine maleate 25
mg/Cap. Bot. 100s.
Use: Decongestant, antihistamine.
HISTATROL. (Center) Histamine phos-
phate control 1:1000 and 1:10,000.
Dropper vial 2 ml 1:1000 or vial
1:100,000 intradermal.
Use: Skin test control.
HISTA-VADRIN SYRUP. (Scherer)
Phenylpropanolamine HCl 20 mg, chlorpheniramine maleate 2 mg, phenylephrine HCl 2.5 mg, alcohol 2%/5 ml. Bot.
pt.
Use: Decongestant, antihistamine.
HISTA-VADRIN TABLETS. (Scherer)
Phenylpropanolamine HCl 40 mg, chlor-
pheniramine maleate 6 mg, phenyle-
phrine HCl 5 mg/Tab. Bot. 100s.
Use: Decongestant, antihistamine.
HISTA-VADRIN T.D. CAPSULES. (Scher-
er) Phenylpropanolamine HCl 50 mg,
chlorpheniramine maleate 4 mg, bel-
ladonna alkaloids 0.2 mg/Cap. Bot. 50s,
250s.
Use: Decongestant, antihistamine com-
bination.
HISTERONE INJECTION. (Hauck)
Testosterone aqueous susp. 50 mg or
100 mg/ml. Vial 10 ml.
Use: Androgen.
•**HISTIDINE,** U.S.P. XXIII. $C_6H_9N_3O_2$. L-
histidine.
Use: Amino acid.
HISTIDINE MONOHYDROCHLORIDE.
Beta-4-Imidazolyl-1-amino propionic
acid HCl.
Use: I.M., peptic and jejunal ulcers.
HISTINE-1. (Freeport) Diphenhydramine
HCl 10 mg, alcohol 12% to 14%/4 ml.
Bot. 4 oz.
Use: Antihistamine with anticholinergic,
antitussive, antiemetic and sedative
effects.
HISTINE-2. (Freeport) Diphenhydramine
HCl 12.5 mg/5 ml w/alcohol 5%. Bot. 4
oz.
Use: Antihistamine with anticholinergic,
antitussive, antiemetic and sedative

effects.
HISTINE-4. (Freeport) Chlorpheniramine
maleate 4 mg/Tab. Bot. 1000s.
Use: Antihistamine.
HISTINE-8. (Freeport) Chlorpheniramine
maleate 8 mg/TR Tab. Bot. 1000s.
Use: Antihistamine.
HISTINE-12. (Freeport) Chlorpheni-
ramine maleate 12 mg/TR Tab. Bot.
1000s.
Use: Antihistamine.
HISTINE-25. (Freeport) Diphenhydramine
HCl 25 mg/Cap. Bot. 1000s.
Use: Antihistamine with anticholinergic,
antitussive, antiemetic and sedative
effects.
HISTINE-50. (Freeport) Diphenhydramine
HCl 50 mg/Cap. Bot. 1000s.
Use: Antihistamine with anticholinergic,
antitussive, antiemetic and sedative
effects.
HISTINE DM SYRUP. (Ethex) Phenylpropanolamine HCl 12.5 mg,
brompheniramine maleate 2 mg, dextromethorphan HBr 10 mg, parabens,
saccharin. Bot. 120 ml or 480 ml.
Use: Decongestant, antihistamine, antitussive.
HISTJEN CAPSULE. (Jenkins) Phenylpropanolamine HCl 25 mg, pyrilamine
maleate 12.5 mg, prophenpyridamine
maleate 12.5 mg, phenylephrine HCl 2.5
mg/Cap. Bot. 1000s.
Use: Decongestant, antihistamine.
HISTODRIX. (Rugby) Pseudoephedrine
sulfate 120 mg, dexbrompheniramine
maleate 6 mg/Tab. Bot. 1000s.
Use: Decongestant, antihistamine.
HISTOGESIC. (Century) Phenylpropanolamine HCl 25 mg, pyrilamine
maleate 10 mg, chlorpheniramine
maleate 2 mg, terpin hydrate 2.5 gr, acetaminophen 5 gr/Tab. Bot. 100s,
1000s.
Use: Decongestant, antihistamine, expectorant, analgesic.
HISTOLYN-CYL. (Berkeley Biologicals)
Histoplasmin sterile filtrate from yeast
cells of *Histoplasma capsulatum.* Vial
1.3 ml.
Use: Skin test.
•**HISTOPLASMIN.** Diluted, U.S.P. XXIII.
(Parke-Davis) An aqueous solution containing standardized sterile culture filtrate of *Histoplasma capsulatum* grown
on liquid synthetic medium. Vial 1 ml to
give 10 tests.
Use: Diagnostic aid in testing for histoplasmosis.
HISTOR-D. (Hauck) **Timecelle:** Chlor-

pheniramine maleate 8 mg, phenylephrine HCl 20 mg, methscopolamine 2.5 mg. Bot. 100s, 500s. **Syr.:** Chlorpheniramine maleate 2 mg, phenylephrine HCl 5 mg/5 ml w/alcohol 2%. Bot. 16 oz.
Use: Antihistamine, decongestant combination.

HISTOSAL. (Ferndale) Pyrilamine maleate 12.5 mg, phenylpropanolamine HCl 20 mg, acetaminophen 324 mg, caffeine 30 mg/Tab. Bot. 100s.
Use: Antihistamine, decongestant, analgesic.

• **HISTRELIN.** USAN.
Use: LHRH agonist. Treatment of porphyria [Orphan drug]
See: Supprelin, Inj. (Ortho).

HISTRELIN ACETATE.
Use: Central prococious puberty. [Orphan drug]

HIST-SPAN. (Kenyon) Pyrilamine maleate 25 mg, phenylpropanolamine HCl 25 mg, prophenpyridamine maleate 10 mg/TR Cap. Bot. 100s, 1000s.
Use: Antihistamine, decongestant.

HIST-SPAN NO. 2. (Kenyon) Pyrilamine maleate 25 mg, phenylpropanolamine HCl 25 mg, prophenpyridamine maleate 10 mg, phenylephrine HCl 10 mg/TR Cap. Bot. 100s, 1000s.
Use: Antihistamine, decongestant.

HISTUSSIN-HC SYRUP. (Bock) Phenylephrine HCl 5 mg, chlorpheniramine maleate 2 mg, hydrocodone bitartrate 2.5 mg. In 480 ml.
Use: Decongestant, antihistamine, narcotic analgesic.

HITONE. (Lafayette) Barium sulfate suspension 125% w/v. Bot. 2000 ml Case 4s.
Use: Radiopaque agent.

HI-TOR. (Barth's) Vitamins B_{12} 15 mcg, niacin 1.5 mg, B_1 6 mg, B_2 12 mg, B_6 54 mcg, pantothenic acid 150 mcg, choline 3.75 mg, inositol 5.25 mg/Tab. Bot. 100s, 500s, 1000s.
Use: Vitamin supplement.

HI-TOR 900. (Barth's) Vitamins B_1 13.5 mg, B_2 5.2 mg, niacin 15 mg, B_6 0.6 mg, pantothenic acid 1.2 mg, biotin, B_{12} 2.5 mcg, iron 0.9 mg, protein 7.5 Gm, inositol 50 mg, choline 40 mg, aminobenzoic acid 0.15 to 2.4 mg/15 Gm. Bot. 1 lb, 3 lb.
Use: Vitamin/mineral supplement.

HIVAB HIV-1/HIV-2 (rDNA) EIA. (Abbott) Enzyme immunoassay for qualitative detection of antibodies to human immunodeficiency viruses Type 1 or Type 2 in human serum or plasma. Test kits 100s, 1000s.
Use: Diagnostic aid.

HI-VEGI-LIP TABLETS. (Freeda) Pancreatin 2400 mg, lipase 12,000 units, protease 60,000 units, amylase 60,000 units/Tab. Bot. 100s, 250s.
Use: Digestive aid.

HIVID. (Roche) Zalcitamine 0.375 mg or 0.75 mg/Tab. Bot. 100s.
Use: Antiviral (Phase II/III AIDS).

HIV-NEUTRALIZING ANTIBODIES.
Use: AIDS treatment. [Orphan drug]

HIWOLFIA. (Bowman) Rauwolfia 25 mg, 50 mg or 100 mg/Tab. Bot. 100s, 1000s.
Use: Antihypertensive.

HMG-CoA REDUCTASE INHIBITORS.
Use: Antihyperlipidemic agent.
See: Mevacor, Tab. (MSD).
Pravachol, Tab. (Bristol-Myers Squibb).
Zocor, Tab. (MSD).

HMM.
See: Hexamethylmelamine.

HMS LIQUIFILM. (Allergan) Medrysone 1%, Liquifilm (polyvinyl alcohol) 1.4%, benzalkonium Cl, edetate disodium, sodium Cl, potassium Cl, sodium phosphate monobasic monohydrate, sodium phosphate dibasic anhydrous, hydroxypropyl methylcellulose, purified water, sodium hydroxide or hydrochloric acid. Ophth. Susp. Dropper Bot. 5 ml, 10 ml.
Use: Anti-inflammatory, ophthalmic.

HN₂. Mechlorethamine HCl.
Use: Alkylating agent.
See: Mustargen, Pow. (MSD).

H₂OEX. (Fellows) Benzthiazide 50 mg/Tab. Bot. 100s, 1000s.
Use: Diuretic.

HOLD. (Beecham Products) Dextromethorphan HBr 5 mg/Loz. Plastic tube 10 Loz.
Use: Antitussive.

HOLD DM. (Menley & James) Dextromethorphan HBr 5 mg, corn syrup, sucrose. Loz. Pkg. 10s.
Use: Nonnarcotic antitussive.

HOLD LOZENGES (CHILDREN'S FORMULA). (Beecham) Phenylpropanolamine HCl 6.25 mg, dextromethorphan HBr 3.75 mg/Loz. Roll 10s.
Use: Decongestant, antitussive.

HOLOCAINE HYDROCHLORIDE. (Various Mfr.) Phenacaine HCl.
Use: Local anesthetic.

HOMARYLAMINE HYDROCHLORIDE. N-Methyl-3,4-methylenedioxyphenethylamine HCl.

• **HOMATROPINE HYDROBROMIDE,**

U.S.P. XXIII. Ophth. Soln., U.S.P. XXIII.
Benzeneacetic acid, α-hydroxy-, 8-methyl-β-azabicyclo-[3.2.1]-oct-3-yl ester, HBr, endo-(±)-. 1αH, 3αH-Tropan-3α-ol mandelate (ester) HBr. (Various Mfr.) 5% Soln. Bot. 1 ml, 2 ml, 5 ml.
Use: Mydriatic/cycloplegic.
See: AK-Homatropine, Soln. (Akorn).
Homatropine HBr, Soln. (Iolab).
Isopto Homatropine, Soln. (Alcon).
Murocoll, Liq. (Muro).
HOMATROPINE HYDROBROMIDE. (Iolab) 2% Soln. Bot. 1 ml, 5 ml.
Use: Mydriatic/cycloplegic.
HOMATROPINE HYDROCHLORIDE.
Use: Topically, mydriatic/cyclopegic; anticholinergic.
HOMATROPINE METHYLBROMIDE W/COMBINATIONS.
See: Dranochol, Tab. (Marin).
Homapin, Tab. (Mission).
Hycodan, Tab., Pow., Syr. (Du Pont).
Obe-Slim, Tab. (Jenkins).
Panitol H.M.B., Tab. (Wesley).
Spasmatol, Tab. (Pharmed).
Tapuline, Tab. (Wesley).
HOMATROPINE METHYLBROMIDE AND PHENOBARBITAL COMBINATIONS.
See: Gustase-Plus, Tab. (Geriatric).
Lanokalin, Tab. (Lannett).
Spasmed Jr., Tab. (Jenkins).
HOMINEX-1. (Ross) Protein 15 g, fat 23.9 g, carbohydrate 46.3 g, linoleic acid 1800 mg, Fe 9 mg, Na 190 mg, K 675 mg, Ca, vitamins A, B_1, B_2, B_3, B_5, B_6, B_{12}, C, D, E, K, biotin, choline, folic acid, inositol, Cl, Cu, I, Mg, Mn, P, Se, Zn and 480 Cal per 100 g. Methionine free. Pow. Can 350 g.
Use: Enteral nutritional supplement.
HOMINEX-2. (Ross) Protein 30 g, fat 15.5 g, carbohydrate 30 g, Fe 13 mg, Na 880 mg, K 1370 mg, Ca, vitamins A, B_1, B_2, B_3, B_5, B_6, B_{12}, C, D, E, K, biotin, choline, folic acid, inositol, Cl, Cu, I, Mg, Mn, P, Se, Zn and 410 Cal per 100 g. Methionine free. Pow. Can 325 g.
Use: Enteral nutritional supplement.
HOMOCHLORCYCLIZINE. B.A.N. 1-(p-Chlorobenzhydryl)-4-methylhomopiperazine. 1-(4-Chlorobenzhydryl)hexahydro-4-methyl-1,4-diazepine.
Use: Antihistamine.
HOMOGENE-S. (Spanner) Testosterone 25 mg, 50 mg or 100 mg/ml. Vial 10 ml.
Use: Androgen.
•**HOMOSALATE.** USAN.
Use: Ultraviolet sunscreen.
W/Combinations.

See: Coppertone, Prods. (Plough).
HOMPRENORPHINE. B.A.N. N-Cyclopropylmethyl-7,8-dihydro-7α-[1(R)-hydroxy-1-methylpropyl]-0^3O^6-dimethyl-endoethenonormorphine.
Use: Analgesic.
•**HOQUIZIL HCI.** USAN. 2-Hydroxy-2-methylpropyl 4-(6,7-dimethoxy-4-quinazolinyl)-1-piperazinecarboxylate monohydrochloride.
Use: Bronchodilator.
HORMOFOLLIN.
See: Estrone (Various Mfr.).
HORMOPLETE. (Key) Conjugated estrogenic substance 0.25 mg, methyltestosterone 2.5 mg, vitamins A 12,500 IU, D 1000 IU, B_1 10 mg, B_2 3 mg, B_6 2 mg, niacinamide 25 mg, nicotinic acid 5 mg, calcium pantothenate 5 mg, C 75 mg, E 2 IU, B_{12} 2 mcg, ferrous sulfate 50 mg, pancreatin 100 mg, dl-methionine 15 mg, inositol 20 mg, choline bitartrate 40 mg, calcium 60 mg, phosphorus 30 mg, copper 0.45 mg, manganese 0.5 mg, potassium 2 mg, zinc 0.5 mg, magnesium 3 mg/Tab. Bot. 50s, 500s.
Use: Vitamin/mineral/hormone supplement.
W/Homosalate w/combinations.
See: Coppertone, Liq. (Plough).
HOSPITAL FOAM CLEANER. (Health & Medical Techniques) 0-phenylphenol 0.1%, 4-chloro-2-cyclopentyl-phenol 0.08%, lauric diethanolamide 0.2%, triethanolamine dodecylbenzenesulfonate 0.3%. Aerosol spray 19 oz.
Use: Germicidal, disinfectant.
HOSPITAL LOTION. (Paddock) Diisobutylcresoxyethoxy-ethyl dimethyl benzyl ammonium Cl, menthol, lanolin, mineral and vegetable oils. Bot. 4 oz, 8 oz, gal.
Use: Emollient.
12-HOUR ANTIHISTAMINE NASAL DECONGESTANT. (URL) Pseudoephedrine sulfate 120 mg, dexbrompheniramine maleate 6 mg, sugar, sucrose. Tab. Pkg. 10s.
Use: Decongestant, antihistamine.
12-HOUR COLD. (Hudson) Phenylpropanolamine HCl 75 mg, chlorpheniramine maleate 4 mg/Cap. Pkg. 10s.
Use: Decongestant, antihistamine.
HPA-23. (antimoniotungstate) An experimental compound developed at the Pasteur Institute in Paris to stop or slow the reproduction of the Acquired Immune Deficiency Syndrome (AIDS) virus, at least temporarily.
H.P. ACTHAR GEL. (Armour) Repository

corticotropin injection highly purified 40
U.S.P. units/1 ml. Vial 1 ml, 5 ml; 80
U.S.P. units/1 ml. Vial 1 ml, 5 ml.
Use: Corticosteroid.
H-R LUBRICATING JELLY. (Holland-
Rantos) Tube 5 oz.
Use: Lubricating agent.
HRC-PRENATAL TABLETS. (Cenci)
Comprehensive, well-balanced, vitamin-
mineral formula. Tab. Bot. 90s, 500s.
Use: Vitamin/mineral supplement.
HRC-TYLAPRIN ELIXIR. (Cenci) Aceta-
minophen 120 mg, alcohol 7%/5 ml. Bot.
2 oz, 4 oz.
Use: Analgesic.
H.S. NEED. (Hanlon) Chloral hydrate $3\frac{3}{4}$
gr, 7.5 gr/Cap. Bot. 100s.
Use: Sedative.
HSV-1. (Wampole-Zeus) Herpes simplex
virus type I test system. For the qualita-
tive and semi-quantitative detection of
HSV-1 antibody in human serum. Test
100s.
Use: Diagnostic aid.
HSV-2. (Wampole-Zeus) Herpes simplex
virus type II antibody test. For the qualitative and semi-quantitative detection of
HSV-2 antibody in human serum. Test
100s.
Use: Diagnostic aid.
H.T. FACTORATE. (Armour) Antihemophilic factor (human) dried, heat
treated for I.V. administration only. Single-dose vial w/diluent and needles.
Use: Classical hemophilia treatment.
H.T. FACTORATE GENERATION II. (Armour) Antihemophilic factor (human)
dried, heat treated for I.V. administration
only. Single dose vial w/diluent and needles.
Use: Classical hemophilia treatment.
HTSH EIA. (Abbott Diagnostics) Enzyme
immunoassay for the quantitative determination of human thyroid stimulating
hormone (HTSH) in human serum or
plasma.
Use: Diagnostic aid.
HTSH RIABEAD. (Abbott Diagnostics)
Immunoradiometric assay for the quantitative measurement of human thyroid
stimulating hormone (HTSH) in serum.
Use: Diagnostic aid.
**HULK HOGAN MULTI-VITAMINS PLUS
EXTRA C.** (S.G. Labs) Vitamins A 2500
IU, E 15 IU, D_3 400 IU, B_1 1.05 mg, B_2
1.2 mg, B_3 13.5 mg, B_6 1.05 mg, B_{12} 4.5
mcg, C 300 mg, folic acid 300 mcg, su-
crose. Tab. chew. Bot. 60s.
Use: Multi-vitamin supplement.
HUMAN ANTIHEMOPHILIC FACTOR.

See: Antihemophilic factor
HUMAN COAGULATION. Fraction II, IX
and X. B.A.N. A preparation of human
blood containing coagulating factors II,
IX and X.
Use: Treatment of hemophilia B defi-
ciency.
**HUMAN GROWTH HORMONE FUNC-
TION TEST.**
See: R-Gene 10, Inj. (KabiVitrum).
**HUMAN IMMUNODEFICIENCY VIRUS
IMMUNE GLOBULIN.**
Use: AIDS treatment. [Orphan drug]
HUMAN INSULIN. Insulin Human, U.S.P.
XXIII.
Use: Hypoglycemic.
See: Humulin Prods. (Lilly).
HUMAN MEASLES IMMUNE SERUM.
See: Immune Globulin, U.S.P. XXIII.
HUMAN SERUM ALBUMIN.
See: Albumotope (Squibb).
HUMATE-P. (Armour). Pasteurized, puri-
fied lyophilized concentrate of antihe-
mophilic factor (human). Inj. single dose
vial.
Use: Antihemophilic.
HUMATIN CAPSULES. (Parke-Davis)
Paromomycin sulfate 250 mg/Cap. Bot.
16s.
Use: Amebicide.
HUMATROPE. (Lilly) Somatropin (recom-
binant DNA origin). Inj. 5 mg/vial.
Use: Growth hormone.
HUMIBID DM. (Adams) Dextromethor-
phan HBr 30 mg, guaifenesin 600
mg/Tab. Bot. 100s.
Use: Antitussive, expectorant.
HUMIBID L.A. (Adams Labs) Guaifenesin
600 mg/SR Tab. Bot. 100s.
Use: Expectorant.
HUMIBID SPRINKLE. (Adams Labs).
Dextromethorphan HBr 15 mg, guaifen-
esin 300 mg/SR Cap. Bot. 100s.
Use: Expectorant, antitussive.
HUMIST. (Scherer) Sodium Cl 0.65%,
chlorobutanol 0.35%. Soln. Bot. 45 ml.
Use: Nasal decongestant combination.
HUMORSOL. (Merck, Sharp & Dohme)
Demecarium bromide 0.125% or 0.25%
ophthalmic soln. w/benzalkonium Cl
1:5000. Soln. 5 ml Ocumeter.
Use: Agent for glaucoma.
HUMULIN 50/50. (Lilly) Isophane insulin
suspension (50%) and insulin injection
(50%), 100 units/ml Inj. Vial 10 ml.
Use: Antidiabetic agent.
HUMULIN 70/30. (Lilly) Isophane insulin
suspension (70%) and insulin injection
(30%), 100 units/ml/Inj. Bot. 10 ml.
Use: Antidiabetic agent.

HUMULIN L. (Lilly) Lente human insulin (recombinant DNA origin) 100 units/ml. Inj. Bot. 10 ml.
Use: Antidiabetic agent.

HUMULIN N. (Lilly) NPH human insulin (recombinant DNA origin) 100 units/ml. Vial 10 ml.
Use: Antidiabetic agent.

HUMULIN R. (Lilly) Regular human insulin (recombinant DNA origin) 100 units/ml. Vial 10 ml.
Use: Antidiabetic agent.

HUMULIN U. (Lilly) Ultralente human insulin (recombinant DNA origin) 100 units/ml. Inj. Bot. 10 ml.
Use: Antidiabetic agent.

HURRICAINE. (Beutlich) Benzocaine 20%. Liq. or Gel Bot. 30 ml.
Use: Anesthetic, topical.

HURRICAINE GEL. (Beutlich) Benzocaine 20%. Gel Bot. 30 ml.
Use: Anesthetic, topical.

HURRICAINE LIQUID. (Beutlich) Benzocaine 20%. Liq. Bot. 30 ml.
Use: Anesthetic, topical.

HURRICAINE LIQUID PACK. (Beutlich) Benzocaine 20%. Packet UD 0.25 ml. Box 50s.
Use: Anesthetic, topical.

HURRICAINE TOPICAL ANESTHETIC SPRAY. (Beutlich) Benzocaine 20%. Aerosol 60 Gm.
Use: Anesthetic, topical.

HURRICAINE TOPICAL ANESTHETIC SPRAY KIT. (Beutlich) Benzocaine 20%. Kit: Aerosol 60 Gm plus 200 disposable extension tubes.
Use: Anesthetic, topical.

HU-TET. (Hyland) Tetanus immune globulin (human) sterile soln. 16.5%, gamma globulin fraction of the plasma of persons who have been immunized w/tetanus toxoid. Vial syringe 250 units.
Use: Agent for immunization.

HVS 1 & 2. (Chemi-Tech) Benzalkonium Cl in a specially formulated base. Soln. Bot. 15 ml.
Use: Cold sores, fever blisters, herpes virus.

HYACIDE. (Niltig) Benzethonium Cl 0.1%, sodium nitrite 0.55%. Soln. Bot. oz.
Use: Antiseptic.

HYALEX. (Miller) Magnesium salicylate 260 mg, magnesium p-aminobenzoate 163 mg, vitamins A 1500 IU, C 30 mg, D 100 IU, E 3 IU, B_{12} 2 mcg, pantothenic acid 5 mg, zinc 0.7 mg/Tab. Bot. 100s.
Use: Vitamin/mineral supplement.

HYALIDASE.

See: Hyaluronidase (Various Mfr.).

• **HYALURONIDASE INJECTION,** U.S.P. XXIII. Hyalidase, Hydase Enzymes which depolymerize hyaluronic acid. Hyalase, Rondase.
Use: Hypodermoclyses, promotion of diffusion.
See: Alidase, Vial (Searle).
Wydase, Vial (Wyeth-Ayerst).

• **HYALURONIDASE FOR INJECTION,** U.S.P. XXIII.
Use: Spreading factor.

HYAMAGNATE. Hydroxy-Aluminum-Magnesium-Aminoacetate, Sodium-free.

HYBEC FORTE. (Amlab) Vitamins B_1 100 mg, B_2 20 mg, B_6 2.5 mg, niacinamide 25 mg, C 200 mg, B_{12} 10 mcg, calcium pantothenate 5 mg, iron 10 mg, choline bitartrate 24 mg, inositol 10 mg, biotin 5 mcg, liver 50 mg, yeast 100 mg/Tab. Bot. 30s, 100s.
Use: Vitamin/mineral supplement.

HYBOLIN DECANOATE. (Hyrex) Nandrolone decanoate 50 mg or 100 mg/ml in oil. Vial 2 ml.
Use: Anabolic steroid.

HYBOLIN IMPROVED. (Hyrex) Nandrolone phenpropionate 25 mg or 50 mg/ml in oil. Vial 2 ml.
Use: Anabolic steroid.

• **HYCANTHONE.** USAN. 1-[(2-(Diethylamino)-ethyl)-amino]-4-(hydroxymethyl)thioxanthen-9-one.
Use: Schistosomacide.

HYCLORITE. Sodium Hypochlorite soln., U.S.P. XXIII.

HYCODAN. (Du Pont) Hydrocodone bitartrate 5 mg, homatropine methylbromide 1.5 mg/5 ml or Tab. **Syr.:** Bot. pt, gal. **Tab.:** Bot. 100s, 500s.
Use: Antitussive combination.

HYCOFF-A-NN LIQUID. (Saron) Dextromethorphan HBr 15 mg, pseudoephedrine HCl 45 mg, dyphylline 100 mg/15 ml. Alcohol free. Bot. pt.
Use: Antitussive, decongestant, bronchodilator.

HYCOFF X-NN. (Saron) Dextromethorphan HBr 10 mg, pseudoephedrine HCl 30 mg/5 ml. Alcohol and sugar free. Bot. pt.
Use: Antitussive, decongestant.

HYCOMINE COMPOUND TABLETS. (Du Pont) Hydrocodone bitartrate 5 mg, chlorpheniramine maleate 2 mg, phenylephrine HCl 10 mg, acetaminophen 250 mg, caffeine (anhydrous) 30 mg/Tab. Bot. 100s, 500s.
Use: Antitussive, antihistamine, decon-

gestant, analgesic.

HYCOMINE PEDIATRIC SYRUP. (Du Pont) Hydrocodone bitartrate 2.5 mg, phenylpropanolamine HCl 12.5 mg/5 ml. Bot. 480 ml.
Use: Antitussive, decongestant.

HYCOMINE SYRUP. (Du Pont) Hydrocodone bitartrate 5 mg, phenylpropanolamine HCl 25 mg/5 ml. Syr. Bot. pt, gal.
Use: Antitussive, decongestant.

HYCORT CREAM. (Everett) Hydrocortisone 1% in a cream base. Tube oz.
Use: Corticosteroid, topical.

HYCORT OINTMENT. (Everett) Hydrocortisone 1% in ointment base. Tube oz.
Use: Corticosteroid, topical.

HYCORTOLE. (Premo) Hydrocortisone. **Cream:** 0.5%: 5 Gm, 20 Gm; 1%: 5 Gm, 20 Gm, 4 oz; 2.5%: Tube 5 Gm, 20 Gm; **Oint.:** 1% or 2.5%. Tube 5 Gm, 20 Gm.
Use: Corticosteroid, topical.

HYCOTUSS EXPECTORANT. (Du Pont) Hydrocodone bitartrate 5 mg, guaifenesin 100 mg, alcohol 10%(v/v)/5 ml. Bot. 480 ml.
Use: Antitussive, expectorant.

HYDANTOIN DERIVATIVES.
Use: Anticonvulsant.
See: Dilantin, Preps. (Parke-Davis). Diphenylhydantoin Sodium, U.S.P. Ethotoin.
Mesantoin, Tab. (Sandoz).
Phenantoin.

HYDASE.
Use: Hypodermoclyses, promotion of diffusion.
See: Hyaluronidase (Various Mfr.).

HYDELTRASOL INJECTION. (Merck, Sharp & Dohme) Prednisolone sodium phosphate 20 mg/ml w/niacinamide 25 mg, sodium hydroxide to adjust pH, disodium edetate 0.5 mg, sodium bisulfite 1 mg, phenol 5 mg, water for injection q.s. 1 ml. Vial 2 ml, 5 ml.
Use: Corticosteroid.

HYDELTRA-T.B.A. (Merck, Sharp & Dohme) Prednisolone tebutate 20 mg/ml w/sodium citrate 1 mg, polysorbate 80 1 mg, sorbitol soln. 0.5 ml (equivalent to 450 mg d-sorbitol), benzyl alcohol 9 mg, water for injection q.s. 1 ml. Vial 1 ml, 5 ml.
Use: Corticosteroid.

HYDERGINE LC LIQUID CAPSULES. (Sandoz) Ergoloid mesylates 1 mg/Cap. Bot. 100s, 500s. SandoPak 100s, 500s.
Use: Psychotherapeutic agent.

HYDERGINE LIQUID. (Sandoz) Equal parts of dihydroergocornine, dihydroer-

gocristine, dihydroergocryptine. (Ergoloid Mesylates). 1 mg/ml. Bot. 100 ml w/dropper.
Use: Psychotherapeutic agent.

HYDERGINE, ORAL. (Sandoz) Equal parts of dihydroergocornine, dihydroergocristine, dihydroergocryptine (Ergoloid Mesylates). 1 mg/Tab. Bot. 100s, 500s. SandoPak (UD) 100s, 500s.
Use: Psychotherapeutic agent.

HYDERGINE, SUBLINGUAL. (Sandoz) Equal parts of dihydroergocornine, dihydroergocristine, dihydroergocryptine (Ergoloid Mesylates). 0.5 mg or 1 mg/Tab. Bot. 100s, 1000s, SandoPak (UD) 100s.
Use: Psychotherapeutic agent.

HYDEX. (Moore Kirk) Methamphetamine HCl 5 mg or 10 mg/Tab. Bot. 1000s.
Use: CNS stimulant.

HYDORIL. (Cenci) Hydrochlorthiazide 25 mg or 50 mg/Tab. Bot. 100s, 1000s.
Use: Diuretic.

HYDRABAMINE PHENOXYMETHYL PENICILLIN.
See: Penicillin V Hydrabamine.

HYDRACRYLIC ACID BETA LACTONE.
See: Propiolactone.

HYDRALAZINE. (Solopak) Hydralazine HCl 20 mg/ml Inj. Vial 1 ml.
Use: Antihypertensive.

• **HYDRALAZINE HCl,** U.S.P. XXIII. Inj., Tab., U.S.P. XXIII. 1-Hydrazinophthalazine HCl. Phthalazine, 1-hydrazino-, HCl. (Various Mfr.) **10 mg, 25 mg, 50 mg:** Tab. Bot. 100s, 1000s, UD 100s; **100 mg:** Tab. Bot. 100s, 1000s.
Use: Antihypertensive.
See: Apresoline, Amp., Tab. (Ciba). Dralzine, Tab. (Lemmon).
Hydralyn, Tab. (Kenyon).
W/Hydrochlorothiazide.
See: Apresazide, Cap. (Ciba). Apresoline-Esidrix, Tab. (Ciba). Hydralazide, Tab. (Zenith). Hydroserpine Plus, Tab. (Zenith).
W/Reserpine.
See: Dralserp, Tab. (Lemmon). Serpasil-Apresoline, Tab. (Ciba).
W/Reserpine, hydrochlorothiazide (Esidrix).
See: Harbolin, Tab. (Arcum). Ser-Ap-Es, Tab. (Ciba). Unipres, Tab. (Solvay).

• **HYDRALAZINE POLISTIREX.** USAN.
Use: Antihypertensive.

HYDRALYN. (Kenyon) Hydralazine HCl 25 mg, 50 mg/Tab. Bot. 100s, 1000s.
Use: Antihypertensive.

HYDRA MAG TABLETS. (Vale) Alu-

minum hydroxide gel, dried, 195 mg, magnesium trisilicate 195 mg, kaolin 162 mg/Tab. Bot. 1000s.
Use: Antacid.
HYDRAMYN. (LuChem) Diphenhydramine HCl 12.5 mg/5 ml, alcohol 5%. Syr. Bot. pt.
Use: Antihistamine.
HYDRARGAPHEN. B.A.N. 2,2'-(Binaphthalene-3-sulfonyloxyphenylmercury). Phenylmercury 2:2-dinaphthylmethane-3:3-disulfonate.
Use: Antiparasitic; anti-infective.
HYDRASERP. (Geneva) Hydrochlorothiazide 25 mg or 50 mg, reserpine 0.1 mg/Tab. Bot. 100s, 1000s.
Use: Antihypertensive combination.
HYDRASTINE. (Penick) Alkaloid. Bot. oz.
HYDRASTINE HYDROCHLORIDE. (Penick) Pow. Bot. oz.
Use: Uterine hemostatic.
HYDRATE. (Hyrex) Dimenhydrinate 50 mg/ml w/propylene glycol 50%, benzyl alcohol 5%. Amp. 1 ml. Box 25s, 100s; Vial 10 ml.
Use: Antiemetic/antivertigo, antihistamine.
HYDRAZIDE CAPSULES. (Goldline) **25/25:** Hydrochlorothiazide 25 mg, hydralazine 25 mg/Cap. **50/50:** Hydrochlorothiazide 50 mg, hydralazine 50 mg/Cap. Bot. 100s.
Use: Antihypertensive.
HYDRA-ZIDE CAPSULES. (Par Pharm.) Hydralazine HCl 50 mg, hydrochlorothiazide 50 mg/Cap. Bot. 100s, 500s, 1000s.
Use: Antihypertensive.
HYDRAZONE. 3-(4-Methyl-piperazinyliminomethyl)rifamycin SV.
Use: Pulmonary tuberculosis.
See: Rimactane, Cap. (Ciba).
HYDREA. (Squibb Mark) Hydroxyurea. 500 mg/Cap. Bot. 100s.
Use: Antineoplastic agent.
HYDREX. (Trimen) Benzthiazide 50 mg/Tab. Bot. 100s.
Use: Diuretics.
HYDRIODIC ACID. (Various Mfr.).
Use: Expectorant.
HYDRIODIC ACID THERAPY.
See: Aminoacetic Acid HI.
HYDRISEA LOTION. (Pedinol) Dead sea salts concentrate 8%, sodium, potassium, calcium magnesium Cl, propylene glycol stearate, polysorbate 40, silicone oil, coloring agent. Bot. 4 oz.
Use: Hyperkeratotic, emollient.
HYDRISINOL CREME AND LOTION. (Pedinol) Sulfonated hydrogenated cas-

tor oil. **Cream:** Spout Cap Jar 4 oz, lb. **Lot.:** Bot. 8 oz.
Use: Emollient.
HYDRO-12. (Table Rock) Crystalline hydroxocobalamin 1000 mcg/ml Pkg. 10 ml.
Use: Vitamin B_{12} supplement.
HYDRO-BAN CAPSULES. (Whiteworth) Juniper oil 10 mg, uva ursi 50 mg, buchu extract 50 mg, parsley piert extract 50 mg, iron 6 mg/Cap. Bot. 42s.
Use: Diuretic with iron.
HYDROBEXAN. (Keene) Hydroxocobalamin 1000 mcg/ml. Inj. Vial 30 ml.
Use: Vitamin B_{12} supplement.
HYDROCARE CLEANING AND DISINFECTING. (Allergan) Tris(2-hydroxyethyl) tallow ammonium Cl 0.013%, thimerosal 0.0002%, bis(2-hydroxyethyl) tallow ammonium Cl, sodium bicarbonate, dibasic, monobasic and anhydrous sodium phosphate, hydrochloric acid, propylene glycol, polysorbate 80, special soluble polyhema. Soln. Bot. 240 ml, 360 ml.
Use: Soft contact lens disinfective.
HYDROCARE PRESERVED SALINE. (Allergan) Isotonic, buffered, NaCl, sodium hexametaphosphate, sodium hydroxide, boric acid, sodium borate, EDTA 0.01%, thimerosal 0.001%. Soln. Bot. 240 ml, 360 ml.
Use: Soft contact lens rinsing/storage solution.
HYDROCET. (Carnrick) Hydrocodone bitartrate 5 mg, acetaminophen 500 mg/Cap. Bot. 100s, UD Box 4 × 25s.
Use: Narcotic analgesic combination.
HYDROCHLORATE. Same as Hydrochloride.
•**HYDROCHLORIC ACID,** N.F XVII. Diluted, N.F. XVIII. (Various Mfr.) Muriatic Acid, Absolute 38%. Diluted 10%.
Use: Well diluted, achlorhydria; pharmaceutic aid (acidifying agent).
HYDROCHLORIC ACID THERAPY.
Use: Gastric acidifier.
See: Betaine HCl (Various Mfr.). Glutamic Acid HCl (Various Mfr.). Glycine HCl (Various Mfr.).
HYDROCHLOROSERPINE. (Freeport) Hydralazine HCl 25 mg, hydrochlorthiazide 15 mg, reserpine 0.1 mg/Tab. Bot. 1000s.
Use: Antihypertensive combination.
HYDROCHOLERETICS.
See: Bile Salts (Various Mfr.). Dehydrocholic Acid (Various Mfr.). Desoxycholic Acid (Various Mfr.). Ox Bile Extract (Various Mfr.).

HYDROCHOLERETIC COMBINATIONS.
See: G.B.S., Tab. (Forest).
• **HYDROCHLOROTHIAZIDE,** U.S.P. XXI-
II. Tab. U.S.P. XXIII. 2H-1,2,4-Benzothia-
diazine-7-sulfonamide, 6-chloro-3,4-di-
hydro-,1,1-dioxide. 6-Chloro-3,4-dihy-
dro-2H-1,2,4-Benzothiadiazene-7-sulfon
amide 1, 1-dioxide.
Use: Diuretic.
See: Chlorzide, Tab. (Foy).
Delco-Retic, Tab. (Delco).
Diu-Scrip, Cap. (Scrip).
Esidrix, Tab. (Ciba).
Hydromal, Tab. (Mallard).
HydroDiuril, Tab. (Merck, Sharp &
Dohme).
Hydrozide-50, Tab. (Mayrand).
Kenazide-E,-H, Tab. (Kenyon).
Oretic, Tab. (Abbott).
Thiuretic, Tab. (Parke-Davis).
Zide, Tab. (Solvay).
W/Deserpidine.
See: Oreticyl, Tab. (Abbott).
W/Enalapril.
See: Vaseretic, Tab. (Merck, Sharp &
Dohme).
W/Guanethidine monosulfate.
See: Esimil, Tab. (Ciba).
W/Hydralazine HCl.
See: Apresazide, Cap. (Ciba).
Apresoline-Esidrix, Tab. (Ciba).
Hydralazide, Tab. (Zenith).
W/Labetalol.
See: Trandide, Tab. (Glaxo).
W/Lisinopril.
See: Prinzide, Tab. (Merck).
W/Methyldopa.
See: Aldoril, Tab. (Merck, Sharp &
Dohme).
W/Propranolol.
See: Inderide, Tab. (Wyeth-Ayerst).
W/Reserpine.
See: Aquapres-R, Tab. (Castal).
Hydropres, Tab. (Merck, Sharp &
Dohme).
Hydroserp, Tab. (Zenith).
Hydroserpine, Tab. (Geneva).
Hydrotensin-50, Tab. (Mayrand).
Hyperserp, Tab. (Elder).
Mallopress, Tab. (Mallard).
Serpasil-Esidrix, Tab. (Ciba).
W/Reserpine, Hydralazine HCl.
See: Harbolin, Tab. (Arcum).
Hydroserpine Plus, Tab. (Zenith).
SER-AP-ES, Tab. (Ciba).
Unipres, Tab. (Solvay).
W/Spironolactone.
See: Aldactazide, Tab. (Searle).
W/Timolol maleate.
See: Timolide, Tab. (Merck, Sharp &

Dohme).
W/Triamterene.
See: Dyazide, Cap. (SK-Beecham).
HYDROCIL INSTANT. (Solvay) Blond
psyllium coating containing psyllium 3.5
Gm/3.7 Gm dose. Tan granular, instant
mix, sugar-free, low sodium, low potas-
sium powder. UD packets. 3.7 Gm in
30s, 500s, Jar 250 Gm.
Use: Laxative.
HYDRO COBEX. (Pasadena Research)
Hydroxocobalamin 1000 mcg/Vial 30 ml.
Use: Vitamin B_{12} supplement.
HYDROCODONE/APAP. (Pharmics) Hy-
drocodone bitartrate 7.5 mg, aceta-
minophen 500 mg. Tab. Bot. 100s, 500s.
Use: Narcotic analgesic combination.
• **HYDROCODONE BITARTRATE,** U.S.P.
XXIII. Tab., U.S.P. XXIII. Dihy-
drocodeinone bitartrate. 4,5α-Epoxy-3-
methoxy-17-methylmorphinan-6-one
tartrate (1:1) hydrate (2:5).
Use: Antitussive.
See: Dicodethal, Elix. (Lannett).
W/Combinations.
See: Hydrocet, Cap. (Carnrick).
Hydrocodone/APAP, Tab. (Pharmics).
Medipain 5, Cap. (Medi-Plex).
Panacet 5/500, Tab. (ECK Pharm.).
Panasal 5/500, Tab. (ECR Pharm.).
Tyrodone, Liq. (Major).
Vicodin, Tab. (Knoll).
**HYDROCODONE BITARTRATE AND AC-
ETAMINOPHEN CAPSULES.** (Various)
Hydrocodone bitartrate 5 mg, aceta-
minophen 500 mg/Cap. Bot. 100s, 500s.
Use: Narcotic/analgesic combination.
**HYDROCODONE BITARTRATE AND AC-
ETAMINOPHEN TABLETS.** (Watson)
Hydrocodone bitartrate 5 mg, aceta-
minophen 500 mg/Tab. Bot. 30s, 100s,
500s.
Use: Narcotic/analgesic combination.
**HYDROCODONE BITARTRATE AND
PHENYLPROPANOLAMINE HCl PEDI-
ATRIC SYRUP.** (PBI) Phenyl-
propanolamine HCl 12.5 mg, hy-
drocodone bitartrate 2.5 mg/Syr. Bot.
118 ml, pt, gal.
Use: Pediatric antitussive combination.
HYDROCODONE COMP. SYRUP. (Gold-
line) Hydrocodone bitartrate w/homat-
ropine methylbromide, Bot. pt, gal.
Use: Antitussive.
• **HYDROCODONE POLISTIREX.** USAN.
Use: Antitussive.
HYDROCODONE RESIN COMPLEX.
Use: Antitussive.
W/Phenyltoloxamine resin complex.
See: Tussionex, Prods. (Pennwalt).

HYDROCORT. (Kenyon) Hydrocortisone 1%, clioquinol 3%, pramoxine HCl 0.5% in a cream base. Jar 20 Gm.
Use: Corticosteroid combination, topical.

HYDROCORTAMATE HCl. 17-Hydroxycorticoster-one-21-diethylaminoaceate HCl.
Use. Anti-Inflammatory, topical.
See: Ulcortar, Oint. (Ulmer).

HYDROCORTEX. (Kenyon) Hydrocortisone 1% in cream base. Jar 20 Gm.
Use: Corticosteroid, topical.

• **HYDROCORTISONE,** U.S.P. XXIII. Cream, Sterile, Susp., Oint., Gel, Tab., Lot., Enema, U.S.P. XXIII. Pregn-4-ene-3,20-dione, 11,17,21-trihydroxy- (11β)-Hydrocortisone. 11β, 17, 21-Trihydroxypregn-4-ene-3, 20-Dione. Compound F. Cortisoln. (Upjohn) Micronized nonsterile powder for prescription compounding.
Use: Anti-inflammatory, topical.
See: Acticort Lotion 100. (Cummins).
Aeroseb-HC, Aerosol (Herbert).
Alphaderm, Cream (Norwich Eaton).
Caldecort Spray (Pharmacraft).
Cetacort, Lot. (Owen).
Cort-Dome, Cream, Lot., Supp. (Miles Pharm).
Cortef, Tab., Cream, Oint. (Upjohn).
Cortenema, Enema (Solvay).
Cortinal, Tube (Kenyon).
Cortril, Oint. (Pfizer).
Cremesone, Cream (Dalin).
Delacort, Lot. (Mericon).
Dermacort, Cream, Lot. (Solvay).
Dermol HC, Cream, Oint. (Dermol).
Dermolate, Prods. (Schering).
Durel-Cort, Creme, Oint., Lot. (Durel).
Ecosone, Cream (Star).
Eldecort, Cream (ICN).
HC Derma-Pax, Liq. (Recsei).
HI-COR-1.0, Cream, (C & M Pharmacal).
HI-COR-2.5, Cream (C & M Pharmacal).
Hycort, Cream, Oint. (Everett).
Hycortole, Cream, Oint. (Premo).
Hydrocortex, Tube (Kenyon).
Hydrocortone, Tab. (Merck, Sharp & Dohme).
Hytone, Cream, Oint., Lot. (Dermik).
KeriCort-10, Cream (Bristol-Myers Squibb).
Lexocort, Pow., Lot. (Lexington).
Lipo-Adrenal Cortex, Vial (Upjohn).
Maso-Cort, Lot. (Mason).
Microcort, Lot. (Alto Pharm.).
My Cort, Cream (Scrip).

Optef, Soln. (Upjohn).
Proctocort, Oint. (Solvay).
Scalpicin, Liq. (Combe).
Signef, Supp. (Forest Pharm.).
Synacort, Cream (Syntex).
T/Scalp, Liq. (Neutrogena).
Tarcortin, Cream (Reed & Carnrick).
Texacort 25, 50, Lot. (Cooper).
Ulcort, Cream, Lot. (Ulmer).

HYDROCORTISONE W/COMBINATIONS.
See: Achromycin W/Hydrocortisone, Oint., Ophth. Oint. (Lederle).
Acrisan w/Hydrocortisone, Liq. (Recsei).
Bafil, Cream. (Scruggs).
Barseb HC, Scalp Lot. (Barnes-Hind).
Barseb Thera-spray, Aerosol (Barnes-Hind).
Biscolan HC, Supp. (Lannett).
Bro-Parin, Otic Susp. (Riker).
Calmurid HC, Cream (Pharmacia).
Carmol HC, Cream (Ingram).
Coidocort, Cream (Coast).
Cor-Tar-Quin, Cream, Lot. (Miles Pharm).
Cortef, Preps. (Upjohn).
Corticoid, Cream (Jenkins).
Cortin, Cream (C & M Pharm.).
Cortisporin, Prep. (Burroughs Wellcome).
Derma-Cover-HC, Liq., Oint. (Scrip).
Dermarex, Cream (Hyrex-Key).
Dicort, Cream, Supp. (Hickam).
Doak Oil Forte, Liq. (Doak).
Drotic No. 2, Drops (Ascher).
Durel-Cort "V,' Cream, Oint., Lot. (Durel).
Fostril HC, Lot. (Westwood).
HC-Form, Jelly (Recsei).
HC-Jel, Jelly (Recsei).
Heb-Cort., Cream, Lot. (Barnes-Hind).
Heb-Cort MC, Lot. (Barnes-Hind).
Heb-Cort. V, Cream, Lot. (Barnes-Hind).
Hi-Cort N Cream (Blaine).
Hill-Cortac, Cream, Lot. (Hill).
Hydrocort, Tube (Kenyon).
Hysone, Oint. (Mallard).
Kencort, Cream (Kenyon).
Kleer, Spray (Scrip).
Lanvisone, Cream (Lannett).
Loroxide-HC, Lot. (Dermik).
Maso-Form, Cream (Mason).
Mity-quin, Cream (Solvay).
Myci-Cort, Liq., Spray (Misemer).
My-Cort, Drops, Lot., Oint., Spray (Scrip).
Neocort, Oint. (H.V.P.).
Neo-Cort Dome, Cream, Lot., Drops

(Miles Pharm).
Neo Cort Top, Oint. (Standex).
Neo-Domeform-HC, Cream, Lot.,
 Susp. (Miles Pharm).
Nutracort, Cream, Gel, Lot.(Owen).
1 + 1 Creme, 1 + 1-F Creme (Dunhall).
Ophthel, Liq. (Elder).
Ophthocort, Oint. (Parke Davis).
Orlex HC Otic (Baylor).
Oto, Drops (Solvay).
Otobiotic, Soln. (Schering).
Otocalm-H Ear Drops (Parmed).
Otostan H.C. (Standex).
Pyocidin-Otic, Soln. (Berlex).
Racet Forte, Cream (Lemmon).
Racet LCD, Cream (Lemmon).
Rectal Medicone-HC (Medicone).
Sherform-HC, Creme (Sheryl).
Stera-Form, Creme (Mayrand).
Steramine Otic, Drops (Mayrand).
Syntar HC Cream, Oint. (Elder).
Tarcortin, Cream (Reed & Carnrick).
Tar-Quin-HC, Oint. (Jenkins).
Tenda HC, Cream (Dermik).
Terra-Cortril, Preps. (Pfipharmecs).
Theracort, Lot. (C & M Pharm.).
Vanoxide-HC, Lot. (Dermik).
V-Cort, Cream (Scrip).
Vioform-Hydrocortisone, Preps.
 (Ciba).
Vio-Hydrocort, Oint., Cream (Quality
 Generics).
Vytone, Cream, (Dermik).
• **HYDROCORTISONE ACETATE,** U.S.P.
XXIII. Sterile Susp., Lot., Ophth. Oint.,
Ophth. Susp., Oint., Cream, U.S.P. XXI-
II. Pregn-4-ene-3,20-dione, 21-(acety-
loxy)-11,17-dihydroxy-, (11β)-. Hydro-
cortisone 21-acetate. 17-Hydroxycorti-
costerone-21-acetate,comp.F. (Upjohn)
Micronized non-sterile powder for pre-
scription compounding.
Use: Adrenocortical steroid (topical anti-
inflammatory).
See: Anucort-HC, Supp. (G & W Labs).
Anuprep HC, Supp. (Great Southern).
Anusol-HC, Supp. (Parke-Davis).
Caldecort, Cream (Pharmacraft).
Caldecort Light, Cream (Pharmacraft).
Cortef Acetate, Ophth. Oint., Inj. (Up-
 john).
Cortifoam, Aerosol (Reed & Carnrick).
Cortiprel, Cream (Pasadena Re-
 search).
Cortril Acetate, Aqueous Susp., Oint.
 (Pfipharmecs).
Ferncort, Lot. (Ferndale).
Fernisone Inj., Vial (Ferndale).
Gynecort, Oint. (Combe).
Hemril-HC Uniserts, Supp. (Upsher-

Smith).
Hydro-Can (Paddock).
Hydrocort, Vial (Dunhall).
Hydrocortone Acetate, Inj. (Merck,
 Sharp & Dohme).
Hydrosone, Inj. (Sig).
Maximum Strength Corticaine, Cream
 (Whitby).
Maximum Strength Dermarest Dricort
 Creme (Del).
My-Cort, Lot. (Scrip).
Pramosone Cream, Lot. (Ferndale).
Span-Ster, Inj. (Scrip).
Tucks-HC (Parke-Davis).
**HYDROCORTISONE ACETATE W/COM-
BINATIONS.**
See: Anusol-HC, Cream, Supp. (Warn-
 er-Chilcott).
Biotic-Opth W/HC, Oint. (Scrip).
Biotres HC, Cream (Central).
Biscolan HC, Supp. (Lannett).
Carmol HC, Cream (Ingram).
Chloromycetin-Hydrocortisone Ophth.
 Susp. (Parke-Davis).
Coly-Mycin-S Otic, Soln. (Warner-
 Chilcott).
Cor-Oticin, Liq. (Maurry).
Cortaid, Cream, Lot., Oint. (Upjohn).
Cortef Acetate, Inj., Oint., Susp. (Up-
 john).
Corticaine Cream (Glaxo).
Derma Medicone-HC, Oint.
 (Medicone).
Dicort, Supp. (Hickam).
Doctient HC, Supp. (Suppositoria).
Epifoam, Aerosol (Reed & Carnrick).
Estro-V HC, Supp. (Webcon).
Eye-Cort, Soln. (Mallard).
Furacin-HC Otic (Eaton).
Furacin HC Urethral Inserts (Eaton).
Furacort Cream (Eaton).
Komed HC, Lot. (Barnes-Hind).
Lida-Mantle HC, Cream (Miles
 Pharm).
Mantadil, Cream (Burroughs Well-
 come).
Neo-Cortef, Preps. (Upjohn).
Neo-Hytone Cream (Dermik).
Neopolycin-HC, Oint., Ophth. Oint.
 (Merrell Dow).
Ophthocort, Oint. (Parke-Davis).
Proctofoam-HC, Aerosol (Reid and
 Carnrick).
Pyracort, Liq. (Lemmon).
Racet Forte, Cream (Lemmon).
Rectacort, Supp. (Century).
Rectal Medicone-HC, Supp.
 (Medicone).
Wyanoids HC, Supp. (Wyeth-Ayerst).
• **HYDROCORTISONE AND ACETIC ACID**

OTIC SOLUTION, U.S.P. XXIII.
Use: Anti-inflammatory.
•HYDROCORTISONE BUTEPRATE, USAN.
Use: Anti-inflammatory.
•HYDROCORTISONE BUTYRATE, U.S.P. XXIII.
Use: Glucocorticoid.
See. Locoid, 3oln. (Female).
•HYDROCORTISONE CYPIONATE, U.S.P. XXII. Oral Susp., U.S.P. XXII. Hydrocortisone 21-cyclopentanepropionate. Hydrocortisone Cypionate.
Use: Glucocorticoid.
HYDROCORTISONE DIETHYLAMINOACETATE HCl.
See: Hydrocortamate.
HYDROCORTISONE DYPROPIONATE.
See: Cortef, Fluid (Upjohn).
•HYDROCORTISONE HEMISUCCINATE, U.S.P. XXIII.
HYDROCORTISONE I.V.
See: A-Hydro Cort, Vial (Abbott).
Solu-Cortef, Vial (Upjohn).
HYDROCORTISONE/IODOCHLORHYDR OXYQUIN. (Various Mfr.) **Cream:** Hydrocortisone 0.5% or 3%, iodochlorhydroxyquin 3%. 15 Gm, 30 Gm, 480 Gm.
Oint.: Hydrocortisone 1%, iodochlorhydroxyquin 3%. 20 Gm, 30 Gm.
Use: Corticosteroid, topical.
HYDROCORTISONE/NEOMYCIN. (Various Mfr.) Hydrocortisone 1%, neomycin sulfate 0.5%. Oint. 20 Gm.
Use: Corticosteroid, topical.
HYDROCORTISONE PHOSPHATE.
See: Hydrocortone Phosphate, Inj. (Merck, Sharp & Dohme).
•HYDROCORTISONE SODIUM PHOSPHATE, U.S.P. XXIII. Inj., U.S.P. XXIII. Pregn-4-ene-3,20-dione, 11,17-dihydroxy-21-(phosphonoxy)-, disodium salt, (11β)-. Hydrocortisone 21-(disodium phosphate). Hydrocortisone Sodium Phosphate.
Use: Adrenocortical steroid (anti-inflammatory).
•HYDROCORTISONE SODIUM SUCCINATE, U.S.P. XXIII. Inj., U.S.P. XXIII. Pregn-4-ene-3,20-dione, 31-(3-carboxy-l-oxopropoxy)-11,17-dihydroxy-, (11β)-. Hydrocortisone 21-(sodium succinate). Hydrocortisone Sodium Succinate.
Use: Adrenocortical steroid (anti-inflammatory).
See: A-hydroCort, Vial (Abbott).
Solu-Cortef, Vial (Upjohn).
•HYDROCORTISONE VALERATE, U.S.P. XXIII. Cream, U.S.P. XXIII.
Use: Glucocorticoid.

See: Westcort Cream, Oint. (Westwood-Squibb).
HYDROCORTONE ACETATE SALINE SUSPENSION. (Merck, Sharp & Dohme) Hydrocortisone acetate 25 mg or 50 mg/ml, sodium Cl 9 mg, polysorbate 80 4 mg, sodium carboxymethylcellulose 5 mg/ml, benzyl alcohol 9 mg q.s. water for Injection to 1 ml. Vial 5 ml.
Use: Corticosteroid.
HYDROCORTONE PHOSPHATE INJECTION. (Merck, Sharp & Dohme) Hydrocortisone sodium phosphate equivalent to hydrocortisone 50 mg/ml, creatinine 8 mg, sodium citrate 10 mg/ml, sodium hydroxide to adjust pH, sodium bisulfite 3.2 mg, methylparaben 1.5 mg, propylparaben 0.2 mg, water for injection q.s./ml. Vial 2 ml multiple dose, 10 ml multiple dose. Disposable syringe 2 ml single dose.
Use: Corticosteroid.
HYDROCORTONE TABLETS. (Merck, Sharp & Dohme) Hydrocortisone 10 mg or 20 mg/Tab. Bot. 100s.
Use: Corticosteroid.
HYDROCREAM BASE. (Paddock) Petrolatum, mineral oil, woolwax alcohol, imidazilidinyl urea, methyl apropylparabens. Cream. Jar lb.
Use: Emollient.
HYDRO-CRYSTI 12. (Roberts Hauck) Hydroxocobalamin, crystalline (vitamin B_{12}) 1000 mcg/ml Inj. Vial 30 ml.
Use: Vitamin B_{12} supplement.
HYDRODIURIL. (Merck, Sharp & Dohme) Hydrochlorothiazide **25 mg/Tab.:** Bot. 100s, 1000s, UD 100s; **50 mg/Tab.:** Bot. 100s, 1000s, UD 100s; **100 mg/Tab.:** Bot. 100s.
Use: Diuretic.
HYDRO-D TABLETS. (Blue Cross) Hydrochlorothiazide. 25 mg or 50 mg/Tab. Bot. 1000s.
Use: Diuretic.
HYDRO-ERGOT. (Interstate) Hydrogenated ergot alkaloids 0.5 mg or 1 mg/Tab. Bot. 100s.
Use: Psychotherapeutic agent.
•HYDROFILCON A. USAN.
Use: Contact lens material.
•HYDROFLUMETHIAZIDE, U.S.P. XXIII. Tab., U.S.P. XXIII. 3,4-Dihydro-6-tri-fluoromethyl-7-sulfamoylbenzo-1,2,4-thiadiazine1,1 dioxide,3,4-Dihydro-6-(tri- fluoromethyl)-2H-1,2,4-benzo-thiadiazine-7-sulfonamide-1,1-Dioxide. Di-Ademil; Hydrenox; Naclex; Rontyl.
Use: Edema, hypertension.
See: Diucardin, Tab. (Wyeth-Ayerst).

Saluron, Tab. (Bristol).
W/Reserpine.
See: Salutensin, Tab. (Bristol).
Salutensin-Demi, Tab. (Bristol).
HYDROGEN DIOXIDE.
See: Hydrogen Peroxide.
HYDROGEN IODIDE.
Use: Expectorant.
See: Hydriodic acid.
•**HYDROGEN PEROXIDE CONCEN-
TRATE,** U.S.P. XXIII.
Use: Anti-infective (topical) when dilut-
ed.
**HYDROGEN PEROXIDE SOLUTION
30%.** Perhydrol, hydrogen pioxide. Bot.
0.25 lb, 0.5 lb, 1 lb.
Use: Dentistry, preparing the 3% solu-
tion.
•**HYDROGEN PEROXIDE TOPICAL SO-
LUTION,** U.S.P. XXIII. (Various Mfr.)
(3%). 4 oz, 8 oz, pt.
Use: Anti-infective, topical.
HYDROGESIC. (Edwards) Hydrocodone
bitartrate 5 mg, acetaminophen 500
mg/Cap. Bot. 100s.
Use: Narcotic analgesic combination.
HYDROLOID-G SUBLINGUAL. (Major)
Ergoloid mesylates. **0.5 mg/Tab.:** Dot.
100s, 250s, 500s, UD 100s. **1 mg/Tab.:**
Bot. 100s, 250s, 1000s, UD 100s.
Use: Psychotherapeutic agent.
HYDROLOID-G TABS. (Major) Ergoloid
mesylates 1 mg/Tab. Bot. 100s, 250s,
1000s, UD 100s.
Use: Psychotherapeutic agent.
HYDROMAL. (Mallard) Hydrochloroth-
iazide 50 mg/Tab. Bot. 1000s.
Use: Diuretic.
HYDROMAX SYRUP. (Blue Cross)
Ephedrine sulfate 6.25 mg, theophylline
32.5 mg, hydroxyzine HCl 2.5 mg/5 ml.
Bot. 16 oz.
Use: Bronchodilator.
HYDROMET. (Barre-National) Hy-
drocodone bitartrate 5 mg, homatropine
MBr 1.5 mg/Syr. Bot. pt, gal.
Use: Antitussive.
HYDROMORPHINOL. B.A.N. 7,8-Dihy-
dro-14-hydroxymorphine. Numorphan
Oral.
Use: Narcotic analgesic.
HYDROMORPHONE. B.A.N. 7,8-Dihy-
dromorphinone. Dilaudid hydrochloride.
Use: Narcotic analgesic.
HYDROMORPHONE. 4,5-Epoxy-3-hy-
droxy-17-methylmorphinan-6-one.
Use: Narcotic analgesic.
•**HYDROMORPHONE
HYDROCHLORIDE,** U.S.P. XXIII. Inj.,
Tab., U.S.P. XXIII. Dihydromorphinone

HCl. 4,5α-Epoxy-3-hydroxy-17-methyl-
morphinan-6-one HCl.
Use: Analgesic; narcotic.
See: Dilaudid Prods. (Knoll).
W/sodium citrate, antimony potassium tar-
trate and chloroform. Inj.
See: Dilocol, Liq. (Table Rock).
HYDROMORPHONE SULFATE. 4,5-
Epoxy 3-hydroxy-17-methylmorphinan-
6-one sulfate (2:1).
Use: Narcotic analgesic.
HYDROMOX. (Lederle) Quinethazone 50
mg/Tab. Bot. 100s, 500s.
Use: Diuretic.
HYDROMOX-R. (Lederle) Quinethazone
50 mg, reserpine 0.125 mg/Tab. Bot.
100s, 500s.
Use: Antihypertensive combination.
HYDROPANE. (Halsey) Hydrocodone
bitartrate 5 mg, homatropine methylbro-
mide 1.5 mg. Pt, gal.
Use: Antitussive combination.
HYDROPEL. (C & M Pharmacal) Silicone
30%, hydrophobic starch derivative
10%, petrolatum. Jar. 2 oz, lb.
Use: Emollient.
HYDROPHEN PEDIATRIC SYRUP.
(Rugby) Phenylpropanolamine HCl 12.5
mg, hydrocodone bitartrate 2.5 mg/5 ml.
Bot. 480 ml.
Use: Decongestant, antitussive.
HYDROPHEN SYRUP. (Rugby) Phenyl-
propanolamine HCl 25 mg, hy-
drocodone bitartrate 5 mg/5 ml. Bot. pt,
gal.
Use: Decongestant, antitussive.
HYDROPHED TABLETS. (Rugby) Theo-
phylline 130 mg, ephedrine sulfate 25
mg, hydroxyzine HCl 10 mg/Tab. Bot.
100s, 500s, 1000s.
Use: Antiasthmatic combination.
HYDROPHILIC OINTMENT, U.S.P. XXIII.
Stearyl alcohol, white petrolatum, propy-
lene glycol, sodium lauryl sulfate, water.
Jar lb. (Fougera).
Use: Ointment base.
HYDROPHILIC OINTMENT BASE. Oil in
water emulsion bases. (Emerson) 1 lb.
Use: Ointment base.
See: Aquaphilic Ointment (Medco).
Cetaphil, Cream, Lot. (Texas Pharma-
cal).
Dermovan, Cream (Texas Pharmacal).
Lanaphilic Ointment (Medco).
Monobase, Oint. (Torch).
Polysorb, Oint. (Savage).
Unibase, Oint. (Parke-Davis).
HYDROPINE. (Rugby) Hydroflumethi-
azide 25 mg, reserpine 0.125 mg/Tab.
Bot. 100s.

Use: Antihypertensive combination.
HYDROPINE H.P. TABLETS. (Rugby)
Hydroflumethiazide 50 mg, reserpine
0.125 mg/Tab. Bot. 100s, 500s, 1000s.
Use: Antihypertensive combination.
HYDROPRES-25 & 50. (Merck, Sharp &
Dohme) **25:** Hydrochlorothiazide 25 mg,
reserpine 0.125 mg/Tab. **50:** Hy-
drochlorothiazide 50 mg, reserpine
0.125 mg/Tab. Bot. 100s, 1000s.
Use: Antihypertensive combination.
•**HYDROQUINONE,** U.S.P. XXIII. Cream,
Topical Soln., U.S.P. XXIII. 1,4-Ben-
zenediol.
Use: Depigmenting agent.
See: Artra Skin Tone Cream (Plough).
Black and White Bleaching Cream
(Plough).
Derma-Blanch, Cream (Chattem).
Eldopaque Cream, Oint. (Elder).
Eldopaque Forte Cream, Oint. (Elder).
Eldoquin, Cream, Lot. (Elder).
Esoterica Medicated Cream Prods.
(SK-Beecham).
Melpaque HP, Cream (Stratus).
Melquin HP, Cream (Stratus).
Nuquin HP, Cream, gel (Stratus).
**HYDROQUINONE MONOBENZYL
ETHER.**
See: Benoquin, Oint., Lot. (Elder).
HYDROSAL. (Hydrosal Co.) Aluminum
acetate 5%. **Susp.:** Bot. 16 oz, gal.
Oint.: 54 Gm, 113.4 Gm, Jar 54 Gm,
454 Gm.
HYDROSERP. (Zenith) Hydrochloroth-
iazide 25 mg or 50 mg, reserpine 0.125
mg or 0.1 mg/Tab. Bot. 100s, 1000s.
Use: Antihypertensive combination.
HYDROSERP-50. (Freeport) Hy-
drochlorothiazide 50 mg, reserpine
0.125 mg/Tab. Bot. 1000s.
Use: Antihypertensive combination.
HYDROSERPINE. (Geneva) Hy-
drochlorothiazide 25 mg or 50 mg, re-
serpine 0.125 mg/Tab. Bot. 100s.
Use: Antihypertensive combination.
HYDROSERPINE 25. (Goldline) Hydrochlorothiazide 25 mg, reserpine. Bot.
100s, 1000s.
Use: Antihypertensive combination.
HYDROSERPINE 50. (Goldline) Hy-
drochlorothiazide 50 mg, reserpine. Bot.
100s, 1000s.
Use: Antihypertensive combination.
HYDROSINE 25 TABLETS. (Major) Hydrochlorothiazide 25 mg, reserpine
0.125 mg/Tab. Bot. 100s. Tartrazine.
Use: Antihypertensive combination.
HYDROSINE 50 TABLETS. (Major) Hy-
drochlorothiazide 50 mg, reserpine

0.125 mg/Tab. Bot. 100s.
Use: Antihypertensive combination.
HYDROSONE. (Sig) Hydrocortisone ac-
etate 25 mg or 50 mg/ml. Vial 5 ml.
Use: Corticosteroid.
HYDROTALCITE. B.A.N. Aluminum mag-
nesium hydroxide carbonate hydrate.
Altacite.
Use: Antacid.
HYDROTENSIN-50. (Mayrand) Hy-
drochlorothiazide 50 mg, reserpine
0.125 mg/Tab. Bot. 100s, 1000s.
Use: Antihypertensive combination.
HYDRO-TEX CREAM. (Syosset) Hydro-
cortisone 0.5% or 1%. Greaseless base.
Cream 30 Gm, 60 Gm, 120 Gm.
Use: Corticosteroid, topical.
HYDROTOIN CREAM. (Knight) Hydro-
cortisone 0.5%. Tube 0.5 oz.
Use: Corticosteroid, topical.
HYDRO-T TABS. (Major) Hydrochloroth-
iazide. **25 mg/Tab:** Bot. 100s, 1000s,
UD 100s; **50 mg/Tab:** Bot. 100s, 1000s,
UD 100s; **100 mg/Tab:** Bot. 100s, 250s,
1000s, UD 100s.
Use: Diuretic.
HYDROXAMETHOCAINE. B.A.N. 2-Di-
methyl-aminoethyl 4-butylaminosalicy-
late. Hydroxytetracaine (I.N.N.).
Use: Local anesthetic.
HYDROXINDASOL HCl. 5-Hydroxy-1-(p-
methoxy-benzyl)-2-methyltryptamine
HCl.
HYDROXO-12. (Ortega) Hydroxocobal-
amin (crystalline) 1000 mcg/ ml/Inj. Vial
10 ml, with methyl and propyl parabens.
Use: Vitamin B_{12} supplement.
•**HYDROXOCOBALAMIN,** U.S.P. XXIII.
Inj., U.S.P. XXIII. α-(5,6-Dimethylbenz-
imidazolyl) hydroxocobamide. Vitamin B
12a and B 12b. Hydrovit; Neo-Cytamen.
Use: Treatment of megaloblastic ane-
mia.
See: AlphaRedisol, Inj. (Merck, Sharp &
Dohme).
Alpha-Ruvite, Vial (Savage).
Cobavite L.A., Vial (Lemmon).
Droxomin, Inj. (Solvay).
Hydrobexan, Vial (Keene).
Rubesol-L.A. 1000, Inj. (Central).
Span-12, Inj. (Scrip).
Sytobex-H, Vial (Parke-Davis).
Twelve-Span, Vial (Foy).
**HYDROXOCOBALAMIN,
CRYSTALLINE.** (Various Mfr.) 1000
mcg/ml Inj. 30 ml.
Use: Vitamin B_{12} supplement.
See: Hydroxocobalamin (Various).
Alphamin (Vortech).
AlphaRedisol (MSD).

Codroxomin (Forest).
Hybalamin (Mallard).
Hydrobexan (Keene).
Hydro Cobex (Pasadena).
Hydro-Crysti (Hauck).
Hydroxo-12 (Ortega).
LA-12 (Hyrex).
HYDROXOCOBALAMIN/SODIUM THIO-SULFATE.
Use: Cyanide poisoning antidote. [Orphan drug]
HYDROXY BIS(ACETATO)ALUMINUM.
Aluminum Subacetate Topical Soln, U.S.P. XXIII.
HYDROXYAMPHETAMINE HBr.
Use: Pupil dilator.
See: Paredrine (Pharmics).
2-HYDROXYBENZAMIDE.
See: Salicylamide.
HYDROXYBIS (SALICYLATO) ALUMINUM DIACETATE.
See: Aluminum aspirin.
HYDROXYCHOLECALCIFEROL. (D₃).
Use: Hypocalcemia.
See: Calcifediol.
• **HYDROXYCHLOROQUINE SULFATE,**
U.S.P. XXIII. Tab., U.S.P. XXIII. Ethanol, 2-4-(7-chloro-4-quinolinyl)-amino pentyl ethylamino-, sulfate (1:1) salt. 7-Chloro-4- 4-[ethyl(2-hydroxyethyl)-amino]-1-methyl- butylamino quinoline sulfate. 2-[[4-[(7chloro-4-quinolyl)amino]-pentyl]ethylamino]ethanol Sulfate (1:1).
Use: Antimalarial, lupus erythematosus suppressant.
HYDROXYDIONE SODIUM. 21-Hydroxy-pregnane- dione sodium succinate.
HYDROXYDIONE SODIUM SUCCINATE.
B.A.N. Sodium 21-hydroxypregnane-3,20-dione succinate.
Use: Anesthetic.
• **HYDROXYETHYL CELLULOSE,** N.F. XVIII.
Use: Topical protectant, thickening agent.
See: Gonioscopic, Soln. (Alcon).
HYDROXYETHYL STARCH. (HES).
Use: Plasma volume expander.
See: Hespan, Inj. (DuPont Critical Care).
HYDROXYISOINDOLIN. Under study.
Use: Antihypertensive.
HYDROXYMAGNESIUM ALUMINATE.
Use: Antacid.
See: Magaldrate.
HYDROXYMYCIN. An antibiotic substance obtained from cultures of *Streptomyces paucisporogenes*.
HYDROXYPETHIDINE. B.A.N. Ethyl 4-(3-hydroxy-phenyl)-1-methylpiperidine-

4-carboxylate.
Use: Narcotic analgesic.
• **HYDROXYPHENAMATE.** USAN. 2-Hydroxy-2-phenyl-butyl carbamate.
Use: Tranquilizer.
HYDROXYPROCAINE. B.A.N. 2-Diethylamino-ethyl 4-aminosalicylate.
Use: Local anesthetic.
• **HYDROXYPROGESTERONE CAPROATE,** U.S.P. XXIII. Inj., U.S.P. XXIII. 17α-Hydrogypregn-4-ene-3,20-dione. Pregn-4-ene-3,20-dione,17-[(I-oxohexyl)-oxy]-. (Various Mfr.) **125 mg/ml:** Inj.Vial 10 ml; **250 mg/ml:** Inj.Vial 5 ml.
Use: Progestin.
See: Delalutin, Vial (Squibb).
Duralutin, Inj. (Roberts/Hauck).
Gesterol L.A. 250, Inj. (Forest).
Hy-Gestrone, Vial (Pasadena Research).
Hylutin, Inj. (Hyrex).
Hyprogest 250, Inj. (Keene).
W/Estradiol valerate.
See: Hy-Gestradol, Inj. (Pasadena Research).
Hylutin-Est., Inj. (Hyrex).
• **HYDROXYPROPYL CELLULOSE, LOW-SUBSTITUTED,** N.F. XVIII.
Use: Topical protectant, tablet coating agent.
• **HYDROXYPROPYL METHYLCELLULOSE,** U.S.P. XXIII. Ophth. soln. U.S.P. XXIII. Cellulose, 2-hydroxypropyl methyl ether. Cellulose hydroxypropyl methyl ether. The propylene glycol ether of methylcellulose available in the 2208, 2906 and 2910 forms.
Use: Suspending agent, topical protectant (ophthalmic).
See: Anestacon (Alcon).
Econopred, Susp. (Alcon).
Occucoat, Soln. (Storz).
W/benzalkonium Cl.
See: Gonak, Soln. (Akorn).
Goniosol (Iolab).
Isopto Tears (Alcon).
Ultra Tears, Soln. (Alcon).
• **HYDROXYPROPYL METHYLCELLULOSE PHTHALATE 200731,** N.F. XVIII.
Use: Pharmaceutic aid, tablet coating agent.
• **HYDROXYPROPYL METHYLCELLULOSE PHTHALATE 200824,** N.F. XVIII.
Use: Pharmaceutic aid, tablet coating agent.
• **HYDROXYPROPYL METHYLCELLULOSE PHTHALATE,** N.F. XVIII.
Use: Pharmaceutic aid, tablet coating agent.
HYDROXYSTEARIN SULFATE. Sul-

fonate hydrogenated castor oil.
HYDROXYSTILBAMIDINE. B.A.N. 4,4'-
Diamidino-2-hydroxystilbene.
Use: Treatment of leishmaniasis and
trypanosomiasis.
HYDROXYTOLUIC ACID. B.A.N. 2-Hy-
droxy-m-toluic acid. 3-Methylsalicylic
acid.
Use: Analgesic.
L-5 HYDROXYTRYPTOPHAN. (Bolar)
Use: Postanoxic intention myoclonus.
[Orphan drug]
•**HYDROXYUREA,** U.S.P. XXIII. Cap.,
U.S.P. XXIII. Hydroxycarbamide (I.N.N.).
Use: Antineoplastic agent. Sickle cell
anemia [Orphan drug]
See: Hydrea, Cap. (Squibb Mark).
•**HYDROXYZINE HCl,** U.S.P. XXIII. Inj.,
Syr., Tab., U.S.P. XXIII. 2-[2-[-4-(p-
Chloro-α-phenylbenzyl-)-1-
piperazinyl]ethoxy]ethanol dihydrochlo-
ride. Inj.: (Abbott) 100 mg/2 ml amp. or
Abboject syringe, 500 mg/10 ml vial.
Use: Tranquilizer, antihistamine.
See: Atarax, Syr., Tab. (Roerig).
Hyzine-50, Inj. (Hyrex).
Rezine, Tab. (Marnel).
Vistazine 25, Inj. (Keene).
Vistazine 50, Inj. (Keene).
Vistaril Isoject. (Roerig).
Vistaril, Cap., Susp. (Pfizer Laborato-
ries).
W/Ephedrine sulf., theophylline.
See: Marax DF, Syr. (Roerig).
Marax Tab. (Roerig).
Theo-Drox, Tab. (Quality Generics).
W/Pentaerythritol tetranitrate.
See: Cartrax 10, 20, Tab. (Roerig).
•**HYDROXYZINEPAMOATE,** U.S.P. XXIII.
Cap., Oral Susp., U.S.P. XXIII. 1,1'-
Methylene bis(2-hydroxy-3-naphtha-
lene-carboxylic acid salt of 1-p-
chlorobenzhydryl)-4-[2-2-hydroxy-
ethoxyethyl]piperazine.
2-(2-(4-(piperazine. 2-(2-(4-(p-Chloro-
α-phenyl-benzyl)-1-
piperazinyl)ethoxy)ethanol 4,4-Methyl-
enebis-(3-hydroxy-2-napthoate) (1:1).
Use: Tranquilizer; antihistamine.
See: Hy-Pam 25 Cap. (Lemmon).
Vistaril, Cap., Susp. (Pfizer Laborato-
ries).
HYDRO-Z-50 TABLETS. (Mayrand) Hy-
drochlorothiazide 50 mg/Tab. Bot. 100s,
1000s.
Use: Diuretic.
HY-E-PLEX. (Nutrition) Vitamin E 400
IU/Cap. Vial. Bot. 100s.
Use: Vitamin E supplement.
Hy-FLOW SOLUTION. (CooperVision)

Polyvinyl alcohol with hydroxyethylcellu-
lose, benzalkonium Cl, EDTA. Bot. 60
ml.
Use: Hard contact lens care.
HY-GESTRONE. (Pasadena Research)
Hydroxyprogesterone caproate. **125
mg/ml.:** Vial 10 ml. **250 mg/ml.:** Vial 5
ml.
Use: Progestin.
HYGIENIC POWDER.
See: Bo-Car-Al, Pow. (Calgon).
HYGROTON. (Rorer) Chlorthalidone 25
mg, 50 mg or 100 mg/Tab. Bot. 100s,
1000s, UD 100s.
Use: Diuretic.
HYLIDONE TABS. (Major) Chlorthali-
done. **25 mg or 50 mg/Tab:** Bot. 100s,
250s, 1000s, UD 100s. **100 mg/Tab:**
Bot. 100s, 250s, 500s, 1000s.
Use: Diuretic.
HYLIVER PLUS. (Hyrex) Folic acid 0.4
mg, liver 10 mcg, vitamin B₁₂ 100
mcg/ml. Vial 10 ml with phenol.
Use: Vitamin supplement.
HYLOREL TABLETS. (Fisons) Gua-
nadrel sulfate 10 mg or 25 mg/Tab. Bot.
100s.
Use: Antihypertensive.
HYLUTIN INJECTABLE. (Hyrex) Hydrox-
yprogesterone caproate in oil 250
mg/ml. Vial 5 ml.
Use: Progestin.
HYMAC CREAM. (NMC Labs) Hydrocor-
tisone 0.5% or 1% in cream base. Tube
oz.
Use: Corticosteroid, topical.
HYMAC OINTMENT. (NMC Labs) Hydro-
cortisone 0.5% or 1% in ointment base.
Tube oz.
Use: Corticosteroid, topical.
•**HYMECROMONE.** USAN.
Use: Choleretic.
HY-N.B.P. OINTMENT. (Bowman) Baci-
tracin zinc 400 units, neomycin sulfate 5
mg, polymyxin B sulfate 10,000
units/Gm. Tube ⅛ oz.
Use: Anti-infective, topical.
HYOSCINE HYDROBROMIDE. Scopo-
lamine HBr, U.S.P. XXIII.
Use: Intestinal antispasmodic.
HYOSCINE-HYOSCYAMINE-ATROPINE.
Use: Anticholinergic.
See: Atropine w/hyoscyamine
w/hyoscine.
HYOSCINE METHOBROMIDE. B.A.N.
Use: Treatment of peptic ulcer.
•**HYOSCYAMINE,** U.S.P. XXIII. Tab.,
U.S.P. XXIII. 1αH,5αH-Tropan-3α-ol(−)-
tropate (ester). Levo form of atropine.
Use: Anticholinergic.

See: Bellafoline, Amp., Tab. (Sandoz).
Cysto-Spaz, Tab. (Webcon).
HYOSCYAMINE-ATROPINE-HYOSCINE.
Use: Anticholinergic.
See: Atropine w/hyoscyamine
w/hyoscine.
• **HYOSCYAMINE HYDROBROMIDE,**
U.S.P. XXIII. 1αH,5αH-Tropan-3α-ol(–)-
tropate HBr. Daturine HBr. (Various
Mfr.).
Use: Anticholinergic.
W/Physostigmine salicylate.
See: Pyatromine-H Inj. (Kremers-Ur-
ban).
HYOSCYAMINE HYDROCHLORIDE.
(Various Mfr.).
HYOSCYAMINE MALEATE.
See: Bellafoline, Amp., Tab. (Sandoz).
HYOSCYAMINE SALTS.
Use: Anticholinergic.
W/Atropine salts.
See: Atropine W/Hyoscyamine.
• **HYOSCYAMINE SULFATE,** U.S.P. XXIII.
Flix, Inj., Oral Soln., Tab., U.S.P. XXIII.
1αH,5αH-Tropan-3α-ol-(–)-tropate (es-
ter) sulfate (2:1) dihydrate.
Use: Anticholinergic.
See: Anaspaz, Tab. (Ascher).
Cystospaz-M, Cap. (Webcon).
Donnamar, Tab. (Marnel).
ED-SPAZ, Tab. (Edwards).
Gastrosed, Drops, Tab. (Hauck).
Levsin/SL, Sublingual Tab. (Schwarz
Pharma Kremers Urban).
W/Atropine sulfate, hyoscine HBr, pheno-
barbital.
See: DeTal, Elix., Tab. (DeLeon).
Donnatal, Prods.(Robins).
Hyatal, Elix., Liq. (Kenyon).
Hyonal C.T., Tab. (Paddock).
Maso-Donna, Elix., Tab. (Mason).
Peece, Tab. (Scrip).
Sedamine, Tab. (Dunhall).
Spasaid, Cap. (Century).
Spasmolin, Tab. (Kenyon).
Spasquid, Elix. (Geneva).
W/Atropine sulfate, hyoscine HBr, pheno-
barbital, pepsin, pancreatin, bile salts.
See: Donnazyme, Tab. (Robins).
W/Atropine sulfate. Scopolamine HCl,
phenobarbital.
See: Ultabs, Tab. (Burlington).
W/Belladonna Alkaloids.
See: Belladonna Prods.
W/Butabarbital.
See: Cystospaz-SR, Cap. (Webcon).
W/Methenamine, atropine sulfate, methyl-
ene blue, salol, benzoic acid, gelsemi-
um.
See: Uriprel, Tab. (Pasadena Re-

search).
W/Phenobarbital, simethicone, atropine
sulfate, scopolamine HBr.
See: Kinesed, Tab. (Stuart).
HYOSCYAMUS EXTRACT.
W/A.P.C.
See: Valacet Junior, Tab. (Vale).
W/A.P.C., gelsemium extract.
See: Valacet, Tab. (Vale).
**HYOSCYAMUS PRODUCTS AND PHE-
NOBARBITAL COMBINATIONS.**
Use: Anticholinergic, sedative.
See: Anaspaz PB, Tab. (Pasadena Re-
search).
Donnacin, Elix., Tab. (Pharmex).
Donnatal, Preps. (Robins).
Elixiral, Elix. (Vita Elixir).
Floramine, Tab. (Lemmon).
Gylanphen, Tab. (Lannett).
Kinesed, Tab. (Stuart).
Neoquess, Tab. (O'Neal).
Nevrotose, Cap. (Vale).
Sedajen, Tab. (Jenkins).
HYOSOPHEN TABLETS. (Rugby). At-
ropine sulfate 0.0194 mg, scopolamine
HBr 0.0065 mg, hyoscyamine HBr or
SO₄ 0.1037 mg, phenobarbital 16.2 mg.
Use: Anticholinergic combination.
HYPAQUE-76. (Winthrop Pharm.) Diatri-
zoate meglumine 66%, diatrizoate sodi-
um 10%, iodine 37%, EDTA. Vial 30 ml,
50 ml, 100 ml.
Use: Radiopaque agent.
HYPAQUE-CYSTO. (Winthrop Pharm)
Diatrizoate meglumine 30% soln., iodine
14.1%. 250 ml in 500 ml dilution bottle.
Pediatric: 100 ml in 300 ml dilution bot-
tle.
Use: Radiopaque agent.
HYPAQUE-M 75%. (Winthrop Pharm) Di-
atrizoate meglumine 50%, diatrizoate
sodium 25%, iodine 38.5%, EDTA. Vial
20 ml, 50 ml.
Use: Radiopaque agent.
HYPAQUE-M 90%. (Winthrop Pharm) Di-
atrizoate meglumine 60%, diatrizoate
sodium 30%, EDTA. Vial 50 ml.
Use: Radiopaque agent.
HYPAQUE MEGLUMINE 30%. (Winthrop
Pharm) Diatrizoate meglumine 30%, io-
dine 14.1%. Bot. 100 ml, 300 ml w/ and
w/o I.V. infusion set.
Use: Radiopaque agent.
HYPAQUE MEGLUMINE 60%. (Winthrop
Pharm) Diatrizoate meglumine 60%, io-
dine 28%, EDTA. Vial 20 ml, 30 ml, 50
ml, 100 ml.
Use: Radiopaque agent.
HYPAQUE ORAL. (Winthrop Pharm)

Pow.: Diatrizoate sodium oral pow. containing iodine 600 mg/Gm. Can 250 Gm, Bot. 10 Gm. **Liq.:** Soln. 41.66%. Bot. 120 ml.
Use: Radiopaque agent.
HYPAQUE SODIUM 20%. (Winthrop Pharm) Diatrizoate sodium 20%, iodine 12%, EDTA. Vial 100 ml.
Use: Radiopaque agent.
HYPAQUE SODIUM 25%. (Winthrop Pharm) Diatrizoate sodium 25%, iodine 15%. Bot. 300 ml, w/ and w/out I.V. infusion set.
Use: Radiopaque agent.
HYPAQUE SODIUM 50%. (Winthrop Pharm) Diatrizoate sodium 50%, iodine 30%. **Vial:** 20 ml, 30 ml, 50 ml. **Dilution Bottle:** 200 ml with EDTA.
Use: Radiopaque agent.
HYPERAB. (Cutter) Rabies immune globulin (Human) 150 IU/ml. **Pediatric:** Vial 2 ml. **Adult:** Vial 10 ml.
Use: Agent for immunization.
HYPERHEP. (Cutter) Hepatitis B immune globulin (Human). Vial 250 unit, prefilled syringe 250 unit.
Use: Agent for immunization.
HYPERICIN. (VIMRx Pharm/NIH)
Use: Antiviral, phase I AIDS.
HYPERLIPIDEMIA, AGENTS FOR.
See: Atromid-S (Wyeth-Ayerst).
Choloxin (Flint).
Cholybar (Parke-Davis).
Clofibrate (Various).
Colestid (Upjohn).
Lopid (Parke-Davis).
Lorelco (Merrell Dow).
Mevacor (MSD).
Pravachol (Bristol-Myers Squibb).
Questran (Bristol Labs).
Questran Light (Bristol Labs).
Zocor (MSD).
HYPERLYTE. (American McGaw) Sodium 25 mEq, potassium 40.5 mEq, calcium 5 mEq, magnesium 8 mEq, chloride 33.5 mEq, acetate 40.6 mEq, gluconate 5 mEq, 6050 mOsm/L. Inj. Vial 25 ml fill in 50 ml.
Use: Parenteral nutritional supplement.
HYPERLYTE CR. (American McGaw) Sodium 25 mEq, potassium 20 mEq, calcium 5 mEq, magnesium 5 mEq, chloride 30 mEq, acetate 30 mEq, 5500 mOsm/L. Inj. Super-vial 150 ml, 250 ml fill.
Use: Parenteral nutritional supplement.
HYPERLYTE R. (American McGaw) Sodium 25 mEq, potassium 20 mEq, calcium 5 mEq, magnesium 5 mEq, chloride 30 mEq, acetate 25 mEq, 4200

mOsm/L. Inj. Vial 25 ml fill in 50 ml.
Use: Parenteral nutritional supplement.
HYPEROPTO 5%. (Professional Pharmacal) Sodium Cl 5%. Oint. Tube 3.5 Gm.
Use: Ophthalmic preparation.
HYPEROPTO OINTMENT. (Professional Pharmacal) Sodium HCl 50 mg, D.I. water 150 mg, anhydrous lanolin 150 mg, liquid petrolatum 50 mg, white petrolatum 599 mg, methylparaben 7 mg, propylparaben 3 mg/Gm. Tube 3.5 Gm.
Use: Ophthalmic preparation.
HYPEROSMOLAR AGENTS.
Use: Laxative.
See: Glycerin, USP (Various).
Sani-Supp, Supp. (G & W Labs).
Fleet Babylax, Liq. (Fleet).
HYPERSTAT I.V. INJECTION. (Schering) Diazoxide 300 mg, pH adjusted to approximately 11.6 with sodium hydroxide/20 ml Amp.
Use: Antihypertensive.
HYPERTEN. (Kenyon) Phenobarbital 0.25 gr, nitroglycerin 1/300 gr, sodium nitrate 1 gr, veratrum viride gr/Tab. Bot. 100s, 1000s.
Use: Antihypertensive.
HYPERTENSION DIAGNOSIS.
See: Regitine, Amp., Tab. (Ciba).
HYPERTENSIVE EMERGENCY DRUGS.
See: Sodium Nitroprusside (Elkins-Sinn).
Nipride (Roche Labs).
Nitropress (Abbott).
Diazoxide Injection, USP (Quad).
Hyperstat IV (Schering). Arfonad (Roche).
HYPERTENSION THERAPY.
See: Aldoclor, Tab. (Merck, Sharp & Dohme).
Aldomet, Tab. (Merck, Sharp & Dohme).
Aldomet Ester HCl, Amp. (Merck, Sharp & Dohme).
Aldoril, Tab. (Merck, Sharp & Dohme).
Alkavervir.
Alseroxylon.
Apresoline, Amp., Tab. (Ciba).
Apresoline, Apresoline Esidrix, Amp., Tab. (Ciba).
Arfonad, Amp. (Roche).
Blocadren, Tab. (Merck, Sharp & Dohme).
Corgard, Tab. (Squibb).
Deserpidine.
Dibenzyline HCl, Cap. (SK-Beecham).
Diupres, Tab. (Merck, Sharp & Dohme).
Diutensen and Diutensen-R, Tab. (Wallace).

Dyazide, Cap. (SK-Beecham).
Enduron, Tab. (Abbott).
Enduronyl, Tab. (Abbott).
Enduronyl Forte, Tab. (Abbott).
Esidrix, Tab. (Ciba).
Eutonyl, Tab. (Abbott).
Eutron, Tab. (Abbott).
Exna and Exna-R, Tab. (Robins).
Hesperidin Methyl Chalcone (Various
    Mfr.).
Hexamethonium Cl and Bromide (Vari-
    ous Mfr.).
HydroDiuril, Tab. (Merck, Sharp &
    Dohme).
Hydropres, Tab. (Merck, Sharp &
    Dohme).
Hygroton, Tab. (USV).
Hyperstat, I.V. Inj. (Schering).
Inversine, Tab. (Merck, Sharp &
    Dohme).
Lopressor, Tab. (Geigy).
Metatensin, Tab. (Merrell Dow).
Midamor, Tab. (Merck, Sharp &
    Dohme).
Moderil, Tab. (Pfizer).
Moduretic, Tab. (Merck, Sharp &
    Dohme).
Naturetin, Tab. (Squibb).
Naquival, Tab. (Schering).
Oretic, Tab. (Abbott).
Oreticyl, Tab. (Abbott).
Prinivil, Tab. (Merck).
Priscoline HCl, Preps. (Ciba).
Protoveratrines A & B.
Raudixin, Tab. (Squibb).
Rautrax, Tab. (Squibb).
Rautrax-N, Tab. (Squibb).
Rauwolfia Serpentina (Various Mfr.).
Rauzide, Tab. (Squibb).
Regroton, Tab. (USV).
Renese-R, Tab. (Pfizer).
Rescinnamine, Tab. (Various Mfr.).
Reserpine (Various Mfr.).
Rutin, Tab. (Various Mfr.).
Sectral, Cap. (Wyeth-Ayerst).
Tetraethylammonium Chloride (Vari-
    ous Mfr.).
Timolide, Tab. (Merck, Sharp &
    Dohme).
Vasodilators.
Vasotec, Tab. (Merck, Sharp &
    Dohme).
Veratrum Alba.
Veratrum Viride.
Wytensin, Tab. (Wyeth-Ayerst).
Zaroxolyn, Tab. (Pennwalt).
HYPER-TET. (Cutter) Tetanus immune
    globulin (Human) U.S.P. Vial 250 units,
    Disp. Syringe 250 units.
Use: Immune serum.

HYPERTHYROIDISM.
See: Antithyroid agents.
HY-PHEN TABLETS. (Ascher) Hy-
    drocodone bitartrate 5 mg, aceta-
    minophen 500 mg. Bot. 100s, 500s.
Use: Antitussive, analgesic.
HYPHYLLINE. Dyphylline. (7-Dihydroxy-
    propyl-theophylline).
See: Neothylline, Elix., Amp., Tab.
    (Lemmon).
HYPNOGENE.
See: Barbital (Various Mfr.).
HYPNOMIDATE. (Janssen) Etomidate.
Use: General anesthetic.
HYPNO-SED. (Jenkins) Bromisovalum 1
    gr, carbromal 3 gr, thiamine mononitrate
    9 mg/Tab. Bot. 1000s.
HYPNOTICS.
See: Sedatives.
"HYPO".
See: Sodium Thiosulfate (Various Mfr.).
HYPO-BEE. (Towne) Vitamins B_1 50 mg,
    B_2 20 mg, B_6 5 mg, B_{12} 15 mcg, niaci-
    namide 25 mg, calcium pantothonate 5
    mg, C 300 mg, E 200 IU, iron 10
    mg/Tab. Bot. 30s, 100s.
Use: Vitamin/mineral supplement.
HYPOCHLORITE PREPS.
See: Antiformin.
    Dakin's Soln.
    Hyclorite.
HYPOCLEAR. (Bausch & Lomb) Isotonic
    soln. with sodium Cl 0.9%. Aerosol soln.
    240 ml, 300 ml.
Use: Soft contact lens care.
HYPOGLYCEMIC AGENTS.
See: Chlorpropamide.
    Diabeta, Tab. (Hoechst-Roussel).
    Diabinese, Tab. (Pfizer).
    Dymelor, Tab. (Lilly).
    Glucotrol, Tab. (Roerig).
    Glynase, Tab. (Upjohn).
    Micronase, Tab. (Upjohn).
    Orinase, Tab., Vial (Upjohn).
    Phenformin HCl.
    Tolbutamide.
    Tolinase, Tab. (Upjohn).
α-**HYPOPHAMINE.** Oxytocin.
• **HYPOPHYOSPHOROUS ACID,** N.F. XVI-
    II.
Use: Antioxidant.
HYPOTEARS OPHTHALMIC LIQUID.
    (Iolab Pharm.) Polyvinyl alcohol 1%,
    PEG-400, dextrose, benzalkonium Cl,
    EDTA. Bot. 15 ml, 30 ml.
Use: Ophthalmic lubricant.
**HYPOTEARS OPHTHALMIC
OINTMENT.** (Iolab Pharm.) White
    petrolatum, light mineral oil. Tube 3.5
    Gm.

Use: Ophthalmic lubricant.

HYPO-TEARS PF. (Iolab) Polyvinyl alcohol 1% in PEG 400, dextrose and EDTA. Soln. In 0.6 ml.
Use: Artificial tear solution.

HYPOTENSIVE AGENTS.
See: Hypertension Therapy.

HYPRHO-D. (Cutter) Rho (D) Immune globulin (Human). Pre-filled single dose syringe. Single dose vial. Pkg. 10s.
Use: Immune serum.

HYPRHO-D MINI-DOSE. (Cutter Biological) RH$_O$ (D) Immune Globulin Micro-Dose. Each package contains a single dose syringe.
Use: Immune serum.

HYPROGEST 250. (Keene) Hydroxyprogesterone caproate 250 mg/ml. Inj. Vial 5 ml.
Use: Progestin.

HYPROMELLOSE. B.A.N. A partial mixed methyl and hydroxypropyl ether of cellulose.
Use: Surface active agent.

HYREXIN-50. (Hyrex) Diphenhydramine HCl 50 mg/ml. Vial 10 ml.
Use: Antihistamine.

HYRUNAL. (Kenyon) Rutin 20 mg, mannitol hexanitrate 0.5 gr, phenobarbital 0.25 gr/Tab. Bot. 100s, 1000s.
Use: Antihypertensive combination.

HYRUNAL W/VERATRUM VIRIDE. (Kenyon) Phenobarbital 0.25 gr, mannitol hexanitrate 0.5 gr, rutin 10 mg, veratrum viride 100 mg/Tab. Bot. 100s, 1000s.
Use: Antihypertensive combination.

HYSCORBIC PLUS TABLETS. (Bock) Vitamins E 45 IU, C 600 mg, folic acid 400 mcg, B$_1$ 20 mg, B$_2$ 10 mg, niacinamide 100 mg, B$_6$ 10 mg, B$_{12}$ 25 mcg, pantothenic acid 25 mg, copper 3 mg, zinc 23.9 mg/Tab. Bot. 60s.
Use: Vitamin/mineral supplement.

HYSERP. (Freeport) Reserpine alkaloid 0.25 mg/Tab. Bot. 1000s.
Use: Antihypertensive.

HYSKON. (Pharmacia) Dextran 70 32% in 10% w/v dextrose. Bot. 100 ml, 250 ml.
Use: Diagnostic aid. For distending the uterine cavity and in irrigating and visualizing its surfaces.

HYSONE. (Mallard) Iodochlorhydroxquin 3%, hydrocortisone 0.5%. Tube 15 Gm.
Use: Antifungal, corticosteroid, topical.

HYSTERONE TABS. (Major) Fluoxymesterone 10 mg/Tab. Bot. 100s.
Use: Androgen.

HYSTEROSCOPY FLUID.

Use: Diagnostic aid.
See: Hyskon (Pharmacia).

HYTAKEROL. (Winthrop Pharm) Dihydrotachysterol. **Cap.:** 0.125 mg. Bot. 50s. **Soln.:** 0.25 mg/ml in oil. Bot. 15 ml.
Use: Treatment of tetany and hypoparathyroidism.

HYTINIC. (Hyrex) Polysaccharide-iron complex 150 mg/Cap. Bot. 50s, 500s.
Use: Iron supplement.

HYTINIC INJECTION. (Hyrex) Ferrous gluconate 2.9 mg, liver equivalent to vitamins B$_{12}$ 15 mcg, vitamins B$_2$ 0.75 mg, B$_5$ 1.25 mg, B$_{12}$ equivalent 1 mcg. Vial 30 ml.
Use: Vitamin/mineral supplement.

HYTONE CREAM. (Dermik) Hydrocortisone in cream base. **1%:** Tube 1 oz, Jar 4 oz. **2.5%:** Tube 1 oz, 2 oz.
Use: Corticosteroid, topical.

HYTONE LOTION 1%. (Dermik) Hydrocortisone 1% (10 mg/ml). Bot. 120 ml.
Use: Corticosteroid, topical.

HYTONE LOTION 2.5%. (Dermik) Hydrocortisone 2 1/2% (25 mg/ml) in lotion base. Bot. 60 ml.
Use: Corticosteroid, topical.

HYTONE OINTMENT. (Dermik) Hydrocortisone in ointment base. **1%:** Tube 28.3 Gm, 113.4 Gm. **2.5%:** Tube 28.3 Gm.
Use: Corticosteroid, topical.

HYTRIN. (Abbott/Burroughs Wellcome) Terazosin HCl **1 mg, 2 mg or 5 mg:** Bot. 100s, 500s, UD 100s. **10 mg:** Tab. Bot. 100s, UD 100s.
Use: Antihypertensive.

HYTUSS TABLETS. (Hyrex) Guaifenesin 100 mg/Tab. Bot. 100s, 1000s.
Use: Expectorant.

HYTUSS-2X. (Hyrex) Guaifenesin 200 mg/Cap. Bot. 100s, 1000s.
Use: Expectorant.

HYZINE-50. (Hyrex) Hydroxyzine HCl 50 mg as HCl/ml. Vial 10 ml.
Use: Antianxiety agent.

I

I-131 RADIOLABELED B1 MONOCLONAL ANTIBODY. (Coulter)
Use: Treatment for non-Hodgkin's B-cell lymphoma. [Orphan drug]

IBENZMETHYZIN. Name used for Procarbazine Hydrochloride.

IBERET. (Abbott) Ferrous sulfate 105 mg, ascorbic acid 150 mg, vitamins B$_{12}$ 25 mcg, B$_1$ 6 mg, B$_2$ 6 mg, niacinamide 30 mg, B$_6$ 5 mg/CR Filmtab. Bot. 60s,

500s.
Use: Vitamin/mineral supplement.
IBERET-500. (Abbott) Ascorbic acid 500 mg, ferrous sulfate 105 mg, vitamins B_1 6 mg, B_2 6 mg, B_3 30 mg, B_5 10 mg, B_6 5 mg, B_{12} 25 mcg/CR Filmtab. Bot. 30s, 60s, 500s, UD 100s.
Use: Vitamin/mineral supplement.
IBERET-FOLIC-500 FILMTAB. (Abbott) Ferrous sulfate 105 mg, vitamin C 500 mg, niacinamide 30 mg, calcium pantothenate 10 mg, thiamine mononitrate 6 mg, B_2 6 mg, B_6 5 mg, folic acid 0.8 mg/CR Filmtab. Bot. 100s, 500s.
Use: Vitamin/mineral supplement.
IBERET LIQUID. (Abbott) Ferrous sulfate 78.75 mg, vitamins C 375 mg, B_{12} 18.75 mcg, B_1 4.5 mg, B_2 4.5 mg, B_3 22.5 mg, B_5 7.5 mg, B_6 3.75 mg sorbitol, parabens, alcohol 1%, dexpanthenol 2.5 mg/5 ml. Bot. 240 ml.
Use: Vitamin/mineral supplement.
IBERET-500 LIQUID, ORAL SOLUTION. (Abbott) Ferrous sulfate 78.75 mg, vitamins B_1 4.5 mg, B_2 4.5 mg, B_3 22.5 mg, B_5 7.5 mg, B_6 3.75 mg, B_{12} 18.75 mcg, C 112.5 mg, sorbitol, parabens/5 ml. Bot. 240 ml.
Use: Vitamin/mineral supplement.
IBEROL. (Abbott) Vitamins B_{12} 12.5 mcg, iron (as ferrous sulfate) 105 mg, C 75 mg (as sodium ascorbate), B_1 3 mg, B_2 3 mg, niacinamide 15 mg, B_6 1.5 mg, B_5 3 mg/Filmtab. Bot. 100s.
Use: Vitamin/mineral supplement.
IBEROL-F. (Abbott) Vitamins B_{12} 12.5 mcg, elemental iron (as 525 mg ferrous sulfate) 105 mg, folic acid 0.2 mg, C 75 mg, B_1 3 mg, B_2 3 mg, niacinamide 15 mg, B_6 1.5 mg, calcium pantothenate 3 mg/Filmtab. Bot. 100s.
Use: Vitamin/mineral supplement.
•**IBOPAMINE.** USAN.
Use: Dopaminergic agent (peripheral).
•**IBUFENAC.** USAN. (p-Isobutylphenylacetic acid).
Use: Antirheumatic (anti-inflammatory, analgesic and antipyretic).
See: Dytransin.
IBUPRIN. (Thompson Medical) Ibuprofen 200 mg/Tab. Bot. 50s, 100s.
Use: Nonsteroidal anti-inflammatory agent.
•**IBUPROFEN.**
Use: Nonsteroidal anti-inflammatory drug; analgesic.
See: Haltran, Tab. (Upjohn).
Ifen, Tab. (Everett).
Medipren, Tab., Capl. (McNeil Prods).
Motrin, Tab. (Upjohn).

Nuprin, Tab. (Bristol-Myers).
Rufen, Tab. (Boots).
•**IBUPROFEN ALUMINUM.** USAN.
Use: Anti-inflammatory.
•**IBUPROFEN PICONOL.** USAN.
Use: Topical anti-inflammatory.
IBUPROHM. (Ohm Labs.) Ibuprofen 200 mg. **Tab.**: Bot. 24s, 50s, 100s, 165s, 250s, 500s, 1000s. 400 mg/Bot. 50s, 100s, 500s, 1000s. 200 mg **Cap.**: Bot. 24s, 50s, 100s, 250s.
Use: Nonsteroidal anti-inflammatory agent.
IBU-TAB. (Alra) Ibuprofen 400 mg, 600 mg or 800 mg/Tab. Bot. 100s, 500s, 1000s, UD 100s.
Use: Nonsteroidal anti-inflammatory agent.
•**IBUTILIDE FUMARATE.** USAN.
Use: Cardiac depressant.
ICAPS PLUS. (La Haye Labs) Vitamin A 6000 IU, C 200 mg, E 60 IU, B_2 20 mg, Zn, Cu, Se, Mn. Tab. Bot. 60s, 120s.
Use: Vitamin and mineral supplement.
ICAPS TIME RELEASE. (La Haye Labs) Vitamin A 7000 IU, C 200 mg, E 100 IU, B_2 20 mg, Zn, Cu, Se. Tab. Bot. 60s, 120s.
Use: Vitamin and mineral supplement.
•**ICATIBANT ACETATE.** USAN.
Use: Bradykinin antagonist.
ICE MINT. (Westwood) Stearic acid, synthetic cocoa butter, lanolin oil, camphor, menthol, beeswax, mineral oil, sodium borate, aromatic oils, emulsifiers, water. Jar 4 oz.
Use: Emollient, counterirritant.
I-CHLOR 0.5%. (Americal) Chloramphenicol 5 mg/ml. Bot. 7.5 ml, 15 ml.
Use: Anti-infective, ophthalmic.
•**ICHTHAMMOL,** U.S.P. XXIII. Oint., U.S.P. XXIII. Ichthynate. Isarol Oint. (Lilly) 10% and 20% ointment.
Use: Mild antiseptic in skin disorders.
W/Aluminum acetate, phenol, zinc oxide, boric acid, eucalyptol.
See: Lanaburn, Oint. (Lannett).
W/Aluminum hydroxide, phenol, zinc oxide, camphor, eucalyptol.
See: Almophen, Oint. (Bowman).
W/Benzocaine, resin cerate, carbolic acid, thymol, camphor, juniper tar, hexachlorophene.
See: Boil-Ease Anesthetic Drawing Salve (Commerce).
W/Benzocaine, tetracaine, resin cerate, thymol iodide.
See: Boilaid, Oint. (E. J. Moore).
W/Hydrocortisone acetate, benzocaine, oxyquinoline sulfate, ephedrine HCl.

See: Derma Medicone-HC (Medicone).
W/Naftalan, calamine, amber pet.
See: Naftalan, Oint. (Paddock).
W/Phenol, benzocaine, balsam peru, aluminum exsiccated, cade oil, eucalyptus oil, carbolic acid.
See: Alucaine, Oint. (Jenkins).
ICHTHAMMOL. (NMC) Ichthammol 10% or 20% in a lanolin-petrolatum base. Oint. Tube 28.4 g.
Use: Topical antiseptic.
ICHTHYNATE.
See: Ichthammol.
•**ICOTIDINE.** USAN.
Use: Antagonist (to histamine H_2 and H_1 receptors).
•**ICTASOL.** USAN.
Use: Disinfectant.
ICTOTEST REAGENT TABLETS. (Miles Diagnostic) Reagent Tab. For urinary bilirubin. Bot. 100s.
Use: Diagnostic aid.
ICY HOT BALM. (Vicks) Methyl salicylate 29%, menthol 7.6%. Jar 3.5 oz, 7 oz.
Use: External analgesic.
ICY HOT CREAM. (Vicks) Methyl salicylate 30%, menthol 10%. Tube 0.25 oz, 1.25 oz, 3 oz.
Use: External analgesic.
ICY HOT, EXTRA STRENGTH. (Richardson-Vicks) Methyl salicylate 30%, menthol 10%, ceresin, cyclomethicone, hydrogenated castor oil, PEG-150 distearate, propylene glycol, stearic acid, stearyl alcohol. Stick 52.5 Gm.
Use: Rub, liniment.
ICY HOT STICK. (Vicks) Methyl salicylate 15%, menthol 8%. Stick 1.75 oz.
Use: External analgesic.
I.D.A. CAPSULES. (Goldline) Isometheptene mucate 65 mg, dichloralphenazone 100 mg, acetaminophen 324 mg/Cap. Bot. 100s.
Use: Analgesic.
IDAMYCIN. (Adria) Idarubicin HCl. Vial 5 mg, 10 mg.
Use: Antineoplastic agent.
•**IDARUBICIN HYDROCHLORIDE.** USAN.
Use: Antineoplastic. [Orphan drug]
See: Idamycin (Adria).
•**IDOXURIDINE,** U.S.P. XXIII. Ophth. Oint., Soln., U.S.P. XXIII. 5-Iodo-2'-deoxyuridine. Uridine; Dendroid; Kerecid; Ophthalmidine.
Use: Treatment of herpes simplex; antiviral.
See: Herplex, Ophthalmic Soln. (Allergan).
Stoxil, Ophthalmic Soln., Oint. (SK-Beecham).

I-DROPS. (Americal) Tetrahydrozoline HCl 0.5%. Ophthalmic soln. Bot. 0.5 oz
Use: Ophthalmic vasoconstrictor/mydriatic.
IDU. Idoxuridine.
Use: Ophthalmic antiviral drug.
See: Herplex Liquifilm, Soln. (Allergan).
Stoxil, Soln. (SKF).
Stoxil, Oint. (SKF).
IFEN. (Everett) Ibuprofen 400 mg or 600 mg/Tab. Bot. 100s, 500s.
Use: Nonsteroidal anti-inflammatory drug; analgesic.
•**IFETROBAN.** USAN.
Use: Antithrombotic.
IFEX. (Mead Johnson Oncology) Ifosfamide 1 Gm or 3 Gm. Pow. for Inj. Vial single dose.
Use: Antineoplastic agent.
IFLrA. Interferon Alfa-2a.
Use: Antineoplastic agent.
See: Roferon-A (Roche).
IFN-ALPHA 2. Interferon Alfa-2b.
Use: Antineoplastic agent.
See: Intron A (Schering).
•**IFOSFAMIDE,** U.S.P. XXIII. USAN.
Use: Investigative: Antineoplastic. [Orphan drug]
•**IFOSFAMIDE, STERILE,** U.S.P. XXIII.
I-GENT. (Americal) Gentamicin sulfate 3 mg/ml. Ophthalmic soln. Bot. 5 ml.
Use: Anti-infective, ophthalmic.
IGEPAL Co-430. (General Aniline & Film) Non-oxynol 4.
IGEPAL Co-730. (General Aniline & Film) Non-oxynol 15.
IGEPAL Co-880. (General Aniline & Film) Non-oxynol 30.
IGIV. (Various Mfr.) Immune globulin IV.
Use: Immunomodulator (Phase II/III pediatric HIV), immune serum.
See: Gaminune N, Inj. (Cutter Biological).
Gammagard, Pow. (Hyland).
Gammar-IV, Pow. (Armour).
Iveegam, Pow. (Immuno).
Sandoglobulin, Pow. (American Red Cross, Sandoz).
Venoglobulin-I, Pow. (Alpha Therapeutic).
I-HOMATRINE 5%. (Americal) Homatropine hydrobromide 5%. Ophthalmic soln. Bot. 5 ml.
Use: Cycloplegic mydriatic.
IL-2. (Various Mfr.) Interleukin-2.
Use: Cytokine agent.
•**ILEPCIMIDE.** USAN.
Use: Anticonvulsant.
ILETIN I. (Lilly) Regular and modified insulin products from beef and pork.

Regular: 100 units/ml. Vial 10 ml
Lente: 100 units/ml. Vial 10 ml.
Semilente: 40 units or 100 units/ml.
Vial 10 ml.
NPH: 100 units/ml. Vial 10 ml.
Use: Antidiabetic agent.
ILETIN II. (Lilly) Special insulin products prepared from purified beef or purified pork.
Lente: 100 units/ml. Vial 10 ml.
NPH: 100 units/ml. Vial 10 ml.
Use: Antidiabetic agent.
ILETIN II CONCENTRATED. (Lilly) Purified pork regular insulin 500 units/ml. Vial 20 ml.
Use: Antidiabetic agent.
• **ILMOFOSINE.** USAN.
Use: Antineoplastic.
• **ILONIDAP.** USAN.
Use: Antiinflammatory.
ILOPAN. (Adria) Dexpanthenol 250 mg/ml. Amp. 2 ml, Disp. Syringe 2 ml.
Use: GI stimulant.
ILOPAN- CHOLINE. (Adria) Ilopan 50 mg, choline bitartrate 25 mg/Tab. Bot. 100s, 500s.
Use: GI stimulant.
ILOPERIDONE. (Hoechst-Roussel Pharm.) USAN.
Use: Antipsychotic.
ILOPROST INFUSION SOLUTION.
Use: Raynaud's phenomenon. [Orphan drug]
ILOSONE. (Dista) Erythromycin estolate.
Cap.: (Erythromycin base) 250 mg/Pulv. Bot. 24s, 100s, UD 100s, Blister pkg. 10 × 10s. **Liq.:** 125 mg or 250 mg/5 ml. Bot. 100 ml, 16 fl oz. **Tab.:** 500 mg. Bot. 50s. **Susp.:** 125 mg or 250 mg/5 ml. Bot. 10 ml.
Use: Anti-infective.
ILOSONE CHEWABLE. (Dista) Erythromycin estolate 125 mg or 250 mg/Tab. Bot. 50s.
Use: Anti-infective.
ILOTYCIN GLUCEPTATE I.V. (Dista) Erythromycin gluceptate. Vial. I.V. 1 Gm, vial 30 ml. Box 1s.
Use: Anti-infective.
ILOTYCIN OPHTHALMIC OINTMENT. (Dista) Erythromycin 5 mg/Gm. Tube 3.5 Gm, UD 1 Gm/dose tube. Box 24s.
Use: Anti-infective.
ILOZYME. (Adria) Pancrelipase equivalent to lipase 11,000 units, protease 30,000 units, amylase 30,000 units/Tab. Bot. 250s.
Use: Digestive enzymes.
I-LUBE. (Americal) Petrolatum ophthalmic ointment. Tube 0.125 oz

Use: Ophthalmic lubricant.
I.L.X. B12 ELIXIR. (Kenwood) Liver fraction 98 mg, iron 102 mg, vitamins B_1 5 mg, B_2 2 mg, nicotinamide 10 mg, B_{12} 10 mcg/15 ml, alcohol 8%. Bot. 12 oz
Use: Vitamin/mineral supplement.
I.L.X. B12 TABLETS. (Kenwood) Iron 37.5 mg, vitamins C 120 mg, B_{12} 12 mcg, desiccated liver 130 mg, B_1 2 mg, B_2 2 mg/Tab. Bot. 100s.
Use: Vitamin/mineral supplement.
I.L.X. ELIXIR. (Kenwood) Iron 70 mg, liver concentrate 98 mg, vitamins B_1 5 mg, B_2 2 mg, nicotinamide 10 mg/15 ml, alcohol 8%. Bot. 12 oz.
Use: Vitamin/mineral supplement.
• **IMAFEN HYDROCHLORIDE.** USAN.
Use: Antidepressant.
IMAGENT GI. (Alliance) Perflubron Liq. In 200 ml.
Use: Radiopaque agent.
• **IMAZODAN HYDROCHLORIDE.** USAN.
Use: Cardiotonic.
• **IMCARBOFOS.** USAN.
Use: Anthelmintic.
IMCIROMAB PENTETATE. USAN.
Use: Monoclonal antibody (antimyosin). [Orphan drug]
IMDUR. (Key) Isosorbide mononitrate 60 mg. ER Tab. Bot. 30s, 100s, UD 100s.
Use: Antianginal agent.
IMENOL. (Sig) Guaiacol 0.1 Gm, eucalyptol 0.08 Gm, iodoform 0.02 Gm, camphor 0.05 Gm/ml. Vial 30 ml.
Use: Expectorant.
I-METHORPHINAN LEVORPHANOL.
See: Levo-Dromoran, Amp., Tab., Vial (Roche).
IMFERON. (Fisons) An iron-dextran complex containing iron 50 mg/ml. Amp. 2 ml. Box 10s. Vial (w/phenol 0.5%) 10 ml. Box 2s.
Use: Iron supplement.
IMIDAZOLE CARBOXAMIDE.
Use: Antineoplastic agent.
See: Dacarbazine, Inj. (Various Mfr.). DTIC-Dome, Inj. (Miles Pharm).
• **IMIDECYL IODINE.** USAN. 1-Carboxymethylene-1-(2-ethanol)-2-alkyl(C_7 to C_{17})-2-imidazolinium chloride-tridecyl polyoxyethylene-ethanol-iodine complex.
Use: Anti-infective (topical).
• **IMIDOLINE HYDROCHLORIDE.** USAN. 1-(m-Chlorophenyl)-3-(2-(dimethylamino)ethyl)-2-imidazolidinone hydrochloride.
Use: Tranquilizer.
• **IMIDUREA,** N.F. XVIII.
Use: Antimicrobial.

IMIGLUCERASE.
Use: Treatment for Gaucher's disease.
See: Cerezyme (Genzyme).
•**IMILOXAN HYDROCHLORIDE.** USAN.
Use: Antidepressant.
IMIPEMIDE.
Use: Anti-infective.
See: Imipenem, USAN.
•**IMIPENEM.** USAN.
Use: Antibacterial.
W/Cilastatin sodium.
See: Primaxin, Inj (Merck).
•**IMIPENEM, STERILE, U.S.P..** U.S.P. XXIII.
Use: Antibacterial.
•**IMIPRAMINE HCl, U.S.P.** U.S.P. XXIII.
Inj., Tab., U.S.P. XXIII. 5H-Dibenz [b,f] azepine-5-propanamine, 10,11-dihydro-N,N-dimethyl-, HCl. 5-(3-Dimethylaminopropyl)-10,11,dihydro-5H-dibenz-(b,f) azepine HCl. Praminil. Berkomine, IA-Pram, Impamin, Iprogen, Norpramine, & Tofranil HCl salts.
Use: Antidepressant.
See: Janimine, Tab. (Abbott).
Presamine, Tab. (USV).
Tofranil, Tab., Amp. (Geigy).
W.D.D., Tab. (Solvay).
IMIPRAMINE PAMOATE. bis 5-[3-(Dimethylamino) propyl]-10,11-dihydro-5H-dibenz [b,f] azapine compound (2:1)with 4,4-methylenebis-[3-hydroxy-2-naphthoic acid].
Use: Antidepressant.
See: Tofranil-PM, Cap. (Geigy).
IMIREX. (Glaxo) Sumatriptan.
Use: Serotonin agonist.
IMITREX. (Cerenex) Sumatriptan succinate. 12 mg/ml. Inj. Single-dose vial: 6 mg; Self-dose system kit: 2 unit-of-use syringes, 1 self-dose unit.
Use: Agent for migraine.
IMMUN-AID. (McGaw) A custard flavored liquid containing 18.5 g protein, 60 g carbohydrate, 11 g fat per liter. With appropriate vitamins and minerals. Pow. Packets 123 g. 24s.
Use: Full enteral nutrition for immunocompromised patients.
IMMUNE GLOBULIN, U.S.P. XXIII. Immune Serum Globulin Human. Gammaglobulin fraction of normal human plasma. Vial 10 ml. Tubex 1 ml, 2 ml w/thimerosal 1:10,000.
Use: Modification of active measles, prophylaxis of hepatitis, treatment of immune deficiencies.
See: Gamastan, Vial (Cutter).
Gamimune, Vial (Cutter).
Gammar, Vial (Armour).

Immuglobin, Vial (Savage).
IMMUNE GLOBULIN IM.
Use: Immune serum.
See: Gamimune N, Inj. (Cutter Biological).
Gammagard, Pow. (Hyland).
Gammar-IV, Pow. (Armour).
Iveegam, Pow. (Immuno).
Sandoglobulin, Pow. (American Red Cross, Sandoz).
Venoglobulin-I, Pow. (Alpha Therapeutic).
IMMUNE GLOBULIN IV.
Use: Immune serum. [Orphan drug]
See: Gamimune N, Inj. (Miles).
Gammagard, Pow. (Hyland).
Gammar-IV, Pow. (Armour).
Iveegam, Pow. (Immuno).
Sandoglobulin, Pow. (American Red Cross, Sandoz).
Venoglobulin-I, Pow. (Alpha Therapeutic).
IMMUNE GLOBULIN, Rh$_0$ (D).
See: Gamulin Rh (Parke-Davis).
HypRho-D (Cutter).
RhoGAM (Ortho Diagnostics).
IMMUNE SERUMS.
See: Cytomegalovirus Immune Globulin Intravenous (Human) (Massachusetts Public Health Biologic Laboratories).
Human Measles Immune Serum (Various Mfr.).
Immune Serum Globulin (Human).
Polygam S/D (Baxter Healthcare/American Red Cross).
IMMUNE SERUM (ANIMAL).
See: Botulism Antitoxin, Vial (Lederle).
Diphtheria Antitoxin.
Gas Gangrene Antitoxin.
Tetanus Antitoxin.
Tetanus Antitoxin—Gas Gangrene Combined.
IMMUNE SERUM (HUMAN).
See: Hypertussis, Vial (Cutter).
Poliomyelitis Immune Globulin (Various Mfr.).
IMMUNE SERUM GLOBULINS.
See: Western Equine Encephalitis (WEE) Immune Globulin (Various Mfr.).
Vaccinia Immune Globulin (VIG) (Human) (Various Mfr.).
IMMUNEX CRP. (Wampole) Two-minute latex agglutination slide test for the qualitative detection of C-Reactive protein in serum. Kit 100s.
Use: Diagnostic aid.
IMMUNO-C. (Biomune Systems)
See: BOVINE WHEY PROTEIN CONCENTRATE.

IMMUNOSUPPRESSIVE DRUGS.
See: Sandimmune, Cap., Oral Soln. or
IV Soln. (Sandoz).
Orthoclone OKT3, Inj. (Ortho).
IMODIUM A-D. (McNeil) Loperamide 1
mg/5 ml, alcohol 5.25%.
Use: Antidiarrheal.
IMODIUM CAPSULES. (Janssen) Lop-
eramide 2 mg/Cap. Bot. 100s, 500s, UD
100s.
Use: Antidiarrheal.
IMODIUM LIQUID. (Janssen) Lop-
eramide 0.2 mg/ml. Bot. 120 ml.
Use: Antidiarrheal.
IMOGAM RABIES IMMUNE GLOBULIN.
(Connaught) Rabies immune globulin
(human) 150 IU/ml. Vials 2 ml, 10 ml in
tamper proof box.
Use: Rabies prophylaxis agent.
IMOLAMINE. B.A.N. 4-(2-Diethyl-
laminoethyl)-5-imino-3-phenyl-1,2,4-
oxadiazoline.
Use: Treatment of angina pectoris.
IMOVAX RABIES I.D. (Connaught) Rabies vaccine 0.25 IU/0.1 ml for I.D. administration for pre-exposure treatment
only. Wistar rabies virus strain PM-1503-
3M grown in human diploid cell culture
Vaccine is lypholized inside an ID syringe sealed in vaccum tube. In single
dose syringe w/1 vial diluent.
Use: Rabies prophylaxis agent.
IMOVAX RABIES VACCINE. (Connaught) Merieux rabies vaccine, Wistar
rabies virus strain PM-1503-3M grown in
human diploid cell cultures. Tamper
proof box w/1 ml vaccine, syringe, needles, and 1 vial diluent.
Use: Rabies prophylaxis agent.
IMPACT. (Approved) Belladonna alka-
loids 0.16 mg, phenylpropanolamine
HCl 50 mg, chlorpheniramine maleate 1
mg, pheniramine maleate 12.5 mg/Cap.
Pack 12s, 24s. Vial 15s, 30s, Bot.
1000s.
Use: Anticholinergic/antispasmodic, de-
congestant, antihistamine.
IMPROMEN. (Janssen) Bromperidol de-
canoate.
Use: Antipsychotic.
IMPROMEN DECANOAS. (Janssen)
Bromperidol decanoate.
Use: Antipsychotic.
• **IMPROMIDINE HYDROCHLORIDE.**
USAN.
Use: Diagnostic aid.
IMREG-1. (Imreg)
Use: Immunomodulator.
IMREG-2. (Imreg)
Use: Immunomodulator.

IMURAN. (Burroughs Wellcome) **Tab.**:
Azathioprine 50 mg/Tab. Bot. 100s, UD
100s. **Inj.**: Azathioprine 100 mg/20 ml.
Vial.
Use: Immunosuppressive agent.
IMUTHIOL. (Cannaught) Diethyldithiocar-
bamate.
Use: Immunomodulator.
**INACTIVATED DIAGNOSTIC DIPHTHE-
RIA TOXIN.**
See: Diphtheria Toxin for Schick Test,
U.S.P. XXIII.
INAPSINE. (Janssen) Droperidol 2.5
mg/ml. Amp. 2 ml, 5 ml, 10 ml. Box 10s.
Multi dose Vial w/methylparaben 1.8
mg, propylparaben 0.2 mg, lactic
acid/10 ml. Box 10s.
Use: General anesthetic.
W/Fentanyl citrate.
See: Innovar, Inj. (Janssen).
INCREMIN W/IRON. (Lederle) l-Lysine
HCl 300 mg, vitamins B_{12} 25 mcg, B_1 10
mg, B_6 5 mg, ferric pyrophosphate solu-
ble 30 mg, sorbitol 3.5 Gm, alcohol
0.75%/5 ml. Syr. Bot. 4 fl oz, 16 fl oz.
Use: Vitamin/mineral supplement.
• **INDACRINONE.** USAN.
Use: Antihypertensive, diuretic.
INDALONE.
See: Butopyronoxyl (Various Mfr.).
INDANDIONE DERIVATIVE.
Use: Anticoagulant.
See: Anisindione (Various Mfr.).
• **INDAPAMIDE.** USAN.
Use: Antihypertensive, diuretic.
See: Lozol, Tab. (Rhone-Poulenc Ror-
er).
INDAPAMIDE. (Arcola) Indapamide 2.5
mg. Tab. Bot. 100s, 1000s.
Use: Antihypertensive, diuretic.
• **INDECAINIDE HYDROCHLORIDE.**
USAN.
Use: Cardiac depressant.
See: Decabid (Lilly).
• **INDELOXAZINE HYDROCHLORIDE.**
USAN.
Use: Antidepressant.
INDERAL INJECTION. (Wyeth-Ayerst)
Propranolol HCl 1 mg/ml. Amp. 1 ml.
Box 10s.
Use: Beta-adrenergic blocking agent.
INDERAL-LA. (Wyeth-Ayerst) Propra-
nolol HCl 80 mg, 120 mg or 160 mg/SR
Cap. Bot. 100s, 1000s, UD 100s.
Use: Beta-adrenergic blocking agent.
INDERAL TABLETS. (Wyeth-Ayerst)
Propranolol HCl 10 mg, 20 mg, 40 mg,
60 mg or 80 mg/Tab. Bot. 100s, 1000s,
UD 100s.
Use: Beta-adrenergic blocking agent.

INDERIDE. (Wyeth-Ayerst) Propranolol HCl 40 mg, hydrochlorothiazide 25 mg/Tab. Bot. 100s, 1000s, UD 100s. Propranolol HCl 80 mg, hydrochlorothiazide 25 mg/Tab. Bot. 100s, 1000s, UD 100s.
Use: Antihypertensive combination.

INDERIDE LA CAPSULES. (Wyeth-Ayerst) Propranolol HCl/hydrochlorothiazide Long Acting Caps: 80 mg/50 mg, 120 mg/50 mg or 160 mg/50 mg. Bot. 100s.
Use: Antihypertensive combination.

INDIAN GUM.
See: Karaya Gum.

INDIGO CARMINE. (Hynson, Westcott & Dunning) Sodium indigotindisulfonate 8 mg/ml. Amp. 5 ml. Box 10s, 100s.
Use: Diagnostic aid.
See: Sodium indigotindisulfonate.

INDIGO CARMINE SOLUTION. (Hynson, Westcott & Dunning) Indigotindisulfonate sodium inj. (0.8% aqueous soln. sodium salt of indigotindisulfonic acid) 40 mg/5 ml. Amp. 5 ml, 10s.
Use: Diagnostic aid.

INDIGOTINDISULFONATE SODIUM, U.S.P. XXIII. Inj., U.S.P. XXIII. 1H-Indole-5-sulfonic acid, 2-(1,3-dihydro-4-oxo-5-sulfo-2H-indol-2-ylidene)-2,3-dihydro-3-oxo-, sodium salt. Indigo Carmine, Amp. (Various Mfr.).
Use: Diagnostic aid (cystoscopy).
See: Sodium Indigotindisulfonate.

• **INDIUM IN III ALTUMOMAB PENTETATE.** USAN.
Use: Radiodiagnostic monoclonal antibody. [Orphan drug]

INDIUM IN 111 MURINE MONOCLONAL ANTIBODY FAB TO MYOSIN.
Use: Diagnostic aid in myocarditis. [Orphan drug]

• **INDIUM IN III OXYQUINOLINE.** USAN.
Use: Radioactive agent, diagnostic aid.

• **INDIUM IN 111 PENTETRATE INJECTION,** U.S.P. XXIII.
Use: Diagnostic aid for cardiac output determination.

• **INDIUM IN 111 SATUMOMAB PENDETIDE.** USAN.
Use: Radiodiagnostic monoclonal antibody.

INDOCHRON E-R. (Inwood) Indomethacin 75 mg. SR Cap. Bot. 60s, 100s.
Use: Nonsteroidal anti-inflammatory agent.

INDOCIN. (Merck) Indomethacin. **Cap.:** 25 mg. Bot. 100s, 1000s, UD 100s. Unit-of-use 100s; 50 mg. Bot. 100s, UD 100s.

Supp.: 50 mg. Pkg. 30s. **Oral Susp.:** 25 mg/5 ml, alcohol 1%, sorbitol 0.1%. Bot. 237 ml.
Use: Nonsteroidal anti-inflammatory drug; analgesic.

INDOCIN I.V. (Merck, Sharp & Dohme) Indomethacin sodium trihydrate equivalent to 1 mg indomethacin/Vial. Vial single dose.
Use: Agent for patent ductus arteriosus.

INDOCIN SR. (Merck) Indomethacin 75 mg/SR Cap. Unit-of-Use 30s, 60s.
Use: Nonsteroidal anti-inflammatory drug; analgesic.

• **INDOCYANINE GREEN,** U.S.P. XXIII. Sterile, U.S.P. XXIII. A tricarbocyanine dye. 1H-Benz [e] indolium, 2-[7-[1,3-dihydro-1,1-dimethyl-3-(4-sulfobutyl)-2H-benz [e] indol-2-ylidene]-1,3,5-heptatrienyl]-1,1-dimethyl-3-(4-sulfobutyl)-, hydroxide, inner salt, sodium salt.
Use: Diagnostic aid (cardiac output determination, hepatic function determination).
See: Cardio-Green, Inj. (Beckton-Dickinson).

INDOGESIC. (Century) Acetaminophen 32.5 mg, butalbital 50 mg/Tab. Bot. 100s, 1000s.
Use: Analgesic, sedative/hypnotic.

INDOKLON. Hexafluorodiethyl ether. Flurothyl. Bis-(2,2,2-trifluorethyl)ether.
Use: Shock inducing agent (convulsant).

• **INDOLAPRIL HYDROCHLORIDE.** USAN.
Use: Antihypertensive.

INDO-LEMMON. (Lemmon) Indomethacin 25 mg or 50 mg/Cap. Bot. 100s, 500s, 1000s.
Use: Nonsteroidal anti-inflammatory drug; analgesic.

• **INDOLIDAN.** USAN.
Use: Cardiotonic.

INDOMETH CAPS. (Major) Indomethacin 25 mg or 50 mg/Tab. **25 mg:** Bot. 100s, 1000s. **50 mg:** Bot. 100s, 500s.
Use: Nonsteroidal anti-inflammatory drug; analgesic.

• **INDOMETHACIN,** U.S.P. XXIII. Cap., Supp., Extended-release Cap., Suspension. 1-(p-Chlorobenzoyl)-5-methoxy-2-methyl-indole-3-acetic acid. (Various Mfr.) **Cap.: 25 mg:** 60s, 100s, 500s, 1000s, UD 100s; **50 mg:** 23s, 72s, 100s, 250s, 500s, UD 100s; **SR Cap.:** 75 mg. Bot. 60s, 100s.
Use: Anti-inflammatory agent (nonsteroid).
See: Indochron E-R, Cap. (Inwood).

Indocin, Cap., S.R. Cap., I.V., Oral Susp., Supp. (Merck).
Indo-Lemmon, Cap. (Lemmon).
INDOMETHACIN. (Roxane) Indomethacin 25 mg/5ml. Oral susp. Bot. 500 ml.
Use: Nonsteroidal anti-inflammatory agent.
• **INDOMETHACIN SODIUM.** USAN.
Use: Anti-inflammatory.
INDOMETHACIN SODIUM TRIHYDRATE.
Use: Patent ductus arteriosus.
See: Indocin I.V., Pow. (Merck & Co.).
• **INDOPROFEN.** USAN.
Use: Analgesic, anti-inflammatory.
• **INDORAMIN.** USAN. N-[1-(2-Indol-3-ylethyl)-4-piperidyl]benzamide. 3-[2-(4-Benzamidopiperidino)ethyl]indole.
Use: Antihypertensive.
• **INDORAMIN HYDROCHLORIDE.** USAN.
Use: Antihypertensive.
• **INDORENATE HYDROCHLORIDE.** USAN.
Use: Antihypertensive.
• **INDOXOLE.** USAN.
Use: Antipyretic, anti-inflammatory.
• **INDRILINE HYDROCHLORIDE.** USAN.
Use: Stimulant.
I-NEOCORT. (American) Neomycin sulfate 5 mg, hydrocortisone acetate 15 mg/5 ml. Ophthalmic susp. Bot. 5 ml.
Use: Anti-infective, corticosteroid.
I-NEOSPOR. (American) Polymyxin B sulfate, gramicidin, neomycin sulfate ophthalmic soln. Bot. 10 ml.
Use: Anti-infective.
INFACAPS A & D. (Lannett) Vitamins A 3000 IU, D 800 IU/Cap. Bot. 1000s, 5000s.
Use: Vitamin supplement.
INFALYTE ORAL SOLUTION. (Mead Johnson) Electrolyte mixture with 30 g/L rice syrup solids containing 4.2 calories/fl. oz. In 1 liter.
Use: Nutritional supplement.
INFANT FOODS.
Use: Enteral nutritional therapy.
See: Enfamil (Mead Johnson Nutritional).
Enfamil Human Milk Fortifier (Mead Johnson Nutritionals).
Enfamil Premature 20 Formula (Mead Johnson Nutritionals).
RCF Liquid (Ross).
Similac (Ross).
Similac PM 60/40 Liquid (Ross).
INFANT FOODS, HYPOALLERGENIC.
Use: Enteral nutritional therapy.
See: Alimentation (Ross).

Isomil (Ross).
Isomil SF (Ross).
I-Soyalac (Loma Linda).
Nutramigen (Mead Johnson Nutritionals).
Pregestimil Powder (Mead Johnson Nutritionals).
ProSobee (Mead Johnson Nutritionals).
Soyalac (Loma Linda).
INFANTOL PINK. (Scherer) Paregoric (equivalent) contains opium 15 mg/fl oz, bismuth subsalicylate, calcium carageenan, pectin, zinc phenolsulfonate, alcohol 2%. Susp. Bot. 4 oz, 8 oz, pt.
Use: Antidiarrheal.
INFANT'S NO-ASPIRIN DROPS. (Walgreen) Acetaminophen 80 mg/0.8 ml. Non-alcoholic. Bot. 15 ml.
Use: Analgesic.
INFARUB CREAM. (Whitehall) Methyl salicylate 35%, menthol 10% in vanishing cream base. Tube 1.25 oz, 3.5 oz.
Use: External analgesic.
INFATUSS. (Scott/Cord) Dextromethorphan HBr 7.2 mg, chlorpheniramine maleate 1.1 mg, phenylpropanolamine HCl 4.8 mg, ammonium Cl 50 mg/5 ml. Bot. 4 oz, pt, gal.
Use: Antitussive, antihistamine, decongestant, expectorant.
INFECTROL OINTMENT. (Bausch & Lomb) Dexamethasone 0.1%, neomycin sulfate equivalent to 0.35% neomycin base and 10,000 units polymyxin B sulfate/Gm. White petrolatum, lanolin, mineral oil, parabens. Oint. Tube 3.5, 3.75 Gm.
Use: Steroid/antibiotic ointment.
INFECTROL SUSPENSION. (Bausch & Lomb) Dexamethasone 0.1%, neomycin sulfate equivalent to 0.35% neomycin base and 10,000 units polymyxin B sulfate/ml. Hydroxypropyl methylcellulose, polysorbate 20, benzalkonium chloride. Drop. Bot. 5 ml.
Use: Steroid/antibiotic drops.
InFe D. (Schein) Iron 50/ml (as dextran), sodium chloride 0.9%. Inj. Amp 2 ml. Vial 10 ml.
Use: Parenteral iron supplement.
INFLAMASE FORTE 1% OPHTHALMIC SOLUTION. (Iolab) Prednisolone sodium phosphate 1% (equivalent to prednisolone phosphate 0.91%). Bot. 5 ml, 10 ml, 15 ml.
Use: Corticosteroid, ophthalmic.
INFLAMASE MILD 1/8% OPHTHALMIC SOLUTION. (Iolab) Prednisolone sodi-

um phosphate 0.125% (equivalent to prednisolone phosphate 0.11%). Bot. 5 ml, 10 ml w/dropper.
Use: Corticosteroid, ophthalmic.
•**INFLUENZA VIRUS VACCINE,** U.S.P. XXIII.
Use: Active immunizing agent.
See: Flu-Imune, Inj. (Lederle).
Fluogen, Inj. (Parke-Davis).
Flu-Shield, Inj. (Wyeth-Ayerst).
Fluvirin, Inj. (Adams).
Fluzone, Inj. (Connaught).
INFLUENZAE TYPE B SERUM (RABBIT) ANTIHEMOPHILUS. (Various Mfr.) The sterile suspension of formaldehyde-killed influenza virus, type A, Asian strain grown in the extra-embryonic fluid of chick eggs.
Use: Agent for immunization.
INFLUENZA VIRUS VACCINE. Types A and B. A/Texas/36/91 (H1N1) 15 mcg, A/Beijing/353/89 (H3N2) 15 mcg, B/Panama/45/90 15 mcg/0.5 ml. Vial. 0.5 ml, 5 ml.
Use: Agent for immunization.
See: Flu-Imune, Inj. (Lederle).
Fluogen, Inj. (Parke-Davis).
Flu-Shield, Inj. (Wyeth-Ayerst).
Fluvirin, Inj. (Adams).
Fluzone, Inj. (Connaught).
INFLUENZA VIRUS VACCINE, TRIVALENT TYPES A & B. (Wyeth-Ayerst) a/Taiwan/1/86 (H1N1) 15 mcg, A/Beijing/353/89 (H3N2) 15 mcg, B/Panama/45/90 15 mcg, hemagglutinin antigens per 0.5 ml, with 0.01% thimerosal. Inj. (Split-Virus). Vial 5 ml. Tubex 0.5 ml.
Use: Agent for immunization.
INFRARUB. (Whitehall) Methyl salicylate 35%, menthol 10%. Cream. Jar 37.5, 90 Gm.
Use: Liniment.
INFUMORPH 200. (Elkins-Sinn) Morphine sulfate 10 mg/ml/Inj. Ampuls 20 ml. Preservative free.
Use: Narcotic analgesic.
INFUMORPH 500. (Elkins-Sinn) Morphine sulfate 25 mg/ml/Inj. Ampuls 20 ml. Preservative free.
Use: Narcotic analgesic.
INGADINE TABS. (Major) Guanethidine · sulfate 10 mg or 25 mg/Tab. Bot. 100s, 1000s.
Use: Antihypertensive.
INH. (Ciba) Isoniazid 300 mg/Tab.
Use: Antituberculous agent.
See: Rimactane/INH, Dual Pack (Ciba).
INHAL-AID. (Key)
Use: Drug delivery system for metered dose inhalers.

INHIBACE. (Roche/Glaxo) Cilazapril.
Use: ACE inhibitor.
INNERCLEAN HERBAL LAXATIVE. (Last) Senna leaf powder, psyllium seed, buckthorne, anise seed, fennel seed. Bot. 1 oz, 2 oz.
Use: Laxative.
INNERTABS. (Last) Senna leaf powder and psyllium seed tablets. Bot. 80s, 200s.
Use: Laxative.
INNOGEL PLUS. (Hogil Pharm.) Pyrethrins 0.3%, piperonyl butoxide technical 3%. Gel. Kits contain 3 predosed gel paks and a comb.
Use: Pediculicides.
INNOVAR INJECTION. (Janssen) Fentanyl citrate 0.05 mg, droperidol 2.5 mg/ml. Amp. 2 ml, 5 ml. Box of 10s.
Use: Narcotic analgesic, general anesthetic.
INOCOR LACTATE. (Sanofi Winthrop) Amrinone lactate (base equivalent) 5 mg/ml, sodium metabisulfite 0.25 mg. Amp. 20 ml. Box 5s.
Use: Short-term management of congestive heart failure.
INOPHYLLINE.
See: Aminophylline (Various Mfr.).
INOSINE PRANOBEX. (Newport Pharmaceuticals) Isoprinosine.
Use: Antiviral. [Orphan drug]
INOSIPLEX. (Newport Pharmaceuticals) Isoprinosine.
Use: Antiviral.
INOSIT.
See: Inositol (Various Mfr.).
INOSITOL. 1,2,3,5/4,6-Cyclohexanehexol. Commercial solvents (Bios 1,Hexahydroxycyclohexane, Inosit, Dambose).
Use: Lipotropic.
W/Choline bitartrate, vitamins, minerals.
W/Choline Cl, dl-methionine, vitamin B_{12}.
See: Cho-Meth, Vial (Kenyon).
W/Methionine, choline bitartrate, liver desiccated, vitamin B_{12}.
See: Limvic, Tab. (Briar).
W/Panthenol, choline Cl, vitamins, minerals, estrone, testosterone.
See: Geramine, Inj. (Brown).
W/Panthenol, choline Cl, vitamins, minerals, estrone, testosterone, polydigestase.
See: Geramine, Tab. (Brown).
•**INOSITOL NIACINATE.** USAN. Myo-Inositol hexanicotinate. Meso-inositol hexanicotinate, hexanicotinate. Mesoinositol hexanicotinate. Hexopal; Mesonex.
Use: Peripheral vasodilator.

INOSITOL NICOTINATE. Inositol Niacinate.

INPERSOL W/DEXTROSE. (Abbott Hospital Prods) Dextrose 1.5%, 2.5% or 4.25%, sodium Cl 140.5 mEq, calcium Cl 3.5 mEq, magnesium Cl 1.5 mEq, sodium lactate 445 mEq/100 ml. **1.5% Dextrose:** 1000 ml, 2000 ml. **2.5% Dextrose:** 1000 ml, 2000 ml. **4.25% Dextrose:** 2000 ml.
Use: Peritoneal dialysis solution.

INPERSOL-LM W/DEXTROSE. (Abbott Hospital Prods) Inpersol-LM w/ dextrose 1.5%, 2.5% or 4.25%. **1.5% Dextrose:** 1000 ml, 2000 ml flexible container. **2.5% Dextrose:** 1000 ml, 2000 ml flexible container. **4.25% Dextrose:** 2000 ml flexible container.
Use: Peritoneal dialysis solution.

INPROQUONE. B.A.N. 2,5-Di(aziridin-1-yl)-3,6-dipropoxy-1,4-benzoquinone.
Use: Antineoplastic agent.

INSPIREASE. (Key).
Use: Drug delivery system for metered-dose inhalers.

INSTA-CHAR. (Kerr) **Regular:** Aqueous suspension activated charcoal 50 Gm/8 oz. **Pediatric:** Aqueous suspension activated charcoal 15 Gm/4 oz.
Use: Antidote.

INSTA-GLUCOSE. (ICN) Undiluted USP glucose. UD tube containing liquid glucose 31 Gm.
Use: Glucose elevating agent.

INST-E-VITE. (Barth's) Vitamin E 100 IU or 200 IU/Cap. **100 IU:** Bot 100s, 500s, 1000s. **200 IU:** Bot. 100s, 250s, 500s.
Use: Vitamin E supplement.

INSULATARD NPH HUMAN. (Nordisk-USA) Human insulin isophane suspension 100 IU/ml.
Use: Antidiabetic agent.

• **INSULIN.** U.S.P. XXIII. Inj., U.S.P. XXIII.
Use: Antidiabetic.
See: Iletin Prods. (Lilly).
Insulin Prods. (Squibb).

INSULIN. (Nordisk) Insulatard NPH Mixtard Velosulin.
Use: Antidiabetic agent.

• **INSULIN I-125,** Inj., U.S.P. 23.
Use: Radioactive agent.

• **INSULIN I-131.** USAN.
Use: Radioactive agent.

• **INSULIN, DALANATED.** USAN.
Use: Antidiabetic.

INSULIN, GLOBIN ZINC INJECTION.
Use: Antidiabetic agent.

• **INSULIN HUMAN,** U.S.P. XXIII. Inj., U.S.P. XXIII.
Use: Antidiabetic.

• **INSULIN INJECTION,** U.S.P. XXIII. Insulin, insulin HCl.
Use: Antidiabetic.

INSULIN-LIKE GROWTH FACTOR-1.
Use: Amyotrophic lateral sclerosis. [Orphan drug]

• **INSULIN, NEUTRAL.** USAN.
Use: Antidiabetic.

INSULIN NOVO RAPITARD. Biphasic Insulin Injection, B.A.N.

• **INSULIN, PROTAMINE ZINC SUSPENSION,** U.S.P. XXII. 40 or 100 units/ml. Vials 10 ml.
Use: Antidiabetic.

INSULIN, REGULAR.
Use: Antidiabetic.
See: Regular Iletin I (Beef and Pork), Inj. (Lilly).
Regular Insulin (Pork), Inj. (Novo Nordisk).
Pork Regular Iletin II (Pork), Inj. (Lilly).
Regular Purified Pork Insulin, Inj. (Novo Nordisk).
Velosulin (Pork), Inj. (Novo Nordisk).
Humulin R, Inj. (Lilly).
Humulin BR, Inj. (Lilly).
Novolin R, Inj. (Novo Nordisk).
Velosulin, Inj. (Novo Nordisk).
Novolin R PenFill, Cartridges (Novo Nordisk).

INSULIN, REGULAR CONCENTRATE.
Use: Antidiabetic agent.
See: Semilente Iletin I (Beef or Pork), Inj. (Lilly).
Semilente Insulin (Beef), Inj. (Novo Nordisk).

INSULIN SUSPENSION, ISOPHANE.
Use: Antidiabetic agent.
See: Humulin 50/50, Inj. (Lilly).
Humulin 70/30, Inj. (Lilly).
Mixtard, Inj. (Novo Nordisk).
Novolin 70/30, Inj. (Novo Nordisk).
Novolin 70/30 PenFill, Cartridge (Novo Nordisk).

INSULIN SUSPENSION, LENTE.
Use: Antidiabetic agent.
See: Lente Insulin, Cial (Novo Nordisk).
Lente L, Vial (Novo Nordisk).
Novolin L, Vial (Novo Nordisk).
Lente Iletin I (Beef and Pork), Inj. (Lilly).
Lente Insulin (Beef), Inj. (Novo Nordisk).
Lente Iletin II (Pork), Inj. (Lilly).
Lente Iletin II (Beef), Inj. (Lilly).
Lente Purified Pork Insulin, Inj. (Novo Nordisk).
Humulin L, Inj. (Lilly).
Novolin L, Inj. (Novo Nordisk).

INSULIN SUSPENSION, NPH.
Use: Antidiabetic agent.
See: NPH Iletin I (Beef and Pork), Inj.
(Lilly).
NPH Insulin (Beef), Inj. (Novo
Nordisk).
Beef NPH Iletin II, Inj. (Lilly).
NPH-N Purified (Pork), Inj. (Novo
Nordisk).
Pork NPH Iletin II, Inj. (Lilly).
Insulatard NPH (Pork), Inj. (Novo
Nordisk).
Humulin N, Inj. (Lilly).
Insulatard NPH, Inj. (Novo Nordisk).
Novolin N, Inj. (Novo Nordisk).
Novolin N PenFill, Cartridge (Novo
Nordisk).
INSULIN SUSPENSION, PZI.
Use: Antiadiabetic agent.
Humulin U Ultralente, Inj. (Lilly).
INSULIN SUSPENSION SEMILENTE.
Use: Antidiabetic agent.
See: Semilente Iletin I (Beef or Pork),
Inj. (Lilly).
Semilente Insulin (Beef), Inj. (Novo
Nordisk).
INSULIN SUSPENSION, ULTRALENTE.
Use: Antidiabetic agent.
See: Ultralente Insulin (Beef), Inj. (Novo
Nordisk).
Humulin U Ultralente, Inj. (Lilly).
•**INSULIN ZINC SUSPENSION,** U.S.P.
XXIII.
Use: Antidiabetic.
See: Humulin L, Bot. (Lilly).
Lente Insulin, Vial (Lilly).
Lente Insulin, Vial (Novo Nordisk).
Lente L, Vial (Novo Nordisk).
Novolin L, Vial (Novo Nordisk).
•**INSULIN ZINC SUSPENSION, EXTEND-
ED,** U.S.P. XXIII.
Use: Antidiabetic.
See: Humulin U Ultralente, Bot. (Lilly).
Ultralente U, Vial (Novo Nordisk).
INTAL INHALER. (Fisons) Cromolyn
sodium inhalation aerosol 800 mcg/actu-
ation. Canister 8.1 Gm, 14.2 Gm.
Use: Respiratory inhalant product.
INTAL NEBULIZER SOLUTION. (Fisons)
Cromolyn sodium 20 mg in 2 ml distilled
water for use with a power operated
nebulizer unit. Box 60s, 120s, Amp. 2
ml.
Use: Respiratory inhalant product.
INTEGRIN CAPS. (Sanofi Winthrop)
Oxypertine.
Use: Anxiolytic, tranquilizer.
INTENSOL. (Roxane) A system of con-
centrated solutions of drugs w/calibrated
dropper:

Chlorpromazine HCl 30 mg or 100
mg/ml.
Dexamethasone 1 mg/ml.
Dihydrotachysterol 0.2 mg/ml.
Hydrochlorothiazide 100 mg/ml.
Prednisone 5 mg/ml.
Thioridazine HCl 30 mg or 100 mg/ml.
•**INTERFERON.** USAN. A family of naturally occurring, small protein molecules
with molecular weights of approximately
15,000 to 21,000 daltons. They are
formed by the interaction of animal cells
with viruses capable of conferring on animal cells resistance to virus infection.
Three major classes of interferons have
been identified: alpha, beta, and gam-
ma. Interferon was first derived from hu-
man white blood cells and originally
used in Finland.
Use: Antineoplastic, antiviral. Treatment
of breast cancer lymphoma, multiple
melanoma and malignant melanoma.
See: Intron-A, Inj. (Schering).
•**INTERFERON ALFA-2A.** USAN.
Use: Antineoplastic, antiviral. [Orphan
drug]
See: Roferon-A (Roche).
•**INTERFERON ALFA-2B.** USAN.
Use: Antineoplastic, antiviral. [Orphan
drug]
See: Intron-A (Schering).
•**INTERFERON ALFA-NL.** USAN.
Use: Antiviral, antineoplastic. [Orphan
drug]
See: Wellferon (Burroughs Wellcome).
•**INTEFERON ALFA-N3.** Formerly Leuko-
cyte Interferon.
Use: Antiviral, antineoplastic.
INTERFERON BETA. (Biogen)
Use: Cytokine agent.
See: Betaseron (Berlex).
•**INTERFERON BETA-1a.** USAN.
Use: Immunomodulator.
•**INTERFERON BETA-1b.** USAN.
Use: Immunomodulator.
INTERFERON BETA (RECOMBINANT).
Use: Immune therapy. [Orphan drug]
See: r-IFN-beta.
R-Frone.
•**INTERFERON GAMMA-1B.** USAN.
Use: Antineoplastic, antiviral, im-
munoregulator. [Orphan drug]
See: Actimmune (Genentech).
**INTERLEUKIN-1 ALPHA (HUMAN RE-
COMBINANT).**
Use: Bone marrow transplant, aplastic
anemia. [Orphan drug]
**INTERLEUKIN-1 RECEPTOR ANTAGO-
NIST, HUMAN RECOMBINANT.**
Use: Juvenile rheumatoid arthritis,

graft-v-host disease in transplant patients. [Orphan drug]
INTERLEUKIN-2.
Use: Cytokine agent.
See: Proleukin (Hoffmann-LaRoche/Immunex).
INTERLEUKIN-2, RECOMBINANT LIPOSOME ENCAPSULATED.
Use: Antineoplastic. [Orphan drug]
INTERLEUKIN-2 PEG. (Cetus).
Use: Cytokine agent.
INTERLEUKIN-3, RECOMBINANT HUMAN. (Sandoz).
Use: Cytokine agent. [Orphan drug]
INTESTINAL ANTI-INFLAMMATORY AGENTS.
Use: Ulcerative colitis.
See: Dipentum (Pharmacia).
Rowasa (Solvay).
INTRALIPID 10% I.V. FAT EMULSION.
(KabiVitrum) I.V. fat emulsion containing soybean oil 10%, egg yolk phospholipids 1.2%, glycerin 2.25% and water for injection. I.V. Flask 50 ml, 100 ml, 250 ml, 500 ml.
Use: Parenteral nutritional supplement.
INTRALIPID 20% I.V. FAT EMULSION.
(KabiVitrum) I.V. fat emulsion containing soybean oil 20%, egg yolk phospholipids 1.2%, glycerin 2.25% and water for injection. I.V. Flask 50 ml, 100 ml, 250 ml, 500 ml.
Use: Parenteral nutritional supplement.
INTRANASAL STEROIDS.
See: Decadron Phosphate Turbinaire (Merck & Co.).
Nasalide (Syntex).
Beconase Inhalation (Allen & Hanburys).
Vancenase Nasal Inhaler (Schering).
Beconase AQ Nasal (Allen & Hanburys).
Vancenase AQ Nasal (Schering).
INTRASITE. (Smith & Nephew Solopak) Graft T starch copolymer 2%, water 8%, propylene glycol 20%. Sterile amorphous interactive hydrogel dressing. 25 Gm.
Use: Wound dressing.
INTRAUTERINE PROGESTERONE SYSTEM.
Use: Contraceptive.
See: Progestasert (Alza).
INTRAVAL SODIUM.
See: Pentothal Sodium, Preps. (Abbott).
INTRAVASCULAR PERFLUOROCHEMICAL EMULSION 20%.
Use: Perfluorochemical emulsion.
See: Fluosol.
•**INTRAZOLE.** USAN. 1-(p-Chloroben-

zoyl)-3-(1H-tetrazol-5-ylmethyl) indole.
Use: Anti-inflammatory.
•**INTRIPTYLINE HYDROCHLORIDE.**
USAN.
Use: Antidepressant.
INTROLITE. (Ross) Protein 22.2 g, carbohydrate 70.5 g, fat 18.4 g, sodium 930 mg, potassium 1570 mg/L with 200 mOsm/kg water, with appropriate vitamins and minerals, 0.53 Cal/ml. Liq.
Use: Enteral nutritional supplement.
INTRON-A FOR INJECTION. (Schering) Interferon alfa-2b (IFN-alpha 2; rIFN-α2; α-2-interferon) recombinant as 3 million, 5 million, 10 million, 20 million or 50 million IU/Vial. Subcutaneous or intramuscular injection. Vial 1s w/diluent.
Use: Antineoplastic agent.
INTROPAQUE LIQUID. (Lafayette) Barium sulfate 60% w/v suspension. Bot. gal. Case 4 Bot.
Use: Radiopaque agent.
INTROPIN 200 mg. (DuPont Critical Care) Dopamine HCl 40 mg/ml, sodium bisulfite 1% as an antioxidant. Vial 5 ml. Box 20s; Amp. 5 ml. Box 20s; Prefilled additive Syr. 5 ml. Box 5s.
Use: Vasopressor used in shock.
INTROPIN 400 mg. (DuPont Critical Care) Dopamine HCl 80 mg/ml, sodium bisulfite 1% as an antioxidant. Vial 5 ml. Box 20s.; Prefilled additive Syringe 5 ml. Box 5s.
Use: Vasopressor used in shock.
INTROPIN 800 mg. (DuPont Critical Care) Dopamine HCl 160 mg/ml, sodium bisulfite 1% as an antioxidant. Vial 5 ml. Box 20s.; Prefilled additive syringe 5 ml. Box 5s.
Use: Vasopressor used in shock.
INULIN. (American Critical Care) Purified inulin 5 Gm/50 ml sodium Cl 0.9%, sodium hydroxide to adjust pH. Amp. 50 ml.
Use: Diagnostic aid.
•**INULIN IN SODIUM CHLORIDE INJECTION, U.S.P.** U.S.P. XXIII.
Use: Diagnostic aid.
INVERSINE. (Merck, Sharp & Dohme) Mecamylamine HCl 2.5 mg/Tab. Bot. 100s.
Use: Antihypertensive.
INVERT SUGAR. (Abbott) 10% soln. Bot. 1000 ml.
Use: Parenteral nutritional supplement.
See: Emetrol, Liq. (Rhone-Poulenc Rorer).
Travert, Soln. (Travenol).
INVERT SUGAR-ELECTROLYTE SOLUTIONS.
Use: Intravenous nutritional therapy.

See: Ionosol G and 10% Invert Sugar (Abbott).
Multiple Electrolyte 2 w/5% Invert Sugar (Kendall McGaw).
5% Travert and Electrolyte No. 2 (Baxter).
Ionosol B and 10% Invert Sugar (Abbott).
10% Travert and Electrolyte No. 2 (Baxter).
Multiple Electrolyte 2 w/10% Invert Sugar (Kendall McGaw).
Ionosol D and 10% Invert Sugar (Abbott).
• **INVERT SUGAR INJECTION,** U.S.P. XXIII.
Use: Replenisher (fluid and nutrient).
• **IOBENZAMIC ACID.** USAN. N-3-(3-Amino-2,4,6-triiodobenzoyl)-N-phenyl-β-alanine. Osbil. (Mallinkcrodt).
Use: Contrast medium for cholecystography.
IOCARE BALANCED SALT SOLUTION. (Iolab) Sodium Cl 0.64%, potassium Cl 0.075%, magnesium Cl0.03%, calcium Cl 0.048%, sodium acetate 0.39%, sodium citrate 0.17%, sodium hydroxide or hydrochloric acid. Soln. Bot. 15 ml, 500 ml.
Use: Intraocular irrigation solution.
• **IOCARMATE MEGLUMINE.** USAN.
Use: Diagnostic aid.
• **IOCARMIC ACID.** USAN. 5,5′-(Adipoyldiamino)-bis-(2,4,6-tri-iodo-N-methylisophthalamic acid). Dimer X is a sterile solution of the meglumine salt.
Use: Radiopaque substance.
• **IOCETAMIC ACID,** U.S.P. XXIII. Tab., U.S.P. XXIII. N-Acetyl-N-(3-amino-2,4,6-triiodophenyl)-2-methylalanine. 3-(N-3-Amino-2,4,6-tri-iodophenyl)acetamido-2-methylpropionic acid.
Use: Diagnostic aid (radiopaque medium).
IOCON GEL. (Owen) Polyoxyethylene ethers, coal tar solution, Iopol (a cationic polymer), alcohol 1%, benzalkonium Cl in a non-ionic/amphoteric base. Tube 3.5 oz
Use: Antiseborrheic.
I-OCTADECANOL.
See: Stearyl Alcohol, N.F. XVIII.
• **IODAMIDE.** USAN. 3-Acetamido-5-(acetamido-methyl)-2,4,6-triiodobenzoic acid. α,5-Di(acetamido)-2,4,6-tri-iodo-m-toluic acid.
Use: Radiopaque, diagnostic aid.
• **IODAMIDE MEGLUMIDE.** USAN.
Use: Radiopaque, diagnostic aid.
W/Combinations:

See: Renovue-65, Vial (Squibb).
Renovue-Dip, Vial (Squibb).
IODEX. (Lee) Iodine 4.7% in petrolatum ointment base. Jar 1 oz, 14 oz.
Use: Antiseptic, germicide.
IODEX W/METHYL SALICYLATE. (Lee) Iodine 4.7%, methyl salicylate 4.8% in potrolatum ointmont baoo.
Use: Antiseptic, external analgesic.
• **IODIDE,SODIUM, I-123 CAPSULES,** U.S.P. XXIII.
Use: Diagnostic aid (thyroid function determination).
• **IODIDE, SODIUM, I-123 TABLETS,** U.S.P. XXIII.
Use: Diagnostic aid (thyroid function determination).
• **IODIDE, SODIUM, I-125 CAPSULES,** U.S.P. XXII.
Use: Diagnostic aid (thyroid function determination), radioactive agent.
• **IODIDE, SODIUM, I-125 SOLUTION,** U.S.P. XXII.
Use: Diagnostic aid (thyroid function determination), radioactive agent.
• **IODIDE, SODIUM, I-131 CAPSULES,** U.S.P. XXIII.
Use: Antineoplastic, diagnostic aid (thyroid function determination), radioactive agent.
• **IODIDE, SODIUM, I-131 SOLUTION,** U.S.P. XXIII.
Use: Antineoplastic, diagnostic aid (thyroid function determination), radioactive agent.
• **IODINATED I-125 ALBUMIN INJECTION,** U.S.P. XXIII.
Use: Diagnostic aid (blood volume determination), radioactive agent.
• **IODINATED I-131 ALBUMIN AGGREGATED INJECTION,** U.S.P. XXIII.
Use: Radioactive agent.
• **IODINATED I-131 ALBUMIN INJECTION,** U.S.P. XXIII.
Use: Diagnostic aid (blood volume determination and intrathecal imaging), radioactive agent.
• **IODINATED GLYCEROL.** B.A.N. A mixture of iodinated dimers of glycerol.
Use: Mucolytic expectorant.
See: Organidin, Elix., Soln., Tab. (Wallace).
• **IODINATED GLYCEROL AND CODEINE PHOSPHATE LIQUID.** (Various Mfr.) Codeine phosphate 10 mg, iodinated glycerol 30 mg/Liq. Bot. pt and gal.
• **IODINATED GLYCEROL DM.** (Various Mfr.) Dextromethorphan 10 mg, iodinated glycerol 30 mg/Liq. Bot. 120 ml, pt, gal.

Use: Antitussive, expectorant.
IODINATED HUMAN SERUM ALBUMIN.
See: Albumotope (Squibb).
•**IODINE,** U.S.P. XXIII. Topical Soln.,
Strong Soln., Tincture, U.S.P. XXIII.
Use: Topical anti-infective; source of io-
dine.
See: Kelp, Tab. (Quality Generics).
**IODINE 131: CAPSULES DIAGNOSTIC-
CAPSULES THERAPEUTIC-SOLU-
TION THERAPEUTIC ORAL.**
See: Iodotope (Squibb).
IODINE CACODYLATE, COLLOIDAL.
Cacodyne Iodine.
IODINE COMBINATION.
See: Calcidrine, Syr. (Abbott).
**IODINE I¹²³ MURINE MONOCLONAL
ANTIBODY TO ALPHA-
FETOPROTEIN.** (Immunomedics)
Use: Diagnostic aid. [Orphan drug]
**IODINE I¹²³ MURINE MONOCLONAL
ANTIBODY TO hCG.** (Immunomedics)
Use: Diagnostic aid. [Orphan drug]
**IODINE I¹³¹ 6B-IODOMETHYL-19-NORC-
HOLESTEROL.**
Use: Diagnostic aid. [Orphan drug]
**IODINE I¹³¹ METAIODOBENZYLGUANI-
DINE SULFATE.**
Use: Diagnostic aid. [Orphan drug]
**IODINE I¹³¹ MURINE MONOCLONAL
ANTIBODY TO ALPHA-
FETOPROTEIN.** (Immunomedics)
Use: Antineoplastic. [Orphan drug]
**IODINE I¹³¹ MURINE MONOCLONAL
ANTIBODY TO hCG.** (Immunomedics)
Use: Antineoplastic. [Orphan drug]
**IODINE I¹³¹ MURINE MONOCLONAL
ANTIBODY IgG2a to B CELL.** (Im-
munomedics)
Use: Antineoplastic. [Orphan drug]
IODINE-IODOPHOR.
See: Betadine, Preps. (Purdue Freder-
ick).
Isodine, Preps. (Blair).
IODINE POVIDONE.
See: Efodine, Oint. (Fougera).
Iodophor.
Mallsol, Liq. (Hauck).
IODINE PRODUCTS, ANTI-INFECTIVE.
See: Anayodin.
Betadine, Preps. (Purdue Frederick).
Chiniofon.
Diodoquin, Tab. (Searle).
Diiodo-Hydroxyquinoline (Various
Mfr.).
Isodine, Preps. (Blair).
Prepodyne, Soln., Scrub (West).
Quinoxyl.
Surgidine, Liq. (Continental).
Vioform, Preps. (Ciba).

IODINE PRODUCTS, DIAGNOSTIC.
See: Chloriodized Oil (Various Mfr.).
Ethyl Iodophenylundecylate (Various
Mfr.).
Iodized Oil.
Iodoalphionic Acid (Various Mfr.).
Iodobrassid.
Iodohippurate Sodium (Various Mfr.).
Iodopanoic Acid (Various Mfr.).
Iodophthalein Sodium (Various Mfr.).
Iodopyracet, Preps. (Various Mfr.).
Lipiodol Lafay, Amp., Vial (Savage).
Methiodal Sodium (Various Mfr.).
Pantopaque, Amp. (Lafayette).
Sodium Acetrizoate (Various Mfr.).
Sodium Iodomethamate (Various Mfr.).
Telepaque, Tab. (Sanofi Winthrop).
IODINE PRODUCTS, NUTRITIONAL.
See: Calcium Iodobehenate (Various
Mfr.).
Entodon.
Hydriodic Acid (Various Mfr.).
Iodobrassid (Various Mfr.).
Potassium Iodide (Various Mfr.).
IODINE RATION, (Barth's) Iodine (from
kelp) 0.15 mg, trace minerals/Tab. Bot.
90s, 180s, 360s.
Use: Mineral supplement.
IODINE RATION. (Nion) Iodine (from
kelp) 0.15 mg/3 Tab. Bot. 175s, 500s.
Use: Iodine supplement.
IODINE SOLUBLE.
See: Burnham Soluble Iodine, Soln.
(Burnham).
IODINE SURFACE ACTIVE COMPLEX.
See: Ioprep, Soln. (Arbrook).
•**IODINE TINCTURE, STRONG,** U.S.P.
XXIII.
Use: Anti-infective (topical).
•**IODIPAMIDE,** U.S.P. XXIII. Benzoic acid,
3,3'-[(1,6-dioxo-1,6-hexanediyl)diimi-
no]bis[2,4,6-triiodo-. NN-Di-(3-carboxy-
2,4,6-tri-iodophenyl)-adipamide. Adipi-
odone (I.N.N.).
Use: Pharmaceutic necessity for Iodi-
pamide Meglumine Injection.
•**IODIPAMIDE MEGLUMINE INJECTION,**
U.S.P. XXIII. Benzoic acid, 3,3'-[(1,6-
dioxo-1,6-hexanediyl)diimino] bis [2,4,6-
triiodo-, compound with 1-deoxy-1-
(methylamino)-d-glucitol (1:2).
Use: Diagnostic aid (radiopaque medi-
um).
IODIPAMIDE METHYLGLUCAMINE.
N,N'-Adipyl-bis(3-amino-2,4,6-tri-
iodobenzoic acid). Also sodium salt inj.
W/Diatrizoate methylglucamine.
See: Sinografin, Vial (Squibb).
•**IODIPAMIDE SODIUM I-131.** USAN.
Use: Radioactive agent.

IODIPAMIDE SODIUM INJECTION.
See: Cholografin Sodium, Soln. (Various Mfr.).
•**IODIXANOL.** USAN
Use: Diagnostic aid (radiopaque medium).
IODIZED OIL. A vegetable oil containing not less than 38% and not more than 42% of organically combined iodine.
Use: Diagnostic aid.
See: Lipiodol Lafay, Amp., Vial (Savage).
IODIZED POPPY-SEED OIL.
See: Lipiodol Lafay, Amp., Vial (Savage).
IODOALPHIONIC ACID. 3-(4-Hydroxy-3,5-Diiodo- phenyl)-2-phenylpropionic acid. Biliselectan dikol, pheniodol.
•**IODOANTIPYRINE I-131.** USAN.
Use: Radioactive agent.
IODOBEHENATE CALCIUM. Calcium iododocosanoate.
Use: Antigoitrogenic.
IODOBRASSID. Ethyl Diiodobrassidate. Lipoiodine.
•**IODOCETYLIC ACID I-123.** USAN.
Use: Diagnostic aid.
•**IODOCHOLESTEROL I-131.** USAN.
Use: Radioactive agent.
IODOCHLORHYDROXYQUIN. Clioquinol, U.S.P. XXIII.
IODO CREAM. (Day-Baldwin) Clioquinol 3%. Tube 1 oz, Jar 1 lb.
Use: Antifungal, external.
IODOFORM.(Various Mfr.) Triiodomethane. Pow., Bot. ⅛ oz, 1 oz, 0.25 lb, 1 lb.
Use: Wound dressing agent.
W/Guaiacol, eucalyptol, camphor.
See: Camusol, Vial (Central).
  Guaiphoto, Vial (Foy).
  Imenol, Inj. (Sig).
  Kleer, Vial (Scrip).
  Respirex, Vial (Savage).
IODO H-C. (Day-Baldwin) Clioquinol 3%, hydrocortisone 1%. **Oint.:** Tube 20 Gm, Jar 1 lb. **Cream:** Tube 20 Gm, Jar 1 lb.
Use: Antifungal, corticosteroid.
•**IODOHIPPURATE SODIUM I-123 INJECTION,** U.S.P. XXIII.
Use: Radioactive agent.
•**IODOHIPPURATE SODIUM I-125.** USAN.
Use: Radioactive agent.
See: Hipputope I 125 (Squibb).
•**IODOHIPPURATE, SODIUM I-131 INJECTION,** U.S.P. XXIII. Glycine, N-(2-iodo-[131]1-benzoyl)-, sodium salt.
Use: Diagnostic aid (renal function determination).

See: Hipputope (Squibb).
IODO-HIPPURIC ACID.
See: Hipputope (Squibb).
IODOL. 2,3,4,5-Tetraiodopyrrole.
IODO OINTMENT. (Day-Baldwin) Clioquinol 3%. Tube oz, Jar lb.
Use: Antifungal, external.
IODO-PAK. (SoloPak) Iodine 100 mcg/ml. Inj. Vial 10 ml.
Use: Parenteral nutritional supplement.
IODOPANOIC ACID.
Use: Diagnostic aid (radiopaque medium).
IODOPEN. (Lyphomed) Sodium iodide 118 mcg/ml. Vial 3 ml, 10 ml.
Use: Parenteral nutritional supplement.
IODOPHENE. Iodophthalein.
IODOPHENE SODIUM.
See: Iodophthalein Sodium. (Various Mfr.).
IODOPHOR.
See: Betadine, Preps. (Purdue Frederick).
  Isodine, Preps. (Blair).
IODOPHTHALEIN SODIUM.
Tetraiodophenolphthalein Sodium, Tetraiodophthalein Sodium, Tetiothalein Sodium (Antinosin, Cholepulvis, Cholumbrin, Foriod, Iodophene, Iodorayoral, Nosophene Sodium, Opacin, Photobiline, Piliophen, Radiotetrane).
Use: Radiopaque agent.
IODOPROPYLIDENE GLYCEROL.
See: Organidin, Elix., Tab., Soln. (Wampole).
•**IODOPYRACET I-125.** USAN.
Use: Radioactive agent.
•**IODOPYRACET I-131.** USAN.
Use: Radioactive agent.
See: Diodrast (R)-131
IODOPYRACET INJ. (Diatrast, Diodone, Iopyracil, Neo-Methiodal, NeoSkiodan) 3,5-Diiodo-4-oxo-1(4H)-pyridineacetic Acid 2,2-Iminodiethanol (1:1) Compound.
Use: Radiopaque medium.
IODOPYRACET COMPOUND. Diodrast.
IODOPYRACET CONCENTRATED. Diodrast.
IODOPYRINE. Antipyrine "iodide."
Use: Iodides, analgesic.
•**IODOQUINOL,** U.S.P. XXIII. Tab., U.S.P. XXIII. 8-Quinolinol-5,7-diiodo. Diiodohydroxyquinoline, (Embequin, Enterosept)5,7-Diiodo-8-quinolinol.
Use: Anti-infective.
See: Floraquin (Searle).
  Sebaquin, Shampoo (Summers Labs.).
W/9-Aminoacridine HCl.

See: Vagitric, Cream (Elder).
Yodoxin, Tab., Pow. (Glenwood).
W/Hydrocortisone alcohol.
See: Vytone, Cream (Dermik).
W/Hydrocortisone, coal tar solution.
See: Cor-Tar-Quin, Cream, Lot. (Miles
Pharm).
W/Stilbestrol, sulfadiazine, tartaric acid,
boric acid, etc.
See: Gynben, Vag. Insert, Cream (I. C.
N).
Gynben Insufflate, Pow. (I. C. N).
W/Surfactants.
See: Lycinate, Supp. (Hoechst).
W/Sulfanilamide, diethylstilbestrol.
See: Amide V/S, Vaginal Insert. (Scrip).
D.I.T.I. Creme (Dunhall).
IODOTHIOURACIL. B.A.N. 1,2-Dihydro-
5-iodo-2-thioxopyrimidin-4-one. 5-Iodo-
2-thiouracil.
Use: Antithyroid substance.
IODOTOPE (Diagnostic). (Squibb) Sodi-
um iodide I-131 for oral use. 7, 14, 28,
70, 106 units Ci/Vial of 5, 10, 15, 20
Cap.
Use: Diagnostic aid.
IODOTOPE (Therapeutic). (Squibb)
Sodium iodide I-131. 1 to 50 mCi Cap./7,
14, 28, 70, 106 mCi solution.
Use: Antithyroid agent.
•**IODOXAMIC ACID.** USAN. NN'-(1,16-
Dioxo-4,-7,10,13-tetraoxahexadecane-
1,16-diyl)di-(3-amino-2,4,6-tri-Iodoben-
zoic acid).
Use: Contrast medium.
IODOXYL.
See: Sodium Iodomethamate (Various
Mfr.).
•**IOFETAMINE HYDROCHLORIDE I 123.**
USAN.
Use: Diagnostic aid, radioactive agent.
•**IOGLICIC ACID.** USAN.
Use: Diagnostic aid (radiopaque medi-
um).
•**IOGLUCOL.** USAN.
Use: Diagnostic aid (radiopaque medi-
um).
•**IOGLUCOMIDE.** USAN.
Use: Diagnostic aid.
•**IOGLYCAMIC ACID.** USAN. 3,3-(Digly-
coloyl-diimino)-bis-[2,4,6-triiodobenzoic
acid]. Biligram, Bilivistan.
Use: Radiopaque (cholecystographic
and cholangiographic).
•**IOGULAMIDE.** USAN.
Use: Diagnostic aid (radiopaque medi-
um).
•**IOHEXOL.** USAN.
Use: Diagnostic aid (radiopaque medi-
um).

IOHYDRO CREAM. (Freeport) Hydrocor-
tisone 1%, clioquinol 3%, pramoxine
HCl 0.5%/0.5 oz. Tube 0.5 oz.
Use: Corticosteroid, antifungal, local
anesthetic.
•**IOMEPROL.** USAN
Use: Diagnostic agent, radiopaque.
•**IOMETHIN I-125.** USAN. 4-[[3-(Dimethy-
lamino)propyl]amino]-7-iodo-^{125}I-quino-
line.
Use: Diagnostic aid (neoplasm).
•**IOMETHIN I-131.** USAN. 4-[[3-(Dimethy-
lamino)propyl]amino]-7-iodo-^{131}I-quino-
line.
Use: Diagnostic aid (neoplasm).
IONAMIN. (Pennwalt) Phentermine.
Phenyl-tertiary-butylamine as resin com-
plex 15 mg or 30 mg/Cap. Bot. 100s,
400s.
Use: Anorexiant.
IONAX ASTRINGENT CLEANSER.
(Owen) Isopropyl alcohol 48%,
Owenethers, (polyoxyethylene ethers),
acetone, salicylic acid, allantoin. Bot. 8
oz.
Use: Anti-acne.
IONAX FOAM. (Owen) Polyoxyethylene
ethers, benzalkonium Cl 0.2%, purified
water, isobutane, propylene glycol,
myristamide, DEA, PEG 1000, FD&C
No. 5. Aerosol can 2.5 oz, 5 oz.
Use: Anti-acne.
IONAX SCRUB. (Owen) Polyethylene
granules, polyoxyethylene ethers, alcohol 10%, benzalkonium Cl. Tube 2 oz, 4
oz.
Use: Anti-acne.
IONAZE.
See: Propazolamide.
ION-EXCHANGE RESINS.
See: Polyamine Methylene Resin.
Resins, Sodium Removing.
IONIL PLUS SHAMPOO. (Owen) Sali-
cylic acid 2%, water, sodium laureth sulfate, lauramide dea, quaternium-22, tal-
loweth-60 myristyl glycol, laureth-23, tea
lauryl sulfate, glycol disterate, laureth-4,
tea-abietoyl hydrolyzed collagen,
DMDM hydantoin, tetrasodium EDTA,
sodium hydroxide, fragrance, FD&C;
blue No. 1. Bot. 4 oz, 8 oz.
Use: Antiseborrheic.
IONIL RINSE. (Owen) Conditioners with
benzalkonium Cl in water base. Bot. 16
oz.
Use: Hair rinse.
IONIL SHAMPOO. (Owen) Salicylic acid,
benzalkonium Cl, alcohol 12%, polyoxyethylene ethers. Plasic bot. w/dis-
penser cap 4 oz, 8 oz, 16 oz, 32 oz.

Use: Antiseborrheic.

IONIL T. (Owen) A nonionic/cationic foaming shampoo w/coal tar, salicylic acid, benzalkonium Cl, alcohol 12%, polyoxyethylene ethers. Plastic bot. 4 oz, 8 oz, 16 oz, 32 oz.
Use: Antiseborrheic.

IONIL T PLUS SHAMPOO (Owen) Owentar II (equivalent to 2% coal tar), water, sodium laureth sulfate, lauramide dea, quaternium-22, laureth-23, talloweth-60 myristyl glycol, tea lauryl sulfate, glycol distearate, laureth-4, tea abietoyl hydrolyzed collagen, DMDM hydantoin, disodium EDTA, fragrance, FD&C blue No.1, FD&C; yellow No. 70. Bot. 4 oz, 8 oz.
Use: Antiseborrhic.

IONOSOL D-CM. (Abbott Hospital Prods) Sodium Cl 516 mg, potassium Cl 89.4 mg, calcium Cl anhydrous 27.8 mg, magnesium Cl anhydrous 14.2 mg, sodium lactate 560 mg/100 ml. Bot. 1000 ml.
Use: Parenteral nutrient.

•**IOPAMIDOL,** U.S.P. XXIII.
Use: Diagnostic aid (radiopaque medium).
See: Isovue-300, Inj. (Squibb).
Isovue-370, Inj. (Squibb).
Isovue-M 200, Inj. (Squibb).
Isovue-M 300, Inj. (Squibb).

•**IOPANOIC ACID,** U.S.P. XXIII. Tabs. U.S.P. XXIII. Benzenepropanoic acid, 3-amino-α-ethyl-2,4,6-triiodo-. 2-(3-Amino-2,4,6-tri-iodobenzyl)-butyric acid. 3-Amino-a-ethyl-2,4,6 Triiodohydrocinnamic acid.
Use: Diagnostic aid (radiopaque medium).
See: Telepaque, Tab. (Sanofi Winthrop).

•**IOPENTOL.** USAN.
Use: Diagnostic aid (radiopaque medium).

IOPHEN. (Various Mfr.) Iodinated glycerol 60 mg (30 mg organically bound iodine)/5 ml. Elix. Bot. pt.
Use: Expectorant.

IOPHEN-C. (Various Mfr.) Codeine phosphate 10 mg, iodinated glycerol 30 mg/5 ml. Liq. Bot. 120 ml, pt, gal.
Use: Antitussive, expectorant.

IOPHEN DM ELIXIR. (Various Mfr.) Dextromethorphan HBr 10 mg, iodinated glycerol 30 mg/5 ml Elix. Bot. 120 ml, 480 ml, 760 ml.
Use: Antitussive, expectorant.

•**IOPHENDYLATE,** U.S.P. XXIII. Benzenedecanoic acid, iodo-t-methyl-, ethyl ester.

Use: Diagnostic aid (radiopaque medium).

•**IOPHENDYLATE INJECTION,** U.S.P. XXIII. Ethiodan, Myodil. Ethyl Iodophenylundecylate.
Use: Diagnostic aid (radiopaque medium).
See: Pantopaque. Amp. (LaFayette).

IOPHENOXIC ACID. Tab. a-(2-4,-Triiodo-3-hydroxybenxyl) butyric acid.

IOPHYLLINE. (Various Mfr.) Theophylline 120 mg, iodinated glycerol 30 mg, alcohol 15%. Elixir. Bot. pt.
Use: Antiasthmatic combination.

IOPIDINE. (Alcon) Apraclonidine 0.05%, benzalkonium Cl 0.01%. Dispenser bot. 5 ml.
Use: Agent for glaucoma.

IOPODATE SODIUM.
See Ipodate Sodium.

IOPREP. (Surgikos) Nonylphenoxypolyethylenoxy (4) ethanol and nonylphenoxypolyethyleneoxy (15) ethanol iodine complex 5.5%, nonylphenoxypolyethyleneoxy (30) ethanol 10%. Solution provides 1% available iodine. Plastic bot. gal.
Use: Antiseptic.

•**IOPROCEMIC ACID.** USAN.
Use: Diagnostic aid.

•**IOPRONIC ACID.** USAN.
Use: Diagnostic aid.

•**IOPYDOL.** USAN. 1-(2,3-Dihydroxypropyl)-3,5-diiodo-4(1H)-pyridone.
Use: X-ray contrast medium for bronchography.

•**IOPYDONE.** USAN. 3,5-Diiodo-4-(1H)-pyridone.
Use: X-ray contrast medium for bronchography.

•**IOSEFAMIC ACID.** USAN. 5,5'-(Sebacoyldiimino) bis[2,4,6-triiodo-N-methylisophthalamic acid]
Use: Contrast medium.

•**IOSERIC ACID.** USAN.
Use: Diagnostic aid.

IOSOPAN. (Goldline) Magaldrate 540 mg/5 ml. Liq. Bot. 355 ml.
Use: Antacid.

IOSOPAN PLUS. (Goldline) Magaldrate 540 mg, simethicone 40 mg/5 ml. Liq. Bot. 355 ml.
Use: Antacid.

•**IOSULAMIDE MEGLUMINE.** USAN.
Use: Diagnostic aid.

•**IOSUMETIC ACID.** USAN.
Use: Diagnostic aid.

•**IOTASUL.** USAN.
Use: Diagnostic aid.

•**IOTETRIC ACID.** USAN.

Use: Diagnostic aid.
• **IOTHALAMATE MEGLUMIDE AND IO-THALMATE SODIUM INJECTION,** U.S.P. XXIII.
Use: Diagnostic aid (radiopaque medium).
• **IOTHALAMATE MEGLUMINE INJECTION,** U.S.P. XXIII. Benzoic acid, 3-(acetylamino)-2,4,6-triiodo-5-[(methylamino)carbonyl]-, compound with 1-deoxy-1-(methylamino)-d-glucitol (1:1).
Use: Diagnostic aid (radiopaque medium).
• **IOTHALAMATE SODIUM I-125.** USAN.
Use: Radioactive agent.
• **IOTHALAMATE SODIUM I-131.** USAN.
Use: Radioactive agent.
• **IOTHALAMATE SODIUM INJECTION,** U.S.P. XXIII. Benzoic acid, 3-(acetylamino)-2,4,6-triiodo-5-[(methylamino)carbonyl]-, sodium salt. 5-Acetamido-2,4,6-triiodo-N-methylisophthalamic acid, sodium salt. Sodium lothalamate.
Use: Diagnostic aid (radiopaque medium).
• **IOTHALAMIC ACID,** 3-(acetylamino)-2,4,6-triiodo-5-[(methylamino)carbonyl]-. 5-Acetamino-2,4,6-triiodo N methylisophthalamic acid.
Use: Radiopaque; pharmaceutic necessity for lothalamate Meglumine Injection, lothalamate Meglumine and lothalamate Sodium Injection, and lothalamate Sodium Injection.
IOTHIOURACIL SODIUM. Sodium salt of 5-iodo-2-thiouracil.
• **IOTROL.** USAN.
Use: Radiopaque medium.
• **IOTROXIC ACID.** USAN.
Use: Diagnostic aid (radiopaque medium).
• **IOTYROSINE 1-131.** USAN.
Use: Radioactive agent.
• **IOVERSOL.** USAN.
Use: Diagnostic aid (radiopaque medium).
See: Optiray 350, Inj (Mallinckrodt Medical).
• **IOXAGLATE MEGLUMINE.** USAN.
Use: Diagnostic agent (radiopaque medium).
See: Hexabrix, Inj. (Wallace).
• **IOXAGLATE SODIUM.** USAN.
Use: Diagnostic agent (radiopaque medium).
• **IOXAGLIC ACID.** USAN.
Use: Diagnostic agent (radiopaque medium).
• **IOXILAN.** USAN

Use: Diagnostic agent.
• **IOXOTRIZOIC ACID.** USAN.
Use: Diagnostic aid.
IPATERP. (Fellows) Terpin hydrate 2 gr, ammonium Cl 1 gr, licorice extract 0.5 gr, ipecac 1/10 gr/Tab. Bot. 1000s.
Use: Expectorant, antitussive.
• **IPAZOLIDE FUMARATE.** USAN
Use: Antiarrhythmic.
• **IPECAC,** U.S.P. XXIII. Pow., Syr. U.S.P. XXIII.
Use: Emetic.
W/Combinations.
See: Balmial Cough Syrup, Syr. (Clapp).
Creozets, Loz. (Creomulsion Co.).
Derfort, Cap. (Cole).
Diatrol, Tab. (Otis Clapp).
Ipsatol/DM, Cough Syr. (Key).
Ipsatol, Syr. (Key).
Mallergan, Liq. (Hauck).
Polyectin, Liq. (Amid).
Rubacac, Tab. (Scrip).
Spenlaxo, Tab. (Spencer-Mead).
Terpium, Tab. (Scrip).
• **IPEXIDINE MESYLATE.** USAN.
Use: Dental caries prophylactic.
I-PILOPINE. (Akorn) Pilocarpine HCl 1%. Ophthalmic soln. Bot. 15 ml.
Use: Miotic.
• **IPODATE CALCIUM,** U.S.P. XXIII. Oral Susp., U.S.P. XXIII. Benzenepropanoic acid, 3-[[(dimethylamino)methylene]amino]-2,4,6-triiodo-, calcium salt.
Use: Diagnostic aid (radiopaque medium).
See: Oragrafin calcium, Granules (Squibb).
• **IPODATE SODIUM,** U.S.P. XXIII. Cap., U.S.P. XXIII. Benzenepropanoic acid, 3-[[(dimethylamino)-methylene] amino]-2,4,6-triiodo-, sodium salt.
Use: Diagnostic aid (radiopaque medium).
See: Bilivist, Cap. (Berlex).
Oragrafin sodium, Cap., Vial (Squibb).
IPOL. (Connaught) Supponcion of 3 types of poliovirus (Types 1, 2 and 3) grown in monkey kidney cell cultures. Inj. Single-dose syringe 0.5 ml.
Use: Vaccine.
IPRAN. (Major) Propranolol HCl 10 mg, 20 mg, 40 mg, 60 mg, 80 mg, 90 mg/Tab. **10 mg, 20 mg, 40 mg:** Bot. 100s, 250s, 1000s, UD 100s; **60 mg:** Bot. 100s, 500s; **80 mg:** Bot. 100s, 500s, 1000s, UD 100s; **90 mg:** Bot. 100s, 500s.
Use: Beta-adrenergic blocking agent.

• **IPRATROPIUM BROMIDE.** USAN. 8-Iso-propyl-3-(±)-tropoyloxy-1αH,5αH-tropa-nium bromide. N-Isopro-pylatropinium bromide.
Use: Bronchodilator.
See: Atrovent, Aerosol (Boehringer In-gelheim).

I-PRED. (Akorn) Prednisolone sodium phosphate 0.5% or 1%. Ophthalmic soln. Bot. 5 ml.
Use: Corticosteroid.

I-PREDNICET. (Akorn) Prednisolone ac-etate 1%. Ophthalmic soln. Bot. 5 ml, 10 ml.
Use: Corticosteroid.

• **IPRINDOLE.** USAN. 5-[3-(Dimethy-lamino)-propyl]-6,7,8,9,10,11-hexahy-dro-5H-cyclo-oct[β]-indole. 5-(3-Di-methylaminopropyl)-6,7,8,9,10-11-hexa-hydrocyclooct[β]indole. Prondol hydrochloride.
Use: Antidepressant.

• **IPROCINODINE HYDROCHLORIDE.** USAN.
Use: Antibacterial.

IPROCLOZIDE. B.A.N. 4-Chlorophenoxy-2′-isopro-pylacetohydrazide.
Use: Monoamine oxidase inhibitor.

• **IPROFENIN.** USAN.
Use: Diagnostic aid.

IPRONIAZID. B.A.N. I-isonicotinyl-2-iso-propylhydrazinephosphate. 2′-Isopropy-lisonicotinohydrazide.
Use: Monoamine oxidase inhibitor.

• **IPRONIDAZOLE.** USAN. 2-Isopropyl-1-methyl-5-nitroimidazole. Ipropran (Hoff-man-LaRoche).
Use: Antiprotozoal (Histomonas).

• **IPROPLATIN.** USAN.
Use: Antineoplastic.

IPROVERATRIL. Name used for vera-pamil.

• **IPROXAMINE HYDROCHLORIDE.** USAN.
Use: Vasodilator.

• **IPSAPIRONE HYDROCHLORIDE.** USAN.
Use: Anxiolytic.

IPSATOL COUGH FORMULA LIQUID FOR CHILDREN AND ADULTS. (Ken-wood) Guaifenesin 100 mg, dex-tromethorphan HBr 10 mg, phenyl-propanolamine HCl 9 mg/5 ml. Bot. 118 ml.
Use: Expectorant, antitussive, decon-gestant.

IPV.
Use: Poliomyelitis immunization.
See: Polio Virus Vaccine, Inactivated.

IRCON. (Key) Ferrous fumarate 200 mg/Tab. Bot. 100s.
Use: Iron supplement.

IRCON-FA. (Key) Ferrous fumarate 250 mg, folic acid 1 mg/Tab. Bot. 100s.
Use: Iron supplement.

IRGASAN CF3. Cloflucarban. Under study
Use: Antiseptic.

• **IRIDIUM IR-192.** USAN.
Use: Radioactive agent.
See: Iriditope (Squibb).

IRIGATE. (Ketchum) Bot. 4 oz
Use: Eyewash.

IRIGATE EYE WASH. (Optopics) Sodium Cl, sodium phosphate mono- and diba-sic, benzalkonium Cl, EDTA. Soln. Bot. 118 ml.
Use: Ophthalmic irrigation solution.

IRISIN. A polysaccharide found in several species of iris.

IROCAINE.
See: Procaine HCl (Various Mfr.).

IRODEX. (Keene) Iron dextran complex 50 mg/ml. Vial 10 ml.
Use: Iron supplement.

IROMIN-G. (Mission) Ferrous gluconate 260 mg (iron 30 mg), vitamins B_{12} (crys-talline on resin) 2 mcg, C 100 mg, A ac-etate 4000 IU, D-2 400 IU, B_1 5 mg, B_2 2 mg, B_6 25 mg, niacinamide 10 mg, calci-um pantothenate 1 mg, folic acid 0.8 mg, calcium gluconate 100 mg, calcium lac-tate 100 mg, calcium carbonate 70 mg (calcium 50 mg)/Tab. Bot. 100s.
Use: Vitamin/mineral supplement.

IRON (2+) FUMARATE. Ferrous Fu-marate, U.S.P. XXIII.

IRON (2+) GLUCONATE.
See: Ferrous Gluconate, U.S.P. XXIII.

IRON BILE SALTS.
See: Bilron, Pulvules (Lilly).

IRON CARBONATE COMPLEX.
See: Polyferose.

IRON CHOLINE CITRATE COMPLEX.
See: Chel-Iron, Tab. (Kinney).
Kelex, Tabseals (Nutrition Control).

• **IRON-DEXTRAN INJECTION,** U.S.P. XXIII.
Use: Hematinic.
See: Ferrodex, Inj. (Keene Pharm.).
Hydextran, Inj. (Hyrex).
Imferon, Amp., Vial (Merrell Dow).

IRON-FOLIC ACID-LIVER. (Medwick) Vial 30 ml.

"IRON FOR WOMEN". (Pharmex) Fer-rous fumarate 5 gr/Tab. Bot. 90s.
Use: Iron supplement.

IRON/LIVER COMBINATIONS, INJEC-TION.

See: Rogenic (Forest).
Hemocyte (US Pharm).
Hytinic (Hyrex).
Licoplex DS (Keene).
Hemocyte-V (US Pharm).
Liver-Iron B Complex w/Vitamin B_{12} (Akorn).
IRON/LIVER COMBINATION, ORAL.
See: Arcotinic, Tab. (Arco).
Feocyte, Tab. (Dunhill).
Rogenic, Tab. (Forest).
I-L-X B_{12}, Tab. (Kenwood).
Livitamin, Cap. (SK-Beecham).
Liquid Geritonic (Geriatric Pharm).
I-L-X B_{12} Elixir (Kenwood).
I-L-X Elixir (Kenwood).
Arcotinic Liquid (Arco).
Livitamin Liquid (SK-Beecham).
IRON OXIDE MIXTURE WITH ZINC OX-IDE. Calamine, U.S.P. XXIII.
IRON PEPTONIZED.
See: Saferon, Tab. (Elder).
IRON PRODUCTS, INJECTION.
See: InFeD (Schein).
IRON PROTEIN COMPLEX.
•**IRON SORBITEX.** USAN. A sterile, colloidal solution of a complex of trivalent iron, sorbitol, and citric acid, stabilized with dextrin and sorbitol.
Use: Hematinic.
•**IRON SORBITEX INJECTION,** U.S.P. XXIII. (Formerly iron sorbitol).
Use: Iron supplement.
See: Jectofer, Amp. (Astra).
IRON SULFATE. W/Maalox.
See: Fermalox, Tab. (Rhone-Poulenc Rorer).
IRON W/VITAMIN B_{12} AND IFC.
See: Pronemia Hematinic Capsules (Lederle).
Contrin Capsules (Geneva).
Ferotrinsic Capsules (Rugby).
Livitrinsic-f Capsules (Goldline).
Trinsicon Capsules (Whitby).
Fergon Plus Caplets (Sanofi Winthrop).
TriHEMIC 600 Tablets (Lederle).
Heptuna Plues Capsules (Roerig).
Livitamin w/Intrinsic Factor Capsules (Savage).
Chromagen Capsules (Savage).
IRONCO-B. (Vale) Ferrous sulfate 120.4 mg, manganese sulfate 21.6 mg, dicalcium phosphate 129.6 mg, vitamins B_1 1 mg, B_2 1 mg, niacin 6 mg, D 100 IU/Tab. Bot. 100s, 1000s.
Use: Vitamin/mineral supplement.
IROPHOS D. (Lannett) Dicalcium phosphate anhydrous 330 mg, ferrous sulfate

30 mg, vitamin D 333 IU/Cap. Bot. 500s, 1000s.
Use: Vitamin/mineral supplement.
IROSPAN. (Fielding) Ferrous sulfate 200 mg, vitamin C 150 mg/Cap. Bot. 60s. Tab. Bot. 100s.
Use: Vitamin/mineral supplement.
IRRADIATED ERGOSTEROL.
See: Calciferol.
IRRIGATE. (Professional Pharmacal) Boric acid 1.2%, potassium Cl 0.38%, sodium carbonate 0.014%, benzalkonium Cl 0.01%, disodium edetate 0.05%. Bot. 0.5 oz, 4 oz.
Use: Ocular cleanser.
IRRIGATING SOLUTIONS, PHYSIOLOG-ICAL.
Use: Sterile irrigating solutions.
See: 0.45% Sodium Chloride Irrigation (Abbott).
0.9% Sodium Chloride Irrigation (Abbott).
Tis-U-Sol (Baxter).
Lactated Ringer's Irrigation (Abbott).
Physiolyte (American McGaw).
PhysioSol (Abbott).
IRRIGATING SOLUTIONS, URINARY.
Use: Sterile irrigating solutions.
See: Neosporin G.U. Irrigant (Burroughs Wellcome).
Renacidin (Guardian).
Resectisol (Kendall McGaw).
Sorbitol-Mannitol (Abbott).
Acetic Acid (Various Mfr.).
Glycine (Aminoacetic acid) (Various Mfr.).
Sodium Chloride (Various Mfr.).
Sterile Water (Various Mfr.).
•**IRTEMAZOLE.** USAN.
Use: Uricosuric.
ISACEN.
See: Oxyphenisatin, Preps. (Various Mfr.).
•**ISAMOXOLE.** USAN.
Use: Antiasthmatic.
ISCADOR. (Hiscia).
Use: Antiviral agent.
I-SCRUB. (Spectra) PEG-200 glyceryl monotallawate, disodium laureth sulfosuccinate, cocoamido propyl amine oxide, PEG-78 glyceryl monococoate, benzyl alcohol and EDTA. Soln. Bot. 240 ml.
Use: Ophthalmic cleansing solution.
•**ISEPAMICIN.** USAN.
Use: Antibacterial.
ISG. Immune globulin intramuscular.
Use: Immune serum.
See: Gamastan, Inj. (Cutter Biological).
Gammar, Inj. (Armour).
ISMELIN. (Ciba) Guanethidine monosu-

fate 10 mg or 25 mg/Tab. Bot. 100s.
Use: Antihypertensive.
ISMO. (Wyeth-Ayerst) Isosorbide mononitrate 20 mg/Tab. Bot. 100s, UD 100s.
Use: Antianginal agent.
ISMOTIC. (Alcon Surgical) Isosorbide solution. W/sodium 4.6 mEq, potassium 0.9 mEq/220 ml, alcohol, saccharin, sorbitol. In 220 ml.
Use: Osmotic diuretic.
ISO-ALCOHOLIC ELIXIR.
Use: Vehicle.
ISOAMINILE. B.A.N. (Robins) 4-Dimethylamino-2-isopropyl-2-phenylvaleronitrile. Dimyril citrate.
Use: Antitussive.
ISOAMYLHYDROCUPREINE DIHYDROCHLORIDE.
See: Eucupin Dihydrochloride.
ISOAMYL NITRATE.
See: Amyl Nitrite, U.S.P. XXIII.
ISOAMYNE.
See: Amphetamine (Various Mfr.).
ISO-BID. (Geriatric) Isosorbide dinitrate 40 mg/Cap. Bot. 30s, 100s, 500s.
Use: Antianginal agent.
ISOBORNYL THIOCYANOACETATE, TECHNICAL.
Use: Pediculicide.
See: Barc, Liq. (Commerce).
W/Anhydrous soap.
W/Docusate sodium and related terpenes.
See: Barc, Cream (Commerce).
ISOBUCAINE HYDROCHLORIDE, U.S.P. XXI. 2-Isobutylamino-2-methylpropyl benzoate HCl. 2- (Isobutylamino)-2-methyl-1-propanol benzoate (ester) HCl.
Use: Local anesthetic (dental).
ISOBUCAINE HCl & EPINEPHRINE INJECTION, U.S.P. XXI.
Use: Local anesthetic (dental).
•**ISOBUTAMBEN.** USAN. Isobutyl p-aminobenzoate. Isocaine. Cycloform.
Use: As a surface anesthetic.
•**ISOBUTANE,** N.F. XVIII.
Use: Aerosol propellant.
ISOBUTYLALLYLBARBITURIC ACID.
W/Aspirin, phenacetin, caffeine.
See: Buff-A-Comp, Tab., Cap. (Mayrand).
Fiorinal, Tab., Cap. (Sandoz).
Lanorinal, Cap. (Lannett).
Palgesic, Tab., Cap. (Pan Amer.).
Tenstan, Tab. (Standex).
W/Codeine phosphtate.
See: Fiorinal w/codeine, Cap. (Sandoz).
ISOBUTYL p-AMINOBENZOATE. Isobutamben, U.S.A.N.
ISOBUTYRAMIDE. (Vertex)

Use: Treatment of sickle cell disease and beta-thalassemia. [Orphan drug]
ISOBUZOLE. B.A.N. 5-Isobutyl-2-(4-methoxyben- zenesulphonamido)-1,3,4-thiadiazole. Glysobuzole (I.N.N.).
Use: Oral hypoglycemic agent.
ISOCAINE. Isobutamben, USAN.
ISOCAINE HCl. (Novocol) Mepivacaine 2% with 1:20,000 levonordefrin. Inj. Dental cartridge 1.8 ml.
Use: Local anesthetic.
ISOCAINE W/LEVONORDEFRIN.
Use: Local anesthetic, injectable.
See: Isocaine HCl, Inj. (Novocol).
ISOCAL. (Mead Johnson Nutrition) Lactose-free isotonic liquid containing as a percentage of the calories protein 13% as caseinate and soy protein; fat 37% as soy oil and medium chain triglycerides; carbohydrate 50% as corn syrup solids w/vitamins and minerals for the tube fed patient. Bot. 8 fl oz, 12 fl oz, 32 fl oz.
Use: Enteral nutritional supplement.
ISOCAL HCN. (Mead Johnson Nutrition) High calorie, nitrogen nutritionally complete food. Protein 15%, fat 45%, carbohydrate 40%. Can 8 fl oz.
Use: Enteral nutritional supplement.
ISOCAL HN. (Mead Johnson) ≈ 1 Kcal/ml with protein 44 Gm, fat 45 Gm, carbohydrates 124 Gm/L. In 237 ml.
Use: Enteral nutritional supplement.
ISOCARBOXAZID.
Use: Antidepressant (MAOI).
See: Marplan, Tab. (Roche).
ISOCET. (Rugby) Acetaminophen 325 mg, caffeine 40 mg, butalbital 50 mg/Tab. Bot. 100s.
Use: Nonnarcotic analgesic combinations.
ISOCLOR EXPECTORANT. (Fisons) Codeine phosphate 10 mg, pseudoephedrine HCl 30 mg, guaifenesin 100 mg/5 ml, alcohol 5%. Bot. pt.
Use: Antitussive, decongestant, expectorant.
ISOCLOR LIQUID. (Fisons) Chlorpheniramine maleate 2 mg, pseudoephedrine HCl 30 mg/5 ml, sorbitol. Bot. pt.
Use: Antihistamine, decongestant.
ISOCLOR TABLETS. (Fisons) Chlorpheniramine maleate 4 mg, pseudoephedrine HCl 60 mg/Tab. Bot. 100s.
Use: Antihistamine, decongestant.
ISOCLOR TIMESULE CAPSULES. (Fisons) Chlorpheniramine maleate 8 mg, pseudoephedrine HCl 120 mg/Cap. Bot. 100s, 500s.
Use: Antihistamine, decongestant.
ISOCOCAINE. Pseudocaine.

ISOCOM. (Nutripharm) Isometheptene mucate 65 mg, dichloralphenazone 100 mg, acetaminophen 325 mg/Cap. Bot. 50s, 100s, 250s.
Use: Agent for migraine.

• **ISOCONAZOLE.** USAN.
Use: Antibacterial, antifungal.

ISOCULT TEST FOR BACTERIURIA. (SmithKline Diagnostics)
Use: Diagnostic aid.

ISOCULT TEST FOR CANDIDA. (SmithKline Diagnostics)
Use: Diagnostic aid.

ISOCULT TEST FOR NEISSERIA GONORRHOEAE. (SmithKline Diagnostics)
Use: Diagnostic aid.

ISOCULT TEST FOR N GONORRHOEAE AND CANDIDA. (SmithKline Diagnostics)
Use: Diagnostic aid.

ISOCULT TEST FOR PSEUDOMONAS AERUGINOSA. (SmithKline Diagnostics)
Use: Diagnostic aid.

ISOCULT TEST FOR STAPHYLOCOCCUS AUREUS. (SmithKline Diagnostics)
Use: Diagnostic aid.

ISOCULT TEST FOR THROAT STREPTOCOCCI. (SmithKline Diagnostics)
Use: Diagnostic aid.

ISOCULT TEST FOR TRICHOMONAS VAGINALIS. (SmithKline Diagnostics)
Use: Diagnostic aid.

ISOCULT TEST FOR T VAGINALIS AND CANDIDA. (SmithKline Diagnostics)
Use: Diagnostic aid.

ISO D. (Dunhall) Isosorbide dinitrate.
Cap.: 40 mg. Bot. 100s, 1000s. **Tab.:** 5 mg (sublingual). Bot. 100s.
Use: Antianginal agent.

ISOEPHEDRINE HCl. d-Isoephedrine HCl.
See: Pseudoephedrine HCl.
W/Chlorpheniramine maleate.
See: Isoclor, Tab., Expectorant Timesule, Liq. (Arnar-Stone).
W/Chlorprophenpyridamine maleate.
See: Isoclor, Tab. (Arnar-Stone).
W/Theophylline sodium glycinate, guaifenesin.
See: Iso-Tabs 60 Tab. (Solvay).

D-ISOEPHEDRINE SULFATE.
See: Pseudoephedrine Sulfate.

• **ISOETHARINE.** USAN. 3,4-Dihydroxy α-(I-isopropylamino-propyl)benzyl alcohol. 1-(3,4-Dihydroxy- phenyl)-2-isopropylaminobutan-1-ol. Numotac hydrochloride.
Use: Bronchodilator.

• **ISOETHARINE HYDROCHLORIDE,** U.S.P. XXIII.
Use: Bronchodilator.
See: Bronkosol, Soln. (Sanofi Winthrop).

• **ISOETHARINE INHALATION SOLUTION,** U.S.P. XXIII.
Use: Bronchodilator.

• **ISOETHARINE MESYLATE,** U.S.P. XXIII. Inhalation Aerosol, U.S.P. XXIII.
Use: Bronchodilator.
See: Bronkometer, Aerosol (Sanofi Winthrop).

• **ISOFLUPREDONE ACETATE.** USAN.
Use: Anti-inflammatory.

• **ISOFLURANE,** U.S.P. XXIII.
Use: Anesthetic.

ISOFLUROPHATE.
Use: Glaucoma agent.
See: Floropryl, Oint. (Merck & Co.).

ISOGREGNENONE. Dydrogesterone.
See: Duphaston, Tab. (Philips Roxane).

ISO-IODEIKON.
See: Phentetiothalein Sodium (No Mfr. currently lists).

ISOJECT. (Roerig) A purified, sterile, disposable injection system.
Permapen (benzathine penicillin G) aqueous soln. 1,200,000 units/2 ml. 10s.
Terramycin (oxytetracycline) intramuscular soln. 250 mg/2 ml. 10s.
Use: Injection system.

I-SOL SOLUTION. (DeyLabs) Sodium Cl 0.64%, potassium Cl 0.075%, calcium Cl 0.048%, magnesium Cl 0.03%, sodium acetate 0.39%, sodium citrate 0.17%, sodium hydroxide or hydrochloric acid. Soln. Bot. 20 ml, 200 ml.
Use: Ophthalmic irrigation solution.

ISOLAN. (Elan) Protein 40 g, fat 36 g, carbohydrates 144 g, Na 690 g, K 1.17 g/L, with appropriate vitamins and minerals. Lactose free. Liq. In 237 ml Tetra Pak containers and 1000 ml New Pak closed systems with and without Color Check.
Use: Enteral nutritional supplement.

ISOLATE COMPOUND ELIXIR. (Various Mfr.) Theophylline 45 mg, ephedrine sulfate 12 mg, isoproterenol HCl 2.5 mg, potassium iodide 150 mg, phenobarbital 6 mg/15 ml, alcohol 19%. Elix. Bot. pt, gal.
Use: Antiasmatic combination.

• **ISOLEUCINE,** U.S.P. XXIII. $C_6H_{13}NO_2$, L-isoleucine. DL-Isoleucine. (Pfaltz & Bauer)—Pow. 10 Gm.
Use: Nutrient.

ISOLLYL IMPROVED. (Rugby) Aspirin 325 mg, caffeine 40 mg, butalbital 50 mg/Tab. or Cap. Bot. 100s, 1000s.
Use: Salicylate analgesic, sedative/hypnotic.

ISOLYTE G WITH DEXTROSE. (American McGaw) Sodium 65 mEq, potassium 17 mEq, chloride 150 mEq, NH$_4$ 70 mEq, dextrose 50 Gm, 170 Cal, 555 mOsm/L. Bot. 1000 ml.
Use: Parenteral nutritional supplement.

ISOLYTE H WITH 5% DEXTROSE. (American McGaw) Sodium 70 mEq, potassium 13 mEq, magnesium 3 mEq, chloride 40 mEq, acetate 16 mEq, dextrose 50 Gm, 170 Cal, 370 mOsm/L. Inj. Soln. 1000 ml.
Use: Parenteral nutritional supplement.

ISOLYTE M WITH 5% DEXTROSE. (American McGaw) Sodium 38 mEq, potassium 35 mEq, chloride 44 mEq, phosphate 15 mEq, acetate 20 mEq, dextrose 50 Gm, 175 Cal, 405 mOsm/L. Inj. Soln. 1000 ml.
Use: Parenteral nutritional supplement.

ISOLYTE P WITH 5% DEXTROSE. (American McGaw) Sodium 25 mEq, potassium 19 mEq, magnesium 3 mEq, chloride 23 mEq, phosphate 3 mEq, acetate 23 mEq, dextrose 50 Gm, 175 Cal, 350 mOsm/L. Inj. Soln. 250 ml, 500 ml, 1000 ml.
Use: Parenteral nutritional therapy.

ISOLYTE R WITH 5% DEXTROSE. (American McGaw) Sodium 41 mEq, potassium 16 mEq, calcium 5 mEq, magnesium 3 mEq, chloride 40 mEq, acetate 24 mEq, dextrose 50 Gm, 175 Cal, 380 mOsm/L. Inj. Soln. 1000 ml.
Use: Parenteral nutritional supplement.

ISOLYTE S pH 7.4. (American McGaw) Sodium 140 mEq, potassium 5 mEq, magnesium 3 mEq, chloride 98 mEq, acetate 27 mEq, gluconate 23 mEq, 295 mOsm/L. Inj. Soln. 500 ml, 1000 ml.
Use: Parenteral nutritional supplement.

ISOLYTE S WITH 5% DEXTROSE. (American McGaw) Sodium 140 mEq, potassium 5 mEq, magnesium 3 mEq, chloride 98 mEq, acetate 27 mEq, gluconate 23 mEq, dextrose 50 Gm, 185 Cal, 550 mOsm/L. Inj. Soln. 1000 ml.
Use: Parenteral nutritional supplement.

• **ISOMAZOLE HYDROCHLORIDE.** USAN.
Use: Cardiotonic.

ISOMEPROBAMATE.
See: Carisoprodol (Various Mfr.).

• **ISOMEROL.** USAN.
Use: Antiseptic.

ISOMETHADONE. B.A.N. 6-Dimethylamino-5-methyl-4,4-diphenylhexan-3-one.
Use: Narcotic analgesic.

• **ISOMETHEPTANE MUCATE, DICHLORALPHENAZONE, AND ACETAMINOPHEN,** Cap, U.S.P. 23.

ISOMETHEPTENE/DICHLORALPHENAZONE/ACETAMINOPHEN.
Use: Migraine combinations.
See: Isometheptene/Dichloralphenazone/Acetaminophen, Cap. (Various Mfr.).
Isocam, Cap. (Nutripharm).
Isopap, Cap. (Geneva Marsam).
Midchlor, Cap. (Schein).
Midrin, Cap. (Carnrick).
Migratine, Cap. (Major).

ISOMETHEPTENE MUCATE.
See: Midrin, Cap. (Carnick).
Octinum, Tab. (Knoll).

ISOMETHEPTENE TARTRATE.
See: Tri-Grain, Vial (Pharmex).

ISOMIL. (Ross) Soy protein isolate infant formula containing 20 calories/fl oz.
Pow.: Can 14 oz. **Concentrated Liq.:** Can 13 fl oz. **Ready-to-feed:** Can 32 fl oz. **Nursing Bottles:** Hospital use. Bot. 8 fl oz.
Use: Enteral nutritional supplement.

ISOMIL DF. (Ross) Protein 17.9 g, carbohydrates 67.3 g, fat 36.7 g, Fe 12 mg, Na 293 mg, K 720 mg, with appropriate vitamins and minerals. 676 cal/L. Lactose free. Liq. 960 ml prediluted, ready-to-use cans.
Use: Enteral nutritional supplement.

ISOMIL SF. (Ross) Low osmolar sucrose-free soy protein isolate infant formula containing 20 calories/fl oz. **Concentrated Liq.:** Can 13 fl oz. **Ready-to-feed:** Can 32 fl oz. **Nursing Bottles:** Hospital use. Bot. 8 fl oz.
Use: Enteral nutritional supplement.

ISOMUNE-CK. (Roche Diagnostics) Rapid immunochemical separation method of the heart specific CK-MB isoenzyme for quantitation when used with an appropriate CK substrate reagent. Test kit 100s, 250s.
Use: Diagnostic aid.

ISOMUNE-LD. (Roche Diagnostics) Rapid immunochemical separation method of the heart specific LD-1 isoenzyme for quantitation when used with an appropriate LD substrate reagent. Test kit 40s, 100s.
Use: Diagnostic aid.

• **ISOMYLAMINE HCl.** USAN. 2-(Diethylamino)ethyl 1-isopentylcyclohexanecar-

boxylate HCl.
Use: Smooth muscle relaxant.
ISOMYN.
See: Amphetamine (Various Mfr.).
ISONATE SUBLINGUAL. (Major) Isosorbide 2.5 mg or 5 mg/Sublingual Tab. Bot. 100s, 1000s, UD 100s.
Use: Antianginal agent.
ISONATE TABLETS. (Major) Isosorbide 5 mg, 10 mg, 20 mg or 30 mg/Tab. **5 mg or 10 mg:** Bot. 100s, 1000s, UD 100s. **20 mg or 30 mg:** Bot. 100s, 1000s.
Use: Antianginal agent.
ISONATE TD-CAPS. (Major) Isosorbide 40 mg/TD Cap. Bot. 100s, 1000s.
Use: Antianginal agent.
ISONATE T.R. TABS. (Major) Isosorbide 40 mg/TD Tab. Bot. 100s, 1000s.
Use: Antianginal agent.
ISONIAZID. (Carolina Medical Products) Isoniazid 50 mg/5 ml. Syr. Bot. pt.
Use: Antituberculous agent.
•**ISONIAZID,** U.S.P. XXIII. Inj., Syr., Tab. U.S.P. XXIII. Isonicotinic acid hydrazide, isonicotinyl hydrazide. Cotinazin; I.N.H.; Mybasan; Neumandin; Nicetal; Nydrazid; Pycazide; Rimifon; Tubomel; Vazadrine. (Various Mfr.) 50 mg/Tab. Bot. 100s, 500, 1000s.
Use: Antibacterial (tuberculostatic).
See: Dow-Isoniazid, Tab. (Merrell Dow).
INH, Tab. (Ciba).
Lanlazid, Tab., Syr. (Lannett).
Niconyl, Tab. (Parke-Davis).
Nydrazid, Inj. (Squibb Mark).
Nydrazid, Tab. (Squibb Marsam).
Triniad, Tab. (Kasar).
Uniad, Tab. (Kasar).
W/Calcium paraminosalicylate.
See: Calpas-INH, Tab. (American Chem. & Drug).
W/Calcium p-aminosalicylate, vitamin B_6.
See: Calpas Isoxine, Tab. (American Chem. & Drug).
Calpas-INAH-6, Tab. (American Chem. & Drug).
W/Pyridoxine HCl. (vitamin B_6).
See: Niadox, Tab (Barnes-Hind)
P-I-N Forte, Syr., Tab. (Lannett).
Teebaconin w/B_6 (Consoln. Mid.).
Triniad Plus 30, Tab. (Kasar).
Uniad-Plus, Tab. (Kasar).
W/Pyridoxine HCl, sodium aminosalicylate.
See: Pasna, Tri-Pack 300, Granules (Barnes-Hind).
W/Rifampin.
See: Rimactane/INH DuoPack (Ciba).
W/Sodium aminosalicylate, pyridoxine.
See: Pasna Tri-Pack, Granules

(Barnes-Hind).
ISONICOTINIC ACID HYDRAZIDE.
See: Isoniazid, U.S.P. XXIII. (Various Mfr.).
ISONICOTINYL HYDRAZIDE.
See: Isoniazid, U.S.P. XXIII. (Various Mfr.).
ISONIPECAINE HYDROCHLORIDE.
See: Meperidine Hydrochloride, U.S.P. XXIII. (Various Mfr.).
ISOPAP. (Geneva Marsam) Isometheptene mucate 65 mg, dichloralphenazone 100 mg, APAP 325 mg/Cap. Bot. 100s.
Use: Migraine combination.
ISOPENTAQUINE.
Use: Antimalarial.
•**ISOPHANE INSULIN SUSPENSION,** U.S.P. XXIII.
Use: Hypoglycemic agent.
See: Humulin, Vial (Lilly).
Novolin, Vial (Novo Nordisk).
NPH Insulin, Vial (Novo Nordisk).
NPH Iletin, Vial (Lilly).
ISOPREDNIDENE. B.A.N. 11β,17α,21-Trihydroxy-16-methylenepregna-4,6-diene-3,20-dione.
Use: ACTH inhibitor.
ISOPREGNENONE.
See: Duphaston, Tab. (Philips Roxane).
Dydrogesterone.
ISOPRENALINE. B.A.N. (±)-1-(3,4-Dihydroxy-phenyl)-2-isopropylaminoethanol.
Isopropylnoradrenaline.
Use: Sympathomimetic.
ISOPRINOSINE. (Newport Pharmaceuticals)
Use: Antiviral, immunomodulator.
See: Inosine pranobex, inosiplex, methisoprinol.
•**ISOPROPAMIDE IODIDE,** U.S.P. XXIII. Tab., U.S.P. XXIII. (3-Carbamoyl-3,3-diphenylpropyl) diisopropyl-methylammonium iodide. Tyrimide.
Use: Anticholinergic.
See: Darbid, Tab. (SK-Beecham).
W/Prochlorperazine maleate.
See: Iso-Perazine, Cap. (Lemmon).
ISOPROPHENAMINE HCl. Name used for Clorprenaline HCl.
ISOPROPICILLIN POTASSIUM. Potassium 3,3-dimethyl-6-(2-methyl-2-phenoxypropionamido)-7-oxo-4-thia-1-azabicyclo [3.2.0]heptane-2-carboxylate.
Use: Anti-infective.
•**ISOPROPYL ALCOHOL,** U.S.P. XXIII.
Use: Local anti-infective; pharmaceutic aid (solvent).
•**ISOPROPYL ALCOHOL, AZEOTROPIC,** U.S.P. XXIII.
ISOPROPYL ALCOHOL SPRAY. (Mor-

ton) Isopropyl alcohol w/propellant. Aerosol Can 6 oz.
Use: Isopropyl alcohol.

ISOPROPYLARTERENOL HYDROCHLORIDE.
Use: Asthma, vasoconstrictor and allergic states.

ISOPROPYLARTERENOL SULFATE.
See: Isoproterenol Sulfate.

• **ISOPROPYL MYRISTATE,** N.F. XVIII.
Use: Pharmaceutic aid (emollient).

iso-NORADRENALINE.
See: Isoproterenol.

ISOPROPYL-NORADRENALINE HCl.
See: Isoproterenol HCl, U.S.P. XXIII.

• **ISOPROPYL PALMITATE,** N.F. XVIII.
Use: Pharmaceutic aid (oleaginous vehicle).

ISOPROPYL PHENAZONE. 4-Isopropyl antipyrine. Larodon.

• **ISOPROPYL RUBBING ALCOHOL,** U.S.P. XXIII.
Use: Rubefacient, solvent.

ISOPROTERENOL.
See: Norisidrine (Abbott).
W/Butabarbital, theophylline, ephedrine HCl.
See: Medihaler-Iso, Vial (Riker).

• **ISOPROTERENOL HYDROCHLORIDE,** U.S.P. XXIII. Inhalation, Tab. Inj.; U.S.P. XXIII. 1,2-Benzenediol,4-[1-hydroxy-2-[(1-methylethyl)-amino]ethyl]-, HCl. 3,4-Dihydroxy-α-[(isopropylamino)methyl] benzyl alcohol hydrochloride. Oleudrin-Proternol. 1:5,000 5 ml and 10 ml in Univ. Add. Syr.; 1:5,000 1 mg and 2 mg pintop vials; 1:50,000 10 ml with Abboject Syr. (21G X 1 0.5[dp]).
Use: Adrenergic (bronchodilator).
See: Isuprel HCl, Prods. (Sanofi Winthrop).
Norisodrine, Aerotrol, Syr. (Abbott).
Proternol, Tab. (Key Pharm.).
Vapo-Iso, Soln. (Fisons).
W/Aminophylline, ephedrine sulfate, phenobarbital.
See: Asminorel, Tab. (Solvay).
W/Clopane (clopentamine) HCl, propylene glycol, ascorbic acid.
See: Aerolone Compound, Soln. (Lilly).
W/Phenobarbital sodium, ephedrine sulfate, theophylline hydrous.
See: Iso-asminyl, Tab. (Cole).
W/Phenylephrine bitartrate.
See: Duo-Medihaler, Vial (Riker).

• **ISOPROTERENOL HYDROCHLORIDE AND PHENYLEPHRINE BITARTRATE INHALATION AEROSOL,** U.S.P. XXIII.
Use: Adrenergic (bronchodilator).
See: Duo-Medihaler, Vial (Riker).

• **ISOPROTERENOL INHALATION SOLUTION,** U.S.P. XXIII.
Use: Bronchodilator.

• **ISOPROTERENOL SULFATE,** U.S.P. XXIII. Inhal. Aerosol, Inhal. Soln., U.S.P. XXIII.
Use: Adrenergic (bronchodilator).
See: Medihaler-Iso, Vial (Riker).
W/Calcium iodide (anhydrous), alcohol.
See: Norisodrine, Syr. (Abbott).

ISOPTIN. (Knoll) Verapamil HCl 10 mg/4 ml. Amp. 4 ml.
Use: Calcium channel blocking agent.

ISOPTIN I.V. (Knoll) Verapamil HCl. **Single Dose Vial:** 5 mg/2 ml or 10 mg/4 ml. **Pre-filled Syringe:** 5 mg/2 ml or 10 mg/4 ml.
Use: Calcium channel blocking agent.

ISOPTIN SR TABLETS. (Knoll) Verapamil HCl 240 mg/SR Tab. Bot. 100s.
Use: Calcium channel blocking agent.

ISOPTIN TABLETS. (Knoll) Verapamil HCl 80 mg or 120 mg/Tab. Bot. 100s, 500s, 1000s, UD 10 X 10s.
Use: Calcium channel blocking agent.

ISOPTO ALKALINE. (Alcon) Hydroxypropyl methylcellulose 1%, benzalkonium Cl 0.01%. Sterile ophthalmic soln. Dropper bot. 15 ml.
Use: Artificial tear solution.

ISOPTO ATROPINE. (Alcon) Atropine sulfate 0.5%, 1% or 3% in methylcellulose solution. **0.5% or 3%:** Drop-Tainer 5 ml. **1%:** Drop-Tainer 5 ml, 15 ml.
Use: Cycloplegic mydriatic.

ISOPTO CARBACHOL. (Alcon) Carbachol U.S.P. 0.75%, 1.5%, 2.25% or 3%, in a sterile buffered solution of methylcellulose 1%. **2.25%:** Drop-Tainer 15 ml. **0.75%, 1.5% or 3%:** Drop-Tainer 15 ml, 30 ml.
Use: Agent for glaucoma.

ISOPTO CARPINE. (Alcon) Pilocarpine HCl in stable sterile 0.5% methylcellulose soln. w/isotonicity of lacrimal fluid. **0.25%, 0.5%, 1%, 2%, 3%, 4%, 5%, 6%, 8% or 10%:** Bot. Drop-Tainer 15 ml; **0.5%, 1%, 2%, 3%, 4% or 6%:** Bot. Drop-Tainer 30 ml.
Use: Agent for glaucoma.

ISOPTO CETAMIDE. (Alcon) Sodium sulfacetamide 15% in buffered pH 7.4, methylcellulose 0.5%. Soln. Drop-Tainer 5 ml, 15 ml.
Use: Anti-infective, ophthalmic.

ISOPTO CETAPRED. (Alcon) Sulfacetamide sodium U.S.P. 10%, prednisolone U.S.P. 0.25%, methylcellulose 0.5% in a sterile, buffered and stable

suspension. Drop-Tainer 5 ml, 15 ml.
Use: Anti-infective, ophthalmic.
ISOPTO FRIN. (Alcon) Phenylephrine
HCl 0.12% in a methylcellulose soln.
Drop-Tainer 15 ml.
Use: Ophthalmic vasoconstrictor/mydri-
atic.
ISOPTO HOMATROPINE. (Alcon) Homa-
tropine HBr 2% or 5% in methylcellulose
soln. Drop-Tainer 5 ml, 15 ml.
Use: Cycloplegic mydriatic.
ISOPTO HYOSCINE. (Alcon) Hyoscine
HBr 0.25% in a methylcellulose soln.
Drop-Tainer 5 ml, 15 ml.
Use: Cycloplegic mydriatic.
ISOPTO PLAIN. (Alcon) Hydroxypropyl
methylcellulose 0.5%, benzalkonium Cl
0.01%. Drop-Tainer 15 ml.
Use: Artificial tear solution.
ISOPTO TEARS. (Alcon) Hydroxypropyl
methylcellulose 0.5%, benzalkonium Cl
0.01%. Bot. Drop-Tainer 15 ml, 30 ml.
Use: Artificial tear solution.
ISORDIL SUBLINGUAL. (Wyeth-Ayerst)
Isosorbide dinitrate 2.5 mg, 5 mg or 10
mg/Tab. **2.5 mg:** Bot. 100s, 500s, Clini-
pak 100s. **5 mg:** Bot. 100s, 250s, 500s,
Clinlpak 100s. **10 mg:** Bot. 100s.
Use: Antianginal agent.
ISORDIL TEMBIDS. (Wyeth-Ayerst)
Isosorbide dinitrate 40 mg/Tab. or Cap.
Tab.: Bot. 100s, 500s, 1000s. **Cap.:** Bot.
100s, 500s.
Use: Antianginal agent.
ISORDIL TITRADOSE TABLETS.
(Wyeth-Ayerst) Isosorbide dinitrate 5
mg, 10 mg, 20 mg, 30 mg or 40 mg/Tab.
5 mg.: Bot. 100s, 500s, 1000s, Clinipak
100s. **10 mg:** Bot. 100s, 500s, 1000s,
Clinipak 100s. **20 mg:** Bot. 100s, 500s,
Clinipak 100s. **30 mg:** Bot. 100s, 500s.
Clinipak 100s. **40 mg:** Bot. 100s, Clini-
pak 100s.
Use: Antianginal agent.
ISORGEN-G. (Grafton) Isosorbide 5 mg
or 10 mg/Tab. Bot. 1000s.
Use: Antianginal agent.
• **ISOSORBIDE.** USAN.
Use: Diuretic.
• **ISOSORBIDE CONCENTRATE,** U.S.P.
XXIII.
Use: Diuretic.
• **ISOSORBIDE DINITRATE,** U.S.P. XXIII.
Extended-release Cap., Chewable Tab.,
Extended-release Tab., Sublingual Tab.,
Tab., U.S.P. XXIII. D-Glucitol, 1,4:3,6-di-
anhydro-, dinitrate.
Use: Coronary vasodilator; antianginal.
See: Dilatrate-SR, Cap. (Reed & Carn-
rick).

Iso-Bid, Cap. (Geriatric).
Iso-D, Tab., Cap. (Dunhall).
Isordil, Tab. (Wyeth-Ayerst).
Isordil Tembids Cap., Tab. (Wyeth-Ay-
erst).
Nitromed, Tab. (U.S. Ethicals).
Onset, Tab. (Bock).
Sorbitrate, Tab. (Stuart).
Sorquad, Tab. (Solvay).
W/Phenobarbital.
See: Sorbitrate w/Phenobarbital, Tab.
(Stuart).
• **ISOSORBIDE MONONITRATE.** USAN.
Use: Coronary vasodilator.
See: Imdur, ER Tab. (Key).
ISMO, Tab. (Wyeth-Ayerst).
Monoket, Tab. (Schwarz Pharma Kre-
mers Urban).
• **ISOSORBIDE ORAL SOLUTION,** U.S.P.
XXIII.
Use: Diuretic.
ISOSOURCE. (Sandoz Nutrition) Protein
(Ca and Na caseinate, soy protein iso-
late) 43.2 Gm, carbohydrate (maltodex-
trin) 1755 Gm, fat (MCT, canola oil,
lecithin) 443.9 Gm, Na 760 mg, K 1182
mg, mOsm/kg H_2O 390, Cal/ml 1.2, vita-
mins A, B_1, B_2, B_3, B_5, B_6, B_{12}, C, D, E,
K, FA, biotin, choline, Ca, Cl, Cu, Fe, I,
Mg, Mn, P, Zn, Se, Cr, Mo. Liq. Bot. 250
ml, 1000 ml.
Use: Enteral nutritional therapy.
ISOSOURCE HN. (Sandoz Nutrition) Pro
tein (Ca and Na caseinate, soy protein
isolate) 56.1 Gm, carbohydrate (maltodextrin) 165 Gm, fat (MCT, canola oil,
lecithin) 43.9 Gm, Na 760 mg, K 1772
mg, mOsm/kg H_2O 390, Cal/ml 1.2, vita-
mins A, B_1, B_2, B_3, B_5, B_6, B_{12}, C, D, E,
K, FA, biotin, choline, Ca, P, I, Fe, Mg,
Cu, Zn, Cl, Mn, Se, Cr, Mo. Liq. Bot. 250
ml, 1000 ml.
Use: Enteral nutritional therapy.
• **ISOSTERYL ALCOHOL.** USAN.
Use: Pharmaceutic aid.
• **ISOSULFAN BLUE.** USAN.
Use: Diagnostic aid.
ISOTEIN HN. (Sandoz Nutrition) Vanilla
Flavor. Maltodextrin, delactosed lactal-
bumin, partially hydrogenated soy oil
with BHA, fructose, medium chain
triglycerides, artificial flavor, sodium ca-
seinate, mono and diglycerides, sodium
Cl, vitamins, minerals. Pow. Packet 2.75
oz.
Use: Enteral nutritional supplement.
ISOTHIPENDYL. B.A.N. 10-(2-Dimethy-
lamino-propyl)-10H-pyrido[3,2-b]-
[1,4]benzothiazine.
Use: Antihistamine.

• **ISOTIQUIMIDE.** USAN.
Use: Antiulcerative.
ISOTRATE. (Hauck) Isosorbide dinitrate
40 mg/Timecelle. Bot. 100s, 500s, UD
50s.
Use: Antianginal agent.
• **ISOTRETINOIN.** USAN.
Use: Keratolytic
• **ISOTRETINOIN,** U.S.P. XXIII. 13-cis-
retinoic acid.
Use: Treatment of severe recalcitrant
cystic acne.
See: Accutane, Cap. (Roche).
ISOVEX. (U.S. Chemical) Ethaverine HCl
100 mg/Cap. Bot. 100s, 1000s.
Use: Peripheral vasodilator.
ISOVORIN. (Lederle)
See: L-LEUCOVORIN.
ISOVUE-128. (Squibb Diagnostics)
Iopamidol 26% (12.8% iodine). Inj. Vial
50 ml.
Use: Radiopaque agent.
ISOVUE-200. (Squibb Diagnostics)
Iopamidol 41% (20% iodine). Inj. Vial 50.
Bot. 100 ml, 200 ml.
Use: Radiopaque agent.
ISOVUE 300 INJECTION. (Squibb)
Iopamidol 612 mg, tromethamine 1 mg,
edetate calcium disodium 0.39 mg/ml.
Vial 50 ml, Box 10s. Bot. 100 ml, Box
10s.
Use: Radiopaque agent.
ISOVUE 370 INJECTION. (Squibb)
Iopamidol 755 mg, tromethamine 1 mg,
edetate calcium disodium 0.48 mg/ml.
Vial 50 ml, Box 10s; Bot. 100 ml, Box
10s; 150 ml, Box 10s; 200 ml, Box 10s.
Use: Radiopaque agent.
ISOVUE-M 200 INJECTION. (Squibb)
Iopamidol 408 mg, tromethamine 1 mg,
edetate calcium disodium 0.26 mg/ml.
Vial 20 ml, Box 10s.
Use: Radiopaque agent.
ISOVUE-M 300 INJECTION. (Squibb)
Iopamidol 612 mg, tromethamine 1 mg,
edetate calcium disodium 0.39 mg/ml.
Vial 20 ml, Box 10s.
Use: Radiopaque agent.
• **ISOXEPAC.** USAN.
Use: Anti-inflammatory.
• **ISOXICAM.** USAN.
Use: Anti-inflammatory.
• **ISOXSUPRINE HCl,** U.S.P. XXIII. Inj.,
Tab., U.S.P. XXIII. 1-(p-Hydroxy-
phenyl)-2-(1'-methyl-2-phenoxy ethyl-
amino) propanol-1 HCl. p-Hydroxy-α-[1-
[(1-methyl-2-phenoxyethyl)amino]ethyl]
benzyl alcohol HCl.
Use: Vasodilator.

See: Vasodilan, Tab. (Mead Johnson).
I-SOYALAC. (Loma Linda) P-soy protein
isolate, l-methionine, CHO-sucrose,
tapioca dextrin. F-soy oil, soy lecithin.
Corn free. Protein 20.2 Gm, carbohydrate 63.4 Gm, fat 35.5 Gm, iron 12 mg,
640 Cal/serving (1 qt). Concentrate 390
ml, ready to use 1 qt.
Use: Enteral nutritional supplement.
• **ISRADIPINE.** USAN.
Use: Antagonist (calcium channel).
See: DynaCirc (Sandoz).
I-SULFACET. (American) Sulfacetamide
sodium 10%, 15% or 30% ophthalmic
soln. Bot. 2 ml, 5 ml, 15 ml.
Use: Anti-infective, ophthalmic.
I-SULFALONE SUSPENSION. (Ameri-
can) Sulfacetamide sodium 100 mg,
prednisolone acetate 5 mg. Ophthalmic
susp. Bot. 5 ml, 15 ml.
Use: Anti-infective, ophthalmic.
ISUPREL GLOSSETS. (Sanofi Winthrop)
Isoproterenol HCl 10 mg or 15 mg/Tab.
Bot. 50s.
Use: Bronchodilator.
ISUPREL INHALATION SOLUTION.
(Sanofi Winthrop) Isoproterenol HCl in-
halation soln. 1:200 or 1:100. Bot. 10 ml,
60 ml.
Use: Bronchodilator.
ISUPREL MISTOMETER. (Sanofi
Winthrop) Isoproterenol HCl. Complete
nebulizing unit of aerosol soln. containing 10 ml or 15 ml of isoproterenol HCl
w/inert propellants, alcohol 33%, ascor-
bic acid. Measured dose of approxi-
mately 131 mcg. Aerosol Unit. Bot. 15
ml, 22.5 ml. Refill 15 ml, 22.5 ml.
Use: Bronchodilator.
ISUPREL STERILE INJECTION. (Sanofi
Winthrop) Isoproterenol HCl 0.2 mg, lac-
tic acid 0.12 mg, sodium lactate 1.8 mg,
sodium Cl 7 mg and not more than 1 mg
sodium metabisulfite as preservative/ml
of 1:5000 soln. Amp. 1 ml Box 25s; 5 ml
Box 10s.
Use: Adjunct treatment of shock, car-
diac standstill, etc.
ISUPRENE.
See: Isoproterenol (Various Mfr.).
• **ITAZIGREL.** USAN.
Use: Platelet anti-aggregatory agent.
ITCHAWAY. (Moyco) Zinc undecylenate
20%, undecylenic acid 2%. Pow. Can
1.5 oz.
Use: Antifungal, external.
ITCH-X. (B. F. Ascher & Co.) Pramoxine
HCl 1%, benzyl alcohol 10%, aloe vera
gel. Spray. In 60 ml.
Use: Local anesthetic.

ITOBARBITAL. W/Acetaminophen.
See: Panitol, Tab. (Wesley).
• **ITRACONAZOLE.** USAN, B.A.N.
Use: Antifungal.
See: Sporanox, Cap. (Janssen).
ITRAMIN TOSYLATE. B.A.N. 2-Nitra-
toethylamine toluene-p-sulfonate.
Use: Angina pectoris; vasodilator.
I-TROL. (Akorn) Neomycin sulfate-
polymyxin B sulfate-dexamethasone
0.1%. Ophthalmic susp. Bot. 5 ml.
Use: Anti-infective, ophthalmic.
I-VALEX-1. (Ross) Protein 15 g, fat 23.9
g, carbohyrate 46.3 g, linoleic acid 1800
mg, Fe 9 mg, Na 190 mg, K 675 mg,
with appropriate vitamins and minerals.
480 Cal per 100 g. Leucine free. Pow.
Can 350 g.
Use: Enteral nutritional supplement.
I-VALEX-2. (Ross) Protein 30 g, fat 15.5
g, carbohyrates 30 g, Fe 13 mg, Na 880
mg, K 1370 mg, with appropriate vitamins and minerals. 410 Cal per 100 g.
Leucine free. Pow. Can 325 g.
Use: Enteral nutritional supplement.
IVAREST. (Blistex) Calamine 14%, ben-
zocalne 5%. Cream: 60 Gm. Lot.: 120
ml.
Use: Topical treatment of poison ivy,
oak, sumac.
IVOCORT. (Hauck) Micronized hydrocortisone alcohol 0.5% or 1%. Bot. 4 oz.
Use: Corticosteroid.
IVY-CHEX. (Bowman) Polyvinyl pyrroli-
done-vinyl acetate, benzalkonium Cl
1:1000 in alcohol acetone base. Aerosol
can 4 oz.
Use: Treatment or prevention of poison
ivy, poison oak, poison sumac dermatitis.
IVY DRY. (Ivy) Tannic acid 10%, isopropyl
alcohol 12.5% Liq. 4 oz, Cream 1 oz,
Super 6 oz.
Use: Relief of itching.
IVY-RID. (Hauck) Polyvinyl pyrrolidone-
vinyl acetate, benzalkonium Cl. Spray
can 2.75 oz.
Use: Relief of itching and discomfort of
poison ivy, poison oak and poison
sumac.
IVY SHIELD SKIN PROTECTANT. (Interpro) Deionized water, TEA stearate,
stearamide MEA, ethoxydiglycol, acetic
acid. Cream. Bot. 36 ml, 118 ml, 473 ml.
Use: Poison ivy treatment, topical.
I-WASH. (Akorn) Phosphate buffered
saline soln. Bot. 4 oz, 8 oz.
Use: Eye wash.
I-WHITE. (Akorn) Phenylephrine 0.12%,

polyvinyl alcohol, hydroxyethyl cellulose.
Soln. Bot. 15 ml.
Use: Ophthalmic vasoconstrictor/mydri-
atic.
IZONID TABLETS. (Major) Isoniazid 300
mg/Tab. Bot. 100s.
Use: Antituberculous agent.

J

JALOVIS.
See: Hyaluronidase (Various Mfr.).
JANIMINE. (Abbott) Imipramine HCl 10
mg, 25 mg or 50 mg/Tab. Bot. 100s,
1000s.
Use: Antidepressant.
JAPAN AGAR.
See: Agar (Various Mfr.).
JAPAN GELATIN.
See: Agar (Various Mfr.).
JAPAN ISINGLASS.
See: Agar (Various Mfr.).
JAPANESE ENCEPHALITIS VACCINE.
Use: Vaccine.
See: JE-VAX.
JE-VAX. (Connaught) Japanese en-
cephalitis virus vaccine. Pow. for Inj. sin-
gle-dose vial with 1.3 ml diluent; 10-
dose vial with 11 ml diluent.
Use: Vaccine, viral.
JENAMICIN. (Hauck) Gentamicin sulfate
40 mg/ml. Vial 2 ml.
Use: Antibacterial, aminoglycoside.
JENEST-28. (Organon) 7 white tablets
norethindrone 0.5 mg, ethinyl estradiol
35 mcg; 14 peach tablets norethindrone
1 mg, ethinyl estradiol 35 mcg; 7 inert
tablets. Cyclic dispenser of 28.
Use: Oral contraceptive.
JENSENEX. (Jenkins) Nicotinic acid 50
mg, salicylamide 0.3 Gm, vitamins B_{12}
activity 3 mcg, C 15 mg/Tab. Bot. 1000s.
Use: Vitamin supplement, analgesic.
JEN-VITE. (Jenkins) Vitamins A 5000 IU,
D 1000 IU, B_1 2.5 mg, B_2 2.5 mg, nicoti-
namide 20 mg, B_6 1 mg, calcium pan-
tothenate 5 mg, B_{12} 2 mcg, C 40 mg, E 2
IU/Cap. Bot. 100s, 1000s.
Use: Vitamin supplement.
JERI-BATH. (Dermik) Concentrated
moisturizing bath oil. Plastic Bot. 8 oz.
Use: Bath dermatological.
JETS. (Freeda) Lysine 300 mg, vitamins
C 25 mg, B_{12} 25 mcg, B_6 5 mg, B_1 10
mg/Chew. tab. Bot. 30s, 250s, 500s.
Use: Vitamin supplement.
JEVITY LIQUID. (Ross) Calcium and
sodium caseinates, soy fiber, hydrolyzed
cornstarch, MCT (fractionated coconut

oil) soy oil, corn oil, soy lecithin, vitamins A, B_1, B_2, B_3, B_5 B_6, B_{12}, C, D, E, K, folic acid, biotin, choline, Ca, P, Mg, Fe, Mn, Cu, Zn, I, Cl. In 240 ml.
Use: Enteral nutritional supplement.
JIFFY. (Block) Benzocaine, menthol, eugenol in glycerin-water base with SD alcohol 38-B 76%. Bot. 0.125 oz.
Use: Local anesthetic.
J-LIBERTY. (J Pharmacal) Chlordiazepoxide HCl 5 mg, 10 mg or 25 mg/Cap.
Use: Antianxiety agent.
JOHNSON'S BABY CREAM. (Johnson & Johnson) Dimethicone 2%. Jar 4 oz, 6 oz, Tube 2 oz.
Use: Skin protectant.
JOHNSON'S BABY SUNBLOCK CREAM. (Johnson and Johnson) Octyl methoxycinnamate, octyl salicylate, oxybenzone, titandium dioxide, benzyl alcohol, cetyl alcohol. PABA free. SPF 15. Waterproof. Cream. Bot. 60 Gm.
Use: Sunscreen.
JOHNSON'S BABY SUNBLOCK EXTRA PROTECTION. (Johnson & Johnson) Octyl methoxycinnamate, octyl salicylate, titanium dioxide, oxybenzone, C12-15 alcohols benzoate, cetyl alcohol, EDTA, vitamin E. Lot. Bot. 120 ml.
Use: Sunscreen.
JOHNSON'S BABY SUNBLOCK LOTION. (Johnson & Johnson) **SPF 30:** Benzophenone-3, octyl methoxycinnamate, octyl salicylate, titanium dioxide. PABA free. Waterproof. Bot. 120 ml.
SPF 15: Octyl methoxycinnamate octyl salicylate, oxybenzone, titanium dioxide, benzyl alcohol, cetyl alcohol. PABA free. Waterproof. Bot. 60 Gm.
JOHNSON'S MEDICATED POWDER. (Johnson & Johnson) Bentonite, kaolin, talc, zinc oxide. Pow. Small, Medium, Large.
Use: Diaper rash product.
•**JOSAMYCIN.** USAN.
Use: Antibacterial.
JUNICOID. (Jenkins) Dextromethorphan HBr 5 mg, cocillana compound 88 mg, potassium guaiacolsulfonate 66 mg, citric acid 22 mg/5 ml. Syr. Bot. 3 oz, 4 oz, gal.
Use: Antitussive, expectorant.
JUNIOR-STRENGTH FEVERALL. (Upsher-Smith) Acetaminophen 120 mg or 325 mg/Supp. Pkg 6s.
Use: Analgesic.
JUNIOR STRENGTH PANADOL. (Sterling Health) Acetaminophen 160 mg. Capl. 30s.

Use: Analgesic.
•**JUNIPER TAR,** U.S.P. XXIII. Oil of cade.
Use: Local anti-eczematic.
JUNYER-ALL. (Barth's) Vitamins A 6000 IU, D 400 IU, B_1 3 mg, B_2 6 mg, C 120 mg, niacin 1 mg, E 12 IU, B_{12} 10 mcg, calcium 217 mg, phosphorus 97.5 mg, red bone marrow 10 mg, organic iron 15 mg, iodine 0.1 mg, beef peptone 20 mg/2 Cap. Bot. 10 month, 3 month, 6 month supply.
Use: Vitamin supplement.
JUST TEARS. (Blairex) Benzalkonium chloride 0.01%, EDTA 0.25%, NaCl. Soln. Bot. 15 ml.
Use: Ocular lubricant.
JUVOCAINE.
See: Procaine HCl (Various Mfr.).

K

K-1. Phytonadione.
Use: Vitamin K.
See: Mephyton, Tab. (Merck & Co.).
  Aqua MEPHYTON, Inj. (Merck & Co.).
  KonaKion, Inj. (For IM use only) (Roche).
K-4. Menadiol sodium diphosphate.
Use: Vitamin K.
See: SynKayvite, Tab., Inj. (Roche).
K+8. (Alra) Potassium chloride 8 mEq. ER Tab. Bot. 100s, 500s.
Use: Potassium replacement product.
K+10. (Alra) Potassium Cl 10 mEq/Tab. Bot. 100s, 500s, 1000s.
Use: Potassium supplement.
K 34. Hexachlorophene.
K + CARE. (Alra) Potassium chloride, saccharin. Soln. Pkt. 15, 20, 25 mEq, 30s, 100s.
Use: Potassium replacement product.
KABIKINASE. (Kabi Pharmacia) Streptokinase 250,000 IU, 600,000 IU or 750,000 IU/Vial. Pow. for inj. Vial 5 ml. 1,500,000 IU/Vial. Vial 10 ml.
Use: Thrombolytic enzyme.
KAERGONA.
See: Menadione (Various Mfr.).
•**KALAFUNGIN.** USAN.
Use: Antifungal.
KALLIDINOGENASE. B.A.N. An enzyme that splits kinin and kallidin from kininogen.
Use: Vasodilator.
KALOL. (Jenkins) Boric acid, sodium biborate, sodium Cl, menthol, thymol, oil of eucalyptus, methyl salicylate (synthetic), carbolic acid/Tab. Bot. 1000s.
KALORY-PLUS. (Tyler) Thyroid 3 gr, am-

phetamine sulfate 15 mg, atropine sulfate ¹/₁₈₀ gr, aloin 0.25 gr, phenobarbital 0.25 gr/TR cap. Bot. 100s, 1000s.
Use: Anorexiant.
KAMAGEL. (Towne) Opium 15 mg, colloidal kaolin 6 Gm, pectin 300 mg, milk of bismuth 5 ml/fl oz. Bot. 4 oz.
Use: Antidiarrheal.
KAMFOLENE. (Wade) Camphor, menthol, methyl salicylate, oils turpentine and eucalyptus, carbolic acid 2%, calamine, zinc oxide in lanolin base. Jar 2 oz, lb.
Use: Antiseptic.
KANALKA TABLETS. (Lannett) Phenobarbital sodium 0.25 gr, benzocaine 0.25 gr, magnesium carbonate 2 gr, calcium carbonate 3 gr/Tab. Bot. 100s, 1000s.
Use: Sedative/hypnotic, antacid.
• **KANAMYCIN SULFATE,** U.S.P. XXIII. Caps., Inj., Sterile, U.S.P. XXIII. D-Streptamine, 0-3-amino-3-deoxy-α-d-glucopyranosyl-(1→6)-0-6-amino-6-deoxy-α-d-gluco-pyranosyl-(14)-2-deoxy-, sulfate (1:1). An antibiotic obtained from *Streptomyces kanamyceticus.*
Use: Antibacterial.
See: Kantrex, Cap., Vial (Bristol).
Klebcil, Inj. (Beecham).
KANK-A. (Blistex) Benzocaine 5%, cetylpyridinium chloride, castor oil, benzoin compound. Liq. Bot. 3.75 ml.
Use: Local anesthetic, topical.
KANKEX. (EJ Moore) Benzocaine, tannic acid, benzyl alcohol, diisobutyl-crosoxy-ethoxy-ethyl-dimethyl-benzyl-ammonium Cl, in propylene base. Bot. 0.5 oz w/applicator.
Use: Local anesthetic, topical.
KANTREX. (Bristol) Kanamycin sulfate. **Cap.:** 0.5 Gm. Bot. 20s, 100s. **Vial:** 0.5 Gm/2 ml or 1 Gm/3 ml. **Pediatric Inj.:** 75 mg/2 ml. **Disposable Syringe:** 500 mg/2 ml.
Use: Aminoglycoside.
KAOCASIL. (Jenkins) Kaolin colloidal 60 mg, calcium carbonate 0.1 Gm, magnesium trisilicate 60 mg, bismuth subgallate 15 mg, papain 8 mg, atropine sulfate 1/2000 gr/Tab. Bot. 1000s.
Use: Antacid, antidiarrheal, digestive aid, anticholinergic/antispasmodic.
KAOCHLOR 10% LIQUID. (Adria) Potassium and chloride 20 mEq/15 ml (potassium Cl 10%), alcohol 5%, saccharin, FD&C Yellow No. 5. Bot. pt.
Use: Potassium supplement.
KAOCHLOR-EFF. (Adria) Elemental potassium 20 mEq, chloride 20

mEq/Tab. Supplied by: Potassium Cl 0.6 Gm, potassium citrate 0.22 Gm, potassium bicarbonate 1 Gm, betaine HCl 1.84 Gm, saccharin 20 mg, artificial fruit flavor, tartrazine (color)/Tab. Sugar free. Carton 60s.
Use: Potassium supplement.
KAOCHLOR S-F 10% LIQUID. (Adria) Potassium 20 mEq, chloride 20 mEq/15 ml, saccharin, flavoring, alcohol 5%. Sugar free. Bot. 4 oz, pt.
Use: Potassium supplement.
KAODENE NON-NARCOTIC. (Pfeiffer) Kaolin 3.9 Gm, pectin 194.4 mg/30 ml, bismuth subsalicylate. Alcohol free. Liq. Bot. 120 ml.
Use: Antidiarrheal.
KAODENE WITH CODEINE. (Pfeiffer) Codeine phosphate 32.4 mg, kaolin 3.9 Gm, pectin 194.4 mg, sodium carboxymethylcellulose, bismuth subsalicylate/30 ml. Susp. Bot. 120 ml.
Use: Antidiarrheal.
KAODENE WITH PAREGORIC. (Pfeiffer) Anhydrous morphine 1.5 mg (paregoric 3.75 ml), kaolin 3.9 Gm, pectin 194.4 mg, sodium carboxymethylcellulose, bismuth subsalicylate/30 ml. Alcohol free. Susp. Bot. 120 ml.
Use: Antidiarrheal.
• **KAOLIN,** U.S.P. XXIII. (Various Mfr.).
Use: Adsorbent for diarrhea.
W/Atropine sulfate, phenobarbital.
W/Belladonna, phenobarbital.
See: Bellkata, Tab. (Ferndale).
W/Bismuth compound.
See: Kaomine, Pow. (Lilly).
W/Bismuth subgallate.
See: Diastop, Liq. (Elder).
W/Bismuth subgallate, pectin, zinc phenolsulfonate, opium pow.
See: Diastay, Tab. (Elder).
W/Bismuth subsalicylate, salol, methyl salicylate, benzocaine, pectin.
See: Donnagel, Susp. (Robins).
W/Calcium carbonate, magnesium trisilicate, bismuth subgallate, papain, atropine sulphate.
See: Kaocasil, Tab. (Jenkins).
W/Cornstarch, camphor, zinc oxide, eucalyptus oil.
See: Mexsana, Pow. (Plough).
W/Furazolidone, pectin.
See: Furoxone, Liq. (Eaton).
W/Hyoscyamine sulfate, sodium benzoate, atropine sulfate, hyoscine HBR, pectin.
See: Donnagel, Susp. (Robins).
W/Neomycin sulfate, pectin.
See: Pecto-Kalin, Liq. (Harvey).
W/Opium pow., bismuth subgallate, pectin, zinc phenolsulfonate.

See: Bismuth, Pectin & Paregoric (Lemmon).
W/Opium pow., pectin, hyoscyamine sulfate, atropine sulfate, hyoscine HBr, alcohol.
See: Donnagel P.G., Susp. (Robins).
W/Paregoric, aluminum hydroxide, bismuth subcarbonate, pectin.
See: Kapinal, Tab. (Jenkins).
W/Pectin.
See: Kaopectate, Liq. (Upjohn).
Kapectin, Liq. (Approved).
Pecto-Kalin, Susp. (Lemmon).
Pectokay Mixture (Bowman).
W/Pectin, belladonna alkaloids.
W/Pectin, bismuth subcarbonate.
See: B-K-P Mixture, Liq. (Sutliff & Case).
W/Pectin, bismuth subcarbonate, belladonna.
See: Kay-Pec, Liq. (Case).
W/Pectin, bismuth subcarbonate, opium pow.
See: KBP/O, Cap. (Cole).
W/Pectin, bismuth subsalicylate.
W/Pectin, bismuth subsalicylate, paregoric, zinc sulfocarbolate.
W/Pectin, hyoscyamine sulfate, atropine sulfate, hyoscine HBr.
See: Kapigam, Liq. (Reid-Rowell).
Palsorb Improved, Liq. (Hauck).
W/Pectin, pow. opium extract.
See: Pecto-Kalin, Susp. (Lemmon).
W/Pectin, opium pow., bismuth subgallate, zinc phenolsulfonate.
See: Cholactabs, Tab. (Philips Roxane).
B.P.P., Tab. (Lemmon).
W/Pectin, paregoric (equivalent).
See: Duosorb, Liq. (Reid-Rowell).
Kaoparin, Liq. (McKesson).
Kapectin, Liq. (Approved).
Ka-Pek w/Paregoric, Liq. (APC).
Parepectolin, Susp. (Rhone-Poulenc Rorer).
W/Pectin, zinc phenolsulfonate.
See: Pectocel, Susp. (Lilly).
Pectocomp, Liq. (Lannett).
W/Phenobarbital, atropine sulfate, aluminum hydroxide gel.
See: Kao-Lumin, Tab. (Philips Roxane).
W/Salol, zinc sulfocarbolate, aluminum hydroxide, bismuth subsalicylate, pectin.
See: Wescola Antidiarrheal-Stomach Upset (Western Research).
KAOLIN COLLOIDAL.
W/Bismuth subcarbonate.
See: Bisilad, Susp. (Central).
W/Magnesium trisilicate, aluminum hydroxide dried gel.
See: Kamadrox, Tab. (Elder).

Kathmagel, Tab. (Mason).
W/Opium, pectin, milk of bismuth.
See: Kamagel Liq. (Towne).
W/Paregoric, pectin.
See: Parepectolin, Susp. (Rhone-Poulenc Rorer Consumer).
W/Paregoric, pectin, milk of bismuth, methyl para-hydroxybenzoate, alcohol.
See: Mul-Sed, Susp. (Webcon).
W/Pectin, aromatics.
See: Paocin, Susp. (Beecham-Massengill).
W/Pectin, belladonna alkaloids.
See: Kamabel, Liq. (Towne).
W/Phenobarbital, homatropine methylbromide.
See: Lanokalin, Tab. (Lannett).
KAOLIN W/PECTIN. (Various Mfr.) Kaolin 90 Gm, pectin 2 Gm/30 ml. Susp. Bot. 180, pt, UD 30 ml.
Use: Antidiarrheal combinations.
KAON CL-10 CONTROLLED RELEASE TABLETS. (Adria) Potassium Cl 750 mg/Tab. Bot. 100s, 500s, 1000s. Stat-Pak 100s.
Use: Potassium supplement.
KAON CL 20%. (Adria) Potassium and chloride 40 mEq (to potassium Cl 3 Gm)/15 ml, saccharin, flavoring, alcohol 5%. Bot. pt.
Use: Potassium supplement.
KAON CL CONTROLLED RELEASE TABLETS. (Adria) Potassium Cl 500 mg/Tab., FD&C Yellow No. 5. Bot. 100s, 250s, 1000s.
Use: Potassium supplement.
KAON ELIXIR. (Adria) Elemental potassium 20 mEq (as potassium gluconate 4.68 Gm)/15 ml, aromatics, grape and lemon-lime flavors, alcohol 5%, saccharin. Unit pkg. pt, gal.
Use: Potassium supplement.
KAON TABLETS. (Adria) Elemental potassium 5 mEq obtained from potassium gluconate 1.17 Gm/SC Tab. Bot. 100s, 500s.
Use: Potassium supplement.
KAOPECTATE. (Upjohn) Kaolin 5.85 Gm, pectin 130 mg/oz. Bot. 8 oz, 12 oz, 16 oz, 1 gal, UD pkg. 3 oz.
Use: Antidiarrheal.
KAOPECTATE ADVANCED FORMULA. (Upjohn) Attapulgite 600 mg/15 ml, sucrose. Liq. Bot. 90, 240, 360, 480 ml.
Use: Antidiarrheal combination.
KAOPECTATE CHILDREN'S. (Upjohn) **Chew. Tab.:** Attapulgite 300 mg, sucrose, dextrose. Pkg. 16s. **Liq.:** Attapulgite 600 mg/15 ml. Bot. 180 ml.
Use: Antidiarrheal combination.

KAOPECTATE MAXIMUM STRENGTH. (Upjohn) Attapulgite 750 mg, Capl. Pkg. 12s, 20s.
Use: Antidiarrheal combination.
KAOPECTATE TABLET FORMULA. (Upjohn) Attapulgite 750 mg/Tab. Blister pak 12s, 20s.
Use: Antidiarrheal.
KAOPHEN TABLETS. (Vale) Phenobarbital 6.5 mg, belladonna extract 0.1 mg, kaolin 388.8 mg/Tab. Bot. 100s, 1000s.
Use: Antidiarrheal.
KAO-SPEN. (Century) Kaolin 5.2 g, pectin 260 mg/30 ml. Susp. Bot. 120 ml, pt, gal.
Use: Antidiarrheal.
KAO-TIN. (Major) Kaolin 5.85 Gm, pectin 130 mg/30 ml. Susp. Bot. 120 ml, 240 ml, pt, gal.
Use: Antidiarrheal.
KAPECTIN. (Approved) Kaolin 90 gr, pectin 2 gr/oz. Bot. gal. W/Paregoric Liq. 4 oz.
Use: Antidiarrheal.
KAPECTOLIN. (Various Mfr.) Kaolin 90 Gm, pectin 2 Gm/30 ml. Susp. Bot. 360 ml.
Use: Antidiarrheal.
KAPECTOLIN P.G. (Century) Powdered opium 24 mg, kaolin 6 mg, pectin 142.8 mg, hyoscyamine sulfate 0.1037 mg, atropine sulfate 0.0194 mg, hyoscine hydrobromide 0.0065 mg, sodium benzoate preservative 65 mg Bot. 120 ml, 180 ml, pt, gal.
Use: Antidiarrheal.
KA-PEK. (APC) Kaolin 90 gr, pectin 4.5 gr/fl oz. Bot. 6 oz, gal.
Use: Antidiarrheal.
KA-PEK WITH PAREGORIC. (APC) Paregoric 60 min, kaolin 90 gr, pectin 4.5 gr/fl oz. Bot. 4 oz.
Use: Antidiarrheal.
KAPILIN.
See: Menadione (Various Mfr.).
KARAYA GUM. (Penick) Indian Gum. Sterculia gum,
See: Tri Cootivin (Prof. Lab.).
W/Frangula.
See: Saraka, Gran. (Plough).
W/Psyllium seed, plantago ovata, brewers yeast.
See: Plantamucin Gran. (Elder).
W/Cortex rhamni frangulae.
See: Movicol (Norgine).
W/Refined psyllium mucilloid.
See: Hydrocil regular (Reid-Rowell).
KARAYA POWDER. (Sween) Bot. 3 oz.
Use: Ostomy care product.
KAREON.

See: Menadione (Various Mfr.).
KARIDIUM. (Lorvic) **Tab.:** Sodium fluoride 2.21 mg, sodium Cl 94.49 mg, disintegrant 0.5 mg. Bot. 180s, 1000s. **Liq.:** Sodium fluoride 2.21 mg, sodium Cl 10 mg, purified water q.s./8 drops. Bot. 30 ml, 60 ml.
Use: Dental caries preventative.
KARIGEL. (Lorvic) Fluoride ion 0.5%, pH 5.6. Gel. Bot. 30 ml, 130 ml, 250 ml.
Use: Dental caries preventative.
KARIGEL-N. (Lorvic) Fluoride ion 0.5% in neutral pH gel. Bot. 24 ml, 125 ml.
Use: Dental caries preventative.
• **KASAL.** USAN. Approximately $Na_8AP_2(OH_2(PO_4)_4$ with about 30% of dibasic sodium phosphate; sodium aluminum phosphate, basic.
Use: Food additive.
KASDENOL. (E.J. Moore) Clorpactin WCS-60. Jar 10 Gm.
Use: Germicidal for bleeding gums.
KASOF. (Stuart) Docusate potassium 240 mg/Cap. Bot. 30s, 60s.
Use: Laxative.
KASUGAMYCIN. Under study.
Use: Antibiotic.
KATO. (ICN) Potassium Cl for oral soln. potassium 20 mEq. Carton 30s, 120s.
Use: Potassium supplement.
KAVITON.
See: Menadione, U.S.P. XXIII. (Various Mfr.).
KAY CIEL ELIXIR. (Forest) Potassium Cl 1.5 Gm/15 ml. (20 mEq/15 ml), alcohol 4%. Bot. 120 ml, 473 ml, gal.
Use: Potassium supplement.
KAY CIEL POWDER. (Forest) Potassium chloride 1.5 Gm/Packette. (20 mEq/Packet), 4% alcohol. Box 30s, 100s, 500s.
Use: Potassium supplement.
KAYEXALATE. (Sanofi Winthrop.) Sodium polystyrene sulfonate. Jar lb.
Use: Potassium removing resin.
KAYLIXIR. (Lannett) Potassium (as potassium gluconate) 20 mEq/15 ml, alcohol 5%, saccharin. Elix. Bot. pt, gal.
Use: Potassium supplement.
KBP/O. (Forest) Kaolin 350 mg, pectin 60 mg, powdered opium 3 mg, bismuth subcarbonate 60 mg/Cap. Bot. 100s, 1000s.
Use: Antidiarrheal.
K-C. (Century) Kaolin 5.2 g, pectin 260 mg, bismuth subcarbonate 260 mg/30 ml. Susp. Bot. 120 ml, pt, gal.
Use: Antidiarrheal.
K+CARE ET. (Alra) Potassium bicarbonate 25 mEq/Effervescent tab. Bot. 30s,

100s, 1000s.
Use: Potassium supplement.
K-C LIQUID. (Century) Kaolin 5.2 Gm,
pectin 260 mg, bismuth subcarbonate
260 mg/oz. Bot. 4 oz, pt, gal.
Use: Antidiarrheal.
K-C SUSPENSION. (Century Pharm.)
Kaolin 5.2 Gm, pectin 260 mg, bismuth
subcarbonate 260 mg/30 ml. Bot. 120
ml, pt, gal.
Use: Antidiarrheal.
KC-20 ELIXIR. (Scruggs) Bot. pt, gal.
KCL-20. (Western Research) Potassium
Cl 1.5 Gm (potassium 20 mEq, chloride
20 mEq)/Packet. Box 30s.
Use: Potassium supplement.
K.D.C. VAGINAL CREAM. (Kenyon) Sul-
fanilamide 15%, 9-aminoacridine HCl
0.2%, allantoin 2% in a dispersible base
containing stearic acid, diglycol,
stearate, triethanolamine, propylene gly-
col, lactic acid, water.
Use: Anti-infective, vaginal.
K-DUR 10 & 20. (Key) **10:** Potassium Cl
750 mg (10 mEq)/SR Tab. **20:** Potassium Cl 1500 mg (20 mEq)/SR Tab. Bot.
100s.
Use: Potassium supplement.
KE.
See: Cortisone Acetate (Various Mfr.).
KEDRIN TABLET. (Dolcin) Analgesic
compound. Bot. 100s.
Use: Analgesic.
KEELAMIN. (Mericon) Zinc 20 mg, man-
ganese 5 mg, copper 3 mg/Tab. Bot.
100s.
Use: Mineral supplement.
KEEP-A-WAKE. (Stayner) Vitamins B_1 5
mg, B_2 2 mg, B_{126} activity (cobalamin
concentrate 1.5 mcg), niacinamide 10
mg, caffeine citrate 2.5 gr/Tab. Bot. 24s.
Use: CNS stimulant.
KEFLEX FOR PEDIATRIC DROPS.
(Dista) Cephalexin 100 mg/ml. Dropper
bot. 10 ml.
Use: Antibacterial, cephalosporin.
KEFTAB. (Dista) Cephalexin HCl mono-
hydrate 500 mg/Tab. Bot. 100s.
Use: Antibacterial, cephalosporin.
KEFUROX. (Lilly) Cefuroxime sodium
750 mg or 1.5 Gm/Vial. ADD-VANTAGE
750 mg: Vial 10 ml, Box 25s. Vial 100
ml, Box 10s. **1.5 Gm:** Vial 100 ml, Box
10s. 1.5 Gm Vial, 10s.
Use: Antibacterial, cephalosporin.
KELEX. (Nutrition) Iron choline citrate
360 mg providing approximately 40 mg
of elemental iron/Tabseal. Bot. 90s.
Use: Iron supplement.
KELGIN. Algin.

KELL E. (Canright) di-α Tocopheryl 100
IU, 200 IU or 400 IU. Bot. 100s.
Use: Vitamin E supplement.
KELLOGG'S TASTELESS CASTOR OIL.
(Beecham Products) Castor oil 100%.
Bot. 2 oz.
Use: Laxative.
KELP (Arcum) Tab. Bot. 100s, 1000s.
KELP PLUS. (Barth's) Iodine from kelp
plus 16 trace minerals/Tab. Bot. 100s,
500s, 1000s.
KELP TABLETS. (Faraday) Iodine from
kelp 0.15 mg/Tab. Bot. 100s.
KEMADRIN. (Burroughs Wellcome) Pro-
cyclidine HCl 5 mg/Tab. Bot. 100s.
Use: Antiparkinson agent.
KEMITHAL. Thialbarbital. 5-Allyl-5-cyclo-
hex-2-enyl-2-thiobarbituric acid.
KENAC CREAM. (NMC Labs) Triamci-
nolone acetonide cream 0.025% or
0.1%. Tube 15 Gm, 60 Gm, 80 Gm, Jar
240 Gm.
Use: Corticosteroid, topical.
KENAC OINTMENT. (NMC Labs) Triamcinolone acetonide ointment 0.1%. Tube
15 Gm, 80 Gm.
Use: Corticosteroid, topical.
KENACORT DIACETATE. (Squibb Mark)
Triamcinolone diacetate equivalent to tri-
amcinolone 4 mg, buffered with sodium
citrate, sodium phosphate/5 ml. Bot. 120
ml.
Use: Corticosteroid.
KENAHIST-S.A. (Kenyon) Phenyl-
propanolamine HCl 50 mg, pheniramine
maleate 25 mg, pyrilamine maleate 25
mg/Tab. Bot. 100s, 1000s.
Use: Decongestant, antihistamine.
KENAJECT-40. (Mayrand) Triamcinolone
acetonide 40 mg/ml/Inj. Vial 5 ml.
Use: Corticosteroid.
KENAKION. (Harriett Lane Home of
Johns Hopkins Hospital) Vitamin K-1 oxide.
Use: Vitamin K-induced kernicterus.
KENALOG. (Westwood-Squibb) Triamcinolone acetonide. **0.1% Cream:** Tube 15
Gm, 60 Gm, 80 Gm, Jar 240 Gm, in
aqueous lotion base w/propylene glycol,
cetyl and stearyl alcohols, glyceryl
monostearate, sorbitan monopalmitate,
polyoxyethylene sorbitan monolaurate,
methylparaben, propylparaben, polyethylene glycol monostearate, simethicone,
sorbic acid. **0.5% Cream:** Tube 20 Gm.
0.1% Oint.: (w/base of polyethylene,
mineral oil) Tube 15 Gm, 60 Gm, 80 Gm;
Jar 240 Gm, **0.5% Oint.:** Tube 20 Gm.
0.1% Lot.: Bot. 15ml, 60 ml. **Spray:** 6.6
mg/100 Gm, alcohol 10.3%. Can 23 Gm,

63 Gm.
Use: Corticosteroid, topical.
KENALOG 0.025%. (Westwood-Squibb)
Triamcinolone acetonide. **Cream:** Tube
15 Gm, 80 Gm, Jar 240 Gm. **Lot.:** In
aqueous lotion base w/propylene glycol,
cetyl and stearyl alcohols, glyceryl
monostearate, sorbitan monopalmitate,
polyoxyethylene sorbitan monolaurate,
methylparaben, propylparaben, polyethylene glycol monostearate, simethicone,
sorbic acid, tinted in an isopropyl palmitate vehicle with alcohol (4.7%). Bot. 60
ml. **Oint.:** Plastibase (w/base of polyethylene and mineral oil gel). 15 Gm, 80
Gm, 240 Gm.
Use: Corticosteroid, topical.
KENALOG H. (Westwood-Squibb) Triamcinolone acetonide cream USP 0.1%.
Each Gm of cream provides 1 mg of triamcinolone acetonide in a specially formulated hydrophilic vanishing cream
base containing propylene glycol, dimethicone 350, castor oil, cetearyl alcohol
and ceteareth-20, propylene glycol
stearate, white petrolatum, purified water. Tube 15 Gm, 60 Gm.
Use: Corticosteroid, topical.
KENALOG-10 INJECTION. (Squibb
Mark) Sterile triamcinolone acetonide
suspension 10 mg/ml, sodium Cl for isotonicity, benzyl alcohol 0.9% (w/v) as a
preservative, sodium carboxymethylcellulose 0.75%, polysorbate 80 0.04%.
Sodium hydroxide or HCl acid may be
present to adjust pH to 5 to 7.5. Nitrogen
packed at the time of manufacture. Vial
5 ml.
Use: Corticosteroid.
KENALOG-40 INJECTION. (Squibb
Mark) Sterile triamcinolone acetonide
suspension 40 mg/ml, sodium chloride
for isotonicity, benzyl alcohol 0.9% (w/v)
as a preservative, sodium carboxymethylcellulose 0.75%, polysorbate
80 0.04%. Sodium hydroxide or HCl acid
may be present to adjust pH to 5 to 7.5.
Nitrogen packed at the time of manufacture. Vial 1 ml, 5 ml, 10 ml.
Use: Corticosteroid.
KENALOG IN ORABASE. (Apothecon)
Triamcinolone acetonide 0.1% in
Orabase. Triamcinolone acetonide 1
mg/Gm. Tube 5 Gm.
Use: Corticosteroid.
KENAZIDE-E. (Kenyon) Hydrochlorothiazide 50 mg/Tab. Bot. 100s, 1000s.
Use: Antihypertensive.
KENAZIDE-H. (Kenyon) Hydrochloroth-
iazide 50 mg/Tab. Bot. 100s, 1000s.

Use: Antihypertensive.
KENCORT. (Kenyon) Hydrocortisone
1%, clioquinol 3% in bland, water wash-
able base. Jar lb.
Use: Corticosteroid, antifungal.
KENDALL'S "COMPOUND B."
See: Corticosterone (Various Mfr.).
KENDALL'S "COMPOUND E."
See: Cortisone Acetate (Various Mfr.).
KENDALL'S "COMPOUND F."
See: 17-Hydroxycorticosterone (Vari-
ous Mfr.).
KENDALL'S "DESOXY COMPOUND B."
See: Desoxycorticosterone Acetate
(Various Mfr.).
KENISONE DROPS. (Kenyon) Neomycin
sulfate 6 mg, hydrocortisone 5 mg,
parachlorometaxylenol 0.05%, pramox-
ine HCl 1%, alcohol 4.8%/ml. Bot. 15 ml.
Use: Anti-infective, corticosteroid, otic.
KENONEL. (Marnel) Triamcinolone ace-
tonide 0.1%. Cream. Tube 20 Gm.
Use: Corticosteroid, topical.
KENTONIC. (Kenyon) Vitamins A 25,000
IU, D 1000 IU, B_1 10 mg, B_2 10 mg, B_6 5
mg, B_{126} 5 mg, C 200 mg, niacinamide
100 mg, calcium pantothenate 20
mg/Cap. Bot. 1000s.
Use: Vitamin supplement.
KEN-TUSS. (Kenyon) Dextromethorphan
HBr 10 mg, phenylephrine HCl 5 mg,
chlorpheniramine maleate 2 mg, salicylamide 227 mg, phenacetin 100 mg, caffeine alkaloid 10 mg, ascorbic acid 20
mg/Tab. Bot. 100s, 1000s.
Use: Antitussive, decongestant, antihistamine, analgesic.
KENWOOD THERAPEUTIC LIQUID.
(Kenwood) Vitamins A 10,000 IU, D 400
IU, E 4.5 IU, C 150 mg, B_1 6 mg, B_2 3
mg, niacinamide 60 mg, B_6 1 mg, calcium pantothenate 6 mg, calcium 38 mg,
phosphorus 29 mg, magnesium 6 mg,
manganese 1 mg, potassium 5 mg/15
ml. Bot. 12 oz.
Use: Vitamin/mineral supplement.
KERALYT GEL. (Westwood) Salicylic
acid 6% in a gel base of propylene glycol
w/alcohol 19.4%, hydroxypropyl cellulose, water. Tube 1 oz.
Use: Keratolytic.
KERATOLYTICS.
See: Condylox (Oclassen).
KERI CREME. (Westwood) Cream containing water, mineral oil, talc, sorbitol,
ceresin, lanolin alcohol, magnesium
stearate, glyceryl oleate/glyceryl glycol, isopropyl myristate, methylparaben,
propylparaben, fragrance, quaternium-
15. Tube 2.5 oz.

Use: Emollient.

KERI FACIAL CLEANSER. (Westwood) Water, glycerin, squalane, propylene glycol, glyceryl stearate, PEG-100 stearate, stearic acid, steareth-20, lanolin alcohol, magnesium aluminium silicate, cetyl alcohol, beeswax, PEG-20 sorbitan, beeswax, mothylparabon, propylparaben, quaternium-15, fragrance. Bot. 4 oz.
Use: Therapeutic skin cleanser.

KERI FACIAL SOAP. (Westwood) Sodium tallowate, sodium cocoate, water, mineral oil, octyl hydroxystearate, fragrance, glycerin, titanium dioxide, PEG-75, lanolin oil, docusate sodium, PEG-4 dilaurate, propylparaben, PEG-40 stearate, glyceryl monostearate, PEG-100 stearate, sodium Cl, BHT, EDTA. Bar 3.25 oz.
Use: Therapeutic skin cleanser.

KERI LIGHT LOTION. (Westwood) Water, stearyl alcohol, ceteareath-20, cetearyl octaneoate, glycerin, stearyl heptanoate, stearyl alcohol, Carbomer 934, sodium hydroxide, squalane, methylparaben, propylparaben, fragrance. Bot. 6.5 oz, 13 oz.
Use: Emollient.

KERI LOTION. (Westwood) Mineral oil, lanolin oil, water, propylene glycol, glyceryl stearate, PEG-100 stearate, PEG 40 stearate, PEG-4 dilaurate, laureth-4, parabens, docusate sodium, triethanolamine, quaternium 15, carbomer 934, fragrance. Bot. 6.5 oz, 13 oz, 20 oz.
Use: Emollient.

KERLONE. (Searle) Betaxolol HCl 10 mg or 25 mg/Tab. Bot. 100s, UD 100s.
Use: Beta-adrenergic blocking agent.

KEROCAINE.
See: Procaine HCl (Various Mfr.).

KERODEX. (Wyeth-Ayerst)
No. 51: Water-miscible. Tube 4 oz, Jar lb.
No. 71: Water-repellent. Tube 4 oz, Jar lb.
Use: Emollient.

KEROHYDRIC. A de-waxed, oil-soluble fraction of lanolin.
Use: Emollient, cleanser.
See: Alpha-Keri, Soap, Spray (Westwood).
Keri, Cream, Lot. (Westwood).
W/Docusate sodium, sodium alkyl polyether sulfonate, sodium sulfoacetate, sulfur, salicylic acid, hexachlorophene.
See: Sebulex, Cream, Liq. (Westwood).

KERR INSTA-CHAR. (Kerr) **Regular:** Aqueous suspension activated charcoal

50 Gm/8 oz. **Pediatric:** Aqueous suspension activated charcoal 15 Gm/4 oz.
Use: Antidote.

KERR TRIPLE DYE. (Kerr) Gentian violet, proflavine hemisulfate, brilliant green in water. Dispensing bot. 15 ml. Single Use Dispos-A-Swab 0.65 ml, Box 10s, Case 10 x 50 Box.
Use: Antiseptic.

KESTRONE 5. (Hyrex) Estrone 50,000 units (5 mg/ml) in aqueous soln. Vial 10 ml.
Use: Estrogen.

KETALAR. (Parke-Davis) Ketamine HCl, sodium Cl, benzethonium Cl. **10 mg/ml:** Vial 20 ml, 25 ml and 50 ml. Pkg. 10s; **50 mg/ml:** Vial 10 ml. **100 mg/ml:** Vial 5 ml. Pkg. 10s.
Use: General anesthetic.

• **KETAMINE HCl,** U.S.P. XXIII. Inj., U.S.P. XXIII. (±)-2-(o-Chlorophenyl)-2-(methylamino) cyclohexanone HCl.
Use: Anesthetic.
See: Ketaject, Vial (Bristol).
Ketalar, Inj. (Parke-Davis).

• **KETANSERIN.** USAN.
Use: Serotonin antagonist.

• **KETAZOCINE.** USAN.
Use: Analgesic.

• **KETAZOLAM.** USAN.
Use: Tranquilizer.

• **KETHOXAL.** USAN.
Use: Antiviral.

• **KETIPRAMINE FUMARATE.** USAN. 5-[3-(Diethylamino)propyl]-5,11-dihydro-10H-dibenz[b, f]-azepin-10-one fumarate (1:1).
Use: Antidepressant.

KETOBEMIDONE. B.A.N. 4-(3-Hydroxyphenyl)-1-methyl-4-propionylpiperidine. Cliradon.
Use: Narcotic analgesic.

• **KETOCONAZOLE.** USAN.
Use: Antifungal.

• **KETOCONAZOLE,** U.S.P. XXIII. Tab., U.S.P. XXIII. 1-acetyl-4 (4-((2-2(2,4 dichlorophenyl)-2-(1-H-imidazol-1-yimethyl)-1,3-dioxolan-4-yl)methoxy) phenyl) piperazine.
Use: Broad spectrum antifungal. Treat nephrotoxicity in organ transplants [Orphan drug]
See: Nizoral, Prods. (Janssen).

KETODESTRIN.
See: Estrone (Various Mfr.).

KETO-DIASTIX REAGENT STRIPS. (Miles Diagnostic) Dip and read reagent strip test for glucose and ketones in urine. Two test areas: glucose levels from 30 mg to 5000 mg/dL; Ketone test

(acetoacetic acid) negative 5 mg, 40 mg, 80 mg, 160 mg/dL. Strip Bot. 50s, 100s.
Use: Diagnostic aid.
KETOHEXAZINE. 4, 6-Diethyl-3(2H)-pyridazinono (Lederle).
Use: Hypnotic.
KETOHYDROXYESTRATRIENE.
See: Estrone.
KETOHYDROXYESTRIN.
See: Estrone (Various Mfr.).
KETONE TESTS.
Use: Diagnostic aid.
See: Acetest Reagent, Tab. (Miles Diagnostic).
Chemstrip K, Reagent paper (Boehringer Mannheim).
Ketostix Strips, Reagent Strips (Miles Diagnostic).
KETONEX-1. (Ross) Protein 15 g, fat 23.9 g, carbohydrates 46.3 g, linoleic acid 1800 mg, Fe 9 mg, Na 190 mg, K 675 mg. With appropriate vitamins and minerals. 480 Cal/100 g. Isoleucine, leucine and valine free. Pow. Can 350 g.
Use: Enteral nutritional supplement.
KETONEX-2. (Ross) Protein 30 g, fat 15.5 g, carbohydrates 30 g, Fe 13 mg, Na 880 mg, K 1370 mg. With appropriate vitamins and minerals. 410 Cal/100 g. Isoleucine, leucine and valine free. Pow. Can 325 g.
Use: Enteral nutritional supplement.
• **KETOPROFEN.** USAN. (Various Mfr.) 25 mg, 50 mg, 75 mg. Cap. Bot. 100s, 500s.
Use: Anti-inflammatory.
See: Orudis, Cap. (Wyeth-Ayerst).
Oruvail, Cap. (Wyeth-Ayerst).
• **KETORFANOL.** USAN.
Use: Analgesic.
• **KETOROLAC TROMETHAMINE.** USAN.
Use: Analgesic.
See: Toradol (Syntex).
KETOROLAC TROMETHAMINE.
Use: Ophthalmic non-steroidal anti-inflammatory agent.
See: Acular (Allergan).
KETOSTIX REAGENT STRIPS. (Miles Diagnostic) Sodium nitroprusside, sodium phosphate, glycine. Stick test for ketones in urine (measures acetoacetic acid). Bot. 50s, 100s, UD 20s.
Use: Diagnostic aid.
• **KETOTIFEN FUMARATE.** USAN.
Use: Antiasthmatic.
KEY-PLEX UNIVIAL. (Hyrex) Vitamins B_1 50 mg, B_2 5 mg, B_{126} 1000 mcg, pyridoxine HCl 5 mg, d-panthenol 6 mg, niacinamide 125 mg, ascorbic acid 50 mg/ml. Vial 10 ml.

Use: Parenteral nutritional supplement.
KEY-PRED. (Hyrex) Prednisolone. **25 mg/ml:** Vial 10 ml, 30 ml; **50 mg/ml:** Vial 10 ml.
Use: Corticosteroid.
KEY-PRED-SP. (Hyrex) Prednisolone sodium phosphate 20 mg/ml. Vial 10 ml.
Use: Corticosteroid.
K-G ELIXIR. (Geneva Marsam) Potassium (as potassium gluconate) 20 mEq/15 ml, alcohol 5%. Elix. Bot. pt.
Use: Potassium replacement.
KHAROPHEN.
See: Acetarsone (Various Mfr.).
KHELLIN. 5,8-dimethoxy-2-methyl-4′,5-furano-6,7-chromone.
Use: Coronary vasodilator.
KIDDIE POWDER. (Gordon) Pure fine Italian talc. Can 3.5 oz.
Use: Antifungal.
KIDDIES SIALCO. (Foy) Chlorpheniramine maleate 2 mg, phenylephrine HCl 2.5 mg, acetaminophen 62.5 mg, salicylamide 75 mg/Tab. Bot. 1000s.
Use: Antihistamine, decongestant, analgesic.
KIDDI-VITES, Improved. (Geneva Marsam) Vitamins A 5000 IU, D 500 IU, B_1 1 mg, B_2 1.5 mg, B_{126} 2 mcg, C 50 mg, B_6 1 mg, pantothenate 2 mg, niacinamide 10 mg/Tab. Bot. 100s, 1000s.
Use: Vitamin supplement.
KIDNEY FUNCTION AGENTS.
See: Biotel Kidney (Biotel).
Indigo Carmine Soln. (Various Mfr.).
Inulin, Amp. (Arnar-Stone).
Iodohippurate, Sodium.
Mannitol Soln., Amp. (Merck & Co.).
Methylene Blue (Various Mfr.).
Phenolsulfonphthalein (Various Mfr.).
KIE SYRUP. (Laser) Potassium iodide 150 mg, ephedrine HCl 8 mg/5 ml. Syr. Bot. pt, gal.
Use: Expectorant, decongestant.
KINATE. Hexahydrotetra hydroxybenzoate salt, quinic acid salt.
KINESED. (Stuart) Phenobarbital 16 mg, hyoscyamine sulfate, atropine sulfate 0.12 mg, scopolamine hydrobromide 0.007 mg/Tab. Bot. 100s.
Use: Anticholinergic combination.
KINEVAC. (Squibb) Sincalide 5 mcg/vial. For gallbladder, pancreatic secretion and cholecystography.
Use: Diagnostic aid.
KIN WHITE. (Whiteworth) Triamcinolone acetonide. **Cream:** 0.025% or 1%. Tube 15 Gm, 80 Gm. **Oint.:** 1%. Tube 15 Gm, 80 Gm.
Use: Corticosteroid, topical.

• **KITASAMYCIN.** USAN. An antibiotic substance obtained from cultures of *Streptomyces kitasatoensis*. Under study.
Use: Antibiotic.

KLAVIKORDAL. (U.S. Ethicals) Nitroglycerin 2.6 mg/SR Tab. Bot. 100s, 1000s.
Use: Antihypertensive.

KLB6 COMPLETE. (Nature's Bounty) Vitamins A 833.3 IU, E 5 mg (as IU), B_3 3.3 mg, C 10 mg, soya lecithin 200 mg, kelp 25 mg, cider vinegar 40 mg, wheat bran 83.3 mg, D 66.7 IU, FA 0.067 mg, B_1 0.25 mg, B_2 0.28 mg, B_6 8.3 mg, B_{126} 1 mcg, biotin 0.05 mg/Tab. Bot. 100s.
Use: Vitamin combination.

KLB6 SOFTGELS. (Nature's Bounty) Vitamin B_6 mcg, soya lecithin 100 mg, kelp 25 mg, cider vinegar 80 mg/Capl. Bot. 100s.
Use: Vitamin combination.

K-LEASE. (Adria) Potassium chloride 10 mEq (750 mg). ER Cap. Bot. 100s, 500s, 1000s, 2500s, UD 100s.
Use: Potassium replacement product.

KLEBSIELLA PNEUMONIAE.
W/*Haemophilus influenzae, Neisseria catarrhalis, streptococci, staphylococci, pneumococci,* killed.
See: Mixed Vaccine No. 4 W/H. Influenzae (Lilly).

KLEER COMPOUND. (Scrip) Acetaminophen 300 mg, phenylpropanolamine HCl 35 mg, guaifenesin. Tab. Bot. 100s.
Use: Analgesic, decongestant, expectorant.

KLEER IMPROVED. (Scrip) Atropine sulfate 0.2 mg, chlorpheniramine maleate 5 mg/ml.
Use: Anticholinergic, antihistamine.

KLEER MILD. (Scrip) Phenylpropanolamine HCl 75 mg/Cap. Bot. 100s.
Use: Decongestant.

KLERIST-D. (Nutripharm) **Cap.:** Pseudoephedrine HCl 120 mg, chlorpheniramine maleate 8 mg. Bot. 100s, **Tab.:** Pseudoephedrine HCl 60 mg, chlorpheniramine maleate 4 mg. Bot. 100s.
Use: Decongestant, antihistamine.

KLER-RO LIQUID. (Ulmer) Surgical cleanser and laboratory detergent. Bot. gal.
Use: Antiseptic.

KLER-RO POWDER. (Ulmer) Surgical cleanser and laboratory detergent. Can 2 lb, Bot. 6 lb.
Use: Antiseptic.

KLONOPIN. (Roche) Clonazepam 0.5 mg, 1 mg or 2 mg/Tab. Rx Pak 100s.
Use: Anticonvulsant.

K-LOR. (Abbott) Potassium Cl equivalent to potassium 20 mEq and Cl 20 mEq/2.6 Gm for oral soln. w/saccharin. Pkg. 30s, 100s. 15 mEq/2 Gm Pkg. 100s.
Use: Potassium supplement.

KLOR-CON 8. (Upsher-Smith) Potassium Cl 8 mEq/ER Tab. Bot. 100s, 500s.
Use: Potassium supplement.

KLOR-CON 10. (Upsher-Smith) Potassium Cl 10 mEq/ER Tab. Bot. 100s, 500s.
Use: Potassium supplement.

KLOR-CON/25 POWDER. (Upsher-Smith) Potassium Cl for oral soln 25 mEq/Pkt. Carton 30s, 100s, 250s.
Use: Potassium supplement.

KLOR-CON/EF. (Upsher-Smith) Potassium bicarbonate 25 mEq/Tab. Carton 30s, 100s.
Use: Potassium supplement.

KLOR-CON POWDER. (Upsher-Smith) Potassium Cl for oral soln. 20 mEq/Packet. w/saccharin. Packet 1.5 Gm. Box 30s, 100s.
Use: Potassium supplement.

KLORLYPTUS. (High) Eucalyptus oil, chlorine in a petroleum ointment and light oil base. **Oint.:** Jar oz, lb. **Oil:** Bot. 30 ml, pt.
Use: Topical dressing.

KLORVESS EFFERVESCENT GRANULES. (Sandoz) Potassium 20 mEq, Cl 20 mEq supplied by potassium Cl 1.125 Gm, potassium bicarbonate 0.5 Gm, L-lysine monohydrochloride 0.913 Gm/Packet. w/saccharin. Box 30s.
Use: Potassium supplement.

KLORVESS EFFERVESCENT TABLETS. (Sandoz) Potassium Cl 1.125 Gm, potassium bicarbonate 0.5 Gm, L-lysine HCl 0.913 Gm/Effervescent Tab. Sodium and sugar free. w/saccharin. Pkg. 60s, 1000s.
Use: Potassium supplement.

KLORVESS LIQUID. (Sandoz) Potassium Cl 1.5 Gm (20 mEq)/15 ml, alcohol 0.75%. Bot. pt.
Use: Potassium supplement.

KLOTRIX. (Mead Johnson) Potassium Cl 10 mEq/SR Tab. Bot. 100s, 1000s, UD 100s.
Use: Potassium supplement.

K-LYTE. (Bristol) Potassium bicarbonate and citrate 25 mEq, saccharin. Lime and orange flavors. Effervescent Tab. Pkg. 30s, 100s, 250s.
Use: Potassium supplement.

K-LYTE/CL. (Bristol) Potassium Cl 25

mEq, saccharin. Citrus and fruit punch flavor. Effervescent Tab. Pkg. 30s, 100s, 250s. Bulk powder 225 GM/Can.
Use: Potassium supplement.
K-LYTE/CL 50. (Bristol) Potassium Cl 50 mEq, saccharin. Citrus and fruit punch flavors. Pkg. 30s, 100s.
Use: Potassium supplement.
K-LYTE DS. (Bristol) Potassium bicarbonate and citrate 50 mEq, saccharin. Lime and orange flavor. Effervescent Tab. Pkg. 30s, 100s.
Use: Potassium supplement.
K-NORM. (Pennwalt) Potassium Cl 10 mEq/CR Cap. Bot. 100s, 500s.
Use: Potassium supplement.
KOATE HP. (Miles Inc) A stable dried concentrate of Anti-hemophilic Factor. When reconstituted, contains heparin ≤ 5 U/ml, PEG ≤ 1500 ppm, glycine ≤ 0.05 M, polysorbate 80 ≤ 25 ppm, TNBP ≤ 5 ppm, calcium chloride ≤ 3 mM, aluminum ≤ 1 ppm, histidine ≤ 0.06 M, albumin (human) ≤ 10 mg/ml. Includes Sterile Water for Injection, double-ended transfer needle, filter needle and administration set. Pow. Bot. 250, 500, 1000 and 1500 IU Factor VIII activity (approximate).
Use: Anti-hemophilic agent.
KODONYL EXPECTORANT. (Blue Cross) Bromodiphenhydramine HCl 3.75 mg, diphenhydramine HCl 8.75 mg, ammonium Cl 80 mg, potassium guaiacolsulfonate 80 mg, menthol 0.5 mg/5 ml. Bot. 16 oz.
Use: Antihistamine, expectorant.
KOGENATE. (Miles) Recombinant antihemophilic factor (Factor VIII). Pow. for inj.
Use: Antihemophilic agent.
KOLEPHRIN CAPLETS. (Pfeiffer) Pseudoephedrine HCl 30 mg, chlorpheniramine maleate 2 mg, acetaminophen 325 mg/Capl. Bot. 36s.
Use: Decongestant, antihistamine, analgesic.
KOLEPHRIN/DM CAPLETS. (Pfeiffer) Pseudoephedrine HCl 30 mg, chlorpheniramine maleate 2 mg, dextromethorphan HBr 10 mg, acetaminophen 325 mg/Capl. Bot. 30s.
Use: Decongestant, antihistamine, antitussive, analgesic.
KOLEPHRIN GG/DM EXPECTORANT. (Pfeiffer) Dextromethorphan HBr 10 mg, guaifenesin 150 mg/5 ml. Alcohol free. Bot. 120 ml.
Use: Antitussive, expectorant.
KOLEPHRIN NN LIQUID. (Pfeiffer)

Phenylpropanolamine HCl 12.5 mg, pyrilamine maleate 10 mg, dextromethorphan HBr 7.5 mg/5 ml. Alcohol free. Bot. 120 ml.
Use: Decongestant, antihistamine, antitussive.
• **KOLFOCON A.** USAN.
Use: Contact lens material (hydrophobic).
• **KOLFOCON B.** USAN.
Use: Contact lens material (hydrophobic).
• **KOLFOCON C.** USAN.
Use: Contact lens material (hydrophobic).
• **KOLFOCON D.** USAN.
Use: Contact lens material (hydrophobic).
KOLYUM LIQUID. (Pennwalt) Potassium ion 20 mEq, chloride ion 3.4 mEq from potassium gluconate 3.9 Gm, potassium Cl 0.25 Gm/15 ml or 5 Gm/15 ml. w/saccharin, sorbitol. Liq.: Bot. pt, gal.
Use: Potassium supplement.
KONAKION. (Roche) Phytonadione-synthetic vitamin K-$_1$, polysorbate 80, phenol, propylene glycol, sodium acetate, glacial acetic acid. Amp. 2 mg/0.5 ml or 10 mg/1 ml. Box 10s.
Use: Prevention and treatment of hypoprothrombinemia.
KONDON'S NASAL JELLY. (Kondon) Tube 20 Gm w/ephedrine alkaloid. Tube 20 Gm.
Use: Nasal decongestant.
KONDREMUL. (Fisons) Mineral oil 55%, Irish moss. Emulsion Bot. pt.
Use: Laxative.
W/Phenolphthalein 2.2 gr/Tbsp. Bot. pt.
W/Cascara 0.66 Gm/15 ml. Bot. 14 oz.
KONSTO. (Freeport) Docusate sodium 100 mg/Cap. Bot. 1000s.
Use: Laxative.
KONSYL POWDER. (Konsyl Pharm) Psyllium hydrophyllic mucilloid. Canister 300 Gm, 450 Gm, Packet 6 Gm, Ctn. 25s.
Use: Laxative.
KONSYL-D POWDER. (Konsyl Pharm) Psyllium hydrophilic mucilloid, dextrose. Canister 325 Gm, 500 Gm, Packet 6.5 Gm, Ctn. 25s.
Use: Laxative.
KONSYL-FIBER. (Konsyl Pharm) Calcium polycarbophil 625 mg. Tab. Bot. 90s.
Use: Laxative.
KONSYL-ORANGE. (Konsyl Pharm) Psyllium fiber 3.4 g/Tbsp., orange flavor. Pow. 12 g, 538 g.
Use: Laxative.

KONYNE-80. (Cutter) Factor IX complex, human heat treated. Vial 500 units or 1000 units w/diluent.
Use: Antihemophilic.
KOPHANE COUGH AND COLD FORMULA LIQUID. (Pfeiffer) Phenylpropanolamine HCl 12.5 mg, chlorpheniramine maleate 2 mg, dextromethorphan HBr 10 mg. Bot. 120 ml.
Use: Decongestant, antihistamine, antitussive.
KORIGESIC TABLETS. (Trimen) Phenylephrine HCl 5 mg, chlorpheniramine maleate 4 mg, acetaminophen 325 mg, caffeine 30 mg/Tab. Bot. 100s.
Use: Decongestant, antihistamine, analgesic.
KORO-FLEX. (Holland-Rantos) Improved contouring spring natural latex diaphragm 60 mm-95 mm.
Use: Contraceptive.
KOROMEX COIL SPRING DIAPHRAGM. (Holland-Rantos) Diaphragm made of pure latex rubber, cadmium plated coil spring. Koromex Jelly and Cream/kit. 50 mm-95 mm at graduations of 5 mm.
Use: Contraceptive.
KOROMEX COMBINATION. (Holland-Rantos) Diaphragm 50 mm-95 mm, Koromex Jelly and Cream/Kit.
Use: Contraceptive.
KOROMEX CRYSTAL CLEAR GEL. (Holland-Rantos) Nonoxynol-9 2% in base of purified water, propylene glycol, cellulose gum, boric acid, sorbitol, simethicone w/pH 4.5. Tube 126 Gm w/applicator.
Use: Contraceptive.
KORUM. (Geneva) Acetaminophen 5 gr/Tab. Bot. 1000s.
Use: Analgesic.
KOTABARB. (Wesley) Phenobarbital 1/4 gr/Tab. Bot. 1000s.
Use: Sedative/hypnotic.
KOVITONIC LIQUID. (Freeda) Iron 350 mg, vitamins B_1 5 mg, B_6 10 mg, B_{126} 30 mcg, folic acid 0.1 mg, l-Lysine 10 mg/15 ml, sorbitol. Liq. Bot. 120 ml, 240 ml, pt, gal.
Use: Vitamin/mineral supplement.
K-PEK. (Rugby) Attapulgite 600 mg/15 ml. Susp. Bot. 237 ml, pt, gal.
Use: Antidiarrheal.
K-PHOS M.F. (Beach) Potassium acid phosphate 155 mg, sodium acid phosphate 350 mg/Tab. Bot. 100s, 500s.
Use: Urinary acidifier.
K-PHOS NEUTRAL. (Beach) Dibasic sodium phosphate 852 mg, potassium acid phosphate 155 mg, sodium acid phosphate 130 mg/Tab. Bot. 100s, 500s.
Use: Phosphorus supplement.
K-PHOS NO. 2 (Beach) Potassium acid phosphate 305 mg, sodium acid phosphate, anhydrous 700 mg/Tab. Bot. 100s, 500s.
Use: Urinary acidifier.
K-PHOS ORIGINAL (Beach) Potassium acid phosphate 500 mg/Tab. Bot. 100s, 500s.
Use: Urinary acidifier, phosphorus supplement.
K.P.N. (Freeda) Vitamins C 333 mg, Fe 11 mg, A 2666 IU, D 133 IU, E (as dl-alpha tocopheryl acetate) 10 mg, B_1 2 mg, B_2 2 mg, B_3 10 mg, B_5 3.3 mg, B_6 0.83 mg, B_{126} 2 mcg, C 33 mg, FA 0.13 mg, I, Cu, Mn, K, Mg, Zn 0.03 mg/Tab. Bot. 100s, 250s, 500s.
Use: Multivitamin with calcium and iron.
K-P SUSPENSION. (Century) Kaolin 5.2 Gm, pectin 260 mg/oz. Bot. gal.
Use: Antidiarrheal.
KRONOFED-A-JR. (Ferndale) Pseudoephedrine HCl 60 mg, chlorpheniramine maleate 4 mg/Cap. Bot. 100s, 500s.
Use: Decongestant, antihistamine.
KRONOFED-A KRONOCAPS. (Ferndale) Pseudoephedrine HCl 120 mg, chlorpheniramine maleate 8 mg/Cap. Bot. 100s, 500s.
Use: Decongestant, antihistamine.
KRONOHIST KRONOCAPS. (Ferndale) Chlorpheniramine maleate 4 mg, pyrilamine maleate 25 mg, phenylpropanolamine HCl 50 mg/Cap. Bot. 100s, 1000s.
Use: Antihistamine, decongestant.
• **KRYPTON CLATHRATE Kr 85.** USAN.
Use: Radioactive agent.
• **KRYPTON Kr 81m,** U.S.P. XXIII.
Use: Radioactive agent.
K-TAB. (Abbott) Potassium Cl (10 mEq) 750 mg/ER Tab. Bot. 100s, 1000s, UD 100s.
Use: Potassium supplement.
K.T.V. TABLETS. (Knight) Vitamin B_{126}, minerals. Bot. 50s.
Use: Vitamin/mineral supplement.
KUDROX DOUBLE STRENGTH SUSPENSION. (Schwarz Pharma Kremers Urban) Aluminum hydroxide 500 mg, magnesium hydroxide 450 mg, simethicone 40 mg/5 ml. Bot. 355 ml.
Use: Antacid.
KUTAPRESSIN. (Kremers-Urban) Liver derivative complex composed of peptides and amino acids. Inj. Vial 20 ml.
Use: Liver derivative complex.

KUTRASE. (Kremers-Urban) Amylase 30 mg, protease 6 mg, lipase 25 mg, cellulase 2 mg, l-hyoscyamine sulfate 0.0625 mg, phenyltoloxamine citrate 15 mg/Cap. Bot. 100s, 500s.
Use: Digestive aid.

KU-ZYME. (Kremers-Urban) Amylase 30 mg, protease 6 mg, lipase 75 mg, cellulase 2 mg/Cap. Bot. 100s, 500s.
Use: Digestive aid.

KU-ZYME HP. (Kremers-Urban) Lipase 8000 units, protease 30,000 units, amylase 30,000 units/Cap. Bot. 100s.
Use: Digestive aid.

KWELCOF. (Ascher) Hydrocodone bitartrate 5 mg, guaifenesin 100 mg/5 ml. Bot. pt, UD 5 ml. Pkg. 10s, 100s. Alcohol, dye, sugar, and corn free.
Use: Antitussive, expectorant.

KWELL. (Reed & Carnrick) Lindane 1%.
Lot.: W/Glyceryl monostearate, cetyl alcohol, stearic acid, trolamine, 2-amino-2-methyl-1-propanol, methyl p-hydroxybenzoate, butyl p-hydroxybenzoate, carrageenan. Bot. 2 oz, 16 oz. **Shampoo:** W/Polyethylene sorbitan monostearate, TEA-lauryl sulfate, acetone, purified water. Bot. 2 oz, pt, gal. **Cream:** W/Stearic acid, lanolin, glycerin, 2-amino-2-methyl-1-propanol, perfume, purified water. Tube 2 oz, Jar lb.
Use: Scabicide, pediculicide.

KWIKDERM CREAM. (NMC Labs) Tolnaftate 1%. Cream. Tube 15 Gm.
Use: Antifungal, external.

KWIKDERM SOLUTION. (NMC Labs) Tolnaftate 1%. Soln. Bot. 10 ml.
Use: Antifungal, external.

KWILDANE SHAMPOO. (Major) Gamma benzene hexachloride 1%. Bot. 60 ml, pt, gal.
Use: Pediculicide.

K-Y. (Johnson & Johnson) Glucono delta lactate, sodium hydroxide, glycerin, chlorhexidine gluconate, hydroxyethylcellulose. Jelly Tube 2.7 Gm, 5 Gm (single use), 5 Gm, 60 Gm.
Use: Vaginal and rectal lubricant.

KYODEX REAGENT STRIPS. (Kyoto) A disposable plastic reagent strip for determination of glucose in whole blood. Vial 25s.
Use: Diagnostic aid.

KYOTEST UG REAGENT STRIPS. (Kyoto) Reagent strips for glucose and ketones in urine.
Use: Diagnostic aid.

KYOTEST UGK REAGENT STRIP. (Kyoto) Disposable reagent strip for measurement of glucose and ketones in the urine. Vial 50s, 100s.
Use: Diagnostic aid.

KYOTEST UK REAGENT STRIPS. (Kyoto) Reagent strip for ketones in urine. Vial 50s.
Use: Diagnostic aid.

KYTRIL. (SK-Beecham) Granisetron HCl 1.12 mg/ml. Inj. Single-use vial 1 ml.
Use: Antiemetic (cancer therapy).

L

LA-12. (Hyrex) Hydroxocobalamin 1000 mcg/ml. Vial 30 ml.
Use: Vitamin B_{12} supplement.

•**LABETALOL HYDROCHLORIDE,** U.S.P. XXIII, Inj., Tab, U.S.P. XXIII, USAN.
Use: Antihypertensive.
See: Trandate Inj., Tab. (Glaxo).
W/Hydrochlorothiazide.
See: Trandate HCT, Tab. (Glaxo).

LABSTIX REAGENT STRIPS. (Miles Diagnostic) Urine screening test. Bot 100s.
Use: Diagnostic aid.

LAC-HYDRIN LOTION. (Westwood-Squibb) Lactic acid 12% neutralized w/ammonium hydroxide. Tube 5 oz, 12 oz.
Use: Emollient.

LACLEDE CLEANER. (Laclede) Container. 2 lb.
Use: Detergent for instruments and trays.

LACLEDE DISCLOSING SWAB. (Laclede) Swabs 6″. 100s, 500s, 1000s.
Use: Dental swab.

LACLEDE TOPI-FLUOR A.P.F. TOPICAL CREAM. (Laclede) Fluoride ion 1.23% (from sodium fluoride) in orthophosphoric acid 0.98%. Jar 50 ml, 500 ml, 1000 ml, 2000 ml.
Use: Dental caries preventative.

LACOTEIN. (Christina) Protein digest 5% w/preservatives. Vial 30 ml (w/iodochin), Vial 30 ml.
Use: Protein supplement.

LACRIL ARTIFICAL TEARS. (Allergan) Hydroxypropyl methylcellulose, gelatin A, chlorobutanol 0.5%. Soln. Dropper bot. 15 ml.
Use: Lubricant, ophthalmic.

LACRI-LUBE NP. (Allergan) White petrolatum 55.5%, mineral oil 42.5%, petrolatum/lanolin alcohol 2%. Oint. 0.7 Gm.
Use: Lubricant, ophthalmic.

LACRI-LUBE S.O.P. (Allergan) White petrolatum, mineral oil, nonionic lanolin derivatives, chlorobutanol. UD 0.7 Gm, Tube 3.5 Gm, 7 Gm.

Use: Lubricant, ophthalmic.
LACRISERT. (Merck & Co.) Hydrox-ypropyl cellulose 5 mg/insert. Pkg. 60 UDs, 2 reusable applicators and storage container.
Use: Artificial tear insert, ophthalmic.
LACTAID. (LactAid Inc.) **Liq.:** Beta-D-galactosidase derived from Kluyveromyces lactis yeast (1000 Neutral Lactase units/5 drop dosage) in carrier of glycerol 50%, water 30%, inert yeast dry matter 20%. Units of 4, 12, 30 and 75 one-quart dosages at 5 drops/dose. **Tab.:** Beta-D-galactosidase from Aspergillis oryzae (3300 FCC lactase units/Tab.) In 12s, 100s.
Use: Enteral nutritional supplement.
LACTALBUMIN HYDROLYSATE.
See: Aminonat.
LACTASE ENZYME.
Use: Enteral nutritional therapy.
See: LactAid, Capl. Liq. (LactAid Inc.).
Lactogest, Cap. (Thompson).
Lactrase, Cap. (Schwarz Pharma Kremers Urban).
Dairy Ease, Tabs. (Sanofi Winthrop).
SureLac, Tab. (Caraco).
• **LACTATED RINGER'S INJECTION,** U.S.P. XXIII.
Use: Electrolyte and fluid replenisher, systemic alkalizer.
• **LACTIC ACID,** U.S.P. XXIII. Propanoic acid, 2-hy-droxy.
Use: Pharmaceutic necessity for Sodium Lactate Injection, U.S.P. XXIII.
W/Sodium pyrrolidone carboxylate.
See: LactiCare (Stiefel).
Lactinol, Lot. Creme (Pedinol).
LACTICARE LOTION. (Stiefel) Lactic acid 5%, sodium pyrrolidone carboxylate 2.5% in an emollient lotion base. Bot. 8 oz, 12 oz, w/pump dispenser.
Use: Emollient.
LACTICARE-HC LOTION. (Stiefel) Hydrocortisone lotion 1% or 2.5%. **1%:** Bot 4 oz. **2.5%:** Bot. 2 oz.
Use: Corticosteroid, topical.
LACTINEX. (Becton Dickinson) *Lactobacillus acidophilus & Lactobacillus bulgaricus* mixed culture. Tab. 250 mg, Bot. 50s. Gran. 1 Gm pk. Box 12s.
Use. Antidiarrheal.
LACTINOL. (Pedinol) Lactic acid 10%. Lot. Bot. 237 ml.
Use: Emollient.
LACTINOL-E CREME. (Pedinol) Lactic acid 10%, Vitamin E 3500 IU/30 g. Cream 56.7 g.
Use: Emollient.
LACTOBACILLUS ACIDOPHILUS.

Preparation made from acid-producing bacterium.
Use: Antidiarrheal.
See: Bacid (Ciba).
DoFUS (Miller).
MoreDophilus (Freeda).
Pro-Bionate (Natren).
Superdophilus (Natren).
LACTOBACILLUS ACIDOPHILUS & BULGARICUS MIXED CULTURE.
See: Lactinex, Tab., Gran. (Becton Dickinson).
LACTOBACILLUS ACIDOPHILUS, VIABLE CULTURE.
See: DoFus, Tab. (Miller)
Lactinex Granules, Tab. (Becton Dickinson).
LACTOBIN.
Use: AIDS-associated diarrhea. [Orhan drug]
LACTOCAL-F. (Laser) Vitamin A 8000 IU, D 400 IU, E 30 IU, C 100 mg, folic acid 1 mg, B_1 3 mg, B_2 3.4 mg, nicotinamide 20 mg, B_6 5 mg, B_{12} 12 mcg, calcium 200 mg, iodine 0.15 mg, iron 65 mg, magnesium 10 mg, copper 2 mg, zinc 15 mg/Tab. Bot. 100s, 1000s.
Use: Vitamin/mineral supplement.
LACTOFLAVIN.
See: Riboflavin, U.S.P. XXIII. (Various Mfr.).
LACTOFREE. (Mead Johnson) Protein 14.7 g, carbohydrates 69.3 g, fat 36.7 g, linoleic acid 6 g, Fe 12 mg, Na 200 mg, K 733.3 mg, with appropriate vitamins and minerals. Lactose free. 666.7 cal/L. Pow. Can 400 g.
Use: Enteral nutritional supplement.
• **LACTOSE,** N.F. XVIII. Milk sugar.
Use: Pharmaceutic aid (tablet and capsule diluent).
See: Natur-Aid, pow. (Scott/Cord).
LACTRASE. (Rhone-Poulenc Rorer) Standardized enzyme lactase (β-D-galactosidase) 125 mg dispersed in maltodextrins. Cap. Bot. 100s.
Use: Enteral nutritional suppelement.
LACTRODECTUS MACTANS ANTIVENIN. (Merck & Co.) Antivenin 6000 units per vial (with 1:10,000 thimersol), supplied with a 2.5 ml vial of Sterile Water for Injection and a 1 mg vial (with 1:10,000 thimersol) of normal horse serum (1:10 dilution) for sensitivity testing.
Use: Antivenin (Black Widow spider).
• **LACTULOSE,** U.S.P. XXIII. Concentrate, Soln., U.S.P. XXIII. 4-0-β-D-Galactopyranosyl-D-fructose. Duphalac.
Use: Treatment of hepatic coma and

chronic constipation.
See: Cephulac, Syr. (Merrell Dow).
Chronulac, Liq. (Merrell Dow).
LADAKAMYCIN.
Use: Refractory acute myelogenous leukemia (AML) agent.
See: Azacitidine.
LADOGAL. (Sanofi Winthrop) Danazol.
Use: Androgen.
LADOGAR. (Sanofi Winthrop) Danazol.
Use: Androgen.
L.A.E.20. (Seatrace) Estradiol valerate 20 mg/ml. Vial 10 ml.
Use: Estrogen.
L.A.E. 40. (Seatrace) Estradiol valerate 40 mg/ml. Vial 10 ml.
Use: Estrogen.
LAGOL OIL. (Last) 8 Hydroxyquinoline 0.038% in oil base. Bot. 1 oz, 2 oz, 4 oz, 16 oz.
Use: Cleanser.
LAGOL OINTMENT. (Last) Allantoin 1%, benzocaine 5%. Jar 1 oz, 8 oz, 16 oz, 5 lb.
Use: Topical dressing, local anesthetic.
LAKTOMOL. (Durel) Whole milk, dewaxed lanolin esters. Bot. pt, gal.
Use: Skin conditioner.
LAMISIL. (Sandoz) Terbinafine HCl. 1%. Cream/Tube 15 and 30 Gm.
Use: Antifungal agent.
LAMOTANE-X. (Myers) Trichlorethylamino glycol benzoate (ethylaminobenzoate-chloralhydrate derivative). Bot. 4 oz, 6 oz, 8 oz, pt, qt, gal.
Use: Antiseptic, anesthetic, antipruritic.
•**LAMOTRIGINE.** USAN.
Use: Anticonvulsant.
LAMPIT. Nifurtimox.
Use: Anti-infective.
LAMPRENE. (Geigy) Clofazimine 50 mg or 100 mg/Cap. Bot. 100s.
Use: Leprostatic.
LANABAC. (Lannett) Aspirin 0.3 gr, caffeine 15 mg, potassium bromide 15 mg, sodium bromide 15 mg/Tab. Bot. 1000s.
Use: Analgesic combination.
LANABARB. (Lannett) **No. 1:** Sodium amobarbital ¾ gr, sodium secobarbital gr/Cap. Bot. 500s, 1000s. **No. 2:** Sodium amobarbital 1.5 gr, sodium secobarbital 1.5 gr/Cap. Bot. 500s, 1000s.
Use: Sedative/hypnotic.
LANABIOTIC. (Combe) Polymyxin B sulfate 5000 units, neomycin (as sulfate) 3.5 mg, bacitracin 500 units, lidocaine 40 mg/Gm. Oint. 15 Gm, 30 Gm.
Use: Anti-infective, local anesthetic.
LANABROM ELIXIR. (Lannett) 60 gr of combined bromides of sodium, potassi-

um, strontium, ammonium/fl oz, Bot. pt, gal.
LANABURN OINT. (Lannett) Aluminum basic acetate, phenol, zinc oxide, boric acid, ichthammol, eucalyptol. Jar lb.
LANACANE CREME. (Combe) Benzocaine, chlorothymol, resorcin. Tube 1.25 oz, 2.5 oz, Spray can 3 oz.
Use: Local anesthetic.
LANACILLIN. (Lannett) Penicillin G potassium **200,000 units/5 ml:** Bot. 100 ml. **400,000 units/5 ml:** Bot. 100 ml, 150 ml.
Use: Antibacterial, penicillin.
LANACILLIN VK TABLETS. (Lannett) Potassium phenoxymethyl penicillin 400,000 units (250 mg), 800,000 units (500 mg)/Tab. Bot. 100s.
Use: Antibacterial, penicillin.
LANACILLIN VK POWDER. (Lannett) Potassium phenoxymethyl penicillin. **125 mg/5 ml** (200,000 units), **250 mg/5 ml** (400,000 units). Bot. 100 ml.
Use: Antibacterial, penicillin.
LANACORT 10. (Combe) Hydrocortisone acetate 1% **Cream.** Tube 15, 30 Gm. **Oint.** Tube 15 Gm.
LANACORT CREAM. (Combe) Hydrocortisone acetate 0.5%. Tube 0.5 oz, 1 oz.
Use: Corticosteroid, topical.
LANAMINS. (Lannett) Vitamin combination. Cap. Bot. 100s, 1000s.
Use: Vitamin supplement.
LANAPHILIC OINTMENT. (Medco Lab) Sorbitol, isopropyl palmitate, stearyl alcohol, white petrolatum, lanolin oil, sodium lauryl sulfate, propylene glycol, methylparaben, propylparaben. Jar 16 oz. Also available w/urea 10% or 20%.
Use: Emollient.
LANAPHILIC W/UREA 10%. (Medco Labs) Urea, stearyl alcohol, white petrolatum, isopropyl palmitate, propylene glycol, sorbitol, sodium lauryl sulfate, lactic acid, parabens. Oint. Jar lb.
Use: Emollient.
LANASED. (Lannett) Atropine sulfate 0.03 mg, hyoscyamine 0.03 mg, methenamine 408 mg, methylene blue 5.4 mg, phenyl salicylate 18.1 mg, gelsemium 6.1 mg, benzoic acid 4.5 mg/Tab. Bot. 1000s.
Use: Anticholineric combination.
LANATOSIDE C. B.A.N. 3-(3″-Acetyl-4″-β-glucosyltridigitoxosido)-digoxogenin.
Use: Myocardial stimulant.
LANATRATE. (Lannett) Ergotamine tartrate 1 mg, caffeine alkaloid 100 mg/Tab. Bot. 100s, 500s, 1000s.

Use: Agent for migraine.

LANATUSS. (Lannett) Guaifenesin 100 mg, phenylpropanolamine HCl 5 mg, chlorpheniramine maleate 2 mg, sodium citrate 197 mg, citric acid 60 mg/5 ml. Bot. 120 ml, pt, gal.
Use: Expectorant, decongestant, antihistamine.

LANAURINE. (Lannett) Antipyrine, benzocaine in glycerin. Bot. 0.5 oz, 4 oz.
Use: Otic preparation.

LANAVITE. (Lannett) Vitamins A 5000 IU, D 1000 IU, E 1 IU, B_1 1.5 mg, B_2 2 mg, B_6 0.1 mg, C 37.5 mg, B_{12} 1 mcg, niacinamide 20 mg, calcium pantothenate 1 mg. Cap. Bot. 500s, 1000s.
Use: Vitamin/mineral supplement.

LANAVITE DROPS. (Lannett) Vitamins A 3000 IU, D 400 IU, B_1 1 mg, B_2 1.2 mg, niacinamide 8 mg, C 60 mg/0.6 ml. Dropper bot. 15 ml, 60 ml.
Use: Vitamin supplement.

LANAZETS. (Lannett) Cetylpyridinium 1 mg, benzocaine 5 mg/Loz. Bot. 500s, 1000s.
Use: Mouth and throat preparation.

LANESTRIN. (Lannett) Estrogenic substance natural in aqueus susp. 20,000 units/ml. Vial 30 ml.
Use: Estrogen.

LANIAZID C.T. (Lannett) Isoniazid 300 mg/Tab. Bot. 100s, 1000s.
Use: Antituberculous agent.

LANIAZID SYRUP. (Lannett) Isoniazid 50 mg/5 ml. Bot. 480 ml.
Use: Antituberculous agent.

LANIAZID TABLETS. (Lannett) Isoniazid 50 mg or 100 mg. **50 mg:** Tab. Bot. 100s, 500s. **100 mg:** Tab. Bot. 100s, 500s, 1000s.
Use: Antituberculous agent.

LANNATES ELIXIR. (Lannett) Sodium glycerophosphate 2 gr, calcium glycerophosphate 2 gr, phosphoric acid 1.5 min, wine base/fl oz. Bot. pt, gal.

LANOKALIN. (Lannett) Phenobarbital 15 mg, homatropine methylbromide 5 mg, colloidal kaolin 300 mg/Tab. Bot. 1000s.
Use: Antacid combination.

•**LANOLIN,** Anhydrous, U.S.P. XXIII.
Use: Water-in-oil emulsion ointment base; absorbent ointment base.
See: Kerohydric (Westwood).
W/Coconut oil, pine oil, castor oil, cholesterols, lecithin and parachlorometaxylenol.
See: Sebacide, Liq. (Paddock).
W/Diiosbutylcresoxyethoxyethyl, dimethyl benzyl ammonium Cl, menthol.
See: Hospital Lot. (Paddock).

•**LANOLIN ALCOHOLS,** N.F. XVIII.
Use: Pharmaceutic aid (ointment base ingredient).

•**LANOLIN, MODIFIED,** U.S.P. XXIII.

LANOLINE. (Burroughs Wellcome) Perfumed emollient. Oint. Tube 1.75 oz.
Use: Emollient.

LANO-LO BATH OIL. (Whorton) 8 oz.

LANOLOR. (Numark) Cream. Jar 8 oz, tube 2 oz.

LANOPHYLLIN ELIXIR. (Lannett) Anhydrous theophylline 80 mg, alcohol 20%/15 ml. Bot. pt, gal.
Use: Bronchodilator.

LANOPHYLLIN-GG CAPSULES. (Lannett) Theophylline 150 mg, guaifenesin 90 mg. Cap. Bot. 100s, 500s.
Use: Bronchodilator, expectorant.

LANOPHYLLIN INJ. (Lannett) Theophylline 250 mg/ml. Inj. Vial 10 ml.
Use: Bronchodilator.

LANOPLEX ELIXIR. (Lannett) Vitamins B_1 4 mg, nicotinamide 40 mg, B_6 2 mg/fl oz. Bot. pt, gal.
Use: Vitamin supplement.

LANOPLEX FORTE CAPSULES. (Lannett) Vitamins B_1 25 mg, B_2 12.5 mg, nicotinamide 50 mg, C 250 mg, B_6 3 mg, B_{12} 5 mcg, calcium pantothenate 10 mg/Cap. Bot. 100s, 500s, 1000s.
Use: Vitamin supplement.

LANOPLEX INJECTION. (Lannett) Vitamins B_1 100 mg, B_2 1 mg, B_6 2 mg, niacinamide 50 mg, calcium pantothenate 10 mg, benzyl alcohol 1%, urea 10%, chlorobutanol 0.5%/ml. Vial 30 ml.
Use: Parenteral nutritional supplement.

LANORINAL. (Lannett) Isobutylallybarbituric acid 50 mg, caffeine 40 mg, aspirin 200 mg, phenacetin 130 mg/Cap. or Tab. **Cap.** Bot. 100s, 1000s. **Tab.** Bot. 1000s.
Use: Analgesic combination.

LANOTHAL PILLS. (Lannett) Phenolphthalein 0.5 gr, aloin 0.25 gr, ipecac 1/15 gr, belladonna extract gr/Pill. Bot. 1000s.

LANOXICAPS. (Burroughs Wellcome) Digoxin 0.05 mg, 0.1 mg, 0.2 mg. Soln. in cap. Bot. 100s.
Use: Cardiac glycoside.

LANOXIN. (Burroughs Wellcome) Digoxin. **0.125 mg:** Bot. 100s, 1000s, Unit-of-use 30s, UD 100s. **0.25 mg:** Bot. 100s, 1000s, 5000s, UD 100s, Unit-of-use 30s. **0.5 mg:** Bot. 100s. **Pediatric Elix.:** 0.05 mg/ml, alcohol 10%. Bot. 60 ml. **Inj.:** (w/propylene glycol 40%, alcohol 10%, sodium phosphate 0.3%, anhydrous citric acid 0.08%) Amp. 0.5 mg/2

ml. Amp. 10s, 50s. **Pediatric Inj.**: 0.1
mg/ml. Amp. 1 ml 10s.
Use: Cardiac glycoside.
• **LANREOTIDE ACETATE.** USAN.
Use: Antineoplastic.
• **LANSOPRAZOLE.** USAN.
Use: Gastric acid pump inhibitor; antiul-
cer agent.
LANTRISUL. (Lannett) Sulfamerazine
2.5 gr, sulfadiazine 2.5 gr, sulfamet-
hazine 2.5 gr. **Tab.**: Bot. 100s, 500s,
1000s. **Susp.**: Bot. pt, gal.
Use: Sulfonamide combination.
LANTURIL. (Sanofi Winthrop) Oxyper-
tine.
Use: Anxiolytic, tranquilizer.
LANUM. (Various Mfr.) Lanolin.
LANVISONE CREAM. (Lannett) Hydro-
cortisone 1%, clioquinol 3%. Tube 20
Gm.
Use: Corticosteorid, antifungal (exter-
nal).
• **LAPYRIUM CHLORIDE.** USAN.
Use: Pharmaceutic aid (surfactant).
LARDET. (Standex) Phenobarbital 8 mg,
theophylline 130 mg, ephedrine HCl 24
mg/Tab. Bot. 100s.
Use: Antiasthmatic combination.
LARDET EXPECTORANT. (Standex)
Phenobarbital 8 mg, theophylline 130
mg, ephedrine HCl 24 mg, guaifenesin
100 mg/Tab. Bot. 100s.
Use: Antiasthmatic combination.
LARGON. (Wyeth-Ayerst) Propiomazine
HCl 20 mg/ml w/ sodium formaldehyde
sulfoxylate, sodium acetate buffer. Amp.
1 ml, 2 ml. Pkg. 25s, Tubex syringe 1 ml.
Use: Sedative/hypnotic.
LARIAM. (Roche) Mefloquine HCl 250
mg/Tab. UD 25s.
Use: Antimalarial.
LARODOPA CAPSULES. (Roche) Lev-
odopa 100 mg, 250 mg or 500 mg/Cap.
100 mg: Bot. 100s. **250 mg:** Bot. 100s,
500s. **500 mg:** Bot. 100s, 500s.
Use: Antiparkinson agent.
LARODOPA TABLETS. (Roche) Lev-
odopa 100 mg, 250 mg or 500 mg. **100
mg:** Bot. 100s. **250 mg and 500 mg:**
Bot. 100s, 500s.
Use: Antiparkinson agent.
LAROTID. (Beecham Labs) Amoxicillin.
Cap.: 250 mg: Bot. 100s, 500s, UD
100s, unit-of-use 18s. **500 mg:** Bot. 50s,
500s. **Oral Susp.:** 125 mg or 250 mg (as
trihydrate)/5 ml. Bot. 80 ml, 100 ml, 150
ml. **Pediatric drops:** 50 mg (as trihydrate)/ml. Bot. 15 ml.
Use: Antibacterial, penicillin.
LARYNEX. (Dover) Benzocaine. Sugar,

lactose and salt free. Loz. UD Box 500s.
Use: Local anesthetic.
• **LASALOCID.** USAN.
Use: Coccidiostat.
LASAN NASAL SPRAY. (Eastwood) Bot.
2/3 oz.
LASAN OINTMENT. (Stiefel) Anthralin
0.4% in ointment base. Tube 60 Gm.
Use: Antipsoriatic.
LASIX. (Hoechst) Furosemide. **Tab.**: 20
mg or 40 mg/Tab. Bot. 100s, 500s,
1000s, UD 100s; 80 mg/Tab. Bot. 50s,
500s, UD 100s. **Inj.:** 10 mg/ml. 2
ml/Amp. Box 5s, 50s, 4 ml/Amp. Box 5s,
25s; 10 ml/Amp. Box 5s, 25s; Syringe 2
ml, 4 ml, 10 ml. Box 5s. Single Use Vial
2 ml, 4 ml, 10 ml. **Oral Soln.:** 10 mg/ml.
Alcohol 11.5%. Dropper Bot 60 ml, Bot.
120 ml.
Use: Diuretic.
LASSAR'S PASTE.
See: Zinc Oxide Paste, U.S.P. XXIII.
(Various Mfr.)
LATEST CRP KIT. (Fisher) Measures C-
reactive protein in serum. Kit 1s.
Use: Diagnostic aid.
LAUDEXIUM METHYLSULFATE. B.A.N.
Decamethylene-α, [ω]-bis-(1-(3, 4-
dimethoxybenzyl)-1,-2,3,4-tetrahydro)
6,7-dimethoxy-2-methylisoquinolinium
methosulfate. Laudolissin.
Use: Neuromuscular blocking agent.
• **LAURETH 4.** USAN.
Use: Pharmaceutic aid.
• **LAURETH 9.** USAN. Mixture of poly-
oxyethylene lauryl ethers having a sta-
tistical average of 9 ethylene oxide
groups per molecule.
Use: Surfactant, emulsifier, spermati-
cide.
• **LAURETH 10S.** USAN.
Use: Spermaticide.
• **LAUROCAPRAM.** USAN.
Use: Pharmaceutic aid.
LAURO EYE WASH. (Otis Clapp) Boric
acid, sodium Cl. Bot. 0.5 oz, 4 oz.
Use: Ophthalmic preparation.
LAUROLINIUM ACETATE. B.A.N. 4-
Amino-1-dodecylquinaldinium acetate.
Laurodin.
Use: Surface-active agent.
LAUROMACROGOL 400. Laureth 9.
• **LAURYL ISOQUINOLINIUM BROMIDE.**
USAN.
Use: Anti-infective.
LAURYL SOLUTION. (Knight) Bot. pt.
Use: Vaginal preparation.
LAURYL SULFOACETATE.
See: Lowila, Cake, Liq., Oint. (West-
wood).

LAVACOL. (Parke-Davis Prods) Ethyl alcohol 70%. Bot. pt.

LAVATAR. (Doak) Coal tar distillate 25.5% in a bath oil base. Liq. Bot. 4 oz, pt.
Use: Antipsoriatic, antipruritic.

• **LAVENDER OIL,** N.F. XVIII.
Use: Perfume.

• **LAVOLTIDINE SUCCINATE.** USAN.
Use: Histamine H_2-receptor blocker.

LAVOPTIK EMERGENCY WASH. (Lavoptik) Eye, face, body wash. 32 oz/Emergency station.
Use: Emergency wash.

LAVOPTIK EYE WASH. (Lavoptik) Sodium Cl 0.49%, sodium biphosphate 0.4%, sodium phosphate 0.45%/100 ml w/benzalkonium Cl 0.005%. Bot. 6 oz.
Use: Irrigating agent, ophthalmic.

LAVORIS. (Procter & Gamble) Zinc Cl, glycerin, poloxamer 407, saccharin, polysorbate 80, flavors, clove oil, alcohol, citric acid, water. Bot. 6 oz, 12 oz, 18 oz, 24 oz.
Use: Mouthwash.

LAXATAB. (Freeport) Danthron 75 mg, docusate sodium 100 mg, D-calcium pantothenate 25 mg/Tab. Bot. 1000s.
Use: Laxative.

LAXATIVE CAPS. (Weeks & Leo) Docusate sodium 100 mg, casanthranol 30 mg/Cap. Bot. 30s, 60s.
Use: Laxative.

LAXATIVES.
See: Agar-Gel (Various Mfr.).
Aloe (Various Mfr.).
Aloin (Various Mfr.).
Bile Salts (Various Mfr.).
Bisacodyl, Tab., Supp. (Various Mfr.).
Bisacodyl Tannex (Barnes-Hind).
Carboxymethylcellulose Sodium (Various Mfr.).
Casanthranol, Cap., Tab. (Various Mfr.).
Cascara Sagrada (Various Mfr.).
Cascara Sagrada Fluidextract, Liq. (Parke-Davis).
Cascara Tab. (Various Mfr.).
Castor Oil (Various Mfr.).
Citrucel (SK-Beecham).
Correctol, Tab. (Plough).
Docusate Sodium (Various Mfr.).
Ex-Lax, Tab., Pow. (Ex-Lax. Inc.).
Feen-a-Mint, Gum, Mints (Plough).
Karaya Gum (Penick).
Liquid Petrolatum, Liq. (Various Mfr.).
Magnesia Magma (Various Mfr.).
Maltsupex (Wallace).
Methylcellulose (Various Mfr.).
Mucilloid of Psyllium Seed W/Dextrose

(Searle).
Mylanta Natural Fiber Supplement (J & J-Merck).
Natures Remedy (SK-Beecham).
Nujol, Liq. (Plough).
Oxyphenisatin Acetate (Various Mfr.).
Petrolatum, Liq. (Various Mfr.).
Petrolatum, Liq., Emulsion (Various Mfr.).
Phenolphthalein (Various Mfr.).
Plantago ovata, Coating (Various Mfr.).
Poloxalkol, Cap., Soln. (Various Mfr.).
Prune Concentrate, Tab., Cap. (Various Mfr.).
Prune Preps. (Various Mfr.).
Psyllium Granules W/Dextrose (Med. Chem.).
Psyllium Husk Pow. (Upjohn).
Psyllium Hydrocolloid, Pow. (Stuart).
Psyllium Hydrophilic Mucilloid (Various Mfr.).
Psyllium Seed, Gel, Gran. (Various Mfr.).
Regutol, Tab. (Plough).
Restore (Inagra).
Sakara, Gran. (Plough).
Senna, Alexandrian, Liq., Tab. (Various Mfr.).
Senna, Cassia angustifolia, Tab. (Brayten).
Senna Conc., Standardized, Gran., Tab., Pow.,
Supp. (Various Mfr.).
Senna Fruit Extract, Liq. (Various Mfr.).
Sennosides A&B, Tab. (Dorsey).
Sodium Biphosphate (Various Mfr.).
Sodium Phosphate (Various Mfr.).
Unifiber (Dow B. Hickam).

LAXINATE 100. (Hauck) Dioctyl sodium sulfosuccinate 100 mg/Cap. Bot. 100s, 1000s.
Use: Laxative.

LAX-PILLS. (G & W) Yellow phenolphthalein 90 mg/Tab. Bot. 30s, 60s.
Use: Laxative.

LAYOR CARANG.
See: Agar (Various Mfr.).

• **LAZABEMIDE.** USAN.
Use: Antiparkinsonian agent.

LAZER CREME. (Pedinol) Vitamins E 3500 units, A 100,000 units/oz. Jar 2 oz.
Use: Emollient.

LAZERFORMALYDE SOLUTION. (Pedinol) Formaldehyde 10%, polysorbate 20, hydroxyethyl cellulose. Bot. 3 oz.
Use: Antiperspirant drying agent for presurgical removal of warts or nonsurgical laser treatment of warts.

LAZERSPORIN-C SOLUTION. (Pedinol) Neomycin sulfate 3.5 mg, polymyxin B

sulfate 10,000 units, hydrocortisone 1%.
Bot. 10 ml.
Use: Anti-infective combination, topical.
L-BULGARICUS. (Antidiarrheal).
See: Bacid (Fisons).
Lactinex B (HW&D).
More-Dophilus (Freeda).
**LC-65 DAILY CONTACT LENS CLEAN-
ER.** (Allergan) Daily cleaning solution
for all hard, soft (hydrophilic), Polycon
and Paraperm oxygen gas permeable
contact lenses. Dropper Bot. 0.5 oz, 2
oz.
Use: Contact lens care.
L-CAINE. (Century) Lidocaine HCl. **Inj.:**
1%, 50 ml. **Topical Liq.:** 4%, 50 ml.
Use: Local anesthetic.
L-CAINE E. (Century) Lidocaine HCl 1%
or 2%, epinephrine 1:100,000/ml. Inj. 20
ml, 50 ml.
Use: Local anesthetic.
L-CAINE VISCOUS. (Century) Lidocaine
HCl 2% with sodium carboxymethylcel-
lulose. Soln. Dot. 100 ml.
Use: Local anesthetic.
L-CARNITINE. Amino acid derivative 250
mg/Cap. Bot. 60s.
Use: Vitamin supplement.
See: Vitacarn.
Carnitor (Sigma-Tau).
L.C.D. (Almay) Alcohol extractions of
crude coal tar. Cream, soln. Bot. 4 oz, pt.
Use: Antipsoriatic, antipruritic.
See: Coal Tar Topical Soln., U.S.P.
XXIII.
LCR.
Use: Antineoplastic.
See: Vincristine sulfate.
L-CYSTEINE.
See: Cysteine.
L-DEPRENYL.
See: Selegiline HCl.
LDH REAGENT STRIP. (Miles Diagnos-
tic) A quantitative strip test for LDH in
serum or plasma. Seralyzer reagent
strip. Dot. 25s.
Use: Diagnostic aid.
LEBER TABULAE. (Paddock) Aloe 0.09
Gm, extract of rhei 0.03 Gm, myrrh 0.01
Gm, frangula 5 mg, galbanum 2 mg,
olibanum 3 mg/Tab. Bot. 100s, 500s,
1000s.
LEBER TAURINE. (Paddock) Sodium
salicylate 8 gr, ox bile 2.25 gr, extract of
cascara 1:4 4.5 gr, pancreatin 1.25 gr,
pepsin 1:10,000 ³/₁₀ gr/fl oz. Bot. pt, gal.
LEC-E-PLEX. (Barth's) Vitamin E 100 IU,
200 IU or 400 IU/Cap. w/lecithin. Bot.
100s, 500s, 1000s.
Use: Vitamin E supplement.

• **LECIMIBIDE.** USAN.
Use: Antihyperlipidemic.
LECITHIN. (Various Mfr.) Lecithin. **Cap.:**
520 mg. Bot. 100s, 250s, 1000s; 650
mg. Bot. 90s, 100s, 250s, 500s. **Pow.:**
120 Gm, kg, lb.
Use: Nutritional supplement.
• **LECITHIN,** N.F. XVIII.
Use: Pharmaceutic aid (emulsifying
agent).
(Arcum) 1200 mg/Cap. Bot. 100s,
1000s; Gran. Bot. 8 oz; Pow. Bot. 4 oz.
(Barth's) 8 gr/Cap. Bot. 100s, 500s,
1000s; Gran. Can 8 oz, 16 oz; Pow.
Can 10 oz.
(Cavendish) Tab. (0.5 gr) Bot. 500s.
(Quality Generics) 1200 mg, Cap. 100s.
(De Pree) Cap. Bot. 100s.
(Pfanstiehl) 25 Gm, 100 Gm, 500
Gm/Pkg.
W/Choline base, cephalin, lipositol.
See: Alcolec Cap., Gran. (American
Lecithin).
W/Coconut oil, pine oil, castor oil, lanolin,
cholesterols, parachlorometaxylenol.
See: Sebacide, Liq. (Paddock).
W/Vitamins.
See: Acletin, Cap. (Associated Concen-
trates).
Lec-E-Plex, Cap. (Barth's).
LEDERCILLIN VK. (Lederle) Penicillin V
potassium, saccharin. **Soln.:** 125 mg or
250 mg/5 ml in 100 ml, 150 ml, 200 ml.
Tab.: 250 mg. Bot. 100s, 1000s, UD
10s, Unit of issue 480s; 500 mg. Bot.
100s, 500s, UD 100s.
Use: Antibacterial, penicillin.
LEDERPLEX CAPSULES. (Lederle) Vita-
mins B₁ 2.25 mg, B₂ 2.6 mg, niaci-
namide 30 mg, B₆ 3 mg, calcium pan-
tothenate 15 mg, B₁₂ 9 mcg/Cap. Bot.
100s.
Use: Vitamin/mineral supplement.
LEDERPLEX LIQUID. (Lederle) Vitamins
B₁ 2.25 mg, B₂ 2.6 mg, niacinamide 30
mg, pantothenic acid 15 mg, B₆ 3 mg,
B₁₂ 9 mcg/10 ml. Bot. 12 oz.
Use: Vitamin/mineral supplement.
**LEGATRIN NIGHT LEG CRAMP RELIEF
TABLETS.** (Scholl) Quinine sulfate 130
mg/Cap. Bot. 30s.
Use: Antimalarial; treatment of night leg
cramps.
LEGATRIN RUB. (Columbia) Menthol
4%, benzocaine 2% in a base of 44%
isopropyl alcohol, carbomer 940, propy-
lene glycol, parabens. Gel. 227 g.
Use: Rubs and liniments.
LEGIONELLA. (Wampole-Zeus) Direct

fluorescent test for legionella organisms. Identification of various legionella bacteria in tissue specimens, sputum, cultures.
Use: Diagnostic aid.
LEGIONELLA, INDIRECT. (Wampole-Zeus) Indirect fluorescent antibody test for *Legionella pneumophila.*
Use: Diagnostic aid.
• **LEMON OIL,** N.F. XVIII.
Use: Pharmaceutic aid (flavor).
LENETRAN. Mephenoxalone.
Use: Tranquilizer.
LENICET.
See: Aluminum Acetate, Basic (Various Mfr.).
• **LENIQUINSIN.** USAN. 6,7-Dimethoxy-4-(vera-trylideneamino) quinoline. Under study.
Use: Antihypertensive.
LENIUM MEDICATED SHAMPOO. (Sanofi Winthrop) Selenium sulfide.
Use: Antiseborrheic.
• **LENOGRASTIM.** USAN.
Use: Immunomodulator (granulocyte colony-stimulating factor).
• **LENPERONE.** USAN.
Use: Antipsychotic.
LENS CLEAR. (Allergan) Sterile, isotonic solution surfactant cleaner w/sorbic acid 0.1%, edetate disodium 0.2%. Bot. 15 ml.
Use: Soft contact lens care.
LENS DROPS. (Ciba Vision) Sodium chloride, borate buffer, carbamide, poloxamer 407, EDTA 0.2%, sorbic acid 0.15%. Soln. Bot. 15 ml.
Use: Re-wetting solution.
LENSEN. (Geneva) Diphenhydramine HCl 25 mg or 50 mg/Cap. Bot. 1000s.
LENSEPT DISINFECTING SOLUTION. (Ciba Vision) Micro-filtered hydrogen peroxide with sodium stannate 3%, sodium nitrate, phosphate buffers. Soln. Bot. 237, 355 ml.
Use: Disinfecting solution.
LENSEPT RINSE AND NEUTRALIZER. (Ciba Vision) Sodium chloride, sodium borate decahydrate, boric acid, bovine catalase, sorbic acid, EDTA. Soln. Bot. 237 ml. System includes lens cup and holder.
Use: Rinsing and neutralizing solution.
LENS FRESH. (Allergan) Sterile, buffered, isotonic aqueous soln. W/hydroxyethyl cellulose, sodium Cl, boric acid, sodium borate, sorbic acid 0.1%, edetate disodium 0.2%. Bot. 0.5 oz.
Use: Contact lens care.
LENSINE EXTRA STRENGTH. (Cooper-

Vision) Cleaning agent with benzalkonium Cl 0.01%, EDTA 0.1%. Soln. Bot. 45 ml.
Use: Hard contact lens care.
LENS LUBRICANT. (Bausch & Lomb) Povidone and polyoxyethylene with thimerosal 0.004%, EDTA 0.1% Soln. Bot. 15 ml.
Use: Lens lubricant.
LENS PLUS. (Allergan) Isotonic soln. w/sodium Cl 0.9%. Aerosol 3 oz, 8 oz, 12 oz. Preservative free.
Use: Soft contact lens care.
LENS PLUS DAILY CLEANER. (Allergan) Buffered solution with cocoamphocarboxyglycinate, sodium lauryl sulfate, hexylene glycol, sodium chloride, sodium phosphate, EDTA. Preservative free. Soln. Bot. 15 ml or 30 ml.
Use: Soft contact lens cleansing solution.
LENS PLUS OXYSEPT DISINFECTING SOLUTION. (Allergan) Hydrogen peroxide with sodium stannate 3%, sodium nitrate and phosphate buffer. Soln. Bot. 240 ml.
Use: Contact lens solution.
LENS PLUS OXYSEPT 2 NEUTRALIZING. (Allergan) Catalase with buffering agents used to neutralize the Lens Plus Oxysept 1 disinfecting solution in a chemical lens care system. For soft contact lens. Tabs. Box 12s. Bot. 36s.
Use: Soft contact lens care.
LENS PLUS OXYSEPT RINSE AND NEUTRALIZER. (Allergan) Isotonic with sodium chloride, mono- and dibasic sodium phosphates, catalytic neutralizing agent, EDTA. Soln. Bot. 15 ml.
Use: Soft contact lens care.
LENS PLUS PRESERVATIVE FREE. (Allergan) Isotonic sodium chloride 9%. Soln. Bot. 90, 240, 360 ml.
Use: Soft contact lens care.
LENS PLUS REWETTING DROPS. (Allergan) Sterile, non-preserved isotonic solution w/sodium Cl, boric acid. UD 0.01 oz (30s).
Use: Soft contact lens care.
LENS PLUS REWETTING DROPS. (Allergan) Isotonic solution with sodium chloride and boric acid. Thimerosol and preservative free. Soln. Bot. 0.3 ml (30s).
Use: Soft contact lens care.
LENSRINS. (Allergan) Sterile preserved saline for heat disinfection, rinsing and storage of soft (hydrophilic) contact lenses; rinsing solution for chemical disinfection. Soln. Bot. 8 oz.

Use: Soft contact lens care.
LENS-WET. (Allergan) Isotonic, buffered soln. of polyvinyl alcohol, thimerosal 0.002%, EDTA 0.01%. Bot. 0.5 fl oz.
Use: Contact lens care.
LENTE ILENTIN I. (Lilly) Insulin zinc suspension 100 units/ml. Beef and pork. Inj. Vial. 10 ml.
Use: Antidiabetic agent.
LENTE ILETIN II. (Lilly) Insulin zinc suspension 100 units/ml. Purified pork. Inj. Bot. 10 ml.
Use: Antidiabetic agent.
LENTE INSULIN. Susp. of zinc insulin crystals.
See: Iletin Lente, Vial (Lilly).
LENTE INSULIN. (Novo Nordisk) Insulin zinc susp. 100 units/ml Beef. Inj. Vial 10 ml.
Use: Antidiabetic agent.
LENTE L. (Novo Nordisk) Insulin zinc suspension 100 units/ml. Purified pork. Inj. Vial 10 ml.
Use: Antidiabetic agent.
LENTINAN. (Lenti-Chemico Pharmaceuticals)
Use: Immunomodulator.
LEPROSTATICS.
Use: Bactericidal.
See: Dapsone, Tab. (Jacobus).
   Lamprene, Cap. (Geigy).
LEPROSY THERAPY.
See: Hansen's disease.
LEPTAZOL.
See: Pentylenetetrazol.
•**LERGOTRILE MESYLATE.** USAN.
Use: Enzyme inhibitor.
LERTON OVULES. (Vita Elixir) Caffeine 250 mg/Cap.
Use: Analeptic.
LESCOL. (Sandoz) Fluvastatin sodium 20 mg or 40 mg. Cap. Bot. 30s, 100s.
Use: Antihyperlipidemic.
LESTEROL. (Dram) Nicotinic acid 500 mg/Tab. Bot. 250s.
Use: Antihyperlipidemic.
LETHOPHEROL. (Nutrition) Vitamin E 100 IU/Kapule. Bot. 100s.
Use: Vitamin E supplement.
•**LETIMIDE HCI.** USAN. 3-[2-(Diethylamino)-ethyl]-2H-1,3-benzoxazine-2,4-(3H)-dione monohydrochloride.
Use: Analgesic.
•**LETROZOLE** USAN.
Use: Antineoplastic.
LETUSIN. Naphthalene-2-sulfonate ester of levopropoxyphene. Levopropoxyphene (Lilly).
•**LEUCINE,** U.S.P. XXIII. $C_6H_{13}NO_2$. L-leucine.

Use: Amino acid.
LEUCOMAX. (Various Mfr.).
Use: Cytokine agent.
L-LEUCOVORIN.
Use: Antineoplastic. [Orphan drug]
See: Isovorin.
LEUCOVORIN CALCIUM. (Barr) 25 mg as calcium. Tab. Pkg. 25s.
Use: Folic acid antagonist overdosage.
LEUCOVORIN CALCIUM. (Lederle)
Tab.: 15 mg as calcium. Pkg. 12s, 24s, UD 50s. **Inj.:** 3 mg/ml as calcium w/ benzyl alcohol 0.9%. Amps 1 ml. **Pow. for Inj.:** 50 mg/vial, 100 mg/vial, 350 mg/vial.
Use: Folic acid antagonist overdosage.
•**LEUCOVORIN CALCIUM,** U.S.P. XXIII. Inj., U.S.P. XXIII. L-Glutamic acid, N-[4-[[(2-amino-5-formyl-1,4,5,6,7,8-hexahydro-4-oxo-6-pteridinyl)-methyl]amino] benzoyl]-, calcium salt (1:1), pentahydrate. Folinic acid-S.F. Formyl tetrahydropteroylglutamic acid, a derivative of folic acid as calcium salt. (Various Mfr.)
Tab.: 5 mg. Bot. 30s, 100s, UD 50s.
Use: Antagonist of amithopterin and other folic-acid antagonists. Anti-anemic (folate-deficiency); antidote to folic acid antagonists. Antineoplastic [Orphan drug]
See: Wellcovorin, Inj., Tab. (Burroughs Wellcome).
LEUKEMIA AGENTS.
See: Antineoplastics.
LEUKERAN. (Burroughs Wellcome) Chlorambucil 2 mg/Tab. Bot. 50s.
Use: Antineoplastic agent.
LEUKINE. (Immunex) Sargramostin (GM-CSF).
Use: Adjunct in bone marrow transplantation.
LEUKOCYTE PROTEASE INHIBITOR, RECOMBINANT SECRETORY.
Use: Alpha-1 antitrypsin deficiency; cystic fibrosis. [Orphan drug]
LEUKOCYTE PROTEASE INHIBITOR, SECRETORY.
Use: Bronchopulmonary dysplasia. [Orphan drug]
LEUPEPTIN.
Use: Adjunct to nerve repair. [Orphan drug]
•**LEUPROLIDE ACETATE.** USAN.
Use: Antineoplastic agent; central precocious puberty [Orphan drug]
LEUROCRISTINE.
See: Vincristine Sulfate (Lilly).
LEUROCRISTINE SULFATE (1:1) (SALT). Vincristine Sulfate, U.S.P. XXIII.

LEUSTATIN. (Ortho Biotech) Cladribine. Soln. 1 mg/ml. Vial. 20 ml single-use.
Use: Antineoplastic.
LEVALLORPHAN. B.A.N. 1-3-Hydroxy-N-allylmorphinan.(—)-N-Allyl-3-hydroxymorphinan.
Use: Narcotic antagonist.
LEVAMFETAMINE, F,D,A, (—)-α-Methylphenethylamine.
LEVAMFETAMINE.
See: Levamphetamine succinate.
• **LEVAMISOLE HYDROCHLORIDE,** U.S.P. XXIII. USAN.
Use: Antineoplastic.
• **LEVAMPHETAMINE SUCCINATE.** USAN. (l-isomer), 1-phenyl-2-amino propane succinate. Amphetamine, levo. 1-a-methylphenethylamine succinate.
Use: Anorexiant.
LEVARTERENOL.
Use: Vasopressor (for shock).
See: Levophed, Inj. (Sanofi Winthrop).
LEVARTERENOL BITARTRATE.
See: Norepinephrine Bitartate, U.S.P. XXIII.
LEVATOL. (Reed & Carnick) Penbutolol sulfatel 20 mg. Tab. Bot. 100s.
Use: Beta-adrenergic blocking agent.
• **LEVCROMAKALIM.** USAN.
Use: Antihypertensive; antiasthmatic.
• **LEVCYCLOSERINE.** USAN.
Use: Enzyme inhibitor (Gaucher's disease).
LEVIRON. (Approved) Desiccated liver 7 gr, iron and ammonium citrate 3 gr, vitamins B_1 1 mg, B_2 0.5 mg, B_6 0.5 mg, calcium pantothenate 0.3 mg, niacinamide 2.5 mg, B_{12} 1 mcg/Cap. Bot. 100s, 1000s.
Use: Vitamin/mineral supplement.
LEVLEN 21 TABLETS. (Berlex) Levonorgestrel 0.15 mg, ethinyl estradiol 0.03 mg/Tab. Slidecase 21s, Box 3s.
Use: Oral contraceptive.
LEVLEN 28 TABLETS. (Berlex) Levonorgestrel 0.15 mg, ethinyl estradiol 0.03 mg/Tab. (21 active, 7 inert). Slidecase 28s, Box 3s.
Use: Oral contraceptive.
LEVO-AMPHETAMINE. Alginate (l-isomer) alpha-2-phenylaminopropane succinate.
See: Levamphetamine.
LEVO-AMPHETAMINE SUCCINATE.
See: Pedestal, Cap., Tab. (Len-Tag).
• **LEVOBUNOLOL HYDROCHLORIDE.** USAN.
Use: Antiadrenergic.
• **LEVOBUNOLOL HYDROCHLORIDE,** U.S.P. XXIII, Ophth. (Various Mfr.) 2.5

mg/ml or 5 mg/ml Ophth. Soln. Bot. 5 ml, 10 ml, 15 ml.
Use: Beta-adrenergic blocking agent for glaucoma.
See: Betagan, Ophth. Soln. (Allergan).
• **LEVOCABASTINE HYDROCHLORIDE.** USAN.
Use: Antihistamine.
See: Livostin, Ophth. Susp. (Iolab).
• **LEVOCARNITINE,** U.S.P. XXIII, Oral, USAN.
Use: Carnitine deficiency. [Orphan drug]
See: Carnitor, Liq., Tab. (Sigma Tau). L-Carnitine, Cap. (R & D Labs). Vitacarn, Liq. (Kendall McGaw).
• **LEVODOPA,** U.S.P. XXIII. Cap., Tab., U.S.P. XXIII. L-Tyrosine, 3-hydroxy-. (—)-3-(3,4-Dihydroxyphenyl)-L-alanine. Berkdopa; Brocadopa; Veldopa.
Use: Treatment of the Parkinsonian syndrome.
See: Bio Dopa, Cap. (Bio-Deriv.). Dopar, Cap. (Norwich Eaton). Larodopa, Tab. or Cap. (Roche). Levopa, Cap. (ICN). Parda, Cap. (Parke-Davis).
• **LEVODOPA AND CARBIDOPA.**
Use: Antiparkinson agent.
See: Sinemet-10/100, Tab. (DuPont Pharm).
Sinemet-25/100, Tab. (DuPont Pharm).
Sinemet-25/250, Tab. (DuPont Pharm).
Sinemet CR, SR Tab., (DuPont Pharm).
LEVO-DROMORAN. (Roche) Levorphanol tartrate. **Amp.:** 2 mg/ml w/methyl and propyl parabens, sodium hydroxide to adjust pH. Amp. 1 ml, Box 10s. **Vial:** 2 mg/ml w/phenol 0.45%, sodium hydroxide to adjust pH. Vial 10 ml. **Tab.:** 2 mg. Bot. 100s.
Use: Narcotic analgesic.
LEVO-EPINEPHRINE BITARTRATE.
See: Lyophrin, Soln. (Alcon).
• **LEVOFURALTADONE.** USAN. 1-5-Morpholinomethyl-3-[(5-nitrofurfurylidene)amino]-2-oxazolidinone.
Use: Antibacterial, antiprotozoal.
LEVOID. (Nutrition) Levothyroxine sodium. **Tab.:** 0.1 mg or 0.2 mg. Bot. 90s, 500s. **Inj.:** 0.1 mg/ml w/sodium formaldehyde sulfoxylate 0.1%, phenol 0.5%, sodium hydroxide, glycine buffer. Vial 10 ml.
Use: Thyroid hormone.
• **LEVOMETHADYL ACETATE.** USAN.

Use: Narcotic analgesic.
• **LEVOMETHADYL ACETATE HYDROCHLORIDE.** USAN.
Use: Treatment of heroin addicts. [Orphan drug]
LEVOMETHORPHAN. B.A.N. (—)-3-Methoxy-N-methylmorphinan.
Use: Cough suppressant.
LEVOMORAMIDE. B.A.N. (—)-1-(3-Methyl-4-mor-pholino-2,2-diphenylbutyryl)pyrrolidine.
Use: Narcotic analgesic.
• **LEVONANTRADOL HYDROCHLORIDE.** USAN.
Use: Analgesic.
• **LEVONORDEFRIN,** U.S.P. XXIII. l-1-(1-Aminoethyl)3,4-Dihydroxy benzyl alcohol. Levonordefrin. (-)-α-(1-Aminoethyl)-3,4-dihydroxybenzyl Alcohol.
Use: Adrenergic (vasoconstrictor).
• **LEVONORGESTREL,** U.S.P. XXIII.
Use: Progestin.
See: Norplant (Wyeth-Ayerst).
• **LEVONORGESTREL AND ETHINYL ESTRADIOL TABLETS,** U.S.P. XXIII.
Use: Oral contraceptive.
See: Nordette, Tab. (Wyeth-Ayerst).
LEVOPHED. (Breon) Norepinephrine bitartrate 1 mg/ml Amp. 4 ml.
Use: Vasopressor used in shock.
LEVOPHED BITARTRATE. (Sanofi Winthrop) Norepinephrine bitartrate w/sodium Cl, sodium metabisulfite 1 mg or 2 mg/ml. Amp. 4 ml. Box 10s.
Use: Vasopressor used in shock.
LEVOPHENACYLMORPHAN. B.A.N. (—)-3-Hydroxy-N-phenacylmorphinan.
Use: Narcotic analgesic.
LEVOPROME. (Lederle) Methotrimeprazine 20 mg/ml w/benzyl alcohol 0.9% w/v, disodium edetate 0.065% w/v, sodium metabisulfite 0.3% w/v. Vial 10 ml.
Use: CNS analgesic.
• **LEVOPROPOXYPHENE NAPSYLATE,** U.S.P. XXII. Cap., Oral susp., U.S.P. XXII. 2-Naphthalenesulfonic acid compound with (—)-α-[2-(dimethylamino)-1-methylethyl]-α-phenylphenethyl propionate (1:1) monohydrate. α-1-4-Dimethylamino-1,2-diphenyl-3-methyl-2-b utanol propionate 2-naphthalene-sulfonate hydrate. (—)-α-4-(Dimethylamino)-3-methyl-1,2-diphenyl-2-butanol Propionate (ester) 2-Naphthalensulfonate (salt).
Use: Antitussive.
• **LEVOPROPYLCILLIN POTASSIUM.** USAN. (1) Potassium 3,3-Dimethyl-7-oxo-6-(—)-(2-phenoxybutyramido)-4-

thia-1-azabicyclo[3.2.0]-heptane-2-carboxylate; (2) Potassium 6-(—)-(2-phenoxybutyramido) penicillinate.
Use: Antibacterial.
LEVORA. (Hamilton Pharma) Ethinyl estradiol 0.030 mg, levonorgestrel 0.15 mg. Tab. Bot. 21s, 28s.
Use: Oral contraceptive.
LEVORENINE.
See: Epinephrine, U.S.P. XXIII. (Various Mfr.).
LEVOROXINE. (Bariatric) Sodium levothyroxine 0.05 mg, 0.1 mg, 0.2 mg or 0.3 mg/Tab. Bot. 100s, 500s.
Use: Thyroid hormone.
LEVORPHAN TARTRATE.
• **LEVORPHANOL TARTRATE,** U.S.P. XXIII. Inj., Tab., U.S.P. XXIII. 1-3-Hydroxy-N-methyl-morphinan bitartrate. 17-Methylmorphinan-3-ol Tartrate (1:1).
Use: Narcotic analgesic.
See: Levo-Dromoran, Amp., Tab., Vial (Roche).
LEVO-T. (Lederle) Levothyroxine sodium 0.025, 0.05, 0.075, 0.1, 0.125, 0.15, 0.2 or 0.3 mg. Tab. Bot. 100s (all strengths), 1000s (0.05, 0.1, 0.15 and 0.2 mg only).
LEVOTHROID. (Rhone-Poulenc Rorer) Levothyroxine sodium. **Tab.:** 25 mcg, 50 mcg, 75 mcg, 100 mcg, 125 mcg, 150 mcg, 175 mcg, 200 mcg or 300 mcg/Tab. Bot. 100s, 1000s, UD 100s (except for 25 mcg). **Inj.:** 200 mcg or 500 mcg. Vial 6 ml.
Use: Thyroid hormone.
LEVOTHYROXINE SODIUM. (McGuff) Levothyroxine sodium 500 mcg/Vial (100 mcg/ml reconstituted). Pow. for Inj.
Use: Thyroid hormone.
• **LEVOTHYROXINE SODIUM,** U.S.P. XXII. Tab., U.S.P. XXIII. L-Tyrosine, 0-(4-hydroxy-3,5-diiodo-phenyl)-3,5-diiodo-, monosodium salt, hydrate. Sodium L-3-[4-(4-Hydroxy-3,5-diiodophenoxy)-3,5-di-iodopheny]-alanine.
Use: Thyroid hormone.
See: Cytolen, Tab. (Len-Tag).
   Levoid, Tab., Vial (Nutrition Control Products).
   Levo-T, Tab. (Lederle).
   Levothroid, Tab., Inj. (Rhone-Poulenc Rorer).
   Synthroid, Tab., Inj. (Flint).
W/Mannitol.
See: Levoxine, Inj. (Daniels).
   Synthroid, Inj. (Flint).
W/Sodium liothyronine.
Use: Thyroid hormone.
See: Thyrolar, Tab. (Rhone-Poulenc Rorer).

• **LEVOXADROL HYDROCHLORIDE.**
USAN. l-2(2,2-Diphenyl-1,3-dioxolan-4-yl) piperidine hydrochloride levo form of dioxadrol HCl.
Use: Local anesthetic.
LEVOXINE. (Daniels) **Tab.:** Levothyroxine sodium 25 mcg, 50 mcg, 75 mcg, 100 mcg, 125 mcg, 150 mcg, 175 mcg, 200 mcg or 300 mcg/Tab. Bot. 100s, 1000s. **Pow.:** Levothyroxine sodium 200 mcg or 500 mcg. Vial 10 ml.
Use: Thyroid hormone.
LEVSIN. (Kremers-Urban) L-hyoscyamine sulfate. **Tab.:** 0.125 mg. Bot. 100s, 500s. **Soln.:** 0.125 mg/ml, alcohol 5%. Bot. 15 ml. **Elix.:** 0.125 mg/5 ml, alcohol 20%. Bot. pt. **Inj.:** 0.5 mg/ml. Vial 1 ml, 10 ml.
Use: Anticholinergic/antispasmodic.
LEVSIN-PB DROPS. (Kremers-Urban) Hyoscyamine sulfate 0.125 mg, phenobarbital 15 mg/ml, alcohol 5%. Liq. Bot. 15 ml.
Use: Anticholinergic/antispasmodic, sedative/hypnotic.
LEVSIN W/PHENOBARBITAL. (Schwarz Pharma Kremers Urban) L-hyoscyamine sulfate 0.125 mg, phenobarbital 15 mg/Tab. Bot. 100s, 500s.
Use: Gastrointestinal anticholinergic combination.
LEVSIN/SL. (Schwarz Pharma Kremers Urban) Hyoscyamine sulfate 0.125 mg/Tab. Sublingual. Bot. 100s, 500s.
Use: Gastrointestinal anticholinergic/antispasmodic.
LEVSINEX TIMECAPS. (Kremers-Urban) L-hyoscyamine sulfate 0.375 mg/TR Cap. Bot. 100s, 500s.
Use: Anticholinergic/antispasmodic.
LEVULOSE. Fructose.
LEVULOSE-DEXTROSE.
See: Invert Sugar.
• **LEXITHROMYCIN.** USAN.
Use: Antiviral antibiotic.
LEXOCORT POWDER. (Lexington) Hydrocortisone 0.1% in a talc base. Pkg. 20 Gm.
Use: Corticosteroid, topical.
LEXTRON. (Lilly) Liver-stomach concentrate 50 mg, iron 30 mg, vitamins B_{12} (activity equivalent) 2 mcg, B_1 1 mg, B_2 0.25 mg w/other factors of vitamin B complex present in the liver-stomach concentrate/Pulv. Bot. 84s.
Use: Vitamin supplement.
L-GLUTATHIONE.
See: Glutathione.
L'HOMME. (Geneva) Vitamins A 4000 IU,

D 400 IU, B_1 1 mg, B_2 1.2 mg, B_{12} 2 mcg, calcium pantothenate 5 mg, B_3 10 mg, C 30 mg, calcium 100 mg, phosphorus 76 mg, iron 10 mg, manganese 1 mg, magnesium 1 mg, zinc 1 mg. Bot. 100s.
Use: Vitamin/mineral supplement.
• **LIAROZOLE FUMARATE.** USAN (Janssen).
Use: Antipsoriatic.
• **LIAROZOLE HYDROCHLORIDE.** USAN (Janssen).
Use: Antineoplastic.
LI BAN SPRAY. (Leeming) Synthetic pyrethroid 0.5%, related compounds 0.065%, aromatic petroleum hydrocarbons 0.664%. Bot. 5 oz, Box 6s.
Use: Control of lice, fleas on bedding, furniture, etc. (Not to be used on humans or animals).
• **LIBENZAPRIL.** USAN.
Use: ACE inhibitor.
LIBRAX. (Roche) Clidinium bromide (Quarzan) 2.5 mg, chlordiazepoxide HCl (Librium) 5 mg/Cap. Bot. 100s, 500s, Teledose 100s (10 strips of 10).
Use: Anticholinergic combination.
LIBRITABS. (Roche) Chlordiazepoxide 5 mg, 10 mg or 25 mg/Tab. **5 mg:** Bot. 100s, 500s; **10 mg:** Bot. 100s, 500s; **25 mg:** Bot. 100s.
Use: Antianxiety agent.
LIBRIUM. (Roche) Chlordiazepoxide HCl 5 mg, 10 mg or 25 mg/Cap. Bot. 100s, 500s, Tel-E-Dose (10 strips of 10; 4 cards of 25) in RNP (Reverse Numbered Package).
Use: Antianxiety agent.
LIBRIUM INJECTABLE. (Roche) Chlordiazepoxide HCl 100 mg/dry filled amp. plus special I.M. diluent, 2 ml for I.M. administration/compound w/benzyl alcohol 1.5%, polysorbate 80 4%, propylene glycol 20%, w/maleic acid and sodium hydroxide to adjust pH to approx. 3. Amp. 5 ml w/2 ml diluent, Box 10s.
Use: Antianxiety agent.
LICE-ENZ. (Copley) Pyrethrins 0.3%, piperonylbutoxide 3%. Shampoo. Bot. 60 Gm.
Use: Miscellaneous pediculicides.
LICETROL LIQUID. (Republic) Pyrethrins 0.2%, piperonyl butoxide technical 2%, petroleum distillate 0.8%. Bot. 60 ml, 120 ml.
Use: Pediculicide.
LICOPLEX. (Mills) Desiccated whole bile 2 gr, dried whole pancreatic substance 3/4 gr, dl-methionine 2 gr, choline bitartrate 3 gr/Tab. Bot. 100s.

Use: Bile laxative, cholagogue.

LICOPLEX DS. (Keene) Iron 2.9 mg, vitamins B_{12} equivalent 1 mcg, B_2 0.75 mg, B_3 50 mg, B_5 1.25 mg, B_{12} 15 mcg/ml, procaine 2%. Inj. Vial 30 ml.
Use: Parenteral nutritional supplement.

LICOPLEX DS. (Keene) Cyanocobalamin 15 mcg, liver inj. equivalent to cyanocobalamin activity 1 mcg, ferrous gluconate 25 mg, riboflavin 0.75 mg, calcium pantothenate 1.25 mg, niacinamide 50 mg. Vial 30 ml.
Use: Vitamin/mineral supplement.

• **LICRYFILCON A.** USAN.
Use: Contact lens material.

• **LICRYFILCON B.** USAN.
Use: Contact lens material.

LIDA-MANTLE-HC CREME. (Miles Pharm) Lidocaine 3%, hydrocortisone acetate 0.5% in cream base. Tube oz.
Use: Corticosteroid combination, topical.

• **LIDAMIDINE HYDROCHLORIDE.** USAN.
Use: Antiperistaltic.

LIDEX CREAM. (Syntex) Fluocinonide 0.05%. Cream. In 15 Gm, 30 Gm, 60 Gm, 120 Gm.
Use: Corticosteroid, topical.

LIDEX-E. (Syntex) Fluocinonide 0.05% in aqueous emollient base. Tube 15 Gm, 30 Gm, 60 Gm, 120 Gm.
Use: Corticosteroid, topical.

LIDEX GEL. (Syntex) Fluocinonide 0.05% in gel base. Tube 15 Gm, 30 Gm, 60 Gm, 120 Gm.
Use: Corticosteroid, topical.

LIDEX OINTMENT. (Syntex) Fluocinonide 0.05% in ointment base. Tube 15 Gm, 30 Gm, 60 Gm, 120 Gm.
Use: Corticosteroid, topical.

LIDEX TOPICAL SOLUTION. (Syntex) Fluocinonide 0.05%. Soln. Bot. 20 ml, 60 ml.
Use: Corticosteroid, topical.

• **LIDOCAINE,** U.S.P. XXIII. Oint., Oral topical soln., Sterile, Topical aerosol, U.S.P. XXIII. 2-Diethylamino-2′,6-acetoxylidide. Acetamide, 2-(diethylamino)-N-(2,6-dimethylphenyl)-
Use: Local anesthetic.
See: Dermaflex, Gel (Zila).
Zilactin-L, Liq. (Zila).

• **LIDOCAINE AND EPINEPHRINE INJECTION,** U.S.P. XXIII.
Use: Local anesthetic.
See: L-Caine E, Vial (Century).
Norocaine 1%, 2% w/Epinephrine. (Vortech).
Xylocaine W/Epinephrine, Soln. (Astra).

• **LIDOCAINE HYDROCHLORIDE,** U.S.P. XXIII. Inj., Jelly, Topical Soln., U.S.P. XXIII. Acetamide, 2-(diethylamino)-N-(2,6-dimethylphenyl)-, HCl. 2-Die- thylamino-2′,6-acetoxylidide HCl.
Use: Cardiac depressant (antiarrhythmic), local anesthetic.
(Abbott) **0.2%, 0.4%, 0.8%:** w/5% Dextrose. 250 ml single-dose container; **1%, 2%.** Abboject syringe 5 ml; Vial 1 Gm, 2 Gm. Premixed: 0.2%, 0.4% in 5% dextrose. Inj. containers (flexible or glass) 500 ml. **1%:** 2 ml, 5 ml single-dose amp. **1.5%:** 20 ml single-dose amp. **2%:** 10 ml/20 ml vial (for dilution to prepare I.V. drip soln.) **5%:** w/ 7.5% Dextrose amp. 2 ml.
(Maurry) 2%. Vial.
(Pharmex) 1%, 2%. Vial 50 ml.
Use: Injection for infiltration block anesthesia and I.V. drip for cardiac arrhythmias.
See: Anestacon, Liq. (Webcon).
Ardecaine 1%, 2%, Inj. (Burgin-Arden).
Dolicaine, I.M. (Reid-Rowell).
L-Caine, Inj., Liq. (Century)
Nervocaine, Inj. (Keene).
Norocaine, Inj. (Vortech).
Stanacaine (Standex).
Xylocaine HCl, Preps. (Astra).
W/Benzalkonium Cl.
See: Medi-Quik, Aerosol (Lehn & Fink).
Medi-Quick Pump Spray (Lehn & Fink).
W/Benzalkonium Cl, phenol, menthol, eugenol, thyme oil, eucalyptus oil.
See: Unguentine Spray (Norwich).
W/Cetyltrimethylammonium bromide, hexachlorophene.
See: Aerosept, Aerosol (Dalin).
W/Hydrocortisone, clioquinol.
See: Bafil, Lot. (Scruggs).
Hil-20 Lot. (Reid-Rowell).
W/Dextrose.
W/Methylparaben, sodium Cl.
W/Methyl parasept.
See: L-Caine, Inj. (Century).
W/Methyl parasept, epinephrine.
See: L-Caine-E, Inj. (Century).
W/Orthohydroxyphenyl mercuric Cl, menthol, camphor, allantoin.
See: Kip First Aid preps. (Youngs Drug).
W/Parachlorometaxylenol, phenol, zinc oxide.
See: Unguentine Plus, Cream (Norwich).
W/Polymyxin B sulfate.
See: Lidosporin, Otic soln. (Burroughs-

Wellcome).
• **LIDOCAINE HYDROCHLORIDE AND DEXTROSE INJECTION,** U.S.P. XXIII.
• **LIDOCAINE HYDROCHLORIDE AND EP-INEPHRINE BITARTRATE INJECTION,** U.S.P. XXIII.
• **LIDOCAINE HYDROCHLORIDE AND EP-INEPHRINE INJECTION,** U.S.P. XXIII
• **LIDOFENIN.** USAN.
Use: Diagnostic aid.
• **LIDOFILCON A.** USAN.
Use: Contact lens material.
• **LIDOFILCON B.** USAN.
Use: Contact lens material.
• **LIDOFLAZINE.** USAN. 4-[4,4-bis(p-Fluro-phenyl)-butyl]-1-piperazineaceto-2′,6-xylidide. 4-[3-(4,4-Di-fluorobenzhydryl)propyl]piperazin-1-ylacet-2,6- xylidide.
Use: Cardiovascular agent.
LIDOJECT-1. (Mayrand) Lidocaine HCl 1%. Vial 50 ml.
Use: Local anesthetic.
LIDOJECT-2. (Mayrand) Lidocaine HCl 2%. Vial 50 ml.
Use: Local anesthetic.
LIDOPEN AUTO-INJECTOR. (Survival Technology) Lidocaine HCl 300 mg/3 ml. Auto-injection device.
Use: Antiarrhythmic.
LIDOX CAPS. (Major) Chlordiazepoxide HCl 10 mg, clidinium bromide 2.5 mg. Cap. Bot. 100s, 500s, 1000s, UD 100s.
Use: Anticholinergic combination.
LIDOXIDE. (Interstate) Chlordiazepoxide HCl 5 mg, clidinium bromide 2.5 mg/Tab. Bot. 100s, 500s.
Use: Anticholinergic combination.
LID SCRUBS.
Use: Ophthalmic cleansing solutions.
See: I-Scrub, Soln. (Spectra).
Lid Wipes-SPF, Soln. (Akorn).
OcuClenz, Soln. (Storz/Lederle).
OCuSOFT, Soln. (Cynacon/OCu-SOFT).
LID WIPES-SPF. (Akorn) PEG-200 glyc-eryl monotallowate, PEG-80 glyceryl monococoate, laureth-23, cocoamido propyl amine oxide, NaCl, glycerin, sodi-um dihydrogen phosphate, sodium hy-droxide. Soln. Pads UD 30s.
Use: Ophthalmic cleansing solution.
• **LIFARIZINE.** USAN.
Use: Cerebral anti-ischemic.
LIFER-B. (Burgin-Arden) Cyanocobal-amin 30 mcg, liver inj. 0.1 ml, ferrous gluconate 100 mg, riboflavin 1.5 mg, panthenol 2.5 mg, niacinamide 100 mg, citric acid 16.4 mg, sodium citrate 23.6 mg/ml. Vial 30 ml.

Use: Vitamin/mineral supplement.
LIFE SAVER KIT. (Whiteworth) Ipecac syrup two 1 oz bottles, activated char-coal pow. 1 oz, poison treatment instruc-tion booklet.
Use: Antidote kit.
LIFE SPANNER. (Spanner) Vitamins A 12,500 IU, D 400 IU, E 6 IU, B₁ 10 mg, B₂ 5 mg, B₆ 2 mg, B₁₂ 5 mcg, niaci-namide 50 mg, calcium pantothenate 10 mg, biotin 10 mcg, C 100 mg, hesperidin complex 10 mg, rutin 20 mg, choline bitartrate 40 mg, inositol 30 mg, betaine anhydrous 15 mg, l-lysine monohy-drochloride 25 mg, iron 30 mg, copper 1 mg, manganese 1 mg, potassium 5 mg, calcium 105 mg, phosphorus 82 mg, magnesium 5.56 mg, zinc 1 mg/Cap. Bot. 100s.
Use: Vitamin/mineral supplement.
• **LIFIBRATE.** USAN.
Use: Antihyperlipoproteinemic.
LIFOL-B. (Burgin-Arden) Liver inj. 10 mcg, folic acid 1 mg, cyanocobalamin 100 mcg, phenol 0.5%/ml. Inj. Vial 10 ml.
Use: Nutritional supplement.
LIFOLEX. (Pasadena Research) Liver 10 mcg, cyanocobalamin 100 mcg, folic acid 5 mg/ml. Inj. Vial 10 ml.
Use: Nutritional supplement.
LIGNOCAINE. B.A.N. N-(Diethy-laminoacetyl)-2,6-xylidine. Duncaine; Li-dothesin; Lignostab; Xylocaine; Xylotox.
Use: Local anesthetic.
LILLY BULK PRODUCTS. (Lilly) The fol-lowing products are supplied by Eli Lilly under the U.S.P., N.F. or chemical name as a service to the health professions:
Ammoniated Mercury Oint.
Amyl Nitrite.
Analgesic Balm.
Apomorphine HCl.
Aromatic Elix.
Aromatic Ammonia.
Atropine Sulfate.
Bacitracin Oint.
Belladonna Tincture.
Benzoin.
Boric Acid.
Calcium Gluceptate.
Calcium Gluconate.
Calcium Gluconate with Vitamin D.
Calcium Hydroxide.
Calcium Lactate.
Carbarsone.
Cascara, Aromatic, fluidextract.
Cascara Sagrada fluidextract.
Citrated Caffeine.
Cocaine HCl.

Codeine Phosphate.
Codeine Sulfate.
Colchicine.
Compound Benzoin.
Dibasic Calcium Phosphate.
Diethylstilbestrol.
Ephedrine Sulfate.
Ferrous Gluconate.
Ferrous Sulfate.
Folic Acid.
Glucagon for Inj.
Green Soap Tincture.
Heparin Sodium.
Histamine Phosphate.
Ipecac.
Isoniazid.
Isopropyl Alcohol, 91%.
Liver, Vial for Inj.
Magnesium Sulfate.
Mercuric Oxide, Yellow.
Methadone HCl.
Methenamine for Timed Burning.
Methyltestosterone.
Milk of Bismuth.
Morphine Sulfate.
Myrrh.
Neomycin Sulfate.
Niacin.
Niacinamide.
Nitroglycerin.
Opium (Deodorized).
Ox Bile Extract.
Pancreatin.
Papaverine HCl.
Paregoric.
Penicillin G Potassium.
Phenobarbital.
Phenobarbital Sodium.
Potassium Cl.
Potassium Iodide.
Powder Papers (Glassine).
Progesterone.
Propylthiouracil.
Protamine Sulfate.
Pyridoxine HCl.
Quinidine Gluconate.
Quinidine Sulfate.
Quinine Sulfate.
Riboflavin.
Silver Nitrate.
Sodium Bicarbonate.
Sodium Chloride.
Sodium Salicylate.
Streptomycin Sulfate.
Sulfadiazine.
Sulfapyridine.
Sulfur.
Terpin Hydrate.
Terpin Hydrate and Codeine.
Testosterone Propionate.

Thiamine HCl.
Thyroid.
Tubocurarine HCl.
Tylosterone.
Whitfield's Oint.
Wild Cherry Syrup.
Zinc Oxide.
Zinc Oxide Paste.
LIMARSOL.
See: Acetarsone. (City Chemical).
LIMBITROL. (Roche) Chlordiazepoxide 5 mg, amitriptyline HCl 12.5 mg/Tab. Bot. 100s, 500s, Tel-E-Dose 100s, Prescription pak 50s.
Use: Psychotherapeutic agent.
LIMBITROL DS. (Roche) Chlordiazepoxide 10 mg, amitriptyline HCl 25 mg/Tab. Bot. 100s, 500s, Tel-E-Dose 100s, Prescription pak 50s.
Use: Psychotherapeutic agent.
• **LIME,** U.S.P. XXIII.
Use: Pharmaceutical necessity.
LIME SOLUTION, SULFURATED, U.S.P. XXI.
Use: Scabicide.
LIME SULFUR SOLUTION. Calcium polysulfide, calcium thiosulfate.
Use: Wet dressing.
See: Vlem-Dome, Liq. Concentrate (Miles Pharm).
• **LINAROTENE.** USAN.
Use: Antikeratolytic.
LINCOCIN. (Upjohn) Lincomycin HCl 500 mg/Cap. Bot. 24s, 100s. **Pediatric:** 250 mg/Cap. Bot. 24s.
Use: Anti-infective.
LINCOCIN STERILE SOLUTION. (Upjohn) Lincomycin HCl equivalent to 300 mg or 600 mg lincomycin base, benzyl alcohol 9.45 mg/ml. Vial 2 ml in 5s, 25s, 100s; 10 ml U-Ject.
Use: Anti-infective.
• **LINCOMYCIN.** USAN. Antibiotic produced by *Streptomyces lincolnensis*. Methyl 6,8-Di-deoxy-6-(1-methyl-4-propyl-L-2-pyrrolidine-carboxamido)-1-thio-D-Erythro-α-D-galacto-octopyranoside.
Use: Antibiotic, infections due to gram-positive organisms.
• **LINCOMYCIN HYDROCHLORIDE,** U.S.P. XXIII. Inj., Cap., Sterile, Syr., U.S.P. XXIII. D-erythro-α-D-galacto-Octopyranoside, methyl-6,8-dideoxy-6-[[(1-methyl-4-propyl-2-pyrrolidinyl)carbonyl]amino]-1-thio, HCl.
Use: Antibacterial.
See: Lincocin, Cap., Soln., Syr. (Upjohn).
• **LINDANE,** U.S.P. XXIII. Cream, Lot.,

Shampoo, U.S.P. XXIII. Gamma-benzene-hexachloride, hexachlorocyclohexane.
Fidelity Lab.—Pow. 50%, Pkg. 1 lb, 5 lb.
Imperial—Pow. 50%, Pkg. 1 lb, 4 lb; 12%, Pkg. 1 lb, 4 lb.
Use: Pediculicide, scabicide.
See: Kwell, Cream, Lot., Shampoo (Reed & Carnrick).
LINDORA. (Westwood) Sodium laureth sulfate, water, cocamide DEA, sodium Cl, lactic acid, tetra sodium EDTA, benzophenone-4, FD&C Blue No. 1, fragrance. Bot. 8 oz.
Use: Skin cleanser.
LINODIL CAPSULES. (Sanofi Winthrop) Inositol hexanicotinate.
Use: Hyperlipidemic, peripheral vasodilator.
• **LINOGLIRIDE.** USAN.
Use: Antidiabetic agent.
• **LINOGLIRIDE FUMARATE.** USAN.
Use: Antidiabetic agent.
LINOLENIC ACID W/VIT. E.
See: Petropin, Cap. (Lannett).
LINOMIDE. (Kabi Pharmacia).
Use: Immunomodulator.
• **LINOPIRDINE.** USAN.
Use: Treatment of Alzheimer's disease.
LIORESAL. (Geigy) Baclofen 10 mg or 20 mg/Tab. Bot. 100s, UD 100s.
Use: Muscle relaxant.
LIOTHYRONINE. B.A.N. 3-[4-(4-Hydroxy-3-iodo-phenoxy)-3,5-diiodophenyl]-alanine.(—)-Tri-iodothyronine. Cynomel and Tertroxin sodium derivative.
Use: Thyroid hormone.
• **LIOTHYRONINE I-125.** USAN.
Use: Radioactive agent.
• **LIOTHYRONINE I-131.** USAN.
Use: Radioactive agent.
LIOTHYRONINE RESIN.
• **LIOTHYRONINE SODIUM,** U.S.P. XXIII., Tab. U.S.P. XXIII. L-Tyrosine, 0-(4-hydroxy-3-iodophenyl)-3,5-diiodo-, sodium salt. Sodium L-triiodo-thyronine. Sodium L-4-(3-iodo-4-hydroxphenoxy)-3,5-diiodo-phenylalanine.
Use: Thyroid hormone.
See: Cytomel, Tab. (SK-Beecham).
LIOTHYRONINE SODIUM INJECTION.
Use: Myxedema coma/precoma. [Orphan drug]
• **LIOTRIX,** U.S.P. XXIII. A combination of sodium levothyroxine and sodium 1-triiodothyronine in a ratio of 4 to 1 by weight.
Use: Thyroid hormone.
See: Euthroid, Tab. (Parke-Davis).

Thyrolar, Tab. (Rhone-Poulenc Rorer).
LIPASE. W/Amylase, Protease.
Use: Digestive enzyme.
W/Amylase, bile salts, wilzyme, pepsin, pancreatin, calcium.
See: Enzyme, Tab. (Barth's).
W/Alpha-amylase W-100, proteinase W-300, cellase W-100, estrone, testosterone, vitamins, minerals.
See: Geramine, Tab. (Brown).
W/Alpha-Amylase, proteinasa, cellase.
See: Kutrase (Kremers-Urban).
Ku-Zyme (Kremers-Urban).
W/Amylolytic, proteolytic, cellulolytic enzymes.
See: Arco-Lase, Tab. (Arco).
W/Amylolytic, proteolytic, cellulolytic enzymes, phenobarbital, hyoscyamine sulfate, atropine sulfate.
See: Arco-Lase Plus, Tab. (Arco).
W/Pancreatin, protease, amylase.
See: Dizymes, Cap. (Recsei).
W/Pepsin, homatropine methylbromide, amylase, protease, bile salts.
See: Digesplen, Tab., Elix., Drops (Med. Prod.).
LIPIDIL. (Fournier) Fenofibrate. Cap.
Use: Antihyperlipidemic agent.
LIPIDS.
Use: Intravenous nutritional therapy.
See: Intralipid 10%, Soln. (Clintec).
Intralipid 20%, Soln. (Clintec).
Liposyn II 10%, Soln. (Abbott).
Liposyn II 20%, Soln. (Abbott).
Liposyn III 10%, Soln. (Abbott).
Liposyn III 20%, Soln. (Abbott).
LIPISORB. (Mead Johnson Nutritionals) Protein 35 g/L, fat 48 g/L, carbohydrates 115 g/L, Na 733.3 mg/L, K 1250 mg/L, H_2O 320 mOsm/kg. With appropriate vitamins and minerals. 1 calorie/ml. Vanilla flavored. Pow. Can 1 lb.
Use: Enteral nutritional supplement.
LIPKOTE BY COPPERTONE. (Plough) Padimate O, oxybenzone. SPF 15. Lip balm 4.2 Gm.
Use: Sunscreen.
LIPKOTE SPF 15 ULTRA SUNSCREEN LIPBALM. (Plough) Tube 0.15 oz,
Use: Sunscreen.
LIP MEDEX. (Blistex) Petrolatum, camphor 1%, phenol 0.54%, cocoa butter, dimethyl oxazolidine, lanolin, mixed waxes. Oint. 210 Gm.
Use: Treatment of fever blisters and sore, dry cracked lips.
LIPOCHOLINE. See: Choline dihydrogen citrate. (Various Mfr.).
LIPODERM. (Spirt) Pancreas (porcine) 500 mg, vitamin B_6 3 mg. Cap. Bot.

180s, 500s.
Use: Antipsoriatic.
LIPOFLAVONOID CAPLETS. (Numark)
Vitamins C 100 mg, B_1 0.3 mg, B_2 0.3
mg, B_3 3.3 mg, B_6 0.3 mg, B_{12} 1.7 mcg,
B_5 1.7 mg, choline 111.3 mg,
bioflavonoids 100 mg, inostitol 111.3 mg.
Bot. 100s.
Use: Vitamin supplement.
LIPOFLAVONOID CAPSULES. (Numark)
Choline 111 mg, inositol 111 mg, vita-
mins B_1 0.3 mg, B_2 0.3 mg, B_3 3.3 mg,
B_5 1.7 mg, B_6 0.3 mg, B_{12} 1.7 mcg, C
100 mg, lemon bioflavonoid complex.
Cap. Bot. 100s, 500s.
Use: Vitamin supplement.
LIPOGEN CAPSULES. (Various Mfr.)
Choline 111 mg, inositol 111 mg, Vitamins B_1 0.3 mg, B_2 0.3 mg, B_3 3.3 mg,
B_5 1.7 mg, B_6 0.3 mg, B_{12} 1.7 mcg, C
100 mg/Cap. Bot. 60s, 100s.
Use: Vitamin supplement.
LIPO-K CAPSULES. (Marcen) Epineph-
rine-neutralizing factor 25 units, pancreatic lipotropic factor 1.2 mg, Cy-mu-
copolysaccharides 2.5 mg, choline bitartrate 100 mg, dl-methionine 50 mg,
inositol 25 mg, bile extract 5 mg/Cap.
Bot. 100s, 500s, 1000s.
Use: Treatment of circulatory disturbances.
LIPO-K INJECTABLE. (Marcen) Pancreatic lipotropic factor 1.2 mg, epinephi-
rine-neutralizing factor 25 units, Cy-mu-
copolysaccharides 0.5 mg, sodium citrate 10 mg, inositol 5 mg, phenol
0.5%/ml. Multi-dose Vial 10 ml, 30 ml.
Use: Treatment of circulatory disturbances.
LIPOLYTIC ENZYME.
W/Proteolytic enzyme, amylolytic enzyme,
cellulolytic enzyme, methyl polysiloxane,
ox bile, betaine HCl.
See: Zymme, Cap. (Scrip).
LIPOMUL. (Upjohn) Corn oil 10 Gm/15 ml
w/d-Alpha tocopheryl acetate, butylated
hydroxy-anisole, polysorbate 80, glyceride phosphates, sodium saccharin,
sodium benzoate 0.05%, benzoic acid
0.05%, sorbic acid 0.07%. Bot. pt.
Use: Enteral nutritional supplement.
LIPO-NICIN. (ICN Pharm) Niacin 300 mg,
vitamin C 150 mg, B_1 25 mg, B_2 2 mg,
B_6 10 mg/TR Cap. Bot. 100s.
Use: Peripheral vasodilator.
LIPO-NICIN 100 mg. (ICN Pharm) Nicotinic acid 100 mg, niacinamide 75 mg, vitamins C 150 mg, B_1 25 mg, B_2 2 mg, B_6
10 mg/Tab. Bot. 100s, 500s.
Use: Peripheral vasodilator combina-

tion.
LIPO-NICIN 300 mg TIMED CAPS. (ICN
Pharm) Nicotinic acid 300 mg, vitamins
C 150 mg, B_1 25 mg, B_2 2 mg, B_6 10
mg/TR Cap. Bot. 100s, 500s.
Use: Peripheral vasodilator combination.
LIPONOL CAPSULES. (Rugby) Choline
115 mg, inositol 83 mg, methionine 110
mg, vitamins B_1 3 mg, B_2 3 mg, B_3 10
mg, B_5 2 mg, B_6 2 mg, B_{12} 2 mcg, desiccated liver 56 mg, liver concentrate 30
mg/Cap. Bot. 100s, 500s.
Use: Nutritional supplement.
LIPOSYN. (Abbott Hospital Prods) Intravenous fat emulsion containing safflower oil 10%, egg phosphatides 1.2%,
glycerin 2.5% in water for inj. **10%:** Single-dose container 50 ml, 100 ml, 200
ml, 500 ml; Syringe Pump Unit 50 ml single-dose. **20%:** Single-dose container
200 ml, 500 ml Syringe Pump Unit 25 ml
or 50 ml single-dose.
Use: Parenteral nutritional supplement.
LIPOSYN II. (Abbott Hospital Prods) Intravenous fat emulsion: **10%:** Safflower
oil 5%, soybean oil 5%. Bot. 100 ml, 200
ml, 500 ml. **20%:** Safflower oil 10%, soybean oil 10% w/egg phosphatides 1.2%,
glycerin 2.5%. 200 ml, 500 ml. Bot. Syringe pump unit 25 ml, 50 ml.
Use: Parenteral nutritional supplement.
LIPOSYN III. (Abbott) Oil, soybean, egg
yolk phospholipids. **10%:** 100, 200, 500
ml. **20%:** 100, 500 ml.
Use: Parenteral nutritional supplement.
LIPO-TEARS. (Spectra) Mineral oil,
petrolatum. Preservative free. Drops.
Bot. 1 ml (in 30s).
Use: Ocular lubricant.
LIPOTRIAD CAPLETS. (Numark) Zn 30
mg, vitamin A 5000 IU, C 60 mg, E 30
IU, Cu, Se, B_3 20 mg, B_1 1.5 mg, B_2 1.7
mg, B_6 2 mg, B_{12} 6 mcg, B_5 10 mg,
choline bitartrate, inositol. Bot. 60s.
Use: Vitamin supplement.
LIPOTROPICS WITH VITAMINS.
Use: Nutritional supplement.
See: Lipotriad, Liq. (Numark).
Lipogen, Cap. (Various Mfr.).
Lipotriad, Cap. (Numark).
Lipoflavonoid, Cap. (Numark).
Cholinoid, Cap. (Goldline).
Akoline, C.B., Cap. (Akorn).
Akoline, C.B., Capl. (Akorn).
Liponol, Cap. (Rugby).
Methatropic, Cap. (Goldline).
Cholidase, Tab. (Freeda).
LIPOVITE CAPSULES. (Rugby) Vitamins
B_1 0.3 mg, B_2 0.3 mg, B_3 3.3 mg, B_5

1.67 mg, B$_6$ 0.3 mg, B$_{12}$ 1.67 mcg, choline bitartrate 111 mg/Cap. Bot. 100s, 1000s.
Use: Vitamin B supplement.
LIPOXIDE CAPS. (Major) Chlordiazepoxide HCl 5 mg, 10 mg or 25 mg/Cap. Bot. 100s, 500s, 1000s.
Use: Antianxiety agent.
LIQUAEMIN SODIUM. (Organon) Heparin sodium aqueous soln., benzyl alcohol 1%. **1,000 units/ml:** Vial 10 ml, 30 ml. Box 25s. **5,000 units/ml:** Vial 1 ml, 10 ml. Box 25s. **10,000 units/ml:** Vial 1 ml, 4 ml, Box 25s. **20,000 units/ml:** Vial 1 ml, 2 ml, Box 25s. 5 ml Box 1s. **40,000 units/ml:** Vial 1 ml, Box 25s.
Use: Anticoagulant.
LIQUAEMIN SODIUM-PRESERVATIVE FREE. (Organon) Heparin sodium, preservative free. **1,000 units/ml:** Amp. 1 ml Box 50s. **5,000 units/ml:** Amp. 1 ml Box 50s. **10,000 units/ml:** Amp. 1 ml Box 50s.
Use: Anticoagulant.
LIQUA-GEL. (Paddock) Boric acid, glycerine, propylene glycol, methylparaben, propylparaben, Irish moss extract, methylcellulose. Bot. 4 oz, 16 oz.
LIQUIBID. (Ion) Guaifenesin 600 mg, dye free. SR Tab. Bot. 100s.
Use: Expectorant.
LIQUI-CHAR. (Jones Medical) Acitvated charcoal. **Liq. Bot.:** 12.5 Gm/60 ml, 15 Gm/75 ml. **Squeeze container.:** 25 Gm/120 ml, 50 Gm/240 ml, 30 Gm/120 ml.
Use: Antidote.
LIQUI-DOSS. (Ferndale) Docusate sodium 60 mg, mineral oil. Bot. pt.
Use: Laxative.
LIQUID BAROSPERSE. (Lafayette Pharm.) Barium sulfate 60%. Susp. Bot. 355 ml.
Use: Radiopaque agents.
LIQUID GERITONIC. (Geriatric Pharm.) Fe 105 mg, liver fraction 1 375 mg, B$_1$ 3 mg, B$_2$ 3 mg, B$_3$ 30 mg, B$_6$ 0.3 mg, B$_{12}$ 9 mcg, inositol 60 mg, glycine 180 mg, yeast concentrate 375 mg, Ca, I, K, Mg, Mn, P, alcohol 20%. Liq. Bot. 240 ml, gal.
Use: Iron and liver combination.
LIQUID LATHER. (Ulmer) Gentle wash for hands, body, face, hair. Bot. 8 oz, gal.
Use: Cleanser.
LIQUID PETROLATUM EMULSION.
See: Mineral Oil Emulsion, U.S.P. XXIII.
LIQUID PRED SYRUP. (Muro) Prednisone 5 mg/5 ml in syrup base. Alcohol 5%, saccharin, sorbitol. Bot. 120 ml, 240

ml.
Use: Corticosteorid.
LIQUIFILM FORTE. (Allergan) Enhanced artificial tears w/polyvinyl alcohol 3%, thimerosal 0.002%, edetate disodium in a buffered sterile, isotonic soln. Bot. 0.5 fl oz, 1 fl oz.
Use: Artificial tears.
LIQUIFILM TEARS. (Allergan) Polyvinyl alcohol 1.4%, chlorobutanol 0.5%, sodium Cl, purified water. Bot. 15 ml, 30 ml.
Use: Artificial tears.
LIQUIFILM WETTING SOLUTION. (Allergan) Polyvinyl alcohol, hydroxypropyl methylcellulose, edetate disodium, sodium Cl, potassium Cl, benzalkonium Cl. Bot. 60 ml.
Use: Hard contact lens care.
LIQUIMAT. (Owen) Sulfur 5%, alcohol 22%, in drying makeup base. Plastic Bot. 1.5 oz.
Use: Anti-acne.
LIQUI-NOX. (Alconox) qt, gal.
Use: Anionic and nonionic detergents and wetting agents.
LIQUIPAKE. (Lafayette) Barium sulfate suspension 100% w/v for dilution. Bot. 1850 ml, Case 4s.
Use: Radiopaque agent.
LIQUIPRIN. (SK-Beecham) Acetaminophen 80 mg/1.66 ml, saccharin. Soln. Bot. 35 ml w/dropper.
Use: Analgesic.
LIQUOR CARBONIS DETERGENS.
See: Coal Tar Topical Soln., U.S.P. XXIII. (Various Mfr.).
• **LISADIMATE.** USAN.
Use: Sunscreen.
• **LISINOPRIL.** USAN.
Use: Antihypertensive.
See: Prinivil, Tab. (Merck).
W/Hydrochlorothiazide
See: Prinzide, Tab. (Merck).
LISTEREX SCRUB MEDICATED LOTION. (Warner-Lambert Prods) Salicylic acid 2% Lot. Bot. 4 oz, 8 oz.
Use: Anti-acne.
LISTERINE ANTISEPTIC. (Warner-Lambert Prods) Thymol, eucalyptol, methyl salicylate, menthol. Alcohol 26.9%. Bot. 3 oz, 6 oz, 12 oz, 18 oz, 24 oz, 32 oz.
Use: Mouthwash.
LISTERINE ANTISEPTIC THROAT LOZENGES. (Warner-Lambert Prods) Hexylresorcinol 2.4 mg/Loz. Box 24s.
Use: Throat preparation.
LISTERINE MAXIMUM STRENGTH ANTISEPTIC THROAT LOZENGES. (Warner-Lambert Prods) Hexylresorcinol 4 mg/Loz. Box 24s.

Use: Throat preparation.

LISTERMINT WITH FLUORIDE. (Warner-Lambert Prods) Sodium fluoride 0.02% w/water, alcohol 6.65%, glycerin, poloxamer 407, sodium lauryl sulfate, sodium citrate, sodium saccharin, zinc Cl, citric acid, flavors, colors. Bot. 6 oz, 12 oz, 18 oz, 24 oz, 32 oz.
Use: Mouth preparation, dental caries preventative.

LITE PRED. (Horizon) Prednisolone sodium phosphate 0.125%. Soln. Bot. 5 ml.
Use: Corticosteroid, ophthalmic.

LITHANE. (Miles Pharm) Lithium carbonate 300 mg, tartrazine. Tab. Bot. 100s.
Use: Antipsychotic agent.

•**LITHIUM CARBONATE,** U.S.P. XXIII. ER Cap., Cap., Tab., U.S.P. XXIII. Carbonic acid, dilithium salt.
Use: Antidepressant.
See: Eskalith, Cap., Tab. (SK-Beecham).
　Lithane, Tab. (Miles Pharm).
　Lithobid, Tab. (Ciba).
　Lithotabs, Tab. (Reid-Rowell).

LITHIUM CARBONATE CAPSULES AND TABLETS. (Roxane) Lithium carbonate. **Tab.:** 300 mg. Bot. 100s, 1000s, UD 100s. **Cap.:** 150 mg, 300 mg or 600 mg. Bot. 100s, 1000s, UD 100s.
Use: Antipsychotic agent.

•**LITHIUM CITRATE,** U.S.P. XXIII. Syr. U.S.P. XXIII.
Use: Manic-depressive states.
See: Cibalith-S, Liq. (Ciba).
　Lithonate-S, Liq. (Reid-Rowell).

•**LITHIUM HYDROXIDE,** U.S.P. XXIII. $LiOH.x.H_2O$. Lithium hydroxide monohydrate.
Use: Manic-depressive states.

LITHONATE. (Solvay) Lithium carbonate 300 mg/Cap. Bot. 100s, 1000s, Unit-of-use 90s, 100s, 120s, UD 100s.
Use: Antipsychotic agent.

LITHOSTAT. (Mission) Acetohydroxamic acid 250 mg/Tab. Bot. 120s.
Use: Urinary anti-infective.

LITHOTABS. (Solvay) Lithium carbonate 300 mg/Tab. Bot. 100s, 1000s, UD 100s.
Use: Antipsychotic agent.

LIVEC. (Enzyme Process) Vitamins A 5000 IU, B_1 1.5 mg, B_2 1.7 mg, niacin 20 mg, C 60 mg, B_6 2 mg, pantothenic acid 10 mg, E 30 IU, B_{12} 6 mcg, calcium 250 mg, iron 5 mg, D 400 IU, folacin 0.075 mg/3 Tab. Bot. 100s, 300s.
Use: Vitamin/mineral supplement.

LIVER, B12 AND FOLIC ACID. (Lincoln) Vitamin B_{12} activity 5 mcg, cyanocobalamin 35 mcg, cyanocobalamin 5 mg,

folic acid, w/phenol 0.5%, sodium citrate 0.25%, disodium sequestrene 0.01%, sodium bisulfite 0.025%/ml. Vial 15 ml.
Use: Nutritional supplement.

LIVERBEX. (Spanner) Liver 2 mcg, vitamins B_1, B_2, B_6, B_{12}, niacinamide, pantothenate/ml. Vial 30 ml.
Use: Nutritional supplement.

LIVER COMBO NO. 5. (Rugby) Liver vitamin B_{12} equivalent 10 mcg, crystalline B_{12} 100 mcg, folic acid 0.4 mg/ml. Inj. Vial 10 ml.
Use: Parenteral liver supplement.

LIVER, CRUDE. (Various Mfr.) Vitamin B_{12} 2 mcg/ml. Inj. Vials 30 ml.
Use: Parenteral liver supplement.

LIVER DERIVATIVE COMPLEX.
See: Kutapressin, Inj. (Kremers-Union).

LIVER DESICCATED. Desiccated liver substance.

LIVER EXTRACT. Dry liver extract w/Vitamin B_{12}, folic acid.

LIVER FUNCTION AGENTS.
See. Bromsulphalein, Amp. (Llynson, Westcott & Dunning).
　Iodophthalein (Various Mfr.).
　Sulfobromophthalein Sodium U.S.P. XXIII (Gotham).

LIVERGRAN. (Rawl) Desiccated whole liver 9 Gm, vitamins B_1 18 mg, B_2 36 mg, niacinamide 90 mg, choline bitartrate 216 mg, B_6 3.6 mg, calcium pantothenate 3.6 mg, inositol 90 mg, biotin 6 mcg, vitamins B_{12} 5.4 mcg, methionine 198 mg, arginine 242 mg, cystine 72 mg, glutamic acid 675 mg, histidine 99 mg, isoleucine 333 mg, leucine 495 mg, lysine 297 mg, phenylalanine 189 mg, threonine 333 mg, tryptophan 45 mg, tyrosine 180 mg, valine 306 mg/3 Tsp. Bot. 15 oz.
Use: Nutritional supplement.

LIVER INJECTION. (Various Mfr.). Liver extract for parenteral use.
Use: Parenteral liver supplement.

LIVER INJECTION. (Arcum; Lederle) Vitamin B_{12} 20 mcg/ml. Vial 10 ml.
Use: Nutritional supplement.

LIVER INJECTION, CRUDE. (Lilly) 2 mcg/ml. Vial 30 ml; (Medwick) 2 mcg/ml. Vial 30 ml.
Use: Liver supplement.

LIVER, IRON, FOLIC & COBALT. (Kenyon) Liver refined (B_{12} equivalent) 10 mcg, iron peptonate 59 mg, cobalt gluconate 9 mg, folic acid 5 mg, procaine HCl 1%/2 ml. Vial 30 ml.
Use: Nutritional supplement.

LIVER, IRON, VITAMINS. (Kenyon) Liver (B_{12} equivalent) 1 mcg, iron gluconate

59 mg, niacinamide 50 mg, vitamin B_2 (as 5-phos.) 0.3 mg, B_6 0.3 mg, sodium dicitrate 10 mg/2 ml, procaine HCl 1%. Vial 30 ml.
LIVER, IRON & VITAMINS. (Pharmex) Liver (equivalent to vitamin B_{12} 1 mcg) 100 mg, vitamin B_{12} 5 mcg, B_2 0.3 mg, B_6 0.3 mg, niacinamide 50 mg, iron peptonate 19.5 mg, sodium citrate 1%, phenol 0.5%/3 ml. Vial 30 ml.
Use: Nutritional supplement.
LIVER, IRON, VITAMINS AND AMINO ACIDS. (Kenyon) Liver B_{12} equivalent, 1 mcg, ferrous gluconate 50 mg, B_2 (as 5-phos.) 0.5 mg, d-panthenol 2.5 mg, niacinamide 100 mg, dl-methionine 10 mg, choline Cl 5 mg/2 ml. Vial 30 ml.
Use: Nutritional supplement.
LIVER IRON VITAMINS INJ. (Arcum) Liver inj. (10 mcg B_{12} activity/ml) 0.1 ml, crude liver inj. (2 mcg B_{12} activity/ml) 0.125 ml, green ferric ammonium citrate 20 mg, niacinamide 50 mg, vitamin B_6 0.3 mg, B_2 0.3 mg, procaine HCl 0.5%, phenol 0.5%/2 ml. Vial 30 ml.
Use: Nutritional supplement.
LIVER, IRON, VITAMINS WITH B12. (Kenyon) Liver (B_{12} equivalent) 2 mcg, vitamin B_{12} 15 mcg, ferrous lactate 20 mg, B_1 10 mg, B_2 (as 5-phos.) 9.5 mg, B_6 1 mg, d-panthenol 1 mg, niacinamide 10 mg, choline Cl 0.5 mg/ml. Vial 30.
Use: Nutritional supplement.
LIVER, REFINED. (Medwick) 20 mcg/ml. Vial 10 ml, 30 ml.
Use: Nutritional supplement.
LIVER VASOCONSTRICTOR.
See: Kutapressin, Vial, Amp. (Kremers-Urban).
LIVIFOL. (Dunhall) Vitamin B_{12} activity from liver inj. equivalent to cyanocobalamin 10 mcg, folic acid 1 mg, cyanocobalamin 100 mcg/ml. Vial 10 ml.
Use: Vitamin/mineral supplement.
LIVITAMIN.(Beecham Labs) Ferrous fumarate 100 mg, Vitamins B_1 3 mg, B_2 3 mg, B_6 3 mg, C 100 mg, niacinamide 10 mg, calcium pantothenate 2 mg, B_{12} 5 mcg, copper 0.66 mg, desiccated liver 150 mg/Cap. Bot. 100s.
Use: Vitamin/mineral supplement.
LIVITAMIN CHEWABLE TABLETS. (Beecham Labs) Ferrous fumarate 50 mg, Vitamins C 100 mg, B_1 3 mg, B_2 3 mg, niacinamide 10 mg, B_6 3 mg, calcium pantothenate 2 mg, cyanocobalamin 5 mcg, copper 0.33 mg/Tab. Bot. 100s.
Use: Vitamin/mineral supplement.
LIVITAMIN W/INTRINSIC FACTOR. (Beecham Labs) Desiccated liver 150

mg, ferrous fumarate 100 mg, Vitamins B_1 3 mg, C 100 mg, B_2 3 mg, niacinamide 10 mg, B_{12} 5 mcg, B_6 3 mg, calcium pantothenate 2 mg, copper 0.66 mg, B_{12} w/intrinsic factor 1/3 units/Cap. Bot. 100s.
Use: Vitamin/mineral supplement.
LIVITRINSIC LIQUID. (Beecham Labs) Iron peptonized N.F. 210 mg, liver fraction No. 1 0.5 Gm, Vitamins B_1 3 mg, B_2 3 mg, niacinamide 10 mg, B_6 HCl 3 mg, pantothenic acid 2 mg, B_{12} 5 mcg, copper 0.66 mg/15 ml. Bot. 8 oz, pt, gal.
Use: Vitamin/mineral supplement.
LIVITRINSIC-F CAPSULES. (Goldline) Iron 36.3 mg, vitamins B_{12} 15 mcg, C 75 mg, intrinsic factor concentrate 240 mg, folic acid 0.5 mg/Cap. Bot. 100s, 1000s.
Use: Vitamin/mineral supplement.
LIV-O-REX. (Nutrition) Desiccated liver 1.4 gr, green iron, ammonium citrate 3 gr, Vitamins B_1 1.5 mg, B_2 0.5 mg, calcium pantothenate 0.25 mg, B_6 0.15 mg, niacinamide 10 mg/Cap. Bot. 100s, 1000s.
Use: Vitamin/mineral supplement.
LIVOSTIN. (Iolab) Levocabastine HCl 0.05%, benzalkonium chloride 0.15 mg, propylene glycol, EDTA. Susp. Dropper Bot. 2.5 ml, 5 ml, 10 ml.
Use: Antiallergy agent, ophthalmic.
LIV-O-VITE. (Jenkins) Ferrous fumarate 3 gr (elemental iron 1 gr), desiccated liver 2 gr, thiamine HCl 3 mg, riboflavin 3 mg, cyanocobalamin 3 mcg/Tab. Bot. 1000s.
Use: Vitamin/mineral supplement.
• **LIXAZINONE SULFATE.** USAN.
Use: Cardiotonic (phosphodiesterase inhibitor).
LIXOIL. (Lixoil Labs.) Sulfonated fatty oils and one or more esters of higher fatty acids. Bot. 16 oz.
Use: Dermatologic.
LKV-DROPS. (Freeda) Vitamins A 5000 IU, D 400 IU, E 2 mg, B_1 1.5 mg, B_2 1.5 mg, B_3 10 mg, B_5 2 mg, B_6 2 mg, B_{12} 6 mcg, C 50 mg, biotin 50 mcg/0.6 ml. Bot. 60 ml.
Use: Vitamin supplement.
LLD FACTOR.
See: Vitamin B_{12}, Preps. (Various Mfr.).
L-LEUCOVORIN.
Use: Antineoplastic.
See: Isovorin.
LM-427. Ribabutin.
Use: CDC anti-infective agent.
LMD. (Abbott Hospital Prods) Low molecular weight dextran. LMD 10% w/v in D5-W and LMD 10% w/v in saline 0.9%, 500 ml each.

Use: Plasma volume expander.
LMWD-DEXTRAN 40. (Pharmachem) Normal saline 0.9%, dextrose 10%.
Use: Plasma volume expander.
LOBAC. (Seatrace) Salicylamide 200 mg, phenyltoloxamine 20 mg, acetaminophen 300 mg/Cap. Bot. 100s.
Use: Muscle relaxant, analgesic.
LOBAK TABLETS. (Sanofi Winthrop) Chlormezanone 250 mg, acetaminophen 300 mg/Tab. In 40s, 100s, 1000s.
Use: Antianxiety agent, analgesic.
LOBANA BODY. (Ulmer) Mineral oil, triethanolamine stearate, stearic acid, lanolin, cetyl alcohol, potassium stearate, propylene glycol parabens. Lot. Bot. 120, 240 ml, gal.
Use: Emollient.
LOBANA BODY SHAMPOO. (Ulmer) Bot. 8 oz, gal.
Use: Hair & body cleanser.
LOBANA CONDITIONING SHAMPOO. (Ulmer) Bot. 8 oz, gal.
Use: Shampoo for hair and scalp.
LOBANA DERM-ADE CREAM. (Ulmer) Vitamin A, D, E cream. Jar 2 oz, 8 oz.
Use: Minor skin irritations.
LOBANA LIQUID HAND SOAP. (Ulmer) Dispenser 14 oz, refill 24 oz. Bot. gal.
Use: Cleanser.
LOBANA PERI-GARD. (Ulmer) Water-resistant ointment containing vitamin A & D. Jar 2 oz, 8 oz.
Use: Skin protectant.
LOBANA PERINEAL CLEANSER. (Ulmer) Sprayer 4 oz, 8 oz. Bot. gal.
Use: Urine and fecal cleanser.
LOBELIA FLUIDEXTRACT. W/Hyoscyamus fluidextract, grindelia fluidextract, potassium iodide.
See: L.S. Mixture, Liq. (Paddock).
LOBELINE SULFATE.
See: Lobidram, Tab. (Dram). Nikoban, Loz., Gum. (Thompson).
• **LOBENDAZOLE.** USAN.
Use: Anthelmintic.
• **LOBENZARIT SODIUM.** USAN
Use: Antirheumatic.
LOBIDRAM. (Dram) Lobeline sulfate 2 mg/Tab. Pkg. 15s, 30s.
Use: Withdrawal symptoms of smoking.
LOCOID. (Ferndale) **Cream:** Hydrocortisone butyrate 0.1%. Tube 15 Gm, 45 Gm. **Oint.:** Hydrocortisone butyrate 0.1%. Tube 15 Gm, 45 Gm. **Soln.:** Hydrocortisone butyrate 0.1%, isopropyl alcohol 50%, glycerin, povidone. Bot. 20 ml, 60 ml.
Use: Corticosteroid, topical.

LODINE. (Wyeth-Ayerst) Etodolac 200, 300 or 400 mg/Cap. Bot. 100s, UD 100s.
Use: Nonsteroidal anti-inflammatory agent.
LODOSYN. (Merck & Co.) Carbidopa 25 mg/Tab. Bot. 100s.
Use: Antiparkinson agent.
• **LODOXAMIDE ETHYL.** USAN.
Use: Antiasthmatic, anti-allergic.
• **LODOXAMIDE TROMETHAMINE.** USAN.
Use: Antiasthmatic, anti-allergic, vernal keratoconjunctivitis [Orphan drug]
See: Alomide, Soln. (Alcon).
LODRANE CR. (Poythress) Theophylline anhydrous 100 mg, 200 mg or 300 mg/CR Tab. Bot. 100s, 500s, 1000s, UD 100s, 500s, 1000s.
Use: Bronchodialtor.
LOESTRIN 21 1/20. (Parke-Davis) Norethindrone acetate 1 mg, ethinyl estradiol 20 mcg Tab. Petipac compact 21 Tab. Ctn. 5 compacts or Ctn. 5 refills.
Use: Oral contraceptive.
LOESTRIN 21 1.5/30. (Parke-Davis) Norethindrone acetate 1.5 mg, ethinyl estradiol 30 mg/Tab. Petipac compact. Ctn. 5 compacts or Ctn. 5 refills.
Use: Oral contraceptive.
LOESTRIN Fe 1/20. (Parke-Davis) **White Tab.:** Norethindrone acetate 1 mg, ethinyl estradiol 20 mcg/Tab.; **Brown Tab.:** Ferrous fumarate 75 mg (7 tabs.) Carton 5 petipac compacts 28 Tab., carton of 5 refills 28 Tab.
Use: Oral contraceptive.
LOESTRIN Fe 1.5/30. (Parke-Davis) **Green Tab.:** Norethindrone acetate 1.5 mg, ethinyl estradiol 30 mcg. **Brown Tab.:** Ferrous fumarate 75 mg (7 tabs.). Carton 5 petipac compacts 28 Tab., carton of 5 refills 28 Tab.
Use: Oral contraceptive.
• **LOFEMIZOLE HYDROCHLORIDE.** USAN.
Use: Anti-inflammatory.
LOFENALAC. (Mead Johnson Nutrition) Corn syrup solids 49.2%, casein hydrolysate 18.7% (enzymic digest of casein containing amino acids and small peptides), corn oil 18%, modified tapioca starch 9.57%, protein equivalent 15%, fat 18%, carbohydrate 60%, minerals (ash) 3.6%, phenylalanine 75 mg/100 Gm pow., Vitamins A 1600 IU, D 400 IU, E 10 IU, C 52 mg, folic acid 100 mcg, B$_1$ 0.5 mg, B$_2$ 0.6 mg, niacin 8 mg, B$_6$ 0.4 mg, B$_{12}$ 2 mcg, biotin 0.05 mg, pantothenic acid 3 mg, Vitamin K-1 100 mcg, choline 85 mg, inositol 30 mg, cal-

cium 600 mg, phosphorus 450 mg, iodine 45 mcg, iron 12 mg, magnesium 70 mg, copper 0.6 mg, zinc 4 mg, manganese 1 mg, chloride 450 mg, potassium 650 mg, sodium 300 mg/qt. at normal dilution of 20 k cal/fl oz, Can 2 1/2 lb.
Use: Enteral nutritional supplement.
LOFENE. (Lannett) Diphenoxylate HCl 2.5 mg, atropine sulfate 0.025 mg Bot. 100s, 500s, 1000s.
Use: Antidiarrheal.
•**LOFENTANIL OXALATE.** USAN.
Use: Analgesic, narcotic.
LOFEPRAMINE. B.A.N. 5-3-[N-(4-Chlorophenacyl)methylamino]-propyl-10, 11-dihydrobenz[b,f]azepine. Lopramine (I.N.N.).
Use: Antidepressant.
•**LOFEPRAMINE HYDROCHLORIDE.** USAN.
Use: Antidepressant.
•**LOFEXIDINE HYDROCHLORIDE.** USAN.
Use: Antihypertensive.
LOGEN LIQUID. (Goldline) Diphenoxylate HCl w/atropine sulfate. Bot. 2 oz.
Use: Antidiarrheal.
LOGEN TABLETS. (Goldline) Diphenoxylate HCl, atropine sulfate. Bot. 100s, 500s, 1000s.
Use: Antidiarrheal.
L.O.L. LOTION. (O'Leary) Bot 8 oz, 16 oz.
Use: Anti-acne.
LOMANATE. (Various Mfr.) Diphenoxylate HCl 2.5 mg, atropine sulfate 0.025 mg/5 ml. Bot. 60 ml.
Use: Antidiarrheal.
LOMEFLOXACIN HCl.
Use: Antibiotic, fluoroquinolone.
See: Maxaquin, Tab. (Searle).
•**LOMETRALINE HYDROCHLORIDE.** USAN.
Use: Antipsychotic, antiparkinson agent.
•**LOMETREXOL SODIUM.** USAN.
Use: Antineoplastic.
•**LOMOFUNGIN.** USAN.
Use: Antifungal.
LOMOTIL. (Searle) Diphenoxylate HCl 2.5 mg, atropine sulfate 0.025 mg/Tab. or 5 ml. **Tab.:** Bot. 100s, 500s, 1000s, 2500s, UD 100s. **Liq.:** Bot. w/dropper 2 oz.
Use: Antidiarrheal.
•**LOMUSTINE.** USAN. CCNU; NSC-79037. 1-(2-Chloroethyl)-3-cyclohexyl-1-nitrosourea.
Use: Antineoplastic agent.
See: CeeNu, Cap. (Bristol).

LONALAC. (Mead Johnson Nutrition) Protein as casein 21%, fat as coconut oil 49%, carbohydrate as lactose 30%, vitamins A 1440 IU, B_1 0.6 mg, B_2 2.6 mg, niacin 1.2 mg, calcium 1.69 Gm, phosphorous 1.5 Gm, chloride 750 mg, potassium 1.88 Gm, sodium 38 mg, magnesium 135 mg/qt, Pow, Can 16 oz.
Use: Enteral nutritional supplement.
•**LONAPALENE.** USAN.
Use: Antipsoriatic.
LONG ACTING NASAL SPRAY. (Weeks & Leo) Oxymetazoline HCl 0.05%. Soln. Bot. 0.75 oz.
Use: Nasal decongestant.
LONG ACTING NEO-SYNEPHRINE II NOSE DROPS AND NASAL SPRAY. (Sanofi Winthrop Products) Xylometazoline HCl 0.1% (adult strength) or 0.05% (child strength). Bot. 1 oz, Spray 0.5 oz (adult strength).
Use: Nasal decongestant.
LONG ACTING NEO-SYNEPHRINE II VAPOR SPRAY. (Sanofi Winthrop Products) Xylometazoline HCl 0.1%. Mentholated. Spray Bot. 0.5 fl oz.
Use: Nasal decongestant.
LONITEN. (Upjohn) Minoxidil 2.5 mg or 10 mg/Tab. **2.5 mg:** Unit-of-Use Bot. 100s. **10 mg:** Bot. 500s, Unit-of-Use Bot. 100s.
Use: Antihypertensive.
LONOX. (Geneva Generics) Diphenoxylate HCl 2.5 mg, atropine sulfate 0.025 mg/Tab. Bot. 100s, 500s, 1000s, UD 100s.
Use: Antidiarrheal.
LO/OVRAL. (Wyeth-Ayerst) Norgestrel 0.3 mg, ethinyl estradiol 0.03 mg/Tab. Pilpak dispenser 6s, Tab. 21s.
Use: Oral contraceptive.
LO/OVRAL-28. (Wyeth-Ayerst) Tab. 21s, each containing norgestrel 0.03 mg, ethinyl estradiol 0.03 mg, 7 pink inert. Tab. Pilpak dispenser 6s, Tab 28s.
Use: Oral contraceptive.
•**LOPERAMIDE HCL,** U.S.P. XXIII. Cap., U.S.P. XXIII, Tab., U.S.P. XXIII.
Use: Antiperistaltic.
See: Imodium, Cap. (Ortho).
LOPID. (Parke-Davis) Gemfibrozil. 600 mg/Tab. Bot. 60s.
Use: Antihyperlipidemic agent.
LOPRESSOR. (Geigy) Metoprolol tartrate. **Tab.:** 50 mg or 100 mg. Bot. 100s, 1000s, UD 100s, Gy-Pak 60s, 100s. **Amp.:** 5 mg/5 ml.
Use: Beta-adrenergic blocking agent.
LOPRESSOR HCT. (Geigy) Metoprolol tartrate, hydrochlorothiazide. **Tab.:**

50/25 mg, 100/25 mg or 100/50 mg. Bot. 100s.
Use: Beta-adrenergic blocking agent.
LOPROX. (Hoechst) Ciclopirox olamine 1% in cream base. Tube 15 Gm, 30 Gm, 90 Gm.
Use: Antifungal, external.
LOPURIN. (Boots) Allopurinol 100 mg or 300 mg/Tab. Bot. 100s, 1000s, UD 100s.
Use: Agent for gout.
LORABID. (Lilly). **Cap.:** Loracarbef 200 mg Cap. 30s. **Pow. for Susp.:** 100 mg/5 ml, 200 mg/5 ml Susp. 50 ml, 100 ml.
Use: Antibiotic, cephalosporin.
•**LORACARBEF.** USAN.
Use: Antibacterial.
See: Lorabid, Cap., Pow. (Lilly).
•**LORAJMINE HYDROCHLORIDE.** USAN.
Use: Cardiac depressant.
•**LORATADINE.** USAN.
Use: Antihistamine.
See: Claritin.
•**LORAZEPAM,** U.S.P. XXIII, Tab., Inj., Oral Concentrate. 7-Chloro-5-(o-chlorophenyl)-1,3-dihydro-3-hydroxy-2H-1,4-benzodiazepin-2-one.
Use: Minor tranquilizer.
See: Alzapam, Tab. (Ultra).
    Ativan, Tab., Inj. (Wyeth-Ayerst).
LORAZEPAM. (Purepac) Lorazepam. **0.5 mg:** Tab. Bot. 100s, 500s. **1 mg, 2 mg:** Tab. Bot. 100s, 500s, 1000s.
Use: Antianxiety, sedative/hypnotic.
LORAZEPAM. (Steris Labs) Lorazepam, benzyl alcohol 2%. Inj. 2 mg/ml, 4 mg/ml. Vial 1 ml, 10 ml.
Use: Antianxiety, sedative/hypnotic.
LORAZEPAM INTENSOL. (Roxane) Lorazepam 2 mg/ml. Concentrated oral soln. Dropper Bot. 30 ml.
Use: Antianxiety, sedative/hypnotic.
•**LORBAMATE.** USAN.
Use: Muscle relaxant.
•**LORCAINIDE HYDROCHLORIDE.** USAN.
Use: Cardiac depressant.
LORCET. (UAD Labs) Hydrocodone bitartrate 5 mg, acetaminophen 500 mg/Tab. Bot. 100s.
Use: Narcotic analgesic combination.
LORCET HD. (UAD Labs) Hydrocodone bitartrate 5 mg, acetaminophen 500 mg/Cap. Bot. 100s.
Use: Narcotic analgesic combination.
LORCET PLUS. (UAD Labs) Hydrocodone bitartrate 7.5 mg, acetaminophen 650 mg/Tab. Bot. 100s.
Use: Narcotic analgesic combination.
•**LORECLEZOLE.** USAN.

Use: Antiepileptic.
LORELCO. (Merrell Dow) Probucol 250 mg/Tab. Bot. 120s.
Use: Antihyperlipidemic.
•**LORMETAZEPAM.** USAN.
Use: Sedative/hypnotic.
•**LORNOXICAM.** USAN.
Use: Anti-inflammatory; analgesic.
LOROXIDE. (Dermik) Benzoyl peroxide 5.5%, propylene glycol, cetyl alcohol, hydroxyethylcellulose, kaolin, caramel, talc, cholesterol and related sterols, propylene glycolstearate, polysorbate 20, lanolin alcohol, propylparaben, methylparaben, tetrasodium EDTA, pH buffers, antioxidants, silicone emulsion, silica, decyl oleate, vegetable oil, purcelline oil syn., titanium dioxide, cyclohexanediamine tetraacetic acid, calcium phosphate. Lot. Bot. 25 Gm.
Use: Anti-acne.
LORPHEN. (Geneva) **Cap.:** Chlorpheniramine maleate 8 mg or 12 mg. Bot. 100s. **Tab.:** 4 mg. Bot. 100s.
Use: Antihistamine.
LORPRN. (Russ) Aspirin 325 mg, caffeine 40 mg, butalbital 50 mg/Cap. Bot. 100s
Use: Narcotic analgesic combination.
LORTAB. (Russ) Hydrocodone 2.5 mg, acetaminophen 325 mg/Tab. Bot. 100s, UD 100s.
Use: Narcotic analgesic combination.
LORTAB 5. (Russ) Hydrocodone 5 mg, acetaminophen 500 mg/Tab. Bot. 100s, 500s, UD 100s.
Use: Narcotic analgesic combination.
LORTAB 7. (Russ) Hydrocodone 7.5 mg, acetaminophen 500 mg/Tab. Bot. 100s, UD 100s.
Use: Narcotic analgesic combination.
LORTAB ASA. (Russ) Hydrocodone bitartrate 5 mg, aspirin 500 mg/Tab. Bot. 100s.
Use: Narcotic analgesic combination.
LORTAB LIQUID. (Russ) Hydrocodone 2.5 mg, acetaminophen 120 mg/5 ml w/alcohol 7%. Bot. 1 oz, 4 oz, pt
Use: Narcotic analgesic combination.
•**LORTALAMINE.** USAN.
Use: Antidepressant.
•**LORZAFONE.** USAN.
Use: Minor tranquilizer.
•**LOSARTAN POTASSIUM.** USAN.
Use: Antihypertensive; treatment of CHF (angiotensin II receptor blocker).
LOSEC.
See: Prilosec.
LOSOPAN LIQUID. (Goldline) Magaldrate 540 mg/5 ml. Bot. 12 oz.

Use: Antacid.

LOSOPAN PLUS LIQUID. (Goldline) Magaldrate 540 mg, simethicone 20 mg/5 ml. Bot. 12 oz.
Use: Antacid, antiflatulent.

• **LOSOXANTRONE HYDROCHLORIDE.** USAN.
Use: Antineoplastic.

• **LOSULAZINE HYDROCHLORIDE.** USAN.
Use: Antihypertensive.

LOTALBA CREAM. (Durel) Lotalba 30%, zinc oxide 10%, sulfur potassium 5%, greaseless ointment base 55%. Jar 3 oz, lb.
Use: Anti-acne.

LOTALBA OINTMENT. (Durel) Stabilized white lotion (lotio alba), glycerine, mineral gums. Jar 3 oz, lb.
Use: Anti-acne.

LOTAWIN CAPSULES. (Sanofi Winthrop) Oxypertine.
Use: Anxiolytic, tranquilizer.

• **LOTEPREDNOL ETABONATE.** USAN.
Use: Anti-inflammatory (topical).

LOTENSIN. (Ciba) Benazepril HCl 5 mg, 10 mg, 20 mg, or 40 mg/Tab. Bot. 100s, UD 100s.
Use: Antihypertensive.

LOTIO ALBA. White lotion.
Use: Anti-acne, antiseborrheic.
W/Sulfur, calamine, alcohol.
See: Sulfa-Lo, Lot. (Whorton).

LOTIO ALSULFA. (Doak) Colloidal sulfur 5%. Bot. 4 oz.
Use: Anti-acne, antiseborrheic.

LOTION-JEL. (C.S. Dent) Benzocaine in gel base. Tube 0.2 oz.
Use: Local anesthetic.

LOTOCREME. (C.S. Dent) Bot. 8 oz.
Use: Body rub.

LOTRIMIN. (Schering) Clotrimazole 1%.
Cream: Tube 15 Gm, 30 Gm, 45 Gm, 90 Gm. **Lot.:** Bot. 30 ml. **Soln.:** 1%. Bot. 10 ml, 30 ml.
Use: Antifungal, external.

LOTRIMIN AF. Powder: Miconazole nitrate 2%. Talc. In 90 g. **Spray Liquid:** Miconazole nitrate 2%, SD alcohol 40 17%. In 113 ml. **Spray Powder:** Miconazole nitrate 2%, SD alcohol 40 10%. In 100 g.
Use: Antifungal, external.

LOTRISONE. (Schering) Clotrimazole 1%, betamethasone dipropionate 0.05%/Gm. Tube 15 Gm, 45 Gm.
Use: Antifungal, external.

LOSOTRON PLUS LIQUID. (Various Mfr.) Magaldrate 540 mg, simethicone 20 mg/5 ml. Bot. 360 ml.

Use: Antacid, antiflatulent.

LO-TROP. (Vangard) Diphenoxylate HCl 2.5 mg, atropine sulfate 0.025 mg/Tab. Bot. 100s, 1000s.
Use: Antidiarrheal.

• **LOVASTATIN.** USAN. Butanoic acid, 2-methyl-, 1,2,3,7,8,8a-hexahydro-3,7-dimethyl-8-[2-(tetra-hydro-4-hydroxy-6-oxo-2H-pyran-2-yl)-ethyl]-1-naphthalenyl ester,
[1S-[1α(R*),3α,7β,8β(2S-*,-4S*),8aβ]]-; (2) (S)-2-Methylbutyric acid, 8-ester with (4R,-6R)-6-[2-[(1S,2S,6R,8S,8aR)-1,2,6,7,8,8a-hexahydro-8-hydroxy-2,6-dimethyl-1-naphthyl]ethyl]tetrahydro-4-hydroxy-2H-pyran-2-one.
Use: Antihypercholesteremic.
See: Mevacor, Tab. (Merck & Co.).

LOVE LONGER. (Youngs Drug) Benzocaine 7.5% in water-soluble lubricant base. Tube 0.5 oz.
Use: Local anesthetic.

LOVENOX. (Rhone-Poulenc Rorer) Enoxaparin sodium. 30 mg/0.3 ml. Inj. Pk. 10 prefilled syringes w/26 guage x 1/2-inch needle.
Use: Anticoagulant.

LOWILA CAKE. (Westwood) Sodium lauryl sulfoacetate, dextrin, boric acid, urea, sorbitol, mineral oil, PEG 14 M, lactic acid, cellulose gum, docusate sodium, water, fragrance. Cake 3¾ oz.
Use: Skin cleanser.

LOW-QUEL. (Blue Cross) Diphenoxylate HCl 2.5 mg, atropine sulfate 0.025 mg/Tab. Bot. 100s.
Use: Antidiarrheal.

LOWSIUM. (Rugby) Magaldrate 540 mg/5 ml. Susp. Bot. 360 ml.
Use: Antacid.

LOWSIUM PLUS. (Rugby) **Tab.:** Magaldrate 480 mg, simethicone 20 mg. Bot. 60s. **Susp.:** Magaldrate 540 mg, simethicone 40 mg/5 ml. Bot. 360 ml.
Use: Antacid, antiflatulent.

• **LOXAPINE.** USAN. 2-Chloro-11-(4-methyl-1-piperazinyl) dibenz [b,f] [1,4] oxazepine.
Use: Tranquilizer.

LOXAPINE HYDROCHLORIDE.
Use: Tranquilizer.
See: Daxolin Concentrate, Liq. (Miles Pharm).
Loxitane-C Oral Concentrate (Lederle).
Loxitane, Inj. (Lederle).

• **LOXAPINE SUCCINATE.** USAN. (1)2-Chloro-11-(4-methyl-1-piperazinyl) dibenz-[b,f] [1,4]-oxazepine succinate; (2) Succinic acid compound with 2-

chloro-11-(4-methyl-1-piperazinyl) dibenz-[b,f] [1,4] oxazepine. (Various Mfr.) 5 mg, 10 mg, 25 mg or 50 mg. Cap. Bot. 100s.
Use: Tranquilizer.
See: Loxitane, Cap. (Lederle).
LOXITANE-C. (Lederle) Loxapine HCl oral concentrate 25 mg/ml. Bot. 120 ml w/dropper.
Use: Antipsychotic agent.
LOXITANE CAPSULES. (Lederle) Loxapine succinate. **5 mg/Cap.**: Bot. 100s, UD 10 × 10s. **10 mg, 25 mg or 50 mg/Cap.**: Bot. 100s, 1000s, UD 10 10s.
Use: Antipsychotic agent.
LOXITANE IM. (Lederle) Loxitane HCl (base equivalent) 50 mg/ml. Amp 1 ml. Box 10s.
Use: Antipsychotic agent.
•**LOXORIBINE.** USAN.
Use: Immunostimulant; vaccine adjuvant. [Orphan drug]
L₂OXOTHIAZOLIDINE₄CARBOXYLIC ACID.
Use: Treatment of adult respiratory distress syndrome.
See: Procysteine.
LOZOL. (Rhone-Poulenc Rorer) Indapamide 2.5 mg/Tab. Bot. 100s, 1000s, 2500s, Strip dispenser 100s.
Use: Diuretic, antihypertensive.
L-PAM. p-Di(2-chloroethyl) amino-L-phenylalamine.
Use: An alkylating antineoplastic agent. Under study.
L-SARCOLYSIN.
See: Alkeran, Tab. (Burroughs Wellcome).
L-THREONINE.
Use: Antispasmodic.
L-TRIIODOTHYRONINE SOD.
See: Cytomel, Tab. (SK-Beecham). Liothyronine Sod.
L-TRYPTOPHAN. FDA nationwide recall of all nonprescription supplements containing L-Tryptophan.
LUBAFAX. (Burroughs Wellcome) Surgical lubricant, sterile; water soluble, nonstaining. Foil wrapper 2.7 Gm, 5 Gm. Box 144s.
Use: Surgical lubricant.
LUBATH. (Warner-Lambert Prods) Mineral oil, PPG-15, stearyl ether, oleth-2, nonoxynol-5, fragrance, FD&C Green No. 6. Bot. 4 oz, 8 oz, 16 oz.
Use: Emollient.
LUBINOL. (Purepac) Light, heavy and extra heavy mineral oil. Bot. pt, qt, gal. (Extra heavy Bot.) 8 oz, pt, qt, gal.
Use: Emollient.

LUBRASEPTIC JELLY. (Guardian) Water-soluble amyl phenyl phenol complex 0.12%, phenylmercuric nitrate, 0.007%. Bellows-type tube 10 Gm, 24s.
Use: Urethral instillation, urologic and proctologic exams.
LUBRASOL BATH OIL. (Pharmaceutical Specialties) Mineral oil, lanolin oil, PEG-200 dilaurate, oxybenzone. Bot. 240 ml, 480 ml, gal.
Use: Emollient.
LUBRIDERM CREAM. (Warner-Lambert Prods) Water, mineral oil, petrolatum, glycerin, glyceryl stearate, PEG-100 stearate, squalane, lanolin, lanolin alcohol, lanolin oil, cetyl alcohol, sorbitan laurate, fragrance (if scented), methylparaben, butylparaben, propylparaben, quaternium-15. Tube: (scented) 1.5 oz, 4 oz; (unscented) 4 oz.
Use: Emollient.
LUBRIDERM LOTION. (Warner-Lambert Prods) Water, mineral oil, petrolatum, sorbitol, lanolin, lanolin alcohol, stearic acid, TEA, cetyl alcohol, fragrance (if scented), butylparaben, methylparaben, propylparaben, sodium Cl. Bot. (scented) 4 oz, 8 oz, 16 oz; (unscented) 8 oz, 16 oz.
Use: Emollient.
LUBRIDERM LUBATH OIL. (Warner-Lambert) Mineral oil, PPG-15 stearyl ether, oleth-2, nonoxynol-5. Lanolin free. Bot. 240 ml, pt.
Use: Emollient.
LUBRIN. (Upsher-Smith) Glycerin, laureth 23, PEG 40 stearate, PEG-6-32, PEG-20, caprylic/capric triglyceride. Pkg. 5 inserts.
Use: Vaginal lubricant.
LUBRITEARS. (Bausch & Lomb) White petrolatum, mineral oil, lanolin, chlorobutanol 0.5%. Oint. Tube 3.5 g.
Use: Ocular lubricant.
LUBRITEARS SOLUTION. (Bausch & Lomb) Hydroxypropyl methylcellulose 2906 0.3%, dextran 70 0.1%, EDTA, KCl, NaCl, benzalkonium chloride 0.01%. Bot. 15 ml.
Use: Artificial tears.
•**LUCANTHONE HYDROCHLORIDE.** USAN. 1-[[2-(Diethylamino)ethyl] amino]-4-methylthioxanthen-9-one Monohydrochloride.
Use: Antischistosomal.
LUDENS COUGH DROPS. (Luden's) Honey lemon, honey licorice, menthol, strong flavor menthol, strong flavor eucalyptus or wild cherry flavored loz. Square-pack. Box, bag.

Use: Cough suppressant.
LUDIOMIL. (Ciba) Maprotiline 25 mg, 50 mg or 75 mg/Tab. Bot. 100s, Accu-Pak 100s.
Use: Antidepressant.
• **LUFIRONIL.** USAN.
Use: Collagen inhibitor.
LUFYLLIN. (Wallace) Dyphylline Inj **Amp.:** (500 mg/2 ml) Box 25s. **Elix.:** 100 mg/15 ml; alcohol 20%. Bot. pt, gal. **Tab.:** 200 mg. Bot. 100s, 1000s, UD 100s.
Use: Bronchodilator.
LUFYLLIN-400. (Wallace) Dyphylline 400 mg/Tab. Bot. 100s, 1000s.
Use: Bronchodilator.
LUFYLLIN-EPG. (Wallace) Ephedrine HCl 16 mg, dyphylline 100 mg, phenobarbital 16 mg, guaifenesin 200 mg/Tab. or 10 ml. **Tab.:** Bot. 100s. **Elix.:** (alcohol 5.5%) Bot. pt.
Use: Antiasthmatic combination.
LUFYLLIN-GG. (Wallace) **Tab.:** Dyphylline 200 mg, guaifenesin 200 mg/Tab. Bot. 100s, 1000s. **Elix.:** Dyphylline 100 mg, guaifenesin 100 mg, alcohol 17%/15 ml. Elix. Bot. pt, gal.
Use: Bronchodilator, expectorant.
LUGOL'S SOLUTION. Strong iodine soln, U.S.P. XXIII. (Lyne). Iodine 5 Gm, potassium iodide 10 Gm, in purified water to make 100 ml. Bot. 15 ml. (Wisconsin) Bot. pt.
LUMINAL INJECTION. (Sanofi Winthrop) Phenobarbital 130 mg/ml. Amp 1 ml. Box 100s.
Use: Sedative/hypnotic.
LUMOPAQUE CAPSULES. (Sanofi Winthrop) Tyropanoate sodium.
Use: Radiopaque agent.
LUNG SURFACTANTS.
Use: Surfactant replacement therapy in neonatal respiratory distress syndrome.
See: Exosurf (Burroughs Wellcome). Survanta (Ross).
LUPRON INJECTION. (TAP) Leuprolide acetate 1 mg/0.2 ml. Vial 2.8 ml.
Use: Antineoplastic agent.
LURAMIDE TABS. (Major) Furosemide 20 mg, 40 mg or 80 mg/Tab. Bot. 100s, 1000s.
Use: Diuretic.
LURIDE DROPS. (Hoyt) Sodium fluoride equivalent to 0.125 mg of fluoride/Drop. Plastic dropper bot. 30 ml.
Use: Dental caries preventative.
LURIDE-F LOZI TABLETS. (Colgate-Hoyt) Sodium fluoride in Lozi base tab. available as fluoride. **0.25 mg:** Bot.

120s; **0.5 mg:** Bot. 120s, 1200s; **1 mg:** Bot. 120s, 1000s, 5000s.
Use: Dental caries preventative.
LURIDE PROPHYLAXIS PASTE. (Hoyt) Acidulated phosphate sodium fluoride containing 0.4% fluoride ion w/silicon dioxide abrasive. UD 3 Gm, Jar 50 Gm.
Use: Tooth cleaner.
LURIDE-SF LOZI TABLETS. (Hoyt) Sodium fluoride 1 mg fluoride/Tab. Bot. 120s.
Use: Dental caries preventative.
LURIDE TOPICAL GEL. (Hoyt) Acidulated phosphate sodium fluoride containing fluoride ion 1.2% at pH 3.0 to 4.0 in gel base. Bot. 32 oz, 250 ml.
Use: Dental caries preventative.
LURIDE TOPICAL SOLUTION. (Hoyt) Acidulated phosphate sodium fluoride w/pH 3.2. Bot. 250 ml.
Use: Dental caries preventative.
LURLINE PMS. (Fielding) Acetaminophen 500 mg, pamabrom 25 mg, pyridoxine 50 mg/Tab. Bot. 24s, 50s.
Use: Analgesic combination.
• **LUROSETRON MESYLATE.** USAN.
Use: Antiemetic.
LUROTIN CAPS. (BASF Wyandotte) Beta-carotene 25 mg/Cap. Bot. 100s.
Use: Nutritional supplement.
LUTEOGAN.
See: Progesterone (Various Mfr.).
LUTEOSAN.
See: Progesterone (Various Mfr.).
LUTOCYLOL. (Ciba) Ethisterone.
LUTOLIN-F. (Spanner) Progesterone 25 mg or 50 mg/ml. Vial 10 ml.
Use: Progestin.
LUTOLIN-S. (Spanner) Progesterone 25 mg/ml. Vial 10 ml.
Use: Progestin.
• **LUTRELIN ACETATE.** USAN.
Use: Agonist.
LUTREN.
See: Progesterone (Various Mfr.).
LUTREPULSE. (Ortho) Gonadorelin acetate 0.8 mg or 3.2 mg/vial. Pow. for reconstitution (lyophilized). Vial 10 ml.
Use: Gonadotropin-releasing hormone.
LUTUTRIN.
See: Lutrexin, Tab. (Hynson, Westcott & Dunning).
• **LYAPOLATE SODIUM.** USAN. Sodium ethenesulfonate polymer. Peson (Hoechst).
Use: Anticoagulant.
• **LYCETAMINE.** USAN.
Use: Antimicrobial.
LYCINE HYDROCHLORIDE.
See: Betaine HCl (Various Mfr.).

LYCOLAN ELIXIR. (Lannett) Glycocoll 28 gr, lysine 100 mg in Tokay wine base/15 ml. Bot. pt.
Use: Vitamin supplement.
LYDIA E. PINKHAM HERBAL COMPOUND. (Numark) Vitamin C, iron. Bot. 8 fl oz, 16 fl oz.
LYDIA E. PINKHAM TABLETS. (Numark) Vitamin C, iron, calcium. 72s, 150s.
•**LYDIMYCIN.** USAN.
Use: Antifungal.
LYMECYCLINE. B.A.N. A water-soluble combination of tetracycline, lysine and formaldehyde. Armyl; Mucomycin; Tetralysal.
Use: Antibiotic.
LYMPHAZURIN. (Hirsch) Isosulfan blue 10 mg, sodium monohydrogen phosphate 6.6 mg, potassium dihydrogen phosphate 2.7 mg/ml. Vial 5 ml.
Use: Radiopaque agent.
LYMPHOCYTE IMMUNE GLOBULIN.
Use: Management of rejection in renal transplant.
See: Atgam, Inj. (Upjohn).
LYMPHOGRANULOMA VENEREUM ANTIGEN, U.S.P. XXI. Lymphogranuloma venereum skin test antigen.
Use: Diagnostic aid (dermal reactivity indicator).
•**LYNESTRENOL.** USAN.(1) 19-Nor-17α-pregn-4-en-20-yn-17-ol; (2) 17α-Ethinyl-17β-hydroxyestr-4-ene. Orgametril.
Use: Progestin.
LYNOESTRENOL. Lynestrenol.
LYPHOCIN P. (Lyphomed) Vancomycin HCl 500 mg. Vial 10 ml.
Use: Anti-infective.
LYPHOLYTE. (Lyphomed) Multiple electrolye concentrate. Vial 20 ml, 40 ml, Maxivial 100 ml, 200 ml.
Use: Electrolyte replacement.
LYPHOLYTE II. (Lyphomed) Na$^+$ 35 mEq/L, K$^+$ 20 mEq/L, Ca^{++} 4.5 mEq/L, Mg$^{''}$ 5 mEq/L, Cl 35 mEq/L, acetate 29.5 mEq/L. Single dose flip-top vial 20 ml, 40 ml; flip top vial 100 ml, 200 ml.
Use: Parenteral nutritional supplement.
•**LYPRESSIN NASAL SOLUTION,** U.S.P. XXIII. 8-Lysine vasopressin. Syntopressin.
Use: Antidiuretic.
See: Diapid Nasal Spray (Sandoz).
LYSERGIDE. B.A.N. NN-Diethyl-lysergamide. Lysergic acid diethylamide LSD, Delysid.
Use: Psychotomimetic.
LYSIDIN. Methyl glyoxalidin.
LYSINE. USAN.

Use: Nutrient, rapid weight gain.
•**LYSINE ACETATE,** U.S.P. XXIII. $C_6H_14N_2O_2$-$C_2H_4O_2$
Use: Amino acid.
•**LYSINE MONOHYDROCHLORIDE,** U.S.P. XXIII. $C_6H_14N_2O_2$-HCl
Use: Amino acid.
See: Enisyl, Tab. (Person & Covey).
LYSITONE. (Jenkins) l-Lysine HCl 300 mg, iron peptonate 200 mg, cobalamine concentrate 10 mcg, vitamins B$_1$ 10 mg, niacinamide 20 mg, B$_2$ 2.5 mg, B$_6$ 2 mg, panthenol 2 mg, d-sorbitol 1.83 Gm, alcohol 11%/fl oz. Bot. 3 oz, 8 oz, gal.
Use: Vitamin/mineral supplement.
LYSIVANE.
See: Parsidol, Tab. (Warner-Chilcott).
LYSODREN. (Bristol-Myers/Bristol Oncology) Mitotane 500 mg/Tab. Bot. 100s.
Use: Antineoplastic agent.
•**LYSOSTAPHIN.** USAN. Antibiotic derived from *Staphylococcus staphylolyticus.*
Use: Antibiotic.
LYSURIDE. B.A.N. 9-(3,3-Diethylureido)-4,6,-6a,7,8,9-hexahydro-7-methylindolo[4,3-f,g]-quinoline.
Use: Prophylaxis of migraine.
LYTEERS. (Barnes-Hind) Isotonic, viscous liquid adjusted to pH of tears. Balanced amounts of sodium and potassium ions, cellulose derivative, benzalkonium Cl 0.01%, disodium edetate 0.05%. Bot. 15 ml.
Use: Lubricant, ophthalmic.
LYTREN. (Mead Johnson Nutrition) Water, dextrose, sodium citrate, citric acid, sodium Cl, potassium citrate. Ready-To-Use Bot. 8 fl. oz.
Use: Fluid/electrolyte replacement.

M

MAAGEL. (Approved) Aluminum and magnesium hydroxide. Bot. 12 oz, gal.
Use: Antacid.
MAALOX ANTACID. (Rhone-Poulenc Rorer) Calcium carbonate 1000 mg, sodium ≤ 0.4 mEq. Capl. Bot. 50s.
Use: Antacid.
MAALOX ANTI-DIARRHEAL CAPLETS. (Rhone-Poulenc Rorer) Loperamide HCl 2 mg/Tab. Pkg. 12s.
Use: Anti-diarrheal.
MAALOX DAILY FIBER THERAPY. (Rhone-Poulenc Rorer) Psyllium hydrophilic mucilloid fiber 3.4 g/dose, sucrose and 35 cal/12 g in regular; aspartame, 21 mg/tsp phenylalanine and 9 cal/5.8 g in sugar free. Pow. Can 283 g

(sugar free), 369 g, 3 single-dose (12 g) packets.
Use: Laxative.
MAALOX EXTRA STRENGTH PLUS SUSPENSION. (Rhone-Poulenc Rorer) Magnesium hydroxide 450 mg, aluminum hydroxide 500 mg, simethicone 40 mg/5 ml. Susp. Bot. 148, 355, 769 ml.
Use: Antacid, antiflatulent.
MAALOX EXTRA STRENGTH PLUS TABLETS. (Rhone-Poulenc Rorer) Magnesium hydroxide 350 mg, aluminum hydroxide 350 mg, simethicone 30 mg. Chew. Tab. Bot. 38s, 75s.
Use: Antacid, antiflatulent.
MAALOX EXTRA STRENGTH SUSPENSION. (Rhone-Poulenc Rorer) Aluminum hydroxide 500 mg, magnesium hydroxide 450 mg, simethicone 40 mg, parabens, saccharin, sorbitol/5 ml. Susp. Bot. 148 ml, 355 ml, 769 ml.
Use: Antacid, antiflatulent.
MAALOX EXTRA STRENGTH TABLETS. (Rhone-Poulenc Rorer) Magnesium hydroxide 350 mg, dried aluminum hydroxide gel 350 mg/Tab. Bot. 38s, 75s.
Use: Antacid.
MAALOX HEARTBURN RELIEF LIQUID. (Rhone-Poulenc Rorer) Aluminum hydroxide, magnesium carbonate 140 mg, magnesium carbonate 175 mg, tartrazine, saccharin, magnesium alginate, parabens, sorbitol/5 ml. Bot. 296 ml.
Use: Antacid.
MAALOX HRF. (Rhone-Poulenc Rorer) Aluminum hydroxide/magnesium carbonate codried gel 280 mg, magnesium carbonate 350 mg/10 ml, saccharin, tartrazine. Liq. Bot. 355 ml.
Use: Antacid.
MAALOX PLUS TABLETS. (Rhone-Poulenc Rorer) Magnesium hydroxide 200 mg, dried aluminum hydroxide gel 200 mg, simethicone 25 mg/Tab. Bot. 50s, 100s, 144s.
Use: Antacid, antiflatulent.
MAALOX SUSPENSION. (Rhone-Poulenc Rorer) Magnesium hydroxide 200 mg, aluminum hydroxide 225 mg/5 ml, Susp. Bot. 148 ml, 355 ml, 769 ml.
Use: Antacid.
MAALOX TABLETS. (Rhone-Poulenc Rorer) Magnesium hydroxide 200 mg, dried aluminum hydroxide gel 200 mg/Tab. Bot. 100s.
Use: Antacid.
MAALOX THERAPEUTIC CONCENTRATE SUSPENSION. (Rhone-Poulenc Rorer) Magnesium hydroxide 300 mg, aluminum hydroxide 600 mg/5

ml, Susp. Bot. 355 ml.
Use: Antacid.
MAALOX THERAPEUTIC CONCENTRATE TABLETS. (Rhone-Poulenc Rorer) Magnesium hydroxide 300 mg, aluminum hydroxide 600 mg. Tab. Bot. 48s.
Use: Antacid.
MACPAC. (Norwich Eaton) Nitrofurantoin macrocrystals 50 mg or 100 mg/Cap. UD 28s.
Use: Urinary anti-infective.
MACRISALB (^{131}I) INJECTION. B.A.N. Macroaggregated iodinated (^{131}I) human albumin injection.
Use: Examination of pulmonary perfusion.
MACROAGGREGATED ALBUMIN.
See: Albumotope-LS. (Squibb).
MACROBID (Procter & Gamble) Nitrofurantoin 100 mg (as 25 mg nitrofurantoin macrocrystals and 75 mg nitrofurantoin monohydrate). Cap. Bot. 100s.
Use: Urinary anti-infective.
MACRODANTIN. (Procter & Gamble) Nitrofurantoin macrocrystals **25 mg/Cap.:** Bot. 100s. **50 mg or 100 mg/Cap.:** Bot. 100s, 500s, 1000s, Hospital UD 100s.
Use: Urinary anti-infective.
MACRODEX. (Pharmacia) Dextran 6% w/v in normal saline, 6% w/v in dextrose 5% in water. Bot. 500 ml.
Use: Plasma volume expander.
MACROGOL 400. B.A.N. Polyoxyl stearate.
Use: Surface-active agent.
See: Polyethylene glycol 400.
MACROGOL 4000. B.A.N.
Use: Surface-active agent.
See: Polyethylene glycol 4000.
MACROGOL STEARATE 2000. Polyoxyl 40 Stearate.
MACROTEC. (Squibb) Technetium Tc99m Medronate kit. Vial Kit 10s.
Use: Radiopaque agent.
MACROTIN. W/Phenobarbital, hyoscyamus extract, caulophyllin, helonin, pulsatilla extract.
See: Tranquilans, Tab. (Noyes).
• **MADURAMICIN.** USAN.
Use: Anticoccidal.
• **MAFENIDE.** USAN. α-Aminotoluene-p-sulfonamide. Marfanil [HCl], Sulfomyl [propionate], Sulfamylon [acetate].
Use: Antibacterial.
• **MAFENIDE ACETATE,** U.S.P. XXIII. Cream, U.S.P. XXIII. α-Aminotoluene-p-sulfonamide monoacetate.
See: Sulfamylon Cream (Dow B. Hickam).

MAFENIDE ACETATE SOLUTION.
Use: Prevent graft loss on burn wounds. [Orphan drug]
• **MAFILCON A.** USAN.
Use: Contact lens material.
MAFYLON CREAM. (Sanofi Winthrop) Mafenide acetate.
Use: Burn preparation.
• **MAGALDRATE,** U.S.P. XXIII. Oral Susp., Tab., U.S.P. XXIII. (Wyeth-Ayerst) Monalium Hydrate. Aluminum Magnesium Hydroxide.
Use: Antacid.
See: Iosopan (Goldline).
Monalium Hydrate.
Riopan, Tab., Susp. (Wyeth-Ayerst).
• **MAGALDRATE AND SIMETHICONE.** U.S.P. XXIII, Oral Susp, Tabs., U.S.P. XXIII.
Use: Antacid, antiflatulant.
See: Lowsium. (Rugby).
Lowsium Plus. (Rugby).
Riopan Plus. (Wyeth-Ayerst).
MAGALDRATE PLUS SUSPENSION. (Various Mfr.) Magaldrate 540 mg, simethicone 40 mg/5 ml. Susp. Bot. 360 ml.
Use: Antacid, antiflatulant.
MAGAN. (Adria) Magnesium salicylate (anhydrous) 545 mg/Tab. Bot. 100s, 500s.
Use: Salicylate analgesic.
MAG-CAL TABLETS. (Fibertone) Calcium 416.7 mg (as carbonate), calcium 166.7 mg (as elemental), vitamin D 66.7 IU, magnesium 83.3 mg, copper 0.167 mg, manganese 0.83 mg, potassium 1.67 mg, zinc 0.167 mg/Tab. Bot. 90s, 180s.
Use: Vitamin/mineral supplement.
MAGDROX. (Vita Elixir) Magnesium hydroxide, aluminum hydroxide.
Use: Antacid.
MAGLAGEL. (Kenyon) Magnesium-aluminum hydroxide gel. Bot. 12 oz, pt, gal.
Use: Antacid.
MAG-LUM. (Kenyon) Magnesium trisilicate 7.5 gr, dried aluminum hydroxide gel 4 gr. Tab. Bot. 100s, 1000s.
Use: Antacid.
MAGMA ALBA. (Durel) Sulfurated lime solution (Vleminckx's) 60%, saturated zinc sulfate solution 40%. Jar 3 oz, lb.
Use: Anti-acne.
MAGMALIN LOZENGE. (Vale) Magnesium hydroxide 0.2 Gm, aluminum hydroxide gel, dried 0.2 Gm/Loz. Bot. 1000s.
Use: Antacid.
MAGNACAL LIQUID. (Biosearch) Protein-calcium, sodium caseinate, carbo-hydrate-maltodextrin, sucrose, fat (partially hydrogenated), soy oil, lecithin, mono- and diglycerides. 1.5 Cal/ml, 590 mOsm/kg H_2O. Protein 70 Gm, CHO 250 Gm, fat 80 Gm, sodium 1000 mg, potassium 1250 mg/L. Can 120 ml, 240 ml.
Use: Enteral nutritional supplement.
MAGNALOX LIQUID. (Schein) Aluminum hydroxide 225 mg, magnesium hydroxide 200 mg/5 ml. Liq. Bot. 360 ml.
Use: Antacid.
MAGNALUM. (Richlyn) Magnesium hydroxide 3.75 gr, aluminum hydroxide 2 gr/Tab. Bot. 1000s.
Use: Antacid.
MAGNAPRIN ARTHRITIS STRENGTH TABLETS. (Rugby) Aspirin 325 mg, dried aluminum hydroxide gel 150 mg, magnesium hydroxide 150 mg/Tab. Bot. 100s, 500s.
Use: Analgesic.
MAGNAPRIN TABLETS. (Rugby) Aspirin 325 mg, dried aluminum hydroxide gel 75 mg, magnesium hydroxide 75 mg/Tab. Bot. 100s, 500s.
Use: Analgesic.
MAGNATRIL. (Lannett) Dried aluminum hydroxide gel 4 gr, magnesium trisilicate 7 gr, magnesium hydroxide 2 gr/Tab. Bot. 50s, 100s.
Use: Antacid.
• **MAGNESIA TABLETS,** U.S.P. XXIII.
Use: Antacid.
• **MAGNESIA & ALUMINA ORAL SUSPENSION,** U.S.P. XXIII. (Philips Roxane) Oral Susp. 6 fl oz. 25s.
Use: Antacid.
See: Maalox, Liq. (Rhone-Poulenc Rorer).
• **MAGNESIA & ALUMINA TABLETS,** U.S.P. XXIII.
Use: Antacid.
See: Maalox, Tab. (Rhone-Poulenc Rorer).
MAGNESIA MAGMA. Milk of Magnesia, U.S.P. XXIII.
Use: Antacid, cathartic.
See: Magnesium Hydroxide, Preps.
MAGNESIUM ACETYLSALICYLATE. Apyron, Magnespirin, Magisal, Novacetyl.
Use: Salicylate analgesic.
MAGNESIUM ALUMINATE HYDRATED.
Use: Antacid.
See: Riopan, Susp., Tab. (Wyeth-Ayerst).
MAGNESIUM ALUMINUM HYDROXIDE.
Use: Antacid.
See: Maalox, Susp. (Rhone-Poulenc

Rorer).
Maglagel (Kenyon).
Malogel, Gel (Quality Generics).
Medalox, Gel (Med. Chem.).
W/APC.
　See: Buffadyne, Tab. (Lemmon).
W/Calcium carbonate.
　See: Camalox, Susp. (Rhone-Poulenc
　Rorer).
W/Magnesium trisilicate.
　See: Magnatril Susp. (Lannett).
W/Simethicone.
　See: Maalox Plus, Susp. (Rhone-
　Poulenc Rorer).
• **MAGNESIUM ALUMINUM SILICATE,**
　U.S.P. XXIII.
　Use: Suspending agent.
• **MAGNESIUM CARBONATE,** U.S.P. XXI-
　II. (Baker, J. T.) Pow. 4 oz, 1 lb, 5 lb.
　Use: Antacid.
• **MAGNESIUM CARBONATE AND SODI-
　UM BICARBONATE FOR ORAL SUS-
　PENSION,** U.S.P. XXIII.
　Use: Antacid.
**MAGNESIUM CARBONATE W/COMBI-
　NATIONS.**
　Use: Antacid.
　See: Algicon, Tab. (Rhone-Poulenc
　Rorer).
　Alkets, Tab. (Upjohn).
　Antacid No. 2, Tab. (Bowman).
　Bismatesia, Can (Noyes).
　Bufferin, Tab. (Bristol-Myers).
　Di-Gel, Tab., Liq. (Schering-Plough).
　Dimacid, Tab. (Otis Clapp).
　Kanalka, Tab. (Lannett).
　Magnagel, Liq., Tab. (Hauck).
　Marblen, Susp., Tab. (Fleming).
　Panacarb, Tab. (Lannett).
• **MAGNESIUM CHLORIDE,** U.S.P. XXIII.
　Magnesium Cl hexahydrate.
　Use: Electrolyte replenisher, pharma-
　ceutical necessity for hemodialysis
　and peritoneal dialysis.
　W/Potassium Cl, calcium Cl, red phenol.
　See: Electrolytic replenisher, Vial (In-
　venex).
• **MAGNESIUM CITRATE ORAL SOLU-
　TION,** U.S.P. XXIII. 1,2,3-Propanetricar-
　boxylic acid, hydroxymagnesium salt
　(2:3).
　Use: Cathartic.
• **MAGNESIUM GLUCONATE,** U.S.P.
　XXIII. Tab., U.S.P. XXIII.
　Use: Magnesium supplement.
　See: Almora, Tab. (Forest Pharm.).
MAGNESIUM GLUCONATE. (Western
　Research) Magnesium gluconate 500
　mg/Tab. Bot. 1000s.
　Use: Magnesium supplement.

MAGNESIUM GLYCINATE.
W/Aspirin, magnesium carbonate.
　See: Buffinol, Tab. (Otis Clapp).
W/Gastric mucin, aluminum hydroxide gel.
　See: Mucogel, Tab. (Inwood).
• **MAGNESIUM HYDROXIDE,** U.S.P. XXIII.
　Use: Antacid, cathartic.
　See: Magnesia Magma,
　Milk of Magnesia.
　Phillips' Milk of Magnesia (Sterling
　Health).
　Phillips' Chewable, Tab. (Sterling
　Health).
**MAGNESIUM HYDROXIDE W/COMBI-
　NATIONS.**
　See: Aludrox, Susp., Tab., Vial (Wyeth-
　Ayerst).
　Ascriptin, Tab. (Rhone-Poulenc Ror-
　er).
　Ascriptin A/D, Tab. (Rhone-Poulenc
　Rorer).
　Ascriptin Extra Strength, Tab. (Rhone-
　Poulenc Rorer).
　Ascriptin w/Codeine, Tab. (Rhone-
　Poulenc Rorer).
　Banacid, Tab. (Buffington).
　Camalox, Susp., Tab.(Rhone-Poulenc
　Rorer).
　Delcid, Susp. (Merrell Dow).
　Fermalox, Tab. (Rhone-Poulenc Ror-
　er).
　Gas-Eze, Tab. (E.J. Moore).
　Kolantyl, Gel, Wafer (Merrell Dow).
　Laxsil Liquid, Liq. (Reed & Carnrick).
　Maalox, Susp., Tab. (Rhone-Poulenc
　Rorer).
　Maalox Plus, Susp., Tab. (Rhone-
　Poulenc Rorer).
　Magnatril, Susp., Tab. (Lannett).
　Mylanta, Mylanta II, Liq., Tab. (Stuart).
　Simeco, Liq. (Wyeth-Ayerst).
　WinGel, Liq., Tab. (Sanofi Winthrop
　Products).
MAGNESIUM OROTATE. (Nutrition) 500
　mg/Tab. Bot. 100s.
　See: Magora, Tab. (Miller).
• **MAGNESIUM OXIDE,** U.S.P. XXIII. Cap.,
　Tab., U.S.P. XXIII.
　Use: Pharmaceutic aid (sorbent).
　(Manne) 420 mg/Tab. Bot. 250s, 1000s.
　(Stanlabs) 10 gr/Tab. Bot. 100s, 1000s.
　Use: Pharm. aid (sorbant).
　See: Mag-Ox, Tab.(Blaine).
　Mag-Ox 400, Tab. (Blaine).
　Niko-Mag, Cap. (Scruggs).
　Par-Mag, Cap. (Parmed).
　Uro-Mag, Cap. (Blaine).
W/Calcium, Vitamin D.
　See: Elekap, Cap. (Western Research).
W/Glutamic acid magnesium complex, N-

acetyl-P-aminophenol, ascorbic acid, dl-methionine, lemon bioflavonoid complex, dl-α-tocopheryl acetate, glycine, soybean flour.
See: Ulcimins, Tab. (Miller).
W/Magnesium carbonate, calcium carbonate.
See: Alkets, Tab. (Upjohn).
W/Ox bile (desiccated), hog bile (desiccated.).
See: Hyper-Cholate, Tab. (Hauck).
W/Phenobarbital, atropine sulfate.
See: Magnox, Tab. (Bowman).
• MAGNESIUM PHOSPHATE, U.S.P. XXIII.
Use: Antacid.
• MAGNESIUM SALICYLATE, U.S.P. XXIII. Tab. U.S.P. XXIII.
Use: Analgesic, antipyretic, antirheumatic.
See: Analate, Tab. (Winston).
Efficin, Tab. (Adria).
Magan, Tab. (Adria).
W/Phenyltoloxamine citrate.
See: Mobigesic, Tab. (Ascher).
• MAGNESIUM SILICATE, N.F. XVIII.
Use: Pharmaceutic aid (tablet excipient).
• MAGNESIUM STEARATE, N.Γ. XVIII.
Use: Pharmaceutic aid (lubricant).
• MAGNESIUM SULFATE, U.S.P. XXIII. Inj. U.S.P. XXIII. Epsom salt.
Use: Pow. or crystals cathartic: Inj. anticonvulsant, electrolyte replenisher.
(Abbott)—50% Amp. 2 ml Box 25s, 100s.
Abboject Syringe (20 G X 2.5) 5 ml, 10 ml; 12.5% in Pintop Vial, 8 ml, 20 ml.
(Atlas)—10% Amp. 10 ml Box 100s; 1 Gm/2 ml. Box 100s.
(Baxter)—10%. Vial 10 ml, 20 ml.
(CMC)—1 Gm/2 ml, 10% Amp. 10 ml, 20 ml; 25% Amp. 10 ml 50%. Vial 30 ml.
(Quality Generics)—50% Amp. 2 ml, 100s.
(Lilly)—10% Amp 20 ml Box 6s, 25s; 50% 1 Gm Amp. 2 ml, Box 12s, 100s.
(Parke-Davis)—50% Amp. 2 ml, 10s.
(Trent)—50% Amp. 2 ml, 10 ml. (Various Mfr.) Inj. 12.5% Vial 8 ml; 50% Amps 2 ml, 10 ml; Vial 10 ml, 20 ml, 50 ml; Disp. Syringe 5 ml, 10 ml; 2 ml fill in 5 ml vials.
• MAGNESIUM TRISILICATE, U.S.P. XXIII. Tab., U.S.P. XXIII. Magnesium silicate hydrate.
Use: Antacid.
See: Trisomin, Tab. (Lilly).
MAGNESIUM TRISILICATE W/COMBINATIONS.

See: Alsorb Gel C.T., Gel (Standex).
Arcodex Tablets, Tab. (Arcum).
Banacid, Tab. (Buffington).
Gacid, Tab. (Arcum).
Gaviscon, Tab. (Marion).
Kaocasil, Tab. (Jenkins).
Magnatril, Susp., Tab. (Lannett).
Maracid 2, Tab. (Marin).
Silmagel, Tab. (Lannett).
MAGNESIUM ZINC SHAKE LOTION.
(Durel) Magnesium carbonate, zinc oxide, lime water, menthol, phenol 0.5%. Bot. 8 oz, gal.
Use: Antipruritic, counter-irritant.
MAGNEVIST. (Berlex) Gadopentetate dimeglumine 469.01 mg, meglumine 0.39 mg, diethylenetriamine pentaacetic acid 0.15 mg. Inj. Vial 20 ml.
Use: Radiopaque agent.
MAGNOX SUSPENSION. (Lennod) Aluminum hydroxide 225 mg, magnesium hydroxide 200 mg, saccharin, sorbitol, parabens/5 ml. Bot. 360 ml.
Use: Antacid.
MAGONATE. (Fleming) Magnesium gluconate 500 mg/Tab. Bot. 100s, 1000s.
Use: Magnesium supplement.
MAG-OX 400. (Blaine) Magnesium oxide 400 mg/Tab. Bot. 100s, 1000s.
Use: Antacid.
MAGSAL. (U.S. Chemical) Magnesium salicylate 600 mg, phenyltoloxamine citrate 25 mg/Tab. Bot. 100s.
Use: Analgesic combination.
MAG-TAB SR. (Niche) Magnesium (as lactate) 84 mg/SR Capl. Bot. 60s, 100s.
Use: Mineral and electrolyte.
MAIGRET-50. (Ferndale) Phenylpropanolamine HCl 50 mg/Tab. Bot. 100s.
Use: Nasal decongestant.
MAINTENANCE VITAMIN FORMULA W/MINERALS. (Towne) Vitamins A palmitate 10,000 IU, D 400 IU, B_1 5 mg, B_2 2.5 mg, C 75 mg, niacinamide 40 mg, B_6 1 mg, calcium pantothenate 4 mg, B_{12} 2 mcg, E 2 IU, choline bitartrate 31.4 mg, inositol 15 mg, calcium 75 mg, phosphorous 58 mg, iron 30 mg, magnesium 3 mg, manganese 0.5 mg, potassium 2 mg, zinc 0.5 mg/Cap. Bot. 100s.
Use: Vitamin/mineral supplement.
MAJEPTIL. Thioproperazine. Psychopharmacologic agent; pending release.
MALAGRIDE.
See: Acetarsone.
MALARAQUIN. (Sanofi Winthrop) Chloroquine phosphate.

Use: Antimalarial.
MALATAL TABLETS. (Hauck) Atropine sulfate 0.0194 mg, scopolamine HBr 0.0065 mg, hyoscyamine HBr, SO_4 0.1037 mg, phenobarbital 16.2 mg/Tab. Bot. 1000s.
Use: Anticholinergic/antispasmodic, sedative/hypnotic.
• **MALATHION,** U.S.P. XXIII. Lot., U.S.P. XXIII.
Use: Pediculicide.
• **MALETHAMER.** USAN. Maleic anhydride ethylene polymer.
Use: Antidiarrheal, antiperistaltic.
• **MALIC ACID,** N.F. XVIII.
Use: Pharmaceutic aid (acidifying agent).
MALIC ACID WITH PECTIN.
See: Mallo-Pectin, Liq. (Hauck).
MALLAMINT. (Hauck) Calcium carbonate 420 mg/Tab. Bot. 100s.
Use: Antacid.
MALLAZINE DROPS. (Roberts Hauck) Tetrahydrozoline 0.05%. Soln. 15 ml.
Use: Ophthalmic vasoconstrictor/mydriatic.
MALLERGAN-VC W/CODEINE SYRUP. (Hauck) Phenylephrine HCl 5 mg, promethazine HCl 6.25 mg, codeine phosphate 10 mg/5 ml, alcohol 7%. Syr. Bot. 120 ml.
Use: Decongestant, antihistamine, antitussive.
MALLISOL. (Hauck) Povidone-iodine.
Use: Germicidal, antiseptic surgical scrub.
MALOGEN INJECTION AQUEOUS. (Forest Pharm.) Testosterone. **25 mg/ml:** 10 ml, 30 ml; **50 mg/ml:** 10 ml; **100 mg/ml:** 10 ml.
Use: Androgen.
MALOGEN 100 L.A. IN OIL INJ. (Forest Pharm.) Testosterone enanthate 100 mg/ml. 10 ml.
Use: Androgen.
MALOGEN 200 L.A. IN OIL INJ. (Forest Pharm.) Testosterone enanthate 200 mg/ml. 10 ml.
Use: Androgen.
MALOGEN CYP. (Forest Pharm.) Testosterone cypionate in oil 100 mg or 200 mg/ml. Vial 10 ml.
Use: Androgen.
MALONAL.
See: Barbital (Various Mfr.).
• **MALOTILATE.** USAN.
Use: Liver disorder treatment.
MALOTRONE AQUEOUS INJECTION. (Bluco) Testosterone, USP 25 mg or 50 mg/ml in aqueous susp. Vial 10 ml.

Use: Androgen.
• **MALTODEXTRIN,** N.F. XVIII.
MALTSUPEX. (Wallace) Laxative derived from natural barley malt extract for relief of constipation in children and adults. **Liq.:** Bot. 8 oz, pt. **Pow.:** Jar 8 oz, lb. **Tab.:** Malt soup extract 750 mg/Tab. Bot. 100s.
W/Psyllium seed husks.
Use: Laxative.
See: Syllamalt, Pow. (Wallace).
MAMMOL OINTMENT. (Abbott) Bismuth subnitrate 40%, castor oil 30%, anhydrous lanolin 22%, ceresin wax 7%, balsam Peru 1%. Tube 7/8 oz. Ctn. 12s.
Use: Skin protectant, emollient.
MANCHANIL. (D'Franssia)
Use: Skin bleaching agent.
MANDAMETH. (Major) Methenamine mandelate 0.5 Gm/EC Tab. Bot. 1000s.
Use: Urinary anti-infective.
MANDELAMINE "HAFGRAMS". (Parke-Davis) Methenamine mandelate 0.5 Gm/Tab. Bot. 100s, 1000s, UD 100s.
Use: Urinary anti-infective.
MANDELAMINE 1 GM. (Parke-Davis) Methenamine mandelate 1 Gm/Tab. Bot. 100s, 1000s, UD 100s.
Use: Urinary anti-infective.
MANDELAMINE SUSPENSION FORTE. (Parke-Davis) Methenamine mandelate 500 mg/5 ml. Susp. Bot. 8 oz, pt.
Use: Urinary anti-infective.
MANDELIC ACID.
Use: Urinary anti-infective.
MANDELIC ACID SALTS.
See: Calcium mandelate (Various Mfr.).
MANDELYLTROPEINE.
See: Homatropine Salts (Various Mfr.).
MANDOL. (Lilly) Cefamandole nafate. Vial: **500 mg/10 ml** or **1 Gm/10 ml:** Traypak 25s; **1 Gm/100 ml** or **2 Gm/20 ml:** Traypak 10s; **2 Gm/100 ml:** Traypak 10s; **10 Gm/100 ml:** Traypak 6s; Faspak: 1 Gm or 2 Gm, Pkg 96s. ADD-VANTAGE Vial 1 Gm 25s, 2 Gm 10s.
Use: Antibacterial, cephalosporin.
• **MANGANESE CHLORIDE,** U.S.P. XXIII. Inj., U.S.P. XXIII.
Use: Manganese deficiency treatment.
• **MANGANESE GLUCONATE.** U.S.P. XXIII.
Use: Manganese deficiency.
MANGANESE GLYCEROPHOSPHATE. Glycerol phosphate manganese salt.
Use: Pharmaceutical necessity.
MANGANESE HYPOPHOSPHITE. Manganese (2+) phosphinate.
Use: Pharmaceutical necessity.
• **MANGANESE SULFATE,** U.S.P. XXIII.

Inj., U.S.P. XXIII.
Use: Supplement (trace mineral).
W/Thyroid, ferrous sulfate, ferrous gluconate, sodium ferric pyrophosphate, extract of nux vomica.
See: Hemocrine, Tab. (Hauck).
MANGA-PAK. (SoloPak) Manganese 0.1 mg/ml. Inj. Vial 10 ml, 30 ml.
Use: Parenteral nutritional supplement.
MANIRON. (Bowman) Ferrous fumarate 3 mg/Tab. Bot. 100s, 1000s, 5000s.
Use: Iron supplement.
MANN A.R.P. SOLUTION. (Mann) Bot. pt, qt, 0.5 gal, gal.
Use: Rust preventative, sterilizers.
MANN ASTRINGENT MOUTH WASH CONCENTRATE. (Mann) Bot. 4 oz, qt, 0.5 gal, gal. Also mint flavored. Bot. 4 oz, qt, 0.5 gal, gal.
Use: Mouthwash.
MANNA SUGAR.
See: Mannitol (Various Mfr.).
MANNAN. (Rugby) Purified glucomannan 500 mg/Cap. Bot. 90s.
Use: Nutritional supplement.
MANN BODY DEODORANT. (Mann) Bot. 4 oz, 8 oz, pt, qt.
MANN BREATH DEODORANT. (Mann) Bot. 1 oz, 4 oz, 8 oz, pt, qt, 0.5 gal.
MANN EMOLLIENT. (Mann) Jar. 100 Gm.
Use: Emollient.
MANNEST. (Manne) Conjugated estrogens 0.625 mg, 1.25 mg or 2.5 mg/Tab. Bot. 100s, 200s.
Use: Estrogen.
MANN EUGENOL U.S.P. EXTRA. (Mann) 0.06 lb, 0.13 lb, 0.25 lb, 0.5 lb, 1 lb.
Use: With zinc oxide as protective pack.
MANN GERMICIDAL SOLUTION. (Mann) **Regular:** Bot. gal, 4 gal. **Conc.:** 12.8%. Bot. pt, qt, 0.5 gal, gal.
Use: Germicide.
MANN HAND LOTION. (Mann) Twin pack, gal.
Use: Emollient.
MANN HEMOSTATIC. (Mann) Bot. 1 oz, 4 oz, 8 oz, pt, qt.
Use: Hemostatic.
MANN LIQUID SOAP. (Mann) Concentrated cococastile. Bot. qt, 0.5 gal, gal.
Use: Emollient.
MANN LUBRICANT AND CLEANSER. (Mann) Bot. pt, qt.
Use: Emollient.
MANN SUPERFATTED BAR SOAP. (Mann) Rich in lanolin. Cake. 12s.
Use: Emollient.
MANN TALBOT'S IODINE. (Mann) Glycerin base. Bot. 1 oz, 4 oz, 8 oz, pt, qt.

Use: Antiseptic.
MANN TOPICAL ANESTHETIC. (Mann) Bot. 1 oz, 4 oz, 8 oz, pt. W/stain to indicate area treated. Bot. 1 oz, 4 oz, 8 oz.
Use: Local anesthetic, topical.
MANNITE.
See: Mannitol, U.S.P. XXIII.
•**MANNITOL,** U.S.P. XXIII. Inj. U.S.P. XXIII. Manna Sugar, D-Mannitol, Mannite.
Use: Diagnostic aid (renal function determination), diuretic.
See: Osmitrol (Travenol).
W/Aluminum hydroxide, magnesium hydroxide, glycine, calcium carbonate, peppermint oil.
See: Gas-Eze, Tab. (E.J. Moore).
W/Sorbitol.
See: Cystosol, Liq. (Travenol).
Cytal, Liq. (Cutter).
•**MANNITOL INJECTION,** U.S.P. XXIII. (Abbott) 15% or 20%. Abbo-Vac Single dose container 500 ml.
Use: Diagnostic aid (renal function determination), diuretic.
See: Mannitol Solution, Amp. (Merck & Co.).
MANNITOL HEXANITRATE.
Use: Coronary vasodilator.
See: Vascunitol, Tab. (Apco).
W/Reserpine, rutin, ascorbic acid.
See: Ruhexatal W/Reserpine, Tab. (Lemmon).
MANNITOL HEXANITRATE & PHENOBARBITAL TAB. (Bowman; Quality Generics; Jenkins; Kenyon) Mannitol hexanitrate 0.5 gr, phenobarbital 0.25 gr/Tab. Bot. 1000s. (Kenyon): Bot. 100s, 1000s.
Use: Vasodilator.
MANNITOL HEXANITRATE WITH PHENOBARBITAL COMBINATIONS.
See: Hyrunal, Tab. (Kenyon).
Manotensin,Tab. (Dunhall).
Ruhexatal, Tab. (Lemmon).
Vascused, Tab. (Apco).
Vermantin, Tab. (Trout).
•**MANNITOL IN SODIUM CHLORIDE INJECTION.** U.S.P. XXIII.
Use: Diuretic.
MANNOMUSTINE. B.A.N. 1,6-Di-(2-chloroethyl-amino)-1,6-dideoxy-D-mannitol. Degranol dihydrochloride.
Use: Antineoplastic agent.
MANOTENSIN. (Dunhall) Mannitol hexanitrate 32 mg, phenobarbital 16 mg/Tab. Bot. 100s, 1000s.
Use: Vasodilator combination.
MANTADIL. (Burroughs Wellcome) Chlorocyclizine HCl 2%, hydrocortisone acetate 0.5%, liquid and white petrola-

tum, wax, methylparaben 0.25%. Cream
Tube 15 Gm.
Use: Antipruritic, anti-inflammatory,
anesthetic.
MANTOUX TEST.
See: Tuberculin, U.S.P. XXIII. Test
(Parke-Davis).
MANVENE. 3-Methoxy-16a-methyl-1,3,5:
10-estra-triene-16B,17B-diol.
Use: Antineoplastic agent.
MAOI.
See: MONOAMINE OXIDASE IN-
HIBITORS.
MAOLATE TABLETS. (Upjohn) Chlor-
phenesin carbamate 400 mg/Tab. Bot.
50s, 500s.
Use: Muscle relaxant, mild tranquilizer.
MAOX. (Kenneth Manne) Magnesium ox-
ide 420 mg/Tab. Bot. 250s, 1000s.
Use: Antacid.
MAPAP COLD FORMULA. (Major) Ac-
etaminophen 325 mg, pseudoephedrine
HCl 30 mg, dextromethorphan HBr 15
mg, chlorpheniramine maleate 2 mg.
Tab. Pkg. 24s.
Use: Antitussive combination.
MAPHENIDE. p-Sulphamoylbenzylamine
HCl.
See: Sulfbenzamine HCl.
MAPROFIX.
See: Gardinol Type Detergents (Various
Mfr.).
•**MAPROTILINE.** USAN. N-Methyl-9, 10-
ethanoanthracene-9(10H)-propylamine.
3-(9, 10-Dihydro-9, 10-ethanoanthra-
cen-9-yl)propylmethylamine.
Use: Antidepressant.
See: Ludiomil, Tab. (Ciba).
•**MAPROTILINE HYDROCHLORIDE,**
U.S.P. XXIII. Tab., U.S.P. XXIII. 9,10-
Ethanoathracene-9(10H)- propanamine,
N-methyl-, hydrochloride.
Use: Antidepressant.
MARACID 2. (Marin) Magnesium trisili-
cate 150 mg, aluminum hydroxide dried
gel 90 mg, aminoacetic acid 75 mg/Tab.
Bot.
Use: Antacid, adsorbant.
MARANOX. (C.S. Dent) Acetaminophen
325 mg/Tab. Bot. 8s.
Use: Analgesic.
MARAX DF SYRUP. (Roerig) Hydrox-
yzine HCl 2.5 mg, ephedrine sulfate
6.25 mg, theophylline 32.5 mg, alcohol
5%/5 ml. Color free, dye free. Bot. pt,
gal.
Use: Antiasthmatic combination.
MARAX TAB. (Roerig) Hydroxyzine HCl
10 mg, ephedrine sulfate 25 mg, theophylline 130 mg/Tab. Bot. 100s, 500s.

Use: Antiasthmatic combination.
MARBAXIN 750. (Vortech) Methocar-
bamol 750 mg/Tab. Bot. 500s.
Use: Skeletal muscle relaxant.
MARBEC. (Marlyn) High potency B and C
vitamins. Tab. Bot. 100s, 1000s.
Use: Vitamin supplement.
MARBLEN LIQUID. (Fleming) Magnesium carbonate 400 mg, calcium carbonate 520 mg/5 ml. Bot. 473 ml.
Use: Antacid.
MARBLEN TABLETS. (Fleming) Calcium
carbonate 520 mg, magnesium carbonate 400 mg. Tab. Bot. 100s, 1000s.
Use: Antacid.
MARCAINE. (Sanofi Winthrop) Bupivacaine in sterile isotonic soln. containing
sodium Cl pH adjusted 4.0 to 6.5 w/sodi-
um hydroxide or hydrochloric acid. Multiple-dose vial also contains methylparaben 1 mg/ml as preservative.
0.25%: Amp. 50 ml. Box 5s. Vial: Single
dose 10 ml, 30 ml. Box 10s; multiple
dose 50 ml. Box 1s. **0.5%:** Amp. 30 ml.
Box 1s. Vial: Single dose 10 ml, 30 ml.
Box 10s; multiple dose 50 ml. Box 1s.
0.75%: Amp. 30 ml. Box 5s. Vial (single
dose) 10 ml, 30 ml. Box 10s.
Use: Local anesthetic.
MARCAINE WITH EPINEPHRINE
(1:200,000). (Sanofi Winthrop) **Bupivacaine 0.25%:** with epinephrine
1:200,000 in sterile isotonic soln. containing sodium Cl. Each 1 ml contains
bupivacaine HCl 2.5 mg, epinephrine
bitartrate 0.0091 mg, sodium metabisulfite 0.5 mg, monothioglycerol 0.001 ml,
ascorbic acid 2 mg and edetate calcium
disodium 0.1 mg. In Multiple Dose Vial,
each 1 ml also contains methylparaben
1 mg as antiseptic preservative. pH adjusted to between 3.4 and 4.5 with sodium hydroxide or hydrochloric acid. Amp.
50 ml, 5s, Single Dose Vial 10 ml, 30 ml.
10s, Multiple Dose Vial 50 ml 1s. **Bupivacaine 0.5%:** with epinephrine
1:200,000 in sterile isotonic soln. containing sodium Cl. Each 1 ml contains
bupivacaine HCl 5 mg and epinephrine
bitartrate 0.0091 mg, with sodium
metabisulfite 0.5 mg, monothioglycerol
0.001 ml and ascorbic acid 2 mg, edetate calcium disodium 0.1 mg. In Multiple Dose Vial, each 1 ml also contains
methylparaben 1 mg antiseptic preservative. pH adjusted to between 3.4 and
4.5 with sodium hydroxide or hydrochloric acid. Amp. 3 ml 10s, 30 ml 5s. Single
Dose Vial 10 ml, 30 ml 10s. Multiple
Dose Vial 50 ml 1s. **Bupivacaine**

0.75%: with epinephrine 1:200,000 in sterile isotonic soln. containing sodium Cl. Each 1 ml contains bupivacaine HCl 7.5 mg, epinephrine bitartrate 0.0091 mg with sodium metabisulfite 0.5 mg, monothioglycerol 0.001 ml, ascorbic acid 2 mg as antioxidants, edetate calcium disodium 0.1 mg. pH adjusted to between 3.4 and 4.5 with sodium hydroxide or hydrochloric acid. Amp 30 ml in 5s.
Use: Local anesthetic.

MARCAINE SPINAL. (Sanofi Winthrop) Bupivacaine HCl 15 mg/2 ml (0.75%) and dextrose 165 mg/2 ml (8.25%). Amp. 2 ml, UD pak 10s.
Use: Local anesthetic.

MARCILLIN. (Marnel) **Cap.:** Ampicillin trihydrate 500 mg. Bot. 100s; **Pow. for Susp.:** Ampicillin trihydrate 250 mg/100 ml.
Use: Anti-infective.

MARCOF EXPECTORANT. (Marnel) Hydrocodone bitartrate 5 mg, potassium guaiacolsulfonate 300 mg/5 ml. Liq. Bot. 480 ml.
Use: Narcotic antitussive, expectorant.

MARDON. (Geneva) Propoxyphene HCl. **Cap.:** 32 mg Bot. 100s, 1000s. **65 mg:** Bot. 100s, 500s, 1000s.
Use: Narcotic analgesic.

MARDON COMPOUND. (Geneva) Propoxyphene compound 65 mg, aspirin 3.5 gr, phenacetin 2.5 gr, caffeine 0.5 gr/Cap. Bot. 100s, 500s, 1000s.
Use: Narcotic analgesic combination.

MAREZINE TABLETS. (Himmel) Cyclizine HCl 50 mg/Tab. Bot. 100s. Box 12s.
Use: Anticholinergic.
W/Ergotamine tartrate, caffeine.
See: Migral, Tab. (Burroughs Wellcome).

MARFANIL.
See: Sulfbenzamine HCl (Various Mfr.).

MARGESIC. (Marnel) Butalbital 50 mg, acetaminophen 325 mg, caffeine 40 mg Cap. Bot. 100s.
Use: Analgesic, sedative/hypnotic.

MARHIST. (Marlop) Chlorpheniramine maleate 20 mg, phenylephrine HCl 2.5 mg, methscopolamine nitrate in special base/Cap. Bot. 30s, 100s. Expectorant Bot. 4 oz, pt, gal.
Use: Antihistamine, decongestant, anticholinergic.

MARINE 500 CAPSULES. (Murdock) Omega-3 polyunsaturated fatty acids 500 mg/Cap. containing EPA 90 mg, DHA 60 mg, vitamin E 13 IU/Cap. Bot.

90s.
Use: Nutritional supplement.

MARINE 1000 CAPSULES. (Murdock) Omega-3 polyunsaturated fatty acids 1000 mg/Cap. containing EPA 180 mg, DHA 120 mg, vitamin E 1 IU/Cap. Bot. 60s, 90s, 180s, 300s.
Use: Nutritional supplement.

MARINE LIPID CONCENTRATE. (Vitaline) Omega-3 1200 mg, EPA 360 mg, DHA 240 mg, E 5 IU/Cap., sodium free. Bot. 90s.
Use: Fish oil.

MARINOL CAPSULES. (Roxane) Dronabinol 2.5 mg, 5 mg or 10 mg/Cap. Bot. 25s.
Use: Antiemetic.

MARLIN SALT SYSTEM II. (Marlin) Salt tablets for normal saline 250 mg/Tab. Bot. 200s with bot. 27.7 ml.
Use: Soft contact lens care.

MARLYN FORMULA 50. (Marlyn) Vitamin B_6 w/18 amino acids/Cap. Bot. 100s, 250s, 1000s.
Use: Nutritional supplement.

MARMINE. (Vortech) Dimenhydrinate 50 mg/ml. Inj. Vial 1 ml, 10 ml.
Use: Antiemetic/antivertigo agent.

MARNAL. (Vortech) Aspirin 325 mg, caffeine 40 mg, butalbital 50 mg/Tab. Bot. 100s.
Use: Nonnarcotic analgesic combination.

MARPLAN. (Roche) Isocarboxazid 10 mg/Tab. Bot. 100s.
Use: Antidepressant.

MARTHRITIC. (Marnel) Salsalate 750 mg. Tab. Bot. 100s.
Use: Salicylate analgesic.

• **MASOPROCOL.** USAN.
Use: Antineoplastic.
See: Actinex

MASSE BREAST CREAM. (Advanced Care) Water, glyceryl monostearate, glycerin, cetyl alcohol, lanolin, peanut oil, Span-60, stearic acid, Tween-60, sodium benzoate, propylparaben, methylparaben, potassium hydroxide. Tube 2 oz.
Use: Emollient.

MASSENGILL BAKING SODA FRESHNESS. (SK-Beecham) Sanitized water, sodium bicarbonate. Soln. Bot. 180 ml.
Use: Vaginal preparation.

MASSENGILL FEMININE DEODORANT SPRAY. (Beecham Products) Aerosol Bot. 3 oz.
Use: Vaginal preparation.

MASSENGILL DISPOSABLE DOUCHE. (Beecham Products) Water, S.D. alcohol

40, lactic acid, sodium lactate, octoxymol-9, cetylpyridium Cl, diazolidinyl urea, disodium EDTA, methyl and propyl paraben, fragrance, color. Bot. 6 oz.
Use: Vaginal preparation.
MASSENGILL EXTRA CLEANSING W/PURACLEAN. (SK-Beecham) Vinegar, water, cetylpyridinium chloride, diazolidinyl urea, EDTA. Soln. Bot. 180 ml.
Use: Vaginal preparation.
MASSENGILL LIQUID. (Beecham Products) Lactic acid, S.D. alcohol 40, octoxynol-9, water, sodium lacate. Bot. 4 oz, 8 oz.
Use: Vaginal preparation.
MASSENGILL MEDICATED. (Beecham Products) Povidone iodine 0.3% when added to sanitized fluid. Bot. 6 oz.
Use: Vaginal preparation.
MASSENGILL MEDICATED DOUCHE W/CEPTICIN. (SK-Beecham) Povidone-iodine 12%. Liq. concentrate. Bot. 120 ml, 240 ml.
Use: Vaginal preparation.
MASSENGILL POWDER. (Beecham Products) Sodium Cl, ammonium alum, PEG-8, phenol, methyl salicylate, eucalyptus oil, menthol, thymol, phenol. Jar 4 oz, 8 oz, 16 oz, 22 oz. Packette 10s, 12s.
Use: Vaginal preparation.
MASSENGILL SOFT CLOTH. (SK-Beecham) Hydrocortisone 0.5%, diazolidinyl urea, DMDM hydantoin, isopropyl myristate, methylparaben, polysorbate 60, propylene glycol, propylparaben, sorbitan stearate, steareth-2, steareth-21. Towelettes 10s.
Use: Vaginal preparation.
MASSENGILL UNSCENTED. (SK-Beecham) Water, SD alcohol 40, lactic acid, sodium lactate, octoxynol-9, cetylpyridium chloride, propylene glycol, diazolidinyl urea, parabens, EDTA. Soln. Bot. 180 ml.
Use: Vaginal preparation.
MASSENGILL VINEGAR-WATER DISPOSABLE DOUCHE. (Beecham Products) Water and vinegar solution. Bot. 6 oz.
Use: Vaginal preparation.
MASSENGILL VINGEGAR & WATER EXTRA CLEANSING WITH PURACLEAN. (SK-Beecham) Vinegar, water, cetylpyridinium chloride, diazolidinyl urea, EDTA. Soln. Bot. 180 ml.
Use: Vaginal preparation.
MASSENGILL VINEGAR & WATER EXTRA MILD. (SK-Beecham) Vinegar, water, preservative free. Soln. Bot. 180 ml.

Use: Vaginal preparation.
MASTER FORMULA. (Barth's) Vitamins A 10,000 IU, D 400 IU, C 180 mg, B_1 7 mg, B_2 14 mg, niacin 4.6 mg, B_6 292 mcg, pantothenic acid 210 mcg, B_{12} 25 mcg, biotin 2.9 mcg, E 50 IU, calcium 800 mg, phosphorus 387 mg, iron 10 mg, iodine 0.1 mg, choline 7.78 mg, inositol 11.6 mg, aminobenzoic acid 35 mcg, rutin 30 mg, citrus bioflavonoid complex 30 mg/4 Tab. Bot. 120s, 600s, 1200s.
Use: Vitamin/mineral supplement.
MASTISOL. (Ferndale) Nonirritating medical adhesive. Bot. 4 oz.
Use: Skin dressing adhesive.
MATERNA. (Lederle) Vitamins A 8000 IU, D 400 IU, E 30 IU, C 100 mg, folic acid 1 mg, B_1 3 mg, B_2 3.4 mg, B_6 4 mg, niacinamide 20 mg, B_{12} 12 mcg, calcium 250 mg, iodine 0.3 mg, magnesium 25 mg, iron 60 mg, copper 2 mg, zinc 25 mg/Tab. Bot. 100s.
Use: Vitamin/mineral supplement.
MATRIX METALLOPROTEINASE INHIBITOR.
Use: Corneal ulcers. [Orphan drug]
MATULANE. (Roche) Procarbazine HCl 50 mg/Cap. Bot. 100s.
Use: Antineoplastic agent.
MAURRY'S FUNGICIDE. (Maurry) Nitromersol 37 mg, alcohol 70% - 74%/oz. Bot. oz, pt.
Use: Antifungal, external.
MAXAIR. (Riker) Pirbuterol acetate aerosol 0.2 mg pirbuterol/actuation. Metered dose inhaler 25.6 Gm (300 inhalations).
Use: Sympathomimetic bronchodilator.
MAXAQUIN. (Searle) Lomefloxacin HCl 400 mg/Tab. Bot. 20s, UD 100s.
Use: Antibiotic, fluoroquinolone.
MAX-CARO. (Marlyn) Beta-carotene 15 mg, lecithin. Cap. Bot. 250s.
Use: To reduce severity of photosensitivity reactions in patients with erythropoietic protoporphyria.
MAX EPA CAPSULES. (Various Mfr.) Omega-3 polyunsaturated fatty acids 1000 mg/Cap. containing EPA 180 mg, DHA 60 mg/Cap. Bot. 50s, 60s, 100s.
Use: Fish oil.
MAXIDEX. (Alcon) Dexamethasone 0.1% in a 0.5% soln., methylcellulose vehicle/5 ml. Bot. 5 ml, 15 ml.
Use: Corticosteroid, ophthalmic.
MAXIDEX OINTMENT. (Alcon) Dexamethasone phosphate 0.05%. Tube 3.5 g.
Use: Corticosteroid, ophthalmic.
MAXIFLOR CREAM & OINTMENT. (Her-

bert) Diflorasone diacetate 0.05%. Tubes 15 Gm, 30 Gm, 60 Gm. *Use:* Corticosteroid, topical.

MAXILUBE PERSONAL LUBRICANT. (Mission) Water, silicone oil, glycerin, carbomer 934, triethanolamine, sodium lauryl sulfate, parabens. Jelly 90 Gm. *Use:* Vaginal preparation.

MAXIMUM BAYER ASPIRIN TABLETS AND CAPSULES. (Glenbrook) Aspirin (Acetylsalicylic Acid; ASA) 500 mg. **Tab.:** 10s, 30s, 60s, 100s. **Capl.:** 60s. *Use:* Salicylate analgesic.

MAXIMUM BLUE LABEL. (Vitaline) Vitamins A 833 IU, D 16.7 IU, E 55.1 mg, B_1 16.7 mg, B_2 8.3 mg, B_3 31.7 mg, B_5 66.7 mg, B_6 16.7 mg, B_{12} 16.7 mcg, C 200 mg, folic acid 0.1 mg, zinc 5 mg, Ca, Cr, Cu, I, K, Mg, Mn, Mo, Se, Si, vanadium, biotin 50 mcg, choline, bioflavonoids, inositol, SOD, l-lysine, PABA/Tab. Bot. 180s. *Use:* Vitamin/mineral supplement.

MAXIMUM GREEN LABEL. (Vitaline) Vitamins A 833 IU, D 16.7 IU, E 55.1 mg, B_1 16.7 mg, B_2 8.3 mg, B_3 31.7 mg, B_5 66.7 mg, B_6 16.7 mg, B_{12} 16.7 mcg, C 200 mg, folic acid 0.1 mg, zinc 5 mg, Ca, Cr, I, K, Mg, Mn, Mo, Se, Si, vanadium, biotin 50 mcg, choline, bioflavonoids, inositol, SOD, l-lysine, PABA/Tab. Bot. 180s. *Use:* Vitamin/mineral supplement.

MAXIMUM RED LABEL. (Vitaline) Vitamins A 833 IU, D 66.7 IU, E 55.1 mg, B_1 16.7 mg, B_2 8.3 mg, B_3 31.7 mg, B_5 66.7 mg, B_6 16.7 mg, B_{12} 16.7 mcg, C 200 mg, folic acid 0.1 mg, zinc 5 mg, Ca, Cr, Cu, iron 20 mg, I, K, Mg, Mn, Mo, Se, Si, vanadium, biotin 50 mcg, choline, inositol, bioflavonoids, l-lysine, PABA, SOD/Tab. Bot. 180s. *Use:* Vitamin/mineral supplement.

MAXIMUM STRENGTH ALLERGY DROPS. (Bausch & Lomb) Naphazoline HCl 0.03% soln., benzalkonium chloride 0.01%, methylcellulose 0.5%, EDTA. Bot. 15 ml. *Use:* Ophthalmic vasoconstrictor/mydriatic.

MAXIMUM STRENGTH ANBESOL MOUTH AND THROAT. (Whitehall) **Gel:** Benzocaine 20%, alcohol 60%, carbomer 934 P, polyethylene glycol, saccharin. Tube 7.2 Gm. **Liq.:** Benzocaine 20%, alcohol 60%, saccharin, polyethylene glycol. Bot. 9 ml. *Use:* Mouth and throat product.

MAXIMUM STRENGTH ARTHRITEN. (Alva-Amco) Acetaminophen 250 mg,

magnesium salicylate 250 mg, caffeine anhydrous 32.5 mg, buffered with magnesium carbonate, magnesium oxide, calcium carbonate. Tab. Bot. 40s. *Use:* Nonnarcotic analgesic combination.

MAXIMUM STRENGTH BENADRYL. (Parke-Davis) **Cream:** Diphenhydramine HCl 2%, parabens in a greaseless base. Jar 15 Gm. **Spray, nonaerosol:** Diphenhydramine HCl 2%, alcohol 85%. Bot. 60 ml. *Use:* Antihistamine, topical.

MAXIMUM STRENGTH CLEARASIL CLEARSTICK. *See:* Clearasil.

MAXIMUM STRENGTH CLEARASIL CLEARSTICK FOR SENSITIVE SKIN. *See:* Clearasil.

MAXIMUM STRENGTH COMTREX. *See:* Comtrex.

MAXIMUM STRENGTH CORTAID. (Upjohn) Hydrocortisone 1% in parabens, mineral oil, white petrolatum. Oint. Tube 15 Gm, 30 Gm. *Use:* Corticosteroid combination, topical.

MAXIMUM STRENGTH CORTICAINE. (Whitby) Hydrocortisone acetate 1%, glycerin, menthol, EDTA, parabens. Cream. Tube 30 g. *Use:* Topical corticosteroid.

MAXIMUM STRENGTH DERMAREST DRICORT CREME. (Del) Hydrocortisone (as acetate) 1%, white petrolatum. Cream. Tube 14 g. *Use:* Topical corticosteroid.

MAXIMUM STRENGTH DESENEX ANTIFUNGAL. (Ciba) Miconazole nitrate 2%, EDTA. Cream. Tube 14 g. *Use:* Antifungal agent.

MAXIMUM STRENGTH DEXATRIM. (Thompson) Phenylpropanolamine HCl 75 mg. ER Tab. Pkg. 20s. *Use:* Nonprescription diet aid.

MAXIMUM STRENGTH DEXATRIM WITH VITAMIN C. (Thompson) Phenylpropanolamine HCl, vitamin C 180 mg/Cap. Bot. 20s. *Use:* Nonprescription diet aid.

MAXIMUM STRENGTH DIET AID PLUS VITAMIN C. (O'Connor) Phenylpropanolamine HCl 75 mg, vitamin C 180 mg/Cap. Bot. 20s. *Use:* Nonprescription diet aid.

MAXIMUM STRENGTH DRISTAN. (Whitehall) Pseudoephedrine HCl 30 mg, acetaminophen 500 mg/Cap. Bot. 24s, 48s, 100s. *Use:* Decongestant, analgesic.

MAXIMUM STRENGTH GRAPEFRUIT DIET PLAN W/DIADEX. (O'Connor) Phenylpropanolamine HCl 37.5 mg, grapefruit extract, sugar/Cap. Bot. 20s.
Use: Nonprescription diet aid.

MAXIMUM STRENGTH KERICORT-10. (Bristol-Myers Squibb) Hydrocortisone 1%, parabens, cetyl alcohol, stearyl alcohol. Cream. Tube 56.7 g.
Use: Topical corticosteroid.

MAXIMUM STRENGTH METED. (Gen-Derm) Sulfur 5%, salicylic acid 3%. Shampoo. Bot. 118 ml.
Use: Antiseborrheic combination.

MAXIMUM STRENGTH MIDOL MULTI-SYMPTOM. (Glenbrook) Acetaminophen 325 mg, pyrilamine maleate 12.5 mg/Tab. Bot. 30s.
Use: Nonnarcotic analgesic combination.

MAXIMUM STRENGTH NEOSPORIN. (Burroughs Wellcome) Polymyxin B sulfate 10,000 units, neomycin 3.5 mg, bacitracin 500 units/Gm, white petrolatum. Oint. Tube 15 Gm.
Use: Topical anti-infective.

MAXIMUM STRENGTH NO-ASPIRIN SINUS MEDICATION. (Walgreen) Acetaminophen 500 mg, pseudoephedrine HCl 30 mg/Tab. Bot. 50s.
Use: Analgesic, decongestant.

MAXIMUM STRENGTH NYTOL. (Block) Diphenhydramine HCl 50 mg/Tab., lactose. Pkg. 8s, 16s.
Use: Nonprescription sleep aid.

MAXIMUM STRENGTH ORNEX. (Menley & James) Pseudoephedrine HCl 30 mg, acetaminophen 500 mg/Cap. Bot. 24s, 30s, 48s.
Use: Decongestant, analgesic.

MAXIMUM STRENGTH SINEAID. (McNeil-CPC) Pseudoephedrine HCl 30 mg, acetaminophen 500 mg/Cap. or Tab.
Cap.: Bot. 24s, 50s. **Tab.:** Bot. 24s, 100s.
Use: Decongestant, analgesic.

MAXIMUM STRENGTH SINUTAB NIGHTTIME. (Parke-Davis Consumer) Pseudoephedrine HCl 10 mg, diphenhydramine HCl 8.33 mg, acetaminophen 167 mg/5 ml. Alcohol free. In 120 ml.
Use: Decongestant, antihistamine, analgesic.

MAXIMUM STRENGTH SINUTAB WITHOUT DROWSINESS. (Parke-Davis) Pseudoephedrine HCl 30 mg, acetaminophen 500 mg/Tab. or Cap. **Tab.:** Bot. 24s, 50s. **Cap.:** Bot. 24s.
Use: Decongestant, analgesic.

MAXIMUM STRENGTH SLEEPINAL. (Thompson) **Cap.:** Diphenhydramine HCl 50 mg, lactose. Pkg. 16s. **Soft gel:** diphenhydramine HCl 50 mg, sorbitol. Pkg. 16s.
Use: Sleep aid.

MAXIMUM STRENGTH SUDAFED SEVERE COLD FORMULA. (Burroughs-Wellcome) Dextromethorphan HBr 15 mg, pseudoephedrine HCl 30 mg, acetaminophen 500 mg/Tab. 10s.
Use: Antitussive, decongestant, analgesic.

MAXIMUM STRENGTH THERA-FLU NON-DROWSY.
See: Thera-Flu.

MAXIMUM STRENGTH TYLENOL COUGH LIQUID. (McNeil-CPC) Dextromethorphan HBr 7.5 mg, acetaminophen 250 mg, alcohol 10%. Bot. 120 ml.
Use: Antitussive, analgesic.

MAXIMUM STRENGTH TYLENOL COUGH W/ DECONGESTANT LIQUID. (McNeil-CPC) Pseudoephedrine HCl 15 mg, dextromethorphan HBr 7.5 mg, acetaminophen 250 mg, alcohol 10%. Bot. 120 ml.
Use: Decongestant, antitussive, analgesic.

MAXIMUM STRENGTH TYLENOL FLU GELCAPS. (McNeil-CPC) Acetaminophen 500 mg, pseudoephedrine HCl 30 mg, dextromethorphan HBR 15 mg. Tab. Pkg. 10s.
Use: Antitussive combination.

MAXIMUM STRENGTH TYLENOL SELECT ALLERGY SINUS. (McNeil-CPC) Pseudoephedrine HCl 30 mg, diphenhydramine HCl 25 mg, acetaminophen 500 mg. Cap. Bot. 24s.
Use: Antihistamine, decongestant.

MAXIMUM STRENGTH UNISOM SLEEP-GELS. (Pfizer) Diphenhydramine HCl 50 mg, sorbitol. Cap. Pkg. 8s.
Use: Sleep aid.

MAXIMUM STRENGTH WART REMOVER. (Stiefel) Salicylic acid 17%, alcohol 29%, castor oil, flexible collodion. Liq. 13.3 ml.
Use: Keratolytic.

MAXITON.
See: Amphetamine (Various Mfr.).

MAXITROL OINTMENT. (Alcon) Dexamethasone 0.1%, neomycin 3.5 mg, polymyxin B sulfate 10,000 units/Gm. Tube 3.5 Gm.
Use: Anti-infective, ophthalmic.

MAXITROL OPHTHALMIC SUSPENSION. (Alcon) Dexamethasone 0.1%, neomycin (as sulfate) 3.5 mg, polymyxin

B sulfate 10,000 units/ml. Bot. 5 ml droptainer.
Use: Anti-infective, ophthalmic.
MAXIVATE. (Westwood) Betamethasone dipropionate 0.05%. Cream, Oint. Tube 15 Gm, 45 Gm.
Use: Corticosteroid, topical.
MAXOLON TABLETS. (Beecham Labs) Metoclopramide HCl 10 mg/Tab. Bot. 100s.
Use: GI stimulant.
MAXZIDE. (Lederle) Hydrochlorothiazide 50 mg, triamterene 75 mg/Tab. Bot. 100s, 500s, UD 10 × 10s.
Use: Diuretic, antihypertensive.
MAXZIDE-25 MG. (Lederle) Triamterene 37.5 mg, hydrochlorothiazide 25 mg/Tab. Bot. 100s, UD 100s.
Use: Diuretic combination.
MAYASEN. (Janssen) Astemizole.
Use: Anti-allergenic, antihistamine.
MAYOTIC. (Mayrand) Hydrocortisone 1%, neomycin sulfate 5 mg, polymyxin B sulfate 10,000 units/ml, thimersol 0.01%. Susp. Bot. 10 ml w/dropper.
Use: Otic preparation.
• **MAYTANSINE,** USAN.
Use: Antineoplastic.
MAY-VITA ELIXIR. (Mayrand) Dexpanthenol 10 mg, niacinamide 40 mg, B_6 4 mg, B_{12} 12 mcg, folic acid 1 mg, iron 36 mg, zinc 15 mg, manganese 4 mg/45 ml w/alcohol 13%. Bot. pt.
Use: Vitamin/mineral supplement.
MAZANOR. (Wyeth-Ayerst) Mazindol 1 mg/Tab. Bot. 30s.
Use: Anorexiant.
MAZICON. (Roche) Flumazenil 0.1 mg/ml. Inj. Vial 5 ml, 10 ml.
Use: Antidote.
• **MAZINDOL,** U.S.P. XXIII. Tab., U.S.P. XXIII. 5-(p-Chlorophenyl)-2,3-dihydro-5,H-imidazo [2,1-a]isoindol-5-ol.
Use: Anorexic, appetite suppressant, Duchenne muscular dystrophy [Orphan drug]
See: Mazanor, Tab. (Wyeth-Ayerst). Sanorex, Tab. (Sandoz).
M-CAPS. (Mill-Mark) Methionine 200 mg/Cap. Bot. 50s, 1000s.
Use: Diaper rash product.
MCT OIL. (Mead Johnson) Triglycerides of medium chain fatty acids. Lipid fraction of coconut oil; fatty acid shorter than C-8 <6%, C_8(octanoic) 67%, C_{10}(decanoic) 23%, longer than $C_1$04%. Bot. qt.
Use: Enteral nutritional supplement.
MD-GASTROVIEW. (Mallinckrodt) Diatrizoate meglumine 66%, diatrizoate sodium 10%. Soln. 120 ml, 240 ml.
Use: Radiopaque agent.
MD-60. (Mallinckrodt) Diatrizoate meglumine 52%, diatrizoate sodium 8% (29.2% iodine). Inj. Vial 30 ml, 50 ml.
Use: Radiopaque agent.
MD-76. (Mallinckrodt) Diatrizoate meglumine 66%, diatrizoate sodium 10% (37% iodine). Inj. Vial 50 ml, 100 ml, 150 ml, 200 ml.
Use: Radiopaque agent.
MDP-SQUIBB. (Squibb) Technetium Tc 99 medronate. Reaction vial pkg. 10s.
Use: Radiopaque agent.
MEADININ. Mixture of Amoidin & Amidin alk. of Ammi Majus Linn.
MEASLES CONVALESCENT SERUM.
See: Measles Immune Human Serum.
MEASLES IMMUNE GLOBULIN (HUMAN). Sterile soln. of gamma globulin derived from pooled normal human plasma.
Use: Immune serum.
MEASLES PROPHYLACTIC SERUM.
See: Immune Serum Globulin (Human).
• **MEASLES & MUMPS VIRUS VACCINE LIVE,** U.S.P. XXIII.
Use: Immunizing agent (active).
MEASLES, MUMPS AND RUBELLA VIRUS VACCINE LIVE, U.S.P. XXIII.
MEASLES AND RUBELLA VIRUS VACCINE LIVE, U.S.P. XXIII.
See: M-R-Vax, Inj. (Merck & Co.).
• **MEASLES VIRUS VACCINE, LIVE,** U.S.P. XXIII. Modified live-virus measles vaccine (Schwarz strain).
Use: One-shot vaccine for common measles (rubeola).
Use: Active immunizing agent.
See: Attenuvax, Inj. (Merck & Co.). Lirugen, Inj. (Merrell Dow). M-Vac, Inj. (Lederle).
W/Mumps virus vaccine, rubella virus vaccine.
See: Lirutrin, Vial (Merrell Dow).
W/Rubella virus vaccine.
See: Lirubel, Vial (Merrell Dow). M-R-Vax, Inj. (Merck & Co.).
MEASLES VIRUS VACCINE, LIVE ATTENUATED. Moraten line derived from Enders' attenuated Edmonston strain grown in cell cultures of chick embryos.
See: Attenuvax, Inj. (Merck & Co.).
W/Mumps virus vaccine, rubella virus vaccine.
See: M-M-R., Vial (Merck & Co.).
W/Rubella virus vaccine.
See: M-R-Vax, Inj. (Merck & Co.).
MEASURIN. (Sanofi Winthrop) Aspirin 10 gr./SR Tab. Bot. 60s.

Use: Analgesic.
MEBANAZINE. B.A.N. α-Methylbenzyl-hydrazine. Actomol.
Use: Monoamine oxidase inhibitor.
MEBARAL. (Sanofi Winthrop) Mephobarbital. Tab. **0.5 gr, 0.75 gr or 1.5 gr:** Bot. 250s.
Use. Sedative, anticonvulsant.
• **MEBENDAZOLE,** U.S.P. XXIII. Tab., U.S.P. XXIII. Methyl 5-benzoyl-2-benzimidazolecarbanate.
Use: Anthelmintic.
See: Vermox, Tab. (Janssen).
• **MEBEVERINE HYDROCHLORIDE.** USAN. 4-[Ethyl (p-methoxy-α-methyl-phenethyl) amino] butyl veratrate hydrochloride.
Use: Spasmolytic agent.
MEBEZONIUM IODIDE. B.A.N. 4,4'-Methylenedi-(cy- clohexyltrimethylammonium iodide).
Use: Neuromuscular blocking agent.
MEBHYDROLIN. B.A.N. 5-Benzyl-1,2,3,4-tetrahydro-2-methyl-a-carboline. Fabahistin napadisylate.
Use: Antihistamine.
• **MEBROFENIN.** USAN.
Use: Diagnostic aid (hepatobiliary function determination).
• **MEBUTAMATE.** USAN. 2-Carbamoyloxymethyl-2,3-dimethyl carbamate. Capla.
Use: Hypotensive.
MECAMYLAMINE HYDROCHLORIDE, U.S.P. XXI. Tab., U.S.P. XXI. N, 2, 3, 3-Tetramethyl-2-norbornanamine HCl. 3-Methylaminoiso-camphane HCl. N-Methyl-di-isobornylamine HCl.
Use: Antihypertensive.
See: Inversine, Tab. (Merck & Co.).
• **MECETRONIUM ETHYLSULFATE.** USAN.
Use: Antiseptic.
• **MECHLORETHAMINE HYDROCHLORIDE,** U.S.P. XXIII. Inj. U.S.P. XXIII. 2,2'-Dichloro-n-methyl-diethylamine HCl. Trituration. Dichloren.
Use: Antineoplastic.
See: Mustargen, Vial (Merck & Co.).
MECHOLIN HCl.
See: Methacholine Cl, U.S.P. XXIII.
MECHOLYL OINTMENT. (Gordon) Methacholine Cl 0.25%, methyl salicylate 10% in ointment base. Jar 4 oz, 1 lb, 5 lb.
Use: External analgesic.
MECILLINAM. B.A.N. (2S,5R,6R)-6-(Perhydro-azepin-1-ylmethyleneamino)penicillanic acid.
Use: Antibiotic.

MECLAN. (Ortho Derm) Meclocycline sulfosalicylate 1%. Cream Tube 20 Gm, 45 Gm.
Use: Anti-acne.
MECLASTINE. Clemastine.
• **MECLIZINE HYDROCHLORIDE,** U.S.P. XXIII. Tab., U.S.P. XXIII. 1(p-Chloro-α phonylbonzyl) 1 m-(methylbenzyl)piperazine 2 HCl.
Use: Antinauseant.
See: Antivert, Chew. Tab. (Roerig).
Bonine, Tab. (Roerig).
Dramamine II, Tab. (Upjohn).
Vergon, Cap. (Marnel).
• **MECLOCYCLINE.** USAN. 7-Chloro-4-(dime- thylamino)-1, 4, 4a, 5, 5a, 6, 11, 12a-octahydro-3, 5,10, 12, 12a-pentahydroxy-6-methylene-1, 11-dioxo-2-naphthacenecarboxamide.
Use: Antibiotic.
• **MECLOCYCLINE SULFOSALICYLATE,** U.S.P. XXIII. Cream, U.S.P. XXIII.
Use: Antibiotic.
See: Meclan, Cream (Ortho).
• **MECLOFENAMATE SODIUM,** U.S.P. [XXIII. Cap., U.S.P. XXIII. Benzoic acid, 2-[(2, 6-dichloro-3-methylphenyl) amino], monosodium salt, monohydrate.
Use: Nonsteroidal anti-inflammatory agent.
MECLOFENAMATE SODIUM. (Mylan) Meclofenamate sodium 50 mg or 100 mg/Cap. Bot. 100s, 500s.
Use: Nonsteroidal anti-inflammatory agent.
• **MECLOFENAMIC ACID.** USAN. N-(2,6-Dichloro-m-tolyl)-anthranilic acid.
Use: Anti-inflammatory.
MECLOFENOXATE. B.A.N. 2-Dimethylamino-ethyl 4-chlorophenoxyacetate. Lucidril hydrochloride.
Use: Cerebral stimulant.
MECLOMEN. (Parke-Davis) Meclofenamate sodium monohydrate equivalent to 50 mg or 100 mg meclofenamic acid/Cap. Bot. 100s, 500s (100 mg), UD 100s.
Use: Non-steroidal anti-inflammatory agent.
• **MECLOQUALONE.** USAN. 3-(o-Chlorophenyl)-2-methyl-4 (3 H)-quinazolinone.
Use: Sedative/hypnotic.
• **MECLORISONE DIBUTYRATE.** USAN.
Use: Anti-inflammatory.
• **MECOBALAMIN.** USAN.
Use: Vitamin.
MECLOZINE. B.A.N. 1-(4-Chlorobenzhydryl)-4-(3-methylbenzyl)piperazine. Ancolan dihydrochloride.

Use: Antihistamine.
MECOBALAMIN. B.A.N. α-(5,6-Dimethylbenzimidazol-1-yl)cobamide methyl.
Use: Treatment of vitamin B_{12} deficiency.
MECODRIN.
See: Amphetamine (Various Mfr.).
• **MECRYLATE.** USAN. Methyl 2-cyanoacrylate.
Use: Surgical aid (tissue adhesive).
MECYSTEINE. Methyl Cysteine.
MEDA CAP. (Circle) Acetaminophen 500 mg/Cap. Bot. 25s, 60s, 100s.
Use: Analgesic.
MEDACOTE. (Dal-Med) Pyrilamine maleate 1%, dimethyl polysiloxane, zinc oxide, menthol, camphor in a greaseless base. Lot. Bot. 120 ml.
Use: Antihistamine, topical.
MEDADYNE. (Dal-Med) **Liq.:** Methylbenzethonium chloride, benzocaine, tannic acid, camphor, chlorothymol, menthol, benzyl alcohol, alcohol 61%. Bot. 15 ml, 30 ml. **Throat Spray:** Lidocaine, cetyl dimethyl ammonium chloride, ethyl alcohol. Bot. 30 ml.
Use: Mouth and throat product.
MEDA-HIST EXPECTORANT. (Medwick) Bot. 4 oz, pt, gal.
Use: Decongestant, antitussive.
dep MEDALONE 40 Methylprednisolone acetate in aqueous suspension 40 mg/ml, polyethylene glycol, myristyl-gamma-picolinium Cl. Vial 5 ml.
Use: Corticosteroid.
dep MEDALONE 80 Methylprednisolone acetate in aqueous suspension 80 mg/ml, polyethylene glycol, myristyl-gamma-picolinium Cl. Vial 5 ml.
Use: Corticosteroid.
MEDALOX GEL. (Med. Chem.) Magnesium aluminum hydroxide gel. Bot. 12 oz, pt, gal.
Use: Antacid.
MEDAMINT. (Dal-Med) Benzocaine 10 mg/Loz. Pkg. 12s, 24s.
Use: Mouth and throat product.
MED-APAP ELIXIR. (Medwick) Bot. 4 oz, pt, gal.
MEDA CAP. (Circle) Acetaminophen 500 mg/Cap. Bot. 100s.
Use: Analgesic.
MEDA TAB. (Circle) Acetaminophen 325 mg/Tab. Bot. 100s.
Use: Analgesic.
MEDATUSSIN PEDIATRIC. (Dal-Med) Dextromethorphan HBr 5 mg, guaifenesin 50 mg, potassium citrate, citric acid, sorbitol, saccharin. Syr. Bot. 120 ml.

Use: Antitussive, expectorant.
MEDATUSSIN PLUS COUGH. (Dal-Med) Phenylpropanolamine HCl 25 mg, chlorpheniramine maleate 2 mg, phenyltoloxamine citrate 25 mg, dextromethorphan HBr 20 mg, guaifenesin 100 mg. Bot. pt. gal.
Use: Decongestant, antihistamine, antitussive, expectorant.
MEDA-TUSS PE. (Medwick) Bot. 4 oz, pt, gal.
MEDAZEPAM. B.A.N. 7-Chloro-2,3-dihydro-1-methyl-5-phenyl-1H-1,4-benzodiazepine. Nobrium.
Use: Tranquilizer.
MEDAZYME. (Dal-Med) Cellulase 9 mg, amylase 30 mg, protease 6 mg, lipase 20 mg, simethicone 50 mg/Tab. Bot. 50s, 100s.
Use: Hydrocholeretics.
• **MEDAZEPAM HCl.** USAN. 7-Chloro-2, 3-dihydro-1-methyl-5-phenyl-IH-1, 4-benzodiazepine mono-HCl. Under study.
Use: Tranquilizer.
MEDENT. (Stewart-Jackson) Pseudoephedrine HCl 120 mg, guaifenesin 500 mg/Tab. Bot. 100s.
Use: Decongestant, expectorant.
MEDIATRIC. (Wyeth-Ayerst) Vitamins B_1, B_2 5 mg, B_3 50 mg, B_5 20 mg, B_6 3 mg, B_{12} 2.5 mcg, C 100 mg, iron 9 mg, methyltestosterone 2.5 mg, conjugated estrogens 0.25 mg, methamphetamine HCl 1 mg/Cap. Bot. 100s.
Use: Vitamin/mineral, androgen/estrogen, central nervous system stimulant.
MEDICAINE CREAM. (Walgreen) Benzocaine 3%, resorcinol 2%. Tube 1.25 oz.
Use: Antipruritic.
MEDICATED HEALER. (Walgreen) Strong ammonia soln. 10%, camphor 2.6%. Bot. 6 oz.
Use: Emollient.
MEDICATED POWDER. (Johnson & Johnson) Zinc oxide, talc, fragrance, menthol. Plastic container 3 oz, 6 oz, 11 oz.
Use: Antipruritic.
MEDICONE DERMA. (Medicone) Benzocaine 2%, zinc oxide 13.73%, 8-hydroxyquinoline sulfate 1.05%, ichthammol 1%, menthol 0.48%, petrolatum-lanolin base 79.87%. Oint. Tube 42.5 Gm.
Use: Local anesthetic.
MEDICONE DRESSING. (Medicone) Cod liver oil 125 mg, zinc oxide 125 mg, 8-hydroxyquinoline-sulfate 0.5 mg, benzocaine 5 mg, menthol 1.8 mg/Gm w/petrolatum, lanolin, talcum, paraffin, perfume. Tube 1 oz, 3 oz, Jar lb.

Use: Local anesthetic.

MEDICONE RECTAL. (Medicone) Benzocaine 130 mg, hydroxyquinoline sulfate 16 mg, zinc oxide 195 mg, menthol 9 mg, balsam Peru 65 mg. In a vegetable and petroleum oil base. Supp. 12s, 24s.
Use: Anorectal preparation.

MEDICONE-HC RECTAL. (Medicone) Hydrocortisone acetate 10 mg, benzocaine 2 gr, oxyquinoline sulfate 0.25 gr, zinc oxide 3 gr, menthol 1/7 gr, balsam Peru 1 gr, in a cocoa butter base/Supp. Box 12s.
Use: Anorectal preparation.

MEDICONE SUPPOSITORIES. (Dickinson) Live yeast cell extract, shark liver oil in cocoa butter base 3%. Pkg. 12s.
Use: Anorectal preparation.

MEDI-FLU. (Parke-Davis) Pseudoephedrine HCl 30 mg, chlorpheniramine maleate 2 mg, dextromethorphan HBr 15 mg, acetaminophen 500 mg/Cap. Bot. 20s, 48s.
Use: Decongestant, antihistamine, antitussive, analgesic.

MEDI-FLU LIQUID. (Parke-Davis) Pseudoephedrine HCl 10 mg, dextromethorphan HBr 5 mg, chlorpheniramine maleate 0.67 mg, acetaminophen 167 mg, alcohol 19%. Bot. 180 ml.
Use: Decongestant, antitussive, antihistamine.

MEDIGESIC PLUS. (U.S. Pharm. Corp.) Acetaminophen 325 mg, caffeine 40 mg, butalbital 50 mg/Cap. Bot. 100s.
Use: Analgesic, sedative/hypnotic.

MEDIHALER-DUO.
See: Duo-Medihaler.(Riker).

MEDIHALER-EPI. (Riker) Epinephrine bitartrate 7 mg/ml. Soln. Pkg. Medihaler in inert propellant. Oral adapter w/15 ml. Vial. Refill vial 15 ml.
Use: Antiasthmatic.

MEDIHALER-ISO. (Riker) Isoproterenol sulfate 2 mg/ml. Soln. Oral adapter w/15 ml. Oral adapter w/22.5 ml vial. Refill vial 15 ml and 22.5 ml.
Use: Antiasthmatic.

MEDI-JECT UD VIALS. (Century) Tamper-proof rubber stoppered vial containing 1 ml sterile soln. Single dose use.
See: Ulti-ject disposable syringe prods.
Atropine sulfate 0.4 mg/ml.
Atropine sulfate 1.2 mg/ml.
Scopolamine HBr 400 mcg/ml.

MEDILAX. (Mission) Phenolphthalein 120 mg, aspartame, phenylalanine 1.5 mg/Chew. Tab. Bot. 24s.
Use: Laxative.

MEDIPAIN 5. (Medi-Plex) Hydrocodone bitartrate 5 mg, acetaminophen 500 mg. Cap. Bot. 100s.
Use: Narcotic analgesic combination.

MEDIPAK. (Geneva) First-aid kit.

MEDI-PHITE. (Med Chem.) Vitamins B_1 and B_{12}. Syr. Bot. 4 oz, pt, gal.
Use: Vitamin supplement.

MEDIPLAST. (Beiersdorf) Salicylic acid plaster 40%. Box 25s.
Use: Keratolytic.

MEDIPLEX TABULES. (U.S. Chemical) B-complex, vitamin C, E, trace minerals, zinc/Tab. Bot. 100s.
Use: Vitamin/mineral supplement.

MEDIPREN. (McNeil Prods) Ibuprofen 200 mg/Capl. or Tab. Bot. 6s, 24s, 50s, 100s.
Use: Nonsteroidal anti-inflammatory agent.

MEDIQUE EAR DROPS. (E.J. Moore) Carbamide peroxide in anhydrous glycerol.
Use: Antiseptic, otic.

MEDIQUELL. (Parke-Davis Prods) Dextromethorphan HBr 15 mg/Chewy square. Pkg. 12s, 24s.
Use: Antitussive.

MEDI-QUIK AEROSOL. (Mentholatum) Lidocaine 2.5%, benzalkonium Cl 0.1%, ethanol 38%. Aerosol 3 oz.
Use: Antiseptic, local anesthetic.

MEDI-QUICK ANTIBIOTIC OINTMENT. (Mentholatum) Bacitracin neomycin, polymyxin in ointment base. Tube 0.5 oz.
Use: Anti-infective, topical.

MEDI-SPAS ELIXIR. (Medical Chemicals) Phenobarbital 16.2 mg, hyoscyamine sulfate 0.1037 mg, atropine sulfate 0.0194 mg, hyoscine hydrobromide 0.0065 mg, alcohol 23%/5 ml. Bot. 4 oz, pt, gal.
Use: Anticholinergic/antispasmodic, sedative/hypnotic.

MEDI-TAL. (Medi-Rx) Phenobarbital 16 mg, hyoscyamine sulfate 0.1037 mg, atropine sulfate 0.0194 mg, scopolamine HBr 0.0065 mg, alcohol 23%/5 ml. Bot. pt, gal. Tab. Bot. 100s, 1000s.
Use: Anticholinergic/antispasmodic, sedative/hypnotic.

MEDITUSSIN-X LIQUID. (Hauck) Codeine phosphate 50 mg, ammonium Cl 520 mg, potassium guaiacolsulfonate 520 mg, pyrilamine maleate 50 mg, phenylpropanolamine HCl 50 mg, dl-desoxyephedrine HCl 2 mg, tartar emetic 5 mg, phenyltoloxamine dihydrogen citrate 30 mg/30 ml. Bot. pt, gal.

Use: Antitussive, expectorant, antihistamine.
• **MEDORINONE.** USAN.
Use: Cardiotonic.
MEDOTAR. (Medco Lab) Coal tar 1%, polysorbate 80 0.5%, octoxynol 5, zinc oxide, starch, white petrolatum. Jar lb.
Use: Antipsoriatic, antipruritic.
MEDOTOPES. (Squibb) Radiopharmaceuticals.
See: A-C-D Solution Modified (Squibb).
Acid Citrate Dextrose Anticoagulant Solution Modified (Squibb).
Aggregated Albumin (Squibb).
Albumotope (Squibb).
Angiotensin Immutope Kit (Squibb).
Cobalt-Labeled Vitamin B_{12} (Squibb).
Cobalt Standards for Vitamin B_{12} (Squibb).
Cobatope (Squibb).
Digoxin (^{125}I) Immutope Kit (Squibb).
Gastrin (^{125}I) Immutope Kit (Squibb).
Gold-198 (Squibb).
Hipputope (Squibb).
Human Serum Albumin (Squibb).
Iodine 131: Capsules Diagnostic-Capsules Therapeutic-Solution Therapeutic Oral (Squibb).
Iodinated Human Serum Albumin (Squibb).
Iodo-hippuric Acid (Squibb).
Macroaggregated Albumin (Squibb).
Macrotec (Squibb).
Minitec (Squibb).
Phosphorus-32: Solution Oral, Therapeutic-Sodium Phosphate Solution U.S.P. for oral or IV use therapeutic or diagnostic (Squibb).
Red Cell Tagging Solution (Squibb).
Renotec (Squibb).
Rose Bengal (Squibb).
Rubratope-57: Diagnostic Capsules-Diagnostic Kit (Squibb).
Rubratope-60: Diagnostic Capsules-Diagnostic Kit (Squibb).
Selenomethionine (Squibb).
Sethotope (Squibb).
Technetium 99m (Squibb).
Technetium 99m-Iron-Ascorbate (DTPA) (Squibb).
Technetium 99m Sulfur Colloid Kit (Squibb).
Tesuloid (Squibb).
Thyrostat-FTI (Squibb).
Thyrostat-3 (Squibb).
Thyrostat-4 FTI (Squibb).
MEDRALONE 40. (Keene) Methylprednisolone acetate 40 mg/ml. Vial 5 ml.
Use: Corticosteroid.
MEDRALONE 80. (Keene) Methylprednisolone acetate 80 mg/ml. Vial 5 ml.
Use: Corticosteroid.
• **MEDROGESTONE.** USAN. Formerly Metrogestone. Dimethyl pregna-4, 6 diene-3, 20-dione.
Use: Oral progestin.
See: Colprone (Wyeth-Ayerst).
MEDROL. (Upjohn) Methylprednisolone.
Tab.: 2 mg. Bot. 100s; 4 mg Bot. 30s, 100s, 500s, UD 100s; 8 mg Bot. 25s; 16 mg Bot. 50s; 24 mg Bot. 25s; 32 mg Bot. 25s. **Dosepak:** 4 mg Pkg. 21s. **Alternate Daypak:** 16 mg Pkg. 14s.
Use: Corticosteroid.
• **MEDRONATE DISODIUM.** USAN.
Use: Pharmaceutic aid.
• **MEDRONIC ACID.** USAN.
Use: Pharmaceutic aid.
MEDROSPHOL Hg-197. 1-(Hydroxymercuri-197 Hg)-2-propanol.
See: Merprane.
• **MEDROXALOL.** USAN.
Use: Antihypertensive.
• **MEDROXALOL HYDROCHLORIDE.** USAN.
Use: Antihypertensive.
MEDROXYPROGESTERONE ACETATE. (Lederle) Medroxyprogesterone acetate 10 mg/Tab. Bot. 50s, 250s.
Use: Progestin.
• **MEDROXYPROGESTERONE ACETATE,** U.S.P. XXIII. Sterile Susp., Tab., U.S.P. XXIII. 17 Hydroxy 6α methylpregn 4 ene-3, 20-dione 17-Acetate. (CMC) 50 mg, 100 mg/ml. Vial 5 ml.
Use: Progestin.
See: Amen, Tab. (Carnrick).
Curretab, Tab. (Solvay).
Cycrin, Tab. (ESI Pharma).
depCorlutin (Forest).
Depo-Provera, Vial (Upjohn).
P-Medrate-P.A., Inj. (Solvay).
Provera, Tab. (Upjohn).
• **MEDRYSONE,** U.S.P. XXII. Ophthalmic Susp. U.S.P. XXII. 11 β-Hydroxy-6α-methylpregn-4-ene-3,20-dione.
Use: Topical anti-inflammatory agent.
See: HMS Liquifilm, Ophth. Soln. (Allergan).
MED-TANE ELIXIR. (Medwick) Brompheniramine maleate. Bot. 4 oz, pt, gal.
Use: Antihistamine.
• **MEFENAMIC ACID.** USAN. U.S.P. XXIII. Cap. N-(2,3-Xylyl) anthranilic acid. Ponstan.
Use: Anti-inflammatory agent.
See: Ponstel, Kapseal (Parke-Davis).
• **MEFENIDIL.** USAN.
Use: Cerebral vasodilator.

• **MEFENIDIL FUMARATE.** USAN.
Use: Cerebral vasodilator.
MEFENOREX HCI. USAN. N-(3-chloro-propyl)-α-methylphenethylamineHCl.
Under study.
Use: Anorexiant.
• **MEFEXAMIDE.** USAN.
Use: Stimulant.
• **MEFLOQUINE.** USAN.
Use: Antimalarial.
• **MEFLOQUINE HYDROCHLORIDE.**
USAN.
Use: Antimalarial. [Orphan drug]
See: Lariam (Roche).
MEFOXIN. (Merck & Co.) Sterile cefoxitin sodium 1 Gm or 2 Gm/Vial. **1 Gm:** Vial 10 ml. 10s, 25s, ADD-Vantage Vial Tray 25s. Infusion bottle 100 ml, Tray 10s. Premixed I.V. Soln. in 50 ml. D5W, 24s. **2 Gm:** Vial 20 ml. 10s, 25s, ADD-Vantage Vial, Tray 25s, Infusion bottle 100 ml, Tray 10s. Premixed I.V. Soln. in 50 ml. D5W, 24s. Bulk pkg. 10 Gm/100 ml. Bot.
Use: Antibacterial, cephalosporin.
MEFOXIN IN 5% DEXTROSE. (Merck & Co.) Cefoxitin sodium 1 Gm or 2 Gm in Dextrose in Water 5%. Inj. Viaflex plus containers 50 ml.
Use: Antibacterial, cephalosporin.
MEFRUSIDE. USAN. (FBA) 4-Chloro-N′-methyl-N-(tetrahydro-2-methylfurfuryl)-m-benzenedisulfonamide. Baycaron.
Use: Diuretic.
MEGA-B. (Arco) Vitamins B_1 100 mg, B_2 60 mg, B_6 100 mg, B_{12} 100 mcg, niacinamide 100 mg, folic acid 100 mcg, pantothenic acid 100 mg, d-biotin 100 mcg, PABA 100 mg/Tab. Bot. 30s, 100s, 500s.
Use: Vitamin B supplement.
MEGA B WITH C. (Nature's Bounty) Vitamins B_1 10 mg, B_2 15 mg, B_3 25 mg, B_5 100 mg, B_6 10 mg, B_{12} 25 mcg, C 500 mg, tartrazine, folic acid 400 mcg, biotin 100 mcg, choline bitartrate 125 mg, inositol 250 mg, PABA 50 mg/Tab. Bot. 60s.
Use: Vitamin supplement.
MEGACE. (Mead Johnson Oncology) Megestrol acetate 20 mg or 40 mg/Tab. **20 mg/Tab.:** Bot. 100s; **40 mg/Tab.:** Bot. 100s, 250s, 500s. Megestrol acetate 40 mg/ml, alcohol ≤ 0.06%, sucrose. Susp. Bot. 236.6 ml.
Use: Antineoplastic agent, progestin.
MEGADOSE. (Arco) Vitamins A 25,000 USP units, D 1000 USP units, C 250 mg, E 100 IU, folic acid 400 mcg, B_1 80 mg, B_2 80 mg, niacinamide 80 mg, B_6 80 mg,

B_{12} 80 mcg, biotin 80 mcg, pantothenic acid 80 mg, choline bitartrate 80 mg, inositol 80 mg, para-aminobenzoic acid 80 mg, rutin 30 mg, citrus bioflavonoids 30 mg, betaine HCl 30 mg, glutamic acid 30 mg, hesperidin complex 5 mg, iodine 0.15 mg, calcium gluconate 10 mg, ferrous gluconate 10 mg, magnesium gluconate / mg, manganese gluconate 6 mg, copper gluconate 0.5 mg/Cap. Bot. 100s, 250s.
Use: Vitamin/nutritional supplement.
• **MEGALOMICIN POTASSIUM PHOSPHATE.** USAN.
Use: Antibacterial.
MEGATON. (Hyrex) Dexpanthenol 10 mg, niacinamide 40 mg, vitamins B_6 4 mg, B_{12} 12 mcg, folic acid 1 mg, iron 36 mg, zinc 15 mg, manganese 4 mg, alcohol 13%. Bot. 16 oz.
Use: Vitamin/mineral supplement.
MEGA-VITA. (Saron) Vitamins C 500 mg, niacinamide 500 mg, B_6 50 mg, B_1 25 mg, B_2 10 mg, B_{12} 50 mcg, folic acid 150 mcg, E 200 IU, pantothenic acid 10 mg, A 2500 IU, D 333 IU, magnesium oxide 50 mg, zinc sulfate 50 mg/3 Tab. Bot. 100s.
Use: Vitamin/mineral supplement.
MEGA-VITA HEMATINIC. (Saron) Mega-Vita formula with iron 50 mg, vitamin A 1000 IU, copper 2 mg, manganese 1.8 mg, iodine 0.1 mg, potassium 10 mg/3 Tab.
Use: Vitamin/mineral supplement.
MEGA-VITA TONIC. (Saron) Vitamins B_{12} 25 mcg, B_6 6 mg, niacin 25 mg, aminoacetic acid 750 mg/15 ml, alcohol 17%.
Use: Vitamin supplement.
MEGA VM-80. (Nature's Bounty) Vitamins A 10,000 IU, D 1,000 IU, E 100 mg, B_1 80 mg, B_2 80 mg, B_3 80 mg, B_5 80 mg, B_6 80 mg, B_{12} 80 mcg, C 250 mg, iron 1.2 mg, folic acid 0.4 mg, calcium 4.5 mg, zinc 3.58 mg, choline 80 mg, inositol 80 mg, biotin 80 mcg, PABA 80 mg, rutin, bioflavonoids 30 mg, betaine 30 mg, glutamic acid 30 mg, hesperidin 5 mg, Cu, I, K, Mg, Mn. Tab. Bot. 30s, 60s, 100s.
Use: Vitamins/mineral supplement.
• **MEGESTROL ACETATE,** U.S.P. XXIII. Tab., U.S.P. XXIII. 17 α-acetoxy-6-methylpregna-4,6-diene-3, 20-dione.
Use: Palliative treatment of advanced carcinoma of the breast or endometrium. AIDS-related weight loss [Orphan drug]
See: Megace (Mead Johnson Oncolo-

gy).
Pallace, Tab. (Bristol).
MEGLUMINE, U.S.P. XXIII. 1-Deoxy-1-methyl- amino glucitol. 1-Methylamino-1-deoxy-D-glucitol.
Use: Pharmaceutical aid.
•**MEGLUMINE, DIATRIZOATE INJ.,** U.S.P.
XXIII. N-Meglumine salt of 3, 5 diacetamido-2, 4, 6-triiodo-benzoic acid. Methylglucamine Diatrizoate. D-Glucitol, 1-deoxy-1-(methylamino).
Use: Radiopaque medium.
See: Cardiografin, Vial (Squibb).
Cystografin, Vial (Squibb).
Gastrografin, Soln. (Squibb).
Hypaque-76, Inj. (Sanofi Winthrop).
Hypaque-M 75%, Inj. (Sanofi Winthrop).
Hypaque-M 90%, Inj. (Sanofi Winthrop).
Hypaque Meglumine, Vial (Sanofi Winthrop).
Reno-M-30, -60, Vial (Squibb).
Reno-M-Dip, Vial (Squibb).
W/Meglumine iodipamide.
See: Sinografin, Soln. (Squibb).
W/Sodium diatrizoate.
See: Gastrografin, Soln. (Squibb).
Renografin-60, Inj. (Squibb).
Renografin-76, Inj. (Squibb).
Renovist II, Inj. (Squibb).
•**MEGLUMINE, IODIPAMIDE INJ.,** U.S.P.
XXIII. 1-Deoxy-1-(methyl amino) glucitol, D glucitol, 1-deoxy-1-(methylamino).
Use: Radiopaque medium.
See: Cholografin, Vial (Squibb).
W/Meglumine diatrizoate.
See: Sinografin, Soln. (Squibb).
•**MEGLUMINE, IOTHALAMATE INJ.,** U.S.P. XXIII. 5-Acetamido-2,4,6-triiodo-N-methylisophthalamic acid, N-methylglucamine.
Use: Radiopaque medium.
•**MEGLUTOL.** USAN.
Use: Antihyperlipoproteinemic.
MEJEPTIL.
See: Thioperazine (SK-Beecham).
MELADRAZINE. B.A.N. 2,4-Di(diethylamino)-6- hydrazino-1,3,5-triazine. Lisidonil (+)-tartrate.
Use: Polysynaptic inhibitor.
•**MELAFOCON A.** USAN.
Use: Contact lens material (hydrophilic).
MELANEX. (Neutrogena) Hydroquinone 3% in solution containing alcohol 47.3%. Bot. 1 oz w/Appliderm applicator and pinpoint rod applicator.
Use: Skin bleaching agent.
MELANOMA VACCINE.

Use: Stage III-IV melanoma. [Orphan drug]
MELARSONYL POTASSIUM. B.A.N. Dipotassium 2-[4-(4,6-diamino-1,3,5-triazin-2-ylamino)phenyl]-1,3,2-dithiarsolan-4,5-dicarboxylate. Trimelarsan.
Use: Treatment of trypanosomiasis.
MELARSOPROL. B.A.N. 2-[4-(4,6-Diamino-1,3,5-triazin-2-ylamino)phenyl]-4-hydroxymethyl-1,3,2-dithiarsolan. Mel B.
Use: Treatment of trypanosomiasis.
MELATONIN.
Use: Treatment of circadian rhythm sleep disorders in blind patients. [Orphan drug]
•**MELENGESTROL ACETATE.** USAN.
Use: Antineoplastic, progestin.
MELFIAT-105 UNICELLES. (Solvay) Phendimetrazine tartrate 105 mg/SR Cap. Bot. 100s.
Use: Anorexiant.
MELHORAL CHILD TABLET. (Sanofi Winthrop) Acetylsalicylic acid.
Use: Salicylate analgesic.
MELITOXIN.
See: Dicumarol (Various Mfr.).
•**MELITRACEN HYDROCHLORIDE.** USAN.
Use: Antidepressant.
•**MELIZAME.** USAN.
Use: Sweetener.
MELLARIL CONCENTRATE. (Sandoz) Thioridazine HCl 30 mg/ml, alcohol 3%. Soln. Bot. 4 oz. Concentrate 100 mg/ml. Pk. 4 oz.
Use: Antipsychotic agent.
MELLARIL S. (Sandoz) Thioridazine 25 mg/5 ml or 100 mg/5 ml. Susp. Bot. pt.
Use: Antipsychotic agent.
MELLARIL TABLETS. (Sandoz) Thioridazine HCl 10 mg, 15 mg, 25 mg, 50 mg, 100 mg, 150 mg or 200 mg/Tab. Bot. 100s, 1000s. SandoPak pkg. 100s (except 150 mg).
Use: Antipsychotic agent.
MELLOSE. Methylcellulose.
MELONEX. Metahexamide.
Use: Oral antidiabetic.
•**MELPAQUE HP.** (Stratus) Hydroquinone 4% in a sunblocking base of talc, EDTA, sodium metabisulfite. Cream. Tube 14.2 g, 28.4 g.
Use: Skin bleaching agent.
•**MELPHALAN,** U.S.P. XXIII. Tab., U.S.P. XXIII. L-3- [fb]p[bis(2-Chloroethyl)amino]phenyl alanine. Previously Sarcolysin.
Use: Antineoplastic. [Orphan drug]
See: Alkeran, Tab. (Burroughs Wellcome).

Alkeran, Pow. for Inj. (Burroughs Well-
come).
MELQUIN HP. (Stratus) Hydroquinone
4%, mineral oil, propylparaben, sodium
metabisulfite. Cream. Tube 14.2 g, 28.4
g.
Use: Skin bleaching agent.
• **MEMOTINE HCl.** USAN. 3, 4-Dihydro-1-
[(p-methoxyphenl-oxy)methyl]isoquino-
line HCl.
Use: Antiviral.
• **MEMOTINE HYDROCHLORIDE.** USAN.
Use: Antiviral.
• **MENABITAN HYDROCHLORIDE.**
USAN.
Use: Analgesic.
• **MENADIONE,** U.S.P. XXIII. Inj., U.S.P.
XXIII. 2-Methyl-1,4-naphthoquinone
(Menaphthone, Danitamon K, Aquinone,
Aquaday, Menaquinone).
Use: Orally & I.M., Vitamin K therapy.
W/Ascorbic acid.
See: Rependo, Cap. (Scruggs).
W/Ascorbic acid, hesperidin.
See: Hescor-K, Tab. (Madland).
W/Bioflavonoid citrus compound, ascorbic
acid.
See: C.V.P. W/Vitamin K, Syr., Tab.
(USV Pharm.).
MENADIONE DIPHOSPHATE SODIUM.
See: Menadiol Sodium Diphosphate.
MENADOL. (Rugby) Ibuprofen 200
mg/Tab. Bot. 50s, 100s.
Use: Nonsteroidal anti-inflammatory
agent.
MENADOXIME. B.A.N. Ammonium salt of
2-methylnaphthaquinone-4-oxime O-
carboxymethyl ether. Kapilon Soluble.
Use: Treatment of hypoprothrombine-
mia.
MENAPHTHENE OR MENAPHTHONE.
See: Menadione (Various Mfr.).
MENAQUINONE.
See: Menadione (Various Mfr.).
MENEST. (SK-Beecham) Esterified es-
trogens, conjugated estrogens (equine)
0.3 mg or 0.625 mg/Tab.: Bot. 100s.
1.25 mg/Tab.: Bot. 100s, 1000s; **2.5
mg/Tab.:** Bot. 50s.
Use: Estrogen combination.
MENI-D. (Seatrace) Meclizine 25
mg/Cap. Bot. 100s.
Use: Antiemetic/antivertigo.
• **MENINGOCOCCAL POLYSACCHARIDE
VACCINE GROUP A,** U.S.P. XXIII.
Use: Immunizing agent (active).
**MENINGOCOCCAL POLYSACCHARIDE
VACCINE GROUPS A AND C COM-
BINED,** U.S.P. XXI.
Use: Immunizing agent (active).

W/Groups A, C, Y, W-135 Combined.
See: Menomune, Inj. (Squibb/Con-
naught).
• **MENINGOCOCCAL POLYSACCHARIDE
VACCINE GROUP C,** U.S.P. XXIII.
Use: Immunizing agent (active).
• **MENOCTONE.** USAN. 2-(8-Cyclohexyl-
octyl)-3-hydroxy-1, 4-naphthoquinone.
Under study.
Use: Antimalarial.
• **MENOGARIL.** USAN.
Use: Antineoplastic.
MENOJECT L.A. (Mayrand) Testosterone
cypionate, estradiol cypionate. Vial 10
ml.
Use: Androgen, estrogen combination.
MENOLYN. (Arcum) Ethinyl estradiol
0.05 mg/Tab. Bot. 100s, 1000s.
Use: Estrogen.
MENOMUNE. (Squibb/Connaught)
Meningococcal polysaccharide vaccine,
Groups A, C, Y, W-135. Vial 10 or 50
dose w/diluent.
Use: Agent for immunization.
MENOMUNE-C VACCINE. Group-specif-
ic polysaccharide antigen from Neisseria
meningitis, Group C. Bot. 10 and 50
dose vial.
Use: Agent for immunization.
MENOPLEX TABLETS. (Fiske) Aceta-
minophen 325 mg, phenyltoloxamine cit-
rate 30 mg/ Tab. Bot. 20s.
Use: Analgesic.
• **MENOTROPINS,** U.S.P. XXIII. For Inj.,
U.S.P. XXIII.
Use: Gonadotropin.
See: Pergonal.
MENRIUM. (Roche) **Menrium 5-2:** Chlordiazepoxide 5 mg, water-soluble esteri-
fied estrogens 0.2 mg/Tab. **Menrium 5-
4:** Chlordiazepoxide 5 mg, water-soluble
esterified estrogens 0.4 mg/Tab. **Menri-
um 10-4:** Chlordiazepoxide 10 mg, wa-
ter-soluble esterified estrogens 0.4
mg/Tab. Bot. 100s.
Use: Estrogen.
MENSTRESS CAPS. (Pharmex) Cap.
Bot. 15s.
Use: Cramps.
MENTHOL, U.S.P. XXIII. Cyclohexanol,
5-methyl-2-(1-methylethyl). p-Menthan-
3-ol.
Use: Topical antipruritic, local analgesic, nasal decongestant, antitussive.
See: Benzedrex Inhaler (SK-Beecham).
Blue Gel Muscular Pain Reliever (Rug-
by).
Robitussin Liquid Center Cough
Drops, Loz. (Robins).

Vicks Cough Silencers, Loz. (Vicks).
Vicks Formula 44 Cough Control
  Discs, Loz. (Vicks).
Vicks Inhaler (Vicks).
Vicks Blue Mint, Lemon, Regular and
  Wild Cherry Medicated Cough Drops
  (Vicks).
Vicks Medi-Trating Throat Loz. (Vicks).
Vicks Oracin Regular and Cherry, Loz.
  (Vicks).
Vicks Sinex, Nasal Spray (Vicks).
Vicks Vaporub, Oint. (Vicks).
Vicks Vaposteam, Liq. (Vicks).
Vicks Va-Tro-Nol, Nose Drops (Vicks).
Victors Regular and Cherry, Loz.
  (Vicks).
W/Combinations.
  See: Eucalyptamint, Gel (Ciba).
  Eucalyptamint Maximum Strength,
    Oint. (Ciba).
  Halls Mentho-Lyptus, Prods. (Warner-
    Lambert).
  Listerine Antiseptic, Liq. (Warner-Lam-
    bort).
MENTHOLATUM. (Mentholatum) Men-
  thol 1.35%, camphor 9%, titanium diox-
  ide and fragrance in ointment base of
  petrolatum. Tube 0.4 oz, 1 oz. Jar 1 oz, 3
  oz.
Use: External analgesic.
**MENTHOLATUM DEEP HEATING LO-
TION.** (Mentholatum) Menthol 6%,
  methyl salicylate 20%, lanolin derivative
  in lotion base. Bot. 2 oz, 4 oz.
Use: External analgesic.
MENTHOLATUM DEEP HEATING RUB.
  (Mentholatum) Menthol 5.8%, methyl
  salicylate 12.7%, eucalyptus oil, turpentine oil, anhydrous lanolin, vehicle and
  fragrance. Tube 1.25 oz, 3.33 oz, 5 oz.
Use: External analgesic.
MENTHOLIN. (Apco) Methyl salicylate
  30%, chloroform 20%, hard soap 3%,
  camphor gum 2.2%, menthol 0.8%, al-
  cohol 35%. Bot. 2 oz.
Use: External analgesic.
MENTHYL VALERATE. Validol.
Use: Sedative.
MENTROLZ. (Mayer) Mayercin (Homat-
  ropine methylbromide 0.5 mg and am-
  monium Cl 300 mg), caffeine alkaline 32
  mg, acetophenetidin 150 mg, salicy-
  lamide 225 mg/Tab. Bot. 16s.
Use: Analgesic combination.
• **MEOBENTINE SULFATE.** USAN.
Use: Cardiac depressant.
MEP-40. (Parnell) Methylprednisolone
  acetate 40 mg/ml. Inj. Susp. Vial. 5 ml.
Use: Corticosteroid.
MEPACRINE HYDROCHLORIDE.

Use: Anthelmintic, antimalarial.
  See: Quinacrine HCl, U.S.P. XXIII.
MEPARFYNOL. 2-Ethinylbutanol-2.
  Methylparafynol, methylpentynol.
• **MEPARTRICIN.** USAN.
Use: Antifungal, antiprotozoal.
MEPAVLON.
  See: Meprobamate, U.S.P. XXIII.
MEPAZINE ACETATE & HCl. 10-[1-
  Methyl-3-(piperidyl)methyl] phenoth-
  iazine acetate or HCl.
MEPENZOLATE BROMIDE, U.S.P. XXII.
  Syr., Tab., U.S.P. XXI. N-methyl-3-hy-
  droxypiperidine benzilate methobro-
  mide.
Use: Anticholinergic.
  See: Cantil, Tab., Liq. (Merrell Dow).
W/Phenobarbital.
  See: Cantil w/phenobarbital (Merrell
    Dow).
MEPENZOLATE METHYL BROMIDE.
  Mepenzolate bromide.
Use: Anticholinergic.
MEPERGAN. (Wyeth-Ayerst) Promet-
  hazine HCl 25 mg, meperidine HCl 25
  mg/ml. Inj. Vial 10 ml, Tubex 2 ml. Box
  10s.
Use: Narcotic analgesic combination.
MEPERGAN FORTIS. (Wyeth-Ayerst)
  Meperidine HCl 50 mg, promethazine
  HCl 25 mg/Cap. Bot. 100s.
Use: Narcotic analgesic combination.
• **MEPERIDINE HYDROCHLORIDE,**
  U.S.P. XXIII. Inj., Syr., Tab., U.S.P. XXIII.
  (Various Mfr.) Ethyl-1-methyl-4-
  phenylisonipecotate HCl. (Parke-Davis)
  50 mg/ml, 75 mg/ml or 100 mg/ml as 1
  ml fill in 2 ml Steri-dose syringe. (Dolan-
  tal, Dolantin, Dolosal, Dolvanol, En-
  dolate, Isonipecaine, Pethidine).
Use: Analgesic (narcotic).
  See: Demerol HCl, Prods. (Sanofi
    Winthrop).
W/Acetaminophen.
  See: Demerol APAP, Tab. (Sanofi
    Winthrop).
W/Promethazine HCl.
  See: Mepergan, Preps. (Wyeth-Ayerst).
**MEPERIDINE HCl AND ATROPINE SUL-
FATE.**
Use: General anesthetic.
  See: Atropine and Demerol, Inj.(Sanofi
    Winthrop).
MEPHENESIN. 3-o-Tolyloxypropane-1,2-
  diol. Lissephen; Myanesin; Tolseram
  carbamate.
Use: Skeletal muscle relaxant.
  See: Mervaldin, Tab. (Lannett).
  Myanesin.
W/Acetaminophen, Vitamin C, butabarbi-

tal.
See: T-Caps, Cap. (Burlington).
W/Mephobarbital, hyoscine HBr.
See: Tranquil, Tab. (Kenyon).
W/Pentobarbital.
See: Nebralin, Tab. (Dorsey).
W/Salicylamide, butabarbital sodium.
See: Metrogesic, Tab. (Metro Med).
MEPHENESIN CARBAMATE.
See: Methoxydone.
MEPHENOXALONE. 5-(o-Methoxyphe-
noxy-methyl-)-2-oxazolidinone.
• **MEPHENTERMINE SULFATE,** U.S.P.
XXIII. Inj., U.S.P. XXIII. N,α,α-Trimethyl-
phenethylamine sulfate. Mephine.
Use: Vasoconstrictor and nasal decon-
gestant. Also I.V. or I.M.
See: Wyamine Sulfate Inj. (Wyeth-Ay-
erst).
• **MEPHENYTOIN,** U.S.P. XXIII. Tab.,
U.S.P. XXIII. 5-Ethyl-3-methyl-5-phenyl-
hydantoin.
Use: Anticonvulsant.
See: Mesantoin, Tab. (Sandoz).
• **MEPHOBARBITAL,** U.S.P. XXIII. Tab.,
U.S.P. XXIII. 5-Ethyl-5-phenyl N-methyl-
barbituric acid. 5-Ethyl-1-methyl-5-
phenylbarbituric Acid.
Use: Anticonvulsant, sedative.
See: Mebaral, Tab. (Sanofi Winthrop).
W/Acetaminophen.
See: Koly-Tabs (Scrip).
W/Homatropine methylbromide, atropine
methylnitrate and hyoscine HBr.
W/Mephenesin, hyoscine HBr.
See: Tranquil, Tab. (Kenyon).
MEPHONE.
See: Mephentermine.
MEPHYTON. (Merck & Co.) Phytona-
dione (vitamin K-1) 5 mg/Tab. Bot. 100s.
Use: Prothrombogenic
MEPIBEN. (Schen Labs.) Methylpiperidyl
benzhydryl ether.
Use: Antihistamine.
MEPIPERPHENIDOL BROMIDE. 1-(3
Hydroxy-5-methyl-4-phenylexyl)-1-
methyl piperidium bromide.
Use: Anticholinergic.
MEPIPRAZOLE. B.A.N. 1-(3-
Chlorophenyl)-4-[2-(5-methylpyrazol-3-
yl)ethyl]piperazine.
Use: Psychotropic agent.
• **MEPIVACAINE HCl,** U.S.P. XXIII. Inj.,
U.S.P. XXIII. dl-1-Methyl-2',6-pipe-
coloxylidide monohydrochloride.(±)-1-
Methyl-2,6-pipecoloxylidide Hydrochlo-
ride.
Use: Local anesthetic.
See: Carbocaine, Cartridge, Vial (Cook-
Waite).

Carbocaine, Vial (Sanofi Winthrop).
Cavacaine, Vial (Graham).
Polocaine, Vial (Astra).
MEPIVACAINE HCl. (Goldline) Mepiva-
caine HCl 1%, methylparaben. Inj. Vial
50 ml.
Use: Local anesthetic.
• **MEPIVACAINE HYDROCHLORIDE AND
LEVONORDEFRIN INJ.,** U.S.P. XXIII.
Use: Local anesthetic.
See: Carbocaine, Cartridge, Vial (Cook-
Waite).
• **MEPREDNISONE,** U.S.P. XXIII. 17,21-Di-
hydroxy-16β-methylpregna-1,4-diene-
3,11,20-trione. Betaspred.
Use: Glucocorticoid.
• **MEPROBAMATE,** U.S.P. XXIII. Oral
Susp., Tab., U.S.P. XXIII. 2-Methyl-2-n-
propyl-1,3-propanediol di-carbamate.
2,2-Di(carbamoyloxymethyl)pentane. 2-
Carbamoyloxymethyl-2-methylpentyl
carbamate. Me-pavlon.
Use: Minor tranquilizer, sedative.
See: Arcoban Tab. (Arcum).
Bamate, Tab. (Century).
Equanil Tab., Cap., (Wyeth-Ayerst).
Meprospan, Cap. (Wallace).
Miltown, Tab. (Wallace).
Pax-400,Tab. (Kenyon).
Tranmep, Tab. (Solvay).
W/Acetylsalicylic acid.
See: Equagesic, Tab. (Wyeth-Ayerst).
W/Benactyzine HCl.
See: Deprol, Tab. (Wallace).
W/Estrogens conjugated.
See: Milprem, Tab. (Wallace).
W/Pentaerythritol tetranitrate.
See: Miltrate, Tab. (Wallace).
W/Premarin.
See: PMB 200, Tab. (Wyeth-Ayerst).
W/Tridihexethyl Cl.
See: Milpath, Tab. (Wallace).
Pathibamate—200, 400, Tab. (Leder-
le).
MEPROBAMATE/ASPIRIN. (Various
Mfr.) Aspirin 325 mg, meprobamate 200
mg/Tab. Bot. 100s, 500s.
Use: Nonnarcotic analgesic combina-
tion.
MEPROBAMATE/BENACTYZINE.
Use: Miscellaneous psychotherapeutic
agent.
See: Deprol (Wallace).
MEPROBAMATE, N-ISOPROPYL.
See: Carisoprodol.
MEPROCHOL. B.A.N. (2-Methoxyprop-2-
enyl)-trime-thylammonium bromide. Es-
modil.
Use: Parasympathomimetic.
MEPROGESIC Q. (Various Mfr.) Aspirin

325 mg, meprobamate 200 mg/Tab. Bot. 100s, 500s.
Use: Nonnarcotic analgesic combination.

MEPROLONE TABS. (Major) Methylprednisolone 4 mg/Tab. Bot. 25s, 100s.
Use: Corticosteroid.

MEPRON. (Burroughs Wellcome) Atovaquone. 250 mg/Bot. 200s.
Use: Anti-infective.

MEPROSPAN. (Wallace) Meprobamate in form of coated pellets which release drug continuously for 10 - 12 hours. 200 mg or 400 mg/Cap. Bot. 100s.
Use: Antianxiety agent.

MEPROTHIXOL. B.A.N. 9-(3-Dimethylamino-propyl)-9-hydroxy-2-methoxythiaxanthen.
Use: Analgesic, anti-inflammatory.

• **MEPRYLCAINE HYDROCHLORIDE,** U.S.P. XXII. 2-Methyl-2-propylaminopropyl Benzoate HCl. 2-Methyl-2-(propylamino)-1-propanol benzoate (Ester) Hydrochloride.
Use: Local anesthetic (dental).

• **MEPRYLCAINE HYDROCHLORIDE AND EPINEPHRINE INJ.,** U.S.P. XXII.
Use: Local anesthetic.

• **MEPTAZINOL HYDROCHLORIDE.** USAN.
Use: Analgesic.

MEPYRAMINE. B.A.N. N-4-Methoxybenzyl-N'N-di-methyl-N-2 pyridylethylonodiamine. 2-(N-p-Anisyl-N-2-pyridylamino)ethyldimethylamine. Anthical; Anthisan; Flavelix; Neo-antergan hydrogen maleate.
Use: Antihistamine.

MEPYRAPONE. 2-Methyl-1,2-di-3-pyridyl-1-propane.
See: Metopirone, Tab., Amp. (Ciba).

• **MEQUIDOX.** USAN. 3-Methyl-2-quinozaline-methanol 1,4-dioxide. Under study.
Use: Antibacterial.

MEQUINOLATE. Name used for Proquinolate.

MERAGIDONE SODIUM. The sodium salt of anhydro-N-(beta-methoxy-gamma-hydroxymercuripropyl)-2-pyridone-5-carboxylic acid-theophylline.

• **MERALEIN SODIUM.** USAN.
Use: Topical anti-infective.
See: Sodium Meralein.

MERALLURIDE. B.A.N. Equal amts. of theophylline and methoxyhydroxymercuripropyl succinylurea. [3-[3-(3-Carboxypropionyl)ureido]-2-methoxypropyl]hydroxy-mercury mixture with theophylline.
Use: Diuretic.

MERBAPHEN. 2-(Carboxymethoxy)-3-chlorophenyl (5,5-diethylbarbiturato)mercury.

MERBROMIN. Disodium 2,7-dibrom-4-hydroxy-mercurifluorescein. (Asceptichrome, Chromargyre, Cynochrome, Flavurol, Gallochrome Mercurocol, Mercurophage, Mercurome, Planochrome).
Use: Topical antiseptic.

• **MERCAPTOPURINE,** U.S.P. XXIII. Tab., U.S.P. XXIII. 6-Mercaptopurine. Purine-6-thiol. monohydrate; 6H-purine-6-thione, monohydrate.
Use: Antineoplastic.
See: Purinethol, Tab. (Burroughs Wellcome).

MERCARBOLID. o-Hydroxy-phenylmercuric Cl.

MERCAZOLE.
See: Methimazole, U.S.P. XXIII.

MERCOCRESOLS.
See: Mercresin, Tr. (Upjohn).

• **MERCUFENOL CHLORIDE.** USAN.
Use: Anti-infective.

MERCUPURIN.
See: Mercurophylline Inj. (Various Mfr.).

MERCURANINE.
See: Merbromin (City Chem.).

MERCURIAL, ANTISYPHILITICS. Mercuric Oleate Mercuric Salicylate.

MERCURIC OLEATE. Oleate of mercury.
Use: Parasitic and fungal skin diseases. W/Coal tar crude, salicylic acid, phenol & p-nitrophenol.
See: Prosol, Emulsion (Torch).
Estercol, Emulsion (less p-Nitrophenol) (Torch).

MERCURIC OXIDE OPHTHALMIC OINTMENT, YELLOW.
Use: Local anti-infective.

MERCURIC SALICYLATE. Mercury subsalicylate.
Use: Parasitic and fungal skin diseases.

MERCURIC SUCCINIMIDE. BisSuccinimidato-mercury.

MERCURIC SULFIDE, RED. W/Colloidal sulfur, urea.
See: Teenac Cream, Oint. (Elder).

MERCURIN. Sodium salt of β-methoxy-hydroxy-mercuri propylamide of camphoramic acid. Trimethylcyclopentanedicarboxylic acid. Combined with theophylline is mercurophylline sodium.

MERCUROCAL.
See: Merbromin Soln. (Premo).

MERCUROCHROME. (Various Mfr.) Merbromin 2%. Soln. Bot. 15 ml, 30 ml.
Use: Topical antiseptic.

MERCUROL. (Durel) Oleate of mercury 0.5%, phenol 0.5%, salicylic acid 3%,

coal tar solution 1.2% in Moisturizing hand and body lotion. Bot. 4 oz, pt, gal.
Use: Antipsoriatic, antiseborrheic.
MERCUROME.
See: Merbromin Soln. (City Chem.).
MERCUROPHYLLINE SODIUM. B.A.N. Sodium salt of (beta-methoxygamma-hydroxy-mercuri-propylamide of camphoramic acid) trimethylcyclopentanodi carboxylic acid and theophylline. Mercuzanthin Inj. Amp. 2 ml, Box 6s, 25s, 100s. Tab. Bot. 50s, 100s, 1000s.
Use: Diuretic.
• **MERCURY, AMMONIATED,** U.S.P. XXIII. Oint., Ophth. Oint., U.S.P. XXIII.
Use: Topical anti-infective.
MERCURY BICHLORIDE.
See: Diamond, Tab. (Lilly).
MERCURY COMPOUNDS.
See: Antiseptics, Mercurials.
MERCURY-197-203.
See: Chlormerodrin (Squibb).
MERCURY OLEATE. Mercury (2+) oleate. Pharmaceutic aid.
MERDEX. (Faraday) Docusate sodium 100 mg/Tab. Vial 60 ml.
Use: Laxative.
• **MERISOPROL Hg 197.** USAN.
Use: Diagnostic aid.
• **MERISOPROL ACETATE Hg 197.** USAN.
Use: Radioactive agent.
• **MERISOPROL ACETATE Hg 203.** USAN.
Use: Radioactive agent.
MERITENE POWDER. (Sandoz Nutrition) Vanilla flavor: Specially processed non-fat dry milk, corn syrup solids, sucrose, fructose, calcium caseinate, sodium Cl, natural and artificial flavors, lecithin, vitamins and minerals. Can 1 lb, 4.5 lb, 25 lb. Packet 1.14 oz. Vanilla, chocolate, eggnog, milk chocolate, plain flavors.
Use: Enteral nutritional supplement.
MERODICEIN. Sodium meralein. W/Saligenin.
See: Thantis, Loz. (Hynson, Westcott & Dunning).
• **MEROPENEM.** USAN.
Use: Antibacterial.
MERPRANE. 1-(Hydroxymercuri-197 Hg)-2-propanol.
Use: Diagnostic aid.
MERSOL. (Century) Thimerosal tincture, N.F. 1/1000. 1 oz, 4 oz, pt, gal.
Use: Antiseptic.
MERTHIOLATE. (Lilly) Thimerosal.
Soln: 1:1000: 4 fl. oz, 16 fl oz, gal.
Tincture: 1:1000: alcohol 50%, 0.75 oz, 4 fl oz, 16 fl oz, gal.
Use: Antiseptic.
MERUVAX II. (Merck & Co.) Lyophilized,

live attenuated rubella virus of the Wistar Institute RA 27/3 strain. Each dose contains approximately 25 mcg of neomycin. Single dose Vial w/diluent. Pkg. 1s, 10s.
Use: Agent for immunization. W/Attenuvax.
See: M-R-Vax II, Vial (Merck & Co.). W/Attenuvax, Mumpsvax.
See: M-M-R II, Vial (Merck & Co.). W/Mumpsvax.
See: Biavax II, Vial (Merck & Co.).
MERVALDIN. (Lannett) Formerly Proloxin. Mephenesin. 0.5 Gm/Tab. Bot. 500s, 1000s.
Use: Muscle relaxant.
• **MESALAMINE.** USAN.
Use: Anti-inflammatory.
See: Asacol, DR Tab. (Procter & Gamble).
Pentasa, CR Cap. (Marion Merrell Dow).
Rowasa, Enema, Supp. (Solvay).
MESANTOIN. (Sandoz) (Mephenytoin) Phenantoin, 3-Methyl 5,5-phenylethyl-hydantoin 100 mg/Tab. Bot. 100s.
Use: Anticonvulsant.
MESCOMINE.
See: Methscopolamine bromide (Various Mfr.).
• **MESECLAZONE.** USAN.
Use: Anti-inflammatory.
• **MESIFILCON A.** USAN.
Use: Contact lens material.
• **MESNA.** USAN.
Use: Hemorrhagic cystitis prophylactic. [Orphan drug]
MESNEX. (Mead Johnson Oncology) Mesna 100 mg. Inj. Amp. 2 ml, 4 ml, 10 ml.
Use: Antidote.
• **MESORIDAZINE.** USAN. 10-[2-(1-Methyl-2-piperidyl)ethyl]-2-(methyl-sulfinyl)phenothiazine. Lidanil.
Use: Tranquilizer.
• **MESORIDAZINE BESYLATE,** U.S.P. XXIII. Inj., Oral Soln., Tab., U.S.P. XXIII. 10-2-(1-methyl-2-piperidyl)-ethyl-2-(methylsulfinyl)phenothiazine monobenzenesulfonate.
Use: Antipsychotic agent.
See: Serentil, Amp., Liq., Tab. (Boehringer-Ingelheim).
MESTANOLONE. B.A.N. 17 β-Hydroxy-17αmethyl-5αandrostan-3-one. Androstalone.
Use: Anabolic steroid.
• **MESTEROLONE.** USAN.
Use: Androgen.
MESTIBOL. Monomestrol.

MESTINON. (ICN Pharm) Pyridostigmine bromide 60 mg/Tab. Bot. 100s, 500s. Timespan 180 mg/Tab. Bot. 100s, 500s.
Use: Cholinergic muscle stimulant.
MESTINON INJECTABLE. (ICN Pharm) Pyridostigmine bromide 5 mg/ml, w/methyl and propyl parabens 0.2%, sodium citrate 0.02%, pH adjusted to approximately 5 w/citric acid, sodium hydroxide. Amp. 2 ml. Box 10s.
Use: Cholinergic muscle stimulant.
MESTINON SYRUP. (ICN Pharm) Pyridostigmine bromide 60 mg/5 ml, alcohol 5%. Bot. pt.
Use: Cholinergic muscle stimulant.
MESTINON TIMESPAN. (ICN Pharm) Pyridostigmine bromide 180 mg/Timespan Tab. Bot. 100s.
Use: Cholinergic muscle stimulant.
• **MESTRANOL,** U.S.P. XXIII. 17 αEthynylestradiol 3-methyl ether. 3-Methoxy-19-nor-17-alpha-pregna-1,3,5(10)-trien-20-yn-17-ol. 19 Norpregna-1,3,5(10)trien-20-yn-17-ol,3-methoxy-, (17α)-.
Use: Estrogenic compound.
W/Ethynodiol Diacetate.
See: Ovulen, Tab. (Searle).
Ovulen-21, Tab. (Searle).
Ovulen-28, Tab. (Searle).
W/Norethindrone.
See: Norinyl, Tab. (Syntex).
Norinyl-1 Fe 28 (Syntex).
Ortho-Novum, Tab. (Ortho).
W/Norethindrone, ferrous fumarate.
See: Ortho Novum Fe-28, Fe-28, 1 mg Fe-28, Tab. (Ortho).
W/Norethynodrel.
See: Enovid, Tab. (Searle).
Enovid-E, Tab. (Searle).
Enovid-E 21, Tab. (Searle).
MESULPHEN. B.A.N. 2,7-Dimethylthianthren. Mitigal; Sudermo.
Use: Treatment of skin infections.
• **MESUPRINE HYDROCHLORIDE.** USAN.
Use: Vasodilator, smooth muscle relaxant.
METABALM. (Noyes) Menthol, camphor, thymol, methyl salicylate, clove and cassia oil in a nonstaining vanishing base. Tube oz.
Use: Antipruritic, counter-irritant.
METABOLIN. (Thurston) Vitamins A 833 IU, D 66 IU, B_1 833 mcg, B_2 500 mcg, B_6 0.083 mcg, calcium pantothenate 833 mcg, niacinamide 5 mg, folic acid 0.066 mcg, niacinamide 5 mg, p-aminobenzoic acid 0.416 mcg, inositol 833 mcg, B_{12} 500 mcg, C 5 mg, calcium 33.1 mg,

phosphorus 14.6 mg, iron 2.5 mg, iodine 0.15 mg/Tab. Bot. 100s, 500s, 1000s.
Use: Vitamin/mineral supplement.
• **METABROMSALEN.** USAN. 3,5-Dibromosalicylanilide.
Use: Germicide, disinfectant.
METABUTETHAMINE HYDROCHLORIDE. 2- Isobutylaminoethyl m-aminobenzoid HCl. 2-(Isobutylamino)ethanol m-Aminobenzoate (Ester) Monohydrochloride.
Use: Local anesthetic.
METABUTOXYCAINE HYDROCHLORIDE. 2′-Diethylaminoethyl 3-Amino-2-butoxybenzoate Hydro- Cl.
Use: Local anesthetic.
METACARAPHEN HYDROCHLORIDE. Netrin.
METACETAMOL. B.A.N. 3-Acetamidophenol.
Use: Analgesic.
METACORDRALONE.
See: Prednisolone. (Various Mfr.).
METACORTALONE.
See: Meticortelone, Susp. (Schering).
METACORTANDRACIN.
See: Prednisone, Tab. (Various Mfr.).
METACORTIN.
See: Meticorten, Tab. (Schering).
META-DELPHENE. Diethyltoluamide U.S.P. XXIII.
METAGLYCODOL. 2-m-Chlorophenyl-3-methyl-2,3-butanediol.
Use: Central nervous system depressant.
METAHEXAMIDE. B.A.N. N-Cyclohexyl-N′-(3-amino-4-methylbenzene Sulfonyl) urea. Euglycin. Melanex.
Use: Hypoglycemic agent.
METAHYDRIN. (Merrell Dow) Trichlormethiazide 2 mg or 4 mg/Tab. Bot. 100s.
Use: Diuretic.
• **METALOL HYDROCHLORIDE.** USAN. 4′-[1-Hydroxy-2-(methylamino)-propyl] methanesulfonanilide hydrochloride. Under study.
Use: Adrenergic β receptor antagonist.
METALONE T.B.A. (Foy) Prednisolone tertiary butylacetate 20 mg, sodium citrate 1 mg, polysorbate 80 1 mg, d-sorbitol 450 mg/ml, benzyl alcohol 0.9%, water for inj. Vial 10 ml.
Use: Corticosteroid.
METAMFEPRAMONE (I.N.N.). Dimepropion, B.A.N.
METAMUCIL. (Procter & Gamble) Psyllium hydrophilic mucilloid, sodium 1 mg, potassium 31 mg/Dose. **Regular Flavor:** w/ dextrose. Jar 7 oz, 14 oz, 21 oz. Packette 5.4 Gm. Box 100s. **Orange**

and **Strawberry Flavors:** w/flavoring, sucrose and coloring. Jar 7 oz, 14 oz, 21 oz.
Use: Laxative.
METAMUCIL INSTANT MIX. (Procter & Gamble) Psyllium hydrophilic mucilloid with citric acid, sucrose, potassium bicarbonate, sodium bicarbonate. Powder when combined with water forms an effervescent, flavored liquid. **Lemon Lime Flavor:** w/calcium carbonate. Cartons of 16, 30 or 100 packets of 3.4 Gm **Orange Flavor:** w/flavoring and coloring. Ctn. 16 or 30 packets of 3.4 Gm.
Use: Laxative.
METAMUCIL, SUGAR FREE. (Procter & Gamble) Psyllium hydrophilic mucilloid in sugar-free formula. **Regular Flavor:** Jar 3.7 oz, 7.4 oz, 11.1 oz. Packet 3.4 Gm. Box 100s. **Orange Flavor:** Jar 3.7 oz, 7.4 oz, 11.1 oz.
Use: Laxative.
METANDREN. (Ciba) Methyltestosterone. **Linguet:** 5 mg or 10 mg Bot. 100s. **Tab.:** 10 mg or 25 mg Bot. 100s.
Use: Androgen.
METAPHENYLBARBITURIC ACID.
See: Mephobarbital.
METAPHYLLIN.
See: Aminophylline (Various Mfr.).
METAPREL INHALENT SOLUTION 5%. (Sandoz) Metaproterenol sulfate 50 mg/ml. Bot. 10 ml w/dropper.
Use: Bronchodilator.
METAPREL METERED DOSE INHALER. (Sandoz) Metaproterenol sulfate 225 mg, micronized powder in inert propellant/15 ml. Metered dose inhaler. (Approx. 0.65 mg/inhalation).
Use: Bronchodilator.
METAPREL SYRUP. (Sandoz) Metaproterenol sulfate 10 mg/5 ml. Bot. pt.
Use: Bronchodilator.
METAPREL TABLETS. (Sandoz) Metaproterenol sulfate 10 mg or 20 mg/Tab. Bot. 100s.
Use: Bronchodilator.
• **METAPROTERENOL SULFATE,** U.S.P. XXIII. Inhalation Aerosol, Inhalation Soln., Syrup, Tab., U.S.P. XXIII. 1,-(3,5-Dihydroxyphenyl)-2-isopropyl-aminoethanol sulfate, Alupent.
Use: Bronchodilator.
See: Alupent Inhalation (Geigy).
Metaprel, Tab., Inhalation, Syr. (Sandoz).
Prometa, Syr. (Muro).
METARAMINOL BITARTRATE, U.S.P. XXI. Inj., U.S.P. XXI. 1-α-(1-Aminoethyl)-m-hydroxybenzyl alcohol bitartrate. Ben-

zenemethanol, a-(1 aminoethyl)-3-hydroxy-R-(R*,R*)-2,3-dihydroxybutandioate (1:1) (salt).
Use: Sympathomimetic amine (vasopressor).
See: Aramine, Amp., Vial (Merck & Co.).
METASEP. (MiLance) Parachlorometaxylenol 2%, isopropyl alcohol 9%. Shampoo 120 ml.
Use: Antiseborrheic.
METASTRON. (Medi-Physics/Amersham) Strontium-89 Cl 10.9 to 22.6 mg/ml. Inj. Vial 10 ml.
Use: Radiopharmaceutical.
METATENSIN. (Merrell Dow) Trichlormethiazide 2 mg or 4 mg, each containing reserpine 0.1 mg/Tab. Bot. 100s.
Use: Antihypertensive.
METAXALONE.
Use: Skeletal muscle relaxant.
See: Skelaxin (Carnrick).
METAZOCINE. B.A.N. 1,2,3,4,5,6-Hexahydro-8-hydroxy-3,6, 11-trimethyl-2,6-methano-3-benzazocine.
Use: Narcotic analgesic.
METCARAPHEN HYDROCHLORIDE. 2-Diethylaminoethyl-1-(3′,4di-methylphenyl) cyclopentanecarboxylate HCl.
METED, MAXIMUM STRENGTH (Gen-Derm) Sulfur 5%, salicylic acid 3%. Shampoo. Bot. 118 ml.
Use: Antiseborrheic combination.
• **METENEPROST.** USAN.
Use: Oxytocic, prostaglandin.
METETHOHEPTAZINE. Ethyl hexahydro-1,3-dimethyl-4-phenyl-1H-azepine-4-carboxylate.
Use: Analgesic.
• **METFORMIN.** USAN. 1,1-Dimethyl-biguanide. Diguanil; Glucophage; Metiguanide; Obin [HCl].
Use: Oral hypoglycemic.
METHACHOLINE BROMIDE. Mecholin bromide. (2-Hydroxypropyl)-trimethylammonium bromide acetate. Mecholyl Bromide.
Use: Cholinergic.
• **METHACHOLINE CHLORIDE,** U.S.P. XXIII. (2-Hydroxypropyl)-trimethylammonium Cl acetate. Methylacetyl choline. Amechol.
Use: Cholinergic.
See: Mecholyl Cl, Amp. (J.T. Baker). Provocholine, Amp. (Roche).
METHACHOLINE CHLORIDE.
Use: Diagnostic aid.
See: Provocholine, pow. for reconstitution. (Roche).
• **METHACRYLIC ACID COPOLYMER,**

N.F. XVIII.
Use: Pharmaceutic aid (tablet coating agent).
• **METHACYCLINE.** USAN. 6-Deoxy-6-demethyl-6-methylene-5-oxytetracycline.
Use: Antibiotic.
See: Rondomycin, Cap., Syr. (Wallace).
METHADONE HCL DISKETS. (Lilly) Methadone HCl 40 mg/Dispersible Tab. Bot. 100s.
Use: Narcotic agonist analgesic.
METHADONE HCL INTENSOL. (Lilly) Methadone HCl 10 mg/ml. Oral concentrate. Bot. 30 mg.
Use: Narcotic agonist analgesic.
• **METHADONE HYDROCHLORIDE,** U.S.P. XXIII. Inj., Oral Concentrate, Tab., U.S.P. XXIII. 6-Dimethylamino-4,4-diphenyl-3-heptanone hydrochloride. 3 Heptanone, 6-(dimethylamino)-4,4-diphenyl hydrochloride. Amidon HCl, Butalgin, Diaminon HCl, Hoechst 10820, Miadone, Physeptone HCl, Polamidon HCl.
Use: Narcotic analgesic, narcotic abstinence syndrome suppressant.
See: Dolophine HCl, Preps. (Lilly).
• **METHADYLACETATE.** USAN. 6-(Dimethylamino)-4,4-diphenyl-3-heptanol acetate (ester). 1-Ethyl-4-dimethylamino-2,2-diphenylpentyl acetate. Acetyl-methadol (I.N.N.).
Use: Narcotic analgesic.
• **METHAFILCON B.** USAN.
Use: Contact lens material.
METHAGUAL. (Gordon) Guaiacol 2%, methyl salicylate 8% in petrolatum. Oint. 2 oz, lb.
Use: External analgesic.
METHALAMIC ACID. Name used for lothalamic acid, U.S.P. XXIII.
METHALGEN. (Alra) Camphor, menthol, mustard oil, methyl salicylate in nongreasy cream base. Bot. 2 oz, Jar 4 oz, lb.
Use: External analgesic.
METHALLATAL. 5-Ethyl-5-(2-methylallyl)-2-thiobarbituric acid.
METHALLENESTRIL. B.A.N. 3-(6-Methoxy-2-naphthyl)-2,2-dimethylpentanoic acid.
Use: Estrogen.
• **METHALLIBURE.** USAN. 1-Methyl-6-(1-methylallyl)-2,5-dithiobiurea.
Use: Suppression of pituitary, ovarian, and adrenal function.
• **METHALTHIAZIDE.** USAN. 3-[(Allylthio)methyl]-6-chloro-3,4-dihydro-2-methyl-2H-1,2,4-benzothiadiazine-7-sulfon-

amide 1,1-dioxide.
Use: Hypotensive, diuretic.
METHAMINODIAZEPOXIDE. Chlordiazepoxide HCl, U.S.P. XXIII.
See: Librium, Cap., Amp. (Roche).
METHAMOCTOL. 2-Methyl-6-(methylamino)-2-heptanol.
Use: Adrenergic.
METHAMPHAZONE. B.A.N. 4-Amino-6-methyl-2-phenyl-3(2H)-pyridazone.
Use: Analgesic, antirheumatic.
• **METHAMPHETAMINE HYDROCHLORIDE,** U.S.P. XXIII Deoxyephedrine hydrochloride; N-α-Dimethyl-phenethylamine hydrochloride.
Use: Central nervous system stimulant.
See: Desoxyn, Gradumets, Tab. (Abbott).
Methampex, Tab. (Lemmon).
Methamphetamine HCl, Tab. (Various Mfr.).
W/Pamabrom, pyrilamine maleate, homatropine methylbromide, hyoscyamine sulfate, scopolamine HBr.
See: Aridol, Tab. (MPL).
W/Pentobarbital sodium, vitamins, minerals.
See: Fotamin, Tab. (Mission)
METHAMPHETAMINE-dl HCl.
See: dl-METHAMPHETAMINE HCl.
METHAMPYRONE.
See: Dipyrone.
METHANDIENONE. B.A.N. 17 β-Hydroxy-17 α-methylandrosta-1,4-dien-3-one. Dianabol.
Use: Anabolic steroid.
METHANDRIOL. Methylandrostenediol. (Various Mfr.) 17-alpha-methyl-D⁵-androstene-3-beta, 17 beta-diol. Diolostene, Mestenediol, Methanabol, Spenbolic.
See: Anabol, Inj. (Keene Pharm.).
METHANDRIOL DIPROPIONATE.
See: Andriol Inj. (Solvay).
Arbolic, Inj. (Burgin-Arden).
Crestabolic, Vial (Nutrition).
Durandrol, Vial (Pharmex).
Probolik (Hickam).
METHANDROSTENOLONE. D¹-17 α-methyltestosterone. 17 α-Methyl-17 β-hydroxyandrosta-1,4-dien-3one. 17 β-Hydroxy-17-methylandrosta-1,4-dien-3-one.
See: Dianabol, Tab. (Ciba).
METHANTHELINIUM BROMIDE. B.A.N. 2-Diethyl-aminoethyl xanthen-9-carboxylate methobromide. Banthine Bromide.
Use: Anticholinergic.
• **METHANTHELINE BROMIDE,** U.S.P.

XXII. Sterile, Tab., U.S.P. XXII. Diethyl (2-hydroxyethyl)methyl-ammonium bromide xanthene-9-carboxylate.
Use: Parasympatholytic, anticholinergic.
See: Banthine, Vial, Tab. (Searle). W/Phenobarbital.
See: Banthine w/Phenobarbital, Tab. (Searle).
METHAPHENILENE. B.A.N. 2-(N-Phenyl-N-2-thenylamino)ethyldimethylamine. Diatrin [hydrochloride].
Use: Antihistamine.
METHAPHOR. (Borden) Protein hydrolysate (l-leucine, l-isoleucine, l-methionine, l-phenylalanine, l-tyrosine); methionine, camphor, benzethonium Cl, in Dermabase vehicle/Oint. Tube 1.5 oz.
Use: Dermatologic, amino acid preparation.
METHAPYRILENE FUMARATE. 2-[[2-(Dimethylamino)ethyl]-2-thenylamino] pyridine fumarate (2:3).
NOTE: Due to legislation, products are being reformulated to exclude oral use of this drug. This drug is no longer official in the U.S.P.
Use: Antihistamine.
METHAPYRILENE HYDROCHLORIDE, 2-[[2-(Dimethylamino)-ethyl]-2-thenylamino] pyridine hydrochloride. (Thenylpyramine, Teralin). Blue Line— Elixir 200 mg/fl oz. Bot. pt, gal. Kenyon-Vial 20 mg/ml.
NOTE: Due to legislation, products are being reformulated to exclude oral use of this drug. This drug is no longer official in the U.S.P.
Use: Antihistamine.
METHAPYRILENE HYDROCHLORIDE W/COMBINATIONS.
NOTE: Due to legislation, products are being reformulated to exclude oral use of this drug.
METHARBITONE. B.A.N. 5,5-Diethyl-1-methylbarbituric acid.
Use: Anticonvulsant.
METHATROPIC CAPSULES. (Goldline) Choline 115 mg, inositol 83 mg, methionine 110 mg, vitamins B_1 3 mg, B_2 3 mg, B_3 10 mg, B_5 2 mg, B_6 2 mg, B_{12} 2 mcg, desiccated liver 56 mg, liver concentrate 30 mg/Cap. Bot. 100s, 1000s.
Use: Nutritional supplement.
METHAZINE. (Pharmex) Promethazine HCl 50 mg/ml. Vial 10 ml.
Use: Antihistamine.
• **METHAZOLAMIDE,** U.S.P. XXIII. Tab. U.S.P. XXIII. N-(4-Methyl-2-sulfamoyl-D^2-1,3,4-thiadiazolin-5-ylidene)ac-

etamide. Acetamide, N-5-(aminosulfonyl)-3-methyl-1,3,4-thiadiazol-2(3H)-ylidene-. 5-Acetylimino-4-meth-yl-1,3,4-thiadiazoline-2-sulfonamide.
Use: Carbonic anhydrase inhibitor.
See: Neptazane.
Neptazane, Tab. (Lederle).
METH-CHOLINE CAPSULES, (Schein) Choline 115 mg, inositol 83 mg, methionine 110 mg, vitamins B_1 3 mg, B_2 3 mg, B_3 10 mg, B_5 2 mg, B_6 2 mg, B_{12} 2 mcg, desiccated liver 56 mg, liver concentrate 30 mg/Cap. Bot. 100s, 250s, 1000s.
Use: Nutritional supplement.
METH-DIA-MER SULFA TABLETS. Trisulfapyrimidines Tab., U.S.P. XXIII.
Use: Triple sulfonamide therapy.
See: Chemozine, Tab. (Tennessee Pharm.).
Neotrizine, Tab. (Lilly).
Terfonyl, Susp., (Squibb).
Triple Sulfa, Tab. (Various Mfr.).
METH-DIA-MER SULFONAMIDES.
Use: Triple sulfonamide therapy. W/Sulfacetamide.
See: Sulfa-Plex Vaginal Cream (Solvay).
W/Sulfacetamide, hexestrol.
See: Vagi-Plex, Cream (Solvay).
METH-DIA-MER SULFONAMIDES SUSPENSION, Trisulfapyrimidines Oral Suspension, U.S.P. XXIII.
Use: Triple sulfonamide therapy.
See: Chemozine, Susp. (Tennessee Pharm.).
Neotrizine, Susp. (Lilly).
Terfonyl, Susp. (Squibb).
Triple Sulfa, Susp. (CMC).
METHDILAZINE, U.S.P. XXIII. Tab., U.S.P. XXIII. 10-(1-Methylpyrrolidin-3-yl-methyl)phenothiazine. Dilosyn (hydrochloride).
See: Tacaryl Chew. Tab. (Westwood).
• **METHDILAZINE HCl,** U.S.P. XXIII. Syrup, Tab., U.S.P. XXIII. 10-(1-Methyl-pyrro-lidinyl)phenothiazine HCl.
Use: Antipruritic.
See: Tacaryl, Tab. (Westwood).
• **METHENAMINE,** U.S.P. XXIII. Elix., Tab., U.S.P. XXIII. (Hexamethyleneamine, Cystamin, Cystogen, Hexamine, Hexa-methylenetetramine.).
Use: Antibacterial (urinary).
METHENAMINE W/COMBINATIONS.
Use: Urinary anti-infective.
See: Cystamine, Tab. (Tennessee Pharm.).
Cystex, Tab. (Numark).
Cystised, Tab. (Jenkins).
Cystitol, Tab. (Briar).

Cysto, Tab. (Freeport).
Hexalol, Tab. (Central).
Lanased, Tab. (Lannett).
Prosed/DS, Tab. (Star).
Urimar-T, Tab. (Marnel).
Urisan-P, Tab. (Sandia).
Urised, Tab. (Webcon).
Uritrol, Tab. (Kenyon).
Urogesic Blue, Tab. (Edwards).
Uro Phosphate, Tab. (Poythress).
UTA, Tab. (Bentex).
U-Tract, Tab. (Bowman).
U-Tran, Tab. (Scruggs).
**METHENAMINE AND MONOBASIC
SODIUM PHOSPHATE TABLETS,**
U.S.P. XXIII.
Use: Antibacterial (urinary).
**METHENAMINE ANHYDROMETHYL-
ENE CITRATE.** Formanol, Uropurgol,
Urotropin.
• **METHENAMINE HIPPURATE,** U.S.P.
XXII. Tab., U.S.P. XXII. A 1:1 complex of
methenamine and hippuric acid.
Use: Urinary antiseptic.
See: Hiprex, Tab. (Merrell Dow).
Urex, Tab.(Riker).
• **METHENAMINE MANDELATE,** U.S.P.
XXIII. Tab., For Oral Soln., Oral Susp.;
U.S.P. XXIII.
Use: Urinary antibacterial.
See: Mandacon, Tab. (Webcon).
Mandalay, Tab. (Beutlich).
Mandelamine, Tab., Susp. (Parke-
Davis).
Mandelamine "Hafgram" Tab. (Parke-
Davis).
Mandelets, Tab. (Quality Generics).
Methavin, Tab. (Star).
Renelate, Tab. (Forest Pharm.).
**METHENAMINE MANDELATE W/COM-
BINATIONS.**
Use: Antibacterial (urinary).
See: Mandex, Tab. (Vale).
Pyrisul Plus, Tab. (Kenyon).
Thiacide, Tab. (Beach).
Urisedamine, Tab. (Webcon).
• **METHENOLONE ACETATE.** USAN. 17
β-Hydroxy-1-methyl-5 α-androst-1-en-3-
one acetate. Primobolan.
Use: Anabolic agent.
• **METHENOLONE ENANTHATE.** USAN.
17β-Hydroxy-1-methyl-5αandrost-1-en-
3-one heptanoate. Nibal injection. Pri-
mobolan.
Use: Anabolic.
METHEPONEX. (Rawl) Choline 0.54 Gm,
dl-methionine 1.80 Gm, inositol 0.27
Gm, whole desiccated liver 8.10 Gm, vit-
amins B_1 18 mg, B_2 36 mg, niacinamide
90 mg, B_6 3.6 mg, calcium pantothenate

3.6 mg, biotin 10.8 mcg, B_{12} 5.4 mcg
and amino acid/daily therapeutic dose.
Cap. Bot. 100s, 500s.
Use: Antidiabetic, nutritional supple-
ment.
METHEPTAZINE. Methyl hexahydro-1, 2-
dimethyl-4-phenyl-1H-azepine-4-car-
boxylate.
Use: Analgesic.
METHERGINE. (Sandoz) Methyler-
gonovine maleate. **Amp.:** 0.2 mg/ml, tar-
taric acid 0.25 mg, sodium Cl 3 mg/ml.
SandoPak 20s, 100s. **Tab.:** 0.2 mg. Bot.
100s, 1000s, SandoPak pkgs. 100s.
Use: Hormone.
METHESTROL.
See: Promethestrol (Various Mfr.).
METHETHARIMIDE BEMEGRIDE. 3-
Methyl-3-ethyl glutarimide.
• **METHETOIN.** USAN. 5-Ethyl-1-methyl-5-
phenylimidazoline-2,4-dione. Deltoin.
Use: Anticonvulsant.
METHIBON CAPSULES. (Barrows)
Choline dihydrogen citrate 278 mg, dl-
methionine 111 mg, inositol 83.3 mg, vit-
amin B_{12} 2 mcg, liver concentrate, des-
iccated liver 86.6 mg/Cap. Bot. 100s.
Use: Antidiabetic, nutritional supple-
ment.
• **METHICILLIN SODIUM, STERILE,** U.S.P.
XXIII., Inj., U.S.P. XXIII. Sodium 2,6-
Dimethoxyphenyl penicillin.
Dimethoxyphenyl penicillin sodium
Use: Antibiotic.
See: Celbenin, Vial (Beecham Labs).
Staphcillin, Vial (Bristol).
• **METHIMAZOLE,** U.S.P. XXIII. Tab.,
U.S.P. XXIII. 1-Methylimidazole-2-thiol.
Mercazole. 2H-imidazole-2-thione, 1,3-
dihydro-1-methyl.
Use: Thyroid inhibitor (5 mg to 20 mg).
See: Tapazole, Tab. (Lilly).
Thiamazole (I.N.N.).
METHIODAL SODIUM, U.S.P. XXI. Inj.,
U.S.P. XXIII. Sodium
monoiodomethanesulfonate. Abrodil,
Radiographol, Diagnorenol.
Use: Radiopaque.
METHIOKAPS. (Vale) dl-methionine 200
mg/Cap. Bot. 1000s.
Use: Diaper rash product.
METHIOMEPRAZINE HCl. dl-10-(3-Di-
methyl-amino-2-methylpropyl)-2-
methylthiophenothiazine HCl. (SK-
Beecham).
Use: Antiemetic.
• **METHIONINE,** U.S.P. XXIII. **Note:** Also
see Racemethionine, U.S.P. XXIII.
Use: Amino acid.
METHIOPLEX. (Lincoln) Methionine 25

mg, vitamins B_1 50 mg, niacinamide 100 mg, B_2 2 mg, choline 50 mg, B_6 2 mg, panthenol 2 mg, benzyl alcohol 1%, distilled water q.s./ml. Vial 30 ml.
Use: Nutritional supplement.
• **METHISAZONE.** USAN. N-methylisatin-β-thi-osemicarbazone. 1-Methylindoline-2,3-dione 3-thiosemicarbazone. Marboran.
Use: Antiviral drug.
METHITURAL SODIUM. 5-(1-Methylbutyl)-5-[2-(methylthio)ethyl]-2-thiobarbituric acid sodium salt.
Use: Hypnotic; sedative.
METHIXENE. B.A.N. 9-(1-Methyl-3-piperidyl-methyl)- thiaxanthen. Tremonil (hydrochloride).
Use: Treatment of the Parkinsonian syndrome.
METHNITE. (Kenyon) Methscopolamine nitrate 2.5 mg/Tab. Bot. 100s, 1000s.
Use: Antispasmodic.
• **METHOCARBAMOL,** U.S.P. XXIII. Cap., Tab., U.S.P. XXIII. 1,2-Propanediol, 3-(2-methoxy phenoxy)-, 1-carbamate. (2-Hydroxy-3-o-methoxyphenoxypropyl) carbamate. 3-(o-Methoxyphenoxy)-1,2-propanediol1-carbamate. (Various Mfr.)
Tab.: 500 mg or 750 mg. Bot. 100s, 500s; **Inj.:** 100 mg/ml Vial 10 ml.
Use: Skeletal muscle relaxant.
See: Delaxin, Tab. (Ferndale).
Robaxin, Tab., Inj. (Robins).
W/Aspirin.
See: Robaxisal, Tab. (Robins).
METHOCARBAMOL/ASA. (Various Mfr.) Methocarbamol 400 mg, aspirin 325 mg/Tab. Bot. 15s, 30s, 40s, 100s, 500s, 1000.
Use: Skeletal muscle relaxant combination.
METHOCEL. Methylcellulose.
• **METHOHEXITAL,** U.S.P. XXIII.
Use: Pharmaceutical necessity for Methohexital Sodium for Injection.
• **METHOHEXITAL SODIUM FOR INJECTION,** U.S.P. XXIII. Alpha-(dl)-5-allyl-1-methyl-5-(1-methyl-2-pentynyl) barbituric sodium 2,4,6(lH,-3H,5H)-pyrimidinetrione,.
1-methyl-5-(1-methyl-2-pentynyl)-5-(2-propenyl)-, (±) monosodium salt.
Use: General anesthetic (intravenous).
See: Brevital, Amp., Pow. (Lilly).
METHOHEXITONE. B.A.N. α-5-Allyl-1-methyl-5- (1-methylpent-2-ynyl)barbituric acid.
Use: Anesthetic.
METHOIN. B.A.N. 5-Ethyl-3-methyl-5-phenylhydantoin. 5-Ethyl-3-methyl-5-

phenylimidazoline-2,4-dione. Mephenytoin (I.N.N.).
Use: Anticonvulsant.
• **METHOPHOLINE HCl.** USAN. 1-(p-Chlorophenethyl)-2-methyl-6, 7-dimethoxy-1,2,3,4-tetrahydroisoquinoline HCl.
Use: Analgesic.
See: Versidyne.
METHOPTO 0.25%. (Professional Pharmacal) Methylcellulose pow. 2.5 mg (0.25% soln.), boric acid 12 mg, potassium Cl 7.3 mg, benzalkonium Cl 0.04 mg, glycerin 12 mg/ml w/sodium carbonate to adjust pH and purified water. Bot. 15 ml, 30 ml.
Use: Artificial tear solution.
METHOPTO FORTE 0.5%. (Professional Pharmacal) Methylcellulose pow. 5 mg (0.5% soln.), boric acid 12 mg, potassium Cl 7.3 mg, benzalkonium Cl 0.4 mg, glycerin 12 mg/ml w/sodium carbonate to adjust pH and purified water. Bot. 15 ml.
Use: Artificial tear solution.
METHOPTO FORTE 1%. (Professional Pharmacal) Methylcellulose pow. 10 mg (1% soln.), boric acid 12 mg, potassium Cl 7.3 mg, benzalkonium Cl 0.04 mg, glycerin 12 mg/ml w/sodium carbonate to adjust pH and purified water. Bot. 15 ml.
Use: Artificial tear solution.
METHOPYRAPHONE.
See: Metopirone, Tab., Amp. (Ciba).
METHORATE.
See: Dextromethorphan HBr.
METHORBATE S.C. (Standex) Methenamine 40.8 mg, atropine sulfate 0.03 mg, hyoscyamine sulfate 0.03 mg, salol 18.1 mg, benzoic acid 4.5 mg, methylene blue 5.4 mg/Tab. Bot. 100s.
Use: Urinary anti-infective.
d-METHORPHAN HBr.
See: Dextromethorphan HBr (Various Mfr.).
METHORPHINAN. Racemorphan HBr. Dromoran.
METHOSERPIDINE. B.A.N. 10-Methoxy-deserpidine.
Use: Hypotensive.
• **METHOTREXATE,** U.S.P. XXIII. Tab., U.S.P. XXIII. Amethopterin. 4-Amino-10-methylfolic acid. N-[p-[[(2,4-Diamino-6-pteridinyl)-methyl]-methylamino]benzoyl] glutamic acid. L-glutamic acid, N-[4-[[(2,4-diamino-6-pteridinyl)methyl]-me-thylamino]benzoyl]. (Various Mfr.) Tab. 2.5 mg. Bot. 36s, 100s, UD 20s.
Use: Leukemia in children, antineoplas-

tic, antipsoriatic, juvenile rheumatoid arthritis [Orphan drug]
See: Rheumatrex, Tab. (Lederle).
METHOTREXATE. (Lederle) **Inj.**: 25 mg/ml as sodium, benzyl alcohol 0.9%, sodium Cl 0.26% and water for inj. Vials 2 ml or 10 ml. **Pow. for Inj.**: 20 mg/vial as sodium. Single-use vials.
Use: Antipsoriatic.
• **METHOTREXATE SODIUM FOR INJEC-TION.** U.S.P. XXIII. 4-Amino-N^{10}-methyl-pteroylglutamic acid sodium. (Lederle) 2.5 mg/ml Vial 2 ml; 25 mg/ml. Vial 2 ml w/preservatives; 20 mg, 50 mg, 100 mg Vial cryodesiccated, preservative free; 50 mg, 100 mg, 200 mg Vial; 25 mg/ml solution preservative free.
Use: Leukemia therapy, psoriasis, osteogenic sarcoma [Orphan drug]
See: Folex, Inj. (Adria) Folex PFS. Inj. (Adria) Methotrexate, Inj., Pow. (Lederle).
Mexate, Inj. (Bristol).
METHOTREXATE USP WITH LAURO-CAPRAM.
Use: Topical treatment of **Mycosis fungoides.** [Orphan drug]
• **METHOTRIMEPRAZINE,** U.S.P. XXIII. Inj., U.S.P. XXIII. 2-Methoxy-10-(3-dimethylamino-2-methyl-propyl)phenothiazine. (—)-10-(3-(Dimethyl-amino)-2-methyl-propyl)-2-methoxyphenothiazine. Levomepromazine (I.N.N.) Veractil.
Use: Tranquilizer, non-addicting analgesic.
See: Levoprome, Amp., Vial (Lederle).
METHOXAMINE HCl.
Use: Vasopressor used in shock.
See: Vasoxyl (Burroughs Wellcome).
• **METHOXSALEN,** U.S.P. XXIII. Cap., U.S.P. XXIII.
Use: Topical pigmenting agent.
See: Meloxine, (Upjohn).
Oxsoralen, Cap., Lot. (Elder).
Oxsoralen-Ultra, Cap. (Elder).
8-METHOXSALEN.
Use: Treatment of diffuse systemic sclerosis, rejection of cardiac allografts. [Orphan drug]
See: Uvadex.
• **METHOXSALEN TOPICAL SOLUTION,** U.S.P. XXIII. 8-Methoxypsoralen. 8-Hydroxy-4′,5,6,7-furocoumarin, ammoidin, xanthotoxin. 7H-Furo[3,2-g][1] benzopyran-7-one,2-methoxy-9-methoxy-7H-Furo[3,2-g][1]benzopyran-7-one.
Use: Topical pigmenting agent.
METHOXYDONE.
See: Mephenoxalone (Various Mfr.).

• **METHOXYFLURANE,** U.S.P. XXIII. 2,2-Dichloro-1,1-difluoroethyl methyl ether.
Use: General inhalation anesthetic.
See: Penthrane, Liq. (Abbott).
METHOXYPHENAMINE HYDROCHLO-RIDE, U.S.P. XXI. o-Methoxy-N, α-dimethylphenethylamino HCl.
Use: Adrenergic (bronchodilator).
W/Chlorpheniramine maleate, acetophenetidin, acetylsalicylic acid, caffeine.
See: Pyrroxate, Cap., Tab. (Upjohn).
W/Dextromethorphan HCl, orthoxine, sodium citrate.
See: Orthoxicol, Syr. (Upjohn).
W/Dextromethorphan HBr, phenylephrine HCl, chlorpheniramine maleate.
See: Statuss, Syr., Cap. (Elder).
W/Medrol.
See: Medrol, Tab. (Upjohn).
METHOXYPROMAZINE MALEATE. 10-[3-(Dime-thylamino)propyl]-2-methoxyphenothiazine maleate. Tentone.
Use: CNS depressant.
METHOXYPSORALEN, ORAL.
Use: Psoralen.
See: Oxsoralen (Elder).
Oxsoralen-Ultra (Elder).
8-MOP (Elder).
• **METHSCOPOLAMINE BROMIDE,** U.S.P. XXII. Tab., U.S.P. XXII. Inj. U.S.P. XXI. Epoxytropine tropate methylbromide, scopolamine methylbromide, hyoscine methylbromide. 6β, 7β Epoxy-3α-hydroxy-8-methyl-1αH, 5αH-tropanium bromide(–)-Tropate.
Use: Anticholinergic.
See: Pamine, Tab., Vial (Upjohn).
Scoline, Tab.(Westerfield).
W/Amobarbital.
See: Scoline-Amobarbital, Tab. (Westerfield).
W/Butabarbital Sodium, dried aluminum hydroxide gel and magnesium trisilicate.
See: Eulcin, Tab. (Leeds Pharmacal).
W/Phenobarbital.
See: Pamine PB, Preps. (Upjohn).
Synt-PB, Tab. (Scrip).
W/Phenylpropanolamine HCl, chlorpheniramine maleate.
See: Bobid, Cap. (Boyd).
Symptrol, Cap. (Saron).
METHSCOPOLAMINE NITRATE. Scopolamine Methyl Nitrate, Preps. (Various Mfr.) Mescomine.
See: Cenahist, Cap. (Century).
Dallergy, Cap., Tab., Syr. (Laser).
Extendryl, Cap., Tab., Syr. (Fleming).

Histaspan-D, Cap. (Rhone-Poulenc Rorer).
Sanhist T.D. 12, Tab. (Sandia).
Scotnord, Tab. (Scott/Cord).
Sinovan, Timed Cap. (Drug Ind.).
Spasmid, Elix., Tab. (Dalin).
• **METHSUXIMIDE**, U.S.P. XXIII. Cap., U.S.P. XXIII. N,2-Dimethyl-2-phenylsuccinamide Mesuximide (I.N.N.).
Use: Anticonvulsant.
See: Celontin Kapseal (Parke-Davis).
METHYCLODINE. (Rugby) Methyclothiazide 5 mg, deserpidine 0.25 mg/Tab. Bot. 100s.
Use: Antihypertensive, diuretic.
• **METHYCLOTHIAZIDE**, U.S.P. XXIII. Tab., U.S.P. XXIII. 6-Chloro-3-chloromethyl-2-methyl-7-sulfamyl-3,4-dihydro-1,2,4-benzothiadiazine-1,1-dioxide. 6-Chloro-3-(chloromethyl)-3,4-dihydro-2-methyl-2H-1,2,4-benzothiadiazine-7-sulfonamide 1,1-Dioxide.
Use: Diuretic, antihypertensive.
See: Enduron, Tab. (Abbott) Methyclodine, Tab. (Rugby).
W/Deserpidine.
See: Enduronyl, Tab. (Abbott).
Enduronyl Forte, Tab. (Abbott).
W/Pargyline HCl.
See: Eutron, Tab. (Abbott).
METHYLACETYLCHOLINE.
See: Methacholine.
METHYL ALCOHOL, N.F. XVIII.
Use: Pharmaceutic acid (solvent).
METHYLAMPHETAMINE HYDROCHLORIDE & SULFATE.
See: Desoxyephedrine HCl (Various Mfr.).
6-METHYLENANDROSTA-1,4-DIENE-3,17-DIONE.
Use: Antineoplastic. [Orhan drug]
METHYLANDROSTENEDIOL.
See: Hybolin, Vial (Hyrex).
Methandriol.
W/Adrenal cortex extract, Vitamin B_{12}.
See: Geri-Ace, Inj. (Brown).
W/Carboxymethylcellulose sodium, thimerosal.
See: Cenabolic, Vial (Century).
W/Pentylenetetrazol, nicotinic acid, l-lysine, dl-methionine, ethinyl estradiol, thiamine, pyridoxine, riboflavin, vitamins B_{12}, A, D, ascorbic acid.
See: Ardiatric, Tab. (Burgin-Arden).
• **METHYLBENZETHONIUM CHLORIDE,** U.S.P. XXIII. Lotion, Oint., Pow., U.S.P. XXIII. Benzyl-dimethyl-2[2-(p-1,1,3-tetramethyl-butyl-cresoxy)ethoxy]-ethyl ammonium Cl. (p-Tertiary octyl cresoxy ethoxy ethyl dimethyl-benzyl ammonium

Cl). Benzyldimethyl[2[2-[[4-(1,1,3,3-tetramethylbutyl)tolyl]oxy]ethoxy]-ethyl]ammonium Cl.
Use: Bactericide, local anti-infective.
See: Ammorid, Oint. (Kinney).
Benephen, Prods. (Halsted).
Cuticura Acne Cream (Purex).
Cuticura Medicated First Aid Cream (Purex).
Diaparene Prods. (Glenbrook).
Fordustin, Pow. (Sween).
Surgi-Kleen, Liq. (Sween).
W/Cod liver oil.
See: Benephen, Prods. (Halsted).
Sween Cream (Sween).
W/Magnesium stearate.
See: Mennen Baby Pow. (Mennen).
W/Phenol, acetanilid, zinc oxide, calamine and eucalyptol.
See: Taloin, Oint. (Warren-Teed).
W/Phenylmercuric acetate, methylparaben.
See: Lorophyn, Supp. (Eaton).
Norforms, Aerosal, Supp. (Norwich).
W/Zinc oxide, calamine, eucalyptol.
See: Taloin, Tube (Warren-Teed).
METHYLBENZTROPINE.
See: Ethybenztropine (Sandoz).
METHYLBROMTROPIN MANDELATE.
See: Homatropine Methylbromide, U.S.P. XXIII.
• **METHYLCELLULOSE,** U.S.P. XXIII. Ophth. Soln., Oral Soln., Tab., U.S.P. XXIII. Cellulose methylether. Mellose.
Use: Suspending agent.
See: Cellothyl, Tab. (International Drug).
Cologel, Soln. (Lilly).
Isopto-Plain, Liq. (Alcon).
Melozets, Wafer (Calgon).
W/Benzocaine, vitamins, minerals, niacinamide.
See: Rite-Diet, Cap. (E.J. Moore).
W/Boric acid, glycerine, propylene glycol, methylparaben, propylparaben, irish moss extract.
See: Canfield Lubricating Jelly (Paddock).
W/Carboxymethylcellulose.
See: Ex-Caloric, Wafer (Eastern Research).
W/Dicyclomine HCl, magnesium trisilicate, aluminum hydroxide-magnesium carbonate, dried.
See: Triactin Tab. (Norwich).
W/Dicyclomine HCl, aluminum hydroxide and magnesium hydroxide.
See: Triactin Liq. (Norwich).
W/Phenylphrine HCl.
See: Vernacel (Professional Pharma-

cal).
W/Phenylephrine HCl, benzalkonium Cl.
See: Efricel % (Professional Pharma-
cal).
W/Polysorbate 80, boric acid.
See: Lacril Artificial Tears (Allergan).
METHYLCHROMONE. B.A.N. 3-Methyl-
(4H)-chromen-4-one.
Use: Coronary vasodilator.
METHYLCYSTEINE. B.A.N. Methyl 2-
amino-3-mercaptoproprionate. Mecys-
teine (I.N.N.) Acdrile; Visclair [hydrochlo-
ride]
Use: Vasoconstrictor.
METHYL CYSTEINE HYDROCHLORIDE.
Cysteine methyl ester hydrochloride.
Use: Mucolytic agent.
METHYLDESORPHINE. B.A.N. 6-
Methyl-D⁶-deoxymorphine.
Use: Narcotic analgesic.
• **METHYLDOPA,** U.S.P. XXIII. Oral Susp.,
Tab. U.S.P. XXIII. Levo-3-(3,4-dihydrox-
yphenyl)-2-methylalanine.
Use: Antihypertensive.
See: Aldomet, Tab. (Merck & Co.).
• **METHYLDOPA AND CHLOROTHIAZIDE
TABLETS,** U.S.P. XXIII.
Use: Antihypertensive.
See: Aldoclor, Tab. (Merck & Co.).
• **METHYLDOPA AND HY-
DROCHLOROTHIAZIDE TABLETS,**
U.S.P. XXIII.
Use: Antihypertensive.
See: Aldoril, Tab. (Merck & Co.).
**METHYLDOPA/HYDROCHLOROTHIA-
ZIDE.** (Mylan) Methyldopa 250 mg, hy-
drochlorothiazide 15 mg or 25 mg/Tab.
Bot. 100s, 1000s.
Use: Antihypertensive.
**METHYLDOPA/HYDROCHLOROTHIA-
ZIDE.** (Rugby) Methyldopa 500 mg, hy-
drochlorothiazide 50 mg/Tab. Bot. 100s.
Use: Antihypertensive.
• **METHYLDOPATE HCl,** U.S.P. XXIII. Inj.
U.S.P. XXIII. (Merck & Co.) Ethyl ester of
levo-3-(3,4-dihydroxyphenyl)-2-methyl-
lalanine HCl. l-Tyrosine, 3-hydroxy-
α-methyl-,ethyl ester hydrochloride-.
Use: Antihypertensive agent.
See: Aldomet Ester HCl, Inj. (Merck &
Co.).
METHYLDOPATE HCl. (Lyphomed)
Methyldopate HCl 250 mg/5 ml. Inj. Vial.
6 ml.
Use: Antihypertensive.
• **METHYLENE BLUE,** U.S.P. XXIII. Inj.
U.S.P. XXIII. (Various Mfr.) Methylthion-
ine Cl. 3,7-Bix-(Dimethyl-amino)phenza-
thionium Cl.
Use: Antimethemoglobinemic, antidote

to cyanide poisoning.
See: Urolene Blue, Tab. (Star).
Wright's Stain, Liq. (Hynson, Westcott
& Dunning).
METHYLENE BLUE W/COMBINATIONS.
See: Hexalol, Tab. (Central).
Lanased, Tab. (Lannett).
Urised, Tab. (Webcon).
U-Tract, Tab. (Bowman).
• **METHYLENE CHLORIDE,** N.F. XVIII.
Use: Pharmaceutic aid (solvent).
METHYLERGOMETRINE. B.A.N. N-(+)-
1-(Hydroxymethyl)propyl-(+)-ly-
sergamide.
Use: Uterine stimulant.
• **METHYLERGONOVINE MALEATE,**
U.S.P. XXIII. Inj., Tab., U.S.P. XXIII.
9,10-Didehydro-N-[(S)-1-(hydrox-
ymethyl) propyl]-6-methylergoline-8-car-
boxamide maleate (1:1).
Use: Oxytocic.
See: Methergine, Amp., Tab. (Sandoz).
**METHYLETHYLAMINO-PHENYL-
PROPANOL HCl.**
See: Nethamine HCl. (Various Mfr.).
**METHYLGLUCAMINE DIATRIZOATE,
INJ.,** A water-soluble radiopaque iodine
cpd. N-methylglucamine salt of Diatri-
zoate.
See: Diatrizoate (Various Mfr.).
Diatrizoate Meglumine Inj., U.S.P. XXI-
II.
METHYLGLUCAMINE IODIPAMIDE, INJ.
See: Meglumine Iodipamide, Inj., U.S.P.
XXIII. (Various Mfr.).
W/Diatrizoate methylglucamine.
See: Sinografin, Vial (Squibb).
**METHYLGLYOXAL-BIS-GUANYLHY-
DRAZONE.** Methyl GAG.
METHYLHYDRAZINE-N.
See: N-METHYLHYDRAZINE.
**METHYLISATIN-N BETA-THIOSEMI-
CARBAZONE.**
See: N-METHYLISATIN BETA-
THIOSEMICARBAZONE.
• **METHYL ISOBUTYL KETONE,** N.F. XVI-
II. 4-Methyl-2-pentanone.
Use: Pharmaceutic aid (alcohol denatu-
rant).
METHYLISO-OCTENYLAMINE.
See: Isometheptene HCl (Various Mfr.).
METHYLMERCADONE. Name used for
Nifuratel.
METHYL NICOTINATE.
W/Histamine dihydrochloride, oleoresin
capsicum, glycomonosalicylate.
See: Akes-N-Pain Rub, Oint. (Moore).
W/methyl salicylate, menthol.
See: Musterole Deep Strength Oint.
(Schering-Plough).

W/Methyl salicylate, menthol, camphor, dipropylene glycol salicylate, cassia oil, oleoresins capsicum, ginger.
See: Arthaderm, Lot. (Paddock).
Scrip-Gesic, Oint. (Scrip).
METHYLONE. (Paddock) Methylprednisolone acetate 40 mg/ml. Vial 5 ml.
Use: Corticosteroid.
• **METHYL PALMOXIRATE.** USAN.
Use: Antidiabetic.
• **METHYLPARABEN,** N.F. XVIII. (Various Mfr.) Methyl p-hydroxybenzoate. Methyl Chemosept.
Use: Pharmaceutic aid (antifungal preservative).
• **METHYLPARABEN SODIUM.** USAN. N.F. XVIII.
Use: Antifungal preservative (Pharmaceutic aid).
METHYLPARAFYNOL. 3-Methyl-pentyne-1-ol-3. Oblivon, Somnesin.
METHYLPENTYNOL. B.A.N. 3-Methylpent-1-yn-3-ol. Atempol, Insomnol, Meparfynol, Methylparafynol, Oblivon, Somnesin and Oblivon-C Carbamate.
Use: Tranquilizer.
METHYLPHENETHYLAMINE. 1-alpha-Methylphenethylamine.
See: Amphetamine HCl (Various Mfr.).
• **METHYLPHENIDATE HCl,** U.S.P. XXIII. Tab., Extended-release Tab., U.S.P. XXIII. Methyl a-phenyl-2-piperidine-acetate hydrochloride. (Various Mfr.) **Tab.:** 5 mg, 10 mg or 20 mg. Bot. 100s, 1000s; **SR Tab.:** 20 mg. Bot. 100s.
Use: CNS stimulant.
See: Ritalin HCl, Tab., Vial (Ciba).
METHYLPHENIDYLACETATE HCl. Methyl 1-phenyl-2-piperidylacetate.
See: Methylphenidate HCl (Various Mfr.).
METHYLPHENOBARBITAL. N-Methyl-5-ethyl-5-phenylbarbituric Acid.
See: Mephobarbital.
d-METHYLPHENYLAMINE SULFATE.
See: Dextroamphetamine Sulfate, U.S.P. XXIII. (Various Mfr.).
METHYL PHENYLETHYLHYDANTOIN.
See: Mesantoin, Tab. (Sandoz).
METHYLPHENYLSUCCINIMIDE.
See: Milontin, Kapseal, Susp. (Parke-Davis).
METHYLPHYTYL NAPHTHOQUINONE.
Use: Vitamin K supplement.
See: Phytonadione.
METHYL POLYSILOXANE.
See: Mylicon, Tab., Drops (Stuart).
Phasil, Tab. (Reed & Carnrick).
Silain, Tab. (Robins).

Simethicone.
METHYLPRED-40. (Seatrace) Methylprednisolone acetate 40 mg/ml. Vial 5 ml, 10 ml.
Use: Corticosteroid.
• **METHYLPREDNISOLONE,** U.S.P. XXIII. Tab., U.S.P. XXIII. 11 α,17,21-Trihydroxy-6-α-methyl progna 1,4 diene-3,20-dione. Medrone, Metastab.
Use: Glucocorticoid.
See: A-Methapred, Inj. (Abbott).
Dura-Meth, Inj. (Foy).
Medralone 40, Inj. (Keene).
Medralone 80, Inj. (Keene).
Medrol, Tab. (Upjohn).
W/Neomycin sulfate.
See: Neo-Medrol, Oint. (Upjohn).
W/Sodium succinate.
See: Solu-Medrol, Vial (Upjohn).
• **METHYLPREDNISOLONE ACETATE,** U.S.P. XXIII. Cream, for Enema, Sterile Susp., U.S.P. XXIII. 6-α-methylprednisolone-21-acetate.
Use: Glucocorticoid.
See: Adlone, Inj. (UAD).
Depo-Medrol, Inj., Rectal (Upjohn).
Depo-Pred., Vial (Hyrex).
Medrol Preps., Cream, Oint. (Upjohn).
Mepred-40, Susp. (Savage).
Mepred-80, Susp. (Savage).
Neo-Medrol, Preps. (Upjohn).
Rep-Pred, Vial (Central).
• **METHYLPREDNISOLONE ACETATE FOR ENEMA,** U.S.P. XXIII.
Use: Glucocorticoid.
• **METHYLPREDNISOLONE HEMISUCCINATE,** U.S.P. XXIII.
Use: Adrenocortical steroid.
• **METHYLPREDNISOLONE SODIUM PHOSPHATE.** USAN.
Use: Glucocorticoid.
• **METHYLPREDNISOLONE SODIUM SUCCINATE,** U.S.P. XXIII. For Inj., U.S.P. XXIII. Methylprednisolone 21-(Hydrogen Succinate) sodium salt.
Use: Adrenocorticoid steroid.
See: Solu-Medrol, Mix-O-Vial (Upjohn).
• **METHYLPREDNISOLONE SULEPTANATE.** USAN.
Use: Adrenocortical steroid, anti-inflammatory.
METHYLPROMAZINE. 10-(3-Dimethylaminopropyl)-2-methylphenethiazine.
4-METHYLPYRAZOLE.
Use: Methanol or ethylene glycol poisoning. [Orphan drug]
METHYLPYRIMAL.
See: Sulfamerazine (Various Mfr.).
METHYLROSANILINE CHLORIDE.
Use: Anthelmintic, anti-infective.

See: Gentian Violet, U.S.P. XXIII. (Various Mfr.).

• **METHYL SALICYLATE,** N.F. XVIII. (Various Mfr.) Oil of wintergreen.
Use: Pharmaceutic aid (flavor).

METHYL SALICYLATE W/COMBINATIONS.
Use: Rubefacient rub (external).
See: Analbalm, Liq. (Central).
Analgesic Balm (Various Mfr.).
Analgesic Ointment "Lannett," Oint. (Lannett).
Banalg, Liniment (Forest).
Chloral-Methylol, Oint. (Ulmer).
Cydonol, Lot. (Gordon).
Emul-o-balm, Liq. (Pennwalt).
Gordobalm, Oint. (Gordon).
Guaiamen, Cream (Lannett).
Listerine Antiseptic, Liq. (Warner-Lambert).
Musterole, Oint. (Schering-Plough).
Pain Bust-R II, Cream (Continental).
Sloan's Liniment, Liq. (Warner-Lambert).
Stimurub, Cream (Otis Clapp).

METHYL SULFANIL AMIDOISOXAZOLE.
Sulfamethoxazole.
See: Gantanol, Tab., Susp. (Roche Lab.).

• **METHYLTESTOSTERONE,** U.S.P. XXIII. Tab., Cap., U.S.P. XXIII. Buccal, Tab. 17-Methyltestosterone. 17β-Hydroxy-17-methylandrost-4-en-3-one. (Anertan, Glasso-Sterandryl, Testoviron). (Various Mfr.) 10 mg or 25 mg. **Tab.:** Bot. 100s, 1000s. **Tab. Buccal:** 10 mg. Bot. 100s.
Use: Androgen.
See: Android-10 or 25, Tab. (ICN Pharm).
Arcosterone, Tab. (Arcum).
Metandren, Linguet, Tab. (Ciba).
Neo-Hombreol-M, Tab. (Organon).
Oreton-M, Tab., Buccal Tab. (Schering).
Ostone, Tab. (Solvay).
Testred, Cap. (ICN).
Virilon, Cap. (Star).

METHYLTESTOSTERONE W/COMBINATIONS.
Use: Androgen.
See: Android-5, 10 or 25, Tab. (Brown).
Estritone, Tab. (Kenyon).
Mediatric, Cap., Liq., Tab. (Wyeth-Ayerst).
Premarin w/Methyltestosterone, Tab. (Wyeth-Ayerst).
Virilon, Cap. (Star).

METHYLTHIONINE CHLORIDE. Name used for Methylene Blue.

METHYLTHIONINE HCl. Name used for

Methylene Blue.

METHYLTHIOURACIL, U.S.P. XXI. 6-Methyl-2-thi-ouracil. 4-Methyl-2-thiouracil. Antibason, Methiocil.
Use: Thyroid inhibition.

METHYL VIOLET.
See: Gentian Violet, Crystal Violet, Methylrosanaline Cl.

METHYNDAMINE. Name used for Tetrydamine.

• **METHYNODIOL DIACETATE.** USAN.
Use: Oral progestin.

• **METHYPRYLON,** U.S.P. XXII. Cap., Tab., U.S.P. XXII. 3,3-Diethyl-5-methyl-2,4-piperidinedione.
Use: Hypnotic.
See: Noludar, Cap., Tab. (Roche).

• **METHYSERGIDE.** USAN.
Use: Vasoconstrictor.

• **METHYSERGIDE MALEATE,** U.S.P. XXII. Tab., U.S.P. XXIII. N-[1-(Hydroxymethyl)propyl]-1-methyl-D-lysergamide bimaleate. 1-Methyl-D-lysergic acid butanolamide. (+)-9,10 Didchydro N [1 (hydroxymethyl)-propyl]-1,6-dimethylergoline-8β-carboxamide Maleate (1:1).
Use: Analgesic (specific in migraine).
See: Sansert, Tab. (Sandoz).

• **METIAMIDE.** USAN. Histamine H_2 antagonist. 1-Methyl-3-[2-(5-methylimidazol-4-ylmethylthio)ethyl]thiourea.
Use: Treatment for peptic ulcer.

• **METIAPINE.** USAN.
Use: Antipsychotic.

METICLOPINDOL. Name used for Clopidol.

METICORTEN. (Schering) Prednisone 1 mg/Tab. Bot. 100s.
Use: Corticosteroid.

METIMYD OPHTHALMIC OINT. STERILE. (Schering) Prednisolone acetate 0.5% (5 mg), sulfacetamide sodium 10% (100 mg). Tube 0.125 oz.
Use: Corticosteroid, sulfonamide (topical).

METIMYD OPHTHALMIC SUSP. STERILE. (Schering) Prednisolone acetate 5 mg, sulfacetamide sodium 100 mg/ml. Bot. dropper 5 ml.
Use: Corticosteroid, sulfonamide (topical).

• **METIOPRIM.** USAN.
Use: Antibacterial.

• **METIPRANOLOL HCl.** USAN.
Use: Antibacterial.

• **METIZOLINE.** F.D.A. 2-[(2-Methylbenzo[b]-thien-3-yl)methyl]-2-imidazoline.
Use: Nasal decongestant.
See: Benazoline.

• **METIZOLINE HYDROCHLORIDE.**
USAN.
Use: Adrengeric.
• **METKEPHAMID ACETATE.** USAN.
Use: Analgesic.
METOCLOPRAMIDE. 4-Amino-5-chloro-
N-(2-diethylaminoethyl)-2-methoxyben-
zamide. Primperan is the hydrochloride.
• **METOCLOPRAMIDE**
HYDROCHLORIDE, U.S.P. XXIII, Tab.,
Inj., U.S.P. XXIII. 4-Amino-5-chloro-n-[2-
(diethyl-amino)-ethyl]-o-anisamide dihy-
drochloride hydrate. 4-amino-5-chloro-
N-[2-(diethylamino) ethyl]-2-methoxy-
benzamide monohydrochloride
monohydrate.
Use: Antiemetic.
See: Reclomide, Tab. (Ultra).
Reglan, Amp. (Robins).
METOCLOPRAMIDE INTENSOL. (Rox-
ane) Metoclopramide HCl 10 mg/ml.
Concentrated soln. Dropper Bot. 10 ml,
30 ml.
Use: Gastrointestinal stimulant.
• **METOCURINE IODIDE,** U.S.P. XXIII. Inj.,
U.S.P. XXIII. (+)-O,O′-Dimethylchondro-
curarine di-iodide.
Use: Skeletal muscle relaxant.
See: Metubine Iodid, Vial (Lilly).
METOFOLINE. B.A.N. 1-(4-
Chlorophenethyl)-1,2,3,4-tetrahydro-
6,7-dimethoxy-2-methylisoquinoline.
Use: Analgesic.
METOFURONE. Name used for Ni-
furmerone.
• **METOGEST.** USAN.
Use: Hormone.
• **METOLAZONE.** USAN. 7-Chloro-1,2,3,4-
tetrahydro-2-methyl-4-oxo-3-o-tolyl-6-
quinazolinesulfonamide.
Use: Diuretic, antihypertensive.
See: Diulo, Tab. (Searle).
Mykrox, Tab. (Fisons).
Zaroxolyn, Tab. (Pennwalt).
• **METOPIMAZINE.** USAN. 10-[3-(4-Car-
bamoyl-piperidino)propyl]-2-methane-
sulfonylphenothiazine.
Use: Antiemetic.
METOPON. B.A.N. Methyldihydromorphi-
none 7,8-Dihydro-5-methylmorphinone.
Use: Analgesic.
• **METOPRINE.** USAN.
Use: Antineoplastic agent.
• **METOPROLOL.** USAN. (±)-1-Isopropy-
lamino-3-p-(2-methoxyethyl)phe-
noxypropan-2-ol.
Use: Beta-adrenergic blocking agent.
• **METOPROLOL FUMARATE.** USAN.
Use: Antihypertensive.

• **METOPROLOL SUCCINATE.** USAN.
Use: Antihypertensive; antianginal;
treatment of myocardial infarction.
See: Toprol XL, Extended release Tab.
(Astra).
• **METOPROLOL TARTRATE,** U.S.P. XXIII.
Inj., Tab., U.S.P. XXIII.
Uoo: Beta adrenergic blocking agent.
See: Lopressor, Tab. (Geigy).
METOPROLOL TARTRATE. (Geneva)
Tab.: 50 mg or 100 mg. Bot. 100s,
1000s, UD 100s. **Inj.:** 1 mg/ml. Amp. 5
ml.
Use: Beta-adrenergic blocking agent.
• **METOPROLOL TARTRATE AND HY-
DROCHLOROTHIAZIDE,** U.S.P. XXIII,
Tab., U.S.P. XXIII.
Use: Antihypertensive.
See: Lopressor HCT 100/50, Tab.
(Geigy).
Lopressor HCT 100/25, Tab. (Geigy).
Lopressor HCT 50/25, Tab. (Geigy).
METOQUINE.
Use: Antimalarial.
See: Quinacrine HCl.
• **METOQUIZINE.** USAN. 4,7-Dimethyl-9-
(3,5-dimethyl-pyrazole-1-carboxamido)-
4,6,6a,7,8,9,10,-10a-octahydroindolo-
[4,3-fg]quinoline.
Use: Anti-ulcer agent, anticholinergic.
• **METOSERPATE HYDROCHLORIDE.**
USAN.
Use: Sedative.
METRETON OPHTHALMIC SOLUTION.
(Schering) Prednisolone sodium phos-
phate 5.5 mg/ml. Bot. 5 ml.
Use: Corticosteroid, ophthalmic.
METRIC 21. (Fielding) Metronidazole 250
mg/Tab. Bot. 100s.
Use: Anti-infective.
• **METRIZAMIDE.** USAN. 2-[3-Acetamido-
2, 4, 6-triiodo-5-(N-methylacetamido)
benzamido]-2-deoxy-D- glucopyranose.
Use: Myelography, diagnostic aid (ra-
diopaque medium).
See: Amipaque, Inj. (Sanofi Winthrop).
• **METRIZOATE SODIUM.** USAN.
Use: Diagnostic aid (radiopaque medi-
um).
See: Sodium metrizoate.
METRODIN. (Serono) Urofollitropin 0.83
mg containing 75 IU follicle stimulating
hormone activity/Amp; and 2.2 ml sodi-
um Cl injection/Amp.
Use: Ovulation stimulant.
METROGEL. (Curatek) Metronidazole
0.75%. Gel Tube 30 Gm.
Use: Anti-acne.
METROGEL-VAGINAL. (Curatek)

Metronidazole 0.75%, carbomer 934P, EDTA, parabens and propylene glycol. Gel/Tube (with applicator) 70 Gm.
Use: Anti-infective.
METROGESIC. (Metro Med) Salicylamide 325 mg, acetaminophen 162 mg, phenacetin 65 mg/Tab. Bot. 100s.
Use: Analgesic.
METROGESTONE. 6,17-Dimethylpregna-4,6-diene-3, 20-dione.
Use: Progestin.
METRO I.V. (Kendall-McGaw) Metronidazole 500 mg/100 ml. Inj. Vial 100 ml. Plastic containers 100 ml.
Use: Antibacterial.
METROJEN. (Jenkins) Metrate 1 mg, triple barb 12 mg (representing 33⅓% each, pentobarbital, sodium butabarbital, sodium phenobarbital)/Tab. Bot. 1000s.
Use: Sedative/hypnotic.
• **METRONIDAZOLE,** U.S.P. XXIII. Inj., Tab., U.S.P. XXIII. 1-(2-Hydroxethyl)-2-methyl-5-nitromidazole. 2-Methyl-5-nitromidazole-1-ethanol.
Use: Antitrichomonal. [Orphan drug]
See: Flagyl, Tab. (Searle).
    Flagyl I.V., Vial (Searle).
    Flagyl I.V. RTU, Vial (Searle).
    MetroGel-Vaginal, Gel (Curatek).
    Metronid, Tab. (Ascher).
    Metryl, Tab., Vial (Lemmon).
• **METRONIDAZOLE HYDROCHLORIDE.** USAN.
Use: Antibacterial.
See: Flagyl I.V. (Searle).
• **METRONIDAZOLE PHOSPHATE.** USAN.
Use: Antibacterial, antiprotozoal.
METRONIDAZOLE REDI-INFUSION. (Elkins-Sinn) Metronidazole 500 mg/100 ml Vial.
Use: Amebicide.
METROZOLE. (Metro Med) Metronidazole 250 mg or 500 mg/Tab. **250 mg:** Bot. 100s, 250s; **500 mg:** Bot. 100s.
Use: Anti-infective, amebicide.
METRYL. (Lemmon) Metronidazole 250 mg/Tab. Bot. 100s, 250s, 500s, UD 100s.
Use: Anti-infective, amebicide.
METRYL 500. (Lemmon) Metronidazole 500 mg/Tab. Bot. 100s, 500s.
Use: Anti-infective, amebicide.
METUBINE IODIDE. (Lilly) Metocurine iodide 2 mg/ml. Vial 20 ml.
Use: Skeletal muscle relaxant.
• **METUREDEPA.** USAN. Formerly Dimethyl urethimine. Ethyl [bis(2,2-dimethyl-aziridinyl)-phosphinyl]-carba-

mate. Turloc.
Use: Antineoplastic.
METUSSIN. (Faraday) Dextromethorphan. Bot. 4 oz.
Use: Antitussive.
METUSSIN JR. (Faraday) Dextromethorphan. Bot. 4 oz.
Use: Antitussive.
• **METYRAPONE,** U.S.P. XXIII. Tab., U.S.P. XXIII. 2-Methyl-1,2-di-3-pyridyl-1-propanone.
Use: Diagnostic aid (pituitary function determination).
See: Metopirone, Tab. (Ciba).
METYRAPONE DITARTRATE. 2-Methyl-1,2-di-3-pyridyl-1-propanone ditartrate. Methopyramone.
Use: Diagnostic aid.
    Adrenocortical enzyme inhibitor.
See: Metopirone, Amp. (Ciba).
• **METYRAPONE TARTRATE.** USAN.
Use: Diagnostic aid.
METYRAPONE TARTRATE INJECTION. 2-methyl-1,2-di-3-pyridyl-1-propanone tartrate (1:2).
Use: Diagnostic aid.
• **METYROSINE,** U.S.P. XXIII. Cap., U.S.P. XXIII. L-Tyrosine, a-methyl-,(-)-.
Use: Antihypertensive.
See: Demser (Merck, Sharp & Dohme).
METYZOLINE. B.A.N. 3-(2-Imidazolin-2-yl-methyl)-2-methylbenzo[b]thiophene Eunasin [hydrochloride.]
Use: Vasoconstrictor.
MEVACOR. (Merck) Lovastatin Tab. **10 mg:** Bot. 60s; **20 mg:** Bot. 30s, 60s, 90s, 100s, 180s, 10,000s, UD 100s; **40 mg:** Bot. 60s, 90s, 10,000s.
Use: Antihyperlipidemic.
MEVINOLIN.
See: Lovastatin.
MEXATE-AQ. (Bristol-Myers/Bristol Oncology) Preservative-free liquid. Methotrexate 50 mg, 100 mg or 250 mg/Vial.
Use: Antineoplastic agent.
MEXENONE. B.A.N. 2-Hydroxy-4-methoxy-4'-methylbenzophenone. Uvistat.
Use: Protection of skin from sunlight.
• **MEXILETINE HYDROCHLORIDE,** U.S.P. XXIII, Cap., U.S.P. XXIII.
Use: Cardiac depressant (antiarrhythmic).
See: Mexitil, Cap. (Boehringer Ingelheim).
MEXITIL. (Boehringer Ingelheim) Mexiletine HCl 150 mg, 200 mg or 250 mg/Cap. Bot. 100s, UD 100s.
Use: Antiarrhythmic agent.

• **MEXRENOATE POTASSIUM.** USAN.
Use: Aldosterone antagonist.
MEXSANA MEDICATED POWDER.
(Schering-Plough) Corn starch, kaolin,
triclosan, zinc oxide. Can 3 oz, 6.25 oz,
11 oz.
Use: Diaper rash product.
MEXTRA. (Kenyon) Prednisolone 0.5
mg, acetylsalicylic acid 5 gr/Tab. Bot.
100s, 1000s.
Use: Corticosteroid, analgesic.
MEXTRAFOR. (Kenyon) Acetylsalicylic
acid 5 gr, prednisolone 1.5 mg/Cap. Bot.
100s, 1000s.
Use: Corticosteroid, analgesic.
MEYENBERG GOAT MILK. (Jackson-
Mitchell) Evaporated and powdered
cans of goat milk. Foil pack 4 oz. (makes
one quart).
Use: Cows' milk allergies.
MEZLIN. (Miles Pharm) Mezlocillin sodi-
um. Vial 1 Gm, 2 Gm 3 Gm, 4 Gm. Infu-
sion Bot. 2 Gm, 3 Gm, 4 Gm.
Use: Antibacterial, penicillin.
• **MEZLOCILLIN.** USAN. 6-[D2-(Methylsul-
fonyl-2-oxoimidazolin-1-ylcarboxamido)-
2-phenylacetamido]penicillanic acid.
Use: Antibiotic.
• **MEZLOCILLIN SODIUM, STERILE,**
U.S.P. XXIII.
Use: Antibiotic.
See: Mezlin, Inj. (Miles Pharm).
MG-OROATE. (Miller) Magnesium (as
magnesium orotate) 33 mg/Tab. Bot.
100s.
Use: Magnesium supplement.
MG 217 MEDICATED CONDITIONER.
(Triton) Coal tar solution 2%. Bot. 120
ml.
Use: Antiseborrheic.
MG 217 MEDICATED FORMULA. (Tri-
ton) Coal tar solution 5%, colloidal sulfur
1.5%, salicylic acid 2% in a special base
of cleansers, wetting agents and lanolin.
Shampoo 120 ml, 240 ml.
Use: Antiseborrheic, antipruritic.
MG 400. (Triton) Colloidal sulfur in Guy-
Base II 5%, salicylic acid 3%. Shampoo.
Bot. 240 ml, pt.
Use: Antiseborrheic.
Mg-PLUS PROTEIN. (Miller) Magnesium-
protein complex made w/specially isolat-
ed soy protein 133 mg/Tab. Bot. 100s.
Use: Magnesium supplement.
MIACALCIN. (Sandoz) Calcitonin salmon
100 IU/ml: Inj. Amp. 1 ml. **200 IU/ml:** Vial
2 ml.
Use: Hormone.
MI-ACID GELCAPS. (Major) Calcium car-

bonate 311 mg, magnesium carbonate
232 mg, parabens, EDTA. Bot. 50s.
Use: Antacid.
MI-ACID LIQUID. (Major) Aluminum hy-
droxide 200 mg, magnesium hydroxide
200 mg, simethicone 20 mg/5 ml. Bot.
355 ml, 780 ml.
Use: Antacid, antiflatulent.
MI-ACID II LIQUID. (Major) Aluminum hy-
droxide 400 mg, magnesium hydroxide
400 mg, simethicone 40 mg/5 ml. Bot.
355 ml.
Use: Antacid, antiflatulent.
MIADONE.
See: Methadone HCl. (Various Mfr.).
• **MIANSERIN HCl.** USAN. 1,2,3,4,10,14b-
Hexahydro-2-methyldibenzo[c,f]pyrazi-
no-[1,2-a]-azepine monohydrochloride.
Under study.
Use: Antiserotonin, antihistamine.
MIAQUIN.
See: Camoquin, Tab. (Parke-Davis).
• **MIBOLERONE.** USAN.
Use: Anabolic, androgen.
See: Cheque (Upjohn).
MICASORB. W/Red Veterinary Petrola-
tum.
See: RV Plus, Oint. (Elder).
MICATIN. (Advanced Care) Miconazole
nitrate 2%. **Cream:** Tube 0.5 oz, 1 oz.
Spray powder: Aerosol 3 oz. **Spray Liq-
uid Aerosol:** Bot. 3.5 oz.
Use: Antifungal, topical.
MI-CEBRIN. (Dista) Vitamins B_1 10 mg,
B_2 5 mg, B_6 1.7 mg, pantothenic acid 10
mg, niacinamide 30 mg, B_{12} (activity
equiv.) 3 mcg, C 100 mg, E 5.5 IU, A
10,000 IU, D 400 IU, iron 15 mg, copper
1 mg, iodine 0.15 mg, manganese 1 mg,
magnesium 5 mg, zinc 1.5 mg/Tab. Pkg.
60s, 100s, 1000s, Blister pkg. 10 × 10s.
Use: Vitamin/mineral supplement.
MI-CEBRIN T. (Dista) Vitamins B_1 15 mg,
B_2 10 mg, B_6 2 mg, pantothenic acid 10
mg, niacinamide 100 mg, B_{12} 7.5 mcg,
C 150 mg, E 5.5 IU, A 10,000 IU, D 400
IU, iron 15 mg, copper 1 mg, iodine 0.15
mg, manganese 1 mg, magnesium 5
mg, zinc 1.5 mg/Tab. Bot. 30s, 100s,
1000s, Blister pkg. 10 × 10s.
Use: Vitamin/mineral supplement.
MICOFUR. Anti 5-Nitro-2-Furaldoxime,
Nifuroxime.
Use: Antifungal, antibacterial (topical).
See: Tricofuron, Vaginal Pow., Supp.
(Eaton).
• **MICONAZOLE,** U.S.P. XXIII. Inj., U.S.P.
XXIII. 1-[2,4-Dichloro-β-(2,4-
dichlorobenzyloxy)phenethyl]imidazole.
Use: Antifungal agent.

See: Monistat IV, Inj. (Janssen).
• **MICONAZOLE NITRATE,** U.S.P. XXIII.
   Cream, Vaginal Supp., Pow., U.S.P. XXI-
   II. 1-[2,4-Dichloro-β-[(2,4-dichloroben-
   zyl)-oxy]-phenylmethyl]imidazole
   mononitrate. (Various Mfr.) 2% Vaginal
   cream. Tube 45 Gm with applicator.
   Use: Antifungal.
   See: Breezee Mist Antifungal, Pow.
   (Pedinol).
   Fungoid Tincture, Soln. (Pedinol).
   Maximum Strength Desenex Antifun-
   gal, Cream (Ciba).
   Monistat, Cream, supp. (Ortho).
   Monistat-3, Vaginal supp. (Ortho).
   Monistat-7, Vaginal cream, supp. (Ad-
   vanced Care).
   Monistat-Derm, Prods. (Ortho).
   Nibustat Prods. (Ortho).
   Zeasorb-AF, Pow. (Stiefel).
MICONAZOLE NITRATE. (Copley) Mi-
   conazole nitrate 2%. Cream. Tube 45 g
   (100 mg/dose for 7 doses).
   Use: Antifungal, vaginal.
MICONAZOLE NITRATE. (Taro) Micona-
   zole nitrate 2%, benzoic acid, mineral
   oil, apricot kernel oil. Cream. Tube 15 g,
   30 g.
   Use: Antifungal agent.
MICOREN. (Geigy) n-Crotonyl α-Ethyl-
   aminobutyric acid diethylamine and n-
   crotonyl α-propylaminobutyric acid di-
   ethylamide in aqueous soln. A respira-
   tory stimulant; pending release.
MICRAININ. (Wallace) Meprobamate 200
   mg, aspirin 325 mg/Tab. Bot. 100s.
   Use: Analgesic combination.
MICRhoGAM. (Ortho Diagnostic) Rh₀ (D)
   immune globulin (Human) micro dose.
   Single-dose prefilled syringe. Pkg. 5s,
   25s.
   Use: Agent for immunization.
MICRIDIUM. (Johnson & Johnson)
   Phenacridane (9-(p-hexyloxphenyl)-10-
   methyl-acridinium Cl).
   Use: Skin disorders in infants and chil-
   dren.
MICRIN PLUS. (Johnson & Johnson) Wa-
   ter, S.D. alcohol 38-B, glycerin, polox-
   amer 407, flavor, sodium saccharin, glu-
   tamic acid buffer, cetylpyridinium Cl, FD
   & C Yellow #5, Blue #1. Bot. 12 oz, 24
   oz.
   Use: Mouth preparation.
MICROBUBBLE CONTRAST AGENT.
   Use: Aid in ID of intracranial tumors.
   [Orphan drug]
MICROCULT-GC TEST. (Miles Diagnostic) Miniaturized culture test for the de-
   tection of *Neisseria Gonorrhoeae.* Test

Kit 25s.
   Use: Diagnostic aid.
**MICROFIBRILLAR COLLAGEN HEMO-
   STAT.**
   Use: Hemostatic, topical.
   See: Avitene (Alcon).
MICRO-GUARD. (Sween) Antimicrobial
   skin cream. Tube 0.5 oz, Jar 2 oz.
   Use: Antifungal, external.
MICRO-K EXTENCAPS. (Robins) Potas-
   sium Cl (8 mEq) 600 mg/Cap. Bot. 100s,
   500s, Dis-Co pack 100s.
   Use: Potassium supplement.
MICRO-K 10 EXTENCAPS. (Robins)
   Potassium Cl 750 mg (10 mEq)/Cap.
   Bot. 100s, 500s, Dis-co UD 100s.
   Use: Potassium supplement.
MICRO-K LS. (Robins) Potassium Cl 20
   mEq (1500 mg). Extended release
   Susp. Packet 30s, 100s.
   Use: Potassium supplement.
MICROLIPID. (Biosearch) Fat emulsion
   50%, safflower oil, polyglycerol esters of
   fatty acids, soy lecithin, xanthan gum,
   ascorbic acid. Cal 4500, fat 500 Gm/L,
   80 mOsm/Kg. H₂O. 120 ml.
   Use: Enteral nutritional supplement.
MICRONASE TABLETS. (Upjohn) Gly-
   buride 1.25, 2.5 or 5 mg/Tab. **1.25 mg:**
   Bot. 100s. **2.5 mg:** Bot. 100s, UD 100s.
   5 mg: Bot. 100s, 500s, 1000s, Box
   100s, Unit-of-Use Bot. 30s.
   Use: Antidiabetic.
MICRONEFRIN. (Bird) Racemic methy-
   laminoethanol catechol HCl 2.25 Gm,
   sodium Cl, sodium bisulfite, potassium
   metabisulfite 0.99 Gm, chlorobutanol 0.5
   Gm, benzoic acid 0.5 Gm, propylene
   glycol 8 mg/100 ml. Bot 15 ml, 30 ml.
   Use: Antiasthmatic.
MICRONOR. (Ortho) Norethindrone 0.35
   mg/Tab. Dialpak 28s.
   Use: Oral contraceptive.
MICROSOL. (Star) Sulfamethizole 0.5
   Gm or 1 Gm/Tab. Bot. 100s, 1000s.
   Use: Urinary anti-infective.
MICROSOL-A. (Star) Phenazopyridine
   50 mg, sulfamethizole 0.5 Gm/Tab. Bot.
   100s, 1000s.
   Use: Urinary anti-infective.
MICROSTIX CANDIDA. (Miles Diagnos-
   tic) Test for *candida* species in vaginal
   specimens. Box 25s.
   Use: Diagnostic aid.
MICROSTIX-3 REAGENT STRIPS.
   (Miles Diagnostic) For recognition of ni-
   trite in urine and for semi-quantitation of
   bacterial growth. Bot. 25s w/25 incuba-
   tion pouches.
   Use: Diagnostic aid.

MICROTRAK CHLAMYDIA TRACHOMA-TIS DIRECT SPECIMEN TEST. (Syva) To detect and identify chlamydia trachomatis. Slide test 60s.
Use: Diagnostic aid.

MICROTRAK HSV 1/HSV 2 CULTURE CONFIRMATION/TYPING TEST. (Syva) For identification and typing of herpes simplex in tissue culture. Test kit 1s.
Use: Diagnostic aid.

MICROTRAK NEISSERIA GONORRHEA CULTURE TEST. (Syva) For endocervical, urethral, rectal and pharyngeal cultures. Test kit 85s.
Use: Diganostic aid.

MICRURUS FULVIUS ANTIVENIN. (Wyeth-Ayerst) Inj. Combination package: One vial antivenin, one vial diluent (Bacteriostatic Water for Injection 10 ml.).
Use: Antivenin.

MICTONE 25. (Kenyon) Bethanechol Cl 25 mg/Tab. Bot. 100s, 1000s.
Use: Cholinergic stimulant.

• **MIDAFLUR.** USAN. 4-Amino-2,2,5,5-tetrakis-(trifluoromethyl)-3-imidazoline.
Use: Sedative.

MIDAHIST EXPECTORANT. (Vangard) Codeine phosphate 10 mg, phenyl-propanolamine HCl 18.75 mg, guaifenesin 100 mg/5 ml, alcohol 7.5%. Bot. pt, gal.
Use: Antitussive, decongestant, expectorant.

MIDAMALINE HCl. N-(5-chloro-2-benz-imidazolylmethyl)-N-phenyl-N′N-di-methyl-ethylene-diamine HCl.
Use: Local anesthetic.

MIDAMOR. (Merck & Co.) Amiloride 5 mg/Tab. Bot. 100s.
Use: Diuretic, antihypertensive.

MIDANEED. (Hanlon) Vitamins A 5000 IU, D 500 IU, B_1 5 mg, B_2 3 mg, B_6 0.5 mcg, B_{12} 5 mcg, C 100 mg, niacinamide 10 mg, calcium pantothenate 5 mg/Cap. Bot. 100s.
Use: Vitamin supplement.

MIDATANE DC EXPECTORANT. (Vangard) Brompheniramine maleate 2 mg, guaifenesin 100 mg, phenylephrine HCl 5 mg, phenylpropanolamine HCl 5 mg, codeine phosphate 10 mg/5 ml, alcohol 3.5% Bot. pt, gal.
Use: Antihistamine, expectorant, decongestant, antitussive.

MIDATAPP TR TABLETS. (Vangard) Brompheniramine maleate 12 mg, phenylephrine HCl 15 mg, phenyl-propanolamine HCl 15 mg/Tab. Bot. 100s, 500s, 1000s.
Use: Antihistamine, decongestant.

• **MIDAZOLAM HYDROCHLORIDE.** USAN.
Use: Injectable anesthetic.
See: Versed, Inj. (Roche).

MIDCHLOR. (Schein) Isometheptene mucate 65 mg, dichloralphenazone 100 mg, acetaminophen 325 mg/Cap. Bot. 100s.
Use: Migraine combination.

• **MIDAZOLAM MALEATE.** USAN.
Use: Anesthetic.

• **MIDODRINE HYDROCHLORIDE.** USAN.
Use: Antihypertensive, vasoconstrictor. [Orphan drug]

MIDOL 200. (Glenbrook) Ibuprofen 200 mg/Tab. Bot. 8s, 16s, 32s.
Use: Nonsteroidal anti-inflammatory drug; analgesic.

MIDOL FOR CRAMPS CAPLETS. (Glenbrook) Aspirin 500 mg, caffeine 32.4 mg, cinnamedrine HCl 14.9 mg/Tab. In 8s, 16s, 32s.
Use: Analgesic combination.

MIDOL IB. (Sterling Health) Ibuprofen 200 mg. Tab. Bot. 50s.
Use: Nonsteroidal anti-inflammatory agent.

MIDOL MAXIMUM STRENGTH. (Glenbrook) Cinnamedrine HCl 14.9 mg, aspirin 500 mg, caffeine 32.4 mg/Tab. Bot. 12s, 30s, 60s.
Use: Analgesic combination.

MIDOL MULTI-SYMPTOM, MAXIMUM STRENGTH. (Sterling Health) Acetaminophen 500 mg, pyrilamine maleate 15 mg. Capl. Bot. 32s.
Use: Analgesic combination.

MIDOL MULTI-SYMPTOM, REGULAR STRENGTH. (Sterling Health) Acetaminophen 325 mg, pyrilamine maleate 12.5 mg. Capl. Bot. 16s, 30s.
Use: Analgesic combination.

MIDOL MULTI-SYMPTOM MENSTRUAL, MAXIMUM STRENGTH. (Sterling Health) Acetaminophen 500 mg, caffeine 60 mg, pyrilamine maleate 15 mg. Capl. Pkg. 16s.
Use: Analgesic combination.

MIDOL ORIGINAL FORMULA. (Glenbrook) Cinnamedrine HCl 14.9 mg, aspirin 454 mg, caffeine 32.4 mg/Tab. Bot. 30s, 60s. Strip pack 12s.
Use: Analgesic combination.

MIDOL PM. (Sterling Health) Acetaminophen 500 mg, diphenhydramine 25 mg. Capl. Pkg. 16s.
Use: Analgesic combination.

MIDOL PMS. (Glenbrook) Aceta-

minophen 500 mg, pamabrom 25 mg, pyrilamine maleate 15 mg/Capl. Bot. 16s, 32s.
Use: Analgesic combination.
MIDOL, TEEN. (Sterling Health) Acetaminophen 400 mg, pamabrom 25 mg/Cap. Pkg. 16s.
Use: Analgesic combination.
MIDRIN. (Carnrick) Isometheptene mucate 65 mg, acetaminophen 325 mg, dichloralphenazone 100 mg/Cap. Bot. 50s, 100s.
Use: Agent for migraine.
•**MIFOBATE.** USAN.
Use: Antiatherosclerotic.
•**MIGLITOL.** USAN.
Use: Antidiabetic.
MIGRAINE AGENTS.
See: Sansert, Tab. (Sandoz).
Ergostat, Tab. (Parke-Davis).
Medihaler Ergotamine, Aerosol (3M).
D.H.E. 45, Inj. (Sandoz).
MIGRAINE COMBINATIONS.
See: Isometheptene/Dichloralphenazone/Acetaminophen. (Various Mfr.).
Isocom, Cap. (Nutripharm).
Isopap, Cap. (Geneva Marsam).
Midchlor, Cap. (Schein).
Midrin, Cap. (Carnrick).
Migratine, Cap. (Major).
MIGRATINE. (Major) Isometheptene mucate 65 mg, dichloralphenazone 100 mg, acetaminophen 325 mg/Cap. Bot. 100s, 250s.
Use: Migraine combination.
MIH.
Use: Antineoplastic agent.
See: Matulane (Roche).
MIKAMYCIN. B.A.N. An antibiotic produced by *Streptomyces mitakoensis.* Mikamycin B is Ostreogrycin B.
•**MILACEMIDE HYDROCHLORIDE.** USAN.
Use: Anticonvulsant, antidepressant.
MILD SILVER PROTEIN.
See: Silver Protein, Mild.
•**MILENPERONE.** USAN.
Use: Antipyschotic.
MILES NERVINE. (Miles) Diphenhydramine HCl 25 mg/Tab. Pkg. 12s, Bot. 30s.
Use: Sleep aid.
•**MILIPERTINE.** USAN. 5,6-Dimethoxy-3-[2-[4(o-methoxy-phenyl)-1-piperazinyl]ethyl]-2-methyl-indole.
Use: Tranquilizer.
MILKINOL. (Kremers-Urban) Mineral oil in an emulsifying base. Bot. 240 ml.
Use: Laxative.

•**MILK OF BISMUTH,** U.S.P. XXIII. (Various Mfr.) Bismuth hydroxide, bismuth subcarb.
Use: Orally, intestinal disturbances.
W/Paregoric, kaolin & pectin, methyl parahydroxybenzoate.
See: Mul-Sed, Liq. (Webcon).
•**MILK OF MAGNESIA,** U.S.P. XXIII. (Various Mfr.). Magnesia (Magnesium hydroxide) 325 mg, 390 mg. **Tab.:** 250s, 1000s; **Liq.:** 120 ml, 360 ml, 720 ml, pt, qt, gal, UD 10 ml, 15 ml, 20 ml, 30 ml, 100 ml, 180 ml, 400 ml. **Susp.:** Pt, qt, gal, UD 15 and 30 ml.
Use: Antacid.
See: Magnesium hydroxide.
MILK OF MAGNESIA-CONCENTRATED.
(Roxane) Magnesium hydroxide. Liq. Bot. 100 ml, 180 ml, 400 ml, UD 10 ml, 15 ml, 20 ml, 30 ml.
Use: Antacid.
MILLAZINE. (Major) Thioridazine. **10 mg or 15 mg/Tab.:** Bot. 100s; **25 mg/Tab.:** Bot. 100s, 1000s; **100 mg, 150 mg or 200 mg/Tab.:** Bot. 100s, 500s.
Use: Antipsychotic agent.
MILONTIN. (Parke-Davis) Phensuximide 0.5 Gm/Kapseal. Bot. 100s.
Use: Anticonvulsant.
MILOPHENE. (Milex) Clomiphene citrate 50 mg/Tab. 30s, UD 30s.
Use: Ovulation stimulant.
MILPAR. (Sanofi Winthrop) Magnesium hydroxide, mineral oil.
Use: Antacid, laxative.
•**MILRINONE.** USAN.
Use: Cardiotonic.
See: Primacor.
MILROY ARTIFICIAL TEARS. (Milton Roy) Bot. 22 ml.
Use: Artificial tear solution.
MILTOWN. (Wallace) Meprobamate. **200 mg/Tab.** Bot. 100s. **400 mg/Tab.** Bot. 100s, 500s, 1000s. **600 mg/Tab.** Bot. 100s.
Use: Antianxiety agent.
See: Meprospan (Wallace).
MILTOWN 600. (Wallace) Meprobamate 600 mg/Tab. Bot. 100s, 100s.
Use: Antianxiety agent.
•**MIMBANE HYDROCHLORIDE.** USAN.
1-Methyl-yohimbane HCl.
Use: Analgesic.
•**MINAPRINE.** USAN.
Use: Psychotropic.
•**MINAPRINE HYDROCHLORIDE.** USAN.
Use: Antidepressant.
•**MINAXOLONE.** USAN.
Use: Anesthetic.

MINCARD. Aminometradine. 1-Allyl-3-ethyl-6-aminotetrahydropyrimidine-dione.
Use: Diuretic.

MINEPENTATE. B.A.N. 2-(2-Dimethylamino- ethoxy)ethyl 1-phenylcyclopentanecarboxylate.
Use: Treatment of the Parkinsonian syndrome.

MINERAL ICE, THERAPEUTIC. (Bristol-Myers Products) Menthol 2%, ammonium hydroxide, carbomer 934, cupric sulfate, isopropyl alcohol, magnesium sulfate, thymol. Gel. Tube 105 Gm, 240 Gm, 480 Gm.
Use: Liniment.

MINERAL-CORTICOIDS.
See: Desoxycorticosterone salts (Various Mfr.).

• MINERAL OIL, U.S.P. XXIII.
Use: Cathartic, pharmaceutic aid (solvent, oleaginous vehicle).
See: Petrolatum, Liq.

• MINERAL OIL EMULSION, U.S.P. XXIII.
Use: Cathartic.

• MINERAL OIL ENEMA, U.S.P. XXIII.
Use: Cathartic.

• MINERAL OIL, LIGHT, N.F. XVIII.
Use: Vehicle.

• MINERAL OIL, LIGHT, TOPICAL, U.S.P. XXIII.

MINIBEX. (Faraday) Vitamins B_1 6 mg, B_2 3 mg, B_6 0.5 mg, C 50 mg, niacinamide 10 mg, calcium pantothenate 3 mg, B_{12} 2 mcg, folic acid 0.1 mg/Cap. Bot. 100s, 250s, 1000s.
Use: Vitamin supplement.

MINIDYNE 10%. (Pedinol) Povidone iodine 10%, citric acid, sodium phosphate dibasic. Soln. Bot. 15 ml.
Use: Antiseptic, germicide.

MINI-GAMULIN Rh. (Armour) Rho (D) Immune Globulin (Human) in one-sixth the quantity contained in a standard dose.
Use: Agent for immunization.

MINIPRESS. (Pfizer Laboratories) Prazosin HCl 1 mg, 2 mg or 5 mg/Cap. **1 mg, 2 mg:** Bot. 250s, 1000s, UD 100s; **5 mg:** Bot. 250s, 500s, UD 100s.
Use: Antihypertensive.

MINITEC. (Squibb) Sodium pertechnetate Tc 99 m generator.
Use: Radiopaque agent.

MINITEC GENERATOR (COMPLETE WITH COMPONENTS). (Squibb) Medotopes Kit.
Use: Diagnostic aid.

MINITRAN TRANSDERMAL DELIVERY SYSTEM. (Riker) Nitroglycerin 9 mg.

Patch 33s.
Use: Antianginal.

MINIT-RUB. (Bristol-Myers) Methyl salicylate 15%, methol 3.5%, camphor 2.3% in anhydrous base. Tube 1.5 oz, 3 oz.
Use: External analgesic.

MINIZIDE. (Pfizer Laboratories) Prazosin HCl and polythiazide. **Minizide 1:** Prazosin 1 mg, polythiazide 0.5 mg/Cap. **Minizide 2:** Prazosin 2 mg, polythiazide 0.5 mg/Cap. **Minizide 5:** Prazosin 5 mg, polythiazide 0.5 mg/Cap. Bot. 100s.
Use: Antihypertensive.

MINOCIN. (Lederle) Minocycline HCl **Cap., pellet-filled 50 mg:** Bot. 100s, UD 10 × 10s; **100 mg:** Bot. 50s, 100s, UD 10 10s. **I.V.:** 100 mg/Vial. **Oral Susp.:** 50 mg/5 ml, propylparaben 0.1%, butylparaben 0.06%, alcohol 5% v/v. Bot. 2 oz.
Use: Antibacterial, tetracycline.

• MINOCROMIL. USAN.
Use: Antiallergic.

• MINOCYCLINE. USAN.
Use: Antibacterial.
See: Minocyn (Lederle).

• MINOCYCLINE HYDROCHLORIDE, U.S.P. XXIII. Cap., Oral Susp., Sterile, Tab., U.S.P. XXIII. 4,7-bis-(Dimethylamino)-1,4,4a,5,5a,6,11,12a-octahydro-3,10, 12,12a,tetrahydroxy-1,11-dioxo-2-naph- thacenecarboxamide. (Warner Chilcott) Cap. **50 mg:** Bot. 100s; **100 mg:** Bot. 50s.
Use: Antibiotic. [Orphan drug]
See: Dynacin, Cap. (Medicis Dermatologics).
Minocin, Cap., Syr., Vial (Lederle).

MINODYL. (Quantum) Minoxidil 2.5 mg or 10 mg/Tab. Bot. 100s, 500s.
Use: Antihypertensive.

MINOXIDIL. (Danbury) Minoxidil 2.5 mg/Tab. Bot. 100s, 500s, 1000s.
Use: Antihypertensive.

MINOXIDIL. (Rugby) Minoxidil 10 mg/Tab. Bot. 500s.
Use: Antihypertensive.

• MINOXIDIL, U.S.P. XXIII. Tab., U.S.P. XXIII. 2,4-diamino-6-piperidinopyrimide-3-oxide. (Various Mfr.) 2.5 mg, 10 mg. Tab. Bot. 100s, 500s, 1000s.
Use: Antihypertensive peripheral vasodilator.
See: Loniten, Tab. (Upjohn).

MINOXIDIL, TOPICAL.
Use: Treatment of male pattern baldness.
See: Rogaine, Soln. (Upjohn).

MINTEZOL. (Merck & Co.) Thiabendazole. **Susp.:** 500 mg/5 ml. Bot. 120 ml.

Chew. Tab.: 500 mg. Pkg. 36s.
Use: Anthelmintic.
MINTO-CHLOR SYRUP. (Vale) Codeine sulfate 10 mg, potassium citrate 219 mg, alcohol 2%. Gal.
Use: Antitussive, expectorant.
MINT-O-FECTANT. (Lannett) Mint odor, phenol coefficient 5. Bot. pt, gal, 5 gal, 55 gal drum.
Use: Laxative.
MINTOX. (Major) Aluminum hydroxide 200 mg, magnesium hydroxide 200 mg. Tab. Bot. 100s.
Use: Antacid.
MINTOX PLUS EXTRA STRENGTH LIQ-UID. (Major) Aluminum hydroxide 500 mg, magnesium hydroxide 450 mg, simethicone 40 mg/5 ml. Bot. 355 ml.
Use: Antacid, antiflatulent.
MINTOX PLUS TABLETS. (Major) Aluminum hydroxide 200 mg, magnesium hydroxide 200 mg, simethicone 25 mg. Chew. Tab. 100s.
Use: Antacid, antiflatulent.
MINTOX SUSPENSION. (Major) Aluminum hydroxide 225 mg, magnesium hydroxide 200 mg, parabens, saccharin, sorbitol/5 ml. Susp. Bot. 355 ml, 780 ml.
Use: Antacid, antiflatulent.
MINT SENSODYNE. (Block) Potassium nitrate 5%, saccharin, sorbitol. Toothpaste. Tube 28.3 Gm.
Use: Toothpaste for sensitive teeth.
MINUTE-GEL. (Oral-B) Acidulated phosphate fluoride 1.23% Gel. Bot. 16 oz.
Use: Dental caries preventative.
MIOCHOL. (Iolab) Acetylcholine Cl 20 mg, mannitol 60 mg, Sterile Water for Inj. 2 ml/2 ml univial. 1:100 intraocular.
Use: Agent for glaucoma.
MIOCHOL-E. (Iolab) Acetylcholine Cl 1:100, mannitol 2.8% when reconstituted. Soln. In 2 ml Univials and System Paks.
Use: Agent for glaucoma.
• **MIOFLAZINE HYDROCHLORIDE.** USAN.
Use: Vasodilator.
MIOSTAT INTRAOCULAR SOLUTION. (Alcon Surgical) Carbochol 0.01%. Vial 1.5 ml. Pkg. 12s.
Use: Agent for glaucoma.
MIOTICS, CHOLINESTERASE IN-HIBITORS.
Use: Agents for glaucoma.
See: Humorsal, Soln. (Merck & Co.).
Eserine Sulfate, Oint. (Various Mfr.).
Isopto Eserine, Soln. (Alcon).
Eserine Salicylate, Soln. (Alcon).
Phospholine Iodide, Pow. (Wyeth-Ay-

erst).
Floropryl, Oint. (Merck & Co.).
• **MIPAFILCON A.** USAN.
Use: Contact lens material.
MIRADON. (Schering) Anisindione 50 mg/Tab. Bot. 100s.
Use: Anticoagulant.
MIRAFLOW EXTRA STRENGTH. (Ciba Vision) Isopropyl alcohol 20%, poloxamer 407, amphoteric 10. Thimerosal free. Soln. Bot. 15 ml.
Use: Contact lens care.
MIRAL. (Geneva) Dexamethasone 0.75 mg/Tab. Bot. 100s, 1000s.
Use: Corticosteroid.
MIRASEPT. (CooperVision) Mirasept disinfecting solution, Mirasept rinsing, neutralizing solution w/lens case.
Use: Soft contact lens care.
• **MIRFENTANIL HYDROCHLORIDE.** USAN.
Use: Analgesic.
• **MIRINCAMYCIN HYDROCHLORIDE.** USAN.
Use: Antibacterial, antimalarial.
• **MIRTAZAPINE.** USAN.
Use: Antidepressant.
MISCELLANEOUS URINE TESTS.
Use: Diagnostic aid.
See: Nitrazine Paper (Apothecon).
Phenistix Reagent Strips (Miles Diagnostic)
• **MISONIDAZOLE.** USAN.
Use: Antiprotozoal (trichomonas).
• **MISOPROSTOL.** USAN.
Use: Anti-ulcerative.
MISSION PRENATAL. (Mission) Ferrous gluconate 260 mg (iron 30 mg), vitamins C 100 mg, B_1 5 mg, B_6 3 mg, B_2 2 mg, niacinamide 10 mg, d-calcium pantothenate 1 mg, B_{12} 2 mcg, A (acetate) 4000 IU, D-2 400 IU, calcium carbonate 70 mg, calcium gluconate 100 mg, calcium lactate 100 mg (calcium 50 mg), zinc 15 mg/Tab. Bot. 100s.
Use: Vitamin/mineral supplement.
MISSION PRENATAL F.A. (Mission) Ferrous gluconate 260 mg (iron 30 mg), vitamins C 100 mg, B_1 5 mg, B_6 10 mg, B_2 2 mg, niacinamide 10 mg, B_{12} 2 mcg, folic acid 0.8 mg, A acetate 4000 IU, D2 400 IU, calcium carbonate 70 mg, calcium gluconate 100 mg, calcium lactate 100 mg, (calcium 50 mg), d-calcium pantothenate 1 mg/Tab. Bot. 100s.
Use: Vitamin/mineral supplement.
MISSION PRENATAL H.P. (Mission) Ferrous gluconate 260 mg (iron 30 mg), vitamins C 100 mg, B_1 5 mg, B_6 25 mg, B_2 2 mg, niacinamide 10 mg, calcium pan-

tothenate 1 mg, B_{12} 2 mcg, folic acid 1 mg, A 4000 IU, D 400 IU, calcium carbonate 70 mg, calcium gluconate 100 mg, calcium lactate 100 mg/Tab. Bot. 100s.
Use: Vitamin/mineral supplement.

MISSION PRENATAL-RX. (Mission) Vitamins A 8000 IU, D 400 IU, C 240 mg, B_1 4 mg, B_2 2 mg, B_3 20 mg, B_5 10 mg, B_6 20 mg, B_{12} 8 mcg, folic acid 1 mg, iron 60 mg, calcium 175 mg, iodine 0.3 mg, zinc 15 mg, copper 2 mg/Tab. Bot. 100s.
Use: Vitamin/mineral supplement.

MISSION PRESURGICAL. (Mission) Vitamins C 500 mg, B_1 2.5 mg, B_2 2.6 mg, B_3 30 mg, B_5 16.3 mg, B_6 3.6 mg, B_{12} 9 mcg, A 5000 USP units, D-2 400 USP units, E 45 IU, ferrous gluconate 233 mg, zinc 22.5 mg/Tab. Bot. 100s.
Use: Vitamin/mineral supplement.

MISSION SURGICAL SUPPLEMENT. (Mission) Vitamins C 500 mg, B_1 2.5 mg, B_2 2.6 mg, B_3 30 mg, B_5 16.3 mg, B_6 3.6 mg, B_{12} 9 mcg, A 5000 USP units, D 400 USP units, E 45 USP units, iron 27 mg, zinc 22.5 mg/Tab. Bot. 100s.
Use: Vitamin/mineral supplement.

MITHRACIN. (Miles Pharm) Plicamycin 2500 mcg/Vial. Unit vial 10s.
Use: Antineoplastic agent, antihypercalcemic.

MITHRAMYCIN.
Use: Antineoplastic agent.
See: Plicamycin.

• **MITINDOMIDE.** USAN.
Use: Antineoplastic agent.

MITOBRONITOL. B.A.N. 1,6-Dibromo-1,6-dideoxy-D-mannitol. Myelobromol.
Use: Antineoplastic agent.

• **MITOCARCIN.** USAN. Antibiotic derived from *Streptomyces* species.
Use: Antineoplastic agent.

MITOCLOMINE. B.A.N. NN-Di-(2-chloroethyl)-4-me-thoxy-3-methyl-1-naphthylamine.
Use: Antineoplastic agent.

• **MITOCROMIN.** USAN. Produced by *Streptomyces virdochromogenes.*
Use: Antineoplastic agent.

• **MITOGILLIN.** USAN. An antibiotic obtained from a "unique strain" of *Aspergillus restrictus.*
Use: Antitumorigenic antibiotic.

MITOGUAZONE. (CTRC Research)
Use: Treatment of diffuse non-Hodgkin's lymphoma. [Orphan drug]

• **MITOMALCIN.** USAN. Produced by *Streptomyces malayensis.* Under study.
Use: Antineoplastic.

• **MITOMYCIN,** U.S.P. XXIII. For Inj., U.S.P.

XXIII. In literature as Mitomycin C. Antibiotic isolated from *Streptomyces caespitosis.*
Use: Antibiotic.
See: Mutamycin, Inj. (Bristol).

MITOPODOZIDE. B.A.N. 2'-Ethyl-podophyllohydrazide.
Use: Antineoplastic agent.

• **MITOSPER.** USAN. Substance derived from *Aspergillus* of the glaucus group.
Use: Antineoplastic.

• **MITOTANE,** U.S.P. XXIII. Tab. U.S.P. XXIII. 1,1-Di-chloro-2-(o-chlorophenyl)-2-(p-chlorophenyl)-ethane. Lysodren. Benzene,1-chloro-2-[2,2-dichloro-l-(4-chlorophenyl)ethyl]-.
Use: Antineoplastic agent.
See: Lysodren, Tab. (Bristol).

MITOTENAMINE. B.A.N. 5-Bromo-3-[N-(2-chloro-ethyl)ethylaminomethyl]benzo[b]thiophen.
Use: Antineoplastic agent.

MITOTIC INHIBITORS.
See: Alkaban-AQ (Quad).
Oncovin, Inj. (Lilly).
Velban, Pow. (Lilly).
Velsar, Pow. (Adria).
VePesid, Inj., Cap. (Bristol-Myers Oncology).
Vinblastine Sulfate, Inj. Pow. (Various Mfr.).
Vincasar PFS, Inj. (Adria).
Vincristine Sulfate, Inj. (Various Mfr.).

• **MITOXANTRONE HYDROCHLORIDE.** USAN.
Use: Antineoplastic agent. [Orphan drug]
See: Novantrone (Lederle).

MITRAN. (Hauck) Chlordiazepoxide HCl 10 mg/Cap. Bot. 100s.
Use: Antianxiety agent.

MITROLAN. (Robins) Calcium polycarbophil equivalent to polycarbophil 500 mg/Tab. Blister Pak 36s, 100s.
Use: Laxative.

• **MIVACURIUM CHLORIDE.** USAN.
Use: Blocking agent (neuromuscular).

MIXED RESPIRATORY VACCINE.
Use: Bacterial vaccine.
See: MRV, Inj. (Hollister-Stier, Miles).

• **MIXIDINE.**
Use: Vasodilator (coronary).

MIXTURE 612. Dimethyl Phthalate Solution, Compound.

M-KYA. (Nature's Bounty) Quinine sulfate 64.8 mg, vitamin E 400 IU, lecithin/Cap. Bot. 50s.
Use: Antimalarial preparations.

MLT-ASPIRIN. (Kenyon) Acetylsalicylic acid 7.5 gr/multi-layered Tab. Bot. 100s,

1000s.
Use: Salicylate analgesic.
M-M-R II. (Merck & Co.) Lyophilized preparation of live attenuated measles virus vaccine (Attenuvax), live attenuated mumps virus vaccine (Mumpsvax), live attenuated rubella virus vaccine (Meruvax II). See details under Attenuvax, Mumpsvax and Meruvax II. Single dose vial w/diluent. Pkg. 1s, 10s.
Use: Agent for immunization.
MOBAN. (DuPont) Molindone HCl. **Liq.:** 20 mg/ml concentrate. Bot. 4 oz/w dropper. **Tab.:** 5 mg, 10 mg, 25 mg, 50 mg or 100 mg/Tab. Bot. 100s.
Use: Antipsychotic agent.
MOBENOL.
See: Tolbutamide, U.S.P. XXIII.
MOBIDIN. (Ascher) Magnesium salicylate, anhydrous 600 mg/Tab. Bot. 100s, 500s.
Use: Antiarthritic agent.
MOBIGESIC. (Ascher) Magnesium salicylate 325 mg, phenyltoloxamine citrate 30 mg/ Tab. Bot. 50s, 100s, Pkg. 18s.
Use: Analgesic combination.
MOBISYL CREME. (Ascher) Trolamine salicylate in vanishing creme base. Tubes 100 Gm.
Use: External analgesic.
MOCCASIN BITE.
See: Antivenin, Snake, Polyvalent (Wyeth-Ayerst).
• **MOCLOBEMIDE.** USAN.
Use: Antidepressant.
MOCTANIN. (Ascot) Synthetic esterfied glycerol. Bot. 120 ml.
Use: Gallstone-solubilizing agent.
MODAFINIL. (Cephalon)
Use: Treatment of daytime sleepiness in narcolepsy. [Orphan drug]
• **MODALINE SULFATE.** USAN. 2-Methyl-3-piperidinopyrazine monosulfate.
Use: Antidepressant.
MODANE. (Adria) Phenolphthalein 130 mg/Tab. Pkg. 10s, 30s. Bot. 100s.
Use: Laxative.
MODANE BULK. (Adria) Powdered mixture of equal parts of psyllium and dextrose. Container 14 oz.
Use: Laxative.
MODANE MILD. (Adria) Phenolphthalein 60 mg/Tab. Bot. 10s, 30s, 100s.
Use: Laxative.
MODANE PLUS. (Adria) Phenolphthalein 60 mg, docusate sodium 100 mg/Tab. Bot. 100s, Box 10s, 30s.
Use: Laxative.
MODANE SOFT. (Adria) Docusate sodium 100 mg/Cap. UD Pkg. 30s.

Use: Laxative.
MODANE VERSABRAN. (Adria) Psyllium hydrophilic mucilloid in wheat bran base. Dose 3.4 Gm, Bot. 10 oz.
Use: Laxative.
• **MODECAINIDE.** USAN.
Use: Cardiac depressant.
MODERIL. (Pfizer Laboratories) Rescinnamine 0.25 mg or 0.5 mg Tab. Bot. 100s.
Use: Antihypertensive.
MODICON 21. (Ortho) Norethindrone 0.5 mg, ethinyl estradiol 35 mcg/Tab. Dialpak 21s.
Use: Oral contraceptive.
MODICON 28. (Ortho) Norethindrone 0.5 mg, ethinyl estradiol 35 mcg/Tab., 7 inert Tab. Dialpak 28s.
Use: Oral contraceptive.
MODINAL.
See: Gardinol Type Detergents (Various Mfr.).
MODRASTANE. (Sanofi Winthrop) Trilostane 30 mg or 60 mg/Cap. Bot. 100s.
Use: Adrenal steroid inhibitor.
MODUCAL. (Mead Johnson Nutrition) Maltodextrin. Pow. Can 13 oz.
Use: Enteral nutritional supplement.
MODURETIC. (Merck & Co.) Hydrochlorothiazide 50 mg, amiloride 5 mg/Tab. Bot. 100s, UD 100s.
Use: Diuretic, antihypertensive.
MOENOMYCIN. Phosphorus-containing glycolipide antibiotic. Active against gram-positive organisms. Under study.
• **MOFEGILINE HYDROCHLORIDE.** USAN.
Use: Treatment of Parkinson's disease.
M.O., HALEY'S. (Sanofi Winthrop Products).
See: Haley's M.O., Liq. (Sanofi Winthrop).
MOI-STIR. (Kingswood Lab) Dibasic sodium phosphate, magnesium Cl, calcium Cl, sodium Cl, potassium Cl, sorbitol, sodium carboxymethylcellulose, methyl and propyl parabens. Soln. 120 ml with pump spray.
Use: Saliva substitute.
MOISTURE DROPS. (Bausch & Lomb) Hydroxypropyl methylcellulose, dextran 70. Soln. Bot. 0.5 oz, 1 oz.
Use: Artificial tear solution.
MOISTUREL LOTION. (Westwood) Petrolatum, glycerin, dimethicone steareth-2, cetyl alcohol, benzyl alcohol, laureth-23, carbomer-934, magnesium aluminum silicate, quaternium-15. Lot. Bot. 240 ml.

Use: Emollient.
MOLAR PHOSPHATE.
W/Fluoride ion.
See: Coral Prods. (Lorvic).
Karigel, Gel. (Lorvic).
• **MOLGRAMOSTIM.** USAN.
Use: Hematopoietic (granulocyte macrophage colony-stimulating factor).
• **MOLINAZONE.** USAN. 3-Morpholino-1,2,3-benzotriazin-4(3H)-one.
Use: Analgesic.
• **MOLINDONE HYDROCHLORIDE.** USAN.
Use: Antipsychotic.
See: Lidone, Cap. (Abbott).
Lidone Concentrate, Liq. (Abbott).
Moban, Tab. (DuPont).
MOL-IRON TABLETS. (Schering) Ferrous sulfate 195 mg, (equivalent 39 mg elemental iron)/Tab. Bot. 100s.
Use: Iron supplement.
W/Vitamin C (Schering) Ferrous sulfate 195 mg, ascorbic acid 75 mg/Tab. Bot. 100s.
MOLLIFENE EAR DROPS. (Pfeiffer) Glycerin, camphor, cajaput oil, eucalyptus oil, thyme oil. Soln. Bot. 24 ml.
Use: Otic preparation.
• **MOLSIDOMINE.** USAN.
Use: Antianginal, vasodilator.
MOLYBDENUM SOLUTION. (American Quinine) Molybdenum 25 mcg/ml (as 46 mcg/ml ammonium molybdate tetrahydrate). Inj. Vial 10 ml.
Use: Parenteral nutritional supplement.
MOLYCU. (Burns) Meprobamate 400 mg, copper 60 mg/ml.
Use: Antidote.
MOLY-PAK. (SoloPak) Molybdenum 25 mcg. Inj. Vial 10 ml.
Use: Parenteral nutritional supplement.
MOLYPEN. (Lyphomed) Ammonium molybdate tetrahydrate 46 mcg/ml. Vial 10 ml.
Use: Parenteral nutritional supplement.
MOMENTUM. (Whitehall) Aspirin 500 mg, phenyltoloxamine citrate 15 mg/Tab. Bot. 24s, 48s.
Use: Analgesic.
• **MOMETASONE FUROATE.** USAN. (1) Pregna-1,4-diene-3,20-dione, 9,21-dichloro-17-[(2-furanylcarbonyl)oxy]-11-hydroxy-16-methyl-, (11β,16α)-; (2) 9,21-Dichloro-11β,17-dihydroxy-16α-methylpregna-1,4-diene-3,20-dione 17-(2-furoate).
Use: Topical corticosteroid.
See: Elocon Cream, Oint., Lot. (Schering).

MONACETYL PYROGALLOL. Eugallol. Pyrogallol Monoacetate.
Use: Keratolytic.
MONALIUM HYDRATE. Hydrated magnesium aluminate. Magalorate.
See: Riopan, Tab., Susp. (Wyeth-Ayerst).
• **MONENSIN.** USAN. (1) 2-[5-Ethyltetrahydro-5-[tetrahydro-3-methyl-5-[tetrahydro-6-hydroxy-6-(hydroxymethyl)-3,5-dimethyl-2H-pyran-2-yl]-2-furyl]-2-furyl]-9-hydroxy-β-methoxy-α,a,2,8,-tetramethyl-1,6-dioxaspiro[4,5]decane-7-butyric acid. Coban (as sodium salt)(Lilly).
Use: Antiprotozoal, antibacterial, antifungal.
MONISTAT DUAL-PAK. (Ortho) Miconazole nitrate suppositories and cream.
200 mg/Supp.: Pkg. 3s w/applicator; **Cream 2%.:** Tube 15 Gm, 30 Gm, 90 Gm.
Use: Antifungal, vaginal.
MONISTAT 3 VAGINAL SUPPOSITORIES. (Ortho) Miconazole nitrate 200 mg/Supp. Pkg. 3s w/applicator.
Use: Antifungal, vaginal.
MONISTAT IV. (Janssen) Miconazole 10 mg/ml, PEG 40, castor oil, lactate, methylparaben, propylparaben, water. Amp. 20 ml.
Use: Antifungal.
MONISTAT 5. (Advanced Care) Miconazole nitrate 100 mg in a 1 g base mixture of adapa solidus, cateth-20 and colloidal silicone dioxide. Tampons. 5s with applicator. *Only available in California.*
Use: Antifungal.
MONISTAT 7 VAGINAL CREAM. (Advanced Care) Miconazole nitrate 2% in water-miscible cream. Tube 45 Gm w/dose applicator.
Use: Antifungal, vaginal.
MONISTAT 7 VAGINAL SUPPOSITORIES. (Advanced Care) Miconazole nitrate 100 mg/Supp. Pkg. 7s w/applicator.
Use: Antifungal, vaginal.
MONISTAT 7 COMBINATION PACK. (Advanced Care) **Vaginal Supp.:** Miconazole nitrate 100 mg. In 7s with applicator; **Topical Cream:** Miconazole nitrate 2%. Tube 9 g.
Use: Antifungal, vaginal.
MONISTAT-DERM CREAM. (Ortho) Miconazole nitrate 2%, pegoxol 7 stearate, peglicol 5 oleate, mineral oil, benzoic acid, butylated hydroxyanisole. Tube 15 Gm, 30 Gm, 90 Gm.
Use: Antifungal, external.
MONISTAT-DERM LOTION. (Ortho Derm) Miconazole nitrate 2%, pegoxol 7

stearate, peglicol 5 oleate, mineral oil, benzoic acid, butylated hydroxyanisole. Squeeze bot. 30 ml, 60 ml.
Use: Antifungal, external.
MONOAMINE OXIDASE INHIBITORS.
Use: Antidepressant.
See: Parnate, Tab. (SK-Beecham).
    Marplan, Tab. (Roche).
    Nardil, Tab. (Parke-Davis).
• **MONO AND DI-ACETYLATED MONO-GLYCERIDES,** N.F. XVIII. A mixture of glycerin esterfied mono- and di-esters of edible fatty acids followed by direct acetylation.
Use: Plasticizer.
• **MONO AND DI-GLYCERIDES,** N.F. XVIII. A mixture of mono- and di-esters of fatty acids from edible oils.
Use: Fatty acids, emulsifying agent.
MONOBASE. (Torch) Water-washable emulsion vehicle of fatty alcohols, natural wax, PEG. Consistency maintained over wide temperature range. Jar lb.
Use: Emollient.
• **MONOBENZONE,** U.S.P. XXIII. Oint., U.S.P. XXI. Cream, U.S.P. XXIII. p-(Benzyloxy)phenol.
Use: Depigmenting agent.
See: Benoquin, Oint., Lot. (Elder).
MONOBENZYL ETHER OF HYDRO-QUINONE.
See: Benoquin, Oint., Lot. (Elder).
MONOBROMISOVALERYLUREA.
See: Bromisovalum. (Various Mfr.).
MONOCAPS TABLETS. (Freeda) Iron 41 mg, vitamins A 10,000 IU, D 400 IU, E 15 IU, B_1 15 mg, B_2 15 mg, B_3 41 mg, B_5 15 mg, B_6 15 mcg, B_{12} 15 mcg, C 125 mg, folic acid 0.1 mg, biotin 15 mg, PABA, lysine, linoleic acid, Ca, Cu, I, K, Mg, Mn, Se, Zn/Tab. Bot. 100s, 250s, 500s.
Use: Vitamin/mineral supplement.
MONOCETE SOLUTION. (Pedinol) Monochloracetic acid 80% w/color. Bot. 15 ml.
Use: Cauterizing agent.
MONO-CHLOR. (Gordon) Mono-chloroacetic acid 80%. Bot. 15 ml.
Use: Cauterizing agent.
MONOCHLOROACETIC ACID.
Use: Cauterizing agent.
See: Monocete, Soln. (Pedinol).
    Mono-Chlor, Soln. (Gordon).
MONCHLOROPHENOL-PARA.
See: Camphorated para-chlorophenol, Liq. (Novocol).
MONOCID. (SK-Beecham) Cefonicid sodium 500 mg or 1 Gm/10 ml. Vial 1 Gm/100 ml piggyback. Pharmacy Bulk

Vial equivalent to 10 Gm.
Use: Antibacterial, cephalosporin.
MONOCLATE. (Armour) Monoclonal antibody derived stable lyophilized concentrate of Factor VIII: R heat-treated. With albumin (human) 1% to 2%, mannitol 0.8%, histadine 1.2 mM. Inj. Vial 1 ml single dose with diluent.
Use: Antihemophilic.
MONOCLATE-P. (Armour). Stable concentrate of Factor VIII: C. With albumin (human) 1% to 2%, mannitol 0.8%, histadine 1.2 mMol, < 50 ng/100 AHF activity mouse protein. Pow. for Inj.
Use: Antihemophilic.
MONOCLONAL ANTIBODIES (MURINE OR HUMAN) B-CELL LYMPHOMA.
Use: B-cell lymphoma. [Orphan drug]
MONOCLONAL ANTIBODIES PM-81.
Use: Adjunctive treatment for leukemia. [Orphan drug]
MONOCLONAL ANTIBODIES PM-81 AND AML$_2$-23.
Use: Leukemic bone marrow transplantation. [Orphan drug]
MONOCLONAL ANTIBODY 17-1A.
Use: Pancreatic cancer. [Orphan drug]
MONOCLONAL ANTIBODY TO CD4, 5a8. (Biogen)
Use: Post-exposure prophylaxis for HIV. [Orphan drug]
MONOCLONAL ANTIBODY (HUMAN) AGAINST HEPATITIS B VIRUS.
Use: Prophylaxis in hepatitis B reinfection in liver transplants. [Orphan drug]
MONOCLONAL ANTIBODY FOR LUPUS NEPHRITIS. (Medclone)
Use: Immunization agent. [Orphan drug]
MONOCTANOIN.
Use: Gallstone solubilizing agent. [Orphan drug]
See: Moctanin, Inf. (Ethiteck).
MONOCYCLINE HYDROCHLORIDE.
See: Minocin I.V., Syr., Cap. (Lederle).
MONO-DIFF TEST. (Wampole)
Use: Mononucleosis test.
MONODOX. (Oclassen) Doxycycline monohydrate equivalent to **50 mg** doxycycline. Cap. Bot. 100s or **100 mg** doxycycline. Cap. Bot. 50s, 250s.
Use: Tetracycline.
MONODRAL. (Sanofi Winthrop) Penthienate.
Use: Anticholinergic.
• **MONOETHANOLAMINE,** N.F. XVIII. 2-Aminoethanol.
Use: Pharmaceutic aid (surfactant).
MONO-GESIC TABLETS. (Central) Salsalate (salicylsalicylic acid) 750 mg/Tab.

Bot. 100s, 500s.
Use: Salicylate analgesic.
MONOIODOMETHANESULFONATE SODIUM.
See: Methiodal Sodium, U.S.P. XXIII.
MONOJECT. (Sherwood) Liquid glucose (dextrose 40%). Gel. Tube UD 25 Gm.
Use: Glucose-elevating agent.
MONOJEL. (Sherwood) Glucose 40% in UD 25 Gm.
Use: Glucose-elevating agent.
MONOKET. (Schwarz Pharma Kremers Urban) Isosorbide mononitrate 10 mg or 20 mg. Tab. Bot. 60s, 100s, 180s, UD 100s.
Use: Antianginal agent.
MONO-LATEX. (Wampole) Two minute latex agglutination slide test for the qualitative or semiquantitative detection of infectious mononucleosis heterophile antibodies in serum or plasma. Test kit 20s, 50s, 1000s.
Use: Diagnostic aid.
MONOLAURIN.
Use: Treatment of congenital primary ichthyosis. [Orphan drug]
See: Glylorin.
MONOMERCAPTOUNDECAHYDRO-CLOSO-DO DECABORATE SODIUM.
Use: Treatment of glioblastoma multiforme. [Orphan drug]
MONONINE. (Armour) Factor IX 100 IU/ml with nondetectable levels of Factors II, VII and X with histidine $\approx$ 10 mM, mannitol $\approx$ 3%, mouse protein $\leq$ 50 ng/100 IU Factor IX activity units. Pow. for inj. (lyophilized). Single-dose vials with diluent.
Use: Antihemophilic agent.
MONONUCLEOSIS TESTS.
Use: Diagnostic aid.
See: Mono-Diff Test (Wampole).
  Mono-Latex (Wampole).
  Mono-Lisa (Medical Technology).
  Mono-Plus (Wampole).
  Monospot (Ortho Diagnostics).
  Monosticon (Organon Teknika).
  Monosticon Dri-Dot (Organon Teknika).
  Mono-Sure Test (Wampole).
  Mono-Test (Wampole).
  Mono-Test (FTB) (Wampole).
MONOPAR. Stilbazium Iodide.
Use: Anthelmintic.
MONOPHEN. 2-(4-Hydroxy-3,5-diiodobenzyl)-cyclohexane carboxylic acid.
Use: Orally, cholecystography.
MONO-PLUS. (Wampole) To diagnose infectious mononucleosis from serum,

plasma or fingertip blood. Test kits of 24s.
Use: Diagnostic aid.
• **MONOPRIL.** (Mead Johnson) Fosinopril sodium. 10 mg or 20 mg/Tab., lactose. In 100s, UD 100s.
Use: Antihypertensive.
• **MONOSODIUM GLUTAMATE,** N.F. XVIII.
MONOSODIUM PHOSPHATE.
See: Sodium Biphosphate, U.S.P. XXIII.
MONOSPOT. (Ortho Diagnostics) Diagnosis of infectious mononucleosis. Test kit 20s.
Use: Diagnostic aid.
MONOSTEARIN. (Various Mfr.) Glyceryl monostearate.
MONOSTICON DRI DOT. (Organon Technica) Diagnosis of infectious mononucleosis. Test kit 40s, 100s.
Use: Diagnostic aid.
MONO-SURE TEST. (Wampole) One-minute hemagglutination slide test for the differential qualitative detection and quantitative determination of infectious mononucleosis heterophile antibodies in serum or plasma. Kit 20s.
Use: Diagnostic aid.
MONOSYL. (Arcum) Secobarbital sodium 1 gr, butabarbital 0.5 gr/Tab. Bot. 100s, 1000s.
Use: Sedative/hypnotic.
MONOTARD HUMAN INSULIN. (Squibb/Novo) Human insulin zinc 100 units/ml. Susp. Vial 10 ml.
Use: Antidiabetic.
• **MONOTHIOGLYCEROL,** N.F. XVIII. 3-Mercapto-1,2-propanediol.
Use: Pharmaceutic aid (preservative).
MONO-VACC. (Lincoln) Device used for vaccination against smallpox. Box 12 without vaccine or 20 sterile units with vaccine.
Use: Diagnostic biological.
MONO-VACC TEST O.T. (Connaught) 5 tuberculin units by the mantoux method. Multiple puncture disposable device. Box 25s (tamper-proof).
Use: Tuberculin test.
MONOXYCHLOROSENE. A stabilized, buffered, organic hypochlorous acid derivative.
See: Oxychlorosene (Guardian Chem.).
MONSEL SOLUTION. (Wade) Bot. 2 oz, 4 oz.
Use: Styptic solution.
8-MOP. (ICN Pharm) Methoxsalen 10 mg/Cap. Pkg. 8s.
Use: Psoralens.
• **MORANTEL TARTRATE.** USAN. (E)-1,4,5,6-Tetrahydro-1-methyl-2-

[2(3)methyl-2-thienyl-vinyl]pyrimidine tartrate.
Use: Anthelmintic.
MORANYL.
See: Suramin Sodium.
MORAZONE. B.A.N. 2:3-Dimethyl-4-(3-methyl-2-phenylmorpholinomethyl)-1-phenylpyrazol-5-one.
Use: Analgesic.
MORCO. (Archer-Taylor) Cod liver oil ointment, zinc oxide, benzethonium Cl, benzocaine 1%. 1.5 oz, lb.
Use: Antiseptic, antipruritic.
MORE-DOPHILUS. (Freeda) Acidophilus-carrot derivative 4 billion units/Gm Pow. Bot. 120 Gm.
Use: Antidiarrheal.
• **MORICIZINE.** USAN.
Use: Antiarrhythmic.
See: Ethmozine (DuPont).
• **MORNIFLUMATE.** USAN.
Use: Anti-inflammatory.
MOROLINE. (Schering-Plough) Petrolatum. Jar 1.75 oz, 3.75 oz, 15 oz.
Use: Skin protectant, lubricant.
MOROXYDINE. B.A.N. 4-Morpholine-carboxymidoyl guanidine. N-(Guanidino-formimidoyl)-morpholine.
Use: Antiviral.
MORPEN TABS. (Major) Ibuprofen 400 mg or 600 mg/Tab. Bot. 500s.
Use: Nonsteroidal anti-inflammatory drug; analgesic.
MORPHERIDINE. B.A.N. Ethyl1-(2-morpholino-ethyl)-4-phenylpiperidine-4-carboxylate. Morpholino-ethylnorpethidine.
Use: Narcotic analgesic.
MORPHINE ACETATE.
W/Terpin hydrate, ammonium hypophosphite, potassium guaiacol-sulfonate.
See: Broncho-Tussin Soln. (First Texas).
MORPHINE AND ATROPINE SULFATES TABLETS.
Use: Analgesic, parasympatholytic.
MORPHINE HYDROCHLORIDE. (Various Mfr.) Pow. Bot. 1 oz, 5 oz.
Use: Analgesic.
• **MORPHINE SULFATE,** U.S.P. XXIII. Inj., U.S.P. XXIII. (Various Mfr.) Flake or Pow. Bot. 1/8 oz, 1 oz, 5 oz, H.T. gr, gr, 0.25 gr, 0.5 gr, 1 gr.
Use: Narcotic analgesic, sedative. [Orphan drug]
See: Infumorph 200 & 500, Inj. (Elkins-Sinn).
MS Contin, CR Tab. (Purdue Frederick).
OMS Concentrate, Soln. (Upsher-Smith).

Oramorph SR Tab. (Roxane).
Roxanol, Supp. (Roxane).
Roxanol Rescudose, Soln. (Roxane).
W/Tartar emetic, bloodroot, ipecac, squill, wild cherry.
See: Pectoral, Preps. (Noyes).
MORPHINE SULFATE. (IMS) **25 mg/ml:** Inj. 4, 10, 20, 40 ml *Select-A-Jet* syringe systems. **50 mg/ml:** Inj. 10, 20, 40 ml *Select-A-Jet* syringe systems.
Use: Narcotic analgesic.
• **MORRHUATE SODIUM INJECTION,** U.S.P. XXIII.
Use: Sclerosing agent.
MORTON SALT SUBSTITUTE. (Morton Salt) Potassium Cl, fumaric acid, tricalcium phosphate, monocalcium phosphate. Sodium: < 0.5 mg/5 Gm (0.02 mEq/5 Gm), potassium 2800 mg/5 Gm (72 mEq/5 Gm) 88.6 Gm.
Use: Salt substitute.
MORTON SEASONED SALT SUBSTITUTE. (Morton Salt) Potassium chloride, spices, sugar, fumaric acid, tricalcium phosphate, monocalcium phosphate. Sodium < 1 mg/5 Gm (< 0.04 mEq/5 Gm), potassium 2165 mg/5 Gm (56 mEq/5 Gm). Bot. 85.1 Gm.
Use: Salt substitute.
MOSCO. (Medtech) Salicylic acid. Jar 0.4 oz, 0.8 oz.
Use: Keratolytic.
MOTILIUM. (Janssen) Domperidone maleate.
Use: Antiemetic.
MOTION AID TABLETS. (Vangard) Dimenhydrinate 50 mg/Tab. Bot. 100s, 1000s, UD 10×10s.
Use: Antiemetic/antivertigo.
MOTION CURE. (Wisconsin Pharm.) Meclizine 25 mg/Chew. Tab. 12s.
Use: Antiemetic/antivertigo.
MOTION SICKNESS AGENTS.
See: Antinauseants.
Bucladin, Softab Tab. (Stuart).
Dramamine, Preps. (Searle).
Emetrol, Liq. (Rhone-Poulenc Rorer).
Marezine, Tab., Amp. (Burroughs Wellcome).
Scopolamine HBr (Various Mfr.).
MOTOFEN. (Carnrick) Difenoxin HCl 1 mg, atropine sulfate 0.025 mg/Tab. Bot. 100s.
Use: Antidiarrheal.
• **MOTRETINIDE.** USAN.
Use: Keratolytic.
MOTRIN. (Upjohn) Ibuprofen. **Tab: 300 mg** Bot. 500s, Unit-0f-Use 60s; **400 mg** Bot. 500s, Unit-of-Use 100s, UD 100s; **600 mg** Bot. 500s, Unit-of-Use 100s, UD

100s, **800 mg** Bot. 500s, Unit-of-Use
100s, UD 100s.
Use: Nonsteroidal anti-inflammatory
drug; analgesic.
MOTRIN, CHILDREN'S. (McNeil-CPC)
Ibuprofen 100 mg/5 ml, sucrose. Susp.
Bot. 120 ml, 480 ml.
Use: Nonsteroidal anti-inflammatory
agent, analgesic.
MOTRIN IB. (Upjohn) Ibuprofen **200
mg/Tab.** or **Capl.** Bot. 24s, 50s, 100s,
165s.
Use: Nonsteroidal anti-inflammatory
agent.
MOTRIN IB SINUS. (Upjohn) Pseu-
doephedrine HCl 30 mg, ibuprofen 200
mg. Capl. Pkg. 20s, Bot. 40s.
Use: Decongestant, nonsteroidal anti-
inflammatory agent.
MOUTHKOTE. (Parnell) Xylitol, sorbitol,
Muco protective Factor (MPF) Yerba
Santa, saccharin. Alcohol free. Spray.
Bot. 60, 240 ml and UD 5 ml.
Use: Saliva substitute.
MOUTHKOTE F/R. (Parnell) Sodium fluo-
ride 0.04%, benzyl alcohol, sorbitol,
menthol, EDTA. Rinse. Bot. 237 ml.
Use: Topical fluoride.
MOUTHKOTE O/R. (Parnell) Benzyl alco-
hol 1%, sorbitol, sodium chloride, men-
thol, EDTA. Soln. Bot. 60 ml, 240 ml.
Use: Mouth and throat product.
MOUTHKOTE P/R. (Parnell) **Oint.:**
Diphenhydramine. Tube 15 g. **Spray:**
Diphenhydramine HCl 1.25%, EDTA,
saccharin. Bot. 60 ml, 240 ml.
Use: Mouth and throat product.
• **MOXALACTAM DISODIUM.** USAN.
Use: Antibiotic.
See: Moxam, Inj. (Lilly).
• **MOXALACTAM DISODIUM FOR INJEC-
TION,** U.S.P. XXIII.
Use: Anti-infective.
MOXAM. (Lilly) Moxalactam disodium.
Vial 1 Gm/10 ml Traypak 10s; Vial 2
Gm/20 ml Traypak 10s; Vial 10 Gm/100
ml Traypak 6s.
Use: Antibacterial, cephalosporin.
• **MOXAZOCINE.** USAN.
Use: Analgesic, antitussive.
MOXIPRAQUINE. B.A.N. 8- [fb]6-[4-(3-
Hydroxy-butyl)piperazin-1-yl]hexylamino
-6-methoxy-quinoline.
Use: Protozoacide.
• **MOXNIDAZOLE.** USAN.
Use: Antiprotozoal.
MOXY COMPOUND. (Major) Theo-
phylline 130 mg, ephedrine 25 mg, hy-
droxyzine HCl 10 mg/Tab. Bot. 100s.
Use: Antiasthmatic compound.

MOYCO FLUORIDE RINSE. (Moyco) Flu-
oride 2%. Flavor. Bot. 128 oz. with
pump.
Use: Dental caries preventative.
6-MP. 6-Mercaptopurine.
Use: Antimetabolite.
See: Purinethol, Tab. (Burrough-Well-
come).
M-PREDNISOL-40. (Pasadena) Methyl-
prednisolone acetate 40 mg/ml. Inj.
Susp. Vial 5 ml.
Use: Corticosteroid.
M-PREDNISOL-80. (Pasadena) Methyl-
prednisolone acetate 80 mg/ml. Inj.
Susp. Vial 5 ml.
Use: Corticosteroid.
MRV. (Hollister-Stier) 2000 million organ-
isms/ml from Staphylococcus aureus
(1200 million), Streptococcus, viradens
and non-hemolytic (200 million), Strep-
tococcus pneumoniae (150 million),
Branhamella catarrhalis (150 million),
Klebsiella pneumoniae (150 million), Hemophilus influenzae (150 million). Inj.
Vial 20 ml.
Use: Agent for immunization.
M-R-VAX II. (Merck & Co.) Live attenuated measles virus vaccine (ATTENU-
VAX) and live attenuated rubella virus
vaccine (MERUVAX II). See details un-
der Attenuvax and Meruvax II. Single
dose vial w/diluent. Pkg. 1s, 10s.
Use: Agent for immunization.
MS CONTIN. (Purdue Frederick) Mor-
phine. **CR Tab.: 15 mg or 100 mg:** Bot.
100s, UD 100s. **30 mg:** Bot. 50s, 100s,
250s, Card 25s. **60 mg or 200 mg:** Bot.
100s, UD 25s.
Use: Narcotic analgesic.
MSIR TABLETS. (Purdue Frederick) Mor-
phine 15 mg or 30 mg/IR Tab. Bot. 50s.
Use: Narcotic analgesic.
MSL-109. (Sandoz) Monoclonal antibody.
Use: Antiviral.
MCT. Mitomycin.
Use: Antibiotic.
See: Mutamycin, Pow. (Bristol-Myers
Oncology).
MSTA. (Squibb/Connaught) Mumps skin
test antigen. Vial 1 ml.
Use: Diagnostic aid.
M.T.E.-4. (Lyphomed) Zinc 1 mg, copper
0.4 mg, chromium 4 mcg, manganese
0.1 mg/ml. Vial 3 ml, 10 ml, MD Vial 30
ml.
Use: Mineral supplement.
M.T.E.-4 CONCENTRATED. (Lyphomed)
Zinc 5 mg, copper 1 mg, chromium 10
mcg, manganese 0.5 mg/ml. Vial 1 ml,
MD Vial 10 ml.

Use: Mineral supplement.

M.T.E.-5. (Lyphomed) Zinc 1 mg, copper 0.4 mg, chromium 4 mcg, manganese 0.1 mg, selenium 20 mcg/ml. Vial 10 ml.
Use: Mineral supplement.

M.T.E.-5 CONCENTRATED. (Lyphomed) Zinc 5 mg, copper 1 mg, chromium 10 mcg, manganese 0.5 mg, selenium 60 mcg/ml. Vial 1 ml, MD vial 10 ml.
Use: Mineral supplement.

M.T.E.-6. (Lyphomed) Zinc 1 mg, copper 0.4 mg, chromium 4 mcg, manganese 0.1 mg, selenium 20 mcg, iodide 25 mcg/ml. Vial 10 ml.
Use: Mineral supplement.

M.T.E.-6 CONCENTRATE. (Lyphomed) Zinc 5 mg, copper 1 mg, chromium 10 mcg, manganese 0.5 mg, selenium 60 mcg, iodide 75 mcg/ml. Vial 1 ml. MD vial 10 ml.
Use: Mineral supplement.

M.T.E.-7. (LyphoMed) Zinc 1 mg copper 0.4 mg, manganese 0.1 mg, chromium 4 mcg, selenium 20 mcg, iodide 25 mcg, molybdenum 25 mcg/ml. Vial 10 ml.
Use: Mineral supplement.

MTP-PE. (Ciba-Geigy) Muramyl-tripeptide.
Use: Immunomodulator.

MTX.
Use: Antineoplastic, antipsoriatic.
See: Methotrexate.

MUC 9 + 4 PEDIATRIC. (Lyphomed) Vitamin A 2300 IU, D 400 IU, E 7 mg, B$_1$ 1.2 mg, B$_2$ 1.4 mg, B$_3$ 17 mg, B$_5$ 5 mg, B$_6$ 1 mg, B$_{12}$ 1 mcg, C 80 mg, biotin 20 mcg, folic acid 0.14 mg, K 200 mcg/5 ml, mannitol 375 mg. Pow. Vial. 10 ml.
Use: Parenteral nutritional supplement.

MUCILLOID OF PSYLLIUM SEED. W/Dextrose.
See: Metamucil, Liq. (Searle).

MUCIN.
See: Gastric Mucin (Wilson).

MUCIN, VEGETABLE. W/Yeast or alkalized.
See: Plantamucin, Granules (Elder).

MUCOMYST. (Bristol) A sterile 20% solution of acetylcysteine for nebulization or direct instillation into the lung as a mucolytic agent. Approved as antidote for acetaminophen overdose. Vial. **4 ml:** Ctn. 12s; **10 ml:** Ctn. 3s with dropper; **30 ml:** Ctn. 3s.
Use: Respiratory inhalant.

MUCOMYST-10. (Bristol) A sterile 10% solution of acetylcysteine for nebulization or direct instillation into the lung as a mucolytic agent. Approved as antidote for acetaminophen overdose. Vial. **4 ml:**

Ctn. 12s; **10 ml:** Ctn. 3s with dropper; **30 ml:** Ctn. 3s.
Use: Respiratory inhalant.

MUCOLYTICS.
Use: Respiratory inhalant products.
See: Mucomyst, Soln. (Mead Johnson).

MUCOPLEX. (ICN) Vitamins B$_2$ 1.5 mg, B$_{12}$ 5 mcg, liver fraction 750 mg/Tab. Bot. 100s, 250s.
Use: Vitamin B combination, oral.

MUCOSAL 10 & 20 SOLUTION. (Dey) Acetylcysteine sodium salt 10% or 20%. Soln. Vial 4 ml Box 12s.
Use: Respiratory inhalant.

MUDD. (Chattem) Natural hydrated magnesium aluminum silicate. Topical preparation.
Use: Cleansing agent.

MUDRANE. (Poythress) Aminophylline (anhydrous) 130 mg, phenobarbital 8 mg, ephedrine HCl 16 mg, potassium iodide 195 mg/Tab. Bot. 100s, 1000s.
Use: Antiasthmatic combination.

MUDRANE-2. (Poythress) Potassium iodide 195 mg, aminophylline (anhydrous) 130 mg/Tab. Bot. 100s.
Use: Antiasthmatic combination.

MUDRANE GG. (Poythress) Aminophylline (anhydrous) 130 mg, ephedrine HCl 16 mg, guaifenesin 100 mg, phenobarbital 8 mg/Tab. Bot. 100s, 1000s.
Use: Antiasthmatic combination.

MUDRANE GG-2. (Poythress) Guaifenesin 100 mg, aminophylline (anhydrous) 130 mg/Tab. Bot. 100s.
Use: Antiasthmatic combination.

MUDRANE GG ELIXIR. (Poythress) Theophylline 20 mg, ephedrine HCl 4 mg, guaifenesin 26 mg, phenobarbital 2.5 mg/5 ml, alcohol 20%. Bot. pt, 0.5 gal.
Use: Antiasthmatic combination.

MULTABOLIC. (Kenyon) Adrenal cortex extract 50 mg, vitamin B$_{12}$ 30 mcg, methylandrostenediol 10 mg, liver "pink", B$_{12}$ equivalent. 10 mcg/ml. Vial 10 ml.
Use: Nutritional supplement.

MULTA-GEN 12 +E. (Bowman) Vitamin A 5000 IU, D 400 IU, B$_1$ 2 mg, B$_2$ 2 mg, B$_6$ 0.5 mg, B$_{12}$ 3 mcg, C 37.5 mg, E 15 IU, folic acid 0.2 mg, nicotinamide 20 mg/Cap. Bot. 60s, 500s, 1000s.
Use: Vitamin supplement.

MULTALAN. (Lannett) Vitamin A 5000 IU, D 400 IU, B$_1$ 2.5 mg, B$_2$ 2.5 mg, B$_6$ 0.5 mg, B$_{12}$ 2 mcg, C 50 mg, niacinamide 20 mg, calcium pantothenate 5 mg/Cap. Bot. 500s, 1000s.
Use: Vitamin supplement.

MULTE-PAK-4. (SoloPak) Zinc 1 mg, copper 0.4 mg, manganese 0.1 mg, chromium 4 mg/ml. Vial 3 ml, 10 ml, 30 ml.
Use: Mineral supplement.

MULTE-PAK-5. (SoloPak) Zinc 1 mg, copper 0.4 mg, manganese 0.1 mg, chromium 4 mg, selenium 20 mcg/ml. Vial 3 ml, 10 ml.
Use: Mineral supplement.

MULTI-B-PLEX. (Forest) Vitamins B_1 100 mg, B_2 1 mg, nicotinamide 100 mg, pantothenic acid 10 mg, B_6 10 mg/ml. Vial 10 ml, 30 ml.
Use: Vitamin supplement.

MULTI-B-PLEX CAPSULES. (Forest) Vitamins B_1 50 mg, B_2 5 mg, niacinamide 50 mg, calcium pantothenate 5.4 mg, B_6 0.2 mg, C 150 mg, B_{12} 1 mcg/Cap. Bot. 100s, 1000s.
Use: Vitamin supplement.

MULTI-DAY. (Nature's Bounty) Vitamins A 5000 IU, D 400 IU, E 30 mg, B_1 1.5 mg, B_2 1.7 mg, B_3 20 mg, B_5 10 mg, B_6 2 mg, B_{12} 6 mcg, C 60 mg, FA 0.4 mg. Tab. Bot. 100s, 365s.
Use: Multivitamins.

MULTI-DAY PLUS IRON. (Nature's Bounty) Fe 18 mg, A 5000 IU, D 400 IU, E 15 mg, B_1 1.5 mg, B_2 1.7 mg, B_3 20 mg, B_6 2 mg, B_{12} 6 mcg, C 60 mg, FA 0.4 mg, tartrazine. Tab. Bot. 100s, 365s.
Use: Multivitamin.

MULTI-DAY PLUS MINERALS. (Nature's Bounty). Fe 18 mg, A 5000 IU, D 400 IU, E 30 mg, B_1 1.5 mg, B_2 1.7 mg, B_3 20 mg, B_5 10 mg, B_6 2 mg, B_{12} 6 mcg, C 60 mg, FA 0.4 mg, Ca, Cl, Cr, Cu, I, K, Mg, Mn, Mo, P, Se, Zn, K 50 mcg, biotin 30 mcg. Tab. Bot. 100s.
Use: Multivitamin.

MULTI-DAY W/CALCIUM AND EXTRA IRON TABLETS. (Nature's Bounty). Fe 27 mg, A 5000 IU, D 400 IU, E 30 mg, B_1 1.5 mg, B_2 1.7 mg, B_3 20 mg, B_5 10 mg, B_6 2 mg, B_{12} 6 mcg, C 60 mg, FA 0.4 mg, Ca. Tab. Bot. 100s.
Use: Multivitamins with iron and other supplements.

MULTI-GERM OIL. (Viobin) Corn, sunflower and wheat germ oils. Bot. 4 oz, 8 oz, pt, qt.
Use: Enteral nutritional supplement.

MULTI-JETS. (Kirkman) Vitamins A 10,000 IU, D_2 400 IU, B_1 20 mg, B_2 8 mg, C 120 mg, niacinamide 10 mg, calcium pantothenate 5 mg, B_6 0.5 mg, E 50 IU, desiccated liver 100 mg, dried debittered yeast 100 mg, choline bitartrate 62 mg, inositol 30 mg, dl methionine 30 mg, B_{12} 7 mcg, iron 2.6 mg, calcium (dical phosphate) 58 mg, phosphorus (dical phosphate) 45 mg, iodine (potassium iodide) 0.114 mg, magnesium sulfate 1 mg, copper sulfate 1.99 mg, manganese sulfate 1.11 mg, potassium Cl iodide 79 mg/Tab. Bot. 100s.
Use: Vitamin/mineral supplement.

MULTILEX TABLETS. (Hugby) Iron 15 mg, vitamins A 10,000 IU, D 400 IU, E 5.5 mg, B_1 10 mg, B_2 5 mg, B_3 30 mg, B_5 10 mg, B_6 1.7 mg, B_{12} 3 mcg, C 100 mg, zinc 1.5 mg, Cu, I, Mg, Mn/Tab. Bot. 100s, 1000s.
Use: Vitamin/mineral supplement.

MULTILEX T/M TABLETS. (Rugby) Iron 15 mg, vitamins A 10,000 IU, D 400 IU, E 5.5 mg, B_1 15 mg, B_2 10 mg, B_3 100 mg, B_5 10 mg, B_6 2 mg, B_{12} 7.5 mcg, C 150 mg, Cu, I, Mg, Mn, Zn/Tab. Bot. 100s, 500s, 1000s.
Use: Vitamin/mineral supplement.

MULTILYTE. (Inter-Hermes Pharm) Vitamins A 5000 IU, D 400 IU, E 15 mg, B_1 3 mg, B_2 3.4 mg, B_3 36 mg, B_5 14 mg, B_6 4.4 mg, B_{12} 6 mcg, C 120 mg, FA 0.4 mg, Zn 10.5 mg, biotin 100 mcg, Ca, K, Mg, Mn, phenylalanine. Tab. Pkg. 12s.
Use: Multivitamin w/minerals.

MULTILYTE-20. (Lyphomed) Sodium 25 mEq/L, potassium 20 mEq/L, calcium 5 mEq/L, magnesium 5 mEq/L, chloride 30 mEq/L, acetate 25 mEq/L, gluconate 5 mEq/L. Vial 25 ml fill in 50 ml.
Use: Fluid/electrolyte replacement.

MULTILYTE-40. (Lyphomed) Sodium 25 mEq/L, potassium 40.5 mEq/L, calcium 5 mEq/L, magnesium 8 mEq/L, chloride 33.5 mEq/L, acetate 40.6 mEq/L, gluconate 5 mEq/L. Vial 25 ml fill in 50 ml.
Use: Fluid/electrolyte replacement.

MULTI-MINERAL TABLETS. (Nature's Bounty) Ca 166.7 mg, P 75.7 mg, I 25 mcg, Fe 3 mg, Mg 66.7 mg, Cu 0.33 mg, Zn 2.5 mg, K 12.5 mg, Mn 8.3 mg/Tab. Bot. 100s.
Use: Vitamin/mineral supplement.

MULTIPALS. (Faraday) Vitamins A 5000 IU, D 400 IU, C 50 mg, B_1 3 mg, B_6 0.5 mg, B_2 3 mg, calcium pantothenate 5 mg, niacinamide 20 mg, B_{12} 2 mcg/Tab. Bot. 100s, 250s, 1000s.
Use: Vitamin supplement.

MULTIPALS-M. (Faraday) Vitamins A 6000 IU, D 400 IU, B_1 3 mg, B_2 3 mg, B_6 0.5 mg, B_{12} 5 mcg, C 60 mg, E 2 IU, niacinamide 20 mg, calcium pantothenate 5 mg, iron 10 mg, iodine 0.15 mg, copper 1 mg, magnesium 6 mg, manganese 1 mg, potassium 5 mg/Tab. Bot.

100s, 250s, 1000s.
Use: Vitamin/mineral supplement.
MULTIPLE TRACE ELEMENT. (American Regent) Zinc sulfate 1 mg, copper sulfate 0.4 mg, manganese sulfate 0.1 mg, chromium Cl 4 mg/ml. Inj. Soln. Vial 10 ml.
Use: Mineral supplement.
MULTIPLE TRACE ELEMENT CONCENTRATED. (American Regent) Zinc sulfate 5 mg, copper sulfate 1 mg, manganese sulfate 0.5 mg, chromium Cl 10 mcg/ml. Inj. Soln. Vial 10 ml.
Use: Mineral supplement.
MULTIPLE TRACE ELEMENT NEONATAL. (American Regent) Zn 1.5 mg, Cu 0.1 mg, Mn 25 mcg, Cr 0.85 mcg/ml. Vial 2 ml single dose.
Use: IV nutritional therpay.
MULTIPLE TRACE ELEMENT PEDIATRIC. (American Regent) Zinc sulfate 0.5 mg, copper sulfate 0.1 mg, manganese sulfate 0.03 mg, chromium Cl 1 mcg/ml. Inj. Soln. Vial 10 ml.
Use: Mineral supplement.
MULTIPLE VITAMIN MINERAL FORMULA. (Kirkman) Vitamins A 5000 IU, D_2 400 IU, C 50 mg, B_1 2.5 mg, B_2 2.5 mg, B_6 0.5 mg, B_{12} 1 mcg, niacinamide 15 mg, calcium pantothenate 5 mg, E 0.1 IU, calcium 100 mg, iron 7.5 mg, magnesium 2.5 mg, potassium 2.5 mg, zinc 0.15 mg, manganese 0.5 mg, iodine 0.07 mg/Tab. Bot. 100s.
Use: Vitamin/mineral supplement.
MULTIPLE VITAMINS CHEWABLE. (Kirkman) Vitamins A 5000 IU, D 400 IU, C 50 mg, B_1 3 mg, B_2 2.5 mg, B_6 1 mg, B_{12} 1 mcg, niacinamide 20 mg/Tab. Bot. 100s.
Use: Vitamin supplement.
MULTIPLE VITAMINS W/IRON. (Kirkman) Vitamins A 5000 IU, D 400 IU, C 50 mg, B_1 3 mg, B_2 2.5 mg, B_6 1 mg, B_{12} 1 mcg, niacinamide 20 mg, iron 10 mg/Tab. Bot. 100s.
Use: Vitamin/mineral supplement.
MULTI 75. (Fibertone) Vitamins A 25,000 IU, D 500 IU, E 150 mg, B_1 75 mg, B_2 75 mg, B_3 75 mg, B_5 75 mg, B_6 75 mg, B_{12} 75 mcg, C 250 mg, FA 0.4 mg, Ca, Fe, Biotin, I, Mg, Zn, Cu, PABA, K, Mn, Cr, Si, choline bitartrate, inosol, rutin, lemon flavonoid complex, hesperidin, betaine, glutamic acid HCl/TR Tab. Bot. 50s, 100s, 250s.
Use: Vitamin/mineral supplement.
MULTISTIX 2 REAGENT STRIPS. (Miles Diagnostic) Urinalysis reagent strip test for nitrite and leukocytes. Bot. 100s.

Use: Diagnostic aid.
MULTISTIX 7. (Miles Diagnostic) Urinalysis reagent strip test for glucose ketone, blood, pH, protein, nitrite and leukocytes. Box 100s.
Use: Diagnostic aid.
MULTISTIX 8. (Miles Diagnostic) Urinalysis reagent strip test for detecting glucose, ketone, blood, pH, protein, nitrite, bilirubin and leukocytes. Box. 100s.
Use: Diagnostic aid.
MULTISTIX 8 SG REAGENT STRIPS. (Miles Diagnostic) Urinalysis reagent strip test for glucose, ketone, specific gravity, blood, pH, protein nitrite, leukocytes. Box 100s.
Use: Diagnostic aid.
MULTISTIX 9 REAGENT STRIPS. (Miles Diagnostic) Urinalysis reagent strip test for glucose, bilirubin, ketone, blood, pH, protein, urobilinogen, nitrite, leukocytes. Box 100s.
Use: Diagnostic aid.
MULTISTIX 9 SG REAGENT STRIPS. (Miles Diagnostic) Urinalysis reagent strip test for glucose, bilirubin, ketone, specific gravity, blood, pH, protein, nitrite and leukocytes. Box 100s.
Use: Diagnostic aid.
MULTISTIX 10 SG REAGENT STRIPS. (Miles Diagnostic) Reagent strip test for glucose, bilirubin, ketone, specific gravity, blood, pH, protein, urobilinogen, nitrite and leukocytes in urine. Box 100s.
Use: Diagnostic aid.
MULTISTIX-N. (Miles Diagnostic) Glucose, protein, pH, blood, ketones, bilirubin, urobilinogen, nitrate, leukocytes. Kit. 100s.
Use: In vitro diagnostic aid.
MULTISTIX-N S.G. REAGENT STRIPS. (Miles Diagnostic) Urinalysis reagent strip test for pH, protein, glucose, ketones, bilirubin, blood nitrite, urobilinogen and specific gravity. Bot. 100s.
Use: Diagnostic aid.
MULTISTIX REAGENT STRIPS. (Miles Diagnostic) Urinalysis reagent strip test for pH, protein, glucose, ketone, bilirubin and blood. Box 100s.
Use: Diagnostic aid.
MULTISTIX S. G. REAGENT STRIPS. (Miles Diagnostic) Urinalysis reagent strip test for pH, glucose, protein, ketones, bilirubin, blood and urobilinogen. Box. 100s.
Use: Diagnostic aid.
MULTITEST CMI. (Connaught) One disposable applicator pre-loaded with seven glycerinated liquid antigens and glyc-

erin negative control. 10 units/box.
Use: Diagnostic aid.

MULTI-THERA TABLETS. (Nature's Bounty) Vitamins A 5500 IU, D 400 IU, E 30 mg, B_1 3 mg, B_2 3.4 mg, B_3 30 mg, B_5 10 mg, B_6 3 mg, B_{12} 9 mcg, C 120 mg, folic acid 0.4 mg, biotin 15 mcg/Tab. Bot. 100s.
Use: Vitamin supplement.

MULTI-THERA-M. (Nature's Bounty) Iron 27 mg, vitamins A 5500 IU, D 400 IU, E 30 mg, B_1 3 mg, B_2 3.4 mg, B_3 30 mg, B_5 10 mg, B_6 3 mg, B_{12} 9 mcg, C 120 mg, folic acid 0.4 mg, biotin 15 mcg, zinc 15 mg, Ca, Cl, Cr, Cu, I, K, Mg, Mn, Mo, Se/Tab. Bot. 130s.
Use: Vitamin/mineral supplement.

MULTITRACE-5 CONCENTRATE. (American Regent) Zinc sulfate 5 mg, copper sulfate 1 mg, manganese sulfate 0.5 mg, chromium Cl 10 mcg, selenium 60 mcg. Inj. Soln. Vial 1 ml and 10 ml.
Use: Mineral supplement.

MULTI-VIT DROPS. (Barre) Vitamins A 500 IU, D 400 IU, E 5 mg, B_1 0.5 mg, B_2 0.6 mg, B_3 8 mg, B_6 0.4 mg, B_{12} 2 mcg, C 35 mg/ml. Bot. 50 ml.
Use: Vitamin supplement.

MULTI-VITA. (PBI) Vitamins A 1500 IU/ml, D 400 IU, E 5 mg, B_1 0.5 mg, B_2 0.6 mg, B_3 8 mg, B_6 0.4 mg, B_{12} 2 mcg, C 35 mg, alcohol free. Drop. Bot. 50 ml.
Use: Multivitamin.

MULTI-VITA DROPS. (My-K Labs) Vitamins A 1500 IU, D 400 IU, E 5 mg, B_1 0.5 mg, B_2 0.6 mg, B_3 8 mg, B_6 0.4 mg, B_{12} 2 mcg, C 35 mg/ml. Alcohol free. Bot. 50 ml.
Use: Vitamin/mineral supplement.

MULTI-VITA DROPS W/FLOURIDE. (My-K Labs) Fluoride 0.5 mg, vitamins A 1500 IU, D 400 IU, E 5 mg, B_1 0.5 mg, B_2 0.6 mg, B_3 8 mg, B_6 0.4 mg, B_{12} 2 mcg, C 35 mg/ml. Alcohol free. Bot. 50 ml.
Use: Vitamin supplement; dental caries preventative.

MULTI-VITA DROPS W/IRON. (My-K Labs) Iron 10 mg, vitamins A 1500 IU, D 400 IU, E 5 mg, B_1 0.5 mg, B_2 0.6 mg, B_3 8 mg, B_6 0.4 mg, C 35 mg/ml. Alcohol free. Bot. 50 ml.
Use: Vitamin/mineral supplement.

MULTIVITAMIN AND FLUORIDE DROPS. (Major) Vitamins F 0.25 mg, A 1500 IU, D 400 IU, E 5 mg, B_1 0.5 mg, B_2 0.5 mg, B_3 8 mg, B_6 0.4 mg, B_{12} 2 mg, C 35 mg/Drop. Bot. 50 ml.
Use: Vitamin supplement; dental caries preventative.

MULTI-VITAMIN INFUSION (NEONATAL FORMULA).
Use: Nutritional supplement for low birth weight infants. [Orphan drug]

MULTI-VITAMINS CAPSULES. (Forest) Vitamins A 5000 IU, D 400 IU, B_1 1.5 mg, B_2 2 mg, B_6 0.1 mg, C 37.5 mg, calcium pantothenate 1 mg, niacinamide 20 mg/Cap. Bot. 100s, 1000s, 5000s.
Use: Vitamin supplement.

MULTIVITAMINS ROWELL. (Solvay) Vitamins A 5000 IU, D 400 IU, B_1 2.5 mg, B_2 2.5 mg, C 50 mg, niacinamide 20 mg, B_6 0.5 mg, calcium pantothenate 5 mg, B_{12} 2 mcg, E 10 IU/Cap. Bot. 100s, UD 100s.
Use: Vitamin supplement.

MULTIZINE.
See: Trisulfapyrimidines Tab., U.S.P. XXIII.

MULTOREX. (Approved) Vitamins A 6000 IU, D 1250 IU, C 50 mg, E 5 IU, B_1 3 mg, B_2 3 mg, B_6 0.5 mg, niacinamide 20 mg, calcium pantothenate 5 mg, B_{12} 5 mcg, calcium 59 mg, phosphorus 45 mg/Cap. Bot. 100s, 250s, 1000s.
Use: Vitamin/mineral supplement.

MULVIDREN-F. (Stuart) Fluoride 1 mg, vitamins A 4000 units, D 400 units, C 75 mg, B_1 2 mg, B_2 2 mg, B_6 1.2 mg, B_{12} 3 mcg, calcium pantothenate 3 mg, niacinamide 10 mg/Softab Tab. Bot. 100s.
Use: Vitamin supplement, dental caries preventative.

MUMPS SKIN TEST ANTIGEN. (Connaught) Suspension of killed mumps virus, 40 complement fixing units/ml. Vial 1 ml. (test 10s).
Use: Diagnostic aid.

•**MUMPS SKIN TEST ANTIGEN,** U.S.P. XXIII. (Lilly). Antigen made from allantoic fluid of chick embryos. Vial 1 ml (test 10s).
Use: Diagnostic aid (dermal reactivity indicator).

MUMPSVAX. (Merck & Co.) Live mumps virus vaccine, Jeryl Lynn strain. Single-dose vial w/diluent Pkg. 1s, 10s.
Use: Agent for immunization.
W/Attenuvax, Meruvax II.
See: M-M-R II, Inj. (Merck & Co.).
W/Meruvax II.
See: Biavax II (Merck & Co.).

•**MUMPS VIRUS VACCINE LIVE,** U.S.P. XXIII.
Use: Active immunizing agent.
See: Mumpsvax, Inj. (Merck & Co.).

MUMPS VIRUS VACCINE, LIVE ATTENUATED. Jeryl Lynn (B Level) strain. W/Measles virus vaccine, rubella virus

vaccine.
See: Lirutrin, Vial (Merrell Dow).
M-M-R, Inj. (Merck & Co.).
• **MUPIROCIN.** USAN.
Use: Topical antibacterial.
See: Bactroban, Oint. (Beecham).
MURIATIC ACID.
See: Hydrochloric Acid, N.F. XVIII.
MURI-LUBE. (Lyphomed) Mineral Oil
"Light." Vial 2 ml, 10 ml.
Use: Lubricant for surgery.
MURINE EAR DROPS. (Ross) Car-
bamide peroxide 6.5% in anhydrous
glycerin. Bot. 0.5 oz.
Use: Otic preparation.
MURINE EAR WAX REMOVAL SYSTEM.
(Ross) Carbamide peroxide 6.5% in an-
hydrous glycerin w/ear washing syringe.
Bot. 0.5 oz. and ear washer 1 oz.
Use: Otic preparation.
MURINE EYE DROPS. (Ross) Polyvinyl
alcohol 0.5%, povidone 0.6%, benzalko-
nium chloride, dextrose, EDTA, NaCl.
Soln. Plastic dropper bot. 0.5 oz, 1 oz.
Use: Artificial tear solution.
MURINE PLUS EYE DROPS. (Ross)
Tetrahydrozoline HCl 0.05%, boric acid,
sodium borate, edetate disodium 0.1%,
benzalkonium Cl 0.01%. Bot. 0.5 oz, 1
oz.
Use: Vasoconstrictor, ophthalmic.
MURINE REGULAR FORMULA. (Ross)
Sodium chloride, potassium chloride,
sodium phosphate, glycerin, benzalkoni-
um chloride 0.01%, EDTA 0.05%/Drop.
Bot. 15, 30 ml.
Use: Ophthalmic.
MURO #128 OINTMENT. (Bausch &
Lomb) Sodium Cl 5% in sterile ointment
base. Tube 3.5 Gm.
Use: Hyperosmolar agent.
MURO #128 SOLUTION. (Bausch &
Lomb) Sodium Cl 5%. Soln. Bot. 15 ml,
30 ml.
Use: Hyperosmolar agent.
MURO #128 2% SOLUTION. (Bausch &
Lomb) Sodium Cl 2%. Soln. Dropper
bot. 15 ml.
Use: Hyperosmolar agent.
MUROCEL SOLUTION. (Bausch &
Lomb) Methylcellulose 1%. Soln. Bot. 15
ml.
Use: Artificial tear solution.
MUROCOLL-2. (Bausch & Lomb)
Phenylephrine HCl 10%, scopolamine
HBR 0.3% Bot. 5 ml.
Use: Mydriatic, cycloplegic.
MUROMONAB-CD3.
Use: Immunosuppressive agent.
See: Orthoclone OKT3, Inj. (Ortho).

MUROPTIC-5. (Optopics) Sodium Cl, hy-
pertonic 5%. Soln. Bot. 15 ml.
Use: Hyperosmolar agent.
MURO'S OPCON A SOLUTION. (Bausch
& Lomb) Naphazoline HCl 0.025%,
pheniramine maleate 0.3%. Bot. 15 ml.
Use: Decongestant, antihistamine (oph-
thalmic).
MURO'S OPCON SOLUTION. (Bausch &
Lomb) Naphazoline HCl 0.1%. Bot. 15
ml.
Use: Decongestant, ophthalmic.
MURO TEARS SOLUTION. (Bausch &
Lomb) Hydroxypropyl methylcellulose,
dextran 40. Soln. Bot. 15 ml.
Use: Artificial tear solution.
MUSCLE ADENYLIC ACID. (Various
Mfr.) Active form of adenosine 5-
monophosphate.
See: Adenosine 5-monophosphate,
Preps. (Various Mfr.).
MUSCLE RELAXANTS.
See: Arduan (Organon).
Curare (Various Mfr.).
Flexeril, Tab. (Merck, Sharp &
Dohme).
Flaxedil Triethiodide, Vial (Davis &
Geck).
Lioresal, Tab. (Geigy).
Mephenesin (Various Mfr.).
Meprobamate (Various Mfr.).
Metubine Iodine, Vial (Lilly).
Neostig, Tab. (Freeport).
Norflex, Tab. (Riker).
Nuromax (Burroughs Wellcome).
Parafon Forte, Tab. (McNeil).
P-A-V, Cap. (Amid).
Rela, Tab. (Schering).
Robaxin, Tab., Inj. (Robins).
Soma, Tab., Cap. (Wallace).
Succinylcholine Cl (Various Mfr.).
d-Tubocurarine Cl (Various Mfr.).
MUS-LAX. (Jones Medical) Chlorzoxa-
zone 250 mg, acetaminophen 300
mg/Cap. Bot. 100s.
Use: Skeletal muscle relaxant.
MUSTARAL OIL.
See: Allyl Isothiocyanate.
MUSTARGEN. (Merck & Co.)
Mechlorethamine HCl 10 mg/Vial, sodi-
um Cl q.s. 100 mg/Vial. Treatment set
vial 4s.
Use: Nitrogen mustard.
MUSTEROLE. (Schering-Plough) **Regu-
lar:** Camphor 4%, menthol 2%. Jar 0.9
oz. **Extra Strength:** Camphor 5%, men-
thol 3%. Jar 0.9 oz., Tube 1 oz, 2.25 oz.
Use: External analgesic.
MUSTEROLE DEEP STRENGTH.
(Schering-Plough) Methyl salicylate

30%, menthol 3%, methyl nicotinate 0.5%. Jar 1.25 oz, Tube 3 oz.
Use: External analgesic.

MUSTEROLE EXTRA STRENGTH. (Schering-Plough) Camphor 5%, menthol 3%, methyl salicylate, lanolin, oil of mustard, petrolatum. 27, 30, 67.5 Gm.
Use: Rub/liniment.

MUSTIN.
See: Mechlorethamine HCl, Sterile, U.S.P.

MUSTINE. B.A.N. NN-Di-(2-chloroethyl) methylamine. Chlormethine (I.N.N.).
Use: Antineoplastic agent.

MUTALIN. (Spanner) Protein and iodine. Vial 30 ml.

MUTAMYCIN. (Bristol-Myers/Bristol Oncology) Mitomycin 5 mg, 20 mg or 40 mg/Vial.
Use: Antineoplastic agent.

•**MUZOLIMINE.** USAN.
Use: Diuretic, antihypertensive.

M.V.C. 9 + 3. (Lyphomed) Multivitamin injection for IV infusion. Vial 5 ml, 10 ml, 50 ml.
Use: Vitamin supplement.

M.V.I.-12. (Armour) **Vial 1:** Vitamins A 1 mg, D 5 mcg, E 10 mg, C 100 mg, B_1 3 mg, B_2 3.6 mg, B_6 4 mg, niacinamide 40 mg, dexpanthenol 15 mg/5 ml. **Vial 2:** Biotin 60 mcg, folic acid 400 mcg, Vitamin B_{12} 5 mcg/5 ml. Vials 1 and 2 used together. Box 25s, Ctn. 100s. Vial.
Use: Parenteral nutritional supplement.

M.V.I. PEDIATRIC. (Armour) Vitamin A 0.7 mg, D 10 mcg, E 7 mg, C 80 mg, B_1 1.2 mg, B_2 1.4 mg, B_6 1 mg, B_{12} 1 mcg, potassium 200 mcg, niacinamide 17 mg, dexpanthenol 5 mg, biotin 20 mcg, folic acid 140 mcg/Vial. Box 25s, 5 dose multiple-dose vial, Box 5s.
Use: Parenteral nutritional supplement.

MYADEC. (Parke-Davis) Fe 30 mg, vitamins A 9000 IU, D 400 IU, E 30 mg, B_1 10 mg, B_2 10 mg, B_3 20 mg, B_5 20 mg, B_6 1 mg, B_{12} 1 mcg, C 80 mg, biotin 20 mcg, folic acid 0.14 mg, K 200 mcg/5 ml, mannitol 375 mg. Pow. vial. 10 ml.
Use: Parenteral nutritional supplement.

MYAGEN. Bolasterone.
Use: Anabolic agent.

MYAMBUTOL. (Lederle) Ethambutol HCl. Tab. **100 mg:** Bot. 100s. **400 mg:** Bot. 100s, 1000s, UD 10 × 10s.
Use: Antituberculous agent.

MYANESIN.
See: Mephenesin (Various Mfr.).

MYAPAP DROPS. (My-K) Acetaminophen 80 mg/0.8 ml. Bot. 15 ml w/dropper.

Use: Analgesic.

MYAPAP ELIXIR. (My-K) Acetaminophen 160 mg/5 ml. Bot. 4 oz, pt, gal.
Use: Analgesic.

MYAPAP WITH CODEINE ELIXIR. (My-K) Acetaminophen 120 mg, codeine phosphate 12 mg/5 ml. Bot. 4 oz, pt, gal.
Use: Analgesic, antitussive.

MYBANIL. (My-K) Codeine phosphate 10 mg, bromodiphenhydramine HCl 12.5 mg/5 ml, alcohol 5%. Bot. 4 oz, pt, gal.
Use: Antitussive, antihistamine.

MYCADEC DM DROPS. (My-K) Pseudoephedrine 25 mg, carbonoxamine maleate 2 mg, dextromethorphan HBr 4 mg. Bot. 30 ml.
Use: Decongestant, antihistamine, antitussive.

MYCADEC DM SYRUP. (My-K) Carbinoxamine maleate 4 mg, pseudoephedrine HCl 60 mg, dextromethorphan HBr 15 mg/5 ml, alcohol 0.6%. Bot. 4 oz, pt, gal.
Use: Antihistamine, decongestant, antitussive.

MYCADEC DROPS. (My-K) Pseudoephedrine HCl 25 mg, dextromethorphan HBr 4 mg, carbinoxamine maleate 2 mg/ml. Bot. 30 ml.
Use: Decongestant, antitussive, antihistamine.

MYCARTAI. (Sanofi Winthrop) Pentaerythritol tetranitrate.
Use: Coronary vasodilator.

MYCELEX. (Miles Pharm) Clotrimazole. **Topical Cream:** 1%. Tube 15 Gm, 30 Gm, 90 Gm (2 × 45 Gm). **Topical Soln.:** 1%. Bot. 10 ml, 30 ml.
Use: Antifungal, external.

MYCELEX-7. (Miles) **Vaginal Tab.:** Clotrimazole 100 mg. Pkg. 7s with applicator; **Vaginal Cream:** Clotrimazole 1%. Tube 45 g (7 day therapy) with applicator.
Use: Antifungal, vaginal.

MYCELEX-G. (Miles Pharm) Clotrimazole. **Vaginal Tab.:** 100 mg. Pkg. 7s w/applicator. **Cream:** 1%. Tube 45 Gm, 90 Gm.
Use: Antifungal, vaginal.

MYCELEX-G 500. (Miles Pharm) Clotrimazole 500 mg/Vaginal Tab. w/applicator.
Use: Antifungal, vaginal.

MYCELEX OTC. (Miles Inc.) Clotrimazole 1%, benzyl alcohol 1%. Cream. Tube 15 Gm.
Use: Topical anti-infective.

MYCELEX TROCHES. (Miles Pharm.) Clotrimazole 10 mg/Troche 70s, 140s.
Use: Mouth/throat product.

MYCELEX TWIN PACK. (Miles Pharm) Clotrimazole 500 mg/Vaginal Tab. w/applicator. Topical cream 1%. Tube 7 Gm.
Use: Antifungal, vaginal.

MYCHEL-S. (Rachelle) Sterile chloramphenicol sodium succinate. Vial 1 Gm/15 ml. Box 5s.
Use: Anti-infective.

MYCIFRADIN. (Upjohn) Neomycin sulfate 125 mg/5 ml (equivalent to 87.5 mg neomycin). Oral soln. Bot. pt.
Use: Anti-infective.

MYCIGUENT. (Upjohn) Neomycin sulfate. **Cream:** 5 mg/Gm. Tube 0.5 oz. **Oint.:** 5 mg/Gm. Tube 0.5 oz, 1 oz, 4 oz.
Use: Anti-infective, topical.

MYCINETTES. (Pfeiffer) Benzocaine 15 mg, cetylpyridinium Cl, terpin hydrate, sodium citrate, sorbitol in a demulcent base. Loz. 12s.
Use: Local anesthetic, antiseptic, expectorant.

MYCINETTE SORE THROAT. (Pfeiffer) Phenol 1.4%, alum 0.5%, alcohol free Spray 180 ml.
Use: Mouth/throat product.

MYCI-SPRAY. (Misemer) Phenylephrine HCl 0.25%, pyrilamine maleate 0.15%/ml. Bot. 20 ml.
Use: Decongestant, antihistamine.

MYCITRACIN. (Upjohn) Bacitracin 500 units, neomycin sulfate 5 mg, polymyxin B sulfate 5000 units/Gm. Oint.: Tube 0.5 oz. Box 36s; 1 oz; UD ¹/₃₂ oz Box 144s.
Use: Anti-infective, topical.

MYCITRACIN PLUS. (Upjohn) Polymyxin B sulfate 5000 units/Gm, neomycin 3.5 mg/Gm, bacitracin 500 units/Gm, lidocaine 40 mg, white petrolatum. Tube Oint. 15 Gm.
Use: Topical anti-infective.

MYCITRACIN TRIPLE ANTIBIOTIC MAXIMUM STRENGTH. (Upjohn) Polymyxin B sulfate 5000 units/Gm, neomycin 3.5 mg/Gm, bacitracin 500 units/Gm, parabens, mineral oil, white petorlatum. Oint. Tube 30 Gm, UD 0.94 Gm.
Use: Topical anti-infective.

MYCO BIOTIC II. (Moore) Triamcinolone acetonide 0.1%, nystatin 100,000 units per Gm, aqueous vanishing base, white petrolatum. 15, 30, 60 Gm, Jar 1 lb.
Use: Corticosteroid/antibiotic combination, topical.

MYCOBUTIN. (Adria) Rifabutin. 150 mg/Cap. Bot. 100s.
Use: Antituberculous.

MYCODONE SYRUP. (My-K) Hydrocodone bitartrate 5 mg, homatropine MBr 1.5 mg/5 ml. Bot. 4 oz, pt, gal.

Use: Antitussive.

MYCOGEN II CREAM. (Goldline) Nystatin 100,000 units, triamcinolone acetonide 1 mg/Gm. Cream Tube 15 Gm, 30 Gm, 60 Gm, 120 Gm, lb.
Use: Antifungal, corticosteroid combination.

MYCOLOG II CREAM AND OINTMENT. (Squibb) Triamcinolone acetonide 1 mg, nystatin 100,000 units/Gm. Ointment base w/Plastibase (polyethylene, mineral oil). Tube 15 Gm, 30 Gm, 60 Gm, Jar 120 Gm.
Use: Antifungal, corticosteroid

MYCOGEN II OINTMENT. (Goldline) Nystatin 100,000 units, triamcinolone acetonide 1 mg/Gm. Oint. Tube 15 Gm, 30 Gm, 60 Gm.
Use: Antifungal, corticosteroid combination. combination.

MYCOMIST. (Gordon) Chlorophyll, formalin, benzalkonium Cl. Bot. 4 oz, plastic Bot. 1 oz.
Use: Antifungal for clothing

•**MYCOPHENOLATE MOFETIL.** USAN.
Use: Immunomodulator.

•**MYCOPHENOLIC ACID.** USAN. (E)-6-(4-Hydroxy-6-methoxy-7-methyl-3-oxo-5-phthalanyl)-4-methyl-4-hexenoic acid.
Use: Antineoplastic agent.

MYCOPLASMA PNEUMONIA IFA IgM TEST. (Wampole-Zeus) Indirect fluorescent assay for IgM antibodies to *Mycoplasma pneumoniae.* Box test 100s.
Use: Diagnostic aid.

MYCOPLASMA PNEUMONIA IFA TEST. (Wampole-Zeus) Indirect fluorescent assay for antibodies to *Mycoplasma pneumoniae.* Box test 100s.
Use: Diagnostic aid.

MYCOSTATIN. (Apothecon) Nystatin. **Tab.:** 500,000 units. Bot. 100s. **Cream:** 100,000 units/Gm in aqueous base. Tube 15 Gm, 30 Gm. **Oint.:** 100,000 units/Gm in Plastibase (polyethylene and mineral oil). Tube 15 Gm, 30 Gm. **Susp.:** 100,000 units/ml. In vehicle containing sucrose 50%, saccharin < 1% alcohol. Bot. 60 ml, 473 ml. **Troche:** 200,000 units. 30s. **Vaginal Tab:** 100,000 units, lactose 0.95 Gm, ethyl cellulose, stearic acid, starch. Pkg. 15s, 30s. **Pow.:** (topical) 100,000 units/Gm in talc. Shaker bot. 15 Gm.
Use: Antifungal.

MYCOSTATIN PASTILLES. (Bristol-Myers Oncology) Nystatin, 200,000 units/Troche. 30s.
Use: Antifungal.

MYCO TRIACET. (Various Mfr.) Triamci-

nolone acetonide 0.1%, neomycin sulfate 0.25%, gramicidin 0.25 mg, nystatin 100,000 units/Gm. **Cream:** 15 Gm, 30 Gm, 60 Gm, 480 Gm. **Oint.:** 15 Gm, 30 Gm, 60 Gm.
Use: Corticosteroid, antifungal.
MYCO TRIACET II CREAM & OINTMENT. (Lemmon) Nystatin 100,000 units, triamcinolone acetonide 1 mg/Gm. **Cream:** White petrolatum and mineral oil. Tube 15 Gm, 30 Gm, 60 Gm. **Oint.:** Tube 15 Gm, 30 Gm, 60 Gm.
Use: Antifungal, corticosteroid.
MYCOTUSSIN EXPECTORANT. (My-K) Pseudoephedrine HCl 60 mg, hydrocodone bitartrate 5 mg, guaifenesin 200 mg/5 ml, alcohol 12.5%. Bot. 4 oz, pt, gal.
Use: Decongestant, antitussive, expectorant.
MYCOTUSSIN LIQUID. (My-K) Pseudoephedrine HCl 60 mg, hydrocodone bitartrate 5 mg/5 ml, alcohol 5%. Bot. 4 oz, pt, gal.
Use: Decongestant, antitussive.
MYDACOL. (My-K) Vitamins B_1 5 mg, B_2 2.5 mg, niacinamide 50 mg, B_6 1 mg, B_{12} 1 mcg, pantothenic acid 10 mg, iodine 100 mcg, iron 15 mg, magnesium 2 mg, zinc 2 mg, choline 100 mg, manganese 2 mg/30 ml. Bot. pt, gal.
Use: Vitamin/mineral supplement.
MYDFRIN OPHTHALMIC 2.5%. (Alcon) Phenylephrine HCl 2.5%, benzalkonium Cl 0.01%, EDTA, sodium bisulfite. Drop-Tainers. 3 ml, 5 ml.
Use: Mydriatic.
MYDRIACYL. (Alcon) N-Ethyl-2-phenyl-N-(4-pyridyl-methyl) hydracrylamide. Tropicamide 0.5% or 1%, benzalkonium Cl 0.01%, EDTA. Sterile aqueous soln. 15 ml Drop-Tainer.
Use: Cycloplegic mydriatic.
MYDRIATICS.
Parasympatholytic Types
Atropine Salts (Various Mfr.).
Homatropine Hydrobromide (Various Mfr.).
Scopolamine Salts (Various Mfr.).
Sympathomimetic Types
Amphetamine Sulfate 3% (Various Mfr.).
Clopane HCl, Liq. (Lilly).
Ephedrine Sulfate (Various Mfr.).
Epinephrine HCl (Various Mfr.).
Neo-Synephrine HCl, Preps. (Sanofi Winthrop).
Phenylephrine HCl. (Various Mfr.).
MYELIN.
Use: Multiple sclerosis. [Orphan drug]

MYELO-KIT. (Sanofi Winthrop) Omnipaque 180 or 240 in various sizes and one sterile myelogram tray.
Use: Radiopaque agent.
MYFEDRINE. (Pharmaceutical Basics) Pseudoephedrine 30 mg/5 ml. Liq. Bot. 473 ml.
Use: Decongestant.
MYFEDRINE PLUS SYRUP. (My-K) Pseudoephedrine HCl 30 mg, chlorphenir- amine maleate 2 mg/5 ml. Bot. 4 oz, pt, gal.
Use: Decongestant, antihistamine.
MYFED SYRUP. (My-K) Triprolidine HCl 1.25 mg, pseudoephedrine HCl 30 mg/5 ml. Bot. 4 oz, pt, gal.
Use: Antihistamine, decongestant.
MYGEL LIQUID. (Geneva Generics) Aluminum hydroxide 200 mg, magnesium hydroxide 200 mg, simethicone 20 mg, sodium 1.38 mg/5 ml. Liq. Bot. 360 ml.
Use: Antacid, antiflatulent.
MYGEL SUSPENSION. (Geneva) Aluminum hydroxide 200 mg, magnesium hydroxide 200 mg, simethicone 20 mg/5 ml. Bot. 360 ml.
Use: Antacid, antiflatulent.
MYGEL II SUSPENSION. (Geneva) Aluminum hydroxide 400 mg, magnesium hydroxide 400 mg, simethicone 40 mg/5 ml. Bot. 360 ml.
Use: Antacid, antiflatulent.
MYHISTINE DH. (My-K) Codeine phosphate 10 mg, chlorpheniramine maleate 2 mg, pseudoephedrine HCl 30 mg/5 ml. Liq. Bot. 4 oz, pt, gal.
Use: Antitussive, antihistamine, decongestant.
MYHISTINE ELIXIR. (My-K) Chlorpheniramine maleate 2 mg, phenylephrine HCl 5 mg/5 ml, alcohol 5%. Liq. Bot. 4 oz, pt, gal.
Use: Antihistamine, decongestant.
MYHISTINE EXPECTORANT. (My-K) Codeine phosphate 10 mg, guaifenesin 100 mg, pseudoephedrine HCl 30 mg/5 ml, alcohol 7.5%. Liq. Bot. 4 oz, pt, gal.
Use: Antitussive, expectorant, decongestant.
MYHYDROMINE PEDIATRIC. (My-K) Phenylpropanolamine HCl 12.5 mg, hydrocodone bitartrate 2.5 mg/5 ml. Bot. pt, gal.
Use: Decongestant, antitussive.
MYHYDROMINE SYRUP. (My-K) Phenylpropanolamine HCl 25 mg, hydrocodone bitartrate 5 mg/5 ml. Bot. 4 oz, pt, gal.
Use: Decongestive, antitussive.
MYIDIL. (My-K) Triprolidine HCl 1.25

mg/5 ml, alcohol 4%. Syr. Bot. 120 ml, pt, gal.
Use: Antihistamine.

MYIDONE TABS. (Major) Primidone 250 mg/Tab. Bot. 100s, 1000s.
Use: Anticonvulsant.

MYIDYL SYRUP. (My-K) Triprolidine HCl 1.25 mg/5 ml, alcohol 4%. Bot. 4 oz, pt, gal.
Use: Antihistamine.

MYKACET CREAM. (NMC Labs) Nystatin 100,000 units, triamcinolone acetonide 0.1%/Gm. Tube 15 Gm, 30 Gm, 60 Gm.
Use: Antifungal, corticosteroid.

MY-K ELIXIR. (My-K) Potassium 20 mEq/15 ml, alcohol 5%, saccharin. Bot. pt, gal.
Use: Potassium supplement.

MY-K FORMULA 77D. (My-K) Phenylpropanolamine HCl 12.5 mg, dextromethorphan HBr 10 mg, guaifenesin 100 mg/5 ml, alcohol 10%. Liq. Bot. 180 ml.
Use: Decongestant, antitussive, expectorant.

MY-K FORMULA 77 LIQUID. (My-K) Doxylamine succinate 3.75 mg, dextromethorphan HBr 7.5 mg/5 ml, alcohol 10%. Liq. Bot. 180 ml.
Use: Antihistamine, antitussive.

MYKINAC CREAM. (NMC Labs) Nystatin 100,000 units/Gm in cream base. Tube 15 Gm, 30 Gm.
Use: Antifungal.

MY-K NASAL SPRAY. (My-K) Oxymetazoline HCl 0.05%. Bot. 0.5 oz.
Use: Nasal decongestant.

MYKROX. (Fisons) Metolazone 0.5 mg/Tab. Bot. 100s, 500s, 1000s.
Use: Diuretic.

MYLAGEN GELCAPS. (Goldline) Calcium carbonate 311 mg, magnesium carbonate 232 mg. Pkg. 24s.
Use: Antacid.

MYLAGEN LIQUID. (Goldline) Magnesium hydroxide 200 mg, aluminum hydroxide 200 mg, simethicone 20 mg/5 ml. Bot. 355 ml.
Use: Antacid, antiflatulent.

MYLAGEN II LIQUID. (Goldline) Aluminum hydroxide 400 mg, magnesium hydroxide 400 mg, simethicone 40 mg/5 ml. Bot. 355 ml.
Use: Antacid, antiflatulent.

MYLANTA. (J & J-Merck) Calcium carbonate 600 mg. Loz. 18s, 50s.
Use: Antacid.

MYLANTA DOUBLE STRENGTH. (J & J-Merck) **Chew. Tab.:** Magnesium hydrox-

ide 400 mg, aluminum hydroxide dried gel 400 mg, simethicone 40 mg, Bot. 24s, 60s. **Liq.:** Magnesium hydroxide 400 mg, aluminum hydroxide dried gel 400 mg, simethicone 40 mg, sorbitol/5 ml. Bot. 150 ml, 360 ml. **Susp.:** Magnesium hydroxide 400 mg, aluminum hydroxide dried gel 400 mg, simethicone 40 mg, sodium 0.05 mEq/5 ml. Bot. 150 ml, 360 ml, 720 ml, UD 30, 150 ml.
Use: Antacid.

MYLANTA GAS. (J & J-Merck) Simethicone **40 mg:** Chew. Tab. Bot. 100s, UD 100s; **80 mg:** Chew. Tab. Pkg. 12s, Bot. 48s, 100s, UD 100s.
Use: Antiflatulent.

MYLANTA GAS, MAXIMUM STRENGTH. (J & J-Merck) Simethicone 125 mg/Chew. Tab. Pkg. 12s, Bot. 60s.
Use: Antiflatulent.

MYLANTA GELCAPS. (J & J-Merck) Calcium carbonate 311 mg, magnesium carbonate 232 mg. Bot. 24s, 50s.
Use: Antacid.

MYLANTA LIQUID. (J & J-Merck) Magnesium hydroxide 200 mg, aluminum hydroxide 200 mg, simethicone 20 mg, sodium 0.68 mg/5 ml. Bot. 150 ml, 360 ml, 720 ml, UD 30 ml.
Use: Antacid, antiflatulent.

MYLANTA NATURAL FIBER SUPPLEMENT. (J & J-Merck) Psyllium hydrophilic mucilloid fiber 3.4 g/dose, sucrose, orange flavor. Pow. Can 390 g.
Use: Laxative.

MYLANTA SOOTHING ANTACIDS. (J & J-Merck) Calcium carbonate 600 mg, corn syrup, sucrose. Loz. Pkg. 18s. Bot. 50s.
Use: Antacid.

MYLANTA TABLETS. (J & J-Merck) Magnesium hydroxide 200 mg, aluminum hydroxide 200 mg, simethicone 20 mg, sodium 0.77 mg, sorbitol/Chew. Tab. Bot. 12s, 40s, 48s, 100s, 180s.
Use: Antacid, antiflatulent.

MYLANTA-II LIQUID. (J & J-Merck) Magnesium hydroxide 400 mg, aluminum hydroxide 400 mg, simethicone 40 mg, sodium 1.14 mg, sorbitol/5 ml. Bot. 0.5 oz, 12 oz, UD 30 ml, 100s.
Use: Antacid, antiflatulent.

MYLANTA-II TABLETS. (J & J-Merck) Magnesium hydroxide 400 mg, aluminum hydroxide 400 mg, simethicone 40 mg, sodium 1.3 mg/Chew. Tab. Box 24s, 60s.
Use: Antacid, antiflatulent.

MYLASE 100. Alpha-amylase.
See: Diastase.

W/Prolase, cellulase, calcium carbonate, magnesium glycinate.
See: Zylase Tab. (Vitarine).
MYLERAN. (Burroughs Wellcome) Busulfan 2 mg/Tab. Bot. 25s.
Use: Alkylating agent.
MYLICON. (Stuart) Simethicone 40 mg.
Chew. Tab.: Bot. 100s, 500s, UD 100s.
Drops: 40 mg/0.6 ml. Bot. 30 ml.
Use: Antiflatulent.
MYLICON-80. (Stuart) Simethicone 80 mg/Chew. Tab. Bot. 100s, Box 12s, 48s, UD 100s.
Use: Antiflatulent.
MYLICON-125. (Stuart) Simethicone 125 mg/Chew. Tab. In 12s, 50s.
Use: Antiflatulent.
MYLOCAINE 2% VISCOUS SOLUTION. (My-K) Lidocaine HCl 2%. Bot. 100 ml.
Use: Local anesthetic.
MYLOCAINE 4% SOLUTION. (My-K) Lidocaine HCl 4%. Bot. 50 ml, 100 ml.
Use: Local anesthetic.
MYMETHASONE ELIXIR. (My-K) Dexamethasone 0.5 mg/5 ml, alcohol 5%. Bot. 100 ml, 240 ml.
Use: Corticosteroid.
MYMINIC EXPECTORANT. (Pennex) Phenylpropanolamine HCl 12.5 mg, guaifenesin 100 mg/5 ml, alcohol 5%. Bot. 4 oz, pt, gal.
Use: Decongestant, expectorant.
MYMINIC PEDIATRIC. (My-K) Phenylpropanolamine HCl 12.5 mg, guaifenesin 100 mg/5 ml, alcohol 5%. Liq. Bot. 4 oz, pt, gal.
Use: Decongestant, expectorant.
MYMINIC SYRUP. (My-K) Phenylpropanolamine HCl 12.5 mg, chlorphenir- amine maleate 2 mg/5 ml. Alcohol free. Bot. 4 oz, pt, gal.
Use: Decongestant, antihistamine.
MYMINICOL LIQUID. (Pennex) Phenylpropanolamine HCl 12.5 mg, chlorpheniramine maleate 2 mg, dextromethorphan HBr 10 mg/5 ml. Liq. Bot. 4 oz, pt, gal.
Use: Decongestant, antihistamine, antitussive.
MYNATAL FC. (ME Pharm.) Calcium 250 mg, iron 60 mg, vitamin A 5000 IU, D 400 IU, E 30 IU, B_1 3 mg, B_2 3.4 mg, B_3 20 mg, B_5 10 mg, B_6 10 mg, B_{12} 12 mcg, C 100 mg, folic acid 1 mg, biotin 30 mcg, zinc 25 mg, I, Mg, Cr, Cu, Mo, Mn. Capl. Bot. 100s.
Use: Vitamin-mineral supplement.
MYNATAL PN FORTE. (ME Pharm.) Iron 60 mg, vitamin A 5000 IU, D 400 IU, E 30 IU, C 80 mg, B_1 3 mg, B_2 3.4 mg, B_3

20 mg, B_6 4 mg, B_{12} 12 mcg, folic acid 1 mg, calcium 250 mg, zinc 25 mg, I, Mg, Cu. Capl. Bot. 100s.
Use: Vitamin-mineral supplement.
MYNATAL Rx. (ME Pharm.) Calcium 200 mg, iron 60 mg, vitamin A 4000 IU, D 400 IU, E 15 mg, B_1 1.5 mg, B_2 1.6 mg, B_3 17 mg, B_5 7 mg, B_6 4 mg, B_{12} 2.5 mcg, C 80 mg, folic acid 1 mg, biotin 0.03 mg, zinc 25 mg, Mg, Cu. Capl. Bot. 100s.
Use: Vitamin-mineral supplement.
MYNATE 90 PLUS. (ME Pharm.) Calcium 250 mg, iron 90 mg, vitamin A 4000 IU, D 400 IU, E 30 IU, B_1 3 mg, B_2 3.4 mg, B_3 20 mg, B_6 20 mg, B_{12} 12 mcg, C 120 mg, folic acid 1 mg, zinc 25 mg, DSS 50 mg, I, Cu. Capl. Bot. 100s.
Use: Vitamin-mineral supplement.
MYO-B. (Sig) Adenosine-5-monophosphoric acid, vitamin B_{12}. Vial 10 ml.
MYOCALM. (Parmed) Acetaminophen 8 gr, salicylamide 2 gr, phenyl- toloxamine citrate 40 mg/Tab. Bot. 100s, 1000s.
Use: Analgesic, antihistamine.
MYOCHRYSINE. (Merck & Co.) Sterile aqueous soln. of gold sodium thiomalate 25 mg or 50 mg/ml, benzyl alcohol 0.5%. Amp. 1 ml, Vial 50 mg/ml, 10 ml.
Use: Antirheumatic agent.
MYODIL.
See: Iophendylate Inj., U.S.P. XXIII.
MYODINE C LIQUID. (My-K) Iodinated glycerol 30 mg, codeine phosphate 10 mg/5 ml. Bot. pt, gal.
Use: Expectorant, antitussive.
MYODINE DM LIQUID. (My-K) Iodinated glycerol 30 mg, dextromethorphan HBr 10 mg/5 ml. Bot. pt, gal.
Use: Expectorant, antitussive,
MYODINE LIQUID. (My-K) Iodinated glycerol 60 mg/5 ml. Bot. pt, gal.
Use: Expectorant.
MYOFLEX CREME. (Rhone-Poulenc Rorer) Trolamine salicylate 10% in a vanishing cream base. Tube 2 oz, 4 oz, Jar 8 oz, lb, Pump dispenser 3 oz.
Use: External analgesic.
MYOLIN. (Roberts Hauck) Orphenadrine citrate 30 mg/ml. Inj. Vial 10 ml.
Use: Skeletal muscle relaxant.
MYORGAL. Mysuran. Ambenonium Cl.
Use: Cholinergic.
MYOTALIS. (Vita Elixir) Digitalis 1.5 gr/EC Tab.
Use: Digitalis therapy.
MYOTONACHOL. (Glenwood) Bethanechol Cl 10 mg or 25 mg/Tab. Bot. 100s.
Use: Urinary tract product.

MYOTOXIN. (Vita Elixir) #1: Digitoxin 0.1 mg/Tab. #2: Digitoxin 0.2 mg/Tab.
Use: Cardiac glycoside.

MYPHENTOL ELIXIR. (My-K) Phenobarbital 16.2 mg, hyoscyamine SO₄ or HBr 0.1037 mg, atropine sulfate 0.0194 mg, scopolamine HBr 0.0065 mg/5 ml, alcohol 23%. Bot. 4 oz, pt, gal.
Use: Anticholinergic/antispasmodic, sedative/hypnotic.

MYPHETANE DC COUGH SYRUP. (Pennex) Codeine phosphate 10 mg, brompheniramine maleate 2 mg, phenylpropanolamine HCl 12.5 mg/5 ml, alcohol 1.2%. Bot. 4 oz, gal. *Use:* Antitussive, antihistamine, decongestant.

MYPHETANE DX COUGH SYRUP. (Various Mfr.) Brompheniramine maleate 2 mg, pseudoephedrine HCl 30 mg, dextromethorphan HBr 10 mg/5 ml, alcohol 0.95%. Bot. 4 oz, pt, gal.
Use: Antihistamine, decongestant, antitussive.

MYPHETANE ELIXIR. (My-K) Brompheniramine maleate 2 mg/5 ml, alcohol 3%.
Use: Antihistamine.

MYPHETAPP ELIXER. (My-K) Brompheniramine maleate 2 mg, phenylpropanolamine HCl 12.5 mg/5 ml, alcohol 2.3%. Bot. 4 oz, pt.
Use: Antihistamine, decongestant.

MYPROIC ACID SYRUP. (My-K) Valproic acid 250 mg (as sodium valproate)/5 ml. Bot. pt.
Use: Anticonvulsant.

MYRALACT. B.A.N. N-(2-Hydroxyethyl)tetradecylammonium lactate.
Use: Antiseptic.

MYRIATIN DROPS. (Sanofi Winthrop) Atropine methonitrate BP.
Use: Antispasmodic.

MYRISTICA OIL.
Use: Flavor.

•**MYRISTYL ALCOHOL.**, N.F. XVIII.
MYRISTYL-PICOLINIUM CHLORIDE.
See: Wet Tone, Soln. (Riker).

MYRJ 45. (ICI Americas) Mixture of free polyoxyethylene glycol and its mono- and di-stearates. *Polyoxyl 8 stearate.
Use: Surface-active agent.

MYRJ 52 and 52S. (ICI Americas) Polyoxyethylene 40 stearate. Mixture of free polyoxyethylene glycol and its mono- and di-stearates.
Use: Surface-active agent.

MYRJ 53. (ICI Americas) Polyoxyl 50 stearate.
Use: Surface-active agent.

MYROPHINE. B.A.N. O³-Benzyl-O⁶-tetradecanoylmorphine.
Use: Narcotic analgesic.

MYSOLINE. (Wyeth-Ayerst) Primidone, saccharin. **Tab.**: 50 mg Bot. 100s, 500s; 250 mg. Bot. 100s, 1000s, UD 100s. **Susp.**: 250 mg/5 ml. Bot. 8 oz.
Use: Anticonvulsant.

MYSTECLIN-F. (Squibb) Tetracycline 250 mg, amphotericin B 50 mg/Cap. Bot. 16s, 100s, Unimatic 100s.
Use: Antibacterial, tetracycline.

MYSTECLIN-F SYRUP. (Squibb) Tetracycline 125 mg, potassium metaphosphate, amphotericin B 25 mg/5 ml. Bot. 240 ml.
Use: Antibacterial, tetracycline.

MYSURAN. Ambenonium Cl.
Use: Cholinergic muscle stimulant.
See: Mytelase Cl, Cap. (Winthrop-Breon).

MYTELASE. (Sanofi Winthrop) Ambenonium Cl 10 mg/Cap. Bot. 100s.
Use: Cholinergic muscle stimulant.

MYTICIN G CREME AND OINTMENT.
See: G-MYTICIN CREME AND OINTMENT.

MYTOMYCIN-C. (IOP)
Use: Treatment of refractory glaucoma as an adjunct to AB externo glaucoma surgery. [Orphan drug]

MYTREX. (Savage) Triamcinolone acetonide 0.1%, nystatin 100,000 units/Gm. Cream, Oint. 15 Gm, 30 Gm, 60 Gm, 120 Gm.
Use: Topical corticosteroid, antifungal.

MYTUSSIN AC COUGH. (Pennex) Guaifenesin 100 mg, codeine phosphate 10 mg/5 ml, alcohol 3.5%. Bot. 4 oz, pt, gal.
Use: Expectorant, antitussive.

MYTUSSIN DM EXPECTORANT. (Pennex) Guaifenesin 100 mg, dextromethorphan HBr 10 mg/5 ml, alcohol 1.6%. Bot. 4 oz, pt, gal.
Use: Expectorant, antitussive.

MYTUSSIN DAC SYRUP. (My-K) Guaifenesin 100 mg, pseudoephedrine HCl 30 mg, codeine phosphate 10 mg/5 ml. Bot. 4 oz, pt, gal.
Use: Expectorant, decongestant, antitussive.

MYTUSSIN SYRUP. (My-K) Guaifenesin 100 mg/5 ml, alcohol 3.5%. Bot. 4 oz, pt, gal.
Use: Expectorant.

MYVEROL. (Eastman) Glyceryl monostearate.

N

NA-ANA-TAL. (Churchill) Phenobarbital 0.25 gr, phenacetin 2 gr, aspirin 3 gr, nicotinic acid 50 mg/Tab. Bot. 100s, Liq. Bot. 16 oz.
Use: Sedative/hypnotic, analgesic.

•**NABAZENIL.** USAN.
Use: Anticonvulsant.

•**NABITAN HYDROCHLORIDE.** USAN.
Use: Analgesic.

•**NABOCTATE HYDROCHLORIDE.** USAN.
Use: Antiglaucoma agent.

•**NABUMETONE.** USAN.
Use: Anti-inflammatory.
See: Relafen (Beecham Labs.).

N-ACETYL-p-AMINOPHENOL. Acetaminophen, U.S.P. XXIII.

N^1-ACETYLSULFANILAMIDE.
See: ACETYLSULFANILAMIDE

NACREM. (Jenkins) Ammonium Cl 1.5%, menthol, methyl salicylate, camphor, eucalyptus oil. Tube 0.25 oz.
Use: Sinus congestion, hay fever.

•**NADIDE.** USAN. 3-Carbamoyl-1-β-D-ribofuranosylpyridinium hydroxide. Nicotinamide adenine dinucleotide. 1-(3-Carbamoylpyridinio)-βD-ribofuranoside 5-(adenosine-5'-pyrophosphate). Ensopride. Codehydrogenase I.
Use: Treat alcoholism and drug addiction.

NADINOLA (DELUXE) FOR OILY SKIN. (Strickland) Hydroquinone 2%. Bot. 1.25 oz, 2.25 oz.
Use: Skin bleaching agent.

NADINOLA FOR DRY SKIN. (Strickland) Hydroquinone 2%. Bot. 1.25 oz, 2.25 oz.
Use: Skin bleaching agent.

NADINOLA (ULTRA) FOR NORMAL SKIN. (Strickland) Hydroquinone 2%. Bot. 1.25 oz, 3.75 oz, Tube 1.85 oz.
Use: Skin bleaching agent.

•**NADOLOL,** U.S.P. XXIII. Tab., U.S.P. XXIII.
Use: Antihypertensive and antianginal beta-blocker.
See: Corgard, Tab.

NADOLOL. (Various Mfr.) Tab.: **20 mg:** 100s, UD 100s. **40 mg, 80 mg:** 100s, 1000s, UD 100s. **120 mg:** 100s, 1000s. **160 mg:** 100s.
Use: Beta-adrenergic blocker.(Princeton).

•**NADOLOL AND BENDROFLUMETHIAZIDE,** U.S.P. XXIII. Tab.
Use: Antihypertensive and antianginal beta-blocker.

NAEPAINE HYDROCHLORIDE. 2-(Pentylamino)- ethanol-p-aminobenzoate HCl.
Use: Local anesthetic.

•**NAFAMOSTAT MESYLATE.** USAN.
Use: Anticoagulant.

•**NAFARELIN ACETATE.** USAN.
Use: Agonist, central precocious puberty [Orphan drug].
See: Synarel (Syntex).

NAFAZAIR. (Various Mfr.) Naphazoline HCl 0.1%. Soln. Bot. 15 ml.
Use: Ophthalmic vasoconstrictor.

NAFAZAIR A. (Bausch & Lomb) Naphazoline HCl 0.025%, pheniramine maleate 0.3%, benzalkonium chloride 0.01%, EDTA, boric acid, sodium borate. Bot. 15 ml.
Use: Ophthalmic decongestant combination.

NAFCIL. (Bristol) Nafcillin sodium pow. for inj. Sodium 2.9 mEq/Gm. Vial 500 mg, 1 Gm, 2 Gm; Bulk vial 10 Gm; Piggyback vial 1 Gm, 2 Gm.
Use: Anti-bacterial, penicillin.

•**NAFCILLIN, SODIUM,** U.S.P. XXIII. Cap., Inj., Oral Soln, Sterile, Tab., U.S.P. XXIII. 4-Thia-1-azabicyclo[3.2.0]-heptane-2-carboxylic acid, 6-[[(2-ethoxy-1-naphthalenyl)carbonyl]amino]-3,3-dimethyl-7-oxo-monosodium salt, monohydrate,[2S-[2α,5α,6β]]. Monosodium 6-(2-ethoxy-1-naphthamido)-3,3-dimethyl-7-oxo-4-thia-1-azabicyclo [3.2.0.] heptane-2-carboxylate monohydrate. Sodium 6-(2-ethoxy-1-naphthamido)-penicillanate.
Use: Antibiotic.
See: Nafcil, Inj. (Bristol).
Unipen, Vial, Cap., Pow., Tab. (Wyeth-Ayerst).

NA-FEEN. (Pacemaker) Fluoride 1 mg/Dose. Tab. Bot. 100s, 500s, 1000s; Liq. 2 oz.
Use: Dental caries preventative.

•**NAFENOPIN.** USAN. 2-Methyl-2-[p-(1,2,3,4-tetrahydro-1-naphthyl)phenoxy]propionic acid.
Use: Hypolipidemic.

•**NAFIMIDONE HYDROCHLORIDE.** USAN.
Use: Anticonvulsant.

•**NAFLOCORT.** USAN.
Use: Adrenocortical steroid.

•**NAFOMINE MALEATE.** USAN.
Use: Muscle relaxant.

•**NAFOXIDINE HYDROCHLORIDE.** USAN.
Use: Anti-estrogen.

•**NAFRONYL OXALATE.** USAN. 2-(Diethylamino)ethyl tetrahydro-α-(1-naph-

thyl-methyl)2-furanpropionate oxalate. Dusodril.
Use: Vasodilator.
NAFTALAN.
W/Ichthyol, calamine, amber petrolatum.
See: Nagtalan, Oint. (Paddock).
• **NAFTALOFOS.** USAN.
Use: Anthelmintic.
NAFTAZONE. B.A.N. 1,2-Naphthaquinone 2-semicarbazone.
Haemostop.
Use: Hemostatic.
NAFTIDROFURYL. B.A.N. 2-Diethylaminoethyl 2-(1-naphthylmethyl)-3-(tetrahydro-2-furyl)propionate. Praxilene [oxalate].
Use: Vasodilator.
• **NAFTIFINE HYDROCHLORIDE.** USAN.
Use: Antifungal.
See: Naftin, Cream (Herbert).
NAFTIN. (Herbert) Naftifine HCl 1%.
Cream. 2 Gm, 15 Gm, 30 Gm.
Use: Antifungal, external.
NAGANOL.
See: Suramin Sodium. Naphuride Sodium.
NAGEST. Times Tabs. (Leeds) Phenylpropanolamine HCl 40 mg, phenylephrine HCl 10 mg, phenyltoloxamine di hydrogen citrate 15 mg, chlorpheniramine maleate 5 mg/SA Tab. Bot. 50s, 100s.
Use: Decongestant, antihistamine.
NAILICURE. (Purepac) Denatonium benzoate in a clear nail polish base. Bot. 0.33 oz.
Use: Nail biting deterrent.
NAIL PLUS. (Faraday) Gelatin Cap. Bot. 100s, 200s.
• **NALBUPHINE HYDROCHLORIDE.** USAN. (−)-17-(cyclobutylmethyl)-4, 5a-epoxymorphinan-3, 6a, 14-triol, hydrochloride.
Use: Analgesic.
See: Nubain, Vial (DuPont).
NALDECON-CX ADULT LIQUID. (Apothecon) Phenylpropanolamine 12.5 mg, guaifenesin 200 mg, codeine phosphate 10 mg/10 ml. Alcohol free. Bot. 4 oz, pt.
Use: Decongestant, expectorant, antitussive.
NALDECON-DX ADULT LIQUID. (Apothecon) Phenylpropanolamine HCl 12.5 mg, guaifenesin 200 mg, dextromethorphan HBr 10 mg/10 ml, saccharin, sorbitol. Alcohol free. Bot. 4 oz, pt.
Use: Decongestant, expectorant, antitussive.

NALDECON-DX CHILDREN'S SYRUP. (Apothecon) Phenylpropanolamine HCl 6.25 mg, dextromethorphan HBr 5 mg, guaifenesin 100 mg/5 ml. Bot. 4 oz, 16 oz.
Use: Decongestant, antitussive, expectorant.
NALDECON-DX PEDIATRIC DROPS. (Apothecon) Phenylpropanolamine HCl 6.25 mg, guaifenesin 50 mg, dextromethorphan HBr 5 mg/ml, alcohol free, saccharin, sorbitol. Bot. 30 ml.
Use: Decongestant, expectorant, antitussive.
NALDECON-EX CHILDREN'S SYRUP. (Apothecon) Phenylpropanolamine HCl 6.25 mg, guaifenesin 100 mg/5 ml, saccharin, sorbitol. Bot. 118 ml, 480 ml.
Use: Decongestant, expectorant.
NALDECON-EX PEDIATRIC DROPS. (Apothecon) Phenylpropanolamine HCl 6.25 mg, guaifenesin 50 mg/ml. Bot. 30 ml. w/dropper.
Use: Decongestant, expectorant.
NALDECON PEDIATRIC DROPS. (Bristol) Chlorpheniramine maleate 0.5 mg, phenyltoloxamine citrate 2 mg, phenylpropanolamine HCl 5 mg, phenylephrine HCl 1.25 mg/ml. Bot. 30 ml.
Use: Antihistamine, decongestant.
NALDECON PEDIATRIC SYRUP. (Bristol) Chlorpheniramine maleate 0.5 mg, phenyltoloxamine citrate 2 mg, phenylpropanolamine HCl 5 mg, phenylephrine HCl 1.25 mg/5 ml, sorbitol. Bot. 16 oz.
Use: Antihistamine, decongestant.
NALDECON SENIOR DX. (Apothecon) Dextromethorphan HBr 10 mg guaifenesin 200 mg/5 ml, saccharin, sorbitol, alcohol free. Liq. Bot. 118 ml.
Use: Nonnarcotic antitussive, expectorant.
NALDECON SENIOR EX. (Apothecon) Guaifenesin 200 mg/5 ml, saccharin, sorbitol. Liq. Bot. 118 ml.
Use: Expectorant.
NALDECON SYRUP. (Bristol) Chlorpheniramine maleate 2.5 mg, phenyltoloxamine citrate 7.5 mg, phenylpropanolamine HCl 20 mg, phenylephrine HCl 5 mg/5 ml, sorbitol. Bot. pt.
Use: Antihistamine, decongestant.
NALDECON TABLETS. (Bristol) Phenylephrine HCl 10 mg, phenylpropanolamine HCl 40 mg, phenyltoloxamine citrate 15 mg, chlorpheniramine maleate 5 mg/SR Tab. w/half each ingredient in inner and half in outer layer. Bot. 100s, 500s.
Use: Decongestant, antihistamine.

NALDEGESIC TABLETS. (Bristol) Pseudoephedrine HCl 15 mg, acetaminophen 325 mg/Tab. Bot. 100s.
Use: Decongestant, analgesic.
NALDELATE DX ADULT LIQUID. (Barre-National) Phenylpropanolamine HCl 12.5 mg, dextromethorphan HBr 10 mg, guaifenesin 200 mg, Bot. 120 ml or 480ml.
Use: Decongestant, antitussive, expectorant.
NALDELATE PEDIATRIC SYRUP. (Various Mfr.) Phenylpropanolamine 5 mg, phenylephrine 1.25 mg, chlorpheniramine maleate 0.5 mg, phenyltoloxamine citrate 2 mg/5 ml. Bot. 120 ml, pt, gal.
Use: Decongestant, antihistamine.
NALDELATE SYRUP. (Various Mfr.) Phenylpropanolamine HCl 20 mg, phenylephrine HCl 5 mg, chlorpheniramine maleate 2.5 mg, phenyltoloxamine citrate 7.5 mg/5 ml, sorbitol. Syr. Bot. pt.
Use: Decongestant, antihistamine.
NALFON. (Dista) Fenoprofen calcium.
Cap.: 200 mg. Rx Pak 100s. **300 mg.** Rx Pak 100s, Bot. 500s.
Use: Nonsteroidal anti-inflammatory drug; analgesic.
NALGEST. (Major) Phenylpropanolamine HCl 40 mg, phenylephrine HCl 10 mg, chlorpheniramine maleate 5 mg, phenyltoloxamine citrate 15 mg/Tab. Bot. 100s, 250s, 1000s.
Use: Decongestant, antihistamine.
NALGEST PEDIATRIC. (Major) Phenypropanolamine HCl 5 mg, phenylephrine HCl 1.25 mg, chlorpheniramine maleate 0.5 mg, phenyltoloxamine citrate 2 mg, sorbitol/Drop. Bot. 30 ml.
Use: Decongestant, antihistamine.
• **NALIDIXATE SODIUM.** USAN. Sodium 1-ethyl-1,4-dihydro-7-methyl-4-oxo-1,8-naphthyridine-3-carboxylate monohydrate. Under study.
Use: Antibacterial.
• **NALIDIXIC ACID,** U.S.P. XXIII. Oral Susp., Tab., U.S.P. XXIII. 1-Ethyl-7-methyl-1,8-naphthyridin-4-one-3-carboxylic acid, 1-Ethyl-1,4-dihydro-7-methyl-4-oxo-1,8-naphthyridine-3-carboxylic Acid.
Use: Antibacterial.
See: NegGram, Capl., Susp. (Sanofi Winthrop).
NALLPEN. (Beecham Labs) Nafcillin sodium monohydrate 500 mg, 1 Gm or 2 Gm/Vial. Inj. Piggyback 1 Gm, 2 Gm, Bulk 10 Gm.

Use: Antibacterial, penicillin.
• **NALMETRENE.** USAN.
Use: Antagonist to narcotics.
NALORPHINE. B.A.N. N-Allylnormorphine. Lethidrone [hydrobromide]
Use: Narcotic analgesic.
NALOXONE. B.A.N. (–)-17-Allyl-4,5α-epoxy-3,14-dihydroxymorphinan-6-one.
Use: Narcotic antagonist.
See: Narcan (DuPont).
• **NALOXONE HYDROCHLORIDE,** U.S.P. XXIII. Inj. U.S.P. XXIII. Morphinan-6-one, 4,5-epoxy-3,14-dihy- droxy-17-(2-propenyl)-,hydrochloride.
Use: Narcotic antagonist.
See: Narcan, Amp. (DuPont).
NALSA SPRAY. (Jenkins) Methapyrilene HCl 0.2%, naphazoline HCl 0.05%, cetylpyridinium Cl 0.02%, thimerosal 0.005%. Spray Bot. 20 ml.
Use: Antihistamine, decongestant.
NALSPAN. (PBI) Phenylpropanolamine HCl 20 mg, phenylephrine HCl 5 mg, chlorpheniramine maleate 2.5 mg, phenyltoloxamine citrate 7.5 mg/ml, alcohol free. Syr. Bot. pt.
Use: Decongestant, antihistamine.
• **NALTREXONE.** USAN.
Use: Antagonist to narcotics. [Orphan drug]
See: Trexal, Tab. (DuPont).
NAMAZENE. Phenothiazine.
NAMOL XENYRATE. 2-(4-Biphenylyl) butyric acid, compound with 2-dimethylamino- ethanol.
See: Namoxyrate.
• **NAMOXYRATE.** USAN. 2-[4-Biphenylyl]butyric acid cpd. w/2-dimethylaminoethanol. Namol Xenyrateprevious name.
Use: Analgesic.
See: Namol Xenyrate (Warner-Chilcott).
NAMURON.
See: Cyclobarbital Calcium (Various Mfr.).
NANDROBOLIC L.A. (Forest) Nandrolone decanoate 100 mg/ml. Vial 2 ml, Box 5s.
Use: Anabolic steroid.
NANDROLONE. B.A.N. 17β-Hydroxyestr-4-en-3-one. 17β-Hydroxy-19-norandrost-4-en-3-one. Nortesterone (I.N.N.).
Use: Anabolic steroid.
• **NANDROLONE CYCLOTATE.** USAN.
Use: Anabolic.
• **NANDROLONE DECANOATE,** U.S.P. XXIII. Inj., U.S.P. XXIII. 17β-Hydroxyestr-4-en-3-one-decanoate.

Use: Androgen.
See: Anabolin LA-100, Vial (Alto).
Androlone-D, Inj. (Keene).
Androlone-D 50, Inj. (Keene).
Deca-Durabolin, Amp., Vial (Organon).
Hybolin Decanoate, Inj. (Hyrex).
• **NANDROLONE PHENPROPIONATE,**
U.S.P. XXI. Inj. U.S.P. XXI. 19-nor-17-
beta-Hydroxy-3-ketoandrost-4-ene-17-
phenylpropionate. Norandrostenolone
phenylpropionate. 17β-Hydroxyestr-4-
en-3-one Hydrocinnamate.
Use: Androgen.
See: Anabolin IM, Vial (Alto).
Androlone, Inj. (Keene).
Androlone 50, Inj. (Keene).
Durabolin Inj. (Organon).
Hybolin Improved, Vial (Hyrex).
Nandrolin, Inj. (Solvay).
• **NANTRADOL HCL.** USAN.
Use: Analgesic.
NAOTIN. (Drug Products) Sodium nicoti-
nate. Amp. (equivalent to 10 mg nicotinic
acid/ml) 10 ml, Box 25s, 100s.
Use: Vitamin B$_3$ supplement.
• **NAPACTADINE HYDROCHLORIDE.**
USAN.
Use: Antidepressant.
• **NAPAMEZOLE HYDROCHLORIDE.**
USAN.
Use: Antidepressant.
NAPAMIDE CAPS. (Major) Disopyramide
phosphate 100 mg or 150 mg/Cap. Bot.
100s, 500s, UD 100s.
Use: Antiarrhythmic.
NAPHAZOLE-A. (Major) Naphazoline
HCl 0.025%, pheniramine maleate
0.3%, benzalkonium chloride 0.01%,
EDTA. Bot. 15 ml.
Use: Ophthalmic decongestant combi-
nation.
• **NAPHAZOLINE HYDROCHLORIDE,**
U.S.P. XXIII. Nasal Soln., Ophthalmic
Soln., U.S.P. XXIII. IH-Imidazole, 4,5-di-
hydro-2-(1-naphthalenylmethyl)-,mono-
hydrochloride, 2-(1-Naphthylmethyl)-2-
imidazoline HCl. (Various Mfr.) 0.1%
Soln. Bot. 15 ml.
Use: Adrenergic.
See: AK-Con, Soln., (Akorn).
Albalon, Soln., (Allergan America).
Allerest Eye Drops, Soln. (Pharma-
craft).
Comfort Eye Drops, Soln., (Pilkington
Barnes Hind).
Clear Eyes, Drops (Abbott).
Degest 2, Soln., (Pilkington Barnes
Hind).
Estivin II, Soln. (Alcon).
Maximum Strength Allergy Drops

(Bausch & Lomb).
Muro's Opcon, Soln. (Bausch &
Lomb).
Nafazair, Soln. (Bausch & Lomb.
Naphcon, Drops (Alcon).
Privine HCl, Soln., Spray (Ciba).
VasoClear, Soln., (Iolab).
Vasocon Regular, Liq. (Iolab).
W/Antazoline phosphate, boric acid,
phenylmercuric acetate, sodium Cl, sodi-
um carbonate anhydrous.
See: Antazoline-V, Soln. (Rugby).
Vasocon-A Ophthalmic, Soln. (Iolab).
W/Antazoline phosphate, polyvinyl alco-
hol.
See: Albalon-A Liquifilm, Ophth. (Aller-
gan).
W/Methapyrilene HCl, cetylpyridinum Cl,
thimerosal.
See: Vapocyn II Nasal Spray (Solvay).
W/Pheniramine maleate.
See: AK-Con-A, Soln., (Akorn).
Nafazair A, Soln., (Bausch & Lomb).
Naphazole-A, Soln., (Major).
Naphcon A, Liq. (Alcon).
Naphoptic-A, Soln. (Optopics).
W/PEG 300, benzalkonium Cl
See: Allergy Drops (Bausch & Lomb).
W/Phenylephrine HCl, pyrilamine maleate,
phenylpropanolamine HCl.
See: 4-Way Nasal Spray (Bristol-My-
ers).
W/Polyvinyl alcohol.
See: Albalon, Ophth. Soln. (Allergan).
Albalon Liquifilm, Ophth. Soln. (Aller-
gan).
**NAPHAZOLINE HCl & ANTAZOLINE
PHOSPHATE.** (Various Mfr.) Naphazo-
line HCl 0.05%, antazoline phosphate
0.5%. Soln. 5 ml, 15 ml.
Use: Ophthalmic decongestant, antihis-
tamine.
**NAPHAZOLINE HCl & PHENIRAMINE
MALEATE.** (Various Mfr.) Naphazoline
HCl 0.025%, pheniramine maleate
0.3%. Soln. Bot. 15 ml.
Use: Ophthalmic decongestant, antihis-
tamine.
NAPHAZOLINE PLUS. (Parmed) Napha-
zoline HCl 0.025%, pheniramine
maleate 0.3%, benzalkonium chloride
0.01%, EDTA. Bot. 15 ml.
Use: Ophthalmic decongestant combination.
NAPHCON. (Alcon) Naphazoline HCl
0.012%, benzalkonium Cl 0.01%. Drop-
Tainer Bot. 15 ml.
Use: Ophthalmic vasoconstrictor/mydri-
atic.

NAPHCON A. (Alcon) Naphazoline HCl 0.025%, pheniramine maleate 0.3%. Bot. 15 ml.
Use: Ophthalmic decongestant combination.

NAPHCON FORTE. (Alcon) Naphazoline HCl 0.1%, benzalkonium Cl 0.01%, disodium edetate/ml. Drop-Tainer Bot. 15 ml.
Use: Ophthalmic vasoconstrictor/mydriatic.

NAPHOLINE. (Horizon) Naphazoline HCl 0.1%. Soln. Bot. 15 ml.
Use: Ophthalmic vasoconstrictor/mydriatic.

NAPHOPTIC-A. (Optopics) Naphazoline HCl 0.025%, pheniramine maleate 0.3%, benzalkonium chloride, boric acid, EDTA, sodium borate. Bot. 15 ml.
Use: Ophthalmic decongestant combination.

NAPHTHYL-b SALICYLATE. Betol, Naphthosalol, Salinaphthol.
Use: G.I. & G.U., antiseptic.

NAPHURIDE SODIUM. Suramin Sodium.

NAPROSYN. (Syntex) Naproxen. **Oral susp.:** 125 mg/5 ml, sorbitol. Bot. pt. **250 mg/Tab.:** Bot. 100s, 500s, UD 100s; **375 mg/Tab.:** Bot. 100s, 500s, UD 100s; **500 mg/Tab.:** Bot. 100s, 500s, UD 100s.
Use: Nonsteroidal anti-inflammatory drug; analgesic.

NAPROXEN, U.S.P. XXIII. Tab., U.S.P. XXIII. (+)-6- Methoxy-αmethyl-2-naphthaleneacetic acid. (+)-2-(6 Methoxy-2-naphthyl)propionic acid. (Various Mfr.) **250 mg, 375 mg, 500 mg.** Bot. 100s, 500s, 1000s, UD 100s.
Use: Anti-inflammatory, analgesic, antipyretic.
See: Naprosyn, Susp., Tab. (Syntex).

NAPROXEN. (Roxane) 125 mg/5ml, sorbitol, sucrose, pineapple-orange flavor. Oral Susp. 500 ml, UD 15 ml and 20 ml.
Use: Anti-inflammatory, analgesic, antipyretic.

• **NAPROXEN SODIUM,** U.S.P. XXIII. Tab., U.S.P. XXIII. (Various Mfr.) 250 mg or 500 mg. Tab. Bot. 100s, 500s.
Use: Anti-inflammatory, analgesic, antipyretic.
See: Aleve, Tab. (Procter & Gamble). Anaprox, Tab. (Syntex). Anaprox DS, Tab. (Syntex).

• **NAPROXOL.** USAN. (–)-6-Methoxy-β-methyl-2-naphthaleneethanol.
Use: Anti-inflammatory; analgesic; antipyretic.

NAQUA. (Schering) Trichlormethiazide 2 mg or 4 mg/Tab. Bot. 100s, 1000s.

Use: Diuretic.
W/Reserpine.
See: Naquival, Tab. (Schering).

• **NARANOL HCl.** USAN. 8,9,10,11,11α,-12-Hexahydro-8,10-dimethyl-7 αH-naphtho[1',2:5,-6]pyrano-[3,2-c]pyridin-7-α-ol HCl.
Use: Tranquilizer.

• **NARASIN.** USAN.
Use: Growth stimulant.

• **NARATRIPTAN HYDROCHLORIDE.** USAN.
Use: Migraine

NARCAN. (DuPont) Naloxone HCl. **0.02 mg/ml:** Amp. 2 ml. **0.4 mg/ml:** Amp. 1 ml, Box 10s. Prefilled syringe 1 ml, Tray 10s; Multiple dose vials 10 ml, Box 1s. **1 mg/ml:** Amp. 2 ml, Box 10s; Multiple dose vial 10 ml, Box 1s.
Use: Narcotic antagonist.

NARDIL. (Parke-Davis) Phenelzine sulfate 15 mg/Tab. Bot. 100s.
Use: Antidepressant.

NASABID. (Abana) Pseudoephedrine HCl 90 mg, guaifenesin 250 mg. Cap. Bot. 100s.
Use: Decongestant, expectorant.

NASACORT. (Rhone-Poulenc Rorer) Each actuation: Triamcinolone acetonide 55 mcg. Cannister 15 mg w/nasal adapter.
Use: Intranasal steroid.

NASADENT. (Scherer) Sodium metaphosphate, glycerin, distilled water, dicalcium phosphate dihydrate, sodium carboxymethylcellulose, oil of spearmint, sodium benzoate, saccharin.
Use: Ingestible dentifrice.

NASAHIST B INJECTABLE. (Keene) Brompheniramine maleate 10 ml/Vial. For IM, IV and SC administration.
Use: Antihistamine.

NASAHIST CAPSULES. (Keene) Phenylpropanolamine HCl 40 mg, phenylephrine HCl 10 mg, chlorpheniramine maleate 12 mg/Cap. Bot. 100s.
Use: Decongestant, antihistamine.

NaSal SALINE NASAL. (Sanofi Winthrop.) Sodium Cl 0.65%. Drops, Spray. Bot. 15 ml.
Use: Nasal moisturizer.

NASALCROM NASAL SOLUTION. (Fisons) Cromolyn sodium 40 mg/ml, benzalkonium Cl 0.01%, EDTA 0.01%. Metered dose spray. Delivers 5.2 mg/spray. Complete pkg. 13 ml. Refill 13 ml.
Use: Nasal antiallergic.

NASALIDE. (Syntex) Flunisolide 0.025% soln. Pump. Bot. 25 ml.

Use: Intranasal steroid.
NASAL SALINE. (Sanofi Winthrop Products) Nasal spray and drops. Sodium Cl 0.65% buffered w/phosphates, preservatives. Bot. 15 ml. Spray Bot. 15 ml.
Use: Nasal moisturizer.
NASATAB LA. (Medi-Plex) Guaifenesin 400 mg, pseudoephedrine HCl 120 mg LA Tab. Bot. 30s, 100s.
Use: Expectorant, decongestant.
NASOPHEN. (Premo) Phenylephrine HCl 0.25% or 1%. Bot. pt.
Use: Decongestant.
NATABEC. (Parke-Davis) Vitamins A 4000 IU, D 400 IU, B_1 3 mg, B_2 2 mg, B_6 3 mg, C 50 mg, B_{12} 5 mcg, B_3 10 mg, elemental calcium 240 mg, elemental iron 30 mg/Kapseal. Bot. 100s.
Use: Vitamin/mineral supplement.
NATABEC-F.A. (Parke-Davis) Same as Natabec, plus folic acid 0.1 mg/Kapseal, magnesium, bisulfites. Bot. 100s.
Use: Vitamin/mineral supplement.
NATABEC Rx.(Parke-Davis) Same as Natabec, plus folic acid 1 mg/Kapseal. Bot. 100s.
Use: Vitamin/mineral supplement.
NATABEC WITH FLUORIDE. (Parke-Davis) Same formula as Natabec, plus elemental fluoride 1 mg/Kapseal. Bot. 100s.
Use: Vitamin supplement, dental caries preventative.
NATACOMP-FA TABLETS. (Trimen) Calcium 250 mg, iron 60 mg, vitamins A 8000 IU, D 400 IU, E 30 mg, B_1 3 mg, B_2 3.4 mg, B_3 20 mg, B_5 10 mg, B_6 12 mg, B_{12} 12 mcg, C 120 mg, folic acid 1 mg, Cu, I, Mg, zinc 15 mg/Tab. Bot. 100s, 500s.
Use: Vitamin/mineral supplement.
NATACYN. (Alcon) Natamycin (5%) 50 mg/ml. Bot. 15 ml.
Use: Antifungal agent, ophthalmic.
NATAFORT FILMSEAL. (Parke-Davis) Vitamins A 6000 IU, D 400 IU, C 120 mg, B_1 3 mg, B_2 2 mg, B_6 15 mg, B_{12} 6 mcg, niacin 20 mg, folic acid 1 mg, E 30 IU, calcium 350 mg, magnesium 100 mg, zinc 25 mg, iodine 0.15 mg, iron 65 mg/Tab. Bot. 100s.
Use: Vitamin/mineral supplement.
NATALINS. (Mead Johnson Nutrition) Vitamins A 5000 IU, D 400 IU, E 30 IU, C 90 mg, B_1 1.7 mg, B_2 2 mg, B_6 4 mg, B_{12} 8 mcg, niacin 20 mg, folic acid 0.8 mg, iodine 150 mcg, calcium 200 mg, iron 45 mg, magnesium 100 mg/Tab. Bot. 100s, 1000s. Drum 36,000.
Use: Vitamin/mineral supplement.

NATALINS RX. (Mead Johnson Nutrition) Vitamins A 8000 IU, D 400 IU, E 30 IU, C 90 mg, B_1 2.55 mg, B_2 3 mg, B_6 10 mg, B_{12} 8 mcg, niacin 20 mg, folic acid 1 mg, pantothenic acid 15 mg, biotin 0.05 mg, calcium 200 mg, iron 60 mg, magnesium 100 mg, copper 2 mg, zinc 15 mg, iodine 150 mcg/Tab. Bot. 100s, 1000s.
Use: Vitamin/mineral supplement.
• **NATAMYCIN,** U.S.P. XXIII. Ophth. Susp., U.S.P. XXIII. An antibiotic produced by *Streptomyces natalensis.* Pimafucin.
Use: Antibiotic.
See: Natacyn, Susp. (Alcon).
NATA-SAN. (Sandia) Vitamins A 4000 IU, D 400 IU, B_1 5 mg, B_2 4 mg, B_6 10 mg, nicotinic acid 10 mg, C 100 mg, B_{12} activity 5 mcg, ferrous fumarate 200 mg (elemental iron 65 mg), calcium carbonate 500 mg (calcium 196 mg), copper (sulfate) 0.5 mg, magnesium (sulfate) 0.1 mg, manganese (sulfate) 0.1 mg, potassium (sulfate) 0.1 mg, zinc (sulfate) 0.5 mg/Tab. Bot. 100s, 1000s.
Use: Vitamin/mineral supplement.
NATA-SAN F.A. (Sandia) Vitamins A 4000 IU, D 400 IU, B_1 5 mg, B_2 4 mg, B_6 10 mg, nicotinic acid 10 mg, C 100 mg, B_{12} activity 5 mcg, folic acid 1 mg, iron 65 mg, calcium 200 mg, copper (sulfate) 0.5 mg, magnesium (sulfate) 0.1 mg, manganese (sulfate) 0.1 mg, potassium (sulfate) 0.1 mg, zinc (sulfate) 0.5 mg/Tab. Bot. 100s, 1000s.
Use: Vitamin/mineral supplement.
NATODINE. (Faraday) Iodine in organic form as found in kelp 1 mg/Tab. Bot. 100s, 250s.
NATRAPEL. (Tender) Citronella 10% in 15% Aloe Vera base.
Use: Insect repellent.
NATRICO. (Drug Products) Potassium nitrate 2 gr, sodium nitrite 1 gr, nitroglycerin 0.25 gr, crataegus oxycantha 0.25 gr/Pulvoid. Bot. 100s, 1000s.
Use: Antihypertensive.
NATURACIL. (Mead Johnson Nutrition) Psyllium seed husks 3.4 Gm, carbohydrate 9.6 Gm, sodium 11 mg, 54 cal./2 pieces. Carton 24s, 40s.
Use: Laxative.
NATUR-AID. (Scott/Cord) Lactose, pectin and Carob-lemon juice. Pow. 90%. Bot. 8 oz.
Use: Increase in normal intestinal flora.
NATURAL DIURETIC WATER TABLET. (Amlab) Buchu leaves 1 gr, uva ursi 1 gr, trilicum 1 gr, parsley 1 gr, juniper berries 1 gr, asparagus 1 gr, alfalfa powder 1 gr/Tab. Bot. 100s.

Use: Diuretic.

NATURAL LUNG SURFACTANT.
See: Survanta (Ross Laboratories).

NATURAL VEGETABLE POWDER. (Various Mfr.) Psyllium hydrophilic mucilloid 3.4 Gm, dextrose, sodium < 10 mg, 14 Cal/Dose. Pow. 210 Gm, 420 Gm, 630 Gm.
Use: Laxative.

NATURAL VITAMIN A IN OIL.
See: Oleovitamin A, U.S.P.

NATURALYTE. (UBI) Sodium 45 mEq, potassium 20 mEq, chloride 35 mEq, citrates 48 mEq, dextrose 25 g/L. Soln. Bot. 240 ml, 1 L.
Use: Minerals/electrolytes, oral.

NATURE'S AID LAXATIVE TABS. (Walgreen) Docusate sodium 100 mg, yellow phenolphthalein 65 mg/Tab. Bot. 60s.
Use: Laxative.

NATURE'S BOUNTY 1. (Nature's Bounty) Calcium 50 mg, iron 10 mg, vitamins A 10,000 IU, D 400 IU, E 30 mg, B_1 25 mg, B_2 25 mg, B_3 50 mg, B_5 50 mg, B_6 50 mg, B_{12} 50 mcg, C 250 mg, folic acid 0.4 mg, biotin 50 mcg, choline, inositol, PABA, P, I, Cr, Mg, Zn 15 mg, Mn, Se, Cu, K, Cl, Mo/TR Tab. Bot. 30, 60s.
Use: Vitamin/mineral supplement.

NATURE'S REMEDY TABLETS. (SK-Beecham) Aloe 100 mg, cascara sagrada 150 mg/FC Tab. Foil backed blister pkg. Box 12s, 30s, 60s.
Use: Laxative.

NATURE'S TEARS. (Rugby) Hydroxypropyl methylcellulose 2906 0.3%, dextran 70 0.1%, KCl, NaCl, EDTA. Soln. Bot. 15 ml.
Use: Artificial tears.

NATURETIN. (Princeton) Bendroflumethiazide. **5 mg/Tab.:** Bot. 100s, 1000s. **10 mg/Tab.:** Bot. 100s.
Use: Diuretic.

NATURIL. (Kenyon) Pow. uva ursi extract 0.5 gr, pow. buchu leaves extract 0.5 gr, pow. corn silk extract 0.5 gr, pow. juniper extract 0.25 gr, caffeine 0.25 gr/Tab. Bot. 100s, 1000s.

NATUR-LAX TABLETS. (Faraday) Rhubarb root, cape aloes, cascara sagrada extract, mandrake root, parsley, carrot. Protein coated tab. Bot. 100s.
Use: Laxative.

NAUS-A-TORIES. (Table Rock) Pyrilamine maleate 25 mg, secobarbital 30 mg/Supp. Box 12s.
Use: Antiemetic.

NAUS-A-WAY. (Hauck) Fructose, dextrose, orthophosphoric acid w/controlled hydrogen ion concentration. Soln. Bot.

473 ml.
Use: Antiemetic/antivertigo agent.

NAUSETROL. (Various Mfr.) Fructose, dextrose, orthophosphoric acid with controlled hydrogen ion concentration. Soln. Bot. 4 oz, pt, gal.
Use: Antiemetic/antivertigo agent.

NAVANE. (Hoerig) Thiothixene. **Cap.:** 1 mg, 2 mg, 5 mg, 10 mg or 20 mg. Bot. 100s, 1000s, UD 100s. **Liq.:** 5 mg/ml. Bot. 1 oz, 4 oz. **IM soln.:** 2 mg/ml. Vial 2 ml. Pkg. 10s.
Use: Antipsychotic agent.

NAVANE CONCENTRATE. (Roerig) Thiothixene HCl 5 mg/ml, alcohol 7%. Soln. Bot. 30 ml, 120 ml with dropper.
Use: Antipsychotic agent.

NAVANE INTRAMUSCULAR FOR INJECTION. (Roerig) Thiothixene HCl 5 mg/ml. Lyophilized for reconstitution with 2.2 ml sterile water. Vial 2 ml. Pkg. vial 10s.
Use: Antipsychotic agent.

NAVELBINE. (Burroughs Wellcome) Vinorelbine tartrate 30 mg/m². Inj. Vial.
Use: Antineoplastic.

NAVIDRIX (NAVIDREX, CYCLOPENTHIAZIDE). Cyclopenthiazide. 3-Cyclopentylmethyl derivative of hydrochlorothiazide.
Use: Diuretic.

NAZAFAIR. (Various Mfr.) Naphazoline HCl 0.1%. Soln. Bot. 15 ml.
Use: Ophthalmic vasoconstrictor/mydriatic.

N-CHLORO COMPOUND ANTISEPTICS.
See: Antiseptic, N-Chloro Compounds.

N D CLEAR. (Seatrace) Chlorpheniramine maleate 8 mg, pseudoephedrine HCl 120 mg/T.D. Cap. Bot. 100s, 1000s.
Use: Antihistamine, decongestant.

N-DIETHYL META-TOLUAMIDE.
W/Red Veterinary Petrolatum.
See: RV Pellent, Oint. (Elder).

N-DIETHYLVANILLAMIDE.
See: Ethamivan, Inj. (Various Mfr.)

ND-GESIC. (Hyrex) Acetaminophen 300 mg, pyrilamine maleate 12.5 mg, chlorpheniramine maleate 2 mg, phenylephrine HCl 5 mg/Tab. Bot. 100s, 1000s.
Use: Analgesic, antihistamine, decongestant.

nDNA. (Wampole-Zeus) Anti-native DNA test by IFA. Confirmatory test for active SLE. Test 48s.
Use: Diagnostic aid.

ND-STAT. (Hyrex) Brompheniramine maleate 10 mg/ml. Vial 10 ml.
Use: Antihistamine.

NEALBARBITONE. B.A.N. 5-Allyl-5-

neopentylbarbituric acid. Censedal; Nevental.
Use: Hypnotic; sedative.
• **NEBACUMAB.** USAN.
Use: Anti-endotoxin monoclonal antibody. [Orphan drug]
NEBCIN. (Lilly) Tobramycin sulfate. **Inj.:** 80 mg/2 ml. Vial 2 ml. **Pow. (after reconstitution):** 30 mg/ml or 40 mg/ml. Vial 1.2 Gm. **Pediatric Inj.:** 20 mg/2 ml. Vial 2 ml. **Hyporets:** 60 mg/1.5 ml or 80 mg/2 ml.
Use: Antibacterial, aminoglycoside.
• **NEBIVOLOL.** USAN.
Use: Antihypertensive (beta-blocker).
• **NEBRAMYCIN.** USAN. A complex of antibiotic substances produced by *Streptomyces tenebrarius.*
Use: Antibacterial.
NEBUPENT. (Lyphomed) Pentamidine isethionate 300 mg. Aerosol single dose vial.
Use: Anti-infective.
NEBU-PREL. (Mahon) Isoproterenol sulfate 0.4%, phenylephrine HCl 2%, propylene glycol 10%. Liq. Vial 10 ml.
Use: Bronchodilator.
NECHLORIN. (Interstate) Chlorpheniramine 5 mg, phenylpropanolamine 40 mg, phenylephrine 20 mg, phenyltoloxamine 15 mg/Tab. Bot. 100s.
Use: Antihistamine, decongestant.
• **NEDOCROMIL.** USAN.
Use: Antiallergic (prophylactic).
• **NEDOCROMIL CALCIUM.** USAN.
Use: Antiallergic (prophylactic).
See: Tilade.
• **NEDOCROMIL SODIUM.** USAN.
Use: Antiallergic (prophylactic).
See: Tilade, Aerosol (Fisons).
N.E.E.. (Lexis) Ethinyl estradiol 35 mcg, norethindrone 1 mg/Tab. 6 pcks. 21s, 28s.
Use: Oral contraceptive.
• **NEFAZODONE HYDROCHLORIDE.** USAN.
Use: Antidepressant.
See: Serzone.
• **NEFLUMOZIDE HYDROCHLORIDE.** USAN.
Use: Antipsychotic.
• **NEFOCON A.** USAN.
Use: Hydrophobic contact lens material.
• **NEFOPAM HCl.** USAN. 3,4,5,6-Tetrahydro-5-methyl-1-phenyl-1H-2,5-benzoxazocine HCl.
Use: Muscle relaxant.
NEGACIDE. (Sanofi Winthrop) Nalidixic acid.
Use: Urinary anti-infective.

NEGGRAM. (Winthrop-Breon) Nalidixic acid. **1 Gm/Capl.:** Bot. 100s, UD Pack 100s; **250 mg/Capl.:** Bot. 56s. **500 mg/Capl.:** Bot. 56s, 500s, 1000s, UD Pack 100s; Susp. **250 mg/5 ml:** Bot. pt.
Use: Urinary anti-infective.
• **NELEZAPRINE MALEATE.** USAN.
Use: Muscle relaxant.
NELOVA 0.5/35. (Warner-Chilcott) Ethinyl estradiol 35 mcg, norethindrone 0.5 mg/Tab. 6 Pcks. 21 day and 28 day w/ 7 inert tabs.
Use: Oral contraceptive.
NELOVA 1/35E. (Warner Chilcott) Norethindrone 1 mg, ethinyl estradiol 35 mcg/Tab. 21 day and 28 day (with 7 inert tabs.).
Use: Oral contraceptive.
NELOVA 1/50 M. (Warner-Chilcott) Norethindrone 1 mg, mestranol 50 mcg/Tab. 21 day and 28 day (with 7 inert tabs.).
Use: Oral contraceptive.
NELOVA 10/11. (Warner Chilcott) **Phase 1-** Norethindrone 0.5 mg, ethinyl estradiol 35 mcg/Tab., 10 tabs.; **Phase 2-** Norethindrone 1 mg, ethinyl estradiol 35 mcg/Tab., 11 tabs. 21 day and 28 day (with 7 inert tabs.).
Use: Oral contraceptive.
NELULEN. (Watson Labs) **1/35 E Tab.:** Ethynodiol diacetate 1 mg, ethinyl estradiol 35 mcg. Pcks 21s, 28s. **1/50 E Tab.:** Ethynodiol diacetate 1 mg, ethinyl estradiol 50 mcg. Pcks. 21s, 28s.
Use: Oral contraceptive.
NEMAZINE. 3-(p-Chlorophenyl)-4-imino-2-oxo-1- imidazolidine acetonitrile. Under study.
Use: Anti-inflammatory.
• **NEMAZOLINE HYDROCHLORIDE.** USAN.
Use: Nasal decongestant.
NEMBUTAL ELIXIR. (Abbott) Pentobarbital 18.2 mg/5 ml, alcohol 18%. Bot. pt, gal.
Use: Sedative/hypnotic.
NEMBUTAL SODIUM. (Abbott) Pentobarbital sodium. **Inj.:** 50 mg/ml. Amp 2 ml; Vial 20 ml, 50 ml. Box 5s. **Cap.:** 50 mg: Bot. 100s, 500s. Display pack 100s. **Supp.:** 30 mg, 120 mg or 200 mg. Box 12s.
Use: Sedative/hypnotic.
NEOARSPHENAMINE. Sodium 3,3'-diamino-4,4-dihy-droxyarsenobenzene-N-methanal sulfoxylate. (Neosalvarsan, Neoarsenobenzol).
NEO-BENZ-ALL. (Xttrium) Benzalkonium Cl 20.1%. Packet 25 ml 15s. To make

gal of 1:750 soln. Also Aqueous Neo-Benz-All 1:750 soln. Packet 20 ml, 50s.
Use: Antiseptic, germicidal.
NEO BESEROL. (Sanofi Winthrop) Aspirin, methocarbamol.
Use: Salicylate analgesic, skeletal muscle relaxant.
NEOCALAMINE. (Various Mfr.) Red ferric oxide 30 Gm, yellow ferric oxide 40 Gm, zinc oxide 930 Gm.
Use: Astringent, antiseptic.
NEO-CALGLUCON. (Sandoz) Glubionate calcium 1.8 Gm/5 ml. Syr. Bot. pt.
Use: Calcium supplement.
NEO-CASTADERM. (Lannett) Resorcin, boric acid, acetone, phenol, alcohol 9%. Liq. Bot. 1 oz, 4 oz, 16 oz.
Use: Antifungal, external.
NEO-CHOLEX. (Lafayette) Fat emulsion containing 40%/w/v pure vegetable oil. Bot. 60 ml.
Use: Produce maximum cholecystokinetic activity in roentgen study.
NEOCIDIN. (Major) Polymyxin B sulfate 10,000 units, neomycin sulfate 1.75 mg, gramicidin 0.025 mg/ml. Soln. Bot. 10 ml.
Use: Anti-infective, ophthalmic.
NEOCINCHOPHEN. B.A.N. Ethyl 6-methyl-2-phenylquinolin-4-carboxylate. Novatophan.
Use: Analgesic, antipyretic and in gout.
NEO-COBEFRIN. levo-Nordefrin. 1-2,4-dihydroxyphenyl-3-hydroxy-2-isopropylamine.
Use: Vasoconstrictor.
NEO-CORTEF CREAM. (Upjohn) Hydrocortisone acetate 10 mg (1%), neomycin sulfate 5 mg (0.5%), methylparaben 1 mg, butylparaben 4 mg, polysorbate 80, propylene glycol, cetyl palmitate, glyceryl monostearate, emulsifier/Gm. When necessary, pH adjusted with sulfuric acid. Tube 20 Gm.
Use: Corticosteroid, anti-infective, external.
NEO-CORTEF OINTMENT. (Upjohn) **0.5%:** Hydrocortisone acetate 5 mg, neomycin sulfate 5 mg, methylparaben 0.2 mg, butylparaben 1.8 mg in a bland base of white petrolatum, microcrystalline wax, mineral oil, cholesterol/Gm. Tube 20 Gm. **1%:** Hydrocortisone acetate 10 mg, neomycin sulfate 5 mg/Gm. Oint. Tube 5 Gm, 20 Gm.
Use: Corticosteroid, anti-infective.
NEO-CULTOL. (Fisons) Refined mineral oil jelly. Chocolate flavored. Bot. 6 oz.
Use: Laxative.
NEOCURB. (Pasadena Research)

Phendimetrazine tartrate 35 mg/Tab. Bot. 100s, 1000s.
Use: Anorexient.
NEOCYLATE. (Central) Potassium salicylate 280 mg, aminobenzoic acid 250 mg/Tab. Bot. 100s, 1000s.
Use: Salicylate analgesic.
NEOCYTEN. (Central) Orphenadrine citrate 30 mg/ml. Vial 10 ml.
Use: Skeletal muscle relaxant.
NEODECADRON OPHTHALMIC SOLUTION. (Merck & Co.) Dexamethasone sodium phosphate equivalent to 1 mg dexamethasone phosphate, neomycin sulfate equivalent to 3.5 mg neomycin base/ml, polysorbate 80, sodium bisulfite 0.1%, benzalkonium Cl 0.02%. Ocumeter ophthalmic dispenser 5 ml.
Use: Corticosteroid, anti-infective.
NEODECADRON OPHTHALMIC OINTMENT. (Merck & Co.) Dexamethasone sodium phosphate equivalent to 0.5 mg dexamethasone phosphate, neomycin sulfate equivalent to 3.5 mg neomycin base/Gm, white petrolatum, mineral oil. Tube 3.5 Gm.
Use: Corticosteroid, anti-infective.
NEODECADRON TOPICAL CREAM. (Merck & Co.) Dexamethasone sodium phosphate equivalent to 1 mg dexamethasone phosphate, neomycin sulfate equivalent to 3.5 mg neomycin base/Gm, stearyl alcohol, cetyl alcohol, mineral oil, polyoxyl 40 stearate, sorbitol soln, methyl polysilicone emulsion, creatinine, disodium edetate, sodium citrate, sodium hydroxide to adjust pH, purified water, methylparaben 0.15%, sodium bisulfite 0.25%, sorbic acid 0.1%. Tube 15 Gm, 30 Gm.
Use: Corticosteroid, anti-infective.
NEODECYLLIN. (Penick) Neomycin undecylenate.
Use: Anti-infective.
NEO-DEXAIR. (Bausch & Lomb) Dexamethasone sodium phosphate 0.1%, neomycin sulfate 0.35%, polysorbate 80, EDTA, benzalkonium Cl 0.02%, sodium bisulfite 0.1%. Soln. Bot. 5 ml.
Use: Corticosteroid, anti-infective, ophthalmic.
NEO-DEXAMETH. (Major) Dexamethasone sodium phosphate 0.1%, neomycin sulfate 0.35%, benzalkonium Cl 0.01%, EDTA, polysorbate 80, sodium bisulfite. Soln. Bot. 5 ml.
Use: Corticosteroid, anti-infective, ophthalmic.
NEODRENAL.
See: Isoproterenol.

NEO-DURABOLIC. (Hauck) Nandrolone decanoate injection. **50 mg/ml** or **100 mg/ml:** Vial 2 ml. **200 mg/ml:** Vial 1 ml.
Use: Anabolic steroid.

NEO-FRADIN. (Pharma-Tek) Neomycin sulfate 125 mg/5 ml. Soln. Bot. 480 ml.
Use: Amebicide.

NEO FRANOL. (Sanofi Winthrop) Theophylline monohydrate.
Use: Bronchodilator.

NEOGESIC TABLETS. (Vale) Aspirin 194.4 mg, acetaminophen 129.6 mg, caffeine 32.4 mg/Tab. Bot. 1000s.
Use: Analgesic combination.

NEOLOID. (Lederle) Castor oil 36.4% (emulsified) (w/w). Bot. 4 oz.
Use: Laxative.

NEOMAC OINTMENT. (NMC Labs) Triple antibiotic. Oint. Tube 0.5 oz, 1 oz.
Use: Anti-infective, external.

NEO-MIST NASAL SPRAY. (A.P.C.) Phenylephrine HCl 0.5%, cetalkonium Cl 0.02%. Spray Bot. 20 ml.
Use: Decongestant, antiseptic.

NEO-MIST PEDIATRIC 0.25% NASAL SPRAY. (A.P.C.) Phenylephrine HCl 0.25%, cetalkonium Cl 0.02%. Squeeze Bot. 20 ml.
Use: Decongestant, antiseptic.

NEOMIXIN. (Hauck) Bacitracin zinc 400 units, neomycin sulfate 3.5 mg, polymyxin B sulfate 5000 units in petrolatum base/Gm. Tube 15 Gm.
Use: Anti-infective, external.

NEOMYCIN. B.A.N. An antibiotic produced by a strain of *Streptomyces fradiae*. Expedil, Mycifradin, Myciguent, Neomin, Nivemycin [sulfate].
Use: Anti-infective.

NEOMYCIN BASE.
Use: Antibiotic.
W/Combinations.
See: Maxitrol, Oint., Susp. (Alcon).
　　Neo-Cort-Dome, Cream, Lot. (Miles Pharm).
　　Neotal, Oint. (Hauck).

NEOMYCIN-HYDROCORTISONE CREAM. (Day-Baldwin) Neomycin 5 mg/Gm, hydrocortisone 0.5% or 1% Tube 0.5 oz, 1 oz.
Use: Anti-infective, corticosteroid.

NEOMYCIN-HYDROCORTISONE OINTMENT. (Day-Baldwin) Neomycin 5 mg/Gm, hydrocortisone 0.5%. Tube 1 oz; w/hydrocortisone 1%: 20 Gm, 1 oz.
Use: Anti-infective, corticosteroid.

• **NEOMYCIN PALMITATE.** USAN.
Use: Antibiotic.
See: Biozyme, Oint. (Armour).

• **NEOMYCIN AND POLYMYXIN B SUL-FATES, BACITRACIN, AND HYDRO-CORTISONE ACETATE OINTMENT,** U.S.P. XXIII.
Use: Antibiotic, antifungal.

• **NEOMYCIN AND POLYMYXIN B SUL-FATES, BACITRACIN, AND HYDRO-CORTISONE ACETATE OPHTHALMIC OINTMENT,** U.S.P. XXIII.
Use: Antibiotic, antifungal.

• **NEOMYCIN AND POLYMYXIN B SUL-FATES AND BACITRACIN OINTMENT,** U.S.P. XXIII.
Use: Antibiotic.

• **NEOMYCIN AND POLYMYXIN B SUL-FATES AND BACITRACIN OPH-THALMIC OINTMENT,** U.S.P. XXIII.
Use: Antibiotic.

• **NEOMYCIN AND POLYMYXIN B SUL-FATES, BACITRACIN ZINC, AND HY-DROCORTISONE ACETATE OPH-THALMIC OINTMENT,** U.S.P. XXIII.
Use: Antibiotic, anti-inflammatory.

• **NEOMYCIN AND POLYMYXIN B SUL-FATES, BACITRACIN ZINC, AND HY-DROCORTISONE OINTMENT,** U.S.P. XXIII.
Use: Antibiotic, anti-inflammatory.

• **NEOMYCIN AND POLYMYXIN B SUL-FATES, BACITRACIN ZINC, AND HY-DROCORTISONE OPHTHALMIC OINTMENT,** U.S.P. XXIII.
Use: Antibiotic, anti-inflammatory.

• **NEOMYCIN AND POLYMYXIN B SUL-FATES, BACITRACIN ZINC, AND LIDO-CAINE OINTMENT,** U.S.P. XXIII.
Use: Antibiotic, anesthetic.
See: Lanabiotic, Oint. (Combe).

• **NEOMYCIN AND POLYMYXIN B SUL-FATES AND BACITRACIN ZINC OINT-MENT,** U.S.P. XXIII.
Use: Local anti-infective.

• **NEOMYCIN AND POLYMYXIN B SUL-FATES AND BACITRACIN ZINC OPH-THALMIC OINTMENT,** U.S.P. XXIII.
Use: Ophthalmic antibiotic.

NEOMYCIN AND POLYMYXIN B SUL-FATES AND BACITRACIN ZINC TOPI-CAL AEROSOL, U.S.P. XXI.
Use: Antibiotic.

NEOMYCIN AND POLYMYXIN B SUL-FATES AND BACITRACIN ZINC TOPI-CAL POWDER, U.S.P. XXI.
Use: Antibiotic.

• **NEOMYCIN AND POLYMYXIN B SUL-FATES CREAM,** U.S.P. XXIII.
Use: Antibiotic.

• **NEOMYCIN AND POLYMYXIN B SUL-FATES AND DEXAMETHASONE OPH-THALMIC OINTMENT,** U.S.P. XXIII.
(Various Mfr.) Tube 3.5 g.

Use: Antibiotic, anti-inflammatory.
• **NEOMYCIN AND POLYMYXIN B SUL-FATES AND DEXAMETHASONE OPH-THALMIC SUSPENSION,** U.S.P. XXIII. (Various Mfr.) 5 ml, 10 ml.
Use: Antibiotic, anti-inflammatory.
• **NEOMYCIN AND POLYMYXIN B SUL-FATES AND GRAMICIDIN CREAM,** U.S.P. XXIII.
Use: Antibiotic.
• **NEOMYCIN AND POLYMYXIN B SUL-FATES, GRAMICIDIN, AND HYDRO-CORTISONE ACETATE CREAM,** U.S.P. XXIII.
Use: Antibiotic, anti-inflammatory.
• **NEOMYCIN AND POLYMYXIN B SUL-FATES AND GRAMICIDIN OPH-THALMIC SOLUTION,** U.S.P. XXIII.
Use: Antibiotic.
• **NEOMYCIN AND POLYMYXIN B SUL-FATES AND HYDROCORTISONE AC-ETATE CREAM,** U.S.P. XXIII.
Use: Antibiotic, anti-inflammatory.
• **NEOMYCIN AND POLYMYXIN B SUL-FATES AND HYDROCORTISONE AC-ETATE OPHTHALMIC SUSPENSION,** U.S.P. XXIII.
Use: Antibiotic, anti-inflammatory.
• **NEOMYCIN AND POLYMYXIN B SUL-FATES AND HYDROCORTISONE OPHTHALMIC SUSPENSION,** U.S.P. XXIII. (Various Mfr.) 7.5 ml.
Use: Antibiotic, anti-inflammatory.
• **NEOMYCIN AND POLYMYXIN B SUL-FATES AND HYDROCORTISONE OTIC SOLUTION,** U.S.P. XXIII.
Use: Antibiotic, anti-inflammatory.
• **NEOMYCIN AND POLYMYXIN B SUL-FATES AND HYDROCORTISONE OTIC SUSPENSION,** U.S.P. XXIII.
Use: Antibiotic, anti-inflammatory.
• **NEOMYCIN AND POLYMYXIN B SUL-FATES OPHTHALMIC OINTMENT,** U.S.P. XXIII.
Use: Antibiotic.
• **NEOMYCIN AND POLYMYXIN B SUL-FATES AND PREDNISOLONE AC-ETATE OPHTHALMIC SUSPENSION,** U.S.P. XXIII.
Use: Antibiotic, anti-inflammatory.
• **NEOMYCIN AND POLYMYXIN B SUL-FATES SOLUTION FOR IRRIGATION,** U.S.P. XXIII.
Use: Irrigating solution, topical antibacterial.
• **NEOMYCIN AND POLYMYXIN B SUL-FATES OPHTHALMIC SOLUTION,** U.S.P. XXIII.
Use: Ophthalmic antibiotic.
• **NEOMYCIN SULFATE,** U.S.P. XXIII.

Cream, Oint., Ophth. Oint., Oral Soln., Sterile, Tab., U.S.P. XXIII. An antibiotic from Streptomyces fradiae: (Upjohn) Pow. micronized for compounding. Bot. 100 Gm.
Use: Antibacterial.
See: Mycifradin Sulfate, Tab., Soln. (Upjohn).
Myciguent, Oint., Ophth. Oint., Cream (Upjohn).
Neo-fradin, Soln. (Pharma-Tek).
Neo-Tabs (Pharma-Tek).
W/Combinations.
See: AK-Spore, Preps. (Akorn).
Bacitracin Neomycin, Oint. (Various Mfr.).
Baximin, Oint. (Quality Generics).
Biotres HC, Oint. (Central).
B.N.P., Ophthalmic Oint. (Solvay).
B.P.N., Oint. (Norwich).
Bro-Parin, Otic Susp. (Riker).
Coracin, Oint. (Hauck).
Cordran-N, Oint., Lot. (Dista).
Cor-Oticin, Liq. (Maurry).
Cortisporin, Preps. (Burroughs Wellcome).
Epimycin A, Oint. (Delta).
Hi-Cort N, Cream (Blaine).
Hysoquen Oint. (Solvay).
Maxitrol, Ophth., Oint., Susp. (Alcon).
Mity-Mycin, Oint. (Solvay).
Mycifradin Sulfate Sterile, Vial (Upjohn).
Mycitracin, Oint., Ophth. Oint. (Upjohn).
My-Cort, Oint., Cream, Soln. (Scrip).
Necort, Oint. (A.V.P.).
Neo-Cort Dome, Otic Soln. (Miles Pharm).
Neo-Cortef, Preps. (Upjohn).
Neo-Decadron, Ophth., Topical (Merck & Co.).
Neo-Delta-Cortef, Preps. (Upjohn).
Neo-Hydeltrasol, Oint., Soln. (Merck & Co.).
Neo-Hytone, Cream (Dermik).
Neo-Medrol, Preps. (Upjohn).
Neo-Nysta-Cort, Oint. (Miles Pharm).
Neo-Oxylone, Oint. (Upjohn).
Neosone, Ophth. Oint. (Upjohn).
Neosporin, Preps. (Burroughs Wellcome).
Neotal, Ophth. Oint. (Hauck).
Neo-Thrycex, Oint. (Commerce).
Ocutricin, Preps. (Bausch & Lomb).
Otobione, Soln. (Schering).
Otoreid-HC, Liq. (Solvay).
P.B.N., Oint. (Jenkins).
Spectrocin, Oint. (Squibb Mark).
Statrol Sterile, Ophthalmic Oint. (Al-

con).
Tigo, Oint. (Burlington).
Tri-Bow, Oint. (Bowman).
Tricidin, Oint. (Amlab).
Trimixin, Oint. (Hance).
Triple Antibiotic, Oint. (Kenyon).
• **NEOMYCIN SULFATE AND BACI-
TRACIN OINTMENT,** U.S.P. XXIII.
Use: Antibiotic.
• **NEOMYCIN SULFATE AND BACI-
TRACIN ZINC OINTMENT,** U.S.P.
XXIII.
Use: Antibiotic.
• **NEOMYCIN SULFATE AND DEXAM-
ETHASONE SODIUM PHOSPHATE
CREAM,** U.S.P. XXIII.
Use: Antibiotic, anti-inflammatory.
• **NEOMYCIN SULFATE AND DEXAM-
ETHASONE SODIUM PHOSPHATE
OPHTHALMIC OINTMENT,** U.S.P.
XXIII.
Use: Antibiotic, anti-inflammatory.
• **NEOMYCIN SULFATE AND DEXAM-
ETHASONE SODIUM PHOSPHATE
OPHTHALMIC SOLUTION,** U.S.P.
XXIII. (Various Mfr.) 5 ml.
Use: Antibiotic, anti-inflammatory.
• **NEOMYCIN SULFATE AND FLUOCI-
NOLONE ACETONIDE CREAM,** U.S.P.
XXIII.
Use: Antibiotic, anti-inflammatory.
• **NEOMYCIN SULFATE AND FLUO-
ROMETHOLONE OINTMENT,** U.S.P.
XXIII.
Use: Antibiotic, anti-inflammatory.
• **NEOMYCIN SULFATE AND FLURAN-
DRENOLIDE,** U.S.P. XXIII. Cream, Lot.,
Oint., U.S.P. XXIII.
Use: Antibiotic, anti-inflammatory.
See: Cordran Prods. (Dista).
• **NEOMYCIN SULFATE AND GRAMICIDIN
OINTMENT,** U.S.P. XXIII.
Use: Antibiotic.
• **NEOMYCIN SULFATE AND HYDRO-
CORTISONE,** U.S.P. XXIII. Cream,
Oint., U.S.P. XXIII.
Use: Antibiotic, anti-inflammatory.
• **NEOMYCIN SULFATE AND HYDRO-
CORTISONE ACETATE,** U.S.P. XXIII.
Cream, Lot., Oint., Ophth. Oint., Ophth.
Susp., U.S.P. XXIII.
Use: Antibiotic, anti-inflammatory.
• **NEOMYCIN SULFATE AND METHYL-
PREDNISOLONE ACETATE CREAM,**
U.S.P. XXIII.
Use: Antibiotic, anti-inflammatory.
**NEOMYCIN SULFATE, POLYMYXIN B
SULFATE AND GRAMICIDIN SOLU-
TION.** (Various Mfr.) Polymyxin B sul-
fate 10,000 units/g, neomycin sulfate

1.75 mg/g, gramicidin 0.025 mg/ml. Bot.
10 ml.
Use: Antibiotic, ophthalmic.
• **NEOMYCIN SULFATE AND PRED-
NISOLONE ACETATE OINTMENT,**
U.S.P. XXIII.
Use: Antibiotic, anti-Inflammatory.
• **NEOMYCIN SULFATE AND PRED-
NISOLONE ACETATE OPHTHALMIC
OINTMENT,** U.S.P. XXIII.
Use: Antibiotic, anti-inflammatory.
• **NEOMYCIN SULFATE AND PRED-
NISOLONE ACETATE OPHTHALMIC
SUSPENSION,** U.S.P. XXIII.
Use: Antibiotic, anti-inflammatory.
• **NEOMYCIN SULFATE AND PRED-
NISOLONE SODIUM PHOSPHATE
OPHTHALMIC OINTMENT,** U.S.P.
XXIII.
Use: Antibiotic, anti-inflammatory.
• **NEOMYCIN SULFATE, SULFAC-
ETAMIDE SODIUM, AND PRED-
NISOLONE ACETATE OPHTHALMIC
OINTMENT,** U.S.P. XXIII.
Use: Antibiotic, anti-inflammatory.
• **NEOMYCIN SULFATE AND TRIAMCI-
NOLONE ACETONIDE CREAM,** U.S.P.
XXIII.
Use: Antibiotic, anti-Inflammatory.
• **NEOMYCIN SULFATE AND TRIAMCI-
NOLONE ACETONIDE OPHTHALMIC
OINTMENT,** U.S.P. XXIII.
Use: Antibiotic, anti-inflammatory.
• **NEOMYCIN UNDECYLENATE.** USAN.
Use: Antibacterial.
See: Neodecyllin (Penick).
NEOMYCORSONE.
See: Neosone, Oint. (Upjohn).
NEO NOVALDIN. (Sanofi Winthrop) Dipy-
rone.
Use: Analgesic.
NEOPAP. (PolyMedica) Acetaminophen
125 mg/Supp. In 12s.
Use: Analgesic.
NEOPHAM 6.4%. (KabiVitrum) Essential
and non-essential amino acids 6.4%. Inj.
250 ml, 500 ml.
Use: Parenteral nutritional supplement.
NEO PHYRIN DROPS. (Sanofi Winthrop)
Phenylephrine HCl.
Use: Decongestant.
See: Phenylephrine HCl.
NEO PICATYL. (Sanofi Winthrop) Glyco-
biarsoln.
Use: Amebicide.
NEOPLASTIC AGENTS.
See: Folic acid antagonists. Leukemia
agents.
NEOQUESS TABLETS. (Forest) L-
Hyoscyamine sulfate 0.125 mg/Tab. Bot.

1000s.
Use: Anticholinergic/antispasmodic.
NEOQUINOPHAN.
See: Neocinchophen (Various Mfr.).
NEO QUIPENYL. (Sanofi Winthrop) Primaquine phosphate.
Use: Antimalarial.
NEORESPIN. (Murdock) Ephedrine HCl 25 mg/TR Cap. Bot. 30s.
Use: Bronchodilator.
NEOSAR. (Adria) Cyclophosphamide. For inj. **100 mg:** Cyclophosphamide 100 mg, sodium Cl 45 mg/Vial. Pkg. 12s. **200 mg:** Cyclophosphamide 200 mg, sodium Cl 90 mg/Vial. Pkg. 12s. **500 mg:** Cyclophosphamide 500 mg, sodium Cl 225 mg/Vial. Pkg 12s.
Use: Antineoplastic agent.
NEO-SKIODAN.
Iodopyracet, Diodrast.
NEOSPORIN CREAM. (Burroughs Wellcome) Polymyxin B sulfate, neomycin sulfate. Tube 0.5 oz, foil packet 1/32 oz. Ctn. 144s.
Use: Anti-infective, external.
NEOSPORIN G.U. IRRIGANT. (Burroughs Wellcome) Neomycin sulfate 40 mg, polymyxin B sulfate 200,000 units/ml. Amp. 1 ml. Box 10s, 50s, Multiple dose vial 20 ml.
Use: Genitourinary irrigant.
NEOSPORIN OINTMENT. (Burroughs Wellcome) Polymyxin B sulfate 5000 units, bacitracin zinc 400 units, neomycin sulfate 5 mg/Gm. Tube 0.5 oz, 1 oz. Foil packet 1/32 oz. Box 144s.
Use: Anti-infective, external.
NEOSPORIN, MAXIMUM STRENGTH (Burroughs Wellcome) Polymyxin B sulfate 10,000 units, neomycin 3.5 mg, bacitracin 500 units/Gm, white petrolatum. Oint. Tube 15 Gm.
Use: Topical anti-infective.
NEOSPORIN OPHTHALMIC OINTMENT, STERILE. (Burroughs Wellcome) Polymyxin B sulfate 10,000 units, bacitracin zinc 400 units, neomycin sulfate 3.5 mg/Gm, special white petrolatum base.. Tube 3.5 Gm.
Use: Anti-infective, ophthalmic.
NEOSPORIN OPHTHALMIC SOLUTION, STERILE. (Burroughs Wellcome) Polymyxin B sulfate 10,000 units, neomycin sulfate 1.75 mg, gramicidin 0.025 mg/ml, alcohol 0.5%, thimerosal 0.001%, propylene glycol, polyoxyethylene-polyoxypropylene compound, sodium Cl. Bot 10 ml. Drop-dose.
Use: Anti-infective, ophthalmic.
NEOSPORIN PLUS. (Burroughs Wellcome) **Cream:** 10,000 units polymyxin B sulfate, 3.5 mg neomycin and 40 mg lidocaine per g. 0.25% methylparaben, mineral oil, white petrolatum. Tube 15 g.
Oint.: 10,000 units polymyxin B sulfate, 500 units bacitracin zinc, 3.5 mg neomycin and 40 mg lidocaine per g. In a white petrolatum base. Tube 15 g.
Use: Topical anti-infective.
NEOSTIGMINE AND ATROPINE SULFATE.
Use: Cholinergic muscle stimulant.
See: Neostigmine Min-I-Mix (IMS).
NEOSTIBOSAN. Ethylstibamine.
NEOSTIGMINE BROMIDE, U.S.P. XXI. Tab., U.S.P. XXI. Benzenaminium, 3-[[(dimethylamino)-carbonyl]oxy]-N,N,N-trimethyl-, bromide. (m-Hydroxyphenyl)trimethylammonium bromide dimethylcarbamate.
Use: Cholinergic.
See: Prostigmin Bromide, Tab. (Roche).
NEOSTIGMINE METHYLSULFATE, U.S.P. XXI. Inj., U.S.P. XXI. Benzenaminium, 3-[[(dimethylamino)carbonyl]-oxy]-N,N,N-trimethyl-, methyl sulfate. (m-Hydroxyphenyl) trimethylammonium methylsulfate dimethylcarbamate.
Use: Parasympathomimetic agent, cholinergic.
See: Prostigmin methylsulfate, Vial (Roche Lab.).
NEOSTIGMINE MIN-I-MIX. (MIS) Atropine sulfate 1.2 mg, neostigmine methysulfate 2.5 mg. Inj. Vial.
Use: Cholinergic muscle stimulant.
Use: Ophthalmic vasoconstrictor/mydriatic.
NEO-STREPSAN.
See: Sulfathiazole (Various Mfr.).
NEO-SYNALAR CREAM. (Syntex) Fluocinolone acetonide 0.025%, neomycin sulfate 0.5%, in a water-washable aqueous base, methylparaben and propylparaben as preservatives. Cream. Tube 15 Gm, 30 Gm, 60 Gm.
Use: Corticosteroid, anti-infective.
NEO-SYNEPHRINE 10% PLAIN. (Sanofi Winthrop.) Phenylephrine HCl 10%. Soln. Bot. 5 ml.
Use: Ophthalmic vasoconstrictor/mydriatic.
NEO-SYNEPHRINE HYDROCHLORIDE. (Sanofi Winthrop) Phenylephrine HCl. **Spray:** 0.25% children and adult, 0.5% adult. **Regular:** Squeeze bot. 0.5 oz. **0.5% mentholated:** Squeeze bot. 0.5 oz. **Drops:** 0.125% infant; 0.25% children and adult; 0.5% adult; 1% adult extra strength. Bot. 1 oz; 0.25% and 1%

also bot. 16 oz. **Jelly:** 0.5%. Tube 18.75 Gm.
Use: Nasal decongestant.
NEO-SYNEPHRINE HYDROCHLORIDE.
(Sanofi Winthrop) Phenylephrine HCl.
Amp.: 1%, Carpuject sterile cartridge-needle unit 10 mg/ml. (1 ml fill in 2 ml cartridge) w/22 gauge, 1.25 inch needle. Dispensing Bin 50s; Vial 1 ml Box 25s.
Ophthalmic: 2.5%, Mono-Drop Bot. 15 ml; 10% Mono-Drop Bot. 5 ml.; 10% viscous soln., Mono-Drop Bot. 5 ml.
Use: **Amp.:** Vasopressor used in shock; **Ophth.:** Vasoconstrictor/ mydriatic.
NEO-SYNEPHRINE VISCOUS OPH-THALMIC. (Sanofi Winthrop) Phenylephrine HCl 10%. Soln. Bot. 5 ml.
Use: Ophthalmic vasoconstrictor/mydriatic.
NEO-TABS. (Pharma-Tek) Neomycin sulfate 500 mg (equivalent to 350 mg neomycin base/Tab. Bot. 100s.
Use: Amebicide.
NEOTAL. (Hauck) Zinc bacitracin 400 units, polymyxin B sulfate 5000 units, neomycin sulfate 5 mg, petrolatum and mineral oil base/Gm. Tube 3.5 Gm.
Use: Anti-infective, ophthalmic.
NEO-THRYCEX OINT. (Commerce) Bacitracin, neomycin sulfate, polymyxin B sulfate. Tube 0.5 oz.
Use: Anti-infective, external.
NEOTHYLLINE. (Lemmon) Dyphylline.
200 mg/Tab.: Bot. 100s, 1000s. **400 mg/Tab.:** Bot. 100s, 500s.
Use: Bronchodilator.
NEOTHYLLINE-GG. (Lemmon) Dyphylline 200 mg, guaifenesin 200 mg/Tab. Bot. 100s, 1000s.
Use: Bronchodilator, expectorant.
NEOTRACE-4. (Lyphomed) Zinc 1.5 mg, copper 0.1 mg, chromium 0.85 mcg, manganese 25 mcg/ml. Vial 2 ml.
Use: Mineral supplement.
NEOTRICIN HC. (Bausch & Lomb) Hydrocortisone acetate 1%, neomycin sulfate 3.5 mg, bacitracin zinc 400 units, polymyxin B sulfate 10,000 units in a white petrolatum and mineral oil base. Oint. Tube 3.5 g.
Use: Antibiotic, corticosteroid, ophthalmic.
NEOTRICIN OPHTHALMIC OINTMENT.
(Bausch & Lomb) Polymyxin B sulfate 10,000 units, neomycin sulfate 3.5 mg, bacitracin 400 units/Gm. In 3.5 Gm.
Use: Anti-infective, ophthalmic.
NEOTRICIN OPHTHALMIC SOLUTION.
(Bausch and Lomb) Polymyxin B sulfate 10,000 units, neomycin sulfate 1.75 mg,

gramicidin 0.025 mg/ml. Dropper bot. 10 ml.
Use: Anti-infective, ophthalmic.
NEO-TROBEX INJECTION. (Forest) Vitamins B_1 150 mg, B_6 10 mg, riboflavin 5-phosphate sodium 2 mg, niacinamide 150 mg, panthenol 10 mg, choline Cl 20 mg, inositol 20 mg/ml. Vial 30 ml.
NEOTROL. (Horizon) Phenylephrine HCl 0.25%, pyrilamine maleate 0.2%, cetalkonium Cl 0.05%, tyrothricin 0.03%, phenylmercuric acetate 1:50,000. Soln. Squeeze Bot. 20 ml.
Use: Decongestant, antihistamine.
NEO-VADRIN STRESS FORMULA VITA-MINS PLUS ZINC. (Scherer) Vitamins E 45 IU, C 600 mg, folic acid 400 mcg, B_1 20 mg, B_2 10 mg, B_{12} 25 mcg, biotin 45 mcg, pantothenic acid 25 mg, copper 3 mg, zinc 23.9 mg/Tab. Bot. 60s.
Use: Vitamin/mineral supplement.
NEO-VADRIN TIME RELEASE VIT. C.
(Scherer) Vitamin C 500 mg/Cap. Bot. 50s, 100s.
Use: Vitamin C supplement.
NEO-VADRIN VITAMIN B_6
TR. (Scherer) Vitamin B_6 100 mg/Cap. Bot. 100s.
Use: Vitamin B_6 supplement.
NEOVAL. (Blue Cross) Vitamins A 10,000 IU, D 400 IU, B_1 10 mg, B_2 5 mg, B_6 2 mg, B_{12} 3 mcg, C 100 mg, E 5 mg, pantothenic acid 10 mg, niacinamide 30 mg, iron 15 mg, copper 1 mg, magnesium 5 mg, manganese 1 mg, zinc 1.5 mg, iodine 0.15 mg/Tab. Bot. 100s.
Use: Vitamin/mineral supplement.
NEOVAL T. (Blue Cross) Vitamins A 10,000 IU, D 400 IU, B_1 15 mg, B_2 10 mg, B_6 2 mg, C 150 mg, B_{12} 7.5 mcg, E 5 mg, pantothenic acid 10 mg, E 5 mg, niacinamide 100 mg, iron 15 mg, magnesium 5 mg, manganese 1 mg, zinc 1.5 mg, copper 1 mg/Tab. Bot. 1000s.
Use: Vitamin/mineral supplement.
NEO WHITE OINTMENT. (Whiteworth) Triple antibiotic ointment. Tube 0.5 oz, 1 oz.
Use: Anti-infective, external.
NEPHRAMINE. (Kendall-McGaw) Amino acid concentration 5.4%, nitrogen 0.65 Gm/100 ml. **Essential amino acids:** Isoleucine 560 mg, leucine 880 mg, lysine 640 mg, methionine 880 mg, phenylalanine 880 mg, threonine 400 mg, tryptophan 200 mg, valine 640 mg, histidine 250 mg/100 ml. **Nonessential amino acids:** Cysteine <20 mg/100 ml, sodium 5 mEq, acetate 44 mEq, chloride 3 mEq/L, sodium bisulfite. Inj. 250 ml.

Use: Parenteral nutritional supplement.
NEPHRIDINE.
See: Epinephrine (Various Mfr.).
NEPHRO-CALCI. (R & D) Calcium carbonate 1.5 Gm/Chew. Tab. (600 mg calcium). Bot. 100s, 200s, 500s, 1000s.
Use: Calcium supplement.
NEPHROCAPS CAPSULES. (Fleming) Vitamins B_1 1.5 mg, B_2 1.7 mg, B_3 20 mg, B_5 5 mg, B_6 10 mg, B_{12} 6 mcg, C 100 mg, folic acid 1 mg, biotin 150 mcg/Cap. Bot. 100s.
Use: Vitamin supplement.
NEPHRO-DERM. (R&D Labs) Eucerin, camphor, menthol, petrolatum, parabens, vitamin B_{12}, mineral oil. Cream. Jar 28.35 Gm, 113.6 Gm.
Use: Ointment/lotion base.
NEPHRO-FER. (R&D Labs) Ferrous fumarate 350 mg iron (iron 115 mg)/Tab. Bot. 100s.
Use: Iron-containing product, oral.
NEPHRO-FER RX. (R & D) Iron 106.9 mg, folic acid 1 mg. Tab. Bot. 120s.
Use: Iron with vitamin supplement.
NEPHRON INHALANT AND VAPORIZER. (Nephron) Racemic epinephrine HCl 2.25%. Bot. 0.25 oz, 0.5 oz, 1 oz.
Use: Bronchodilator.
NEPHRO-VITE B & C. (R & D) Vitamins B_1 1.5 mg, B_2 1.7 mg, B_3 20 mg, B_5 10 mg, B_6 10 mg, B_{12} 6 mcg, C 60 mg, folic acid 800 mcg, biotin 300 mcg/Tab. Bot. 100s.
Use: Vitamin/mineral supplement.
NEPHRO-VITE RX. (R & D) Vitamins B_1 1.5 mg, B_2 1.7 mg, B_3 20 mg, B_5 10 mg, B_6 10 mg, B_{12} 6 mcg, C 60 mg, folic acid 1 mg, d-biotin 300 mcg, magnesium < 0.3 mg, lactose/Tab. Bot. 100s.
Use: Vitamin/mineral supplement.
NEPHRO-VITE RX + FE. (R & D) Iron 100 mg, Vitamins B_1 1.5 mg, B_2 1.7 mg, B_3 20 mg, B_5 10 mg, B_6 10 mg, B_{12} 6 mcg, C 60 mg, folic acid 1 mg, d-biotin 300 mcg, lactose/Tab. Bot. 120s.
Use: Iron with vitamin supplement.
NEPHROX. (Fleming) Aluminum hydroxide 320 mg, mineral oil 10%/5 ml. Bot. pt.
Use: Antacid.
NEPTAZANE. (Lederle) Methazolamide 25 mg or 50 mg/Tab. Bot. 100s.
Use: Carbonic anhydrase inhibitor.
•**NEQUINATE.** USAN.
Use: Coccidiostat.
NEQUINATE (I.N.N.). Methyl Benzoquate. B.A.N.
NERAVAL. Methitural Sodium 5-(1-

Methylbutyl)-5-[2-(methylthio)ethyl]-2-thiobarbiturate.
Use: General anesthetic.
NERVINE NIGHTTIME SLEEP-AID. (Miles Labs) Diphenhydramine HCl 25 mg/Tab. Bot. 12s, 30s, 50s.
Use: Sleep aid.
NERVOCAINE. (Keene) Lidocaine HCl 1% or 2%. Inj. Vial 50 ml.
Use: Local anesthetic.
NESACAINE. (Astra) Chloroprocaine HCl 1% or 2%, methylparaben, EDTA. Inj. Vial 30 ml.
Use: Local anesthetic.
NESACAINE-CE. (Astra) **Conc. 2%:** Chloroprocaine HCl 20 mg/ml in a sterile soln. containing sodium bisulfite, sodium Cl, HCl. Vial 30 ml. **Conc. 3%:** Chloroprocaine HCl 30 mg/ml in a sterile soln. containing sodium bisulfite, sodium Cl, HCl. Vial 30 ml.
Use: Local anesthetic.
NESACAINE-MPF. (Astra) Chloroprocaine HCl 2% or 3%. EDTA or preservative-free. Inj. Vial 30 ml.
Use: Local anesthetic.
NESA NINE CAP. (Standex) Vitamins A 5000 IU, D 400 IU, C 37.5 mg, B_1 1.5 mg, B_2 2 mg, niacinamide 20 mg, B_6 0.1 mg, calcium pantothenate 1 mg, E 2 IU/Cap. Bot. 100s.
Use: Vitamin supplement.
NESDONAL SODIUM.
See: Thiopental Sodium U.S.P. XXIII. Pentothal Sodium, Prods. (Abbott).
NESTABS. (Fielding) Vitamins A 8000 IU, D 400 IU, E 30 mg, C 120 mg, B_1 3 mg, B_2 3 mg, B_3 20 mg, B_6 3 mg, B_{12} 8 mcg, calcium 200 mg, iron 36 mg, folic acid 0.8 mg, zinc 15 mg, I/Tab. Bot. 100s.
Use: Vitamin/mineral supplement.
NESTABS FA TABLETS. (Fielding) Vitamins A 8000 IU, D 400 IU, E 30 mg, C 120 mg, B_1 3 mg, B_2 3 mg, B_3 20 mg, B_6 3 mg, B_{12} 8 mcg, calcium 200 mg, iron (as elemental iron) 36 mg, folic acid 1 mg, zinc 15 mg, I/Tab. Bot. 100s.
Use: Vitamin/mineral supplement.
NESTREX. (Fielding) Pyridoxine 25 mg/Tab., dextrose. Bot. 100s.
Use: Vitamin B_6 supplement.
NETHAMINE. Etafedrine HCl. 1-N-ethylephedrine HCl, 2-methylethylamino-1-phenylpropanol HCl.
W/Codeine phosphate, phenylephrine HCl, sodium citrate, doxylamine succinate.
See: Mercodol with Decapryn. Syr. (Merrell Dow).
•**NETILMICIN SULFATE,** U.S.P. XXIII. Inj.,

U.S.P. XXIII.
Use: Antibacterial.
See: Netromycin (Schering).
• **NETRAFILCON A.** USAN.
Use: Contact lens material (hydrophilic).
NETRIN. Under Study.
Use: Anticholinergic.
See: Metcaraphen HCl.
NETROMYCIN. (Schering) Netilmicin 100 mg/ml. Inj. Vial 1.5 ml Box 10s, 25s. Multi-dose vial 15 ml Box 5s. Disposable Syringe 1.5 ml Box 10s.
Use: Antibacterial, aminoglycoside.
NEULACTIL.
See: Pericyazine.
NEUPOGEN. (Amgen). Filgrastim (G-CSF) 300 mcg/ml. Vial 1 ml, 1.6 ml.
Use: Colony stimulating factor.
NEURONTIN. (Parke-Davis) Gabapentin 100 mg, 300 mg, 400 mg; lactose. Cap. Bot. 100s, UD 50s.
Use: Anticonvulsant.
NEUROSIN.
See: Calcium glycerophosphate (Various Mfr.).
NEUT [SODIUM BICARBONATE 4% ADDITIVE SOLUTION]. (Abbott) Sodium bicarbonate 4%. Vial (2.4 mEq each of sodium and bicarbonate), disodium edetate anhydrous 0.05% as stabilizer. Pintop Vial 5 ml, 10 ml. Box 25s, 100s.
Use: Parenteral nutritional supplement.
NEUTRAL ACRIFLAVIN.
See: Acriflavin (Various Mfr.).
NEUTRALIN. (Dover) Calcium carbonate, magnesium oxide/Tab. Sugar, lactose and salt free. UD Box 500s.
Use: Antacid.
NEUTRAL INSULIN INJECTION. B.A.N. A solution of insulin buffered at pH 7 Insulin Novo Actrapid; Nuso.
Use: Hypoglycemic agent.
NEUTRAL PROTAMINE HAGEDORN-INSULIN.
See: Insulin, N.P.H. Iletin (Lilly).
• **NEUTRAMYCIN.** USAN. A neutral macrolide antibiotic produced by a variant strain of *Streptomyces rimosus.*
Use: Antibacterial, antibiotic.
NEUTREXIN. (US Bioscience) Trimetrexate glucuronate 25 mg. Pow. for Inj. (lyophilized). Vial 5 ml w/wo 50 mg leucovorin.
Use: Anti-infective.
NEUTROFLAVIN.
See: Acriflavine (Various Mfr.).
NEUTROGENA ACNE MASK. (Neutrogena) Benzoyl peroxide 5% in sebum absorbing facial mask vehicle. Tube 2 oz.
Use: Anti-acne.
NEUTROGENA BABY CLEANSING FORMULA SOAP. (Neutrogena) Triethanolamine, glycerin, stearic acid, tallow, coconut oil, castor oil, sodium hydroxide, oleic acid, laneth-10 acetate, cocamide DEA, nonoxynol 14, PEG-4 octoate. Bar 105 Gm.
Use: Skin cleanser.
NEUTROGENA BODY LOTION. (Neutrogena) Glyceryl stearate, isopropyl myristate, PEG-100 stearate, butylene glycol, imidazolidinyl urea, carbomer-934, parabens, sodium lauryl sulfate, triethanolamine, cetyl alcohol. Lot. Bot. 240 ml.
Use: Emollient.
NEUTROGENA BODY OIL. (Neutrogena) Isopropyl myristate, sesame oil, PEG-40 sorbitan peroleate, parabens. Bot. 240 ml.
Use: Emollient.
NEUTROGENA CHEMICAL-FREE SUNBLOCKER. (Neutrogena) Titanium dioxide, parabens, diazolidinyl urea, shea butter. SPF 17. Lot. Bot. 120 ml.
Use: Sunscreen.
NEUTROGENA CLEANSING FOR ACNE-PRONE SKIN. (Neutrogena) TEA-stearate, triethanolamine, glycerin, sodium tallowate, sodium cocoate, TEA-oleate, sodium ricinoleate, acetylated lanolin alcohol, cocamide DEA, TEA lauryl sulfate, tocopherol. Bar 105 Gm.
Use: Skin cleanser.
NEUTROGENA DRYING. (Neutrogena) Witch hazel, isopropyl alcohol, propylene glycol, carbomer 940, triethanolamine, EDTA, parabens, benzophenone-2, tartrazine. Gel. Tube 22.5 g.
Use: Anti-acne.
NEUTROGENA DRY SKIN SOAP. (Neutrogena) Triethanolamine, stearic acid, tallow, glycerin, coconut oil, castor oil, sodium hydroxide, oleic acid, laneth-10 acetate, cocamide DEA, nonoxynol 14, PEG-14 octoate, BHT, O-tolyl biguanide. Bar 105 Gm, 165 Gm. Scented or unscented.
Use: Skin cleanser.
NEUTROGENA GLOW SUNLESS TANNING. (Neutrogena) Octyl methoxycinnamate, cetyl alcohol, diazolidinyl urea, parabens, EDTA. SPF 8. Lot. Bot. 120 ml.
Use: Sunscreen.
NEUTROGENA INTENSIFIED DAY MOISTURE. (Neutrogena) Octyl

methoxycinnamate, 2-phenylbenzimidazole sulfonic acid, titanium dioxide, cetyl alcohol, diazolidinyl urea, parabens, EDTA. SPF 15. Cream 67.5 g.
Use: Moisturizer, sunscreen.

NEUTROGENA LIP MOISTURIZER. (Neutrogena) Octyl methoxycinnamate, benzophenone-3, corn oil, castor oil, mineral oil, lanolin oil, petrolatum, lanolin, stearyl alcohol. SPF 15. Lip balm 4.5 g.
Use: Lip moisturizer, sunscreen.

NEUTROGENA MOISTURE SPF 5. (Neutrogena) Octyl methoxycinnamate, petrolatum, cetyl alcohol, parabens, diazolidinyl urea, EDTA, cetyl alcohol. Lot. Bot 60 ml, 120 ml.
Use: Moisturizer, sunscreen.

NEUTROGENA MOISTURE SPF 15. (Neutrogena) Octyl methoxycinnamate, benzophenone-3, glycerine, PEG 100 stearate, dimethicone, PEG-6000 monostearate, triethanolamine, parabens, imidazolidinyl urea, carbomer 954, PABA free. Lot. Bot. 120 ml.
Use: Sunscreen.

NEUTROGENA NON-DRYING CLEANSING. (Neutrogena) Glycerin, caprylic/capric triglyceride, PEG-20 almond glycerides, cetyl recinoleate, isohexadecane, TEA-cocoyl glutamate, methyl glucose sesquistearate, stearyl alcohol, cetyl alcohol, EDTA, dipotassium glycyrrhizate, stearyl glycyrrhetinate, bisabolol, parabens, acrylates/C 10-30 alkyl acrylate crosspolymer, triethanolamine, diazolidinyl urea. Lot. Bot. 165 ml.
Use: Skin cleanser.

NEUTROGENA NORWEGIAN FORMULA EMULSION. (Neutrogena) Glycerin base 2%. Pump dispenser 5.25 oz.
Use: Emollient.

NEUTROGENA NORWEGIAN FORMULA HAND CREAM. (Neutrogena) Glycerin base 41%. Tube 2 oz.
Use: Emollient.

NEUTROGENA OILY SKIN FORMULA SOAP. (Neutrogena) Triethanolamine, glycerin, fatty acids. Bar 3.5 oz.
Use: Skin cleanser.

NEUTROGENA ORIGINAL FORMULA SOAP. (Neutrogena) Triethanolamine, glycerin, fatty acids. Bar 3.5 oz, 5.5 oz.
Use: Skin cleanser.

NEUTROGENA SOAP. (Neutrogena) TEA-stearate, triethanolamine, glycerin, sodium tallowate, sodium cocoate, sodium ricinoleate, TEA-oleate, cocamide DEA, tocopherol. Bar 105 Gm, 165 Gm.

Use: Skin cleanser.

NEUTROGENA SUNBLOCK. (Neutrogena) SPF 8: Octyl methoxycinnamate, menthyl anthranilate, titanium dioxide, mineral oil. Cream 67.5 g. **SPF 15:** Octyl methoxycinnamate, octyl salicylate, menthyl anthranilate, mineral oil, titanium dioxide, propylparaben. Cream 67.5 g. **SPF 25:** Octyl methoxycinnamate, benzophenone-3, octyl salicylate, castor oil, cetearyl alcohol, propylparaben, shea butter. Stick 12.6 g. **SPF30:** Octocrylene, octyl methoxycinnamate, menthyl anthranilate, zinc oxide, mineral oil, vitamin E. Cream 67.5 g.
Use: Sunscreen.

NEUTROGENA SUNSCREEN. (Neutrogena) Ethylhexyl p-methoxycinnamate 7%, oxybenzone 4%, titanium dioxide 2%. Tube 3 oz.
Use: Sunscreen.

NEUTROGENA T/GEL. (Neutrogena) Coal tar extract 2%. Shampoo. Bot. 132 ml.
Use: Antiseborrheic.

NEUTROGENA T/SAL. (Neutrogena) Salicylic acid 2%, solubilized coal tar extract 2%. Shampoo. Bot. 135 ml.
Use: Antiseborrheic shampoo.

• **NEVIRAPINE.** USAN.
Use: Antiviral.

NEW-DECONGEST. (Goldline) **Syr.:** Phenylpropanolamine HCl 20 mg, phenylephrine HCl 5 mg, chlorpheniramine maleate 2.5 mg, phenyltoloxamine citrate 7.5 mg/5 ml. Bot. pt, gal. **TR Tab.:** Phenylpropanolamine HCl 40 mg, phenylephrine HCl 10 mg, chlorpheniramine maleate 5 mg, phenyltoloxamine citrate 15 mg. Bot. 100s, 500s, 1000s.
Use: Decongestant, antihistamine.

NEW-DECONGEST PEDIATRIC SYRUP. (Goldline) Phenylpropanolamine HCl 5 mg, phenylephrine HCl 1.25 mg, chlorpheniramine maleate 0.5 mg, phenyltoloxamine citrate 2 mg/5 ml. Syr. Bot. pt, gal.
Use: Decongestant, antihistamine.

NEW DECONGESTANT. (Goldline) Phenylpropanolamine HCl 40 mg, phenylephrine HCl 10 mg, chlorpheniramine maleate 5 mg/ SR Tab. Bot. 100s, 1000s.
Use: Decongestant, antihistamine.

• **NEXERIDINE HYDROCHLORIDE.** USAN.
Use: Analgesic.

NG-29.
Use: Diagnostic aid. [Orphan drug]

N.G.T. (Geneva Generics) Triamcinolone

acetonide 0.1%, nystatin 100,000 units/Gm. Cream. Tube 15 Gm.
Use: Topical corticosteroid, antifungal.
NIA-BID. (Geriatric Pharm.) Niacin 400 mg/TR Cap. Bot. 100s.
Use: Vitamin supplement.
NIACAL. (Bowman) Calcium lactate 324 mg, niacin 25 mg/Tab. Peppermint flavor. Bot. 100s, 1000s.
Use: Vasodilator, vitamin supplement.
NIACAMIDE.
See: Nikethamide (Various Mfr.).
NIACELS. (Hauck) Niacin 400 mg/TR Cap. Bot. 100s.
Use: Vitamin B$_3$ supplement.
• **NIACIN,** U.S.P. XXIII. Inj., Tab., U.S.P. XXIII. 3-Pyridinecarboxylic acid.
Use: Vitamin B-complex component.
See: Efacin, Tab. (Person & Covey).
   Niac, Cap. (Cole).
   Nicobid, Cap. (Rhone-Poulenc Rorer).
   Nicolar, Tab. (Rhone-Poulenc Rorer).
   Nico-400 (Marion).
   Ni Cord XL, Cap. (Scott/Cord).
   Nicotinex, Elix.(Fleming).
   Span Niacin 300, Tab. (Scrip).
NIACIN W/COMBINATIONS.
See: Adenocrest, Vial (Pharmex).
   Lipo-Nicin, Tab., Cap. (Brown).
   Vasostim, Cap. (Dunhall).
• **NIACINAMIDE,** U.S.P. XXIII. Inj., Tab., U.S.P. XXIII. 3-Pyridinecarboxamide. Nicotinic acid amide. Nicotinamide.
Use: Enzyme co-factor vitamin.
See: Niacinamide (Various Mfr.).
W/Pentylenetetrazol, thiamine HCl, cyanocobalamin, alcohol.
See: Cenalene, Tab., Elix. (Central).
W/Potassium iodide.
See: Iodo-Niacin, Tab. (Cole).
W/Riboflavin.
See: Riboflavin and Niacinamide, Amp. (Lilly).
NIACINAMIDE HI.
W/Potassium iodide.
See: Iodo-Niacin, Tab. (Cole).
NIACOR. (Upsher-Smith) Niacin 500 mg/Tab. Bot. 100s.
Use: Vitamin supplement.
NIALAMIDE. B.A.N. N-Benzyl-α(isonicotinoyl hydrazine)propionamide. Isonicotinic Acid 2-[2-(Benzylcarbamoyl)ethyl]hydrazide.
Use: Monoamine oxidase inhibitor, antidepressant.
NIALEXO-C. (Hauck) Niacin 50 mg, vitamin C 30 mg/Tab. Bot. 100s.
Use: Vitamin supplement.
NIARB SUPER. (Miller) Magnesium 100 mg, vitamin C 200 mg, niacinamide 200

mg (as ascorbate)/Tab. Bot. 100s.
Use: Vitamin/mineral supplement.
NIAZIDE. (Major) Trichlormethiazide 4 mg/Tab. Bot. 100s, 1000s.
Use: Diuretic.
NIAZO. Neotropin.
Use: Urinary antiseptic.
• **NIBROXANE.** USAN.
Use: Antimicrobial.
NICAMETATE. B.A.N. 2-Diethylaminoethyl nicotinate. Euclidan. [dihydrogen citrate].
Use: Peripheral vasodilator.
NICAMINDON.
See: Nicotinamide (Various Mfr.).
• **NICARDIPINE HYDROCHLORIDE.** USAN.
Use: Vasodilator.
See: Cardene (DuPont).
N'ICE. (Beecham Products) Menthol 5 mg/Loz. in sugarless sorbitol base. Pkg. 8s, 16s.
Use: Local anesthetic.
N'ICE W/VITAMIN C DROPS. (SK-Beecham Consumer) Ascorbic acid 60 mg, menthol, sorbitol, tartrazine/Loz. Pks. 16s.
Use: Vitamin supplement, local anesthetic.
• **NICERGOLINE.** USAN. 8β-(5-Bromonicotinoyl-oxy-methyl)-10-methoxy-1,6-dimethylergolline.
Use: Vasodilator.
NICERITROL. B.A.N. Pentaerythritol tetranicotinate.
Use: Treatment of hypercholesterolemia.
NICHOLS SYPHON POWDER. (Last) Sodium bicarbonate, sodium Cl, sodium borate. Pouch 12.2 Gm (add to 32 oz. water to yield isotonic soln.).
NICLOCIDE. (Miles Pharm) Niclosamide 500 mg/Chew. Tab. Box 4s.
Use: Anthelmintic.
• **NICLOSAMIDE.** USAN. 2',5-Dichloro-4-nitro-salicylanilide. Yomesan.
Use: Anthelmintic.
See: Niclocide, Tab. (Miles).
NICO-400. (Jones Medical) Niacin 400 mg/Cap. Bot. 100s.
Use: Vitamin B$_3$ supplement.
NICOBID. (Rhone-Poulenc Rorer) Nicotinic acid 125 mg, 250 mg or 500 mg/Tempule TR Cap. Bot. 100s, 500s.
Use: Vitamin B$_3$ supplement.
NICOBION.
See: Nicotinamide (Various Mfr.).
NICOCODINE. B.A.N. O^3-Methyl-O^6-nicotinoylmorphine.
Use: Narcotic analgesic.

NICODERM. (Marion Merrell Dow) Total nicotine content 36 mg or 114 mg/patch. 14 systems/box.
Use: Smoking deterrent.

NICODICODINE. B.A.N. 7,8-Dihydro-0³-methyl-O⁶-nicotinoylmorphine.
Use: Antitussive.

NICODUOZIDE. A mixture of nicothazone and isoniazid.

NICOLAR. (Rhone-Poulenc Rorer) Niacin 500 mg/Tab. Bot. 100s.
Use: Vitamin B₃ supplement.

NICOMORPHINE. B.A.N. 3,6-Dinicotinoylmorphine.
Use: Narcotic analgesic.

• **NICORANDIL.** USAN.
Use: Coronary vasodilator.

NI CORD XL CAPS. (Scott/Cord) Nicotinic acid 400 mg/Cap. Bot. 100s, 500s.
Use: Vitamin B₃ supplement.

NICORETTE. (SK-Beecham) Nicotine polacrilex 2 mg/Chew. piece. Box 96s.
Use: Smoking deterrent.

NICORETTE DS. (SK-Beecham) Nicotine polacrilex 4 mg/Chew. gum. Box 96s.
Use: Smoking deterrent.

NICOTAMIDE.
See: Nicotinamide (Various Mfr.).

NICOTHAZONE. Nicotinaldehyde thiosemicarbazone.

NICOTILAMIDE.
See: Nicotinamide (Various Mfr.).

NICOTINAMIDE. Niacinamide, U.S.P. XXIII. Vitamin B₃, Aminicotin, Dipegyl, Nicamindon, Nicotamide, Nicotilamide, Nicotinic Acid Amide.

NICOTINAMIDE ADENINE DINU-CLEOTIDE. Name used for Nadide.

NICOTINE TRANSDERMAL SYSTEMS.
Use: Smoking deterrent.
See: Habitrol (Basel Pharm.)
Nicoderm (Marion Merrell Dow).
Nicotrol (Parke-Davis).
Prostep (Lederle).

• **NICOTINE POLACRILEX.** USAN.
Use: Smoking deterrent.
See: Nicorette (Marion Merrell Dow).

NICOTINEX ELIXIR. (Fleming) Niacin 50 mg/5 ml, alcohol 14%. Bot. pt, gal.
Use: Vitamin B₃ supplement.

NICOTINIC ACID. Niacin, U.S.P. XXIII.

NICOTINIC ACID W/COMBINATIONS.
See: Niacin w/Combinations (Various Mfr.).

NICOTINIC ACID AMIDE. Niacinamide, U.S.P. XXIII.
See: Niacinamide (Various Mfr.).

• **NICOTINYL ALCOHOL.** USAN. 3-Pyridine-methanol. beta-Pyridylcarbinol.
Use: Vasodilator.

NICOTINYL TARTRATE. 3-Pyridinemethanol tartrate.
See: Roniacol Timespan, Tab. (Roche).

NICOTROL. (Parke-Davis) Total nicotine content 8.3 mg, 16.6 mg or 24.9 mg/patch. 14 systems/box.
Use: Smoking deterrent.

NICOUMALONE. B.A.N. 3-[2-Acetyl-1-(4-nitro-phenyl)ethyl]-4-hydroxycoumarin. Acenocoumarol (I.N.N.) Sinthrome.
Use: Anticoagulant.

NICO-VERT. (Edwards) Niacin 50 mg, dimenhydrinate 25 mg/Cap. Bot. 100s.
Use: Antiemetic/antivertigo.

NIDROXYZONE. 5-Nitro-2-furaldehyde-2-(2-hydroxy-ethyl)semicarbazone.

NIDRYL. (Geneva Generics) Diphenhydramine 12.5 mg/5 ml. Elix. Bot. 120 ml.
Use: Antihistamine.

NIERALINE.
See: Epinephrine (Various Mfr.).

• **NIFEDIPINE,** U.S.P. XXIII. Cap., U.S.P. XXIII. Dimethyl1,4-dihydro-2,6-dimethyl-4-(2-nitrophenyl)pyridine-3,5-dicarboxylate.
Use: Coronary vasodilator, interstitial cystitis. [Orphan drug]
See: Adalat, Cap. (Miles Pharm).
Adalat CC, ER Tab. (Miles Pharm).
Procardia, Cap. (Pfizer).

NIFENAZONE. B.A.N. 2,3-Dimethyl-4-nicotinamido-1-phenyl-5-pyrazolone. Thylin.
Use: Anti-inflammatory, analgesic.

NIFEREX. (Central) **Elix.:** Iron 100 mg/5 ml polysaccharide-iron complex, alcohol 10%. Sugar and dye free. Bot. 8 oz.
Tab.: Iron 50 mg. Bot. 100s.
Use: Iron supplement.

NIFEREX-150. (Central) Polysaccharide iron complex equivalent to iron 150 mg/Cap. Bot. 100s, 1000s.
Use: Iron supplement.

NIFEREX-150 FORTE CAPSULES. (Central) Elemental iron as polysaccharide-iron complex 150 mg, folic acid 1 mg, vitamin B₁₂ 25 mcg/Cap. Bot. 100s, 1000s.
Use: Iron supplement.

NIFEREX FORTE ELIXIR. (Central) Iron 100 mg, folic acid 1 mg, vitamin B₁₂ 25 mcg/5 ml. Bot. 4 oz.
Use: Iron supplement.

NIFEREX-PN. (Central) Iron 60 mg, folic acid 1 mg, vitamins C 50 mg, B₁₂ 3 mcg, A 4000 IU, D 400 IU, B₁ 3 mg, B₂ 3 mg, B₆ 2 mg, B₃ 10 mg, zinc sulfate 80 mg, calcium carbonate 312 mg/Tab, sorbitol. Bot. 100s, 1000s.
Use: Vitamin/mineral supplement.

NIFEREX-PN FORTE TABLETS. (Central) Calcium 250 mg, iron 60 mg, vitamins A 5000 IU, D 400 IU, E 30 mg, B_1 3 mg, B_2 3.4 mg, B_3 20 mg, B_6 4 mg, B_{12} 12 mcg, C 80 mg, folic acid 1 mg, Cu, I, Mg, zinc 25 mg/Tab. Bot. 100s.
Use: Vitamin/mineral supplement.
NIFEREX W/VITAMIN C. (Central) Iron 50 mg, vitamin C 269 mg (as ascorbic acid 100 mg, as sodium ascorbate 169 mg)/Tab. Bot. 50s.
Use: Vitamin/mineral supplement.
• **NIFLURIDIDE.** USAN.
Use: Ectoparasiticide.
• **NIFUNGIN.** USAN. Substance derived from *Aspergillus giganteus.*
• **NIFURADENE.** USAN. 1-[(5-Nitrofurfurylidene)-amino]-2-imidazolidinone.
Use: Antibacterial.
• **NIFURALDEZONE.** USAN. 5-Nitro-2-furaldehyde semioxamazone. Furamazone (Eaton).
Use: Antibacterial.
• **NIFURATEL.** USAN. 5-[(Methylthio)methyl]-3-[(5-nitro furfurylidene)-amino]-2-oxazolidinone. Macmiror, Magmilor, Polmiror. Under study.
Use: Antibacterial, antifungal, trichomonacidal.
• **NIFURATRONE.** USAN. N-(2-Hydroxyethyl)-α-(5-nitro-2-furyl)nitrone.
Use: Antibacterial.
• **NIFURDAZIL.** USAN. 1-(2-Hydroxyethyl)-3-[(5-nitrofurfurylidene)-amino]-2-imidazolidinone.
Use: Antibacterial.
NIFURETHAZONE. 5-Nitro-2-furaldehyde-2-[2-(dimethylamino)ethyl] semicarbazone.
Use: Antibacterial.
• **NIFURIMIDE.** USAN. (±)4-Methyl-1-[(5-nitro-fur-furylidene)amino]-2-imidazolidinone.
Use: Antibacterial.
• **NIFURMERONE.** USAN. Chloromethyl 5-nitro-2-furyl ketone. Metofurone.
Use: Antimycotic agent.
NIFUROXIME. 5-Nitro-2-fural-doxime. (Z)-5-Nitro-2-furaldehyde Oxime.
Use: Antifungal, antibacterial (topical), antiprotozoal.
See: Micofur.
W/Furazolidone.
See: Tricofuron, Pow., Supp. (Eaton).
• **NIFURPIRINOL.** USAN.
Use: Antibacterial.
• **NIFURQUINAZOL.** USAN. 2,2′-[[2-(5-Nitro-2-furyl)-4-quinazolinyl]imino]diethanol. Under study.

Use: Antibacterial.
• **NIFURSOL.** USAN. 3,5-Dinitrosalicylic acid (5-nitrofurfurylidene) hydrazide.
Use: Histomonocide, vet. growth stimulant.
NIFURTIMOX. B.A.N. Tetrahydro-3-methyl-4-(5-ni-trofurfurylideneamino)-1,4-thiazine 1,1-dioxide.
Use: Treatment of trypanosomiasis.
NIGHTTIME PAMPRIN. (Chattem) Diphenhydramine HCl 50 mg, acetaminophen 650 mg. Pow. Pkg. 4s.
Use: Sleep aid.
NIGRIN. Streptonigrin.
Use: Antineoplastic.
NIKO-MAG. (Scruggs) Magnesium oxide 500 mg/Cap. Bot. 100s, 1000s.
Use: Antacid.
NIKOTIME TD CAPS. (Major) Niacin 125 mg or 250 mg/TD Cap. Bot. 100s, 1000s.
Use: Vitamin B_3 supplement.
NILAIN. (A.V.P.) Aspirin 227 mg, acetaminophen 227 mg, caffeine 32.4 mg/Cap. Bot. 100s.
Use: Analgesic combination.
NILCOL ELIXIR. (Health Care Industries) Phenylpropanolamine 25 mg, chlorpheniramine maleate 2 mg, guaifenesin 100 mg, dextromethorphan HBr 15 mg/15 ml.
Use: Decongestant, antihistamine, expectorant, antitussive.
NILCOL TABLETS. (Health Care Industries) Phenylpropanolamine 50 mg, chlorpheniramine maleate 4 mg, guaifenesin 200 mg, dextromethorphan HBr 30 mg/Tab. Bot. 100s.
Use: Decongestant, antihistamine, expectorant, antitussive.
NILSPASM. (Parmed) Phenobarbital 50 mg, hyoscyamine sulfate 0.31 mg, atropine sulfate 0.06 mg, scopolamine hydrobromide 0.0195 mg/Tab. Bot. 100s, 1000s.
Use: Sedative/hypnotic, anticholinergic/antispasmodic.
NILSTAT OINTMENT & CREAM. (Lederle) Nystatin 100,000 units/Gm. **Cream base** w/Emulsifying wax, isopropyl myristate, glycerin, lactic acid, sodium hydroxide, sorbic acid 0.2%. Tube 15 Gm, Jar 240 Gm. **Oint. base:** w/light mineral oil, Plastibase 50 W. Tube 15 Gm.
Use: Antifungal, external.
NILSTAT ORAL. (Lederle) Nystatin 500,000 units/FC Tab. Bot. 100s, UD 10 × 10s.
Use: Antifungal.

NILSTAT ORAL SUSPENSION. (Lederle) Nystatin 100,000 units/ml, methylparaben 0.12%, propylparaben 0.03%, cherry flavor. Bot. 60 ml w/dropper, 16 fl oz.
Use: Antifungal.

NILSTAT POWDER. (Lederle) Nystatin pow. 150 million, 1 billion or 2 billion units/Bot.
Use: Antifungal.

NIL TUSS. (Minnesota Pharm.) Dextromethorphan HBr 10 mg, chlorpheniramine maleate 1.25 mg, phenylephrine HCl 5 mg, ammonium Cl 83 mg/5 ml. Syr. Bot. pt.
Use: Antitussive, antihistamine, decongestant, expectorant.

NIL VAGINAL CREAM. (Century) Sulfanilamide 15%, 9-aminoacridine HCl 0.2%, allantoin 1.5%. Bot. 4 oz. w/applicator.
Use: Anti-infective, vaginal.

• **NILVADIPINE.** USAN.
Use: Antagonist (calcium channel).

• **NIMAZONE.** USAN. 3-(p-Chlorophenyl)-4-imino-2-oxo-1-imidazolidineacetonitrile.
Use: Anti-inflammatory.

NIMBUS. (NMS Pharm.) Monoclonal antibody-based enzyme immunoassay. Screens for urinary chorionic gonadotropin. Pkg. 10s, 25s, 50s.
Use: Diagnostic aid.

• **NIMIDANE.** USAN.
Use: Acaricide.

• **NIMODIPINE.** USAN.
Use: Vasodilator.
See: Nimotop, Cap. (Miles Inc.).

NIMORAZOLE. B.A.N. 4-[2-(5-Nitroimidazol-1-yl)ethyl]morpholine. Nitrimidazine. Naxogin; Nulogyl.
Use: Treatment of trichomoniasis.

NIMOTOP. (Miles Inc.) Nimodipine 30 mg Liq. Cap. Bot. UD 100s.
Use: For neuorlogical deficits due to spasm following subarachnoid hemorrhage.

NINE-VITA. (Robinson) Vitamins A 5000 IU, D 1000 IU, B_1 1.5 mg, B_2 2 mg, niacinamide 20 mg, B_6 0.1 mg, calcium pantothenate 1 mg, C 37.5 mg, E 2 IU/Cap. Bot. 100s, 1000s, Bulk Pack 5000s.
Use: Vitamin supplement.

NIONG. (U.S. Ethicals) Nitroglycerin 2.6 mg or 6.5 mg/CR Tab. Bot. 100s.
Use: Antianginal.

NIPENT. (Parke-Davis) Pentostatin 10 mg/Pow. Vial. Single dose.
Use: Antineoplastic.

NIRATRON. (Progress) Chlorpheni-

ramine maleate 4 mg/Tsp. Bot. pt.
Use: Antihistamine.

• **NIRIDAZOLE.** USAN. 1-(5-Nitrothiazol-2-yl)-imidazolidin-2-one. Ambilhar.
Use: Treatment of schistosomiasis.

NIRON. (Mills) Niacinamide 150 mg, vitamins B_1 10 mg, B_2 6 mg, B_{12} 25 mcg, iron 30 mg/PA Tab. Bot. 100s.
Use: Vitamin/mineral supplement.

• **NISBUTEROL MESYLATE.** USAN.
Use: Bronchodilator.

• **NISOBAMATE.** USAN. (1) 2-(Hydroxymethyl)-2,3-dimethylpentyl isopropylcarbamate carbamate (ester); (2)2-sec-Butyl-2-methyl-1,3-propanediol carbamate isopropylcarbamate.
Use: Minor tranquilizer, sedative, hypnotic.

• **NISOLDIPINE.** USAN.
Use: Vasodilator.

• **NISOXETINE.** USAN.
Use: Antidepressant.

• **NISTERIME ACETATE.** USAN.
Use: Androgen.

NITE TIME COLD FORMULA. (Barre-National) Pseudoephedrine HCl 10 mg, doxylamine succinate 1.25 mg, dextromethorphan HBr 5 mg, acetaminophen 167 mg, alcohol 25%. Liq. Bot. 180 ml, 300 ml.
Use: Decongestant, antihistamine, antitussive, analgesic.

• **NITHIAMIDE.** USAN.
Use: Antibacterial.

• **NITRAFUDAM HYDROCHLORIDE.** USAN.
Use: Antidepressant.

• **NITRALAMINE HYDROCHLORIDE.** USAN. 2-[[o-Chloro-α-(nitromethyl)benzyl]-thio] ethyl-amine HCl.
Use: Fungicide.

• **NITRAMISOLE HYDROCHLORIDE.** USAN.
Use: Anthelmintic.

• **NITRAZEPAM.** USAN. 1,3-Dihydro-7-nitro-5-phenyl-2H-1,4-benzodiazepin-2-one. Mogadon.
Use: Hypnotic, sedative.

NITRAZINE PAPER. (Squibb) Phenaphthazine. Sodium dinitrophenyl-azo-naphthol disulfonate. Determines pH of a solution, in pH 4.5-7.5 range. 15 ft. roll with dispenser and color chart.
Use: Diagnostic aid.

NITRAZONE. (Kenyon) Nitrofurazone.
Cream: 2% in a water soluble base. Tube oz. **Soluble Dressing:** 0.2% in a water soluble base of polyethylene glycol.
Use: Burn preparation.

NIT REMOVAL SYSTEM.
See: Step 2 (GenDerm).
• **NITRENDIPINE.** USAN.
Use: Antihypertensive.
• **NITRIC ACID,** N.F. XVIII.
Use: Pharmaceutic aid (acidifying agent).
NITRIC ACID SILVER. Silver Nitrate, U.S.P. XXIII.
NITRIC OXIDE. (Anaquest)
Use: Treatment of primary pulmonary hypertension in the newborn. [Orphan drug]
NITRO-BID. (Marion Merrell Dow) Nitroglycerin 2.5 mg, 6.5 mg or 9 mg/TR Cap. Bot. 60s, 100s.
Use: Antianginal.
NITRO-BID IV. (Marion Merrell Dow) Nitroglycerin 5 mg/ml. Inj. Vial 1 ml box 10s; 5 ml Box 10s; 10 ml Box 5s.
Use: Antianginal.
NITRO-BID OINTMENT. (Marion Merrell Dow) Nitroglycerin (glyceryl trinitrate) 2%, lactose in lanolin and petrolatum base. Tube 20 Gm, 60 Gm, UD pak 100s.
Use: Antianginal.
NITRO-BID PLATEAU CAPS. (Marion Merrell Dow) Nitroglycerin 2.5 mg, 6.5 mg or 9 mg/SR Cap. Bot. 60s, 100s.
Use: Antianginal.
NITROCAP. (Freeport) Nitroglycerin 2.5 mg/TR Cap. Bot. 100s.
Use: Antianginal.
NITROCINE TIMECAPS. (Kremers-Urban) Nitroglycerin 2.5 mg, 6.5 mg or 9 mg/SR Cap. Bot. 100s.
Use: Antianginal.
• **NITROCYCLINE.** USAN. 4-(Dimethylamino)-1-4,4α, 5,5α,6,11,12α-octahydro-3,10,12,12α-tetrahydroxy-7-nitro-1,11-dioxo-2-naphthacenecarboxamide.
Use: Antibiotic.
• **NITRODAN.** USAN.
Use: Anthelmintic.
NITRODISC. (Searle) Nitroglycerin. Transcutaneous nitroglycerin discs releasing 5 mg/24 hr, 7.5 mg/24 hr or 10 mg/24 hr. Carton 30s, 100s (7.5 mg/24 hr).
Use: Antianginal.
NITRO-DUR. (Key Pharm) Nitroglycerin. Transdermal system releasing 2.5 mg, 5 mg, 7.5 mg, 10 mg or 15 mg/24 hours. Carton 30s.
Use: Antianginal.
NITROFAN CAPS. (Major) Nitrofurantoin 50 mg or 100 mg/Cap. Bot. 100s, 500s.
Use: Urinary anti-infective.
NITROFOR-50. (Kenyon) Nitrofurantoin 50 mg/Tab. Bot. 100s, 1000s.

Use: Urinary anti-infective.
NITROFOR-100. (Kenyon) Nitrofurantoin 100 mg/Tab. Bot. 100s, 1000s.
Use: Urinary anti-infective.
• **NITROFURANTOIN,** U.S.P. XXIII. Tab., Cap., Inj., U.S.P. XXIII. 2,4-Imidazolidinedione, 1-[[(5-nitro-2-fura- nyl)methylene]-amino]-. 1-[(5-Nitrofur- furylidene)amino]hydantoin. 1-(5-Nitro-furfurlyideneamino)imidazoline-2,4-dione. Berkfurin; Furadantin; Urantoin.
Use: Antibacterial for urinary tract infections.
See: Furadantin, Preps. (Norwich Eaton).
Furalan, Tab. (Lannett).
Macrobid, Cap. (Procter & Gamble).
Nitrex, Tab. (Star).
Nitrofor-50, Tab. (Kenyon).
Nitrofor-100, Tab. (Kenyon).
Nitrofurantoin sodium, Vial (Norwich Eaton).
Urotoin, Tab. (Scruggs).
NITROFURANTOIN MACROCRYSTALS. (Various Mfr.) 25 mg (Schein only), 50 mg or 100 mg. Cap. Bot. 30s, 100s, 500s, 1000s.
Use: Urinary anti-infective.
See: Macrodantin, Cap. (Norwich Eaton).
• **NITROFURAZONE,** U.S.P. XXIII. Cream, Oint., Topical Soln., U.S.P. XXIII. 5-Nitro-2-furaldehyde semicarbazone. (Various Mfr.) **Top. Soln:** 0.2%. Bot. Pt., gal. **Oint.:** 0.2%. Tube 480 g.
Use: Bacteriostatic for surface wounds.
See: Furacin, Preps. (Roberts).
Nitrazone, Cream, Soln., Dressing (Kenyon).
Nitrozone, Oint. (Century).
W/Allantoin, stearic acid.
See: Eldezol, Oint. (Elder).
NITROGARD. (Parke-Davis) Transmucosal controlled-released nitroglycerin 1 mg, 2 mg or 3 mg/Tab. Bot. 100s.
Use: Antianginal.
• **NITROGEN,** N.F. XVIII.
Use: Pharmaceutic aid (air displacement).
NITROGEN MONOXIDE. Laughing Gas, Nitrous Oxide.
Use: Inhalation anesthetic, analgesic.
NITROGEN MUSTARD.
See: Mustargen, Vial (Merck & Co.).
NITROGEN MUSTARD DERIVATIVES.
See: Leukemia Agents.
Leukeran, Tab. (Burroughs-Wellcome).
Mustargen HCl, Vial (Merck & Co.).
Triethylene Melamine, Tab. (Lederle).

NITROGLYCERIN. (Various Mfr.) 5 mg/ml. Inj. Vial 5 ml, 10 ml.
Use: Antianginal.
• **NITROGLYCERIN, DILUTED,** U.S.P. XXIII.
Use: Vasodilator.
NITROGLYCERIN IN 5% DEXTROSE. (Various Mfr.) **25 mg, 100 mg:** Inj. Soln. 250 ml. **50 mg:** Inj. Soln. 250, 500 ml. **200 mg:** Inj. Soln. 500 ml.
Use: Antianginal.
• **NITROGLYCERIN INJECTION,** U.S.P. XXIII. (Abbott) 25 mg/ml. Vial 5 ml, 10 ml.
Use: Vasodilator, treatment of angina.
See: Tridil, Inj. (American Critical Care).
NITROGLYCERIN, INTRAVENOUS.
See: Nitro-Bid IV (Marion Merrell Dow). Tridil (Du Pont).
• **NITROGLYCERIN OINTMENT,** U.S.P. XXIII.
Use: Vasodilator.
• **NITROGLYCERIN TABLETS,** U.S.P. XXIII. 1,2,3-Propanetriol, trinitrate. (Various Mfr.) Glyceryl Trinitrate, Glonoin, Nitroglycerol, Trinitrin, Trinitroglycerol Tab.
Use: Vasodilator.
See: Niglycon, Tab. (Consoln. Midland).
Niong, Tab. (U.S. Ethicals).
Nitrobid, Cap. (Marion Merrell Dow).
Nitrocels, Cap. (Winston).
Nitrodyl, Cap. (Bock).
Nitrogard (Parke-Davis).
Nitroglyn, Tab. (Key Pharm.).
Nitrol Oint. (Kremers-Urban).
Nitro-Lyn, Cap. (Lynwood).
Nitrong, Tab. (Wharton).
Nitrospan, Cap. (Rhone-Poulenc Rorer).
Nitrotym, Cap. (Kenyon).
Nitro, TD Cap. (Fleming).
Trates, Cap. (Solvay).
Vasoglyn, Unicelles (Solvay).
W/Butabarbital.
See: Nitrodyl-B, Cap. (Bock).
Nitrotym-Plus, Cap. (Kenyon).
NITROGLYCERIN TRANSDERMAL.
Use: Vasodilator.
See: Deponit 5 and 10 (Wyeth-Ayerst).
Nitrodisc (Searle).
NTS (Bolar).
Transderm-Nitro (Ciba).
NITROGLYCEROL.
See: Nitroglycerin (Various Mfr.).
NITROGLYN. (Key) Nitroglycerin 2.5 mg, 6.5 mg or 9 mg/SR Cap. Bot. 100s.
Use: Antianginal.
NITROL IV. (Rhone-Poulenc Rorer) Nitroglycerin 0.8 mg/ml. Amp. 1 ml Box 25s; 10 ml Box 10s; 30 ml Box 5s.

Use: Antianginal.
NITROL IV CONCENTRATE. (Rhone-Poulenc Rorer) Nitroglycerin for infusion 50 mg/10 ml. Amp. Box 10s.
Use: Antianginal.
NITROLAN. (Elan) Protein 60 g, fat 40 g, carbohydrates 160 g, sodium 690 mg, potassium 1.17 g/L, lactose free. With appropriate vitamins and minerals. Liq. In 237 ml Tetra Pak containers and 1000 ml New Pak closed systems with and without Color Check.
Use: Enteral nutritional supplement.
NITROLIN. (Schein) Nitroglycerin 2.5 mg or 9 mg/SR Cap. **2.5 mg:** Bot. 100s. **9 mg:** Bot. 60s.
Use: Antianginal.
NITROLINGUAL SPRAY. (Rhone-Poulenc Rorer) Nitroglycerin lingual aerosol 0.4 mg/metered dose. Canister 13.8 Gm containing 200 metered doses.
Use: Antianginal.
NITROL OINTMENT. (Adria) Nitroglycerin 2% in lanolin and petrolatum base. Tube 30 Gm, 60 Gm, Pack 6s.
Use: Antianginal.
NITRO-LYN. (Lynwood) Nitroglycerin 2.5 mg/Cap. Bot. 100s.
Use: Antianginal.
NITROMANNITE.
See: Mannitol Hexanitrate (Various Mfr.).
NITROMANNITOL.
See: Mannitol Hexanitrate (Various Mfr.).
NITROMED. (U.S. Ethicals) Nitroglycerin 2.6 mg or 6.5 mg/CR Tab. Bot. 100s.
Use: Antianginal.
• **NITROMERSOL,** U.S.P. XXIII. Topical Soln., U.S.P. XXIII. Tincture, U.S.P. XXI. 4-Nitro-3-hydroxy mercuri-o-cresol anhydride. 5-Methyl-2-nitro-7-oxa-8-mercurabicyclo (4.2.0) octa-1,3,5-triene. Metaphen.
Use: Local anti-infective.
• **NITROMIDE.** USAN. 3,5-Dinitrobenzamide.
Use: Coccidiostat, antibacterial.
• **NITROMIFENE CITRATE.** USAN.
Use: Anti-estrogen.
NITRONET. (U.S. Ethicals) Nitroglycerin 2.6 mg or 6.5 mg/CR Tab. Bot. 100s.
Use: Antianginal.
NITRONG OINTMENT. (Wharton) Nitroglycerin 2%. Oint. Tube 30 Gm, 60 Gm with dose applicator.
Use: Antianginal.
NITRONG TABLETS. (Wharton) Nitroglycerin 2.6 mg, 6.5 mg or 9 mg/CR Tab. Bot. 30s, 60s (9 mg), 100s.

Use: Antianginal.
NITROPHENOL-p.
See: p-NITROPHENOL.
NITROPRESS. (Abbott Hospital Prods.)
Sodium nitroprusside 50 mg/2 ml. Vial.
Use: Antihypertensive.
NITROPRUSSIDE SODIUM.
Use: Antihypertensive.
See: Nipride, Pow. for Inj. (Roche).
Nitropress, Pow. for Inj. (Abbott).
Sodium Nitroprusside, Pow. for Inj.
(Various Mfr.).
• **NITROSCANATE.** USAN.
Use: Anthelmintic.
NITROSOUREAS.
Use: Alkylating agent (antineoplastic).
See: CeeNu (Bristol Myers Oncology).
BiCNU (Bristol Myers Oncology).
Zanosar (Upjohn).
Thiotepa (Lederle).
NITROSTAT. (Parke-Davis) Nitroglycerin
0.15 mg, 0.3 mg, 0.4 mg or 0.6 mg/Tab.
Bot. 25s, 100s, UD 100s.
Use: Antianginal.
NITROSTAT IV. (Parke-Davis) Nitroglyc-
erin for infusion. **0.8 mg/ml:** Amp. 10 ml.
5 mg/ml: Amp. 10 ml, Vial 10 ml. **10
mg/ml:** Vial 10 ml.
Use: Antianginal.
NITROUS ACID, SODIUM SALT. Sodium
Nitrite, U.S.P. XXIII.
• **NITROUS OXIDE,** U.S.P. XXIII. Laughing
Gas. Nitrogen Monoxide.
Use: General anesthetic (inhalation).
NITROXOLINE. B.A.N. 8-Hydroxy-5-ni-
troquinoline. Nibiol.
Use: Antibacterial.
• **NIVAZOL.** USAN. 2'-(p-Fluorophenyl)-
2H-17α-pregna-2,4-dien-20-yno [3,2-
c]pyrazol-17-ol.
Use: Glucocorticoid.
NIVEA MOISTURIZING. (Beiersdorf)
Cream: Mineral oil, petrolatum, lanolin
alcohol, glycerin, microcrystalline wax,
paraffin, magnesium sulfate, decy-
loleate, octyl dodecanol, aluminum
stearate, citric acid, magnesium
stearate. In 120 Gm, 180 Gm, 300 Gm,
480 Gm. **Lot.:** Mineral oil, lanolin, isopropyl myristate, cetearyl alcohol, glyceryl stearate, acrylamide/sodium acrylate copolymer, simethicone, methy-
chloroisothiazolinone, methylisothiazolinone. In 180 ml, 300
ml, 450 ml.
Use: Emollient.
NIVEA MOISTURIZING CREME SOAP.
(Beiersdorf) Sodium tallowate, sodium
cocoate, glycerin, petrolatum, titanium
dioxide, NaCl, octyldodecanol,

macadamia nut oil, aloe, sodium thiosulfate, lanolin alcohol, pentasodium pentetate, EDTA, BHT, beeswax. Bar 90 g,
150 g.
Use: Skin cleanser.
NIVEA OIL. (Beiersdorf) Emulsion of neu-
tral aliphatic hydrocarbons. **Liq.:** Bot. 2
oz, 4 fl oz, pt, qt. **Cream:** Tube 1 oz, 2⅓
oz, Jar 4 oz, 6 oz, 1 lb, 5 lb. tin. **Soap:**
Bath or toilet size.
Use: Emollient.
See: Basic, soap (Beiersdorf).
NIVEA SUN. (Beiersdorf) Octyl
methoxycinnamate, octyl salicylate,
benzophenone-3, 2-phenylbenzimida-
zole-5-sulfonic acid. Lot. Bot. 120 ml.
Use: Sunscreen.
• **NIVIMEDONE SODIUM.** USAN.
Use: Anti-allergic.
NIX CREME RINSE. (Burroughs Well-
come) Permethrin 1%. Bot. 2 oz.
Use: Pediculicide.
• **NIZATIDINE.** USAN.
Use: Anti-ulcerative (Histamine H$_2$-re-
ceptor antagonist).
See: Axid, Cap. (Lilly).
NIZORAL CREAM. (Janssen) Ketocona-
zole 2% cream. Tube 15 Gm, 30 Gm.
Use: Antifungal, external.
NIZORAL SUSPENSION. (Janssen) Ke-
toconazole 20 mg/ml. Saccharin. Bot. 4
oz.
Use: Antifungal.
NIZORAL TABLETS. (Janssen) Keto-
conazole 200 mg/Tab. Bot. 100s. Box of
10 strips of 10 tablets.
Use: Antifungal.
N-METHYLHYDRAZINE.
Use: Antineoplastic.
See: Procarbazine.
**N-METHYLISATIN BETA-THIOSEMI-
CARBAZONE.** Under study.
Use: Smallpox protection.
N-MULTISTIX. (Miles Diagnostic) Glu-
cose, protein, pH, blood, ketones, biliru-
bin, urobilinogen, nitrate, leukocytes. Kit
100s.
Use: In vitro diagnostic aid.
N-MULTISTIX S. G. REAGENT STRIPS.
(Miles Diagnostic) Urinalysis reagent
strip test for pH, protein, glucose, ke-
tones, bilirubin, blood, nitrite, urobilino-
gen and specific gravity. Bot. 100s.
Use: Diagnostic aid.
N, N-DIETHYLVANILLAMIDE.
See: Ethamivan, Inj. (Various Mfr.)
NO-ASPIRIN. (Walgreen) Aceta-
minophen 325 mg/Tab. Bot. 100s.
Use: Analgesic.
NO-ASPIRIN EXTRA STRENGTH. (Wal-

green) Acetaminophen 500 mg/Tab. or Cap. **Tab.**: Bot. 60s, 100s. **Cap.**: Bot. 50s, 100s.
Use: Analgesic.

•**NOBERASTINE.** USAN.
Use: Antihistamine.

•**NOCODAZOLE.** USAN.
Use: Antineoplastic.

NODOZ. (Bristol-Myers) Caffeine 100 mg, aspartame, phenylalanine 15 mg, spearmint flavor. Chew. Tab. Pkg. 12s, 30s.
Use: Analeptic.

NO-DROWSINESS ALLEREST. (Fisons) Pseudoephedrine HCl 30 mg, acetaminophen 325 mg/Tab. Bot. 20s.
Use: Decongestant, analgesic.

NO DROWSINESS SINAREST. (Fisons) Pseudoephedrine HCl 30 mg, acetaminophen 500 mg/Tab. Bot. 24s.
Use: Decongestant, analgesic.

•**NOGALAMYCIN.** USAN.
Use: Antineoplastic.

NO-HIST CAPSULES. (Dunhall) Phenylephrine HCl 5 mg, phenylpropanolamine HCl 40 mg, pseudoephedrine HCl 40 mg/Cap. Bot. 100s.
Use: Decongestant.

NO-HIST-S SYRUP. (Dunhall) Phenylephrine HCl 5 mg, phenylpropanolamine HCl 40 mg, pseudoephedrine HCl 40 mg/5 ml. Bot. pt.
Use: Decongestant.

NOKANE. (Wren) Salicylamide 4 gr, N-acetyl-p-aminophenol 4 gr, caffeine 0.5 gr/Tab. Bot. 40s.
Use: Analgesic combination.

NOLAHIST. (Carrnick) Phenindamine tartrate 25 mg/Tab. Bot. 100s.
Use: Antihistamine.

NOLAMINE. (Carrnick) Chlorpheniramine maleate 4 mg, phenindamine tartrate 24 mg, phenylpropanolamine HCl 50 mg/Tab. Bot. 100s, 250s.
Use: Antihistamine, decongestant.

NOLEX LA. (Carrnick). Phenylpropanolamine 75 mg, guaifenesin 400 mg/SR Tab. Bot. 100s.
Use: Decongestant, expectorant.

•**NOLINIUM BROMIDE.** USAN.
Use: Anti-ulcerative, antisecretory.

NOLVADEX. (Zeneca) Tamoxifen citrate equivalent to 10 mg tamoxifen/Tab. Bot. 60s, 250s.
Use: Antineoplastic agent.

NOMETIC. Diphenidol.
Use: Antiemetic.

NOMIFENSINE. B.A.N. 8-Amino-1,2,3,4-tetrahydro-2-methyl-4-phenylisoquinoline.

Use: Thymoleptic and central nervous system stimulant.

Note: Some products withdrawn from market due to incidence of hemolytic anemia.

NO MORE BURN. (Johnson & Johnson) Lidocaine HCl 2.3%, benzethonium Cl 0.13%, aloe. Spray bot. 89 ml.
Use: Local anesthetic, topical.

NO MORE GERMIES SOAP. (Johnson & Johnson) Triclosan 0.25%, PEG, EDTA. Bar 237 ml.
Use: Antiseptic and germicide.

NO MORE GERMIES TOWELETTES. (Johnson & Johnson) Benzalkonium chloride, aloe vera gel, EDTA, methylparaben, SD alcohol 40 15%. Pkg. 24 individually wrapped.
Use: Antiseptics and germicides.

NO MORE ITCHIES. (Johnson & Johnson) Hydrocortisone 1%, SD alcohol 40-B 45%. Spray bot. 67 ml.
Use: Topical corticosteroid.

NO MORE OUCHIES. (Johnson & Johnson) Lidocaine HCl 2.3%, benzethonium Cl 0.13%. Spray bot. 89 ml.
Use: Local anesthetic, topical.

NONAMIN. (Western Research) Calcium 100 mg, chloride 90 mg, magnesium 50 mg, zinc 3.75 mg, iron 4.5 mg, copper 0.5 mg, iodine 37.5 mcg, potassium 49 mg, phosphorus 100 mg/Tab. Bot. 1000s.
Use: Mineral supplement.

NON-DROWSY CONTAC SINUS. (SK Beecham) Pseudoephedrine HCl 30 mg, acetaminophen 500 mg. Cap. Bot. 24s.
Use: Decongestant combination.

NONE. (Forest) Heparin sodium 1000 units/ml. No preservatives. Amps 5 ml. Box 25s.
Use: Anticoagulant.

NONOXYNOL. (Ortho) Nonylphenoxypolyethoxyethanol.
Use: Spermicide.
See: Emko, Preps. (Emko).

•**NONOXYNOL 4.** USAN. Nonylphenoxypoly-ethyleneoxyethanol. Igepal CO-430. Under study.
Use: Nonionic surfactant.

•**NONOXYNOL 9,** U.S.P. XXIII. Poly (ethylene glycol) p-nonylphenyl ether. Igepal CO-630.
Use: Spermatocide.
See: Because, Foam (Schering). Conceptrol, Cream, Gel (Ortho). Delfen, Foam (Ortho). Emko Prods. (Emko-Schering). Encare, Insert (Eaton-Merz).

Gynol II, Jelly (Ortho).
Intercept, Inserts (Ortho).
Ortho-Creme, Cream (Ortho).
Ortho-Gynol, Jelly (Ortho).
• **NONOXYNOL 10,** U.S.P. XXIII.
Use: Spermatocide.
• **NONOXYNOL 15.** USAN. Nonylphenoxy-
poly-ethyleneoxyethanol. Igepal CO-
880. Under study.
Use: Nonionic surfactant.
• **NONOXYNOL 30.** USAN. Nonylphenoxy-
poly-ethyleneoxyethanol. Under study.
Use: Nonionic surfactant.
NONSPECIFIC PROTEIN THERAPY.
See: Protein, Nonspecific Therapy.
**NONSTEROIDAL INFLAMMATORY
AGENTS, OPHTHALMIC.**
See: Ocufen (Allergan).
Profenal (Alcon).
Voltaren (Ciba Vision Ophthalmics).
**NONYLPHENOXYPOLYETHOXY
ETHANOL.** Nonoxynol.
Use: Spermicide.
See: Delfen Vaginal Foam (Ortho).
• **NORACYMETHADOL HCl.** USAN. α-4,
4-Diphenyl-6-methylamino-3-heptanol
acetate HCl.
Use: Analgesic agent.
• **NORBOLETHONE.** USAN. 13-Ethyl-17-
hydroxy-18, 19-dinor-17αa-pregn-4-en-
3-one.
Use: Anabolic.
NORBUTRINE. D.A.N. 2-Cyclobuty-
lamino-1-(3,4-dihydroxyphenyl) ethanol.
Use: Bronchodilator.
NORCET TABLETS. (Holloway) Hy-
drocodone bitartrate 5 mg, acetaminophen 500 mg/Tab. Bot. 100s.
Use: Narcotic analgesic combination.
NORCODEINE. B.A.N. N-Demethyl-O³-
methylmor-phine.
Use: Narcotic analgesic.
NORCURON. (Organon) Vecuronium
bromide 10 mg/5 ml. **With diluent:** Vial 5
ml lyophilized powder and 5 ml ampul of
sterile water for injection. Box 10s. **Without diluent:** Vial 5 ml lyophilized powder. Box 10s. **Prefilled syringe:** Vial 10
ml lyophilized powder and 10 ml syringe
w/bacteriostatic water for injection. Box
10s.
Use: Muscle relaxant, adjunct to anesthesia.
NORCYCLINE. 6-Demethyl-6-deoxyte-
tracycline. Bonomycin. Sancycline.
Use: Anti-infective.
NORDETTE. (Wyeth-Ayerst) Levonorgestrel 0.15 mg, ethinyl estradiol
0.03 mg/Tab. 6 Pilpak dispensers, 21
day and 28 day w/ 7 inert tabs.

Use: Oral contraceptive.
NOREL PLUS CAPSULES. (U.S. Pharmaceutical Corp.) Chlorpheniramine
maleate 4 mg, phenyltoloxamine dihydrogen citrate 25 mg, phenylpropanolamine HCl 25 mg, acetaminophen 325 mg/Cap. Bot. 100s.
Use: Antihistamine, decongestant, analgesic.
• **NOREPINEPHRINE BITARTRATE,**
U.S.P. XXIII. Inj., U.S.P. XXIII. 1,2-Ben-
zenediol, 4-(2-amino-1-hydroxyethyl)-,
2,3-dihydroxybutanedioate (1:1) (Salt),
monohydrate l-a-(Aminomethyl)3,4-di-
hydroxybenzyl alcohol bitartrate.
Use: Adrenergic (vasopressor).
See: Levophed Bitartrate, Soln., Amp.
(Sanofi Winthrop).
NORETHANDROLONE, B.A.N. 17-Al-
phaethyl-17-hydroxynorandrostenone,
17-Hydroxy-19-nor-17α- pregn-4-en-3-
one. Nileyar.
Use: Anabolic steroid.
NORETHIN 1/50 M. (Roberts) Norethin-
drone 1 mg, mestranol 50 mcg/Tab. 21
day and 28 day (with 7 inert tabs.).
Use: Oral contraceptive.
NORETHIN 1/35 E. (Roberts) Norethin-
drone 1 mg, ethinyl estradiol 35 mg/Tab.
21 day and 28 day (with 7 inert tabs.).
Use: Oral contraceptive.
• **NORETHINDRONE,** U.S.P. XXIII. Tab.,
U.S.P. XXIII. 19-Norpregn-4-en-20-yn-3-
one, 17-hydroxy-, (17α)-. 17-Hydroxy-
19-nor-17-alpha-pregn-4-en-20-yn-3-
one.
Use: Progestin.
See: Micronor, Tab. (Ortho).
Norlutin, Tab. (Parke-Davis).
Nor-QD, Tab. (Syntex).
W/Ethinyl estradiol.
See: Brevicon 21 and 28, Tab. (Syntex).
GenCept, Tab. (Gencon).
Jenest-28, Tab. (Organon).
Modicon 21 and 28, Tab. (Ortho).
Ortho-Novum 21 and 28, Prods. (Or-
tho).
Ovcon-35, Tab. (Mead Johnson).
Ovcon-50, Tab. (Mead Johnson).
W/Mestranol.
See: Norinyl, Prods. (Syntex).
Ortho-Novum, Prods. (Ortho).
W/Mestranol, ferrous fumarate.
See: Norinyl-I Fe 28, Prods. (Syntex).
• **NORETHINDRONE ACETATE,** U.S.P.
XXIII. Tab., U.S.P. XXIII. 19-Norpregn-4-
en-20-yn-3-one, 17-(acetyloxy)-, (17α)-,
17α-Ethinyl-19-nortestosterone. 17-Hy-
droxy-19-nor-17α-pregn-4-en-20-yn-3-
one Acetate.

Use: Progestin.
See: Aygestin, Tab. (Wyeth-Ayerst).
Norlutate, Tab. (Parke-Davis).
• **NORETHINDRONE ACETATE AND ETHINYL ESTRADIOL TABLETS,** U.S.P. XXIII.
Use: Oral contraceptive.
See: Brevicon, Tab. (Syntex).
Cootoot, Tab. (Squibb).
Loestrin, Prods. (Parke-Davis).
Norinyl, Prods. (Syntex).
Norlestrin, Prods. (Parke-Davis).
• **NORETHINDRONE AND ETHINYL ESTRADIOL TABLETS,** U.S.P. XXIII.
Use: Oral contraceptive.
• **NORETHINDRONE AND MESTRANOL TABLETS,** U.S.P. XXIII.
Use: Oral contraceptive.
NORETHISTERONE. B.A.N. 17β-Hydroxy-19-norpregn-4-en-20-yn-3-one. 17α-Ethynyl-17β-hydroxyoestr-4-en-3-one. 17α-Ethynyl-19-nor-testosterone. Micronor; Noriday; Primolut N; Norlutin-A [acetate].
Use: Progestin.
• **NORETHYNODREL,** U.S.P. XXIII. 17-Hydroxy-19-nor-17α-pregn-5(10)-en-20-yn-3-one.
Use: Progesterone agent.
See: Enovid, Prods. (Searle).
NORFLEX. (3M Pharm) Orphenadrine citrate 100 mg/SR Tab. Bot. 100s, 500s.
Use: Skeletal muscle relaxant.
NORFLEX INJECTABLE. (3M Pharm) Orphenadrine citrate 30 mg, sodium bisulfite 2 mg, sodium Cl 5.8 mg, water for injection qs 2 ml. Amp. 2 ml 6s, 50s.
Use: Skeletal muscle relaxant.
• **NORFLOXACIN.** USAN.
Use: Quinolone antibacterial.
See: Chibroxin, Ophth. Soln. (Merck).
Noroxin, Tab. (Merck & Co.).
• **NORFLURANE.** USAN. 1,1,1,2-Tetrafluoroe-thane. Under study.
Use: Inhalation anesthetic.
NORFORMS. (Fleet) PEG 20, PEG 6, PEG 20 palmitate, lactic acid, methylbenzethonium Cl/Supp. Unscented and herbal scent. Box 6s, 12s, 24s.
Use: Vaginal preparation.
NORGESIC FORTE TABLETS. (Riker) Orphenadrine citrate 50 mg, aspirin 770 mg, caffeine 60 mg/Tab. Bot. 100s, 500s, UD 100s.
Use: Skeletal muscle relaxant, salicylate analgesic.
NORGESIC TABLETS. (Riker) Orphenadrine citrate 25 mg, aspirin 385 mg, caffeine 30 mg/Tab. Bot. 100s, 500s, UD 100s.

Use: Skeletal muscle relaxant, salicylate analgesic.
• **NORGESTIMATE.** USAN.
Use: Progestin.
W/ Ethinyl estradiol.
See: Ortho-Cyclen, Tab. (Ortho).
Ortho Tri-Cyclen, Tab. (Ortho).
• **NORGESTOMET.** USAN.
Use: Progestin.
• **NORGESTREL,** U.S.P. XXIII. Tab., U.S.P. XXIII. 18,19-Dinorpregn-4-en-20-yn-3-one, 13-ethyl-17-hydroxy,-(17 α)-(+)-. (±)-13-Ethyl-17-hydroxy-18, 19-dinor-17α-pregn-4-en-20-yn-3-one. (±)-13-Ethyl-17α-ethynyl-17-hydroxygon-4-en-3-one.
Use: Oral contraceptive.
See: Ovrette, Tab. (Wyeth-Ayerst).
• **NORGESTREL AND ETHINYL ESTRADIOL TABLETS,** U.S.P. XXIII.
Use: Oral contraceptive.
See: Lo/Ovral, Tab. (Wyeth-Ayerst).
Ovral-Prep. (Wyeth-Ayerst).
NORINYL 1 + 35. (Syntex) Norethindrone 1 mg, ethinyl estradiol 0.035 mg/Tab. Wallette 21 and 28 day (7 inert tabs).
Use: Oral contraceptive.
NORINYL 1 + 50. (Syntex) Norethindrone1 mg, mestranol 0.05 mg/Tab. Wallette 21 and 28 day (7 inert tabs).
Use: Oral contraceptive.
NORINYL 2 MG. (Syntex) Norethindrone 2 mg, mestranol 0.1 mg/Tab. Memorette Disp. of 20s. Refill folders of 20s.
Use: Oral contraceptive.
NORISODRINE AEROTROL. (Abbott) Norisodrine HCl (isoproterenol HCl) 0.25% (2.8 mg/ml) in inert chlorofluorohydrocarbon propellants, alcohol 33%, ascorbic acid 0.1% as preservative. Aerotrol 15 ml. Box 12s.
Use: Bronchodilator.
NORISODRINE WITH CALCIUM IODIDE SYRUP. (Abbott) Isoproterenol sulfate 3 mg, calcium iodide, anhydrous 150 mg/5 ml, alcohol 6%. Bot. pt.
Use: Bronchodilator.
NORLAC RX. (Solvay) Calcium 200 mg, iron 60 mg, vitamins A 8000 IU, D 400 IU, E 30 mg, B₁ 2 mg, B₂ 2 mg, B₃ 20 mg, B₆ 4 mg, B₁₂ 8 mcg, C 90 mg, folic acid 1 mg, Cu, I, Mg, zinc 15 mg/Tab. Bot. 100s, Unit-of-use 100s.
Use: Vitamin/mineral supplement.
NORLESTRIN-21 1/50 TABLETS. (Parke-Davis) Norethindrone acetate 1 mg, ethinyl estradiol 50 mcg/Tab. (yellow). Compact 21s. Pkg. 5 compacts. Pkg. 5 refills; Ctn. 10 ×5 refills.
Use: Oral contraceptive.

NORLESTRIN-28 1/50 TABLET. (Parke-Davis) Norethindrone acetate 1 mg, ethinyl estradiol 50 mcg/Tab. (yellow). Compact 21 yellow, 7 white (inert) tablets. Pkg. 5 compacts. Pkg. 5 refills; Ctn. 10×5 refills.
Use: Oral contraceptive.

NORLESTRIN-21 2.5/50 TABLETS. (Parke-Davis) Norethindrone acetate 2.5 mg, ethinyl estradiol 50 mcg/Tab. (pink). Compact 21s. Pkg. 5 compacts. Pkg. 5 refills; Ctn. 10×5 refills.
Use: Oral contraceptive.

NORLESTRIN Fe 1/50 TABLETS. (Parke-Davis) Norethindrone acetate 1 mg, ethinyl estradiol 50 mcg/Tab. (yellow). Compact 21 yellow tab., 7 brown 75 mg ferrous fumarate tab. Pkg. 5 compacts. Pkg. 5 refills; ctn. 10×5 refills.
Use: Oral contraceptive.

NORLESTRIN Fe 2.5/50 TABLETS. (Parke-Davis) Norethindrone acetate 2.5 mg, ethinyl estradiol 50 mcg/Tab. (pink). Compact 21 pink tab., 7 brown 75 mg ferrous fumarate tab. Pkg. 5 compacts. Pkg. 5 refills; Ctn. 10×5 refills.
Use: Oral contraceptive.

NORLEVORPHANOL. B.A.N. ( ) 3-hydroxymorphinan.
Use: Narcotic analgesic.

NORLUTATE. (Parke-Davis) Norethindrone acetate 5 mg/Tab. Bot. 50s.
Use: Progestin.

NORLUTIN. (Parke-Davis) Norethindrone 5 mg/Tab. Bot. 50s.
Use: Progestin.

NORMADERM CREAM & LOTION. (Doak) Buffered lactic acid in vanishing bases. **Cream:** Jar 3¾ oz, 16 oz. **Lot.:** Bot. 4 oz, 16 oz, 128 oz.
Use: Emollient, acid restorer for skin.

NORMAL HUMAN SERUM ALBUMIN. Albumin Human, U.S.P. XXIII.

NORMAL SALINE.
See: 0.2% Sodium chloride (Solopak).
0.45% sodium chloride (1/2 normal saline) (Various Mfr.).
0.9% Sodium chloride (Normal saline) (Various Mfr.).
3% Sodium chloride (Various Mfr.).
5% Sodium chloride (Various Mfr.).

NORMALINE KIT. (Apothecary Products) Salt tablets for normal saline 250 mg/Tab. Preservative free. 200s with Bot. 27.7 ml.
Use: Ophthalmic preparation.

NORMETHADONE. B.A.N. 6-Dimethylamino-4,4-di-phenylhexan-3-one.
Use: Narcotic analgesic.

NORMETHANDRONE. (Parke-Davis)

17-α-methyl-19-nortestoster-one.
17β-Hydroxy-17-methylestr-4-en-3-one. Methalutin.

NORMODYNE. (Schering) Labetalol HCl. **Inj.:** 5 mg/ml. Amp. 20 ml, 40 ml, 60 ml. **Tab.:** 100 mg, 200 mg or 300 mg. Bot. 100s, 500s, UD 100s. Calendar pak 56s.
Use: Antihypertensive.

NORMOL. (Alcon Lenscare) Sterile, isotonic solution of thimerosal 0.004%, chlorhexidine gluconate 0.005%, edetate disodium 0.1%. Bot. 8 oz.
Use: Soft contact lens care.

NORMORPHINE. B.A.N. N-Demethylmorphine.
Use: Narcotic analgesic.

NORMOSOL-M in D5-W. (Abbott Hospital Prods) Dextrose 5 Gm, sodium Cl 234 mg, potassium acetate 128 mg, magnesium acetate 21 mg, sodium bisulfite 30 mg/100 ml. Bot. 500 ml, 1000 ml in Abbo-Vac (glass) or Life Care (flexible) containers.
Use: Parenteral nutritional supplement.

NORMOSOL-R; NORMOSOL-R pH 7.4; 500 ml., 1000 ml. NORMOSOL-R D5-W. (Abbott Hospital Prods) Sodium Cl 526 mg, sodium acetate ??? mg, sodium gluconate 502 mg, potassium Cl 37 mg, magnesium Cl 14 mg pH of Normosol-R and Normosol R in D5-W adjusted with HCl/100 ml. Bot. 1000 ml, 500 ml. in Life Care (flexible) containers.
Use: Parenteral nutritional supplement.

NORMOTENSIN. (Marcen) I.M. soln. for inj. Mucopolysaccharide 20 mg, sodium nucleate 25 mg, epinephrine neutralizing factor 25 units, sodium citrate 10 mg, inositol 5 mg, phenol 0.5%/ml. Multidose vial 10 ml, 30 ml.
Use: Antihypertensive.

NOROLON. (Sanofi Winthrop) Chloroquine phosphate.
Use: Antimalarial.

NOROXIN. (Merck & Co.) Norfloxacin 400 mg/Tab. Bot. 100s, UD 20s, UD 100s.
Use: Urinary anti-infective.

NORPACE. (Searle) Disopyramide phosphate 100 mg or 150 mg/Cap. Bot. 100s, 500s, 1000s, UD 100s.
Use: Antiarrhythmic.

NORPACE CR. (Searle) Disopyramide phosphate 100 mg or 150 mg/CR Cap. Bot. 100s, 500s, UD 100s.
Use: Antiarrhythmic.

NORPHYL. (Vita Elixir) Aminophylline 100 mg/Tab.
Use: Bronchodilator.

NORPIPANONE. B.A.N. 4,4-Diphenyl-6-

piperidinohexan-3-one.
Use: Analgesic.
NORPLANT. (Wyeth-Ayerst) Levonorgestrel 36 mg. Implant kit 6s..
Use: Progestin contraceptive system.
NORPRAMIN. (Merrell Dow) Desipramine HCl 10 mg, 25 mg, 50 mg, 75 mg, 100 mg or 150 mg/Tab. **10 mg:** Bot. 100o; **25 mg:** Dot. 100s, 1000s, UD 100s; **50 mg:** Bot. 100s, 1000s, UD 100s; **75 mg:** Bot. 100s; **100 mg:** Bot. 100s. **150 mg:** Bot. 50s.
Use: Antidepressant.
NOR-Q.D. (Syntex) Norethindrone 0.35 mg/Tab. Dispenser 42s.
Use: Oral contraceptive.
NORTESTERIONATE. 19-Nortestosterone cyclopentylpropionate.
NORTRIPTYLINE. (Schein) 10 mg, 25 mg, 50 mg or 75 mg. Cap. Bot. 100s; **25 mg:** Bot. 500s also.
Use: Antidepressant.
• **NORTRIPTYLINE HCl,** U.S.P. XXIII. Oral Soln., Cap. U.S.P. XXIII. 5-(3-Methylaminopropylidene)-10,11- dihydro-5H-dibenzo [a,d] cycloheptene HCl. 10,11-Dihydro-N-methyl-5H-dibenzo(a,d)cycloheptene-D^5, a propylamine Hydrochloride.
Use: Antidepressant.
See: Aventyl HCl, Liq., Pulvule (Lilly). Pamelor, Cap., Liq. (Sandoz).
NORVAL. Docusate sodium.
Use: Laxative.
NORVASC. (Pfizer) Amlodipine **2.5 mg:** Bot. 100s; **5 mg:** Bot. 100s; **10 mg:** Bot. 100s.
Use: Calcium channel blocker.
NORWICH EXTRA STRENGTH. (Procter & Gamble) Aspirin 500 mg/Tab. Bot. 150s.
Use: Salicylate, analgesic.
NORZINE. (Purdue Frederick) **Tab. or Supp.:** Thiethylperazine maleate 10 mg. Bot. 100s. Supp. Pkg 12s. **Inj.:** Thiethylperazine maleate 5 mg/ml. Amp. 2 ml.
Use: Antiemetic/antivertigo agent.
NOSALT. (SK-Beecham) Potassium Cl, potassium bitartrate, adipic acid, mineral oil, fumaric acid. Sodium <10 mg/5 Gm (0.43 mEq/5 Gm), potassium 2502 mg/5 Gm(64 mEq/5 Gm). Pkg. 330 Gm.
Use: Salt substitute.
NOSALT SEASONED. (SK-Beecham) Potassium Cl, dextrose, onion and garlic, spices, lactose, cream of tartar, paprika, silica, disodium inosinate, disodium guanylate, turmeric. Sodium < 5 mg/5 Gm (0.2 mEq/5 Gm), potassium

1328 mg/5 Gm (34 mEq/5 Gm). Pkg. 240 Gm.
Use: Salt substitute.
NOSCAPINE HCl. I-Narcotine hydrochloride.
Use: Antitussive.
See: Conar Prods. (Beecham Labs).
W/Chlorpheniramine maleate, phenylephrine HCl, N-acetyl-p-aminophenol, salicylamide, vitamin C.
See: Noscaps, Cap. (Table Rock).
W/Phenylephrine HCl.
See: Conar Liq. (Beecham Labs).
W/Phenylephrine HCl, guaifensin.
See: Conar, Expectorant (Beecham Labs).
NOSCAPS. (Table Rock) Noscapine 7.5 mg, chlorpheniramine maleate 1 mg, phenylephrine HCl 5 mg, N-acetyl-p-aminophenol 150 mg, salicylamide 150 mg, vitamin C 20 mg/Cap. Bot. 100s, 500s.
Use: Antihistamine, decongestant, analgesic, vitamin C.
• **NOSIHEPTIDE.** USAN.
Use: Growth stimulant.
NOSKOTE. (Schering-Plough) Oxybenzone 3%, homosalate 8%. SPF 8. Cream 13.2 Gm, 30 Gm.
Use: Sunscreen.
NOSKOTE SUNBLOCK. (Schering-Plough) Padimate O 8%, oxybenzone 3%, benzyl alcohol. SPF 15. Cream. Tube 30 Gm.
Use: Sunscreen.
NOSTRIL. (Boehringer I) Phenylephrine HCl 0.25% or 0.5%, benzalkonium Cl 0.004% in buffered aqueous soln. Bot. 15 ml, pump spray.
Use: Decongestant.
NOSTRILLA. (Boehringer I) Oxymetazoline HCl 0.05%, benzalkonium Cl 0.02%. Bot. 15 ml, pump spray.
Use: Decongestant.
NOVACET. (Genderm) Sodium sulfacetamide 100 mg, sulfur 50 mg, propylene glycol, isopropyl myristate, propylene glycol stearate, benzyl alcohol, EDTA. Lot. Bot. 30 ml.
Use: Anti-acne.
NOVA-DEC. (Rugby) Iron 20 mg, vitamins A 10,000 IU, D 400 IU, E 30 mg, B_1 10 mg, B_2 10 mg, B_3 100 mg, B_5 20 mg, B_6 5 mg, B_{12} 6 mcg, C 250 mg, folic acid 0.4 mg, Cu, I, Mg, Mn, zinc 20 mg/Tab. Bot. 100s.
Use: Vitamin/mineral supplement.
NOVADYNE EXPECTORANT. (Various Mfr.) Pseudoephedrine 30 mg, codeine phosphate 10 mg, guaifenesin 100 mg,

alcohol 7.5%. Bot. 120 ml, pt, gal.
Use: Decongestant, antitussive, expectorant.
NOVAFED A CAPSULES. (Marion Merrell Dow) Pseudoephedrine HCl 120 mg, chlorpheniramine maleate 8 mg/CR Cap. Bot. 100s.
Use: Decongestant, antihistamine.
NOVAFED CAPSULES. (Marion Merrell Dow) Pseudoephedrine HCl 120 mg/CR Cap. Bot. 100s.
Use: Decongestant.
NOVAGEST EXPECTORANT W/CODEINE. (Major) Pseudoephedrine HCl 30 mg, codeine phosphate 10 mg, guaifenesin 100 mg/5 ml, alcohol 8.2%. Liq. Bot. 118 ml.
Use: Decongestant, antitussive, expectorant.
NOVAHISTINE DH. (SK-Beecham) Pseudoephedrine HCl 30 mg, codeine phosphate 10 mg, chlorpheniramine maleate 2 mg/5 ml, alcohol 5%, saccharin, sorbitol. Bot. 1 oz, pt.
Use: Decongestant, antitussive, antihistamine.
NOVAHISTINE DMX. (SK-Beecham) Pseudoephedrine HCl 30 mg, dextromethorphan HBr 10 mg, guaifenesin 100 mg/10 ml, alcohol 10%, saccharin, sorbitol, sugar. Bot. 4 oz.
Use: Decongestant, antitussive, expectorant.
NOVAHISTINE ELIXIR. (Lakeside) Phenylephrine HCl 5 mg, chlorpheniramine maleate 2 mg/5 ml, alcohol 5%, sorbitol. Bot. 4 oz, 8 oz.
Use: Decongestant, antihistamine.
NOVAHISTINE EXPECTORANT. (SK-Beecham) Pseudoephedrine HCl 30 mg, codeine phosphate 10 mg, guaifenesin 100 mg/5 ml, alcohol 7.5%, saccharin, sorbitol. Bot. 4 oz, pt.
Use: Decongestant, antitussive, expectorant.
NOVALDIN. (Sanofi Winthrop) Dipyrone Available as Tab., Amp., Drops.
Use: Analgesic.
NOVAMIDON.
See: Aminopyrine (Various Mfr.).
NOVAMINE. (Clintec Nutrition) Amino acid concentration 11.4%, for infusion. Nitrogen 1.8 Gm/100 ml. Essential amino acids (mg/100 ml): Isoleucine 570, leucine 790, lysine 900, methionine 570, phenylalanine 790, threonine 570, tryptophan 190, valine 730. Nonessential amino acids (mg/100 ml): Alanine 1650, arginine 1120, histidine 680, proline 680, serine 450, tyrosine 30, glycine

790, glutamic acid 570, aspartic acid 330, acetate 114 mEq/L, sodium metabisulfite 30 mg/100 ml. In 250 ml, 500 ml, 1 L.
Use: Parenteral nutritional supplement.
NOVAMINE 15%. (Clintec Nutrition) Amino acids 15%: Lysine 1.18 Gm, leucine 1.04 Gm, phenylalanine 1.04 Gm, valine 960 mg, isoleucine 749 mg, methionine 749 mg, threonine 749 mg, tryptophan 250 mg, alanine 2.17 Gm, arginine 1.47 Gm, glycine 1.04 Gm, histidine 894 mg, proline 894 mg, glutamic acid 749 mg, serine 592 mg, aspartic acid 434 mg, tyrosine 39 mg, nitrogen 2.37 Gm/100 ml. Inj. 500 ml, 1000 ml.
Use: Parenteral nutritional supplement.
NOVAMINE WITHOUT ELECTROLYTES. (Clintec Nutrition) Amino acid concentration 8.5%, for infusion. Nitrogen 1.35 Gm/100 ml. Essential amino acids (mg/100 ml): Isoleucine 420, leucine 590, lysine 673, methionine 420, phenylalanine 590, threonine 420, tryptophan 140, valine 550. Nonessential amino acids (mg/100 ml): Alanine 1240, arginine 840, histidine 500, proline 500, serine 340, tyrosine 20, glycine 590, glutamic acid 420, aspartic acid 250, acetate 88 mEq/L, sodium bisulfite 30 mg/100 ml. In 500 ml, 1 L.
Use: Parenteral nutritional supplement.
NOVANTRONE. (Lederle) Mitoxantrone HCl 2 mg base/ml. Inj. Vial 10 ml, 12.5 ml, 15 ml.
Use: Antineoplastic agent.
NOVATOPHAN.
See: Neocinchophen (Various Mfr.).
NOVATROPINE.
See: Homatropine Methylbromide (Various Mfr.).
• **NOVOBIOCIN CALCIUM,** U.S.P. XXIII. Oral Susp., U.S.P. XXIII.
Use: Antibacterial.
See: Cathomycin Calcium.
NOVOBIOCIN MONOSODIUM SALT.
Use: Antibacterial.
See: Sodium Novobiocin.
• **NOVOBIOCIN SODIUM,** U.S.P. XXIII. Cap., U.S.P. XXIII.
Use: Antibacterial.
See: Albamycin, Cap. (Upjohn). Cathomycin Sodium.
NOVOCAIN. (Sanofi Winthrop) Procaine HCl soln. **1%:** Amp. 2 ml, Box 25s. 6 ml, Box 50s; Vial 30 ml, Box 10s. **2%:** Vial 30 ml, Box 10s.
Use: Local anesthetic.
NOVOCAIN FOR SPINAL ANESTHESIA. (Sanofi Winthrop) Procaine HCl 10%

soln. Amp. 2 ml. Box 25s.
Use: Spinal anesthesia.
NOVOLIN 70/30. (Novo Nordisk) Isophane susp. 70% (human), regular in-
sulin 30% (human, semi-synthetic) 100
units/ml. Inj. Vial 10 ml.
Use: Antidiabetic agent.
NOVOLIN 70/30 PENFILL. (Novo
Nordisk) Isophane insulin suspension
and insulin injection 100 U per ml human
insulin. Cartridge 1.5 ml.
Use: Antidiabetic agent.
NOVOLIN L. (Novo Nordisk) Human in-
sulin (semi-synthetic) 100 units/ml. An
insulin-zinc suspension (Lente). Inj. Vial
10 ml.
Use: Antidiabetic agent.
NOVOLIN N. (Novo Nordisk) Human in-
sulin NPH (semisynthetic) 100 units/ml.
Isophane insulin suspension (insulin
w/protamine and zinc). Inj. Vial 10 ml.
Use: Antidiabetic agent.
NOVOLIN N PENFILL. (Novo Nordisk)
Isophane insulin suspension (NPH) 100
U per ml human insulin. Cartridge. 1.5
ml.
Use: Antidiabetic agent.
NOVOLIN R. (Novo Nordisk) Human in-
sulin, regular (semisynthetic) 100
units/ml. Inj. Vial 10 ml.
Use: Antidiabetic agent.
NOVOLIN R PENFILL. (Novo Nordisk)
Semisynthetic human regular insulin
100 units/ml. Inj. 1.5 ml cartridges.
Use: Antidiabetic agent.
NOXIPTYLINE, B.A.N. 3-(2-Dimethyl-
laminoethyloxy-imino)dibenzo[a,d]cyclo-
hepta-1,4-diene.
Use: Antidepressant.
NOXYTHIOLIN. B.A.N. N-Hydrox-
ymethyl-N'-methylthiourea. Noxyflex.
Use: Antifungal agent.
**NOXZEMA ANTISEPTIC CLEANSER
SENSITIVE SKIN FORMULA.** (Noxell)
Benzalkonium Cl 0.13%. Bot. 4 oz, 8 oz.
Use: Skin cleanser.
**NOXZEMA ANTISEPTIC SKIN
CLEANSER.** (Noxell) SD-40 alcohol
63%. Bot. 4 oz, 8 oz.
Use: Skin cleanser.
**NOXZEMA ANTISEPTIC SKIN
CLEANSER EXTRA STRENGTH FOR-
MULA.** (Noxell) SD-40 alcohol 36%,
isopropyl alcohol 34%. Bot. 4 oz, 8 oz.
Use: Skin cleanser.
NOXZEMA CLEAR-UPS. (Noxell) Sali-
cylic acid 0.5% on pads. Jar 50s.
Use: Anti-acne.
**NOXZEMA CLEAR UPS ACNE MEDI-
CINE MAXIMUM STRENGTH LOTION.**

(Noxell) Benzoyl peroxide 10%. Bot. 1
oz. Vanishing formula.
Use: Anti-acne.
**NOXZEMA CLEAR UPS MAXIMUM
STRENGTH.** (Noxell) Salicylic acid 2%
on pads. Jar 50s.
Use: Anti-acne.
NOXZEMA MEDICATED SKIN CREAM.
(Noxell) Menthol, camphor, clove oil, eu-
calyptus oil, phenol. Jar 2.5 oz, 4 oz, 6
oz, 10 oz. Tube 4.5 oz. Bot. 6 oz., 14 oz.
Pump Bottle 10.5 oz.
Use: Counterirritant.
NOXZEMA ON-THE-SPOT. (Noxell) Ben-
zoyl peroxide 10% in vanishing and tint-
ed lotion. Bot. 0.25 oz.
Use: Anti-acne.
NP-27 AEROSOL. (Thompson Medical)
Tolnaftate 1%, alcohol 14.9%. Spray
Can 100 ml.
Use: Antifungal, external.
NP-27 CREAM. (Thompson Medical) Tol-
naftate 1% in cream base. Tube 45 Gm.
Use: Antifungal, external.
NP-27 LIQUID. (Thompson Medical) Tol-
naftate 1%. Plastic bot. 2 oz.
Use: Antifungal, external.
NPH ILETIN I. (Lilly) Insulin from beef and
pork. 100 units/ml. Inj. Vial 10 ml.
Use: Antidiabetic agent.
NPH INSULIN. (Novo Nordisk) Isophane
insulin suspension (NPH) 100 units per
ml beef. Vial. 10 ml.
Use: Antidiabetic agent.
NPH-N. (Novo Nordisk) Purified pork in-
sulin 100 units/ml in isophane insulin
suspension (insulin w/protamine and
zinc). Inj. Vial 10 ml.
Use: Antidiabetic agent.
**N-TRIFLUOROACETYLADRIAMYCIN-
14-VALERATE.** (Anthra Pharm)
Use: Antineoplastic.
NTS TRANSDERMAL SYSTEM. (Bolar)
Nitroglycerin transdermal system 5
mg/24 hours or 15 mg/24 hours. Box
30s.
Use: Antianginal agent.
NTZ LONG-ACTING. (Sanofi Winthrop.)
Oxymetazoline HCl 0.05%, benzalkoni-
um Cl and phenylmercuric acetate
0.002% as preservatives. Drops. Bot. 1
oz. Spray Bot. 1 oz.
Use: Decongestant.
NUBAIN. (DuPont) Nalbuphine HCl, sodi-
um metabisulfite 0.1%. **10 mg/ml:** Amp
1 ml. Vial 10 ml. Box 1s. **20 mg/ml:** Amp
1 ml. Syringe 1 ml calibrated. Vial 10 ml.
Use: Narcotic analgesic.
NU-BOLIC. (Seatrace) Nandrolone phenpropionate 25 mg/ml. Vial 5 ml.

Use: Anabolic steroid.

NUCITE.
See: Inositol (Various Mfr.).

NUCLEIC ACID ANTAGONISTS.
Use: Antineoplastic agent.
See: Leukeran, Tab. (Burroughs Well-come).
Mustargen, Vial (Merck & Co.).
Myleran, Tab. (Burroughs Wellcome).
Purinethol, Tab. (Burroughs Well-come).
Triethylene Melamine, Tab. (Lederle).

NUCOFED. (Beecham Labs) Codeine phosphate 20 mg, pseudoephedrine HCl 60 mg/5 ml or Cap. Syrup is alcohol-free. **Liq.:** Bot. pt. **Cap.:** Bot. 60s.
Use: Antitussive, decongestant.

NUCOFED EXPECTORANT.
(Roberts/Hauck) Codeine phosphate 20 mg, pseudoephedrine HCl 60 mg, guaifenesin 200 mg/5 ml, alcohol 12.5%, saccharin. Bot. 480 ml.
Use: Antitussive, decongestant, expectorant.

NUCOFED PEDIATRIC EXPECTORANT.
(Roberts) Codeine phosphate 10 mg, pseudoephedrine HCl 30 mg, guaifenesin 100 mg/5 ml, alcohol 6%. Bot. pt.
Use: Antitussive, decongestant, expectorant.

NUCOTUSS EXPECTORANT. (Barre-National) Pseudoephedrine HCl 60 mg, codeine phosphate 20 mg, guaifenesin 200 mg/5 ml, alcohol 12.5%, winter-green flavor. Liq. Bot. 480 ml.
Use: Decongestant, antitussive, expectorant.

NUCOTUSS PEDIATRIC EXPECTO-RANT. (Barre-National) Pseu-doephedrine HCl 30 mg, codeine phosphate 10 mg, guaifenesin 100 mg/5 ml, strawberry flavor. Liq. Bot. 480 ml.
Use: Decongestant, antitussive, expectorant.

• **NUFENOXOLE.** USAN.
Use: Antiperistaltic.

NU-IRON. (Mayrand) Polysaccharide-iron complex. **Cap.:** Elemental iron 150 mg. Bot. 100s. **Elix.:** Elemental iron 100 mg/5 ml. Bot. 8 oz.
Use: Iron supplement.

NU-IRON 150. (Mayrand) Polysaccha-ride-Iron complex 100 mg/5 ml, alcohol 10%. Elix. 237 ml.
Use: Iron supplement.

NU-IRON PLUS ELIXIR. (Mayrand) Poly-saccharide iron complex 100 mg, folic acid 1 mg, vitamin B$_{12}$ 25 mcg/5 ml, al-cohol 10%. Bot. 8 oz.
Use: Vitamin/mineral supplement.

NU-IRON-V. (Mayrand) Polysaccharide iron 60 mg, folic acid 1 mg, ascorbic acid 50 mg, vitamins B$_{12}$ 3 mcg, A 4000 IU, D 400 IU, B$_1$ 3 mg, B$_2$ 3 mg, niacinamide 10 mg, B$_6$ 2 mg/Tab, calcium carbonate. Bot. 100s.
Use: Vitamin/mineral supplement.

NULLAPONS. (General Aniline & Film) The whole group of chelating agents re-lated to ethylenediaminetetraacetic acid. Pkg. according to demand.
Use: Sequestering agent.

NULLO. (Chattem Consumer) Water-sol-uble chlorophyllin copper complex 33.3 mg/Tab. Bot. 30s, 60s, 135s.
Use: Systemic deodorizer.

NUL-TACH. (Davis & Sly) Potassium 16 mg, magnesium 13 mg, ascorbic acid 250 mg/Tab. Bot. 100s.
Use: Paroxysmal tachycardia.

NULYTELY. (Braintree) PEG 3350 420 Gm, sodium bicarbonate 5.72 Gm, sodi-um chloride 11.2 Gm, potassium chlo-ride 1.48 Gm. Pow. Jugs. 4 L.
Use: Laxative.

NUMORPHAN. (DuPont) Oxymorphone HCl. **1 mg/ml.:** Amp. 1 ml. Box 10s. **1.5 mg/ml.:** Amp. 1 ml, Box 10s. Vial 10 ml, Box 1s. **Rectal Supp.:** 5 mg. Box 6s.
Use: Narcotic analgesic.

NUMOTIZINE CATAPLASM. (Hobart) Guaiacol 0.26 Gm, beechwood creosote 1.302 Gm, methyl salicylate 0.26 Gm/100 Gm. Jar 4 oz.
Use: External analgesic.

NUMOTIZINE COUGH SYRUP. (Hobart) Guaifenesin 5 gr, ammonium Cl 5 gr, sodium citrate 20 gr, menthol 0.04 gr/fl oz. Bot. 3 oz, pt, gal.
Use: Expectorant.

NUMZIDENT. (Purepac) Benzocaine, clove oil, peppermint oil. Gel 0.5 oz.
Use: Topical anesthetic for mouth.

NUM-ZIT. (Purepac) Benzocaine, men-thol, glycerin, methylparaben, alcohol 12%. Liq. Bot. 22.5 ml.
Use: Topical anesthetic for mouth.

NUM-ZIT GEL. (Purepac) Benzocaine, menthol. Tube 10 Gm.
Use: Topical anesthetic for mouth.

NUNOL.
See: Phenobarbital (Various Mfr.).

NUPERCAINAL. (Ciba) **Cream:** Dibu-caine 0.5%, acetone, sodium bisulfite 37%. Tube 1.5 oz. **Oint.:** Dibucaine 1%, sodium bisulfite 0.5%. Tube 1 oz, 2 oz.
Use: Topical anesthetic.

NUPERCAINAL. (Ciba Consumer) Co-coa butter 2.1 Gm, zinc oxide 0.25 Gm, acetone, sodium bisulfite 0.25

Gm/Supp. Box 12s, 24s.
Use: Anorectal preparation.
NUPRIN CAPLETS. (Bristol-Myers)
Ibuprofen 200 mg/Capl. Bot. 100s.
Use: Nonsteroidal anti-inflammatory
drug; analgesic.
NUPRIN TABLETS. (Bristol-Myers)
Ibuprofen 200 mg/Tab. Blister Pak 8s.
Bot. 24s, 50s, 200s.
Use: Nonsteroidal anti-inflammatory
drug; analgesic.
NUQUIN HP. (Stratus) **Cream:** 4% hydro-
quinone, 30 mg dioxybenzone, 20 mg
oxybenzone per g. Vanishing base.
Stearyl alcohol, EDTA, sodium
metabisulfite. Tube 14.2 g , 28.4 g, 56.7
g. **Gel:** 4% hydroquinone, 30 mg dioxybenzone per g. Alcohol, sodium
metabisulfite, EDTA. Tube 14.2 g, 28.4
g.
Use: Skin bleaching agent.
NUROMAX. (Burroughs Wellcome) Doxacurium chloride 1 mg/ml. Inj. Vial 5 ml.
Use: Neuromuscular blocking agent.
NURSOY. (Wyeth-Ayerst) Vitamins A
2500 IU, D-3 400 IU, C 55 mg, B_1 0.67
mg, B_2 1 mg, E 9 IU, niacin 9.5 mEq, B_6
0.4 mg, B_{12} 2 mcg, pantothenic acid 3
mg, K-1 0.1 mg, folic acid 50 mcg,
choline 85 mg, inositol 26 mg, I, biotin,
Ca, P, Na, K, Mg, Mn, Cl, Cu, Zn/qt of
formula. Concentrated liq. Can 13 oz.
Ready to feed Can 32 oz. Ready to feed
Hospital Bot. 4 oz. Pow. Can 1 lb.
Use: Enteral nutritional supplement.
NU-SALT. (Cumberland Pkg.) Potassium
Cl, potassium bitartrate, calcium silicate,
natural flavor derived from yeast. Sodium 0.85 mg/5 Gm (< 0.04 mEq/5 Gm),
potassium 2640 mg/5 Gm (68 mEq/5
Gm). Pkg. 90 Gm.
Use: Salt substitute.
NU-TEARS. (Optopics) Polyvinyl alcohol
1.4%, EDTA, NaCl, benzalkonium chloride, potassium chloride. Soln. Bot. 15
ml.
Use: Artificial tears.
NU-TEARS II. (Optopics) Polyvinyl alcohol 1%, PEG-400 1%, EDTA, benzalkonium chloride. Soln. Bot. 15 ml.
Use: Artificial tears.
NU-THERA. (Kirkman) Vitamins A 10,000
IU, D 400 IU, B_1 10 mg, B_2 5 mg, niacinamide 100 mg, B_6 1 mg, B_{12} 5 mcg, C
150 mg, calcium 103 mg, phosphorus
80 mg, iron 10 mg, magnesium 5.5 mg,
manganese 1 mg, potassium 5 mg, zinc
1.4 mg/Cap. Bot. 100s.
Use: Vitamin/mineral supplement.
•**NUTMEG OIL,** N.F. XVIII.

Use: Pharmaceutic aid (flavor).
NUTRACORT. (Owen/Galderma) Hydro-
cortisone 1%. **Cream:** Jar 4 oz. Tube 30
Gm, 60 Gm. **Lot.:** Bot. 2 oz, 4 oz.
Use: Corticosteroid, topical.
NUTRADERM. (Owen/Galderma) Oil-in-
water emulsion. **Lot.:** Plastic bot. 8 oz,
16 oz. **Cream:** Tube 1.5 oz, 3 oz, Jar lb.
Use: Emollient.
NUTRADERM BATH OIL. (Owen/Galder-
ma) Mineral oil, PEG-4 dilaurate, lanolin
oil, butylparaben, benzophenone-3, fragrance, D & C Green No. 6. Bot. 8 oz.
Use: Emollient.
NUTRALORIC. (Nutraloric) A chocolate,
vanilla or strawberry flavored liquid containing, when mixed with whole milk to
make 1 L, 91.7 g protein, 175 g carbohydrates, 125 g fat, 875 mg sodium,
3166.7 mg potassium, 2.2 calories/ml.
Pow. Can 480 g.
Use: Enteral nutritional supplement.
NUTRAMENT DRINK BOX. (Drackett)
Protein 10 Gm, fat 7 Gm, carbohydrate
35 Gm, vitamins, minerals/240 calo-
ries/8 oz. Drink Box.
Use: Enteral nutritional supplement.
NUTRAMENT LIQUID. (Drackett) Protein
16 Gm, fat 10 Gm, carbohydrates 52
Gm, vitamins, minerals/360 calories/12
oz. Can.
Use: Enteral nutritional supplement.
NUTRAMIGEN. (Mead Johnson Nutrition) Hypoallergenic formula that supplies 640 calories/qt. Protein 18 Gm, fat
25 Gm, carbohydrates 86 Gm, vitamins
A 2000 IU, D 400 IU, E 20 IU, C 52 mg,
folic acid 100 mcg, B_1 0.5 mg, B_2 0.6
mg, niacin 8 mg, B_6 0.4 mg, B_{12} 2 mcg,
biotin 50 mcg, pantothenic acid 3 mg, K-
1 100 mcg, choline 85 mg, inositol 30
mg, calcium 600 mg, phosphorus 400
mg, iodine 45 mcg, iron 12 mg, magnesium 70 mg, copper 0.6 mg, zinc 5 mg,
manganese 200 mcg, chloride 550 mg,
potassium 700 mg, sodium 300 mg/qt of
formula (4.9 oz pow.). Can 16 oz,
390ml concentrate and 1 qt ready-to-
use.
Use: Enteral nutritional supplement.
NUTRAMIN. (Thurston) Vitamins A 666
IU, D 66 IU, B_1 666 mcg, B_2 333 mcg,
niacinamide 2 mg, folic acid 0.0444
mcg, calcium 16.6 mg, phosphorus 8.33
mg, iron 1.33 mg, iodine 0.15 mg/Tab.
Bot. 200s, 500s, 1000s.
Use: Vitamin/mineral supplement.
NUTRAMIN GRANULAR. (Thurston) Vitamins A 333 IU, D 333 IU, B_1 3.3 mg, B_2
1.6 mg, niacinamide 10 mg, folic acid

0.133 mg, calcium 250 mg, phosphorus 115 mg, iron 6.6 mg, iodine 0.15 mg/5 Gm. Bot. 10 oz, 32 oz.
Use: Vitamin/mineral supplement.
NUTRA-PLEX. (Medi-Plex) Vitamin B_1 0.17 mg, B_2 0.19 mg, B_3 2.2 mg, B_5 1.1 mg, B_6 0.2 mg, B_{12} 0.7 mcg, zinc 1.7 mg/5 ml, Mn, Mg, alcohol 13.5%. Liq. Bot. 480 ml.
Use: B vitamin combination.
NUTRAPLUS. (Owen) Urea 10% in emollient cream base or lotion base with preservatives. **Cream:** Tube 3 oz, Jar lb. **Lot.:** Bot. 8 oz, 16 oz.
Use: Emollient.
NUTRA-SOOTHE. (Pertussin) Colloidal oatmeal and light mineral oil. Emollient bath preparation. Pow. Pkts. 9s.
Use: Bath dermatologic.
NUTRA TEAR. (Dakryon) Vitamin B_{12} 0.05% in polyvinyl alcohol-containing ocular wetting solution, benzalkonium chloride 0.004%, EDTA. Drop. Bot. 15 ml.
Use: Ophthalmic lubricant.
NUTRAVIMS. (Approved) Vitamins A 6000 IU, D 1250 IU, C 50 mg, E 5 IU, B_{12} 5 mcg, B_1 3 mg, B_2 3 mg, B_6 0.5 mg, niacinamide 20 mg, calcium pantothenate 5 mg, zinc 1.5 mg, manganese 1 mg, iodine 0.15 mg, potassium 5 mg, magnesium 4 mg, iron 15 mg, calcium 59 mg, phosphorus 45 mg/Cap. Bot. 100s, 250s, 1000s.
Use: Vitamin/mineral supplement.
NUTREN 1.0 LIQUID. (Clintec Nutrition) Potassium and sodium caseinate, maltodextrin, sucrose, MCT, corn oil, lecithin, vitamins A, B_1, B_2, B_3, B_5, B_6, B_{12}, C, D, E, K, folic acid, biotin, choline, Ca, Cl, Cu, Fe, I, Mg, Mn, P, Zn. 250 ml.
Use: Enteral nutritional supplement.
NUTREN 1.5 LIQUID. (Clintec Nutrition) Casein, maltodextrin, corn syrup, sucrose, MCT, corn oil, vitamins A, B_1, B_2, B_3, B_5, B_6, B_{12}, C, D, E, K, folic acid, biotin, choline, Ca, Cl, Cu, Fe, I, Mg, Mn, P, Zn. 250 ml.
Use: Enteral nutritional supplement.
NUTREN 2.0 LIQUID. (Clintec Nutrition) Casein, maltodextrin, corn syrup, sucrose, MCT, corn oil, vitamins A, B_1, B_2, B_3, B_5, B_6, B_{12}, C, D, E, K, folic acid, biotin, choline, Ca, Cl, Cu, Fe, I, Mg, Mn, P, Zn. 250 ml.
Use: Enteral nutritional supplement.
NUTREX. (Holloway) Calcium 162 mg, iron 27 mg, vitamins A 5000 IU, D 400 IU, E 30 mg, B_1 2.25 mg, B_2 2.6 mg, B_3 20 mg, B_5 10 mg, B_6 3 mg, B_{12} 9 mcg, C

90 mg, folic acid 0.4 mg, Cu, I, K, Mg, Mn, P, zinc 22.5 mg, biotin 45 mcg/Tab. Bot. 100s.
Use: Vitamin/mineral supplement.
NUTRICON TABLETS. (Pasadena) Calcium 200 mg, iron 20 mg, vitamins A 2500 IU, D 200 IU, E 11 mg, B_1 1.5 mg, B_2 1.5 mg, B_3 10 mg, B_5 5 mg, B_6 2 mg, B_{12} 5 mcg, C 50 mg, folic acid 0.4 mg, Cu, I, Mg, zinc 3.75 mg, biotin/Tab. Bot. 120s.
Use: Vitamin/mineral supplement.
NUTRI-E. (Nutri Lab.) Vitamin E. **Cream:** 200 IU/Gm. Jar 1 oz, 2 oz. **Oil:** 1 oz. **Oint.:** 200 IU/Gm. Tube 1 oz, 1.5 oz. **Cap.:** 200 IU. Bot. 80s; 400 IU. Bot. 60s, 100s; 800 IU. Bot. 55s.
Use: Vitamin E supplement.
NUTRIGANIC. (Commerce) Multi-vitamin with minerals and amino acids. Tab. Bot. 50s.
Use: Vitamin/mineral supplement.
NUTRILAN. (Elan) A vanilla, chocolate or strawberry flavored liquid containing 38 g protein, 37 g fat, 143 g carbohydrates, 632.5 mg Na, 1.073 g K/L. With appropriate vitamins and minerals. In 237 ml Tetra Pak containers.
Use: Enteral nutritional supplement.
NUTRILIPID. (Kendall McGaw) Soybean oil intravenous fat emulsion. **10%:** Calories 1.1/ml. In 250 ml, 500 ml. **20%:** Calories 2/ml. In 250 ml, 500 ml.
Use: Parenteral nutritional supplement.
NUTRILYTE. (American Regent) Acetate 2.03 mEq, potassium 2.03 mEq, chloride 1.68 mEq, sodium 1.25 mEq, magnesium 0.4 mEq, calcium 0.25 mEq, gluconate 0.25 mEq per ml, ≈ 6212 mOsml/L. Concentrated soln. Bot. 20 ml, 100 ml.
Use: Intravenous nutritional therapy.
NUTRILYTE II. (American Regent) Acetate 1.475 mEq, potassium 1 mEq, chloride 1.75 mEq, sodium 1.75 mEq, magnesium 0.25 mEq, calcium 0.225 mEq per ml, ≈ 6212 mOsml/L. Concentrated soln. Bot. 20 ml, 100 ml.
Use: Intravenous nutritional therapy.
NUTRI-PLEX TABLETS. (Faraday) Vitamins B_1 5 mg, B_2 5 mg, B_6 5 mg, pantothenic acid 25 mg, B_{12} 12.5 mcg, niacinamide 50 mg, iron gluconate 30 mg, choline bitartrate 50 mg, inositol 50 mg, PABA 15 mg, C 150 mg/2 Tab. Bot. 100s, 250s.
Use: Vitamin/mineral supplement.
NUTRISOURCE MODULAR SYSTEM. (Sandoz Nutrition) Individual Nutrisource modules available: protein,

amino acids, amino acids-high branched
chain, carbohydrate, lipid-medium chain
triglycerides, lipid-long branched chain
triglycerides, vitamins, minerals. Cans of
liquid. Packets of powder.
Use: Enteral nutritional supplement.
NUTRI-VAL. (Marcen) Vitamins A 5000
IU, D 500 IU, B_1 10 mg, B_2 5 mg, B_{12} activity 5 mcg, B_6 5 mcg, C 50 mg, hesperidin 5 mg, niacinamide 15 mg, folic
acid 0.2 mg, calcium pantothenate 50
mg, choline bitartrate 50 mg, betaine
HCl 25 mg, lipo-K 0.4 mg, duodenum
substance 50 mg, pancreas substance
50 mg, inositol 25 mg, Cy-yeast hydrolysates 50 mg, rutin 5 mg, 1-lysine
HCl 5 mg, E 5 IU, Ossonate (glucuronic
complex) 8 mg, glutamic acid 30 mg,
lecithin 5 mg, iron 20 mg, iodine 0.15
mg, calcium 50 mg, phosphorus 40 mg,
boron 0.1 mg, copper 1 mg, manganese
1 mg, magnesium 1 mg, potassium 5
mg, zinc 0.5 mg, biotin 0.02 mg/Cap.
Bot. 100s, 500s, 1000s.
Use: Vitamin/mineral supplement.
**NUTRI-VITE NATURAL MULTIPLE VITA-
MIN AND MINERALS.** (Faraday) Vitamins A 15,000 IU, D 400 IU, B_1 1.5 mg,
B_2 3 mg, B_{12} 15 mcg, niacin 500 mcg,
B_6 20 mcg, choline 1.75 mg, folic acid 13
mcg, pantothenic acid 50 mcg, p-
aminobenzoic acid 12 mcg, inositol 1.72
mg, C 60 mg, citrus bioflavonoids 15
mg, E 50 IU, iron gluconate 15 mg, calcium 192 mg, phosphorus 85 mg, iodine
0.15 mg, red bone marrow 30 mg/3 Tab.
Protein coated Tab. Bot. 100s, 250s.
Use: Vitamin/mineral supplement.
NUTRIZYME. (Enzyme Process) Vitamins A 5000 IU, D 400 IU, C 60 mg, B_1
1.5 mg, B_2 1.7 mg, niacinamide 20 mg,
B_6 2 mg, pantothenate 10 mg, B_{12} 6
mcg, E 30 IU, iron 10 mg, copper 1 mg,
zinc 1 mg, Folacin 0.025 mg/Tab. Bot.
90s, 250s.
Use: Vitamin/mineral supplement.
NUTROFEM-II. (Life's Finest) Calcium
250 mg, iron 9 mg, vitamins A 2500 IU,
D 200 IU, E 10 mg, B_1 0.75 mg, B_2 0.85
mg, B_3 10 mg, B_5 5 mg, B_6 1 mg, B_{12} 3
mcg, C 30 mg, folic acid 0.2 mg, Cu, Mg,
zinc 7.5 mg, biotin/Tab. Bot. 60s, 90s,
180s.
Use: Vitamin/mineral supplement.
NUTROPIN. (Genentech) Somatropin 5
mg ($\approx$ 13 IU)/vial, mannitol 45 mg, benzyl alcohol 0.9%; 10 mg ($\approx$ 26 IU)/vial,
mannitol 90 mg, benzyl alcohol 0.9%.
Pow. for inj. (lyophilized). Vials with 10
ml diluent.

Use: Growth hormone.
NUZINE OINTMENT. (Hobart) Guaiacol
1.66 Gm, oxyquinoline sulfate 0.42 Gm,
zinc oxide 2.5 Gm, glycerine 1.66 Gm,
lanum (anhydrous) 43.76 Gm, petrolatum 50 Gm/100 Gm. Tube 1 oz.
Use: Anorectal preparation.
NYCOFF. (Dover) Dextromethorphan
HBr/lab. UD Box 500s. Sugar, lactose
and salt free.
Use: Antitussive.
NYCO-WHITE. (Whiteworth) Nystatin,
neomycin, gramcidin, triamcinolone.
Cream. Tube 15 Gm, 30 Gm, 60 Gm.
Use: Anti-infective, external.
NYCO-WORTH. (Whiteworth) Nystatin.
Cream Tube 15 Gm.
Use: Anti-infective, external.
NYCRALAN. (Lannett) Vitamin B_1 10 mg,
calcium lactate 10 gr/Tab. Bot. 100s.
Use: Vitamin/mineral supplement.
NYDRAZID INJECTION. (Apothecon)
Isoniazid 100 mg/ml, chlorobutanol
0.25%, sodium hydroxide or hydrochloric acid to adjust pH. Vial 10 ml.
Use: Antituberculous agent.
• **NYLESTRIOL.** USAN. 3-Cyclopentyloxy-
19-nor-17 α-pregna-1,3,5(10)-trien-20-
yne-16, 17β-diol.
Use: Estrogen.
NYLIDRIN HYDROCHLORIDE, U.S.P.
XXII. Inj., Tab., U.S.P. XXII. p-Hydroxy-
a-[1-[(1-methyl-3-phenyl-propyl)-
amino]ethyl]benzyl alcohol HCl.
Use: Peripheral vasodilator.
See: Arlidin, Tab. (Rhone-Poulenc Rorer).
NYQUIL COUGH/COLD, CHILDREN'S.
(Richardson-Vicks) Pseudoephedrine
HCl 10 mg, chlorpheniramine maleate
0.67 mg, dextromethorphan HBr 5 mg/5
ml, sucrose, alcohol free, cherry flavor.
Liq. 120 ml.
Use: Decongestant, antihistamine, antitussive.
NYQUIL LIQUICAPS. (Richardson-Vicks)
Pseudoephedrine HCl 30 mg, diphenhydramine HCl 25 mg, dextromethorphan
HBr 15 mg, acetaminophen 250
mg/Cap. Bot. 20s.
Use: Decongestant, antihistamine,
analgesic, antitussive.
**NYQUIL NIGHTTIME COLD/FLU MEDI-
CINE.** (Richardson-Vicks) Pseudoephedrine HCl 10 mg, doxylamine
succinate 2.1 mg, dextromethorphan
HBr 5 mg, acetaminophen 167 mg/5 ml,
alcohol 10%, sucrose, saccharin (cherry
flavor), tartrazine (regular flavor). Liq.
Bot. 295 ml.
Use: Decongestant, antihistamine, anti-

tussive, analgesic.

NYQUIL NIGHT TIME COLD MEDICINE LIQUID. (Vicks Health Care) Dextromethorphan HBr 30 mg, pseudoephedrine HCl 60 mg, doxylamine succinate 7.5 mg, acetaminophen 1000 mg/oz, alcohol 25%. Regular and cherry flavors. Regular flavor contains FDC Yellow #5 tartrazine. Bot. 6 oz, 10 oz, 14 oz.
Use: Antitussive, decongestant, antihistamine, analgesic.

NYQUIL NIGHTTIME HEAD COLD ALLERGY FORMULA, CHILDREN'S. (Richardson-Vicks) pseudoephedrine HCl, chlorpheniramine maleate per 5 ml, 0.67 mg, alcohol free, sorbitol, sucrose, grape flavor. Liq. Bot. 120 ml.
Use: Upper respiratory combination.

NYRAL. (Vale) Cetylpyridinium Cl 0.5 mg, benzocaine 5 mg/Loz. w/parabens. Pkg. 100s, 1000s.
Use: Antiseptic.

NYSACETOL. (Kenyon) N-Acetyl-p-aminophenol 5 gr/Tab. Bot. 100s, 1000s.
Use: Analgesic.

•**NYSTATIN,** U.S.P. XXIII. Cream, For Oral Susp., Lot., Oint., Topical Pow., Oral Susp., Tab., Vaginal Supp., Vaginal Tab., U.S.P. XXIII. An antifungal antibiotic derived from cultures of *Streptomyces noursei.* (Various Mfr.) 100,000 units/ml.
Oral Susp. Bot. 5 ml, 60 ml, 480 ml.
Vaginal Tab. Pkg. 15s or 30s.
Use: Antifungal.
See: Mycostatin Preps. (Apothecon).
Nilstat, Tab., Cream, Oint., Pow. (Lederle).
Nilstat, Oral Drops (Lederle).
Nilstat, Vaginal Tab. (Lederle).
Nystatin, Bulk Pow. (Paddock).
Nystex, Cream, Oint., Susp. (Savage).
O-V Statin, Tab. (Squibb Mark).
W/Clioquinol.
See: Nystaform, Oint. (Miles Pharm).
W/Demethylchlortetracycline.
See: Declostatin, Tab., Cap. (Lederle).
W/Gramicidin, neomycin, triamcinolone.
See: Mycolog, Cream, Oint. (Squibb).
W/Tetracycline phosphate buffered.
See: Achrostatin-V, Cap. (Lederle).
W/Tetracycline phosphate complex.
See: Tetrex-F, Cap. (Bristol).

•**NYSTATIN AND CLOROQUINOL OINTMENT,** U.S.P. XXII.
Use: Antifungal.
See: Nystaform, Oint. (Miles Pharm).

•**NYSTATIN AND TRIAMCINOLONE ACETONIDE CREAM,** U.S.P. XXIII.
Use: Antifungal, anti-inflammatory.

•**NYSTATIN AND TRIAMCINOLONE ACETONIDE OINTMENT,** U.S.P. XXIII.
Use: Antifungal, anti-inflammatory.

•**NYSTATIN, NEOMYCIN SULFATE, GRAMICIDIN AND TRIAMCINOLONE ACETONIDE,** U.S.P. XXIII. Cream, Oint., U.S.P. XXIII.
Use: Antifungal, antibacterial, anti-inflammatory.
See: Mycolog, Prods. (Squibb).

NYSTEX CREAM & OINTMENT. (Savage) Nystatin 100,000 units/Gm. Tube 15 Gm, 30 Gm.
Use: Anti-infective, external.

NYSTEX ORAL SUSPENSION. (Savage) Nystatin 100,000 units/ml in suspension. Bot. 60 ml.
Use: Antifungal.

NYTCOLD MEDICINE. (Rugby) Pseudoephedrine HCl 10 mg, doxylamine succinate 1.25 mg, dextromethorphan HBr 5 mg, acetaminophen 167 mg, alcohol 25%, glucose, saccharin, sucrose, cherry flavor. Liq. Bot. 177 ml.
Use: Decongestant, antihistamine, antitussive, analgesic.

NYTIME COLD MEDICINE. (Rugby) Acetaminophen 1000 mg, doxylamine succinate 7.5 mg, pseudoephedrine HCl 60 mg, dextromethorphan HBr 30 mg/30 ml, alcohol 25%. Bot. 6 oz, 10 oz.
Use: Analgesic, antihistamine, decongestant, antitussive.

NYTOL. (Block) Diphenhydramine HCl 25 mg/Tab. Bot. 16s, 32s, 72s.
Use: Sleep aid.

NYTOL, MAXIMUM STRENGTH. (Block) Diphenhydramine HCl 50 mg, lactose. Tab. Bot. 8s.
Use: Nonprescription sleep aid.

O

O.A.D. (Sween) Ostomy deodorant. Bot. 1.25 oz, 4 oz, 8 oz.
Use: Ostomy appliance deodorant.

OASIS. (Zitar) Artificial saliva. Bot. 6 oz.
Use: To relieve xerostomia.

OATMEAL, GUM FRACTION.
See: Aveeno, Preps. (Cooper).

OBACIN. (Kenyon) Phendimetrazine tartrate 35 mg/Tab. Bot. 100s, 1000s.
Use: Anorexiant.

OBALAN. (Lannett) Phendimetrazine tartrate 35 mg/Tab. Bot. 100s, 1000s.
Use: Anorexiant.

OBE-NIX. (Holloway) Phentermine HCl 30 mg/Cap. (equivalent to 24 mg base)

Bot. 100s.
Use: Anorexiant.
OBEPAR. (Tyler) Vitamins A 3000 IU, D
300 IU, B₁ 3 mg, B₂ 2 mg, nicotinamide
10 mg, B₆ 3 mg, calcium pantothenate 2
mg, B₁₂ 3 mcg, C 37.5 mg, calcium 150
mg, iron 5 mg, magnesium 1 mg, man-
ganese 0.1 mg, potassium 1 mg, zinc
0.15 mg/Cap. Bot. 100s.
Use: Vitamin/mineral supplement.
OBEPHEN. (Hauck) Phentermine HCl 30
mg (equivalent to 24 mg base) Cap. Bot.
1000s.
Use: Anorexiant.
OBESITY AGENTS.
See: Anti-Obesity Agents (Various Mfr.).
OBESTIN-30. (Ferndale) Phentermine
HCl 30 mg/Cap. Bot. 100s, 1000s.
Use: Anorexiant.
OBE-TITE. (Scott/Cord) Phendimetrazine
tartrate 35 mg/Tab. Bot. 100s, 500s.
Use: Anorexiant.
OBETROL. (Obetrol) Dextroamphetamine saccharate, amphetamine aspartate, amphetamine sulfate, dextroamphetamine sulfate in equal parts. 10 mg
or 20 mg tab. Bot. 100s, 500s, 1000s.
Use: Diet aid.
OBETROL-10 TABS. (Obetrol) Dex-
troamphetamine saccharate 2.5 mg,
amphetamine asparate 2.5 mg, amphet-
amine sulfate 2.5 mg, dextroampheta-
mine sulfate 2.5 mg/Tab. Bot. 100s,
500s, 1000s.
Use: Diet aid.
OBETROL-20 TABS. (Obetrol) Metham-
phetamine saccharate 5 mg, ampheta-
mine asparate 5 mg, amphetamine sulfate 5 mg, dextroamphetamine sulfate 5
mg/Tab. Bot. 100s, 500s, 1000s.
Use: Diet aid.
OBEZINE. (Western Research)
Phendimetrazine tartrate 35 mg/Tab.
Handicount 28 (36 bags of 28s).
Use: Anorexiant.
• **OBIDOXIME CHLORIDE.** USAN. 1,1′-
(Oxydime-thylene)-bis-[4-formylpyridini-
um]dichloride dioxime.
Use: Cholinesterase reactivator.
OB-NATAL. (Armen Pharm.) Prenatal vit-
amins and minerals/TR Tab. Bot. 100s.
Use: Vitamin/mineral supplement.
OB-NATAL PLUS. (Armen Pharm.) Pre-
natal vitamins and minerals. Tab. Bot.
100s.
Use: Vitamin/mineral supplement.
OBRICAL. (Canright) Calcium lactate
500 mg, vitamins D 400 IU, ferrous sul-
fate exsiccated 35 mg, B₁ 1 mg, B₂ 1
mg, C 10 mg/Tab. Bot. 100s, 1000s.

Use: Vitamin/mineral supplement.
OBRICAL-F. (Canright) Ferrous sulfate
50 mg, calcium lactate 500 mg, vitamins
D 400 IU, B₁ 1 mg, B₂ 1 mg, C 10 mg,
folic acid 0.67 mg/Tab. Bot. 100s, 1000s.
Use: Vitamin/mineral supplement.
OBRITE. (Milton Roy) Contact lens and
eye glass cleaner. Plastic spray Bot. 30
ml, 55 ml.
Use: Contact lens and eye glass care.
OB-TINIC. (Hauck) Iron 65 mg, vitamins A
6000 IU, D 400 IU, E 30 IU, B₁ 1.1 mg,
B₂ 1.8 mg, B₃ 15 mg, B₆ 2.5 mg, B₁₂ 5
mcg, C 60 mg, folic acid 1 mg, Ca/Tab.
Bot. 100s.
Use: Vitamin/mineral supplement.
OBTUNDIA CALAMINE CREAM. (Otis
Clapp) Zinc oxide, calamine, camphorat-
ed meta-cresoln. Tube 2 oz. Aid pak
0.11 oz, Foil pak 36s. Unit box 0.11 oz,
foil pak 6s.
Use: Antipruritic, skin protectant.
OBTUNDIA FIRST AID SPRAY. (Otis
Clapp) Camphorated meta-cresoln.
Aerosol can 2.5 oz.
Use: Antiseptic.
OBTUNDIA SURGICAL DRESSING.
(Otis Clapp) Camphorated meta-
cresoln. Bot. 0.5 oz, 4 oz. Swab pad Box
10s, Aid pak 100s.
Use: Antiseptic.
OBY-TRIM. (Rexar) Phentermine HCl 30
mg/Cap. Bot. 1000s.
Use: Anorexiant.
O-CAL F.A. (Pharmics) Iron 66 mg, calci-
um 200 mg, vitamins A 5000 IU, C 90
mg, D 400 IU, B₆ 4 mg, B₁ 3 mg, B₂ 3
mg, niacinamide 20 mg, B₁₂ 12 mcg,
folic acid 1 mg, sodium fluoride 1.1 mg,
iodine 0.15 mg, magnesium 100 mg,
copper 2 mg, zinc 15 mg/Tab. Bot. 100s.
Use: Vitamin/mineral supplement.
OCAPERIDONE. (Janssen) USAN.
Use: Antipsychotic.
OCCLUSAL-HP. (Genderm) Salicylic
acid 17%. Bot. 10 ml.
Use: Keratolytic.
OCCUCOAT. (Storz) Hydroxypropyl
methylcellulose 2%. Soln. Syringe 1 ml
with cannula.
Use: Ophthalmic preparation.
OCEAN. (Fleming) Sodium Cl 0.65%,
benzyl alcohol. Bot. 45 ml, pt.
Use: Nasal membrane moisturizer.
OCEAN PLUS. (Fleming) Caffeine 2.5%,
benzyl alcohol. Bot. 15 ml.
OCL SOLUTION. (Abbott Hospital Prods)
Oral colonic lavage soln. Sodium Cl 146
mg, sodium bicarbonate 168 mg, sodi-
um sulfate decahydate 1.29 Gm, potas-

sium Cl 75 mg, PEG-3350 6 Gm,
polysorbate-80 30 ml/100 ml. 1.35 L 3-
pack units.
Use: Laxative.
• **OCRYLATE.** USAN. Octyl 2-cyano-acry-
late.
Use: Surgical aid (tissue adhesive).
• **OCTABENZONE.** USAN. 2-Hydroxy-4-
(octyloxy) benzophenone. Spectra-Sorb
UV 531. Under study.
Use: Sunscreen agent.
OCTACOSACTRIN. B.A.N. α⁻ Corti-
cotrophin.
Use: Corticotrophic peptide.
OCTADECANOIC ACID.
See: Stearic Acid, N.F. XVIII.
OCTADECANOIC ACID, SODIUM SALT.
See: Sodium Stearate, N.F. XVIII.
OCTADECANOIC ACID, ZINC SALT.
See: Zinc Stearate, N.F. XVIII.
OCTADECANOL-I.
See: Stearyl Alcohol, N.F. XVIII.
OCTAMIDE. (Adria) Metoclopramide 10
mg/Tab. Bot. 100s, 500s.
Use: GI stimulant.
OCTAMIDE PFS. (Adria) Metoclopramide
HCl per ml. 5 mg, preservative free. Vial.
Single dose; 2, 10, 30 ml.
Use: GI stimulant.
• **OCTANOIC ACID.** USAN.
Use: Antifungal.
OCTAPEPTIDE SEQUENCE.
Use: An antiviral agent.
See: Flumadine (Roche).
OCTAPHONIUM CHLORIDE. B A N
Benzyldiethyl-2-[4-(1,1,3,3-tetramethyl-
butyl)phenoxy]-ethylammonium Cl. Oc-
taphen; Phenoctide.
Use: Antiseptic.
OCTAREX. (Approved) Vitamins A 5000
IU, D 1000 IU, B₁ 1.5 mg, B₂ 2 mg, B₆
0.1 mg, calcium pantothenate 1 mg,
niacinamide 20 mg, C 37.5 mg, E 1 IU,
B₁₂ 1 mcg/Cap. Bot. 100s, 1000s.
Use: Vitamin/mineral supplement.
OCTATROPINE METHYLBROMIDE.
B.A.N. Anisotropine methylbromide. 2-
Propyl-pentanoylmethyltropinium bro-
mide. 8-Methyl-O-(2-
propylvaleryl)tropinium bromide.
Use: Anticholinergic.
OCTAVERINE. B.A.N. 6,7-Dimethoxy-1-
(3,4,5-triethoxyphenyl)isoquinoline.
Use: Antispasmodic.
OCTAVIMS. (Approved) Vitamins A 6000
IU, D 1250 IU, C 50 mg, E 5 IU, B₁ 3 mg,
B₂ 3 mg, B₆ 0.5 mg, niacinamide 20 mg,
calcium pantothenate 5 mg, B₁₂ 5 mcg,
calcium 59 mg, phosphorus 45 mg/Cap.
Bot. 100s, 250s, 1000s.

Use: Vitamin/mineral supplement.
• **OCTAZAMIDE.** USAN.
Use: Analgesic.
• **OCTENIDINE HYDROCHLORIDE.**
USAN.
Use: Anti-infective, topical.
• **OCTENIDINE SACCHARIN.** USAN.
Use: Dental plaque inhibitor.
• **OCTICIZER.** USAN. 2-Ethylhexyl
diphenyl phosphate. Santicizer 141
(Monsanto). SCAN Spray-On. (Johnson
& Johnson).
Use: Pharmaceutic aid (plasticizer).
OCTOCAINE HCl. (Novocol) Lidocaine
HCl 2%, epinephrine 1:50,000 or
1:100,000. Inj. Dent. Cartridge 1.8 ml.
Use: Local anesthetic.
• **OCTOCRYLENE.** USAN.
Use: Ultraviolet screen.
• **OCTODRINE.** USAN. 1,5-Dimethylhexy-
lamine. Under study.
Use: Vasoconstrictor, local anesthetic.
OCTOFOLLIN.
See: Benzestrol, U.S.P. XXIII.
• **OCTOXYNOL 9,** N.F. XVIII.
Use: Surfactant.
• **OCTREOTIDE.** USAN.
Use: Antisecretory (gastric).
• **OCTREOTIDE ACETATE.** USAN.
Use: antidiarrheal, gastrointestinal tu-
mor; antihypotensive, carcinoid crisis;
growth hormone suppressant,
acromegaly.
• **OCTRIPTYLINE PHOSPHATE.** USAN.
Use: Antidepressant.
• **OCTRIZOLE.** USAN.
Use: Ultraviolet screen.
**N-OCTYL BICYALOHEPTENE DICAR-
BOSIMIDE.** W/N-N-diethyl-m-tolu-
amide, 2,3,4,5-bis-(delta-2-butylene)
tetrahydrofurfural, Di-n-propyl isocin-
chomeronate, other isomers, iso-
propanol.
See: Bansum, Bot. (Summers).
• **OCTYLDODECANOL,** N.F. XVIII.
Use: Pharmaceutic aid (oleaginous ve-
hicle).
**OCTYLPHENOXY POLY-
ETHOXYETHANOL.** A mono-ether of a
polyethylene glycol. Igepal CA 630 (An-
tara).
W/Phenylmercuric acetate, methyl-
paraben, sodium borate.
See: Lorophyn jelly, Supp. (Eaton).
W/Lactic acid, sodium lactate.
See: Jeneen premeasured liquid
douche (Norwich).
OCUCLEAR EYE. (Schering) Oxymeta-
zoline HCl 0.025%. Bot. 15 ml, 30 ml.
Use: Vasoconstrictor/mydriatric, oph-

thalmic.

OCUCLENZ. (Storz/Lederle) Disodium oleamido PEG-2 sulfosuccinate, cocoamphodiacetate, poloxamer 185, poloxamer 188, parabens, citric acid, EDTA. Soln. Bot. 120 ml.
Use: Ophthalmic cleansing solution.

OCUCOAT PF. (Storz Ophthalmics) Dextran 70 0.1%, hydroxypropyl methycellulose. Preservative free. Drops. In 0.5 ml single-dose containers.
Use: Ocular lubricant.

OCUFEN. (Allergan) Flurbiprofen sodium 0.03%. Bot. 2.5 ml, 5 ml, 10 ml w/dropper.
Use: Topical nonsteroidal anti-inflammatory drug, ophthalmic.

•**OCUFILCON A.** USAN.
Use: Contact lens material.

•**OCUFILCON B.** USAN.
Use: Contact lens material.

•**OCUFILCON C.** USAN.
Use: Contact lens material.

OCUFILCON E. USAN.
Use: Contact lens material.

OCUFLOX. (Allergan) Ofloxacin 3 mg/ml. Soln. Bot. 5 ml.
Use: Antibiotic, ophthalmic.

•**OCULAR LUBRICANTS.**
Use: Ophthalmic.
See: Akwa Tears (Akorn).
Artificial Tears (Rugby).
Dey-Lube (Dey).
Dry Eyes (Bausch & Lomb).
Duolube (Bausch & Lomb).
Duratears Naturale (Alcon).
Hypotears (Iolab).
Lacri-Lube NP (Allergan).
Lacri-Lube S.O.P. (Allergan).
Lipo-Tears (Spectra).
LubriTears (Bausch & Lomb).
OcuCoat PF (Storz Ophthalmics).
Puralube (Fougera).
Refresh PM (Allergan).
Tears Renewed (Akorn).
Vit-A-Drops (Vision Pharm).

OCU-LUBE. (Bausch & Lomb) Petrolatum sterile, preservative and lanolin free. Tube 3.5 Gm.
Use: Ophthalmic lubricant.

OCUMETER.
See: Decadron Phosphate, Preps. (Merck & Co.).
Humorsol, Ophth. Soln. (Merck & Co.).
Neo-Decadron, Preps. (Merck & Co.).

OCUSERT. (Ciba) Pilocarpine ocular therapeutic system.
Pilo-20: Releases 20 mcg pilocarpine/hour for one week. Pkg. 8s.
Pilo-40: Releases 40 mcg pilocarpine/hour for one week. Pkg. 8s.
Use: Agent for glaucoma.

OCUSOFT. (Cynacon/Ocusoft) PEG-80 sorbitan laurate, sodium trideceth sulfate, PEG-150 distearate, cocoamido propyl hydroxysultaine, lauroamphocarboxyglycinate, sodium laureth-13 carboxylate, PEG-15 tallow polyamine, quaternium-15. Soln. Pads UD 30s, Bot. 120 ml.
Use: Ophthalmic cleansing solution.

OCUSULF-10. (Optopics) Sodium sulfacetamide 10%. Soln. Bot. 2 ml, 15 ml.
Use: External bacterial eye infections.

OCUTRICIN. (Bausch & Lomb) **Oint.:**
Polymyxin B sulfate 10,000 units, bacitracin zinc 400 units, neomycin sulfate 3.5 mg. Tube 3.5 g. **Soln.:** Polymyxin B sulfate 10,000 units, neomycin sulfate 1.75 mg, gramicidin 0.025 mg/ml. Dropper bot. 10 ml.
Use: Antibiotic, ophthalmic.

OCUVITE. (Lederle) Formerly distributed by Storz.

ODALATE. (Kenyon) Chlorpheniramine maleate 8 mg, phenylpropanolamine HCl 50 mg, atropine sulfate 0.36 mg/Cap. Bot. 100s, 1000s.
Use: Antihistamine, decongestant, anticholinergic/antispasmodic.

ODARA. (Lorvic) Alcohol 48%, carbolic acid less than 2%, zinc Cl, potassium iodide, glycerin, methyl salicylate, oil eucalyptus, tincture myrrh. Concentrated Liq. Bot. 8 oz.
Use: Mouthwash, gargle.

ODONIL. (Kenyon) dl-Methionine 200 mg/Cap. Bot. 100s, 1000s.
Use: Diaper rash product.

OESTERGON.
See: Estradiol (Various Mfr.).

OESTRADIOL.
See: Estradiol (Various Mfr.).

OESTRASID.
See: Dienestrol (Various Mfr.).

OESTRIN.
See: Estrone (Various Mfr.).

OESTRIOL SODIUM SUCCINATE.
B.A.N. Oestra-1,3,5(10)-triene-3,16α,17β-di(sodium succinate).
Use: Treatment of thrombocytopenic hemorrhage.

OESTRIOL SUCCINATE. B.A.N. Oestra-1,3,5-(10)-triene-3,16α,17β-triol 16,17-di(hydrogen succinate).
Use: Treatment of thrombocytopenic hemorrhage.

OESTROFORM.
See: Estrone (Various Mfr.).

OESTROMENIN.

See: Diethylstilbestrol (Various Mfr.).
OESTROMON.
See: Diethylstilbestrol (Various Mfr.).
OFF-EZY CORN & CALLOUS REMOVER. (Del) Salicylic acid 17% in a collodion-like vehicle of 65% ether and 21% alcohol. Kit. 13.5 ml with callous smoother and 3 corn cushions.
Use: Keratolytic.
OFF-EZY CORN REMOVER. (Commerce) Salicylic acid 13.57% in flexible collodion base, ether 65%, alcohol 21%. Bot. 0.45 oz.
Use: Keratolytic.
OFF-EZY WART REMOVER. (Commerce) Salicylic acid 17% in flexible collodion base, ether 65%, alcohol 21%. Bot. 13.5 ml.
Use: Keratolytic.
•**OFLOXACIN.** USAN.
Use: Antibacterial. [Orphan drug]
See: Floxin (Ortho).
Ocuflox, Ophth. Soln. (Allergan).
•**OFORNINE.** USAN.
Use: Antihypertensive.
OGEN. (Abbott) Estropipate. **Tab. 0.625:** Estropipate 0.75 mg/Tab. Bot. 100s. **Tab. 1.25:** Estropipate 1.5 mg/Tab. Bot. 100s. **Tab. 2.5:** Estropipate 3 mg/Tab. Bot. 100s. **Tab 5.:** Estropipate 6 mg/Tab. Bot. 100s.
Use: Estrogen.
OGEN VAGINAL CREAM. (Abbott) Estropipate 1.5 mg/Gm. Tube 1.5 oz w/applicator.
Use: Estrogen, vaginal.
OILATUM SOAP. (Stiefel) Polyunsaturated vegetable oil 7.5%. Bar 120 g, 240 g.
Use: Skin cleanser.
OIL OF CAMPHOR W/COMBINATIONS.
See: Sloan's Liniment, Liq. (Warner-Lambert).
OIL OF CLOVES W/ALCOHOL.
See: Buckley "Z.O.", Liq. (Crosby).
OIL OF OLAY DAILY UV PROTECTANT. (Procter & Gamble) SPF 15. **Cream:** Titanium dioxide, ethylhexyl p-methoxycinnamate, 2-phenylbenzimidazole-5-sulfonic acid, glycerin, triethanolamine, imidazolidinyl urea, parabens, carbomer, PEG-10, EDTA, castor oil, tartrazine. Scented and unscented. 51 g. **Lot.:** Ethylhexyl p-methoxycinnamate, 2-phenylbenzimidazole-5-sulfonic acid, titanium dioxide, cetyl alcohol, imidazolidinyl urea, parabens, EDTA, castor oil, tartrazine. Bot. 105 g, 157.7 g.
Use: Sunscreen.
OIL OF PINE W/COMBINATIONS.

See: Sloan's Liniment, Liq. (Warner-Lambert).
OIL-O-SOL. (Health Care Industries) Corn oil 52%, castor oil 40.8%, camphor 6.8%, hexylresorcinol 0.1%. Bot. 1 oz, 2 oz, 4 oz.
Use: Antiseptic.
OINTMENT BASE, WASHABLE.
See: Absorbent Base (Upsher-Smith). Cetaphil, Cream, Lot. (Owen). Velvachol, Cream (Owen).
•**OINTMENT, HYDROPHILIC,** U.S.P. XXIII.
Use: Pharmaceutical aid (oil-in-water emulsion ointment base).
•**OINTMENT, WHITE,** U.S.P. XXIII.
Use: Pharmaceutical aid (oleaginous ointment base).
•**OINTMENT, YELLOW,** U.S.P. XXIII.
Use: Ointment base.
•**OLAFLUR.** USAN.
Use: Dental caries prophylactic.
OLAMINE.
See: Ethanolamine.
•**OLANZAPINE.** USAN.
Use: Antipsychotic (postsynaptic dopamine).
•**OLAQUINDOX.** B.A.N. 2-(2-Hydroxyethylcarbamoyl)-3-methylquinoxaline 1,4-dioxide.
Use: Growth promoter, bactericide, veterinary medicine.
OLDEROL. (Doral) Vitamins B_1 15 mg, B_2 10 mg, niacinamide 100 mg, B_6 5 mg, B_{12} 4 mcg, calcium pantothenate 20 mg, folic acid 150 mcg, C 750 mg, E 30 IU/Cap. Bot. 60s.
Use: Vitamin/mineral supplement.
OLEANDOMYCIN. B.A.N. An antibiotic from *Streptomyces antibioticus.*
Use: Antibiotic.
OLEANDOMYCIN PHOSPHATE. Phosphate of an antibacterial substance produced by *Streptomyces antibioticus.*
Use: Anti-infective.
OLEANDOMYCIN SALT OF PENICILLIN.
See: Pen-M (Pfizer) Under study.
OLEANDOMYCIN, TRIACETYL. Troleandomycin, U.S.P. XX.
•**OLEIC ACID,** N.F. XVIII. 9-Octadecanoic acid.
Use: Pharmaceutical aid (emulsion adjunct).
•**OLEIC ACID I-131.** USAN.
Use: Radioactive agent.
•**OLEIC ACID I-125.** USAN.
Use: Radioactive agent.
OLEOVITAMIN A, Vitamin A, U.S.P. XXIII.
•**OLEOVITAMIN A & D,** U.S.P. XXIII. Cap., U.S.P. XXIII.
Use: Vitamin A & D therapy.

See: Super-D, Perles, Liq. (Upjohn).
• **OLEOVITAMIN D, SYNTHETIC.**
Use: Vitamin D supplement.
See: Viosterol in Oil.
• **OLEYL ALCOHOL,** N.F. XVIII. (Z)-9-Oc-
tadecen-1-ol.
Use: Emulsifying agent, emollient.
• **OLIVE OIL,** N.F. XVIII.
Use: Emollient, pharmaceutical aid (set-
ting retardant for dental cements).
• **OLSALAZINE SODIUM.** USAN.
Use: Maintenance of remission of ulcer-
tiave colitis in patients intolerant of sul-
fasalazine.
See: Dipentum (Pharmacia).
• **OLVANIL.** USAN.
Use: Analgesic.
OM 401.
Use: Sickle cell disease. [Orphan drug]
OMBRE EXTRA STRENGTH. (E.J.
Moore) Vitamins A palmitate, D, B_1, B_2,
B_6, B_{12}, niacinamide, calcium pan-
tothenate, ascorbic acid/Tab. Bot. 50s,
100s.
Use: Vitamin/mineral supplement.
**OMEGA-3 (N-3) POLYUNSATURATED
FATTY ACIDS.** From cold water fish
oils.
Use: Dietary supplement to reduce risk
of coronary artery disease.
See: Cardi-Omega 3, Cap. (Thompson
Medical).
Marine 500, 1000, Cap. (Murdock).
Max EPA, Cap. (Various Mfr.).
Promega, Cap. (Parke-Davis).
Proto-Chol, Cap. (Squibb).
Sea-Omega 50, Cap. (Rugby).
OMEGA OIL. (Block) Methyl nicotinate,
methyl salicylate, capsicum oleoresin,
histamine dihydrochloride, isopropyl al-
cohol 44%. Bot. 2.5 oz, 4.85 oz.
Use: External analgesic.
• **OMEPRAZOLE.** USAN.
Use: Inhibitor of gastric acid secretion.
See: Prilosec (Merck, Sharp & Dohme)
• **OMEPRAZOLE SODIUM.** USAN.
Use: Gastric acid secretory depressant.
OMNICOL. (Delta) Dextromethorphan
HBr 15 mg, chlorpheniramine maleate 4
mg, phenylephrine HCl 5 mg, phenin-
damine tartrate 4 mg, salicylamide 227
mg, acetaminophen 100 mg, caffeine al-
kaloid 10 mg, ascorbic acid 25 mg/Tab.
Bot. 100s. Bot. pt.
Use: Antitussive, antihistamine, decon-
gestant, analgesic.
OMNIHEMIN. (Delta) Iron 110 mg, vitamins C 150 mg, B_{12} 7.5 mcg, folic acid 1
mg, zinc 1 mg, copper 1 mg, manganese 1 mg, magnesium 1 mg/Tab. or

5 ml. **Cap.:** Bot. 100s; **Soln.:** Bot. pt.
Use: Vitamin/mineral supplement.
OMNIHIB. (SK-Beecham) Purified capsular polysaccharide 10 mcg, tetanus toxoid 24 mcg/0.5 ml, sucrose 8.5%. Pow.
for Inj. (lyophilized). Vial w/ 0.6 ml syringe of diluent.
Use: Agent for immunization.
OMNI-M TABLETS. (Blue Cross) Vitamins, minerals. Bot. 100s.
Use: Vitamin/mineral supplement.
OMNINATAL. (Delta) Iron 60 mg, copper
2 mg, zinc 15 mg, vitamins A 8000 IU, D
400 IU, C 90 mg, calcium 200 mg, folic
acid 1.5 mg, B_1 2.5 mg, B_2 3 mg, niacinamide 20 mg, pyridoxine HCl 10 mg,
pantothenic acid 15 mg, B_{12} 8 mcg/Tab.
Bot. 100s.
Use: Vitamin/mineral supplement.
OMNIPAQUE. (Sanofi Winthrop) Iohexol
(46.4% iodine). Nonionic contrast medium. **180 mg/ml:** Vial 10 ml, 20 ml. **240
mg/ml:** Vial 10 ml, 100 ml. Bot. 200 ml.
300 mg/ml: Vial 10 ml, 30 ml, 50 ml, 100
ml. **350 mg/ml:** Vial 50 ml, 100 ml. Bot.
200 ml.
Use: Radiopaque agent.
OMNIPEN. (Wyeth-Ayerst) Ampicillin, anhydrous 250 mg or 500 mg/Cap. Bot.
100s, 500s.
Use: Antibacterial, penicillin.
OMNIPEN. (Wyeth-Ayerst) Ampicillin trihydrate 125 mg or 250 mg/5 ml when reconstituted. Pow. for oral susp. **125
mg/5 ml:** Bot. 100 ml, 150 ml, 200 ml.
250 mg/5 ml: Bot. 100 ml, 150 ml, 200
ml, UD 5 ml × 20.
Use: Antibacterial, penicillin.
OMNIPEN-N. (Wyeth-Ayerst) Ampicillin
sodium pow. for inj. 125 mg, 250 mg,
500 mg, 1 Gm or 2 Gm/Vial. Pkg. 10s.
Piggyback units 500 mg, 1 Gm, 2 Gm,
Bulk 10 Gm/Vial. Pkg. 1s.
Use: Antibacterial, penicillin.
OMNISCAN. (Sanofi Winthrop) Gadodiamide 287 mg, caldiamide sodium 12
mg/ml. Inj. Vial 10 ml, 20 ml, 15 ml fill in
20 ml vials.
Use: Radiopaque agent.
OMNITABS. (Blue Cross) Vitamins A
5000 IU, D 400 IU, C 50 mg, B_1 3 mg, B_2
2.5 mg, niacin 20 mg, B_6 1 mg, B_{12} 1
mcg, pantothenic acid 0.9 mg/Tab. Bot.
100s.
Use: Vitamin supplement.
OMNITABS WITH IRON. (Blue Cross) Vitamins A 5000 IU, D 400 IU, B_1 3 mg, B_2
2.5 mg, B_6 1 mg, B_{12} 1 mcg, C 50 mg,
niacinamide 20 mg, calcium pantothenate 1 mg, iron 15 mg/Tab. Bot. 100s.

Use: Vitamin/iron supplement.

OMNITRATE. (Kenyon) Vitamins A 6000 IU, D 600 IU, E 0.1 mg, B_1 1 mg, B_2 0.1 mg, B_6 0.1 mg, C 37.5 mg, B_{12} 1 mcg, niacinamide 15 mg, folic acid 0.067 mg, hesperidin 50 mg, calcium carbonate 400 mg, iron-ferrous iodide dried 20 mg, magnesium 15 mg, iodine 0.15 mg, manganese 3 mg, zinc 3 mg/3 Cap. Bot. 1000s.
Use: Vitamin/mineral supplement.

OMS CONCENTRATE. (Upsher-Smith) Morphine sulfate 20 mg/ml. Soln. 30, 120 ml.
Use: Narcotic analgesic.

ONCASPAR. (Enzon) Pegaspargase 750 IU/ml in a phosphate buffered saline solution. Inj. In single-use vials.
Use: Antineoplastic agent.

ONCORAD OV103.
Use: Ovarian cancer. [Orphan drug]

ONCOVIN SOLUTION. (Lilly) Vincristine sulfate for inj. 1 mg/ml, 2 mg/2 ml or 5 mg/5 ml. Ctn. 10s. Hyporets 1 mg/Pkg 3s; 2 mg/Pkg 3s.
Use: Antineoplastic agent.

ONCOSCINT CR/OV. (Cytogen)
See: SATUMOMAB PENDETIDE.

•**ONDANSETRON HCl.** USAN.
Use: Antiemetic (cancer chemotherapy).
See: Zofran (Cerenex).

ONDROX. (Unimed) Vitamin A 333 IU, beta carotene 1667 IU, E 16.7 IU, C 41.7 mg, folic acid 66.7 mcg, B_1 0.25 mg, B_2 0.28 mg, B_3 3.3 mg, B_6 0.33 mg, B_{12} 1 mcg, D 100 IU, biotin 5 mcg, B_5 1.7 mg, I, Fe, Ca, Mg, Cu, Zn 2.5 mg, P, K, vitamin K, Cr, Mn, Mo, Se, Omega 3 oils, V, B, Si, citrus bioflavonoids, sodium benzoate, potassium sorbate, BHT, inositol, propyl gallate, l-acetylcysteine, l-glutathione, l-methionine, l-glutamine, taurine. SR Tab. Bot. 60s, 180s.
Use: Vitamin and mineral supplements.

ONE-A-DAY ESSENTIAL. (Miles Inc.) Vitamins A 5000 IU, E 30 IU, C 60 mg, folic acid 0.4 mg, B_1 1.5 mg, B_2 1.7 mg, niacin 20 mg, B_6 2 mg, B_{12} 6 mcg, pantothenic acid 10 mg, D 400 IU/Tab. Sodium free. Bot. 100s.
Use: Vitamin supplement.

ONE-A-DAY MAXIMUM FORMULA. (Miles Inc.) Vitamins A 5000 IU, E 30 IU, C 60 mg, folic acid 0.4 mg, B_1 1.5 mg, B_2 1.7 mg, niacin 20 mg, B_6 2 mg, B_{12} 6 mcg, K 50 mcg, D 400 IU, pantothenic acid 10 mg, iron 18 mg, calcium 129.6 mg, phosphorus 100 mg, iodine 150 mcg, magnesium 100 mg, copper 2 mg,

chromium 10 mcg, selenium 10 mcg, molybdenum 10 mcg, manganese 2.5 mg, potassium 37.5 mg, biotin 30 mcg, chloride 34 mg, zinc 15 mg/Tab. Bot. 30s, 60s, 100s.
Use: Vitamin/mineral supplement.

ONE ONLY VITAMIN TABLETS. (Robinson) Vitamins A 5000 IU, D 400 IU, B_1 2 mg, B_2 2.5 mg, B_6 1 mg, B_{12} 1 mcg, niacinamide 20 mg, panthenol 1 mg/Tab. Bot. 100s, 250s, 1000s.
Use: Vitamin supplement.

ONE ONLY VITAMIN TABLETS WITH IRON. (Robinson) Vitamins A 5000 IU, D 400 IU, B_1 2 mg, B_2 2.5 mg, C 50 mg, B_6 1 mg, B_{12} 1 mcg, niacinamide 20 mg, calcium pantothenate 1 mg, iron 15 mg/Tab. Bot. 100s, 250s, 1000s.
Use: Vitamin/mineral supplement.

ONE-TABLET-DAILY. (Various Mfr.) Vitamins A 5000 IU, D 400 IU, E 30 mg, B_1 1.5 mg, B_2 1.7 mg, B_3 20 mg, B_5 10 mg, B_6 2 mg, B_{12} 6 mcg, C 60 mg, folic acid 0.4 mg. Tab. Bot. 30s, 100s, 250s, 365s, 1000s.
Use: Multivitamin.

ONE TABLET DAILY. (Various Mfr.) Vitamins A 5000 IU, D 400 IU, E 30 mg, B_1 1.5 mg, B_2 1.7 mg, B_3 20 mg, B_5 10 mg, B_6 2 mg, B_{12} 6 mcg, C 60 mg, folic acid 0.4 mg/Tab. Bot. 100s, 250s, 365s.
Use: Vitamin supplement.

ONE TABLET DAILY PLUS IRON. (Various Mfr.) Iron 18 mg, vitamins A 5000 IU, D 400 IU, E 15 mg, B_1 1.5 mg, B_2 1.7 mg, B_3 20 mg, B_6 2 mg, B_{12} 6 mcg, C 60 mg, folic acid 0.4 mg/Tab. Bot. 100s, 250s, 365s.
Use: Vitamin/mineral supplement.

ONE TABLET DAILY WITH IRON. (Various Mfr.) Iron 18 mg, A 5000 IU, D 400 IU, E 30 mg, B_1 1.5 mg, B_2 1.7 mg, B_3 20 mg, B_6 2 mg, B_{12} 6 mcg, C 60 mg, folic acid 0.4 mg. Bot. 100s, 250s, 365s.
Use: Multivitamin w/iron.

1000-BC, IM OR IV. (Solvay) Vitamins B_1 25 mg, B_2 2.5 mg, B_6 5 mg, panthenol 5 mg, B_{12} 500 mcg, niacinamide 75 mg, C 100 mg/ml. Vial 10 ml.
Use: Vitamin supplement.

1+1-F CREME. (Dunhall) Hydrocortisone 1%, pramoxine HCl 1%, iodochlorhydroxyquin 3%. Tube 30 Gm.
Use: Corticosteroid, local anesthetic, antifungal.

1-2-3 OINTMENT NO. 20. (Durel) Burow's solution, lanolin, zinc oxide (Lassar's paste). Jar oz, 1 lb, 6 lb.
Use: Anti-inflammatory agent, topical.

1-2-3 OINTMENT NO. 21. (Durel) Burow's

solution 1 part, lanolin 2, zinc oxide (Lassar's paste) 1.5, cold cream 1.5. Jar oz, 1 lb, 6 lb.
Use: Anti-inflammatory agent, topical.
ONOTON TABLETS. (Sanofi Winthrop) Pancreatin, hemicellulose, ox bile extracts.
Use: Digestive aid.
ONTOSEIN.
See: Orgotein (Diagnostic Data).
ONY-CLEAR. (Pedinol) Triacetin, cetylpyridinium chloride, chloroxylenol, benzlkonium chloride, alcohol. Spray, aerosol. 45, 60 ml.
Use: Topical anti-infective.
OPCON. (Bausch & Lomb) Naphazoline HCl 0.1%. Bot. 15 ml.
Use: Vasoconstrictor/mydriatic, ophthalmic.
OPCON-A. (Bausch & Lomb) Naphazoline HCl 0.025%, pheniramine maleate 0.3%. Bot. 15 ml.
Use: Vasoconstrictor/mydriatic, antihistamine (ophthalmic).
O,P'-DDD.
Use: Miscellaneous antineoplastic.
See: Lysodren (Bristol-Myers Oncology).
OPERAND. (Redi-Products) **Aerosal:** Iodine 0.5%. 90 ml. **Skin cleanser:** Iodine 1%. 90 ml. **Oint.:** Iodine 1%. 30 Gm, lb, packette 1.2 Gm and 2.7 Gm. **Perineal wash conc.:** Iodine 1%. 240 ml. **Prep soln.:** Iodine 1%. 60 ml, 120 ml, 240 ml, pt, qt. **Soln:** Prep pad 100s, swab stick 25s. **Surgical scrub:** Povidone-iodine 7.5%. 60 ml, 120 ml, 240 ml, pt, qt, gal, packette 22.5 ml. **Whirlpool conc.:** Iodine 1%. gal.
Use: Antiseptic, germicide.
OPERAND DOUCHE. (Redi-Products) Povidone-iodine. Soln. 60 ml, 240 ml, UD 15 ml.
Use: Vaginal preparation.
o-PHENYLPHENOL. W/ Amyl complex, phenylmercuric nitrate.
See: Lubrasptic Jelly (Guardian).
OPHTHACET. (Vortech) Sodium sulfacetamide 10%. Soln. 15 ml.
Use: Ophthalmic.
OPHTHAINE HCl. (Apothecon) Proparacaine HCl 0.5%, glycerin 2.45%, chlorobutanol 0.2%, benzalkonium Cl, sodium hydroxide or hydrochloric acid to adjust pH. Soln. Bot. w/dropper 15 ml.
Use: Local anesthetic, ophthalmic.
OPHTHALGAN. (Wyeth-Ayerst) Glycerin ophthalmic soln. w/chlorobutanol (chloral derivative 0.55%) as preservative. Bot. 7.5 ml w/dropper screw cap.

Use: Hyperosmolar preparation.
OPHTHALMIC ALPHA ADRENERGIC BLOCKING AGENTS.
See: Rev-Eyes (Storz/Lederle).
OPHTHA P/S. (Misemer) Prednisolone acetate 0.5%, sodium sulfacetamide 10%, hydroxyethylcellulose, EDTA, polysorbate 80, sodium thiosulfate, benzalkonium chloride 0.025%. Susp. Bot. 5 ml.
Use: Ophthalmic.
OPHTHA P/S OPHTHALMIC SUSPENSION. (Misemer) Sodium sulfacetamide 10%, prednisolone acetate 0.5%. Bot. 5 ml w/dropper.
Use: Steroid/sulfonamide combination, ophthalmic.
OPHTHETIC STERILE OPHTHALMIC SOLUTION. (Allergan) Proparacaine HCl 0.5%, benzalkonium Cl, glycerin, sodium Cl, purified water. Dropper bot. 15 ml.
Use: Local anesthetic, ophthalmic.
OPHTHIFLUOR. (Deklerht) Fluorescein sodium 10%. Inj. Amp. 5 ml.
Use: Diagnostic aid, ophthalmic.
OPHTHOCORT. (Parke-Davis) Hydrocortisone acetate 0.5%, chloramphenicol 1%, polymyxin B sulfate 10,000 units/Gm Oint. Tube 3.5 Gm.
Use: Corticosteroid, anti-infective (ophthalmic).
OPIPRAMOL. B.A.N. 5- 3-[4-(2-Hydroxyethyl)-piperazin-1-yl]propyl - dibenz[b,f]azepine.
Use: Antidepressant.
• **OPIPRAMOL HYDROCHLORIDE.** USAN. 4-[3-(5H-Dibenz[b,f]azepin-5yl)-propyl]-1-piperazine-ethanol dihydrochloride.
Use: Antidepressant, tranquilizer.
• **OPIUM,** U.S.P. XXIII.
Use: Pharmaceutical necessity for powdered opium.
OPIUM ALKALOIDS, TOTAL, AS THE HYDROCHLORIDE SALT.
See: Pantopon, Amp. (Roche).
OPIUM AND BELLADONNA. (Wyeth-Ayerst) Powdered opium 60 mg, extract of belladonna 0.25 gr/Supp. Box 20s.
Use: Narcotic analgesic, anticholinergic/antispasmodic.
• **OPIUM POWDER,** U.S.P. XXIII.
Use: Pharmaceutical necessity for Paregoric.
W/Albumin tannate, colloidal kaolin, pectin.
See: Ekrised, Tab. (Hauck).
W/Atropine sulfate, alcohol.
See: Stopit Liq. (Scrip).

W/Belladonna extract.
See: B & O, Supp. (Webcon).
W/Bismuth subgallate, kaolin, pectin, zinc phenolsulfonate.
See: Diastay, Tab. (Elder).
W/Kaolin, pectin, bismuth subcarbonate.
See: KBP/O, Cap. (Cole).
W/Kaolin, pectin, hyoscyamine sulfate, atropine sulfate, hyoscine HBr.
See: Donnagel-PG, Susp. (Robins).
•**OPIUM TINCTURE,** U.S.P. XXIII.
W/Homatropine MBr, Pectin.
See: Dia-Quel, Liq. (I.P.C.).
W/Pectin.
See: Opecto, Elix. (Bowman).
Parelixir, Liq. (Purdue Frederick).
OPIUM TINCTURE, CAMPHORATED.
Use: Antidiarrheal.
See: Paregoric, U.S.P. XXIII.
W/Glycyrrhiza fluid extract, tartar emetic, glycerin.
See: Brown Mixture.
OPTI-BON EYE DROPS. (Barrows) Phenylephrine HCl, berberine sulfate, boric acid, sodium Cl, sodium bisulfite, glycerine, camphor water, peppermint water, thimerosal 0.004%. Bot. 1 oz.
Use: Ophthalmic preparation.
OPTICAPS. (Approved) Vitamins A 32,500 IU, D 3250 IU, B_1 15 mg, B_2 5 mg, B_6 0.5 mg, C 150 mg, E 5 IU, calcium pantothenate 3 mg, niacinamide 150 mg, B_{12} 20 mcg, iron 11.26 mg, choline bitartrate 30 mg, inositol 30 mg, pepsin 32.5 mg, diastase 32.5 mg, calcium 30 mg, phosphorus 25 mg, magnesium 0.7 mg, Fr. dicalcium phosphate 110 mg, manganese 1.3 mg, potassium 0.68 mg, zinc 0.45 mg, hesperidin compound 25 mg, biotin 20 mcg, Brewer's yeast 50 mg, wheat germ oil 20 mg, hydrolized yeast 81.25 mg, protein digest. 47.04 mg, amino acids 34.21 mg/Cap. Bot. 30s, 60s, 90s, 1000s.
Use: Vitamin/mineral supplement.
OPTICARE PMS. (Standard Drug) Vitamin A 2083 IU, E 16.7 IU, D_3 16.7 IU, folic acid 33.3 mcg, B_1 4.2 mg, B_2 4.2 mg, B_3 4.2 mg, B_5 4.2 mg, B_6 50 mg, B_{12} 10.4 mcg, biotin 10.4 mcg, choline bitartrate 52 mg, inositol 4.2 mg, PABA 4.2 mg, C 250 mg, bioflavonoids 41.7 mg, rutin 4.2 mg, Ca 20.8 mg, Mg 41.7 mg, I 12.5 mg, Fe 2.5 mg, Cu 0.08 mg, Zn 4.2 mg, Mn 1.7 mg, K 7.9 mg, Se 16.7 mcg, Cr 16.7 mcg, amylase activity 2500 USP units, protease activity 2500 USP, lipase activity 200 USP units, betaine acid HCl 16.7 mg, tartrazine. Tab. Bot. 15s.
Use: Multivitamin/mineral supplement

w/iron.
OPTI-CLEAN. (Alcon) Polysorbate 21, polymeric cleaning beads, thimerosal 0.004%, EDTA 0.1%. Bot 12 ml, 20 ml.
Use: Contact lens care.
OPTI-CLEAN II. (Alcon) Isotonic polymeric cleaning agent, hydroxyethylcellulose, polysorbate 21, EDTA 0.1%, polyquaternium-1 0.001%. Thimerosal free. Bot. 12 ml, 20 ml.
Use: Contact lens care.
OPTICYL. (Optopics) Tropicamide 0.5%, 1%. Soln. Bot. 2 ml, 15 ml.
Use: Mydriatic/cycloplegic.
OPTI-FREE. (Alcon) Citrate buffer, NaCl, EDTA 0.05%, polyquaternium-1 0.001%. Soln. 120 ml, 240 ml, 360 ml.
Use: Ophthalmic.
OPTIGENE. (Pfeiffer) Sodium Cl, sodium phosphate mono- and dibasic, benzalkonium Cl, EDTA. Soln. Bot. 118 ml.
Use: Ophthalmic irrigation solution.
OPTIGENE 3. (Pfeiffer) Tetrahydrozoline HCl 0.05%. Soln. Bot. 15 ml.
Use: Vasoconstrictor/mydriatic, ophthalmic.
OPTILETS-500. (Abbott) Vitamins B_1 15 mg, B_2 10 mg, niacinamide 100 mg, calcium pantothenate 20 mg, B_6 5 mg, C 500 mg, A 10,000 IU, D 400 IU, E 30 IU, B_{12} 12 mcg/Filmtab. Bot. 100s, 130s.
Use: Vitamin/mineral supplement
OPTILETS-M-500. (Abbott) Vitamins C 500 mg, niacinamide 100 mg, calcium pantothenate 20 mg, B_1 15 mg, A 10,000 IU, B_2 10 mg, B_6 5 mg, D 400 IU, B_{12} 12 mcg, E 30 IU, iron 20 mg, magnesium 80 mg, zinc 1.5 mg, copper 2 mg, manganese 1 mg, iodine 0.15 mg/Filmtab. Bot. 100s.
Use: Vitamin/mineral supplement.
OPTIMINE. (Schering) Azatadine maleate 1 mg/Tab. Bot. 100s.
Use: Antihistamine.
OPTIMYD. (Schering) Prednisolone phosphate 0.5%, sodium sulfacetamide 10%, sodium thiosulfate. Soln-Sterile. Drop bot. 5 ml.
Use: Steroid/sulfonamide combination, ophthalmic.
OPTI-ONE MULTI-PURPOSE. (Alcon) EDTA 0.05%, polyquaternium-1 0.001%, sodium chloride. Buffered, isotonic. Soln. 118 ml, 237 ml, 355 ml, 473 ml.
Use: Soft contact lens care.
OPTI-ONE REWETTING. (Alcon) EDTA 0.05%, polyquaternium-1 0.001%, sodium chloride. Buffered, isotonic. Drops. Bot. 10 ml.
Use: Soft contact lens care.

OPTIPRANOLOL. (Bausch & Lomb) Metipropranolol HCl 0.3%. Bot. 5 ml, 10 ml.
Use: Agent for glaucoma.
OPTIRAY. (Mallinckrodt) Ioversol.
Use: Radiopaque agent.
OPTIRAY 350. (Mallinckrodt Medical) Ioversol 74%, iodine 35%, tromethamine 3.6 mg, EDTA 0.2 mg/ml. Inj. 30 and 50 ml glass vials, 75 ml fill in 150 ml glass bottles, 100 ml fill in 150 ml glass bottles, 150 ml glass bottles, 200 ml fill in 250 ml glass bottles, 30 and 50 ml hand-held plastic syringes, 50 ml fill in 125 ml power injector plastic syringes, 100 ml fill in 125 ml power injector plastic syringes and 125 ml power injector plastic syringes.
Use: Radiopaque agent.
OPTISED SOLN. (Ketchum) Zinc sulfate 0.025%, phenylephrine HCl 0.12%. Bot. 15 ml.
Use: Decongestant combination, ophthalmic.
OPTI-SOFT. (Alcon) Isotonic soln of sodium Cl, borate buffer, EDTA 0.1%, polyquaternium-1 0.001%. Thimerosal free. Soln. Bot. 237 ml, 355 ml.
Use: Soft contact lens care.
OPTI-SOFT ESPECIALLY FOR SENSITIVE EYES. (Alcon) Buffered, isotonic. EDTA 0.1%, polyquaternium-1 0.001%, NaCl, borate buffer. For lenses w/ ≤ 45% water content. Soln. Bot. 118 ml, 237 ml, 355 ml.
Use: Soft contact lens care.
OPTI-TEARS. (Alcon) Isotonic solution with dextran, sodium Cl, potassium Cl, hydroxypropyl methylcellulose, EDTA 0.1%, polyquaternium-1 0.01%. Thimerosal free. Soln. Bot. 15 ml.
Use: Contact lens care.
OPTIVITE FOR WOMEN. (Optimox) Vitamins A 2083 IU, D 16.7 IU, E 14 mg, B_1 4.2 mg, B_2 4.2 mg, B_3 4.2 mg, B_5 4.2 mg, B_6 50 mg, B_{12} 10.4 mcg, C 250 mg, iron 2.5 mg, folic acid 0.03 mg, zinc 4.2 mg, choline 52 mg, inositol 10 mg, Cr, Cu, I, K, Mg, Mn, Se, citrus bioflavonoids, PABA, rutin, pancreatin, biotin/Tab. Bot. 180s.
Use: Vitamin/mineral supplement.
OPTIVITE P.M.T. (Optimox) Vitamins A 2083 IU, D 16.7 IU, E 16.7 mg, B_1 4.2 mg, B_2 4.2 mg, B_3 4.2 mg, B_5 4.2 mg, B_6 50 mg, B_{12} 10.4 mcg, C 250 mg, iron 2.5 mg, FA 0.03 mg, Zn 4.2 mg, choline bitartrate 52 mg, Cr, Cu, I, K, Mg, Mn, Se, bioflavonoids, betaine, PABA, rutin, pancreatin, biotin/Tab. Bot. 180s.

Use: Geriatric vitamin/mineral supplement.
OPTI-ZYME ENZYMATIC CLEANER FOR SENSITIVE EYES. (Alcon Lenscare) Pork pancreatin tablets. Pak 8s, 24s, 36s, 56s.
Use: Contact lens care.
OPTO-MIST. (Ketchum) Sodium propionate, sodium Cl, camphor, peppermint oil. Bot. 0.5 oz.
ORA5. (McHenry) Copper sulfate, iodine, potassium iodide, alcohol 1.5%. Liq. Bot. 3.75 ml, 30 ml.
Use: Mouth preparation.
ORABASE. (Colgate-Hoyt) Gelatin, pectin, sodium carboxymethylcellulose in hydrocarbon gel w/polyethylene and mineral oil. 0.75 gm Packet Box 100s. Tube 5 Gm, 15 Gm.
Use: Mouth preparation.
ORABASE BABY. (Colgate-Hoyt) Benzocaine 7.5%, saccharin, alcohol free, fruit flavor. Gel. 7.2 Gm.
Use: Mouth and throat product.
ORABASE GEL. (Colgate-Oral) Benzocaine 15%, ethyl alcohol, tannic acid, salicylic acid, saccharin. Gel. 7 g.
Use: Mouth preparation.
ORABASE HCA. (Colgate-Hoyt) Hydrocortisone acetate 0.5% in paste base. Packet 0.75 Gm Box 100s. Tube 5 Gm.
Use: Corticosteroid mouth preparation.
ORABASE LIP HEALER. (Colgate-Hoyt) Benzocaine 5%, allantoin 1%, menthol 0.5%, petrolatum, lanolin, camphor, phenol. Cream. 10 Gm.
Use: Mouth and throat product.
ORABASE-O. (Colgate-Hoyt) Benzocaine 20% in a polyethylene, mineral oil base. Gel. In 15 Gm.
Use: Local anesthetic.
ORABASE PLAIN. (Colgate-Hoyt) Gelatin, pectin & sodium carboxymethylcellulose in polyethylene and mineral gel. Paste. 5, 15 Gm.
Use: Mouth and throat product.
ORABASE WITH BENZOCAINE. (Colgate-Hoyt) Benzocaine 20% in gel base. Packet 0.75 Gm, Box 100s. Tube 5 Gm, 15 Gm.
Use: Local anesthetic.
ORACAP CAPSULES. (Vangard) Phenylpropanolamine HCl 75 mg, chlorpheniramine maleate 12 mg/Cap. Bot. 100s, 1000s.
Use: Decongestant, antihistamine.
ORACIT. (Carolina Medical Prod.) Sodium citrate 490 mg, citric acid 640 mg/5 ml, (sodium 1 mEq/ml equivalent to 1 mEq bicarbonate), alcohol 0.25%. Soln.

Bot. pt, UD 15, 30 ml.
Use: Systemic alkalinizer.
ORADERM LIP BALM. (Schattner) Sodium phenolate, sodium tetraborate, phenol, base containing an anionic emulsifier. ⅛ oz.
Use: Local anesthetic, antiseptic.
ORADEX-C. (Commerce) Cetylpyridinium Cl 2.5 mg, benzocaine 10 mg/Troche. Bot. 10s.
Use: Antiseptic, local anesthetic.
ORAFIX MEDICATED. (SK-Beecham) Allantoin 0.2%, benzocaine 2%. Tube 0.75 oz.
Use: Local anesthetic, denture adhesive.
ORAFIX ORIGINAL. (SK-Beecham) Tube 1.5 oz, 2.5 oz, 4 oz.
Use: Denture adhesive.
ORAFIX SPECIAL. (SK-Beecham) Tube 1.4 oz, 2.4 oz.
Use: Denture adhesive.
ORA-FRESH. (A.V.P.) Sugar-free, non-alcoholic, nontoxic, flavored mouthwash. UD cup 1 oz, Bot. 4 oz, 16 oz.
Use: Mouth preparation.
ORAGEST S.R. (Major) Phenylpropanolamine HCl 75 mg, chlorpheniramine maleate 12 mg/SR Cap. Bot. 100s, 250s, 1000s, UD 100s.
Use: Decongestant, antihistamine.
ORAGRAFIN CALCIUM GRANULES. (Squibb) Ipodate calcium (61.7% iodine) 3 Gm/8 Gm Pkg. 25 × 1 dose pkg.
Use: Radiopaque agent.
ORAGRAFIN SODIUM CAPSULES. (Squibb) Ipodate sodium (61.4% iodine) 0.5 Gm/Cap. Bot. 100s, 144s. Unimatic pkg. 100s. Card 6s. Box 25s.
Use: Radiopaque agent.
ORAHESIVE POWDER. (Hoyt) Gelatin, pectin, sodium carboxymethylcellulose. Bot. 25 Gm.
Use: Denture adhesive.
ORAHIST TR. (Vangard) Chlorpheniramine maleate 8 mg, phenylpropanolamine HCl 50 mg, isopropamide iodide 2.5 mg/TR Cap. Bot. 100s, 1000s.
Use: Antihistamine, decongestant.
ORAJEL. (Commerce) Benzocaine 10% in a special base. Tube 0.2 oz, 0.5 oz.
Use: Local anesthetic.
ORAJEL BABY. (Commerce) Benzocaine 7.5% in a special base. Tube 0.5 oz.
Use: Local anesthetic.
ORAJEL BRACE-AID ORAL HYGIENIC RINSE. (Commerce) Carbamide peroxide 10% in anhydrous glycerin. Tube oz.

Use: Mouth preparation.
ORAJEL D. (Commerce) Benzocaine in a special anti-irritant base. Tube 0.5 oz.
Use: Local anesthetic.
ORAJEL MAXIMUM STRENGTH. (Commerce) Benzocaine 20% in special base. Tube ⅓ oz, ¾₆ oz.
Use: Local anesthetic.
ORAJEL MOUTH-AID. (Commerce) Benzocaine 20%, benzalkonium Cl 0.12%, zinc Cl 0.1% in special emollient base. Tube 0.33 oz.
Use: Local anesthetic, antibacterial.
ORAJEL PERIOSEPTIC. (Del Pharm.) Carbamide peroxide 15%, saccharin, methylparaben, EDTA. Liq. Bot. 13.3 ml.
Use: Local anesthetic.
ORAL-B MUPPETS FLUORIDE TOOTHPASTE. (Oral-B) Fluoride 0.22%. Pump 4.3 oz.
Use: Dental caries preventative.
ORALCID.
See: Acetarsone.
ORAL CONTRACEPTIVES.
See: Demulen, Tab. (Searle).
Desogen, Tab. (Organon).
Enovid-E, Tab. (Searle).
GenCept, Tab. (Gencon).
Jenest-28, Tab. (Organon).
Loestrin, Prods. (Parke-Davis).
Lo/Ovral, Prods. (Wyeth-Ayerst).
Miconor, Tab. (Ortho).
Modicon, Prods. (Ortho).
Nelulen, Tab. (Watson Labs).
Norethin 1/35 E Tab. (Roberts).
Norethin 1/50 M Tab. (Roberts).
Nordette, Tab. (Wyeth-Ayerst).
Norinyl, Prods. (Syntex).
Norlestrin, Prods. (Parke-Davis).
Norquen, Tab. (Syntex).
Ortho Cept, Tab. (Ortho).
Ortho-Cyclen, Tab. (Ortho).
Ortho Tri-Cyclen, Tab. (Ortho).
Ortho-Novum, Prods. (Ortho).
Ovcon-35, Tab. (Mead Johnson).
Ovcon-50, Tab. (Mead Johnson).
Ovral, Tab. (Wyeth-Ayerst).
Ovrette, Tab. (Wyeth-Ayerst).
Ovulen, Tab. (Searle).
Triphasil, Tab. (Wyeth-Ayerst).
ORAL DROPS/CANKER SORE RELIEF. (Weeks & Leo) Carbamide peroxide 10% in anhydrous glycerin base. Bot. 30 ml.
Use: Mouth preparation.
ORALONE DENTAL. (Thames) Triamcinolone acetonide 0.1%. Paste 5 Gm.
Use: Corticosteroid, topical.
•**ORAL REHYDRATION SALTS,** U.S.P. XXIII.

ORAMIDE. (Major) Tolbutamide 0.5 Gm/Tab. Bot. 100s, 1000s.
Use: Antidiabetic agent.

ORAMINIC II. (Vortech) Brompheniramine maleate 10 mg per ml/Inj. Vial. 10 ml multidose.
Use: Antihistamine.

ORAMORPH SR. (Roxane) SR Tab.: Morphine sulfate 30 mg, lactose. 50s, 100s, 250s, UD 100s. SR Tab.: Morphine sulfate 60 mg, lactose. 100s, UD 25s. SR Tab.: Morphine sulfate 100 mg, lactose. 100s, UD 25s.
Use: Narcotic analgesic.

• **ORANGE FLOWER OIL,** N.F. XVII.
Use: Flavor, perfume, vehicle.

• **ORANGE FLOWER WATER,** N.F. XVIII.
Use: Flavor, perfume.

• **ORANGE OIL,** N.F. XVIII.
Use: Flavor.

• **ORANGE PEEL TINCTURE, SWEET,** N.F. XVIII.
Use: Flavor.

• **ORANGE SPIRIT, COMPOUND,** N.F. XVIII.
Use: Flavor.

• **ORANGE SYRUP,** N.F. XVIII.
Use: Flavored vehicle.

ORANYL. (Otis Clapp) Pseudoephedrine HCl 30 mg/Tab. Sugar, caffeine, lactose and salt free. Safety pack 500s.
Use: Decongestant.

ORANYL PLUS. (Otis Clapp) Acetaminophen, pseudoephedrine HCl/Tab. Caffeine, sugar, lactose and salt free.
Use: Analgesic, decongestant.

ORAP. (McNeil Pharm) Pimozide 2 mg/Tab. Bot. 100s.
Use: Antipsychotic agent.

ORAPHEN-PD. (Great Southern) Acetaminophen 120 mg per 5 ml, alcohol 5%, cherry flavor. Elix. 120 ml.
Use: Acetaminophen.

ORARSAN.
See: Acetarsone.

ORASEPT. (Pharmakon Labs) Tannic acid 114.9 mg, methylbenzethonium HCl 14.4 mg, benzocaine 14.4 mg, ethyl alcohol 61%/ml, camphor, menthol, benzyl alcohol, spearmint oil, cassia oil. Liq. Bot. 15 ml, 30 ml.
Use: Mouth and throat preparation.

ORASEPT, ORAL. (Pharmakon Labs.) Tannic acid 114.9 mg, methylbenzethonium HCl 14.4 mg, benzocaine 14.4 mg, ethyl alcohol 61% per ml, camphor, menthol, benzyl alcohol, spearmint oil, oil of cassia. Liq. Bot. 15, 30 ml.
Use: Mouth and throat preparation.

ORASEPT, THROAT. (Pharmakon Labs)

Benzocaine 10.16 mg, methylbenzethonium CL 10.51 mg per ml, ethanol 67.36% in a sorbitol solution of 70%, glycerin, menthol, peppermint, saccharin. Throat spray. 45 ml.
Use: Mouth and throat preparation.

ORASONE. (Solvay) Prednisone **1 mg, 5 mg, 10 mg or 20 mg/Tab.**: Bot. 100o, 1000s, UD 100s. **50 mg/Tab.**: Bot. 100s, UD 100s.
Use: Corticosteroid.

ORATECT. (MGI) Benzocaine 15% in SD alcohol 65.8%, wintergreen flavor. Gel. Tube 10.5 Gm.
Use: Mouth and throat preparation.

ORATUSS TR. (Vangard) Caramiphen edisylate 20 mg, chlorpheniramine maleate 8 mg, phenylpropanolamine HCl 50 mg, isopropamide iodide 2.5 mg/TR Cap. Bot. 100s, 500s.
Use: Antitussive, antihistamine, decongestant, anticholinergic/antispasmodic.

ORAZINC. (Mericon) Zinc sulfate 220 mg/Cap. Bot. 100s, 1000s.
Use: Mineral supplement.

ORBENIN. Sodium cloxacillin.
Use: Antibiotic.

ORBIFERROUS. (Orbit) Ferrous fumarate 300 mg, vitamins B_{12} 12 mcg, C 50 mg, B_1 3 mg, defatted desiccated liver 50 mg/Tab. Bot. 60s, 500s.
Use: Vitamin/mineral supplement.

ORBIT. (Spanner) Vitamins A 6250 IU, D 400 IU, B_1 3 mg, B_2 3 mg, B_6 2 mg, B_{12} 5 mcg, C 75 mg, niacinamide 20 mg, calcium pantothenate 10 mg, E 15 IU, biotin 15 mcg, iron 20 mg/Tab. Bot. 100s.
Use: Vitamin/mineral supplement.

ORCIPRENALINE. B.A.N. 1-(3,5-Dihydroxyphenyl)-2-isopropylaminoethanol.
Use: Bronchodilator.

• **ORCONAZOLE NITRATE.** USAN.
Use: Antifungal.

ORDRINE. (Vitarine) Chlorpheniramine maleate 12 mg, phenylpropanolamine HCl 75 mg/SR Cap. Bot. 100s, 1000s.
Use: Antihistamine, decongestant.

ORDRINE AT EXTENDED RELEASE. (Vitarine) Phenylpropanolamine HCl 75 mg, caramiphen edisylate 40 mg, sucrose. Cap. Bot. 50s, 100s, 500s.
Use: Cough preparation.

ORETIC. (Abbott) Hydrochlorothiazide 25 mg or 50 mg/Tab. Bot. 100s, 1000s, UD 100s.
Use: Diuretic.

ORETICYL 25 and 50. (Abbott) **25:** Hydrochlorothiazide 25 mg, deserpidine

0.125 mg/Tab. Bot. 100s. **50:** Hydrochlorothiazide 50 mg, deserpidine 0.125 mg/Tab. Bot. 100s.
Use: Antihypertensive combination.
ORETON METHYL. (Schering) Methyltestosterone. **Buccal Tab.:** 10 mg, Bot. 100s. **Tab.:** 10 mg or 25 mg. Bot. 100s.
Use: Androgen.
OREXIN. (Roberts) Vitamins B₁ 10 mg, B₆ 5 mg, B₁₂ 25 mcg/Softab Tab. Bot. 100s.
Use: Vitamin supplement.
ORGLAGEN TABLETS. (Goldline) Orphenidrine citrate 100 mg/Tab. Bot. 100s, 1000s.
Use: Skeletal muscle relaxant.
•**ORGOTEIN.** USAN. A group of soluble metalloproteins isolated from liver, red blood cells, and other mammalian tissues.
Use: Anti-inflammatory.
ORGOTEIN. (Diagnostic Data) Pure water soluble protein with a compact conformation maintained by 4 Gm atoms of chelated divalent metals, produced from bovine liver as a Cu-Zn mixed chelate having superoxide dismutase activity. Ontosein, Palosein.
ORIGINAL ECLIPSE SUNSCREEN. (Eclipse) padimate O, glyceryl PABA, SPF 10. Lot. Bot. 120 ml.
Use: Sunscreen.
ORIGINAL SENSODYNE. (Block) Strontium chloride hexahydrate 10%, saccharin, sorbitol. Toothpaste. Tube 59.5 Gm.
Use: Mouth and throat preparation.
ORIMUNE TRIVALENT. (Lederle) Poliovirus vaccine. Live, Oral, Trivalent. Sabin strains Types 1, 2, and 3. Dose of 0.5 ml Dispette disposable pipette 1 dose. 10s. Pkg. 5s, 20s, 50s.
Use: Agent for immunization.
ORINASE. (Upjohn) Tolbutamide 250 mg or 500 mg/Tab. **250 mg:** Bot. 100s; **500 mg:** Bot. 200s, 500s, 1000s, UD Box 100s, Unit-of-Use Bot. 50s, 100s.
Use: Antidiabetic agent.
ORINASE DIAGNOSTIC. (Upjohn) Tolbutamide sodium 1 Gm/Vial. Pow. for inj. Vial with 20 ml amp diluent.
Use: Diagnostic aid.
ORISUL. (Ciba) Sulfaphenazole. A sulfonamide under study.
•**ORMAPLATIN.** USAN.
Use: Antineoplastic.
ORMAZINE. (Hauck) Chlorpromazine HCl 25 mg/ml. Vial 10 ml.
Use: Antipsychotic agent.
•**ORMETROPRIM.** USAN. (1)2,4-Diamino-5-(6-methylveratryl)pyrimidine; (2)2,4-diamino-5-(4,5-dimethoxy-2-methylbenzyl)pyrimidine.
Use: Antibacterial.
ORNADE. (SK-Beecham) Phenylpropanolamine HCl 75 mg, chlorpheniramine maleate 12 mg/Spansule. Bot. 50s, 500s, UD 100s.
Use: Decongestant, antihistamine.
ORNEX. (SK-Beecham) Acetaminophen 325 mg, phenylpropanolamine HCl 12.5 mg/Capl. Blister Pak 24s, 48s. Bot. 100s. Dispensary pak 792s.
Use: Analgesic, decongestant.
ORNEX, MAXIMUM STRENGTH. (Menley & James) Pseudoephedrine HCl, acetaminophen 500 mg. Cap. Bot. 24s, 30s, 48s.
Use: Upper respiratory combination.
•**ORNIDAZOLE.** USAN.
Use: Anti-infective.
ORNIDYL. (Marion Merrell Dow) Eflornithine HCl 200 mg/ml. Inj. Vial. 100 ml.
Use: Antiprotozoal.
•**ORPANOXIN.** USAN.
Use: Anti-inflammatory.
ORPENEED VK. (Hanlon) Penicillin, buffered 400,000 units/Tab. Bot. 100s.
Use: Antibacterial, penicillin.
•**ORPHENADRINE CITRATE,** U.S.P. XXII. Inj., U.S.P. XXIII. N,N-Dimethyl-2-(0-methyl-α-phenyl-benzyloxy)-ethylamine. N,N-Dimethyl-2-((o-methyl α phenyl benzyl)oxy)-ethylamine Citrate (1:1). (Various Mfr.) Inj. 30 mg/ml. Amps 2 ml, vial 10 ml. **Tab.:** 100 mg. Bot. 30s, 100s, 500s, 1000s.
Use: Skeletal muscle relaxant, antihistamine.
See: Banflex (Forest Pharm.).
Flexoject (Mayrand).
Flexon, Inj. (Keene).
Myolin (Roberts Hauck).
Norflex, Tab., Amp. (3M Pharm).
Orphanate, Inj. (Hyrex).
W/Aspirin, phenacetin, caffeine.
See: Norgesic, Tab. (Riker).
Norgesic Forte, Tab. (Riker).
ORPHENADRINE HYDROCHLORIDE. N,N-Dimethyl-2-(o-methyl-α-phenylbenzyloxy)ethylamine.
See: Disipal, Tab. (Riker).
W/Comb.
See: Estomul, Liq., Tab. (Riker).
ORPHENGESIC. (Various Mfr.) Orphenadrine citrate 25 mg, aspirin 385 mg, caffeine 30 mg/Tab. Bot. 100s, 500s, UD 100s.
Use: Skeletal muscle relaxant, salicylate analgesic.
ORPHENGESIC FORTE. (Various Mfr.)

Orphenadrine citrate 50 mg, aspirin 770 mg, caffeine 60 mg/Tab. Bot. 100s, 500s.
Use: Skeletal muscle relaxant, salicylate analgesic.

ORTAC-DM LIQUID. (Ion) Dextromethorphan 10 mg, phenylephrine HCl 5 mg, guaifenesin 100 mg/5 ml. Bot. 4 oz.
Use: Antitussive, decongestant, expectorant.

ORTAL SODIUM. Sodium 5-ethyl-5-hexylbarbiturate. Hexethal sodium.

ORTEDRINE.
See: Amphetamine (Various Mfr.).

ORTEGA OTIC M. (Ortega) Hydrocortisone 1%, neomycin sulfate 5 mg, polymyxin B sulfate 10,000 units per ml. Soln. 10 ml w/dropper.
Use: Otic preparation.

ORTHESIN.
See: Benzocaine.

ORTHO ALL-FLEX DIAPHRAGM. (Ortho) Diaphragm kit (all flex arcing spring) in plastic compact, sizes 55, 60, 65, 70, 75, 80, 85, 90, 95 mm.
Use: Contraceptive.

ORTHOCAINE.
See: Orthoform (No mfr. listed).

ORTHO-CEPT. (Ortho) Desogestrel 0.15 mg, ethinyl estradiol 0.03 mg. Tab. Pkg. 28s w/ 7 inert tab. and 21s.
Use: Oral contraceptive.

ORTHOCLONE OKT3. (Ortho) Muromonab-CD3 5 mg per 5 ml. Inj. 5 ml amps.
Use: Immunosuppressive drug.

ORTHOCLONE OKT3 STERILE SOLUTION. (Ortho) Orthoclone OKT3 is murine monoclonal antibody to the T3 antigen of human T cells which function as immunosuppressant. Amp. 5 ml.
Use: Immunosuppressive agent.

ORTHO-CREME CONTRACEPTIVE CREAM. (Advanced Care) Nonoxynol-9 2% in nonfatty acid cream base. Tube 70 Gm w/measured dose applicator. Refill tube 70 Gm, 115 Gm.
Use: Contraceptive.

ORTHO-CYCLEN. (Ortho) Norgestimate 250 mcg, ethinyl estradiol 35 mcg. Tab. Pkg. 21s, 28s.
Use: Oral contraceptive.

ORTHO DIAPHRAGM. (Ortho) Diaphragm kit, coil spring sizes 50, 55, 60, 65, 70, 75, 80, 85, 90, 95, 100, 105 mm.
Use: Contraceptive.

ORTHO DIAPHRAGM-WHITE. (Ortho) Diaphragm kit, flat spring sizes 55, 60, 65, 70, 75, 80, 85, 90, 95 mm.

Use: Contraceptive.

ORTHO DIENESTROL CREAM. (Ortho) Dienestrol 0.01%. Tube 78 Gm with or without applicator.
Use: Estrogen.

ORTHOFLAVIN. (Enzyme Process) Vitamins C 150 mg, E 25 mg/Tab. Bot. 100s, 250s.
Use: Vitamin supplement.

ORTHOFORM. (No mfr. listed.) Menthyl 3-amino-4-hydroxybenzoate.
Use: Local anesthetic.

W/Tyrothricin. (Columbus) Tyrothricin 0.5 mg, tetracaine HCl 0.5%, epinephrine 1/1000 Soln. 2%/Gm. Oint., Tube oz.
Use: Anti-infective, ophthalmic.

ORTHO-GYNOL CONTRACEPTIVE JELLY. (Advanced Care) p-diisobutyl-phenoxy-polyethoxy-ethanol 1%, in water-dispersible jelly at pH 4.5. Tube 81 Gm w/measured-dose applicator. Tube 81 Gm, 126 Gm.
Use: Contraceptive.

ORTHOHYDROXYPHENYLMERCURIC CHLORIDE. (O-chloromercuriphenol).
Use: Antiseptic.

W/Benzocaine, ephedrine HCl.
See: Myrimgacaine, Liq. (Upjohn).

W/Benzocaine, parachlorometaxylenol, benzalkonium Cl, phenol.
See: Unguentine Aerosol (Norwich).

W/Benzoic acid, salicylic acid.
See: NP-27 Liq. (Norwich).

W/Benzoic acid, salicylic acid, sec.-amyltricresols.
See: Salicresin, Liq.(Upjohn).

W/Zinc acetate, salicylic acid, phenol.
See: Zemacol, Medicated Skin Lotion (Norwich).

ORTHO-NOVUM 1/35-21. (Ortho) Norethindrone 1 mg, ethinyl estradiol 0.035 mg/Tab. Dialpak 21s.
Use: Oral contraceptive.

ORTHO-NOVUM 1/35-28. (Ortho) Norethindrone 1 mg, ethinyl estradiol 0.035 mg/Tab. w/7 inert Tab. Dialpak 28s.
Use: Oral contraceptive.

ORTHO-NOVUM 1/50-21. (Ortho) Norethindrone 1 mg, mestranol 50 mcg/Tab. Dialpak 21s.
Use: Oral contraceptive.

ORTHO-NOVUM 1/50-28. (Ortho) Norethindrone 1 mg, mestranol 50 mcg/Tab. w/7 inert Tab. Dialpak 28s.
Use: Oral contraceptive.

ORTHO-NOVUM 7/7/7/-21 TABLETS. (Ortho) Norethindrone 0.5 mg, ethinyl estradiol 0.035 mg/Tab.; norethindrone

0.75 mg, ethinyl estradiol 0.035 mg/Tab.;
norethindrone 1 mg, ethinyl estradiol
0.035 mg/Tab. Dialpak 21s.
Use: Oral contraceptive.
ORTHO-NOVUM 7/7/7/-28 TABLETS.
(Ortho) Same as Ortho-Novum 7/7/7/-21
w/7 inert tab. Dialpak 28s.
Use: Oral contraceptive.
ORTHO-NOVUM 10/11-21 TABLETS.
(Ortho) Norethindrone 0.5 mg, ethinyl
estradiol 0.035 mg/Tab; norethindrone 1
mg, ethinyl estradiol 0.035 mg/Tab. Dialpak 21s.
Use: Oral contraceptive.
ORTHO-NOVUM 10/11-28 TABLETS.
(Ortho) Norethindrone 0.5 mg, ethinyl
estradiol 0.035 mg/Tab; norethindrone 1
mg, ethinyl estradiol 0.035 mg/Tab; w/in-
ert tab. Dialpak 28s.
Use: Oral contraceptive.
ORTHO PERSONAL LUBRICANT. (Advanced Care) Greaseless, water soluble
and non-staining aqueous hydrocolloid
gel. Acid buffered to vaginal pH. Tube 2
oz, 4 oz.
Use: Lubricant.
ORTHO TRI-CYCLEN. (Ortho) 7 white
tablets containing norgestimate 0.18
mg, ethinyl estradiol 35 mcg; 7 light blue
tablets containing norgestimate 0.215
mg, ethinyl estradiol 35 mcg; 7 blue
tablets containing norgestimate 0.25
mg, ethinyl estradiol 35 mcg. Tab. Pkg.
21s, 28s.
Use: Oral contraceptive.
ORTHOXICOL COUGH SYRUP.
(Roberts) Phenylpropanolamine HCl 8.3
mg, chlorpheniramine maleate 1.3 mg,
dextromethorphan HBr 6.7 mg, alcohol
8%, sorbitol, parabens. Bot. 60 ml, 120
ml, 480 ml.
Use: Decongestant, antihistamine, antitussive.
ORTHOXINE. Methoxyphenamine.
ORTICALM.
Use: Hypotensive, tranquilizer.
See: Serpasil, Prod. (Squibb).
OR-TOPTIC M. (Ortega) Prednisolone
acetate 0.5%, sodium sulfacetamide,
hydroxyethylcellulose, EDTA, polysorbate 80, sodium thiosulfate, 0.025%
benzalkonium chloride. Susp. 5 ml drop
bot.
Use: Ophthalmic.
OR-TYL. (Ortega) Dicyclomine HCl 10
mg/ml. Inj. Vial. 10 ml.
Use: Antispasmodic.
ORUDIS. (Wyeth-Ayerst) Ketoprofen 25
mg, 50 mg or 75 mg/Cap. Bot. **25 mg or
50 mg:** 100s; **75 mg:** 100s, 500s, UD

100s.
Use: Nonsteroidal anti-inflammatory
drug; analgesic.
ORVUS.
See: Gardinol Type Detergents (Various
Mfr.).
OSARSAL.
See: Acetarsone.
OS-CAL 250. (Marion) Oyster shell pow-
der as calcium 250 mg, vitamin D 125 IU
and trace minerals (Cu, Fe, Mg, Mn, Zn,
silica)/Tab. Bot. 100s, 240s, 500s,
1000s.
Use: Calcium/vitamin D supplement.
OS-CAL 500. (SK-Beecham) Calcium
500 mg/Tab. Bot. 60s, 120s.
Use: Calcium supplement.
OS-CAL + D. (SK-Beecham) Calcium
carbonate 625 mg, vitamin D 125
units/Tab. Bot. 100s.
Use: Calcium/vitamin D supplement.
OS-CAL 500 + D. (SK-Beecham) Calcium
carbonate 1250 mg, vitamin D 125
units/Tab. Bot. 60s.
Use: Calcium/vitamin D supplement.
OS-CAL 500 CHEWABLE TABLETS.
(Marion) Calcium 500 mg/Tab. Bot. 60s
Use: Calcium supplement.
OS-CAL-FORTE. (Marion) Calcium 250
mg, iron 5 mg, magnesium 1.6 mg, manganese 0.3 mg, zinc 0.5 mg, vitamin A
1668 IU, D 125 IU, B_1 1.7 mg, B_2 1.7
mg, B_6 2 mg, niacinamide 15 mg, C 50
mg, E 0.83 IU/Tab. Bot. 100s.
Use: Vitamin/mineral supplement.
OS-CAL FORTIFIED. (SK-Beecham) Formerly distributed by Marion.
OS-CAL PLUS. (SK-Beecham) Calcium
250 mg, vitamins D 125 IU, A 1666 IU, C
33 mg, B_2 0.66 mg, B_1 0.5 mg, B_6 0.5
mg, niacinamide 3.33 mg, zinc 0.75 mg,
manganese 0.75 mg, iron 16.6 mg/Tab.
Bot. 100s.
Use: Vitamin/mineral supplement.
OSMITROL. (Travenol) Mannitol in water.
5%: 1000 ml; **10%:** 500 ml, 1000 ml;
15%: 150 ml, 500 ml; **20%:** 250 ml, 500
ml. Mannitol in 0.3% sodium **5%:** 1000
ml. Mannitol in 0.45% sodium **20%:** 500
ml.
Use: Osmotic diuretic.
See: Mannitol.
OSMOGLYN. (Alcon Surgical) Glycerin
50% in flavored aqueous vehicle. Plastic
bot. 6 oz.
Use: Osmotic diuretic.
OSMOLITE. (Ross) Isotonic liquid food
containing 1.06 calories/ml. Two quarts
(2000 calories) provides 100% US RDA
vitamins and minerals for adults and

children. Osmolality: 300 mOsm/kg water. Ready-to-Use: Bot. Can 8 fl oz, 32 fl oz.
Use: Enteral nutritional supplement.

OSMOLITE HN. (Ross) High nitrogen isotonic liquid food containing 1.06 calories/ml; 1400 calories provides 100% US RDA vitamins and minerals for adults and children. Osmolality: 300 mOsm/kg water. Ready-to-Use: Bot. 8 fl oz. Can 8 fl oz, 32 fl oz.
Use: Enteral nutritional supplement.

OSMOTIC DIURETICS.
See: Mannitol (Various Mfr.).
Osmitrol (Baxter).
Ureaphil (Abbott).
Glyrol (Iolab Pharm).
Osmoglyn (Alcon).
Ismotic (Alcon).

OSPOLOT. Tetrahydro-2-(p-sulfamolyphenyl)-1,2-thiazine-1,1-dioxide.
Use: Anticonvulsant drug; pending release.

OSSONATE CAPSULE. (Marcen) Cartilage mucopolysaccharide extract, chondroitin sulfate 50 mg/Cap. Bot. 100s, 500s, 1000s.

OSSONATE-PLUS, CAPS. (Marcen) Ossonate-mucopolysaccharide extract 50 mg, acetaminophen 300 mg, salicylamide 200 mg/Cap. Bot. 100s, 500s, 1000s.
Use: Anti-arthritic agent.

OSSONATE-PLUS, INJ. (Marcen) Ossonate cartilage mucopolysaccharide extract 12.5 mg, casein hydrolysates 80 mg, sulfur 20 mg, sodium citrate 5 mg, benzyl alcohol 0.5%, phenol 0.5%/ml. Multidose 10 ml vial.
Use: Skeletal muscle relaxant, pain reliever.

OSSONATE-75. (Marcen) Chondroitin sulfate 37.5 mg, benzyl alcohol 0.5%, phenol 0.5%, sodium citrate 5 mg/ml. Vial 10 ml.
Use: Infantile and atopic eczemas, drug allergies, dermatoses associated with intestinal toxemias.

OSTEOCALCIN. (Arcola) Calcitonin-salmon 200 IU, phenol 5 mg/ml. Inj. Vial 2 ml.
Use: Hormone for regulation of calcium and bone metabolism.

OSTEO-D. (Lemmon)
See: SECALCIFEROL.

OSTEOLATE INJECTION. (Fellows) Sodium thiosalicylate 50 mg, benzyl alcohol 2%/ml. Vial 30 ml.
Use: Salicylate analgesic.

OSTEON/D. (Pasadena Research) Calci-

um 600 mg, phosphorus 400 mg, magnesium 240 mg, vitamin D 400 IU/6 Tab. Bot. 180s.
Use: Vitamin/mineral supplement.

OSTI-DERM LOTION. (Pedinol) Aluminum sulfate, phenol, zinc oxide, camphor, glycerin, sorbitol, magnesium carbonate, bentonite 670, cabosil, acetic acid Ielcoloid HVF, Tween 20, calcium carbonate. Lot. Bot. 42.5 g.
Use: Antipruritic, astringent.

OSTIDERM ROLL-ON. (Pedinol) Aluminum chlorohydrate, aluminum sulfate, glycerin, phenol, camphor, alcohol, sorbitol, calcium carbonate, bentonite, hydroxypropylcellulose, polysorbate-20, EDTA, diazolidinyl urea, sodium benzoate, potassium sorbate. Bot. 88.7 ml.
Use: Antipruritic, astringent.

OSTO-K. (Parthenon) Potassium 1 mEq (39 mg from gluconate, Cl and citrate), vitamin C 25 mg, sodium 0.52 mg/Tab. Bot. 60s.
Use: Potassium/vitamin C supplement.

OSTREOGRYCIN. B.A.N. Antimicrobial substances produced by *Streptomyces ostreogriseus*. (Specific substances are designated by a terminal letter; thus, Ostreogrycin B) Ostreocin is a mixture of Ostreogrycins B and G; Ostreogrycin B is Mikamycin B.

OSVARSAN.
See: Acetarsone.

OTIC-CARE. (Parmed) Hydrocortisone 1%, neomycin sulfate 5 mg, polymyxin B sulfate 10,000 units/ml, glycerin, hydrochloric acid, propylene glycol, potassium metabisulfate. Soln.
Use: Otic preparation.

OTIC DOMEBORO. (Miles Pharm) Acetic acid 2%, aluminum acetate solution. Plastic dropper bot 2 oz.
Use: Otic preparation.

OTIC-HC. (Hauck) Chloroxylenol 1 mg, pramoxine HCl 10 mg, hydrocortisone alcohol 10 mg, benzalkonium Cl 0.2 mg/ml. Bot. 12 ml.
Use: Anti-infective, otic.

OTIC-NEO-CORT DOME.
See: Neo-Cort Dome Otic Soln. (Miles Pharm).

OTIC-PLAIN. (Hauck) Chloroxylenol 1 mg, pramoxine HCl 10 mg, benzalkonium Cl 0.2 mg/ml. Bot. 12 ml.
Use: Anti-infective, otic.

OTIC SOLUTION NO. 1. (Foy) Hydrocortisone alcohol 10 mg, pramoxine HCl 10 mg, benzalkonium Cl 0.2 mg, acetic acid glacial 20 mg/ml w/propylene glycol q.s.
Use: Anti-infective, otic.

OTOBIOTIC OTIC SOLUTION. (Schering) Polymyxin B, hydrocortisone in propylene glycol and glycerin vehicle w/edetate disodium, sodium bisulfite, anhydrous sodium sulfite, purified water. Bot. w/dropper 15 ml.
Use: Otic preparation.
OTOCAIN. (Holloway) Benzocaine 20%, benzethonium Cl 0.1%, glycerin 1%, polyethylene glycol. Soln. Bot. 15 ml.
Use: Local anesthetic, otic.
OTOCALM-H EAR DROPS. (Parmed) Pramoxine HCl 10 mg, hydrocortisone alcohol 10%, p-Chloro-m-Xylenol 1 mg, benzalkonium Cl 0.2 mg, acetic acid glacial 20 mg, propylene glycol/ml. Bot. 10 ml.
Use: Anti-infective, otic.
OTOCORT STERILE SOLUTION. (Lemmon) Neomycin sulfate equivalent to 3.5 mg neomycin base, polymyxin B sulfate 10,000 units, hydrocortisone 10 mg/ml, propylene glycol, glycerin, potassium metabisulfite, HCl, purified water. Bot. 10 ml.
Use: Anti-infective, otic.
OTOCORT STERILE SUSPENSION. (Lemmon) Neomycin sulfate equivalent to 3.5 mg neomycin base, polymyxin B sulfate 10,000 units, hydrocortisone 10 mg/ml, cetyl alcohol, propylene glycol, polysorbate 80, thimerosal, water for injection. Bot. 10 ml.
Use: Anti-infective, otic.
OTOGESIC HC SOLUTION. (Metro Med) Polymyxin B sulfate 10,000 IU, neomycin sulfate 3.5 mg, hydrocortisone 10 mg/ml, potassium metabisulfite 0.1%. Bot. 10 ml.
Use: Anti-infective, otic.
OTOGESIC HC SUSPENSION. (Metro Med) Polymyxin B sulfate 10,000 units, neomycin sulfate 3.5 mg, hydrocortisone 10 mg/ml, benzalkonium Cl 0.01%. Bot. 10 ml.
Use: Anti-infective, otic.
OTOMYCIN-HPN. (Misemer) Polymyxin B sulfate 10,000 units, neomycin sulfate 3.5 mg, hydrocortisone 10 mg/ml. Bot. w/dropper 10 ml.
Use: Anti-infective, otic.
OTRIVIN. (Geigy) Xylometazoline HCl. **Nasal Drops:** 0.1% w/sodium Cl, phenylmercuric acetate 1:50,000. Dropper bot. 20 ml. **Nasal Spray:** 0.1% w/potassium phosphate monobasic, potassium Cl, sodium phosphate dibasic, sodium Cl, benzalkonium Cl 1:5000. Plastic squeeze spray 15 ml. **Ped. Nasal Soln. Drops:** 0.05%. Bot. 20 ml.

Use: Nasal decongestant.
OUABAIN OCTAHYDRATE. Ouabain, U.S.P. XXIII.
OUTGRO. (Whitehall) Chlorobutanol 5%, tannic acid 25%, isopropyl alcohol 83%. Bot. 13 oz.
Use: Ingrown toenail preparation.
OVARIAN EXTRACT. Aqueous extract of whole ovaries of cattle.
Use: Estrogen.
OVARIAN SUBSTANCE. (Various Mfr.) Whole ovarian substance from cattle, sheep or swine.
Use: Estrogen.
OVASTAT. (Medac)
See: TREOSULFAN.
OVCON-35. (Mead Johnson Nutrition) Norethindrone 0.4 mg, ethinyl estradiol 0.035 mg/Tab. Ctn. 6×21s.
Use: Oral contraceptive.
OVCON-35, 28 day. (Mead Johnson Nutrition) Norethindrone 0.4 mg, ethinyl estradiol 0.035 mg, w/7 inert tab/Carton 6×28s.
Use: Oral contraceptive.
OVCON-50. (Mead Johnson Nutrition) Norethindrone 1 mg, ethinyl estradiol 0.05 mg/Tab. Ctn. 6×21s.
Use: Oral contraceptive.
OVCON-50, 28 day. (Mead Johnson Nutrition) Norethindrone 1 mg, ethinyl estradiol 0.05 mg, w/7 inert tab/Carton. 6×28s.
Use: Oral contraceptive.
OVIDE. (GenDerm) Malathion 0.5%. Lot. Bot. 59 ml.
Use: Scabicide/pediculicide.
OVIFOLLIN.
See: Estrone (Various Mfr.).
OVLIN. (Sig) **Tab.:** Ethinyl estradiol 0.02 mg, conjugated estrogens 0.2 mg/Tab. Bot. 100s, 1000s. **Inj.:** Estrone 2 mg, estradiol 0.05 mg, vitamin B$_{12}$ 1000 mcg/ml. Vial 30 ml.
Use: Estrogen.
OVOCYLIN DIPROPIONATE. (Ciba) Estradiol dipropionate.
Use: Estrogen.
OVRAL. (Wyeth-Ayerst) Norgestrel 0.5 mg, ethinyl estradiol 0.05 mg/Tab. 6 Pilpak dispensers, 21 Tab. Tripak 63s.
Use: Oral contraceptive.
OVRAL-28. (Wyeth-Ayerst) Norgestrel 0.5 mg, ethinyl estradiol 0.05 mg/Tab. w/7 inert Tab. Pilpak dispenser 6s containing 21 Tab, 7 inert Tab.
Use: Oral contraceptive.
OVRETTE. (Wyeth-Ayerst) Norgestrel 0.075 mg/Tab. 6 Pilpak dispenser, Tab. 28s.

Use: Oral contraceptive.

OVUGEN. (BioGenex) In vitro diagnostic test for measurement of LH urine to determine ovulation. Kits. 6s, 10s.
Use: Ovulation test.

OVUKIT SELF-TEST. (Monoclonal Antibodies) Monoclonal antibody-based enzyme immunoassay test for hLH in urine. Kit 6, 9 day.
Use: Ovulation test.

OVULATION STIMULANTS.
See: Clomid (Merrell Dow).
Serophene (Serono).
Metrodin (Serono).

OVULATION TESTS.
See: Answer Ovulation (Carter).
Clearplan Easy (Whitehall).
OvuQUICK Self-Test (Monoclonal Antibodies).
Color Ovulation Test (Bioamerica).
Conceive Ovulation Predictor (Quidel).
First Response Ovulation Predictor Test Kit (Carter Products).
Fortel Home Ovulation Test (Bioamerica).
OvuGen (BioGenex).
OvuKIT Self-Test (Monoclonal Antibodies).

OVULEN-21. (Searle) Ethynodiol diacetate 1 mg, mestranol 0.1 mg/Tab. Compack Disp. 21s, 6×21, 2421. Refill 21s, 1221.
Use: Oral contraceptive.

OVULEN-28. (Searle) Ethynodiol diacetate 1 mg, mestranol 0.1 mg/Tab. w/7 inert Tab. Compack 28s: 21 active tab., 7 placebo tab. Compack dispenser 28s. Box 6×28. Refill 28s, Box 1228.
Use: Oral contraceptive.

OVUSTICK SELF-TEST. (Monoclonal Antibodies) Home test for ovulation. Test kit 10s.
Use: Diagnostic aid.

OXABID. (Jamieson-McKames) Magnesium oxide 140 mg or magnesium oxide heavy 400 mg/Cap. Bot. 100s.
Use: Antacid.

•**OXACILLIN, SODIUM,** U.S.P. XXIII. Cap., Inj., Soln., Sterile, U.S.P. XXIII. 5-Methyl-3-phenyl-4-isoxazolyl penicillin. Sodium 3,3-Dimethyl-6-(5-methyl-3-phenyl-4-isoxazole-carboxamido)-7-oxocarboxylate.
Use: Antibiotic.
See: Bactocill, Cap., Vial (Beecham Labs).
Prostaphilin, Preps. (Bristol).
Sodium oxacillin.

OXADIMEDINE HCl. N-(2-Benzoxazolyl)-N-benzyl-N′,N-dimethylethylenediamine

HCl.
Use: Antiarrhythmic.

OXAFURADENE. Name used for Nifuradene.
Use: Platelet aggregation agent.

•**OXAGRELATE.** USAN.
Use: Platelet aggregation agent.

OXALIPLATIN. (Axion)
Use: Treatment of ovarian cancer. [Orphan drug]

•**OXAMARIN HYDROCHLORIDE.** USAN. 6,-7-bis[2-(Diethylamino)-ethoxy]-4-methylcoumarin dihydrochloride.
Use: Systemic hemostat.

•**OXAMISOLE HYDROCHLORIDE.** USAN.
Use: Immunoregulator.

•**OXAMNIQUINE,** U.S.P. XXIII. Cap., U.S.P. XXIII. 6-Hydroxymethyl-2-isopropylaminomethyl-7-nitro-1,2,3,4-tetrahydroquino-line.
Use: Treatment of schistosomiasis.
See: Vansil, Cap. (Pfizer Laboratories).

OXANAMIDE. 2-Ethyl-3-propyl glycidamide.
Use: Tranquilizer.

•**OXANDROLONE,** U.S.P. XXIII. Tab., U.S.P. XX (1) Dodecahydro-3-hydroxy-6-(hydroxy-methyl)-3,3α,-6-trimethyl-1H-benz[e]indene-7-acetic acid, α-lactone. (2) 17 β-hydroxy-17-methyl-2-oxa-5α-androstan-3-one.
Use: Anabolic. [Orphan drug]
See: Anavar, Tab. (Searle).

•**OXANTEL PAMOATE.** USAN.
Use: Anthelmintic.

•**OXAPROTILINE HYDROCHLORIDE.** USAN.
Use: Antidepressant.

•**OXAPROZIN.** USAN. 3-(4,5-Diphenyloxazol-2-yl)-propionicacid.
Use: Anti-inflammatory.
See: Daypro.

•**OXARBAZOLE.** USAN.
Use: Antiasthmatic.

•**OXATOMIDE.** USAN.
Use: Anti-allergic, antiasthmatic.

•**OXAZEPAM,** U.S.P. XXIII. Cap., Tab., U.S.P. XXIII. 7-Chloro-1,3-dihydro-3-hydroxy-5-phenyl-2H-1,4-benzodia-zepin-2-one. Serenid-D.
Use: Sedative.
See: Serax, Cap., Tab. (Wyeth-Ayerst).

OXAZOLINDINEDIONES.
See: Paradione (Abbott).
Tridione (Abbott).

OX BILE EXTRACT. Purified oxgall.
See: Bile Extract, Ox.

OXELADIN. B.A.N. 2-(2-Diethylaminoethoxy)-ethyl 2-eethyl-2-phenyl-

butyrate. Pectamol citrate.
Use: Cough suppressant.
• **OXENDOLONE.** USAN.
Use: Antiandrogen (benign prostatic hypertrophy).
• **OXETHAZAINE.** USAN. 2,2'-[(2-Hydroxyethyl)imino]bis-[N-(α,α- dimethylphenethyl)-N-methylacetamide].
Use: Local anesthetic.
• **OXETORONE FUMARATE.** USAN.
Use: Analgesic specific for migraine.
• **OXFENDAZOLE.** USAN.
Use: Anthelmintic.
See: Synanthic (Syntex).
• **OXFENICINE.** USAN.
Use: Vasodilator.
OX GALL.
See: Bile Extract, Ox.
• **OXIBENDAZOLE.** USAN.
Use: Anthelmintic.
• **OXICONAZOLE NITRATE.** USAN.
Use: Antifungal.
See: Oxistat Cream (Glaxo Dermatology)
Oxistat Lotion (Glaxo).
OXIDIZED BILE ACIDS.
See: Bile Acids, Oxidized.
• **OXIDIZED CELLULOSE,** U.S.P. XXIII.
Absorbable cellulose. Cellulosic acid.
Use: Local hemostatic.
• **OXIDOPAMINE.** USAN.
Use: Adrenergic.
OXI-FREEDA. (Freeda) Vitamin A 5000 IU, E 150 mg, B_3 40 mg, C 100 mg, B_1 20 mg, B_2 20 mg, B_5 20 mg, B_6 20 mg, B_{12} 10 mcg, chelated Zn 15 mg, Se 50 mcg, Se, glutathione 40 mg, L-cysteine 75 mg. Tab. Bot. 100s, 250s.
Use: Vitamin combinations, miscellaneous.
• **OXIFUNGIN HYDROCHLORIDE.** USAN.
Use: Antifungal.
• **OXILORPHAN.** USAN.
Use: Antagonist to narcotics.
• **OXIMONAM.** USAN.
Use: Antibacterial.
• **OXIMONAM SODIUM.** USAN.
Use: Antibacterial.
OXINE.
See: Oxyquinoline sulfate (Various Mfr.).
• **OXIPEROMIDE.** USAN.
Use: Antipsychotic.
OXIPOR VHC PSORIASIS LOTION.
(Whitehall) Coal tar soln. 48.5%, salicylic acid 1%, benzocaine 2%, alcohol 81%. Bot. 1.9 oz, 4 oz.
Use: Antipsoriatic.
• **OXIRAMIDE.** USAN.
Use: Cardiac depressant.

OXISTAT. (Glaxo Derm.) Oxiconazole nitrate 1%. **Cream:** Tube 15 Gm, 30 Gm; **Lotion:** Bot. 30 ml.
Use: Antifungal, external.
• **OXISURAN.** USAN. (Methyl-sulfinyl)-methyl-2-pyridyl ketone.
Use: Antineoplastic agent.
• **OXMETIDINE HYDROCHLORIDE.** USAN.
Use: Antagonist to histamine receptors.
• **OXMETIDINE MESYLATE.** USAN.
Use: Antagonist to histimine receptors.
• **OXOGESTONE PHENPROPIONATE.** USAN. **#1:** 20β-Hydroxy-19-norpregn-4-en-3-one hydrocinnamate. **#2:** 20β-hydroxy-19-nor-4-pregnen-3-one 20-phenylpropionate.
Use: Progestin.
OXOLAMINE. (Arcum) Crystalline hydroxycobalamin 1000 mcg/ml. Vial 10 ml.
Use: Vitamin B_{12} supplement.
OXOPHENARSINE HYDROCHLORIDE.
2-Amino-4-arsenophenol hydrochloride.
L-2-OXOTHIAZOLIDINE₄-CARBOXYLIC ACID.
Use: Treatment of adult respiratory distress syndrome. [Orphan drug]
See: Procysteine.
OXOTHIAZOLIDINE CARBOXYLATE. (Clintec Nutritional/Ben Venise Labs) Phase I restoration of glutathione depletion in HIV, ARC, AIDS; prevention of inflammation-induced HIV replication.
Use: Immunomodulator.
OXPENTIFYLLINE. B.A.N. 3,7-Dimethyl-1-(5-oxohexyl)xanthine. Pentoxifylline (I.N.N.).
Use: Vasodilator.
See: Trental (Hoechst).
OXPHENERIDINE. 1-(β-phenyl-β-hydroxy-ethyl)-4-carbethoxy-4-phenylpiperidine.
• **OXPRENOLOL HCl,** U.S.P. XXIII, USAN. Extended release tab., U.S.P. XXIII. 1-[o-(Allyloxy)-phenoxy]-3-(isopropylamino)-2-propanol HCl. Trasicor. Under study.
Use: Beta-adrenergic receptor blocking agent.
OXSORALEN LOTION. (ICN Pharm) Methoxsalen 1% in an inert lotion vehicle of alcohol 71%, propylene glycol, acetone, water. Bot. oz.
Use: Psoralen, topical.
OXSORALEN-ULTRA. (ICN Pharm) Methoxsalen 10 mg/Cap. Bot. 50s, 100s.
Use: Psoralen.
• **OXTRIPHYLLINE,** U.S.P. XXIII. Oral

Soln, ER Tab., U.S.P. XXIII. Choline theophyllinate.
Use: Bronchodilator.
See: Choledyl, Tab., Elix. (Parke-Davis).
W/Guaifenesin.
See: Brondecon, Tab., Elix. (Parke-Davis).

OXY-5 ACNE-PIMPLE MEDICATION. (SK-Beecham) Benzoyl peroxide 5% in lotion base. Bot. fl oz.
Use: Anti-acne.

OXY 5 TINTED. (SK-Beecham) Benzoyl peroxide 5%, titanium dioxide, sodium PCA, cetyl alcohol, silica, iron oxides, propylene glycol, citric acid, sodium laurel sulfate, stearyl alcohol, parabens. Lot. Bot. 30 ml.
Use: Anti-acne.

OXY-10 COVER MAXIMUM STRENGTH ACNE-PIMPLE MEDICATION. (SK-Beecham) Benzoyl peroxide 10%. Lot. Bot. oz.
Use: Anti-acne.

OXY-10 MAXIMUM STRENGTH ACNE-PIMPLE MEDICATION. (SK-Beecham) Benzoyl peroxide 10% in lotion base. Bot. fl oz.
Use: Anti-acne.

OXY 10 WASH. (SK-Beecham) Benzoyl peroxide 10%. Liq. Bot. 120 ml.
Use: Anti-acne.

OXY-10 WASH ANTIBACTERIAL SKIN WASH. (SK-Beecham) Benzoyl peroxide 10%. Bot. 4 fl oz.
Use: Anti-acne.

• **OXYBENZONE,** U.S.P. XXIII. 2-Hydroxy-4-methoxybenzophenone. Methanone, (2-hydroxy-4-methoxyphenyl)phenyl-. Cyasorb UV 9 (Lederle).
Use: Ultraviolet screen.
W/Dioxybenzone, benzophenone.
See: Solbar, Lot. (Person & Covey).

OXYBENZONE WITH COMBINATIONS.
See: Coppertone, Prods. (Schering-Plough).
Noskote, Cream (Schering-Plough).
Shade, Prods. (Schering-Plough).
Sunger, Prods. (Schering-Plough).
Super Shade, Lot. (Schering-Plough).

OXYBUPROCAINE. B.A.N. 2-Diethylaminoethyl 4-amino-3-butoxybenzoate. Novesine hydrochloride.
Use: Local anesthetic.

• **OXYBUTYNIN CHLORIDE,** U.S.P. XXIII. Syr., Tab., U.S.P. XXIII. 4-Diethylamino-2-butynyl-α-phenylcyclo-hexanegly-colate hydrochloride.
Use: Anticholinergic.
See: Ditropan Syr., Tab. (Marion Lab.).

Oxybutynin Cl (Mead Johnson).

OXYCEL. (Deseret) Cellulosic acid in absorbable hemostatic agent prepared from cellulose. Resembles ordinary surgical gauze or cotton. Pledget 2 × 1 1 in. 10s. Pad 3 3 in. 8 ply. 10s. Strip 5 0.5 in. 4 ply. 18 2 in. 4 ply. 10s. 36 0.5 in. 4 ply.
Use: Hemostatic, topical.

OXYCET. (Halsey) Oxycodone HCl 5 mg, acetaminophen 325 mg/Tab. Bot. 100s, 500s, Hospital pack 250s.
Use: Narcotic analgesic combination.

OXY-CHINOL. (Ferndale) Potassium oxyquinoline sulfate 1 gr/Tab. Bot. 100s, 1000s.
Use: Deodorizer, bacteriostatic.

• **OXYCHLOROSENE.** USAN. Monoxychlorosene. Hydrocarbon derivative containing fourteen carbons and hypochlorous acid. The hydrocarbon chain also has a phenyl substituent which in turn holds a sulfonic acid group.
Use: Anti-infective, topical.
See: Clorpactin, Prod. (Scrip).

• **OXYCHLOROSEN SODIUM.** USAN. Sodium salt of the complex derived from hypochlorous acid and tetradecylbenzene sulfonic acid. Action of active chlorine.
Use: Anti-infective, topical.

OXYCINCHOPHEN. B.A.N. 3-Hydroxy-2-phenyl-quinoline-4-carboxylic acid.
Use: Uricosuric.

OXY CLEAN LATHERING FACIAL. (SK-Beecham) Sodium tetraborate decahydrate dissolving particles in a base of surfactant cleaning agents. Soap free. Scrub 79.5 Gm.
Use: Anti-acne.

OXY CLEAN MEDICATED CLEANSER AND PADS. (SK-Beecham) **Cleanser and reg. strength pads:** Salicylic acid 0.5%, SD alcohol 40 B 40%, citric acid, menthol, sodium lauryl sulfate. **Max. strength pads:** Salicylic acid 2%, SD alcohol 40 B 50%, citric acid, menthol, sodium lauryl sulfate. Cleanser 120 ml Pad. 50s.
Use: Anti-acne.

OXY CLEAN MEDICATED PADS FOR SENSITIVE SKIN. (SK-Beecham) Salicylic acid 0.5%, SD alcohol 40B 16%. Jar 50s.
Use: Anti-acne.

OXY CLEAN SCRUB. (SK-Beecham) Sodium tetraborate decahydrate dissolving particles in a base of surfactant cleaning agents, soap free. Lot. Bot. 79.5 Gm.
Use: Anti-acne.

OXY CLEAN SOAP. (SK-Beecham) Salicylic acid 3.5%, sodium borate. Bar 97.5 Gm.
Use: Anti-acne.
• **OXYCODONE.** USAN. 7,8-Dihydro-14-hydroxy-O³-methylmorphinone. Dihydrohydroxycodeineone Eucodal hydrochloride; Proladone pectinate.
Use: Narcotic analgesic.
OXYCODONE AND ASPIRIN. (Various Mfr.) Oxycodone HCl 4.5 mg, oxycodone terephthalate 0.38 mg, aspirin 325 mg/Tab. Bot. 100s, 500s.
Use: Narcotic analgesic combination.
• **OXYCODONE AND ACETAMINOPHEN CAPSULES,** U.S.P. XXIII.
Use: Analgesic.
• **OXYCODONE AND ACETAMINOPHEN TABLETS,** U.S.P. XXIII.
Use: Analgesic.
• **OXYCODONE HYDROCHLORIDE,** U.S.P. XXIII, Oral Soln. (1)(–)-4,5α-Epoxy-14-hydroxy-3-methoxy-17-methylmorphinan-6-ono, (2)() 14 Hydroxydi-hydrocodeinone.
Use: Narcotic analgesic.
See: Dihydrohydroxycodeinone HCl.
W/Acetaminophen, oxycodone terephthalate.
See: Percocet-5, Tab. (DuPont).
Tylox, Cap. (McNeil).
• **OXYCODONE TEREPHTHALATE,** U.S.P. XXIII.
Use: Analgesic.
OXY COVER. (SK-Beecham) Benzoyl peroxide 10%. Cream. 30 Gm.
Use: Anti-acne.
OXYETHYLATED TERTIARY OCTYLPHENOL-FORMALDEHYDE POLYMER.
See: Triton WR-1339 (Rohm & Haas).
OXYETHYLENE OXYPROPYLENE POLYMER.
See: Poloxalkol.
W/Danthron, B₁, carboxymethyl cellulose.
See: Evactol, Cap. (Delta).
OXYFEDRINE. B.A.N. L-3-[(β-Hydroxy-α-methyl-phen-ethyl-amino]-3′-methoxypropiophenone. Ildamen hydrochloride.
Use: Coronary vasodilator.
• **OXYFILCON A.** USAN.
Use: Contact lens material.
• **OXYGEN,** U.S.P. XXIII.
Use: Medicinal.
• **OXYGEN 93 PERCENT,** U.S.P. XXIII.
Use: Medicinal.
OXY MEDICATED SOAP. (SK Beecham) Triclosan 1%, bentonite, cocoam-

phodipropionate, iron oxides, glycerin, magnesium silicate, sodium borohydride, sodium cocoate, sodium tallowate, talc, EDTA, titanium dioxide. Bar. 97.5 g.
Use: Anti-acne.
OXYMESTERONE. B.A.N. 4,17β-Dihydroxy-17α-methylandrost-4-en-3-one. 4-Hydroxy-17α-methyl-testosterone. Oranabol.
Use: Anabolic steroid.
OXYMETAZOLINE. B.A.N. 2-(4-t-Butyl-3-hydroxy-2,6-dimethylbenzyl)-2-imidazoline. Afrin and Hazol hydrochloride.
Use: Vasoconstrictor.
OXYMETAZOLINE HCl.
Use: Ophthalmic Soln.
Ophthalmic vasoconstrictors/mydriatics.
See: Ocuclear (Schering-Plough).
Visine (Pfizer).
• **OXYMETAZOLINE HYDROCHLORIDE,** U.S.P. XXIII. Nasal Soln., U.S.P. XXIII. Phenol, 3-[(4,5-dihydro-1H-imidazol-2-yl-)methyl]-6-(1,1-dimethyl-ethyl)-2,4-dimethyl-, monohydrochloride. 6-Tertbutyl-3-(2-imidazolin-2-ylmethyl)-2,4-dimethylphenol HCl.
Use: Decongestant, adrenergic.
See: Afrin, Nasal Spray, Soln. (Schering).
Duration Nasal Spray (Schering-Plough).
Duration Nose Drops (Schering-Plough).
Duration Nose Drops for Children (Schering-Plough).
St. Joseph Nasal Spray for Children (Schering-Plough).
St. Joseph Nose Drops for Children (Schering-Plough).
• **OXYMETHOLONE,** U.S.P. XXIII. Tab., U.S.P. XXIII. 17-beta-Hydroxy-2-(hydroxymethylene)-17-methyl-5α-androstan-3-one.
Use: Androgen.
See: Anadrol, Tab. (Syntex).
• **OXYMORPHONE HCl,** U.S.P. XXIII. Inj., Supp., U.S.P. XXIII. 14-Hydroxydihydromorphinone HCl. 4,5α-Epoxy-3,14-dihydroxy-17-methylmorphinan-6-one Hydrochloride.
Use: Analgesic, narcotic. [Orphan drug]
See: Numorphan Amp., Vial, Supp. (DuPont).
OXY NIGHT WATCH. (SK-Beecham) Salicylic acid 1%, cetyl alcohol, silica, propylene glycol, stearyl alcohol, sodium laureth sulfate, parabens, EDTA. Lot. Bot. 60 ml.

Use: Anti-acne.

• **OXYPERTINE.** USAN. 5,6-Dimethoxy-2-methyl-3-[2-(4-phenyl-1-piperazinyl)ethyl]indole. 1-[2-(5,6-Dimethoxy-2-methylindol-3-yl)ethyl]-4-phenylpiperazine. Integrin hydrochloride.
Use: Psychotropic.

• **OXYPHENBUTAZONE,** U.S.P. XXIII. Tab., U.S.P. XXIII. 1-(p-Hydroxyphenyl)-2-phenyl-4-butyl-3,5-pyrazolidine-dione. Oxazolidin. 4-Butyl-1-(p-hydroxyphenyl)-2-phenyl 3,5-pyrazolidinedione monohydrate.
Use: Antiarthritic, anti-inflammatory analgesic, antipyretic.
See: Oxalid, Tab. (USV Labs.).

• **OXYPHENCYCLIMINE HCI,** U.S.P. XXII. Tab., U.S.P. XXII. 1-Methyl-1,4,5,6-tetrahydro-2-pyrimidylmethyl-alpha-cyclohexyl-alpha-phenylglycolate HCl. (1,4,5,6-Tetrahydro-1-methyl-2-pyrimidinyl)methyl α-phenylcyclohexane-glycolate monohydrochloride.
Use: Antispasmodic.
See: Daricon, Tab. (Beecham Labs).
W/Hydroxyzine HCl.
See: Enarax, Tab. (Beecham Labs).
W/Phenobarbital.
See: Daricon-PB, Tab. (Beecham Labs).

OXYPHENISATIN. B.A.N. 3,3-Di-(4-hydroxyphenyl)-indolin-2-one. Bydolax; Contax diacetate.
Use: Laxative.

• **OXYPHENISATIN ACETATE.** USAN. 3,3-bis(p-Hydroxyphenyl)2-indolinone diacetate. Diacetoxydiphenylisatin, Acetphenolisatin, Acetylphenylisatin, Diacetoxyphenyloxindol, Bisatin, Phenylisatin bis-(acetoxyphenyl) oxindol.
Use: Laxative.
See: Endophenolphthalein (Roche).
Isacen (No Mfr. currently lists).
Prulet, Tab. (Mission).
Prulet Liquitab. (Mission).

OXYPHENUDRINE. α-[fb][(p-Hydroxy-α-methylphenethyl)amino]methylprotocatechuyl alcohol.

• **OXYPURINOL.** USAN. 4,6-Dihydroxypyrazolo(3,4-d)pyrimidine. 1H-Pyrazolo[3,4-d]pyrimidine-4,6-diol.
Use: Xanthine oxidase inhibitor.

• **OXYQUINOLINE.** USAN.
Use: Disinfectant.

OXYQUINOLINE BENZOATE. (Merck) Pkg. lb. 8-Hydroxyquinoline benzoate.
W/Alkyl aryl sulfonate, disodium edetate, aminacrine HCl, copper sulfate, sodium sulfate.

See: Triva, Vaginal Jelly, Pow. (Boyle).
W/Benzoic acid, salicylic acid, sodium tetradecyl sulfate.
See: NP-27 Cream (Norwich).

• **OXYQUINOLINE SULFATE,** N.F. XVIII. 8-Hydroxyquinoline sulfate.
Use: Disinfectant.
See: Chinosol, Tab., Pow., Vial (Vernon).

OXYQUINOLINE SULFATE W/COMBINATIONS.
See: Oxyzal Wet Dressing, Soln. (Gordon).
Rectal Medicone, Oint. (Medicone).
Rectal Medicone-HC, Oint. (Medicone).
Rectal Medicone Unguent, Oint. (Medicone).
Trapens, Tab. (Mills).
Triticoll, Tab. (Western Research).
Triva, Douche Pow. (Boyle).

OXY RESIDON'T. (SK-Beecham) Triclosan 0.6%, diazolidinyl urea. Liq. Bot. 240 ml.
Use: Antiseptic and germicide.

OXY-SCRUB. (SK-Beecham) Abradant cleanser containing dissolving abradant particles of sodium tetraborate decahydrate. Tube 2.65 oz.
Use: Anti-acne.

OXYSEPT. (Allergan) **Disinfecting Soln.:** Hydrogen peroxide 3%, sodium stannate, sodium nitrate, phosphate buffer. Bot. 240 ml or 360 ml. **Neutralizer Tab.:** Catalase, buffering agents. In 12s (w/ Oxytab cup) or 36s.
Use: Soft contact lens care.

OXYSEPT 1. (Allergan) Microfiltered hydrogen peroxide 3% w/sodium stannate and sodium nitrate, preservative free, buffered. Soln. Bot. 355 ml.
Use: Contact lens product.

OXYSEPT 2. (Allergan) Catalase (catalytic neutralizing agent), EDTA, sodium Cl, mono- and dibasic sodium phosphates. Buffered, preservative free. Soln. In 15 ml single-use containers (25s).
Use: Contact lens product.

OXYTETRACLOR. (Kenyon) Oxytetracycline HCl 250 mg/Cap. Bot. 100s, 1000s.
Use: Anti-infective, tetracycline.

• **OXYTETRACYCLINE,** U.S.P. XXIII. Inj., Sterile, Tab., U.S.P. XXIII.
Use: Antibiotic.
See: Oxytetraclor, Cap. (Kenyon).
Terramycin, Prods. (Pfizer Laboratories).

• **OXYTETRACYCLINE AND HYDROCOR-**

TISONE ACETATE OPHTHALMIC SUS-PENSION, U.S.P. XXIII.
Use: Antibiotic, anti-inflammatory.
• **OXYTETRACYCLINE AND NYSTATIN CAPSULES,** U.S.P. XXIII.
Use: Antibiotic, antifungal.
• **OXYTETRACYCLINE AND NYSTATIN FOR ORAL SUSPENSION,** U.S.P. XXII.
Use: Antibiotic, antifungal.
• **OXYTETRACYCLINE AND PHENAZOPYRIDINE HYDROCHLO-RIDES AND SULFAMETHIZOLE CAP-SULES,** U.S.P. XXIII.
Use: Antibiotic, urinary analgesic, anti-spasmodic, anti-infective.
• **OXYTETRACYCLINE CALCIUM,** U.S.P. XXIII. Oral Susp., U.S.P. XXIII.
Use: Antibiotic.
• **OXYTETRACYCLINE HYDROCHLO-RIDE,** U.S.P. XXIII. Cap., Inj., Sterile, U.S.P. XXIII. 5-Hydroxytetracycline HCl. An antibiotic from *Streptomyces rimosus.*
Use: Antibiotic, antirickettsial.
See: Dalimycin, Cap. (Dalin).
   Oxlopar, Cap. (Parke-Davis).
   Oxy-Kesso-Tetra, Cap. (McKesson).
   Terramycin HCl, Preps. (Pfizer Laboratories, Pfipharmecs).
   Uri-tet, Cap. (American Urologicals).
   Urobiotic (Roerig).
• **OXYTETRACYCLINE HYDROCHLO-RIDE AND HYDROCORTISONE OINT-MENT,** U.S.P. XXIII.
Use: Antibiotic, anti-inflammatory.
• **OXYTETRACYCLINE HYDROCHLO-RIDE AND POLYMYXIN B SULFATE,** U.S.P. XXIII.
Use: Antibiotic.
• **OXYTETRACYCLINE HYDROCHLO-RIDE AND POLYMYXIN B SULFATE OPHTHALMIC OINTMENT,** U.S.P. XXIII.
Use: Antibiotic.
• **OXYTETRACYCLINE HYDROCHLO-RIDE AND POLYMYXIN B SULFATE TOPICAL POWDER,** U.S.P. XXIII.
Use: Antibiotic.
• **OXYTETRACYCLINE HYDROCHLO-RIDE AND POLYMYXIN B SULFATE VAGINAL TABLETS,** U.S.P. XXIII.
Use: Antibiotic.
OXYTETRACYCLINE-POLYMYXIN B.
Mix of oxytetracycline HCl and polymyxin B sulfate.
Use: Antibiotic.
See: Terramycin HCl w/Polymyxin B. Sulfate, Oint., Tab., Pow. (Pfizer Laboratories, Pfipharmecs).

OXYTOCICS.
See: Ergot Preps.
• **OXYTOCIN INJECTION,** U.S.P. XXIII.
Use: Oxytocic.
See: Pitocin, Amp. (Parke-Davis).
   Syntocinon, Amp. (Sandoz).
• **OXYTOCIN NASAL SOLUTION,** U.S.P. XXIII.
Use: Oxytocic.
OXYTOCIN, SYNTHETIC.
See: Pitocin, Amp. (Parke-Davis).
   Syntocinon, Amp. (Sandoz).
   Syntocinon Nasal Spray (Sandoz).
OXY WASH. (SK-Beecham) Benzoyl peroxide 10%. Liq. Bot. 120 ml.
Use: Anti-acne.
OXYZAL WET DRESSING. (Gordon) Benzalkonium Cl 1:2000, oxyquinoline sulfate, distilled water. Dropper bot. 1 oz, 4 oz.
Use: Minor skin irritations.
OYSCO. (Rugby) Elemental calcium 500 mg/Tab. Bot. 60s.
Use: Calcium supplement.
OYSCO D. (Rugby) Ca 250 mg, D 125 IU. Tab. Bot. 100s, 250s, 1000s.
Use: Calcium and vitamin D supplement.
OYST-CAL 500. (Goldline) Calcium carbonate 1.25 Gm (calcium 500 mg)/Tab. Bot. 60s, 120s.
Use: Calcium supplement.
OYST-CAL-D. (Goldline) Calcium 250 mg, vitamin D 125 IU/Tab. Bot. 100s, 1000s.
Use: Calcium/vitamin D supplement.
OYSTER CALCIUM. (Nature's Bounty) Ca 275 mg, D 200 IU, A 800 IU. Tab. Bot. 100s.
Use: Calcium and vitamin supplement.
OYSTER SHELL CALCIUM-500. (Vangard) Calcium carbonate 1.25 Gm, (calcium 500 mg). Tab. Bot. 100s, UD 100s, 640s.
Use: Minerals and electrolytes, oral.
OYSTER SHELLS.
See: Os-Cal, Tab. (Marion).
W/Vitamin D-2.
See: Ostrakal, Tab. (Elder).
OYSTERCAL 500. (Nature's Bounty) Calcium carbonate 1.25 Gm (calcium 500 mg)/Tab. Bot. 100s.
Use: Calcium supplement.
OYSTERCAL-D. (Nature's Bounty) Calcium 250 mg, vitamin D 125 IU/Tab. Bot. 100s, 250s.
Use: Calcium/vitamin D supplement.
• **OZOLINONE.** USAN.
Use: Diuretic.

P

P₁E₁; P₂E₁; P₃E₁; P₄E₁; P₆E₁. (Alcon) Pilocarpine HCl 1%, 2%, 3%, 4% or 6% respectively, with epinephrine bitartrate 1%. Plastic dropper vial 15 ml.
Use: Agent for glaucoma.

P.A.A.M. (Kenyon) Acetylsalicylic acid 5 gr, para-aminobenzoic acid 5 gr, vitamin C 50 mg/Tab. Bot. 100s, 1000s.
Use: Salicylate analgesic, vitamin combination.

PABA-"5". (Durel) P-amino benzoic acid in quick-drying moisturizing base. Bot. 4 oz.
Use: Sunscreen.

P AND S LIQUID. (Baker/Cummins) Bot. 4 oz, 8 oz.
Use: Antiseborrheic.

P AND S PLUS. (Baker/Cummins) Coal tar solution 8% (crude coal tar 1.6%, ethyl alcohol 6.4%), salicylic acid 2%. Gel 105 Gm.
Use: Tar-containing preparation, topical.

P AND S SHAMPOO. (Baker/Cummins) Salicylic acid 2%, lactic acid 0.5% Bot. 4 oz.
Use: Antiseborrheic.

PABALAN. (Lannett) Potassium para-amino benzoate 5 gr, potassium salicylate 5 gr, ascorbic acid 50 mg/Tab. Bot. 100s, 1000s.

PABALATE. (Robins) Sodium salicylate 300 mg, sodium aminobenzoate 300 mg/EC Tab. Bot. 100s, 500s.
Use: Antirheumatic.

PABALATE-SF. (Robins) Potassium salicylate 300 mg, potassium aminobenzoate 300 mg/Tab. Bot. 100s, 500s.
Use: Antirheumatic.

PABAQUINONE CREAM. (Dermohr Pharmacal) Hydroquinone 4%, amyl dimethyl paba 3% in creamy base. Tube oz.
Use: Skin-bleaching agent.

PABA-SALICYLATE. (Various Mfr.) Sodium salicylate, p-aminobenzoate, vitamin C/Tab. Bot. 100s, 500s.
Use: Salicylate analgesic, vitamin combination.

PABA SODIUM. (Various Mfr.). Sodium p-aminobenzoate.
Use: Vitamin supplement.

PABASONE. (Pinex) Sodium salicylate 5 gr, para-aminobenzoic acid 5 gr, ascorbic acid 20 mg/Tab. Bot. 100s.
Use: Salicylate analgesic, vitamin combination.

P-A-C. Preparations of phenacetin, aspirin, caffeine.

See: A.P.C. Preparations, Empirin Preparations.

p-ACETYLAMINOBENZALDEHYDE THIOSEMICARBAZONE. (Amithiozone, Antib, Berculon A, Benzothiozon, Conteben, Myuizone, Neustab, Tebethion, Thiomicid, Thioparamizone, Thiacetazone)
Use: Antituberculous.

P-A-C REVISED FORMULA ANALGESIC. (Upjohn) Aspirin 400 mg, caffeine 32 mg/Tab. Bot. 100s, 1000s.
Use: Salicylate analgesic.

PACEMAKER PROPHYLAXIS PASTES WITH FLUORIDE. (Pacemaker) Silicone dioxide and diatomaceous earth, sodium fluoride 4.4%. Light abrasive, cinnamon/cherry. Medium abrasive, orange. Heavy abrasive, mint. Paste Bot. 8 oz.
Use: Dental caries preventative.

PACKER'S PINE TAR LIQUID SHAMPOO. (Rydelle) Bot. 6 fl oz.
Use: Antiseborrheic.

PACKER'S PINE TAR SOAP. (Rydelle) Bar 3.3 oz.
Use: Tar-containing preparation, topical.

PACLIN G. (Geneva) Penicillin G potassium. **Tab.: 100 M units or 200 M units:** Bot. 1000s. **250 M units or 400 M units:** Bot. 100s, 1000s.
Use: Antibacterial, penicillin.

PACLIN VK. (Geneva) Penicillin phenoxymethyl 125 mg or 250 mg/Tab. Bot. 100s, 1000s.
Use: Antibacterial, penicillin.

• **PACLITAXEL.** USAN.
Use: Antineoplastic.
See: Taxol.

• **PADIMATE A.** USAN.
Use: Ultraviolet screen.

• **PADIMATE O.** USAN.
Use: Ultraviolet screen.
See: Coppertone Prods. (Schering-Plough).
Eclipse Prods. (Dorsey).
Escalol 506 (Van Dyk).
Noskote Prods. (Schering-Plough).
Pabafilm (Owen).
Shade Prods. (Schering-Plough).
Sunger Prods. (Schering-Plough).
Super Shade, Prods. (Schering-Plough).
Tropical Blend Sunscreen Lot. (Schering-Plough).

PAH.
See: Sodium Aminohippurate Inj. (Various Mfr.).

PAIN-A-LAY. (Glessner) Antiseptic, anesthetic soln. Bot. 4 oz w/sprayer, Bot. 4

oz, 8 oz, 1 pt.
Use: Mouth and throat product.
PAIN AND FEVER CAPSULES. (Lederle) Acetaminophen 500 mg/Cap. Bot. 50s, 100s.
Use: Analgesic.
PAIN AND FEVER LIQUID. (Lederle) Acetaminophen 160 mg/5 ml (children's strength). Unit-of-use 4 oz, Bot. 16 oz.
Use: Analgesic.
PAIN AND FEVER TABLETS. (Lederle) Acetaminophen 325 mg or 500 mg/Tab.
325 mg: Bot. 100s, 1000s; **500 mg:** Bot. 50s, 100s.
Use: Analgesic.
PAIN BUST-R II. (Continental) Methyl salicylate 17%, menthol 12%. Cream. Jar 90 g.
Use: Rub and liniments.
PAIN-EZE. (E.J. Moore) Benzocaine, menthol, peppermint oil. Tube ⅛ oz, oz.
Use: Local anesthetic.
PAIN RELIEF, ASPIRIN FREE. (Hudson) Acetaminophen 325 mg/Tab. Bot. 100s, 200s.
Use: Analgesic.
PAIN RELIEF OINTMENT. (Walgreen) Methyl salicylate 15%, menthol 10%. Tube 1.5 oz, 3 oz.
Use: External analgesic.
PAIN RELIEVER. (Rugby) Acetaminophen 250 mg, aspirin 250 mg, caffeine 65 mg/Tab. Bot. 100s, 1000s.
Use: Analgesic combination.
PAIN RELIEVERS-TENSION HEADACHE RELIEVERS. (Weeks & Leo) Acetaminophen 325 mg, phenyltoloxamine citrate 30 mg/Tab. Bot. 40s, 100s.
Use: Analgesic combination.
PALBAR NO. 2. (Hauck) Atropine sulfate 0.012 mg, scopolamine HBr 0.005 mg, hyoscyamine HBr 0.018 mg, phenobarbital 32.4 mg/Tab. Bot. 100s.
Use: Anticholinergic/antispasmodic, sedative/hypnotic.
• **PALDIMYCIN.** USAN.
Use: Antibacterial.
PALESTROL.
See: Diethylstilbestrol (Various Mfr.).
PALGESIC. (Pan American) Isobutylallylbarbituric acid ¾ gr, phenacetin 2 gr, aspirin 3 gr, caffeine gr/Tab. or Cap. Bot. 100s.
Use: Sedative/hypnotic, salicylate analgesic.
PALINUM.
Use: Sedative/hypnotic.
See: Cyclobarbital Calcium (Various Mfr.).

PALMIDROL. N-(2-Hydroxyethyl)palmitamide.
PALMITATE-A 5000. Vitamin A 5000 IU. Tab. 100s.
Use: Vitamin supplement.
• **PALMOXIRATE SODIUM.** USAN.
Use: Antidiabetic.
PALS. (Palisades) Chlorophyllin copper complex 100 mg. Tab. Bot. 30s, 100s, 1000s, UD 30s.
Use: Systemic deodorizer.
PAM.
See: Melphalan.
PAM-L.
See: L-PAM.
PAMABROM. 2-Amino-2-methyl-1-propanol salt of 8-bromotheophyllinate.
W/Acetaminophen.
See: Pamprin, Tab. (Chattem Labs.).
W/Acetaminophen, pyrilamine maleate.
See: Cardui, Tab. (Chattem Labs.).
Sunril, Cap. (Emko).
W/Pyrilamine maleate, homatropine methylbromide, hyoscyamine sulfate, scopolamine HBr, methamphetamine HCl.
See: Aridol, Tabs. (MPL).
• **PAMATOLOL SULFATE.** USAN.
Use: Anti-adrenergic.
PAMELOR. (Sandoz) Nortriptyline HCl. Cap or Liq. **Cap.:** 10 mg, 25 mg, 50 mg or 75 mg base. **10 mg:** Bot. 100s, SandoPak 100s; **25 mg:** Bot. 100s, 500s, SandoPak 100s; **50 mg:** Bot. 100s, SandoPak 100s. **75 mg:** Bot. 100s. **Liq.:** Nortriptyline HCl equivalent to 10 mg base/5 ml. Bot. pt.
Use: Antidepressant.
• **PAMIDRONATE DISODIUM.** USAN.
Use: Bone resorption inhibitor.
PAMINE. (Upjohn) Methscopolamine bromide 2.5 mg/Tab. Bot. 100s, 500s.
Use: Anticholinergic/antispasmodic.
p-AMINOBENZENE-SULFONY-LACETYLIMIDE.
See: Sulfacetamide.
p-AMINOBENZOIC ACID, SALTS.
See: p-Aminobenzoate potassium and p-Aminobenzoate sodium.
p-AMINOSALICYLIC ACID SALTS.
See: Aminosalicylic Acid Salts.
PAMPRIN. (Chattem) Acetaminophen 400 mg, pamabrom 25 mg, pyrilamine maleate 15 mg/Tab. Bot. 24s, 48s.
Use: Analgesic combination.
PAMPRIN EXTRA STRENGTH MULTI-SYMPTOM RELIEF FORMULA TABLETS. (Chattem) Acetaminophen 400 mg, pamabrom 25 mg, pyrilamine maleate 15 mg/Tab. Bot. 12s, 24s, 48s.

Use: Analgesic combination.
PAMPRIN MAXIMUM CRAMP RELIEF FORMULA CAPLETS. (Chattem) Acetaminophen 500 mg, pamabrom 25 mg, pyrilamine maleate 15 mg/Tab. Bot. 8s, 16s, 32s.
Use: Analgesic combination.
PAMPRIN MAXIMUM CRAMP RELIEF FORMULA CAPSULES. (Chattem) Pamabrom 25 mg, acetaminophen 500 mg, pyrilamine maleate 15 mg/Cap. Pkg. 8s, 16s, 32s.
Use: Analgesic combination.
PANACARB. (Lannett) Bismuth subnitrate, sodium bicarbonate, magnesium carbonate, papain, diastase/Tab. Bot. 1000s.
Use: Antacid.
PANACET 5/500. (ECR Pharm) Hydrocodone bitartrate 5 mg, acetaminophen 500 mg. Tab. Bot. 100s.
Use: Narcotic analgesic combination.
PANADEINE CO. TABLETS. (Sanofi Winthrop) Paracetamol, codeine.
Use: Narcotic analgesic combination.
PANADEINE TABLETS. (Sanofi Winthrop) Paracetamol, codeine.
Use: Narcotic analgesic combination.
• **PANADIPLON.** USAN.
Use: Anxiolytic.
PANADO. (Sanofi Winthrop) Paracetamol, codeine.
Use: Narcotic analgesic combination.
PANADOL. (Glenbrook) Acetaminophen 500 mg/Tab. or Cap. **Tab:** Bot. 2s, 30s, 60s, 100s; **Cap:** Bot. 10s, 24s, 48s.
Use: Analgesic.
PANADOL CHILDREN'S. (Glenbrook) Acetaminophen. **Tab.:** 80 mg. Bot. 30s. **Liq.:** 80 mg/0.8 ml. Bot. 2 oz, 4 oz. **Drops:** 80 mg/0.5 oz. Bot. 0.5 oz.
Use: Analgesic.
PANADOL, INFANTS' DROPS. (Glenbrook) Acetaminophen 100 mg/ml. Bot. 15 ml with 0.8 ml dropper.
Use: Analgesic.
PANADOL JR. (Glenbrook) Acetaminophen 160 mg/Caplet. Box. 30s.
Use: Analgesic.
PANADYL. (Misemer) Pyrilamine maleate 25 mg, phenylpropanolamine HCl 50 mg, pheniramine maleate 25 mg/Tab. Bot. 100s, 1000s.
Use: Antihistamine, decongestant.
PANADYL FORTE. (Misemer) Phenylpropanolamine HCl 50 mg, phenylephrine HCl 25 mg, chlorpheniramine maleate 8 mg/Tab. Bot. 100s.
Use: Antihistamine, decongestant.
PANAFIL. (Rystan) Papain pow. 10%,

urea 10%, chlorophyllin copper complex 0.5%, hydrophilic base. Oint. Tube oz, Jar lb.
Use: Topical enzyme preparation.
PANAFIL WHITE OINTMENT. (Rystan) Papain 10,000 units enzyme activity, hydrophilic base/Gm, urea 10%. Tube oz.
Use: Topical enzyme preparation.
PANALGESIC CREAM. (Poythress) Methyl salicylate 35%, menthol 4%. Jar 4 oz.
Use: External analgesic.
PANALGESIC LIQUID. (Poythress) Methyl salicylate 55.01%, menthol 1.25%, camphor 3.1%, in alcohol 22%, emollients, color. Bot. 4 oz, pt, 0.5 gal.
Use: External analgesic.
PANASAL 5/500. (ECR Pharm) Hydrocodone bitartrate 5 mg, aspirin 500 mg. Tab. Bot. 100s.
Use: Narcotic analgesic combination.
PANASOL. (Seatrace) Prednisone 5 mg/Tab. Bot. 100s.
Use: Corticosteroid.
PANASOL-S. (Seatrace) Prednisone 1 mg/Tab. Bot. 100s, 1000s.
Use: Corticosteroid.
PANASORB DROPS. (Sanofi Winthrop) Paracetamol, codeine.
Use: Narcotic analgesic combination.
PANASORB ELIXIR. (Sanofi Winthrop) Paracetamol, codeine.
Use: Narcotic analgesic combination.
PANASORB SUPPOSITORIES. (Sanofi Winthrop) Paracetamol, codeine.
Use: Narcotic analgesic combination.
PANASORB TABLETS. (Sanofi Winthrop) Paracetamol.
Use: Analgesic.
PANC-500. (Freeda) Hesperidin 100 mg, citrus bioflavonoids 100 mg, rutin 50 mg, vitamin C 500 mg/Tab. Bot. 100s, 250s, 500s.
Use: Vitamin supplement.
• **PANCOPRIDE.** USAN.
Use: Antiemetic; antianxiety agent; peristaltic stimulant.
PANCREASE. (McNeil Pharm) Enteric coated pancrelipase capsules. **Regular:** Lipase 4000 units, amylase 20,000 units, protease 25,000 units/Cap. Bot. 100s, 250s; **MT4:** Lipase 4000 units, amylase 12,000 units, protease 12,000 units/Cap. Bot. 100s; **MT10:** Lipase 10,000 units, amylase 30,000 units, protease 30,000 units/Cap. Bot. 100s; **MT16:** Lipase 16,000 units, amylase 48,000 units, protease 48,000 units/Cap. Bot. 100s; **MT 25:** Lipase 25,000 units, amylase 70,000 units, pro-

tease 55,000 units. Cap. Bot. 100s; **MT 32:** Lipase 32,000 units, amylase 90,000 units, protease 70,000 units. Cap. Bot. 100s.
Use: Digestive enzymes.
PANCREATIC ENZYME.
W/Pepsin, ox bile.
See: Nu' Leven, Nu' Leven Plus, Tab. (Lemmon).
PANCREATIC SUBSTANCE. Substance from fresh pancreas of hog or ox, containing the enzymes amylopsin, trypsin, steapsin.
W/Bile extract, dl-methionine, choline bitartrate.
See: Licoplex, Tab. (Mills).
W/Bile salts, lipase.
See: Cotazym-B, Tab. (Organon).
W/Bile, whole (desiccated), oxidized bile acids, homatropine methylbromide.
See: Pancobile, Tab. (Solvay).
W/Lipase.
See: Cotazym, Cap., Packet (Organon).
• **PANCREATIN,** U.S.P. XXIII. Cap., Tab., U.S.P. XXIII. Pancreatic enzymes obtained from hog or cattle pancreatic tissue.
Use: Digestant.
See: Depancol, Tab. (Warner-Chilcott).
Elzyme, Tab. (Elder).
Panteric, Tab. (Parke Davis).
PANCREATIN W/COMBINATIONS.
See: Entozyme, Tab. (Robins).
Nu'Leven, Tab. (Lemmon).
Pepsatal, Tab. (Kenyon).
Ro-Bile, Tab. (Solvay).
Sto-Zyme, Tab. (Jalco).
Zypan, Tab. (Standard Process).
• **PANCRELIPASE,** U.S.P. XXIII. Cap., Tab., U.S.P. XXIII. Formerly Lipancreatin. Preparation of hog pancreas with high content of steapsin and adequate amounts of pancreatic enzymes.
Use: Pancreatic enzymes preparation; digestive aid.
See: Accelerase, Cap. (Organon).
Cotazym, Cap., Packet (Organon).
Viokase, Pow., Tab. (Robins).
W/Mixed conjugated bile salts, cellulase.
See: Accelerase, Cap. (Organon).
Cotazym-B, Tab. (Organon).
PANCREOZYMIN. B.A.N. A hormone obtained from duodenal mucosa.
Use: Diagnostic aid.
PANCRETIDE. (Baxter) Pancreatic polypeptide in normal saline.
Use: Fibrinolytic conditions.
PANCURONIUM.
See: Pancuronium Bromide (Organon).
• **PANCURONIUM BROMIDE.** USAN. (1)

1,1'-(3α,17β-Dihydroxy-5α-androstan-2β,16β-ylene)bis-[1-methylpiperidinium]dibromide diacetate: (2) 2β,16β-dipiperidino-5α-androstane-3α, 17 β-diol diacetate dimethobromide. (Various Mfr.)
1 mg/ml: Vials 10 ml; **2 mg/ml:** Vials, amps, syringes 2 ml or 5 ml.
Use: Skeletal muscle relaxant.
See: Pavulon, Inj. (Organon).
PANEX. (Hauck) Acetaminophen 325 mg/Tab. Bot. 1000s.
Use: Analgesic.
PANEX 500. (Hauck) Acetaminophen 500 mg/Tab. Bot. 1000s.
Use: Analgesic.
PANHEMATIN. (Abbott) Hemin 313 mg/43 ml when reconstituted. Vial 100 ml.
Use: Agent for acute intermittent porphyria.
PANIDAZOLE. B.A.N. 2-Methyl-5-nitro-1-[2-(4-pyridyl)ethyl]imidazole.
Use: Amebicide.
PANITOL. (Wesley) Allylisobutyl barbituric acid 15 mg, acetaminophen 300 mg/Tab. Bot. 100s, 1000s.
Use: Sedative/hypnotic, analgesic.
PANITOL H.M.B. (Wooloy) Panitol formula plus homatropine methylbromide 2.5 mg/Tab. Bot. 100s, 1000s.
Use: Sedative/hypnotic, analgesic, anticholinergic/antispasmodic.
PANMYCIN. (Upjohn) Tetracycline HCl 250 mg/Cap. Bot. 100s, 1000s.
Use: Antibacterial, tetracycline.
See: Panmycin, Cap. (Upjohn).
PANOXYL ACNE GEL. (Stiefel) Benzoyl peroxide 5% or 10%, alcohol 20%, polyoxyethylene lauryl ether 6% in a hydroalcoholic gel base. Tube 2 oz, 4 oz.
Use: Anti-acne.
PANOXYL AQ ACNE GEL. (Stiefel) Benzoyl peroxide 2.5%, 5% or 10%, polyoxyethylene lauryl ether in an aqueous gel base. Tube 2 oz, 4 oz.
Use: Anti-acne.
PANOXYL BAR-5. (Stiefel) Benzoyl peroxide 5% in a rich-lathering, mild surfactant cleansing base. Bar 4 oz.
Use: Anti-acne.
PANOXYL BAR-10. (Stiefel) Benzoyl peroxide 10% in rich-lathering, mild surfactant cleansing base. Bar 4 oz.
Use: Anti-acne.
PANPARNIT HYDROCHLORIDE.
Caramiphen HCl.
Use: Antiparkinson agent.
PANSCOL. (Baker/Cummins) Salicylic acid 3%, lactic acid 2%, phenol (less than 1%). **Oint.:** Jar 3 oz. **Lot.:** Bot. 4 oz.

Use: Emollient.

•**PANTHENOL,** U.S.P. XXIII. Alcohol corresponding to pantothenic acid. Pantothenol. Pantothenylol. (±)-2,4-Dihydroxy-N-(3-hydroxypropyl)-3,3-dimethylbutyramide.
Use: Treatment of paralytic ileus and postoperative distention.
See. Ilopan, Amp., Vial (Warren-Teed).
Panadon, Cream (Gordon Labs.).
Panthoderm Cream (USV Pharm).

PANTHENOL W/COMBINATIONS.
See: Geriatrazole Prod., Vial (Kenyon).
Lifer-B, Liq. (Burgin-Arden).
Nutricol, Cap., Inj. (Nutrition Control).
Vi-Testrogen, Vial (Pharmex).

PANTHODERM CREAM. (Rhone-Poulenc Rorer) Dexpanthenol 2% in water-miscible cream. Tube 1 oz, Jar 2 oz, lb.
Use: Emollient.

PANTOCAINE.
See: Tetracaine HCl. (Various Mfr.).

PANTOCRIN-F. (Spanner) Plurigland, ovarian, anterior and posterior pituitary, adrenal, thyroid extracts. Vial 30 ml.

PANTOPAQUE. (Alcon Surgical) Iophendylate, ethyl iodophenylundecanoate. Amp. 3 ml 3s; 6 ml 6s; 1 ml 2s.
Use: Radiopaque agent.

•**PANTOPRAZOLE.** USAN.
Use: Antiulcer (gastric H$^+$/K$^+$-ATPase inhibitor).

PANTOTHENIC ACID. As calcium or sodium salt.
Use: Vitamin B$_5$ supplement.
See: Vitamin preparations.

PANTOTHENIC ACID SALTS.
See: Calcium Pantothenate.
Sodium Pantothenate.

PANTOTHENOL.
See: Panthenol, Preps. (Various Mfr.).

PANTOTHENYL ALCOHOL.
See: Panthenol, Preps. (Various Mfr.).

PANTOTHENYLOL.
See: Panthenol, Preps. (Various Mfr.).

PANVITEX GERIATRIC CAPSULES.
(Forest Pharm.) Safflower oil 340 mg, vitamins A 10,000 IU, D 400 IU, B$_1$ 5 mg, B$_6$ 1 mg, B$_2$ 2.5 mg, B$_{12}$ activity 2 mcg, C 75 mg, niacinamide 40 mg, calcium pantothenate 4 mg, E 2 IU, inositol 15 mg, choline bitartrate 31.4 mg, calcium 75 mg, phosphorus 58 mg, iron 30 mg, manganese 0.5 mg, potassium 2 mg, zinc 0.5 mg, magnesium 3 mg/Cap. Bot. 100s, 1000s.
Use: Vitamin/mineral supplement.

PANVITEX GERIATRIC INJ. (Forest Pharm.) Testosterone 10 mg, vitamins

B$_{12}$ 100 mcg, B$_1$ 50 mg, nicotinamide 50 mg, B$_6$ 5 mg, estrone 0.5 mg, liver injection equivalent in B$_{12}$ activity of cyanocobalamin 2 mcg, lidocaine 20 mg, panthenol 10 mg, B$_2$ 5 mg/ml. Vial 30 ml.
Use: Vitamin/hormone supplement.

PANVITEX PLUS MINERALS CAPSULES. (Forest Pharm.) Vitamins A 5000 IU, D 400 IU, B$_1$ 3 mg, B$_2$ 2.5 mg, niacinamide 20 mg, B$_6$ 1.5 mg, calcium pantothenate 5 mg, B$_{12}$ 2.5 mcg, C 50 mg, E 3 IU, calcium 215 mg, phosphorus 166 mg, iron 13.4 mg, magnesium 7.5 mg, manganese 1.5 mg, potassium 5 mg, zinc 1.4 mg/Cap. Bot. 100s, 1000s.
Use: Vitamin/mineral supplement.

PANVITEX PRENATAL CAPSULES.
(Forest Pharm.) Ferrous fumarate 150 mg, cobalamin concentration 2 mcg, vitamins A 6000 IU, D 400 IU, B$_1$ 1.5 mg, B$_2$ 2.5 mg, niacinamide 15 mg, B$_6$ 3 mg, C 100 mg, calcium 250 mg, calcium pantothenate 5 mg, folic acid 0.2 mg/Cap. Bot. 100s, 1000s.
Use: Vitamin/mineral supplement.

PANVITEX T-M. (Forest Pharm.) Vitamins A 10,000 IU, D 400 IU, B$_1$ 10 mg, B$_6$ 1 mg, B$_2$ 5 mg, B$_{12}$ 5 mcg, C 150 mg, niacinamide 100 mg, calcium 103 mg, phosphorus 80 mg, iron 10 mg, manganese 1 mg, potassium 5 mg, zinc 1.4 mg, magnesium 5.56 mg/Cap. Bot. 100s, 1000s.
Use: Vitamin/mineral supplement.

PAP. (Abbott Diagnostics) Enzyme immunoassay for measurement of prostatic acid phosphatase. Test kit 100s.
Use: Diagnostic aid.

P.A.P. No. 1. (Jenkins) Phenobarbital 15 mg, acid acetylsalicylic 0.23 Gm, acetophenetidin 0.15 Gm/Tab. Bot. 1000s.
Use: Sedative/hypnotic, analgesic.

PAPA-CARIA. (Jenkins) Magnesium carbonate 100 gr, calcium carbonate 50 gr, sodium bicarbonate 120 gr, bismuth subnitrate 50 gr, cerium oxalate 25 gr, magnesium trisilicate 70 gr, powder ginger 4 gr, papain 11 gr, pancreatin 5.5 gr/oz. Pkg. 2 oz.
Use: Digestive aid.

PAPADEINE #3. (Vangard) Codeine phosphate 30 mg, acetaminophen 300 mg/Tab. Bot. 100s, 1000s.
Use: Narcotic analgesic combination.

•**PAPAIN,** U.S.P. XXIII. Tab. for Topical Soln., U.S.P. XXIII. A proteolytic substance derived from *Carlica papaya.*
Use: Proteolytic enzyme.
See: Papase, Tab. (Parke-Davis).

Softlens Enzymatic Contact Lens
Cleaner (Allergan).
PAPAIN W/COMBINATIONS.
See: Bilate, Tab. (Central).
Cerophen, Tab. (Wendt-Bristol).
Digenzyme, Tab. (Burgin-Arden).
Kaocasil, Tab. (Jenkins).
Panacarb, Tab. (Lannett).
Panafil, Oint. (Rystan).
PAP-A-LIX. (Freeport) n-Acetyl-
aminophenol 120 mg, alcohol 10%/5 ml.
Bot. 4 oz, gal.
Use: Analgesic.
• **PAPAVERINE HYDROCHLORIDE,**
U.S.P. XXIII. Inj., Tab., U.S.P. XXIII. 6,7-
Dimethoxy-l-veratrylisoquinoline Hy-
drochloride.
Use: Smooth muscle relaxant.
See: BP-Papaverine, Cap. (Burlington).
Cerespan, Cap. (Rhone-Poulenc Ror-
er).
Cirbed, Cap. (Boyd).
Delapav, Time Cap. (Dunhall).
Myobid, Cap. (Laser).
P-200, Cap. (Boots).
Pavabid, Cap. (Marion).
Pavacap, Unicells (Solvay).
Pavacaps, Cap. (Freeport).
Pavacen Cenules, Cap. (Central).
Pavaclor, Cap. (Pasadena Research).
Pavadel, Cap. (Canright).
Pavadyl, Cap. (Dock).
Pavakey 300, Cap. (Key).
Pavakey S.A., Cap. (Key).
Pava-lyn, Cap. (Lynwood).
Pava Par, Cap. (Parmed).
Pavasule, Cap. (Jalco).
Pavatest T.D., Cap. (Fellows-Testa-
gar).
Pavatym, Cap. (Everett).
Pavatran T.D. Cap. (Mayrand).
Paverolan, Lanacap (Lannett).
Vasocap, Cap. (Keene).
Vazosan, Tab. (Sandia).
W/Codeine sulfate.
See: Copavin, Pulvule, Tab. (Lilly).
W/Codeine sulfate, aloin, sodium salicy-
late.
See: Copavin Compound, Elix. (Lilly).
W/Codeine sulfate, emetine HCl,
ephedrine HCl.
See: Golacol, Syr. (Arcum).
W/Phenobarbital.
See: Pavadel-PB, Cap. (Canright).
PAPAVERINE TOPICAL GEL.
Use: Sexual dysfunction in spinal cord
injury patients. [Orphan drug]
PAPAVEROLINE. B.A.N. 1-(3,4-Dihy-
droxybenzyl)-6,7-dihydroxyisoquinoline.
Use: Vasodilator.

PAPLEX ULTRA. (Medicis) Salicylic acid
26% in flexible collodion. Bot. 15 ml.
Use: Keratolytic.
PARA-AMINOBENZOIC ACID.
Aminobenzoic Acid, U.S.P. XXIII.
See: Paba-"5", Lot. (Durel).
Pabanol, Lot. (Elder).
Presun, Lot., Gel (Westwood).
W/Acetylsalicylic acid, vitamin C.
See: P.A.A.M., Tab. (Kenyon).
PARA-AMINOSALICYLATE, SODIUM.
See: Aminosalicylate Sodium.
PARA-AMINOSALICYLIC ACID. Aminos-
alicylic Acid, U.S.P. XXIII.
Use: Tuberculosis infections. [Orphan
drug]
PARABAXIN. (Parmed) Methocarbamol
500 mg or 750 mg/Tab. Bot. 100s.
Use: Skeletal muscle relaxant.
PARABROM.
See: Pyrabrom.
PARABROMIDYLAMINE.
See: Brompheniramine, Dimetane,
Preps. (Robins).
PARACAIN.
See: Procaine Hydrochloride (Various
Mfr.).
PARACARBINOXAMINE MALEATE.
Carbinoxamine.
PARACET FORTE TABS. (Major) Chlor-
zoxazone, acetaminophen. Bot. 100s,
1000s.
Use: Skeletal muscle relaxant.
PARACETALDEHYDE.
See: Paraldehyde, U.S.P. XXIII.
PARACETAMOL. B.A.N. 4-Acetami-
dophenol.
Use: Analgesic; antipyretic.
PARACHLORAMINE
HYDROCHLORIDE. Meclizine HCl,
U.S.P. XXIII.
See: Bonine, Tab. (Pfizer).
PARACHLOROMETAXYLENOL.
Use: Phenolic antiseptic.
See: D-Seb, Liq. (Cooper).
Nu-Flow, Liq. (Cooper).
W/9-aminoacridine HCl, methyl-dode-
cylbenzyl-trimethyl ammonium Cl,
pramoxine HCl, hydrocortisone, acetic
acid.
See: Drotic No. 2, Drops (Ascher).
W/Benzocaine.
See: TPO 20 (DePree).
W/Coconut oil, pine oil, castor oil, lanolin,
cholesterols, lecithin.
See: Sebacide, Liq. (Paddock).
W/Hydrocortisone, pramoxine HCl, benza-
lkonium Cl, acetic acid.
See: Oto Drops (Solvay).
W/Lidocaine, phenol, zinc oxide.

See: Unguentine Plus, Cream (Norwich).
W/Pramoxine HCl, hydrocortisone, benzalkonium Cl, acetic acid.
See: My Cort Otic #2, Drops (Scrip).
Steramine Otic, Drops (Mayrand).
W/Resorcinol, sulfur.
See: Rezamid, Lot. (Dermik).

• **PARACHLOROPHENOL,** U.S.P. XXIII.
Camphorated, U.S.P XX. Phenol, 4-chloro. p-Chlorophenol.
Use: Topical antibacterial.
W/Camphor.
See: Camphorated parachlorophenol.

PARACODIN.
See: Dihydrocodeine.

PARADIONE CAPSULES. (Abbott) Paramethadione 150 mg or 300 mg/Cap.
Bot. 100s.
Use: Anticonvulsant.

PARADYNE. (Spanner) Dipyrone injection 50%. Vial 10 ml.

PARAEUSAL LIQUID. (Paraeusal) Liq.
Bot. 2 oz, 6 oz, 12 oz.
Use: Minor skin irritations.

PARAEUSAL SOLID. (Paraeusal) Oint.
Jar 1 oz, 2 oz, 16 oz.
Use: Minor skin irritations.

• **PARAFFIN,** N. F. XVII.
Use: Stiffening agent.

• **PARAFFIN, SYNTHETIC,** N.F. XVIII.

PARAFLEX. (McNeil Pharm.) Chlorzoxazone 250 mg/Tab. Bot. 100s.
Use: Skeletal muscle relaxant.

PARAFON FORTE DSC. (McNeil Pharm.) Chlorzoxazone 500 mg/Capl.
Bot. 100s, 500s, UD 100s.
Use: Skeletal muscle relaxant.

PARAFORM. Paraformaldehyde. (No Mfr. listed).

PARAFORMALDEHYDE.
Use: Essentially the same as formaldehyde.
See: Formaldehyde (Various Mfr.).
Trioxymethylene (an incorrect term for paraformaldehyde).

PARAGLYCYLARSANILIC ACID. N-Carbamylmethyl-p-aminobenzenearsonic acid, the free acid of tryparsamide.

PARAHIST HD LIQUID. (Pharmics) Phenylephrine HCl 5 mg, chlorpheniramine maleate 2 mg, hydrocodone bitartrate 1.67 mg, alcohol free. Bot. 473 ml.
Use: Decongestant, antihistamine, antitussive.

PARA-JEL. (Approved) Benzocaine 5%, cetyl dimethyl benzyl ammonium Cl.
Tube 0.25 oz.
Use: Local anesthetic.

• **PARALDEHYDE,** U.S.P. XXIII. Sterile, U.S.P. XXI. 1,3,5-Trioxane, 2,4,6-trimethyl-.2,4,6-Trimethyl-s-trioxane.
Paracetaldehyde. Bot. 0.25 lb, 1 lb. Amp.
Use: I.M., I.V. or orally; hypnotic and sedative.
See: Paral, Cap., Liq., Amp. (Forest).

PARAL ORAL. (Forest) Paraldehyde 30 ml. Bot. 12s, 25s.
Use: Sedative/hypnotic.

PARAMEPHRIN.
See: Epinephrine (Various Mfr.).

• **PARAMETHADIONE,** U.S.P. XXII. Cap., Oral Soln., U.S.P. XXII. 2,4-Oxazolidinedione, 5-methyl-3,5-dimethyl-.5-Ethyl-3,5-dimethyl-2,4-oxazolidenedione.
Use: Anticonvulsant.
See: Paradione, Cap., Soln. (Abbott).

• **PARAMETHASONE ACETATE,** U.S.P. XXIII. Tab., U.S.P. XXIII. 16α-Methyl-6α-fluoroprednisolone-21-acetate.6α-Fluoro-11β,17,21-trihydroxy-16α-methylpregna-1,4-diene-3,20-dione 21-Acetate.
Use: Glucocorticoid.
See: Haldrone, Tab. (Lilly).

PARA-MONOCHLOROPHENOL.
See: Camphorated para-chlorophenol, Liq. (Novocol).

• **PARANYLINE HYDROCHLORIDE.**
USAN.
Use: Anti-inflammatory.

• **PARAPENZOLATE BROMIDE.** USAN.
Use: Anticholinergic.

PARAPLATIN. (Bristol-Myers Oncology) Carboplatin 50 mg, 150 mg or 450 mg. Inj. Vial.
Use: Antineoplastic agent.

PARAROSANILINE EMBONATE.
Pararosaniline pamoate.

• **PARAROSANILINE PAMOATE.** USAN.
Bis-[tris(p-Aminophenyl)methylium] (4,4′-methylenebis[3-hydroxy-2-naphthoate])hydrate. Under study.
Use: Antischistosomal agent.

PARASYMPATHOLYTIC AGENTS.
Cholinergic blocking agents.
See: Anticholinergic Agents.
Antispasmodics.
Mydriatics.
Parkinsonism.

PARASYMPATHOMIMETIC AGENTS.
See: Cholinergic Agents.

PARATHAR. (Rhone-Poulenc Rorer) Teriparatide acetate hPTH activity 200 units with gelatin 20 mg pow. for inj. Vial 10 ml w/10 ml vial diluent.
Use: Diagnostic aid.

PARATHYROID THERAPY. Dihydro-tachysterol, U.S.P. XXIII. Tachysterol.
See: Hytakerol, Soln., Cap. (Sanofi Winthrop).
Parathyroid Injection (Various Mfr.).
PARATROL LIQUID. (Walgreen) Pyrethrins 0.2%, piperonyl butoxide technical 2%, deodorized kerosene 0.8%. Bot. 2 oz.
Use: Pediculicide.
PARAZONE. (Interstate) Chlorzoxazone 250 mg, acetaminophen 300 mg/Tab. Bot. 100s, 1000s.
Use: Skeletal muscle relaxant, analgesic.
• **PARBENDAZOLE.** USAN. Methyl 5-butyl-2-benzimidazolecarbamate. Helmatac. Under study.
Use: Anthelmintic.
PARBUTOXATE. β-Dimethylaminoethyl-3-amino-4-butoxybenzoate.
PARCILLIN. (Parmed) Crystalline potassium penicillin G 240 mg, 400,000 units/Tab. Bot. 100s, 1000s. Pow. for syr. 400,000 units/Tsp. 80 ml.
Use: Antibacterial, penicillin.
• **PARCONAZOLE HYDROCHLORIDE.** USAN.
Use: Antifungal.
PAR DECON. (Par) Phenylpropanolamine HCl 40 mg, phenylephrine HCl 10 mg, chlorpheniramine maleate 5 mg, phenyltoloxamine citrate 15 mg/Tab. Bot. 100s, 500s, 1000s.
Use: Antihistamine/decongestant.
PAR GLYCEROL. (Pharmaceutical Resources) Iodinated glycerol 60 mg (organically bound iodine 30 mg)/5 ml with alcohol 21.75%, peppermint oil, corn syrup and saccharin. Caramel-mint flavor. Bot. pt.
Use: Expectorant.
PAREDRINE. (Pharmics) Hydroxyamphetamine HBr 1%, boric acid 2%, thimerosal 1:50,000. Bot. 15 ml.
Use: Pupil dilation.
• **PAREGORIC,** U.S.P. XXIII. (Various Mfr.).
Use: Antiperistaltic.
W/Bismuth subgallate, kaolin, pectin.
See: Dysenaid Jr., Tab. (Jenkins).
W/Glycyrrhiza fluidextract, antimony potassium tartrate.
See: Brown Mixture, Liq. (Lilly).
W/Kaolin (colloidal), aluminum hydroxide, bismuth subcarbonate, pectin.
See: Kapinal, Tab. (Jenkins).
W/Kaolin, pectin.
See: Kaoparin, Susp. (McKesson).
Parepectolin, Susp. (Rhone-Poulenc Rorer Consumer).

W/Kaolin, pectin, bismuth subsalicylate, zinc sulfocarbonate.
W/Milk of bismuth, kaolin, pectin.
See: Mul-Sed, Liq. (Webcon).
W/Pectin, kaolin.
See: Parepectolin, Susp. (Rhone-Poulenc Rorer).
W/Zinc sulfocarbolate, phenyl salicylate, bismuth subsalicylate, pepsin.
See: C M with Paregoric, Liq. (Beecham Labs).
Corrective Mixture with Paregoric (Beecham Labs).
PAREMYD. (Allergan) Hydroxyamphetamine HBr 1%, tropicamide 0.25%. Soln. Bot. 5 ml, 15 ml.
Use: Mydriatic/cycloplegic.
PARENABOL. Boldenone undecylenate.
PAREPECTOLIN. (Rhone-Poulenc Rorer) Attapulgite 600 mg/15 ml. Liq. Bot. 240 ml.
Use: Antidiarrheal.
• **PAREPTIDE SULFATE.** USAN.
Use: Antiparkinsonian.
PAR ESTRO. (Parmed) Conjugated estrogens 1.25 mg/Tab. Bot. 100s.
Use: Estrogen.
PARETHOXYCAINE HCl.
W/Zirconium oxide, calamine.
See: Zotox, Spray, Cream (Commerce).
PAR-F. (Pharmics) Iron 60 mg, calcium 250 mg, vitamins C 120 mg, A 5000 IU, D 400 IU, B₁ 3 mg, B₂ 3.4 mg, B₁₂ 12 mcg, B₆ 12 mg, niacinamide 20 mg, iodine 0.15 mg, magnesium 100 mg, copper 2 mg, zinc 15 mg, E 30 IU, folic acid 1 mg/Tab. Bot. 100s.
Use: Vitamin/mineral supplement.
PARHIST SR. (Parmed) Phenylpropanolamine HCl 75 mg, chlorpheniramine maleate 12 mg/Cap. Bot. 100s, 1000s.
Use: Decongestant, antihistamine.
PARKELP. (Phillip R. Park) Pacific sea kelp. **Tab.:** Bot. 100s, 200s, 500s, 800s. **Gran.:** Bot. 2 oz, 7 oz, 1 lb, 3 lb.
Use: Iodine supplement.
PARKINSONISM, AGENTS for. Parasympatholytic agents.
See: Akineton, Tab., Inj. (Knoll).
Artane, Elix., Tab., Sequels (Lederle).
Benztropine Mesylate, Tab. (Various Mfr.).
Caramiphen HCl.
Cogentin, Tab., Amp. (Merck & Co.).
Dopar, Cap. (Norwich Eaton).
Eldepryl, Tab. (Somerset).
Kemadrin, Tab. (Burroughs Wellcome).
Larodopa, Tab. (Roche).

Lodosyn, Tab. (Merck & Co.).
Parlodel, Tab., Cap. (Sandoz).
Permax, Tab. (Lilly).
Sinemet, Tab. (Du Pont Pharma).
Symmetrel, Cap., Syr. (DuPont).
Trihexyphenidyl HCl (Various Mfr.).
Trihexy-2 (Geneva).
PARLODEL. (Sandoz) Bromocriptine mesylate. **Tab.:** 2.5 mg. Bot. 30s, 100s.
Cap.: 5 mg. Bot. 30s, 100s.
Use: Antiparkinson agent.
PARMETH. (Parmed) Promethazine HCl 50 mg/Cap. Bot. 100s, 1000s.
Use: Antihistamine, antiemetic/antivertigo agent.
PARMINYL. W/Salicylamide, phenacetin, caffeine, acetaminophen.
See: Dolopar, Tab. (O'Neal).
PAR-NATAL-FA. (Parmed) Vitamins A 4000 IU, D 400 IU, thiamine HCl 2 mg, riboflavin 2 mg, pyridoxine HCl 0.8 mg, ascorbic acid 50 mg, niacinamide 10 mg, iodine 0.15 mg, folic acid 0.1 mg, cobalamin concentrate 2 mcg, iron 50 mg, calcium 240 mg/Cap. Bot. 100s, 1000s.
Use: Vitamin/mineral supplement.
PAR-NATAL PLUS 1 IMPROVED.
(Parmed) elemental calcium 200 mg, elemental iron 65 mg, vitamins A 4000 IU, D 400 IU, E 11 mg, B_1 1.5 mg, B_2 3 mg, B_3 20 mg, B_6 10 mg, B_{12} 12 mcg, C 120 mg, folic acid 1 mg, zinc 25 mg, Cu/Tab. Bot. 100s, 500s.
Use: Vitamin/mineral supplement.
PARNATE. (SK-Beecham) Tranylcypromine sulfate 10 mg/Tab. Bot. 100s.
Use: Antidepressant.
PARODONTAX DENTAL CREAM. (E.J. Moore) Sodium bicarbonate plus five natural herbs. Tube 60 Gm.
Use: Dental caries preventative.
PARODYNE.
See: Antipyrine (Various Mfr.).
PAROLEINE.
See: Petrolatum Liquid (Various Mfr.).
•**PAROMOMYCIN SULFATE,** U.S.P. XX.
Cap., Syr., U.S.P. XXIII. An antibiotic substance obtained from cultures of certain *Streptomyces* species, one of which is *Streptomyces rimosus.*
Use: Antiamebic.
PAROTHYL. (Interstate) Meprobamate 400 mg, tridihexethyl Cl 25 mg/Tab. Bot. 100s.
Use: Antianxiety agent, anticholinergic/antispasmodic.
PAROXETINE HCl.
Use: Antidepressant.
See: Paxil, Tab. (SK-Beecham).

PAROXYL.
See: Acetarsone (Various Mfr.).
PARPANIT.
See: Caramiphen HCl (Various Mfr.).
PARSIDOL. (Parke-Davis) Ethopropazine HCl 10 mg or 50 mg/Tab. Bot. 100s.
Use: Antiparkinson agent.
PARSLEY CONCENTRATE.
W/Garlic concentrate.
See: Allimin, Tab. (Mosso).
PAR-Supp. (Parmed) Estrone 0.2 mg, lactose 50 mg/Vaginal Supp. Pkg. 12s.
Use: Vaginitis.
PARTAPP TD. (Parmed) Phenylpropanolamine HCl 15 mg, phenylephrine HCl 15 mg, brompheniramine maleate 12 mg/TD Tab. Bot. 1000s.
PARTEN. (Parmed) Acetaminophen 10 gr/Tab. Bot. 100s, 1000s.
Use: Analgesic.
•**PARTRICIN.** USAN. Antibiotic produced by *Streptomyces aureofaciens.*
Use: Antifungal, antiprotozoal.
PARTUSS. (Parmed) Dextromethorphan hydrobromide 60 mg, potassium guaiacolsulfonate 8 gr, chlorpheniramine maleate 6 mg, ammonium Cl 8 gr, tartar emetic $^1/_{12}$ gr, chloroform 2 min/30 ml. Bot. 4 oz, pt, gal.
Use: Antitussive, expectorant, antihistamine.
PARTUSS "A". (Parmed) Acetaminophen 5 gr, salicylamide 2 gr, caffeine 0.5 gr, atropine sulfate 0.12 mg, guaifenesin 100 mg, phenylpropanolamine HCl 25 mg/Tab. Bot. 1000s.
Use: Analgesic, anticholinergic/antispasmodic, expectorant, decongestant.
PARTUSS A.C. (Parmed) Guaifenesin 100 mg, pheniramine maleate 7.5 mg, codeine phosphate 10 mg, alcohol 3.5%/5 ml. Bot 4 oz.
Use: Expectorant, antihistamine, antitussive.
PARTUSS LA. (Parmed) Phenylpropanolamine HCl 75 mg, guaifenesin 400 mg/LA Tab. Bot. 100s, 500s.
Use: Decongestant, expectorant.
PARVLEX. (Freeda) Iron 100 mg, vitamins B_1 20 mg, B_2 20 mg, B_3 20 mg, B_5 1 mg, B_6 10 mg, B_{12} 50 mcg, C 50 mg, folic acid 0.1 mg, Cu, Mn/Tab. Bot. 100s, 250s, 500s.
Use: Vitamin/mineral supplement.
P.A.S. ACID. (Kasar) Para-aminosalicylic acid 500 mg/Tab. Bot. 1000s.
Use: Antituberculous agent.
PAS-C. (Hellwig) Pascorbic. p-aminosalicylic acid 0.5 Gm with vitamin C/Tab.

Bot. 1000s.
Use: Antituberculous agent.
PASDIUM. (Kasar) Sodium aminosalicylate 0.5 Gm or 1 Gm/Tab. Bot. 1000s.
Use: Antituberculous agent.
PASSIFLORA. Dried flowering and fruiting tops of Passiflora incarnata.
W/Phenobarbital, extract hyoscyamus.
See: Somlyn w/Pb, Cap. (Scrip).
W/Phenobarbital, jamaica dogwood.
See: Sominol, Phenobarbital, Tab. (O'Neal).
W/Phenobarbital, valerian, hyoscyamus.
See: Aluro, Tab. (Foy).
PASIJEN. (Jenkins) Passiflora 1 gr, valerian 1 gr, extract henbane 1/8 gr (total alkaloids 0.00019 gr), phenobarbital 0.25 gr/Tab. Bot. 1000s.
Use: Anticholinergic/antispasmodic, sedative/hypnotic.
PASTEURELLA TULARENSIS ANTIGEN. 10,000 million organisms/ml.
(Lederle)—Vial 5 ml, 20 ml.
Use: Diagnostic aid.
PATENT DUCTUS ARTERIOSUS, AGENTS FOR.
See: Indocin, I.V., Inj. (Merck & Co.).
Prostin VR Pediatric, Inj. (Upjohn).
PATH. (Parker) Buffered neutral formalin soln. 10%. Bot. 1 gal, 5 gal. Jar 4 oz.
Use: Tissue specimen fixative.
PATHILON. (Lederle) Tridihexethyl chloride 25 mg/Tab. Bot. 100s.
Use: Anticholinergic/antispasmodic.
PATHOCIL. (Wyeth-Ayerst) Sodium dicloxacillin monohydrate. Monohydrate sodium salt of 6[3-(2,6-dichlorophenyl)-5-methyl-4-isoxazolyl]penicillin. **250 mg/Cap.:** Bot. 100s. **500 mg/Cap.:** Bot. 50s. **Pow. for oral susp.:** 62.5 mg/5 ml. Bot. to make 100 ml.
Use: Antibacterial, penicillin.
• **PAULOMYCIN.** USAN.
Use: Antibacterial.
PAVABID HP. (Marion Merrell Dow) Papaverine HCl 300 mg/Capl. Bot. 60s.
Use: Peripheral vasodilator.
PAVABID PLATEAU. (Marion Merrell Dow) Papaverine HCl 150 mg/TR Cap. Bot. 100s, 250s, 1000s, UD 100s.
Use: Peripheral vasodilator.
PAVACAPS. (Freeport) Papaverine HCl 150 mg/TR Cap. Bot. 1000s.
Use: Peripheral vasodilator.
PAVACEN CENULES. (Central) Papaverine HCl 150 mg/TR Cap. Bot. 100s.
Use: Peripheral vasodilator.
PAVADEL. (Canright) Papaverine HCl 150 mg/Cap. Bot. 100s, 1000s.

Use: Peripheral vasodilator.
PAVADEL PB. (Canright) Papaverine HCl 150 mg, phenobarbital 45 mg/Cap. Bot. 100s.
Use: Peripheral vasodilator.
PAVADYL CAPSULES. (Bock) Papaverine HCl 150 mg/Cap. Bot. 100s.
Use: Peripheral vasodilator.
PAVAGEN. (Rugby) Papaverine 150 mg/TR Cap. Bot. 500s, 1000s, UD 100s.
Use: Peripheral vasodilator.
PAVA-LYN. (Lynwood) Papaverine HCl 150 mg/Cap. Bot. 100s.
Use: Peripheral vasodilator.
PAVASED. (Hauck) Papaverine HCl 150 mg/Cap. Bot. 100s, 500s.
Use: Peripheral vasodilator.
PAVATINE TABS. (Major) Papaverine 300 mg/Tab. Bot. 100s.
Use: Peripheral vasodilator.
PAVATINE T.D. CAPS. (Major) Papaverine 150 mg/TD Cap. Bot. 100s, 1000s.
Use: Peripheral vasodilator.
PAVATYM. (Everett) Papaverine HCl 150 mg/TR Cap. Bot. 100s, 1000s, UD 100s.
Use: Peripheral vasodilator.
PAVEROLAN. (Lannett) Papaverine 150 mg/Lanacap. Bot. 100s, 1000s.
Use: Peripheral vasodilator.
PAVRIN-T.D. (Kenyon) Papaverine HCl 150 mg/Cap. Bot. 100s, 1000s.
Use: Peripheral vasodilator.
PAVULON. (Organon) Pancuronium bromide. **1 mg/ml:** Vial 10 ml, Box 25s. **2 mg/ml:** Amp. 2 ml, 5 ml, Box 25s.
Use: Muscle relaxant, adjunct to anesthesia.
PAX-400. (Kenyon) Meprobamate 400 mg/Tab. Bot. 100s, 1000s.
Use: Antianxiety agent.
PAXAREL. (Circle) Acetylcarbromal 250 mg/Tab. Bot. 100s.
Use: Sedative/hypnotic.
PAXIL. (SK-Beecham) Paroxetine 20 mg or 30 mg. Tab. **20 mg:** Bot. 30s, 100s, UD 100s; **30 mg:** Bot. 30s.
Use: Antidepressant.
PAXIPAM. (Schering) Halazepam 20 mg or 40 mg/Tab. Bot. 100s, UD 100s.
Use: Antianxiety agent.
• **PAZINACLONE.** USAN.
Use: Antianxiety.
PAZO OINTMENT. (Bristol-Myers) Benzocaine 0.8%, zinc oxide 4%, ephedrine sulfate 0.2%, camphor 2.18% in lanolin-petrolatum base. Tube 1 oz, 2 oz.
Use: Anorectal preparation.
PAZO SUPPOSITORIES. (Bristol-Myers) Benzocaine 15.44 mg, ephedrine sulfate 3.86 mg, zinc oxide 77.2 mg, camphor

42.07 mg/Supp. Box 12s, 24s.
Use: Anorectal preparation.
• **PAZOXIDE.** USAN.
Use: Antihypertensive.
PB 100. (Schlicksup) Phenobarbital 1.5
gr/Tab. Bot. 1000s.
Use: Sedative/hypnotic.
PBZ. (Geigy) Tripelennamine HCl. **Tab.:**
25 mg Bot. 100s. 50 mg Bot. 100s,
1000s. **Elix.:** Tripelennamine citrate
(equivalent to HCl 25 mg)/5 ml. Bot. 473
ml.
Use: Antihistamine.
PBZ-SR. (Geigy) Tripelennamine HCl 100
mg/SR Tab. Bot. 100s.
Use: Antihistamine.
PCE DISPERTAB TABLETS. (Abbott)
Erythromycin particles 333 mg/Tab. Bot.
60s, 500s.
Use: Anti-infective.
p-CHLOROMETAXYLENOL.
W/Benzocaine, benzyl alcohol, propylene
glycol.
See: 20-Caine Burn Relief (Alto).
W/Hydrocortisone, pramoxine HCl.
See: Orlex HC, Otic (Baylor).
p-CHLOROPHENOL.
See: Parachlorophenol.
PCMX.
See: Parachlorometaxylenol.
PDP LIQUID PROTEIN. (Wesley Pharm.)
Protein 15 Gm (from protein hy-
drolysates), cal 60/30 ml. Bot. pt, qt, gal.
Use: Protein supplement.
PEACOCK'S BROMIDES. (Natcon) **Liq.:**
Potassium bromide 6 gr, sodium bro-
mide 6 gr, ammonium bromide 3 gr/5 ml.
Bot. 8 oz. **Tab.:** Potassium bromide 3 gr,
sodium bromide 3 gr, ammonium bro-
mide 1.5 gr. Bot. 100s.
Use: Sedative/hypnotic.
• **PEANUT OIL,** N.F. XVIII.
Use: Pharmaceutic aid (solvent, oleagi-
nous vehicle).
PECAZINE. B.A.N. 10-(1-Methyl-3-
piperidylmethyl)-phenothiazine.
Use: Tranquilizer.
PECILOCIN. B.A.N. An antibiotic pro-
duced by Paecilomyces variotin banier
(var. antibioticus). 1-(8-Hydroxy-6-
methyldodeca-trans trans cis-2,4,6-tri-
enoyl)-2-pyrrolidone.
See: Variotin.
PECTAMOL. (British Drug House) Di-
ethylaminoethoxyethyl-a,a-di-
ethylphenylacetate citrate. Bot. 4 fl oz,
16 fl oz, 80 fl oz, 160 fl oz.
Use: Antitussive.
• **PECTIN,** U.S.P. XXIII. (Various Mfr.).
Use: Protectant, pharmaceutic aid (sus-

pending agent).
PECTIN W/COMBINATIONS.
See: Diatrol, Tab. (Otis Clapp).
Donnagel Susp. (Robins).
Donnagel-PG, Susp. (Robins).
Furoxone, Liq., Tab. (Eaton).
Infantol Pink, Liq. (Scherer).
Kaopectate, Liq. (Upjohn)
Kapigam, Liq. (Solvay).
Kapinal, Tab. (Jenkins).
KBP/O, Cap. (Cole).
Parepectolin, Susp. (Rhone-Poulenc
Rorer Consumer).
Pectocomp, Liq. (Lannett).
Pectokay, Liq. (Bowman).
PECTOCOMP. (Lannett) Pectin 4 gr,
kaolin 90 gr, zinc phenolsulfonate 1 1/8
gr/fl oz. Bot. pt, gal.
Use: Antidiarrheal.
PEDAMETH. (Forest) Racemethionine.
Cap.: 200 mg. Bot. 50s, 500s. **Liq.:** 75
mg/5 ml. Bot. pt.
Use: Diaper rash product.
PEDENEX. (Approved) Caprylic acid,
zinc undecylenate, sodium propionate.
Tube 1.5 oz. Foot pow. spray 5 oz.
Use: Antifungal, external.
PEDIACARE ALLERGY FORMULA.
(McNeil-CPC) Chlorpheniramine
maleate 1 mg/5 ml, sorbitol, sucrose.
Grape flavor. Syr. Bot. 120 ml.
Use: Antihistamine.
PEDIA CARE COUGH-COLD. (McNeil-
CPC) **Chew. Tab.:** Pseudoephedrine
HCl 15 mg, chlorpheniramine maleate 1
mg, dextromethorphan HBr 5 mg, aspar-
tame (phenylalanine 6 mg), dextrose,
sucrose. Fruit flavor. Pkg. 16s. **Liq.:**
Pseudoephedrine HCl 15 mg, chlor-
pheniramine maleate 1 mg, dex-
tromethorphan HBr 5 mg/5 ml, sorbitol,
sucrose. Alcohol free. Cherry flavor. Syr.
Bot. 120 ml.
Use: Decongestant, antihistamine, anti-
tussive.
**PEDIACARE INFANTS' DECONGES-
TANT.** (McNeil) Pseudoephedrine HCl
7.5 mg/0.8 ml. Cherry flavor. Syr. Bot. 15
ml.
Use: Decongestant.
PEDIA CARE NIGHTREST LIQUID. (Mc-
Neil-CPC) Pseudoephedrine HCl 15 mg,
chlorpheniramine maleate 1 mg, dextromethorphan HBr 7.5 mg/5 ml, sorbitol, sucrose. Alcohol free. Cherry flavor. Syr. Bot. 120 ml.
Use: Decongestant, antihistamine, anti-
tussive.
PEDIACOF SYRUP. (Sanofi Winthrop)
Codeine phosphate 5 mg, phenyle-

phrine HCl 2.5 mg, chlorpheniramine maleate 0.75 mg, potassium iodide 75 mg/5 ml, sodium benzoate 0.2%, alcohol 5%. Syr. Bot. 16 fl oz.
Use: Antitussive, decongestant, antihistamine, expectorant.

PEDIAFLOR FLUORIDE DROPS. (Ross) Fluoride 0.5 mg/ml as sodium fluoride 1.1 mg/ml. Bot. 50 ml.
Use: Dental caries preventative.

PEDIALYTE. (Ross) Sodium 45 mEq, potassium 20 mEq, chloride 35 mEq, citrate 30 mEq, dextrose 25 Gm/L. 100 calories/L. **Plastic Bot.:** 8 fl oz. (unflavored), 32 fl oz. (unflavored, fruit). **Nursing Bot.:** Hospital use. Bot. 8 fl oz.
Use: Minerals/electrolytes, oral.

PEDIAMYCIN DROPS. (Ross) Erythromycin ethylsuccinate for oral suspension 100 mg/2.5 ml. Bot. 50 ml (Dropper enclosed).
Use: Anti-infective.

PEDIAPRED ORAL LIQUID. (Fisons) Prednisolone sodium phosphate 6.7 mg/5 ml. Bot. 4 oz.
Use: Corticosteroid.

PEDIASURE. (Ross) Protein 30 Gm (Na caseinate, whey protein concentrate), carbohydrate 109.8 Gm (hydrolyzed cornstarch, sucrose), fat 49.8 Gm (hioleic safflower oil, soy oil, MCT actionated coconut oil], mono- and diglycerides, soy lecithin), sodium 380 mg, potassium 1308 mg/L, vitamins A, B_1, B_2, B_3, B_5, B_6, B_{12}, C, D, E, K, inositol, Cl, Ca, P, Mg, I, Mn, Cu, Zn, Fe, biotin, choline, folic acid. < 310 MOSM/kg H_2O, 1 cal/ml. Gluten free. Vanilla flavor. Ready-to-use can 240 ml.
Use: Enteral nutritional supplement.

PEDIATRIC COUGH SYRUP. (Weeks & Leo) Ammonium Cl 300 mg, sodium citrate 600 mg/oz. Bot. 4 oz.
Use: Expectorant.

PEDIATRIC MAINTENANCE SOLUTION. (Abbott) I.V. solution w/dose calculated according to age, weight, clinical condition. Bot. 250 ml.
Use: Fluids, electrolyte and nutrient replenisher.

PEDIATRIC MULTIPLE TRACE ELEMENT. (American Regent) Zinc (as sulfate) 0.5 mg, copper (as sulfate) 0.1 mg, manganese (as sulfate) 0.03 mg, chromium (as chloride) 1 mcg/ml. Soln. Vial 10 ml.
Use: Parenteral nutritional supplement.

PEDIATRIC TRIBAN. (Great Southern) Trimethobenzamide HCl 100 mg, benzocaine 2%/Supp. Pkg. 10s.

Use: Antiemetic/antivertigo.

PEDIATROL (B13). (Kenyon) Vitamins B_{12} 25 mcg, B_1 10 mg/5 ml. Bot. pt, gal.
Use: Vitamin supplement.

PEDIAZOLE SUSPENSION. (Ross) Erythromycin ethylsuccinate 200 mg, sulfisoxazole acetyl 600 mg/5 ml. Bot. Granules reconstituted to 100 ml, 150 ml, 200 ml.
Use: Anti-infective.

PEDI-BATH SALTS. (Pedinol) Colloidal sulfur, potassium iodide, balsam peru, sodium hyposulfate, sodium bicarbonate, pine needle oil. Bot. 170 Gm.
Use: Bath dermatological, emollient.

PEDI-BOOT MIST KIT. (Pedinol) Cetyl pyridinium Cl, triacetin, chloroxylenol. Bot. 2 oz.
Use: Fungicide, sanitizer, deodorizer for shoes.

PEDI-BORO SOAK PAKS. (Pedinol) Astringent wet dressing w/aluminum sulfate, calcium acetate, coloring agent. Box 12s, 100s.
Use: Minor skin irritations.

PEDI-CORT V CREME. (Pedinol) Clioquinol 3%, hydrocortisone 1%. Tube 20 Gm.
Use: Antifungal, corticosteroid.

PEDICRAN WITH IRON. (Scherer) Vitamin B_{12} (crystallized) 25 mcg, ferric pyrophosphate, soluble (elemental iron 30 mg) 250 mg, thiamine mononitrate 10 mg, nicotinamide 10 mg, alcohol 1%/5 ml. Bot. 4 oz, pt.
Use: Vitamin/mineral supplement.

PEDICULICIDES/SCABICIDES.
See: A-200, Shampoo (Beecham).
A-200 Pyrinate, Gel (Beecham).
Barc, Liq. (Commerce Drug).
Blue, Gel (Various Mfr.).
Elimite, Cream (Herbert).
Eurax, Preps. (Westwood Squibb).
G-well, Preps. (Goldline).
Kwell, Preps. (Reed & Carnrick).
Licetrol 400, Liq. (Republic).
Lindane, Preps. (Various Mfr.).
Nix, Liq. (Burroughs Wellcome).
Ovide, Lot. (GenDerm).
Pronto Concentrate, Shampoo (Commerce Drug).
Pyrinyl, Liq. (Various Mfr.).
R & C, Shampoo (Reed & Carnrick).
RID, Liq. (Leeming).
Scabene, preps. (Stiefel).
Step 2, Liq. (GenDerm).
Tisit, Preps. (Pfeiffer).
Tisit Blue, Gel (Pfeiffer).
Triple X Kit, Liq. (Carter Products).
PEDI-DRI FOOT POWDER. (Pedinol)

Aluminum chlorohydroxide, zinc undecylenate, menthol, formaldehyde. Spout Cap Bot. 2 oz.
Use: Antiperspirant, deodorant, fungicidal foot powder.

PEDIOTIC. (Burroughs Wellcome) Hydrocortisone 1%, neomycin 3.5 mg (as sulfate), polymyxin B sulfate 10,000 units/ml. Susp. Bot 7.5 ml with dropper.
Use: Corticosteroid, anti-infective, otic.

PEDI-PRO FOOT POWDER. (Pedinol) Aluminum chlorhydroxide, menthol, zinc undecylenate, chloroxylenol. Bot. 2 oz.
Use: Fungicide, antiperspirant, deodorant.

PEDITUSS COUGH. (Major) Phenylephrine HCl 2.5 mg, chlorpheniramine maleate 0.75 mg, codeine phosphate 5 mg, potassium iodide 75 mg/5 ml, alcohol 5%, saccharin, sorbitol, sucrose. Syr. Bot. pt., gal.
Use: Decongestant, antihistamine, narcotic antitussive, expectorant.

PEDI-VIT A CREME. (Pedinol) Vitamin A 100,000 units/oz. Jar 2 oz, 16 oz, 5 lb.
Use: Emollient.

PEDOLATUM. (King) Salicylic acid, sodium salicylate. Oint. Pkg. 0.5 oz.
Use: External analgesic.

PEDRIC SENIOR. (Vale) Acetaminophen 320 mg.
Use: Analgesic.

PEDTE-PAK-4. (SoloPak) Zinc 1 mg, copper 0.1 mg, manganese 0.025 mg, chromium 1 mcg. Vial 3 ml.
Use: Parenteral nutritional supplement.

PEDTRACE-4. (Lyphomed) Zinc 0.5 mg, copper 0.1 mg, chromium 0.85 mcg, manganese 0.25 mg/ml. Vial 3 ml, 10 ml.
Use: Parenteral nutritional supplement.

PEDVAXHIB. (Merck & Co.) Purified capsular polysaccharide, *Neisseria meningitidis* OMPC 250 mcg/dose when reconstituted, sodium chloride 0.9%, lactose 2 mg, thimerosal 1:20,000. Pow. for Inj. Single-dose vial with vial of aluminum hydroxide diluent.
Use: Agent for immunization.

PEEWEE'S CHILDREN'S CHEWABLE VITAMINS. (Mission) Vitamin A 2500 IU, D 400 IU, E 15 IU, C 60 mg, folic acid 0.3 mg, B_1 1.05 mg, B_2 1.2 mg, B_3 13.5 mg, B_6 1.05 mg, B_{12} 4.5 mcg, iron 15 mg/Tab. Sugar. Bot. 100s.
Use: Vitamin/mineral supplement.

• **PEFLOXACIN.** USAN.
Use: Antibacterial.

• **PEFLOXACIN MESYLATE.** USAN.
Use: Antibacterial.

PEGADEMASE BOVINE.
Use: Modified enzyme for use in ADA deficiency. [Orphan drug]
See: Adagen (Enzon).

PEGANONE. (Abbott) Ethotoin 250 mg/Tab. or 500 mg/Cap. Bot. 100s.
Use: Anticonvulsant.

• **PEGASPARGASE.** USAN
Use: Antineoplastic. [Orphan drug]
See: Oncaspar, Inj. (Enzon).

PEGLICOL 5 OLEATE. USAN.
Use: Emulsifying agent.

PEG-GLUCOCEREBROSIDASE. (Enzon)
Use: Treatment of Gaucher's disease. [Orphan drug]

PEG-INTERLEUKIN-2. (Cetus)
Use: Treatment of immunodeficiency in T-cell defects. [Orphan drug]

PEG-L-ASPARAGINASE. (Enzon)
Use: Antineoplastic. [Orphan drug]

P.E.G. OINTMENT. (Medco Lab) Polyethylene glycol. Jar 16 oz.
Use: Water soluble ointment base.

• **PEGOTERATE.** USAN.
Use: Suspending agent.

• **PEGOXOL 7 STEARATE.** USAN.
Use: Emulsifying agent.

PELAMINE. (Major) Tripelennamine HCl 50 mg/Tab. Bot. 100s, 1000s.
Use: Antihistamine.

• **PELANSERIN HYDROCHLORIDE.** USAN.
Use: Antihypertensive.

PELENTAN. Ethyl Biscoumacetate. (No Mfr. currently lists).

• **PELIOMYCIN.** USAN. An antibiotic derived from *Streptomycin luteogriseus.*
Use: Antineoplastic agent.

• **PELRINONE HYDROCHLORIDE.** USAN.
Use: Cardiotonic.

• **PEMEDOLAC.** USAN.
Use: Analgesic.

• **PEMERID NITRATE.** USAN. 4-[3-(Dimethylimino)propoxy]-1,2,2,6,6-pentamethylpiperidine dinitrate.
Use: Antitussive.

• **PEMOLINE.** USAN. 2-amino-5-phenyl-4-azolin-4-one.
Use: Childhood attention-deficit syndrome (hyperkinetic syndrome).
See: Cylert Prods. (Abbott).

PEMPIDINE. B.A.N. 1,2,2,6,6-Pentamethylpiperidine.
Use: Hypotensive.

PENAGEN-VK. (Grafton) Penicillin V. **Tab.:** 250 mg. Bot. 100s. **Pow.:** 250 mg/100 ml.
Use: Antibacterial, penicillin.

• **PENAMECILLIN.** USAN. Acetoxymethyl

6-phenyl-acetamidopenicillanate.
Use: Antibiotic.
• **PENBUTOLOL.** USAN.(–)-1-tert-Buty-
lamino-3-(2-
cyclopentylphenoxy)propan-2-ol.
Use: Beta adrenergic blocking agent.
See: Levatol (Reed and Carnrick).
• **PENCICLOVIR.** USAN.
Use: Antiviral.
PENDECAMAINE. B.A.N. NN-Dimethyl-
(3-palmitamidopropyl)glycine betaine.
Use: Surface active agent.
PENECARE. (Reed & Carnrick) **Cream:**
Isostearic acid, lactic acid, stearic acid,
PPG-12/SMDI copolymer, steareth-21,
steareth-2, mineral oil, magnesium alu-
minum silicate, imidurea. Tube. 120 g.
Lot.: Isostearic acid, lactic acid, stearic
acid, steareth-21, PPG-12/SMDI copoly-
mer, steareth-2, magnesium aluminum
silicate, imidurea. Bot. 240 ml.
Use: Emollient.
PENECORT CREAM. (Herbert) Hydrocortisone 1% or 2.5%, benzyl alcohol,
petrolatum, stearyl alcohol, propylene
glycol, isopropyl myristate, polyoxyl 40
stearate, carbomer 934, sodium lauryl
sulfate, edetate disodium w/sodium hy
droxide to adjust pH, purified water. **1%:**
Tube 30 Gm, 60 Gm. **2.5%:** Tube 30
Gm.
Use: Corticosteroid
PENETHAMATE HI.
See: Benzylpenicillin 2-diethy-
laminoethyl ester HI.
PENETHAMATE HYDRIODIDE. B.A.N.
2 Diethylaminoethyl 6-phenylacetami-
dopenicillanate hydriodide. Benzylpeni-
cillin 2-diethylaminoethyl ester hydrio-
dide.
Use: Treatment of respiratory tract in-
fections.
PENETREX. (Rhone-Poulenc Rorer)
Enoxacin 200 mg or 400 mg/Tab. Bot.
50s.
Use: Antibacterial, fluoroquinolone.
• **PENFLURIDOL.** USAN. 1-[4,4-bis(p-
Fluorophenyl)butyl]-4-(4-chloro-α,α,α-tri-
fluoro-m-tolyl)-4-piperidi-nol. 4-(4-
Chloro-3-trifluoromethylphenyl)-1-[4,4-
di-(4-fluorophenyl)butyl]piperidin-4-ol.
Use: Tranquilizer.
PENFONYLIN.
See: Pentid, Prods. (Squibb).
• **PENICILLAMINE,** U.S.P. XXIII. Cap.,
Tab., U.S.P. XXIII. (Merck & Co.) D-3-
Mercaptovaline. Cuprimine.
Use: Metal complexing agent, cystin-
uria, rheumatoid arthritis.
See: Cuprimine, Cap. (Merck & Co.).

Depen, Tab. (Wallace).
PENICILLIN. Unless clarified, it means an
antibiotic substance or substances produced by growth of the molds *Penicillium notatum* or *P. chrysogenum.*
Use: Antibacterial.
PENICILLIN ALUMINUM. Aluminum 3,3-
dimethyl-7-oxo-6-(2-phenylacetamido)-
4-thia-1-azabicyclo-[3.2.0]-heptane-2-
carboxylate.
Use: Antibacterial, penicillin.
PENICILLIN CALCIUM. Calcium 3,3-di-
methyl-7-oxo-6-(2-phenylacetamido)-4-
thia-1-azabicyclo-[3.2.0]-heptane-2-car-
boxylate. U.S.P. XIII.
Use: Antibacterial, penicillin.
PENICILLIN, DIMETHOXY-PHENYL. Me-
thicillin Sodium.
Use: Antibacterial, penicillin.
See: Staphcillin, Vial (Bristol).
• **PENICILLIN G BENZATHINE,** U.S.P.
XXIII. Sterile Susp., Oral Susp., Sterile,
Tab. U.S.P. XXIII. Benzathine penicillin
G.
Use: Antibiotic.
See: Bicillin, Tab. (Wyeth-Ayerst).
Bicillin Long-Acting (Wyeth-Ayerst).
Permapen, Aqueous Susp. (Pfizer
Laboratories).
**PENICILLIN G BENZATHINE & PRO-
CAINE COMBINED.**
Use: Antibacterial, penicillin.
See: Bicillin C-R, Inj. (Wyeth-Ayerst).
Bicillin C-R 900/300, Inj. (Wyeth-Ay-
erst).
• **PENICILLIN G POTASSIUM,** U.S.P. XXIII.
Cap., Inj., for Oral Soln., Sterile, Tab.,
Tab. for Oral Soln., U.S.P. XXIII. (Potas-
sium Penicillin, Benzyl Penicillin Pot.).
Use: Antibiotic.
See: Arcocillin, Preps. (Arcum).
Biotic-T-500, Tab. (Scrip).
Cryspen 400, Tab. (Knight).
Deltapen, Syr., Tab. (Trimen).
G-Recillin-T, Tab. (Solvay).
Hyasorb, Tab. (Key Pharm.).
K-Cillin, Prods.(Mayrand).
Lanacillin, Pow. (Lannett).
Palocillin-S, Pow. (Hauck).
Palocillin-5, Tab. (Hauck).
Parcillin, Tab. (Parmed).
Pensorb, Tab. (Kenyon).
Pentids, Syr., Tab. (Squibb Mark).
Pfizerpen, Tab., Syr. (Pfizer Laborato-
ries).
Pfizerpen, Inj. (Roerig).
**PENICILLIN G POTASSIUM W/COMBI-
NATIONS.**
See: Lanacillin "200,000", "400,000"
(Lannett).

Pentid, Prods. (Squibb).

**PENICILLIN G PROCAINE COMBINA-
TIONS.**
See: Bicillin C-R, Tubex (Wyeth-Ay-
erst).
Bicillin C-R 900/300 Inj. (Wyeth-Ay-
erst).
Duracillin Г.Λ., Λmp. (Lilly).
Duracillin Fortified, Vial (Lilly).
• **PENICILLIN G PROCAINE AND DIHY-
DROSTREPTOMYCIN SULFATE IN-
TRAMAMMARY INFUSION,** U.S.P.
XXIII.
Use: Antibiotic.
• **PENICILLIN G PROCAINE, DIHY-
DROSTREPTOMYCIN SULFATE,
CHLORPHENIRAMINE MALEATE,
AND DEXAMETHASONE SUSPEN-
SION, STERILE,** U.S.P. XXIII.
Use: Antibiotic, antihistamine, anti-in-
flammatory.
• **PENICILLIN G PROCAINE, DIHY-
DROSTREPTOMYCIN SULFATE, AND
PREDNISOLONE SUSPENSION,
STERILE,** U.S.P. XXIII.
Use: Antibiotic, anti-inflammatory.
• **PENICILLIN G PROCAINE AND DIHY-
DROSTREPTOMYCIN SULFATE SUS-
PENSION, STERILE,** U.S.P. XXIII.
Use: Antibiotic.
• **PENICILLIN G PROCAINE, NEOMYCIN
AND POLYMYXIN B SULFATES, AND
HYDROCORTISONE ACETATE TOPI-
CAL SUSPENSION,** U.S.P. XXIII.
Use: Antibiotic, anti-inflammatory.
• **PENICILLIN G PROCAINE AND NOVO-
BIOCIN SODIUM INTRAMAMMARY IN-
FUSION,** U.S.P. XXIII.
Use: Antibiotic.
• **PENICILLIN G PROCAINE W/ALU-
MINUM STEARATE SUSPENSION,
STERILE,** U.S.P. XXIII.
Use: Antibiotic.
• **PENICILLIN G, PROCAINE, STERILE,**
U.S.P. XXIII. Sterile Susp., Intramamma-
ry infusion, U.S.P. XXIII. Procaine Peni-
cillin.
Use: Antibiotic.
W/Parenteral, aqueous susp., (Procaine
Penicillin, for Aqueous Inj.,) Procaine
Penicillin and buffered Penicillin for
aqueous, Inj.
See: Crysticillin A.S., Vial (Squibb).
Diurnal-Panicillin (Upjohn).
Duracillin A.S., Preps. (Lilly).
Pfizerpen-A.S. (Roerig).
Tu-Cillin, Inj. (Solvay).
Wycillin, Susp. (Wyeth-Ayerst).
Parenteral, in oil w/aluminum mono-
stearate. Penicillin Procaine in Oil Inj.

• **PENICILLIN G SODIUM FOR
INJECTION,** U.S.P. XXIII. (Various Mfr.)
Sodium Benzylpenicillin.
Use: Antibiotic.
• **PENICILLIN G SODIUM, STERILE,**
U.S.P. XXIII.
Use: Antibiotic.
**PENICILLIN HYDRADAMINE PHE
NOXYMETHYL.** 3,3-Dimethyl-7-oxo-6-
(2-phenoxyacetamido)-4-thia-1-azabicy-
clo[3.2.0]heptane-2-carboxylic acid
compound with N,N′-bis[(1,2,3,4,-
4a,9,10,10a-octahydro-7-isopropyl-
1,4a-dimethyl-1-phenanthryl)methyl]eth-
ylenediamine.
Use: Antibiotic.
PENICILLIN N. Adicillin, B.A.N.
Use: Antibiotic.
PENICILLIN O CHLOROPROCAINE. 6-
[2-(Allylthio)acetamido]-3-3-dimethyl-7-
oxo-4-thia-1-azabicyclo-[3.2.0]heptane-
2-carboxylic acid compound with 2-(di-
ethylamino)ethyl
4-amino-2-chlorbenzoate (1:1).
Use: Antibacterial, penicillin.
PENICILLIN O, SODIUM. Allylmercap-
tomethyl penicillin.
Use: Antibacterial.
PENICILLIN, PHENOXYETHYL.
Use: Antibacterial, penicillin.
See: Phenethicillin, Penicillin potassium
152.
**PENICILLIN PHENOXYMETHYL BENZA-
THINE.**
Use: Antibacterial, penicillin.
See: Penicillin V Benzathine.
**PENICILLIN PHENOXYMETHYL HY-
DRABAMINE.**
Use: Antibacterial, penicillin.
See: Penicillin V Hydrabamine.
• **PENICILLIN S BENZATHINE AND PENI-
CILLIN G PROCAINE SUSPENSION,
STERILE,** U.S.P. XXIII.
Use: Antibiotic.
• **PENICILLIN V,** U.S.P. XX for Oral Susp.,
Tab. U.S.P. XXIII. Phenoxymethyl peni-
cillin. A biosynthetic penicillin formed by
fermentation, with suitable precursors of
Penicillin notatum.
Use: Antibiotic.
See: Biotic Pow. (Scrip).
Compocillin-V, Water, Susp. (Ross).
Ledercillin VK (Lederle).
Penagen-VK, Tab., Pow. (Gafton).
Robicillin-VK (Robins).
Uticillin VK (Upjohn).
V-Cillin, Preps. (Lilly).
V-Pen, Tab. (Century).
• **PENICILLIN V BENZATHINE,** U.S.P. XXI-

II. Oral Susp., U.S.P. XXIII.
Use: Antibiotic.
See: Pen-Vee, Prods. (Wyeth-Ayerst).
PENICILLIN V HYDRABAMINE. Hydrabamine phenoxymethyl penicillin.
Use: Antibacterial, penicillin.
See: Compocillin V Hydrabamine, Oral Susp. (Ross).
• **PENICILLIN V POTASSIUM,** U.S.P. XXIII. Oral Soln., Tab., U.S.P. XXIII.
Use: Antibiotic.
See: Beepen VK, Tab., Syr. (Beecham Labs).
Betapen VK., Soln., Tab. (Bristol).
Biotic-V-Powder (Scrip).
Bopen, V-K, Tab. (Boyd).
Dowpen VK, Tab. (Merrell Dow).
Lanacillin VK, Tab., Pow. (Lannett).
Ledercillin VK, Oral Soln., Tab. (Lederle).
LV, Tab (Elder).
Pen-Vee-K, Soln., Tab. (Wyeth-Ayerst).
Pfizerpen VK, Pow., Tab. (Pfizer Laboratories).
Phenethicillin Potassium.
Repen-VK, Tab., Oral Susp. (Solvay).
Robicillin VK, Tab., Soln. (Robins).
Ro Cillin VK, Soln., Tab. (Solvay).
Saropen-VK (Saron).
SK-Penicillin VK, Soln., Tab. (SK-Beecham).
Suspen, Liq. (Circle).
Uticillin VK, Tab., Soln. (Upjohn).
V-Cillin K, Tab., Oral Soln. (Lilly).
Veetids, Soln., Tab. (Squibb Mark).
PENICILLINASE. B.A.N. An enzyme that hydrolyzes penicillin, obtained from several strains of bacteria (*B.cereus*). Vial (1000 units) 20 ml.
Use: Clinical lab use only.
PENIDURAL.
Use: Antibacterial.
See: Benzathine Penicillin. B.A.N.
PEN-KERA CREME WITH KERATIN BINDING FACTOR. (Ascher) Bot. 8 oz.
Use: Emollient.
PENNTUSS. (Pennwalt) Codeine (as polistirex) 10 mg, chlorpheniramine maleate 4 mg/5 ml. Bot. pt.
Use: Antitussive, antihistamine.
PENSORB. (Kenyon) Crystalline penicillin G potassium 250,000 units, buffered w/calcium carbonate/Tab. Bot. 100s, 1000s.
Use: Antibacterial, penicillin.
• **PENTABAMATE.** USAN. 3-Methyl-2,4-pentanediol dicarbamate.
Use: Tranquilizer.
PENTA-CAP #1. (Kenyon) Pentaerythritol

tetranitrate 30 mg/Cap. Bot. 90s, 100s, 1000s.
Use: Antianginal.
PENTA-CAP PLUS. (Kenyon) Pentaerythritol tetranitrate 30 mg, amobarbital 50 mg/Cap. Bot. 100s, 1000s.
Use: Antianginal.
PENTACOSACTRIDE. D-Ser^1-Nle^4-(Val-NH$_2$)$^{25-\beta}$1 25corticotrophin.
Use: Corticotrophic peptide.
See: Norleusactide (I.N.N.).
PENTACYNIUM METHYLSULPHATE. B.A.N. 4-2-[(5-Cyano-5,5-diphenylpentyl)dimethylammonio]ethyl-4-methylmorpholinium di(methylsulfate).
Use: Hypotensive.
• **PENTAERYTHRITOL TETRANITRATE,** U.S.P. XXIII. Diluted, U.S.P. XXIII.
Use: Vasodilator.
See: Angijen Green, Tab. (Jenkins).
Arcotrate Nos. 1 and 2, Tab. (Arcum).
Dilac-80, Cap. (Ascher).
Duotrate-45, Cap. (Marion).
Kortrate, Cap. (Arnid).
Maso-Trol, Tab. (Mason).
Metranil, Cap. (Meyer).
Nitrin, Tab. (Vale).
Penta-Cap No. 1, Cap. (Kenyon).
Penta-E, Tab. (Recsei).
Pentafin, Granucap, Tab. (Solvay).
Penta-Tal Nos. 1 and 2, Tab. (Kenyon).
Pentetra, Tab. (Paddock).
Pentylan, Tab. (Lannett).
Pentylan w/Phenobarbital, Tab. (Lannett)
Peritrate, Tab. (Parke-Davis).
Petro-20 mg, Tab. (Foy).
Reithritol, Tab. (Bowman).
Tentrate, Tab. (Tennessee Pharm.).
Tetracap-30, Cap. (Freeport).
Tetracap-80, Cap. (Freeport).
Tetratab, Tab. (Freeport).
Tetratab No. 1, Tab. (Freeport).
Tranite, Cap., Tab. (Westerfield).
Vasolate, Cap. (Parmed).
Vasolate-80, Cap. (Parmed).
PENTAERYTHRITOL TETRANITRATE, DILUTED, U.S.P. XXIII.
Use: Vasodilator.
PENTAERYTHRITOL TETRANITRATE W/COMBINATIONS.
See: Angijen S.C., Tab. (Jenkins).
Arcotrate No. 3, Tab. (Arcum).
Bitrate, Tab. (Arco).
Dimycor, Tab. (Standard Drug).
Penta-Cap Plus, Cap. (Kenyon).
Penta-Tal Nos. 3 and 4, Tab. (Kenyon).
Pentetra w/Phenobarbital, Tab. (Paddock).
Pentylan w/Phenobarbital, Tab. (Lan-

nett).

Peritrate w/Nitroglycerin, Tab. (Parke-Davis).

Respet, Tab. (Westerfield).

• **PENTAFILCON A.** USAN.
Use: Contact lens material.

• **PENTAGASTRIN.** USAN. N-t-Butyloxy-carbonyl-β-alanyl-l -tryptophyl-l -me-thionyl-L-aspartyl-L-phenylalanine amide.
Use: Gastric acid secretion stimulant.
See: Peptavlon, Amp. (Wyeth-Ayerst).

PENTALAMIDE. B.A.N. 2-Pentyloxyben-zamide.
Use: Treatment of fungal infections.

• **PENTALYTE.** USAN.
Use: Electrolyte combination.

PENTAM 300. (Lyphomed) Pentamidine isethionate 300 mg/Vial.
Use: Anti-infective.

PENTAMETHONIUM BROMIDE. B.A.N.
Pentamethylenedi(trimethylammonium bromide).
Use: Hypotensive.

PENTAMETHONIUM IODIDE. B.A.N.
Pentamethylenedi(trimethylammonium iodide).
Use: Hypotensive.

PENTAMETHYLENETETRAZOL.
See: Pentylenetetrazol, U.S.P.

PENTAMIDINE. B.A.N. 4,4'-(Pentameth-ylenedioxy)-dibenzamidine.
Use: Treatment of trypanosomiasis.

PENTAMIDINE ISETHIONATE. (Abbott) 300 mg. Inj., lyophilized. Single-dose fliptop vials.
Use: Anti-infective.
See: Pentam 300, Inj. (Lyphomed).

PENTAMIDINE ISETHIONATE (INHALA-TION).
Use: Anti-infective. [Orphan drug]

PENTAMOXANE HCl. 2-Isoamylamino-methyl-1,4-benzodioxane HCl.
Use: Tranquilizing agent.

• **PENTAMUSTINE.** USAN.
Use: Antineoplastic.

PENTAPHONATE. Dodecyltriph-enylphosphonium pentachloropheno-late.
Use: Anti-infective.

PENTAPIPERIDE. B.A.N. 1-Methyl-4-(3-methyl-2-phenylvaleryloxy)piperidine.
Use: Anticholinergic.

PENTAPIPERIDE METHYLSULFATE. 4'-(1-Methylpiperidyl)-2-phenyl-3-methyl-valerate dimethylsulfate. Valpipamate Methylsulfate.
Use: Anticholinergic.

• **PENTAPIPERIUM METHYLSULFATE.** USAN.

Use: Anticholinergic.

PENTAPYRROLIDINIUM BITARTRATE.
See: Pentolinium Tartrate.

PENTAQUINE. B.A.N. 8-(5-Isopropy-laminopentyl-amino)-6-methoxyquino-line.
Use: Antimalarial.

PENTAQUINE PHOSPHATE. 8-[[5-(Iso-propyl-amino)pentyl]amino]-6-methoxyquinoline phosphate.

PENTARCORT. (Dalin) Hydrocortisone alcohol 0.5%, coal tar solution 2%, clio-quinol 3%, diperodone HCl 0.25%, vita-mins A 850 IU, D 85 IU/Gm. Tube 15 Gm.
Use: Corticosteroid, anti-infective, topi-cal.

PENTASA. (Marion Merrell Dow) Mesalamine 250 mg. CR Cap. Bot. 240s, UD 80s.
Use: Ulcerative colitis, proctosigmoiditis or proctitis.

PENTASODIUM COLISTINMETHANE-SULFONATE. Sterile Colistimethate Sodium, U.S.P. XXIII.

• **PENTASTARCH.** USAN.
Use: Leukopheresis adjunct (red cell sedimenting agent). [Orphan drug]

PENTA-STRESS. (Penta) Vitamins A 10,000 IU, D 500 IU, B_1 10 mg, B_2 10 mg, B_6 1 mg, calcium pantothenate 5 mg, nicainamide 50 mg, C 100 mg, E 2 IU, B_{12} 3.3 mcg/Cap. Bot. 90s, 1000s, Jar 250s.
Use: Vitamin supplement.

PENTA-TAL. (Kenyon) Pentaerythritol tetranitrate 10 mg or 20 mg/Tab. Bot. 100s, 1000s.
Use: Antianginal.

PENTA-TAL #3, #4. (Kenyon) Pentaery-thritol tetranitrate 10 mg or 20 mg, phe-nobarbital 15 mg/Tab. Bot. 100s, 1000s.
Use: Antianginal.

PENTAVALENT GAS GANGRENE. Anti-toxin.

PENTA-VIRON. (Penta) Calcium carbon-ate 500 mg, ferrous fumarate 100 mg, vitamins C 50 mg, D 167 IU, A 3.333 IU, B_1 3.3 mg, B_2 3.3 mg, B_6 2 mg, calcium pantothenate 1.6 mg, niacinamide 16.7 mg, E 2 IU/Cap. Bot. 100s, 1000s, Jar 250s.
Use: Vitamin supplement.

PENTAZINE. (Century) Promethazine ex-pectorant. Bot. 4 oz, 16 oz, gal.
Use: Antihistamine.

PENTAZINE INJ. (Century) Promet-hazine 50 mg/ml. Inj. Vial 10 ml.
Use: Antihistamine.

PENTAZINE W/CODEINE. (Century)

Promethazine expectorant. Bot. 4 oz, 16 oz, gal.
Use: Antihistamine.
• **PENTAZOCINE,** U.S.P. XXIII. 2,6-Methano-3-benzazocin-8-ol, 1,2,3,4,5,6-hexahydro-6,11-dimethyl-3-(3-methyl-2-butenyl)-1,2,3,-4,5,6-Hexahydro-cis-6,11-dimethyl-3-(3-methyl-2-butenyl)-2, 6-methano-2-benzazocin-8-ol.
Use: Analgesic.
• **PENTAZOCINE HYDROCHLORIDE,** U.S.P. XXIII. Tab., U.S.P. XXIII.
Use: Analgesic.
W/ Acetaminophen.
See: Talacen, Cap. (Sanofi Winthrop).
• **PENTAZOCINE HYDROCHLORIDE AND ASPIRIN TABLETS,** U.S.P. XXIII.
Use: Analgesic.
See: Talwin Compound, Tab. (Sanofi Winthrop).
• **PENTAZOCINE LACTATE INJECTION,** U.S.P. XXIII.
Use: Analgesic.
See: Talwin Injection, Inj. (Sanofi Winthrop).
• **PENTAZOCINE AND NALOXONE HYDROCHLORIDE TABLETS.** U.S.P. XXIII.
Use: Analgesic.
See: Talwin NX, Tab. (Sanofi Winthrop).
• **PENTETATE CALCIUM TRISODIUM.** USAN.
Use: Chelating agent (plutonium).
• **PENTETATE CALCIUM TRISODIUM Yb 169.** USAN.
Use: Radioactive agent.
• **PENTETATE INDIUM DISODIUM IN 111.** USAN.
Use: Diagnostic aid, radioactive agent.
• **PENTETIC ACID.** U.S.P. XXIII. USAN.
Use: Diagnostic aid.
PENTETRA-PARACOTE. (Paddock) Pentaerythritol tetranitrate 30 mg or 80 mg/Cap. Bot. 100s, 500s, 1000s.
Use: Antianginal.
PENTHIENATE. B.A.N. 2-Diethylaminoethyl α-cyclopentyl-α-(2-thienyl).
Use: Antispasmodic.
PENTHIENATE BROMIDE. Diethyl (2-Hydroxyethyl) methylammonium bromide α-cyclopentyl-2-thio- pheneglycolate.
PENTHRANE. (Abbott Hospital Prods.) Methoxyflurane. Bot. 15 ml, 125 ml.
Use: General anesthetic.
PENTHRICHLORAL. B.A.N. 5,5-Di(hydroxymethyl)-2-trichloromethyl-1,3-dioxan.
Use: Hypnotic; sedative.
• **PENTIAPINE MALEATE.** USAN.

Use: Antipsychotic.
PENTIDS. (Squibb Mark) Potassium Penicillin G buffered with calcium carbonate. **Tab.:** 125 mg (200,000 units). Bot. 100s. **Syr.:** 125 mg (200,000 units)/5 ml. Bot. 100 ml, 200 ml.
Use: Antibacterial, penicillin.
PENTIFYLLINE. B.A.N. 1-Hexyl-3,7-dimethyl-xanthine.
Use: Vasodilator.
PENTINA. (Freeport) Rauwolfia serpentina, 100 mg/Tab. Bot. 1000s.
Use: Antihypertensive.
• **PENTISOMICIN.** USAN.
Use: Anti-infective.
• **PENTIZIDONE SODIUM.** USAN.
Use: Antibacterial.
• **PENTOBARBITAL,** U.S.P. XXIII. Elixir, U.S.P. XXI. (Various Mfr.) 5-Ethyl-5-(1-methylbutyl) barbituric acid.
Use: Sedative.
See: Nembutal, Elix., Gradumets (Abbott) Penta, Tab. (Dunhall).
PENTOBARBITAL COMBINATIONS.
Use: Sedative/hypnotic.
See: Cafergot-PB, Supp., Tab. (Sandoz).
Nembutal, Preps. (Abbott).
Quad-Set, Tab. (Kenyon).
• **PENTOBARBITAL, SODIUM,** U.S.P. XXII. Cap. Elixir, Inj.: U.S.P. XXIII. 2,4,6,(1H,3H,5H)-Pyrimidinetrione, 5-ethyl-5-(1-methyl-butyl)-, monosodium salt. Sodium 5-Ethyl-5-(1-methylbutyl) barbiturate. Embutal. (Various Mfr.) 100 mg. Cap. Bot. 1000s.
Use: Hypnotic, sedative.
See: Maso-Pent, Tab. (Mason).
Nembutal Sodium, Preps. (Abbott).
Night-Caps, Cap. (Bowman).
W/Adiphenine HCl, phamasorb, aluminum hydroxide.
See: Spasmasorb, Tab. (Hauck).
W/Atropine sulfate, hyoscine HBr, hyoscyamine sulfate.
See: Eldonal, Elix., Tab., Cap. (Canright).
W/Ephedrine.
See: Ephedrine and Nembutal-25, Cap. (Abbott).
W/Ergotamine tartrate, caffeine alkaloid, bellafoline.
See: Cafergot-P.B., Tab. (Sandoz).
W/Homatropine methylbromide, dehydrocholic acid, ox bile extract.
See: Homachol, Tab. (Lemmon).
W/Pyrilamine maleate.
See: A-N-R, Rectorette (Hauck).
W/Seco-, buta-, phenobarbital.
W/Vitamin compounds, d-methampheta-

mine HCl.
See: Fetamin, Tab. (Mission).
PENTOBARBITAL SODIUM. (Wyeth-Ayerst) 50mg/ml. Inj. Tubex 2 ml.
Use: Hypnotic, sedative.
PENTOBARBITAL, SOLUBLE.
See: Pentobarbital Sodium, U.S.P.
PENTOL TABS. (Major) Pentaerythritol tetranitrate. **10 mg/Tab.:** Bot. 1000s; **20 mg/Tab.:** Bot. 100s, 1000s; **80 mg/SA Tab.:** Bot. 250s, 1000s.
Use: Antianginal.
PENTOLINIUM TARTRATE. Pentamethylene-1:5-bis (1'-methylpyrrolidinium bitartrate). N,N-Pentamethylenedi-(1-methylpyrrolidinium hydrogen tartrate. Pentapyrrolidinium Bitartrate.
Use: Antihypertensive.
• **PENTOMONE.** USAN.
Use: Prostate growth inhibitor.
• **PENTOPRIL.** USAN.
Use: Enzyme inhibitor (angiotensin-converting).
PENTOSAN SODIUM POLYSULPHATE.
Use: Treatment of interstitial cystitis. [Orphan drug]
See: Elmiron.
• **PENTOSTATIN.** USAN.
Use: Leukemia. [Orphan drug]
PENTOTHAL. (Abbott) **Pow. for Inj.:** Thiopental sodium 20 mg/ml. In 1, 2.5, 5 g kits, 400 mg syringes; 25 mg/ml. In 1, 2.5, 5 g, 500 mg kits, 250, 400, 500 mg syringes. **Rectal Susp.:** Thiopental sodium 400 mg/g. In 2 g syringe.
Use: Anesthetic.
• **PENTOXIFYLLINE.** USAN. Oxpentifylline. B.A.N.
Use: Oral hemorrheologic agent for peripheral vascular disease.
See: Trental (Hoechst).
PENTRAX SHAMPOO. (Rydell) Tar extract 8.75%, detergents, conditioning agents. Bot. 4 oz, 8 oz.
Use: Antiseborrheic.
• **PENTRINITROL.** USAN.
Use: Vasodilator.
PENT-T-80. (Mericon) Pentaerythritol tetranitrate 80 mg/T.D. Cap. Bot. 100s, 1000s.
Use: Antianginal.
PENTYLAN. (Lannett) Pentaerythritol tetranitrate 10 mg or 20 mg/Tab. Bot. 100s, 500s, 1000s.
Use: Antianginal agent.
PEN-V. (Goldline) Penicillin 250 mg or 500 mg/Tab. Bot. 100s, 1000s.
Use: Antibacterial, penicillin.
PEN-VEE K. (Wyeth-Ayerst) Potassium phenoxymethyl penicillin. 250 mg or 500

mg/Tab. Bot. 100s, 500s, Redipak 100s.
Use: Antibacterial, penicillin.
PEN-VEE K FOR ORAL SOLUTION. (Wyeth-Ayerst) Penicillin V potassium. **125 mg/5 ml:** Bot. 100 ml, 200 ml. **250 mg/5 ml:** Bot. 100 ml, 150 ml, 200 ml.
Use: Antibacterial, penicillin.
PEPCID. (Merck & Co.) Famotidine. **Tab.:** 20 mg or 40 mg. Bot. 30s, UD 100s. **Oral Susp.:** 40 mg/5 ml. Bot. 10 doses. **I.V.:** Single dose vial 10 mg/ml or 20 mg/2 ml; Multi-dose vial 40 ml.
Use: Histamine H_2 antagonist.
• **PEPLOMYCIN SULFATE.** USAN.
Use: Antineoplastic.
• **PEPPERMINT,** N.F. XVIII. Oil, Water, N.F. XVIII.
Use: Pharmaceutic aid (flavor), antitussive, expectorant, nasal decongestant.
See: Vicks Prods. (Vicks).
• **PEPPERMINT OIL,** N.F. XVIII.
Use: Pharmaceutic aid (flavor).
• **PEPPERMINT SPIRIT,** U.S.P. XXIII.
Use: Digestive aid, flavor, perfume.
• **PEPPERMINT WATER,** N.F. XVIII.
Use: Vehicle.
PEPSAMAR COMP. TABLETS. (Sanofi Winthrop) Aluminum hydroxide, magnesium hydroxide.
Use: Antacid.
PEPSAMAR ESP LIQUID. (Sanofi Winthrop) Aluminum hydroxide, glycerin.
Use: Antacid.
PEPSAMAR ESP TABLETS. (Sanofi Winthrop) Aluminum hydroxide, magnesium hydroxide, mannitol powder.
Use: Antacid.
PEPSAMAR HM TABLETS. (Sanofi Winthrop) Aluminum hydroxide, starch.
Use: Antacid.
PEPSAMAR LIQUID. (Sanofi Winthrop) Aluminum hydroxide.
Use: Antacid.
PEPSAMAR SUSPENSION. (Sanofi Winthrop) Aluminum hydroxide, magnesium hydroxide, sorbitol.
Use: Antacid.
PEPSAMAR TABLETS. (Sanofi Winthrop) Aluminum hydroxide.
Use: Antacid.
PEPSATAL. (Kenyon) Pepsin 200 mg, pancreatin 200 mg, bile salts 100 mg, dehydrocholic acid 30 mg, desoxycholic acid 30 mg/Tab. Bot. 100s, 1000s.
Use: Digestive aid.
PEPSICONE GEL. (Sanofi Winthrop) Aluminum hydroxide, magnesium hydroxide, simethicone.
Use: Antacid, antiflatulent.
PEPSICONE TABLET. (Sanofi Winthrop)

Aluminum hydroxide, magnesium hydroxide, simethicone.
Use: Antacid, antiflatulent.
PEPSIN.
Use: Digestive aid.
PEPSIN W/COMBINATIONS.
See: Biloric, Cap. (Arcum).
Donnazyme, Tab. (Robins).
Entozyme, Tab. (Robins).
Enzobile, Tab. (Hauck).
Gourmase-PB, Cap. (Solvay).
Kanulase, Tab. (Dorsey).
Leber Taurine, Liq. (Paddock).
Nu'Leven, Tab. (Lemmon).
Pepsatal, Tab. (Kenyon).
Ro-Bile, Tab. (Solvay).
Zypan, Tab. (Standard Process).
PEPSIN LACTATED, ELIXIR.
See: Peptalac, Liq. (Bowman).
• **PEPSTATIN.** USAN.
Use: Enzyme inhibitor (pepsin).
PEPTAMEN LIQUID. (Clintec Nutrition)
Enzymatically hydrolyzed whey proteins, maltodextrin, starch, MCT, sunflower oil, lecithin, vitamins A, B_1, B_2, B_3, B_5, B_6, B_{12}, C, D, E, K, folic acid, biotin, choline, Ca, Cl, Cu, Fe, I, Mg, Mn, P, Zn. Can 500 ml.
Use: Enteral nutritional supplement.
PEPTAVLON. (Wyeth-Ayerst) Pentagastrin 0.25 mg, sodium Cl/ml. For evaluation of gastric acid secretion. Amp. 2 ml, Ctn. 10s.
Use: Diagnostic aid.
PEPTENZYME. (Reed & Carnrick) Alcohol 16%. Pleasantly aromatic. Bot. pt.
Use: Pharmaceutic aid.
PEPTO-BISMOL LIQUID. (Procter & Gamble) Bismuth subsalicylate 262 mg/15 ml. Bot. 4 oz, 8 oz, 12 oz, 16 oz.
Use: Antidiarrheal.
PEPTO-BISMOL MAXIMUM STRENGTH LIQUID. (Procter & Gamble) 524 mg/15 ml. Bot. 120 ml, 240 ml, 360 ml.
Use: Antidiarrheal.
PEPTO-BISMOL TABLETS. (Procter & Gamble) Bismuth subsalicylate 262.5 mg/Chew. Tab. Pkg. 24s, 42s.
Use: Antidiarrheal.
PERANDREN PHENYLACETATE. (Ciba) Testosterone phenylacetate.
Use: Androgen.
PERATIZOLE. B.A.N. 1-[-[(2,4-Dimethylthiazol-5-yl)butyl]-4-(4-methylthiazol-2-yl)piperazine.
Use: Antihypertensive agent.
PERCAINE.
Use: Local anesthetic.
See: Dibucaine HCl, U.S.P.
PERCHLORACAP. (Mallinckrodt) Potas-

sium perchlorate 200 mg/Cap. Bot. 100s.
Use: Radiographic adjunct.
PERCHLORETHYLENE.
See: Tetrachlorethylene, U.S.P. XXIII.
PERCHLORPERAZINE.
See: Compazine, Preps. (SK-Beecham).
PERCOCET. (DuPont) Oxycodone HCl 5 mg, acetaminophen 325 mg/Tab. Bot. 100s, 500s, UD 250s.
Use: Narcotic analgesic combination.
PERCODAN. (DuPont) Oxycodone HCl 4.5 mg, oxycodone terephthalate 0.38 mg, aspirin 325 mg/Tab. Bot. 100s, 500s, 1000s, UD 250s.
Use: Narcotic analgesic combination.
W/Hexobarbital.
See: Percobarb, Cap. (DuPont).
PERCODAN-DEMI. (DuPont) Oxycodone HCl 2.25 mg, oxycodone terephthalate 0.19 mg, aspirin 325 mg/Tab. Bot. 100s.
Use: Narcotic analgesic combination.
PERCOGESIC. (Vicks) Acetaminophen 325 mg, phenyltoloxamine citrate 30 mg/Tab. Bot. 24s, 50s, 90s.
Use: Analgesic, antihistamine.
PERCOMORPH LIVER OIL. (May be blended with 50% other fish liver oils; each Gm contains vitamins A 60,000 IU & D 8500 IU).
See: Oleum Percomorphum.
PERCY MEDICINE. (Merrick Medicine) Bismuth subnitrate 959 mg, calcium hydroxide 21.9 mg/10 ml, alcohol 5%.
Use: Antidiarrheal.
PERDIEM. (Rhone-Poulenc Rorer) Blend of psyllium 82%, senna 18% as active ingredients in granular form. Sodium content (0.08 mEq) 1.8 mg/rounded tsp. (6 Gm). Canister 100 Gm, 250 Gm, UD 6 Gm.
Use: Laxative.
PERDIEM FIBER. (Rhone-Poulenc Rorer) Psyllium 100% as active ingredient in granular form. Sodium content (0.08 mEq) 1.8 mg/rounded tsp. (6 Gm). Canister 100 Gm, 250 Gm, UD 6 Gm.
Use: Laxative.
PERE-DIOSATE. (Towne) Docusate sodium 100 mg, casanthranol 30 mg/Cap. Bot. 100s.
Use: Laxative.
PERESTAN. (Interstate) Docusate sodium 100 mg, casanthranol 30 mg/Cap. Bot. 100s, 1000s.
Use: Laxative.
• **PERFILCON A.** USAN.
Use: Contact lens material.
See: Permalens (CooperVision).

- **PERFLUBRON.** USAN.
  Use: Contrast agent; temporary blood substitute.
  See: Imagent GI, Liq. (Alliance).
  PERFLUOROCHEMICAL EMULSION.
  Use: To prevent deficient blood supply to the heart muscle.
  See: Fluosol, Emulsion (Alpha Therapeutics).
- **PERFOSFAMIDE.** USAN.
  Use: Antineoplastic. [Orphan drug]
  PERGALEN.
  See: Sodium Apolate.
- **PERGOLIDE MESYLATE.** USAN.
  Use: Dopamine agonist.
  PERGONAL (MENOTROPINS). (Serono) Follicle stimulating hormone (FSH) and luteinizing hormone (LH). **75 IU:** Unit contains 1 Amp. FSH/LH and 1 Amp. sodium Cl diluent. Pkg. 10s. **150 IU:** Unit contains 1 Amp. FSH/LH and 1 Amp. sodium Cl diluent.
  Use: Gonadotropin.
  PERGRAVA. (Arcum) Vitamins A 2000 IU, D 300 IU, B_1 2 mg, B_2 2 mg, nicotinamide 10 mg, B_6 2 mg, B_{12} 5 mcg, C 60 mg, calcium 40 mg/Cap. Bot. 100s, 1000s.
  Use: Vitamin/mineral supplement.
  PERGRAVA NO. 2. (Arcum) Vitamins A 2000 IU, D 300 IU, B_1 2 mg, B_2 2 mg, nicotinamide 10 mg, B_6 2 mg, C 60 mg, calcium lactate monohydrate 200 mg, ferrous gluconate 31 mg, folic acid 0.1 mg/Cap. Bot. 100s, 1000s.
  Use: Vitamin/mineral supplement.
- **PERHEXILINE.** USAN. 2-(2,2-Dicyclohexylethyl)- piperidine.
  Use: Treatment of angina pectoris.
- **PERHEXILINE MALEATE.** USAN. 2-(2,2-Dicyclohexylethyl) piperidine maleate.
  Use: Cardiovascular agent.
  PERHYDROL.
  See: Hydrogen Peroxide 30% (Various Mfr.).
  PERI SOFCAP. (Alton) Docusate sodium with peristim. Bot. 100s, 1000s.
  Use: Laxative.
  PERIACTIN. (Merck & Co.) Cyproheptadine HCl 4 mg/Tab. Bot. 100s.
  Use: Antihistamine.
  PERIACTIN SYRUP. (Merck & Co.) Cyproheptadine HCl 2 mg/5 ml, alcohol 5%, sorbic acid 0.1%. Bot. 473 ml.
  Use: Antihistamine.
  PERI-CARE. (Sween) Vitamins A and D in petroleum ointment base. Tube 0.5 oz, 1.75 oz. Jar 2 oz, 5 oz, 8 oz.
  Use: Emollient.

PERI-COLACE. (Mead Johnson) **Cap.:** Docusate sodium 100 mg, casanthranol 30 mg/Cap. Bot. 30s, 60s, 250s, 1000s, UD 100s. **Syr.:** Docusate sodium 60 mg, casanthranol 30 mg/15 ml, ethyl alcohol 10%. Bot. 8 oz, pt.
Use: Laxative.
PERICYAZINE. B.A.N. 2-Cyano-10-[3-(4-hydroxy-piperidino)propyl]phenothiazine. Neulactil.
Use: Tranquilizer.
PERIDEX. (Procter & Gamble) Chlorhexidine gluconate 0.12%, alcohol 11.6%, glycerin, PEG-40 sorbitan diisostearate, flavor, sodium saccharin, FD&C blue No. 1, water. Bot. pt.
Use: Mouth preparation.
PERIDIN-C. (Beutlich) Hesperidin methyl chalcone 50 mg, hesperidin complex 150 mg, ascorbic acid 200 mg/Tab. Bot. 100s, 500s.
Use: Vitamin supplement.
PERI-DOS. (Goldline) Docusate sodium 100 mg, casanthranol 30 mg/Cap. Bot. 30s, 60s, 100s, 1000s.
Use: Laxative.
PERIES. (Xttrium) Medicated pads w/witch hazel, glycerin. Jar pad 40s.
Use: Hygienic wipe and local compress.
PERIMED. (Olin) Hydrogen peroxide 1.5%, povidone-iodine 6%, saccharin. Pouch 20 ml.
Use: Mouth and gum preparation.
PERINDOPRIL ERBUMINE.
Use: Antihypertensive.
See: Aceon, Tab. (Ortho).
PERIO-EZE-20. (Moyco) Oral paste.
Use: Analgesic for pain of gums and mucosa.
PERIPHERAL VASODILATOR COMBINATIONS.
Use: Vasodilator.
See: Lipo-Nicin/100 mg, Tab. (Brown).
Lipo-Nicin/250 mg, Tab. (Brown).
Lipo-Nicin/300 mg, TR Tab. (Brown).
PERISTOMAL COVERING.
See: Stomahesive, Wafer (Squibb).
PERITIME-80. (Kenyon; Werner) Pentaerythritol tetranitrate 80 mg/Cap. Bot. 100s.
Use: Antianginal.
PERITINIC. (Lederle) Elemental iron 100 mg, docusate sodium 100 mg, vitamins B_1 7.5 mg, B_2 7.5 mg, B_6 7.5 mg, B_{12} 50 mcg, C 200 mg, niacinamide 30 mg, folic acid 0.05 mg, pantothenic acid 15 mg/Tab. Bot. 60s.
Use: Vitamin/mineral supplement, laxative.
PERITRATE. (Parke-Davis) Pentaerythri-

tol tetranitrate. **10 mg/Tab.**: Bot. 100s, 1000s. **20 mg/Tab.**: Bot. 100s, 1000s, UD 100s. **40 mg/Tab.**: Bot. 100s. *Use:* Antianginal.

PERITRATE S.A. (Parke-Davis) Pentaerythritol tetranitrate 80 mg (20 mg in immediate release layer, 60 mg in sustained release base)/Tab. Bot. 100s, 1000s, UD 100s. *Use:* Antianginal.

PERI-WASH. (Sween) Bot. 4 oz, 8 oz, 1 gal, 5 gal, 30 gal, 55 gal. *Use:* Anorectal preparation.

PERI-WASH II. (Sween) Bot. 4 oz, 8 oz, 1 gal, 5 gal, 30 gal, 55 gal. *Use:* Anorectal preparation.

•**PERLAPINE.** USAN. 6-(4-Methyl-1-piperazinyl) Morphanthridine. *Use:* Hypnotic.

PERLATAN. *See:* Estrone (Various Mfr.).

PERMANGANIC ACID, POTASSIUM SALT. Potassium Permanganate, U.S.P. XXIII

PERMAPEN. (Roerig) Benzathine penicillin G 1,200,000 units/ml. Disp. syringe 2 ml. *Use:* Antibacterial, penicillin.

PERMAX. (Athena Neurosciences) Pergolide mesylate. *Use:* Antiparkinson agent.

•**PERMETHRIN.** USAN. Synthetic pyrethrin. *Use:* Pediculicide for treatment of head lice, ectoparasiticide. *See:* Nix, Cream (Burroughs Wellcome).

PERMITIL. (Schering) Fluphenazine HCl. **2.5 mg or 5 mg/Tab:** Bot. 100s. **10 mg/Tab.**: Bot. 1000s. *Use:* Antipsychotic agent.

PERMITIL ORAL CONCENTRATE. (Schering) Fluphenazine HCl 5 mg/ml. Bot. 120 ml w/calibrated dropper. Hospital use. *Use:* Antipsychotic agent.

PERNOX LOTION. (Westwood) Microfine granules of polyethylene 20%, sulfur 2%, salicylic acid 2% in a combination of soapless cleansers and wetting agents. Bot. 6 oz. *Use:* Anti-acne.

PERNOX MEDICATED LATHERING SCRUB CLEANSER. (Westwood) Polyethylene granules 26%, sulfur 2%, salicylic acid 1.5% w/soapless surface-active cleansers and wetting agents. Regular or lemon. Tube 2 oz, 4 oz. *Use:* Anti-acne.

PERNOX SHAMPOO. (Westwood) Sodium laureth sulfate, water, lauramide DEA, quaternium 22, PEG-75 lanolin/hydrolyzed animal protein, fragrance, sodium Cl, lactic acid, sorbic acid, disodium EDTA, FD&C yellow No. 6 and blue No. 1. Bot. 8 oz. *Use:* Cleanser and conditioner for oily hair.

PEROXIDASE. W/Glucose oxidase, potassium, iodide. *See:* Diastix Reagent Strips (Miles Diagnostic).

PEROXIDE, DIBENZOYL. Benzoyl Peroxide, Hydrous.

PEROXIDES. *See:* Hydrogen Peroxide (Various Mfr.). Urea Peroxide. Zinc Peroxide.

PEROXIN A5. (Dermol) Benzoyl peroxide 5%. Gel. Tube 45 g. *Use:* Anti-acne.

PEROXIN A10. (Dermol) Benzoyl peroxide 10%. Gel. Tube 45 g. *Use:* Anti-acne.

PEROXYL MOUTHRINSE. (Hoyt) Hydrogen peroxide 1.5% in mint flavored base, alcohol 6%. Bot. 8 oz. *Use:* Mouth preparation.

•**PERPHENAZINE,** U.S.P. XXIII. Inj., Oral Soln., Syr., Tab., U.S.P. XXIII. 2-Chloro-10-[3-[4-(2-hydroxyethyl)-piperazinyl]propyl]-phenothiazine. 4-(3-(2-Chloro-phenothiazin-1-yl)propyl)-1-piperazine-ethanol. *Use:* Antiemetic, tranquilizer. *See:* Trilafon, Prods. (Schering).

•**PERPHENAZINE/AMITRIPTYLINE TABLETS,** U.S.P. XXIII. (Various, eg, Bolar, Geneva, Goldline, Lemmon, Par, Rugby, Schein, Zenith). Perphenazine (mg): 2, 8; Amitriptyline (mg): 10, 25. Bot. 21s, 100s, 500s, 1000s; Bot. 100s, 500s, 1000s. *Use:* Miscellaneous psychotherapeutic agents. *See:* Etrafon, Prods. (Schering). Triavil, Tab. (Merck & Co.).

PERSA-GEL. (Ortho Derm) Benzoyl peroxide 5% or 10%, acetone base. Tube 1.5 oz, 3 oz. *Use:* Anti-acne.

PERSA-GEL W. (Ortho Derm) Benzoyl peroxide 5% or 10% in water base. Tube 1.5 oz, 3 oz. *Use:* Anti-acne.

PERSANGUE. (Arcum) Ferrous gluconate 192 mg, vitamins C 150 mg, B_1 3 mg, B_2 3 mg, B_{12} 50 mcg/Cap. Bot. 100s, 500s. *Use:* Vitamin/mineral supplement.

PERSANTINE. (Boehringer Ingelheim) Dipyridamole 25 mg, 50 mg or 75 mg/Tab. **25 mg or 50 mg:** Bot. 100s, 1000s, UD 100s. **75 mg:** Bot. 100s, 500s, UD 100s.
Use: Antiplatelet agent.
PERSANTINE IV. (DuPont-Merck) Dipyridamole. Inj. For evaluation of coronary artery disease.
Use: Diagnostic aid.
• **PERSIC OIL,** N.F. XVII.
Use: Vehicle.
PERTECHNETIC ACID, SODIUM SALT. Sodium Pertechnetate Tc 99 m Solution.
PERTOFRANE. (Rhone-Poulenc Rorer) Desipramine HCl 25 mg or 50 mg/Cap. Bot. 100s, 1000s.
Use: Antidepressant.
PERTROPIN. (Lannett) Linolenic acid 7 min/Cap. Bot. 100s.
Use: Oral nutritional supplement.
PERTSCAN-99m. (Abbott Diagnostics) Radiodiagnostic. Inj. Tc-99m.
Use: Diagnostic aid.
PERTUSSIN ALL-NIGHT PM. (Pertussin Labs) Acetaminophen 167 mg, doxylamine succinate 1.25 mg, pseudoephedrine HCl 10 mg, dextromethorphan HBr 5 mg/5 ml, alcohol 25%. Liq. Bot. 240 ml.
Use: Analgesic, antihistamine, decongestant, antitussive.
PERTUSSIN CS. (Canaan Labs) Dextromethorphan HBr 3.5 mg, guaifenesin 25 mg/5 ml, 8.5% alcohol. Bot. 90 ml.
Use: Antitussive, expectorant.
PERTUSSIN ES. (Pertussin) Dextromethorphan HBr 15 mg/5 ml, alcohol 9.5%, sugar, sorbitol. Liq. Bot. 120 ml.
Use: Antitussive.
PERTUSSIN SYRUP. (Canaan Labs) Dextromethorphan HBr 15 mg/5 ml, alcohol 9.5%. Bot. 3 oz, 6 oz.
Use: Antitussive.
• **PERTUSSIS VACCINE,** U.S.P. XXIII. (Various Mfr.).
Use: Active immunization against whooping cough.
• **PERTUSSIS VACCINE, ADSORBED,** U.S.P. XXIII. Vial 7.5 ml.
Use: Active immunizing agent.
PERTUSSIS VACCINE AND DIPHTHERIA AND TETANUS TOXOIDS, COMBINED.
Use: Active immunizing agent.
See: Acel-Imune, Vial (Lederle). Tri-Immunol, Vial (Lederle). Triple Antigen, Vial (Wyeth-Ayerst). Tri-Solgen, Vial, Hyporet (Lilly).
PERUVIAN BALSAM.

Use: Local protectant, rubefacient.
W/Benzocaine, zinc oxide, bismuth subgallate, boric acid.
See: Anocaine, Supp. (Hauck).
W/Benzocaine, zinc oxide, 8-hydroxyquinoline benzoate, menthol. Unit-of-Use 90s. **50 mg:** Bot. 100s, 1000s, UD 100s. **75 mg:** Bot. 100s.
See: Hemorrhoidal Oint. (Towne).
W/Ephedrine sulfate, belladonna extract, zinc oxide, boric acid, bismuth oxyiodide, subcarbonate.
See: Wyanoids, Preps. (Wyeth-Ayerst).
W/Lidocaine, bismuth subgallate, zinc oxide, aluminum subacetate.
See: Xylocaine, Supp. (Astra).
W/Oxyquinoline sulfate, pramoxine HCl, zinc oxide.
See: Zyanoid, Oint. (Elder).
PESON. Sodium Lyapolate. Polyethenesulfonate sodium.
Use: Anticoagulant.
PETERSON'S OINTMENT. (Peterson) Carbolic acid, camphor, tannic acid, zinc oxide. Tube w/pipe 1 oz. Jar 16 oz. Can 1.4 oz, 3 oz.
Use: Anorectal preparation.
PETHADOL TABLETS. (Halsey) Meperidine HCl 50 mg or 100 mg/Tab. Bot. 100s, 1000s.
Use: Narcotic analgesic.
PETHIDINE HYDROCHLORIDE.
See: Meperidine HCl, U.S.P. XXIII.
PETN.
See: Pentaerythritol tetranitrate.
PETRICHLORAL. Pentaerythritol chloral. 1,1′,1″,1-(Neopentanetetrayltetraoxy)tetrakis [2,2,2-trichloroethanol].
Use: Sedative.
PETRO-20. (Foy) Pentaerythritol tetranitrate 20 mg/Tab. Bot. 100s, 1000s.
Use: Antianginal.
• **PETROLATUM,** U.S.P. XXIII.
Use: Ointment base.
See: Lipkote, Stick (Schering-Plough).
• **PETROLATUM GAUZE,** U.S.P. XXIII.
Use: Surgical aid.
• **PETROLATUM, HYDROPHILIC,** U.S.P. XXIII.
Use: Absorbent ointment base; topical protectant.
See: Lipkote (Schering-Plough).
PETROLATUM, LIQUID. Mineral Oil, U.S.P. XXIII. Light Mineral Oil, U.S.P. XXIII. Adepsine Oil, Glymol, Liquid Paraffin, Parolein, White Mineral Oil, Heavy Liquid Petrolatum.
Use: Laxative.
See: Clyserol Oil Retention Enema (Fuller Labs).

Fleet Mineral Oil Enema (Fleet).
Mineral Oil (Various Mfr.).
Nujol, Liq. (Schering-Plough).
Saxol (Various Mfr.).
PETROLATUM, LIQUID, EMULSION.
Use: Lubricant, laxative.
See: Milkinol, Liq. (Kremers-Urban).
W/Agar-Gel.
See: Agoral Plain, Liq. (Parke-Davis).
Petrogalar, Preps. (Wyeth-Ayerst).
W/Cascara.
See: Petrogalar w/Cascara, Emulsion
(Wyeth-Ayerst).
W/Docusate sodium.
See: Milkinol, Liq. (Kremers-Urban).
W/Irish moss, casanthranol.
See: Neo-Kondremul (Fisons).
W/Milk of magnesia.
See: Haley's M. O., Liq. (Sanofi
Winthrop Products).
W/Phenolphthalein.
See: Agoral, Emulsion (Parke-Davis).
Petrogalar w/Phenolphthalein, Emul-
sion (Wyeth-Ayerst).
Phenolphthalein in liquid Petrolatum
Emulsion.
PETROLATUM, RED VETERINARIAN.
(Elder) Also known as RVP.
See: Rubrapet, Oint. (Medco).
W/Micasorb.
See: RV Plus, Oint. (Elder).
W/N-diethyl metatoluamide.
See: RV Pellent, Oint. (Elder).
W/Zinc oxide, 2-ethoxyethyl p-methoxycin-
namate.
See: RV Paque, Oint. (Elder).
•**PETROLATUM, WHITE,** U.S.P. XXIII.
Use: An oleaginous ointment base, topi-
cal protectant.
See: Moroline, Oint. (Schering-Plough).
PETRO-PHYLIC SOAP. (Doak) Hy-
drophilic Petrolatum. Cake 4 oz.
Use: Emollient, anti-infective, external.
PF4RIA. (Abbott Diagnostics) Platelet
factor 4 radioimmunoassay for the quan-
titative measurement of total PF4 levels
in plasma.
Use: Diagnostic aid.
PFEIFFER'S ALLERGY. (Pfeiffer) Chlor-
pheniramine maleate 4 mg/Tab. Bot.
24s.
Use: Antihistamine.
PFEIFFER'S COLD SORE. (Pfeiffer)
Gum benzoin 7%, camphor, menthol,
thymol, eucalyptol, alcohol 85%. Lot.
Bot. 15 ml.
Use: Cold sores, fever blisters, cracked
lips.
PFIZERPEN-AS. (Roerig) Procaine peni-
cillin G 3,000,000 units in aqueous

susp./Vial. Carton 5s. Multi-Vial Pack,
Carton 100s.
Use: Antibacterial, penicillin.
PFIZERPEN FOR INJECTION. (Roerig)
Potassium penicillin G, buffered. **Multi-
Vial Pack:** 1,000,000 units or 5,000,000
units/Vial. Carton 10s, 100s; **Individual
Vial:** 20,000,000 units/Vial 1s, 10s.
Use: Antibacterial, penicillin.
PFIZERPEN VK TABLETS. (Pfizer Labo-
ratories) Penicillin V potassium 250 mg
or 500 mg/Tab. **250 mg:** Bot. 1000s. **500
mg:** Bot. 100s.
Use: Antibacterial, penicillin.
PGA. See: Folic Acid, U.S.P. XXIII.
PGE.
Use: Prostaglandin.
See: Alprostadil.
PHacid. (Baker/Cummins) Bot. 8 oz.
Use: Shampoo.
PHADIATOP RIA TEST. (Pharmacia) De-
termination of IgE antibodies specific to
inhalant allergens in human serum. Kit
60s.
Use: Diagnostic aid.
PHANACOL COUGH. (Pharmakon)
Phenylpropanolamine HCl 25 mg, dextromethorphan HBr 10 mg, guaifenesin
100 mg, acetaminophen 325 mg/5 ml.
Syrup. Bot. 118 ml, 236 ml.
Use: Antitussive, expectorant.
PHANADEX COUGH SYRUP. (Phar-
makon) Phenylpropanolamine HCl 25
mg, pyrilamine maleate 40 mg, dextromethorphan HBr 15 mg, guaifenesin
100 mg/5 ml, sugar, potassium citrate,
citric acid. Syr. Bot. 118 ml, 236 ml.
Use: Decongestant, antihistamine, antitussive, expectorant.
PHANATUSS COUGH SYRUP. (Pharmakon Labs) Dextromethorphan HBr 10
mg, guaifenesin 85 mg, potassium citrate 75 mg, citric acid 35 mg/5 ml, sor-
bitol, menthol. Syr. Bot. 118 ml.
Use: Antitussive, expectorant.
PHANQUONE. B.A.N. 4,7-Phenanthro-
line-5,6-quinone. Phanquinone (I.N.N.).
Use: Treatment of amebiasis.
See: Entobex.
pH ANTISEPTIC SKIN CLEANSER.
(Walgreen) Alcohol 63%. Bot. 16 oz.
Use: Astringent, cleanser.
PHARAZINE. (Halsey) Bot. 4 oz, 16 oz,
gal.
Use: A series of cough and cold prod-
ucts.
PHARMADINE. (Sherwood Pharm.)
Povidone-iodine. **Oint.:** Pkt. 1 Gm, 1.5
Gm, 2 Gm, 30 Gm, 1 lb. **Perineal wash:**
240 ml. **Skin cleanser:** 240 ml. **Soln.:**

15 ml, 120 ml, 240 ml, pt, qt. **Soln.,**
swabs: 100s. **Soln., swabsticks:** 1 or
3/packet in 250s. **Spray:** 120 Gm. **Sur-**
gical scrub: 30 ml, pt, qt, gal, foil-pack
15 ml. **Surgical scrub sponge/brush:**
25s. **Swabsticks, lemon glycerin:**
100s. **Whirlpool soln.:** gal.
Use: Antiseptic.
PHARMAFLUR. (Pharmics) Sodium fluoride 2.21 mg. Tab. Bot. 1000s.
Use: Dental caries preventative.
PHARMALGEN. (Pharmacia) Freeze-
dried hymenopteria venom/venom protein from honey bee, yellow jacket, yellow hornet, white-faced hornet, wasp,
mixed vespid. Diagnostic kit: 5 × 1 ml
Vial. Treatment kit: 6 × 1 ml vial or 1 ×
1.1 mg multiple dose vial. Starter Kit: 6 ×
1 ml, pre-diluted 0.01 mcg to 100
mcg/ml.
Use: Diagnostic aid, treatment kit.
PHARMALGEN RAST STANDARDIZED
ALLERGENIC EXTRACTS-POLLENS.
(Pharmacia) 100,000 allergenic
units/Vial. Box 5 x 1 ml.
Use: Diagnostic aid, treatment kit.
PHAZYME. (Reed & Carnrick) Sime-
thicone 60 mg/Tab. Bot. 50s, 100s,
1000s.
Use: Antiflatulent.
PHAZYME-95. (Reed & Carnrick) Sime-
thicone 95 mg/Tab. Bot. 100s.
Use: Antiflatulent.
PHAZYME 125. (Reed & Carnrick) Sime-
thicone 125 ml. Cap. Bot. 50s.
Use: Antiflatulent.
PHAZYME DROPS. (Reed & Carnrick)
Simethicone 40 mg/0.6 ml, saccharin.
Bot. 30 ml w/dropper.
Use: Antiflatulent.
• **PHEMFILCON A.** USAN.
Use: Contact lens material.
PHENACAINE HYDROCHLORIDE,
U.S.P. XXI. N,N′-Bis(p-ethoxy-phenyl)
acetamidine HCl, monohydrate.
Use: Local anesthetic (ophthalmic).
W/Atropine, phenol, nut gall, zinc oxide.
See: Tanicaine, Oint., Supp. (Upjohn).
W/Cod liver oil.
See: Morusan Oint. (Beecham Labs).
W/Ephedrine. (Upjohn) Phenacaine HCl
1%, epinephrine 1:25,000. Ophth. oint.
Tube 1 dr.
W/Mercarbolide. (Upjohn) Holocaine HCl
2%, mercarbolide 1:3000. Ophth. oint.,
Tube w/applicator tip, 1 dr.
PHENACAL. (NeuroGenesis/Matrix) D,L-
phenylalanine 500 mg, L-glutamine 15
mg, L-tyrosine 25 mg, L-carnitine 10 mg,
L-arginine pyroglutamate 10 mg, L-or-

nithine/L-aspartate 10 mg, chromium
0.033 mg, selenium 0.012 mg, vitamin
B_1 0.33 mg, B_2 5 mg, B_3 3.3 mg, B_5 0.33
mg, B_6 0.33 mg, B_{12} 1 mcg, E 5 IU, biotin 0.05 mg, folic acid 0.066 mg, iron 1
mg, zinc 2.5 mg, calcium 35 mg, iodine
0.25 mg, copper 0.33 mg, magnesium
25 mg/Cap. Bot. 42s, 180s.
Use: Oral nutritional supplement.
• **PHENACEMIDE,** U.S.P. XXIII. Tab.,
U.S.P. XXIII. Phenylacetylurea.
Use: Anticonvulsant.
See: Phenurone, Tab. (Abbott).
PHENACETIN. Acetophenetidin. Ethoxy-
acetanilide.
Use: Antipyretic, analgesic.
NOTE: This drug has been withdrawn
from the market due to liver and kid-
ney toxicity. This drug is no longer
official in the U.S.P.
PHENACETYLCARBAMIDE.
See: Phenurone, Tab. (Abbott).
PHENACETYLUREA.
See: Phenurone, Tab. (Abbott).
PHENACRIDANE. (9(p-Hexloxphenyl)-
10-methyl-acridinium Cl).
See: Micridium (Johnson & Johnson).
PHENACTROPINIUM CHLORIDE.
B.A.N. N-Phenacylhomatropinium Cl.
Trophenium.
Use: Hypotensive.
PHENACYL HOMATROPHINIUM HCI.
Not available.
PHENADOXONE. B.A.N. 6-Morpholino-
4,4-diphenyl-heptan-3-one. Heptalgin
hydrochloride.
Use: Analgesic, hypnotic.
PHENAGESIC. (Dalin) Phenylephrine
HCl 10 mg, phenylpropanolamine HCl
50 mg, pyrilamine maleate 25 mg,
pheniramine maleate 25 mg, acetyl-p-
aminophenol 300 mg/Tab. or 5 ml. **Tab.:**
Bot. 50s. **Syr.:** (without acetaminophen):
Bot. 6 oz, pt.
Use: Decongestant, antihistamine,
analgesic.
PHENAGLYCODOL. B.A.N. 2-p-
Chlorophenyl-3-methyl-2,3-butanediol.
2-(4-Chlorophenyl)-3-methylbutane-2,3-
diol.
Use: Central nervous system depres-
sant.
PHENAHIST INJECTABLE. (T.E.
Williams) Atropine sulfate 0.2 mg,
phenylpropanolamine HCl 12.5 mg,
chlorpheniramine maleate 5 mg/ml. Vial
10 ml.
Use: Anticholinergic/antispasmodic, de-
congestant, antihistamine.
PHENAHIST-TR TABLETS. (T.E.

PHENAZOPYRIDINE HCl

Williams) Phenylephrine HCl 25 mg, phenylpropanolamine HCl 50 mg, chlorpheniramine maleate 8 mg, hyoscyamine sulfate 0.143 mg, atropine 0.0362 mg, scopolamine HBr 0.012 mg. Tab. Bot. 100s.
Use: Decongestant, antihistamine, anticholinergic/antispasmodic.
PHENALZINE DIHYDROGEN SULFATE.
See: Nardil, Tab. (Parke-Davis).
PHENAMAZOLINE HCl. 2-(Anilinomethyl)-2-imidazoline HCl.
Use: Vasoconstrictor.
PHENAMETH DM. (Major) Promethazine HCl 6.25 mg, dextromethorphan HBr 15 mg/5 ml, alcohol. Syr. Bot. 120 ml.
Use: Antihistamine, antitussive.
PHENAMETH TABLETS. (Major) Promethazine 25 mg. Tab. Bot. 1000s.
Use: Antihistamine, antiemetic.
PHENAMETH VC W/CODEINE. (Major) Phenylephrine HCl 5 mg, promethazine HCl 6.25 mg, codeine phosphate 10 mg/5 ml, alcohol 7%. Syr. Bot. pt, gal.
Use: Decongestant, antihistamine, antitussive.
PHENAMETH W/CODEINE. (Major) Promethazine HCl 6.25 mg, codeine phosphate 10 mg/5 ml, alcohol 7%. Syr. Bot. 4 oz, pt, gal.
Use: Antihistamine, antitussive.
PHENAMPROMIDE. B.A.N. N-(1-Methyl-2-piperidinoethyl)propionanilide.
Use: Analgesic.
PHENANTOIN. Mephenytoin. N-Methyl-5,5-phenylethylhydantoin.
See: Mesantoin, Tab. (Sandoz).
PHENAPAP. (Rugby) Pseudoephedrine HCl 30 mg, chlorpheniramine 2 mg, acetaminophen 325 mg. Tab. Bot. 30s, 100s, 1000s.
Use: Decongestant, antihistamine, analgesic.
PHENAPHEN-650 WITH CODEINE. (Robins) Codeine phosphate 30 mg, acetaminophen 650 mg. Tab. Bot. 50s, Dis-Co packs 4 × 25s.
Use: Narcotic analgesic combination.
PHENAPHTHAZINE. Sodium dinitro phenylazonaphthol disulfonate.
See: Nitrazine Paper, Roll (Squibb).
PHENARSONE SULFOXYLATE. (5-Arsono-2-hydroxyanilino)methanesulfinic acid disodium salt.
Use: Antiamebic.
PHENASPIRIN COMPOUND. (Davis & Sly) Phenobarbital 0.25 gr, aspirin 3.5 gr. Cap. Bot. 1000s.
Use: Sedative/hypnotic, salicylate analgesic.

PHENASPIRIN COMPOUND CAPSULES. (Lannett) Aspirin 3.5 gr, phenobarbital 0.25 gr. Cap. Bot. 1000s, 5000s.
Use: Salicylate analgesic, sedative/hypnotic.
PHENATE T.D. (Hauck) Phenylpropanolamine HCl 40 mg, chlorpheniramine maleate 4 mg, acetaminophen 325 mg. CR Tab. Bot. 100s, 1000s.
Use: Decongestant, antihistamine, analgesic.
PHENATIN. (Jenkins) Acetophenetidin 0.2 Gm, acetylsalicylic acid 0.25 Gm, caffeine 30 mg, camphor monobromated 0.1 Gm. Tab. Bot. 1000s.
Use: Analgesic combination.
PHENATIN TD CAPSULE. (Jenkins) Phenylpropanolamine HCl 50 mg, chlorpheniramine maleate 1 mg, pheniramine maleate 12.5 mg, atropine sulfate 0.025 mg, scopolamine HBr 0.014 mg, belladonna alkaloids (total) 0.16 mg, hyoscyamine sulfate 0.122 mg. Cap. Bot. 1000s.
Use: Decongestant, antihistamine, anticholinergic/antispasmodic.
PHENATUSS. (Dalin) Codeine phosphate 10 mg, chlorpheniramine maleate 2 mg, phenylephrine HCl 5 mg, guaifenesin 100 mg, 1-menthol 1 mg/5 ml. Bot. 4 oz, pt, gal.
Use: Antitussive, antihistamine, decongestant, expectorant.
PHENAZINE. (Jenkins) Phendimetrazine bitartrate 50 mg/ml. Vial 10 ml.
Use: Anorexiant.
PHENAZINE. (Keene) Promethazine HCl 25 mg or 50 mg. Vial 10 ml.
Use: Antihistamine, antiemetic.
PHENAZOCINE. B.A.N. 1,2,3,4,5,6-Hexahydro-6,11-dimethyl-3-phenethyl-2,6-methano-3-benzazocin-8-ol.
Use: Analgesic; antipyretic.
PHENAZOCINE HBr. 1,2,3,4,5,6-Hexahydro-8-hydroxy-6,11-dimethyl-3-phenethyl-2,6-methano-3-benzazo-cine HBr.
Use: Analgesic.
PHENAZODINE. (Lannett) Phenazopyridine HCl 100 mg or 200 mg. Tab. Bot. 100s, 500s, 1000s.
Use: Urinary tract product.
PHENAZONE.
See: Antipyrine (Various Mfr.).
•**PHENAZOPYRIDINE HCl,** U.S.P. XXIII. Tab., U.S.P. XXIII. 2,6-Diamino-3-phenylazopyridine HCl.
Use: Analgesic (urinary tract).
See: Azogesic, Tab. (Century).

Azo-Pyridon, Tab. (Solvay).
Azo-Standard, Tab. (Webcon).
Azo-Sulfizin (Solvay).
Phen-Azo, Tab. (Vanguard).
Phenazodine, Tab. (Lannett).
Pyridin, Tab. (Parke-Davis).
Uri-Pak (Westerfield).
PHENAZOPYRIDINE HCI W/COMBINA-TIONS.
See: Azo Gantanol, Tab. (Roche).
Azo Gantrisin, Tab. (Roche).
Azosulfisoxazole (Various Mfr.).
Pyridium Plus, Tab.(Parke-Davis).
Thiosulfil-A, Tab. (Wyeth-Ayerst).
Thiosulfil-A Forte, Tab. (Wyeth-Ayerst).
Triurisul, Tab. (Sheryl).
Uridium, Tab. (Ferndale; Pharmex).
Urisan-P, Tab. (Sandia).
Uritral, Cap. (Central).
Urobiotic, Cap. (Pfizer).
Urogesic, Tab. (Edwards).
Urotrol, Tab. (Mills).
PHENBENICILLIN. B.A.N. 6-(α-Phe-noxyphenyl-acetamido)pencillanic acid. α-Phenoxybenzylpenicillin.
Use: Antibiotic.
• **PHENBUTAZONE SODIUM GLYCERATE.** USAN. 4-Butyl-3-hy-droxy-1,2-diphenyl-3-pyrazolin-5-one sodium salt compound with glycerol.
Use: Anti-inflammatory.
PHENBUTRAZATE. B.A.N. 2-(3-Methyl-2-phenylmorpholino)ethyl 2-phenyl-butryate.
Use: Appetite suppressant.
PHENCAP. (Jenkins) Phenyl-propanolamine HCI 50 mg, chlorpheniramine maleate 8 mg, atropine sulfate 1/180 gr. Cap. Bot. 1000s.
Use: Decongestant, antihistamine, anticholinergic/antispasmodic.
• **PHENCARBAMIDE.** USAN. S-2-Diethyl-ammoethyl diphenylthiocarbamate.
Use: Spasmolytic agent.
See: Escorpal (Farben-Fabriken).
PHENCHLOR-EIGHT. (Freeport) Chlorpheniramine maleate 8 mg. TR Cap. Bot. 1000s.
Use: Antihistamine.
PHENCHLOR SHA. (Rugby) Phenyl-propanolamine HCI 50 mg, phenylephrine HCI 25 mg, chlorpheniramine maleate 8 mg, hyoscyamine sulfate 0.19 mg, atropine sulfate 0.04 mg, scopolamine HBr. Tab. Bot. 100s, 500s.
Use: Decongestant, antihistamine, anticholinergic.
PHENCHLOR-TWELVE. (Freeport) Chlorpheniramine maleate 12 mg. TR

Cap. Bot. 1000s.
Use: Antihistamine.
• **PHENCYCLIDINE HYDROCHLORIDE.** USAN. 1-(1-Phenylcyclohexyl)piperidine HCI.
Use: Anticholinergic.
• **PHENDIMETRAZINE TARTRATE,** U.S.P. XXIII. Cap., Tab., U.S.P. XXIII. d-3,4-Di-methyl-2-phenylmorpholine bitartrate.
Use: Anorexic.
See: Adipost, Cap. (Ascher).
Adphen, Tab. (Ferndale).
Anorex, Cap., Tab. (Dunhall).
Bacarate, Tab. (Solvay).
Bontril PDM, Tab. (Carnrick).
Bontril Slow Release, Cap. (Carnrick).
Delcozine, Tab. (Delco).
Di-Ap-Trol, Tab. (Foy).
Elphemet, Tab. (Canright).
Limit, Tab. (Bock).
Melfiat, Tab. (Solvay).
Melfiat 105, Cap. (Solvay).
Obacin, Tab. (Kenyon).
Obalan, Tab. (Lannett).
Obepar, Tab. (Parmed).
Obe-Tite, Tab. (Scott/Cord).
Phenazine, Inj. (Jenkins).
Phen-70, Tab. (Parmed).
Phenzine, Tab. (Hauck).
Prelu-2, Cap. (Boehringer Ingelheim).
Reducto, Tab. (Arcum).
Rexigen Forte, SR Cap. (Ion).
Slim-Tabs, Tab. (Wesley).
Statobex, Prods. (Lemmon).
Stodex, Tab., Cap. (Jalco).
Trimtabs, Tab. (Mayrand).
PHENDRY. (LuChem) Diphenhydramine HCI 12.5 mg/5 ml, alcohol 14%. Elix. Bot. pt, gal.
Use: Antihistamine.
PHENDRY CHILDREN'S ALLERGY MEDICINE. (LuChem) Diphenhydramine HCI 12.5 mg/5 ml, alcohol 14%. Elix. Bot. 120 ml.
Use: Antihistamine.
• **PHENELZINE SULFATE,** U.S.P. XXIII. Tab., U.S.P. XXIII. Phenethylhydrazine sulfate. Monoamine oxidase inhibitor, betaphenylethyl-hydrazinedihydrogen sulfate.
Use: Antidepressant.
See: Nardil, Tab. (Parke-Davis).
PHENERBEL-S. (Rugby) Phenobarbital 40 mg, errgotamine tartrate 0.6 mg, l-alkaloids of belladonna 0.2 mg. Tab. Bot. 100s.
Use: Sedative/hypnotic, anticholinergic.
PHENERGAN-D. (Wyeth-Ayerst) Promethazine HCI 6.25 mg, pseudoephedrine HCI 60 mg. Tab. Bot. 100s.

Use: Antihistamine, decongestant.
PHENERGAN FORTIS. (Wyeth-Ayerst) Promethazine HCl 25 mg/5 ml, alcohol 1.5%. Bot. pt.
Use: Antihistamine.
PHENERGAN INJECTION. (Wyeth-Ayerst) Promethazine HCl 25 mg or 50 mg/ml. Inj. Amp. 1 mg Pkg. 5s, 25s, Tubex 10s.
Use: Antihistamine.
PHENERGAN PLAIN. (Wyeth-Ayerst) Promethazine HCl 6.25 mg/5 ml, alcohol 7%, saccharin. Syr. Bot. 120 ml, 180 ml, 240 ml, pt, gal.
Use: Antihistamine.
PHENERGAN SUPPOSITORIES. (Wyeth-Ayerst) Promethazine HCl 12.5 mg, 25 mg or 50 mg. Supp. Box. 12s, Redipak.
Use: Antihistamine.
PHENERGAN SYRUP PLAIN. (Wyeth-Ayerst) Promethazine HCl 6.25 mg/5 ml. Bot. 4 oz, 6 oz, 8 oz, pt, gal.
Use: Antihistamine.
PHENERGAN TABLETS. (Wyeth-Ayerst) Promethazine HCl 12.5 mg, 25 mg or 50 mg. Tab. Bot. 100s. Redipak 100s.
Use: Antihistamine.
PHENERGAN VC. (Wyeth-Ayerst) Promethazine HCl 6.25 mg, phenylephrine HCl 5 mg/5 ml, alcohol 7%. Bot. 4 oz, 6 oz, 8 oz, pt, gal.
Use: Antihistamine, decongestant.
PHENERGAN VC WITH CODEINE. (Wyeth-Ayerst) Promethazine HCl 6.25 mg, codeine phosphate 10 mg, phenylephrine HCl 5 mg/5 ml, alcohol 7%. Bot. 4 oz, 6 oz, 8 oz, pt, gal.
Use: Antihistamine, antitussive, decongestant.
PHENERGAN WITH CODEINE. (Wyeth-Ayerst) Promethazine HCl 6.25 mg, codeine phosphate 10 mg/5 ml. Bot. 4 oz, 6 oz, 8 oz, pt, gal.
Use: Antihistamine, antitussive.
PHENERGAN WITH DEXTROMETHORPHAN. (Wyeth-Ayerst) Promethazine HCl 6.25 mg, dextromethorphan HBr 15 mg/5 ml, alcohol 7%. Bot. 4 oz, 6 oz, pt, gal.
Use: Antihistamine, antitussive.
PHENERIDINE. 1-(β-Phenyl-b-ethyl)-4-carbethoxy-4-phenylpiperidine. Ethyl 1-phenethyl-4-phenyl-isonipecotate.
Use: Analgesic.
PHENETHICILLIN. B.A.N. 6-(α-Phenoxypropion-amido)penicillanic acid. Broxil [potassium salt].
Use: Antibiotic.
PHENETHYL ALCOHOL. B.A.N. 2-

Phenylethanol.
Use: Antiseptic.
I-PHENETHYLBIGUANIDE MONOHYDROCHLORIDE. Phenformin HCl.
PHENETRON. (Lannett) Chlorpheniramine maleate 4 mg. Tab. Bot. 1000s.
Use: Antihistamine.
PHENETRON COMPOUND TABLETS. (Lannett) Chlorpheniramine maleate 2 mg, aspirin 390 mg, caffeine 30 mg. Tab. Bot. 1000s.
Use: Antihistamine, salicylate analgesic.
PHENETRON INJECTABLE. (Lannett) Chlorpheniramine maleate. Amp. (10 mg/ml) 1 ml 25s, 100s, Vial 30 ml; (100 mg/ml) Vial 5 ml.
Use: Antihistamine.
PHENETRON SYRUP. (Lannett) Chlorpheniramine maleate 2 mg/5 ml. Bot. pt, gal.
Use: Antihistamine.
PHENETURIDE. B.A.N. (2-Phenylbutyryl)urea. Ethylphenacemide (I.N.N.) Benuride.
Use: Anticonvulsant.
PHENEX-1. (Ross) Protein 15 g, fat 23.9 g, carbohydrates 46.3 g, linoleic acid 1800 mg, Fo 9 mg, Na 190 mg, K 675 mg, Cal 480/100 g. With appropriate vitamins and minerals. Phenylalanine free. Pow. Can 350 g.
Use: Enteral nutritional supplement.
PHENEX-2. (Ross) Protein 30 g, fat 15.5 g, carbohydrates 30 g, Fe 13 mg, Na 880 mg, K 1370 mg, Cal 410/100 g. With appropriate vitamins and minerals. Phenylalanine free. Pow. Can 325 g.
Use: Enteral nutritional supplement.
PHENFORMIN HCl. Imidodicarbonimidic diamide, nN-(2-phenylethyl)-monohydrochloride. N^1-β-Phenylbiguanide HCl.
Use: Hypoglycemic.
Note: Withdrawn from market in 1978. Available under IND exemption.
PHENGLUTARIMIDE. B.A.N. 2-(2-Diethylaminoethyl)-2-phenylglutarimide. Aturbane HCl.
Use: Treatment of the Parkinsonian syndrome.
PHENHIST DH W/CODEINE. (Rugby) Pseudoephedrine HCl 30 mg, chlorpheniramine maleate 2 mg, codeine phosphate 10 mg/5 ml, alcohol 5%. Liq. Bot. 120 ml, 480 ml.
Use: Decongestant, antihistamine, antitussive.
PHENHIST EXPECTORANT. (Rugby) Pseudoephedrine HCl 30 mg, codeine

phosphate 10 mg, guaifenesin 100 mg/5 ml, alcohol 7.5%. Liq. Bot. 118 ml, pt, gal.
Use: Decongestant, antihistamine, antitussive.
PHENIFORM.
See: Phenformin HCl.
PHENINDAMINE TARTRATE, 2,3,4,9-Tetrahydro-2-methyl-9 phenyl-1 H-indeno-[2,1-c] pyridine bitartrate. 2,3,4,9-Tetrahydro-2-methyl-9-phenyl-lH-indeno-(2,1-c)pyridine Tartrate (1:1).
Use: Antihistamine.
See: Nolahist, Tab. (Carnrick).
Thephorin, Tab. (Roche).
W/Chlorpheniramine maleate, phenylpropanolamine HCl.
See: Nolamine, Tab. (Carnrick).
W/Phenylephrine HCl, aspirin, caffeine, aluminum hydroxide, magnesium carbonate.
See: Dristan, Tab. (Whitehall).
W/Phenylephrine HCl, caramiphen ethanedisulfonate.
See: Dondril, Tab. (Whitehall).
W/Phenylephrine HCl, chlorpheniramine maleate, drytane.
See: Comhist, Tab., Elix. (Baylor).
W/Phenylephrine HCl, chlorpheniramine maleate, belladonna alkaloids.
See: Comhist L.A., Cap. (Baylor Labs.).
W/Phenylephrine HCl, pyrilamine maleate, chlorpheniramine maleate, dextromethorphan HBr.
See: Histalet, Histalet-DM, Histalet-Forte, Syr. (Solvay).
PHENIODOL.
See: Iodoalphionic Acid (Various Mfr.).
PHENIPRAZINE. B.A.N.
α-Methylphenethylhydrazine. Cavodil [hydrochloride].
Use: Monoamine oxidase inhibitor.
PHENIPRAZINE HCl. (α-Methyl-phenethyl)-hydrazine monohydrochloride.
Use: Antihypertensive.
PHENIRAMINE MALEATE. 2-[a-[2-(Dimethyl- amino)ethyl]benzyl]-pyridine bimaleate. Prophen- pyridamine.
Use: Antihistamine.
See: Inhiston, Tab. (Schering-Plough).
W/Combinations.
Allerstat, Cap. (Lemmon).
Chexit, Tab. (Sandoz Consumer).
Citra Forte, Cap., Syr. (Boyle).
Decobel, Cap. (Lannett).
Kenahist-S.A., Tab. (Kenyon).
Partuss AC (Parmed).
Phenagesic, Tab., Syr. (Dalin).
Poly-Histine Cap., Elix., Lipospan

(Bock).
T.A.C., Cap. (Towne).
Thor, Cap. (Towne).
Trigelamine, Oint. (E.J. Moore).
Tritussin, Syr. (Towne).
PHENOBARBITAL. (Pharmaceutical Associates) 15 mg/5 ml. Elixir. Bot. Pt, UD 5 ml, 10 ml, 20 ml.
Use: Sedative, hypnotic, anticonvulsant.
•**PHENOBARBITAL,** U.S.P. XXIII. Elixir, Tab., U.S.P. XXIII. 2,4,6(1H,3H,%H)
Pyrimidinetrione, 5-ethyl-5-phenyl. 5-Ethyl-5-phenylbarbituric acid.
Phenylethylbarbituric acid, phenylethylmalonylurea, Barbenyl, Dormiral, Duneryl, Neurobarb, Numol, Phenonyl, Somonal. (Various Mfr.) **Tab.: 15 mg, 30 mg:** Bot. 100s, 1000s, 5000s, UD 100s; **60 mg:** Bot. 100s, 1000s, UD 100s; **100 mg:** 100s, 1000s. **Elixir:** 20 mg/5 ml. Bot. Pt, gal, UD 5 ml, UD 7.5 ml.
Use: Anticonvulsant, hypnotic, sedative.
See: Henomint, Elix. (Bowman).
Hypnette, Supp., Tab. (Fleming).
Orprine, Liq. (Pennwalt).
Pheno-Square, Tab. (Hauck).
Sedadrops, Liq. (Merrell Dow).
Solfoton, Tab., Cap. (ECR Pharm.).
PHENOBARBITAL W/AMINOPHYLLINE.
See: Aminophylline (Various Mfr.).
PHENOBARBITAL W/ATROPINE SULFATE.
See: Atropine Sulfate (Various Mfr.).
P.A., Tab. (Scrip).
PHENOBARBITAL W/BELLADONNA.
See: Belladonna Products and Phenobarbital Combinations.
PHENOBARBITAL WITH CENTRAL NERVOUS SYSTEM STIMULANTS.
See: Arcotrate No. 3, Tab. (Arcum).
Bronkolixir, Elix. (Sanofi Winthrop).
Bronkotab, Tab. (Sanofi Winthrop).
Quadrinal, Susp., Tab. (Knoll).
Sedamine, Tab. (Dunhall).
Spabelin, Elix., Tab. (Arcum).
PHENOBARBITAL COMBINATIONS.
See: Aminophylline w/Phenobarbital, Combinations.
Aspirin-Barbiturate, Combinations.
Atropine-Hyoscine-Hyoscyamine Combinations.
Atropine Sulfate w/Phenobarbital.
Belladonna Extract Combinations.
Belladonna Products and Phenobarbital Combinations.
Homatropine Methylbromide and Phenobarbital Combinations.
Hyoscyamus Products and Phenobarbital Combinations.

Mannitol Hexanitrate w/Phenobarbital
Combinations.

Mephenesin and Barbiturates Combinations.

Phenobarbital w/Central Nervous System Stimulants.

Secobarbital Combinations.

Sodium Nitrite Combinations.

Theobromine w/Phenobarbital Combinations.

Theophylline w/Phenobarbital Combinations.

Veratrum Viride w/Phenobarbital Combinations.

PHENOBARBITAL W/HOMATROPINE METHYLBROMIDE.
See: Homatropine Methylbromide and Phenobarbital Combinations.

PHENOBARBITAL W/HYOSCYAMUS.
See: Hyoscyamus Products and Phenobarbital Combinations.

PHENOBARBITAL W/MANNITOL HEXANITRATE.
Use: Anticonvulsant, sedative/hypnotic.
See: Mannitol Hexanitrate w/Phenobarbital Combinations.

•PHENOBARBITAL SODIUM, U.S.P. XXII. Inj., Sterile, U.S.P. XXIII. Tab., U.S.P. XXI. Sodium 5-ethyl-5-phenylbarbiturate. 2,4,6(1H,3H,5H)-Pyrimidinetrione, 5-ethyl-5 phenyl, monosodium salt. (Sodium Phenylethylbarbiturate, Soluble Phenobarbital). (Various Mfr.) 130 mg/ml. Inj. Tubex 1 ml, vial 1 ml.
Use: Anticonvulsant, sedative, hypnotic.
See: Luminal Sodium, Inj. (Sanofi Winthrop).

PHENOBARBITAL SODIUM. (Wyeth-Ayerst) Inj. **30 mg/ml, 60 mg/ml:** Tubex 1 ml; **65 mg/ml:** Vial 1 ml; **130 mg/ml:** Tubex 1 ml, vial 1 ml.
Use: Anticonvulsant, sedative, hypnotic.

PHENOBARBITAL SODIUM IN PROPYLENE GLYCOL. Vitarine. Amp. 0.13 Gm: 1 ml, Box 25s, 100s.
Use: Anticonvulsant, hypnotic, sedative.

PHENOBARBITAL AND THEOBROMINE COMBINATIONS.
See: Theobromine w/Phenobarbital Combinations.

PHENOBARBITAL W/THEOPHYLLINE.
See: Theophylline w/Phenobarbital Combinations.

PHENOBARBITAL W/VERATRUM VIRIDE.
See: Veratrum Viride w/Phenobarbital Combinations.

PHENO-BELLA. (Ferndale) Belladonna extract 10.8 mg, phenobarbital 16.2 mg/Tab. Bot. 100s, 1000s.

Use: Anticholinergic/antispasmodic, sedative/hypnotic.

PHENOBUTIODIL. B.A.N. w-(2,4,6-Triiodophenoxy)-butyric acid. Vesipaque (Warner-Lambert).
Use: Radiopaque substance.

PHENOJECT-50. (Mayrand) Promethazine HCl 50 mg/ml. Inj. Vial 10 ml.
Use: Antihistamine, antiemetic.

•PHENOL, U.S.P. XXIII. Liq., U.S.P. XXIII. (Various Mfr.) Carbolic acid.
Use: Pharmaceutic aid (preservative), topical antipruritic.
W/Aluminum hydroxide, zinc oxide, camphor, eucalyptol, ichthammol, thyme oil.
See: Almophen, Olnt. (Bowman).
W/Benzocaine, ichthammol, balsam peru, alum exsiccated, cade oil, oil eucalyptus, carbolic oil.
See: Alucaine, Oint. (Jenkins).
W/Benzocaine, triclosan.
See: Solarcaine Pump Spray (Schering-Plough).
W/Dextromethorphan.
See: Chloraseptic DM Lozenges (Eaton).
W/Resorcinol,
See: Black & White Ointment (Schering-Plough).
W/Resorcinol, boric acid, basic fuchsin, acetone.
See: Castellani's Paint, Liq. (Various Mfr.).

•PHENOLATE SODIUM. USAN.
Use: Disinfectant.

PHENOLAX. (Upjohn) Phenolphthalein 64.8 mg/Wafer. Bot. 100s.
Use: Laxative.

•PHENOL, LIQUEFIED, U.S.P. XXIII.
Use: Topical antipruritic.

•PHENOLPHTHALEIN, U.S.P. XXIII. Tab., U.S.P. XXIII. (Various Mfr.) 3,3-Bis(p-hydroxyphenyl)phthalide. Pkg. 1 oz, 0.25 lb., 1 lb.
Use: Cathartic.
See: Alophen, Pill (Parke-Davis).
Espotabs, Tab. (Combe).
Evac-U-Lax, Wafer (Hauck).
Evasof, Tab. (Lemmon).
Ex-Lax, Prods. (Sandoz Consumer).
Feen-A-Mint, Tab., Gum (Schering-Plough).
Phenolax, Wafer (Upjohn).
Veracolate, Tab. (Numark).

PHENOLPHTHALEIN W/COMBINATIONS.
See: Bilocomp, Tab. (Lannett).
Correctol, Tab. (Schering-Plough).
Disolan, Cap. (Lannett).
Evac-Q-Kit, Tab., Supp. (Warren-

Teed).
Dual Formula Feen-A-Mint Pills (Schering-Plough).
Feen-A-Mint, Gum, Mint, Pill (Schering-Plough).
4-Way Cold Tab. (Bristol-Myers).
Lanothal Pills (Lannett).
PHENOLPHTHALEIN IN LIQUID PETRO-LATUM EMULSION. (Various Mfr.).
See: Petrolatum, Liq.
• **PHENOLPHTHALEIN YELLOW,** U.S.P. XXIII.
Use: Cathartic.
PHENOLSULFONATES.
See: Sulfocarbolates.
PHENOLSULFONIC ACID. Sulfocarbolic acid.
Note: Used in Sulphodine, Tab. (Strasenburgh).
PHENOLTETRABROMOPHTHALEIN. Disulfonate Disodium.
See: Sulfobromophthalein Sodium, U.S.P. XXIII.
PHENOLZINE SULFATE. β-Phenylethylhydrazine hydrogen sulfate.
PHENOMORPHAN. B.A.N. 3-Hydroxy-N-phenethylmorphinan.
Use: Narcotic analgesic.
PHENO NUX TABLETS. (Vale) Phenobarbital 16.2 mg, nux vomica extract 8.1 mg, calcium carbonate 194.4 mg/Tab. Bot. 1000s.
Use: Sedative/hypnotic, antacid.
PHENOPERIDINE. B.A.N. Ethyl 1-(3-hydroxy-3-phenylpropyl)-4-phenylpiperidine-4-carboxylate. Operidine HCl.
Use: Narcotic analgesic.
PHENOPTIC. (Optopics) Phenylephrine HCl 2.5%. Soln. Bot. 2 ml, 5 ml, 15 ml.
Use: Ophthalmic vasoconstrictor/mydriatic.
PHENOTHIAZINE. Thiodiphenylamine.
PHENOTURIC. (Truett) Phenobarbital 40 mg/5 ml. Elix. Bot. pt, gal.
Use: Sedative/hypnotic.
PHENOXINE. (Lannett) Phenylpropanolamine HCl 25 mg/Tab. Bot. 1000s.
Use: Diet aid.
• **PHENOXYBENZAMINE HCl,** U.S.P. XXI. Cap., U.S.P. XXI. N-Phenoxyisopropyl-N-benzyl-beta-chlorethylamine HCl. N-(2-Chloroethyl)-N-(1-methyl-2-phenoxyethyl)benzylamine HCl.
Use: Antihypertensive.
See: Dibenzyline, Cap. (SK-Beecham).
PHENOXYMETHYL PENICILLIN.
See: Penicillin V.
PHENOXYMETHYL PENICILLIN POTASSIUM.

See: Penicillin V Potassium.
PHENOXYNATE. Mixture of phenylphenols 17-18%, octyl and related alkylphenols 2-3%.
See: Surtenol, Liq. (Guardian Chem.).
PHENOXYPROPAZINE. B.A.N. (1-Methyl-2-phenoxyethyl)hydrazine. Drazino hydrogen maleate.
Use: Monoamine oxidase inhibitor.
PHENPROBAMATE. B.A.N. 3-Phenylpropyl carbamate. Gamaquil.
Use: Skeletal muscle relaxant.
• **PHENPROCOUMON,** U.S.P. XXII. Tab., U.S.P. XXII. 3-(α-Ethylbenzyl)-4-hydroxycoumarin. 4-Hydroxy-3-(1-phenylpropyl)coumarin. Marcoumar.
Use: Anticoagulant.
See: Liquamar, Tab. (Organon).
PHEN-70. (Parmed) Phendimetrazine tartrate 70 mg/Tab. Bot. 100s, 1000s.
Use: Anorexiant.
• **PHENSUXIMIDE,** U.S.P. XXII. Cap., U.S.P. XXII. N-Methyl-2-phenylsuccinimide.
Use: Anticonvulsant.
See: Milontin, Preps. (Parke-Davis).
PHENTAL. (Geneva) Belladonna alkaloids, phenobarbital 0.25 gr/Tab. Bot. 1000s.
Use: Anticholinergic/antispasmodic, sedative/hypnotic.
PHENTAMINE. (Major) Phentermine HCl 30 mg/Cap. (equivalent to 24 mg base). Bot. 100s.
Use: Anorexiant.
• **PHENTERMINE.** USAN. α,α-Dimethylphenethylamine. Phenyl-tertiary-butylamine. Duromine (an ion-exchange resin complex).
Use: Anorexiant.
See: Adipex, Tab. (Lemmon).
Adipex-8 C.T., Cap. (Lemmon).
Adipex-P, Cap. (Lemmon).
Fastin, Cap. (Beecham Labs).
Parmine, Cap. (Parmed).
Tora, Tab. (Solvay).
Unifast Unicelles, Cap. (Solvay).
Wilpowr, Cap. (Foy).
PHENTERMINE AS RESIN COMPLEX.
See: Ionamin, Cap. (Pennwalt).
• **PHENTERMINE HYDROCHLORIDE,** U.S.P. XXIII. Cap., Nasal Jelly, Tab., U.S.P. XXIII. Benzeneethanamine, α,α-dimethyl-, HCl.
Use: Anorexiant.
See: Zantryl, Cap. (Ion).
PHENTETIOTHALEIN SODIUM. Iso-lodeikon.
Use: Radiopaque agent.
PHENTOLAMINE HYDROCHLORIDE.

m-[n-(2-lmi-dazolin-2-ylmethyl)-p-toluidi-no]phenol HCl.
Use: Antihypertensive.
See: Regitine HCl, Tab. (Ciba).

• **PHENTOLAMINE MESYLATE,** U.S.P. XXIII. For Inj., U.S.P. XXIII. Phenol, 3-[[(4,5-dihydro-1H-lmidazol-2-yl)methyl]-(4-methyl-phenyl)amino]-, monomethanesulfonate (salt). m-[N-(2-Imidazolin-2-ylmethyl)-p-toluidino]-phenol methanesulfonate.
Use: Anti-adrenergic.
See: Regitine Inj. (Ciba).

PHENTOLAMINE METHANESUL-FONATE. Phentolamine mesylate, U.S.P. XXIII.

PHENTOLOX w/APAP. (Richlyn) Phenyltoloxamine citrate 30 mg, acetaminophen 325 mg/Tab. Bot. 1000s.
Use: Antihistamine, analgesic.

PHENTOX COMPOUND. (My-K Labs) Phenylpropanolamine HCl 20 mg, phenylephrine HCl 5 mg, chlorphenlramine maleate 2.5 mg, phenyltoloxamine citrate 7.5 mg/5 ml. Bot. pt, gal.
Use: Decongestant, antihistamine.

PHENTYDRONE. 1,2,3,4-Tetrahydrofluoren-9-one.
Use: Systemic fungicide.

PHENURONE. (Abbott) Phenacemide 0.5 Gm/Tab. Bot. 100s.
Use: Anticonvulsant.

N-PHENYLACETAMIDE.
See: Acetanilid (Various Mfr.).

PHENYLACETYLUREA.
See: Phenurone, Tab. (Abbott).

• **PHENYLAMINOSALICYLATE.** USAN. Phenyl 4 aminosalicylate. Fenamisal (I.N.N.) Phenypastebamin.
Use: Tuberculostatic.

• **PHENYLALANINE,** U.S.P. XXIII. $C_9H_{11}NO_2$ as L-phenylalanine.
Use: Amino acid.
See: Phenylketonuria therapy.

PHENYLALANINE MUSTARD.
See: Melphalan, U.S.P. XXIII. analgesic.

PHENYLAZO-DIAMINO-PYRIDINE.
See: Phenazopyridine (Various Mfr.).

PHENYLAZO-DIAMINO-PYRIDINE HCl or HBr.
See: Phenazopyridine HCl or HBr (Various Mfr.).

PHENYLAZO-DIAMINOPYRIDINE HY-DROCHLORIDE.
See: Rodine, Tab. (Paddock).

PHENYLAZO SULFISOXAZOLE. (A.P.C.) Sulfisoxazole 0.5 Gm, phenylazopyridine 50 mg/Tab. Bot. 1000s.
Use: Antibacterial, sulfonamide, urinary

PHENYLAZO TABLETS. (A.P.C.) Phenylazodiamino-pyridine HCl 1.5 gr/Tab. Bot. 1000s.
Use: Urinary analgesic.

PHENYLBUTYRATE SODIUM.
Use: Treatment of blood disorders. [Orphan drug]

PHENYLCARBINOL.
See: Benzyl Alcohol, N.F. XVIII.

PHENYLCINCHONINIC ACID. Name used for cinchophen.

• **PHENYLEPHRINE HYDROCHLORIDE,** U.S.P. XXIII. Inj., Nasal Soln., Ophth. Soln., U.S.P. XXIII. Benzenemethanol, 3-hydroxy-α-[(methylamino)-methyl]-, hydrochloride (S)-. l-m-Hydroxy-a-[(methylamino)methyl]-benzyl alcohol hydrochloride. (Neophryn). (Various Mfr.) Soln. **2.5%:** Bot. 2 ml, 5 ml, 15 ml; **10%:** Bot. 1 ml, 2 ml, 5 ml, 15 ml.
Use: Sympathomimetic agent, vasoconstrictor, mydriatic.
See: AK-Dilate (Akorn).
   AK-Nefrin (Akorn).
   Alcon-Efrin, Soln. (Webcon).
   Allerest Nasal Spray (Pharmacraft).
   Coricidin Decongestant Nasal Mist (Schering).
   Ephrine, Spray (Walgreen).
   Isopto Frin (Alcon).
   Mydtrin 2.5% (Alcon).
   Neo-Synephrine HCl, Preps. (Sanofi Winthrop Products).
   Phenoptic (Optopics).
   Prefrin Liquifilm Ophth. Soln. (Allergan).
   Pyracort-D, Spray (Lemmon).
   Relief (Allergan).
   Sinarest, Nasal Spray (Pharmacraft).
   Super-Anahist Nasal Spray (Warner-Lambert).
W/Combinations.
See: Acotus, Liq. (Whorton).
   Anodynos Forte, Tab. (Buffington).
   Bellafedrol A-H, Tab. (Lannett).
   Bur-Tuss Expectorant (Burlington).
   C.D.M. Expectorant Liq. (Lannett).
   Cenahist, Cap. (Century).
   Cenaid, Tab. (Century).
   Chlor-Trimeton Expectorant (Schering).
   Chlor-Trimeton Expectorant w/Codeine (Schering).
   Conar, Susp., Expectorant (Beecham Labs).
   Conar-A, Tab., Susp. (Beecham Labs).
   Congespirin, Tab. (Bristol-Myers).
   Coricidin Demilets (Schering).
   Dallergy, Syr., Cap., Tab., Inj. (Laser).

Demazin, Syr. (Schering).
Dimetane Decongestant, Tab., Elix. (Robins).
Dimetane Expectorant, Liq. (Robins).
Dimetane Expectorant-DC, Liq. (Robins).
Dimetapp, Elix., Extentabs (Robins).
Doktors, Drops, Spray (Scherer).
Eldatapp, Tab., Liq. (Elder).
Emagrin Forte, Tab. (Clapp).
Entex, Prods. (Norwich Eaton).
Eye-Gene, Soln. (Pearson).
4 Way Tab., Spray (Bristol-Myers).
Furacin Nasal Soln. (Eaton).
Histabid, Cap. (Meyer).
Histapp Prods. (Upsher-Smith).
Histaspan-D, Cap. (Rhone-Poulenc Rorer).
Histaspan-Plus, Cap. (Rhone-Poulenc Rorer).
Mydfrin Ophthalmic, Liq. (Alcon).
Na-Co-Al, Tab. (High).
Nasahist, Cap. (Keene).
Pediacof, Syr. (Sanofi Winthrop).
Phenoptic, Soln. (Muro).
Phenylzin Drops, Ophth. Soln. (CooperVision).
Prefrin-A Ophth. Soln. (Allergan).
Prefrin-Z Ophth. Soln. (Allergan).
Pyraphed, Soln. (Lemmon).
Pyristan, Cap., Elix. (Arcum).
Queledrine, Syr. (Abbott).
Rhinall, Liq. (Scherer).
Rhinex DM, Tab. (Lemmon).
Rymed, Prods. (Edwards).
Sinex, Nasal Spray (Vicks).
Singlet, Tab. (Merrell Dow).
Spectab, Tab. (Solvay).
Spec-T Sore Throat-Decongestant Loz. (Squibb).
Sucrets Cold Decongestant Loz. (Calgon).
Tearefrin, Liq. (CooperVision).
Trind, Liq. (Mead Johnson).
Trind-DM, Liq. (Mead Johnson).
Tri-Ophtho, Soln. (Maurry).
Turbilixir, Liq. (Burlington).
Turbispan Leisurecaps, Cap. (Burlington).
Tussar-DM, Liq. (Rhone-Poulenc Rorer).
Tympagesic, Liq. (Adria).
Vacon, Liq. (Scherer).
Valihist, Cap. (Clapp).
Vasocidin, Ophth. Soln. (CooperVision).
Vasosulf, Ophth. Soln. (Iolab).
•**PHENYLETHYL ALCOHOL,** U.S.P. XXIII.
Betaphenylethanol. Benzylcarbinol. (Various Mfr.) Phenethyl Alcohol.

Use: Antibacterial; preservative (ophthalmic).
PHENYL-ETHYL-HYDRAZINE, beta.
Phenelzine dihydrogen sulfate.
See: Nardil, Tab. (Parke-Davis).
PHENYLETHYLMALONYLUREA.
See: Phenobarbital (Various Mfr.).
PHENYL FENFSIN L.A. (Goldline)
Phenylpropanolamine HCl 75 mg, guaifenesin 400 mg/Tab. Bot. 100s, 500s.
Use: Decongestant, expectorant.
PHENYLGESIC TABS. (Goldline)
Phenyltoloxamine citrate 30 mg, acetaminophen 325 mg/Bot. 100s, 1000s.
Use: Antihistamine, analgesic.
PHENYLIC ACID.
See: Phenol, U.S.P. XXIII.
PHENYLKETONURIA THERAPY.
See: Lofenalac, Pow. (Mead Johnson).
Phenistix Reagent Strips (Miles Diagnostic).
•**PHENYLMERCURIC ACETATE,** N.F. XVIII. (Various Mfr.)
(Acetato)phenylmercury. Bot. 1 lb, 5 lb, 10 lb.
Use: Preservative (bacteriostatic).
W/9-Aminoacridine HCl, tyrothricin, urea, lactose.
See: Trinalis, Vaginal Supp. (Webcon).
W/Benzocaine, chlorothymol, resorcin.
See: Lanacane Creme (Combe).
W/Boric acid, polyoxyethylenenonylphenol or oxyquinoline benzoate.
See: Koromex, Preps. (Holland-Rantos).
W/Methylbenzethonium Cl.
See: Norforms, Aerosol, Supp. (Norwich).
PHENYLMERCURIC BORATE. (F. W. Berk) Pkg. Custom packed.
W/Benzyl alcohol, benzocaine, butyl p-aminobenzoate.
See: Dermathyn, Oint. (Davis & Sly).
PHENYLMERCURIC CHLORIDE.
Chlorophenylmercury.
•**PHENYLMERCURIC NITRATE,** N.F. XVIII. (Merphenyl Nitrate, Phenmerzyl Nitrate) A.P.L.—Oint. 1:1500, 1 oz, 4 oz, lb. Chicago Pharm.-Loz. w/benzocaine. Bot. 100s, 1000s. Ophth. Oint., 1:3000, Tube ⅛ oz. Soln. 1:20,000, Bot. pt, gal. Vaginal supp., 1:5000, Box 12s.
Use: Bacteriostatic.
See: Preparation H, Oint., Supp. (Whitehall).
W/Amyl, phenylphenol complex.
See: Lubraseptic Jelly (Guardian).
W/Undecylenic acid.
See: Bridex, Oint. (Briar).

PHENYLMERCURIC PICRATE.
Use: Germicide.
PHENYLPHENOL-o.
W/Amyl complex, phenylmercuric nitrate.
See: Lubraseptic Jelly. (Guardian).
• **PHENYLPROPANOLAMINE HY-**
DROCHLORIDE, U.S.P. XXIII. Extend-
ed-release Cap., U.S.P. XXIII. (±)-
Norephedrine HCl. 2-Amino-1-phenyl-1-
propanol (Mydriatine).
Use: Sympathomimetic.
See: Maximum Strength Dexatrim, ER
Tab. (Thompson).
Obestat, Cap. (Lemmon).
Obestat 150, Cap. (Lemmon).
Propadrine HCl, Preps. (Merck & Co.).
Propagest, Tab. (Carnrick).
Spray-U-Thin (Caprice Greystoke).
PHENYLPROPANOLAMINE HCl
W/COMBINATIONS.
See: Allerest, Prods. (Pharmacraft).
Allerstat, Cap. (Lemmon).
A.R.M., Tab. (SK-Beecham).
Bayer, Prods. (Glenbrook).
BQ Cold, Tab. (Bristol-Myers).
Breacol Cough Medication, Liq. (Glen-
brook).
Bur-I uss Expectorant (Burlington).
Chexit, Tab. (Sandoz Consumer).
Comtrex, Cap., Liq., Tab. (Bristol-My-
ers).
Congespirin, Liq., Tab. (Bristol-Myers).
Contac, Prods. (SK-Beecham).
Cophene No. 2, Cap. (Dunhall).
Coricidin Cough Formula (Schering).
Coricidin ``D'' Decongestant, Tab.
(Schering).
Coricidin Sinus Headache, Tab.
(Schering).
Coryban-D, Cap. (Leeming).
Decobel, Cap. (Lannett).
Dex-A-Diet, Prods. (O'Connor).
Dezest, Cap. (Geneva).
Dimetane Expectorant, Liq. (Robins).
Dimetapp, Elix., Extentabs (Robins).
Drinophen, Cap. (Lannett).
Entex, Cap., Liq. (Norwich Eaton).
Entex LA, Tab. (Norwich Eaton).
Halls Mentho-Lyptus Cough Formula,
Liq. (Warner-Lambert).
Histabid, Cap. (Glaxo).
Histalet Forte T. D., Tab. (Solvay).
Hista-Vadrin, Syr., Tab., Cap. (Scher-
er).
Kleer Compound, Tab. (Scrip).
Meditussin-X, Liq. (Hauck).
Naldecon, Drop, Syr., Tab. (Bristol).
Nasahist, Cap., Inj. (Keene).
Nolamine, Tab. (Carnrick).
Ornade, Cap. (SK-Beecham).

Ornex, Cap. (SK-Beecham).
Panadyl, Tab., Cap. (Misemer).
Partuss-A, Tab. (Parmed).
Partuss T.D., Tab. (Parmed).
Pyristan, Cap., Elix. (Arcum).
Rhinex DM, Liq. (Lemmon).
Rymed, Prods. (Edwards).
Sanhist TD, Tab., Vial (Sandia).
Santussin, Cap., Susp. (Sandia).
Sinarest, Tab. (Pharmcraft).
Sine-Off, Tab. (SK-Beecham).
Sinulin, Tab. (Carnrick).
Spec-T Sore Throat-Decongestant,
Loz. (Squibb).
St. Joseph Cold Tablets for Children
(Schering-Plough).
Sto-Caps, Cap. (Jalco).
Sucrets Cold Decongestant Loz. (Cal-
gon).
Triaminic, Preps. (Sandoz Consumer).
Triaminicin, Chew. Tab. (Sandoz Con-
sumer).
Triaminicol, Syr. (Sandoz Consumer).
Turbilixir, Liq. (Burlington).
Turbispan Leisurecaps, Cap. (Burling-
ton).
Tusquelin, Syr. (Circle).
Tussagesic, Susp., Tab. (Sandoz Con-
sumer).
U.R.I., Cap., Liq. (ICN).
PHENYLPROPANOLAMINE HCl &
GUAIFENESIN TABLETS. (Various
Mfr.) Phenylpropanolamine HCl 75 mg,
guaifenesin 400 mg. Tab. Bot. 100s,
500s.
Use: Decongestant, expectorant.
PHENYLPROPANOLAMINE HCl & HY-
DROCODONE SYRUP. (PBI) Phenyl-
propanolamine HCl 25 mg, hy-
drocodone bitartrate 5 mg. Bot. 480 ml.
Use: Decongestant, antitussive.
• **PHENYLPROPANOLAMINE POLIS-**
TIREX. USAN.
Use: Adrenergic (vasoconstrictor).
PHENYLPROPYLMETHYLAMINE HY-
DROCHLORIDE. Vonedrine HCl
PHENYL SALICYLATE. Salol.
W/Atropine sulfate, hyoscyamine,
methenamine, methylene blue, gelsemi-
um, benzoic acid.
See: Lanased, Tab. (Lannett).
Renalgin, Tab. (Meyer).
U-Tract, Tab. (Bowman).
W/Euphorbia extract and various oils.
See: Rayderm Oint. (Velvet Pharma-
cal).
W/Methenamine, methylene blue, benzoic
acid, hyoscyamine alkaloid, atropine sul-
fate.
See: Urised, Tab. (Webcon).

UTA, Tab. (ICN).
W/Methenamine, sodium biphosphate, methylene blue, hyoscyamine, alkaloid.
See: Urostat Forte, Tab. (Elder).
PHENYL-TERT-BUTYLAMINE.
See: Phentermine.
PHENYLTHILONE. 2-Ethyl-2-phenyl-3,5-thiomorpho-linedione.
Use: Anticonvulsant.
PHENYLTOLOXAMINE. B.A.N. N-2-(2-Benzylphen-oxy)ethyldimethylamine. o-Benzylphenyl-2-dimethyl-aminoethyl ether.
Use: Antihistamine.
PHENYLTOLOXAMINE CITRATE. N,N-Dimethyl-2-[(alpha-phenyl-o-tolyl)oxy]ethylamine citrate.
Use: Antihistamine.
See: Volaxin Modified, Tab. (Elder).
PHENYLTOLOXAMINE CITRATE W/COMBINATIONS.
See: Dengesic, Tab. (Scott-Alison).
Dilone, Tab. (Vicks).
Meditussin-X, Liq. (Hauck).
Myocalm, Tab. (Parmed).
Naldecon, Preps. (Bristol).
Poly-histine Prods. (Bock).
Quadrahist, Tab. (Pharmex).
S.A.C. Sinus, Tab. (Towne).
Scotgesic, Elix., Cap. (Scott/Cord).
PHENYLTOLOXAMINE RESIN W/COMBINATIONS.
See: Tussionex, Cap., Liq., Tab. (Pennwalt).
PHENYLZIN. (CooperVision) Zinc sulfate 0.25%, phenylephrine HCl 0.12%. Bot. 15 ml.
Use: Ophthalmic decongestant combination.
• **PHENYRAMIDOL HCL.** USAN. 2(β-Hydroxyphen-ethylamino)pyridine HCl. α-[(2-Pyridylamino)(-methyl]-benzyl alcohol hydrochloride.
Use: Analgesic.
PHENYTHILONE. 2-Ethyl-2-phenyl-3, 5-thiamorpho-linedione.
• **PHENYTOIN,** U.S.P. XXIII. Oral Susp., Tab., U.S.P. XXIII. 2,4-Imidazolidinedione, 5,5-diphenyl-. 5,5-Di-phenylhydantoin. Diphenylhydantoin.
Use: Anticonvulsant.
See: Dilantin Prods. (Parke-Davis).
Di-phenyl, TR Cap. (Drug. Ind.).
Ekko, Cap. (Fleming).
Toin, Unicelles (Solvay).
• **PHENYTOIN SODIUM,** U.S.P. XXIII. Extended Cap., Inj., Prompt Cap., U.S.P. XXIII. Sterile, U.S.P. XXI. 2,4-Imidazolidinedione, 5,5-diphenyl-, monosodium salt. 5,5-Diphenylhydantoin sodium salt.

Diphenylhydantoin sodium. Alepsin, Dihydan soluble, Diphentoin, Silantin Sodium, Epanutin, Eptoin, Phenytoin soluble, Solantoin, Solantyl, Denyl Sodium, Soluble Phenytoin (5,5-diphenyl-hydantoinate Sodium).
Use: Anticonvulsant, cardiac depressant (anti-arrhythmic).
See: Dilantin Sodium, Preps. (Parke-Davis).
Diphenylan Sodium, Cap. (Lannett).
Ekko Jr. and Sr., Cap. (Fleming).
PHENYTOIN SODIUM WITH PHENO-BARBITAL.
Use: Anticonvulsant.
See: Dilantin with Phenobarbital Kapseals, Cap. (Parke-Davis).
PHEOCHROMOCYTOMA, AGENTS FOR.
See: Demser, Cap. (Merck & Co.).
Dibenzyline, Cap. (SK-Beecham).
Regitine, Inj. (Ciba Pharm.).
PHERAZINE DM. (Halsey) Promethazine 6.25 mg, dextromethorphan HBr 15 mg, alcohol 7%/5 ml. Bot. 4 oz, 6 oz, pt, gal.
Use: Antihistamine, antitussive.
PHERAZINE VC WITH CODEINE SYRUP. (Halsey) Phenylephrine HCl 5 mg, promethazine HCl 6.25 mg, codeine phosphate 10 mg, alcohol 7%/5 ml. Bot. pt, gal.
Use: Decongestant, antihistamine, antitussive.
PHERAZINE VC SYRUP. (Halsey) Phenylephrine HCl 5 mg, promethazine HCl 6.25 mg, alcohol 7%/5 ml. Bot. pt, gal.
Use: Decongestant, antihistamine.
PHERAZINE W/CODEINE. (Halsey) Promethazine HCl 6.25 mg, codeine phosphate 10 mg/5 ml, alcohol 7%, sorbitol, sucrose. Syr. Bot. 120 ml, pt, gal.
Use: Antihistamine, antitussive.
PHETHARBITAL. 5,5-Diethyl-1-phenyl-barbituric acid.
PHETHENYLATE. 5-Phenyl-5-(2-thienyl)hydantoinate. Also sodium salt.
PHICON. (T.E. Williams) Pramoxine HCl 0.5%, vitamin A 7500 IU, E 2000 IU/30 Gm. Cream. Tube 60 Gm.
Use: Local anesthetic, external.
PHICON F. (T.E. Williams) Undecylenic acid 8%, pramoxine HCl 0.05%. Cream. 60 Gm.
Use: Antifungal, external.
PHILLIPS' CHEWABLE. (Sterling Health) Magnesium hydroxide 311 mg. Tab. 100s, 200s.
Use: Laxative, antacid.
PHILLIP'S LAXATIVE GELCAPS. (Ster-

ling Health) Phenolphthalein 90 mg, docusate sodium 83 mg Bot. 30s.
Use: Laxative.

PHILLIPS' LAXCAPS. (Sterling Health) Docusate sodium 83 mg, phenolphthalein 90 mg/Cap. Bot. 8s, 24s, 48s.
Use: Laxative.

PHILLIPS' MILK OF MAGNESIA. (Sterling Health) Magnesium hydroxide. Reg. and Mint. Bot. 4 oz, 12 oz, 26 oz; Tab. Bot. 30s, 100s, 200s.
Use: Laxative, antacid.

PHILLIPS' MILK OF MAGNESIA CONCENTRATED. (Sterling Health) Magnesium hydroxide 800 mg/5 ml, sorbitol, sugar. Liq. Bot. 240 ml.
Use: Antacid.

PHISH OMEGA. (Pharmics) Natural salmon oil concentrate containing EPA 120 mg, DHA 100 mg/Cap. Bot. 60s.
Use: Fish oil.

PHISH OMEGA PLUS. (Pharmics) Natural fish oil concentrate containing EPA 300 mg, DHA 200 mg/Cap. Bot. 60s.
Use: Fish oil.

pHisoDerm. (Sanofi Winthrop) Sodium octoxynol-2 ethane sulfonate, white petrolatum, water, mineral oil (with lanolin alcohol and oleyl alcohol), sodium benzoate, octoxynol-3 tetrasodium EDTA, methylcellulose, hydrochloric acid. **Regular:** Bot. 5 oz, 9 oz, 16 oz. **Dry type:** Bot. 5 oz, pt. Wall dispenser pt. **Oily type:** Bot. 5 oz, 16 oz. **Lightly Scented:** Bot. 5 oz, 9 oz, 16 oz. **For Baby:** Bot. 5 oz, 9 oz.
Use: Skin cleanser, conditioner.

pHisoDerm GENTLE CLEANSING BAR. (Sanofi Winthrop) Sodium tallowate, sodium cocoate, petrolatum, glycerin, lanolin, sodium Cl, BHT, trisodium EDTA, titanium dioxide. Bar 99 Gm.
Use: Skin cleanser.

pHisoHex. (Sanofi Winthrop) Entsufon sodium, hexachlorophene 3%, petrolatum, lanolin cholesterols, methylcellulose, polyethylene glycol, polyethylene glycol monostearate, lauryl myristyl diethanolamide, sodium benzoate, water, pH adjusted with hydrochloric acid. Emulsion, Bot. 5 oz, pt, gal. Wall dispensers pt. Unit packets 0.25 oz. Box 50s, Pedal operated dispenser 30 oz.
Use: Antiseptic, germicide skin cleanser.

pHisoMed. (Sanofi Winthrop) Hexochlorophene.
Use: Antiseptic, germicide.

pHisoPUFF. (Sanofi Winthrop) Nonmedicated cleansing sponge. Box sponge

1s.
Use: Skin cleanser.

PHISTOL. (Kenyon) Vitamins A 10,000 IU, D 1000 IU, B_1 5 mg, B_2 3 mg, B_6 1 mg, C 100 mg, calcium pantothenate 5 mg, niacinamide 25 mg/Cap. Bot. 100s, 1000s.
Use: Vitamin supplement.

PHOLEDRINE. B.A.N. 4-(2-Methylaminopropyl)-phenol. Veritain; Veritol.
Use: Sympathomimetic.

PHOSCHOL. (Advanced Nutritional Technology) Phosphatidycholine (highly purified lecithin). **Softgel:** 200 mg, 565 mg or 900 mg. Bot. 100s, 300s. **Liq. Conc.:** 3000 mg/5 ml. Bot. 240 ml, 480 ml.
Use: Oral nutritional supplement.

PHOSCOLIC ACID. 2,2′-Phosphinicodilacetic acid.
Use: Adjuvant.

PHOS-FLUR ORAL RINSE SUPPLEMENT. (Colgate-Hoyt) Acidulated phosphate sodium fluoride 0.05%, fluoride 1 ml/5 ml. Bot. 250 ml, 500 ml, gal.
Use: Dental caries preventative.

PHOSLO. (Braintree) Calcium acetate 667 mg (calcium 169 mg)/Tab. Bot. 200s.
Use: Minerals and electrolytes, oral.

PHOSPHACAL-D. (Lannett) Dicalcium phosphate anhydrous 330 mg, vitamin D 333 IU/Cap. Bot. 500s, 1000s.
Use: Vitamin/mineral supplement.

PHOSPHATE.
See: Potassium Phosphate, Inj. (Abbott).
Sodium Phosphate, Inj. (Abbott).

PHOSPHENTASIDE. Adenosine-5-monophosphate. Adenylic acid.
W/Vitamin B_{12}, niacin.
See: Denylex Gel, Vial (Westerfield).
W/Vitamin B_{12}, niacin, B_1.
See: Adenolin, Vial (Lincoln).

PHOSPHOCOL P32. (Mallinckrodt) Chromic phosphate P32: 10 or 15 mCi with a concentration of up to 5 mCi/ml and specific activity of up to 5 mCi/mg at time of standardization. Susp. Vial 5 ml.
Use: Radiopharmaceutical.

PHOSPHOCYSTEAMINE.
Use: Cystinosis. [Orphan drug]

PHOSPHOLINE IODIDE. (Wyeth-Ayerst) Echothiophate Iodide for Ophthalmic Solution. Sterile echothiophate iodide powder w/potassium acetate 40 mg, diluent: chlorobutanol 0.5%, mannitol 1.2%, boric acid 0.06%, sodium phosphate exsiccated 0.026% for preparing 0.03%, 0.06%, 0.125% and 0.25% potencies/5 ml of sterile eye drops. Pack-

age: 1.5 mg for 0.03%; 3 mg for 0.06%;
6.25 mg for 0.125%; 12.5 mg for 0.25%.
Use: Agent for glaucoma.
PHOSPHOLIPIDS, SOY.
See: Granulestin Concentrate, Gran.
(Associated Concentrates).
**PHOSPHORATED CARBOHYDRATE
SOLUTION.**
See: Emetrol, Liq. (Bock).
Naus-A-Way, Soln. (Hauck).
Nausetrol, Soln. (Various Mfr.).
• **PHOSPHORIC ACID,** N.F. XVIII.
Use: Solvent.
• **PHOSPHORIC ACID, DILUTED,** N.F.
XVIII.
Use: Pharmaceutic aid (solvent).
PHOSPHORUS.
Use: Phosphorus replacement.
See: Uro-KP-Neutral, Tab. (Star).
K-Phos Neutral, Tab. (Beach).
Neutra-Phos, Cap., Pow. (Willen).
Neutra-Phos-K, Cap., Pow. (Willen).
PHOSPHO-SODA. (Fleet) Sodium
biphosphate 48 Gm, sodium phosphate
18 Gm/100 ml. Bot. 1.5 oz, 3 oz, 8 oz.
Flavored, unflavored.
Use: Laxative.
PHOSPHOTEC. (Squibb) Technetium Tc
99m pyrophosphate kit. 10 vials/kit.
Use: Radiodiagnostic.
PHOTOPLEX SUNSCREEN. (Herbert)
Butyl methoxydibenzoylmethane 3%,
padimate O 7%. Lot. 120 ml.
Use: Sunscreen.
PHRENILIN FORTE CAPSULES. (Carn-
rick) Acetaminophen 650 mg, butalbital
50 mg/Cap. Bot. 100s.
Use: Analgesic, sedative/hypnotic.
PHRENILIN TABLETS. (Carnrick) Butal-
bital 50 mg, acetaminophen 325
mg/Tab. Bot. 100s.
Use: Sedative/hypnotic, analgesic.
PHRENILIN WITH CODEINE #3. (Carnrick) Acetaminophen 325 mg, butalbital
50 mg, codeine phosphate 30 mg/Cap.
Bot. 100s.
Use: Narcotic analgesic combination,
sedative/hypnotic.
**PHRESH 3.5 FINNISH CLEANSING LIQ-
UID.** (3M Products) Water, cocamidopropyl betaine, lactic acid, polyoxyethylene distearate, polyoxyethylene monostearate, hydroxyethyl cellulose, sodium
phosphate, methylparaben. Bot. 6 oz.
Use: Soapless cleansing agent.
pH-STABIL CREAM. (Hermal) Skin protection cream. Bot. 8 oz. Tube 2 oz.
Use: Skin protectant.
PHTHALAMAQUIN. (Penick) Quinetolate.

Use: Antiasthmatic.
**PHTHALAZINE, I-HYDRAZINO-, MONO-
HYDRO-CHLORIDE.** Hydralazine Hy-
drochloride, U.S.P. XXIII.
PHTHALYLSULFACETAMIDE. 4'-
(Acetylsulfamoyl) phthalanilic acid. En-
terosulfon.
PHYLCARDIN.
See: Aminophylline (Various Mfr.).
PHYLLINDON.
See: Aminophylline (Various Mfr.).
PHYLLOCONTIN. (Purdue Frederick)
Aminophylline 225 mg/CR Tab. Bot.
100s.
Use: Bronchodilator.
PHYLLOQUINONE. 2-Methyl-3-phytyl-
1,4-naphthoquinine, vitamin K.
See: Phytonadione, U.S.P., Inj., Tab.
(Various Mfr.).
Vitamin K-1 (Various Mfr.).
PHYLORINOL. (Schaffer) Phenol 0.6%,
boric acid, strong iodine solution, sor-
bitol 70% solution, sodium copper
chlorophyll.
Use: Mouth and throat product.
**PHYSIOLOGICAL IRRIGATING SOLU-
TION.**
See: TIS-U-SOL, Soln. (Travenol).
Physiosol, Soln. (Abbott).
Physiolyte, Soln. (American McGaw).
PHYSIOLYTE. (American McGaw) Sodi-
um Cl 530 mg, sodium acetate 370 mg,
sodium gluconate 500 mg, potassium Cl
37 mg, magnesium Cl 30 mg/100 ml.
Soln. Bot. 500 ml, 2 L, 4 L.
Use: Irrigating solution.
PHYSIOSOL IRRIGATION. (Abbott Hos-
pital Prods.) Bot. 250 ml, 500 ml, 1000
ml glass or Aqualite (semi-rigid) contain-
ers.
Use: Irrigating solution.
• **PHYSOSTIGMINE,** U.S.P. XXIII. Pyrrolo
[2,3-b] indol-5-ol methylcarbamate (ester), (3as-cis). 1,2,3a β,8,8aβ-Hexahy-
dro-1,3a,8-trimethyl-pyrrolo[2,3-b]-indol-
5yl-methylcarbamate. An alkaloid.
Use: Parasympathomimetic agent.
• **PHYSOSTIGMINE SALICYLATE,** U.S.P.
XXIII. Inj., Ophth. Soln., U.S.P. XXIII.
Pyrrolo[2,3-b]indol-5-ol,1,2,3,3a,8,8a-
hexahydro-1,3a,8-trimethyl-, methylcarbamate (ester), (3aS-cis)-,mono(2-hy-
droxybenzoate). Physostigmine mono-
salicylate. Eserine salicylate.
(Forest)—Pow., Tube 1 gr, 5 gr, 15 gr.
Use: Parasympathomimetic agent,
Friedreich's and other inherited ataxi-
as [Orphan drug]
See: Antilirium, Amp. (Forest).
Isopto-Eserine, Ophthalmic, Soln. (Al-

con).
W/Atropine sulfate.
See: Atrophysine, Inj. (Lannett).
W/I-Hyoscyamine HBr.
See: Phyatromine-H, Amp., Vial (Kremers-Urban).
W/Pilocarpine, methylcellulose.
See: Isopto P-ES, Soln. (Alcon).
• **PHYSOSTIGMINE SULFATE,** U.S.P. XXIII. Ophth. Oint., U.S.P. XXIII. Pyrrolo[2,3-b]indol-5-ol, 1,2,3,3a, 8,8a-hexahydro-1,3a,8-trimethyl-, methylcarbamate (ester), (3aS-cis)-,sulfate (2:1).
Use: Cholinergic (ophthalmic).
• **PHYTATE PERSODIUM.** USAN.
Use: Pharmaceutic aid.
• **PHYTATE SODIUM.** USAN. Sodium salt of inositol hexaphosphoric acid.
Use: Chelating agent (calcium).
PHYTIC ACID. Inositol hexophosphoric acid.
PHYTOMENADIONE. B.A.N. 2-Methyl-3-phytyl-1,4-naphthaquinone. Vitamin K Konakion; Mephyton.
Use: Antidote to anticoagulants.
PHYTONADIOL SODIUM DIPHOSPHATE. Disodium salt of 2-methyl-3-phytyl-1,4-naphthohydroquinone $0^1,0^4$-diphosphoric acid.
• **PHYTONADIONE,** U.S.P. XXIII. Inj., Tab., U.S.P. XXIII. Vitamin K 1,4-Naphthalenediono, 2-methyl-3-(3,7,11,15-tetramethyl-2-hexadecenyl)-,[R-[R*,R*-(E)]]-. Phylloquinone. 2-Methyl-3-phytyl-1,4-naphthoquinone.
Use: Prothrombogenic.
See: Aquamephyton, Inj. (Merck & Co.).
Konakion, Amp. (Roche).
Mephyton, Tab. (Merck & Co.).
• **PICENADOL HYDROCHLORIDE.** USAN.
Use: Analgesic.
PICLOXYDINE. B.A.N. NN'-Di-(p-Chlorophenyl-guanidinoformimidoyl)-piperazine. 1,4-Di-(4-chloro-phenyl-guanidinoformimidoyl)piperazine.
Use: Bactericide; fungicide.
• **PICOTRIN DIOLAMINE.** USAN.
Use: Keratolytic.
PICRIC ACID, TRINITROPHENOL.
See: Butesyn Picrate, Oint. (Abbott).
Silver Salts (Various Prods.).
PICROTOXIN. Cocculin.
Use: Respiratory stimulant.
P.I.D.
See: Phenindione (Various Mfr.).
PIFARNINE. USAN.
Use: Anti-ulcerative.
PIFENATE. B.A.N. Ethyl 2,2-diphenyl-3-(2-piperidyl)propionate.
Use: Analgesic.

PILAGAN. (Allergan) Pilocarpine nitrate 1%, 2% or 4%. Soln. Bot. 15 ml.
Use: Agent for glaucoma.
PILE-GON. (E.J. Moore) Bismuth subgallate, balsam peru, zinc oxide, cod liver oil in petrolatum base. Tube 1.25 oz.
Use: Anorectal preparation.
PILOCAR. (Iolab) Pilocarpine HCl 0.5%, 1%, 2%, 3%, 4% or 6%. Bot. 15 ml; Twinpack 2 × 15 ml 0.5%, 1%, 2%, 3%, 4% or 6%; 1 ml Dropperettes 1%, 2%, 3% or 4%. Box 12s.
Use: Agent for glaucoma.
• **PILOCARPINE,** U.S.P. XXIII. Ocular system U.S.P. XXIII.
Use: Ophthalmic cholinergic, miotic.
See: Ocusert Pilo-20 and Pilo-40 (Ciba).
• **PILOCARPINE HYDROCHLORIDE,** U.S.P. XXIII. Ophth. Soln., U.S.P. XXIII. (Various Mfr.) Pilocarpine muriate.
Use: Cholinergic 0.5% to 8.0% soln. topically as a miotic, xerostomia and keratoconjunctivitis sicca [Orphan drug]
See: Almocarpine (Wyeth-Ayerst).
Isopto-Carpine, Ophthalmic (Alcon).
Mi-Pilo, Soln.(Barnes-Hind).
Pilocar, Soln. (CooperVision).
Pilomiotin, Soln. (CooperVision).
Piloptic, Soln. (Muro).
Salagen, Tab. (MGI Pharma).
W/Epinephrine HCl.
See: E-Carpine, Inj. (Alcon).
Epicar, Ophthalmic Soln. (Barnes-Hind).
W/Epinephrine bitartrate, mannitol, benzalkonium Cl.
See: E-Pilo, Soln. (CooperVision).
W/Physostigmine salicylate, methylcellulose.
See: Isopto P-ES, Soln. (Alcon).
• **PILOCARPINE NITRATE,** U.S.P. XXIII. Ophth. Soln., U.S.P. XXIII.
Use: Cholinergic (ophthalmic).
See: P.V. Carpine (Allergan).
W/Phenylephrine HCl.
Use: Parasympathomimetic agent.
See: Pilofrin Liquifilm, Ophthalmic (Allergan).
PILOPINE. (International Pharm.) Pilocarpine HCl 1%, 2% or 4%. Soln. Bot. 15 ml.
Use: Agent for glaucoma.
PILOPINE HS GEL. (Alcon) Pilocarpine HCl 4%. Tube 5 Gm.
Use: Agent for glaucoma.
PILOPTIC-1. (Optopics) Pilocarpine HCl 1%. Soln. Bot. 15 ml.
Use: Agent for glaucoma.

PILOPTIC-2. (Optopics) Pilocarpine HCl 2%. Soln. Bot. 15 ml.
Use: Agent for glaucoma.
PILOSTAT. (Bausch & Lomb) Pilocarpine HCl 1%, 2% or 4%. Soln. Bot. 15 ml, twin pack 15 ml.
Use: Agent for glaucoma.
PIMA SYRUP (Fleming) Potassium iodide 5 gr/5 ml. Bot. pt, gal.
Use: Expectorant.
• **PIMAGEDINE HYDROCHLORIDE.** USAN.
Use: Treatment of diabetic complications (advanced glycosylation end-product formation inhibitors).
• **PIMETINE HYDROCHLORIDE.** USAN. 4-Benzyl-1-(2-dimethylaminoethyl)piperidine HCl.
Use: Cardiovascular drug (anticholesteremic).
PIMINODINE. B.A.N. 1-(3-Phenylamino) propyl-4-phenylpiperidine-4-carboxylic acid ethyl ester. Ethyl 4-phenyl-1-(3-phenylaminopropyl)piperidine-4-carboxylate.
Use: Narcotic analgesic.
PIMINODINE ESYLATE. Ethyl 1-(30 anilinopropyl)-4-phenylisonipecotate monoethanesulfonate.
Use: Analgesic.
PIMINODINE ETHANESULFONATE. Ethyl-4-phenyl-1-[3-(phenylamino)propyl]-piperidine-4-carboxylate ethanesulfonate.
Use: Narcotic analgesic.
• **PIMOBENDAN.** USAN.
Use: Cardiotonic.
• **PIMOZIDE,** U.S.P. XXIII, Tab., USAN. 1-[1-[4,4-bis(p-Fluorophenyl)butyl]-4-piperidyl]-2-benzimidazoline. Orap.
Use: Tranquilizer.
See: Orap, Tab. (McNeil Pharm).
• **PINACIDIL.** USAN.
Use: Antihypertensive.
• **PINADOLINE.** USAN.
Use: Analgesic.
• **PINDOLOL,** U.S.P. XXIII. Tab., U.S.P. XXIII. 1-(Indol-4-yloxy)-3-(isopropyl-amino)-2-propanol.
Use: Beta-adrenergic blocking agent.
See: Visken (Sandoz).
• **PINE NEEDLE OIL,** N.F. XVIII.
Use: Perfume; flavor.
PINE TAR, U.S.P. XXI.
Use: Local anti-eczematic; rubefacient.
PINEX CONCENTRATE COUGH SYRUP. (Last) Dextromethorphan HBr 7.5 mg/5 ml (after diluting 3 oz. concentrate to make 16 oz. solution). Bot. 3 oz.
Use: Antitussive.

PINEX COUGH SYRUP. (Last) Dextromethorphan HBr 7.5 mg/5 ml. Bot. 3 oz, 6 oz.
Use: Antitussive.
PINEX REGULAR. (Pinex) Potassium guaiacolsulfonate, oil of pine and eucalyptus, extract of grindelia, alcohol 3%/30 ml. Syr. Bot. 3 oz, 6 oz. Also cherry flavored 3 oz. Super and concentrated 3 oz.
Use: Expectorant.
• **PINOXEPIN HCl.** USAN.
Use: Tranquilizer.
PIN-RID. (Apothecary) **Soft gelcap.:** Pyrantel pamoate 180 mg (equivalent to 62.5 mg pyrantel base). Pkg. 24s; **Liq.:** Pyrantel pamoate 144 mg/ml (equivalent to 50 mg/ml pyrantel base). Bot. 30 ml.
Use: Anthelmintic.
PIN-X. (Effcon) Pyrantel base (as pamoate) 50 mg/ml. Liq. Bot. 30 ml.
Use: Anthelmintic.
PIPAMAZINE. B.A.N. 1-[3-(2-Chlorophenothiazin-10-yl)-propyl] isonipecotramide. 10-[3-(4-Carbamoylpiperidino)propyl]-2-chlorophenothiazine. Mornidine.
Use: Antiemetic.
• **PIPAMPERONE.** USAN. 1'-[3-(p-Fluorobenzoyl)propyl][1,4-bipiperidine]-4-carboxamide. Under study.
Use: Tranquilizer.
• **PIPAZETHATE.** USAN. 2-(2-Piperidinoethoxy)-ethyl pyrido[3,2-b][1,4]benzothiazine-10-carboxylate. Selvigon HCl.
Use: Cough suppressant.
PIPAZETHATE HYDROCHLORIDE. 2-(2-Piperidinoethoxy)ethyl-10-H-pyrido [3,2-b]-[1,4]benzothiazine-10-carboxylate HCl.
Use: Antitussive.
• **PIPECURONIUM BROMIDE.** (Gedeon Richter, Hungary; Organon) USAN.
Use: Muscle relaxant.
PIPENZOLATE BROMIDE. B.A.N. 1-Ethyl-3-piperidyl benzilate methylbromide. 3-Benziloyloxy-1-ethyl-1-methylpiperidinium bromide.
Use: Anticholinergic.
• **PIPERACILLIN SODIUM, STERILE,** U.S.P. XXIII.
Use: Antibacterial.
W/ Tazobactam
See: Zosyn, Inj. (Lederle).
• **PIPERAMIDE MALEATE.** USAN. 4'-[4-[3-(Dimethylamino)propyl]-1-piperazinyl]acetanilide dimaleate.
Use: Antiparasitic.
• **PIPERAZINE,** U.S.P. XXIII.

Use: Anthelmintic.
PIPERAZINE CALCIUM EDETATE.
B.A.N.
[Dihydrogen(ethylenedinitrilo)tetraacetato]-calcium piperazine salt. Perin.
Use: Anthelmintic.
•**PIPERAZINE CITRATE,** U.S.P. XXIII.
Syr., Tab., U.S.P. XXIII. Piperazine, 2-
hydroxy-1,2,3-propanetricarboxylate
(3:2) hydrate. Piperazine citrate (3:2) hydrate. Piperazine Citrate Telra Hydrous
Tripiperazine Dicitrate.
Use: Anthelmintic.
See: Bryrel, Syr. (Sanofi Winthrop).
Pipril, Liq. (Kenyon).
Ta-Verm, Syr., Tab. (Table Rock).
Vermago, Syr. (Westerfield).
•**PIPERAZINE EDETATE CALCIUM.**
USAN. Dihydrogen
[(ethylenedinitrilo)tetraacetato]calciate(2-) compound with piperazine (1:1).
Perin.
Use: Anthelmintic
PIPERAZINE ESTRONE SULFATE.
See: Estropipitate.
PIPERAZINE HEXAHYDRATE. Tivazine.
PIPERAZINE PHOSPHATE.
Use: Anthelmintic.
PIPERAZINE TARTRATE.
See: Razine Tartrate, Tab. (Paddock).
PIPERIDINE PHOSPHATE.
Use: Psychlatric drug.
PIPERIDINOETHYL BENZILATE HCl. No
products listed.
PIPERIDOLATE. B.A.N. 1-Ethyl-3-
piperidyl diphenylacetate.
Use: Parasympatholytic.
PIPERIDOLATE HYDROCHLORIDE. 1-
Ethyl-3-piperidyl diphenylacetate HCl.
Use: Anticholinergic.
PIPEROCAINE. B.A.N. 3-(2-
Methylpiperidino)-propyl benzoate.
Use: Local anesthetic.
PIPERONYL BUTOXIDE. B.A.N. 5-[2-(2-
Butoxy-ethoxy)ethoxymethyl]-6-propyl-
1,3-benzodioxole.
Use: Pediculicide.
W/ Pyrethrins.
See: InnoGel Plus (Hogil Pharm.).
Tegrin-LT, Shampoo/Cond. (Block).
PIPEROXAN. B.A.N. 2-Piperidinomethyl-
1,4-benzodioxan.
Use: Adrenergic blocking agent.
PIPEROXAN HYDROCHLORIDE. 2-(1-
Piperidylmethyl)-1,4-benzodioxan HCl.
Fourneau 933. Benzodioxane. Diagnosis of hypertension.
Use: Diagnostic aid.
PIPERPHENIDOL HCl. 5-Methyl-4-
phenyl-1-(1-piperidyl)-3-hexanol HCl.

PIPETHANATE HCl. 2-Piperidinoethyl
benzilate HCl.
Use: Tranquilizer.
•**PIPOBROMAN,** U.S.P. XXII. Tab., U.S.P.
XXII. 1,4-Bis(3-bromopropionyl)piperazine. D2,a-thiazolidine-acetate.
Use: Antineoplastic.
See: Vercyte, Tab. (Abbott).
•**PIPOSULFAN.** USAN. 1,4-Dihydracryloylpiperazine dimethanesulfonate.
Use: Antineoplastic agent.
PIPOTHIAZINE. B.A.N. 2-Dimethylsulfamoyl-10-3-[4-(2-hydroxyethyl)piperidino]propyl phenothiazine.
Use: Neuroleptic.
•**PIPOTIAZINE PALMITATE.** USAN.
Use: Antipsychotic.
See: Piportil (Ives).
•**PIPOXOLAN HCl.** USAN. 5,5-Diphenyl-
2-(2- piperidinoethyl)-1,3-dioxolan-4-one
HCl. Rowapraxin.
Use: Muscle relaxant.
PIPRACIL. (Lederle) Piperacillin sodium
2 Gm, 3 Gm, 4 Gm or 40 Gm/Vial, 2 Gm,
3 Gm or 4 Gm/Infusion Bottle. Sterile.
Use: Antibacterial, penicillin.
PIPRADOL. B.A.N. α-2-Piperidylbenzhydrol.
Use: Central nervous system stimulant.
PIPRIL. (Kenyon) Piperazine citrate 0.5
Gm/5 ml. Bot. pt, gal.
Use: Anthelmintic.
PIPRINHYDRINATE. B.A.N.
Diphenylpyraline salt of 8-chlorotheopylline. 4-Benzyhydryloxy-1-methylpiperidine salt of 8-chlortheophylline. Kolton;
Mepedyl.
Use: Antihistamine.
•**PIPROZOLIN.** USAN. Ethyl 3-ethyl-4-
oxo-5-piperidino D2, alpha-thiazolidineacetate.
Use: Choleretic.
•**PIQUINDONE HYDROCHLORIDE.**
USAN.
Use: Antipsychotic.
•**PIQUIZIL HCl.** USAN. Isobutyl 4-(6,7-
dimethoxy-4-quinazolinyl)-1-piperazinecarboxylate monohydrochloride.
Use: Bronchodilator.
•**PIRACETAM.** USAN. 2-Oxopyrrolidin-1-
ylacetamide. Nootropyl.
Use: Cerebral stimulant, myoclonus
[Orphan drug]
•**PIRANDAMINE HYDROCHLORIDE.**
USAN.
Use: Antidepressant.
•**PIRAZMONAM SODIUM.** USAN.
Use: Antimicrobial.
•**PIRAZOLAC.** USAN.
Use: Antirheumatic.

• **PIRBENICILLIN SODIUM.** USAN.
Use: Antibacterial.
• **PIRBUTEROL ACETATE.** USAN. 2-tert-
Butylamino-1-(5-hydroxy-6-hydrox-
ymethyl-2-pyridyl)ethanol acetate.
Use: Bronchodilator.
• **PIRBUTEROL HYDROCHLORIDE.**
USAN.
Use: Bronchodilator.
• **PIRENPERONE.** USAN.
Use: Tranquilizer.
• **PIRENZEPINE HYDROCHLORIDE.**
USAN.
Use: Antiulcerative.
• **PIRETANIDE.** USAN.
Use: Diuretic.
See: Arlix, Prods. (Hoechst).
• **PIRFENIDONE.** USAN.
Use: Anti-inflammatory, antipyretic.
PIRIDAZOL.
See: Sulfapyridine, Tab. (Various Mfr.).
• **PIRIDICILLIN SODIUM.** USAN.
Use: Antibacterial.
PIRIDOCAINE HCl. Beta-(2-Piperidyl)
ethyl-o-aminobenzoate.
PIRIDOXILATE. B.A.N. The reciprocal
salt of (5-hydroxy-4-hydroxymethyl-6-
methyl-3-pyridyl)-meth-oxyglycolic acid
with [4,5-bis(hydroxymethyl)-2-methyl-3-
pyridyl] oxyglycolicacid (1:1). GLYO-6.
Use: Treatment of angina.
• **PIRIDRONATE SODIUM.** USAN.
Use: Regulator (calcium).
• **PIRIPROST.** USAN.
Use: Antiasthmatic.
• **PIRIPROST POTASSIUM.** USAN.
Use: Antiasthmatic.
PIRITON.
See: Chlorpheniramine (Various Mfr.).
PIRITRAMIDE. B.A.N. 4-(4-Carbamoyl-4-
piperidino-piperidino)-2,2-diphenylbuty-
ronitrile. Dipodolor.
Use: Analgesic.
• **PIRITREXIM ISETHIONATE.** USAN.
Use: Antiproliferative agent. [Orphan
drug]
• **PIRLIMYCIN HYDROCHLORIDE.** USAN.
Use: Antibacterial.
• **PIRMAGREL.** USAN.
Use: Inhibitor (thromboxane syn-
thetase).
• **PIRMENOL HYDROCHLORIDE.** USAN.
Use: Cardiac depressant.
• **PIRNABINE.** USAN.
Use: Antiglaucoma agent.
• **PIROCTONE.** USAN.
Use: Antiseborrheic.
• **PIROCTONE OLAMINE.** USAN.
Use: Antiseborrheic.

PIRODAVIR. (Janssen) USAN.
Use: Antiviral agent.
• **PIROGLIRIDE TARTRATE.** USAN.
Use: Antidiabetic.
• **PIROLATE.** USAN.
Use: Antiasthmatic.
• **PIROLAZAMIDE.** USAN.
Use: Cardiac depressant.
• **PIROXANTRONE HYDROCHLORIDE.**
USAN.
Use: Antineoplastic.
• **PIROXICAM,** U.S.P. XXIII. Cap., U.S.P.
XXIII. N-pyridyl-methyl-hydroxy-(ben-
zothiazine-1 idioxide)carboxamide. (Var-
ious Mfr.) 10 mg or 20 mg. Cap. Bot.
100s, 500s.
Use: Anti-inflammatory.
See: Feldene, Cap. (Pfizer).
• **PIROXICAM CINNAMATE.** USAN.
Use: Anti-inflammatory.
• **PIROXICAM OLAMINE.** USAN.
Use: Anti-inflammatory, analgesic.
• **PIROXIMONE.** USAN.
Use: Cardiotonic.
• **PIRPROFEN.** USAN.
Use: Anti-inflammatory.
See: Rengasil (Geigy).
• **PIRQUINOZOL.** USAN.
Use: Anti-allergic.
PIRSIDOMINE. (Hoechst AG) USAN.
Use: Vasodilator.
PISO's. (Pinex) Ipecac, ammonium Cl,
menthol in syrup base. Bot. 3 oz, 5 oz.
Use: Expectorant.
PITAYINE.
See: Quinidine, Preps. (Various Mfr.).
PITOCIN. (Parke-Davis) Oxytocin
w/chlorobutanol 0.5%, acetic acid to ad-
just pH. Amp. 5 units/0.5 ml; 10 units/1
ml. Box 10s, Steri-dose syringe; 10
units/1 ml 10s.
Use: Oxytocic.
PITRESSIN SYNTHETIC. (Parke-Davis)
Vasopressin w/chlorobutanol 0.5%, pH
adjusted with acetic acid. Amp. 0.5 ml
(10 pressor units), 1 ml (20 pressor
units). Box 10s.
Use: Posterior pituitary hormones.
PITTS CARMINATIVE. (Commerce) Bot.
2 oz.
Use: Antiflatulent.
PITUITARY, ANTERIOR. The anterior
lobe of the pituitary gland supplies pro-
tein hormones classified under following
headings.
See: Corticotropin, Preps. (Various
Mfr.).
Gonadotropin, Preps. (Various Mfr.).
Growth Hormone.
Thyrotropic Principle.

PITUITARY FUNCTION TEST.
See: Metopirone, Tab. (Ciba).
PITUITARY, POSTERIOR, HORMONES.
(a) Vasopressin. Pressor principle, β-hypophamine, postlobin-V.
See: Pitressin, Amp. (Parke-Davis).
(b) Oxytocin. Oxytocic principle. α-hypophamine, postiobin-O.
See: Oxytocin, Inj. (Various Mfr.).
Pitocin, Amp. (Parke-Davis).
Syntocinon, Amp. (Sandoz).
• **PITUITARY, POSTERIOR, INJECTION,** U.S.P. XXIII.
Use: Hormone (antidiuretic).
See: Pituitrin, Obstetrical, Amp. (Parke-Davis).
Pituitrin, Surgical, Amp. (Parke-Davis).
• **PIVAMPICILLIN HYDROCHLORIDE.** USAN.
Use: Antibacterial.
• **PIVAMPICILLIN PAMOATE.** USAN.
Use: Antibacterial.
• **PIVAMPICILLIN PROBENATE.** USAN.
Use: Antibacterial.
PIVAZIDE. N-Benzyl-N'-pivaloylhydrazine. Tersavid.
PIVHYDRAZINE. B.A.N. 1-Benzyl-2-pivaloyl hydrazine.
Use: Monoamine oxidase inhibitor.
PIVMECILLINAM. B.A.N. Pivaloyloxymethyl (2S,5R,6R)-6-(perhydroazepin-1-ylmethyleneamino)-penicillanate.
Use: Antibiotic.
• **PIVOPRIL.** USAN.
Use: Antihypertensive.
PIX CARBONIS.
See: Coal Tar, Preps. (Various Mfr.).
PIX JUNIPERI.
Use: Sunscreen, moisturizer.
See: Juniper Tar, Comp. (Various Mfr.).
PIZOTIFEN. B.A.N. 4-(9,10-Dihydrobenzo[4,5]-cyclohepta[1,2-b]thien-4-ylidene)-1-methylpiperidine.
Use: Prophylaxis of migraine.
• **PIZOTYLINE.** USAN. 4-(9,10-Dihydro-4H-benzo[4,5]-cyclohepta[1,2-b]thien-4-ylidene)-1-methylpiperdine.
Use: Anabolic, antidepressant, migraine prophylactic.
PLACEBO CAPSULES. (Cowley) No. 3 orange red; No. 4 yellow. Bot. 1000s.
Use: Placebo.
PLACEBO TABLETS. (Cowley) 1 gr white; 2 gr white; 3 gr white, red or yellow, pink, orange; 4 gr white; 5 gr white. Bot. 1000s.
Use: Placebo.
PLACENTA.
See: Gonadotropins, Chorionic, Inj.

(Various Mfr.).
PLACIDYL. (Abbott) Ethchlorvynol. **200 mg/Cap.:** Bot. 100s. **500 mg/Cap.:** Bot. 100s, 500s, UD 100s. **750 mg/Cap.:** Bot. 100s.
Use: Sedative/hypnotic.
• **PLAGUE VACCINE,** U.S.P. XXIII. (Cutter) 2000 million killed *Pasteurella pestis*/ml. Vial 2 ml, 20 ml.
Use: S.C. vaccination, active immunizing agent.
PLANOCAINE.
See: Procaine HCl, Preps. (Various Mfr.).
PLANOCHROME.
See: Merbromin, Soln. (Various Mfr.).
PLANTAGO, OVATA COATING.
See: Effersyllium, Prods. (Stuart).
Konsyl, Pow. (Burton, Parsons).
L.A. Formula, Pow. (Burton, Parsons).
Metamucil, Pow. (Searle).
W/Psyllium seed, gum karaya, Brewer's yeast.
See: Plantamucin, Gran. (Elder).
W/Vitamin B₁.
See: Siblin, Gran. (Parke-Davis).
• **PLANTAGO SEED,** U.S.P. XXIII. Psyllium Seed, Plantain Seed.
Use: Fecal softener.
PLANT PROTEASE CONCENTRATE.
See: Ananase, Tab. (Rhone-Poulenc Rorer).
PLAQUENIL SULFATE. (Winthrop-Breon) Hydroxychloroquine sulfate 200 mg/Tab. (equivalent to base 155 mg). Bot. 100s.
Use: Antimalarial, antirheumatic.
PLAQUENIL TABLET. (Sanofi Winthrop.) Hydroxychloroquine sulfate.
Use: Antimalarial, antirheumatic.
PLASBUMIN-5. (Cutter) Normal serum albumin (Human) 5% U.S.P. fractionated from normal serum plasma, heat treated against hepatitis virus. Albumin 12.5 Gm/250 ml. Vial 50 ml. Bot. with IV set 250 ml, 500 ml.
Use: Plasma protein fraction.
PLASBUMIN-25. (Cutter) Normal serum albumin (Human) 25% U.S.P. fractionated from normal serum plasma, heat treated against hepatitis virus. Albumin 12.5 Gm/50 ml. Vial 20 ml. Bot. with IV set 50 ml, 100 ml.
Use: Plasma protein fraction.
PLASMA.
See: Normal Human Plasma (Various Mfr.).
PLASMA EXPANDERS OR SUBSTITUTES.
See: Dextran 6% and LMD 10% (Ab-

bott).

Macrodex, Soln. (Pharmacia).

PLASMA-LYTE A INJECTION. (Travenol) Sodium 140 mEq, potassium 5 mEq, magnesium 3 mEq, chloride 98 mEq, acetate 27 mEq, gluconate 23 mEq/L w/pH adjusted to 7.4. Plastic bot. 500 ml, 1000 ml.
Use: Parenteral nutritional supplement.

PLASMA-LYTE 148 INJECTION. (Travenol) Sodium 140 mEq, potassium 5 mEq, magnesium 3 mEq, chloride 98 mEq, acetate 27 mEq, gluconate 23 mEq/L. Plastic bot. 500 ml, 1000 ml.
Use: Parenteral nutritional supplement.

PLASMA-LYTE M and 5% DEXTROSE INJECTION. (Travenol) Sodium 40 mEq, potassium 16 mEq, calcium 5 mEq, magnesium 3 mEq, chloride 40 mEq, acetate 12 mEq, lactate 12 mEq/L. Plastic bot. 500 ml, 1000 ml.
Use: Parenteral nutritional supplement.

PLASMA-LYTE R and 5% DEXTROSE INJECTION. (Travenol) Sodium 140 mEq, potassium 10 mEq, calcium 5 mEq, magnesium 3 mEq, chloride 103 mEq, acetate 47 mEq, lactate 8 mEq/L. Bot. 500 ml, 1000 ml.
Use: Parenteral nutritional supplement.

PLASMA-LYTE 56 and 5% DEXTROSE. (Travenol) Sodium 40 mEq, potassium 13 mEq, magnesium 3 mEq, chloride 40 mEq, acetate 16 mEq/L. Plastic bot. 500 ml, 1000 ml.
Use: Parenteral nutritional supplement.

PLASMA-LYTE 148 AND 5% DEXTROSE. (Travenol) Dextrose 50 Gm, calories 190, sodium 140 mEq, potassium 5 mEq, magnesium 3 mEq, chloride 98 mEq, acetate 27 mEq, 547 mOsm, gluconate 23 mEq/L. Soln. Bot. 500 ml, 1000 ml.
Use: Parenteral nutritional supplement.

PLASMA-LYTE 56 IN WATER. (Travenol) Sodium 40 mEq, potassium 13 mEq, magnesium 3 mEq, chloride 40 mEq, acetate 16 mEq/L. Plastic bot. 500 ml, 1000 ml.
Use: Parenteral nutritional supplement.

PLASMA-LYTE R INJECTION. (Travenol) Sodium 140 mEq, potassium 10 mEq, calcium 5 mEq, magnesium 3 mEq, chloride 103 mEq, acetate 47 mEq, lactate 8 mEq/L. Bot. 1000 ml.
Use: Parenteral nutritional supplement.

PLASMANATE. (Cutter) Plasma protein fraction (Human) 5%. U.S.P. Vial 50 ml. Bot. 250 ml, 500 ml with set.
Use: Plasma protein fraction.

PLASMA-PLEX. (Armour) Plasma pro-

tein fraction 5%. Inj. Vial 250 ml, 500 ml.
Use: Plasma protein fraction.

• **PLASMA PROTEIN FRACTION,** U.S.P. XXIII. (Hyland) For the plasma protein preparation obtained from human plasma using the Cohn fractionation technic. Bot. 250 ml.
Use: Blood-volume supporter.
See: Plasmanate, Soln. (Cutter).
Plasma-Plex, Soln. (Armour).
Plasmatein (Abbott).

PLASMATEIN. (Alpha Therapeutic) Plasma protein fraction 5%. Inj. Vial w/injection set 250 ml, 500 ml.
Use: Plasma protein fraction.

PLASMIN. B.A.N. The proteolytic enzyme derived from the activation of plasminogen. Actase is Plasmin (Human).

PLASMINOGEN. B.A.N. The specific substance derived from plasma which, when activated, has the property of lysing fibrinogen, fibrin, and some other proteins.

PLASMOCHIN NAPHTHOATE. Pamaquine naphthoate.
Use: Antimalarial.

• **PLATELET CONCENTRATE,** U.S.P. XXIII.
Use: Platelet replenisher.

PLATELET FACTOR 4. (Abbott Diagnostics) Radioimmunoassay for quantitative measurement of total PF4 levels in plasma. Test kit 100s.
Use: Diagnostic aid.

PLATINOL. (Bristol-Myers/Bristol Oncology) Cisplatin 10 mg or 50 mg/Vial.
Use: Antineoplastic agent.

PLATINOL-AQ. (Bristol-Myers Oncology) Cisplatin (CDDP) 1 mg/ml. Inj. Vial. 50 ml, 100 ml.
Use: Antineoplastic agent.

• **PLAURACIN.** USAN.
Use: Growth stimulant.

PLEGISOL. (Abbott Hospital Prods) Calcium Cl dihydrate 17.6 mg, magnesium Cl hexahydrate 325.3 mg, potassium Cl 119.3 mg, sodium Cl 643 mg/100 ml. Approximately 260 mOsm/L. Single Dose Container 1000 ml without sodium bicarbonate.
Use: Cardioplegic solution.

PLENDIL. (Merck & Co.) **ER Tab.:** Felodipine 5 mg. Bot. 30s, 100s, UD 100s. **Tab.:** Felodipine 10 mg. Bot. 30s, 100s, UD 100s.
Use: Calcium channel blocking agent.

PLEWIN TABLETS. (Sanofi Winthrop) Glycobiarsol, chloroquine phosphate.
Use: Amebicide.

PLEXOLAN CREAM. (Last) Zinc oxide,

lanolin. Tube 1.25 oz, 3 oz. Jar 16 oz.
Use: Skin protectant.

PLEXON. (Sig) Testosterone 10 mg, estrone 1 mg, liver 2 mcg, pyridoxine HCl 10 mg, panthenol 10 mg, inositol 20 mg, choline Cl 20 mg, vitamin B_2 2 mg, B_{12} 100 mcg, procaine HCl 1%, niacinamide 100 mg/ml. Vial 10 ml.
Use: Hormone, vitamin/mineral supplement.

PLIAGEL. (Alcon) Sodium Cl, potassium Cl, poloxamer 407, sorbic acid 0.25%, EDTA 0.5%. Soln. Bot. 25 ml.
Use: Soft contact lens care.

• **PLICAMYCIN,** U.S.P. XXIII. Inj. U.S.P. XXIII. Antibiotic derived from *Streptomyces agrillaceus* & *S. tanashiensis.*
Use: Antineoplastic.
See: Mithracin, Pow. (Miles Pharm).

• **PLOMESTANE.** USAN.
Use: Antineoplastic (aromatase inhibitor).

PLOVA. (Washington Ethical) Psyllium mucilloid. Pow. (flavored) 12 oz., (plain) 10 0.5 oz.
Use: Laxative.

PLURAVIT DROPS. (Sanofi Winthrop) Multivitamin.
Use: Vitamin supplement.

PMB 200. (Wyeth-Ayerst) Premarin (Conjugated Estrogens, U.S.P.) 0.45 mg, meprobamate 200 mg/Tab. Bot. 60s.
Use: Estrogen, antianxiety agent.

PMB 400. (Wyeth-Ayerst) Premarin (Conjugated Estrogens, U.S.P.) 0.45 mg, meprobamate 400 mg/Tab. Bot. 60s.
Use: Estrogen, antianxiety agent.

P.M.P. COMPOUND. (Mericon) Chlorpheniramine maleate 4 mg, phenylephrine HCl 15 mg, salicylamide 300 mg, scopolamine methylnitrate 0.8 mg/Tab. Bot. 100s, 1000s.
Use: Antihistamine, decongestant, analgesic.

PMP EXPECTORANT. (Mericon) Codeine phosphate 10 mg, phenylephrine HCl 10 mg, guaifenesin 40 mg, chlorpheniramine maleate 2 mg/5 ml. Bot. gal.
Use: Antitussive, decongestant, expectorant, antihistamine.

PNEUMOCOCCAL VACCINE, POLYVALENT. Purified capsular polysaccharides from 23 pneumococcal types.
Use: Agent for immunization.
See: Pneumovax 23, Inj. (Merck & Co.)
Pnuimune 23, Inj. (Merck & Co.).

PNEUMOCOCCI.
W/*Haemophilus influenzae, Neisseria catarrhalis, streptococci, Klebsiella pneumoniae, staphylococci, pneumococci,* killed.
See: Mixed Vaccine No. 4 w/H. Influenzae, Inj. (Lilly).

PNEUMOMIST. (ECR Pharm) Guaifenesin 600 mg. SR Tab. Bot. 100s.
Use: Expectorant.

PNEUMONIA VACCINE, KILLED DIPLOCOCCUS.
W/*Neisseria catarrhalis, Klebsiella pneumoniae, streptococci, staphylococci.*
See: Combined Vaccine No. 4 w/Catarrhalis, Inj. (Lilly).

PNEUMONIAE VACCINE, KILLED KLEBSIELLA.
W/*Neisseria catarrhalis, Diplococcus pneumoniae, streptococci, staphylococci.*
See: Combined Vaccine No. 4 w/Catarrhalis, Inj.(Lilly).

PNEUMOTUSSIN HC. (ECR Pharm) Hydrocodone bitartrate 5 mg, guaifenesin 100 mg/5 ml Syrup. Bot. 120 ml, 480 ml.
Use: Narcotic antitussive, expectorant.

PNEUMOVAX 23. (Merck & Co.) Pneumococcal vaccine polyvalent 0.5 ml/dose. Vial 5 dose, 1 dose X 5s.
Use: Agent for Immunization.

PNS UNNA BOOT. (Pedinol) Non-sterile gauze bandage 10 yds × 3″. Box 12s.
Use: Ambulatory procedure in treatment of leg ulcers and varicosities.

PNU-IMUNE 23. (Lederle) Pneumococcal vaccine 0.5 ml dose. Vial dose 5s. Lederject disposable syringe 5 × 1 dose.
Use: Agent for immunization.

• **POBILUKAST EDAMINE.** USAN.
Use: Asthma.

POCHLORIN. Prophyrinic and chlorophyllic compound.
Use: Anti-hypercholesteremic agent.

POD-BEN-25. (C & M Pharmacal) Podophyllin 25% in benzoin tincture. Bot. 1 oz.
Use: Keratolytic.

PODIASPRAY. (Dalin) Undecylenic acid, salicylic acid, dichlorophene. Spray-on pow. 6 oz.
Use: Fungicide, germicide.

PODIODINE. (A.V.P.) Germicidal surgical scrub and solution.
Use: Germicide.

PODOBEN. (American) Podophyllum resin extract 25%. Bot. 5 ml.
Use: Keratolytic.

PODOCON-25. (Paddock) Podophyllum resin 25% in benzoin tincture. Soln. 15 ml.
Use: Keratolytic.

• **PODOFILOX.** USAN.

Use: Cytotoxic, topical.
See: Condylox (Oclassen).
PODOFIN. (Syosset Labs) Podophyllum resin 25% in benzoin tincture. Liq. Bot. 7.5 ml.
Use: Keratolytic.
PODOPHYLLIN.
See: Podophyllum resin.
• **PODOPHYLLUM,** U.S.P. XXIII.
Use: Caustic.
W/Oxgall, cascara sagrada, dandelion root, tincture nux vomica.
See: Oxachol, Liq. (Philips Roxane).
• **PODOPHYLLUM RESIN,** U.S.P. XXIII. Topical Soln., U.S.P. XXIII. (Various Mfr.) Podophyllin. Pkg. 1 oz, 0.25 lb, 1 lb.
Use: Caustic.
See: Podoben, Liq. (Maurry).
W/Salicylic acid.
See: Ver-Var, Soln. (Owen).
POINT-TWO MOUTHRINSE. (Hoyt) Sodium fluoride 0.2% in a flavored neutral liquid. Bot. 120 ml.
Use: Dental caries preventative.
POISON ANTIDOTE KIT. (Bowman) Charcoal suspension. Bot. 2 oz, 4s. Ipecac syrup, Bot. 1 oz, 1/Kit.
Use: Antidote.
• **POISON IVY EXTRACT, ALUM PRECIPITATED.** USAN. An aqueous suspension of a pyridine extract of poison ivy which is precipitated with alum and adjusted to standard concentrations.
Use: Ivy poisoning counteractant.
See: Aqua Ivy, Inj. (Miles Pharm).
Poisonivi, Extract (Cutter).
Poisonok, Extract (Cutter).
POISON IVY AND OAK PROPHYLAXIS. (Hollister-Stier) Allergenic extract for oral administration. Dropper Bot. 15 ml Pkg. 3s. Strength 1:25, 1:50, 1:100.
Use: Hyposensitization of patients allergic to poison ivy and poison oak.
• **POISON OAK EXTRACT.** USAN.
Use: Anti-allergic.
POISON OAK-N-IVY ARMOR. (Tec Labs) Trioctyl citrate, mineral oil, monostearyl citrate, beeswax, 4-chloro-3,5-xylenol. Lot. Bot. 59.1 ml.
Use: Topical poison ivy treatment.
• **POLACRILLIN.** USAN. Methacrylic acid with divinylbenzene. A synthetic ion-exchange resin, supplied in the hydrogen or free acid form. Amberlite IRP-64 (Rohm and Haas).
Use: Pharmaceutic aid.
• **POLACRILLIN POTASSIUM,** N.F. XVIII. A synthetic ion-exchange resin, prepared through the polymerization of methacrylic acid and divinylbenzene,

further neutralized with potassium hydroxide to form the potassium salt of methacrylic acid and divinylbenzene. Supplied as a pharmaceutical-grade ion-exchange resin in a particle size of 100- to 500-mesh.
Use: Pharmaceutic aid (tablet disintegrant).
See: Amberlite IRP-88 (Rohm and Haas).
POLADEX TABS. (Major) Dexchlorpheniramine maleate. **4 mg/Tab.:** Bot. 100s, 250s, 1000s; **6 mg/Tab.:** Bot. 100s, 1000s.
Use: Antihistamine.
POLAMETHENE RESIN CAPRYLATE. The physiochemical complex of the acid-binding ion exchange resin, polyamine-methylene resin and caprylic acid.
POLARAMINE. (Schering) Dexchlorpheniramine maleate (d-isomer of Chlor-Trimeton). **Repetab:** 4 mg/Tab. Bot. 100s; 6 mg/Tab. Bot. 100s, 1000s. **Syr.:** 2 mg/5 ml. Bot. 16 oz.
Use: Antihistamine.
POLARAMINE EXPECTORANT. (Schering) Dexchlorpheniramine maleate 2 mg, pseudoephedrine sulfate 20 mg, guaifenesin 100 mg/5 ml, alcohol 7.2%. Bot. 16 oz.
Use: Antihistamine, decongestant, expectorant.
POLDEMAN AD SUSPENSION. (Sanofi Winthrop) Kaolin.
Use: Antidiarrheal.
POLDEMAN SUSPENSION. (Sanofi Winthrop) Kaolin.
Use: Antidiarrheal.
POLDEMICINA SUSPENSION. (Sanofi Winthrop) Kaolin.
Use: Antidiarrheal.
• **POLICAPRAM.** USAN.
Use: Pharmaceutic aid (tablet binder).
POLIDENT DENTU-GRIP. (Block) Carboxymethylcellulose gum, ethylene oxide polymer. Pkg. 0.675 oz, 1.75 oz, 3.55 oz.
Use: Denture adhesive.
POLIDEXIDE. B.A.N. Dextran cross-linked with epichlorhydrin and 0-substituted with 2-diethylaminoethyl groups, some of them quaternized with diethylaminoethyl Cl. Secholex hydrochloride.
Use: Antihypercholesterolemic agent.
• **POLIFEPROSAN 20.** USAN.
Use: Pharmaceutic aid (biodegradable polymer for controlled drug delivery).
• **POLIGEENAN.** USAN. 3,6-Anhydro-4-O-β-D-galactopyranosyl-α-D-galactopyra-

nose 2,4′-bis(potassium/sodium sulfate)-(1-3)-polysaccharide. Polysaccharide produced by limited hydrolysis of carragheen from red algae.
Use: Enzyme inhibitor.
• **POLIGLECAPRONE 25.** USAN.
Use: Pharmaceutic aid (surgical suture material, absorbable).
• **POLIGLECAPRONE 90.** USAN.
Use: Pharmaceutic aid (surgical suture coating, absorbable).
• **POLIGLUSAIN.** USAN.
Use: Wound healing; hemostatic.
• **POLIGNATE SODIUM.** USAN.
Use: Enzyme inhibitor.
POLI-GRIP. (Block) Karaya gum, magnosium oxide in petrolatum mineral oil base, peppermint and spearmint flavor. Tube 0.75 oz, 1.5 oz, 2.5 oz.
Use: Denture adhesive.
POLIOMYELITIS IMMUNE GLOBULIN (HUMAN). (Various Mfr.) Preparation of gamma globulin primarily assayed for content of poliomyelitis antibodies in accordance with standard procedures licensed by National Institutes of Health.
POLIOMYELITIS VACCINE.
(Squibb/Connaught) (Purified, Salk Type IPV) Amp. 5 x 1 ml. Vial 10 dose.
Use: Agent for immunization.
• **POLIOMYELITIS VACCINE INACTIVATED,** U.S.P. XXIII.
Use: Active immunizing agent.
POLIOVIRUS VACCINE, INACTIVATED.
(Squibb/Connaught) Amp. 1 ml. Box 5s. Vial 10 dose. Subcutaneous administration.
Use: Agent for immunization.
• **POLIOVIRUS VACCINE LIVE ORAL,**
U.S.P. XXIII. Poliovirus vaccine, live, oral, type I, II or III. Poliovirus vaccine, live, oral, trivalent.
Use: Active immunizing agent.
See: Orimune Trivalent I, II & III, Vial (Lederle).
POLIOVIRUS VACCINE, LIVE, ORAL, TRIVALENT. Immunization against polio strains 1, 2 & 3.
Use: Agent for immunization.
See: Orimune (Lederle).
• **POLIPROPENE 25.** USAN.
Use: Pharmaceutic aid.
• **POLIXETONIUM CHLORIDE.** USAN. (Allergan). Poly[oxyethylene(dimethyliminio) ethylene(dimethyliminio)ethylene dichloride].
Use: Preservative.
POLOCAINE. (Astra) Mepivacaine 1%, 1.5% or 2%. Inj. Vial 30 ml, 50 ml.
Use: Local anesthetic.

POLOCAINE 3% INJECTION. (Astra) Mepivacaine HCl 3%. Astrapak 1.8 ml, Box 100 cartridges.
Use: Local anesthetic.
POLORIS POULTICES. (Block) Benzocaine 7.5 mg, capsicum 4.6 mg in poultice base. Pkg. 5 unit, 12 unit.
Use: Local anesthetic.
• **POLOXALENE.** USAN. Liquid nonionic surfactant polymer of polyoxypropylene polyoxyethylene type.
Use: Surfactant.
POLOXALKOL. B.A.N. A polymer of ethylene oxide, propylene oxide and propylene glycol.
Use: Surface active agent.
POLOXALKOL. Polyoxyethylene polyoxypropylene polymer.
See: Magcyl, Cap. (Elder).
W/Casanthrol.
See: Casakol, Cap. (Upjohn).
W/Phenylephrine HCl, dextrose soln.
See: Isohalent, Soln. (Elder).
• **POLOXAMER,** N.F. XVIII.
Use: Surfactant.
• **POLOXAMER 182 D.** USAN.
Use: Pharmaceutic aid (surfactant).
• **POLOXAMER 182 LF.** USAN.
Use: Food additive; pharmaceutic aid.
• **POLOXAMER 188.** USAN.
Use: Cathartic; sickle cell crisis, severe burns [Orphan drug]
• **POLOXAMER 188 LF.** USAN.
Use: Pharmaceutic aid (surfactant).
• **POLOXAMER 331.** USAN.
Use: Food additive (surfactant); AIDS-related toxoplasmosis [Orphan drug]
POLOXAMER-IODINE.
See: Prepodyne, Soln. (West).
POLOXYL LANOLIN. B.A.N. A polyoxyethylene condensation-product of anhydrous lanolin. Aqualose.
Use: Emollient.
POLY I; POLY C12U.
Use: AIDS, antineoplastic. [Orphan drug]
POLYAMINE-METHYLENE RESIN.
See: Exorbin (Various Mfr.).
POLYAMINE RESIN.
See: Polyamine-Methylene Resin (Various Mfr.).
POLYANETHOL SULFONATE, SODIUM.
See: Grobax, Vial (Roche Diagnostics).
POLYANHYDROGLUCOSE. Polyanhydroglucuronic acid.
See: Dextran, Inj., Soln. (Various Mfr.).
POLYBASE. (Paddock) Preblended polyethylene glycol suppository base for incorporation of medications where a water soluble base is indicated. Jar 1 lb, 5

lb.
Use: Suppository base.
POLYBENZARSOL. Benzocal.
POLY-BON DROPS. (Barrows) Vitamins A 3000 IU, D 400 IU, C 60 mg, B_1 1 mg, B_2 1.2 mg, niacinamide 8 mg/0.6 ml. Bot. 50 ml.
Use: Vitamin supplement.
•**POLYBUTESTER.** USAN.
Use: Surgical suture material.
•**POLYBUTILATE.** USAN.
Use: Surgical suture coating.
POLYCARBOPHIL. A synthetic, loosely crosslinked, hydrophilic resin of the poly-carboxylic type. Sorboquel.
Use: Laxative.
POLYCILLIN. (Bristol) Ampicillin trihy-drate. **250 mg/Cap.:** Bot. 100s, 500s, 1000s, UD 100s. **500 mg/Cap.:** Bot. 100s, 500s, UD 100s. **Pediatric Drops:** 100 mg/ml. Dropper bot. 20 ml.
Use: Antibacterial, penicillin.
POLYCILLIN-N. (Bristol) Sodium ampi-cillin 125 mg, 250 mg, 500 mg, 1 Gm or 2 Gm/Vial. Pkg. 1s, 10s. Piggyback vial 500 mg, 1 Gm, 2 Gm. Bulk vial 10 Gm.
Use: Antibacterial, penicillin.
POLYCILLIN ORAL SUSPENSION. (Bristol) Ampicillin trihydrate. **125 mg/5 ml:** Bot. 80 ml, 100 ml, 150 ml, 200 ml, UD 5 ml. **250 mg/5 ml:** Bot. 80 ml, 100 ml, 150 ml, 200 ml, UD 5 ml. **500 mg/5 ml:** Bot. 100 ml, UD 5 ml.
Use: Antibacterial, penicillin.
POLYCILLIN-PRB ORAL SUSPENSION. (Bristol) Ampicillin trihydrate 3.5 Gm, probenecid 1 Gm/Bot. Bot 9s.
Use: Antibacterial, penicillin.
POLYCITRA-K. (Willen) Potassium cit-rate monohydrate 1100 mg, citric acid monohydrate 334 mg, potassium ion 10 mEq/5 ml. Bot. 4 oz, pt.
Use: Systemic alkalinizer.
POLYCITRA-K CRYSTALS. (Willen) Potassium citrate monohydrate 3300 mg, citric acid 1002 mg, potassium ion 30 mEq, equivalent to 30 mEq bicarbon-ate/UD pkg. Box 100s.
Use: Systemic alkalinizer.
POLYCITRA-LC. (Willen) Potassium cit-rate monohydrate 550 mg, sodium cit-rate dihydrate 500 mg, citric acid mono-hydrate 334 mg, potassium ion 5 mEq, sodium ion 5 mEq/5 ml. Bot. 4 oz, pt.
Use: Systemic alkalinizer.
POLYCITRA SYRUP. (Willen) Potassium citrate monohydrate 550 mg, sodium cit-rate dihydrate 500 mg, citric acid mono-hydrate 334 mg, potassium ion 5 mEq, sodium ion 5 mEq/5 ml. Bot. 4 oz, pt.

Use: Systemic alkalinizer.
POLYCOSE. (Ross) **Pow.:** Glucose poly-mers derived from controlled hydrolysis of corn starch. Calories 380, carbohy-drate 94 Gm, water 6 Gm, sodium 110 mg, potassium 10 mg, chloride 223 mg, calcium 30 mg, phosphorus 5 mg/100 Gm. Can 12.3 oz. Case 6s. **Liq.:** Calo-ries 200, carbohydrate 50 Gm, water 70 Gm, sodium 70 mg, potassium 6 mg, chloride 140 mg, calcium 20 mg, phos-phorus 3 mg/100 ml. Bot. 4 oz. Case 48s.
Use: Enteral nutritional supplement.
POLYCYCLINE INTRAVENOUS.
See: Bristacycline, Cap., Vial (Bristol).
•**POLYDEXTROSE.** USAN.
Use: Food additive.
POLYDINE OINTMENT. (Century) Povi-done iodine in ointment base. Jar 1 oz, 4 oz, lb.
Use: Anti-infective, external.
POLYDINE SCRUB. (Century) Povidone iodine in scrub solution. Bot. 1 oz, 4 oz, 8 oz, pt, gal.
Use: Antiseptic.
POLYDINE SOLUTION. (Century) Povi-done iodine solution. Bot. 1 oz, 4 oz, 8 oz, pt, gal.
Use: Antiseptic.
•**POLYDIOXANONE.** USAN.
Use: Surgical aid.
POLY ENA TEST SYSTEM FOR RNP AND SM. (Wampole-Zeus) Qualitative identification of auto antibodies to ex-tractable nuclear antigens in human serum by gel precipitation technique. Aid in the diagnosis of SLE, MCTD, PSS, SS. Box test 48s.
Use: Diagnostic aid.
POLY ENA TEST SYSTEM FOR RNP, SM, SSA AND SSB. (Wampole-Zeus) Qualitative identification of auto antibod-ies to extractable nuclear antigens in hu-man serum by gel precipitation tech-niques. Aid in the diagnosis of SLE, MCTD, PSS, SS. Box test 96s.
Use: Diagnostic aid.
POLY ENA TEST SYSTEM FOR SSA AND SSB. (Wampole-Zeus) Qualitative identification of auto antibodies to ex-tractable nuclear antigens in human serum by gel precipitation techniques. Aid in the diagnosis of SLE, MCTD, PSS, SS. Box test 48s.
Use: Diagnostic aid.
POLYESTRADIOL PHOSPHATE.
See: Estradurin, Amp. (Wyeth-Ayerst).
•**POLYETHADENE.** USAN. 1,2:3,4-Diepoxybutane polymer with ethylen-

imine. Erythritol anhydride polyethyleneimine polymer.
Use: Antacid.
•POLYETHYLENE EXCIPIENT, N.F. XVII.
Use: Pharmaceutic aid (stiffening agent).
•POLYETHYLENE GLYCOL 300, 400, 600, 1500, 1540, 4000 AND 6000, N.F. XVIII. Oint., N.F. XVIII.
Use: Water-soluble ointment and suppository base; tablet excipient.
See: P.E.G., Oint. (Medco).
•POLYETHYLENE GLYCOL 3350 AND ELECTROLYTES FOR ORAL SOLUTION, U.S.P. XXIII.
Use: Rehydration.
•POLYETHYLENE GLYCOL MONOETHYL ETHER, U.S.P. XXIII.
•POLYETHYLENE OXIDE, N.F. XVIII.
Use: Pharmaceutical aid.
•POLYFEROSE. USAN. An iron carbohydrate chelate containing approximately 45% of iron in which the metallic (Fe) ion is sequestered within a polymerized carbohydrate derived from sucrose.
Use: Hematinic.
POLY-F FLUORIDE DROPS. (Major) Fluoride 0.5 mg, vitamins A 1500 IU, D 400 IU, E 5 mg, B_1 0.5 mg, B_2 0.6 mg, B_3 8 mg, B_6 0.4 mg, B_{12} 2 mcg, C 35 mg/ml. Drops. Bot. 50 ml.
Use: Vitamin/mineral supplement.
POLYGAM. (American Red Cross) Protein 50 mg/ml (90% gammaglobulin), sodium chloride = 0.15 M, glucose 20 mg, polyethylene glycol 2 mg, glycine 0.3 M, albumin (human) 3 mg/ml. Inj. Single-use bot. 0.5 g, 2.5 g, 5 g, 10 g.
Use: Immune serum.
POLYGAM S/D. (Baxter Healthcare/American Red Cross) Protein 50 mg (90% gamma globulin), albumin (human) 3 mg, glycine 22.5 mg, glucose 20 mg, polyethylene glycol 2 mg, tri(n-butyl) phosphate 1 mcg, octoxynol 9 1 mcg, polysorbate 80 100 mcg/ml. Inj. Single-use vials 2.5 g, 5 g, 10 g.
Use: Immune serum.
POLYGELINE. B.A.N. A polymer of urea and polypeptides derived from denatured gelatin.
Use: Restoration of blood volume.
•POLYGLACTIN 370 & 910. USAN. Lactic acid polyester with glycolic acid.
Use: Synthetic absorbable suture.
•POLYGLYCOLIC ACID. USAN. Poly-(oxycarbonylmethylene).
Use: Surgical aid.
See: Dexon Sterile Suture (David & Geck).

•POLYGLYCONATE. USAN.
Use: Surgical Aid.
POLY-HISTINE CS. (Bock) Brompheniramine maleate 2 mg, phenylpropanolamine HCl 12.5 mg, codeine phosphate 10 mg/5 ml, alcohol 0.95%. Bot. pt.
Use: Antihistamine, decongestant, expectorant.
POLY-HISTINE-D CAPSULES. (Bock) Phenylpropanolamine HCl 50 mg, phenyltoloxamine citrate 16 mg, pyrilamine maleate 16 mg, pheniramine maleate 16 mg/Cap. Bot. 100s.
Use: Decongestant, antihistamine.
POLY-HISTINE-D ELIXIR. (Bock) Phenylpropanolamine HCl 12.5 mg, phenyltoloxamine citrate 4 mg, pyrilamine maleate 4 mg, pheniramine 4 mg/5 ml, alcohol 4%. Bot. pt.
Use: Antihistamine, decongestant.
POLY-HISTINE DM. (Bock) Dextromethorphan HBr 10 mg, phenylpropanolamine HCl 12.5 mg, brompheniramine maleate 2 mg/5 ml. Bot. pt.
Use: Antitussive, decongestant, antihistamine.
POLY-HISTINE-D PED CAPS. (Bock) Phenylpropanolamine HCl 25 mg, phenyltoloxamine citrate 8 mg, pheniramine maleate 8 mg, pyrilamine maleate 8 mg/Cap. Bot. 100s.
Use: Decongestant, antihistamine.
POLY-HISTINE ELIXIR. (Bock) Phenyltoloxamine citrate 4 mg, pyrilamine maleate 4 mg, pheniramine maleate 4 mg/5 ml, alcohol 4%. Elix. Bot. pt.
Use: Antihistamine.
•POLYMACON. USAN. Poly(2-hydroxyethyl methacrylate).
Use: Contact lens material.
POLYMERIC OXYGEN.
Use: Sickle cell anemia. [Orphan drug]
•POLYMETAPHOSPHATE P-32. USAN
Use: Radioactive agent.
POLYMETHINE BLUE DYE. (3,3'-Diethylhiadicarbocyanine iodide).
POLYMONINE. A formaldehyde polymer of N-methylmonoanisylamine.
POLYMOX. (Bristol) Amoxicillin trihydrate. Cap.: 250 mg. Bot. 100s, 500s, UD 100s; 500 mg. Bot. 50s, 100s, 500s, UD 100s. Oral Susp.: 125 mg or 250 mg/5 ml. Bot. 80 ml, 100 ml, 150 ml. Dosatrol 125 mg or 250 mg/Bot. 5 ml. Ped. Drops: 50 mg/ml. Bot. 15 ml.
Use: Antibacterial, penicillin.
POLYMYXIN. B.A.N. Generic term for an-

tibiotics obtained from fermentations of various media by strains of *Bacillus polymyxa.*
Use: Polymyxins A, B and D active against susceptible gram-negative bacteria.
POLYMYXIN B. (Various Mfr.) (No Pharmaceutical Form Available) Antimicrobial substances produced by *Bacillus polymyxa.*
W/Bacitracin zinc, neomycin sulfate, benzalkonium Cl.
See: Biotres, Oint. (Central).
• **POLYMYXIN B SULFATE,** U.S.P. XXIII.
Otic Soln., Sterile, U.S.P. XXIII.
Use: Antibiotic.
See: Aerosporin, Pow., Soln. (Burroughs Wellcome).
• **POLYMYXIN B SULFATE AND BACITRACIN ZINC TOPICAL AEROSOL,** U.S.P. XXIII.
Use: Antibiotic.
• **POLYMYXIN B SULFATE AND BACITRACIN ZINC TOPICAL POWDER,** U.S.P. XXIII.
Use: Antibiotic.
• **POLYMYXIN B SULFATE AND HYDROCORTISONE OTIC SOLUTION,** U.S.P. XXIII.
Use: Antibiotic, anti-inflammatory.
POLYMYXIN B SULFATE STERILE.
(Roerig) Polymyxin B sulfate 500,000 units/Vial 20 ml for reconstitution.
Use: Anti-infective.
POLYMYXIN B SULFATE W/COMBINATIONS.
See: AK-Poly-Bac Oint. (Akorn).
AK-Spore, Preps. (Akorn).
Aquaphor, Oint. (Beiersdorf).
Cortisporin, Preps. (Burroughs Wellcome).
Epimycin A, Oint. (Delta).
Maxitrol, Oint., Ophthalmic Oint. (Upjohn).
Mycitracin, Oint., Ophthalmic Oint. (Upjohn).
Neomixin, Oint. (Hauck).
Neosporin, Preps. (Burroughs Wellcome).
Neosporin G.U. Irrigant, Amp. (Burroughs Wellcome).
Neotal, Oint. (Hauck).
Neo-Thrycex, Oint. (Commerce).
Ocutricin, Preps. (Bausch & Lomb).
Otobiotic, Soln. (Schering).
Otoreid-HC, Liq. (Solvay).
P.B.N., Oint. (Jenkins).
Polysporin, Oint., Ophthalmic Oint. (Burroughs Wellcome).
Polytrim Ophth. Soln. (Allergan).

Pyocidin-Otic, Soln. (Berlex).
Statrol, Liq. (Alcon).
Statrol Sterile Ophthalmic Oint. (Alcon).
Terramycin, Preps. w/Polymyxin (Pfizer).
Tigo, Oint. (Burlington).
Tribotic, Oint. (Burgin Arden).
Tribiotic Plus, Oint. (Thompson).
Trimixin, Oint. (Hance).
Triple Antibiotic Oint. (Kenyon).
POLYMYXIN E.
See: Colistin sulfate.
POLYMYXIN-NEOMYCIN-BACITRACIN OINTMENT. (Various Mfr.).
Use: Antibiotic for treatment of gram-positive and gram-negative organisms.
POLYNOXYLIN. B.A.N. Poly[methylenedi(hydroxymethyl)urea]Anaflex; Ponoxylan.
Use: Antibacterial, anti-inflammatory.
POLYNOXYLIN. Poly[methylenedi(hydroxymethyl)urea]. Anaflex.
POLYOXYETHYLENE 8 STEARATE.
Myrj 45. (ICI U.S.), Polyoxyl 8 Stearate.
POLYOXYETHYLENE (20) SORBITAN MONOLEATE.
See: Polysorbate 80, U.S.P. XXIII. (Various Mfr.).
POLYOXYETHYLENE 20 SORBITAN TRIOLEATE. Tween 85. (ICI U.S.), Polysorbate 85.
POLYOXYETHYLENE 20 SORBITAN TRISTEARATE. Tween 65. (ICI U.S.), Polysorbate 65.
POLYOXYETHYLENE 40 MONOSTEARATE.
Polyoxyl 40 Stearate.
See: Myrj 52 & Myrj 52S (ICI U.S.).
• **POLYOXYETHYLENE 50 STEARATE,** N.F. XVIII.
Use: Surfactant; emulsifying agent.
POLYOXYETHYLENEONYLPHENOL.
W/Alkyldimethylbenzylammonium Cl, methylrosaniline Cl, polyethylene glycol tert-dodecylthioether.
See: Hyva, Vaginal Tab. (Holland-Rantos).
POLYOXYETHYLENE LAURYL ETHER.
W/Benzoyl peroxide, ethyl alcohol.
See: Benzagel, Gel (Dermik).
Desquam-X, Preps. (Westwood).
W/Hydrocortisone, sulfur.
See: Fostril HC, Lot. (Westwood).
W/Sulfur.
See: Fostril, Lot. (Westwood).
Proseca, Oint. (Westwood).
POLYOXYETHYLENE NONYL PHENOL.
W/Sodium edetate, docusate sodium, 9-

aminoacridine HCl.
See: Vagisec Plus, Supp. (Schmid).
POLYOXYETHYLENE SORBITAN MONOLAURATE. Polysorbate 20, N.F. XVIII.
W/Ferrous gluconate.
See: Simron, Cap. (Marion Merrell Dow).
W/Ferrous gluconate, vitamins.
See: Simron Plus, Cap. (Marion Merrell Dow).
• **POLYOXYL 8 STEARATE.** USAN. Polyoxyethylene 8 stearate.
Use: Surfactant.
See: Myrj 45 (Atlas).
• **POLYOXYL 10 OLEYL ETHER,** N.F. XVIII.
Use: Pharmaceutic aid (surfactant).
• **POLYOXYL 20 CETOSTEARYL ETHER,** N.F. XVIII.
Use: Pharmaceutic aid (surfactant).
• **POLYOXYL 35 CASTOR OIL,** N.F. XVIII.
Use: Pharmaceutic aid (surfactant, emulsifying agent).
• **POLYOXYL 40 HYDROGENATED CASTOR OIL,** N.F. XVIII.
Use: Pharmaceutic aid (surfactant, emulsifying agent).
• **POLYOXYL 40 STEARATE,** N.F. XVIII.
Macrogic Stearate 2,000 (I.N.N.) Polyoxyethylene 40 monostearate.
Use: Pharmaceutic aid (surfactant).
Use: Hydrophilic oint., surfactant; surface-active agent.
See: Myrj 52 (Atlas).
Myrj 52S (Atlas).
W/Polyethylene glycol, chlorobutanol.
See: Blink-N-Clean (Allergan).
POLY-PRED LIQUIFILM. (Allergan) Prednisolone acetate 0.5%, neomycin sulfate equivalent to 0.35% neomycin base, polymyxin B sulfate 10,000 units/ml, polyvinyl alcohol 1.4%, thimerosal 0.001%. Dropper bot. 5 ml, 10 ml.
Use: Corticosteroid, anti-infective, ophthalmic.
• **POLYPROPYLENE GLYCOL,** N.F. XVIII.
An addition polymer of propylene oxide and water.
Use: Pharmaceutic aid (suspending agent).
POLYSACCHARIDE-IRON COMPLEX.
Use: Iron-containing products, oral.
See: Niferex (Central).
Hytinic (Hyrox).
Niferex-150 (Central).
Nu-Iron (Mayrand).
Nu-Iron 150 (Mayrand).
POLYSEPT. (Dalin) Polymyxin B sulfate 5000 units, bacitracin 400 units,

neomycin sulfate 5 mg, diperodon HCl 10 mg/Gm. Tube 0.5 oz.
Use: Anti-infective, external.
POLYSONIC LOTION. (Parker) Multi-purpose ultrasound lotion with high coupling efficiency. Bot. 8.5 oz, gal.
Use: For diagnostic and therapeutic medical ultrasound.
• **POLYSORBATE 20,** N.F. XVIII. (Atlas) Tween 20. Polyoxyethlene 20 sorbitan monolaurate.
Use: Surface-active agent.
• **POLYSORBATE 40,** N.F. XVIII. (Atlas) Tween 40. Polyoxyethylene 20 sorbitan monopalmitate.
Use: Surface-active agent.
• **POLYSORBATE 60,** N.F. XVIII. (Atlas) Tween 60. Polyoxyethylene 20 sorbitan monosteurate.
Use: Surface-active agent.
• **POLYSORBATE 65.** USAN. (Atlas) Tween 65. Polyoxyethylene 20 sorbitan tristearate.
Use: Surface-active agent.
• **POLYSORBATE 80,** N.F. XVIII. Polyoxyethylene (20) Sorbitan Monooleate.
Use: Surfactant.
• **POLYSORBATE 85.** USAN. (Atlas) Polyoxyethylene 20 sorbitan trioleate. Tween 85.
Use: Surface-active agent.
POLYSORB HYDRATE. (Fougera) Sorbitan sesquinoleate in a wax and petrolatum base. Cream. Tube 56.7 Gm, lb.
Use: Emollients.
POLYSPORIN OINTMENT. (Burroughs Wellcome) Polymyxin B sulfate 10,000 units, bacitracin zinc 500 units/Gm in special white petrolatum base. Tube 3.75 Gm.
Use: Anti-infective, external.
POLYSPORIN OPHTHALMIC OINTMENT. (Burroughs Wellcome) Polymyxin B sulfate, 10,000 units, bacitracin zinc 500 units. Tube 3.5 g.
Use: Antibiotic, ophthalmic.
POLYSPORIN POWDER. (Burroughs Wellcome) Polymyxin B 10,000 units, zinc bacitracin 500 units, lactose base/Gm. Shaker vial 10 Gm.
Use: Anti-infective, external.
POLYSULFIDES. Polythionate.
POLYTABS-F CHEWABLE VITAMIN. (Major) Fluoride 1 mg, vitamins A 2500 IU, D 400 IU, E 15 mg, B_1 1.05 mg, B_2 1.2 mg, B_3 13.5 mg, B_6 1.05 mg, B_{12} 4.5 mcg, C 60 mg, folic acid 0.3 mg/Tab. Bot. 100s, 1000s.
Use: Vitamin/mineral supplement.
POLYTAR BATH. (Stiefel) A 25% polytar

blend of four different vegetable and mineral tars in an emulsion base. Bot. 8 fl oz.

Use: Tar-containing bath dermatological.

POLYTAR SHAMPOO. (Stiefel) A neutral soap containing 1% Polytar in a surfactant shampoo. Buffered. Plastic Bot. 6 fl oz, 12 fl oz, gal.

Use: Antiseborrheic.

POLYTAR SOAP. (Stiefel) A neutral soap containing 1% Polytar. Cake 4 oz.

Use: Tar-containing preparation.

POLYTEF. (Ethicon) Poly(tetrafluoroethylene). PTFE.

Use: Prosthetic aid.

• **POLYTHIAZIDE,** U.S.P. XXIII. Tab., U.S.P. XXIII. 2-Methyl-3,4-dihydro-3,(2,2,2-Trifluoroethylthiomethyl)-6-chloro-7-sulfamyl-1,2,4-benzothiadiazine, 1,1-dioxide. 6-Chloro-3,4-dihydro-2-methyl-3-[[(2,2,2,-trifluoroethyl)thio]-methyl]-2H-1,2,4-Benzothiadiazine-7- sulfonamide 1,1-dioxide.

Use: Diuretic; antihypertensive.

See: Renese Tab. (Pfizer Laboratories). W/Prazosin.

See: Minizide, Cap. (Pfizer Laboratories). W/Reserpine.

See: Renese-R, Tab. (Pfizer Laboratories).

POLYTINIC. (Pharmics) Elemental iron 100 mg, vitamin C 300 mg, folic acid 1 mg/tab. Bot. 100s.

Use: Vitamin/mineral supplement.

POLYTRIM. (Allergan) Polymyxin B sulfate 10,000 units/Gm or ml, trimethoprim 1 mg/ml. Drop. Bot. 10 ml.

Use: Anti-infective, ophthalmic.

POLYTUSS-DM. (Rhode) Dextromethorphan HBr 15 mg, chlorpheniramine maleate 1 mg, guaifenesin 25 mg/5 ml. Bot. 4 oz, 8 oz.

Use: Antitussive, antihistamine, expectorant.

• **POLYURETHANE FOAM.** USAN.

Use: Prosthetic aid.

POLYVIDONE.

See: Polyvinylpyrrolidone.

POLY-VI-FLOR 0.5 mg CHEWABLE TABS. (Mead Johnson Nutrition) Vitamins A 2500 IU, D 400 IU, E 15 IU, C 60 mg, B_1 1.05 mg, B_2 1.2 mg, niacin 13.5 mg, B_6 1.05 mg, B_{12} 4.5 mcg, fluoride 0.5 mg, folic acid 0.3 mg/Chew. tab. Bot. 100s. **With Iron:** Above formula plus iron 12 mg, copper 1 mg, zinc 10 mg/Tab. Bot. 100s.

Use: Vitamin/mineral supplement, den-

tal caries preventative.

POLY-VI-FLOR 1 mg CHEWABLE TABLETS. (Mead Johnson Nutrition) Vitamins A 2500 IU, D 400 IU, E 15 IU, C 60 mg, B_1 1.05 mg, B_2 1.2 mg, niacin 13.5 mg, B_6 1.05 mg, B_{12} 4.5 mcg, fluoride 1 mg, folic acid 0.3 mg/Chew. tab. Bot. 100s, 1000s. **With Iron.** Above formula plus iron 12 mg, copper 1 mg, zinc 10 mg/Tab.

Use: Vitamin/mineral supplement, dental caries preventative.

POLY-VI-FLOR 0.25 mg DROPS. (Mead Johnson Nutrition) Vitamins A 1500 IU, D 400 IU, E 5 IU, C 35 mg, B_1 0.5 mg, B_2 0.6 mg, B_6 0.4 mg, niacin 8 mg, B_{12} 2 mcg, fluoride 0.25 mg/ml. Dropper bot. 50 ml.

Use: Vitamin/mineral supplement, dental caries preventative.

POLY-VI-FLOR 0.5 mg DROPS. (Mead Johnson Nutrition) Vitamins A 1500 IU, D 400 IU, E 5 IU, C 35 mg, B_1 0.5 mg, B_2 0.6 mg, B_6 0.4 mg, niacin 8 mg, B_{12} 2 mcg, fluoride 0.5 mg/ml. Dropper bot. 30 ml, 50 ml.

Use: Vitamin/mineral supplement, dental caries preventative.

POLY-VI-FLOR 0.25 mg w/IRON DROPS. (Mead Johnson Nutrition) Vitamins A 1500 IU, D 400 IU, E 5 IU, C 35 mg, B_1 0.5 mg, B_2 0.6 mg, B_6 0.4 mg, niacin 8 mg, fluoride 0.25 mg, iron 10 mg/ml. Bot. 50 ml.

Use: Vitamin/mineral supplement, dental caries preventative.

POLY-VI-FLOR 0.5 mg W/IRON DROPS. (Mead Johnson Nutrition) Vitamins A 1500 IU, D 400 IU, E 5 IU, C 35 mg, B_1 0.5 mg, B_2 0.6 mg, B_6 0.4 mg, niacin 8 mg, fluoride 0.5 mg, iron 10 mg/ml. Dropper bot. 50 ml.

Use: Vitamin/mineral supplement, dental caries preventative.

POLY-VI-FLOR TABS CHEW. (Mead Johnson Nutritional) Fluoride 0.5 mg, vitamins A 2500 IU, D 400 IU, E 15 mg, B_1 1.05 mg, B_2 1.2 mg, B_3 13.5 mg, B_6 1.05 mg, B_{12} 4.5 mcg, C 60 mg, folic acid 0.3 mg, Cu, iron 12 mg, zinc 10 mg, sucrose. Tab. Bot. 100s.

Use: Vitamin/mineral supplement, dental caries preventative.

POLYVINOX. B.A.N. Poly(butyl vinyl ether). Shostakovsky Balsam.

Use: Skin application.

• **POLYVINYL ACETATE PHTHALATE,** N.F. XVIII.

Use: Pharmaceutical aid (coating agent).

• **POLYVINYL ALCOHOL,** U.S.P. XXIII.

Ethanol, homopolymer.
Use: Viscosity-increasing agent; pharmaceutic necessity for ophthalmic solution dosage form.
See: Liquifilm Forte (Allergan).
Liquifilm Tears (Allergan).
W/Hydroxypropyl methylcellulose.
See: Liquifilm Wetting Soln. (Allergan).
POLYVINYLPYRROLIDONE, POLYVIDONE, POVIDONE.
W/Acetrizoate Sodium
See: Salpix, Vial (Ortho).
POLYVINYLPYRROLIDONE VINYLACETATE COPOLYMERS.
See: Ivy-Rid, Spray (Hauck).
W/Benzalkonium.
See: Ivy-Chex, Aerosol (Bowman).
POLY-VI-SOL CHEWABLE TABS. (Mead Johnson Nutrition) Vitamins A 2500 IU, E 15 IU, D 400 IU, C 60 mg, B_1 1.05 mg, B_2 1.2 mg, niacin 13.5 mg, B_6 1.05 mg, B_{12} 4.5 mcg, folic acid 0.3 mg/Chew. tab. Bot. 100s. Circus Shape Tab. Bot. 100s. **With Iron:** Above formula plus Iron 12 mg, zinc 8 mg/Tab. Bot. 100s. Circus shape Tab. Bot. 100s.
Use: Vitamin/mineral supplement.
POLY-VI-SOL DROPS. (Mead Johnson Nutrition) Vitamins A 1500 IU, D 400 IU, C 35 mg, B_1 0.5 mg, B_2 0.6 mg, E 5 IU, B_6 0.4 mg, niacin 8 mg, B_{12} 2 mcg/ml. Bot. 30 ml, 50 ml with calibrated "Safti-Dropper."
Use: Vitamin supplement.
POLY-VI-SOL W/IRON DROPS. (Mead Johnson Nutrition) Vitamins A 1500 IU, D 400 IU, E 5 IU, C 35 mg, B_1 0.5 mg, B_2 0.6 mg, B_6 0.4 mg, niacin 8 mg, iron 10 mg/ml. Bot. 50 ml.
Use: Vitamin/mineral supplement.
POLY-VI-SOL W/IRON TABLETS, CHEWABLE. (Mead Johnson) Iron 12 mg, vitamins A 2500 IU, D 400 IU, E 15 mg, B_1 1.05 mg, B_2 1.2 mg, B_3 13.5 mg, B_6 1.05 mg, B_{12} 4.5 mcg, C 60 mg, folic acid 0.3 mg, Cu, zinc 8 mg/ tab. Bot. 100s. Circus shape. 60s, 100s.
Use: Vitamin/mineral supplement.
POLY-VI-SOL W/MINERALS. (Mead Johnson Nutritional) Iron 12 mg, vitamins A 2500 IU, D 400 IU, E 15 mg, B_1 1.05 mg, B_2 1.2 mg, B_3 13.5 mg, B_6 1.06 mg, B_{12} 4.5 mcg, C 60 mg, folic acid 0.3 mg, Cu, zinc 8 mg/Chew. tab. Bot. 60s, 100s.
Use: Vitamin/mineral supplement.
POLYVITAMINS.
See: Vitamin preparations.
POLY-VITAMINS W/FLUORIDE. (Various Mfr.) **Tab.:** Fluoride 0.5 mg, vitamins A

2500 IU, D 400 IU, E 15 mg, B_1 1 mg, B_2 1.2 mg, B_3 13.5 mg, B_6 1 mg, B_{12} 4.5 mcg, C 60 mg, folic acid 0.3 mg/Tab. Bot. 100s, 1000s.
Use: Vitamin/mineral supplement, dental caries preventative.
POLY VITAMINS W/FLUORIDE TABLETS CHEWABLE. (Various Mfr.) Fluoride 1 mg, vitamins A 2500 IU, D 400 IU, E 15 mg, B_1 1.05 mg, B_2 1.2 mg, B_3 13.5 mg, B_6 1.05 mg, B_{12} 4.5 mcg, C 60 mg, folic acid 0.3 mg. Bot. 100s, 1000s.
Use: Vitamin/mineral supplement, dental caries preventative.
POLYVITAMIN WITH IRON. (Rugby) Iron 10 mg, vitamins A 1500 IU, D 400 IU, E 5 mg, B_1 0.5 mg, B_2 0.6 mg, B_3 8 mg, B_6 0.4 mg, C 35 mg/ml. Dropper bot. 50 ml.
Use: Vitamin/mineral supplement.
POLYVITAMIN W/IRON FLUORIDE. (Rugby) Fluoride 1 mg, vitamins A 2500 IU, D 400 IU, E 15 mg, B_1 1.05 mg, B_2 1.2 mg, B_3 13.5 mg, B_6 1.05 mg, B_{12} 4.5 mcg, C 60 mg, folic acid 0.3 mg, iron 12 mg/Tab. Bot. 100s, 1000s.
Use: Vitamin/mineral supplement, dental caries preventative.
POLYVITAMIN W/FLUORIDE. (Rugby) Fluoride 0.5 mg, vitamins A 1500 IU, D 400 IU, E 5 mg, B_1 0.5 mg, B_2 0.6 mg, B_3 8 mg, B_6 0.4 mg, B_{12} 2 mcg, C 35 mg/ml. Dropper bot. 50 ml.
Use: Vitamin/mineral supplement, dental caries preventative.
POLYVITE WITH FLUORIDE. (Geneva Generics) Fluoride 0.25 mg, vitamins A 1500 IU, D 400 IU, E 5 mg, B_1 0.5 mg, B_2 0.6 mg, B_3 8 mg, B_6 0.4 mg, B_{12} 2 mcg, C 35 mg/ml. Dropper bot. 50 ml.
Use: Vitamin/mineral supplement, dental caries preventative.
• **PONALRESTAT.** USAN.
Use: Aldose reductase inhibitor.
PONARIS. (Jamol) Nasal emollient of mucosal lubricating and moisturizing botanical oils. Cajeput, eucalyptus, peppermint in iodized cottonseed oil. Bot. 1 oz w/dropper.
Use: Nasal moisturizer.
PONDIMIN. (Robins) Fenfluramine HCl 20 mg/Tab. Bot. 100s, 500s.
Use: Anorexiant.
PONSTEL KAPSEALS. (Parke-Davis) Mefenamic acid 250 mg/Cap. Bot. 100s.
Use: Nonsteroidal anti-inflammatory drug; analgesic.
PONTOCAINE 2% AQUEOUS SOLUTION. (Sanofi Winthrop) Tetracaine HCl 20 mg, chlorobutanol 4 mg/ml of 2%

soln. Bot. 30 ml, Box 12s. Bot. 118 ml, Box 6s.
Use: Local anesthetic.
PONTOCAINE 0.5% SOLUTION FOR OPHTHALMOLOGY. (Sanofi Winthrop) Tetracaine HCl 5 mg, sodium Cl 7.5 mg, chlorobutanol 4 mg/ml of 0.5% solution. Bot. 15 ml, Pkg. 12s. Bot. 59 ml Pkg. 6s.
Use: Local anesthetic.
PONTOCAINE CREAM. (Sanofi Winthrop) Tetracaine HCl, equivalent to 1% tetracaine HCl base, in a bland, water-miscible cream with methylparaben and sodium metabisulfite as preservatives. Tube 1 oz. Pkg. 6s.
Use: Local anesthetic.
PONTOCAINE EYE OINTMENT. (Sanofi Winthrop) Tetracaine 0.5% in a base of white petrolatum and light mineral oil. Tube 1/8 oz. Pkg. 12s.
Use: Local anesthetic.
PONTOCAINE HYDROCHLORIDE. (Sanofi Winthrop) Niphanoid (instantly soluble) form consisting of a network of extremely fine, highly purified particles, resembling snow. Amp. 20 mg, Box 100s. 1% isotonic, isobaric solution: Tetracaine HCl 10 mg, sodium Cl 6.7 mg, acetone sodium bisulfite not more than 2 mg/ml. Amp. 2 ml, Box 25s.
Use: Local anesthetic.
PONTOCAINE HYDROCHLORIDE IN DEXTROSE (Hyperbaric) SOLUTIONS. (Sanofi Winthrop) **0.2%:** Tetracaine HCl 2 mg/ml in a sterile solution containing dextrose 6%. Amp. 2 ml, 10s. **0.3%:** Tetracaine HCl 3 mg/ml in a sterile solution containing dextrose 6%. Amp. 5 ml, 10s.
Use: Local anesthetic.
PONTOCAINE OINTMENT. (Sanofi Winthrop) Tetracaine 0.5% and menthol in an ointment consisting of white petrolatum and white wax. Tube 1 oz.
Use: Local anesthetic.
PO-PON-S. (Shionogi) Vitamins A 2000 IU, D 100 IU, E 5 mg, B_1 5 mg, B_2 3 mg, B_3 35 mg, B_5 15 mg, B_6 4 mg, B_{12} 6 mcg, C 100 mg, Ca, P/Tab. Bot. 60s, 240s.
Use: Vitamin/mineral supplement.
POPPY-SEED OIL, The ethyl ester of the fatty acids of the poppy w/iodine.
See: Lipiodol, Ascendant & Lafay, Amps., Vial (Savage).
PORCELANA SKIN BLEACHING AGENT. (Jeffrey Martin) **Regular:** Hydroquinone 2%. Jar 2 oz, 4 oz. **Sunscreen:** Hydroquinone 2%, octyl dimethyl PABA 2.5%. Jar 4 oz.

Use: Skin bleaching agent.
• **PORFIMER SODIUM.** USAN.
Use: Antineoplastic.
• **PORFIROMYCIN.** USAN.
Use: Antibacterial; antineoplastic.
PORK NPH ILETIN II. (Lilly) Purified pork insulin 100 units/ml in isophane insulin suspension (insulin w/ protamine and zinc). Inj. Bot. 10 ml.
Use: Antidiabetic agent.
PORK REGULAR ILETIN II. (Lilly) Insulin 100 units/ml. Purified pork. Inj. Vial 10 ml.
Use: Antidiabetic agent.
PORK THYROID, DEFATTED.
See: Tuloidin, Tab. (Solvay).
• **POROFOCON A.** USAN.
Use: Contact lens material.
• **POROFOCON B.** USAN.
Use: Cabcurve lens (soft lenses).
PORTABIDAY. (Washington Ethical) Concentrated soln. of alkylamine lauryl sulfate, a mild detergent with pH approx. 6 for use with Portabiday Vaginal Cleansing Kit. Bot. 3 oz.
Use: Vaginal preparation.
PORTAGEN. (Mead Johnson Nutrition) A nutritionally complete dietary powder containing as a % of the calories protein 14% as caseinate, fat 41% (medium chain triglycerides 86%, corn oil 14%), carbohydrate 45% as corn syrup solids and sucrose, vitamins A 5000 IU, D 500 IU, E 20 IU, C 52 mg, B_1 1 mg, B_2 1.2 mg, B_6 1.4 mg, B_{12} 4 mcg, niacin 13 mg, folic acid 0.1 mg, choline 83 mg, biotin 0.05 mg, calcium 600 mg, phosphorus 450 mg, magnesium 133 mg, iron 12 mg, iodine 47 mcg, copper 1 mg, zinc 6 mg, manganese 0.8 mg, chloride 550 mg, sodium 300 mg, potassium 800 mg, pantothenic acid 6.7 mg, K-1 0.1 mg/Qt. 20 Kcal/fl oz. Can 1 lb.
Use: Enteral nutritional supplement.
POSITIVE AND NEGATIVE HCG URINE CONTROLS. (Wampole) Positive and negative human urine controls for Wampole urine pregnancy tests. 1 set, 1 vial each.
Use: Diagnostic aid.
POSKINE. B.A.N. O-Propionylhyoscine. Proscopine hydrobromide.
Use: Central nervous system depressant.
POSLAM PSORIASIS OINTMENT. (Last) Sulfur 5%, salicylic acid 2%. Jar 1 oz.
Use: Antipsoriatic.
POSTAFENE.
See: Bonamine, Tab. (Pfizer).
POSTERIOR PITUITARY HORMONES.

See: Pituitrin (S) (Parke-Davis).
Pitressin Synthetic (Parke-Davis).
Pitressin Tannate in Oil (Parke-Davis).
Diapid (Sandoz).
Concentraid (Ferring Labs).
DDAVP (Rhone-Poulenc Rorer).
• **POSTERIOR PITUITARY INJECTION,**
U.S.P. XXIII.
Use: Hormone (antidiuretic).
POSTLOBIN-O.
See: Pituitary, Posterior, Hormone (b).
POSTLOBIN-V.
See: Pituitary, Posterior, Hormone (a).
POSTURE. (Wyeth-Ayerst) Calcium
phosphate 300 mg or 600 mg/Tab. Bot.
60s.
Use: Calcium supplement.
POSTURE D 600. (Wyeth-Ayerst) Calci-
um phosphate 600 mg, vitamin D 125
IU/Tab. Bot. 60s.
Use: Calcium/vitamin D supplement.
POTABA. (Glenwood) Potassium p-
aminobenzoate. **Cap.:** 0.5 Gm. Bot.
250s, 1000s. **Pow.:** 100 Gm. 1 lb. **Tab.:**
0.5 Gm. Bot. 100s, 1000s. **Envule:** 2
Gm. Box 50s.
Use: Para aminobenzoic acid supple-
ment.
POTABLE-AQUA IODINE. (Wisconsin)
Tab. Bot. 50s.
Use: Water purification.
POTABLE AQUA KIT. (Wisconsin)
Tetraglycine hydroperiodide 16.7%
(6.68% titrable iodine). Tab. Bot. 50s
with collapsible gallon container.
Use: Water purification.
POTACHLOR 10%. (My-K Labs) Potassi-
um and chloride 20 mEq/15 ml. With al-
cohol 5%. Bot. pt, gal. With alcohol
3.8%. Bot. pt, gal, UD 15 ml and 30 ml.
Use: Potassium supplement.
POTACHLOR 20%. (My-K Labs) Potassi-
um and chloride 40 mEq/15 ml, alcohol
free. Liq. Bot. pt, gal.
Use: Potassium supplement.
POTASALAN ELIXIR. (Lannett) Potassi-
um Cl 10%, alcohol 4%. Bot. pt, gal.
Use: Potassium supplement.
• **POTASH, SULFURATED,** U.S.P. XXIII.
Use: Pharmaceutical aid (source of sul-
fide).
**POTASSIC SALINE LACTATED INJEC-
TION.**
Use: Fluid and electrolyte replenisher.
• **POTASSIUM ACETATE,** U.S.P. XXIII. Inj.,
U.S.P. XXIII. Acetic acid, potassium salt.
(Various Mfr.) **Inj.:** (Abbott) 40 mEq, 20
ml in 50 ml Vial.
Use: Electrolyte replenisher; to avoid Cl
when high concentration of potassium

is needed.
POTASSIUM ACID PHOSPHATE.
See: K-Phos, Tab. (Beach).
Uro-K, Tab. (Star).
**POTASSIUM ACID PHOSPHATE/SODI-
UM ACID PHOSPHATE.**
Use: Urinary tract product.
See: K-Phos M.F. (Beach).
K-Phos No. 2 (Beach).
• **POTASSIUM ASPARTATE AND MAGNE-
SIUM ASPARTATE.** USAN.
Use: Nutrient.
• **POTASSIUM BENZOATE,** N.F. XVIII.
Use: Preservative.
• **POTASSIUM BICARBONATE,** U.S.P.
XXIII.
Use: Electrolyte replenisher.
• **POTASSIUM BICARBONATE EFFER-
VESCENT TABLETS FOR ORAL SO-
LUTION,** U.S.P. XXIII.
Use: Potassium supplement.
• **POTASSIUM BICARBONATE AND
POTASSIUM CHLORIDE FOR EFFER-
VESCENT ORAL SOLUTION,** U.S.P.
XXIII.
Use: Potassium supplement.
• **POTASSIUM BICARBONATE AND
POTASSIUM CHLORIDE EFFERVES-
CENT TABLETS FOR ORAL SOLU-
TION,** U.S.P. XXIII.
Use: Potassium supplement.
• **POTASSIUM BICARBONATE AND SODI-
UM BICARBONATE AND CITRIC ACID
EFFERVESCENT TABLETS FOR
ORAL SOLUTION,** U.S.P. XXIII
Use: Potassium supplement.
POTASSIUM BITARTRATE.
Use: Cathartic.
POTASSIUM BROMIDE.
W/Aspirin, caffeine, sodium bromide.
See: Lanabac, Tab. (Lannett).
W/Sodium bromide, strontium bromide,
ammonium bromide.
See: Lanabrom, Elix. (Lannett).
• **POTASSIUM CARBONATE,** U.S.P. XXIII.
Use: Potassium therapy.
• **POTASSIUM CHLORIDE,** U.S.P. XXIII.
Extended-Release Cap., Extended-Re-
lease Tab., In Dextrose Inj., Inj., Oral
Soln., For Oral Soln., U.S.P. XXIII. Elixir,
U.S.P. XXI.
Use: Potassium deficiency, hy-
popotassemia.
Ampules:
(Abbott) **Ampules:** 20 mEq, 10 ml; 40
mEq, 20 ml. **Pintop Vials:** 10 mEq, 5
ml in 10 ml; 20 mEq, 10 ml in 20 ml;
30 mEq, 12.5 ml in 30 ml; 40 mEq,
12.5 ml in 30 ml. **Fliptop Vials:** 20
mEq, 10 ml in 20 ml; 40 mEq, 20 ml

in 50 ml. **Univ. Add. Syr.**: 5 mEq/5 ml, 20 mEq/10 ml, 30 mEq/20 ml, 40 mEq/20 ml (Lilly) **Amp.** (40 mEq) 20 ml, 6s, 25s.
Capsules:
See: K-Norm, Cap. (Pennwalt).
Micro-K Extencaps, Cap. (Robins).
Liquid·
See: Cena-K, Liq. (Century).
Choice 10 and 20, Soln. (Whiteworth).
Kaochlor, Preps. (Adria).
Kaon-C1 20%, Liq. (Adria).
Kay Ciel, Elix. (Berlex).
Klor-Con, Liq. (Upsher-Smith).
Klorvess, Liq. (Dorsey).
Klotrix, Tab. (Mead Johnson).
K-Lyte/C1, Tab. (Bristol).
Pan-Kloride, Liq. (U.S. Products).
Potassine, Liq. (Recsei).
Taside, Liq. (Solvay).
Powder:
See: Kaochlor-Eff, Gran. (Adria).
Kato, Pow. (Ingram).
Kay Ciel, Pow. (Berlex).
K-Lor, Pow. (Abbott).
K-Lyte/Cl, Pow. (Bristol).
Potage, Pow. (Lemmon).
Tablets:
See: K⁺8, ER Tab. (Alra).
Kaon, Tab. (Adria).
Kaon Controlled Release Tab. (Adria).
Klorvess Effervescent Tab. (Dorsey).
K-Lyte/Cl 50, Tab. (Bristol).
K-Tab, Tab. (Abbott).
Micro-K Extencap (Robins).
Slow-K, Tab. (Ciba).
Ten-K, Cap. (Geigy).
POTASSIUM CHLORIDE. (Roxane) **Oral soln.:** Potassium Cl, sugar free. 40 mEq/30 ml. Bot. 6 oz, 500 ml, 1 L, 5 L 20%. 80 mEq/30 ml. Bot. 500 ml, 1 L, 5 L. **Pow.:** 20 mEq/4 Gm. Pkt. 30s, 100s.
Use: Potassium supplement.
• **POTASSIUM CHLORIDE IN DEXTROSE AND SODIUM CHLORIDE INJECTION,** U.S.P. XXIII.
• **POTASSIUM CHLORIDE IN LACTATED RINGER'S AND DEXTROSE INJEC-TION,** U.S.P. XXIII.
• **POTASSIUM CHLORIDE IN SODIUM CHLORIDE INJECTION,** U.S.P. XXIII.
• **POTASSIUM CHLORIDE K 42.** USAN.
Use: Radioactive agent.
POTASSIUM CHLORIDE WITH POTAS-SIUM GLUCONATE.
See: Kolyum, Prods. (Pennwalt).
• **POTASSIUM CHLORIDE, POTASSIUM BICARBONATE, AND POTASSIUM CITRATE EFFERVESCENT TABLETS FOR ORAL SOLUTION,** U.S.P. XXIII.

POTASSIUM CHLORIDE SOLUTION, (Lederle) Potassium Cl 10% or 20%. Sugar free. Bot. 16 oz, gal.
Use: Potassium supplement.
• **POTASSIUM CITRATE,** U.S.P. XXIII. **ER Cap., XXII.** Tripotassium Citrate.
Use: Systemic alkalizer. [Orphan drug]
See. Urocit-K, Tab. (Mission).
W/Sodium citrate.
See: Bicitra, Liq. (Willen).
W/Sodium citrate, citric acid.
See: Polycitra-K, Crystals, Liq. (Willen).
Polycitra-LC, Liq.(Willen).
• **POTASSIUM CITRATE AND CITRIC ACID ORAL SOLUTION,** U.S.P. XXIII.
POTASSIUM CLAVULANATE/AMOXI-CILLIN.
Use: Antibacterial, penicillin.
See: Amoxicillin and Potassium Clavu-lanate.
POTASSIUM CLAVULANATE/TICAR-CILLIN.
Use: Antibacterial, penicillin.
See: Ticarcillin and Clavulanate Potas-sium.
POTASSIUM ESTRONE SULFATE.
W/Estrone.
See: Dura-Keelin, Vial (Pharmex).
W/Micro crystalline estrone.
See: Estrones Duo-Action, Vial (Med. Chem.).
• **POTASSIUM GLUCALDRATE.** USAN.
Use: Antacid.
• **POTASSIUM GLUCONATE,** U.S.P. XXIII. Elixir, Tab., U.S.P. XXIII. Monopotassium D-gluconate.
Use: Electrolyte replenisher.
See: Kalinate, Elix. (Bock).
Kaon, Elixir, Tab. (Warren-Teed).
• **POTASSIUM GLUCONATE AND POTAS-SIUM CHLORIDE ORAL SOLUTION,** U.S.P. XXIII.
Use: Replacement therapy.
• **POTASSIUM GLUCONATE AND POTAS-SIUM CHLORIDE FOR ORAL SOLU-TION,** U.S.P. XXIII.
Use: Replacement therapy.
POTASSIUM GLUCONATE ELIXIR.
(Mills) Elemental potassium as potassi-um gluconate 20 mEq, base w/sorbitol soln./Tab. Bot. 8 oz.
Use: Potassium supplement.
POTASSIUM GLUCONATE ELIXIR. (Var-ious Mfr.) Potassium 40 mEq provided by potassium gluconate 9.36 Gm/30 ml, alcohol 5%. Bot. pt, Patient-Cup 15 ml.
Use: Potassium supplement.
• **POTASSIUM GLUCONATE, POTASSIUM CITRATE, AND AMMONIUM CHLO-RIDE ORAL SOLUTION,** U.S.P. XXIII.

Use: Replacement therapy.
• **POTASSIUM GLUCONATE AND POTAS-SIUM CITRATE ORAL SOLUTION,** U.S.P. XXIII.
Use: Replacement therapy.
POTASSIUM GLUTAMATE. The monopotassium salt of l-glutamic acid.
POTASSIUM G PENICILLIN.
See: Penicillin G Potassium, U.S.P. XXIII.
• **POTASSIUM GUAIACOLSULFONATE,** U.S.P. XXIII. Sulfoguaiacol. Potassium Hydroxymethoxybenzenesulfonate. Used in many cough preps.
Use: Expectorant.
See: Conex, Liq. (Westerfield).
Pinex Regular, Syr. (Pinex).
POTASSIUM GUAIACOLSULFONATE W/COMBINATIONS.
See: Cheralin, Syr. (Lannett).
Cherralex, Syr. (Barre).
Efricon Expectorant (Lannett).
Eucapine, Syr. (Lannett).
Formadrin, Liq. (Kenyon).
Guahist, Vial (Hickam).
Guaicohist, Vial (Pharmex).
Guaiodol-Plus, Vial (Kenyon).
Partuss, Liq. (Parmed).
Tusquelin, Syr. (Circle).
POTASSIUM HETACILLIN.
See: Versapen K, Inj., Cap. (Bristol).
• **POTASSIUM HYDROXIDE,** N.F. XVIII.
Use: Pharmaceutical aid (alkalinizing agent).
• **POTASSIUM IODIDE,** U.S.P. XXIII. Tab., Oral Soln., U.S.P. XXIII.
Use: Expectorant; antifungal; source of iodine.
See: Pima, Syr., Expectorant (Fleming).
SSKI, Liq. (Upsher-Smith).
POTASSIUM IODIDE W/COMBINATIONS.
See: Diastix, Reagent Strips (Miles Diagnostic).
Elixophyllin-KI, Elix. (Berlex).
Iodo-Niacin, Tab. (Cole).
KIE, Syr., Tab. (Laser).
Mudrane, Tab. (Poythress).
Mudrane-2, Tab. (Poythress).
Quadrinal, Tab., Susp. (Knoll).
POTASSIUM IODIDE AND NIACINAMIDE.
See: Iodo-Niacin, Tab. (Cole).
POTASSIUM MENAPHTHOSULPHATE.
B.A.N. Dipotassium 2-methyl-1,4-disulp-natonaphthalene. Vikastab [dihydrate]
Use: Vitamin K analogue.
• **POTASSIUM METABISULFITE,** N.F. XVIII.
• **POTASSIUM METAPHOSPHATE,** N.F.

XVIII.
Use: Buffering agent.
POTASSIUM p-AMINOBENZOATE.
See: Potaba, Preps. (Glenwood).
W/Potassium salicylate.
See: Pabalate-SF, Tab. (Robins).
W/Pyridoxine.
See: Potaba Plus 6, Cap., Tab. (Glenwood).
POTASSIUM p-AMINOSALICYLATE.
See: Paskalium, Preps. (Glenwood).
POTASSIUM PENICILLIN G .
Use: Antibiotic.
See: Penicillin G, Potassium U.S.P. XXIII.
POTASSIUM PENICILLIN V.
Use: Antibiotic.
See: Phenoxymethyl Penicillin Potassium, U.S.P. XXIII.
POTASSIUM PERCHLORATE.
Use: Radiopaque agent.
See: Perchloracap (Mallinckrodt).
• **POTASSIUM PERMANGANATE,** U.S.P. XXIII. Tab. for Topical Soln., U.S.P. XXI.
Permanganic acid, potassium salt.
Use: Topical anti-infective.
POTASSIUM PHENETHICILLIN.
Phenethicillin Potassium, U.S.P. XXIII.
Use: Antibiotic.
POTASSIUM PHENOXYMETHYL PENI-CILLIN.
Use: Antibiotic.
See: Penicillin V Potassium, U.S.P. XXIII.
• **POTASSIUM PHOSPHATE,** DIBASIC, U.S.P. XXIII. Inj., U.S.P. XXIII.
Use: Calcium regulator.
• **POTASSIUM PHOSPHATE, MONOBA-SIC,** N.F. XVIII. Dipotassium hydrogen phosphate. Solution by Various Mfr. **Inj.:** (Abbott) 15 mM, 5 ml in 10 ml Vial; 45 mM, 15 ml in 20 ml Vial.
Use: Buffering agent, source of potassium.
POTASSIUM REAGENT STRIPS. (Miles Diagnostic) Quantitative dry reagent strip test for potassium in serum or plasma. Bot. 50s.
Use: Diagnostic aid.
POTASSIUM-REMOVING RESINS.
See: Sodium Polystyrene Sulfonate (Various Mfr.).
SPS (Carolina Medical Products Co.).
Kayexalate (Sanofi Winthrop.)
POTASSIUM RHODANATE.
See: Potassium Thiocyanate.
POTASSIUM SALICYLATE.
See: Neocylate, Tab. (Central).
W/Mephenesin, colchicine alkaloid.
W/Potassium bromide, methapyrilene HCl,

vitamins.
See: Alva-Tranquil, Cap., Tab., T.D. Tab. (Alva/Amco).
W/Potassium p-aminobenzoate.
See: Pabalate-SF, Tab. (Robins).
POTASSIUM SALT.
See: Potassium Sorbate, N.F. XVIII.
•**POTASSIUM SODIUM TARTRATE,** U.S.P. XXIII.
Use: Cathartic.
•**POTASSIUM SORBATE,** N.F. XVIII. 2,4-Hexadienoic Acid, Potassium Salt.
Use: Preservative (antimicrobial).
POTASSIUM SULFOCYANATE. Potassium Rhodanate.
See: Potassium Thiocyanate (Various Mfr.).
POTASSIUM THERAPY.
See: Kaon, Elix., Tab. (Warren-Teed).
Potassium Chloride, Preps. (Various Mfr.).
Slow-K, Tab. (Ciba).
Ten-K, Cap. (Geigy).
POTASSIUM THIOCYANATE. Potassium sulfocyanate, Potassium Rhodanate.
POTASSIUM THIPHENCILLIN. Potassium 6-(phenylmercaptoacetamido)penicillanate.
Use: Anti-infective.
POTASSIUM TROCLOSENE. (Monsanto) Potassium dichloroisocyanurate. Dichloro-s-triazine-2,4,6(1H,3H,5H)trione Potassium derivative.
Use: Anti-infective.
•**POVIDONE,** U.S.P. XXIII. 2-Pyrrolidinone, 1-ethyl, homopolymer.
Use: Dispersing and suspending agent.
•**POVIDONE I-125.** USAN.
Use: Radioactive agent.
•**POVIDONE I-131.** USAN.
Use: Radioactive agent.
•**POVIDONE-IODINE,** U.S.P. XXIII., Topical Aerosol Soln., Oint., Cleansing Soln., Topical Soln., U.S.P. XXIII. Poly(1-(2-oxo-1-pyrrolidinyl)-ethylene) Iodine Complex.
Use: Local anti-infective.
See: Betadine, Preps. (Purdue-Fredrick).
BPS, Preps. (AVP).
Efo-Dine (Fougera).
Femidine, Liq. (AVP).
Isodine, Preps. (Blair).
Massengill Medicated, Liq. (SK-Beecham).
POVIDONE-IODINE COMPLEX.
See: Betadine, Preps. (Purdue-Frederick).
Isodine, Preps. (Blair).
POYALIVER STRONGER. (Forest

Pharm.) Liver inj. (equivalent to 10 mcg B_{12}), vitamin B_{12} 100 mcg, folic acid 10 mcg, niacinamide 1%/ml. Vial 10 ml.
Use: Parenteral nutritional supplement.
POYAMIN JEL INJECTION. (Forest Pharm.) Cyanocobalamin 1000 mcg/ml. Vial 10 ml.
Use: Parenteral nutritional supplement.
POYAPLEX. (Forest Pharm.) Vitamins B_1 100 mg, niacinamide 100 mg, B_6 10 mg, B_2 1 mg, panthenol 10 mg, B_{12} 5 mcg/ml. Vial 10 ml, 30 ml.
Use: Parenteral nutritional supplement.
P.P.D. TUBERCULIN.
See: Tuberculin, Purified Protein Derivative, U.S.P. (Various Mfr.).
P.P. FACTOR (PELLAGRA PREVENTIVE FACTOR).
See: Nicotinic Acid, Preps. (Various Mfr.).
•**PPG-15 STEARYL ETHER.** USAN.
Use: Pharmaceutic aid (surfactant).
PPI-002.
Use: Malignant mesothelioma. [Orphan drug]
PR-122 (REDOX-PHENYTOIN). (Pharmatec)
Use: Anticonvulsant. [Orphan drug]
PR-225 (REDOX-ACYCLOVIR). (Pharmatec)
Use: Treatment of Herpes simplex encephalitis in AIDS. [Orphan drug]
PR-239 (REDOX-PENICILLIN G). (Pharmatec)
Use: Treatment of AIDS-associated neurosyphilis. [Orphan drug]
PR-320 (MOLECUSOL-CARBAMAZEPINE). (Pharmatec)
Use: Anticonvulsant. [Orphan drug]
•**PRACTOLOL.** USAN. 4′-[2-Hydroxy-3-(iso- propylamino)propoxy]acetanilide.
Use: Antiadrenergic (β-receptors).
PRAJMALIUM BITARTRATE. B.A.N. N-Propylaj-malinium hydrogen tartrate.
Use: Treatment of heart arrhythmias.
PRALIDOXIME. B.A.N. 2-Hydroxyiminomethyl-1-methylpyridinium.
Use: Antagonist to cholinesterase inhibitors.
•**PRALIDOXIME CHLORIDE,** U.S.P. XXIII. Sterile, Tabs: U.S.P. XXIII. Pyridinium, 2-[(hydroxyimino)methyl]-1-methyl-,chloride. 2-Formyl-1-methylpyridinium Chloride Oxime. Pam.
Use: Cholinesterase reactivator.
See: Protopam Chloride, Tab., Vial (Wyeth-Ayerst).
•**PRALIDOXIME IODIDE.** USAN. 2-Pyridine aldoxime methiodide.
Use: Cholinesterase reactivator.

See: Protopam Iodide (Wyeth-Ayerst).
• **PRALIDOXIME MESYLATE.** USAN.
Use: Cholinesterase reactivator.
PRALIDOXIME METHIODIDE.
See: Pralidoxime Iodide (Various Mfr.).
PRAMEGEL ANTIPRURITIC GEL. (Gen-Derm) Pramoxine HCl 1%, menthol 0.5% in base w/benzyl alcohol. Bot. 4 oz.
Use: Local anesthetic.
PRAMET FA. (Ross) Vitamins A 4000 IU, D-2 400 IU, C 100 mg, B_1 3 mg, B_2 2 mg, B_6 5 mg, B_{12} 3 mcg, niacinamide 10 mg, calcium pantothenate 0.92 mg, iodine 100 mcg, calcium 250 mg, copper 0.15 mg, iron 60 mg, folic acid 1 mg/Gradumet. Bot. 100s.
Use: Vitamin/mineral supplement.
PRAMILET FA. (Ross) Vitamins A 4000 IU, B_1 3 mg, B_2 2 mg, B_6 3 mg, B_{12} 3 mcg, C 60 mg, D 400 IU, calcium panthothenate 1 mg, niacinamide 10 mg, calcium 250 mg, copper 0.15 mg, iodine 0.1 mg, iron 40 mg, magnesium 10 mg, zinc 0.085 mg, folic acid 1 mg/Filmtab. Bot. 100s.
Use: Vitamin/mineral supplement.
PRAMIRACETAM SULFATE.
Use: Adjunct to electroconvulsive therapy. [Orphan drug]
PRAMIVERINE. B.A.N. 4,4-Diphenyl-N-isopropylcyclohexylamine.
Use: Spasmolytic.
PRAMOCAINE (I.N.N.). Pramoxine, B.A.N.
Use: Allergic dermatitis.
PRAMOSONE CREAM 0.5%. (Ferndale) Hydrocortisone acetate 0.5%, pramoxine HCl 1% in cream base. Tube 1 oz, 4 oz. Jar 4 oz, lb.
Use: Corticosteroid, local anesthetic.
PRAMOSONE CREAM 1%. (Ferndale) Hydrocortisone acetate 1%, pramoxine HCl 1% in cream base. Tube 1 oz, 4 oz. Jar 4 oz, lb.
Use: Corticosteroid, local anesthetic.
PRAMOSONE CREAM 2.5%. (Ferndale) Hydrocortisone acetate 2.5%, pramoxine HCl 1% in cream base. Tube 1 oz, 4 oz. Jar lb.
Use: Corticosteroid, local anesthetic.
PRAMOSONE LOTION 0.5%. (Ferndale) Hydrocortisone acetate 0.5%, pramoxine HCl 1% in lotion base. Bot. 1 oz, 4 oz, 8 oz.
Use: Corticosteroid, local anesthetic.
PRAMOSONE LOTION 1%. (Ferndale) Hydrocortisone acetate 1%, pramoxine HCl 1% in lotion base. Bot. 2 oz, 4 oz, 8 oz.

Use: Corticosteroid, local anesthetic.
PRAMOSONE LOTION 2.5%. (Ferndale) Hydrocortisone acetate 2.5%, pramoxine HCl 1% in lotion base. Bot 2 oz, gal.
Use: Corticosteroid, local anesthetic.
PRAMOSONE OINTMENT 1%. (Ferndale) Hydrocortisone acetate 1%, pramoxine HCl 1% in ointment base. Tube 1 oz, 4 oz. Jar 4 oz, lb.
Use: Corticosteroid, local anesthetic.
PRAMOXINE. B.A.N. 4-[3-(4-Butoxyphenoxy)-propyl]morpholine. Pramocaine (I.N.N.).
Use: Local anesthetic.
• **PRAMOXINE HYDROCHLORIDE,** U.S.P. XXIII. Cream, Jelly, U.S.P. XXIII. 4-[3-(p-Butoxyphenoxy)propyl]morpholine HCl.
See: Local anesthetic.
See: Itch-X, Spray (B. F. Ascher & Co.).
Prax, Lot. (Ferndale).
Proctofoam, Aerosol (Reed & Carnrick).
Tronothane HCl, Cream, Jel (Abbott).
PRAMOXINE HCl W/COMBINATIONS.
See: Anti-Itch, Lot. (Towne).
Dermarex, Cream (Hyrex).
Gentz, Jelly, Wipes (Philips Roxane).
1 + 1 Creme (Dunhall).
1 + 1-F Creme (Dunhall).
Otocalm-H Ear Drops (Parmed).
Perifoam, Aerosol (Rowell Labs.).
Proctofoam-HC, Aerosol (Reed-Carnrick).
Sherform-HC, Oint. (Sheryl).
Steraform Creme (Mayrand).
Steramine Otic, Drops (Mayrand).
PRAMPINE. B.A.N. O-Propionylatropine, PAMN methonitrate.
Use: Treatment of peptic ulcer.
• **PRANOLIUM CHLORIDE.** USAN.
Use: Cardiac depressant.
PRAVACHOL. (Bristol-Myers Squibb). Pravastatin sodium **10 mg or 20 mg:** Tab. Bot. 100s, UD 100s; **40 mg:** Tab. Bot. 100s.
Use: Antihyperlipidemic agent.
PRAVASTIN SODIUM.
Use: Antihyperlipidemic agent.
See: Pravachol (Bristol-Myers Squibb).
PRAX CREAM. (Ferndale) Pramoxine HCl 1% in cream base. Tube 1 oz. Jar 4 oz, lb.
Use: Local anesthetic.
PRAX LOTION. (Ferndale) Pramoxine HCl 1%. Bot. 15 ml, 120 ml.
Use: Local anesthetic.
• **PRAZEPAM,** U.S.P. XXIII. Cap., Tab. U.S.P. XXIII. 7-Chloro-1-(cyclopropyl-methyl)-1,2-dihydro-5-phenyl-2H-1, 4-benzodiazepin-2-one. (Various Mfr.)

Tab.: 5 mg or 10 mg. Bot. 100s, 500s;
Cap.: 5 mg or 10 mg. Bot. 100s, 500s.
Use: Muscle relaxant.
See: Centrax, Cap. (Parke-Davis).
•**PRAZIQUANTEL,** U.S.P. XXIII, Tab. 2-Cyclohexylcarbonyl-1,3,4,6,7,11b-hexahydro-2H-pyrazino[2,1-a]-isoquinolin-4-ono.
Use: Anthelmintic.
See: Biltricide, Tab. (Miles Pharm).
PRAZITONE. B.A.N. 5-Phenyl-5-(2-piperidyl)-methylbarbituric acid.
Use: Antidepressant.
•**PRAZOSIN HYDROCHLORIDE,** U.S.P. XXIII. Cap., U.S.P. XXIII. 1-(4-Amino-6,7-dimethoxy-2-quinazoliny)-4-(2-furoyl)piperazine monohydrochloride. (Various Mfr.) 1 mg, 2 mg, 5 mg. Cap. Bot. 30s, 60s, 90s, 100s, 120s, 250s, 500s, 1000s, UD 100s.
Use: Antihypertensive.
See: Minipress, Cap. (Pfizer Laboratories).
PRE-ATTAIN LIQUID. (Sherwood) Sodium caseinate, maltodextrin, corn oil, soy lecithin, vitamins A, B_1, B_2, B_3, B_5, B_6, B_{12}, C, D, E, K, folic acid, Ca, Cl, Cu, Fe, I, Mg, Mn, P, Zn. Can 250 ml, closed system 1000 ml.
Use: Enteral nutritional supplement.
PRECEF FOR INJECTION. (Bristol) Ceforanide 500 mg or 1 Gm/Vial or piggyback.
Use: Antibacterial, cephalosporin.
PRECISION HIGH NITROGEN DIET. (Sandoz Nutrition) Vanilla flavor: Maltodextrin, pasteurized egg white solids, sucrose, natural and artificial flavors, medium chain triglycerides, partially hydrogenated soybean oil, polysorbate 80, mono and diglycerides, vitamins, minerals. Pow. Packet 2.93 oz.
Use: Enteral nutritional supplement.
PRECISION LR DIET. (Sandoz Nutrition) Orange flavor: Maltodextrin,pasteurized egg white solids, sucrose, medium chain triglycerides, partially hydrogenated soybean oil with BHA, citric acid, natural and artificial flavors, mono and diglycerides, polysorbate 80, FD & C Yellow No. 5 and No. 6, vitamins, minerals. Pow. Packet 3 oz.
Use: Enteral nutritional supplement.
PREDAJECT. (Mayrand) Prednisolone acetate 50 mg/ml. Vial 10 ml.
Use: Corticosteroid.
PREDALONE 50. (Forest) Prednisolone acetate 50 mg/ml. Vial 10 ml.
Use: Corticosteroid.
PREDAMIDE OPHTHALMIC. (Maurry) Sodium sulfacetamide 10%, prednisolone acetate 0.5%, hydroxyethyl cellulose, polysorbate 80, sodium thiosulfate, benzalkonium Cl 0.025%. Bot. 5 ml, 15 ml.
Use: Anti-infective, corticosteroid, ophthalmic.
PREDCOR INJECTION. (Hauck) Prednisolone acetate 25 mg or 50 mg/ml. Vial 10 ml.
Use: Corticosteroid.
PRED-FORTE. (Allergan) Prednisolone acetate 1%, benzalkonium Cl polysorbate 80, boric acid, sodium citrate, sodium bisulfite, sodium Cl, edetate disodium, hydroxypropyl methylcellulose, purified water. Susp. Plastic dropper bot. 1 ml, 5 ml, 10 ml, 15 ml.
Use: Corticosteroid, ophthalmic.
PRED-G. (Allergan) Prednisolone acetate 1%, gentamicin sulfate 0.3%. Bot. 2 ml, 5 ml, 10 ml.
Use: Corticosteroid, anti-infective, ophthalmic.
PRED-G S.O.P. (Allergan) Prednisolone acetate 0.6%, gentamicin sulfate 0.3%, chlorobutanol 0.5%. Oint. Tube 3.5 g.
Use: Antibiotic, corticosteroid, ophthalmic.
PREDICORT-AP. (Dunhall) Prednisolone sodium phosphate 20 mg, prednisolone acetate 80 mg/ml. Vial 10 ml.
Use: Corticosteroid.
PREDICORT-RP. (Dunhall) Prednisolone sodium phosphate equivalent to prednisolone phosphate 20 mg, niacinamide 25 mg/ml. Vial 10 ml.
Use: Corticosteroid.
PRED MILD. (Allergan) Prednisolone acetate 0.12%, benzalkonium Cl, polysorbate 80, boric acid, sodium citrate, sodium bisulfite, sodium Cl, edetate disodium, hydroxypropyl methylcellulose, purified water. Susp. Bot. 5 ml, 10 ml.
Use: Corticosteroid, ophthalmic.
•**PREDNAZATE.** USAN.
Use: Anti-inflammatory.
•**PREDNICARBATE.** USAN.
Use: Glucocorticoid.
See: Dermatop, Cream (Hoechst-Roussel).
PREDNICEN-M. (Central) Prednisone 5 mg/Tab. Bot. 100s, 1000s.
Use: Corticosteroid.
•**PREDNIMUSTINE.** USAN.
Use: Antineoplastic. [Orphan drug]
PREDNISOLAMATE. B.A.N. Prednisolone 21-diethylaminoacetate. Deltacortril DA hydrochloride.
Use: Corticosteroid.

• **PREDNISOLONE,** U.S.P. XXIII. Cream, Tab., U.S.P. XXIII. Pregna-1,4-diene-3,20-dione, 11,17,21-trihy-droxy-, (11β)-11β,17,21-Trihydroxypregna-1,4-diene-3,20 dione. Metacortandralone.
Use: Adrenocortical steroid (anti-inflammatory).
See: Cordrol, Tab. (Vita Elixir).
   Delta-Cortef, Tab. (Upjohn).
   Fernisolone, Tab., Inj. (Ferndale).
   Orasone, Tab. (Solvay).
   Orasone 50, Tab. (Solvay).
   Prednis, Tab. (USV Labs.).
W/Aluminum hydroxide gel, dried.
See: Predoxide, Tab. (Hauck).
W/Aspirin.
See: Sarogesic, Tab. (Saron).
W/Chloramphenicol.
See: Chloroptic-P, Ophthalmic Oint. (Allergan).
W/Neomycin sulfate.
   Neo-Deltef, Drops (Upjohn).
W/Sulfacetamide sodium, methyloollulose.
See: Isopto Cetapred, Susp. (Alcon).
W/Sulfacetamide sodium.
See: Cetapred Ophthalmic Oint. (Alcon).
• **PREDNISOLONE ACETATE,** U.S.P. XXIII, Ophth., Sterile Susp., U.S.P. XXIII. Pregna-1,4-diene-3,20-dione, 21-(acetyloxy)-11,17-dihydroxy-,(11β)-
Use: Adrenocortical steroid (anti-inflammatory).
See: Econopred, Susp. (Alcon).
   Key-Pred, Inj. (Hyrex).
   Nisolone, Vial (Ascher).
   Predicort, Amp. (Dunhall).
   Pred, Preps. (Allergan).
   Pred-Forte, Ophthalmic Susp. (Allergan).
   Savacort-50, 100, Vial (Savage).
   Sigpred, Inj. (Sig).
   Steraject, Vial (Mayrand).
   Sterane, Inj. (Pfizer Laboratories).
PREDNISOLONE ACETATE W/COMBINATIONS.
See: Blephamide Liquifilm, Soln. (Allergan).
   Blephamide S.O.P., Ophthalmic, Oint. (Allergan).
   Cetapred Opthalmic Oint. (Alcon).
   Dua-Pred, Inj. (Solvay).
   Isopto Cetapred Susp. (Alcon).
   Metimyd, Ophthalmic Susp., Oint. (Schering).
   Neo-Delta-Cortef, Preps. (Upjohn).
   Panacort R-P, Vial (Ferndale).
   Prednefrin, Mild, Susp. (Allergan).
   Sulphrin Ophth. Oint. (Bausch &

Lomb).
   Tri-Ophtho, Ophthalmic (Maurry).
   Vasocidin, Preps. (Iolab).
PREDNISOLONE ACETATE AND PREDNISOLONE SODIUM PHOSPHATE.
(Various Mfr.) Prednisolone acetate 80 mg, prednisolone sodium phosphate 20 mg/ml. Inj. Susp. Vial 10 ml.
Use: Corticosteroid.
• **PREDNISOLONE ACETATE OPHTHALMIC SUSPENSION,** U.S.P. XXIII.
See: Prednisolone Acetate.
PREDNISOLONE BUTYLACETATE. 1,4-Pregnadiene-3,20-dione-11β,17α,21-triol-tert-butyl-acetate.
Use: Corticosteroid.
See: Hydeltra-T.B.A., Vial (Merck & Co.).
PREDNISOLONE CYCLOPENTYLPROPIONATE. d^1,4-Pregnadiene-3,20-dione-11, 17a-diol-21-cy-clopentylpropionate(prednisolone-21 cyclopentylpropionate).
Use: Corticosteroid.
• **PREDNISOLONE HEMISUCCINATE, U.S.P..** U.S.P. XXIII. Pregna-1,4-diene-3,20-dione, 21-(3-carboxy-1-oxopropoxy)-11, 17-dihydroxy-, (11β)-.
Use: Adrenocortical steroid (anti-inflammatory).
• **PREDNISOLONE SODIUM PHOSPHATE,** U.S.P. XXIII. Inj., Ophth. Soln.: U.S.P. XXIII. Pregna-1,4-diene-3,20-dione, 11,17-dihydroxy-21-(phosphonoxy)-,disodium salt, (11) . (Various Mfr.) 0.125%, 1% Soln. Bot. 5 ml, 15 ml.
Use: Adrenocortical steroid (anti-inflammatory).
See: AK-Pred, Soln. (Akorn).
   Alto-Pred Soluble, Vial (Alto).
   Hydeltrasol, Inj. (Merck & Co.).
   Inflamase Forte, Ophthalmic Soln. (Iolab).
   Inflamase, Ophthalmic Soln. (Iolab).
   Key-Pred SP, Inj. (Hyrex).
   Liquid Pred, Inj. (Muro).
   Metreton, Ophthalmic Soln. Sterile (Schering).
   Pediapred, Liq. (Fisons).
   P.S.P. IV (Four), Inj. (Solvay).
   Savacort-S, Inj. (Savage).
W/Neomycin sulfate.
See: Neo-Hydeltrasol, Ophthalmic Soln., Ophthalmic Oint. (Merck & Co.).
W/Niacinamide, disodium edetate, sodium bisulfite, phenol.
See: P.S.P. IV, Inj. (Solvay).
W/Prednisolone acetate.
See: Panacort R-P, Vial (Ferndale).
   Solu-Pred, Vial (Kenyon).

W/Sodium Sulfacetamide.
See: Optimyd, Soln. (Schering).
Vasocidin, Liq. (Iolab).
PREDNISOLONE TERTIARY-BUTYLAC-ETATE.
See: Prednisolone Tebutate, U.S.P. XXIII.
PREDNISOL T.B.A (Pasadena Research) Prednisolone tebutate 20 mg/ml. Vial 10 ml.
Use: Corticosteroid.
• **PREDNISOLONE TEBUTATE SUSPENSION, STERILE,** U.S.P. XXIII. Pregna-1,4-diene-3,20-dione, 11,17-dihydroxy-21-(3,3-dimethyl-1-oxobutyl)oxy-, (11β).
Use: Adrenocorticol steroid.
See: Hydeltra-T.B.A., Vial (Merck & Co.).
Metalone, Vial (Foy).
• **PREDNISONE,** U.S.P. XXIII. Oral Soln., Syrup, Tabs., U.S.P. XXIII. Pregna-1,4-diene-3,11,20-trione, 17,21-dihydroxy-. D1,4-Pregnadiene-17α,21-diol-3,11-20-trione. 1-Dehydro-cortisone, Metacortandracin. 17,21-Dihydroxypregna-1,4-diene-3,11,20-trione.
Use: Glucocorticoid.
See: Delta-Dome, Tab. (Miles Pharm).
Deltasone, Tab. (Upjohn).
Keysone, Tab.(Hyrex).
Meticorten, Tab. (Schering).
Maso-Pred, Tab. (Mason).
Orasone, Tab. (Solvay).
Sterapred, Tab. (Mayrand).
W/Chlorpheniramine maleate.
See: Histone, Tab. (Blaine).
W/Phenylephrine HCl.
See: Prednefrin-S, Soln. (Allergan).
PREDNISONE INTENSOL ORAL SOLUTION. (Roxane) Prednisone concentrated oral solution 5 mg/ml. Bot. 30 ml w/calibrated dropper.
Use: Corticosteroid.
• **PREDNIVAL.** USAN. 11 beta, 17, 21-Trihydroxypregna-1,4-diene-3,20-dione 17 valerate.
Under study.
Use: Topical anti-inflammatory.
PREDNYLIDENE. B.A.N. 11β,17α,21-Trihydroxy-16-methylenepregna-1,4-diene-3,20-dione. Dacortilene; Decortilen.
Use: Corticosteroid.
PREDSULFAIR. (Pharmafair) **Drops:** Prednisolone acetate 0.5%, sodium sulfacetamide 10%, hydroxypropyl methylcellulose, polysorbate 80 0.5%, sodium thiosulfate, benzalkonium Cl 0.01%. Bot. 5 ml, 15 ml. **Oint.:** Prednisolone acetate 0.5%, sodium sulfacetamide 10%, mineral oil, white petrolatum, lanolin,

parabens. In 3.5 Gm.
Use: Corticosteroid, anti-infective, ophthalmic.
PREFLEX FOR SENSITIVE EYES. (Alcon Lenscare) Isotonic, aqueous solution of sorbic acid sodium phosphates, sodium Cl, tyloxapol, hydroxyethyl cellulose, polyvinyl alcohol. Bot. 1.5 oz.
Use: Soft contact lens care.
PREFRIN LIQUIFILM. (Allergan) Phenylephrine HCl 0.12%, antipyrine 0.1%, polyvinyl alcohol 1.4%, benzalkonium Cl 0.004%, edetate disodium. Bot. 0.7 fl oz.
Use: Ophthalmic decongestant.
PREFRIN-A. (Allergan) Phenylephrine 0.12%, pyrilamine maleate 0.1%, antipyrine 0.1%, benzalkonium Cl, sodium bisulfite, edetate disodium. Bot. 15 ml.
Use: Ophthalmic antihistamine, decongestant.
PREGESTIMIL. (Mead Johnson Nutrition) Protein hydrolysate formula supplies 640 calories/qt. protein 18 Gm, fat 26 Gm, carbohydrate 86 Gm, vitamins A 2000 IU, D 400 IU, E 15 IU, C 52 mg, folic acid 100 mcg, thiamine 0.5 mg, riboflavin 0.6 mg, niacin 8 mg, B_6 0.4 mg, B_{12} 2 mcg, biotin 0.05 mg, pantothenic acid 3 mg, K-1 100 mcg, choline 85 mg, inositol 30 mg, calcium 600 mg, phosphorus 400 mg, iodine 45 mcg, iron 12 mg, magnesium 70 mg, copper 0.6 mg, zinc 4 mg, manganese 0.2 mg, chloride 550 mg, potassium 700 mg, sodium 300 mg/Qt. (20 Kcal/fl oz.). Pow. Can lb.
Use: Enteral nutritional supplement.
PREGNASLIDE LATEX HCG TEST WITH FAST TRAK SLIDES. (Wampole) Latex agglutination slide test for the qualitative detection of human chorionic gonadotropin in urine. Test 24s. Test kit 96s.
Use: Diagnostic aid.
PREGNENINOLONE.
See: Ethisterone.
• **PREGNENOLONE.** F.D.A. 3-beta-Hydroxypregn-5-en-20-one. Synthetic steroid intermediate. 3-Hydroxy-20-keto-pregene-5.
Use: Treatment of rheumatoid arthritis.
• **PREGNENOLONE SUCCINATE.** USAN. 3-Hydroxy-5-pregnen-20-one, hydrogen succinate.
Use: Glucocorticoid.
PREGNOSIS SLIDE TEST. (Roche Diagnostics) Latex agglutination inhibition slide test. 50s, 200s.
Use: Diagnostic aid.
PREGNOSPIA. (Organon Technica) Mon-

oclonal antibody-based enzyme immunoassay. 25s, 100s.
Use: Diagnostic aid.
PREGNYL. (Organon) Human chorionic gonadotropin 10,000 IU/Vial w/diluent 10 ml, mannitol, benzyl alcohol. Vial 10 ml.
Use: Chorionic gonadotropin.
PRE-H CAL. (T.E. Williams) Calcium 95 mg, iron 51.5 mg, vitamins A 4000 IU, D 400 IU, B_1 3 mg, B_2 3 mg, B_5 3 mg, B_6 5 mg, B_{12} 2.5 mcg, C 50 mg, folic acid 0.5 mg, Cu/Tab. Bot. 60s.
Use: Vitamin/mineral supplement.
PREJECT PREINJECTION TOPICAL ANESTHETIC. (Hoyt) Benzocaine 20% in polyethylene glycol base. Jar 2 oz.
Use: Local anesthetic.
PRELAN. (Lannett) Vitamins A 4000 IU, B_1 0.5 mg, B_2 2 mg, niacin 10 mg, B_6 3 mg, B_{12} 2 mcg, D 400 IU, C 50 mg, calcium 200 mg, iron 30 mg/Tab. Bot. 100s.
Use: Vitamin/mineral supplement.
PRELAN F.A. TABLETS. (Lannett) Vitamin A 4000 IU, B_1 0.5 mg, B_2 2 mg, niacin 10 mg, B_6 3 mg, B_{12} 2 mcg, D 400 IU, C 50 mg, calcium 200 mg, iron 30 mg, folic acid 1 mg/Tab. Bot. 100s.
Use: Vitamin/mineral supplement.
PRELESTRIN. (Pasadena Research) Conjugated estrogens 0.625 mg or 1.25 mg/Tab. Bot. 100s, 1000s.
Use: Estrogen.
PRELONE SYRUP. (Muro) Prednisolone 15 mg/5 ml, alcohol 5%, saccharin. Cherry flavor. 240 ml.
Use: Corticosteroid.
PRELU-2. (Boehringer Ingelheim) Phendimetrazine tartrate 105 mg/Cap. Bot. 100s.
Use: Anorexiant.
PREMARIN. (Wyeth-Ayerst) Conjugated estrogens tablets. Water-soluble conjugated estrogens derived from natural sources. 0.3 mg, 0.625 mg, 0.9 mg, 1.25 mg or 2.5 mg/Tab.: Bot. 100s, 1000s. 0.625 mg or 1.25 mg: 5000s, UD 100s. Cycle packs 25s.
Use: Estrogen.
PREMARIN INTRAVENOUS. (Wyeth-Ayerst) Conjugated Estrogens U.S.P., for Injection. Vial 25 mg/5 ml w/diluent. (Vial also contains lactose 200 mg, sodium citrate 12.5 mg, simethicone 0.2 mg). Diluent contains benzyl alcohol 2%, Water for Injection, U.S.P.
Use: Estrogen.
PREMARIN VAGINAL CREAM. (Wyeth-Ayerst) Conjugated Estrogens, U.S.P. 0.625 mg/1 Gm w/cetyl esters wax, cetyl

alcohol, white wax, glyceryl monostearate, propylene glycol monostearate, methyl stearate, phenylethyl alcohol, sodium lauryl sulfate, glycerin, mineral oil. Tube w/applicator 1.5 oz. (42.5 Gm). Tube refill.
Use: Estrogen.
PREMARIN W/MEPROBAMATE.
See: PMB 200 and 400, Tab. (Wyeth-Ayerst).
PREMARIN W/METHYLTESTOS-TERONE. (Wyeth-Ayerst) Premarin (Conjugated Estrogens, U.S.P.) 1.25 mg, methyltestosterone 10 mg/Yellow Tab. Premarin 0.625 mg, methyltestosterone 5 mg/Red Tab. Bot. 100s, 1000s.
Use: Estrogen, androgen combination.
W/Methyltestosterone, methamphetamine HCl, vitamins.
See: Mediatric, Cap., Liq., Tab. (Wyeth-Ayerst).
PREMATE-200. (Major) Meprobamate 200 mg, tridihexethyl Cl 25 mg/Tab. Bot. 100s.
Use: Antianxiety agent, anticholinergic.
PREMATE-400. (Major) Meprobamate 400 mg, tridihexethyl Cl 25 mg/Tab. Bot. 100s.
Use: Antianxiety agent, anticholinergic.
PREMENSTRUAL TENSION.
See: Motion Sickness.
Pamabrom (Various Mfr.).
Pyranisamine Bromotheophyllinate (Various Mfr.).
PREMSYN PMS CAPLETS. (Chattem) Acetaminophen 500 mg, pamabrom 25 mg, pyrilamine maleate 15 mg/Capl. Bot. 20s, 40s.
Use: Analgesic, diuretic, antihistamine.
• **PRENALTEROL HYDROCHLORIDE.** USAN.
Use: Adrenergic.
PRENATAL. (Kenyon) Vitamins A 100 IU, D 500 IU, B_1 1 mg, C 25 mg, B_2 1 mg, niacinamide 3 mg, iron 39 mg, calcium 140 mg, phosphorus 62 mg, potassium iodide 0.065 mg, copper sulfate 1 mg, cobalt sulfate 1 mg, magnesium oxide 10 mg, manganese sulfate 14 mg, potassium sulfate 11 mg, sodium sulfate 0.4 mg, zinc oxide 0.4 mg, fluoride 1 mg/Tab. Bot. 100s, 1000s.
Use: Vitamin/mineral supplement.
PRENATAL FOLIC ACID + IRON. (Everett) Vitamins, minerals, folic acid 1 mg/Tab. Bot. 100s.
Use: Vitamin/mineral supplement.
PRENATAL MR 90. (Ethex) Calcium 250 mg, iron 90 mg, vitamin A 4000 IU, D 400 IU, E 30 mg, B_1 3 mg, B_2 3.4 mg, B_3

20 mg, B_6 20 mg, B_{12} 12 mcg, C 120 mg, folic acid 1 mg, Zn 25 mg, I, Cu, DSS. Tab. Bot. 100s.
Use: Vitamin supplement.
PRENATAL NO. 2. (Kenyon) Vitamins A 4000 IU, B_1 2 mg, B_2 2 mg, B_6 0.8 mg, C 50 mg, niacinamide 10 mg, iodide 0.15 mg, folic acid 0.1 mg, B_{12} concentrate 2 mcg, iron 50 mg, calcium 240 mg/Cap. Bot. 100s, 1000s.
Use: Vitamin/mineral supplement.
PRENATAL ONE. (Major) Vitamins A 8000 IU, D 400 IU, E 30 mg, C 90 mg, folic acid 1 mg, B_1 2.5 mg, B_2 3 mg, niacin 20 mg, B_6 10 mg, B_{12} 12 mcg, calcium 200 mg, iodine, iron 65 mg, magnesium, zinc 35 mg/Tab. Bot. 100s, 500s.
Use: Vitamin/mineral supplement.
PRENATAL-S. (Goldline) Calcium 200 mg, iron 60 mg, vitamins A 8000 IU, D 400 IU, E 30 mg, B_1 1.7 mg, B_2 2 mg, B_3 20 mg, B_6 4 mg, B_{12} 8 mcg, C 60 mg, folic acid 0.8 mg, I, Mg, zinc 25 mg/Tab. Bot. 100s, 1000s.
Use: Vitamin/mineral supplement.
PRENATAL WITH FOLIC ACID. (Geneva Generics) Calcium 200 mg, iron 60 mg, vitamins A 8000 IU, D 400 IU, E 30 mg, B_1 1.7 mg, B_2 2 mg, B_3 20 mg, B_6 4 mg, B_{12} 8 mcg, C 60 mg, folic acid 0.8 mg, I, Mg/Tab. Bot. 100s.
Use: Vitamin/mineral supplement.
PRENATAL WITH FOLIC ACID. (Vitarine) Vitamins A 6000 IU, D 400 IU, E 30 IU, folic acid 1 mg, C 60 mg, B_1 1.1 mg, B_2 1.8 mg, B_6 2.5 mg, B_{12} 5 mcg, niacin 15 mg, calcium 125 mg, iron 65 mg/Tab. Bot. 100s, 1000s.
Use: Vitamin/mineral supplement.
PRENATE 90 TABLETS. (Bock) Vitamins A 8000 IU, D 400 IU, E 30 mg, C 120 mg, folic acid 1 mg, B_1 3 mg, B_2 3.4 mg, B_6 20 mg, B_{12} 12 mcg, niacinamide 20 mg, docusate sodium, calcium 250 mg, iodine, iron 90 mg, Cu, zinc 20 mg/FC Tab. Bot. 100s, 1000s.
Use: Vitamin/mineral supplement.
PRENAVITE. (Rugby) Calcium 200 mg, iron 60 mg, vitamins A 8000 IU, D 400 IU, E 30 mg, B_1 1.7 mg, B_2 2 mg, B_3 20 mg, B_6 4 mg, B_{12} 8 mcg, C 60 mg, folic acic 0.8 mg, I, Mg/Tab., sodium free. Bot. 100s, 500s.
Use: Vitamin/mineral supplement.
PRENISTAT. (Pharmex) Prednisolone sodium phosphate 20 mg, niacinamide 25 mg/ml. Vial 10 ml.
Use: Corticosteroid.
•**PRENYLAMINE.** USAN. N-(3,3-Diphenyl-

propyl)-α-methylphenethylamine. Segontin; Synadrin lactate.
Use: Coronary vasodilator.
PREPARATION H. (Whitehall) Phenylmercuric nitrate 1:10,000, live yeast cell derivative 2000 units skin respiratory factor, shark liver oil 3%. Supp. w/PEG 600 dilaurate. **Oint.:** Tube 1 oz, 2 oz. Supp. 12s, 24s, 36s, 48s. **Cream:** Tube 27 g, 54 g.
Use: Anorectal preparation.
PREPARATION H CLEANSING TISSUES. (Whitehall) Propylene glycol, phenoxyethanol, parabens, citric acid, alcohol free. In travel pack, 40s.
Use: Anorectal preparation.
PREPCAT. (Lafayette) Barium sulfate 1.2% w/w suspension. Bot. 480 ml, Case Bot. 24s.
Use: Radiopaque agent.
PREPCAT 2000. (Lafayette) Barium sulfate 1.2% w/w suspension. Bot. 2000 ml, Case Bot. 4s.
Use: Radiopaque agent.
PREPCORT CREAM. (Whitehall) Hydrocortisone 0.5%. Tube 0.5 oz, 1 oz.
Use: Corticosteroid.
PRE-PEN. (Kremers-Urban) Benzylpenicilloyl-polylysine 0.25 ml/Amp.
Use: Diagnostic aid.
PRE-PEN/MDM. (Kremers Urban)
See: BENZYLPENICILLIN, BENZYLPENICILLOIC, BENZYLPENILLOIC ACID.
PREPIDIL. (Upjohn) Dinoprostone 0.5 mg/Gel. Syringes (with 2 shielded catheters 10 and 20 mm tip) 3 Gm.
Use: Agent for cervical ripening.
PREPODYNE. (West) Titratable iodine. **Soln.:** 1%. Bot. pt, gal. **Scrub:** 0.75%. Bot. 6 oz, gal. **Swabs:** Saturated with soln. Pkt. 1s, Box 100s. **Swabsticks:** Saturated with soln. Pkt. 1s, Box 50s. Pkt. 3s, Box 75s.
Use: Topical antiseptic.
PRESALIN. (Hauck) Aspirin 260 mg, salicylamide 120 mg, acetaminophen 120 mg, aluminum hydroxide 100 mg/Tab. Bot. 50s.
Use: Analgesic combination, antacid.
PRESSOR AGENTS.
See: Sympathomimetic agents.
PRESSOROL. (Travenol) Metaraminol bitartrate. Vial 10 ml (10 mg/ml).
Use: Vasopressor.
PRESUN 4 CREAMY. (Bristol-Myers) Padimate O 1.4%, alcohol, titanium dioxide. Waterproof lotion. Bot. 4 oz.
Use: Sunscreen.
PRESUN 8 CREAMY. (Bristol-Myers)

Padimate O 5%, oxybenzone 2%. Waterproof. Bot. 4 oz.
Use: Sunscreen.
PRESUN 8 LOTION. (Bristol-Myers) Padimate O 7.3%, oxybenzone 2.3%, SD alcohol 40 60%. Bot. 4 oz.
Use: Sunscreen.
PRESUN 15 CREAMY. (Bristol-Myers) Padimate O 8%, oxybenzone 3%, benzyl alcohol. Waterproof. Bot. 4 oz.
Use: Sunscreen.
PRESUN 15 FACIAL SUNSCREEN. (Bristol-Myers) Padimate O (Octyl dimethyl PABA) 8%, oxybenzone 3%. Bot. 2 oz.
Use: Sunscreen.
PRESUN 15 FACIAL SUNSCREEN STICK. (Bristol-Myers) Octyl dimethyl PABA 8%, oxybenzone 3%. Stick 0.42 oz.
Use: Sunscreen.
PRESUN 15 LIP PROTECTOR. (Bristol Myers) Padimate O 8%, oxybenzone 3%. Stick 4.5 Gm.
Use: Sunscreen.
PRESUN 15 LOTION. (Bristol-Myers) Padimate O 5%, PABA 5%, oxybenzone 3%, SD alcohol 40 58%. Bot. 4 oz.
Use: Sunscreen.
PRESUN 15 SENSITIVE SKIN SUNSCREEN. (Bristol-Myers) Octyl methoxycinnamate, oxybenzone, octyl salicylate, cetyl alcohol, PABA free, waterproof, SPF 15. Cream. Bot. 120 ml.
Use: Sunscreen.
PRESUN 23. (Bristol-Myers) Padimate O, octyl methoxycinnamate, oxybenzone, octyl salicylate, SD alcohol 40 19%, waterproof. Spray mist. Bot. 105 ml.
Use: Sunscreen.
PRESUN 29 SENSITIVE SKIN SUNSCREEN. (Bristol-Myers) Octyl methoxycinnamate, oxybenzone, octyl salicylate. SPF 29. Waterproof. Bot. 4 oz.
Use: Sunscreen.
PRESUN 39 CREAMY SUNSCREEN. (Bristol-Myers) Padimate O, oxybenzone, cetyl alcohol, waterproof. Cream. Bot. 120 ml.
Use: Sunscreen.
PRESUN ACTIVE. (Bristol-Myers) Octyl methoxycinnamate, oxybenzone, octyl salicylate, 69% SD alcohol 40. PABA free. Waterproof. SPF 15, 30. Gel. 120 g.
Use: Sunscreen.
PRESUN FOR KIDS CREAM. (Bristol-Myers) Octyl methoxycinnamate, oxybenzone, octyl salicylate, cetyl alcohol,

PABA free, waterproof SFP 29. Cream. Bot. 120 ml.
Use: Sunscreen.
PRESUN FOR KIDS SPRAY. (Bristol-Myers) Padimate O, octyl methoxycinnamate, oxybenzone, octyl salicylate, SD alcohol 40 19%, waterproof, SPF 23. Spray Bot. 105 ml.
Use: Sunscreen.
PRESUN MOISTURIZING. (Bristol-Myers) Octyl dimethyl PABA, oxybenzone, cetyl alcohol, diazolidinyl urea. SPF 46. Lot. Bot. 120 ml.
Use: Sunscreen.
PRESUN MOISTURIZING SUNSCREEN WITH KERI, SPF 15. (Bristol-Myers) Octyl dimethyl PABA, oxybenzone, cetyl alcohol, diazolidinyl urea. Waterproof. Lot. 120 ml.
Use: Sunscreen.
PRESUN MOISTURIZING SUNSCREEN WITH KERI, SPF 25. (Bristol-Myers) Octyl methoxycinnamate, oxybenzone, octyl salicylate, petrolatum, cetyl alcohol, diazolidinyl urea. Waterproof. Lot. 120 ml.
Use: Sunscreen.
PRESUN SPRAY MIST. (Bristol-Myers) Octyl dimethyl PABA, octyl methoxycinnamate, oxybenzone, octyl salicylate, 19% SD alcohol 40, C12-15 alcohols benzoate. Waterproof. SPF 23. 120 ml.
Use: Sunscreen.
PRETAMAZIUM IODIDE. B.A.N. 4-(Biphenyl-4-yl)-3-ethyl-2-[4-(pyrrolidin-1-yl)styryl]thiazolium iodide.
Use: Treatment of enterobiasis.
PRETEND-U-ATE. (Vitalax) Enriched candy-appetite pacifier. Pkg. 20s.
Use: Diet aid.
PRETHCAMIDE. Mixture of crotethamide and cropropamide. Micoren (Geigy).
PRETT'S DIET AID. (MiLance) Alginic acid 200 mg, sodium carboxymethylcellulose 100 mg, sodium bicarbonate 70 mg/Chow. Tab. Bot. 60s.
Use: Nonprescription diet aid.
PRETTY FEET & HANDS. (SK-Beecham) Lotion 3 fl oz.
Use: Emollient.
PRETZ-PAK. (Parnell) Benzyl alcohol 3.5%, polyethylene glycols, carboxymethylcellulose, urea, poloxamer, *Mucoprotective Factor* yerba santa, allantoin, aluminum chlorhydroxy allantoin. Oint. Tube 15 g.
Use: Operative and postoperative care in intranasal and endoscopic surgery.
PREVIDENT DISCLOSING DROPS. (Hoyt) Erythrosine sodium 1%. Bot. 1

oz.
Use: Disclosing dental plaque.
PREVIDENT DISCLOSING TABLET.
(Hoyt) Erythrosine sodium 1%/Tab. UD
strip 1000s.
Use: Disclosing dental plaque.
PREVIDENT PROPHYLAXIS PASTE.
(Hoyt) Sodium fluoride containing 1.2%
fluoride ion w/pumice and alumina abrasives. Cup 2 Gm, Box 200s. Jar 9 oz.
Use: Dental caries preventative.
PREVIEW. (Lafayette) Barium sulfate
60% w/v suspension. Bot. 355 ml, Case
24 bot.
Use: Radiopaque agent.
PREVIEW 2000. Barium sulfate 60% w/v
suspension. Bot. 2000 ml, Case 4 Bot.
Use: Radiopaque agent.
PREVISION. Mestranol, U.S.P. XXIII.
PREXONATE TABLETS. (Tennessee
Pharm.) Vitamins A acetate 5000 IU, D
500 IU, B_6 2 mg, B_1 5 mg, B_2 2 mg, C
100 mg, B_{12} 2.5 mcg, calcium pantothenate 1 mg, niacinamide 15 mg, folic
acid 1 mg, iron 45 mg, calcium 500 mg,
intrinsic factor 3 mg/Tab. Bot. 100s,
1000s.
Use: Vitamin/mineral supplement.
• **PREZATIDE COPPER ACETATE.** USAN.
Use: Immunomodulator.
PRID SALVE. (Walker Pharmacal)
Ichthammol, Phenol, Lead Oleate,
Rosin, Beeswax, Lard. Tin 20 Gm.
Use: Drawing salve.
• **PRIDEFINE HYDROCHLORIDE.** USAN.
Use: Antidepressant.
• **PRILOCAINE AND EPINEPHRINE IN-
JECTION,** U.S.P. XXIII.
Use: Local anesthetic.
• **PRILOCAINE HYDROCHLORIDE,** U.S.P.
XXIII. Inj., U.S.P. XXIII. 2-(Propylamino)-
o-propionotolidide HCl.
Use: Local anesthetic.
See: Citanest Hydrochloride, Vial, Amp.
(Astra).
PRILOSEC. (Merck, Sharp and Dohme)
Omeprazole 20 mg/Cap. Bot. 30s, UD
100s.
Use: Duodenal ulcer, gastroesophageal
reflux disease, hypersecretory conditions.
PRIMACAINE. 2′-Diethylamino-ethyl-2-
butoxy-3-aminobenzoate HCl.
Use: Local anesthetic.
PRIMACOR. (Sterling Winthrop) Inj. 1
mg/ml. Single-dose vial 10 ml, 20 ml;
Carpuject sterile cartridge-needle units 5
ml.
Use: A cardiotonic agent.
See: Milrinone.

PRIMADERM. (Arrow Medical) Cod liver
oil concentrate (Vitamins A and D), zinc
oxide in a mentholated petrolatum-lanolin base. Oint. In 30 Gm, 60 Gm.
Use: Burn preparation.
PRIMADERM-B. (Arrow Medical) Benzocaine, zinc oxide, cod liver oil in a petrolatum-lanolin base. Oint. 30 Gm, 60 Gm.
Use: Burn preparation.
• **PRIMAQUINE PHOSPHATE,** U.S.P.
XXIII. Tab., U.S.P. XXIII. 1,4-Pentanediamine, N-(6-methoxy-8-quinolinyl)-,
phosphate (1:2). (Sanofi Winthrop). Tab.
26.3 mg, Bot. 100s.
Use: Prevents relapses in nearly all
cases of vivax malaria.
PRIMAQUINE PHOSPHATE. (Sterling
Winthrop)
Use: Treatment of PCP associated with
AIDS. [Orphan drug]
PRIMATENE. (Whitehall) Theophylline
130 mg, ephedrine HCl 24 mg/Tab. Bot.
24s, 60s.
Use: Antiasthmatic combination.
PRIMATENE MIST SOLUTION. (Whitehall) Epinephrine 0.2 mg, alcohol 34%.
Bot. 0.5 oz. Spray.
Use: Bronchodilator.
PRIMATENE MIST SUSPENSION.
(Whitehall) Epinephrine bitartrate 0.3
mg. Bot. 10 ml w/mouthpiece. Spray.
Use: Bronchodilator.
PRIMATENE M. TABLETS. (Whitehall)
Theophylline 118 mg, ephedrine HCl 24
mg, pyrilamine maleate 16.6 mg/Tab.
Bot. 24s, 60s.
Use: Bronchodilator, antihistamine.
PRIMATENE P TABLETS. (Whitehall)
Theophylline 118 mg, ephedrine HCl 24
mg, phenobarbital 8 mg/Tab. Bot. 24s,
60s.
Use: Bronchodilator, sedative/hypnotic.
**PRIMATUSS COUGH MIXTURE 4 LIQ-
UID.** (Rugby) Doxylamine succinate
3.75 mg, dextromethorphan HBr 7.5
mg/5 ml, alcohol 10% Liq. Bot. 180 ml.
Use: Antihistamine, antitussive.
**PRIMATUSS COUGH MIXTURE 4D LIQ-
UID.** (Rugby) Pseudoephedrine HCl 20
mg, dextromethorphan HBr 10 mg,
guaifenesin 67 mg/5 ml, alcohol 10%.
Liq. Bot. 120 ml.
Use: Decongestant, antitussive, expectorant.
PRIMAXIN. (Merck & Co.) Imipenem (anhydrous equivalent), cilastatin w/sodium
bicarbonate buffer. **250-250:** ADD-Vantage Vial, Tray 10s, 25s. Tray 10 infusion
bottles. **500-500:** ADD-Vantage Vial,
Tray 10s, 25s. Tray 10 infusion bottles.

Use: Anti-infective.

PRIMAXIN I.M. (Merck) Imipenem (anhydrous equivalent), cilastatin w/ sodium bicarbonate buffer. Pow. for Inj. Vials 500 mg/500 mg, 750 mg/750 mg.
Use: Anti-infective.

PRIMAXIN I.V. (Merck) Imipenem (anhydrous equivalent), cilastatin w/ sodium bicarbonate buffer. Pow. for Inj. Vials, infusion bot., ADD-Vantage vials 250 mg/250 mg, 500 mg/500 mg.
Use: Anti-infective.

• **PRIMIDOLOL.** USAN.
Use: Anti-anginal; cardiac depressant.

• **PRIMIDONE,** U.S.P. XXIII. Tab., Oral Susp., U.S.P. XXIII. 4,6(1H,5H)-Pyrimidinedione, 5-ethyldihydro-5-phenyl-5-Ethyldihydro-5-phenyl-4,6(1H,5H)-pyrimidinedione. Tab. 250 mg Bot. 100s, 1000s.
Use: Anticonvulsant.

PRIMOSTRUM. A prep. of primiparous colostrum.

PRINCIPEN '125' FOR ORAL SUSPENSION. (Squibb) Ampicillin trihydrate 125 mg/5 ml, saccharin. Reconstitution to 80 ml, 100 ml, 150 ml, 200 ml, UD 5 ml 100s.
Use: Antibacterial, penicillin.

PRINCIPEN '250' CAPSULES. (Squibb) Ampicillin 250 mg/Cap. Bot. 100s, 500s, UD 100s.
Use: Antibacterial, penicillin.

PRINCIPEN '250' FOR ORAL SUSPENSION. (Squibb) Ampicillin trihydrate 250 mg/5 ml, saccharin. Reconstitution to 80 ml, 100 ml, 150 ml, 200 ml, UD 5 ml 100s.
Use: Antibacterial, penicillin.

PRINCIPEN '500' CAPSULES. (Squibb) Ampicillin trihydrate 500 mg/Cap. 100s, 500s, UD 100s.
Use: Antibacterial, penicillin.

PRINCIPEN WITH PROBENECID. (Squibb) Ampicillin (as trihydrate) 3.5 Gm, probenecid 1 Gm/regimen. Single dose bot., 9s.
Use: Antibacterial, penicillin.

PRINIVIL. (Merck) Lisinopril **2.5 mg/Tab.:** Bot. 30s, 100s, UD 100s. **5 mg/Tab.:** Bot. 1000s, 10,000s, 90s, 100s, UD 100s. **10 mg or 20 mg/Tab.:** Bot. 1000s, 10,000s, 30s, 90s, 100s, UD 100s. **40 mg/Tab.:** Bot. 100s.
Use: Antihypertensive.

• **PRINOMIDE TROMETHAMINE.** USAN.
Use: Antirheumatic.

• **PRINOXODAN.** USAN.
Use: Cardiotonic.

PRINZIDE. (Merck & Co.) Lisinopril 10 or

20 mg, hydrochlorothiazide 12.5 mg/Tab or lisinopril 20 mg, hydrochlorothiazide 25 mg/Tab. Bot. 30s, 100s.
Use: Antihypertensive.

PRISCOLINE. (Ciba) Tolazoline HCl 25 mg/ml, tartaric acid 0.65%, chlorobutanol 0.5%. Vial 10 ml.
Use: Antihypertensive.

PRISILIDENE HYDROCHLORIDE. *See:* Alphaprodine HCl (Various Mfr.).

PRISTINAMYCIN. B.A.N. An antibiotic produced by Streptomyces pristina spiralis.
Use: Anti-infective.

PRIVADORN. *See:* Bromisovalum (Various Mfr.).

PRIVINE. (Ciba Consumer) Naphazoline HCl. **Nasal Soln.:** 0.05%. Bot. 20 ml w/dropper. **Nasal Spray:** 0.05%. Bot. 15 ml.
Use: Decongestant.

• **PRIZIDILOL HYDROCHLORIDE.** USAN.
Use: Antihypertensive.

PRO-50. (Dunhall) Promethazine HCl 50 mg/ml. Vial 10 ml.
Use: Antihistamine, antiemetic.

PRO-ACET DOUCHE CONCENTRATE. (Pro-Acet) Lactic, citric, and acetic acids, sodium lauryl sulfate, lactose, dextrose and sodium acetate. Pkg. polyethylene envelope 10 ml. Contents of 1 envelope to be diluted with 2 quarts of water. Douche 6 oz, 12 oz. Travel Packet 10 ml.
Use: Vaginal preparation.

• **PROADIFEN HYDROCHLORIDE.** USAN. 2-(Diethylamino)ethyl-2,2-diphenyl-valerate hydrochloride.
Use: Drug potentiator.

PROBALAN. (Lannett) Probenecid 0.5 Gm/Tab. Bot. 100s, 1000s.
Use: Agent for gout.

PROBAMPACIN SUSPENSION. (Goldline) Bot. 60 ml.
Use: Antibacterial, penicillin.

PRO-BANTHINE. (Schiapparelli Searle) Propantheline bromide **7.5 mg/Tab.:** Bot. 100s. **15 mg/Tab.:** Bot. 100s, 500s, UD 100s.
Use: Anticholinergic/antispasmodic.

PROBARBITAL SODIUM. 5-Ethyl-5-isopropylbarbiturate sodium.

PROBAX. (Fischer Pharmaceuticals) Propolis 2%, petrolatum, mineral oil, lanolin. Gel. Tube 3.5 Gm.
Use: Mouth and throat preparation.

PROBEC-T. (Stuart) Vitamins B_1 15 mg, B_2 10 mg, niacinamide 100 mg, B_6 5 mg, B_{12} 5 mcg, C 600 mg. Bot. 60s.
Use: Vitamin/mineral supplement.

PROBEN. (Richlyn) Probenecid 500 mg, colchicine 0.5 mg/Tab. Bot. 1000s.
Use: Agent for gout.
PROBEN-C. (Rugby) Probenecid 500 mg, colchicine 0.5 mg/Tab. Bot. 100s, 1000s.
Use: Agent for gout.
• **PROBENECID,** U.S.P. XXIII. Tabs., U.S.P. XXIII. Benzoic acid, 4-[(dipropylamino)sulfonyl]-p-(Dipropylsulfamoyl) benzoic acid.
Use: Uricosuric.
See: Benemid, Tab. (Merck & Co.).
Probalan, Tab. (Lannett).
W/Ampicillin.
See: Amcill-GC, Oral Susp. (Parke-Davis).
Polycillin-PRB, Liq. (Bristol).
Principen w/Probenecid, Cap. (Squibb).
W/Ampicillin trihydrate.
See: Probampacin (Biocraft).
• **PROBENECID AND COLCHICINE,** U.S.P. XXIII.
Use: Uricosuric combination for chronic gouty arthritis.
See: Colbenemid, Tab. (Merck & Co.).
PROBENZAMIDE. 0-Propoxybenzamide. (Warner-Lambert).
• **PROBICROMIL CALCIUM.** USAN.
Use: Anti-allergenic.
PRO-BIONATE. (Natren) *Lactobacillus acidophilus* strain NAS 2 billion units/Gm. **Pow.** 52.5 g, 90 g. **Cap.** Bot. 30s, 60s.
Use: Antidiarrheal.
• **PROBUCOL,** U.S.P. XXIII. (1) Acetone bis(3,5-di-tertbutyl-4-hydroxyphenyl) mercaptole; (2) 4,4′-(iso-propylidenedithio)-bis[2,6-di-tert-butylphenol].
Use: Anticholesteremic.
See: Lorelco, Tab. (Merrell Dow).
• **PROCAINAMIDE HYDROCHLORIDE,** U.S.P. XXIII. Cap., Inj., Tab., Ext. Rel. Tab., U.S.P. XXIII. Benzamide, 4-amino-N-[2-(diethylamino)ethyl]-HCl. p-Amino-N-[2-(diethylamino)ethyl]benzamide HCl.
Use: Cardiac depressant in arrhythmias.
See: Procamide SR, Tab. (Solvay).
Procan SR, Tab. (Parke-Davis).
Pronestyl, Cap., Vial (Princeton).
PROCAINE BASE.
W/Benzyl alcohol, propyl-p-aminobenzoate.
Use: Local anesthetic.
See: Rectocaine, Vial (Moore-Kirk).
W/Butyl-p-aminobenzoate, benzyl alcohol, in sweet almond oil.

See: Anucaine, Amp. (Calvin).
PROCAINE BUTYRATE. p-Aminobenzoyl-di-ethylaminoethanol butyrate.
• **PROCAINE HYDROCHLORIDE,** U.S.P. XXIII. Inj., Sterile, U.S.P. XXIII. Benzoic acid, 4-amino-, 2-(diethylamino)-ethyl ester, HCl. 2-Diethylaminoethyl p-aminobenzoate HCl. Allocaine, Bernocaine, Chlorocaine, Ethocaine, Irocaine, Kerocaine, Syncaine. (Abbott) 1% or 2% solution. Multiple-dose Vial 30 ml.
Use: Local anesthetic.
See: Anucaine, Amp. (Calvin).
Novocain, Amp., Soln. (Sanofi Winthrop).
• **PROCAINE HYDROCHLORIDE AND EPINEPHRINE INJECTION,** U.S.P. XXIII.
Use: Local anesthetic.
PROCAINE HYDROCHLORIDE AND LEVONORDEFRIN INJECTION.
Use: Local anesthetic.
• **PROCAINE PENICILLIN G SUSPENSION, STERILE,** U.S.P. XXIII.
Use: Antibiotic.
See: Crysticillin, Vial (Squibb).
Penicillin G, Procaine (Various Mfr.).
Pfizerpen For Injection (Pfipharmecs).
• **PROCAINE, PENICILLIN G W/ALUMINUM STEARATE SUSPENSION, STERILE,** U.S.P. XXIII.
Use: Antibiotic.
See: Penicillin G Procaine with Aluminum Stearate, Sterile, U.S.P. XXIII.
• **PROCAINE AND PHENYLEPHRINE HYDROCHLORIDES INJECTION,** U.S.P. XXIII.
Use: Local anesthetic (dental).
• **PROCAINE AND TETRACAINE HYDROCHLORIDES AND LEVONORDEFRIN INJECTION,** U.S.P. XXIII.
Use: Local anesthetic (dental).
PROCAINE, TETRACAINE AND NORDEFRIN HYDROCHLORIDES INJECTION.
Use: Local anesthetic.
PROCAINE, TETRACAINE AND PHENYLEPHRINE HYDROCHLORIDES INJECTION.
Use: Anesthetic.
PROCALAMINE INJECTION. (Kendall McGaw) Injection of amino acid 3%, glycerin 3%, electrolytes. Bot. 1000 ml.
Use: Parenteral nutritional supplement.
PRO-CAL-SOF. (Vangard) Docusate calcium 240 mg/Cap. Bot. 100s, 1000s, UD 100s.
Use: Laxative.
PROCAN SR. (Parke-Davis) Procainamide HCl sustained release 250 mg, 500 mg, 750 mg or 1 Gm/Tab. Bot.

100s, 500s (except 1 Gm), UD 100s.
Use: Antiarrhythmic.
PRO-CAP 65. (Foy) Propoxyphene HCl
65 mg, aspirin 227 mg, phenacetin 162
mg, caffeine 32.4 mg/Cap. Bot. 500s.
Use: Narcotic analgesic combination.
• **PROCARBAZINE HCl,** U.S.P. XXI. Cap.,
U.S.P. XXI. Benzamide, N-(1-
methylethyl)-4-[(2-methyl-hy-
drazino)methyl]-HCl. (Roche) Natulan.
Use: Cytostatic, Antineoplastic.
See: Matulane, Cap. (Roche).
PROCARDIA. (Pfizer) Nifedipine 10 mg
or 20 mg/Cap. Bot. 100s, 300s, UD
100s.
Use: Calcium channel blocking agent.
PROCARDIA XL. (Pfizer) Nifedipine 30
mg, 60 mg or 90 mg/SR Tab. **30 mg or
60 mg:** Bot. 100s, UD 100s. **90 mg:** Bot
100s.
Use: Calcium channel blocking agent.
• **PROCATEROL HYDROCHLORIDE.**
USAN.
Use: Bronchodilator.
**PROCEPTION SPERM NUTRIENT
DOUCHE.** (Milex) Ringer type glucose
douche. Bot. ample for 10 douches.
Use: Douche.
• **PROCHLORPERAZINE,** U.S.P. XXIII.
Supp., U.S.P. XXIII. 10H-Phenothiazine,
2-chloro-10-[3-(4-methyl-1-
piperazinyl)propyl]-.
Use: Antiemetic.
See: Compazine, Preps. (SK-
Beecham).
W/Isopropamide.
See: Iso-Perazine, Cap. (Lemmon).
PROCHLORPERAZINE. (G & W Labs)
Prochlorperazine 25 mg, coconut oil,
palm kernel oil. Supp. 12s.
Use: Antiemetic.
• **PROCHLORPERAZINE EDISYLATE,**
U.S.P. XXIII. Inj., Oral Soln., Syr., U.S.P.
XXIII. 10H-Phenothiazine, 2-chloro-10-
[3-(4-methyl-1-piperazinyl)propyl]-1,2-
ethanedisulfonate (1:1).
Use: Tranquilizer, antiemetic.
See: Compazine, Preps. (SK-
Beecham).
**PROCHLORPERAZINE ETHANEDISUL-
FONATE.** Prochlorperazine Edisylate,
U.S.P. XXIII.
Use: Tranquilizing agent.
PROCHLORPERAZINE/ISOPROPAMIDE.
(Various Mfr.) Isopropamide iodide 5
mg, prochlorperazine maleate 10
mg/Cap. Bot. 100s, 500s, 1000s, UD
100s.
Use: Anticholinergic/antispasmodic,
antiemetic/antivertigo agent.

• **PROCHLORPERAZINE MALEATE,**
U.S.P. XXIII. Tab., U.S.P. XXIII. 10H-
Phenothiazine, 2-chloro-10-[3-(4-
methyl-1-piperazinyl)-propyl]-(Z)-2-
butenedio- ate (1:2).
Use: Antiemetic, tranquilizer.
See: Compazine, Preps. (SK-
Beecham).
• **PROCINONIDE.** USAN.
Use: Adrenocortical steroid.
• **PROCLONOL.** USAN. Bis(p-
chlorophenyl)-cyclopropylmethanol. Un-
der study.
Use: Acaricide, fungicide.
**PRO COMFORT ATHLETE'S FOOT
SPRAY.** (Scholl) Tolnaftate 1%. Aerosol
Can 4 oz.
Use: Antifungal, external.
**PRO COMFORT JOCK ITCH SPRAY
POWDER.** (Scholl) Tolnaftate 1%.
Aerosol can 3.5 oz.
Use: Antifungal, external.
PROCRIT. (Ortho Biotech) Epoetin alfa
2000, 3000, 4000 or 10,000 units. Inj.
Vial. 1 ml.
Use: Recombinant human erythropoi-
etin.
PROCTOCORT. (Solvay) Hydrocortisone
1%. Cream 30 Gm w/rectal applicator.
Use: Corticosteroid.
PROCTOCREAM-HC. (Reed & Carnrick)
Hydrocortisone acetate 1%, pramoxine
HCl 1%. Cream 30 Gm.
Use: Corticosteroid, local anesthetic.
PROCTOFOAM. (Reed & Carnrick)
Pramoxine HCl 1% in an anesthetic mu-
coadhesive foam base. Foam. Can. 15
Gm.
Use: Anorectal preparation.
PROCTOFOAM-HC. (Reed & Carnrick)
Hydrocortisone acetate 1%, pramoxine
HCl 1% in hydrophilic foam base. Bot.
aerosol container, Aerosol foam 10 Gm
w/applicator.
Use: Corticosteroid, local anesthetic.
PROCTOFOAM N.S. (Reed & Carnrick)
Pramoxine HCl 1%. Aerosol Bot. 10 Gm
w/applicator.
Use: Local anesthetic.
PRO-CUTE CREAM. (Ferndale) Silicone,
hexachlorophene, lanolin. 2 oz, lb.
Use: Emollient.
PRO-CUTE LOTION. (Ferndale) Hexa-
chlorophene, silicone, lanolin. Bot. 8 oz.
Use: Emollient.
• **PROCYCLIDINE HCl,** U.S.P. XXIII. Tab.,
U.S.P. XXIII. α-Cyclohexyl-α-phenyl-1-
pyrrolidinepropanol HCl.
Use: Skeletal muscle relaxant.

See: Kemadrin, Tab. (Burroughs Well-come).

PROCYSTEINE. (Free Radical Sciences)
See: L₂-Oxothiazolidine₄-carboxylic acid.

PRODERM TOPICAL DRESSING. (Hick-am) Castor oil 650 mg, peruvian balsam 72.5 mg/0.82 cc. Aerosol 4 oz.
Use: Prevention of decubiti.

•**PRODILIDINE HCl.** USAN. (1,2-Di-methyl-3-phenyl-3-pyrrolidyl propionate HCl.
Use: Analgesic.

•**PRODOLIC ACID.** USAN.
Use: Anti-inflammatory.

PRO-EST. (Burgin-Arden) Progesterone 25 mg, estrogenic substance 25,000 IU, sodium carboxymethylcellulose 1 mg, sodium Cl 0.9%, benzalkonium Cl 1:10,000, sodium phosphate dibasic 0.1% in water.
Use: Progestin, estrogen combination.

PRO-ESTRONE. (Pharmex) Estradiol benzoate 2.5 mg, progesterone 12.5 mg/ml. Vial 10 ml.
Use: Estrogen, progestin combination.

•**PROFADOL HCl.** USAN. m-(1-Methyl-3-propyl-3-pyrrolidinyl)phenol HCl.
Use: Analgesic.

PROFAMINA.
See: Amphetamine (Various Mfr.).

PROFASI HP. (Serono) Chorionic go-nadotropin 5000 units or 10,000 units/Vial. With 1 vial product and 1 vial diluent (w/mannitol and benzyl alcohol).
Use: Chorionic gonadotropin.

PROFENAL. (Alcon) Suprofen 1% soln. Drop-Tainer 2.5 ml.
Use: Nonsteroidal anti-inflammatory drug, ophthalmic.

PROFESSIONAL CARE LOTION, EX-TRA STRENGTH. (Walgreen) Zinc ox-ide 0.25% in a lotion base. Bot. 16 oz.
Use: Astringent, antiseptic, skin protec-tant.

PROFIBER LIQUID. (Sherwood) Sodium caseinate, dietary fiber from soy, calci-um caseinate, hydrolyzed cornstarch, corn oil, soy lecithin, vitamins A, B₁, B₂, B₃, B₅, B₆, B₁₂, C, D, E, K, folic acid, bi-otin, choline, Ca, Cl, Cr, Cu, Fe, I, Mg, Mn, Mo, P, Se, Zn. Can 250 ml, closed system 1000 ml.
Use: Enteral nutritional supplement.

PROFILATE HP. (Alpha Therapeutic) A stable freeze-dried concentrate of Anti-hemophilic Factor VIII: C (Human) sus-pended in heptane and heated. Inj. Vial. 10, 25 ml.
Use: Antihemophilic.

PROFILININE HEAT-TREATED. (Alpha Therapeutics) Dried plasma fraction of coagulation factors II, VII, IX and X. He-parin free. Vial, single dose with diluent.
Use: Antihemophilic.

PROFLAVINE.
Use: Topical, antiseptic.

PROFLAVINE DIHYDROCHLORIDE. 3,6-Diaminoacridine dihydrochloride.

PROFLAVINE SULFATE. 3,6-Di-aminoacridine sulfate.

PROFREE/GP. (Allergan) Papain, sodi-um Cl, sodium borate, sodium carbon-ate, edetate disodium. Kit 15s or 24s.
Use: Rigid gas permeable contact lens care.

•**PROGABIDE.** USAN.
Use: Anticonvulsant, muscle relaxant.

PROGELAN. (Lannett) Progesterone 25 mg, 50 mg or 100 mg/ml in oil. Vial 10 ml.
Use: Progestin.

PROGELAN AQUEOUS. (Lannett) Prog-esterone 25 mg or 50 mg, aqueous susp./ml. Vial 10 ml.
Use: Progestin.

PROGENS TABS. (Major) Conjugated estrogens. **0.625 mg/Tab.:** Bot. 100s, 1000s; **1.25 mg/Tab.:** Bot. 1000s; **2.5 mg/Tab.:** Bot. 100s, 1000s.
Use: Estrogen.

PRO-GESIC. (Nastech) Trolamine salicy-late 10%, propylene glycol, methyl-parahydroxybenzoic acid, propyl parahydroxybenzoic acid, EDTA. Liq. Bot. 75 ml.
Use: Rub/liniment.

PROGESTASERT. (Alza) T-shaped in-trauterine device (IUD) unit containing a reservoir of progesterone 38 mg with barium sulfate dispersed in medical grade silicone fluid. In 6s w/inserter.
Use: Contraceptive, progestin.

•**PROGESTERONE,** U.S.P. XXIII. Inj., Sterile Susp. U.S.P. XXIII. 4-Pregnene-3,20-dione. Corpus luteum hormone. Flavolutan, Luteogan, Luteosan, Lutren.
Use: Progestin.
Aqueous. Susp.
See: Progelan Aqueous, Vial (Lannett). Prorone, Inj. (Sig).
In Oil
See: Femotrone, Inj. (Bluco). Lipo-Lutin, Amp. (Parke-Davis). Progelan, Vial (Lannett). Progestin, Vial (Various Mfr.). Prorone, Inj. (Sig).
W/Estradiol benzoate.
See: Pro-Estrone, Vial (Pharmex). W/Estradiol, testosterone, procaine HCl,

procaine base.
See: Hormo-Triad, Vial (Bell).
W/Estrogenic substance.
See: Profoygen Aqueous (Foy).
Progex, Inj. (Pasadena Research).
•**PROGESTERONE INTRAUTERINE
CONTRACEPTIVE SYSTEM,** U.S.P.
XXIII.
Use: Contraceptive.
PROGESTERONE-LIKE.
See: Haloprogesterone.
Norethynodrel.
PROGESTIN. Progesterone (Various
Mfr.).
•**PROGLUMIDE.** USAN. ($\pm$)-4-Benzamido-
N,N-dipropylglutaramic acid. Nulsa
(Wallace).
Use: Anticholinergic.
PROGLYCEM. (Baker Norton) **Cap.:** Dia-
zoxide 50 mg/Cap. Bot. 100s. **Oral
Susp.:** Diazoxide 50 mg/ml. Bot. 30 ml
w/calibrated dropper.
Use: Glucose elevating agent.
PROGRAF. (Fujisawa) **Cap.:** Tacrolimus
1 mg or 5 mg. Bot. 100s; **Inj.:** Tacrolimus
5 mg/ml. In 1 ml amps (10s).
Use: Immunosuppressant
PROGUANIL HYDROCHLORIDE.
See: Chloroguanide Hydrochloride.
Paludrine, Tab. (Wyeth-Ayerst).
PROHANCE. (Squibb Diagnostics)
Gadoteridol 279.3 mg, calteridol calcium
0.23 mg, tromethamine 1.21 mg/ml. Inj.
5 ml fill in 15 ml vials, 10 ml fill in 30 ml
vials, 15 ml fill in 30 ml vials and 20 ml fill
in 30 ml vials.
Use: Radiopaque agent.
PROHEPTAZINE. B.A.N. Hexahydro-1,3-
dimethyl-4-phenyl-1H-azepin-4-ol propionate (ester).
Use: Analgesic.
PROHIBIT. (Connaught) Purified capsular polysaccharide 25 mcg, conjugated
diphtheria toxoid protein 18 mcg/0.5 ml
dose. Inj. Vial 1 dose, 5 dose, 10 dose.
Use: Agent for immunization.
PRO-HYDRO. (Mills) Protein hydrolysates (45% amino acids) 50 gr, iron
46 mg, l-lysine HCl 600 mg, dl-methione
75 mg, niacinamide 30 mg, vitamins B_1
3 mg, B_2 2 mg, B_6 2 mg, B_{12} 3 mcg, C
60 mg, calcium pantothenate 12 mg/6
Tab. Bot. 168s.
W/O Iron. Same formula as above without
iron.
W/Vitamin E. Same formula with vitamin E
30 IU.
Use: Vitamin/mineral supplement.
PROLACTIN RIA. (Abbott Diagnostics)
Quantitative measurement of total circu-

lating human prolactin. Test unit 50s,
100s.
Use: Diagnostic aid.
PROLACTIN RIABEAD. (Abbott Diagnostics) Radioimmunoassay for the
quantitative measurement of prolactin in
human serum and plasma.
Use: Diagnostic aid.
PROLADYL. Pyrrobutamine. 1-Pyrrolidyl-
3-phenyl-4-(p-chlorophenyl)-2-butene
phosphate.
Use: Antihistamine.
PROLASE. Proteolytic enzyme from *Car-
ica papaya.*
See: Papain.
PROLASTIN. (Cutter) Alpha$_1$-proteinase
inhibitor $\geq$ 20 mg alpha$_1$-PI/ml when re-
constituted. W/polyethylene glycol, su-
crose and small amounts of other plas-
ma proteins. Inj. Vial, single dose.
Use: Alpha$_1$-proteinase inhibitor.
PROLENE. (Ethicon) Surgical suture,
nonabsorbable.
PROLENS. (Ketchum) Bot. 2 oz.
Use: Contact lens care.
•**PROLINE,** U.S.P. XXIII. $C_5H_9NO_2$ as L-
proline.
Use: Amino acid.
PROLINTANE. B.A.N. 1-(α-Propy-
lphenethyl)-pyrrolidine. 1-Phenyl-2-
(pyrrolidin-1-yl)pentane. Villescon.
Use: Tonic.
•**PROLINTANE HYDROCHLORIDE.**
USAN.
Use: Antidepressant.
PROLIXIN. (Princeton) Fluphenazine
HCl. **Tab.:** 1 mg. Bot. 50s, 500s; 2.5 mg.
w/tartrazine. Bot. 50s, 500s; 5 mg. w/tar-
trazine. Bot. 500s, UD 100s; 10 mg.
w/tartrazine. Bot. 50s, 500s. **Elixir:** 0.5
mg/ml, alcohol 14%. Dropper Bot. 60 ml.
Bot. pt. **Inj.:** 2.5 mg/ml. Vial 10 ml
w/methyl and propyl parabens. Unimatic
syringe 1 ml, Single dose syringe 25
mg/ml. 10s.
Use: Antipsychotic agent.
PROLIXIN CONCENTRATE. (Princeton)
Fluphenazine HCl 5 mg/ml, alcohol
14%. Bot. 120 ml w/dropper.
Use: Antipsychotic agent.
PROLIXIN DECANOATE. (Princeton)
Fluphenazine decanoate 25 mg/ml (in
sesame oil with benzyl alcohol). Unimat-
ic syringe 1 ml. Vial 5 ml.
Use: Antipsychotic agent.
PROLIXIN ENANTHATE. (Princeton)
Fluphenazine enanthate 25 mg/ml (in
sesame oil with benzyl alcohol). Vial 5
ml.
Use: Antipsychotic agent.

PROLOPRIM. (Burroughs Wellcome) Trimethoprim 100 mg/Tab. Bot. 100s, UD 100s (in sesame oil with benzyl alcohol).
Use: Urinary anti-infective.

PROMACHLOR. (Geneva) Chlorpromazine HCl 10 mg, 25 mg, 50 mg, 100 mg or 200 mg/Tab. Bot. 100s, 1000s
Use: Antiemetic/antivertigo, antipsychotic agent.

• **PROMAZINE HCI,** U.S.P. XXIII. Inj., Oral Soln., Syr., Tab., U.S.P. XXIII. 10-(α-Dimethylamino-n-propyl) phenothiazine HCl. 10-[3-(Dimethylamino)propyl]- phenothiazine monohydrochloride.
Use: Ataraxic, anticholinergic.
See: Sparine, Tab., Inj. (Wyeth-Ayerst).

PROMEGA. (Parke-Davis) Omega-3 (N-3) polyunsaturated fatty acids 1000 mg, containing EPA 350 mg, DHA 150 mg, vitamins E (3% RDA), A, B_1, B_2, B_3, Ca, Fe (< 2% RDA)/Cap., cholesterol and sodium free. Bot. 30s.
Use: Vitamin/mineral supplement.

PROMEGA PEARLS. (Parke-Davis) EPA 168 mg, DHA 72 mg, cholesterol < 2 mg, E 1 IU, < 2% RDA of A, B_1, B_2, B_3, Fe, Ca. Cap. Bot. 60s, 90s.
Use: Fish oil.

PROMETA. (Muro) Metaproterenol sulfate 10 mg/5 ml, with saccharin and sorbitol, strawberry flavor. Syr. Bot. 480 ml.
Use: Bronchodilator.

PROMETHAZINE DC. (Lannett) Phenylephrine HCl 5 mg, promethazine HCl 6.25 mg, alcohol 7%. Syr. Bot. 120 ml, pt, gal.
Use: Decongestant, antihistamine.

PROMETHAZINE DM. (Various Mfr.) Promethazine HCl 6.25 mg, dextromethorphan HBr 15 mg/5 ml, alcohol. Syr. Bot. 120 ml, pt, gal.
Use: Antitussive combination.

PROMETH-50. (Seatrace) Promethazine HCl 50 mg/ml. Vial 10 ml.
Use: Antihistamine, antiemetic/antivertigo.

PROMETH EXPECTORANT. (Medwick) With or without codeine. Bot. 4 oz, pt, gal.
W/Dextromethorphan. Bot. 4 oz, pt, gal.
Use: Antihistamine, antitussive.

PROMETH EXPECTORANT VC. (Medwick) With or without codeine. Bot. 4 oz, pt, gal.
Use: Antihistamine, antitussive.

PROMETH VC W/ CODEINE LIQUID. (Various Mfr.) Phenylephrine HCl 5 mg, promethazine HCl 6.25 mg, codeine phosphate 10 mg, alcohol. Bot. Pt. or gal.

Use: Decongestant, antihistamine, antitussive.

PROMETH WITH CODEINE COUGH SYRUP. (Goldline) Promethazine 6.25 mg, codeine phosphate 10 mg.5 ml, alcohol 7%. Pt, gal.
Use: Antihistamine, antitussive, antivertigo.

PROMETH W/DEXTROMETHORPHAN. (Barre-National) Promethazine HCl 6.25 mg, dextromethorphan HBr 15 mg/5 ml, alcohol. Syr. Bot. 120 ml, pt, gal.
Use: Antihistamine, antitussive.

PROMETHAZINE. B.A.N. 10(2-Dimethylamino-propyl)phenothiazine. Phenergan hydrochloride.
Use: Antihistamine; antiemetic, sedative.

PROMETHAZINE-50. (Kenyon) Promethazine HCl 50 mg, sodium formaldehyde sulfoxylate 0.75 mg, sodium metabisulfite 0.25 mg, disodium EDTA 0.1 mg, calcium Cl 0.04 mg, phenol 5 mg, buffered with sodium acetate/ml. Vial 10 ml.
Use: Antihistamine.

PROMETHAZINE CHLOROTHEOPHYLLINATE.
See: Promethazine Theoclate, B.A.N.

PROMETHAZINE HCI WITH CODEINE. (Various Mfr.) Promethazine HCl 6.25 mg, codeine phosphate 10 mg/5 ml, alcohol 7%. Syr. Bot. 120 ml, pt, gal.
Use: Antihistamine, antitussive.

• **PROMETHAZINE HYDROCHLORIDE,** U.S.P. XXIII. Tab., Syr., Inj., Supp., U.S.P. XXIII. 10H-Phenothiazine-10-ethanamine, N,N-trimethyl-, HCl. 10-(2-Dime- thylaminopropyl)phenothiazine HCl.
Use: Antihistamine, antiemetic.
See: Methazine, Vial (Pharmex).
Pentazine, Expectorant, Vial (Century).
Phenergan, Preps. (Wyeth-Ayerst).
Phenerject, Vial (Mayrand).
Prorex, Vial, Amp. (Hyrex).
Provigan, Inj. (Solvay).
Remsed, Tab. (DuPont).
Sigazine, Inj. (Sig).

PROMETHAZINE HCI W/COMBINATIONS.
Use: Antihistamine, antiemetic/antivertigo.
See: Mepergan, Vial, Cap. (Wyeth-Ayerst).
Phenergan-D, Tab. (Wyeth-Ayerst).
Phenergan VC Expectorant (Wyeth-Ayerst).

PROMETHAZINE THEOCLATE. B.A.N.

Promethazine salt of 8-chlorotheophylline. Promethazine chlorotheophyllinate. Avomine.
Use: Antihistamine; antiemetic; sedative.
PROMETHAZINE VC. (PBI) Promethazine HCl 6.25 mg, phenylephrine HCl 5 mg/5 ml, alcohol 7%. Bot. 4 oz, pt, gal.
Use: Antihistamine, decongestant.
PROMETHAZINE VC WITH CODEINE. (PBI) Promethazine HCl 6.25 mg, phenylephrine HCl 5 mg, codeine 10 mg/5 ml, alcohol 7%. Bot. 4 oz, pt, gal.
Use: Antihistamine, decongestant, antitussive.
PROMETHESTROL. B.A.N. 3,4-Di-(4-hydroxy- 3-methylphenyl)hexane. Methestrol (I.N.N.).
Use: Estrogen.
PROMETHESTROL DIPROPIONATE.
Use: Estrogen.
See: Meprane Dipropionate, Tab. (Reed & Carnrick),
W/Phenobarbital.
See: Meprane-Phenobarbital, Tab. (Reed & Carnrick).
PROMETHIST W/ CODEINE SYRUP. (Rahslog Corp.) Phenylephrine HCl 5 mg, promethazine HCl 6.25 mg, codeine phosphate 10 mg, alcohol. Bot. 120 ml.
Use; Decongestant, antihistamine, antitussive.
PROMETOL. (Viobin) Concentrated wheat germ oil. **3 min/Cap.:** Bot. 100s, 250s. **10 min/Cap.:** Bot. 100s.
PROMINAL.
See: Mephobarbital.
PROMINE. (Major) Procainamide 250 mg, 375 mg or 500 mg/Cap. Bot. 100s, 250s, 1000s, UD 100s (375 mg/Cap. w/500s instead of 250s).
Use: Antiarrhythmic.
PROMINE S.R. (Major) Procainamide. **SR Tab.:** 250 mg. Bot. 100s, 250s; 500 mg. Bot. 100s, 250s, 1000s; 750 mg. Bot. 100s, 250s. **SR Cap.:** 250 mg, 375 mg or 500 mg.
Use: Antiarrhythmic.
PRO-MIN-VITE. (Drug Industries) Vitamins A 10,000 IU, D 1000 IU, E 3 IU, C 100 mg, B_1 10 mg, B_2 3 mg, B_6 2 mg, citrus bioflavonoids 25 mg, calcium pantothenate 10 mg, niacin 20 mg, B_{12} 2 mcg, biotin 0.1 mg, l-lysine 25 mg, iron 20 mg, copper 0.5 mg, manganese 2 mg, molybdenum 0.5 mg, zinc 1 mg, potassium 5 mg, magnesium 5 mg, iodine 0.1 mg/Tab. Bot. 100s, 500s.
Use: Vitamin/mineral supplement.
PROMIST HD. (Russ) Hydrocodone bitar-

trate 2.5 mg, pseudoephedrine HCl 30 mg, chlorpheniramine maleate 2 mg/5 ml, alcohol 5%, menthol, saccharin, sorbitol. Bot. pt.
Use: Antitussive, decongestant, antihistamine.
PROMIST LA. (Russ) Pseudoephedrine HCl 120 mg, guaifenesin 500 mg/Tab. Bot. 100s.
Use: Decongestant, expectorant.
PROMIT. (Pharmacia) Dextran 1 150 mg/ml Inj. Vial 20 ml.
Use: Dextran adjunct.
PRO-MIX R.D.P. (Navaco) Protein 15 Gm (from whey protein), fat 0.8 Gm, carbohydrate 1 Gm, sodium 46 mg, potassium 165 mg, chloride 46 mg, calcium 73.6 mg, phosphorus 64.4 mg, iron 0.3 mg, Cr, Cu, Mg, Mn, Mo, Se, Zn, 72 Cal./5 Tbsp. (20 Gm). Pow. Packet 20 Gm, can 300 Gm.
Use: Enteral nutritional supplement.
PROMOD. (Ross) Protein supplement. Nine scoops provides protein 45 Gm, 100% U.S. RDA. Pow. Can 9.7 oz.
Use: Enteral nutritional supplement.
PROMOXALAN. B.A.N. 2,2-Diisopropyl-1,3-dioxolane-4-methanol. 4-Hydroxymethyl-2,2-di-isopropyl-1,3-dioxolan.
Use: Skeletal muscle relaxant.
PROMPT. (DePree) **Spray:** Benzocaine 1.5%, parachlorometaxylenol 0.5%. Can 5 oz. **Lot.:** Benzocaine 1%, triclosan 0.2%. Bot. 4 oz. **Tab.:** Acetaminophen 5 gr, Bot. 50s, 100s, 200s.
Use: Anesthetic, analgesic.
PROMYLIN ENTERIC COATED MICROZYMES. (Shear/Kershman) Enteric coated pancrelipase. Lipase 4000 units, amylase 20,000 units, protease 25,000 units.
Use: Digestive enzymes.
PRO-NASYL. (Progonasyl Co.) o-lodobenzoic acid 0.5%, triethanolamine 5.5% in a special neutral hydrophilic base compounded from oleic acid, mineral oil, vegetable oil. Bot. 15 ml, 60 ml.
Use: Treatment of sinusitis.
PRONEMIA HEMATINIC. (Lederle) Iron 115 mg, B_{12} 15 mcg, IFC 75 mg, C 150 mg, folic acid 1 mcg. Cap. Bot. 30s.
Use: Iron w/B_{12} and intrinsic factor.
PRONESTYL. (Princeton) Procainamide. **Cap.:** 250 mg. Bot. 100s, 1000s; 375 mg. Bot. 100s; 500 mg. Bot. 100s, 1000s. **Inj.:** 100 mg/ml w/benzyl alcohol 0.9%, sodium bisulfite 0.09%. Vial 10 ml; 500 mg/ml w/methylparaben 0.1%, sodium bisulfite 0.2%. Vial 2 ml. **Tab.:** 250 mg. Bot. 100s, 1000s, Unimatic 100s;

375 mg. Bot. 100s; 500 mg. Bot. 100s, 1000s, Unimatic 100s.
Use: Antiarrhythmic.

PRONESTYL-SR. (Princeton) Procainamide 500 mg/Tab. Bot. UD 100s.
Use: Antiarrhythmic.

PRONETHALOL. B.A.N. 2-Isopropylamino-1-(2-naphthyl)-ethanol. Alderlin hydrochloride.
Use: Adrenergic beta-receptor blocking agent.

PRONETHELOL. (I.C.I.). Adrenergic beta-receptor antagonist; pending release.

PRONTO CONCENTRATE LICE KILLING SHAMPOO KIT. (Commerce) Pyrethrins 0.33%, piperonyl butoxide technical 4%. Bot. 2 oz, 4 oz.
Use: Pediculicide.

PRONTO LICE KILLING SPRAY. (Commerce) 3-phenoxybenzyl d-cis and trans 2,2 dimethyl 3-(2-methylpropenyl) cyclopropanecarboxylate. Spray cans 5 oz.
Use: Pediculicide for inanimate objects.

PROPAC. (Biosearch) Protein 3 Gm (from whey protein), carbohydrate 0.2 Gm, fat 0.3 Gm, chloride 3 mg, potassium 20 mg, sodium 9 mg, calcium 24 mg, phosphorus 12 mg, 16 Cal./Tbsp. (4 Gm). Pow. Packet 19.5 Gm, Can 350 Gm.
Use: Enteral nutritional supplement.

PROPACET 100. (Lemmon) Propoxyphene napsylate 100 mg, acetaminophen 650 mg/Tab. Bot. 100s, 500s, UD 100s.
Use: Narcotic analgesic combination.

PROPAESIN. Propyl p-Aminobenzoate. (Various Mfr.).

• **PROPAFENONE HYDROCHLORIDE.** USAN.
Use: Antiarrhythmic.
See: Rythmol, Tab. (Knoll).

PROPAGEST TABLETS. (Carnrick) Phenylpropanolamine HCl 25 mg/Tab. Bot. 100s.
Use: Decongestant.

PROPAGON-S. (Spanner) Estrone 2 mg or 5 mg/ml. Vial 10 ml.
Use: Estrogen.

PROPAIN HC. (Springbok) Acetaminophen 500 mg, hydrocodone bitartrate 5 mg/Cap. Bot. 100s, 500s.
Use: Narcotic analgesic combination.

PROPAMIDINE. B.A.N. 1,3-Di-(4-amidinophenoxy)-propane. Brolene isethionate.
Use: Bactericide; fungicide.

PROPAMIDINE ISETHIONATE 0.1% OPHTHALMIC SOLN.
Use: Acanthamoeba keratitis. [Orphan

drug]
• **PROPANE,** N.F. XVIII.
Use: Aerosol propellant.

PROPANEDIOL DIACETATE, 1,2.
See: VoSol, Liq. (Wampole).

1,2,3-PROPANETRIOL, TRINITRATE. Nitroglycerin Tab., U.S.P. XXIII.

• **PROPANIDID.** USAN. [4- [Ib] (Diethylcarbamoyl)- methoxy -3-methoxyphenyl] acetic acid propyl ester. Propyl 4-diethylcarbamoylmethoxy-3-methoxyphenylacetate. Epontol.
Use: Systemic anesthetic.

PROPANOLOL. 1-Isopropylamino-3-(l-napthyloxy)propan-2-ol. Propranolol.

• **PROPANTHELINE BROMIDE,** U.S.P. XXIII. Sterile, Tabs., U.S.P. XXIII. 2-Propanaminium, N-methyl-N-(1-methylethyl)-N-[2-](9H-xanthen-9-ylcarbonyl)oxy[ethyl]-, Br.
Use: Anticholinergic.
See: Pro-Banthine, Preps. (Searle).
Spastil, Tab. (Kenyon).
W/Phenobarbital.
See: Probital, Tab. (Searle).
W/Thiopropazate dihydrochloride.
See: Pro-Banthine W/Dartal, Tab. (Searle).

PROPA PH CLEANSING FOR NORMAL/COMBINATION SKIN. (Del Pharm.) Salicylic acid 0.5%, SD alcohol 40, aloe vera gel, EDTA, menthol. Lot. Bot. 180 ml.
Use: Anti-acne.

PROPA PH CLEANSING FOR OILY SKIN. (Del Pharm.) Salicylic acid 0.5%, SD alcohol 40, aloe vera gel, EDTA, menthol. Lot. Bot. 180 ml.
Use: Anti-acne.

PROPA PH CLEANSING FOR SENSITIVE SKIN. (Del Pharm.) Salicylic acid 0.5%, SD alcohol 40, aloe vera gel, EDTA, menthol. Pads. In 45s.
Use: Anti-acne.

PROPA PH CLEANSING MAXIMUM STRENGTH. (Del Pharm.) Salicylic acid 2%, SD alcohol 40, aloe vera gel, EDTA, menthol. Pads. In 45s.
Use: Anti-acne.

PROPA PH FOAMING FACE WASH. (Del Pharm.) Salicylic acid 2%, aloe vera gel, EDTA, menthol. Alcohol, oil and soap free. Liq. Bot. 180 ml.
Use: Anti-acne.

PROPA PH MAXIMUM STRENGTH. (Del Pharm.) Salicylic acid 2%, acetylated lanolin alcohol, cetearyl alcohol, stearyl alcohol, aloe vera gel, EDTA, menthol. Cream. Tube 19.5 g.
Use: Anti-acne.

PROPA PH MEDICATED ACNE CREAM WITH ALOE. (Commerce) Salicylic acid 2%. Tube 1 oz.
Use: Anti-acne.

PROPA PH MEDICATED ACNE STICK WITH ALOE. (Commerce) Salicylic acid 2%. Stick 0.05 oz.
Use: Anti-acne.

PROPA PH MEDICATED CLEANSING PADS WITH ALOE. (Commerce) Salicylic acid 0.5%, SD alcohol 40 25%, aloe. Jar containing 45 pads.
Use: Anti-acne.

PROPA PH PEEL-OFF ACNE MASK. (Del Pharm.) Salicylic acid 2%, tartrazine, parabens, fruit acid complex, aloe vera gel, SD alcohol 40. In 60 ml.
Use: Anti acne.

PROPA PH SKIN CLEANSER WITH ALOE. (Commerce) Salicylic acid USP 0.5%, SD alcohol 40 25%. Bot. 6 oz, 10 oz.
Use: Anti-acne.

• **PROPARACAINE HCl,** U.S.P. XXIII. Ophth. Soln., U.S.P. XXIII. Benzoic acid, 3-amino-4-propoxy-, 2-(diethylamino)ethyl ester, HCl. Proxymetacaine, B.A.N. (Various Mfr.) 0.5% Soln. Bot. 2 ml, 15 ml, UD 1 ml.
Use: Anesthetic (topical, ophthalmic).
See: Alcaine Ophthalmic Soln. (Alcon).
　　AK-Taine, Soln. (Akorn).
　　Fluoracaine, Soln. (Akorn).
　　Ophthaine HCl, Soln. (Squibb Mark).
　　Ophthetic, Ophthalmic Soln. (Allergan).

PROPARACAINE HCl & FLUORESCEIN SODIUM. (Pasadena) Proparacaine HCl 0.5%, fluorescein sodium 0.25%, thimerosal 0.01%, EDTA. Soln. Bot. 5 ml.
Use: Anesthetic (topical, ophthalmic).

PROPARACAINE HCL/PROCAINE HCL.
Use: Injectable anesthetic.
See: Ravocaine and novocain w/Levophed (Cook-Waite).
　　Ravocaine and novocain w/neocobefrin (Cook-Waite).

• **PROPATYL NITRATE.** USAN. 2-Ethyl-2-hydrox-ymethyl-1,3-propanedioltrinitrate. Ettriol Trinitrate. 1,1,1-Trisnitratomethylpropane. Etrynit; Gina. Investigational drug in U.S. but available in England.
Use: Coronary vasodilator.

PROPAZOLAMIDE. 2-Propionylamino-1,3,4-thiadiazole-5-sulfonamide. Ionaze (Lilly).

• **PROPENZOLATE HYDROCHLORIDE.** USAN. 1-Methyl-3-piperidyl-α-phenylcyclohexaneglycolate HCl.
Use: Anticholinergic.

PROPERIDINE. B.A.N. Isopropyl 1-methyl-4-phenyl-piperidine-4-carboxylate.
Use: Narcotic analgesic.

PROPESIN. Name used for Risocaine.

PROPHENE 65. (Halsey) Propoxyphene HCl 65 mg/Cap. Bot. 100s, 500s, 1000s.
Use: Narcotic analgesic.

PROPHENPYRIDAMINE.
See: Pheniramine (Various Mfr.).

PROPHENPYRIDAMINE MALEATE.
See: Pheniramine Maleate.

PROPHENPYRIDAMINE MALEATE W/COMBINATIONS.
See: Histjen, Cap. (Jenkins).
　　Hist-Span No. 2, Cap. (Kenyon).
　　Panadyl, Tab., Cap. (Misemer).
　　Polyectin, Liq. (Amid).
　　Trimahist Elix., Liq. (Tennessee).
　　Vasotus, Liq. (Sheryl).

PRO-PHREE. (Ross) Fat 31 g, carbohydrate 60 g, linoleic acid 2250 mg, Fe 11.9 mg, Na 250 mg, K 875 mg, with appropriate vitamins and minerals, 520 Cal/100 g. Protein free. Pow. Can 350 g.
Use: Enteral nutritional supplement.

PROPHYLLIN. (Rystan) **Pow.:** Sodium propionate 1%, water soluble chlorophyllin 0.0025%. **Oint.:** Sodium propionate 5%, chlorophyll derivatives 0.0125%. Tube 1 oz.
Use: Anti-infective, external.

PROPICILLIN. B.A.N. 6 (α Phenoxybutyramido)-penicillanic acid(1-Phenoxypropyl)penicillin. Brocillin & Ultrapen are the potassium salt.
Use: Antibiotic.

• **PROPIKACIN.** USAN.
Use: Antibacterial.

PROPIMEX-1. (Ross) Protein 15 g, fat 23.9 g, carbohydrate 46.3 g, linoleic acid 1800 mg, Fe 9 mg, Na 190 mg, K 675 mg, with appropriate vitamins and minerals, 480 Cal/100 g. Methionine and valine free. Pow. Can 350 g.
Use: Enteral nutritional supplement.

PROPIMEX-2. (Ross) Protein 30 g, fat 15.5 g, carbohydrate 30 g, Fe 13 mg, Na 880 mg, K 1370 mg, with appropriate vitamins and minerals, 410 Cal/100 g. Methionine and valine free. Pow. Can 325 g.
Use: Enteral nutritional supplement for propionic or methylmalonic acidemia.

PROPINE STERILE OPHTHALMIC SOLUTION. (Allergan) Dipivefrin HCl 0.1%, benzalkonium Cl 0.004%, mannitol, sodium metabisulfite, edetate disodi-

um. Bot. 5 ml, 10 ml, 15 ml.
Use: Agent for glaucoma.
PROPIODAL.
See: Entodon.
• **PROPIOLACTONE.** USAN. 2-Oxe-
tanone; beta-propiolactone, Betaprone.
Hydracrylic acid, β-lactone.
Use: Sterilization of vaccines and tissue
grafts.
• **PROPIOMAZINE.** USAN. 1-[10-(2-Di-
methylaminopropyl)-phenothiazine-2-
yl]-1-propanone.
Dorevane; Indorm.
Use: Sedative.
See: Largon, Amp. (Wyeth-Ayerst).
• **PROPIOMAZINE HYDROCHLORIDE,**
U.S.P. XXII. Inj., U.S.P. XXII. 1-[10-[2-
(Dimethylamino)propyl]- phenothiazin-2-
yl]-1-propanone HCl.
Use: Sedative.
See: Largon, Inj. (Wyeth-Ayerst).
PROPIONATE COMPOUND.
See: Propion Gel (Wyeth-Ayerst).
PROPIONATE SALTS.
See: Copper.
Potassium.
Sodium.
Zinc.
• **PROPIONIC ACID,** N.F. XVIII.
Use: Antimicrobial.
W/Sodium propionate, docusate sodium,
salicylic acid.
See: Prosal, Liq. (Gordon).
Propionate-Caprylate Mixtures.
**PROPIONYL ERYTHROMYCIN LAURYL
SULFATE.**
See: Erythromycin Propionate Lauryl
Sulfate.
• **PROPIRAM FUMARATE.** USAN. N-(1-
Methyl-2-pipe-ridinoethyl)-N-(2-pyridyl)
propionamide fumarate. 1:1.
Use: Analgesic.
PROPISAMINE.
See: Amphetamine (Various Mfr.).
PROPITOCAINE. Prilocaine.
See: Citanest, Soln., Vial, Amp. (Astra).
PROPLEX. (Hyland) Factor IX Complex
(Human), clotting Factor II (prothrom-
bin), VII (proconvertin), IX (PTC, antihe-
mophilic factor B) and X (Stuart-Prower
factor) all dried and concentrated. Vial
30 ml w/Diluent.
Use: Antihemophilic.
PROPLEX T. (Hyland) Factor IX complex,
heat treated. W/Factors II, VII, IX and X.
W/heparin. Dried concentrate. Vial
w/diluent.
Use: Antihemophilic.
• **PROPOFOL.** USAN.
Use: Anesthetic.

See: Diprivan, Inj. (Zeneca).
PROPONADE CAPSULES. (Blue Cross)
Chlorpheniramine maleate 8 mg,
phenylpropanolamine HCl 50 mg, iso-
propamide 2.5 mg/Cap. Bot. 100s.
Use: Antihistamine, decongestant.
PROPOQUIN. Amopyroquin HCl.
Use: Antimalarial.
PROPOXAMIDE. o-Propoxybenzamide.
• **PROPOXYCAINE HYDROCHLORIDE,**
U.S.P. XXIII. 2-(Diethylamino)ethyl-4-
amino-2-propoxybenzoate HCl.
Use: Local anesthetic.
• **PROPOXYCAINE AND PROCAINE HY-
DROCHLORIDES AND LEVONORDE-
FRIN INJECTION,** U.S.P. XXIII.
Use: Local anesthetic (dental).
**PROPOXYCAINE AND PROCAINE HY-
DROCHLORIDES AND NOREPINEPH-
RINE BITARTRATE INJECTION,** U.S.P.
XXIII.
Use: Local anesthetic (dental).
See: Ravocaine Cartridge (Cook-
Waite).
PROPOXYCHLORINOL. Toloxychlorinol.
• **PROPOXYPHENE HCl,** U.S.P. XXIII.
Cap. U.S.P. XXIII. Benzenethanol, α[2-
(dimethylamino)-1-methyl-ethyl]-
α-phenyl, propanoate (ester), HCl.
Use: Analgesic.
See: Darvon, Pulvules (Lilly).
Dolene, Cap. (Lederle).
Progesic, Cap. (Ulmer).
Pro-Pox 65, Cap. (Kenyon).
SK-65, Cap. (SK-Beecham).
**PROPOXYPHENE HCl W/COMBINA-
TIONS.**
Use: Analgesic.
See: Darvon Compound, Pulvule (Lilly).
Darvon Compound-65, Cap. (Lilly).
Darvon With A.S.A., Cap. (Lilly).
Dolene, AP-65, Tab. (Lederle).
Dolene Compound-65, Cap. (Lederle).
Wygesic, Tab. (Wyeth-Ayerst).
• **PROPOXYPHENE HCl AND ACETA-
MINOPHEN TABLETS,** U.S.P. XXIII.
Use: Analgesic.
**PROPOXYPHENE HCl AND APC CAP-
SULES.**
Use: Analgesic.
• **PROPOXYPHENE HCl, ASPIRIN AND
CAFFEINE CAPSULES,** U.S.P. XXIII.
Use: Analgesic.
• **PROPOXYPHENE NAPSYLATE,** U.S.P.
XXIII. Oral Susp., Tab., U.S.P. XXIII.
Use: Analgesic.
See: Darvocet-N (Lilly).
Darvon-N, Tab. (Lilly).
W/Acetaminophen.
See: Darvocet-N, Tab. (Lilly).

• **PROPOXYPHENE NAPSYLATE AND ACETAMINOPHEN TABLETS,** U.S.P. XXIII.
Use: Analgesic.
• **PROPOXYPHENE NAPSYLATE AND ASPIRIN TABLETS,** U.S.P. XXIII.
Use: Analgesic.
• **PROPRANOLOL HYDROCHLORIDE,** U.S.P. XXIII. Inj., Tab., U.S.P. XXIII. 2-Propanol, 1-[(1-methylethyl)amino]-3-(1-naphthalenyloxy)-, HCl. Propanolol HCl. **Oral Soln.** (Roxane): 20 mg or 40 mg/5 ml. Patient cups UD 5 ml (10s). **Concentrated Oral Soln.** (Roxane): 80 mg/ml. Bot. 30 ml w/calibrated dropper.
Use: Antiarrhythmic agent.
See: Betachron E-R, Cap. (Inwood). Inderal, Tab., Inj. (Wyeth-Ayerst).
• **PROPRANOLOL HYDROCHLORIDE AND HYDROCHLOROTHIAZIDE TABLETS,** U.S.P. XXIII.
See: Inderide, Tab. (Wyeth-Ayerst).
PROPRANOLOL HCl INTENSOL. (Roxane) Propranolol HCl 80 mg/ml concentrated oral soln. Bot. 30 ml with dropper.
Use: Beta-adrenergic blocking agent.
PROPULSID. (Janssen) Cisapride 10 mg, 20 mg, lactose/Tab. Bot. 100s.
Use: Prokinetic agent.
PROPYL p-AMINOBENZOATE. (Various Mfr.) Propaesin.
Use: Local anesthetic.
W/Procaine base, benzyl alcohol, phenol.
See: Rectocaine, Vial (Moore-Kirk).
PROPYLDOCETRIZOATE. B.A.N. Propyl 3-diacetylamino-2,4,6-tri-iodobenzoate. Pulmidol.
Use: Radio-opaque substance.
• **PROPYLENE CARBONATE,** N.F. XVII.
Use: Pharmaceutical aid (gelling agent).
• **PROPYLENE GLYCOL,** U.S.P. XXIII. 1-2-Propanediol.
Use: Pharmaceutical aid (humectant, solvent).
• **PROPYLENE GLYCOL ALGINATE,** N.F. XVIII.
Use: Pharmaceutical aid.
• **PROPYLENE GLYCOL DIACETATE,** N.F. XVIII.
Use: Pharmaceutical aid.
PROPYLENE GLYCOL MONO-STEARATE, N.F. XVIII. 1,2-Propanediol monostearate.
Use: Emulsifying agent.
• **PROPYL GALLATE,** N.F. XVIII.
Use: Pharmaceutic aid (antioxidant).
• **PROPYLHEXEDRINE,** U.S.P. XXIII. Inhalant, U.S.P. XXIII. N,α-Dimethylcyclo-

hexaneethylamine. Evetin HCl.
Use: Adrenergic (vasoconstrictor), appetite suppressant, antihistamine.
See: Benzedrex, Inhalant (SK-Beecham Prods).
• **PROPYLIODONE,** U.S.P. XXIII. Sterile Oil Susp., U.S.P. XXIII. 1(4H)-Pyridineacetic acid, 3,5-diiodo-4-oxo-, propyl ester. Sterile oil Susp. (peanut oil). Sterile water susp. Propyl 3,5-diiodo-4-oxopyridine-1-ylacetate. 3,5-Diiodo-1-propoxycarbonylmethyl-4-pyridone.
Use: Radio-opaque substance.
See: Dionosil Oily (Glaxo).
PROPYLNORADRENALINE-ISO.
See: Isoproterenol.
• **PROPYLPARABEN,** N.F. XVIII. Propyl p-hydroxybenzoate. Propyl Chemosept (Chemo Puro).
Use: Pharmaceutic aid (antifungal preservative).
• **PROPYLPARABEN SODIUM,** N.F. XVIII.
Use: Antifungal preservative.
• **PROPYLTHIOURACIL,** U.S.P. XXIII. Tab., U.S.P. XXIII. 4(1H)-Pyrimidinone, 2,3-dihydro-6-propyl-2-thioxopropyl. (Abbott) 50 mg/Tab. Bot. 100s, 1000s. (Lilly) 50 mg/Tab. Bot. 100s, 1000s. (Lederle) 50 mg/Tab. Bot. 100s, 1000s. 50 mg/Tab. Bot. 100s, 1000s, UD 100s.
Use: Thyroid inhibitor.
PROPYPHENAZONE. B.A.N. 4-Isopropyl-2,3-dimethyl-1-phenyl-5-pyrazolone.
Use: Analgesic.
PROQUAMEZINE. B.A.N. 10-(2,3-Bisdimethyl-aminopropyl)phenothiazine. Aminopromazine (I.N.N.) Myspamol.
Use: Bronchial spasmolytic.
• **PROQUAZONE.** USAN. 1-Isopropyl-7-methyl-4-phenyl-2 (1H)-quinazolinone.
Use: Anti-inflammatory.
• **PROQUINOLATE.** USAN.
Use: Coccidiostat.
• **PRORENOATE POTASSIUM.** USAN.
Use: Aldosterone antagonist.
PROREX. (Hyrex) Promethazine HCl 25 mg or 50 mg/ml. Vial 10 ml.
Use: Antihistamine, antiemetic/antivertigo.
PRORONE. (Sig) Progesterone 25 mg/ml. Aqueous or oil susp. Vial 10 ml.
Use: Progestin.
• **PROROXAN HYDROCHLORIDE).** USAN.
Use: Anti-adrenergic.
PROSCAR. (Merck & Co.) Finasteride 5 mg/Tab. Unit-of-use 30s, 100s, UD 100s.
Use: Androgen inhibitor.

•**PROSCILLARIDIN.** USAN. 3β, 14β-Dihydroxy-bufa-4,20,22-trienolide 3-rhamnoside. Talusin, Tradenal.
Use: Cardiac glycoside.

PROSED/DS. (Star) Methenamine 81.6 mg, phenyl salicylate 36.2 mg, methylene blue 10.8 mg, benzoic acid 9 mg, atropine sulfate 0.06 mg, hyoscyamine sulfate 0.06 mg. Tab. Bot. 100s, 1000s.
Use: Urinary anti-infective.

PROSOBEE. (Mead Johnson Nutrition) Milk free formula supplies 640 cal./qt, protein 19.2 Gm, fat 34 Gm, carbohydrate 64 Gm, vitamins A 2000 IU, D 400 IU, E 20 IU, C 52 mg, folic acid 100 mcg, B_1 0.5 mg, B_2 0.6 mg, niacin 8 mg, B_6 0.4 mg, B_{12} 2 mcg, biotin 50 mg, pantothenic acid 3 mg, K-1 100 mcg, choline 50 mg, inositol 30 mg, calcium 600 mg, phosphorus 475 mg, iodine 65 mcg, iron 12 mg, magnesium 70 mg, copper 0.6 mg, zinc 5 mg, manganese 1.6 mg, chloride 530 mg, potassium 780 mg, sodium 230 mg/Qt. (20 Kcal/fl oz). Concentrated liq. can 13 fl oz; Ready-to-use liq. can 8 fl oz, 32 fl oz. Pow., can 14 oz.
Use: Enteral nutritional supplement.

PROSOBEE CONCENTRATE. (Mead Johnson) P-soy protein isolate, l-methionine. CHO. corn syrup solids, soy and coconut oil, lecithin, mono and diglycerides. Protein 20.3 Gm, CHO 65.4 Gm, fat 33.6 Gm, iron 12 mg, 640 cal./serving. Concentrate 390 ml.
Use: Enteral nutritional supplement.

PRO-SOF PLUS. (Vangard) Docusate sodium 100 mg, casanthranol 30 mg/Cap. Bot. 100s, 1000s, UD 32s, 100s.
Use: Laxative.

PRO-SOF SG 100. (Vangard) Docusate sodium 100 mg/Cap. Bot. 100s, 1000s, UD 10×10s.
Use: Laxative.

PRO-SOF SG 200. (Vangard) Docusate sodium 250 mg/Cap. Bot. 100s, 500s, UD pkg. 10×10s.
Use: Laxative.

PRO-SOF SYRUP. (Vangard) Docusate sodium 20 mg/5 ml. Bot. pt.
Use: Laxative.

PRO-SOF w/CASANTHRANOL SG. (Vangard) Cansanthranol 30 mg, docusate sodium 100 mg/Cap. Bot. 100s, 1000s.
Use: Laxative.

PROSOM. (Abbott) Estazolam 1 mg or 2 mg/Tab. Bot. 100s, UD 100s.
Use: Sedative/hypnotic.

PROSTAGLANDIN E. Dinoprostone, B.A.N.
Use: Prostaglandin.

PROSTAGLANDIN E1 ALPHA-CY-CLODEXTRIN.
Use: Arterial occlusive disease. [Orphan drug]

PROSTAGLANDIN F. Dinoprost, B.A.N.
Use: Prostaglandin.

PROSTAGLANDINS.
Use: Abortifacient.
See: Hemabate (Upjohn).
    Prostin E2 (Upjohn).

•**PROSTALENE.** USAN.
Use: Prostaglandin.

PROSTAPHLIN CAPSULES. (Bristol) Sodium oxacillin 250 mg or 500 mg/Cap. Bot. 48s, 100s, Dosatrol Pack 100s.
Use: Antibacterial, penicillin.

PROSTAPHLIN FOR INJECTION. (Bristol) Crystalline oxacillin sodium 250 mg, 500 mg, 1 Gm, 2 Gm or 4 Gm/dry filled Vial. Piggyback vial 1 Gm, 2 Gm, Bulk vial 10 Gm.
Use: Antibacterial, penicillin.

PROSTAPHLIN ORAL SOLUTION. (Bristol) Sodium oxacillin reconstitute for oral soln. 250 mg/5 ml. Bot. 100 ml, Dosa-Trol Pack 25s.
Use: Antibacterial, penicillin.

PROSTEP. (Lederle) Transdermal nicotine 11 or 22 mg/day. Patch 7s.
Use: Smoking deterrent.

PROSTIGMIN. (ICN Pharm) Injectable neostigmine methylsulfate. **1:1000:** 1 mg/ml w/phenol 0.45%. Vial 10 ml. Box 10s. **1:2000:** 0.5 mg/ml. Amp. 1 ml w/methyl and propylparabens 0.2%. Box 10s. Vial 10 ml w/phenol 0.45%. Box 10s. **1:4000:** 0.25 mg/ml Amp. 1 ml w/methyl and propylparabens 0.2%. Box 10s.
Use: Cholinergic muscle stimulant.

PROSTIGMIN BROMIDE TABLETS. (ICN Pharm) Neostigmine bromide 15 mg/Tab. Bot. 100s, 1000s.
Use: Cholinergic muscle stimulant.

PROSTIN/15 M. (Upjohn) Carboprost 250 mcg, tromethamine 83 mcg/ml. Inj. Amp. 1 ml.
Use: Abortifacient.

PROSTIN E2. Dinoprostone, B.A.N.

PROSTIN VR PEDIATRIC. (Upjohn) Alprostadil 500 mcg/ml. Amp. 1 ml. Box 5s.
Use: Agent for patent ductus arteriosus.

PROSTONIC. (Seatrace) Thiamine HCl 10 mg, alanine 130 mg, glutamic acid 130 mg, amino-acetic acid 130 mg/Cap. Bot. 100s.

Use: Palliative relief of benign prostatic hypertrophy

PROTABOLIN. (Pasadena Research) Methandriol dipropionate 50 mg/ml. Vial 10 ml.

PROTAC. (Republic) Benzocaine 10 mg, cetylpyridinium Cl 2.5 mg/Troche. In 10s.
Use: Local anesthetic, antiseptic.

• **PROTAMINE SULFATE,** U.S.P. XXIII. Inj., for inj., U.S.P. XXIII. (Lilly)-Amp. 1%, 5 ml; 1s, 25s; 25 ml 6s.
Use: I.V.; heparin overdosage.

PROTAR PROTEIN. (Dermol) Coal tar 5%. Odor free. Shampoo. Bot. 120 ml.
Use: Antiseborrheic.

PROTARGIN MILD.
See: Silver Protein, Mild (Various Mfr.).

PROTARGOL. (Sterwin) Strong silver protein. Pow. Bot. 25 Gm.
Use: Topical silver antiseptic.

PROTASE. (Kenyon) Standardized amount of extract of proteolytic enzymes from *Carica papaya* with 10,000 units of activity/Tab. Bot. 100s, 1000s.
Use: Digestive enzymes.

PROTEASE.
W/Pancreatin, amylase.
See: Dizymes, Cap. (Recsei).
W/Vitamins B_1, B_{12}.
See: Arcoret, Tab. (Arco).
W/Vitamins B_1, B_{12}, iron.
See: Arcoret W/Iron, Tab. (Arco).

PROTECTOL MEDICATED POWDER. (Daniels) Calcium undecyclenate 15%. Bot. 2 oz.
Use: Diaper rash product.

PROTEGRA SOFTGELS. (Lederle) Vitamins E 200 IU, C 250 mg, beta carotene 3 mg, zinc 7.5 mg, copper, selenium, manganese. Cap. Bot. 50s.
Use: Vitamin combination.

PROTEINASE INHIBITOR, ALPHA 1.
See: Prolastin (Cutter).

PROTEIN C CONCENTRATE.
Use: Protein C deficiency. [Orphan drug]

• **PROTEIN HYDROLYSATE INJECTION,** U.S.P. XXIII.
Use: Fluid and nutrient replenisher.
See: Amigen, Inj. (Baxter Lab.).
Aminogen, Amp., Vial (Christina).
Lacotein, Vial (Christina).
Travamin, Inj. (Travenol).
Virex, Inj. (Burgin-Arden).

PROTEIN HYDROLYSATES ORAL.
Use: Enteral nutritional supplement.
See: Lofenalac, Pow. (Mead Johnson).
Nutramigen, Pow. (Mead Johnson).
Pregestimil, Pow. (Mead Johnson).

Stuart Amino Acids, Pow. (Stuart).
W/Lysine HCl, methionine, niacinamide, calcium pantothenate, vitamin B complex, C, iron.
See: Pro-Hydro, Tab. (Mills).
W/Vitamin B_{12}.
See: Stuart Amino Acids and B_{12}, Tab. (Stuart).

PROTEIN, NONSPECIFIC THERAPY.
See: Lacotein, Vial (Christina).
Mucusol, Amp., Vial (Kremers-Urban).

PROTENATE. (Hyland) Plasma protein fraction (Human) 5%. Inj. Vial 250 ml, 500 ml w/administration set.
Use: Plasma protein fraction.

PROTEOLYTIC ENZYMES.
See: Papase, Tab. (Parke-Davis).
Vardase, Prods. (Lederle). W/Amylolytic enzyme, cellulolytic enzyme, lipolytic enzyme.
See: Arco-Lase, Tab. (Arco).
Kutrase, Cap. (Kremers-Urban).
Kuzyme, Cap. (Kremers-Urban).
Zymmo, Cap. (Scrip). W/Amylolytic enzyme, lipolytic enzyme, cellulolytic enzyme, belladonna extract.
See: Mallenzyme, Tab. (Hauck).
W/Amylolytic, cellulolytic enzymes, lipase, phenobarbital, hyoscyamine sulfate, atropine sulfate.
See: Arco-Lipase Plus, Tab. (Arco).
W/Amylolytic enzyme, homatropine methylbromide, d-sorbitol. (Papain).
See: Converzyme, Liq. (Ascher).
W/Calcium carbonate, glycine, amylolytic and cellulolytic enzymes.
See: Co-Gel, Tab. (Arco).
W/Neomycin palmitrate, hydrocortisone acetate, water-miscible base.
See: Biozyme, Oint. (Armour).

PROTHIONAMIDE. B.A.N. 2-Propylisonicotinthioamide.
Use: Treatment of tuberculosis.

PROTHIPENDYL. B.A.N. 10-(3-Dimethylaminopropyl)pyrido[3,2-b][1,4]benzothiazine.
Use: Tranquilizer; antiemetic.

PROTHIPENDYL HCI. [(4-Dimethylaminopropyl-pyrido(3,2B)Benzothiazine)] HCl-monohydrate.
Use: Sedative.

PROTICULEEN. (Spanner) Vitamin B_{12} activity 10 mcg, folic acid 10 mg, B_{12} crystalline 50 mcg, niacinamide 75 mg/ml. Multiple dose vial 10 ml. I.M. inj.
Use: Parenteral nutritional supplement.

• **PROTIRELIN.** USAN. 1-[N-(5-Oxo-L-prolyl)-L-histidyl]- -prolinamide. 5-oxo-L-histidyl-L-proline amide.
Use: Thyrotropin releasing hormone.

See: Thypinone, Inj. (Abbott).
PROTIRELIN. (UCB Pharm)
Use: Prevention of infant respiratory distress syndrome. [Orphan drug]
PROTOKYLOL. B.A.N. 1-(3,4-Dihydroxyphenyl)-2-(α-methyl-3,4-methylenedioxyphenethylamino)-ethanol.
Use: Sympathomimetic.
PROTOPAM CHLORIDE. (Wyeth-Ayerst) **Emergency kit:** One 1 Gm/20 ml vial of pralidoxime Cl w/one 20 ml amp. diluent, disposable syringe, needle and alcohol swab. **Hospital package:** Six 20 ml vials of 1 Gm each of sterile Protopam Cl powder, without diluent or syringe.
Use: Antidote.
PROTOSAN. (Recsei) Protein 87.5%, lactose 0.5%, fat 1.3%, ash 3.5%, sodium 0.02%. Jar 1 lb, 5 lb.
Use: Nutritional supplement.
PROT-O-SEA. (Barth's) Protein 90%, containing amino acids and minerals. Bot. 100s, 500s.
Use: Nutritional supplement.
PROTOSTAT. (Ortho) Metronidazole 250 mg or 500 mg/Tab. **250 mg:** Bot. 100s. **500 mg:** Bot. 50s.
Use: Amebicide, anti-infective.
PROTOVERATRINE A.
See: Pro-Amid, Tab. (Amid).
PROTOVERATRINES A & B MALEATE.
PROTRAN PLUS. (Vangard) Meprobamate 150 mg, ethoheptazine citrate 75 mg, aspirin 250 mg/ Tab. Bot. 100s. 500s.
Use: Antianxiety agent, analgesic combination.
• **PROTRIPTYLINE HYDROCHLORIDE,** U.S.P. XXIII. Tab., U.S.P. XXIII. N-methyl-5H-dibenzo [α,d]cycloheptene-5-propylamine HCl.
Use: Antidepressant.
See: Vivactil, Tab. (Merck & Co.).
PROTROPIN. (Genentech) Somatrem. Vial 5 mg (13 IU), 10 mg (26 IU). Contains 2 vials somatrem and 2 vials diluent.
Use: Growth hormone.
PROTUSS. Hydrocodone bitartrate 5 mg, potassium guaiacolsulfonate 300 mg/5 ml, saccharin, sorbitol. Liq. Bot. 20 ml, 120 ml, 480 ml.
Use: Antitussive, expectorant.
PROVAL #3. (Solvay) Acetaminophen 325 mg, codeine phosphate 30 mg/Tab. Bot. 100s, 500s.
Use: Narcotic analgesic combination.
PROVATENE. (Solgar) Beta-carotene 15 mg/Soft gel perle. Bot. 60s, 180s.
Use: To reduce photosensitivity in pa-

tients with erythropoeitic protoporphyria.
PROVENTIL. (Schering) Albuterol sulfate 2 mg or 4 mg/Tab. Bot. 100s, 500s.
Use: Bronchodilator.
PROVENTIL INHALER. (Schering) Metered dose aerosol unit containing albuterol in propellants. Each actuation delivers 90 mcg of albuterol. Canister 17 Gm with oral adapter. Box 1s.
Use: Bronchodilator.
PROVENTIL REPETABS. (Schering) Albuterol 4 mg, lactose/Tab. Bot. 100s, 500s.
Use: Bronchodilator.
PROVENTIL SOLUTION. (Schering) Albuterol sulfate solution. **0.5%:** Albuterol sulfate 6 mg/ml. Bot. 20 ml. Box 1s. **0.083%:** Albuterol sulfate 0.83 mg/ml. Bot. 3 ml. Box 100s.
Use: Bronchodilator.
PROVENTIL SYRUP. (Schering) Albuterol sulfate 2 mg/5 ml. Bot. 16 oz.
Use: Bronchodilator.
PROVERA. (Upjohn) Medroxyprogesterone acetate 2.5 mg, 5 mg or 10 mg/Tab. **2.5 mg:** Bot. 25s. **5 mg:** Bot. 25s, 100s. **10 mg:** Bot. 25s, 100s, Dosepak 10s.
Use: Progestin.
PROVOCHOLINE. (Roche) Methacholine Cl for inhalation 100 mg/Vial for reconstitution. Vial 5 ml. Box 1s.
Use: Diagnostic aid.
PROX/APAP. (UAD Labs) Propoxyphene HCl 65 mg, acetaminophen 650 mg/Tab. Bot. 100s, 500s.
Use: Narcotic analgesic combination.
• **PROXAZOLE.** USAN. 5-[(2-Diethylamino)ethyl]-3-(α-ethyl-benzyl)-1,2,4-oxadiazole.
Use: Antispasmodic, analgesic, anti-inflammatory.
• **PROXAZOLE CITRATE.** USAN.
Use: Relaxant (smooth muscle), analgesic, anti-inflammatory.
• **PROXICROMIL.** USAN.
Use: Anti-allergic.
PROXIGEL. (Reed & Carnrick) Carbamide peroxide 11% in a water free gel base. Tube 1.2 oz.
Use: Antiseptic, cleanser.
• **PROXORPHAN TARTRATE.** USAN.
Use: Analgesic; antitussive.
PROXY 65. (Parmed) Propoxyphene HCl 65 mg, acetaminophen 650 mg/Tab. Bot. 100s, 500s.
Use: Narcotic analgesic combination.
PROXYMETACAINE. B.A.N. 2-Diethylaminoethyl 3-amino-4-propoxyben-

zoate.
Use: Local anesthetic.
PROXYPHYLLINE. B.A.N. 7-(2-Hydroxypropyl)-theophylline.
Use: Bronchodilator.
PROZAC. (Dista) Fluoxetine HCl **Pulvules:** 10 mg or 20 mg Bot. 100s. **Liq.:** 20 mg/5 ml Bot. 120 ml.
Use: Antidepressant.
PROZINE-50. (Hauck) Promazine HCl 50 mg/ml. Vial 10 ml.
Use: Antipsychotic agent.
PRUDENTS. (Bariatric) Acetylphenylisatin 5 mg/Tab. Bot. 30s, 100s. Chewable protein and amino acid.
Use: Laxative.
PRULET. (Mission) White phenolphthalein 60 mg/Tab. Strips 12s, 40s.
Use: Laxative.
PRUNE CONCENTRATE. W/cascarin.
See: Prucara, Tab. (ICN).
PRUNE POWDER CONCENTRATED DEHYDRATED.
See: Diacetyldihydroxyphenylisatin. W/Cascara fluidextract aromatic and psyllium husk powder.
See: Casyllium, Pow. (Upjohn).
PRUNE PREPS.
See: Casyllium, Granules (Upjohn).
PRUN-EVAC. (Pharmex) Bot. 30s.
Use: Laxative.
PRURILO. (Whorton) Menthol 0.25%, phenol 0.25%, calamine lotion in special lubricating base. Bot. 4 oz, 8 oz.
Use: Minor skin irritations.
PSEUDO-CAR DM. (Geneva Generics) Pseudoephedrine HCl 60 mg, carbinoxamine maleate 4 mg, dextromethorphan HBr 15 mg/5 ml, alcohol < 0.6%. Bot. pt, gal.
Use: Decongestant, antihistamine, antitussive.
PSEUDO-CHLOR. (Major) Pseudoephedrine HCl 120 mg, chlorpheniramine maleate 8 mg/Cap. Bot. 250s.
Use: Decongestant, antihistamine.
• **PSEUDOEPHEDRINE HYDROCHLORIDE,** U.S.P. XXIII. Syrup, Tab., U.S.P. XXIII. Isoephedrine HCl. α(1-Methylamino)-ethyl benzyl alcohol HCl. (+)-Pseudoephedrine HCl.
Use: Adrenergic (vasoconstrictor).
See: Cenafed, Tab., Syr. (Century).
D-Feda, Cap., Syr. (Dooner).
Novafed, Cap., Liq. (Merrell Dow).
Sinufed, Cap. (Hauck).
Sudafed, Tab., Syr. (Burroughs Wellcome).
Sudafed S.A., Cap. (Burroughs Wellcome).

Ursinus, Inlay Tab. (Sandoz Consumer).
PSEUDOEPHEDRINE HCl W/COMBINATIONS.
See: Actifed, Tab., Syr. (Burroughs Wellcome).
Actifed Allergy, Cap. (Burroughs Wellcome).
Ambenyl-D, Liq. (Marion).
Anatuss DM, Syr., Tab. (Mayrand).
Atridine, Tab. (Interstate).
Banophen, Cap. (Major).
Brexin, Cap., Liq. (Savage).
Congestac, Tab. (SK-Beecham Prods).
CoTylenol, Tab. (McNeil).
CoTylenol Liquid Cold Formula (McNeil).
Deconamine, Cap., Tab., Elix., Syr. (Berlex).
Dimacol, Cap., Liq. (Robins).
Dorocol, Prods. (Sandoz Consumer).
Fedrazil, Tab. (Burroughs Wellcome).
Isoclor, Preps. (American Critical Care).
Kronofed-A, Cap. (Ferndale).
Mapap Cold Formula, Tab. (Major).
Maximum Strength Tylenol Flu, Tab. (McNeil CPC).
Novafed A, Liq., Cap. (Merrell Dow).
Novahistine Sinus, Tab. (Merrell Dow).
Phenergan-D, Tab. (Wyeth-Ayerst).
Robitussin Cold & Cough, Cap. (Robins).
Robitussin-DAC, Liq. (Robins).
Robitussin-PE, Liq. (Robins).
Robitussin Severe Congestion, Cap.(Robins).
Rondec D, Drops; C, Tab.; S, Syr.; T, Filmtab (Ross).
Rondec DM, Drops, Syr. (Ross).
Sine-Aid IB, Cap. (McNeil-CPC).
Sine-Off, Prods. (SK-Beecham Prods).
Sudafed Plus, Tab., Syr. (Burroughs Wellcome).
Triphed, Tab. (Lemmon).
Tussafed Expectorant Liq. (Cavital).
Tylenol Cold Night Time, Liq. (McNeil-CPC).
Tyrodone, Liq. (Major).
• **PSEUDOEPHEDRINE POLISTIREX.** USAN.
Use: Nasal decongestant.
• **PSEUDOEPHEDRINE SULFATE,** U.S.P. XXIII.
Use: Nasal decongestant, adrenergic (bronchodilator).
See: Afrinol Repetabs (Schering).
W/Chlorpheniramine maleate.
See: Chlor-trimeton Decongestant, Tab.

(Schering).
W/Dexbrompheniramine.
See: Disophrol Chronotabs, Tab.
(Schering).
Drixoral S.A., Tab. (Schering).
W/Dexchlorpheniramine.
See: Polaramine Expectorant (Schering).
PSEUDOGEST. (Major) Pseudoephedrine HCl 30 mg or 60 mg/Tab. Bot. 24s, 100s.
Use: Decongestant.
PSEUDOGEST PLUS. (Major) Pseudoephedrine HCl 60 mg, chlorpheniramine maleate 4 mg/Tab. In 24s.
Use: Decongestant, antihistamine.
PSEUDO-HIST. (Holloway) Pseudoephedrine HCl 30 mg, chlorpheniramine maleate 10 mg/Cap. Bot. 100s.
Use: Decongestant, antihistamine.
PSEUDO-HIST EXPECTORANT. (Holloway) Pseudoephedrine 15 mg, hydrocodone bitartrate 2.5 mg, guaifenesin 100 mg, alcohol 5%. Bot. 480 ml.
Use: Decongestant, antitussive, expectorant.
PSEUDOMONAS HYPERIMMUNE GLOBULIN (MUCOID EXOPOLYSACCHARIDE).
Use: Pulmonary infection in cystic fibrosis. [Orphan drug]
PSEUDOMONAS TEST.
Use: Urine test.
See: Isocult for Pseudomonas aeruginosa (SK-Beecham Diagnostics).
PSEUDOMONIC ACID A.
Use: Topical anti-infective.
See: Bactroban (SK-Beecham).
"PSEUDO-PHEDRINE". (Whiteworth) Pseudoephedrine HCl 30 mg/Tab. Bot. 100s, 1000s.
Use: Decongestant.
PSEUDO PLUS. (Weeks & Leo) Pseudoephedrine HCl 60 mg, chlorpheniramine maleate 4 mg/Tab. Bot. 40s.
Use: Decongestant, antihistamine.
PSEUDO SYRUP. (Major) Pseudoephedrine 30 mg/5 ml. Liq. Bot. 120 ml, pt, gal.
Use: Decongestant.
PSILOCYBIN. B.A.N. (Sandoz) 3-(2-Dimethylaminoethyl)indol-4-yl dihydrogen phosphate.
Use: Psychotogenic agent.
PSORALENS.
See: Methoxsalen.
Trioxsalen.
PSORCON. (Dermik) Diflorasone diacetate (0.05%) 0.5 mg/Gm. **Oint.:** Tube 15 Gm, 30 Gm, 60 Gm. **Cream:** Tube 15

Gm, 30 Gm, 60 Gm.
Use: Corticosteroid.
PSORIGEL. (Owen) Coal tar soln. 7.5%, alcohol 33% in hydroalcoholic gel vehicle. Tube 4 oz.
Use: Tar-containing preparation.
PSORINAIL. (Summers) Coal tar solution w/isopropyl alcohol 2.5%, 3-butylene glycol l, acetyl mandelic acid. Liq. Bot. 30 ml.
Use: Antipsoriatic, topical.
PSORION CREAM. (ICN) Betamethasone dipropionate 0.05%, mineral oil, white petrolatum, propylene glycol. Cream. Tube 15 g, 45 g.
Use: Topical corticosteroid.
PSYCHOTHERAPEUTIC DRUGS.
See: Ataraxic Agents.
PSYLLIUM GRANULES.
Use: Laxative.
See: Perdiem Fiber, Gran. (Rhone-Poulenc Rorer Consumer).
W/Dextrose.
See: Muci-lax, Granules (Shionogi).
W/Senna.
See: Perdiem, Granules (Rhone-Poulenc Rorer Consumer).
• **PSYLLIUM HUSK,** U.S.P. XXIII.
Use: Cathartic.
W/Cascara fluidextract aromatic, prune powder.
Use: Cathartic.
See: Casyllium, Pow. (Upjohn).
PSYLLIUM HYDROCOLLOID.
Use: Laxative.
See: Effersyllium, Pow. (Stuart).
• **PSYLLIUM HYDROPHILIC MUCILLOID FOR ORAL SUSPENSION,** U.S.P. XXIII.
Use: Bulk producing laxative.
See: Konsyl, Pow. (Lafayette).
Modane Versabran, Pow. (Adria).
Mucillium, Pow. (Whiteworth).
Mylanta Natural Fiber Supplement, Pow. (J & J-Merck).
Restore (Inagra).
W/Dextrose.
See: Hydrocil Plain (Solvay).
Konsyl-D Pow. (Lafayette).
V-lax, Pow. (Century).
W/Dextrose, casanthranol.
See: Hydrocil Fortified (Solvay).
W/Oxyphenisatin acetate.
See: Plova, Pow. (WEL).
W/Standardized senna concentrate.
See: Senokot w/Psyllium, Pow. (Purdue Frederick).
PSYLLIUM SEED GEL.
Use: Laxative.
W/Planta Ovata, gum Karaya, Brewer's

yeast.
See: Plantamucin, Granules (Elder).
P.T.E.-4. (Lyphomed) Zinc 1 mg, copper
0.1 mg, chromium 1 mcg, manganese
25 mcg/ml. Vial 3 ml.
Use: Mineral supplement.
P.T.E.-5. (Lyphomed) Zinc 1 mg, copper
0.1 mg, chromium 1 mcg, manganese
25 mcg, selenium 15 mcg/ml. Vial 3 ml,
10 ml.
Use: Mineral supplement.
PTEROIC ACID. The compound formed
by the linkage of carbon 6 of 2-amine-4-
hydroxypteridine by means of a methyl-
ene group with the nitrogen of p-
aminobenzoic acid.
PTEROYLGLUTAMIC ACID.
See: Folic Acid, Preps. (Various Mfr.).
PTEROYLMONOGLUTAMIC ACID.
Pteroylglutamic acid.
See: Folic Acid, Preps. (Various Mfr.).
PTFE. (Ethicon) Polytef.
PTU.
See: Propylthiouracil.
PULMOCARE. (Ross) High fat, low-car-
bohydrate liquid diet for pulmonary pa-
tients containing 1500 calories/Liter;
1420 calories provides 100% U.S. RDA
vitamins and minerals. Calorie:Nitrogen
ratio is 150:1. Osmolarity: 490 mosm/Kg
water. Can 8 fl oz.
Use: Enteral nutritional supplement.
**PULMONARY SURFACTANT REPLACE-
MENT.** (Scios Nova)
Use: Prevention & treatment of infant
respiratory distress syndrome. [Or-
phan drug]
**PULMONARY SURFACTANT REPLACE-
MENT, PORCINE.**
Use: Prevention/treatment of respiratory distress syndrome in premature infants. [Orphan drug]
See: Curosurf.
PULMOSIN. (Spanner) Guaiacol 0.1 Gm,
eucalyptol 0.08 Gm, camphor 0.05 Gm,
iodoform 0.02 Gm/2 ml. Multiple dose
vial 30 ml. Inj. I.M.
PULMOZYME. (Genentech) Dornase alfa
1 mg, calcium chloride dihydrate 0.15
mg, NaCl 8.77 mg/ml. Soln. for inhala-
tion. Amps. Single-use 2.5 ml.
Use: Anti-infective.
•**PUMICE,** U.S.P. XXIII.
Use: Abrasive (dental).
PUNCTUM PLUG. (Eagle Vision) Silicone
plug. In 1.6 mm, 2 mm, 2.8 mm. Pkg. 2,
10, 20 plugs, one inserter tool.
Use: Punctal plug.
PURA. (D'Franssia) High potency vitamin
E cream.

Use: Emollient.
PURALUBE. (Fougera) White petrola-
tum, light mineral oil. Oint. Tube 3.5 Gm.
Use: Ophthalmic lubricant.
PURALUBE TEARS. (Fougera) Polyvinyl
alcohol 0.1%, polyethylene glycol 400
1%, EDTA, benzalkonium Cl. Soln. Bot.
15 ml.
Use: Ophthalmic lubricant.
PUREBROM COMPOUND ELIXIR.
(Purepac) Brompheniramine maleate 4
mg/5 ml, phenylephrine HCl, phenyl-
propanolamine HCl, alcohol. Bot. pt, gal.
Use: Antihistamine, decongestant.
PURESEPT MURINE SALINE. (Ross)
Disinfecting soln.: Sterile hydrogen
peroxide solution 3%, sodium stannate,
sodium nitrate, phosphate buffers,
thimerosal free. 237 ml. **Murine Saline
Soln.:** Buffered isotonic solution w/bo-
rate buffers, NaCl, sorbic acid 0.1%,
EDTA 0.1%. 60, 237, 355 ml. Includes
cups and lens holder.
Use: Soft contact lens care.
PURGE EVACUANT. (Fleming) Castor oil
95%. Bot. 1 oz, 2 oz.
Use: Laxative.
PURI-CLENS. (Sween) UD 2 oz. Bot. 8
oz.
Use: Wound deodorizer, cleanser.
PURIFIED OXGALL.
See: Bile Extract, Ox (Various Mfr.)
**PURIFIED PROTEIN DERIVATIVE OF
TUBERCULIN.**
Use: Mantoux TB test.
See: Tuberculin, Old, Vial (Parke-
Davis).
PURINETHOL. (Burroughs Wellcome)
Mercaptopurine 50 mg/Tab. Bot. 25s,
250s.
Use: Antineoplastic agent.
•**PUROMYCIN.** USAN. 3'-(L-α-Amino-p-
methoxy-drocinnamamido)-3-deoxy-
N,N-dimethyladenosine.
Use: Antibiotic.
•**PUROMYCIN HYDROCHLORIDE.**
USAN.
Use: Antineoplastic; antiprotozoal.
PURPLE FOXGLOVE.
See: Digitalis, Preps. (Various Mfr.).
PURPOSE SHAMPOO. (Ortho Derm)
Water, amphoteric-19, PEG-44 sorbitan
laurate, PEG-150 distearate, sorbitan
laurate, boric acid, fragrance, benzyl al-
cohol. Bot. 8 oz.
Use: Shampoo.
PURPOSE SOAP. (Johnson & Johnson)
Sodium tallowate, sodium cocoate, glyc-
erin, NaCl, BHT, EDTA. Bar 108 g, 180
g.

Use: Skin cleanser.

PURSETTES PREMENSTRUAL TABLETS. (Jeffrey Martin) Acetaminophen 500 mg, pamabrom 25 mg, pyrilamine maleate 15 mg/Tab. Bot. 24s.
Use: Analgesic, diuretic, antihistamine.

P.V. CARPINE LIQUIFILM. (Allergan) Pilocarpine nitrate 1%, 2% or 4%, polyvinyl alcohol 1.4%, sodium acetate, sodium Cl, citric acid, menthol, camphor, phenol, eucalyptol, chlorobutanol 0.5%, purified water. Dropper bot. 15 ml.
Use: Agent for glaucoma.

PVP-I OINTMENT. (Day-Baldwin) Povidone-iodine. Tube 1 oz, Jar lb, Foilpac 1.5 Gm.
Use: Antiseborrheic, antiseptic.

P-V-TUSSIN. (Solvay) Hydrocodone bitartrate 2.5 mg, pseudoephedrine HCl 30 mg, chlorpheniramine maleate 2 mg, alcohol 5%. Syrup. Bot. pt, gal.
Use: Antitussive, decongestant, antihistamine.

P-V TUSSIN TABLETS. (Solvay) Hydrocodone bitartrate 5 mg, phenindamine tartrate 25 mg, guaifenesin 200 mg/Tab. Bot. 100s.
Use: Antitussive, antihistamine, expectorant.

PY-CO-PAY TOOTH POWDER. (Block) Sodium Cl, sodium bicarbonate, calcium carbonate, magnesium carbonate, tricalcium phosphate, eugenol, methyl salicylate. Can 7 oz.
Use: Dentifrice.

9-[3-PYDIDYLMETHYL-9-DEAZAGUANINE. (Briocryst Pharm)
Use: Antineoplastic. [Orphan drug]

PYLODATE. (Kenyon) Phenylazodiaminopyridine HCl 100 mg, methenamine mandelate 500 mg/Tab. Bot. 100s, 1000s.
Use: Urinary antiseptic.

PYMA. (Forest Pharm.) **TR Cap.:** Pyrilamine maleate 50 mg, chlorpheniramine maleate 6 mg, pheniramine maleate 20 mg, phenylephrine HCl 15 mg. Bot. 30s, 100s, 1000s. **Inj.:** Chlorpheniramine maleate 5 mg, phenylpropanolamine HCl 12.5 mg, atropine sulfate 0.2 mg/ml. Vial 10 ml.
Use: Antihistamine, decongestant, anticholinergic/antispasmodic.

PYOCIDIN-OTIC SOLUTION. (Forest) Hydrocortisone 5 mg, polymyxin B sulfate 10,000 USP units/ml in a vehicle containing water and propylene glycol. Bot. 10 ml w/sterile dropper.
Use: Corticosteroid, anti-infective otic.

• **PYRABROM.** USAN. Pyrilamine 8-bromotheophyllinate. Glybrom.
Use: Antihistamine.

PYRACOL. (Davis & Sly) Pyrathyn HCl 0.08 Gm, ammonium Cl 0.778 Gm, citric acid 0.52 Gm, menthol 0.006 Gm/fl oz. Bot. pt.

PYRADIN. (Jenkins) Acetophenetidin 4 gr, antipyrine 1 gr, caffeine 1/8 gr, tincture hyoscyamus 8 min. (total alkaloids 0.00032 gr), tincture gelsemium 4 min./Tab. Bot. 1000s.
Use: Analgesic, anticholinergic/antispasmodic.

PYRADONE.
See: Aminopyrine (Various Mfr.).

PYRAMINYL.
See: Pyrilamine Maleate (Various Mfr.).

PYRANILAMINE MALEATE.
See: Pyrilamine Maleate, Preps. (Various Mfr.).

PYRANISAMINE BROMOTHEOPHYLLINATE.
See: Pyrabrom (Various Mfr.).

PYRANISAMINE MALEATE.
See: Pyrilamine Maleate, Preps. (Various Mfr.).

• **PYRANTEL PAMOATE,** U.S.P. XXIII. Oral Susp., U.S.P. XXIII.
Use: Anthelmintic.
See: Antiminth, Oral Susp. (Pfizer Laboratories).
 Pin-Rid, Cap., Liq. (Apothecary).
 Pin-X, Liq. (Effcon).

• **PYRANTEL TARTRATE.** USAN. 1,4,5,6-Tetrahydro-1-methyl-2-[trans-2-(2-thienyl)vinyl]-pyrimidine Tartrate.
Use: Anthelmintic.

PYRATHIAZINE HYDROCHLORIDE. 10-[2-(1-Pyrrolidinyl)ethyl]-phenothiazine.

• **PYRAZINAMIDE,** U.S.P. XXIII. Tab., U.S.P. XXIII. Pyrazinecarboxamide. 2-Carbamyl pyrazine. Pyrazinecarboxamide. Aldinamide, Zinamide. Pyrazinoic acid 0.5 Gm/Tab. Bot. 500s. Lederle-500 mg/Tab. Bot. 500s.
Use: Antibacterial (tuberculostatic).

PYRAZINECARBOXAMIDE. Pyrazinamide, U.S.P. XXIII.

• **PYRAZOFURIN.** USAN.
Use: Antineoplastic.

PYRAZOLINE.
See: Antipyrine (Various Mfr.).

PYRBENZINDOLE.
See: Benzindopyrine Hydrochloride (Various Mfr.).

PYRIBENZAMINE.
See: PBZ, Prods. (Geigy).

PYRICAIN. (Jenkins) Cetylpyridium Cl 4 mg, sodium propionate 10 mg, benzo-

caine 5 mg/Tab. Bot. 1000s.
PYRICARDYL.
See: Nikethamide, Inj. (Various Mfr.).
PYRIDAMOLE TABS. (Major) Dipyri-
damole 25 mg, 50 mg or 75 mg/Tab. **25
mg:** Bot. 1000s, 2500s; **50 mg or 75
mg:** 100s, 1000s.
Use: Antianginal, antiplatelet.
PYRIDATE TABS. (Major) Phenazopyri-
dine 100 mg or 200 mg/Tab. Bot. 1000s.
Use: Urinary analgesic, anti-infective.
PYRIDENE. (Approved) Phenylazodi-
aminopyridine HCl 100 mg/Tab. Bot.
24s, 100s, 1000s.
Use: Urinary tract analgesic.
PYRIDIATE. (Rugby) Phenazopyridine
HCl 100 mg/Tab. Bot. 100s.
Use: Urinary tract product.
**PYRIDINE-BETA-CARBOXYLIC ACID DI-
ETHYL AMIDE.**
See: Nikethamide, Inj. (Various Mfr.).
PYRIDIUM. (Parke-Davis) Phenazopyri-
dine HCl 100 mg or 200 mg/Tab. Bot.
100s, 1000s, UD 100s.
Use: Urinary analgesic, anti-infective.
W/Hyoscyamine HBr, butabarbital.
See: Pyridium Plus, Tab. (Parke-Davis).
• **PYRIDOSTIGMINE BROMIDE,** U.S.P.
XXIII. Syr., Tab., U.S.P. XXIII. Pyridinium
3 [[(dimethylamino) carbonyl]oxy] 1
methyl-, bromide. Dimethyl carbamic es-
ter of 3-hydroxy-1-methylpyridinium bro-
mide.
Use: Cholinergic.
See: Mestinon, Tab., Syr., Amp.
(Roche).
Regonal (Organon).
PYRIDOX. (Oxford) **No. 1:** Pyridoxine HCl
100 mg/Tab. **No. 2:** Pyridoxine HCl 200
mg/Tab. Bot. 100s.
Use: Vitamin B_6 supplement.
PYRIDOXAL. Vitamin B_6. 3-Hydroxy-4-
formyl-5-hydroxy-methyl-2-methylpyri-
dine.
Use: Vitamin B_6 supplement.
PYRIDOXAMINE. Vitamin B_6. 3-Hydroxy-
4-aminomethyl-5-hydroxymethyl-2-
methylpyridine.
Use: Vitamin B_6 supplement.
• **PYRIDOXINE HYDROCHLORIDE,** U.S.P.
XXIII. Inj., Tab., U.S.P. XXIII. Vitamin B_6.
3,4-Pyridinedimethanol, 5-hydroxy-6-
methyl-, hydrochloride. Pyridoxol hy-
drochloride.
Use: Enzyme co-factor vitamin.
See: Hexa Betalin, Amp., Tab., Vial (Lil-
ly).
Hexavibex, Vial (Parke-Davis).
Pan B_6, Tab. (Panray).

PYRIDOXOL. 3-Hydroxy-4,5-hydrox-
ymethyl-2-methylpyridine.
See: Pyridoxine, Vitamin B_6.
**PYRILAMINE BROMOTHEOPHYLLI-
NATE.**
See: Pyrabrom.
W/2-amino-2-methyl-1-propanol.
See: Bromaleate.
• **PYRILAMINE MALEATE,** U.S.P. XXIII.
Tab., U.S.P. XXIII. 2-[[2-(Dimethy-
lamino)ethyl](p-methoxy-benzyl)-
amino]-pyridine maleate (1:1).
Pyranisamine, Pyranilamine, Pyraminyl,
Anisopyradamine. Available: Cap. sus-
tained action, Cream, Ophthalmic Soln.,
Syr., Tab.
Use: Antihistamine.
See: Pyristan, Cap., Elix. (Arcum).
W/Combinations.
See: Antihistamine Cream (Towne).
Anti-Itch Cream (Towne).
Cardui, Tab. (Chattem Labs.).
Corizahist, Tab. (Mason).
Coton, Syr., Tab. (Solvay).
Femicin, Tab. (SK-Beecham).
Histjen, Cap. (Jenkins).
Hist-Span No. 2, Cap. (Kenyon).
Kenahist S.A., Tab. (Kenyon).
Miles Nervine, Tab. (Miles).
Nasal Spray (Ferila).
Prefrin-A Ophth. Soln. (Allergan).
Triaminic Prods. (Sandoz Consumer).
• **PYRIMETHAMINE,** U.S.P. XXIII. Tab.,
U.S.P. XXIII. 2,4-Pyrimidinediamine, 5-
(4-chlorophenyl) 6-ethyl-.2,4-Diamino-5-
(p-chlorophenyl)-6-ethyl-pyrimidine.
Daraprim.
Use: Antimalarial.
See: Daraprim, Tab. (Burroughs Well-
come).
W/Sulfadoxine.
See: Fansidar, Tab. (Roche).
PYRINEX PEDICULICIDE. (Ambix)
Pyrethrins 0.2%, piperonyl butoxide
technical 2%, deodorized kerosene
0.8%. Shampoo. Bot. 118 ml.
Use: Miscellaneous pediculicides.
• **PYRINOLINE.** USAN.
Use: Cardiac depressant.
PYRINYL. (Various Mfr.) Pyrethrins 0.2%,
piperonyl butoxide technical 2%, de-
odorized kerosene 0.8%. Liq. Bot. 60,
120 ml.
Use: Pediculicide.
PYRISTAN. (Arcum) Phenylephrine HCl 8
mg, phenylpropanolamine HCl 15 mg,
chlorpheniramine maleate 3 mg, pyrilamine maleate 10 mg/Cap. Bot. 50s,
500s. Elix. Bot. 4 oz, pt, gal.

Use: Decongestant, antihistamine.

PYRISUL. (Kenyon) Sulfamethylthiadiazole 250 mg, phenylazodiamine pyridine 50 mg/Tab. Bot. 100s, 1000s.

Use: Anti-infective.

PYRISUL-FORTE. (Kenyon) Sulfamethylthiadiazole 500 mg, phenylazodiamine pyridine 50 mg/Tab. Bot. 100s, 1000s.

Use: Anti-infective.

PYRISUL PLUS. (Kenyon) Sulfamethylthiadiazole 250 mg, methenamine mandelate 250 mg, phenylazodiamine pyridine 50 mg/Tab. Bot. 100s, 1000s.

Use: Anti-infective.

PYRITHEN.
See: Chlorothen Citrate (Various Mfr.).

• **PYRITHIONE SODIUM.** USAN.
Use: Antibacterial, topical; antifungal, topical.

• **PYRITHIONE ZINC.** USAN. Bis [1-hydroxy-2-(1H)-pyridinethionato]zinc. Zinc bis(pyridine-2-thiol)1-oxide. Zinc Omadine.
Use: Treatment of seborrhea.
See: Danex Shampoo (Herbert). Zincon Shampoo (Lederle).

PYRITINOL. B.A.N. Di(5-hydroxy-4-hydroxy-methyl-6-methyl-3-pyridylmethyl) disulfide.
Use: Cerebral neuroactivator which increases vigilance and increases or normalizes cerebral metabolism and blood flow.

PYROGALLIC ACID OINTMENT. (Gordon) Pyrogallic acid 25%, chlorobutanol. Jar 1 oz, 1 lb.
Use: Verruca therapy.

PYROGALLOL. Pyrogallic acid.

PYROHEP TABS. (Major) Cyproheptadine HCl 4 mg/Tab. Bot. 250s, 500s.
Use: Antihistamine.

PYROPHENINDANE. 1-(1-Methyl-3-pyrroli-dylmethyl)-3-phenylindane. (Mead Johnson).

• **PYROVALERONE HCl.** USAN. 4'-Methyl-2-(1-pyrrolidinyl)valerophenone HCl.
Use: Central stimulant.

• **PYROXAMINE MALEATE.** USAN.
Use: Antihistamine.

• **PYROXYLIN,** U.S.P. XXI. Soluble guncotton. Cellulose nitrate.
Use: Pharmaceutic necessity for Collodion.

PYRRALAN COMPOUND CAPSULES. (Lannett) Thenylpyramine fumarate 25 mg, acetylsalicylic acid 3.25 gr, phenacetin 2.5 gr, caffeine 0.25 gr/Cap. Bot. 100s, 500s, 1000s.

Use: Antihistamine, analgesic.

PYRRALAN EXPECTORANT. (Lannett) Thenyl-pyramine fumarate 80 mg, ephedrine HCl 30 mg, ammonium Cl 500 mg/fl oz. Bot. pt, gal.
Use: Antihistamine, bronchodilator, expectorant.

PYRRALAN EXPECTORANT "DM.". (Lannett) Same formula as Pyrralan Expectorant w/d-methorphan HBr 10 mg/5 ml. Bot. pt, gal.
Use: Antitussive, antihistamine, bronchodilator, expectorant.

• **PYRROBUTAMINE PHOSPHATE,** U.S.P. XXI. 1-[4-(p-Chlorophenyl)-3-phenyl-2-butenyl]pyrrolidine diphosphate. 1-[α-(p-Chlorobenzyl)cinnamyl]pyrrolidine phosphate (1:2).
Use: Antihistamine.
W/Clopane HCl, Histadyl.
See: Co-Pyronil, Preps. (Lilly).

• **PYRROCAINE.** USAN. 1-Pyrrolidine-aceto-2',6-xylidide. Endocaine.
Use: Local anesthetic.

PYRROCAINE HYDROCHLORIDE. 1-Pyr- rolidineaceto-2',6-xylidide HCl.
Use: Local anesthetic (dental).

PYRROCAINE HYDROCHLORIDE AND EPINEPHRINE INJ.
Use: Local anesthetic (dental).

• **PYRROLIPHENE HYDROCHLORIDE.** USAN. d-α-Benzyl-β-methyl-α-phenyl-1-pyrrolidine-propanol acetate HCl. α-d-2-Acetoxy-1,2-dephenyl-3-methyl-4-pyrrolidinobutane HCl.
Use: Analgesic.

• **PYRROLNITRIN.** USAN. 3-Chloro-4-(3-chloro-2-nitrophenyl)pyrrole. Under study.
Use: Antifungal.

PYRROXATE. (Upjohn) Chlorpheniramine maleate 4 mg, phenylpropanolamine HCl 25 mg, acetaminophen 500 mg/Cap. Blister pkg. 24s. Bot. 500s.
Use: Antihistamine, decongestant, analgesic.

• **PYRVINIUM PAMOATE,** U.S.P. XXIII. Tab., Oral Susp., U.S.P. XXIII. Quinolinium, 6-(dimethyl-amino)-2-[2-(2,5-dimethyl-1-phenyl-1H-pyrrol-3-yl)ethenyl]-1-methyl-, salt with 4,4'-methylenebis[3-hydroxy-2-naphthalenecarboxylic acid]
Use: Anthelmintic.

Q

QB LIQUID. (Major) Theophylline 150 mg, guaifenesin 90 mg. Bot. pt, gal.
Use: Bronchodilator, expectorant.

QT QUICK TANNING SUNTAN BY COPPERTONE. (Schering-Plough) Ethylhexyl p-methoxycinnamate, dihydroxyacetone. SPF 2. Lot. Bot. 120 ml.
Use: Sunscreen, artificial tanner.

QUA-BID. (Quaker City Pharmacal) Papaverine HCl 150 mg. TR Cap. Bot. 100s, 1000s.
Use: Peripheral vasodilator.

• **QUADAZOCINE MESYLATE.** USAN.
Use: Antagonist (opioid).

QUADRA-HISTER. (Schein) Phenylephrine HCl 5 mg, phenyltoloxamine citrate 7.5 mg. Syr. Bot. pt.
Use: Decongestant, antihistamine.

QUADRIHIST. (Pharmex) Pyrilamine maleate, phenyltoloxamine dihydrogen citrate, prophenpyridamine maleate. Tab. Bot. 36s, 1000s.
Use: Antihistamine.

QUADRINAL. (Knoll) Ephedrine HCl 24 mg, phenobarbital 24 mg, theophylline calcium salicylate 130 mg, potassium iodide 320 mg. Tab. Bot. 100s, 1000s.
Use: Bronchodilator, sedative/hypnotic, expectorant.

QUADRODIDE.
See: Quadrinal, Susp., Tab. (Knoll).

QUADRUPLE SULFONAMIDES.
See: Sulfonamides.

QUAD-SET. (Kenyon) Secobarbital 25 mg, pentobarbital 25 mg, butabarbital 25 mg, phenobarbital 25 mg. Tab. Bot. 100s, 1000s.
Use: Sedative/hypnotic.

QUARZAN. (Roche) Clidinium bromide 2.5 mg or 5 mg. Cap. Bot. 100s.
Use: Anticholinergic/antispasmodic.

• **QUAZEPAM.** USAN.
Use: Sedative; hypnotic.
See: Doral (Baker Cummins).

• **QUAZINONE.** USAN.
Use: Cardiotonic.

• **QUAZODINE.** USAN.
Use: Cardiotonic; bronchodilator.

• **QUAZOLAST.** USAN.
Use: Anti-asthmatic.

QUELICIN. (Abbott Hospital Prods) Succinylcholine Cl. **20 mg/ml:** Fliptop vial 10 ml, Abboject Syringe 5 ml; **50 mg/ml:** Amp. 10 ml; **100 mg/ml:** Amp. 10 ml; **Quelicin-500:** 5 ml in Pintop vial 10 ml; **Quelicin-1000:** 10 ml in Pintop vial 20 ml.
Use: Muscle relaxant.

QUELIDRINE COUGH SYRUP. (Abbott) Dextromethorphan HBr 10 mg, chlorpheniramine maleate 2 mg, ephedrine HCl 5 mg, phenylephrine HCl 5 mg, ammonium Cl 40 mg, ipecac fluidextract 0.005 ml, ethyl alcohol 2%/5 ml. Bot. 4 oz.
Use: Antitussive, antihistamine, bronchodilator, decongestant, expectorant.

QUERCETIN. Active constituent of rutin. Quertine.

QUERTINE. Quercetin. 3,3′,4,5,7-Pentahydroxy-flavone.
Use: Bioflavonoid supplement.

QUESTRAN. (Bristol) Cholestyramine resin 4 Gm active ingredient/9 Gm Powder Packet. Box packet 50s. Can 378 Gm (42 dose).
Use: Antihyperlipidemic, antipruritic.

QUESTRAN LIGHT. (Bristol Labs) Anhydrous cholestyramine 4 Gm/Packet or scoopful. Pow. for Oral Susp. Can 210 Gm (42 doses), carton packet 5 Gm (60s).
Use: Antihyperlipidemic.

QUIAGEL. (Rugby) Kaolin 6 Gm, pectin 142.8 mg, hyoscyamine sulfate 0.1037 mg, atropine sulfate 0.0194 mg, scopolamine HBr 0.0065 mg/30 ml. Susp. Bot. pt, gal.
Use: Antidiarrheal.

QUIAGEL PG. (Rugby) Powdered opium 24 mg, kaolin 6 Gm, pectin 142.8 mg, hyoscyamine sulfate 0.1037 mg, atropine sulfate 0.0194 mg, scopolamine HBr 0.0065 mg/30 ml, alcohol 5%. Susp. Bot. 180 ml, pt, gal.
Use: Antidiarrheal.

QUIAGEN SOFT GELATIN CAPS. (Goldline) Theophylline, glyceryl guaiacolate. Bot. 100s, 500s.
Use: Bronchodilator.

QUIBRON. (Bristol) Theophylline (anhydrous) 150 mg, guaifenesin 90 mg. Cap. Bot. 100s, 1000s, Box 100s individually wrapped.
Use: Antiasthmatic combination.

QUIBRON-300. (Bristol) Theophylline (anhydrous) 300 mg, guaifenesin 180 mg. Cap. Bot. 100s.
Use: Antiasthmatic combination.

QUIBRON PLUS. (Bristol) Ephedrine HCl 25 mg, theophylline (anhydrous) 150 mg, butabarbital 20 mg, guaifenesin 100 mg. Bot. 100s.
Use: Antiasthmatic combination.

QUIBRON PLUS ELIXIR. (Bristol-Myers Squibb) Theophylline 150 mg, ephedrine HCl 25 mg, guaifenesin 100 mg, butabarbital 20 mg, alcohol 15%.

Elix. Bot. Pt.
Use: Antiasthmatic combination.
QUIBRON-T DIVIDOSE TABLETS. (Bristol) Theophylline anhydrous 300 mg. Tab. Dividose design breakable into 100, 150 or 200 mg portions. Immediate release. Bot. 100s.
Use: Antiasthmatic
QUIBRON-T/SR DIVIDOSE TABLETS. (Bristol) Theophylline anhydrous 300 mg. Tab. Dividose design breakable into 100 mg, 150 mg or 200 mg portions. Sustained release. Bot. 100s.
Use: Antiasthmatic.
QUICK-K. (Western Research) Potassium bicarbonate 650 mg (6.5 mEq) potassium. Tab. Bot. 30s, 100s.
Use: Potassium supplement.
QUICK PEP. (Thompson) Caffeine 150 mg, dextrose 300 mg. Tab. Bot. 32s.
Use: Analeptic.
QUIEBAR. (Nevin) Butabarbital sodium. **Spantab:** 1.5 gr. TR Spantab. Bot. 50s, 500s. **Elix.:** 30 mg/5 ml. Bot. pt, gal. **Tab.:** 15 mg. Bot. 100s, 1000s; 30 mg. Bot. 1000s. **A.C. Cap.:** Bot. 100s, 500s.
Use: Sedative/hypnotic.
QUIEBEL. (Nevin) Butabarbital sodium 15 mg, belladonna extract 15 mg. Cap. Bot. 100s, 1000s. Elix. pt, gal.
Use: Sedative/hypnotic, anticholinergic/antispasmodic.
QUIECOF. (Nevin) Dextromethorphan HBr 7.5 mg, chlorpheniramine maleate 0.75 mg, guaiacol glyceryl ether 25 mg. Bot. 4 oz, pt, gal.
Use: Antitussive, antihistamine, expectorant.
QUIESS. (Forest) Hydroxyzine HCl 25 mg/ml. Vial 10 ml.
Use: Antianxiety agent, antihistamine.
QUIET NIGHT. (PBI) Pseudoephedrine HCl 10 mg, doxylamine succinate 1.25 mg, dextromethorphan HBr 5 mg, acetaminophen 167 mg/5 ml. Liq. Bot. 180 ml, 300 ml.
Use: Decongestant, antihistamine, antitussive, analgesic.
QUIET TIME. (Whiteworth) Acetaminophen 600 mg, ephedrine sulfate 8 mg, dextromethorphan HBr 15 mg, doxylamine succinate 7.5 mg, alcohol 25 mg/30 ml. Bot. 180 ml.
Use: Analgesic, decongestant, antitussive, antihistamine.
QUIET WORLD. (Whitehall) Acetaminophen 2.5 gr, aspirin 3.5 gr, pyrilamine maleate 25 mg. Tab. Bot. 12s, 30s.
Use: Salicylate analgesic combination, antihistamine.
QUIK-CEPT. (Laboratory Diagnostics) Slide test for pregnancy, rapid latex inhibition test. Kit 25s, 50s, 100s.
Use: Diagnostic aid.
QUIK-CULT. (Laboratory Diagnostics) Slide test for fecal occult blood. Kit 150s, 200s, 300s and tape test
Use: Diagnostic aid.
QUIN-260 TABS. (Major) Quinine sulfate 260 mg. Tab. Bot. 250s.
Use: Antimalarial, nocturnal leg cramps.
QUINACILLIN. B.A.N. 6-(3-Carboxyquinoxaline-2-carboxamideo) penicillanic acid.
Use: Antibiotic.
• **QUINACRINE HYDROCHLORIDE,** U.S.P. XXII. Tab., U.S.P. XXII. 1,4-Pentanediamine,N⁴-(6-chloro-2-methoxy-9-acridinyl)-N¹,N¹-diethyl-, dihydrochloride, dihydrate. 6-Chloro-9-[[4-(diethylamino)-1-methylbutyl]amino] -2-methoxyacridine dihydrochloride.
Use: Anthelmintic, antimalarial.
See: Atabrine HCl, Tab. (Winthrop Pharm).
QUINAGLUTE DURA-TABS. (Berlex) Quinidine gluconate 324 mg. Tab. Bot. 100s, 250s, 500s, UD 100s. Unit-of-use 90s, 120s.
Use: Antiarrhythmic.
QUINALAN GLUCONATE SR TABS. (Lannett) Quinidine gluconate 324 mg. Tab. Bot. 100s, 250s, 500s.
Use: Antiarrhythmic.
QUINALBARBITONE SODIUM. B.A.N. Monosodium derivative of 5-allyl-5-(1-methylbutyl)-barbituric acid.
Use: Hypnotic; sedative.
• **QUINALDINE BLUE.** USAN. 1-Ethyl-2-[3-(1-ethyl-2(1H) quinolylidene) propenyl]-quinolinium Cl. Vernitest reagent. (Fuller)
Use: Diagnostic agent (obstetrics).
QUINAMINOPH TABS. (Goldline) Quinine sulfate 260 mg. Tab. Bot. 100s, 500s.
Use: Antimalarial, nocturnal leg cramps.
QUINAMM. (Merrell Dow) Quinine sulfate 260 mg. Tab. Bot. 100s.
Use: Antimalarial, nocturnal leg cramps.
• **QUINAPRIL HYDROCHLORIDE.** USAN.
Use: Enzyme inhibitor (angiotensin-converting).
See: Accupril, Tab. (Parke-Davis).
• **QUINAZOSIN HYDROCHLORIDE.** USAN. 2-(4-Allyl-1 piperazinyl)-4-amino-6,7-dimethoxy-quinazoline dihydrochloride.
Use: Hypotensive.

• **QUINBOLONE.** USAN. 17-beta-(1-Cyclopenten-1-yloxy)-androsta-1,4-dien-3-one.
Use: Anabolic agent.

• **QUINDECAMINE ACETATE.** USAN. 4,4'-(Deca- methylenediimino) diquinaldine diacetate dihydrate.
Use: Topical anti-infective.

• **QUINDONIUM BROMIDE.** USAN. 2,3-3α,5,6,11,12,12α-Octahydro-8-hydroxy-1H-benzo-[α]-cyclopenta[f]-quinolizinium bromide.
Use: Cardiovascular agent.

• **QUINELORANE HYDROCHLORIDE.** USAN.
Use: Dopaminergic agonist; antidyskinetic; antihyperprolactinemic; antihypertensive.

QUINESTRADOL. B.A.N. 3-Cyclopentyloxyestra-1,3,5(10)-triene-16α,17β-diol.
Use: Estrogen.

• **QUINESTROL,** U.S.P. XXII. Tab., U.S.P. XXII. 3-(Cyclopentyloxy)-19-nor-17-α-pregna-1,3,5(10)-triene-20-yn-17-ol.
Use: Estrogen.
See: Estrovis, Tab. (Parke-Davis).

• **QUINETHAZONE,** U.S.P. XXII. Iab., U.S.P. XXII. 7-Chloro-2-ethyl-6-sulfamyl-1,2,3,4-tetra-hydro-4-quinazolinone. 7-Chloro-2-ethyl-1,2,3,4-tetrahydro-4-oxo-6-quinazolinesulfonamide.
Use: Diuretic.
See: Hydromox, Tab. (Lederle).
W/Reserpine.
See: Hydromox R, Tab. (Lederle).

• **QUINETOLATE.** USAN. 6-(Diethylcarbamoyl)-3-cyclohexene-1-carboxylic acid comp. with 4- ((2-(dime-thylamino) ethyl)amino)6-methoxy- quinoline(2:1) Phthalamaquin (Penick).
Use: Anti-asthmatic.

• **QUINFAMIDE.** USAN.
Use: Anti-amoebic.

• **QUINGESTANOL ACETATE.** USAN. 3-(Cyclopentyloxy)-19-nor-17α-pregna-3,5-dien-20-yn-17-ol acetate. Under study.
Use: Progesterone.

• **QUINGESTRONE.** USAN. 3-(Cyclopentyloxy)pregna-3,5-dien-20-one.
Use: Progesterone.

QUINIDEX EXTENTABS. (Robins) Quinidine sulfate 300 mg. Tab. Bot. 100s, 250s. Dis-co pack 100s.
Use: Antiarrhythmic.

QUINIDEX L-A.
See: Quinidex Extentabs (Robins).

• **QUINIDINE GLUCONATE,** U.S.P. XXIII., Inj., U.S.P. XXIII. Cinchonan-9-ol, 6'-methoxy-,(9s)-, mono-D-gluconate (salt). (Lilly) Amp. (80 mg/ml) 10 ml.
Use: Quinidine therapy; cardiac depressant.
See: Duraquin, Tab. (Parke-Davis).
Quinaglute, Dura-Tab. (Berlex).
Quinalan, Tab. (Lannett).

QUINIDINE POLYGALACTURONATE.
See: Cardioquin Tab. (Purdue Frederick).

• **QUINIDINE SULFATE,** U.S.P. XXIII. Cap., Extended-release Tab., U.S.P. XXIII. Cinchonan-9-ol, 6'-methoxy-,(9s)-, sulfate (2:1) (salt), dihydrate.
Use: Cardiac depressant.
See: Cin-Quin (Solvay).
Quinidex Extentabs (Robins).
Quinora, Tab. (Key).

QUININE ASCORBATE. USAN.
Use: As a deterrent to smoking.

QUININE BISULFATE.
Use: Analgesic, antipyretic, antimalarial.

QUININE DIHYDROCHLORIDE.
Use: Antimalarial.

QUININE ETHYLCARBONATE.
See: Euquinine (Various Mfr.).

QUININE GLYCEROPHOSPHATE. Quinine compound with glycerol phosphate.

• **QUININE SULFATE,** U.S.P. XXIII. Cap., Tab., U.S.P. XXIII. Cinchonan-9-ol,6'-methoxy (8α,9R) sulfate (2:1) (salt) di hydrate.
Use: Antimalarial.
See: Quinamm, Tab. (Merrell Dow).
Quine, Cap. (Solvay).
W/Aminophylline.
See: Strema, Cap. (Foy).
W/Atropine sulfate, emetine HCl, aconitine, camphor monobromate.
See: Coryza, Tab. (Bowman).
W/Niacin, vitamin E.
See: Myodyne, Tab. (Paddock).

QUININE AND UREA HYDROCHLORIDE.
Use: Sclerosing agent.

QUINISOCAINE (I.N.N.). Dimethisoquin, B.A.N.

QUINNONE CREAM. (Dermohr Pharmacal) Hydroquinone 4% in creamy base. Tube 1 oz.
Use: Skin bleaching agent.

QUINOPHAN.
See: Cinchophen (Various Mfr.).

QUINORA. (Key) Quinidine sulfate 300 mg. Tab. Bot. 100s, 1000s, UD 100s.
Use: Antiarrhythmic.

QUINOXYL.
See: Chiniofon

• **QUINPIROLE HYDROCHLORIDE.**

USAN.
Use: Antihypertensive.
QUINPRENALINE. Quinterenol Sulfate.
QUIN-RELEASE. (Major) Quinidine gluconate 324 mg. SR Tab. Bot. 100s, 250s, 500s, UD 100s.
Use: Antiarrhythmic.
QUINCANA PLUS. (Mennen) Undecylenic acid 2%, zinc undecylenate 20%. Pow. 81 Gm, 165 Gm.
Use: Antifungal, external.
QUINTABS. (Freeda) Vitamins A 10,000 IU, D 400 IU, E 25 mg, B_1 25 mg, B_2 25 mg, B_3 100 mg, B_5 25 mg, B_6 25 mg, B_{12} 25 mcg, C 300 mg, folic acid 0.1 mg, inositol 50 mg, PABA 30 mg. Tab. Bot. 100s, 250s, 500s.
Use: Vitamin supplement.
QUINTABS-M. (Freeda) Iron 15 mg, Vitamins A 10,000 IU, D 400 IU, E 41.3 mg, B_1 30 mg, B_2 30 mg, B_3 150 mg, B_5 30 mg, B_6 30 mg, B_{12} 30 mcg, C 300 mg, folic acid 0.4 mg, Ca, Cu, K, Mg, Mn, Se, Zn, PABA.Sodium free. Tab. Bot. 100s, 250s, 500s.
Use: Vitamin/mineral supplement.
• **QUINTERENOL SULFATE.** USAN. 8-Hydroxy-alpha-[(isopropylamino)methyl]-5-quinolinemethanol sulfate (2:1).
Use: Bronchodilator.
• **QUINUCLIUM BROMIDE.** USAN.
Use: Antihypertensive.
• **QUINUPRISTIN.** USAN.
Use: Antibacterial agent.
• **QUIPAZINE MALEATE.** USAN. 2-(1-Piperazinyl) quinoline maleate.
Use: Oxytocic.
QUIPENYL NAPHTHOATE.
See: Pamaquine naphthoate.
Plasmochin naphthoate.
QUIPHILE. (Geneva Generics) Quinine sulfate 260 mg. Tab. Bot. 100s.
Use: Antimalarial.
Q-VEL SOFTGELS. (Ciba Consumer) Quinine sulfate 64.8 mg, vitamin E 400 IU (as dl-alpha tocopheryl acetate), lecithin/Cap. Bot. 30s.
Use: Antimalarial, nocturnal leg cramps.

R

R-3 SCREEN TEST. (Wampole) A three-minute latex-eosin slide test for the qualitative detection of rheumatoid factor activity in serum. Kit 100s.
Use: Diagnostic aid.
• **RABIES IMMUNE GLOBULIN,** U.S.P. XXIII.
Use: Immunizing agent (passive).

RABIES PROPHYLAXIS.
See: Imovax Rabies Vaccine (Merieux Institute).
Imovax Rabies I.D. Vaccine (Merieux Institute).
Hyperab (Cutter).
Imogam (Merieux Institute).
Antirabies Serum (Solvay).
• **RABIES VACCINE,** U.S.P. XXIII. (Lilly) 1 dose Vial of 1.1 ml. The suspending fluid consists of cysteine HCl 0.1%, lactose 5%, gelatin 0.2%, dibasic potassium phosphate 0.25%. Vaccine preserved w/thimerosal 1:10,000. (Lederle) 1000 units/Vial. Antirabies Serum.
Use: Immunizing agent, active.
R & C SHAMPOO. (Reed & Carnrick) Pyrethrin shampoo. Bot. 2 oz, 4 oz.
Use: Pediculicide.
R & C SPRAY III. (Reed & Carnrick) Spray containing pyrethroid (sumethrin) 0.382%, other isomers 0.018%, petroleum distillate 4.255%. Aerosol Container 5 oz.
Use: Pediculicide.
RACEMETHIONINE, U.S.P. XXI. Cap., Tab., U.S.P. XXI. Dl-2-Amino-4-(methylthio)butyric acid. Methionine.
Use: Acidifier (urinary).
See: Amurex, Cap. (Solvay).
Odonil, Cap. (Kenyon).
Pedameth. Cap., Liq. (Forest).
RACEMETHIONINE W/COMBINATIONS.
See: Aminomin, Vial (Pharmex).
Aminovit, Vial (Hickam).
Ardiatric, Tab. (Burgin-Arden).
Cho-Meth, Vial (Kenyon).
Geriatrazole, Vial (Kenyon).
Geriatro-B, Vial (Kenyon).
Hi-Pro Wafers, Tab. (Mills).
Licoplex, Tab. (Mills).
Limvic, Tab. (Briar).
Lipo-K, Cap. (Marcen).
Lychol-B, Inj. (Burgin-Arden).
Minoplex, Vial (Savage).
Pro-Hydro, Tab. (Mills).
Vio-Geric, Tab. (Solvay).
Vio-Geric-H, Tab. (Solvay).
Vi-Testrogen, Vial (Pharmex).
RACEMETHORPHAN. B.A.N. (±)-3-Methoxy-N-methylmorphinan
Use: Narcotic analgesic.
RACEMIC CALCIUM PANTOTHENATE.
See: Calcium Pantothenate, Racemic.
RACEMIC DESOXY-NOR-EPHEDRINE.
See: Amphetamine (Various Mfr.).
RACEMIC EPHEDRINE HCI.
Racephedrine HCl.
RACEMIC PANTOTHENIC ACID.
See: Vitamin, Preps.

RACEMORAMIDE. B.A.N. (±)-1-(3-Methyl-4-morpholino-2,2-diphenylbutyryl)pyrrolidine.
Use: Narcotic analgesic.
RACEMORPHAN HBr. B.A.N. (±)-3-Hydroxy-N-methylmorphinan.
Use: Narcotic analgesic.
RACEPHEDRINE HYDROCHLORIDE. (Upjohn) dl-a-[1-(Methylamino)ethyl]benzyl alcohol HCl.
Cap.: ⅜ gr. Bot. 40s, 250s, 1000s.
Soln.: 1%. Bot. 1 fl oz, pt, gal.
Use: Vasoconstrictor, nasal decongestant.
See: Ephedrine Combinations
W/Aminophylline, phenobarbital.
See: Amodrine, Tab. (Searle).
W/Theophylline sodium glycinate, phenobarbital.
See: Synophedal, Tab. (Central).
• **RACEPHENICOL.** USAN.
Use: Antibacterial.
• **RACEPINEPHRINE HYDROCHLORIDE,** U.S.P. XXIII. Inhalation Soln., U.S.P. XXIII.
Use: Bronchodilator.
RADIOACTIVE ISOTOPES.
See: Medotope, Prods. (Squibb).
Radio-Gold, Soln.
Radio-Iodinated Serum Albumin (Human).
Sodium Radio-Chromate, Inj.
Sodium Radio-Iodide, Soln.
Sodium Radio Phosphate, Soln.
RADIOACTIVE ISOTOPES.
See: Aggregated Radioiodinated Albumin, Human I-131.
Chlormerodrin Hg-197, Inj.
Chlormerodrin Hg-203, Inj.
Cyanocobalamin Co-57, Cap.
Cyanocobalamin Co-60, Cap.
Gold Au-198, Inj.
Radiodinated Serum Albumin, Human I-125.
Radiodinated Serum Albuminia, Human I-131.
Selenomethionine Se-75, Inj.
Sodium Chromate Cr-51, Inj.
Sodium Iodide I-125, Soln., Cap.
Sodium Iodide I-131, Soln., Cap.
Sodium Phosphate P-32, Cap., Inj.
Sodium Rose Bengal I-131, Inj.
Strontium Nitrate Sr-85, Inj.
Technetium Tc-99m, Kit, Inj.
Triolein I-131, Cap., Soln.
Xenon Xe-133, Inj.
RADIOGOLD (^{198}Au), SOLUTION. Gold Au-198 Injection, U.S.P. XXIII.
Use: Irradiation therapy.
See: Auretope, Vial (Squibb).

RADIO-IODIDE (^{131}I), SODIUM.
Use: Radioactive isotopes.
See: Iodotope (Squibb).
Radiocaps (Abbott).
RADIO-IODINATED (^{131}I) SERUM ALBUMIN. (Human), Iodinated I-131 Albumin Injection, U.S.P. XXIII.
RADIO-IODINATED SERUM ALBUMIN (Human),(^{125}I).
See: Albumotope (^{125}I) (Squibb).
RADIOPHARMACEUTICALS.
See: Iodotope (Squibb).
Sodium Iodide L 131 (Mallinckrodt).
Sodium Phosphate P 32 (Mallinckrodt).
Phosphocol P 32 (Mallinckrodt).
RADIO-PHOSPHATE (^{32}P), SODIUM.
Use: Radioactive isotopes.
RADIOSELENOMETHIONINE 75 Se. Selenomethionine Se 75.
RADIOTOLPOVIDONE I-131. Tolpovidone I-131.
See: Raovin (Abbott).
• **RAFOXANIDE.** USAN.
Use: Anthelmintic.
RAGUS. (Miller) Magnesium 27 mg, vitamin C 100 mg, calcium 580 mg, phosphorus 450 mg, l-lysine 25 mg, dl-methionine 50 mg, A 5000 IU, D 400 IU, E 10 mg, B_1 20 mg, B_2 3 mg, B_6 5 mg, B_{12} 9 mcg, niacinamide 80 mg, pantothenic acid 5 mg, iron 20 mg, copper 1 mg, manganese 2 mg, potassium 10 mg, zinc 2 mg, iodine 0.1 mg/3 Tab. Bot. 100s.
Use: Vitamin/mineral supplement.
R A LOTION. (Medco Lab) Resorcinol 3%, calamine, starch, sodium borate, bentonite, alcohol 43%. Plastic bot. 4 oz, 8 oz, 16 oz.
Use: Anti-acne.
• **RAMIPRIL.** USAN.
Use: Antihypertensive, enzyme inhibitor (angiotensin-converting).
See: Altace (Hoechst-Roussel)
• **RAMOPLANIN.** USAN.
Use: Antibacterial.
RAMSES. (Schmid) Nonoxynol 9 5%. Vaginal jelly. 150 Gm.
Use: Spermicide.
RAMSES BENDEX. (Schmid) Flexible cushioned diaphragm; arcing spring. 65-90 mm. Pkg. w/Ramses Vaginal Jelly Tube 1 oz, 3 oz.
Use: Contraceptive.
RAMSES DIAPHRAGM. (Schmid) Flexible cushioned diaphragm 50-95 mm. Pkg. diaphragm, tube of Ramses Vaginal Jelly. Pkg. diaphragm alone.

Use: Contraceptive.
RAMSES EXTRA. (Schmid) Condom with nonoxynol 9 5.6%. In 12s.
Use: Contraceptive.
RAMSES JELLY. (Schmid) Nonoxynol 9. Tube w/applicator 5 oz.
Use: Contraceptive.
RANDOLECTIL. (Farbenfabriken Bayer) Butaperazine.
Use: Psychotropic agent.
RANESTOL. Triclofenol piperazine.
Use: Anthelmintic.
• **RANIMYCIN.** USAN.
Use: Antibacterial.
RANITIDINE.
Use: Histamine H$_2$ antagonist.
See: Zantac, Tab., Inj., Syr. (Glaxo and Roche).
• **RANITIDINE BISMUTH CITRATE.** USAN.
Use: Anti-ulcer agent (histamine H$_2$-receptor blocker).
• **RANITIDINE HYDROCHLORIDE.** USAN. U.S.P. XXIII
Use: Histamine H$_2$ anatagonist.
See: Zantac, Inj., Tab., Syr. (Glaxo Pharm.).
• **RANITIDINE HYDROCHLORIDE IN SODIUM CHLORIDE INJECTION.** U.S.P. XXIII
Use: Histamine H$_2$ anatagonist.
See: Zantac Inj. Premixed (Glaxo Pharm.).
• **RANOLAZINE HYDROCHLORIDE.** USAN.
Use: Antianginal.
RAPID TEST STREP. (SmithKline Diagnostics) Latex slide agglutination test for identification of group A Streptococci. In 25s, 100s.
Use: Diagnostic aid.
RASTINON. Tolbutamide, U.S.P. XXIII.
RATTLESNAKE BITE THERAPY.
See: Antivenin, Snake Polyvalent (Wyeth-Ayerst).
RAUDILAN PB TABLETS. (Lannett) Rauwolfia serpentina root 50 mg, phenobarbital 15 mg/Tab. Bot. 100s, 500s, 1000s.
Use: Antihypertensive.
RAUDIXIN. (Princeton) Rauwolfia whole root w/tartrazine. 50 mg or 100 mg/Tab. Bot. 100s, 1000s.
Use: Antihypertensive.
RAUNEED. (Hanlon) Rauwolfia 50 mg or 100 mg/Tab. Bot. 100s.
Use: Antihypertensive.
RAUNESCINE. (Penick) An alkaloid of Rauwolfia serpentina. Under study.
Use: Antihypertensive.

RAUNORMINE. (Penick) 11-Desmethoxy reserpine.
RAURINE. (Westerfield) Reserpine. **Tab.:** 0.1 mg. Bot. 100s. **Delayed Action Cap.:** 0.5 mg. Bot. 100s.
Use: Antihypertensive.
RAUSERFIA. (New Eng. Phr. Co.) Rauwolfia serpentina 50 mg or 100 mg/Tab. Bot. 100s.
Use: Antihypertensive.
RAUTINA. (Fellows) Rauwolfia serpentina whole root 50 mg or 100 mg/Tab. Bot. 1000s.
Use: Antihypertensive.
RAUVAL. (Vale) Rauwolfia whole root 50 mg or 100 mg/Tab. Bot. 100s, 500s, 1000s.
Use: Antihypertensive.
RAUVERAT. (Kenyon) Rauwolfia serpentina whole root pow. 50 mg, veratrum viride extract equivalent to total alkaloids 1.1 mg/Tab. Bot. 100s, 1000s.
Use: Antihypertensive.
RAUVERID. (Forest) Rauwolfia serpentina pow. whole root 50 mg/Tab. Bot. 100s.
Use: Antihypertensive.
RAU-VER-TIN. (Kenyon) Rauwolfia serpentina 40 mg, veratrum viride 25 mg, rutin 20 mg, mannitol hexanitrate 30 mg/Tab. Bot. 100s, 1000s.
Use: Antihypertensive.
RAUWOLFIA CANESCENS ALKALOID.
See: Harmonyl, Tab. (Abbott).
RAUWOLFIA SERPENTINA ACTIVE PRINCIPLES (ALKALOIDS). Deserpidine, Rescinnamine.
See: Reserpine, Inj. (Various Mfr.).
RAUWOLFIA SERPENTINA ALKALOIDAL EXTRACT.
See: Alseroxylon (Various Mfr.).
• **RAUWOLFIA SERPENTINA,** U.S.P. XXIII. Powder, Tab., U.S.P. XXIII.
Use: Antihypertensive.
See: Raudixin, Tab. (Princeton).
  Rauja, Tab. (Table Rock).
  Raumason, Tab. (Mason).
  Rauneed, Tab. (Hanlon).
  Rauval, Tab. (Vale).
  Rawfola, Tab. (Foy).
  Serfia, Tab. (Westerfield).
  Serfolia, Tab. (Hauck).
  T-Rau, Tab. (Tennessee Pharm.).
  Wolfina, Tab. (Westerfield).
W/Bendroflumethiazide.
See: Rautrax-N, Tab. (Princeton).
  Rauzide, Tab. (Princeton).
W/Bendroflumethiazide, potassium Cl (400).
See: Rautrax, Tab. (Princeton).

W/Mannitol hexanitrate, rutin.
See: Maxitate W/Rauwolfia, Tab. (Pennwalt).
W/Phenobarbital.
See: Raudilan PB, Tab. (Lannett).
RAUWOLSCINE. An alkaloid of *Rauwolfia canescens.* Under study.
Use: Antihypertensive.
RAUZIDE. (Princeton) Rauwolfia serpentina pow. 50 mg, bendroflumethiazide 4 mg, tartrazine/Tab. Bot. 100s.
Use: Antihypertensive.
RAVOCAINE. (Cook-Waite) Propoxycaine HCl 4 mg, procaine 20 mg, norepinephrine bitartrate equivalent to 0.033 mg levophed base, sodium Cl 3 mg, acetone sodium bisulfite not more than 2 mg. Cartridge 1.8 ml.
Use: Local anesthetic.
RAVOCAINE AND NOVOCAIN WITH LEVOPHED. (Cook-Waite) Propoxycaine HCl 7.2 mg, procaine 36 mg, norepinephrine 0.12 mg, acetone sodium bisulfite 1.8 ml. Inj. Dental Cartridge.
Use: Local anesthetic.
RAVOCAINE AND NOVOCAIN WITH NEO-COBEFRIN. (Cook-Waite) Propoxycaine HCl 7.2 mg, procaine 36 mg, levonordefrin 0.09 mg, acetone sodium bisulfite 1.8 ml. Inj. Dental cartridge.
Use: Local anesthetic.
RAWFOLA. (Foy) Rauwolfia serpentina 50 mg/Tab. Bot. 1000s.
Use: Antihypertensive.
RAWL VITE. (Rawl) Vitamins A 10,000 IU, D 500 IU, B_1 10 mg, B_2 5 mg, B_6 1 mg, calcium pantothenate 5 mg, nicotinamide 50 mg, C 125 mg, E 2.5 IU/Tab. Bot. 100s.
Use: Vitamin supplement.
RAWL WHOLE LIVER VITAMIN B COMPLEX. (Rawl) Whole liver 500 mg, amino acids found in the whole liver, vitamins B_1 1 mg, B_2 2 mg, niacinamide 5 mg, choline Cl 12 mg, B_6 0.2 mg, calcium pantothenate 0.2 mg, inositol 5 mg, biotin 0.6 mcg, B_{12} 0.3 mcg/Cap. Bot. 100s, 500s.
Use: Vitamin/mineral supplement.
RAY BLOCK. (Del-Ray) Octyl dimethyl PABA 5%, benzophenone-3 3%, SD alcohol. Lot. Bot. 118.3 ml.
Use: Sunscreen.
RAY-D. (Nion) Vitamin D 400 IU, thiamine mononitrate 1 mg, riboflavin 2 mg, niacin 10 mg, iodine 0.1 mg, calcium 375 mg, phosphorus 300 mg/6 Tab. In base of brewer's yeast. Bot. 100s, 500s.
Use: Vitamin/mineral supplement.

RAYDERM OINTMENT. (Velvet Pharmacal) Euphorbia extract, phenyl salicylate, neatsfoot oil, olive oil, lanolin in emulsion base preserved with methyl and propylparabens. Tube 1.5 oz, Jar lb.
Use: Burn preparation.
RAY-NOX. (Torch) PABA and para-aminobenzoic sodium. Jar 2 oz, 1 lb.
Use: Sunscreen.
•**RAYON, PURIFIED,** U.S.P. XXIII.
Use: Surgical aid.
RAYTHESIN. (Raymer).
See: Propyl p-Aminobenzoate.
RAZEPAM. (Major) Temazepam 15 mg or 30 mg/Cap. Bot. 100s.
Use: Sedative/hypnotic.
RAZOXANE. B.A.N. 1,2-Bis(3,5-dioxopiperazin-1-yl)propane.
Use: Antineoplastic.
RCF. (Ross) Carbohydrate free low iron soy protein formula base. Carbohydrate and water must be added. For infants unable to tolerate the amount or type of carbohydrate in conventional formulas. Can 14 fl oz. (Concentrated liq.).
Use: Enteral nutritional supplement.
REABILAN. (Elan) Protein 31.5 g, fat 39 g, carbohydrates 131.5 g, Na 702 mg, K 1.252 g/L, lactose free. With appropriate vitamins and minerals. Liq. Bot. 375 ml.
Use: Enteral nutritional supplement.
REABILAN HN. (Elan) Protein 58.2 g, fat 52 g, carbohydrates 158 g, Na 1000 mg, K 1661 mg/L, lactose free. With appropriate vitamins and minerals. Liq. Bot. 375 ml.
Use: Enteral nutritional supplement.
REA-LO. (Whorton) Urea in water soluble moisturizing oil base. **Lot.:** 15%. Bot. 4 oz, pt. **Cream:** 30%. Jar 2 oz, 16 oz.
Use: Emollient.
REALPHENE.
See: Acetarsone, Tab. (City Chem.).
•**RECAINAM HYDROCHLORIDE.** USAN.
Use: Antiarrhythmic.
•**RECAINAM TOSYLATE.** USAN.
Use: Antiarrhythmic.
•**RECLAZEPAM.** USAN.
Use: Sedative.
RECLOMIDE. (Major) Metoclopramide HCl 10 mg/Tab. Bot. 100s, 500s, 1000s, UD 100s.
Use: GI stimulant.
RECOMBINANT TISSUE PLASMINOGEN ACTIVATOR.
See: Activase (Genetech).
RECOMBINATE. (Hyland) Concentrated recombinant antihemophilic factor, contains albumin (human) 12.5 mg/ml, polyethylene glycol 1.5 mg, sodium 180

mEq/L, histidine 55 mm, polysorbate-80 1.5 mcg/AHF IU, calcium 0.2 mg/ml. Pow. for inj. Single dose bot. 250 IU, 500 IU, 1000 IU.
Use: Antihemophilic agent.

RECOMBIVAX-HB. (Merck) Hepatitis B vaccine recombinant. **Pediatric:** 2.5 mcg/0.5 ml, 5 mcg/0.5 ml. Single dose vials 0.5 ml and 3 ml (2.5 mcg only); **Adult:** 10 mcg/ml. Vial 3 ml.
Use: Agent for immunization.

RECORTEX 10X IN OIL. (Forest Pharm.) 1000 mcg/ml. Vial 10 ml.

RECOVER. (Commerce) Bot. 2.25 oz.
Use: Skin discoloration cover-up cream.

RECTAGENE II. (Pfeiffer) Bismuth subgallate 2.25%, bismuth resorcin compound 1.75%, benzyl benzoate 1.2%, peruvian balsam 1.8%, zinc oxide 11%, bismuth subiodide, calcium phosphate in a hydrogenated vegetable oil base. Box 12s.
Use: Anorectal preparation.

RECTAGENE MEDICATED RECTAL BALM. Live yeast cell derivative that supplies 2000 units Skin Respiratory Factor/30 g, refined shark liver oil 3%, white petrolatum, lanolin, thyme oil, 1:10,000 phenyl mercuric nitrate. Oint. 56.7 g.
Use: Anorectal preparation.

RECTAL MEDICONE. (Medicone) Benzocaine 2 gr, balsam peru 1 gr, hydroxyquinoline sulfate 0.25 gr, menthol 1/7 gr, zinc oxide 3 gr/Supp. Box 12s, 24s.
Use: Antiseptic, local anesthetic.

RECTAL MEDICONE UNGUENT. (Medicone) Benzocaine 20 mg, oxyquinoline sulfate 5 mg, menthol 4 mg, zinc oxide 100 mg, balsam peru 12.5 mg, petrolatum 625 mg, lanolin 210 mg/Gm. Tube 1.5 oz.
Use: Anorectal preparation.

RECTOCAINE. (Moore Kirk) Phenol 1%, propyl-p-aminobenzoate 7%, benzyl alcohol 7%, procaine 0.5%. Amp. 5 ml.
Use: Local anesthetic, rectal.

RECTULES. (Forest Pharm.) Chloral hydrate 10 or 20 gr in water-soluble base. Supp. Pkg. 12s.
Use: Sedative/hypnotic.

• **RED BLOOD CELLS,** U.S.P. XXIII. Human red blood cells given by IV infusion.
Use: Blood replenisher.

RED CELL TAGGING SOLUTION.
See: A-C-D Solution (Squibb).

RED CROSS TOOTHACHE KIT. (Mentholatum) Complete kit containing toothache drops w/cotton pellets and tweezers.

Use: Local anesthetic.

• **RED FERRIC OXIDE,** N.F. XVIII.
Use: Pharmaceutic aid (color).

RED MERCURIC IODIDE.
See: Auralcaine, Liq. (Truett).

REDITEMP-C. (Wyeth-Ayerst) Ammonium nitrate, water and special additives. Pkg. large and small sizes. 4 × 10s.
Use: For short-term topical cold application.

REDUCTO, IMPROVED. (Arcum) Phendimetrazine bitartrate 35 mg/Tab. Bot. 100s, 1000s.
Use: Anorexiant.

REDUTEMP. (Inter. Ethical Labs.) Acetaminophen 500 mg/Tab. Bot. 60s.
Use: Acetaminophen.

REESE'S PINWORM. (Reese) Pyrantel pamoate 144 mg. Liq. 30 ml.
Use: Anthelmintic.

REFRESH. (Allergan) Polyvinyl alcohol 1.4%, povidone 0.6%, sodium Cl 0.3 ml. UD 30s or 50s (single dose container).
Use: Artificial tear solution.

REFRESH PLUS. (Allergan) Carboxymethylcellulose sodium 0.5%. Preservative free. Soln. 0.3 ml/single use container. In 30s, 50s.
Use: Artificial tear solution.

REFRESH PM. (Allergan) White petrolatum 55%, mineral oil 41.5%, petrolatum, lanolin alcohol 2%, sodium Cl. Tube 0.12 oz.
Use: Ocular lubricant.

REGAIN. (NCI) Protein 15 g, carbohydrates 52 g, fat 7 g, sodium 45 mg, K 75 mg, Ca 200 mg, P 100 mg, Ca, Fe, vitamin B_{12}, Mg, folic acid, fructose. With dietary fiber. 300 calories. Lactose free. Vanilla, strawberry and malt flavors. Bar 85 g.
Use: Enteral nutritional supplement for patients with impaired renal function.

REGITINE. (Ciba) Phentolamine mesylate 5 mg/Vial (w/mannitol 25 mg in lyophilized form). Pkg. 2s, 6s.
Use: Diagnostic aid.

REGLAN. (Robins) Metoclopramide HCl. **Inj.: 10 mg/2 ml:** Amp. 2 ml, 10 ml; **5 mg/ml:** Vial 2 ml, 10 ml, 30 ml. **Syr.:** 5 mg (as monohydrochloride monohydrate)/5 ml. Bot. pt, Dis-Co Pack 10× 10s. **Tab.: 5 mg:** Bot. 100s. **10 mg:** Bot. 100s, 500s, Dis-co Pak 100s.
Use: Antiemetic, GI stimulant.

REGONOL. (Organon) Pyridostigmine bromide 5 mg/ml. Amp 2 ml, Vial 5 ml.
Use: Cholinergic muscle stimulant.

• **REGRAMOSTIM.** USAN.
Use: Biological response modifier; anti-

neoplastic adjunct.

REGROTON. (Rhone-Poulenc Rorer) Chlorthalidone 50 mg, reserpine 0.25 mg/Tab. Bot. 100s, 1000s.
Use: Antihypertensive.

REGROTON DEMI. (Rhone-Poulenc Rorer) Chlorthalidone 25 mg, reserpine 0.125 mg/Tab. Bot. 100s, 1000s.
Use: Antihypertensive.

REGULACE CAPSULES. (Republic) Docusate sodium 100 mg, casanthranol 30 mg/Cap. Bot. 60s, 100s, 1000s.
Use: Laxative.

REGULAR ILETIN I. (Lilly) Insulin 100 units/ml. Beef and pork. Inj. Bot. 10 ml.
Use: Antidiabetic agent-insulin.

REGULAR INSULIN. (Novo Nordisk) Insulin 100 units/ml. Pork. Inj. Vial. 10 ml.
Use: Antidiabetic agent-insulin.

REGULAR PURIFIED PORK INSULIN. (Novo Nordisk) Insulin 100 units/ml. Purified pork. Inj. Vial. 10 ml.
Use: Antidiabetic agent-insulin.

REGULAR STRENGTH BAYER ENTERIC COATED CAPLETS. (Sterling Health) Aspirin 325 mg. Bot. 50s, 100s.
Use: Salicylate.

REGULAR STRENGTH MIDOL MULTI-SYMPTOM. (Glenbrook) Acetaminophen 325 mg, pyrilamine maleate 12.5 mg. Tab. Bot. 30s.
Use: Nonnarcotic analgesic combination.

REGULAX SS. (Republic) Docusate sodium. **100 mg/Cap.:** Bot. 60s, 100s, 1000s; **250 mg/Cap.:** Bot. 100s.
Use: Laxative.

REGULOID, Orange. (Rugby) Psyllium mucilloid 3.4 Gm, sucrose 70%/rounded tsp. Pow. 420 Gm, 630 Gm.
Use: Laxative.

REGULOID SUGAR FREE. (Rugby) Psyllium hydrophilic mucilloid 3.4 Gm, sodium < 0.01 Gm, aspartame phenylalanine 6 mg. Pow. 222, 333 Gm.
Use: Laxative.

REGUTOL. (Schering-Plough) Docusate sodium 100 mg/Tab. Box 30s, 60s, 90s.
Use: Laxative.

REHYDRALYTE. (Ross) Sodium 75 mEq, potassium 20 mEq, chloride 65 mEq, citrate 30 mEq, dextrose 25 Gm/L, 100 calories/L. Ready-to-use Bot. 8 oz.
Use: Fluid/electrolyte replacement.

RELAFEN. (SK Beecham) Nabumetone 500 mg/Tab. Bot. 100s, 500s, UD 100s. Nabumetone 750 mg/Tab. Bot. 100s, 500s, UD 100s.
Use: Nonsteroidal anti-inflammatory agent.

RELAXIN. A purified ovarian hormone of pregnancy (obtained from sows) responsible for pubic relaxation or separation of the symphysis pubis in mammals.
See: Lutrexin, Tab. (Hynson, Westcott & Dunning).

RELEFACT TRH. (Ferring) Protirelin 0.5 mg/ml. Amp. 1 ml Box 5s.
Use: Diagnostic aid.

RELIEF EYE DROPS. (Allergan) Phenylephrine HCl 0.12%, antipyrine 0.1%, polyvinyl alcohol 1.4%, edetate disodium. Bot. 0.3 ml.
Use: Ophthalmic decongestant.

RELIEF SOLUTION. (Allergan) Phenylephrine HCl 0.12%, antipyrine 0.1%. soln. Bot. 20 ml.
Use: Ophthalmic decongestant combination.

• **RELOMYCIN.** USAN. A macrolide antibiotic produced by a variant strain of *Streptomyces hygroscopicus.*
Use: Antibiotic.

REMCOL-C. (Shionogi) Chlorphoniramine maleate 2 mg, dextromethorphan HBr 15 mg, acetaminophen 300 mg/Cap. In 24s.
Use: Antihistamine, antitussive, analgesic.

REMCOL COLD CAPSULES. (Shionogi) Phenylpropanolamine HCl 25 mg, chlorpheniramine maleate 2 mg, acetaminophen 300 mg/Cap. In 24s.
Use: Decongestant, antihistamine, analgesic.

REM COUGH MEDICINE. (Last) Dextromethorphan HBr 5 mg/5 ml. Bot. 3 oz, 6 oz.
Use: Antitussive.

REMEGEL SOFT CHEWABLE ANTACID TABLETS. (Warner-Lambert) Aluminum hydroxide-magnesium carbonate 476.4 mg/Chew. Tab. Pkg. 8s, 24s.
Use: Antacid.

• **REMIPROSTOL.** USAN.
Use: Antiulcer agent.

REMIVOX. (Janssen) Lorcainide HCl.
Use: Antiarrhythmic.

REMOVING CREAM. (O'Leary) Specially formulated to remove Covermark. Jar 4 oz.

• **REMOXIPRIDE HYDROCHLORIDE.** USAN.
Use: Antipsychotic.

REMULAR-S. (Inter. Ethical Labs.) Chloroxazone 250 mg/Tab. Bot. 100s.
Use: Skeletal muscle relaxants.

RENACIDIN. (Guardian) The composition of this powder, as manufactured, is in terms of 156 to 171 Gm citric acid (anhy-

drous) and 21 to 30 Gm d-gluconic acid (as the lactone) w/purified magnesium hydroxycarbonate 75 to 87 Gm, magnesium acid citrate 9 to 15 Gm, calcium (as carbonate) 2 to 6 Gm, water 17 to 21 Gm per 300 Gm. Bot. 25 Gm 6s; 150 Gm, 300 Gm.
Use: Genitourinary irrigant.

RENALTABS-S.C. (Forest Pharm.) Methenamine 40.8 mg, benzoic acid 4.5 mg, phenyl salicylate 18.1 mg, hyoscyamine sulfate ¹/₂₀₀₀ gr, atropine sulfate 0.03 mg, methylene blue 5.4 mg, gelsemium 6.1 mg/Tab. Bot. 1000s.
Use: Urinary anti-infective.

RENAMIN. (Clintec) Sterile hypertonic soln. of essential and non-essential amino acids. Bot. 250 ml, 500 ml.
Use: Parenteral nutritional supplement.

RENANOLONE. 3α-Hydroxypregnane-11,20-dione.
Use: Steroid anesthetic.

RENBU. (Wren) Butabarbital sodium 32.4 mg/Tab. Bot. 100s, 1000s.
Use: Sedative/hypnotic.

RENESE. (Pfizer Laboratories) Polythiazide 1 mg, 2 mg or 4 mg/Tab. Bot. 100s, 1000s.
Use: Diuretic, antihypertensive.

RENESE-R TABLETS. (Pfizer Laboratories) Polythiazide 2 mg, reserpine 0.25 mg/Tab. Bot. 100s, 1000s.
Use: Antihypertensive.

RENGASIL. (Geigy) Pirprofen. Investigational drug.
Use: Anti-inflammatory agent.

RENOFORM.
See: Epinephrine, Preps. (Various Mfr.).

RENOGRAFIN-60,-76. (Squibb Diagnostics) **-60:** Diatrizoate meglumine 52%, sodium diatrizoate 8%, iodine 29.2%. Vial 10 ml, 100 ml, 10s; 30 ml, 50 ml, 25s. **-76:** Diatrizoate meglumine 66%, sodium diatrizoate 10%, iodine 37%. Vial 20 ml, 50 ml, 25s; 100 ml, 200 ml, 10s.
Use: Radiopaque agent.

RENO-M-DIP. (Squibb Diagnostics) Diatrizoate meglumine, iodine 14.1%. 30% for drip infusion pyelography. Inj. Bot. 300 ml. Also w/soln. admin. sets. (Formerly Renografin-Dip).
Use: Radiopaque agent.

RENO-M-30. (Squibb Diagnostics) Diatrizoate meglumine 30%, iodine 14.1%. Vial 50 ml, 100 ml, Box 25s.
Use: Radiopaque agent.

RENO-M-60. (Squibb Diagnostics) Diatrizoate meglumine 60%, iodine 28%. Vial 10 ml, 30 ml, 50 ml, 100 ml.
Use: Radiopaque agent.

RENO-SED. (Vita Elixir) Methenamine 2 gr, salol 0.5 gr, methylene blue ¹/₁₀ gr, benzoic acid ⅛ gr, atropine sulfate ¹/₁₀₀₀ gr, hyoscyamine sulfate ¹/₂₀₀₀ gr/Tab.
Use: Urinary anti-infective.

RENOVIST INJ. (Squibb Diagnostics) Diatrizoate methylglucamine 34.3%, diatrizoate sodium 35%, iodine 37%. Vial 50 ml, Box 25s.
Use: Radiopaque agent.

RENOVIST II. (Squibb Diagnostics) Diatrizoate sodium 29.1%, meglumine diatrizoate 28.5%, iodine 31%. Inj. Vial 30 ml, 60 ml, Box 25s.
Use: Radiopaque agent.

RENOVUE-65. (Squibb Diagnostics) Iodamide meglumide 65%, organically bound iodine 30%, edetate disodium. Vial 50 ml.
Use: Radiopaque agent.

RENOVUE-DIP. (Squibb Diagnostics) Iodamide meglumide 24%, iodine 11.1%. Infusion Bot. 300 ml.
Use: Radiopaque agent.

RENPAP. (Wren) Acetaminophen 4 gr, salicylamide 3 gr, caffeine ⅔ gr, allylisobutylbarbituric acid gr/Tab. Bot. 100s, 1000s.
Use: Salicylate analgesic.

RENTAMINE PEDIATRIC. (Major) Phenylephrine tannate 5 mg, chlorpheniramine tannate 4 mg, carbetapentane tannate, saccharin, sucrose. Pt.
Use: Cough preparation.

RENTUSS. (Wren) **Tab.:** Dextromethorphan HBr 10 mg, guaifenesin 100 mg, phenylephrine HCl 5 mg, phenylpropanolamine HCl 25 mg, chlorpheniramine maleate 2 mg, acetaminophen 300 mg. Bot. 100s, 500s, 1000s. **Syr.:** Same except guaifenesin 50 mg, acetaminophen 120 mg/5 ml. Pt, gal.
Use: Antitussive, expectorant, decongestant, antihistamine, analgesic.

RENU EFFERVESCENT ENZYMATIC CLEANER. (Bausch & Lomb) Subtilisin, polyethylene glycol, sodium carbonate, sodium Cl, tartaric acid. Tab. In 10s, 20s, 30s.
Use: Soft contact lens care.

RENU LIQUID. (Biosearch) P-Ca and Na caseinates, CHO-maltodextrin sucrose, F-partially hydrogenated soy oil, mono and diglycerides, soy lecithin, protein 35 Gm, CHO 125 Gm, fat 40 Gm, sodium 500 mg, potassium 1250 mg/L, 1 Cal/ml, 300 mOsm/kg, H_2O. In 250 ml ready to use.
Use: Enteral nutritional supplement.

RENU MULTI-PURPOSE. (Bausch & Lomb) Isotonic soln. w/sodium Cl, sodium borate, boric acid, poloxamine, polyaminopropyl biguanide 0.00005%, EDTA. Soln. Bot. 240 ml, 360 ml.
Use: Soft contact lens care.
RENU SALINE. (Bausch & Lomb) Isotonic buffered soln. of sodium Cl, boric acid, polyaminopropyl biguanide 0.00003%, EDTA. Soln. Bot. 240 ml, 360 ml.
Use: Soft contact lens care.
RENU THERMAL ENZYMATIC CLEANER. (Bausch & Lomb) Subtilisin, sodium carbonate, sodium Cl, boric acid. Tab. 8s, 16s.
Use: Soft contact lens care.
REPAN. (Everett) Butalbital 50 mg, caffeine 40 mg, acetaminophen 325 mg/Tab. Bot. 100s.
Use: Analgesic combination.
• **REPIRINAST.** USAN.
Use: Antiallergic; antiasthmatic.
REPLENS. (Warner-Lambert) Purified water, glycerin, mineral oil, polycarbophil, carbomer 934P, hydrogenated palm oil, glyceride, methylparaben, sorbic acid. Gel. Appl. 12.
Use: Vaginal preparation.
REPLETE LIQUID. (Clintec Nutrition) K caseinate, Ca caseinate, maltodextrin, sucrose, corn oil, lecithin, vitamins A, B_1, B_2, B_3, B_5, B_6, B_{12}, C, D, F, K, folic acid, biotin, choline, Ca, Cl, Cu, Fe, I, Mg, Mn, P, Zn. In 250 ml.
Use: Enteral nutritional supplement.
REPOSANS-10. (Wesley) Chlordiazepoxide HCl 10 mg/Cap. Bot. 1000s.
Use: Antianxiety agent.
REPRIEVE. (Mayer) Caffeine 32 mg, salicylamide 225 mg, vitamin B_1 50 mg, homatropine methylbromide 0.5 mg/Tab. Bot. 8s, 16s.
Use: Analgesic combination.
• **REPROMICIN.** USAN.
Use: Antibacterial.
• **REPROTEROL HYDROCHLORIDE.** USAN.
Use: Bronchodilator.
REPTILASE-R. (Abbott Diagnostics) Diagnostic for the investigation of fibrin formation and disturbances in fibrin formation due to causes other than thrombin inhibition.
Use: Diagnostic aid.
REQUA'S CHARCOAL TABLETS. (Requa) Wood charcoal 10 gr/Tab. Pkg. 50s. Can 125s.
Use: Antiflatulent.
RESA. (Vita Elixir) Reserpine 0.25

mg/Tab.
Use: Antihypertensive.
RESAID. (Geneva) Phenylpropanolamine HCl 75 mg, chlorpheniramine maleate 12 mg/Cap. Bot. 100s, 1000s.
Use: Decongestant, antihistamine.
RESAID S.R. (Geneva Generics) Phenylpropanolamine HCl 75 mg, chlorpheniramine maleate 12 mg/SR Cap. Bot. 100s, 1000s.
Use: Decongestant, antihistamine.
RESCAPS-D S.R. (Geneva) Phenylpropanolamine HCl 75 mg, caramiphen edisylate 40 mg/Cap. Bot. 100s.
Use: Cough preparation.
RESCINNAMINE. Methyl 18β-Hydroxy-11,17 α-dimethoxy-3β20α-yohimban-16β-carboxylate 3,4,5- Trimeth-oxycinnamate (Ester). Methyl 0-(3,4,5-trimethoxy-cinnamoyl)reserpate.
Use: Antihypertensive.
See: Anaprel.
Moderil, Tab. (Pfizer Laboratories).
RESCON CAPSULES. (Ion) Pseudoephedrine 120 mg, chlorpheniramine maleate 12 mg/TR Cap. Bot. 100s.
Use: Decongestant, antihistamine.
RESCON-DM. (Ion) Dextromethorphan HBr 10 mg, pseudoephedrine HCl 30 mg, chlorpheniramine maleate 2 mg, sugar free. Liq. Bot. 120 ml.
Use: Antitussive, decongestant, antihistamine.
RESCON-GG CAPSULES. (Ion) Pseudoephedrine HCl 120 mg, chlorpheniramine maleate 8 mg/Cap. Bot. 100s.
Use: Decongestant, antihistamine.
RESCON-GG LIQUID. (Ion) Phenylephrine HCl 5 mg, guaifenesin 100 mg/5 ml Bot. 4 oz.
Use: Decongestant, expectorant.
RESCON JR. (Ion) Pseudoephedrine HCl 60 mg, chlorpheniramine maleate 4 mg/Cap. Bot. 100s.
Use: Decongestant, antihistamine.
RESCON LIQUID. (Ion) Phenylpropanolamine HCl 12.5 mg, chlorpheniramine maleate 2 mg/5 ml. Bot. 4 oz.
Use: Decongestant, antihistamine.
RESECTISOL. (Kendall McGaw) Mannitol soln. 5 Gm/1000 ml in distilled water (275 mOsm/L.). In 2000 ml.
Use: Genitourinary irrigant.
RESERPANEED. (Hanlon) Reserpine 0.25 mg/Tab. Bot. 100s, 1000s.
Use: Antihypertensive.
• **RESERPINE,** U.S.P. XXIII. Elix., Inj., Tab., U.S.P. XXIII. Yohimban-16-carboxylic acid, 11,17-dimethoxy-18-[(3,4,5-trimethoxybenzyol)oxy]-, methyl ester.

Pure alkaloid from Rauwolfia serpentina.
Use: Antihypertensive.
See: Arcum R-S, Tab. (Arcum).
Broserpine, Tab. (Brothers).
De Serpa, Tab. (De Leon).
Elserpine, Tab. (Canright).
Maso-Serpine, Tab. (Mason).
Rauloydin, Tab. (Solvay).
Raurine, Tab. (Westerfield).
Reserjen, Tab. (Jenkins).
Reserpaneed, Tab. (Hanlon).
Serpalan, Tab. (Lannett).
Serpasil Preps. (Ciba).
Sertabs, Tab. (Table Rock).
T-Serp, Tab. (Tennessee).
Vio-Serpine, Tab. (Solvay).
Zepine, Tab. (Foy).
RESERPINE W/COMBINATIONS.
See: Demi-Regroton, Tab. (Rhone-
Poulenc Rorer).
Diupres, Tab. (Merck & Co.).
Harbolin, Tab. (Arcum).
Hydromox R, Tab. (Lederle).
Hydropres-25 or -50, Tab. (Merck &
Co.).
Hydroserp, Tab. (Zenith).
Hydroserpine, Tab. (Geneva).
Hydrotensin-50, Tab. (Mayrand).
Mallopress, Tab. (Hauck).
Metatensin, Tab. (Merrell Dow).
Naquival, Tab. (Schering).
Regroton, Tab. (Rhone-Poulenc Ror-
er).
Renese-R, Tab. (Pfizer Laboratories).
Salutensin, Tab. (Bristol).
Ser-Ap-Es, Tab. (Ciba).
Serpasil-Apresoline, Tab. (Ciba).
Serpasil-Esidrix, Tab. (Ciba).
Unipres, Tab. (Solvay).
• **RESERPINE AND CHLOROTHIAZIDE
TABLETS,** U.S.P. XXIII.
Use: Antihypertensive.
• **RESERPINE AND HYDROCHLOROTH-
IAZIDE TABLETS.** U.S.P. XXIII.
Use: Antihypertensive.
• **RESERPINE, HYDRALAZINE HCl and
HYDROCHLOROTHIAZIDE,** U.S.P.
XXIII.
Use: Antihypertensive.
RESINOL MEDICINAL OINTMENT.
(Mentholatum) Zinc oxide 12%,
calamine 6%, resorcinol 2% in a lanolin
and petrolatum base. Jar 3.5 oz, 1.25
oz.
Use: Skin protectant.
**RESIN UPTAKE KIT WITH LIOTHYRO-
NINE I-125 BUFFER SOLUTION.**
See: Thyrostat-3 (Squibb).
RESINS, ANTACID.
See: Polyamine methylene Resins.

RESOL. (Wyeth-Ayerst) Sodium 50 mEq,
potassium 20 mEq, Cl 50 mEq, citrate
34 mEq, calcium 4 mEq, magnesium 4
mEq, phosphate 5 mEq, glucose 20
Gm/L. Contains 80 calories/L. Ctn. 32 fl
oz.
Use: Fluid/electrolyte replacement.
RESOLVE/GP DAILY CLEANER. (Aller-
gan) Buffered solution with cocoampho-
carboxyglycinate, sodium lauryl sulfate,
hexylene glycol, alkyl ether sulfate, fatty
acid amide surfactant cleaning agents,
preservative free. Soln. Bot. 30 ml.
Use: Contact lens product.
RESONIUM-A. (Sanofi Winthrop) Sodium
polystyrene sulfonate.
Use: Potassium removing resin.
RESORCIN.
See: Resorcinol (Various Mfr.).
• **RESORCINOL,** U.S.P. XXIII. Compound
Oint., U.S.P. XXIII. 1,3-Benzenediol.
Use: Topical antifungal.
• **RESORCINOL AND SULFUR LOTION.**
U.S.P. XXIII.
Use: Scabicide, parasiticide, antifungal.
RESORCINOL W/COMBINATIONS.
See: Acnomel, Cake, Cream. (SK-
Beecham).
Bicozene, Cream (Ex-Lax).
Biscolan, Supp. (Lannett).
Black and White Ointment, (Schering-
Plough).
Castaderm, Preps. (Lannett).
Clearasil, Stick (Vicks).
Lanacane Creme (Combe).
Mazon, Oint. (SK-Beecham).
RA Lot. (Medco).
Rezamid Lot. (Dermick).
• **RESORCINOL MONOACETATE,** U.S.P.
XXIII. (Various Mfr.) Resorcin acetate.
Use: Antiseborrheic, keratolytic.
See: Euresol, Liq. (Knoll).
W/Salicylic acid, ethyl alcohol, castor oil.
See: Resorcitate w/oil, Lot. (Almay).
W/Salicylic acid, LCD, betanaphthol, cas-
tor oil, isopropyl alcohol.
See: Neomark, Liq. (C&M Pharm.).
RESORCINOLPHTHALEIN SODIUM.
See: Fluorescein Sodium, U.S.P. XXIII.
(Various Mfr.).
W/Oil. Resorcinol monoacetate 1.5%, sali-
cylic acid 1.5%, castor oil 1.5%, ethyl al-
cohol 81%. Bot. 8 fl oz.
Use: Topical antiseborrheic.
RESOURCE. (Sandoz Nutrition) Ca and
Na caseinates, soy protein isolate 37
Gm, sugar, hydrolyzed cornstarch 140
Gm, corn oil, soy lecithin 37 Gm, Na 890
mg, K 1600 mg, A, B_1, B_2, B_3, B_5. B_6,
B_{12}, C, D, E, K, folic acid, Ca, P, I, Fe,

Mg, Cu, Zn, Mn, Cl, gluten free, vanilla, chocolate, strawberry flavor. Liq. Bot. 237 ml.
Use: Enteral nutritional therapy.
RESOURCE INSTANT CRYSTALS.
(Sandoz Nutrition) Vanilla flavor: maltodextrin, sucrose, hydrogenated soy oil, sodium caseinate, calcium caseinate, soy protein isolate, potassium citrate, polyglycerol esters of fatty acids, artificial flavors, vitamins and minerals. Instant Crystals 1.5 oz. or 2 oz. packets.
Use: Enteral nutritional supplement.
RESOURCE PLUS. (Sandoz Nutrition) Ca and Na caseinates, soy protein isolate 54.9 Gm, maltodextrin, sucrose 200 Gm, corn oil, lecithin 53.3 Gm, Na 899 mg, K 1740 mg, A, B_1, B_2, B_3, B_5. B_6, B_{12}, C, D, E, K, folic acid, biotin, choline, Ca, P, I, Fe, Mg, Cu, Zn, Cl, Mn, gluten free, vanilla, chocolate, strawberry flavor. Liq. Bot. 8 oz.
Use: Enteral nutritional therapy.
RESPA-1ST. (Respa) Pseudoephedrine HCl 60 mg, guaifenesin 600 mg. SR Tab. Bot. 100s.
Use: Decongestant, expectorant.
RESPA-DM. (Respa) Dextromethorphan HBr 30 mg, guaifenesin 600 mg. SR Tab. Bot. 100s.
Use: Antihistamine, expectorant.
RESPA-GF. (Respa) Guaifenesin 600 mg. SR Tab. Bot. 100s.
Use: Expectorant.
RESPAHIST. (Respa). Pseudoephedrine HCl 60 mg, brompheniramine maleate 6 mg. SR Cap. Bot 100s.
Use: Decongenstant, antihistamine.
RESPAIRE-60 SR. (Laser) Pseudoephedrine HCl 60 mg, guaifenesin 200 mg/S.R. Cap. Bot. 100s, 1000s.
Use: Decongestant, expectorant.
RESPAIRE-120 SR. (Laser) Pseudoephedrine HCl 120 mg, guaifenesin 250 mg/SR Cap. Bot. 100s, 1000s.
Use: Decongestant, expectorant.
RESPALOR. (Mead Johnson Nutritional) Protein 75 g, carbohyrate 146 g, fat 70 g, Na 1248 mg, K 1456 mg, Fe 12.5 mg, cal 1498/L. Lactose free. Vanilla flavor. With appropriate vitamins and minerals. Liq. Bot. 237 ml.
Use: Enteral nutritional support.
RESPBID. (Boehringer Ingelheim) Theophylline 250 mg or 500 mg/Tab. Bot. 100s.
Use: Bronchodilator.
RESPIHALER DECADRON PHOSPHATE. (Merck & Co.).
See: Decadron phosphate, respihaler

(Merck & Co.).
RESPIRACULT. (Medical Tech. Corp.) Culture test for group A beta-hemolytic streptococci. In 10s.
Use: Diagnostic aid.
RESPIRALEX. (Medical Tech. Corp.) Latex agglutination test to detect group A streptococci in throat and nasopharynx. Kit 1s.
Use: Diagnostic aid.
RESPIRATORY SYNCYTIAL VIRUS IMMUNE GLOBULIN (HUMAN).
Use: Prophylaxis against respiratory tract infection. [Orphan drug]
RESPORAL. (Pioneer Pharm.) Pseudoephedrine sulfate 120 mg, dexbrompheniramine maleate/Tab. Bot. 10s, 20s, 30s, 50s, 100s, 1000s.
Use: Upper respiratory combination.
RESPORAL TR TABLETS. (Pioneer Pharm) Pseudoephedrine sulfate 120 mg, dexbrompheniramine maleate 6 mg. In 10s, 20s, 30s, 50s, 100s, 1000s.
Use: Decongestant, antihistamine.
RES-Q. (Boyle) Activated charcoal 50%, magnesium hydroxide 25%, tannic acid (Universal antidote). Pkg. 0.5 oz.
Use: Antidote.
REST EASY. (Walgreen) Acetaminophen 1000 mg, pseudoephedrine HCl 60 mg, dextromethorphan HBr 30 mg, doxylamine succinate 7.5 mg/30 ml. Bot. 6 oz, 16 oz.
Use: Analgesic, decongestant, antitussive, antihistamine.
RESTORE. (Inagra) Psyllium hydrophilic mucilloid fiber 3.4 g/12 g dose, orange flavor, saccharin, sucrose. Pow. 390 g, 538 g. Also available sugar free with aspartame, phenylalanine 30 mg/tsp, saccharin. Pow. 300 g, 425 g.
Use: Laxative.
RESTORIL. (Sandoz) Temazepam 7.5 mg, lactose. Cap. Bot. 100s. ControlPak 25s, UD 100s.
Use: Sedative/hypnotic.
RETIN-A CREAM. (Ortho) Tretinoin 0.1%, 0.05% or 0.025%. Tube 20 Gm, 45 Gm.
Use: Anti-acne.
RETIN-A GEL. (Ortho) Tretinoin 0.01% or 0.025%, alcohol 90%. Tube 15 Gm, 45 Gm.
Use: Anti-acne.
RETIN-A LIQUID. (Ortho) Tretinoin (retinoic acid, Vitamin A acid) 0.05%, polyethylene glycol 400, butylated hydroxytoluene and alcohol 55%. Bot. 28 ml.
Use: Anti-acne.

RETINOIC ACID. Tretinoin, U.S.P. XXIII.
Use: Keratolytic.
See: Retin A Prods. (Ortho).
RETINOIC ACID ALL- TRANS. Tretinoin,
U.S.P. XXIII.
Use: Acute promyelocytic leukemia.
[Orphan drug]
RETINOIC ACID, 9-CIS.
Use: Acute promyelocytic leukemia.
[Orphan drug]
RETINOL. B.A.N. 3,7-Dimethyl-9-(2,6,6-
trimethyl-cyclohex-1-enyl)nona-2,4,6,8-
all-trans-tetraen-1-ol.
See: Vitamin A alcohol.
RETINOL. (Nature's Bounty) Vitamin A
100,000 IU, glycol stearate, mineral oil,
propylene glycol, lanolin oil, propylene
glycol stearate SE, lanolin alcohol,
retinol, parabens, EDTA. Cream. Tube
60 g.
Use: Emollient.
RETROVIR. (Burroughs Wellcome) Zi-
dovudine 100 mg/Cap. Bot. 100s.
Use: Antiviral agent.
REVERSOL. (Organon) Edrophonium
chloride 10 mg/ml. Inj. Vial. 10 ml.
Use: Cholinergic muscle stimulant.
REV-EYES. (Storz/Lederle) Dapiprazole
HCl 25 mg. Pow. Vial. 5 ml.
Use: Ophthalmic alpha adrenergic
blocking agent.
REVS CAFFEINE T.D. CAPSULES. (Vi-
tarine) Caffeine 250 mg/Cap. Bot. 100s,
1000s.
Use: CNS stimulant.
REXAHISTINE. (Econo-Rx) Phenylephrine HCl 5 mg, chlorpheniramine
maleate 1 mg, menthol 1 mg, sodium
bisulfite 0.1%, alcohol 5%/5 ml. Bot. Gal.
Use: Decongestant, antihistamine.
REXAHISTINE DH. (Econo-Rx) Codeine
phosphate 10 mg, phenylephrine HCl 10
mg, chlorpheniramine maleate 2 mg,
menthol 1 mg, alcohol 5%/5 ml. Bot. gal.
Use: Antitussive, decongestant, antihis-
tamine.
REXAHISTINE EXPECTORANT. (Econo-
Rx) Codeine phosphate 10 mg, phenyle-
phrine HCl 10 mg, chlorpheniramine
maleate 2 mg, guaifenesin 100 mg,
menthol 1 mg, alcohol 5%/5 ml. Bot.
Gal.
Use: Antitussive, decongestant, antihis-
tamine, expectorant.
REXIGEN. (Ion) Phendimetrazine tartrate
35 mg/Tab. Bot. 100s.
Use: Anorexiant.
REXIGEN FORTE CAPSULES. (Ion)
Phendimetrazine tartrate 105 mg/SR
Cap. Bot. 100s.

Use: Anorexiant.
REZAMID LOTION. (Summers) Sulfur
5%, resorcinol 2% in a base of SD-40 al-
cohol, zinc oxide, talc, propylene glycol,
sodium bisulfate, EDTA, parabens. Lot.
56.7 g.
Use: Anti-acne.
REZINE. (Marnel) Hydroxyzine HCl 10
mg or 25 mg. Tab. Bot. 100s.
Use: Antianxiety agent.
RF LATEX TEST. (Laboratory Diagnostics) Rapid latex agglutination test for the
qualitative screening and semi-quantita-
tive determination of rheumatoid factor.
Kit 100s.
Use: Diagnostic aid.
R-FRONE. (Serono)
See: INTERFERON BETA (RECOMBI-
NANT).
R-GEL. (Healthline Labs) Capsaicin
0.025%, EDTA. Gel. Tube 15 ml, 30 ml.
Use: Topical analgesic.
R-GEN. (Owen) Purified water, ampho-
teric 2, hydrolyzed animal protein, lau-
ramine oxide, methylparaben, benzalko-
nium Cl, tetrasodium, EDTA, propyl-
paraben, fragrance. Bot. 8 oz.
Use: Protein shampoo.
R-GEN ELIXIR. (Goldline) Iodinated glyc-
erol 60 mg/5 ml. Bot. pt.
Use: Expectorant.
R-GENE 10. (KabiVitrum) Arginine HCl
10% (950 mOsm/L) with Cl ion 47.5
mEq/100 ml. Inj. 500 ml.
Use: Pituitary (growth hormone) func-
tion test.
R-HCTZ-H. (Lederle) Reserpine 0.1 mg,
hydrochlorothiazide 15 mg, hydralazine
HCl 25 mg/Tab. Bot. 100s, 500s.
Use: Antihypertensive.
RHEABAN. (Leeming) Colloidal activated
attapulgite 750 mg/Tab. In 12s.
Use: Antidiarrheal.
RHEABAN MAXIMUM STRENGTH.
(Pfizer) Activated attapulgite 750 mg.
Capl. Pkg. 12s.
Use: Antidiarrheal.
RHEOMACRODEX. (Pharmacia) Dextran
40 10% in sodium Cl 0.9% or in dextrose
5%. Soln. Bot. 500 ml.
Use: Plasma expander.
RHESONATIV. (KabiVitrum) Human im-
munoglobulin anti-Rh₀ (D) 0.2 Gm,
glycine 20 mg, diluent (water for injec-
tion) 2 ml.
Use: Immune serume.
RHEUMASAL. (Jenkins) Sodium salicy-
late 5 gr, potassium iodide 1 gr, gelsemi-
um extract 0.25 gr, cimicifuga extract 1/8
gr/Tab. Bot. 1000s.

Use: Salicylate analgesic.

RHEUMATEX. (Wampole) Latex agglutination test for the qualitative detection
and quantitative determination of
rheumatoid factor in serum. Kit 100s.
Use: Diagnostic aid.

RHEUMATOID FACTOR TESTS.
See: Rheumanosticon Dri-Dot
(Organon Teknika).

RHEUMATON. (Wampole) Two-minute
hemagglutination slide test for the qualitative and quantitative determination of
rheumatoid factor in serum or synovial
fluid. Test kit 20s, 50s, 150s.
Use: Diagnostic aid.

RHEUMATREX DOSE PACK. (Lederle)
Methotrexate 2.5 mg. Tab. Pkg. 5, 7.5,
10, 12.5, 15 mg/week dose packs.
Use: Antipsoriatic.

RHINALL DROPS. (Scherer) Phenylephrine HCl 0.25%, sodium bisulfite. Bot.
oz.
Use: Decongestant.

RHINALL SPRAY. (Scherer) Phenylephrine HCl 0.25%. Bot. oz.
Use: Decongestant.

RHINALL 10. (Scherer) Phenylephrine
HCl 0.2%. Drop. Dot. oz.
Use: Decongestant.

RHINATATE. (Major) Phenylephrine tannate 25 mg, chlorpheniramine tannate 8
mg, pyrilamine tannate 25 mg/Tab. Bot.
100s, 250s.
Use: Upper respiratory combination.

RHINOCAPS. (Ferndale) Aspirin 162 mg,
acetaminophen 162 mg, phenylpropanolamine HCl 20 mg/Cap. Bot.
100s.
Use: Analgesic, decongestant.

RHINOCORT. (Astra) Budesonide 32
mcg/actuation (200 sprays). Can 7 g
with nasal adapter.
Use: Intranasal steroid.

RHINOGESIC. (Vale) Phenylephrine HCl
5 mg, chlorpheniramine maleate 2 mg,
salicylamide 250 mg, acetaminophen
150 mg/Tab. Bot. 100s, 1000s.
Use: Decongestant, antihistamine,
analgesic.

RHINOGESIC-GG. (Vale) Phenylephrine
HCl 5 mg, chlorpheniramine maleate 2
mg, salicylamide 250 mg, acetaminophen 150 mg, guaifenesin 100
mg/Tab. Bot. 100s, 1000s.
Use: Decongestant, antihistamine,
analgesic, expectorant.

RHINOLAR. (McGregor) Phenylpropanolamine HCl 75 mg, chlorpheniramine maleate 8 mg, methscopolamine
nitrate 2.5 mg/SR Cap. Dye Free. Bot.

60s.
Use: Decongestant, antihistamine, anticholinergic.

RHINOLAR-EX. (McGregor) Phenylpropanolamine HCl 75 mg, chlorpheniramine maleate 8 mg/SR Cap. Dye free.
Bot. 60s.
Use: Decongestant, antihistamine.

RHINOLAR-EX 12. (McGregor) Phenylpropanolamine HCl 75 mg, chlorpheniramine maleate 12 mg/SR Cap. Dye
free. Bot. 60s.
Use: Decongestant, antihistamine.

RHINOSYN. (Great Southern) Pseudoephedrine HCl 60 mg, chlorpheniramine maleate 4 mg, alcohol 0.45%,
sucrose. Syr. Bot. 120 ml, pt.
Use: Decongestant, antihistamine.

RHINOSYN-DM LIQUID. (Great Southern) Pseudoephedrine HCl 30 mg, chlorpheniramine maleate 2 mg, dextromethorphan HBr 15 mg, alcohol
1.4%, sucrose. Bot. 120 ml.
Use: Decongestant, antihistamine, antitussive.

RHINOSYN-DMX SYRUP. (Great Southern) Dextromethorphan HBr 15 mg,
guaifenesin 100 mg, alcohol 1.4%. Bot.
120 ml.
Use: Antitussive, expectorant.

RHINOSYN-X LIQUID. (Great Southern)
Pseudoephedrine HCl 30 mg, dextromethorphan HBr 10 mg, guaifenesin
100 mg, alcohol 7.5%. Bot. 120 ml.
Use: Decongestant, antitussive, expectorant.

RHODANATE.
See: Potassium Thiocyanate.

RHODANIDE. More commonly Rhodanate, same as thiocyanate.
See: Potassium thiocyanate.

• **RHo (D) IMMUNE GLOBULIN,** U.S.P.
XXIII.
See: Gamulin Rh, Vial (Parke-Davis).

RHo(D) IMMUNE GLOBULIN (HUMAN).
Use: Immune thrombocytopenic purpura. [Orphan drug]

RhoGAM. (Ortho Diagnostic) Rh$_o$ (D) im-
mune globulin (human). Single-dose vial
Pkg. 5s; Prefilled syringe Pkg. 5s, 25s.
Use: Agent for immunization.

RHULIGEL. (Rydelle) Phenylcarbinol 2%,
menthol 0.3%, camphor 0.3%, SD alcohol 23A 31%. Gel 60 Gm.
Use: Topical poison ivy product.

RHULISPRAY. (Rydelle) Phenylcarbinol
0.67%, calamine 4.7%, menthol
0.025%, camphor 0.25%, benzocaine
1.15%, alcohol 28.8%. Aerosol 120 Gm.
Use: Topical poison ivy product.

RHYTHMIN. (Sidmak) Procainamide 250 mg or 500 mg/SR Tab. Bot. 100s, 500s, 1000s.
Use: Antiarrhythmic.
•**RIBAMINOL.** USAN. Ribonucleic acid compound, 2-(diethylamino)-ethanole. Under study.
Use: Learning and memory enhancer.
•**RIBAVIRIN,** U.S.P. XXIII. Soln. for inhalation.
Use: Antiviral. [Orphan drug]
See: Virazole, Inj. (ICN).
•**RIBOFLAVIN,** U.S.P. XXIII. Inj., Tab., U.S.P. XXIII. Vitamins B_2, G, yellow enzyme, lactoflavin.
Use: Vitamin (enzyme orco-factor).
W/Nicotinamide. (Lilly) Riboflavin 5 mg, nicotinamide 200 mg/ml Amp. 1 ml, Box 100s.
Use: I.M., I.V.; Vitamin B therapy.
W/Vitamins.
See: Vitamin Preparations.
RIBOFLAVIN, METHYLOL.
•**RIBOPRINE.** USAN. N-(3-Methyl-2-butenyl) adrenosin.
Use: Antineoplastic agent.
RIBOZYME INJECTION. (Fellows) Riboflavin-5-Phosphate Sodium 50 mg/ml Vial 10 ml.
RICIN (BLOCKED) CONJUGATED MURINE MCA. (Immunogen)
Use: Antineoplastic. [Orphan drug]
RICINOLEATE SODIUM.
See: Preceptin, Gel (Ortho).
RICOLON SOLUTION. (Sanofi Winthrop) Ricolon concentrate.
Use: Leucocytotic preparation.
RID. (Leeming) Piperonyl butoxide 3%, pyrethrins 0.3%, petroleum distillate 1.2%, benzyl alcohol 2.4%. Bot. 2 oz, 4 oz.
Use: Pediculicide.
RID-A-PAIN WITH CODEINE. (Pfeiffer) Codeine phosphate 1 mg, acetaminophen 97.2 mg, aspirin 226.8 mg, caffeine 32.4 mg, salicylamide 32.4 mg/Tab. In 24s, 48s.
Use: Narcotic analgesic combination.
RIDENOL. (R.I.D.) Acetaminophen 80 mg/5 ml. Syr. Bot. 120 ml.
Use: Analgesic.
RID LICE CONTROL SPRAY. (Leeming) Synthetic pyrethroids 0.5%, related compounds 0.065%, aromatic petroleum hydrocarbons 0.664%. Can 5 oz.
Use: Pediculicide.
RID LICE ELIMINATION SYSTEM.
(Leeming) Rid lice killing shampoo, nit removal comb, Rid lice control spray and instruction booklet/unit.
Use: Pediculicide.
RID LICE SHAMPOO-KIT. (Leeming) Pyrethrins 0.3%, piperonyl butoxide 3%. Bot. 2 oz, 4 oz.
Use: Pediculicide.
RIDAURA CAPSULES. (Smith Kline & French) Auranofin 3 mg/Cap. Bot. 60s.
Use: Antirheumatic.
•**RIDOGREL.** USAN.
Use: Thromboxane eynthetase inhibitor.
•**RIFABUTIN.** USAN.
Use: Antituberculous; MAC disease [Orphan drug]
See: Mycobutin.
RIFADIN. (Marion Merrell Dow) Rifampin. **150 mg/Cap.:** Bot. 30s. **300 mg/Cap.:** Bot. 30s, 60s, 100s. **600 mg/Inj.:** Vials.
Use: Antituberculous agent.
RIFAMATE. (Merrell Dow) Rifampin 300 mg, isoniazid 150 mg/Cap. Bot. 60s.
Use: Antituberculous agent.
•**RIFAMETANE.** USAN.
Use: Antibacterial.
•**RIFAMIDE.** USAN.
Use: Antibacterial.
RIFAMPICIN. B.A.N. 3-(4-Methylpiperazin-1-ylimino-methyl)rifamycin SV.
Use: Antibiotic.
See: Rifadin, Cap. (Merrell Dow).
Rimactane, Cap. (Ciba).
•**RIFAMPIN,** U.S.P. XXIII. Cap., U.S.P. XXIII. Hydrazone 3-(4-Methyl-piperazinylimino-methyl rifamycin SV.
Use: Antibacterial (tuberculostatic). [Orphan drug]
See: Rifadin, Cap, Inj. (Marion Merrell Dow).
Rifomycin (Various Mfr.).
Rimactane, Cap. (Ciba).
•**RIFAMPIN AND ISONIAZID CAPSULES,** U.S.P. XXIII.
Use: Antibacterial (tuberculostatic).
RIFAMPIN, ISONIAZID, PYRAZINAMIDE.
Use: Antibacterial (tuberculostatic). [Orphan drug]
RIFAMYCIN. B.A.N. Rifamycin SV, an antibiotic produced by certain strains of *Streptomyces mediterranei.* 3-[[(4-Methyl-1-piperazinyl)imino]-methyl]-.
Use: Antibacterial (tuberculostatic).
See: Rifampin, U.S.P. XXIII.
•**RIFAPENTINE.** USAN.
Use: Antibacterial.
RIFATER. (Marion Merrell Dow) Rifampin 120 mg, isoniazid 50 mg, pyrazinamide 300 mg. Tab. 60s, UD 100s.
Use: Antituberculous agent.
RIFAXIMIN. USAN.
Use: Antibacterial.

R-IFN-BETA. (Biogen)
See: INTERFERON BETA (RECOMBI-
NANT).
RIFN-ALPHA 2.
Use: Miscellaneous antineoplastic.
RIG.
Use: Rabies prophylaxis product.
See: Hyperab (Cutter).
Imogam (Merieux).
Roferon-A (Roche).
RILUZOLE. (Rhone-Poulenc Rorer)
Use: Treatment of amyotrophic lateral
sclerosis. [Orphan drug]
RIMACTANE. (Ciba) Rifampin 300
mg/Cap. Bot. 30s, 60s, 100s.
Use: Antituberculous agent.
RIMACTANE/INH. (Ciba) Dual pack: 60
Rimactane 300 mg/Cap., 30 Isoniazid
300 mg/Tab.
Use: Antituberculous agent.
RIMADYL. (Roche)
Use: Nonsteroidal anti-inflammatory
agent.
See: Carprofen.
• **RIMANTADINE HCl.** USAN. Alpha-
methyl-1-adamantanemethylamine HCl.
Use: Antiviral.
See: Flumadine, Tab., Syr. (Forest).
• **RIMCAZOLE HYDROCHLORIDE.**
USAN.
Use: Antipsychotic.
• **RIMEXOLONE.** USAN.
Use: Anti-inflammatory.
RIMITEROL. B.A.N. erythro-3,4-Dihy-
droxy-α-(2-piperidyl)benzyl alcohol.
Use: Bronchodilator.
• **RIMITEROL HYDROBROMIDE.** USAN.
α-(3,4-Dihydroxy-phenyl)-2-
piperidinemethanol HBr.
Use: Bronchodilator.
RIMSO-50. (Research Industries) Di-
methyl sulfoxide in a 50% aqueous soln.
Bot. 50 ml.
Use: Interstitial cystitis, intravesical in-
stillation.
RINADE. (Econo Med) Chlorpheniramine
maleate 8 mg, phenylephrine HCl 20
mg, methscopolamine nitrate 2.5
mg/Cap. Bot. 120s.
Use: Antihistamine, decongestant, anti-
cholinergic.
RINADE-BID. (Econo Med) Chlorpheni-
ramine maleate 8 mg, pseudoephedrine
HCl 120 mg/SR Cap. Dye free. Bot.
100s.
Use: Antihistamine, decongestant.
RINGER'S-DEXTROSE INJECTION.
(Various Mfr.) Dextrose 50 Gm/l, Na 147,
K 4, C 4.5, Cl 156. 500, 1000 ml.
Use: Intravenous nutritional therapy.

• **RINGER'S INJECTION,** U.S.P. XXIII.
Lactated, U.S.P. XXIII. (Abbott) 250 ml,
500 ml, 1000 ml; (Invenex) 250 ml, 500
ml, 1000 ml; Abbo-Vac glass or flexible
containers, Vial 50 ml Pkg. 25s. (Lilly)
Amp. 20 ml, Pkg. 6s. (Cutter) Bot. 500
ml, 1000 ml.
Use: Fluid and electrolyte replenisher,
irrigating soln.
W/Dextrose. (Cutter) 5% soln. Bot. 1000
ml.
• **RINGER'S INJECTION, LACTATED,**
U.S.P. XXIII.
Use: Fluid and electrolyte replenisher.
• **RINGER'S IRRIGATION,** U.S.P. XXIII.
(Abbott) 500 ml, 1000 ml.
Use: Irrigation soln.
RIOPAN. (Whitehall) Magaldrate. **Tab.:**
Magaldrate 480 mg, sodium < 0.1
mg/Tab. In 60s, 100s. **Susp.:** Magal-
drate 540 mg, sodium 0.1 mg/5 ml. Bot.
6 oz, 12 oz. Individual Cup 30 ml each.
Use: Antacid.
**RIOPAN PLUS DOUBLE STRENGTH
SUSPENSION.** (Whitehall) Magaldrate
1080 mg, simethicone 40 mg/5 ml. Bot.
360 ml.
Use: Antacid, antiflatulent.
**RIOPAN PLUS DOUBLE STRENGTH
TABLETS.** (Whitehall) Magaldrate 1080
mg, simethicone 20 mg. Chew. Tab. Bot.
60s.
Use: Antacid, antiflatulent.
RIOPAN PLUS SUSPENSION. (White-
hall) Magaldrate 540 mg, simethicone
40 mg/5 ml. Bot. 360 ml.
Use: Antacid, antiflatulent.
RIOPAN PLUS TABLETS. (Whitehall)
Magaldrate 480 mg, simethicone 20 mg.
Chew. Tab. Bot. 50s, 100s.
Use: Antacid, antiflatulent.
• **RIOPROSTIL.** USAN.
Use: Gastric antisecretory.
• **RIPAZEPAM.** USAN.
Use: Tranquilizer (minor)
• **RISEDRONATE SODIUM.** USAN.
Use: Regulator (calcium).
• **RISOCAINE.** USAN.
Use: Anesthetic (local).
• **RISOTILIDE HYDROCHLORIDE.** USAN.
Use: Antiarrhythmic.
RISPERDAL. (Janssen) Risperidone 1
mg, 2 mg, 3 mg, 4 mg. Tab. Bot. 60s,
blister pack 100s.
Use: Antipsychotic agent.
RISPERIDONE.
Use: Antipsychotic.
See: Risperdal, Tab. (Janssen).
• **RISTIANOL PHOSPHATE.** USAN.

Use: Immunoregulator.
RISTOCETIN. B.A.N. An antibiotic from species of Actinomycetes *Norcardia lurida.*
Use: Antibiotic.
RITALIN HYDROCHLORIDE. (Ciba) Methylphenidate HCl. 5 mg, 10 mg, 20 mg Tab. Bot. 100s.
Use: CNS stimulant.
RITALIN-SR. (Ciba) Methylphenidate HCl 20 mg/SR Tab. Bot. 100s.
Use: CNS stimulant.
• **RITANSERIN.** USAN.
Use: Serotonin antagonist.
RITE-DIET. (E.J. Moore) Methylcellulose, benzocaine, vitamins A, D, B_1, B_2, C plus iron, calcium, potassium, niacinamide/Cap. Bot. 42s.
Use: Diet aid with vitamins.
• **RITODRINE.** USAN. Erythro-p-Hydroxy-α-[1-[(p-hydroxyphenethyl)amino]ethyl] benzyl alcohol
Use: Smooth muscle relaxant.
See: Prempar HCl.
Yutopar, Tab., Inj. (Astra).
• **RITODRINE HYDROCHLORIDE,** U.S.P. XXIII. Inj., Tab., U.S.P. XXIII.
Use: Relaxant (smooth muscle).
• **RITOLUKAST.** USAN.
Use: Antiasthmatic.
RMS SUPPOSITORIES. (Upsher-Smith) Morphine sulfate 5 mg, 10 mg, 20 mg or 30 mg/Supp. Box 12s.
Use: Narcotic analgesic.
ROBAFEN. (Major) Guaifenesin 100 mg/5 ml, alcohol 3.5%. Syr. Bot. 118 ml, 240 ml, pt, gal.
Use: Expectorant.
ROBAFEN AC COUGH. (Major) Guaifenesin 100 mg, codeine phosphate 10 mg/5 ml, alcohol 3.5%, parabens. Syrup. Bot. 473 ml.
Use: Expectorant, narcotic antitussive.
ROBAFEN-CF. (Major) Phenylpropanolamine HCl 12.5 mg, dextromethorphan HBr 10 mg, guaifenesin 100 mg, alcohol 4.75%. Bot. 118 ml.
Use: Antitussive, expectorant combination.
ROBAFEN DAC. (Major) Pseudoephedrine 30 mg, codeine phosphate 10 mg, guaifenesin 100 mg, alcohol 1.4%. Bot. Pt.
Use: Decongestant, antitussive, expectorant.
ROBAFEN DM. (Major) Dextromethorphan HBr 10 mg, guaifenesin 100 mg/5 ml, alcohol 1.4%. Syrup. Bot. 473 ml.
Use: Nonnarcotic antitussive, expectorant.

ROBANUL.
See: Robinul, Preps. (Robins).
ROBATHOL BATH OIL. (Pharmaceutical Specialties) Cottonseed oil, alkyl aryl polyether alcohol. Lanolin free. Bot. 240 ml, 480 ml, gal.
Use: Bath dermatological.
ROBAXIN. (Robins) Methocarbamol. **Tab.:** 500 mg, Bot. 100s, 500s, UD 100s. **Inj.:** 1 Gm/10 ml of a 50% aqueous soln. of polyethylene glycol 300. Vial 10 ml.
Use: Skeletal muscle relaxant.
ROBAXIN-750. (Robins) Methocarbamol 750 mg/Tab. Bot. 100s, 500s, Dis-Co Pak 100s.
Use: Skeletal muscle relaxant.
ROBAXISAL. (Robins) Methocarbamol (Robaxin) 400 mg, aspirin 325 mg/Tab. Bot. 100s, 500s, Dis-Co pack 100s.
Use: Muscle relaxant, analgesic.
• **ROBENIDINE HYDROCHLORIDE.** USAN.
Use: Coccidiostat.
ROBIMYCIN. (Robins) Erythromycin 250 mg/Tab. Bot. 100s, 500s.
Use: Antibacterial, erythromycin.
ROBINUL. (Robins) Glycopyrrolate 1 mg/Tab. Bot. 100s, 500s.
Use: Anticholinergic.
ROBINUL FORTE TABLETS. (Robins) Glycopyrrolate 2 mg/Tab. Bot. 100s.
Use: Anticholinergic.
ROBINUL INJECTABLE. (Robins) Glycopyrrolate 0.2 mg/ml, benzyl alcohol 0.9%. Vial 1 ml, 2 ml, 5 ml, 20 ml.
Use: Anticholinergic.
ROBITET. (Robins) Tetracycline HCl. Cap. **250 mg:** Bot. 100s, 1000s; **500 mg:** Bot. 100s, 500s.
Use: Antibacterial.
ROBITUSSIN. (Robins) Guaifenesin 100 mg/5 ml, alcohol 3.5%. Bot 1 oz, 4 oz, 8 oz, 1 pt, gal. UD 5 ml, 10 ml, 15 ml.
Use: Expectorant.
ROBITUSSIN A-C. (Robins) Guaifenesin 100 mg, codeine phosphate 10 mg/5 ml, alcohol 3.5%, saccharin, sorbitol. Bot. 2 oz, 4 oz, pt, gal.
Use: Expectorant, antitussive.
ROBITUSSIN-CF. (Robins) Guaifenesin 100 mg, phenylpropanolamine HCl 12.5 mg, dextromethorphan HBr 10 mg/10 ml, alcohol 4.75%, saccharin, sorbitol. Syr. Bot. 4 oz, 8 oz, 12 oz, pt.
Use: Expectorant, decongestant, antitussive.
ROBITUSSIN COLD & COUGH LIQUI-GELS. (Robins) Guaifenesin 200 mg, pseudoephedrine HCl 30 mg, dex-

tromethorphan HBr 10 mg, sorbitol.
Cap. Bot. 20s.
Use: Antitussive and expectorant.
ROBITUSSIN COUGH CALMERS.
(Robins) Dextromethorphan HBr 5 mg,
corn syrup, sucrose, cherry flavor. Loz.
Pkg. 16s.
Use: Nonnarcotic antitussive.
ROBITUSSIN COUGH DROPS. (Robins
Consumer) Menthol 7.4 mg, eucalyptus
oil, sucrose, corn syrup, cherry and
menthol eucalyptus flavor. Loz. Pkg. 9s,
25s, menthol 10 mg, eucalyptus oil, su-
crose, corn syrup, honey-lemon flavor.
Loz. Pkg. 9s, 25s.
Use: Nonnarcotic antitussive.
ROBITUSSIN-DAC. (Robins) Guaifenesin 100 mg, pseudoephedrine HCl 30
mg, codeine phosphate 10 mg/5 ml, alcohol 1.9%, saccharin, sorbitol. Syr. Bot.
4 oz, pt.
Use: Expectorant, decongestant, antitussive.
ROBITUSSIN DIE CO. (Robins) Guaifon-
esin 100 mg, alcohol 3.5%/5 ml. Syr. UD
pack 5 ml, 10 ml, 15 ml; (10 x 10s).
Use: Expectorant.
ROBITUSSIN-DM. (Robins) Guaifenesin
100 mg, dextromethorphan HBr 10 mg/5
ml. Syr. Bot. 4 oz, 8 oz, pt, gal, UD 5 ml,
10 ml (100s).
Use: Expectorant, antitussive.
**ROBITUSSIN LIQUID CENTER COUGH
DROPS.** (Robins) Menthol 10 mg, eu-
calyptus oil, parabens, sorbitol, sucrose.
Loz. Pkg. 20s.
Use: Mouth and throat products.
**ROBITUSSIN MAXIMUM STRENGTH
COUGH & COLD FOROMULA.**
(Robins) Dextromethorphan HBr 15 mg,
pseudoephedrine HCl 30 mg, alcohol
1.4%, glucose. Liq. Bot. 240 ml.
Use: Antitussive, decongestant.
ROBITUSSIN NIGHT RELIEF. (Robins)
Acetaminophen 108.3 mg, pseu-
doephedrine HCl 10 mg, pyrilamine
maleate 8.3 mg, dextromethorphan HBr
5 mg, alcohol-free, saccharin, sorbitol.
Bot. 300 ml.
Use: Analgesic, decongestant, antihist-
amine, antitussive.
ROBITUSSIN-PE. (Robins) Guaifenesin
100 mg, pseudoephedrine HCl 30 mg/5
ml, alcohol 1.4%, saccharin. Syr. Bot. 4
oz, 8 oz, pt.
Use: Expectorant, decongestant.
ROBITUSSIN PEDIATRIC. (Robin's)
Dextromethorphan HBr 7.5 mg/5 ml, alcohol free, saccharin, sorbitol, cherry flavor. Liq. Bot. 120, 240 ml.

Use: Nonnarcotic antitussive.
**ROBITUSSIN PEDIATRIC COUGH &
COLD FORMULA.** (Robins) Dextromethorphan HBr 7.5 mg, pseu-
doephedrine HCl 15 mg/5 ml. Liq. Bot.
120 ml.
Use: Antitussive, decongestant.
**ROBITUSSIN SEVERE CONGESTION
LIQUI-GELS.** (Robins) Guaifenesin 200
mg, pseudoephedrine HCl 30 mg, sor-
bitol. Cap. Pkg. 24s.
Use: Expectorant combination.
ROBOMOL/ASA TABS. (Major) Metho-
carbamol w/ASA. Bot. 100s, 500s.
Use: Skeletal muscle relaxant, analgesic.
ROCALTROL. (Roche) Calcitriol 0.25
mcg or 0.5 mcg/Cap. **0.25 mcg:** Bot.
30s, 100s. **0.5 mcg:** Bot. 100s.
Use: Management of hypocalcemia in
patients undergoing chronic renal dialysis.
• **ROCASTINE HYDROCHLORIDE.**
USAN.
Use: Antihistamine.
ROCEPHIN. (Roche) Ceftriaxone sodium
250 mg, 500 mg, 1 Gm, or 2 Gm/Vial to
be reconstituted for IV or IM administra-
tion. Box 10s. Piggyback Bot. 1 Gm or 2
Gm Box 10s. Bulk Pharmacy Container
10 Gm Box 1s. ADD-Vantage Vial 1 Gm
or 2 Gm Box 10s. Frozen Premix 1 Gm
or 2 Gm Iso-osmotic in 50 ml plastic container, not to be stored above -20 de-
grees C.
Use: Antibacterial, cephalosporin.
• **ROCURONIUM BROMIDE.** USAN.
Use: Adjunct to anesthesia (nondepo-
larizing neuromuscular blocker).
• **RODOCAINE.** USAN.
Use: Local anesthetic.
ROENTGENOGRAPHY.
See: Iodine Products, Diagnostic.
ROFERON-A. (Roche) Interferon alfa-2a,
recombinant as 3 million, 9 million or 18
million IU/Vial in injectable soln. Avail-
able as sterile pow. in 18 million IU
w/diluent. Subcutaneous or intramuscu-
lar inj. 3 million IU/ml Box 10s. 18 million
IU/0.5 ml Box 1s.
Use: Antineoplastic agent.
• **ROFLURANE.** USAN. 2-Bromo-1, 1,2-tri-
fluoroethyl methyl ether.
Use: General anesthetic.
ROGAINE. (Upjohn) Minoxidil 20 mg/ml
Topical Soln. Bot. 60 ml w/applicator.
Use: Male pattern baldness.
ROGENIC. (Forest) **SC Tab.:** Iron 60 mg,
vitamin C 100 mg, B_6 6 mg, B_{12} 25 mcg,
desiccated liver. Bot. 100s, 1000s.

Use: Vitamin/mineral supplement.

• **ROGLETIMIDE.** USAN. Pyridoglutethimide.
Use: Antineoplastic (aromatase inhibitor).

ROLAIDS CALCIUM RICH. (Warner-Lambert) Calcium carbonate 412 mg, magnesium hydroxide 80 mg. Chew. Tab. 12s, 36s, 75s, 150s.
Use: Antacid.

ROLATUSS EXPECTORANT LIQUID. (Huckaby) Phenylephrine HCl 5 mg, chlorpheniramine maleate 2 mg, codeine phosphate 9.85 mg, ammonium Cl 33.3 mg, alcohol 5%. Bot. 480 ml.
Use: Decongestant, antitussive, antihistamine, expectorant.

ROLATUSS W/HYDROCODONE. (Major) Phenylpropanolamine HCl 3.3 mg, phenylephrine HCl 5 mg, pyrilamine maleate 3.3 mg, pheniramine maleate 3.3 mg, hydrocodone bitartrate 1.67 mg. Liq. Bot. 480 ml.
Use: Decongestant, antitussive, antihistamine.

• **ROLETAMIDE.** USAN. 3′,4,5-Trimethoxy-3-(3-pyrrolin-1-yl)acrylophenone.
Use: Hypnotic.

• **ROLGAMIDINE.** USAN.
Use: Antidiarrheal.

ROLICAP. (Arcum) Vitamins A acetate 5000 IU, D_2 400 IU, B_1 3 mg, B_2 2.5 mg, B_6 10 mg, C 50 mg, niacinamide 20 mg, B_{12} 1 mcg/Chew. Tab. Bot. 100s, 1000s.
Use: Vitamin supplement.

ROLICYPRAM. B.A.N. (+)-5-Oxo-N-(trans-2-phenylcyclopropyl)-L-pyrrolidine-2-carboxamide.
Use: Antidepressant.

• **ROLICYPRINE.** USAN. (+)-5-Oxo-N-(trans-2-phenylcyclopropyl)-L-2-pyrrolidinecarboxamide.
Use: Antidepressant.

• **ROLIPRAM.** USAN.
Use: Tranquilizer.

• **ROLITETRACYCLINE, STERILE,** U.S.P. XXII. Inj., U.S.P. XXII. N-(Pyrrolidinomethyl) tetracycline. 4-(Dimethylamino)-1,4,4a,5,5a,6,11,12a-octahydro-3,6,10,12,12a-pentahydroxy-6-methyl-1,11-dioxo-N-(1-pyrrolidinylmethyl)-2-naphthacenecarboxamide. Tetrex PMT nitrate Inj. Syntetrin Inj. (Bristol) Velacycline (Squibb).
Use: Antibacterial.

• **ROLITETRACYCLINE NITRATE.** USAN. Tetrim.
Use: Antibacterial.

• **ROLODINE.** USAN. 4-(Benzylamino)-2-

methyl-7H-pyrrolo-[2,3-d]-pyrimidine.
Use: Muscle relaxant.

ROMACH ANTACID TABLETS. (Last) Magnesium carbonate 400 mg, sodium bicarbonate 250 mg/Tab. Strip pack 60s, 500s.
Use: Antacid.

ROMAZICON. (Hoffman-LaRoche) Flumazenil 0.1 mg/ml. Inj. vials 5 and 10 ml.
Use: Antidotes.

ROMEX COUGH & COLD CAPSULES. (APC) Guaifenesin 65 mg, dextromethorphan HBr 10 mg, chlorpheniramine maleate 1.5 mg, pyrilamine maleate 12.5 mg, phenylephrine HCl 5 mg, acetaminophen 160 mg/Cap. Bot. 21s.
Use: Expectorant, antitussive, antihistamine, decongestant.

ROMEX COUGH & COLD TABLETS. (APC) Dextromethorphan HBr 7.5 mg, phenylephrine HCl 2.5 mg, ascorbic acid 30 mg. Box 15s.
Use: Antitussive, decongestant.

ROMEX TROCHES & LIQUID. (APC) **Troche:** Polymyxin B sulfate 1000 units, benzocaine 5 mg, cetalkonium Cl 2.5 mg, gramicidin 100 mcg, chlorpheniramine maleate 0.5 mg, tyrothricin 2 mg. Pkg. 10s. **Liq.:** Guaifenesin 200 mg, dextromethorphan HBr 60 mg, chlorpheniramine maleate 12 mg, phenylephrine HCl 30 mg/fl oz. Bot. 4 oz.
Use: Antibacterial, antihistamine, expectorant, antitussive, decongestant.

ROMYCIN. (Roberts) Erythromycin 2%, SD alcohol 40-A 66%. Topical Soln. Bot. 60 ml.
Use: Anti-acne.

RONDAMINE-DM. (Major) Pseudoephedrine 25 mg/ml, carbinoxamine maleate 2 mg/ml, dextromethorphan HBr 4 mg/ml. Drop. 30 ml.
Use: Cough preparation.

RONDEC ORAL DROPS. (Ross) Carbinoxamine maleate 2 mg, pseudoephedrine HCl 25 mg/ml. Bot. 30 ml w/dropper.
Use: Antihistamine, decongestant (pediatric).

RONDEC SYRUP. (Ross) Carbinoxamine maleate 4 mg, pseudoephedrine HCl 60 mg/5 ml. Syr. Bot. 4 oz, pt.
Use: Antihistamine, decongestant (pediatric).

RONDEC-DM ORAL DROPS. (Ross) Carbinoxamine maleate 2 mg, pseudoephedrine HCl 25 mg/ml, dextromethorphan HBr 4 mg/ml, alcohol 6%. Bot. 30

ml w/dropper.
Use: Antihistamine, decongestant, antitussive.
RONDEC-DM SYRUP. (Ross) Carbinoxamine maleate 4 mg, pseudoephedrine HCl 60 mg, dextromethorphan HBr 15 mg/5 ml, alcohol 6%. Bot. 4 oz, pt.
Use: Antihistamine, decongestant, antitussive.
RONDEC TABS FILM. (Ross) Pseudoephedrine HCl 60 mg, carbinoxamine maleate 4 mg, lactose/Tab. Bot. 100s, 500s.
Use: Upper respiratory combination.
RONDEC-TR. (Ross) Carbinoxamine 8 mg, pseudoephedrine HCl 120 mg/SR Tab. Bot. 100s.
Use: Antihistamine, decongestant.
• **RONIDAZOLE.** USAN.
Use: Antiprotozoal.
• **RONNEL.** USAN. Fenchlorphos.
Use: Insecticide (systemic).
See: Korlan (Dow).
Irolene (Dow).
RONVET. (Geneva) Erythromycin stearate 250 mg/Tab. Bot. 100s.
Use: Antibacterial
• **ROPINIROLE HYDROCHLORIDE.** USAN.
Use: Antiparkinsonian agent.
• **ROPITOIN HYDROCHLORIDE.** USAN.
Use: Cardiac depressant.
• **ROPIZINE.** USAN.
Use: Anticonvulsant.
ROQUINIMEX.
Use: Antineoplastic. [Orphan drug]
See: Linomide.
ROSA GALLICAL.
See: Estivin, Soln. (Alcon).
ROSANILINE DYES.
See: Fuchsin, Basic (Various Mfr.). Methylrosaniline Cl, Soln., Inj. (Various Mfr.).
• **ROSARAMICIN.** USAN.
Use: Antibacterial.
• **ROSARAMICIN BUTYRATE.** USAN.
Use: Antibacterial.
• **ROSARAMICIN PROPIONATE.** USAN.
Use: Antibacterial.
• **ROSARAMICIN SODIUM PHOSPHATE.** USAN.
Use: Antibacterial.
• **ROSARAMICIN STEARATE.** USAN.
Use: Antibacterial.
ROSE BENGAL. (Akorn) Rose bengal 1%. Bot. 5 ml.
Use: Diagnostic for staining dead ocular tissue.
• **ROSE BENGAL SODIUM I-125.** USAN.
Use: Radioactive agent.

• **ROSE BENGAL SODIUM I-131 INJECTION,** U.S.P. XXIII. Sodium 4,5,6,7-Tetrachloro-2′,-4,5,7-tetraiodofluorescein.
Use: Diagnostic aid (hepatic function).
ROSE BENGAL STRIPS. (Barnes-Hind) Rose bengal 1.3 mg. For disclosing corneal injury and pathology. Strip box 100s.
Use: Diagnostic aid.
ROSE-C LIQUID. (Barth's) Vitamin C 300 mg, rose hip extract/Tsp. Dropper Bot. 2 oz, 8 oz.
Use: Vitamin C supplement.
ROSE HIPS. (Burgin-Arden) Vitamin C 300 mg, in base of sorbitol. Bot. 4 oz, 8 oz.
Use: Vitamin C supplement.
ROSE HIPS VITAMIN C. (Kirkman) Vitamin C. **100 mg/Tab:** Bot. 100s, 250s. **250 mg or 500 mg/Tab:** Bot. 100s, 250s, 500s.
Use: Vitamin C supplement.
• **ROSE OIL,** N.F. XVIII.
Use: Perfume.
ROSETS. (Akorn) Rose bengal 1.3 mg/strip. Pkg. 100s.
Use: Diagnostic agent, ophthalmic.
• **ROSE WATER, STRONGER,** N.F. XVIII.
Use: Perfume.
• **ROSE WATER OINTMENT,** U.S.P. XXIII
Use: Emollient, ointment base.
ROSIN, U.S.P. XXI.
Use: Stiffening agent, pharmaceutical necessity.
• **ROSOXACIN.** USAN.
Use: Antibacterial, antigonococcal.
See: Rosoxacin, Pow. (Sanofi Winthrop).
ROSS SLD. (Ross) Low-residue nutritional supplement for patients restricted to a clear liquid feeding or with fat malabsorption disorders. Packet 1.35 oz. Ctn. 6s. Case 4 ctn. Can 13.5 oz. Case 6s.
Use: Nutritional supplement.
ROTALEX TEST. (Medical Tech. Corp.) Latex slide agglutination test for detection of rotavirus in feces. Kit 1s.
Use: Diagnostic aid.
ROTAZYME II. (Abbott Diagnostics) Enzyme immunoassay for detection of rotavirus antigen in feces. Test kit 50s.
Use: Diagnostic aid.
• **ROTOXAMINE.** USAN. (–)-2-[p-Chloro-α-[2-(dimethylamino)ethoxy]-benzyl] pyridine.
Use: Antihistamine.
ROWASA. (Solvay) **Rectal Susp.:** Mesalamine 4 Gm/60 ml. In units

of 7 disposable bot. **Supp.**: Mesalamine 500 mg. Box 12s, 24s.
Use: Ulcerative colitis, proctosigmoiditis, proctitis.

• **ROXADIMATE.** USAN.
Use: Sunscreen.

ROXANOL ORAL SOLUTION. (Roxane) Morphine sulfate concentrated oral soln, sugar-free and alcohol free. **20 mg/ml:** Bot. 30 ml or 120 ml w/calibrated dropper. **100 mg/5 ml:** Bot. 240 ml w/calibrated spoon.
Use: Narcotic analgesic.

ROXANOL RECTAL. (Roxane) Morphine sulfate 5, 10, 20, 30 mg. Supp. 12s.
Use: Narcotic agonist analgesic.

ROXANOL 100. (Roxane) Morphine sulfate 100 mg/5 ml. Soln. Bot. 240 ml.
Use: Narcotic agonist analgesic.

ROXANOL RESCUDOSE. (Roxane) Morphine sulfate. **Supp.** 5, 10, 20, 30 mg. Pkg. 12s. **Oral Soln.:** 10 mg/2.5 ml, UD 2.5 ml.
Use: Narcotic agonist analgesic.

ROXANOL SR TABLETS. (Roxane) Morphine sulfate 30 mg/SR Tab. Bot. 50s, 250s, UD 100s.
Use: Narcotic analgesic.

ROXANDOL UD. (Roxane) Morphine sulfate 20 mg/5 ml. Soln. Bot. 100, 500 ml.
Use: Narcotic agonist analgesic.

• **ROXARSONE.** USAN. 3-Nitro-4-hydroxyphenylarsonic acid.
Use: Coccidiostat and antibacterial.

• **ROXATIDINE ACETATE HYDROCHLORIDE.** USAN.
Use: Antiulcer agent.

ROXICET ORAL SOLUTION. (Roxane) Oxycodone HCl 5 mg, acetaminophen 325 mg/5 ml. Bot. 5 ml, 500 ml.
Use: Narcotic analgesic.

ROXICET 5/500. (Roxane) Oxycodone HCl 5 mg, acetaminophen 500 mg/Cap. Bot. 100s, 500s, UD 100s.
Use: Narcotic analgesic combination.

ROXICET TABLETS. (Roxane) Oxycodone HCl 5 mg, acetaminophen 325 mg, 0.4% alcohol/Tab. Bot. 100s, UD 4 X 25s.
Use: Narcotic analgesic.

ROXICODONE. (Roxane) **Liq.:** Oxycodone HCl 5 mg/5 ml. Bot. 500 ml. **Tab.:** Oxycodone HCl 5 mg. Bot. 100s, UD 4 X 25s.
Use: Narcotic analgesic.

ROXILOX. (Roxane) Oxycodone 5 mg, acetaminophen 500 mg/Cap. Bot. 100s.
Use: Narcotic analgesic combination.

ROXIPRIN TABLETS. (Roxane) Oxycodone HCl 4.5 mg, oxycodone terephthalate 0.38 mg, aspirin 325 mg/Tab. Bot. 100s, 1000s, UD 4 X 25s.
Use: Narcotic analgesic.

• **ROXITHROMYCIN.** USAN.
Use: Antibacterial.

R-S LOTION. (Hill) No. 2: Sulfur 8%, resorcinol monoacetate 4%. Bot. 2 oz.
Use: Topical drying medication.

R-TANNAMINE. (Qualitest) Phenylephrine tannate 25 mg, chlorpheniramine tannate 8 mg, pyrilamine tannate 25 mg/Tab. Bot. 100s.
Use: Upper respiratory combination.

R-TANNAMINE PEDIATRIC. (Qualitest) Phenylephrine tannate 5 mg, chlorpheniramine tannate 2 mg, pyrilamine tannate 12.5 mg. Pt.
Use: Upper respiratory combination.

R-TANNATE TABLETS. (Various Mfr.) Phenylephrine tannate 25 mg, chlorpheniramine tannate 8 mg, pyrilamine tannate 25 mg. In 100s.
Use: Decongestant, antihistamine.

R-TANNATE PEDIATRIC SUSPENSION. (Various Mfr.) Phenylephrine tannate 5 mg, chlorpheniramine tannate 2 mg, pyrilamine tannate 12.5 mg, saccharin. In 480 ml.
Use: Decongestant, antihistamine.

RUBACELL. (Abbott Diagnostics) Passive hemagglutination (PHA) test for the detection of antibody to rubella virus in serum or recalcified plasma.
Use: Diagnostic aid.

RT-PA.
Use: Tissue plasminogen.
See: Activase (Genetech).

RU 486.
Use: Antiprogesterone.
See: Mifepristone.

RUBACELL II. (Abbott) Passive hemagglutination (PHA) test to detect antibody to rubella in serum or recalcified plasma. In 100s, 1000s.
Use: Diagnostic aid.

RUBAQUICK DIAGNOSTIC KIT. (Abbott Diagnostics) Rapid passive hemagglutination (PHA) for the detection of antibodies to rubella virus in serum specimens.
Use: Diagnostic aid.

RUBA-TECT. (Abbott Diagnostics) Hemagglutination inhibition test for the detection and quantitation of rubella antibody in serum. In 100s.
Use: Diagnostic aid.

RUBAZYME. (Abbott Diagnostics) Enzyme immunoassay for 1 gG antibody to rubella virus. Test kit 100s, 1000s.
Use: Diagnostic aid.

RUBAZYME-M. (Abbott Diagnostics) Enzyme immunoassay for IgM antibody to rubella virus in serum. Test kit 50s.
Use: Diagnostic aid.

• **RUBELLA & MUMPS VIRUS VACCINE, LIVE,** U.S.P. XXIII.
Use: Active immunizing agent.
See: Biavax II, Inj. (Merck & Co.).

RUBELLA & RUBEOLA VACCINE. (Merck & Co.) M-R-VAX II. Inj. Vial.
Use: Vaccine, viral.

• **RUBELLA VIRUS VACCINE, LIVE,** U.S.P. XXIII.
Use: Active immunizing agent.
See: Cendevax, Inj. (SK-Beecham). Meruvax, Inj. (Merck & Co.).
W/Measles vaccine.
See: M-R-Vax, Inj. (Merck & Co.).
W/Measles vaccine, mumps vaccine.
See: M-M-R, Inj. (Merck & Co.).

RUBELLA VIRUS VACCINE, LIVE ATTENUATED. Live attenuated strain of rubella virus HPV-77.
Use: Agent for immunization.
W/Measles vaccine.
See: Lirubel, Vial (Merrell Dow).
W/Measles vaccine, mumps vaccine.
See: Lirutrin, Vial (Merrell Dow).

RUBEOLA VACCINE. Inj. Vial. 1 & 10 dose.
Use: Vaccine, viral.
See: Attenuvax (Merck & Co.).

RUBEX. (Bristol-Myers Oncology) Doxorubicin HCl 10 mg, lactose 50 mg. Pow. Vial.
Use: Antineoplastic.

• **RUBIDIUM CHLORIDE Rb 82,** Inj., U.S.P. 23.
Use: Radioactive agent.

• **RUBIDIUM CHLORIDE Rb 86.** USAN.
Use: Radioactive agent.

• **RUBIDIUM CHLORIDE.** USAN.

RUBRAPLEX. (Lannett) Vitamins B_1 2.5 mg, B_2 2 mg, B_6 0.5 mg, B_{12} 5 mcg, calcium pantothenate 1 mg, niacinamide 20 mg/Cap. Bot. 100s, 1000s.
Use: Vitamin supplement.

RUBRATOPE-57. (Squibb) Cyanocobalamin Co 57 Capsules; Soln U.S.P.
Use: Vitamin supplement.

RUBRAVITE LIQUID. (Lannett) Vitamins B_1 10 mg, B_{12} 25 mcg/5 ml. Bot. pt.
Use: Vitamin supplement.

RUFEN. (Boots) Ibuprofen 400 mg, 600 mg or 800 mg/Tab. Bot. 100s, 500s, UD 100s.
Use: Nonsteroidal anti-inflammatory drug; analgesic.

RUFOCROMOMYCIN. B.A.N. An antibiotic produced by Streptomyces ru-fochromogenus.
Use: Antibacterial.

RUFOLEX. (Lannett) Vitamins B_1 1.5 mg, B_2 1.5 mg, B_6 1 mg, B_{12} 5 mcg, C 50 mg, niacinamide 10 mg, ferrous fumarate 200 mg, d-sorbitol 200 mg, folic acid 0.25 mg/Cap. Bot. 100s.
Use: Vitamin/mineral supplement.

RU-LETS M 500. (Rugby) Vitamin C 500 mg, niacinamide 100 mg, calcium pantothenate 20 mg, B_1 15 mg, B_2 10 mg, B_6 5 mg, A 10,000 IU, B_{12} 12 mcg, D 400 IU, E 30 mg, magnesium 80 mg, iron 20 mg, copper 2 mg, zinc 1.5 mg, manganese 1 mg, iodine 0.15 mg/Tab. Bot. 100s.
Use: Vitamin/mineral supplement.

RULOX. (Rugby) **#1 Tab.:** Aluminum hydroxide 200 mg, magnesium hydroxide 200 mg. **#2 Tab.:** Aluminum hydroxide 400 mg, magnesium hydroxide 400 mg. Bot. 100s, 1000s.
Use: Antacid.

RULOX PLUS SUSPENSION. (Rugby) Aluminum hydroxide 500 mg, magnesium hydroxide 450 mg, simethicone 40 mg/5 ml. Bot. 355 ml.
Use: Antacid.

RULOX PLUS TABLETS. (Rugby) Aluminum hydroxide 200 mg, magnesium hydroxide 200 mg, simethicone 25 mg. Chew. Tab. Bot. 50s.
Use: Antacid.

RULOX SUSPENSION. (Rugby) Aluminum hydroxide 225 mg, magnesium hydroxide 200 mg/5 ml. Susp. Bot. 360 ml, 769 ml, gal.
Use: Antacid.

RUM-K. (Fleming) Potassium Cl 10 mEq/5 ml in butter/rum flavored base. Bot. pt, gal.
Use: Potassium supplement.

RUST INHIBITOR.
See: Anti-Rust, Tab. (Sanofi Winthrop). Sodium Nitrite, Tab. (Various Mfr.).

• **RUTAMYCIN.** USAN. From strain of *Streptomyces rutgersensis.* Under study.
Use: Antifungal antibiotic.

RUTGERS 612.
See: Ethohexadiol. (Various Mfr.).

RUTIN. (Various Mfr.) 3-Rhamnoglucoside of 5,7,3',4-tetrahydroxyflavonol. Eldrin, globulariacitrin, myrticalorin, oxyritin, phytomelin, rutoside, sophorin. Tab. 20 mg, 50 mg, 60 mg, 100 mg.
Use: Vascular disorders.

RUTIN COMBINATIONS.
See: Hexarutan, Tab. (Westerfield). Hyrunal, Tab. (Kenyon).

Vio-Geric-H, Tab. (Solvay).
RUTOSIDE.
See: Rutin, Tab. (Various Mfr.).
RU-TUSS DE. (Boots) Pseudoephedrine HCl 120 mg, guaifenesin 600 mg/Tab. Bot. 100s.
Use: Decongestant, expectorant.
RU-TUSS II. (Boots) Phenyl propanolamine HCl 75 mg, chlorpheniramine maleate 12 mg/Cap. Bot. 100s.
Use: Decongestant, antihistamine.
RU-TUSS EXPECTORANT. (Boots) Pseudoephedrine HCl 30 mg, dextromethorphan HBr 10 mg, guaifenesin 100 mg/5 ml, alcohol 10%. Bot. pt.
Use: Decongestant, antitussive, expectorant.
RU-TUSS LIQUID. (Boots) Phenylephrine HCl 30 mg, chlorpheniramine maleate 2 mg/30 ml, alcohol 5%. Bot. pt.
Use: Decongestant, antihistamine.
RU-TUSS TABLETS. (Boots) Phenylephrine HCl 25 mg, phenylpropanolamine HCl 50 mg, chlorpheniramine maleate 8 mg, hyoscyamine sulfate 0.19 mg, atropine sulfate 0.04 mg, scopolamine hydrobromide 0.01 mg/Tab. Bot. 100s, 500s.
Use: Decongestant, antihistamine, anticholinergic/antispasmodic.
RU-TUSS w/HYDROCODONE. (Boots) Hydrocodone bitartrate 1.67 mg, phenylephrine HCl 5 mg, phenylpropanolamine HCl 3.3 mg, pheniramine maleate 3.3 mg, pyrilamine maleate 3.3 mg/5 ml, alcohol 5%. Bot. 473 ml.
Use: Antitussive, decongestant, antihistamine.
RU-VERT M. (Solvay) Meclizine HCl 25 mg/Tab. Bot. 100s.
Use: Antiemetic, antivertigo.
RVPAQUE. (ICN Pharm.) Red petrolatum, zinc oxide, cinoxate, in water-resistant base. Tube 15 g, 37.5 g.
Use: Sunscreen.
RYMED. (Edwards) Pseudoephedrine HCl 30 mg, guaifenesin 250 mg/Cap. Bot. 100s.
Use: Decongestant, expectorant.
RYMED LIQUID. (Edwards) Pseudoephedrine HC1 30 mg, guaifenesin 100 mg/5 ml, alcohol 1.4%. Bot. pt.
Use: Decongestant, expectorant.
RYMED-TR. (Edwards) Phenylpropanolamine HCl 75 mg, guaifenesin 400 mg/Tab. Bot. 100s.
Use: Decongestant, expectorant.
RYNA. (Wallace) Chlorpheniramine 2 mg, pseudoephedrine HCl 30 mg/5 ml. Bot. 4 oz, pt.

Use: Antihistamine, decongestant.
RYNA-C. (Wallace) Codeine phosphate 10 mg, pseudoephedrine HCl 30 mg, chlorpheniramine maleate 2 mg, saccharin, sorbitol/5 ml. Bot. 4 oz, pt.
Use: Antitussive, decongestant, antihistamine.
RYNA-OX. (Wallace) Guaifenesin 100 mg, pseudoephedrine HCl 30 mg, codeine phosphate 10 mg, alcohol 7.5%, saccharin, sorbitol/5 ml. Bot. 4 oz, pt.
Use: Expectorant, decongestant, antitussive.
RYNATAN. (Wallace) **Tab.:** Phenylephrine tannate 25 mg, chlorpheniramine tannate 8 mg, pyrilamine tannate 25 mg. Bot. 100s, 500s. **Pediatric Susp.:** Phenylephrine tannate 5 mg, chlorpheniramine tannate 2 mg, pyrilamine tannate 12.5 mg/5 ml. Bot. pt.
Use: Decongestant, antihistamine.
RYNATUSS. (Wallace) Carbetapentane tannate 60 mg, chlorpheniramine tannate 5 mg, ephedrine tannate 10 mg, phenylephrine tannate 10 mg/Tab. Bot. 100s, 500s.
Use: Decongestant, antihistamine.
RYNATUSS PEDIATRIC SUSPENSION. (Wallace) Carbetapentane tannate 30 mg, chlorpheniramine tannate 4 mg, ephedrine tannate 5 mg, phenylephrine tannate 5 mg, saccharin, tartrazine/5 ml. Susp. Bot. 8 oz, pt.
Use: Decongestant, antihistamine.
RYTHMOL. (Knoll) Propafenone HCl 150 mg, 225 mg or 300 mg. Tab. **50 mg or 300 mg:** Bot. 100s, 500s. **225 mg:** Bot. 100s, UD 100s.
Use: Antiarrhythmic.

S

S-2 INHALANT & NEBULIZERS. (Nephron) Racemic epinephrine HCl 1.25%. Bot. 0.25 oz, 0.5 oz, 1 oz.
Use: Bronchodilator.
SAAVE+. (NeuroGenesis/Matrix) Vitamin D 40 mg, L-phenylalanine, L-glutamine 25 mg, vitamins A 333.3 IU, B$_1$ 2.417 mg, B$_2$ 0.85 mg, B$_3$ 33 mg, B$_5$ 15 mg, B$_6$ 3 mg, B$_{12}$ 5 mcg, folic acid 0.067 mg, C 100 mg, E 5 IU, biotin 0.05 mg, calcium 25 mg, chromium 0.01 mg, iron 1.5 mg, magnesium 25 mg, zinc 2.5 mg/Cap. Yeast and preservative free. Bot. 42s, 180s.
Use: Vitamin/mineral supplement.
SABIN VACCINE.

Use: Vaccine, viral.
See: Orimune (Lederle).
SAC-500. (Western Research) Vitamin C 500 mg/Timed Release Cap. Bot. 1000s.
Use: Vitamin supplement.
SACARASA.
See: SUCRASE (yeast-derived).
S-A-C TABLETS. (Lannett) Acetaminophen 150 mg, salicylamide 230 mg, caffeine 30 mg/Tab. Bot. 36s, 100s, 1000s.
Use: Nonnarcotic analgesic combinations.
• **SACCHARIN,** N.F. XVIII. 1,2-Benzisothiazolin-3-one-1, 1-dioxide.
(Merck)—Pkg. 1 oz, 0.25 lb, 1 lb.
(Squibb) Tabs. 0.25, 0.5 gr. Bot. 500s, 1000s; 1 gr. Bot. 1000s.
Use: Sweetening agent when sugar is contraindicated.
See: Necta Sweet, Tab. (Norwich Eaton).
• **SACCHARIN CALCIUM,** U.S.P. XXIII. 1,2-Benzisothiazolin-3-one 1, 1-dioxide calcium salt hydrate (2:7).
Use: Non-nutritive sweetener.
• **SACCHARIN SODIUM,** U.S.P. XXIII. Oral Soln., Tab., U.S.P. XXIII. (Benzosulfimide Sod., Soluble Gluside, Soluble Saccharine) Pow., Bot. 1 oz, 0.25 lb, 1 lb. Tab. usual sizes. (Various Mfr.).
Use: Sweetening agent and test for circulation time of blood.
See: Crystallose, Crystals, Liq. (Jamieson).
Ril Sweet, Liq. (Plough).
Sweeta (Squibb Mark).
SACCHARIN SOLUBLE.
See: Saccharin Sodium, Tab., Pow. (Various Mfr.).
SAFESKIN. (C & M Pharmacal) A dermatologically acceptable detergent for patients who are sensitive to ordinary detergents. No whiteners, brighteners or other irritants. Bot. qt.
Use: Laundry detergent for sensitive skin.
SAFE SUDS. (Ar-Ex) Hypoallergenic, all-purpose detergent for patients whose hands or respiratory membranes are irritated by soaps or detergents. pH 6.8. No enzymes, phosphates, lanolin, fillers, bleaches. Bot. 22 oz.
Use: Laundry detergent for sensitive skin.
SAFE TUSSIN 30. (Kramer) Guaifenesin 100 mg, dextromethorphan HBr 15 mg/5 ml. Liq. Bot. 120 ml.
Use: Nonnarcotic antitussive, expecto-

rant.
SAFETY-COATED ARTHRITIS PAIN FORMULA. (Whitehall) Enteric coated aspirin 500 mg/Tab. Bot. 24s, 60s.
Use: Salicylate analgesic.
SAFFLOWER OIL.
Use: Enteral nutritional supplement.
See: Microlipid (Sherwood).
• **SAFFLOWER OIL,** U.S.P. XXIII.
See: Safflower Oil Caps. (Various Mfr.).
W/Choline bitartrate, soybean lecithin, inositol, natural tocopherols, B_6, B_{12}, and panthenol.
See: Nutricol, Cap., Vial (Nutrition).
• **SAFINGOL.** USAN.
Use: Antineoplastic adjunct; antipsoriatic.
• **SAFINGOL HYDROCHORIDE.** USAN.
Use: Antineoplastic adjunct; antipsoriatic.
SAFROLE. 4-Allyl-1,2-(methylenedioxy) benzene.
SALAC CLEANSER. (Gen Derm) Salicylic acid 2% in a surfactant blend. Liq. Bot. 177 ml.
Use: Anti-acne agent.
SALACETIN.
See: Acetylsalicylic Acid (Various Mfr.).
SAL-ACID. (Pedinol) Salicylic acid 40% in collodion-like vehicle. Plaster. Pkg. 14s.
Use: Keratolytic.
SALACID 25%. (Gordon) Salicylic acid 25% in ointment base. Jar 2 oz, lb.
Use: Keratolytic.
SALACID 60%. (Gordon) Salicylic acid 60% in ointment base. Jar 2 oz.
Use: Keratolytic.
SALACTIC FILM. (Pedinol) Salicylic acid 16.7% in flexible collodion w/color. Applicator bot. 0.5 oz.
Use: Keratolytic.
SALAGEN. (MGI Pharma) Pilocarpine HCl 5 mg. Tab. Bot. 100s.
Use: Mouth and throat product.
• **SALANTEL.** USAN.
Use: Anthelmintic.
SALATAR CREAM. (Lannett) Coal tar soln. 5%, salicylic acid 3%. Jar 4 oz, lb.
Use: Antiseborrheic, keratolytic.
SALAZIDE-DEMI TABLETS. (Major) Hydroflumethiazide 25 mg, reserpine 0.125 mg/Tab. Bot. 100s.
Use: Antihypertensive combination.
SALAZIDE TABS. (Major) Hydroflumethiazide 50 mg, reserpine 0.125 mg/Tab. Bot. 100s, 500s, 1000s.
Use: Antihypertensive combination.
SALAZOSULFAPYRIDINE (I.N.N.). Sulphasalazine. B.A.N.

SALAZOSULPHADIMIDINE. B.A.N. 4'-
(4,6-Dimethylpyrimidin-2-ylsulphamoyl)-
4-hydroxyazo-benzene-3-carboxylic
acid.
Use: Sulfonamide.
SALBUTAMOL. B.A.N. 1-(4-Hydroxy-3-
hydroxy-methylphenyl)-2-(t-buty-
lamino)ethanol.
Use: Bronchodilator.
SALCATONIN. B.A.N. A component of
natural salmon calcitonin.
Use: Treatment of hypercalcemia and
Paget's disease.
SALCEGEL. (Apco) Sodium salicylate 5
gr, calcium ascorbate 25 mg, calcium
carbonate 1 gr, dried aluminum hydrox-
ide gel 2 gr/Tab. Bot. 100s.
Use: Analgesic.
• **SALCOLEX.** USAN.
Use: Analgesic, anti-inflammatory.
• **SALETHAMIDE MALEATE.** USAN. N-[2-
Di-ethyl(amino)ethyl]-salicylamide
maleate. Under study.
Use: Analgesic.
SALETIN.
See: Acetylsalicylic Acid (Various Mfr.).
SALETO. (Hauck) Aspirin 210 mg, aceta-
minophen 115 mg, salicylamide 65 mg,
caffeine anhydrous 16 mg/Tab. Bot. 50s,
100s, 1000s.
Use: Analgesic.
SALETO-200. (Hauck) Ibuprofen 200
mg/Tab. Bot. 1000s, UD 50s.
Use: Nonsteroidal anti-inflammatory
agent; analgesic.
SALETO-400. (Hauck) Ibuprofen 400
mg/Tab. Bot. 100s, 500s.
Use: Nonsteroidal anti-inflammatory
agent; analgesic.
SALETO-600. (Hauck) Ibuprofen 600
mg/Tab. Bot. 100s, 500s.
Use: Nonsteroidal anti-inflammatory
agent; analgesic.
SALETO-800. (Hauck) Ibuprofen 800
mg/Tab. Bot. 100s, 500s.
Use: Nonsteroidal anti-inflammatory
agent; analgesic.
SALETO D. (Hauck) Acetaminophen 240
mg, salicylamide 120 mg, caffeine 16
mg, phenylpropanolamine HCl 18
mg/Cap. Bot. 20s, 50s.
Use: Analgesic, decongestant.
SALFLEX. (Carnrick Labs) Salsalate 500
mg or 750 mg/Tab. Bot. 100s.
Use: Analgesic.
• **SALICYL ALCOHOL.** USAN.
Use: Local anesthetic.
• **SALICYLAMIDE,** U.S.P. XXIII.
Use: Analgesic.
SALICYLAMIDE. B.A.N. (Bryant) o-Hy-

droxybenzamide. Salimed.
Use: Analgesic; antipyretic.
SALICYLAMIDE W/COMBINATIONS.
See: Akes-N-Pain, Cap. (Edward J.
Moore).
Anodynos, Tab. (Buffington).
Anodynos Forte, Tab. (Buffington).
Arthol, Tab. (Towne).
Cenaid, Tab. (Century).
Centuss, MLT Tab. (Century).
Codalan, 1,2,3, Tab. (Lannett).
Dapco, Tab. (Mericon).
Decohist, Cap. (Towne).
Dengesic, Tab. (Scott-Alison).
Duoprin, Tab. (Dunhall).
Emagrin, Tab. (Otis Clapp).
Emersal, Liq. (Medco).
F.C.A.H., Cap. (Scherer).
Lobac, Cap. (Seatrace).
Myocalm, Tab. (Parmed).
Nokane, Tab. (Wren).
Partuss-A, Tab. (Parmed).
Partuss T.D., Tab. (Parmed).
P.M.P. Compound, Tab. (Mericon).
Presalin, Tab. (Hauck).
Renpap, Tab. (Wren).
Rhinex, Tab. (Lemmon).
S-A-C, Tab. (Lannett).
S.A.C., Preps. (Towne).
Saleto, Preps. (Hauck).
Salipap, Tab. (Freeport).
Salocol, Tab. (Hauck).
Salphenyl, Liq., Cap. (Hauck).
Sanger Special, Tab. (Edward J.
Moore).
Scotgesic, Cap., Elix. (Scott/Cord).
Sedacane, Cap. (Edward J. Moore).
Sedalgesic, Tab. (Table Rock).
Sedragesic, Tab. (Lannett).
Sinulin, Tab. (Reed & Carnrick).
Sleep, Tab. (Towne).
Tega-code Cap. (Ortega).
Triaprin-DC, Cap. (Dunhall).
SALICYLANILIDE. N-Phenyl salicy-
lamide.
Use: Antifungal agent.
SALICYLATED BILE EXTRACT. Cholo-
gestin.
• **SALICYLATE MEGLUMINE.** USAN.
Use: Antirheumatic, analgesic.
SALICYLAZOSULFAPYRIDINE.
See: Sulfasalazine, U.S.P. XXIII.
• **SALICYLIC ACID,** U.S.P. XXIII. Collodi-
on, Plaster, Gel, U.S.P. XXIII. Benzoic
acid, 2-hydroxy. Orthohydroxybenzoic
acid. Cryst. Pkg. 1 oz, 0.25 lb, 1 lb; Pow.
Pkg. 0.25 lb, 1 lb.
Use: Keratolytic.
See: Calicylic, Creme (Gordon).
Listrex Scrub, Liq. (Warner-Lambert).

Maximum Strength Wart Remover, Liq. (Stiefel).
OFF-Ezy Corn & Callous Remover, Kit (Del).
Sal-Acid, Plaster (Pedinol).
Salactic Film, Liq. (Pedinol).
Salicylic Acid Acne Treatment, Bar (Stiefel).
Salonil, Cream (Torch).
Salicylic Acid Acne Treatment, Bar (Stiefel)
Sal-Plant, Gel (Pedinol).
Sebulex, Cream (Westwood).
Trans-Plantar, Transdermal patch (Tsumura Medical).
Wart-Off, Liq. (Leeming).
SALICYLIC ACID COMBINATIONS.
See: Acnaveen, Bar (Cooper).
Acno (Cummins).
Akne Drying Lotion, Liq. (Alto).
Clearasil, Preps (Procter & Gamble).
Cuticura (Purex).
Duofilm, Liq. (Stiefel).
Duo-WR, Soln. (Whorton).
Fostex, Cream, Liq. (Westwood).
Foursalco, Tab. (Jenkins).
Ionax, Liq. (Owen).
Ionil, Liq. (Owen).
Ionil T, Liq. (Owen).
Keralyt, Gel (Westwood).
Komed, Lot. (Barnes-Hind).
Neutrogena T/Sal, Shampoo (Neutrogena).
Occlusal HP, Liq. (GenDerm).
Oxy Clean Medicated Pads for Sensitive Skin (SK-Beecham).
Oxy Night Watch, Lot. (SK-Beecham).
Pernox, Lot. (Westwood).
Podiaspray, Aerosol Pow. (Dalin).
Pragmatar, Oint. (Menley & James).
Propa pH, Preps (Del Pharm.).
Salatar, Cream (Lannett).
Sal-Dex, Liq. (Scrip).
Salicylic Acid Soap (Stiefel).
Saligel, Gel (Stiefel).
Salsprin, Tab. (Seatrace).
Sebaveen, Shampoo (Cooper).
Sebucare, Liq. (Westwood).
Sebulex Shampoo, Liq. (Westwood).
Therac, Lot. (C&M Pharm.).
Tinver, Lot. (Barnes-Hind).
Vanseb, Dandruff Shampoo (Herbert).
Vanseb-T Tar Shampoo (Herbert).
Vericin, Oint. (Gordon).
Ver-Var, Soln. (Owen).
Zemacol, Lot. (Norwich).
SALICYLIC ACID CREAM. (Durel) Salicylic acid 5%, in Duromantel cream.
Use: Antiseborrheic, keratolytic.
SALICYLIC ACID SOAP. (Stiefel) Neutral

soap containing salicylic acid 2%. Cake 4 oz.
Use: Antiseborrheic, keratolytic.
SALICYLIC ACID & SULFUR SOAP. (Stiefel) Salicylic acid 3%, sulfur 10% in neutral soap bar. Cake 4.1 oz.
Use: Antiseborrheic, keratolytic.
• **SALICYLIC ACID TOPICAL FOAM,** U.S.P. XXIII.
Use: Keratolytic.
SALICYLSALICYLIC ACID. Salsalate. USAN.
Use: Analgesic.
See: Arcylate, Tab. (Hauck)
Disalcid, Tab. (Riker).
W/Aspirin.
See: Duragesic, Tab. (Meyer).
Persistin, Tab. (Fisons).
SALICYLSULPHONIC ACID. Sulfosalicylic acid. Dextrotest (Miles Diagnostic).
SALIGENIN. (City Chem.) Salicyl alcohol. Bot. 25 Gm, 100 Gm.
W/Merodicein.
See: Thantis, Loz. (Hyson, Westcott & Dunning).
SALINAZID. B.A.N. 2'-Salicylideneisonicotinohydrazide.
Use: Treatment of tuberculosis.
SALINE. (Bausch & Lomb) Buffered Isotonic. Thimerosal 0.001%, boric acid, NaCl, EDTA. Soln. Bot. 355 ml.
Use: Soft contact lens care.
SALINE SOLUTION. (Americal) Saline solution, isotonic, preserved. Bot. 12 oz.
Use: Soaking agent.
SALINE SPRAY. (Americal) Isotonic nonpreserved saline aerosol soln. Bot. 2 oz, 8 oz, 12 oz.
Use: Soft contact lens care.
SALINEX NASAL DROPS. (Muro) Buffered nasal isotonic saline drops. Bot. 15 ml w/dropper.
Use: Nasal moisturizer.
SALINEX NASAL MIST. (Muro) Sodium Cl 0.4%. Drops 15 ml, spray 50 ml.
Use: Nasal moisturizer.
SALIPAP. (Freeport) Salicylamide 5 gr, acetaminophen 5 gr/Tab. Bot. 1000s.
Use: Analgesic.
SALIPRAL. (Kenyon) Allylisobutyl-barbituric acid 3/4 gr, aspirin 3 gr, phenacetin 2 gr, caffeine gr/Tab. Bot. 1000s.
Use: Sedative, analgesic.
SALIPRAL-C. (Kenyon) Same formula as above w/vitamin C/Cap. Bot. 100s, 1000s.
Use: Sedative, analgesic, vitamin C supplement.
SALITHOL LIQUID. (Madland) Balm of methyl salicylate, menthol, camphor.

Bot. pt, gal. Oint. Jar 1 lb, 5 lb.
Use: External analgesic.
SALIVART. (Westport Pharm.) Sodium carboxymethylcellulose 1 gr, sorbitol 3 gr, sodium, potassium, calcium chloride 0.015 gr, magnesium Cl 0.005 gr, dibasic potassium phosphate, nitrogen (as propellant). Spray can 75 ml.
Use: Mouth preparation.
SALIVA SUBSTITUTE. (Roxane) Sorbitol, sodium carboxymethylcellulose, methylparaben. Dye free. Soln. Bot. 120 ml.
Use: Mouth preparation.
SALMEFAMOL. B.A.N. 1-(4-Hydroxy-3-hydroxy-methylphenyl)-2-(4-methoxy-α-methylphenethylamino)ethanol.
Use: Bronchodilator.
•**SALMETEROL XINAFOATE.** USAN.
Use: Bronchodilator.
SALOCOL. (Hauck) Acetaminophen 115 mg, aspirin 210 mg, salicylamide 65 mg, caffeine 16 mg/Tab. Bot. 1000s.
Use: Analgesic.
SAL-OIL-T. (Syosset) Coal tar 10%, salicylic acid 6%, allantoin vegetable oils. Soln. Bot. 60 ml.
Use: Antiseborrheic, keratolytic.
SALONIL. (Torch) Salicylic acid 40%, lanolin. Jar. lb.
Use: Antiseborrheic, keratolytic.
SALPABA W/COLCHICINE. (Madland) Sodium salicylate 0.25 Gm, para-aminobenzoic acid 0.25 Gm, vitamin C 20 mg, colchicine 0.25 mg/Tab. Bot. 100s, 1000s.
Use: Agent for gout.
SALPHENYL CAPSULES. (Hauck) Salicylamide 200 mg, acetaminophen 130 mg, chlorpheniramine maleate 2 mg, phenylephrine HCl 10 mg/Cap. Bot. 100s.
Use: Analgesic, antihistamine, decongestant.
SAL-PLANT. (Pedinol) Salicylic acid 17% in flexible collodion vehicle. Gel. Tube 14 g.
Use: Keratolytic.
•**SALSALATE,** U.S.P. XXIII. Cap., U.S.P. XXIII. USAN.
Use: Analgesic, antipyretic, anti-inflammatory.
See: Disalcid, Tab. (Riker).
Marthritic, Tab. (Marnel).
Salsitab, Tab. (Upsher-Smith).
SALSITAB. (Upsher-Smith) Salsalate 500 mg or 750 mg/Tab. Bot. 100s, 500s, UD 100s.
Use: Analgesic.
SALTEN. (Wren) Salicylamide 10 gr/Tab.

Bot. 100s, 1000s.
Use: Analgesic.
SAL-TROPINE. (Hope Pharm.) Atropine Sulfate 0.4 mg. Tab. Bot. 100s.
Use: Anticholinergic.
SALT REPLACEMENT PRODUCTS.
See: Slo-Salt (Mission).
Slo-Salt-K (Mission).
Sodium Chloride (Various Mfr.).
SALT SUBSTITUTES.
Use: Sodium-free seasoning agent.
See: Adolph's Salt Substitute (Adolph's).
Adolph's Seasoned Salt Substitute (Adolph's).
Morton Salt Substitute (Morton Salt).
Morton Seasoned Salt Substitute (Morton Salt).
NoSalt (SK-Beecham).
Nu-Salt (Cumberland Pkg.).
SALT TABLETS. (Cross) Sodium Cl 650 mg/Tab. Dispenser 500s.
Use: Salt replenisher.
SALURON. (Bristol Labs.) Hydroflumethiazide 50 mg/Tab. Bot. 100s.
Use: Diuretic.
SALUTENSIN. (Bristol Labs.) Hydroflumethiazide 50 mg, reserpine 0.125 mg/Tab. Bot. 100s, 1000s.
Use: Antihypertensive combination.
SALUTENSIN-DEMI. (Bristol Labs.) Hydroflumethiazide 25 mg, reserpine 0.125 mg/Tab. Bot. 100s.
Use: Antihypertensive combination.
SALVARSAN.
Use: Antisyphilitic.
SALVITE-B. (Faraday) Sodium chloride 7 gr, dextrose 3 gr, vitamin B_1 1 mg/Tab. Bot. 100s, 1000s.
SANAMYCIN. B.A.N. Actinomycin.
Use: Antineoplastic agent.
SANCHIA SILICONE PROTECTIVE CREAM. (Otis Clapp) Silicone and lanolin in greaseless cream base. Tube 3 oz, Jar 16 oz.
Use: Protective agent.
SANCURA. (Thompson) Benzocaine, chlorobutanol, chlorothymol, benzoic acid, salicylic acid, benzyl alcohol, cod liver oil, lanolin in a washable petrolatum base. Oint. 30 Gm, 90 Gm.
Use: Local anesthetic.
•**SANCYCLINE.** USAN. 6-Demethyl-6-deoxytetracycline. Formerly Norcycline.
Use: Antibiotic.
SANDIMMUNE. (Sandoz) Cyclosporine. **Oral soln.:** 100 mg/ml. Bot. 50 ml with graduated pipette. **Inj.:** 50 mg/ml Amp. 5 ml.
Use: Immunosuppressive agent.

SANDOGLOBULIN. (Sandoz) Immune globulin: Reconstitution fluid 1 Gm/33 ml; 3 Gm/100 ml; 6 Gm/200 ml.
Use: Immune serum.
SANDOPTAL. Isobutyl allylbarbituric acid.
See: Butalbital.
W/Caffeine, aspirin, phenacetin.
See: Fiorinal, Tab., Cap. (Sandoz).
W/Caffeine, aspirin, phenacetin, codeine phosphate.
See: Fiorinal w/codeine, Cap. (Sandoz).
SANDOPTAL SODIUM.
W/Sodium diethylbarbiturate, sodium phenylethylbarbiturate, scopolamine HBr, dihydroergotamine methanesulfonate.
See: Plexonal (Sandoz).
SANDOSTATIN. (Sandoz) Octreotide acetate 0.05 mg, 0.1 mg, 0.5 mg. Inj. Amp 1 ml.
Use: Adjunctive treatment of certain tumors.
SANESTRO. (Sandia) Estrone 0./ mg, estradiol 0.35 mg, estriol 0.14 mg/Tab. Bot. 100s, 1000s.
Use: Estrogen.
SANGER HER CAPS. (Edward J. Moore) Acetaminophen 227 mg, aspirin 227 mg, caffeine anhydrous 32.4 mg/Cap. Bot. 18s.
Use: Analgesic.
SANGER SPECIAL C-12. (Edward J. Moore) Salicylamide, co. colocynth extract, dried ferrous sulfate, blue cohosh/Tab. Bot. 24s.
SANGER VAGINAL ITCH CREAM. (Edward J. Moore) Benzocaine, dibucaine, tetracaine. Tube 1.25 oz.
Use: Local anesthetic combination.
• **SANGUINARIUM CHLORIDE.** USAN.
Use: Antimicrobial; anti-inflammatory; antifungal.
SANGUIS. (Sig) Liver 10 mcg, vitamin B_{12} 100 mcg, folic acid 1 mcg/ml. Vial 10 ml.
Use: Nutritional supplement.
SANHIST T.D. 5. (Sandia) Phenylpropanolamine HCl 50 mg, chlorpheniramine maleate 5 mg, ascorbic acid 100 mg/Tab. Bot. 100s, 1000s.
Use: Decongestant, antihistamine.
SANHIST T.D. 12. (Sandia) Phenylpropanolamine HCl 50 mg, chlorpheniramine maleate 12 mg, ascorbic acid 100 mg, methscopolamine nitrate 4 mg/Tab. Bot. 100s, 1000s.
Use: Decongestant, antihistamine combination.
SANI-SUPP. (G & W Labs) Glycerin,

sodium stearate. Supp. 10s, 12s, 24s, 25s, 48s, 50s, 100s, 1000s.
Use: Laxative.
SANITUBE. (Sanitube Co.) Calomel 30%, oxyquinoline benzoate, triethanolamine soap in a nonirritating excipient base. Oint. 5 Gm.
Use: Topical agent for prophylaxis of syphilis and gonorrhea.
SANI-VESS. (Forest Pharm.) Papain, sodium bicarbonate, citric acid, tartaric acid, lactose, thymol, aromatics. Pkg. 6 oz.
SANLUOL.
See: Arsphenamine (Various Mfr.).
SANOREX. (Sandoz) Mazindol 1 mg or 2 mg/Tab. Bot. 100s.
Use: Anorexiant.
SANSERT. (Sandoz) Methysergide maleate 2 mg/Tab. Bot. 100s.
Use: Agent for migraine.
SANSTRESS. (Sandia) Vitamins A 25,000 IU, D 400 IU, B_1 10 mg, B_2 5 mg, niacinamide 100 mg, B_6 1 mg, B_{12} 5 mcg, C 150 mg, calcium 103 mg, phosphorus 80 mg, iron 10 mg, copper 1 mg, iodine 0.1 mg, magnesium 5.5 mg, manganese 1 mg, potassium 5 mg, zinc 1.4 mg/Cap. Bot. 100s, 1000s.
Use: Vitamin/mineral supplement.
SANTISEPTIC LOTION. (Santiseptic) Menthol, phenol, benzocaine, zinc oxide, calamine. Bot. 4 oz.
Use: Minor skin irritations.
SANTYL. (Knoll) Proteolytic enzyme derived from *Clostridium histolyticum*. 250 units/Gm. Oint. Tube 15 Gm, 30 Gm.
Use: Topical enzyme preparation.
• **SAPERCONAZOLE.** USAN.
Use: Antifungal.
SAPONATED CRESOL SOLUTION.
See: Cresol (Various Mfr.).
SAPONINS, WATER SOLUBLE.
• **SARAFLOXACIN HYDROCHLORIDE.** USAN.
Use: Anti-infective.
SARAPIN. (High) An aqueous distillate of *Sarracenia purpurea*, pitcher plant, prepared for parenteral administration. Amp. 10 ml, 12s. Multidose vial 50 ml.
Use: Relief of neuromuscular or neuralgic pain.
SARATOGA. (Blair) Boric acid, zinc oxide, eucalyptol, white petrolatum. Oint. Tube 1 oz, 2 oz.
Use: Minor skin irritations.
SARDO BATH OIL CONCENTRATE. (Plough) Mineral oil, isopropyl palmitate. Bot. 3.75 oz, 7.75 oz.
Use: Emollient.

SARDO BATH & SHOWER. (Schering-Plough) Mineral oil, tocopherol. Oil. Bot. 112.5 ml.
Use: Emollient.
SARDOETTES MOISTURIZING TOW-ELETTES. (Plough) Mineral oil, isopropyl palmitate, impregnated towelling material. Individual packets. Box 25s.
Use: Emollient.
•**SARGRAMOSTIM.** USAN.
Use: Treatment of secondary neutropenia; leukopoietic (granulocyte macrophage colony-stimulating factor). [Orphan drug]
See: Leukine (Immune).
Prokine (Hoechst-Roussel).
SARISOL NO. 2. (Halsey) Butabarbital sodium 30 mg/Tab. Bot. 100s, 1000s.
Use: Sedative/hypnotic.
•**SARMOXICILLIN.** USAN.
Use: Antibacterial.
SARNA. (Stiefel) Camphor 0.5%, menthol 0.5%, phenol 0.5% in a soothing emollient base. Bot. 7.4 oz.
Use: Emollient.
SARNA ANTI-ITCH. (Stiefel) Camphor 5%, menthol 5%, carbomer 940, cetyl alcohol, DM DM hydantoin. Foam. Bot. 105 ml.
Use: Emollient.
SAROCYCLINE CAPSULES. (Saron) Tetracycline HCl 250 mg/Cap. Bot. 100s.
Use: Anti-infective, tetracycline.
•**SARPICILLIN.** USAN.
Use: Antibacterial.
SASTID SOAP. (Stiefel) Precipitated sulfur 10%. Bar 4.3 oz.
Use: Anti-acne.
SATUMOMAB PENDETIDE.
Use: Detection of ovarian cancer. [Orphan drug]
See: Oncoscint CR/OV.
SAUREX. (Enzyme Process) Phosphorus 30 mg, pepsin 1:10,000 equal to 100 mg pepsin 1:3000, betaine HCl 125 mg/Tab. Bot. 100s, 250s.
Use: Digestive aid.
SAXOL.
See: Petrolatum Liquid (Various Mfr.).
SCABENE LOTION. (Stiefel) Lindane 1% in lotion base. Bot. 2 oz, 16 oz.
Use: Pediculicide.
SCABENE SHAMPOO. (Stiefel) Lindane 1% in shampoo base. Bot. 2 oz, 16 oz.
Use: Pediculicide.
SCABICIDES.
See: Benzyl Benzoate (Various Mfr.).
Cuprex, Liq. (Calgon).
Eurax, Cream, Lot. (Geigy).

Kwell, Lot., Cream, Shampoo (Reed & Carnrick).
SCADAN SCALP LOTION. (Miles Pharm) Cetyl trimethyl ammonium bromide (cetab) 1%, stearyl dimethyl benzyl ammonium Cl 0.1%. Bot. 4 oz.
Use: Antiseborrheic.
CCALPICIN. (Combo) Hydrocorticone 1%, menthol, SD alcohol 40. Liq. Bot. 45 ml, 75 ml, 120 ml.
Use: Topical corticosteroid.
SCAN. (Parker) Water soluble gel. Bot. 8 oz, gal.
Use: Ultrasound B scan procedures.
SCARLET RED. (Lilly) Oint. 5%. Tube oz.
Use: Wound healing agent.
SCHAMBERG'S. (C & M Pharmacal) Menthol 0.15%, phenol 1%, zinc oxide, peanut oil, lime water. Bot. pt, gal.
Use: Antipruritic, counterirritant.
•**SCHICK TEST CONTROL,** U.S.P. XXIII.
Use: Diagnostic aid.
See: Diphtheria Toxin, Diagnostic, Inactivated, (Various Mfr.).
SCHIRMER TEAR TEST. (Various Mfr.) Sterile tear test strips.
Use: Diagnostic aid, ophthalmic.
SCHLESINGER'S SOLUTION.
See: Morphine HCl (Various Mfr.).
SCLAVO BIOLOGICALS. (Sclavo) A wide variety of generic forms of biological products.
SCLAVO PPD SOLUTION MANTOUX. (Sclavo) Tuberculin purified protein derivative (PPD) multiple puncture device. Test Pkg. 20s, 250s.
Use: Diagnostic aid.
SCLAVOTEST-PPD. (Sclavo) Tuberculin purified protein derivative (PPD) multiple puncture device. Test Pkg. 25s, 100s.
Use: Diagnostic aid.
SCLEREX. (Miller) Inositol 2 Gm, magnesium complex 34 mg, vitamins C 100 mg, calcium succinate 25 mg, A 2500 IU, D 200 IU, E 100 IU, B_1 5 mg, B_2 5 mg, B_6 5 mg, B_{12} 5 mcg, niacin 10 mg, niacinamide 30 mg, pantothenic acid 7.5 mg, folic acid 0.1 mg, iron 10 mg, copper 1 mg, manganese 2 mg, zinc 9 mg, iodine 0.10 mg/3 Tab. Bot. 60s.
Use: Vitamin/mineral supplement.
SCLEROMATE. (Palisades Pharm.) Morrhuate sodium 50 mg/ml. Inj. Vial 30 ml.
Use: Sclerosing agent.
SCLEROSING AGENTS.
See: Morrhuate Sodium (Pasadena Research Labs.).
Scleromate (Palisades Pharm.).
Sotradecol (Elkins-Sinn).
•**SCOPAFUNGIN.** USAN.

Use: Antifungal, antibacterial.
SCOPE. (Procter & Gamble) Cetylpyridinium Cl 0.45%, domiphen bromide 0.005%, SD alcohol 38F 18.5%. Liq. Bot. 180 ml, 360 ml, 540 ml, 720 ml, 960 ml, 1200 ml.
Use: Mouthwash.
SCOPOLAMINE. Hyoscine, l-Scopolamine, Epoxytropine tropate.
See: Hyoscine, Preps. (Various Mfr.).
SCOPOLAMINE AMINOXIDE HBr. W/Acetylcarbromal and bromisovalum.
See: Tranquinal, Tab. (Barnes-Hind).
SCOPOLAMINE HBR. (Invenex) Scopolamine HBr 0.3 mg/ml. Inj. Vial 1 ml.
Use: Preanesthetic sedation, obstetric amnesia, calming agent.
SCOPOLAMINE HBR. (Burroughs Wellcome) Scopolamine HBr 0.86 mg/ml. Inj. amp. 0.5 ml.
Use: Preanesthetic sedation, obstetric amnesia, calming agent.
SCOPOLAMINE HBR. (Various Mfr.) Scopolamine HBr 0.4 mg and 1 mg/ml. Inj. Amp., Vial 1 ml.
Use: Preanesthetic sedation, obstetric amnesia, calming agent.
• **SCOPOLAMINE HYDROBROMIDE,** U.S.P. XXIII. Inj., Ophth. Oint., Ophth. Soln., Tab., U.S.P. XXIII. Benzeneacetic acid, α-(hydroxymethyl)-, 9-methyl-3-oxa-9-azatricyclo [3.3.1.02,4]non-7-yl ester, hydrobromide, trihydrate. 6β, 7β-Epoxy-lαH,5αH-tropan-3α-ol(-)-tropate(ester)hydrobromide trihydrate. Hyoscine HBr.
Use: Sedative & hypnotic, anticholinergic, mydriatic, cyclopegic.
W/Atropine and hyoscyamine.
See: Atropine sulfate tab. Belladonna alkaloids.
W/Butabarbital, chlorpheniramine maleate.
See: Pedo-Sol, Elix., Tab. (Warren).
W/Hydroxypropyl methylcellulose.
See: Isopto HBr, Soln. (Alcon).
W/Hyoscyamine sulfate, atropine sulfate, phenobarbital.
See: Donnacin, Elix., Tab. (Pharmex). Hyonal C.T., Tab. (Paddock). Hytrona, Tab. (Webcon). Nilspasm, Tab. (Parmed). Sedamine, Tab. (Dunhall). Sedapar, Tab. (Parmed). Setamine, Tab. (Reid-Rowell). Spasaid, Cap. (Century).
W/Pamabrom, pyrilamine maleate, homatropine methylbromide, hyoscyamine sulfate, methamphetamine HCl.
See: Aridol, Tab. (MPL).

SCOPOLAMINE HYDROBROMIDE COMBINATIONS.
See: Belladonna Products. Hyoscine HBr. (Various Mfr.).
SCOPOLAMINE METHOBROMIDE.
See: Methscopolamine Bromide, Preps. (Various Mfr.).
SCOPOLAMINE METHYL NITRATE.
See: Methscopolamine Nitrate, Prep. (Various Mfr.).
SCOPOLAMINE SALTS.
See: Belladonna Products. Hyoscine salts.
SCORBEX/12. (Pasadena) Vitamins B_1 20 mg, B_2 3 mg, B_3 75 mg, B_5 5 mg, B_6 5 mg, B_{12} 1000 mcg, C 100 mg/ml. Vial dual compartment 10 ml.
Use: Vitamin supplement.
SCOTAVITE. (Scott/Cord) Vitamins A 25,000 IU, D 400 IU, B_1 10 mg, B_2 10 mg, B_6 5 mg, B_{12} 5 mcg, niacinamide 100 mg, calcium pantothenate 20 mg, C 200 mg, d-alpha tocopheryl 15 IU, acid succinate iodine 0.15 mg/Tab. Bot. 100s, 500s.
Use: Vitamin/mineral supplement.
SCOTCIL. (Scott/Cord) **Tab.:** Potassium penicillin 400,000 units w/calcium carbonate/Tab. Bot. 100s, 500s. **Pow.:** 80 ml, 150 ml.
Use: Antibacterial; penicillin.
SCOTCOF. (Scott/Cord) Doxtromethor phan HBr 6.85 mg, chlorpheniramine maleate 1.8 mg, phenylephrine HCl 4.4 mg, guaifenesin 66 mg, ammonium Cl 30.00 mg, chloroform 0.125 mg, alcohol 4.10%/5 ml. Bot. 4 oz, pt, gal.
Use: Antitussive, antihistamine, decongestant, expectorant.
SCOTGESIC. (Scott/Cord) **Cap.:** Acetaminophen 240 mg, salicylamide 100 mg, phenyltoloxamine dihydrogen citrate 30 mg, butabarbital ⅛ gr/Cap. Bot. 100s, 500s, 1000s. **Liq.:** Butabarbital 12.15 mg, acetaminophen 300 mg, salicylamide 60 mg, phenyltoloxamine citrate 30 mg/15 ml. Bot. 4 oz, pt.
Use: Analgesic, sedative.
SCOTNORD. (Scott/Cord) Chlorpheniramine maleate 8 mg, phenylephrine HCl 20 mg, methscopolamine nitrate 2.5 mg/Cap. Bot. 100s, 500s.
Use: Antihistamine, decongestant combination.
SCOTONIC. (Scott/Cord) Vitamins B_1 10 mg, B_2 5 mg, B_6 1 mg, niacinamide 50 mg, choline Cl 100 mg, inositol 100 mg, B_{12} 25 mcg, calcium 19 mg, iron 50 mg, folic acid 0.15 mg, alcohol 15%, sodium benzoate 0.1%/45 ml. Bot. pt, gal.

Use: Vitamin/mineral supplement.

SCOTREX. (Scott/Cord) Tetracycline 250 mg/Cap. or 5 ml. Cap. Bot. 16s, 100s, 500s. Syr. 2 oz, pt.
Use: Anti-infective.

SCOTT'S EMULSION. (Beecham Products) Vitamins A 1250 IU, D 1400 IU/4 tsp. Bot. 0.25 oz, 12.5 oz.
Use: Vitamin A & D supplement.

SCOT-TUSSIN ALLERGY. (Scot-Tussin) Diphenhydramine HCl 12.5 mg/5 ml, parabens, menthol. Liq. Bot. 120 ml.
Use: Antihistamine.

SCOT-TUSSIN DM COUGH CHASERS. (Scot-Tussin) Dextromethorphan HBr 2.5 mg, dye free, sorbitol. Loz. Pkg. 20s.
Use: Nonnarcotic antitussive.

SCOT-TUSSIN DM LIQUID. (Scot-Tussin) Dextromethorphan HBr 15 mg, chlorpheniramine maleate 2 mg/5 ml, alcohol 10%. Bot. 4 oz, 8 oz. Sugar free.
Use: Antihistamine, decongestant.

SCOT-TUSSIN DM2 SYRUP. (Scot-Tussin) Dextromethorphan HBr 15 mg, guaifenesin 100 mg, alcohol 1.4%/5 ml. Bot. 120 ml, 240 ml.
Use: Antitussive, expectorant.

SCOT-TUSSIN EXPECTORANT. (Scot-Tussin) Guaifenesin 100 mg/5 ml, alcohol 3.5%, saccharin, menthol, sorbitol, dye free. Syr. Bot. pt, gal, 120 ml.
Use: Expectorant.

SCOT-TUSSIN ORIGINAL 5-ACTION COLD MEDICINE. (Scot-Tussin) Phenylephrine HCl 4.2 mg, pheniramine maleate 13.3 mg, sodium citrate 83.3 mg, sodium salicylate 83.3 mg, caffeine citrate 25 mg/5 ml, sugar. Alcohol free. Grape flavor. Syr. Bot. 120 ml.
Use: Decongestant, antihistamine, analgesic.

SCOT-TUSSIN SUGAR-FREE. (Scot-Tussin) Dextromethorphan HBr 15 mg, chlorpheniramine maleate 2 mg/5 ml. Bot. 4 oz, 8 oz, 16 oz, gal.
Use: Antitussive, antihistamine.

SCOTT-TUSSIN SUGAR FREE EXPECTORANT. (Scot-Tussin) Guaifenesin 100 mg/5 ml w/alcohol 3.5%. Dye free, sodium free, sugar free.
Use: Expectorant.

SCOT-TUSSIN SUGAR-FREE 5-ACTION. (Scot-Tussin) Phenylephrine HCl 4.17 mg, pheniramine maleate 13.33 mg, sodium citrate 83.33 mg, sodium salicylate 83.33 mg, caffeine citrate 25 mg/5 ml, non-narcotic, non-alcoholic. Bot. 4 oz, 8 oz, 16 oz, gal.
Use: Decongestant, antihistamine, analgesic combination.

SCOT-TUSSIN WITH SUGAR. (Scot-Tussin) Phenylephrine HCl 4.17 mg, pheniramine maleate 13.3 mg, sodium citrate 83.33 mg, sodium salicylate 83.33 mg, caffeine citrate 25 mg/5 ml. Bot. 4 oz, 8 oz, 16 oz, gal.
Use: Decongestant, antihistamine, analgesic combination.

SCOTUSS. (Scott/Cord) Dextromethorphan 15 mg, chlorpheniramine maleate 1 mg, phenylephrine HCl 5 mg, phenylpropanolamine HCl 5 mg, N-acetyl-P-aminophenol 120 mg, guaifenesin 100 mg, alcohol 8.2%/5 ml. Bot. 4 oz, pt, gal.
Use: Antitussive, antihistamine, decongestant, expectorant combination.

SCOTUSS PEDIATRIC COUGH SYRUP. (Scott/Cord) Dextromethorphan HBr 7.5 mg, guaifenesin 50 mg, chlorpheniramine maleate 0.5 mg, phenylephrine HCl 2.5 mg, acetaminophen 60 mg, phenylpropanolamine HCl 2.5 mg, methylparaben 0.15%, propylparaben 0.05%/5 ml. Bot. 4 oz, pt.
Use: Antitussive, expectorant, antihistamine, decongestant, analgesic.

SCURENALINE.
See: Epinephrine, Prep. (Various Mfr.).

SCUROFORME.
See: Butyl Aminobenzoate (Various Mfr.).

S.D.M. #5. (ICI Americas) Mannitol hexanitrate 7% in lactose.
Use: Vasodilator.

S.D.M. #17. (ICI Americas) Nitroglycerin 10% in lactose.
Use: Vasodilator.

S.D.M. #23. (ICI Americas) Pentaerythritol tetranitrate 20% in lactose.
Use: Vasodilator.

S.D.M. #27. (ICI Americas) Nitroglycerin 10% in propylene glycol.
Use: Vasodilator.

S.D.M. #35. (ICI Americas) Pentaerythritol tetranitrate 35% in mannitol.
Use: Vasodilator.

S.D.M. #37. (ICI Americas) Nitroglycerin 10% in ethanol.
Use: Vasodilator.

S.D.M. #40. (ICI Americas) Isorsorbide dinitrate 25% in lactose.
Use: Vasodilator.

S.D.M. #50. (ICI Americas) Isosorbide dinitrate 50% in lactose.
Use: Vasodilator.

SDZ MSL-109. (Sandoz)
Use: Prophylaxis of cytomegalovirus disease in organ transplants & AIDS. [Orphan drug]

SEA GREENS. (Modern) Iodine 0.25

mg/Tab. Bot. 220s, 460s.
SEALE'S LOTION-MODIFIED. (C & M
Pharm.) Sulfur 6.4%, zinc oxide, ben-
tonite, sodium borate, acetone. Bot. pt.
Use: Anti-acne.
SEA MASTER. (Barth's) Vitamins A
10,000 units, D 400 units/Cap. Bot.
100s, 500s.
Use: Vitamin A & D supplement.
SEA-OMEGA 30. (Rugby) N-3 fat content
(mg) EPA 180, DHA 140. 100s.
Use: Nutritional supplement.
SEA-OMEGA 50. (Rugby) Omega-3
polyunsaturated fatty acid 1000 mg/Cap.
containing EPA 300 mg, DHA 200 mg,
vitamin E 1 IU Bot. 30s, 50s.
Use: Nutritional supplement.
SEA & SKI BABY LOTION FORMULA.
(Carter Products) Octyl-dimethyl PABA.
SPF 2. Lot. Bot. 120 ml.
Use: Sunscreen.
SEA & SKI GOLDEN TAN. (Carter Prod-
ucts) Padimate O. SPF 4. Lot. Bot. 120
ml.
Use: Sunscreen.
SEBA-LO. (Whorton) Acetone-alcohol
cleanser. Bot. 4 oz.
Use: Skin cleanser.
SEBANA SHAMPOO. (Myers) Salicylic
acid 2%. Bot. 4 oz, 8 oz, pt, qt, 0.5 gal.
Use: Antiseborrheic.
SEBANATAR SHAMPOO. (Myers) Sali-
cylic acid 2%, liquor carbonis detergens
3%. Bot. 4 oz, 8 oz, pt, qt, 0.5 gal, gal.
Use: Antiseborrheic.
SEBA-NIL CLEANSING MASK. (Owen)
Astringent face mask containing ben-
tonite, polyethylene, SD alcohol-40, sul-
fated castor oil, titanium dioxide, kaolin,
chromium oxide, methylparaben. Tube
3.7 oz.
Use: Anti-acne.
SEBA-NIL LIQUID. (Owen) Alchol 49.7%,
acetone, polysorbate 20. Liq. Bot. 240
ml, pt.
Use: Anti-acne.
SEBASORB LOTION FOR ACNE. (Sum-
mers) Activated attapulgite 10%,
polysorbate 80, colloidal sulfur 2%, sali-
cylic acid 2%. Bot. 2 oz. w/dispenser
top.
Use: Anti-acne.
SEBEX. (Rugby) Pyrithione zinc 2%.
Shampoo. Bot. 120 ml.
Use: Antiseborrheic.
SEBEX-T. (Rugby) Coal tar soln. 5%, col-
loidal sulfur 2%, salicylic acid 2%.
Shampoo. Bot. 120 ml.
Use: Antiseborrheic.
SEBIZON LOTION. (Schering) Sulfac-

etamide sodium 100 mg, methylparaben
1 mg w/trisodium edetate, sodium thiosulfate, propylene glycol, isopropyl
myristate, propylene glycol monostearate, polyethylene glycol 400 monostearate, water. Tube 3 oz.
Use: Antiseborrheic.
SEBUCARE SCALP LOTION. (Westwood) Laureth-4, salicylic acid 1.5%, alcohol 61%, water, PPG 40 butyl ether,
dihydroabietyl alcohol, fragrance. Bot. 4
oz.
Use: Antiseborrheic.
SEBULEX CREAM SHAMPOO. (Westwood) Same formula as Sebulex in a
cream shampoo. Tube 4 oz.
Use: Antiseborrheic.
SEBULEX SHAMPOO. (Westwood) Sulfur 2%, salicylic acid 2%. Cream 4.2 oz,
Liq. 4 oz.
Use: Antiseborrheic.
SEBULEX WITH CONDITIONERS.
(Westwood) Sulfur 2%, salicylic acid
2%. Bot. 4 oz, 8 oz.
Use: Antiseborrheic.
SEBULON. (Westwood) Pyrithione zinc
2%. Shampoo. Bot. 120 ml, 240 ml.
Use: Antiseborrheic.
SEBUTONE CREAM SHAMPOO. (West-
wood) Tar equivalent to coal tar U.S.P.
5%, sulfur 2%, salicylic acid 2%, in se-
bulytic type surface active soapless
cleansers, wetting agents. Tube 4 oz.
Use: Antiseborrheic, antipsoriatic.
**SEBUTONE THERAPEUTIC TAR SHAM-
POO.** (Westwood) Tar equivalent to
coal tar, U.S.P. 0.5%, sulfur 2%, salicylic
acid 2%, in sebulytic-type surface-active
soapless cleansers, wetting agents. Bot.
4 oz, 8 oz.
Use: Antiseborrheic, antipsoriatic.
SECALCIFEROL.
Use: Treatment of familial hypophos-
phatemic rickets. [Orphan drug]
See: Osteo-D.
SECBUTOBARBITONE. B.A.N. 5-sec-
Butyl-5-ethylbarbituric acid. Butabarbi-
tone.
Use: Sedative/hypnotic.
• **SECOBARBITAL,** U.S.P. XXIII. Elix.,
U.S.P. XXIII. 5-Allyl-5-(methylbutyl)-bar-
bituric acid. Pow., Bot. ⅛ oz, 1 oz.
Use: Hypnotic.
See: Seco-8, Cap. (Fleming).
SECOBARBITAL COMBINATIONS.
See: Efed, Syr., Tab. (Alto).
Monosyl, Tab. (Arcum).
Quad-Set, Tab. (Kenyon).
SECOBARBITAL ELIXIR.
See: Seconal Elix. (Lilly).

• **SECOBARBITAL SODIUM,** U.S.P. XXIII.
Cap., Inj., Sterile, U.S.P. XXIII. Sodium
5-allyl-5-(1-methyl-butyl)-barbiturate.
Quinalbarbitone Sodium. B.A.N. (Various Mfr.) 100 mg. Cap. Bot. 100s, 500s,
1000s.
Use: Sedative/hypnotic.
See: Seco-8, Cap. (Fleming).
Seconal Sodium, Prep. (Lilly).
SECOBARBITAL SODIUM. (Wyeth-Ayerst) 50 mg/ml. Inj. Tubex 2 ml.
Use: Sedative, hypnotic.
• **SECOBARBITAL SODIUM AND AMO-BARBITAL SODIUM CAPSULES,**
U.S.P. XXIII.
Use: Hypnotic, sedative.
See: Tuinal, Cap. (Lilly).
SECONAL SODIUM PULVULES. (Lilly)
Secobarbital sodium 100 mg. Cap. Bot.
100s, UD 100s.
Use: Sedative, hypnotic.
SECRAN LIQUID. (Scherer) Vitamins B_1
10 mg, B_3 10 mg, B_{12} 25 mcg, alcohol
17%. Bot. pt.
Use: Vitamin B supplement.
SECRAN PRENATAL TABS. (Scherer)
Vitamins A acetate 8000 units, D 400 IU,
E 30 IU, C 60 mg, niacinamide 20 mg,
B_2 2 mg, B_1 1.7 mg, B_6 2.5 mg, B_{12} 8
mcg, folic acid 1 mg, calcium 250 mg,
magnesium, elemental zinc 20 mg, iron
60 mg/Tab. Bot. 100s, 240s.
Use: Vitamin/mineral supplement.
SECRETIN. B.A.N. A hormone obtained
from duodenal mucosa.
Use: Diagnostic for pancreatic dysfunction.
SECRETIN FERRING POWDER. (Ferring) Secretin 75 cu/10 ml Vial. 10 cu/ml
when reconstituted with 7.5 ml.
Use: Diagnostic aid.
SECTRAL. (Wyeth-Ayerst) Acebutolol
HCl 200 or 400 mg/ Cap. Bot. 100s, UD
100s.
Use: Antihypertensive.
SEDACANE. (Edward J. Moore) Acetaminophen 120 mg, salicylamide 210 mg,
caffeine 30 mg, calcium gluconate 60
mg/Cap. Bot. 12.
Use: Analgesic combination.
SEDAFORM.
See: Chlorobutanol (Various Mfr.).
SEDAJEN. (Jenkins) Phenobarbital 5/16
gr, passiflora 1.5 gr, hyoscyamus gr (total alkaloids 0.0003 gr)/Tab. Bot. 1000s.
Use: Sedative, antispasmodic.
SEDALGESIC INSERTS. (Table Rock)
Aspirin 195 mg, secobarbital 30 mg/Insert. Box 12s.

Use: Analgesic, sedative.
SEDALGESIC TABLETS. (Table Rock)
Bromisovalum 150 mg, acetaminophen
100 mg, salicylamide 100 mg/Tab. Bot.
100s, 500s.
Use: Sedative/analgesic.
SEDAMINE. (Approved) Phosphorated
carbohydrate soln. Bot. 4 oz.
Use: Antinauseant.
SEDAMINE. (Dunhall) Hyoscyamine sulfate 0.1037 mg, atropine sulfate 0.0194
mg, hyoscine HBr 0.0065 mg, phenobarbital 16.2 mg/Tab. Bot. 100s, 1000s.
Use: Antispasmodic, sedative.
SEDAPAP #3 CAPSULES. (Mayrand)
Acetaminophen 500 mg, butalbital 50
mg, codeine phosphate 30 mg/Cap. Bot.
100s.
Use: Narcotic analgesic combination.
SEDAPAP-10 TABLETS. (Mayrand) Acetaminophen 10 gr, butabarbital 50
mg/Tab. Bot. 100s.
Use: Analgesic, sedative.
SEDAPAR. (Parmed) Atropine sulfate
0.0195 mg, hyoscine HBr 0.0065 mg,
hyoscyamine sulfate 0.1040 mg, phenobarbital 0.25 gr/Tab. Bot. 1000s.
Use: Sedative, antispasmodic.
SEDATANS TABLETS. (Lannett) Tab.
Bot. 100s, 1000s.
SEDATIVE/HYPNOTIC AGENTS.
See: Bromides (Various Mfr.).
Barbiturates (Various Mfr.).
Butisol Sodium (McNeil).
Carbamide (Urea) Compounds (Various Mfr.).
Chloral Hydrate, Preps. (Various Mfr.).
Chlorobutanol (Various Mfr.).
Dalmane, Cap. (Roche).
Intasedol, Elix. (Elder).
Largon, Inj. (Wyeth-Ayerst).
Lotusate, Cap. (Sanofi Winthrop).
Noludar, Tab., Cap. (Roche).
Paraldehyde, Preps. (Various Mfr.).
Phenergan HCl, Preps. (Wyeth-Ayerst).
Placidyl, Cap. (Abbott).
Plexonal, Tab. (Sandoz).
Restoril, Cap. (Sandoz).
Triazolam, Tab. (Various Mfr.).
Valmid, Tab. (Lilly).
Vingesic, Cap. (Amid).
SEDEVAL.
See: Barbital (Various Mfr.).
SEDRAGESIC TABLETS. (Lannett) Acetaminophen 0.325 Gm, salicylamide
0.195 Gm, d-amphetamine sulfate 2.5
mg, hexobarbital 8 mg, secobarbital
sodium 2.7 mg, butabarbital sodium 2.7
mg, phenobarbital 2.7 mg/Tab. Bot.

100s, 1000s.
Use: Analgesic, sedative combination.
SEDRAL. (Vita Elixir) Phenobarbital ⅛ gr, theophylline 2 gr, ephedrine gr/Tab.
Use: Sedative, bronchodilator.
• **SEELAZONE.** USAN.
Use: Anti-inflammatory, uricosuric.
• **SEGLITIDE ACETATE.** USAN.
Use: Antidiabetic
SELDANE. (Marion Merrell Dow) Terfenadine 60 mg/Tab. Bot. 100s.
Use: Antihistamine.
SELDANE-D. (Marion Merrell Dow) Pseudoephedrine HCl 120 mg, terfenadine 60 mg/SR Tab. Lactose. Bot. 100s.
Use: Decongestant, antihistamine.
SELEGILINE HCl.
Use: Antiparkinson agent. [Orphan drug]
See: Eldepryl (Somerset).
SELENICEL. (Pasadena Research) Selenium yeast complex 200 mcg, vitamins C 100 mg, E 100 mg/Cap. Bot. 90s.
Use: Vitamin supplement.
• **SELENIOUS ACID,** U.S.P. XXIII, Inj., U.S.P. XXIII.
SELENIUM. (Nion) Selenium 50 mcg/Tab. Bot. 100s.
Use: Parenteral nutritional supplement.
SELENIUM DISULFIDE.
See: Selenium Sulfide, Deterg., Susp. (Various Mfr.).
• **SELENIUM SULFIDE,** U.S.P. XXIII., Lot. U.S.P. XXIII.
Use: Treatment of dandruff; antifungal, antiseborrheic.
See: Exsel Lotion (Herbert).
Iosel 250, Liq. (Owen).
Selsun, Susp. (Abbott).
Selsun Gold for Women, Shampoo (Ross).
• **SELENOMETHIONINESE 75 INJECTION,** U.S.P. XXII. 2-Amino-4-(methylselenyl) butyric acid (^{75}Se).
Use: Diagnostic aid.
See: Sethotope, Inj. (Squibb).
SELE-PAK. (SoloPak) Selenium 40 mcg/ml. Inj. Vial 10 ml, 30 ml.
SELEPEN. (LyphoMed) Selenium 40 mcg/ml. Inj. Vial 10 ml, 30 ml.
Use: Parenteral nutritional supplement.
SELESTOJECT. (Mayrand) Betamethasone sodium phosphate 4 mg/ml (equivalent to 3 mg betamethasone alcohol). Soln. Vial 5 ml.
Use: Corticosteroid.
• **SELFOTEL.** USAN.
Use: NMDA antagonist.
SELORA POWDER. (Sanofi Winthrop)

Potassium Cl.
Use: Salt substitute.
SELSUN BLUE. (Ross) Selenium sulfide 1% in lotion base. Bot. 4 oz, 7 oz, 11 oz.
Dry, oily, normal extra conditioning, and extra medicated (contains 0.5% menthol) formulas.
Use: Antiseborrheic.
SELSUN GOLD FOR WOMEN. (Ross) Selenium sulfide 1%. Shampoo. Bot. 120 ml, 210 ml, 330 ml.
Use: Antiseborrheic.
SELSUN SUSPENSION. (Abbott) Selenium sulfide 2.5%. Bot. 4 fl oz.
Use: Antiseborrheic.
• **SEMATILIDE HYDROCHLORIDE.** USAN.
Use: Antiarrhythmic.
SEMICID. (Whitehall) Nonoxynol-9 100 mg/Vag. Supp. Box 10s, 20s.
Use: Contraceptive.
SEMPREX-D. (Burroughs Wellcome) Acrivastine 8 mg, pseudoephedrine HCl 60 mg. Cap. Bot. 100s.
Use: Decongestant.
• **SEMUSTINE.** USAN.
Use: Antineoplastic.
SENEXON. (Rugby) Senna concentrate 187 mg/Tab. Sugar. Bot. 100s, 1000s.
Use: Laxative.
SENILAVITE. (Defco) Vitamins A 5000 IU, C 100 mg, D_1 2.5 mg, D_2 2 mg, nicotinamide 10 mg, B_6 1 mg, calcium pantothenate 5 mg, B_{12} w/intrinsic factor concentrate 0.133 IU, ferrous fumarate 150 mg, glutamic acid HCl 150 mg, docusate sodium 50 mg/Cap. Bot. 100s.
Use: Nutritional supplement.
SENILEZOL ELIXIR. (Edwards) Vitamins B_1 0.42 mg, B_2 0.42 mg, B_3 1.67 mg, B_5 0.83 mg, B_6 0.17 mg, B_{12} 0.83 mcg, ferric pyrophosphate 3.3 mg, alcohol 15%. Bot. pt.
Use: Vitamin/mineral supplement.
SENIOR FORMULA CAPSULES. (Life's Finest) Calcium 125 mg, iron 5 mg, vitamins A 2500 IU, D 200 IU, E 15.1 mg, B_1 1.1 mg, B_2 1.2 mg, B_3 15 mg, B_5 7.5 mg, B_6 1.5 mg, B_{12} 4.5 mcg, C 45 mg, folic acid 0.2 mg, Cr, Cu, Mg, Mn, P, Se, zinc 3.75 mg/Cap. Bot. 60s, 90s, 180s.
Use: Vitamin/mineral supplement.
• **SENNA,** U.S.P. XXIII. Fluidextract, Syr., U.S.P. XXIII. Alexandrian.
Use: Cathartic.
See: Casafru, Liq. (Key).
SENNA CONC., STANDARDIZED.
Use: Cathartic.
See: Senokot, Gran., Tab., Supp. (Purdue Frederick).

X-Prep. Pow. (Gray).
W/Docusate sodium.
See: Gentlax S. Tab. (Blair).
Senokap-DSS, Cap. (Purdue Frederick).
Senokot S., Tab. (Purdue Frederick).
W/Guar gum.
See. Gentlax B Tab., Gran. (Blair).
W/Psyllium.
See: Perdiem, Gran. (Rhone-Poulenc Rorer Consumer).
Senokot W/Psyllium Pow. (Purdue Frederick).
SENNA FRUIT EXTRACT, STANDARIZED.
Use: Cathartic.
See: Senokot, Syr. (Purdue Frederick). X-Prep, Liq. (Gray).
SENNA-GEN TABS. (Goldline) Bot. 100s, 1000s.
Use: Laxative.
SENNA POWDER COMPOUND.
(Penick) Comp. licorice pow. Bot. 0.25 lb, 1 lb.
Use: Mild cathartic.
•**SENNOSIDES,** U.S.P. XXIII. Tab., U.S.P. XXIII.
Use: Laxative.
See: Gentle Nature (Sandoz Consumer).
SENNOSIDES A & B.
Use: Laxative.
See: Ex-Lax Gentle Nature (Sandoz).
SENOKOT TABLETS and GRANULES.
(Purdue Frederick) **Gran.:** Standardized senna concentrate. Canister 2 oz, 6 oz, 12 oz. **Tab.:** Bot. 50s, 100s, 1000s, Unit strip pack 100s, Box 20s.
Use: Laxative.
SENOKOT S TABLETS. (Purdue Frederick) Standardized senna concentrate w/docusate sodium. Tab. Bot. 30s, 60s, 1000s.
Use: Laxative.
SENOKOT SUPPOSITORIES. (Purdue Frederick) Standardized senna concentrate. Pkg. 6s.
Use: Laxative.
SENOKOT SYRUP. (Purdue Frederick) Standardized extract senna fruit. Bot. 2 oz, 8 oz.
Use: Laxative.
SENOKOTXTRA. (Purdue Fredrick) Senna concentrate 374 mg/Tab. Bot. 12s.
Use: Laxative.
SENOLAX. (Schein) Senna concentrate 217 mg/Tab. Bot. 100s, 1000s.
Use: Laxative.
SENSITIVE EYES DAILY CLEANER.
(Bausch & Lomb) Isotonic solution, bo-

rate buffer, surfactant cleaner, sodium Cl, hydroxypropyl methylcellulose, sorbic acid 0.25%, EDTA 0.5%, thimerosal free. Soln. Bot. 30 ml.
Use: Soft contact lens care.
SENSITIVE EYES DROPS. (Bausch & Lomb) Isotonic solution with a borate buffer system, sorbic acid 0.1%, EDTA. Soln. Bot. 30 ml.
Use: Soft contact lens care.
SENSITIVE EYES PLUS. (Bausch & Lomb) Boric acid, sodium borate, potassium chloride, sodium chloride, polyaminopropyl biguanide 0.00003%, EDTA 0.025%. Soln. Bot. 355 ml.
Use: Soft contact lens care.
SENSITIVE EYES SALINE. (Bausch & Lomb) Sodium Cl, borate buffer, sorbic acid 0.1%, EDTA. Soln. Bot. 118 ml, 237 ml, 355 ml.
Use: Soft contact lens care.
SENSITIVE EYES SALINE/CLEANING SOLUTION. (Bausch & Lomb) Isotonic solution w/borate buffer, NaCl, poloxamine, sorbic acid 0.15%, EDTA 0.1%. Soln. Bot. 240 ml.
Use: Soft contact lens care.
SENSODYNE FRESH MINT TOOTHPASTE. (Block) Potassium nitrate 5%, sodium monofluorophosphate 0.76%, saccharin, sorbitol, mint flavor. Tube 2.4 oz, 4.6 oz.
Use: Preparation for sensitive teeth.
SENSODYNE-SC TOOTHPASTE.
(Block) Glycerin, sorbitol, sodium methyl cocoyltaurate, PEG-40 stearate, strontium Cl hexahydrate 10%, methyl and propylparabens, tint. Tube 2.1 oz, 4.0 oz.
Use: Preparation for sensitive teeth.
SENSORCAINE. (Astra) Bupivacaine HCl 0.25%, 0.50% or 0.75%. Inj. Amp. 30 ml. Vial 10 ml, 30 ml, 50 ml.
Use: Local anesthetic.
SENSORCAINE W/EPINEPHRINE. (Astra) Bupivacaine HCl 0.5%, epinephrine 1:200,000. Inj. Amp. 30 ml. Vial 30 ml.
Use: Local anesthetic.
•**SEPAZONIUM CHLORIDE.** USAN.
Use: Anti-infective, topical.
•**SEPERIDOL HCl.** USAN. 4-[4-(4-Chloro-α,α,α-trifluoro-m-tolyl)-4-hydroxypiperidino]-4'-fluorobutyrophenone HCl. Under study.
Use: Neuroleptic, antipsychotic.
SEPO. (Otis Clapp) Benzocaine. Loz. Bot. 80s. Safety pack 500s.
Use: Local anesthetic.
•**SEPROXETINE HYDROCHLORIDE.** USAN.

Use: Antidepressant.

SEPTA. (Circle) Bacitracin 400 units, neomycin sulfate 5 mg, polymyxin B sulfate 5000 units/Gm in ointment base. Tube oz.
Use: Anti-infective, topical.

SEPTI-CHEK. (Roche Diagnostics) Blood culture and simultaneous sub-culture system with three media to support clinically significant pathogens. Quick and easy assembly forms a closed system to protect sub-cultures from contamination.
Use: Diagnostic aid.

SEPTIPHENE. 4-Chloro-α-phenyl-o-cresol. Santophen 1. (Monsanto).
Use: Disinfectant.

SEPTI-SOFT. (Vestal) Hexachlorophene 0.25%. Liq. Bot. 240 ml, pt, gal.
Use: Antiseptic, germicide.

SEPTISOL. (Vestal) **Soln.:** Hexachlorophene 0.25%. Bot. 240 ml, qt, gal. **Foam:** Hexachlorophene 0.23%, alcohol 46%. In 180 ml, 600 ml.
Use: Antiseptic, germicide.

SEPTO. (Vita Elixir) Methylbenzethonium Cl, ethanol 2%, menthol.
Use: Antiseptic, germicide.

SEPTRA. (Burroughs Wellcome) Sulfamethoxazole 400 mg, trimethoprim 80 mg/Tab. Bot. 100s, 500s, UD 100s.
Use: Anti-infective.

SEPTRA I.V. (Burroughs Wellcome) **80/400:** Trimethoprim 80 mg, sulfamethoxazole 400 mg/5 ml. Amp. 5 ml, Vial 10 ml, 20 ml, Add-Vantage Vial 5 ml, 10 ml.
Use: Anti-infective.

SEPTRA IV ADD-VANTAGE. (Burroughs Wellcome) Trimethoprim 80 mg, sulfamethoxazole 400 mg/5 ml vial or trimethoprim 160 mg, sulfamethoxazole 800 mg/10 ml vial. Box. 10s.
Use: Anti-infective.

SEPTRA DS. (Burroughs Wellcome) Trimethoprim 160 mg, sulfamethoxazole 800 mg/Tab. Bot. 100s, 250s, UD 100s.
Use: Anti-infective.

SEPTRA GRAPE SUSPENSION. (Burroughs Wellcome) Trimethoprim 40 mg, sulfamethoxazole 200 mg/5 ml. Bot. 473 ml.
Use: Anti-infective.

SEPTRA SUSPENSION. (Burroughs Wellcome) Trimethoprim 40 mg, sulfamethoxazole 200 mg/5 ml. Bot. 100 ml, 473 ml.
Use: Anti-infective.

• **SERACTIDE ACETATE.** USAN. Ala[26]-Gly[27]-SER[31α1-39] corticotrophin acetate.
Use: Corticotrophic peptide, hormone

(adrenocorticotropic).
See: Acthar Gel (Armour).

SER-A-GEN. (Goldline) Hydrochlorothiazide 15 mg, reserpine 0.1 mg, hydralazine HCl 25 mg/Tab. Bot. 100s, 1000s.
Use: Antihypertensive combination.

SERALAZIDE. (Lannett) Hydrochlorothiazide 15 mg, reserpine 0.1 mg, hydralazine HCl 25 mg/Tab. Bot. 100s, 1000s.
Use: Antihypertensive combination.

SERALYZER. (Miles Diagnostic) A system for the measurement of enzymes, potassium levels, blood chemistries and therapeutic drug assays consisting of a reflectance photometer and a series of solid-phase reagent strips.
Use: Diagnostic aid.

SER-AP-ES. (Ciba) Reserpine 0.1 mg, hydralazine HCl 25 mg, hydrochlorothiazide 15 mg/Tab. Bot. 100s, 1000s, Accu-Pak 100s.
Use: Antihypertensive combination.

SERAX. (Wyeth-Ayerst) Oxazepam. **Cap.:** 10 mg, 15 mg, 30 mg. Bot. 100s, 500s, Redipak 25s, 100s. **Tab.:** 15 mg. Bot. 100s.
Use: Antianxiety agent.

SEREEN. (Foy) Chlordiazepoxide HCl 10 mg/Cap. Bot. 500s, 1000s.
Use: Antianxiety agent.

SEREINE. (Optikem) EDTA 0.1%, benzalkonium chloride 0.01%. Soln. Bot. 60 ml.
Use: Hard contact lens care.

SERENE. (Approved) Salicylamide 2 gr, scopolamine aminoxide HBr 0.2 mg/Cap. Bot. 24s, 60s.
Use: Analgesic, sedative.

SERENTIL. (Boehringer Ingelheim) Mesoridazine besylate. **Inj.:** 25 mg/ml Amp. 1 ml **Tab.:** 10 mg, 25 mg, 50 mg, 100 mg. Bot. 100s. **Oral Conc.:** 25 mg/ml dropper.
Use: Antipsychotic.

SEREVENT. (Allen & Hanburys) Salmeterol xinafoate 25 mcg from actuator/actuation. Aerosol. Canister 60 actuations, refills 120 actuations.
Use: Bronchodilator.

SERICINASE. A proteolytic enzyme.

• **SERINE,** U.S.P. XXIII. $C_3H_7NO_3$ as L-serine.
Use: Amino acid.

• **SERMETACIN.** USAN.
Use: Anti-inflammatory.

• **SERMORELIN ACETATE.** USAN.
Use: Growth hormone-releasing factor (human); diagnostic aid (growth fail-

ure). [Orphan drug]

SERNYLAN. Phencyclidine. B.A.N.
1-(1-Phenycyclohexyl)-piperidine HCl.
Use: Anesthetic.

SEROMYCIN. (Lilly) Cycloserine 250
mg/Pulv. Bot. 40s.
Use: Antituberculous agent.

SEROPHENE. (Serono) Clomiphene citrate 50 mg/Tab. Bot. 10s, 30s.
Use: Ovulation stimulant.

**SEROTONIN REUPTAKE INHIBITORS,
SELECTIVE.**
Use: Antidepressant.
See: Paxil, Tab. (SK-Beecham).
Prozac, Liq., Pulv. (Dista).
Zoloft, Tab. (Roerig).

SERPALAN TABLETS. (Lannett) Reserpine alkaloid 0.1 mg, 0.25 mg/Tab. Bot.
100s, 500s, 1000s.
Use: Antihypertensive.

SERPASIL-APRESOLINE. (Ciba) **#1:** Reserpine 0.1 mg, hydralazine HCl 25
mg/Tab. Bot. 100s. **#2:** Reserpine 0.2
mg, hydralazine HCl 50 mg/Tab. Bot.
100s.
Use: Antihypertensive combination.

SERPASIL-ESIDRIX. (Ciba) **#1:** Reserpine 0.1 mg, hydrochlorothiazide 25
mg/Tab. **#2:** Reserpine 0.1 mg, hydrochlorothiazide 50 mg/Tab. Bot. 100s,
1000s.
Use: Antihypertensive combination.

SERPAZIDE TABLETS. (Major) Reserpine 0.1 mg, hydralazine HCl 25 mg, hydrochlorothiazide 15 mg. Bot. 100s,
1000s.
Use: Antihypertensive combination.

**SERRATIA MARCESCENS EXTRACT
(POLYRIBOSOMES).**
Use: Primary brain malignancies. [Or-
phan drug]

SERTABS. (Table Rock) Reserpine 0.25
mg or 0.5 mg/Tab. Bot. 100s, 500s.
Use: Antihypertensive.

SERTINA. (Fellows) Reserpine 0.25
mg/Tab. Bot. 1000s, 5000s.
Use: Antihypertensive.

•**SERTINDOLE.** USAN.
Use: Antipsychotic; neuroleptic.

•**SERTRALINE HYDROCHLORIDE.**
USAN.
Use: Antidepressant.
See: Zoloft (Roerig)

SERUM, ALBUMIN, NORMAL HUMAN.
See: Albumin Human, U.S.P. XXIII.
(Various Mfr.).

**SERUM, ALBUMIN, HUMAN, RADIOIOD-
INATED.**
See: Iodinated. I-125
Albumin Injection, U.S.P. XXIII.

**SERUM, ANTIHEMOPHILUS INFLUEN-
ZAE TYPE B (RABBIT).** Anti-
haemophilus (influenzae Type B Serum,
Rabbit). (Squibb).

SERUM, GLOBULIN (HUMAN), IMMUNE.
See: Globulin Immune Serum (Human),
(Various Mfr.).

SERUM, MEASLES IMMUNE, HUMAN.
See: Measles Virus Vaccine Live,
U.S.P. XXIII.

SERUM PERTUSSIS IMMUNE, HUMAN.
See: Pertussis Vaccine Adsorbed,
U.S.P. XXIII.

SERUTAN. (Beecham Products) Psyllium. **Gran.:** Pkg. 6 oz, 18 oz. **Pow.:** 7 oz,
14 oz, 21 oz. Fruit flavored: 6 oz, 12 oz,
18 oz.
Use: Laxative.

•**SERVIRUMAB.** USAN.
Use: Antiviral.

SERZONE. (Bristol-Myers Squibb)
See: Nefazodone.

•**SESAME OIL,** N.F. XVIII.
Use: Pharm. aid (solvent).

SESAME STREET VITAMINS. (McNeil-
CPC) **For ages 4 and older:** Vitamins A
5000 IU, B_1 1.5 mg, B_{12} 6 mcg, C 60 mg,
D 400 IU, E 30 IU, folic acid 400 mcg, biotin 300 mcg/Chew Tab. Bot. 60s. **For
ages 2-3:** Vitamins A 2500 IU, B_1 0.7
mg, B_2 0.8 mg, B_3 9 mg, B_5 5 mg, B_6 0.7
mg, B_{12} 3 mcg, C 40 mg, D 400 IU, E 10
IU, folic acid 200 mcg, biotin 150
mcg/Chew Tab. Bot. 60s.
Use: Vitamin supplement.

**SESAME STREET VITAMINS AND MIN-
ERALS.** (McNeil-CPC) **For ages 4 and
older:** Vitamins A 5000 IU, B_1 1.5 mg, B_2
1.7 mg, B_3 20 mg, B_5 10 mg, B_6 2 mg,
B_{12} 6 mcg, C 60 mg, D 400 IU, E 30 IU,
folic acid 400 mcg, biotin 300 mcg, calcium 100 mg, iron 18 mg, iodine 150 mcg,
zinc 15 mg, copper 2 mg/Chew Tab. Bot.
60s. **For ages 2-3:** Vitamins A 2500 IU,
B_1 0.7 mg, B_{12} 3 mcg, C 40 mg, D 400
IU, E 10 IU, folic acid 200 mcg, biotin
150 mcg, calcium 80 mg, iron 10 mg, iodine 70 mcg, zinc 8 mg, copper 1
mg/Chew Tab. Bot. 60s.
Use: Vitamin/mineral supplement.

SESTRON. N-Ethyl-3,3'-diphenyl-
dipropylamine. Profenil. (Smith, Miller &
Patch).

SETHOTOPE. (Squibb) Selenomethionine selenium 75; available as 0.25, 1
mCi.

•**SETOPERONE.** USAN.
Use: Antipsychotic.

SEVIRUMAB. USAN.
Use: Monoclonal antibody (antiviral).

•**SEVOFLURANE.** USAN. Fluoromethyl 2,2,2-trifluoro-1-(trifluoromethyl)ethyl ether.
Use: Anesthetic (inhalation).
SFC LOTION. (Stiefel) Soap free. Stearyl alcohol, parabens. Bot. 237 ml, 474 ml.
Use: Skin cleanser.
SHADE. (Schering-Plough) SPF 15. Contains one or more of the following ingredients: Padimate O, oxybenzone, ethyl-hexyl-p-methoxycinnamate. Bot. 118 ml, 120 ml, 240 ml.
Use: Sunscreen.
SHADE CREAM. (O'Leary) Jar 0.25 oz.
Use: Contouring cream.
SHADE SUNBLOCK GEL, 15 SPF. (Schering-Plough) Ethylhexyl p-methoxycinnamate, octyl salicylate, oxybenzone, SD alcohol 40. PABA free. SPF 15. Waterproof. Gel. Bot. 120 Gm.
Use: Sunscreen.
SHADE SUNBLOCK GEL, 25 SPF. (Schering-Plough) Ethylhexyl p-methoxycinnamate, octyl salicylate, homosalate, oxybenzone, SD alcohol 40. PABA free. Gel. Bot. 120 Gm.
Use: Sunscreen.
SHADE SUNBLOCK GEL, 30 SPF. (Schering-Plough) Ethylhexyl p-methoxycinnamate, homosalate, oxybenzone, 73% SD alcohol 40. Bot. 120 g.
Use: Sunscreen.
SHADE SUNBLOCK LOTION, 15 SPF. (Schering-Plough) Ethylhexyl p-methoxycinnamate, oxybenzone, benzyl alcohol, phenethyl alcohol. PABA free. Waterproof. Lot. Bot. 120 ml.
Use: Sunscreen.
SHADE SUNBLOCK LOTION, 30 SPF. (Schering-Plough) Ethylhexyl p-methoxycinnamate, 2-ethylhexyl salicylate, homosalate, oxybenzone, benzyl alcohol, phenethyl alcohol. PABA free. Waterproof. Lot. Bot. 120 ml.
Use: Sunscreen.
SHADE SUNBLOCK LOTION, 45 SPF. (Schering-Plough) Ethylhexyl p-methoxycinnamate, oxybenzone, 2-ethylhexyl salicylate, benzyl alcohol, phenethyl alcohol. PABA free. Waterproof. Lot. Bot. 120 ml.
Use: Sunscreen.
SHADE SUNBLOCK STICK, 30 SPF. (Schering-Plough) Ethylhexyl p-methoxycinnamate, oxybenzone, 2-ethylhexyl salicylate, homosalate. PABA free. Waterproof. Stick. 18 Gm.
Use: Sunscreen.

SHADE UVAGUARD. (Schering-Plough) Octyl methoxycinnamate 7.5%, avobenzone 3%, oxybenzone 3%. Waterproof. SPF 15. Lot. 120 ml.
Use: Sunscreen.
SHEIK ELITE. (Schmid) Condom with nonoxynol 9 5.6%. In 12s.
Use: Contraceptive.
•**SHELLAC,** N.F. XVIII.
Use: Pharmaceutic aid (tablet coating agent).
SHEPARD'S CREAM LOTION. (Dermik) Creamy lotion with no lanolin or mineral oil, for entire body. Scented or unscented. Bot. 8 oz, 16 oz.
Use: Emollient.
SHEPARD'S SKIN CREAM. (Dermik) Scented or unscented, w/no lanolin or mineral oil. Jar 4 oz.
Use: Emollient.
SHERFORM-HC CREME. (Sheryl) Hydrocortisone 1%, pramoxine HCl 0.5%, clioquinol 3%. Oint. Tube 0.5 oz.
Use: Corticosteroid combination.
SHERHIST. (Sheryl) Phenylephrine HCl, pyrilamine maleate/Tab. 100s. Liq. pt.
Use: Decongestant, antihistamine.
SHERNATAL TABLETS. (Sheryl) Phosphorus free calcium, non-irritating iron, trace minerals and essential vitamins. Tab. 100s.
Use: Vitamin/mineral supplement.
SHERRY-JEN TONIC. (Jenkins) Vitamins B_1 8 mg, B_2 4 mg, cyanocobalamin 4 mcg, nicotinamide 20 mg, calcium pantothenate 5 mg, B_6 1 mg, inositol 30 mg, choline bitartrate 60 mg, ferric ammonium citrate 60 mg, alcohol 9%/fl oz. Bot. 4 oz, 8 oz, gal.
Use: Vitamin/mineral supplement.
SHERTUS LIQUID. (Sheryl) Dextromethorphan HBr, chlorpheniramine maleate, phenylephrine HCl, ammonium Cl. Liq. pt.
Use: Antitussive, antihistamine, decongestant, expectorant.
SHOHL'S SOLUTION. Sodium Citrate and Citric Acid Oral Soln, U.S.P. XXIII.
Use: Systemic alkalizer.
SHORT CHAIN FATTY ACID SOLUTION.
Use: Ulcerative colitis. [Orphan drug]
SHOSTAKOVSKY BALSAM. Polyvinox. B.A.N.
SHUR-CLENS. (Calgon Vestal) Poloxamer 188 20%. Soln. Bot. UD 100, 200 ml.
Use: Topical drug, miscellaneous.
SHUR SEAL GEL. (Milex) Nonoxynol-9 6 Gm/5 oz. pre-measured pak. Box 24s.
Use: Contraceptive jelly for use with diaphragm.

SIALCO. (Foy) Chlorpheniramine maleate 4 mg, salicylamide 150 mg, acetaminophen 125 mg, phenylephrine HCl 5 mg/Tab. Bot. 100s, 500s, 1000s.
Use: Antihistamine, analgesic, decongestant.

SIBELIUM. (Janssen) Flunarizine HCl.
Use: Vasodilator.

SIBLIN. (Warner-Lambert Consumer) Water-absorbent material from plantago/Tsp. Box lb.
Use: Laxative.

• **SIBOPIRDINE.** USAN.
Use: Nootropic.

• **SIBUTRAMINE HYDROCHLORIDE.** USAN.
Use: Antidepressant; appetite suppressant.

SICKLE CELL TEST.
Use: Diagnostic aid.
See: Sickledex Test (Ortho Diag.).

SICKLEDEX. (Ortho Diag.) Test kit 12s, 100s.
Use: Diagnostic aid.

SIDEROL. (Doral) Chelated iron ammonium citrate 720 mg, folic acid 400 mcg, vitamins B_{12} 25 mcg, B_1 50 mg, B_6 1 mg, niacin 60 mg, panthenol 10 mg, PABA 6 mg, l-lysine HCl 100 mg, inositol 10 mg, choline citrate 50 mg, methionine 6.25 mg, Cu, Zn, Mn, K, Mg, in base with sorbitol, liver fraction no. 1, beef peptone/ml. Bot. 6 oz.
Use: Vitamin/mineral supplement.

SIGAMINE. (Sig) Cyanocobalamin injection 1000 mcg/ml. Vial 10 ml, 30 ml. Also Sigamine L.A. Vial 10 ml.
Use: Vitamin B_{12} supplement.

SIGAZINE. (Sig) Promethazine HCl 50 mg/ml. Vial 10 ml.
Use: Antihistamine.

SIGESIC.(Rand) Cap. Bot. 100s, 1000s.
Use: Analgesic, sedative.

SIGNA CREME. (Parker) Conductive cosmetic quality electrolyte cream. Bot. 5 oz, 2 L, 4 L.
Use: High conductive electrode cream for diagnostic electrocardiograms.

SIGNA GEL. (Parker) Conductive saline electrode gel. Tube 250 Gm.
Use: Defibrillation, ECG, EMG, electrosurgery.

SIGNA PAD. (Parker) Pre-moistened electrode pads.
Use: ECG procedures.

SIGNATAL C. (Sig) Calcium 230 mg, iron 49.3 mg, vitamins A 4000 IU, D 400 IU, B_1 2 mg, B_2 2 mg, B_6 1 mg, B_{12} 2 mcg, folic acid 0.1 mg, niacinamide 10 mg, C 50 mg, iodine 0.15 mg/S.C. Tab. Bot.

100s, 1000s.
Use: Vitamin/mineral supplement.

SIGNATE. (Sig) Dimenhydrinate 50 mg, propylene glycol 50%, benzyl alcohol 5%/ml. Vial 10 ml.
Use: Antiemetic/antivertigo.

SIGNEF "SUPPS". (Fellows) Hydrocortisone 15 mg/Supp. 12s. w or w/out appl.
Use: Corticosteroid, vaginal.

SIGPRED. (Sig) Prednisolone acetate. Vial 10 ml.
Use: Corticosteroid.

SIGTAB. (Upjohn) Vitamins A 5000 IU, D 400 IU, B_1 10.3 mg, B_2 10 mg, C 333 mg, niacin 100 mg, B_6 6 mg, pantothenic acid 20 mg, folic acid 0.4 mg, B_{12} 18 mcg, E 16.5 mg/Tab. Bot. 30s, 90s, 500s.
Use: Vitamin supplement.

SIGTAB-M. (Roberts) Vitamin A 6000 IU, D_3 400 IU, E 45 IU, C 100 mg, B_3 25 mg, B_1 5 mg, B_2 5 mg, B_6 3 mg, folic acid 400 mcg, B_5 15 mg, K_1 25 mcg, biotin 45 mcg, Ca 200 mg, P 200 mg, iron 18 mg, Mg, Cu 18 mg, zinc, I, Mn, K, Cl, Mo, Se, Cr, Ni, Sn, V, Si, B 15 mg. Tab. Bot.100s.
Use: Vitamin-mineral supplement.

SILACLEAN 20/20. (Professional Supplies) Benzalkonium Cl, EDTA. Soln. Bot. 60 ml.
Use: Hard contact lens care.

• **SILAFILCON A.** USAN.
Use: Contact lens material.

• **SILANDRONE.** USAN. 17 β-(Trimethylsiloxy)-androst-4-en-3-one.
Use: Androgen.

SILEXIN LOZENGES. (Otis Clapp) Dextromethorphan HBr 5 mg, benzocaine 7.9 mg/Loz. 400s.
Use: Antitussive, local anesthetic.

SILEXIN SYRUP. (Otis Clapp) Dextromethorphan HBr, guaifenesin in sugar, salt and alcohol free vehicle. Bot. 1 oz, 4 oz, 16 oz.
Use: Antitussive, expectorant.

SILEXIN TABS. (Otis Clapp) Dextromethorphan HBr, benzocaine/Tab. 400s.
Use: Antitussive, local anesthetic.

• **SILICEOUS EARTH, PURIFIED,** N.F. XVIII.
Use: Filtering medium.

SILICONE. (Dow Chemicals) Dimethicone. Liq., Bot. oz. Bulk Pkg. Oint. See also:
W/Lanolin.
See: Sanchia Silicone Protective Cream (Otis Clapp).
W/Nitro-Cellulose, castor oil.
See: Covicone, Cream (Abbott).

W/Triethylene glycol, mineral oil.
See: Allergex, Liq., Spray (Hollister-
Stier).
- **SILICON DIOXIDE,** N.F. XVIII.
Use: Pharm. aid (suspending agent, an-
ticaking agent, disintegrating agent).
- **SILICONE DIOXIDE, COLLOIDAL,** N.F.
XVIII.
Use: Tablet diluent, suspending & thick-
ening agent.
SILICONE OINTMENT. Dimethicone Di-
methyl polysiloxane.
See: Covicone Cream (Abbott).
SILICONE OINTMENT NO. 2. (C & M
Pharmacal) High viscosity silicone 10%
in a blend of petrolatum and hydropho-
bic starch. Jar 2 oz, lb.
Use: Protective agent.
SILICONE POWDER. (Gordon) Talc with
silicone. Pkg. 4 oz, 1 lb, 5 lb.
Use: Dusting powder to prevent tape
from adhering to clothing.
SILMAGEL. (Lannett) Aluminum hydrox-
ide 2.5 gr, magnesium tricilicate 3.85
gr/Tab. Bot. 1000s, 5000s.
Use: Antacid.
- **SILODRATE.** USAN. Magnesium alumi-
nosilicate hydrate.
Use: Antacid.
SILPHEN COUGH. (Silarx) Diphenhydramine HCl 12.5 mg/5 ml, alcohol 5%,
menthol, sucrose. Syrup. Bot. 118 ml.
Use: Antitussive.
SILTEX. (Edward J. Moore) Camphor,
menthol, allantoin, tincture of benzoin in
lanolin-petrolatum base. Tube 0.25 oz.
Use: Chapped lips, cold sores, fever
blisters.
SILVADENE. (Marion Merrell Dow) Silver
sulfadiazine (10 mg/Gm) 1%, base
w/white petrolatum, stearyl alcohol, iso-
propyl myristate, sorbitan monooleate,
polyoxyl 40 stearate, propylene glycol,
water, methylparaben. Cream Jar 50
Gm, 85 Gm, 400 Gm, 1000 Gm. Tube
20 Gm.
Use: Antimicrobial, topical.
SILVER COMPOUNDS.
See: Silver Iodide, Colloidal.
Silver Nitrate, Preps. (Various Mfr.).
Silver Picrate (City Chem.).
Silver Protein, Mild (Various Mfr.).
Silver Protein, Strong (Various Mfr.).
- **SILVER NITRATE,** U.S.P. XXIII. Ophth.
Soln., Toughened, U.S.P. XXIII. Nitric
acid silver.
Use: Astringent, caustic, antiseptic.
SILVER NITRATE OINTMENT. (Gordon)
Silver nitrate 1% in ointment base. Jar
oz.

Use: Astringent, epithelial stimulant.
- **SILVER NITRATE OPHTHALMIC SOLU-
TION,** U.S.P. XXIII. (Wax Amp.).
Use: Astringent, anti-infective.
Generic Products:
(Gordon)-Soln. 10%, 25%, 50%. Bot.
oz.
(Lilly)—Amp. 1%, 100s.
(Parke-Davis)—Cap. 1%, 100s.
SILVER NITRATE TOPICAL STICKS.
(Graham-Field) Silver nitrate, potassium
nitrate 25%. Appl. 100s.
Use: Cauterizing agent.
- **SILVER NITRATE, TOUGHENED,** U.S.P.
XXIII. Silver nitrate plus 4% silver Cl.
Use: Caustic.
SILVER PICRATE. (City Chem.) 1 oz.
Use: Antiseptic.
SILVER PROTEIN, MILD. Argentum
Vitellinum, Cargentos, Mucleinate Mild,
Protargin Mild.
See: Argyrol Prods. (Iolab).
SILVER PROTEIN, STRONG.
See: Protargol, Pow. (Storling).
- **SILVER SULFADIAZINE.** USAN.
Use: Anti-infective, topical.
See: Silvadene, Cream (Marion Merrell
Dow).
SSD Cream (Boots).
SSD AF Cream (Boots).
Thermazene, Cream (Sherwood).
SIMAAL GEL. (Schein) Aluminum hy-
droxide 200 mg, magnesium hydroxide
200 mg, simethicone 20 mg/5 ml. Liq.
Bot. 360 ml.
Use: Antacid, antiflatulant.
SIMAAL 2 GEL. (Schein) Aluminum hy-
droxide 500 mg, magnesium hydroxide
400 mg, simethicone 40 mg/5 ml. Liq.
Bot. 360 ml.
Use: Antacid, antiflatulant.
- **SIMETHICONE,** U.S.P. XX, Emulsion,
Oral Susp., Tab., U.S.P. XXIII, Cap.,
U.S.P. XXIII. Mixture of liquid dimethyl
polysiloxanes with silica aerogel.
Use: Antiflatulent, pharmaceutic aid (re-
lease agent).
See: Mylicon, Tab., Liq. (Stuart).
Mylicon-80, Tab. (Stuart).
Silain, Tab. (Robins).
Ingredients of:
Mylanta, Tab., Liq. (Stuart).
Phazyme, Tab. (Reed & Carnick).
W/Aluminum hydroxide, magnesium hy-
droxide.
See: Di-Gel, Liq., Tab. (Plough).
Mylanta, Mylanta II, Tab., Liq. (Stuart).
Silain-Gel, Liq. (Robins).
Simeco, Liq. (Wyeth-Ayerst).
Simethox, Liq. (Quality Generics).

W/Enzymes.
See: Phazyme, Tab. (Reed & Carnrick).
W/Hyoscyamine sulfate, atropine sulfate,
hyoscine HBr, butabarbital sodium.
See: Sidonna, Tab. (Reed & Carnrick).
W/Hyoscyamine sulfate, atropine sulfate,
scopolamine HBr, phenobarbital.
See: Kinesed, Chew. Tab. (Stuart).
W/Magnesium aluminum hydroxide.
See: Maalox Plus, Susp. (Rhone-
Poulenc Rorer).
W/Magnesium carbonate.
See: Di-Gel, Tab., Liq. (Plough).
W/Magnesium hydroxide.
See: Laxsil, Liq. (Reed & Carnrick).
W/Magnesium hydroxide, dried aluminum
hydroxide gel.
See: Maalox Plus, Tab. (Rhone-
Poulenc Rorer).
W/Pancreatin.
See: Phazyme, Tab. (Reed & Carnrick).
Phazyme-95, Tab. (Reed & Carnrick).
W/Pancreatin, phenobarbital.
See: Phazyme-PB, Tab. (Reed & Carn-
rick).
SIMILAC 13/SIMILAC 13 WITH IRON.
(Ross) Milk-based infant formula ready-
to-feed containing 13 calories/fl oz., 1.8
mg iron/100 calories. Bot. 4 fl. oz.
Use: Enteral nutritional therapy for in-
fants.
SIMILAC 20/SIMILAC WITH IRON 20.
(Ross) Milk-based infant formula. Stan-
dard dilution (20 cal/fl oz). Similac with
iron: iron 1.8 mg/100 cal. **Pow.:** Can lb.
Concentrated Liq.: Can 13 fl oz.
Ready-to-feed: Can 8 fl oz, 32 fl oz. Bot.
4 fl oz, 8 fl oz.
Use: Enteral nutritional therapy for in-
fants.
SIMILAC 24 LBW. (Ross) Low-iron infant
formula, ready-to-feed, 24 calories/fl oz.
Bot. 4 fl oz.
Use: Enteral nutritional therapy for infants.
SIMILAC 24/SIMILAC 24 WITH IRON.
(Ross) Milk-based infant formula ready-
to-feed (24 cal/fl oz), iron 1.8 mg/100
calories. Bot. 4 fl oz.
Use: Enteral nutritional therapy for in-
fants.
SIMILAC 27. (Ross) Milk-based ready-to-
feed infant formula (27 cal/fl oz). Bot. 4 fl
oz.
Use: Enteral nutritional therapy for infants.
**SIMILAC LOW-IRON LIQUID &
POWDER.** (Ross) Protein 14.3 g, carbohydrates 72 g, fat 36 g, iron 1.5 mg,
with appropriate vitamins and minerals.

Liq.: 390 ml concentrate, 240 ml and 1
qt. ready-to-use, 120 ml and 240 ml
nursettes. **Pow.:** 1 lb.
Use: Enteral nutritional therapy for infants.
**SIMILAC NATURAL CARE HUMAN MILK
FORTIFIER.** (Ross) Liquid fortifier designed to be mixed with human milk or
fed alternately with human milk to low-
birth-weight infants. Supplied as 24 cal/fl
oz. Bot. 4 fl oz.
Use: Enteral nutritional therapy for infants.
SIMILAC PM 60/40. (Ross) Milk-based
formula ready-to-feed or powder with
60:40 whey to casein ratio (20 cal/fl oz).
Bot.: Hospital use 4 fl oz. ready-to-feed.
Pow.: Can lb.
Use: Enteral nutritional therapy for in-
fants.
SIMILAC SPECIAL CARE 20. (Ross) Infant formula ready-to-feed (20 cal/fl oz).
Bot. 4 fl oz.
Use: Enteral nutritional therapy for in-
fants.
SIMILAC SPECIAL CARE 24. (Ross) In-
fant formula ready-to-feed (24 Cal/fl oz).
Bot. 4 fl oz.
Use: Enteral nutritional therapy for in-
fants.
SIMPLET. (Major) Pseudoephedrine HCl
60 mg, chlorpheniramine maleate 4 mg,
acetaminophen 650 mg/Tab. Dye free.
Bot. 100s.
Use: Decongestant, antihistamine,
analgesic.
SIMRON. (SK-Beecham) Iron (supplied
as ferrous gluconate) 10 mg/Cap. Bot.
100s.
Use: Iron supplement.
SIMRON PLUS. (SK-Beecham) Iron 10
mg (supplied as ferrous gluconate), vita-
mins B_{12} 3.33 mcg, ascorbic acid 50 mg,
B_6 1 mg, folic acid 0.1 mg/Cap. Bot.
100s.
Use: Iron supplement.
• **SIMTRAZENE.** USAN. 1,4-Dimethyl-1,4-
diphenyl-2-tetrazene.
Use: Antineoplastic agent.
SIMVASTATIN.
Use: Antihyperlipidemic agent.
See: Zocor (Merck & Co.).
SINAPILS. (Pfeiffer) Phenylpropanolamine HCl 12.5 mg, chlorpheniramine maleate 1 mg, acetaminophen
324 mg, caffeine 32.5 mg/Tab. Bot. 36s.
Use: Decongestant, antihistamine,
analgesic.
SINAREST. (Pharmacraft) Aceta-
minophen 325 mg, chlorpheniramine

maleate 2 mg, phenylpropanolamine HCl 18.7 mg/Tab. Pkg. 20s, 40s, 80s.
Use: Analgesic, antihistamine, decongestant.

SINAREST 12 HOUR. (Ciba Consumer) Oxymetazoline HCl 0.05%. Spray Bot. 15 ml.
Use: Nasal decongestant.

SINAREST DECONGESTANT NASAL SPRAY. (Pharmacraft) Oxymetazoline HCl 0.05%. Bot. 0.5 oz.
Use: Nasal decongestant.

SINAREST, EXTRA-STRENGTH. (Pharmacraft) Acetaminophen 500 mg, chlorpheniramine maleate 2 mg, phenylpropanolamine HCl 18.7 mg/Tab. 24s.
Use: Analgesic, antihistamine, decongestant.

SINAREST, NO DROWSINESS. (Pharmacraft) Pseudoephedrine HCl 30 mg, acetaminophen 500 mg/Tab. Pkg. 20s.
Use: Decongestant, analgesic.

• **SINCALIDE.** USAN.
Use: Choleretic.

SINE-AID IB. (McNeil-CPC) Pseudoephedrine 30 mg, ibuprofen 200 mg. Capl. Pkg. 20s.
Use: Decongestant, analgesic.

SINE-AID MAXIMUM STRENGTH. (McNeil-CPC) Pseudoephedrine HCl 30 mg, acetaminophen 500 mg/Tab.or Cap.
Tab.: Bot. 24s, 100s **Cap.:** Bot. 24s, 50s.
Use: Decongestant, analgesic.

SINE-AID SINUS HEADACHE CAPLETS, EXTRA STRENGTH. (McNeil Prods) Acetaminophen 500 mg, pseudoephedrine HCl 30 mg/Capl. Bot. 24s, 50s.
Use: Analgesic, decongestant.

SINE-AID SINUS HEADACHE TABLETS. (McNeil Prods) Acetaminophen 325 mg, pseudoephedrine HCl 30 mg/Tab. Bot. 24s, 50s, 100s.
Use: Analgesic, decongestant.

• **SINEFUNGIN.** USAN.
Use: Antifungal.

SINEMET CR. (DuPont Pharm.) Carbidopa 25 or 50 mg, levodopa 100 or 200 mg/SR Tab. Bot. 100s, UD 100s.
Use: Antiparkinson agent.

SINEMET 10/100. (DuPont Pharm.) Carbidopa 10 mg, levodopa 100 mg/Tab. Bot. 100s, UD 100s.
Use: Antiparkinson agent.

SINEMET 25/100. (DuPont Pharm.) Carbidopa 25 mg, levodopa 100 mg/Tab. Bot. 100s, UD 100s.
Use: Antiparkinson agent.

SINEMET 25/250. (DuPont Pharm.) Carbidopa 25 mg, levodopa 250 mg/Tab.

Bot. 100s, UD 100s.
Use: Antiparkinson agent.

SINE-OFF MAXIMUM STRENGTH ALLERGY-SINUS FORMULA CAPLETS. (SK-Beecham) Chlorpheniramine maleate 2 mg, pseudoephedrine HCl 30 mg, acetaminophen 500 mg/Cap. Pkg. 20s.
Use: Antihistamine, decongestant, analgesic..

SINE-OFF MAXIMUM STRENGTH NO DROWSINESS FORMULA CAPLETS. (SK-Beecham) Pseudoephedrine HCl 30 mg, acetaminophen 500 mg/Cap. Pkg. 20s.
Use: Decongestant, analgesic.

SINE-OFF TABLETS. (SK-Beecham) Chlorpheniramine maleate 2 mg, phenylpropanolamine HCl 12.5 mg, aspirin 325 mg. Tab. Pkg. 24s, 48s, 100s.
Use: Antihistamine, decongestant, analgesic.

SINEQUAN. (Roerig) Doxepin HCl. **Cap.:** 10 mg/Cap. Bot. 100s, 1000s, UD 100s; 25 mg or 50 mg/Cap. Bot. 90s, 100s, 1000s, UD 100s; 75 mg/Cap. Bot. 100s, 1000s, UD 100s; 100 mg/Cap. Bot. 100s, 1000s, UD 100s; 150 mg/Cap. Bot. 50s, 500s, UD 100s. **Oral Concentrate:** 10 mg/ml. Bot. 120 ml.
Use: Antidepressant.

SINEX. (Vicks) Phenylephrine HCl 0.5%, cetylpyridinium Cl 0.04% w/thimerosal 0.001% preservative. Nasal spray. Bot. 0.5 oz, 1 oz.
Use: Nasal decongestant.

SINEX LONG ACTING. (Vicks) Oxymetazoline HCl 0.05% in aqueous soln. w/thimerosal 0.001%. Nasal spray. Bot. 0.5 oz, 1 oz.
Use: Nasal decongestant.

SINGLET. (Lakeside) Pseudoephedrine HCl 60 mg, chlorpheniramine maleate 4 mg, acetaminophen 650 mg/Tab. Bot. 100s.
Use: Decongestant, antihistamine, analgesic.

SINOCON TR. (Vangard) Phenylpropanolamine HCl 20 mg, phenylephrine HCl 5 mg, phenyltoloxamine citrate 7.5 mg, chlorpheniramine maleate 2.5 mg/Tab. Bot. 100s, 1000s.
Use: Decongestant, antihistamine.

SINO-EZE MLT. (Richlyn) Salicylamide 3.5 gr, acetaminophen 100 mg, phenylephrine HCl 5 mg, chlorpheniramine maleate 2 mg/Tab. Bot. 1000s.
Use: Analgesic, decongestant, antihistamine.

SINOGRAFIN. (Squibb) Meglumine diatri-

zoate 52.7%, meglumine iodipamide 26.8%. Vial 10 ml.
Use: Diagnostic aid.

SINOVAN TIMED. (Drug Industries) Chlorpheniramine maleate 8 mg, phenylephrine HCl 20 mg, methscopolamine nitrate 2.5 mg/Cap. Bot. 100s, 1000s.
Use: Antihistamine, decongestant combination.

SINUBID. (Parke-Davis) Acetaminophen 600 mg, phenylpropanolamine HCl 100 mg, phenyltoloxamine 66 mg/Tab. Bot. 100s.
Use: Analgesic, decongestant, antihistamine.

SINUCOL. (Tennessee Pharm.) Chlorpheniramine maleate 8 mg, phenylephrine HCl 20 mg, methscopolamine nitrate 2.5 mg/Cap. Bot. 100s, 500s. Inj. Vial 10 ml.
Use: Antihistamine, decongestant combination.

SINUESE. (Jenkins) Potassium guaiacol sulfonate 40 mg, sodium iodide 50 mg, menthol, camphor, guaiacol, eucalyptol/ml. Vial 30 ml, 12s.
Use: Expectorant combination.

SINUFED TIMECELLE. (Roberts/Hauck) Pseudoephedrine HCl 60 mg, guaifenesin 300 mg/Cap. Bot. 100s.
Use: Decongestant, expectorant.

SINULIN TABLETS. (Carnrick) Phenylpropanolamine HCl 25 mg, chlorpheniramine maleate 4 mg, acetaminophen 650 mg/Tab. Bot. 20s, 100s. Blister 24s.
Use: Decongestant, antihistamine, analgesic.

SINUMIST-SR. (Hauck) Guaifenesin 600 mg/Tab. Bot. 100s.
Use: Expectorant.

SINUPAN. (Ion) Phenylephrine HCl 40 mg, guaifenesin 200 mg/SR Cap. Bot. 100s.
Use: Decongestant, expectorant.

SINUSEZE. (Amlab) Acetaminophen 325 mg, phenylpropanolamine HCl 25 mg, phenyltoloxamine citrate 22 mg/Tab. Bot. 36s.
Use: Analgesic, decongestant, antihistamine.

SINUS EXCEDRIN. (Bristol-Myers Squibb) Pseudoephedrine HCl 30 mg, acetaminophen 500 mg/Tab or Cap. Bot. 24s, 50s.
Use: Decongestant, analgesic.

SINUS PAIN FORMULA ALLEREST. (Fisons) Pseudoephedrine HCl 30 mg, chlorpheniramine maleate 2 mg, acetaminophen 500 mg. **Cap.:** Bot. 24s, 50s.

Gelcap: Bot. 20s, 40s.
Use: Decongestant, antihistamine, analgesic.

SINUS RELIEF. (Major) Pseudoephedrine HCl 30 mg, acetaminophen 325 mg/Tab. Bot. 24s.
Use: Decongestant, analgesic.

SINUS TABLETS. (Kenyon) Phenacetin 150 mg, acetaminophen 150 mg, phenyltoloxamine dihydrogen citrate 22 mg/Tab. Bot. 100s, 1000s.
Use: Analgesic, antihistamine.

SINUS TABLETS. (Walgreen) Acetaminophen 325 mg, chlorpheniramine maleate 2 mg, pseudoephedrine HCl mg/Tab. Bot. 30s.
Use: Analgesic, antihistamine, decongestant.

SINUSTAT. (Murdock) Pseudoephedrine HCl 60 mg/Cap. Bot. 30s.
Use: Decongestant.

SINUTAB ALLERGY FORMULA. (Parke-Davis) Pseudoephedrine sulfate 120 mg, dexbrompheniramine maleate 6 mg/SR Tab. Sucrose, sugar. Bot. 10s, 20s.
Use: Decongestant, antihistamine.

SINUTAB MAXIMUM STRENGTH. (Parke-Davis Prods) Acetaminophen 500 mg, pseudoephedrine HCl 30 mg, chlorpheniramine maleate 2 mg/Tab., Cap. Blister pack 24s.
Use: Analgesic, decongestant, antihistamine.

SINUTAB MAXIMUM STRENGTH NIGHTTIME SINUS FORMULA. (Parke-Davis Prods) Acetaminophen 1000 mg, diphenhydramine HCl 50 mg, pseudoephedrine 60 mg/oz. Bot. 4 oz.
Use: Analgesic, antihistamine, decongestant.

SINUTAB II MAXIMUM STRENGTH NO DROWSINESS FORMULA. (Parke-Davis Prods) Acetaminophen 500 mg, pseudoephedrine HCl 30 mg/Cap. Pack 24s.
Use: Analgesic, decongestant.

SINUTAB WITHOUT DROWSINESS. (Parke-Davis) Pseudoephedrine HCl 30 mg, acetaminophen 325 mg/Tab. Bot. 12s, 24s, 100s.
Use: Decongestant, analgesic.

SINUTROL. (Weeks & Leo) Phenylpropanolamine HCl 25 mg, phenyltoloxamine citrate 22 mg, acetaminophen 325 mg/Tab. Bot. 40s, 90s.
Use: Decongestant, antihistamine, analgesic.

SINUVENT. (WE Pharm) Phenylpropanolamine 75 mg, guaifenesin 600

mg. LA Tab. Bot. 100s.
Use: Decongestant, expectorant.
SIROIL. (Siroil) Mercuric oleate, cresol, vegetable and mineral oil. Emulsion, Bot. 8 oz.
Use: Antiseptic.
SIR-O-LENE. (Siroil) Tube 4 oz.
Use: Emollient.
• **SIROLIMUS.** USAN.
Use: Immunosuppressant.
• **SISOMICIN.** USAN.
Use: Antibacterial.
• **SISOMICIN SULFATE,** U.S.P. XXIII. Inj., U.S.P. XXIII.
Use: Antibacterial.
SITABS. (Canright) Lobeline sulfate 1.5 mg, benzocaine 2 mg, aluminum hydroxide—magnesium carbonate codried gel 150 mg/Loz. Bot. 100s.
Use: Smoking deterrent.
• **SITOGLUSIDE.** USAN.
Use: Antiprostatic hypertrophy.
SITZMARKS. (Konsyl Pharm.) Radiopaque rings 20/Cap. Bot. 10s.
Use: GI contrast agent.
SIXAMEEN. (Spanner) Vitamins B_1 100 mg, B_6 100 mg/ml. Vial 10 ml.
Use: Vitamin B supplement.
SKEETER STIK. (Outdoor Recreation) Lidocaine 4%, phenol 2%, isopropyl alcohol 45.5% in a propylene glycol base. Stick 1s.
Use: Local anesthetic.
SKELAXIN. (Carnrick) Metaxalone 400 mg/Tab. Bot. 100s, 500s.
Use: Skeletal muscle relaxant.
SKELETAL MUSCLE RELAXANTS.
See: Anectine, Soln., Pow. (Burroughs Wellcome).
Flexeril, Tab. (Merck & Co.).
Mephenesin (Various Mfr.).
Metubine Iodide, Vial (Lilly).
Neostig, Tab. (Freeport).
Paraflex, Tab. (McNeil).
Parafon Forte, Tab. (McNeil).
Quelicin, Fliptop & pintop Vials, Syringe w/lancet, Amp. (Abbott).
Rela, Tab. (Schering).
Robaxin, Tab., Inj. (Robins).
Skelaxin, Tab. (Carnrick).
Soma, Preps. (Wallace).
Sucostrin, Vial, Amp. (Squibb).
Syncurine, Vial (Burroughs Wellcome).
Trancopal, Cap. (Sanofi Winthrop).
d-Tubocurarine Chloride (Various Mfr.).
SK&F 110679. (SK-Beecham)
Use: Growth hormone. [Orphan drug]
SKIN DEGREASER. (Health & Medical

Techniques) Freon 100%. Bot. 2 oz, 4 oz.
Use: Presurgical skin degreaser.
SKIN SHIELD LIQUID BANDAGE. (Del) Dyclonine HCl, benzethonium Cl. Bot. 0.45 oz.
Use: Skin protectant.
SKIN TEST ANTIGEN, MULTIPLE.
See: Multitest CMI (Merieux).
SLEEP II. (Walgreen) Diphenhydramine HCl 25 mg/Tab. Bot. 16s, 32s, 72s.
Use: Sleep aid.
SLEEP CAP. (Weeks & Leo) Diphenhydramine HCl 50 mg/Cap. Bot. 25s, 50s.
Use: Sleep aid.
SLEEP-EZE TABLETS. (Whitehall) Diphenhydramine HCl 25 mg/Tab. Pkg. 12s, 26s, 52s.
Use: Sleep aid.
SLEEP-EZE 3. (Whitehall) Diphenhydramine HCl 25 mg/Tab. Pkg. 12s, 24s.
Use: Sleep aid.
SLEEP TABS. (Towne) Scopolamine aminoxide HBr 0.2 mg, salicylamide 250 mg/Tab. Bot. 36s, 90s.
Use: Sleep aid.
SLEEPWELL 2-NITE. (Rugby) Diphenhydramine HCl 25 mg. Tab. Bot. 72s.
Use: Sleep aid.
SLENDER. (Carnation) Skim milk, vegetable oils, caseinates, vitamins, minerals. **Liq.:** 220 cal/ 10 oz. Can. **Pow.:** 173 or 200 cal mixed w/6 oz skim or low fat milk. Pkg oz.
Use: Diet aid.
SLENDER-X. (Progressive Drugs) Phenylpropanolamine, methylcellulose, caffeine, vitamins/Tab. Pkg. 21s, 42s, 84s. Gum 20s, 60s.
Use: Diet aid.
SLIMETTES. (Blue Cross) Phenylpropanolamine HCl 35 mg, caffeine 140 mg/Cap. Box 20s.
Use: Diet aid.
SLIM-FAST. (Thompson Medical) Meal replacement powder mixed with milk to replace 1, 2 or 3 meals a day.
Use: Diet aid.
SLIM-LINE. (Thompson Medical) Benzocaine, dextrose/Chewing gum. Box 24s.
Use: Diet aid.
SLIM-MINT. (Thompson) Benzocaine 6 mg, lecithin, tartrazine. Pkg. Gum. 24s.
Use: Nonprescription diet aid.
SLIM PLAN PLUS WITHOUT CAFFEINE. (Whiteworth) Phenylpropanolamine HCl 75 mg/Tab. Box 40s.
Use: Diet aid.
SLIM-TABS. (Wesley) Phendimetrazine tartrate 35 mg/Tab. Bot. 1000s.

Use: Anorexiant.

SLOAN'S LINIMENT. (Warner-Lambert Prods) Capsicum oleoresin 0.62%, methyl salicylate 2.66%, oil of camphor 3.35%, turpentine oil 46.76%, oil of pine 6.74%. Bot. 2 oz, 7 oz.
Use: External analgesic.

SLO-BID GYROCAPS. (Rhone-Poulenc Rorer) Theophylline anhydrous 50 mg, 75 mg, 100 mg, 125 mg, 200 mg or 300 mg/TR Cap. Bot. 100s, 1000s, UD 100s.
Use: Bronchodilator.

SLO-NIACIN. (Upsher-Smith) Niacin **250 mg/Tab.** Bot. 100s, 1000s. **500 mg/Tab.** Bot. 100s, UD 100s. **750 mg/Tab.** Bot. 100s.
Use: Vitamin supplement.

SLO-PHYLLIN 80 SYRUP. (Rhone-Poulenc Rorer) Theophylline anhydrous 80 mg/15 ml. Nonalcoholic. Bot. 4 oz, pt, gal, UD 15 ml.
Use: Bronchodilator.

SLO-PHYLLIN GG. (Rhone-Poulenc Rorer) Theophylline anhydrous 150 mg, guaifenesin 90 mg/Cap. or 15 ml syr.
Cap.: Bot. 100s. **Syr.:** Bot. pt.
Use: Bronchodilator, expectorant.

SLO-PHYLLIN GYROCAPS. (Rhone-Poulenc Rorer) Theophylline anhydrous 60 mg, 125 mg, 250 mg/TR Cap. Bot. 100s, 1000s, UD 100s.
Use: Bronchodilator.

SLO-PHYLLIN TABLETS. (Rhone-Poulenc Rorer) Theophylline anhydrous 100 mg, 200 mg/Tab. Bot. 100s, 1000s, UD 100s.
Use: Bronchodilator.

SLO-SALT-K. (Mission) Potassium Cl 150 mg, sodium Cl 410 mg/Tab. Bot. 1000s. Strip 100s.
Use: Potassium/sodium supplement.

SLOW-K. (Ciba) Potassium Cl. Bot. 100s, 1000s, Accu-Pak units 100s. Consumer Pack 100s.
Use: Potassium supplement.

• **SLOW FE.** (Ciba) Dried ferrous sulfate 160 mg/Tab. Bot. 30s, 100s.
Use: Iron supplement.

SLOW-MAG. (Searle) Magnesium 64 mg/DR Tab. Bot. 60s.
Use: Magnesium supplement.

SLT. (Western Research) Sodium levothyroxine 0.1 mg, 0.2 mg or 0.3 mg /Tab. Bot. 1000s.
Use: Hypothyroidism treatment.

SLT LOTION. (C & M Pharmacal) Salicylic acid 3%, lactic acid 5%, coal tar soln. 2%. Bot. 4.3 oz.
Use: Antiseborrheic.

S-M-A FORMULA. (Wyeth-Ayerst) A se-ries of liquid feeding formulas.
Iron Fortified, Infant Formula-Powder.
Iron Fortified, Infant Formula-Ready to Feed.
Iron Fortified, Infant Formula-Liquid.
Lo-Iron, Infant Formula-Liquid.
Lo-Iron, Infant Formula-Powder.
Lo-Iron, Infant Formula-Ready to Feed.
Use: Enteral nutritional therapy for infants.

SMALL FRY CHEWABLE TABS. (Approved) Vitamins A 5000 IU, D 1000 IU, B_{12} 5 mcg, B_1 3 mg, B_2 2.5 mg, B_6 1 mg, C 50 mg, niacinamide 20 mg, calcium pantothenate 1 mg, E 1 IU, l-lysine 15 mg, biotin 10 mg/Tab. Bot. 100s, 250s, 365s.
Use: Vitamin/mineral supplement.

• **SMALLPOX VACCINE,** U.S.P. XXIII.
(Lederle)—Tube 1s, 5s, 10s, vaccinations. 1 vaccination and needle in glass capillary tube. (Wyeth-Ayerst)—Tube 1s, 5s, 10s, vaccinations.
Use: Agent for immunization.

SN-13, 272.
See: Primaquine Phosphate, U.S.P. XXIII. (Various Mfr.).

SNAKEBITE ANTIVENINS.
See: Antivenin (Micurus fulvius) (Wyeth-Ayerst).

SNAKE VENOM.
Use: S.C., I.M., orally; trypanosomiasis.
See: Antivenin. (Wyeth-Ayerst).

SNAPLETS-D. (Baker Cummins) Pseudoephedrine HCl 6.25 mg, chlorpheniramine maleate 1 mg, taste free. Granules 30s.
Use: Pediatric decongestant and antihistamine.

SNAPLETS-DM. (Baker Cummins) Phenylpropanolamine HCl 6.25 mg, dextromethorphan HBr 5 mg, taste free. Granules. 30s.
Use: Pediatric antitussive combination.

SNAPLETS-EX. (Baker Cummins) Phenylpropanolamine HCl 6.25 mg, guaifenesin 50 mg, taste free. Granules 30s.
Use: Pediatric expectorant combination.

SNAPLETS-FR. (Baker Cummins) Acetaminophen 80 mg. Granules Pks. 32 premeasured.
Use: Acetaminophen.

SNAPLETS-MULTI. (Baker Cummins) Phenylpropanolamine HCl 6.25 mg, chlorpheniramine maleate 1 mg, dextromethorphan HBr 5 mg, taste free.

Granules 30s.
Use: Pediatric antitussive combination.
SNOOTIE BY SEA & SKI. (Carter Products) Padimate O. SPF 10. Lot. Bot. 30 ml.
Use: Sunscreen.
SNO-STRIPS. (Akorn) Sterile tear flow test strips, 100s.
Use: Diagnostic aid, ophthalmic.
SOAC-LENS. (Alcon Lenscare) Thimerosal 0.004%, EDTA 0.1%. Bot. 4 oz.
Use: Contact lens care.
SOAKARE. (Allergan) Benzalkonium Cl 0.01%, edetate disodium, NaOH to adjust pH, purified water. Bot. 4 fl oz.
Use: Hard contact lens care.
SOAPS, GERMICIDAL.
See: Dial, Preps. (Armour).
   Fostex, Cake, Cream, Liq. (Westwood).
   pHisoHex, Liq. (Sanofi Winthrop).
   Thylox, Shampoo, Soap (Dent).
SOAP SUBSTITUTES
See: Acne-Dome, Cleanser (Miles Pharm).
   Domerine, Shampoo (Miles Pharm).
   Lowila, Cleanser (Westwood).
   pHisoDerm, Preps. (Sanofi Winthrop).
• **SODA LIME,** N.F. XVIII.
Use: Carbon dioxide absorbant.
SODA MINT.(Bowman) Sodium bicarbonate 5 gr, peppermint oil q.s./Tab. Bot. 100s, 1000s.
SODA MINT. (Lilly) Sodium bicarbonate 5 gr, peppermint oil q.s./Tab. Bot. 100s.
Use: Antacid.
SODASONE. (Fellows) Prednisolone sodium phosphate 20 mg, niacinamide 25 mg/ml. Vial 10 ml.
Use: Corticosteroid.
• **SODIUM ACETATE,** U.S.P. XXIII. Inj., Soln., U.S.P. XXIII. Acetic acid, sodium salt, trihydrate. (Abbott) 40 mEq, 20 ml in 50 ml Fliptop vial.
Use: Alkalinizer; pharmaceutic aid.
SODIUM ACETATE & THEOPHYLLINE.
• **SODIUM ACETAZOLAMIDE.** Acetazolamide Sodium, U.S.P. XXIII.
Use: Carbonic anhydrase inhibitor.
SODIUM ACETOSULFONE. Sodium 2-N-acetylsulfamyl-4,4'-diaminodiphenylsulfone.
Use: Leprostatic agent.
See: Promacetin, Tab. (Parke-Davis).
SODIUM ACETRIZOATE INJECTION.
B.A.N. Sodium 3-acetamino-2,4,6-triiodobenzoate, Diaginol.
Use: Radiopaque substance.
SODIUM ACID PHOSPHATE.

See: Sodium Biphosphate (Various Mfr.).
SODIUM ACTINOQUINOL. 8-Ethoxy-5-quinoline sulfonic acid sodium salt.
Use: Treatment of flash burns (ophthalmic).
See: Uviban.
SODIUM ALGINATE, N.F. XVIII.
Use: Suspending agent.
See: Algin.
   Kelgin (Kelco).
SODIUM AMINOBENZOATE. Sodium p-aminobenzoate.
Use: Dermatomyositis and scleroderma.
SODIUM AMINOPTERIN. Aminopterin sodium.
SODIUM AMINOSALICYLATE.
See: Aminosalicylate Sodium, U.S.P. XXIII.
SODIUM AMOBARBITAL. Amobarbital Sodium, U.S.P. XXIII.
• **SODIUM AMYLOSULFATE.** USAN. Sodium salt of potato amylopectin. Depepsin.
Use: Peptic ulcer.
SODIUM ANAZOLENE. 4-[(4-Anilino-5-sulfo-1-naphthyl)azo]-5-hydroxy-2,7-naphthalene disulfonic acid trisodium salt.
Use: Diagnostic aid.
SODIUM ANOXYNAPHTHONATE.
B.A.N. Sodium 4'-anilino-8-hydroxy-1,1-azonaphthalono-3, 5,6 tri sulfonate.
Use: Investigation of cardiac disease.
See: Anazolene Sodium (I.N.N.).
SODIUM ANTIMONY GLUCONATE. (Pentostam)
Use: Anti-infective agent.
SODIUM APOLATE. B.A.N. Sodium ethenesulfonate polymer.
Use: Anticoagulant.
• **SODIUM ARSENATE AS 74.** USAN.
Use: Radioactive agent.
• **SODIUM ASCORBATE,** U.S.P. XXIII. Monosodium L-ascorbate.
Use: Pharmaceutic necessity for ascorbic acid injection.
See: Cenolate, Inj. (Abbott).
   Sodascorbate, Tab. (Mosso).
   Vitac Injection, Vial (Hickman).
SODIUM AUROTHIOMALATE.
See: Gold Sodium Thiosulfate, U.S.P. XXIII.
• **SODIUM BENZOATE,** N.F. XVIII.
Use: Pharmaceutic aid (antifungal agent, preservative).
SODIUM BENZOATE AND SODIUM PHENYLACETATE.
Use: For urea cycle enzymopathies. [Orphan drug]

See: Ucephan (Kendall-McGaw).
SODIUM BENZYLPENICILLIN. Penicillin
G Sodium, U.S.P. XXIII. Sodium Peni-
cillin G.
Use: Antibiotic.
• **SODIUM BICARBONATE,** U.S.P. XXIII.
Inj., Oral Pow., Tab., U.S.P. XXIII. (Ab-
bott) Inj. **4.2%:** (5 mEq) Infant 10 ml Sy-
ringe (21 G × 1.5 in. needle). **7.5%:**
(44.6 mEq) 50 ml Syringe (18 G 1.5 in.
needle) or 50 ml Amp. **8.4%:** (10 mEq)
Pediatric 10 ml Syringe (21 G 1.5 in.
needle) or (50 mEq) 50 ml Syringe (18 G
1.5 in. needle) or 50 ml Vial.
Use: Antacid, electrolyte replenisher,
systemical alkalizer.
W/Bismuth subcarbonate and Magnesia.
See: Anachloric A, Tab. (Upjohn).
W/Sodium Bitartrate.
See: Ceo-Two, Supp. (Beutlich).
W/Sodium carboxymethylcellulose, alginic
acid.
See: Pretts, Tab. (Marion).
SODIUM BIPHOSPHATE.
Use: Cathartic.
See: Sodium Phosphate Monobasic,
U.S.P. XXIII.
SODIUM BISMUTH TARTRATE.
See: Bismuth Sodium Tartrate, Preps.
SODIUM BISULFITE. Sulfurous acid,
monosodium salt. Monosodium sulfite.
Use: Antioxidant.
• **SODIUM BORATE,** N.F. XVIII.
Use: Pharmaceutic aid (alkalinizing
agent).
SODIUM BUTABARBITAL.
See: Butabarbital Sodium, U.S.P. XXIII.
SODIUM CALCIUM EDETATE. B.A.N.
Calcium chelate of thedisodium salt of
ethylenediamine-NNN'-N-tetra-acetic
acid.
Use: Treatment of lead poisoning.
See: Calcium Disodium Versenate.
SODIUM CALCIUM EDETATE.
See: Calcium Disodium Versenate,
Amp., Tab. (Riker).
• **SODIUM CARBONATE,** N.F. XVIII.
Use: Pharmaceutic aid (alkalinizing
agent).
**SODIUM CARBOXYMETHYLCELLU-
LOSE.** Carboxymethylcellulose Sodi-
um, U.S.P. XXIII. CMC. Cellulose Gum.
SODIUM CELLULOSE GLYCOLATE.
See: Carboxymethylcellulose, sodium
(Various Mfr.).
SODIUM CEPHALOTHIN. Cephalothin
Sodium, U.S.P. XXIII.
Use: Antibiotic.
• **SODIUM CHLORIDE,** U.S.P. XXIII. In-
halation Soln., Inj., Bacteriostatic for Inj.,

Irrigation, Ophth. Oint., Ophth. Soln.,
Tab., Tab. for Soln., U.S.P. XXIII.
Use: Fluid and irrigation, electrolyte replenisher, isotonic vehicle.
• **SODIUM CHLORIDE AND DEXTROSE
TABLETS,** U.S.P. XXIII.
Use: Electrolyte and nutrient replenisher.
• **SODIUM CHLORIDE INJECTION,** U.S.P.
XXIII. (Abbott) Normal saline 0.9% in
150 ml, 250 ml, 500 ml, 1,000 ml cont.;
Partial-fill: 50 ml in 200 ml, 50 ml in 300
ml, 100 ml in 300 ml; **Fliptop vial:** 10 ml,
20 ml, 50 ml, 100 ml; **Bacteriostatic
vial:** 10 ml, 20 ml, 30 ml; 50 mEq, 20 ml
in 50 ml fliptop or pintop vial; 100 mEq,
40 ml in 50 ml fliptop vial; 50 mEq, 20 ml
univ. add. syr.; sodium Cl 0.45%, 500 ml,
1,000 ml; sodium Cl 5%, 500 ml; sodium
Cl irrigating solution, 250 ml, 500 ml,
1,000 ml, 3,000 ml; (Upjohn) sodium Cl
9 mg/ml w/benzyl alcohol 9.45 mg. Vial
20 ml (Sanofi Winthrop) **Carpuject:** 2 ml
fill cartridge, 22 gauge 1 1/4 inch needle
or 25 gauge 5/8 inch needle.
Use: Fluid and irrigation, electrolyte re-
plenisher, isotonic vehicle.
• **SODIUM CHLORIDE Na 22.** USAN.
Use: Radioactive agent.
SODIUM CHLORIDE SUBSTITUTES.
See: Salt substitutes.
SODIUM CHLORIDE TABLETS, U.S.P.
XXIII. (Parke-Davis) Sodium Cl 15 1/2
gr/Tab. Bot. 1000s.
Use: Preparation of normal saline solu-
tion.
SODIUM CHLORIDE THERAPY.
See: Thermolene, Tab. (Lannett).
Thermotabs., Tab. (Calgon).
**SODIUM CHLOROTHIAZIDE FOR IN-
JECTION.** Chlorothiazide Sodium For
Injection, U.S.P. XXIII.
Use: Diuretic.
SODIUM CHOLATE. (City Chem.) Sodi-
um cholate Bot. 100 Gm.
• **SODIUM CHROMATE Cr 51 INJ.,** U.S.P.
XXIII.
Use: Diagnostic aid (blood volume de-
termination).
See: Radio Chromate Cr 51 Sodium.
• **SODIUM CITRATE,** U.S.P. XXIII. 1,2,3-
Propanetricarboxylic acid, 2-hy-droxy-,
trisodium salt. Trisodium citrate. Trisodi-
um citrate dihydrate.
Use: Anticoagulant.
See: Anticoagulant Citrate Dextrose So-
lution, U.S.P. XXIII.
Anticoagulant Citrate Phosphate Dex-
trose Solution, U.S.P. XXIII.
• **SODIUM CITRATE AND CITRIC ACID**

ORAL SOLUTION, U.S.P. XXIII.
Shohl's Solution.
Use: Systemic alkalinizer.
SODIUM CLOXACILLIN.
See: Cloxacillin Sodium, U.S.P. XXIII.
SODIUM COLISTIMETHATE. Colistimethane Sodium, Sterile, U.S.P. XXIII.
Antibiotic produced by *Aerobacillus colistinus.*
SODIUM COLISTIN METHANESULFONATE. Colistimethane Sodium,
U.S.P. XXIII. The sodium methanesulfonate salt of an antibiotic substance
elaborated by *Aerobacillus colistinus.*
Use: Antibiotic.
•**SODIUM DEHYDROACETATE,** N.F.
XVIII.
Use: Pharmaceutic aid (antimicrobial preservative).
SODIUM DEXTROTHYROXINE. Sodium
D-3,3′,5,5-tetraiodothyronine. Sodium
D-3-(4-(4-Hydroxy-3,5-diiodophenoxy)-
3,5-diiodophenyl)-alanine.
Use: Anticholesteremic.
SODIUM DIATRIZOATE. Diatrizoate
Sodium, U.S.P. XXIII.
Use: Radiopaque medium.
SODIUM DIBUNATE. B.A.N. Sodium 2,7-
di-t-butylnaphthalene-1-sulfonate.
Use: Cough suppressant.
SODIUM DICLOXACILLIN. Dicloxacillin
Sodium, U.S.P. XXIII.
Use: Antibiotic.
SODIUM DICLOXACILLIN MONOHYDRATE.
Use: Antibiotic.
See: Pathocil, Prep. (Wyeth-Ayerst).
SODIUM DIHYDROGEN PHOSPHATE.
Sodium Biphosphate, U.S.P. XXIII.
SODIUM DIMETHOXYPHENYL PENICILLIN.
See: Methicillin Sodium (Various Mfr.).
SODIUM DIOCTYL SULFOSUCCINATE.
See: Docusate Sodium, U.S.P. XXIII.
SODIUM DIPHENYLHYDANTOIN.
Phenytoin Sodium, U.S.P. XXIII.
Diphenylhydantoin Sodium.
Use: Anticonvulsant.
SODIUM DIPROTRIZOATE, B.A.N. Sodium 3,5-dipropionamide-2,4,6-tri-
iodobenzoate.
SODIUM EDETATE, Edetate Disodium,
U.S.P. XXIII. Tetrasodium ethylenediaminetetraacetate.
Use: Chelating agent.
See: Vagisec products (Julius Schmid).
SODIUM ETHACRYNATE. Ethacrynate
Sodium for Injection, U.S.P. XXIII.
Use: Diuretic.
•**SODIUM ETHASULFATE.** USAN.

Use: Detergent.
SODIUM ETHYL-MERCURI-THIO-SALICYLATE.
See: Thimerosal (Various Mfr.).
Merthiolate, Preps. (Lilly).
SODIUM FEREDETATE (I.N.N.). Sodium
iron edetate. B.A.N.
SODIUM FLUORESCEIN, Fluorescein
Sodium U.S.P. XXIII. Resorcinolphthalein sodium.
Use: Diagnostic aid (corneal trauma indicator).
•**SODIUM FLUORIDE,** U.S.P. XXIII. Oral
Soln., Tab, U.S.P. XXIII.
Use: Dental caries prophylactic.
See: Fluoride, Tab. (Kirkman).
Fluoride Loz. (Kirkman).
Flura Drops, Drops (Kirkman).
Flura-Loz, Loz. (Kirkman).
Karidium, Liq., Tab. (Lorvic).
Kari-Rinse, Liq. (Lorvic).
Luride, Tab. (Colgate Hoyt).
Mouthkote F/R, Rinse (Parnell).
NaFeon, Tab., Liq. (Pacemaker).
Pediaflor, Drops (Ross).
T-Fluoride, Tab. (Tennessee Pharm.).
W/Vitamins.
See: Fluorac, Tab. (Rhone-Poulenc
Rorer).
Mulvidren-F, Tab. (Stuart).
So-Flo, Tab., Drops (Professional
Pharm.).
W/Vitamins A, D, C.
See: Cari-Tab, Softab. (Stuart).
Tri-Vi-Flor, Drops, Tab. (Mead Johnson).
•**SODIUM FLUORIDE AND PHOSPHORIC
ACID GEL,** U.S.P. XXIII.
Use: Dental caries prophylactic.
•**SODIUM FLUORIDE AND PHOSPHORIC ACID TOPICAL SOLUTION,** U.S.P.
XXIII.
Use: Dental caries prophylactic.
•**SODIUM FLUORIDE F 18,** Inj., U.S.P. 23.
SODIUM FOLATE. Monosodium folate.
Use: Water soluble, hematopoietic vitamin.
SODIUM FORMALDEHYDE SULFOXYLATE, N.F. XVIII. (Various Mfr.)
$H_2C(OH)SO_2Na.$
Use: Reducing agent, preservative.
SODIUM-FREE SALT.
See: Co-Salt, Bot. (Rhone-Poulenc
Rorer).
Diasal, Prep. (Savage).
**SODIUM GAMMA-HYDROXYBUTYRIC
ACID.** Under study.
Use: Anesthetic adjuvant, sleep disorders. [Orphan drug]
SODIUM GENTISATE.

See: Gentisate Sodium.

SODIUM GLUCALDRATE. B.A.N. Sodium gluconatodihydroxyaluminate.
Use: Treatment of gastric hyperacidity.

SODIUM GLUCASPALDRATE, B.A.N.
Octasodium tetrakis (gluconato)-bis (salicylato), μ-diacetatodialuminate(III) dihydrate.
Use: Analgesic.

• **SODIUM GLUCONATE,** U.S.P. XXIII.

SODIUM GLUCOSULFONE INJ. Disodium 1,1'-[Sulfonylbis(p-phenyleneimino)]bis-[D-gluco-2,3,4,5,6-pentahydroxy-1-hexanesulfonate].
Use: Leprostatic.

SODIUM GLUTAMATE.
See: Glutamate.

SODIUM GLYCEROPHOSPHATE. Glycerol phosphate sodium salt.
Use: Pharmaceutic necessity.

SODIUM GLYCOCHOLATE, A BILE SALT.
See: Bile Salts.
W/Phenolphthalein, cascara sagrada extract, sodium taurocholate, aloin.
See: Oxiphen, Tab. (Webcon).
W/Sodium nitrite, blue flag.
See: So-Nitri-Nacea, Cap. (Scrip).
W/Sodium taurocholate, sodium salicylate, phenolphthalein, bile extract, cascara sagrada extract.
See: Glycols, Tab. (Bowman).

SODIUM HEPARIN. Heparin Sodium, U.S.P. XXIII.
Use: Anticoagulant.

SODIUM HEXACYCLONATE. Sodium 1-hydroxy-methylcyclohexaneacetate.

SODIUM HEXOBARBITAL. Sodium 5-(1-cyclohexen-1-yl)-1,5-dimethylbarbiturate.
Use: Intravenous general anesthetic.

SODIUM HYALURONATE.
Use: Ophthalmic.
See: Amo Vitrax (Allergan).
Amvisc (Iolab).
Amvisc Plus (Iolab).
Healon (Kabi Pharmacia Ophthalmics).
W/Chondroitin sulfate.
See: Viscoat, Soln. (Alcon).

SODIUM HYDROGEN CITRATE. (Various Mfr.).

• **SODIUM HYDROXIDE,** N.F. XVIII. Caustic Soda.
Use: Pharmaceutic aid (alkalizing agent).

SODIUM HYDROXYDIONE SUCCINATE. Sodium 21-hydroxypregnane-3,20-dione succinate.

• **SODIUM HYPOCHLORITE SOLUTION,**

U.S.P. XXIII.
Use: Local anti-infective, disinfectant.
See: Antiformin.
Dakin's Soln.
Hyclorite.

SODIUM HYPOPHOSPHITE. Sodium phosphinate.
Use: Pharmaceutic necessity.

SODIUM HYPOSULFITE.
See: Sodium Thiosulfate (Various Mfr.).
W/Potassium guaiacolsufonate.
See: Guaiadol Aqueous, Vial (Medical Chem.).
W/Potassium guaiacolsulfonate, chlorpheniramine maleate, sodium bisulfite.
See: Gomahist, Inj. (Burgin-Arden).
W/Sulfur, sodium citrate, phenol, benzyl alcohol.
See: Sulfo-Iodide, Inj. (Marcen).

SODIUM IODIPAMIDE. Disodium 3,3'-(Adipoyl- diimino) bis-[2,4,6-triiodobenzoate].
Use: Radiopaque medium.

SODIUM IODOMETHAMATE. Disodium 1,4-dihydro-3,5-diiodo-1-methyl-4-oxo-2,6-pyridine dicarboxylate. (Iodoxyl, Pyelecton, Uropac).

SODIUM IODOMETHANE SULFONATE. Methiodal Sodium, U.S.P. XXIII.

SODIUM IOTHALAMATE. Iothalmate Sodium Inj., U.S.P. XXIII.
Use: Radiopaque medium.

SODIUM IOTHIOURACIL. Sodium 5-iodo-2-thiouracil.

SODIUM IPODATE. Ipodate Sodium, U.S.P. XXIII.
Use: Radiopaque.
See: Biloptin.
Oragrafin Sodium, Cap. (Squibb).

SODIUM IRONEDETATE. B.A.N. Iron chelate of the monosodium salt of ethylenediamine-NNN'N-tetra-acetic acid.
Use: Treatment of iron-deficiency anemia.
See: Sodium Feredetate (I.N.N.).

SODIUM ISOAMYLETHYLBARBITURATE.
See: Amytal Sodium, Prep. (Lilly).

• **SODIUM LACTATE INJECTION,** U.S.P. XXIII. Propanoic acid, 2-hydroxy-, monosodium salt. Monosodium lactate. (Abbott) 1/6 Molar, 250 ml, 500 ml, 1,000 ml; 50 mEq, 10 ml in 20 ml fliptop vial.
Use: Fluid and electrolyte replenisher.

• **SODIUM LACTATE SOLUTION,** U.S.P. XXIII.
Use: Replenisher (electrolyte).

• **SODIUM LAURYL SULFATE,** N.F. XVIII.
Sulfuric acid monododecyl ester sodium

salt. Sodium monododecyl sulfate.
Use: Pharmaceutical aid (surfactant).
See: Duponol.
W/Hydrocortisone.
See: Nutracort, Cream, Lot. (Owen).
SODIUM LEVOTHYROXINE. Levothy-
roxine Sodium, U.S.P. XXIII.
SODIUM LIOTHYRONINE. Liothyronine
Sodium, U.S.P. XXIII.
Use: Thyroid hormone.
SODIUM LYAPOLATE. Polyethylene sul-
fonate sodium. Peson (Hoechst). Sodi-
um Apolate, B.A.N.
Use: Anticoagulant.
SODIUM MALONYLUREA.
See: Barbital Sodium (Various Mfr.).
SODIUM MERCAPTOMERIN. Mercap-
tomerin Sodium, U.S.P. XXIII.
Use: Diuretic.
• **SODIUM METABISULFITE,** N.F. XVIII.
SODIUM METHIODAL. Methiodal Sodi-
um, U.S.P. XXIII. Sodium
monoiodomethanesulfonate. Sodium
Iodomethanesulfonate, Inj.
Use: Radiopaque medium.
**SODIUM METHOHEXITAL FOR INJEC-
TION.** Methohexital Sodium for Injec-
tion, U.S.P. XXIII.
Use: General anesthetic.
See: Brevital Sod., Pow. (Lilly).
SODIUM METHOXYCELLULOSE. Mix-
ture of methylcellulose and sodium.
SODIUM METRIZOATE, B.A.N. Sodium
3-acetamido-2,4,6-triiodo-5-(N-methyl-
acetamido) benzoate.
Use: Contrast medium.
• **SODIUM MONOFLUOROPHOSPHATE,**
U.S.P. XXII.
SODIUM MORRHUATE, INJ. Morrhuate
Sodium Inj., U.S.P. XXIII.
Use: Sclerosing agent.
SODIUM NAFCILLIN. Nafcillin Sodium,
U.S.P. XXIII.
Use: Antibacterial.
SODIUM NICOTINATE. Sodium pyridine-
3-carboxylate (Various Mfr.).
W/Adenosine 5 monophosphoric acid.
Use: I.V. nicotinic acid therapy.
SODIUM NITRATE. (Various Mfr.) Gran,
Pkg. lb.
SODIUM NITRATE COMBINATIONS.
See: Hyperlon, Tab. (Kenyon).
Veraphen, Tab. (Davis and Sly).
• **SODIUM NITRITE,** U.S.P. XXIII. Inj.,
U.S.P. XXIII. (Various Mfr.) Gran., Bot.
0.25 lb, 1 lb.
Use: Antidote to cyanide poisoning, an-
tioxidant.
W/Sodium thiosulfate, amyl nitrite.
Use: Vasodilator and antidote to

cyanide poisoning.
See: Cyanide Antidote Pkg. (Lilly).
• **SODIUM NITROPRUSSIDE,** U.S.P. XXIII.
Sterile, U.S.P. XXIII.
Use: Hypotensive agent.
See: Keto-Diastix (Miles Diagnostic).
Nipride, Vial (Roche).
Nitropress, Vial (Abbott).
**SODIUM NORAMIDOPYRINE
METHANESULFONATE.** Dipyrone.
B.A.N.
SODIUM NOVOBIOCIN. Sodium salt of
antibacterial substance produced by
Streptomyces niveus. Novobiocin
monosodium salt.
Use: Antibiotic.
See: Albamycin, Cap., Syr., Vial (Up-
john).
SODIUM ortho-IODOHIPPURATE.
Iodohippurate Sodium, I-131 Injection,
U.S.P. XXIII.
See: Hipputope (Squibb).
• **SODIUM OXYBATE.** USAN. Sodium 4-
hydroxybutyrate.
Use: Adjunct to anesthesia.
SODIUM PANTOTHENATE.
Use: Orally, dietary supplement.
SODIUM PARA-AMINOBENZOATE.
See: p Aminobenzoate, Sodium (Vari-
ous Mfr.).
**SODIUM PARA-AMINOHIPPURATE IN-
JECTION.**
Use: I.V., to determine kidney tubular
excretion function.
SODIUM PARA-AMINOSALICYLATE.
See: p-Aminosalicylate, Sodium (Vari-
ous Mfr.).
SODIUM PENICILLIN G. Penicillin G
Sodium, Sterile, U.S.P. XXIII. Sodium
benzylpenicillin.
SODIUM PENICILLIN O. Sodium-6-[2-
(allylthio)-acetamido]-3,3-dimethyl-7-
oxo-4-thia-1-azabicyclo-[3.2.0]heptane-
2-carboxylate.
SODIUM PENTOBARBITAL. Pentobarbi-
tal Sodium, U.S.P. XXIII.
Use: Hypnotic.
SODIUM PERBORATE. Sodium Perox-
yborate. Sodium peroxyhydrate.
SODIUM PEROXYBORATE.
See: Sodium Perborate. (Various Mfr.).
SODIUM PEROXYHYDRATE.
See: Sodium Perborate. (Various Mfr.).
• **SODIUM PERTECHNETATE Tc 99 m IN-
JECTION,** U.S.P. XXIII. Pertechnetic
acid, sodium salt.
Use: Diagnostic aid (brain scanning;
thyroid scanning).
See: Minitec (Squibb).
SODIUM PHENOBARBITAL. Phenobar-

bital Sodium, U.S.P. XXIII.
Use: Anticonvulsant, hypnotic.
SODIUM PHENYLETHYLBARBITU-RATE. Phenobarbital Sodium, U.S.P. XXIII.
•**SODIUM PHOSPHATE,** U.S.P. XXIII. Dried, Inj., U.S.P. XXIII. Effervescent, U.S.P. XXI. Disodium hydrogen phosphate. (Abbott) 3 mM P and 4 mEq sodium. 15 ml in 30 ml fliptop vial.
Use: Cathartic, buffering agent, source of phosphate.
W/Gentamicin sulfate, monosodium phosphate, sodium Cl, benzalkonium Cl.
See: Garamycin Ophthalmic, Soln. (Schering).
W/Sodium biphosphate.
See: Enemeez, Enema (Armour).
Fleet Enema (Fleet).
Phospho-Soda, Liq. (Fleet).
Saf-tip, Enemas (Fuller).
•**SODIUM PHOSPHATE, DIBASIC,** U.S.P. XXIII.
Use: Laxative.
•**SODIUM PHOSPHATE, DRIED,** U.S.P. XXIII.
Use: Cathartic.
•**SODIUM PHOSPHATE, MONOBASIC,** U.S.P. XXIII. Monosodium Phosphate. Sodium Acid Phosphate, Sodium Dihydrogen Phosphate, Sodium Biphosphate.
Use: Cathartic.
See: Travad, Enema (Flint).
W/Gentamicin sulfate, disodium phosphate, sodium Cl, benzalkonium Cl.
See: Garamycin Ophthalmic Soln. (Schering).
W/Methenamine.
See: Uro-Phosphate, Tab. (Poythress).
W/Methenamine mandelate, levo-hyoscyamine sulfate.
See: Levo-Uroquid, Tab. (Beach).
W/Methenamine, phenyl salicylate, methylene blue, hyoscyamine, alkaloid.
See: Urostat Forte, Tab. (Elder).
W/Sodium acid pyrophos, sodium bicarbonate.
See: Vacuetts, Supp. (Dorsey).
W/Sodium phosphate.
See: Enemeez Enema (Armour).
Fleet Enema (Fleet).
Phospho-Soda, Liq. (Fleet).
Saf-tip Enemas (Fuller).
•**SODIUM PHOSPHATES ENEMA,** U.S.P. XXIII.
Use: Cathartic.
•**SODIUM PHOSPHATES ORAL SOLUTION,** U.S.P. XXIII.
Use: Cathartic.

•**SODIUM PHOSPHATE P32 SOLUTION,** U.S.P. XXIII. Phosphoric -32P acid, disodium salt. Disodium phosphate -32P.
Use: Antineoplastic, antipolycythemic. Diagnostic. aid (ocular tumor localization.).
SODIUM PHYTATE. Nonasodium phytate: Sodium cyclohexanehexyl (hexaphosphate).
Use: Chelating agent.
SODIUM PICOSULPHATE. B.A.N. Disodium 4,4'-(2-pyridyl)methylenedi(phenyl sulfate).
Use: Laxative.
•**SODIUM POLYPHOSPHATE.** USAN.
Use: Pharmaceutic aid.
•**SODIUM POLYSTYRENE SULFONATE,** U.S.P. XXIII, Susp., U.S.P. XXIII. Benzene, ethenyl-, homopolymer, sulfonated, sodium salt. Styrene polymer, sulfonated, sodium salt.
Use: Ion exchange resin (potassium).
See: Kayexalate, Pow. (Sanofi Winthrop).
•**SODIUM PROPIONATE,** N.F. XVIII. 5% Soln. Eye-drops (Crookes-Barnes) Lacrivial 15 ml.
Use: Preservative.
W/Chlorophyll "a"
See: Prophyllin, Pow., Oint. (Rystan).
W/Neomycin sulfate.
See: Otobiotic, Ear Drops (Schering).
W/Propionic acid, docusate sodium, salicylic acid.
See: Prosal, Liq. (Gordon).
SODIUM PSYLLIATE.
Use: Sclerosing agent.
•**SODIUM PYROPHOSPHATE.** USAN.
Use: Pharmaceutic aid.
SODIUM RADIO CHROMATE INJ. Sodium Chromate Cr 51 Inj., U.S.P. XXIII.
SODIUM RADIO IODIDE SOLUTION. Sodium Iodide I-131 Solution, U.S.P. XXIII.
Use: Thyroid tumors, hyperthyroidism, cardiac dysfunction.
SODIUM RADIO-PHOSPHATE, P-32 Soln. Radio-Phosphate P32 Solution. Sodium phosphate P-32 Solution, U.S.P. XXIII.
SODIUM REMOVING RESINS.
See: Resins.
SODIUM RHODANATE.
See: Sodium Thiocyanate.
SODIUM RHODANIDE.
See: Sodium Thiocyanate.
SODIUM SACCHARIN. Saccharin Sodium, U.S.P. XXIII.
Use: Noncaloric sweetener.

• **SODIUM SALICYLATE,** U.S.P. XXIII.
Tab., U.S.P. XXIII.
Use: Analgesic.
W/Iodide (Various Mfr.).
Use: Intravenous injection.
W/Iodide and cholchicine. (Various Mfr.).
Use: I.V., gout.
SODIUM SALICYLATE, NATURAL.
Use: Analgesic.
See: Alysine, Elix. (Merrell Dow).
SODIUM SALICYLATE COMBINATIONS.
See: Apcogesic, Tab. (Apco).
Bisalate, Tab. (Allison).
Bufosal, Gran. (Table Rock).
Corilin, Liq. (Schering).
Nucorsal, Tab. (Westerfield).
Pabalate, Tab. (Robins).
pHisoDan, Liq. (Sanofi Winthrop).
SODIUM SECOBARBITAL. Secobarbital
Sodium, U.S.P. XXIII.
Use: Hypnotic.
**SODIUM SECOBARBITAL AND SODIUM
AMOBARBITAL CAPSULES.**
Use: Sedative.
See: Tuinal, Cap. (Lilly).
• **SODIUM STARCH GLYCOLATE,** N.F.
XVIII.
Use: Pharmaceutic aid (tablet excipient).
• **SODIUM STEARATE,** N.F. XVIII. Octadecanoic acid, sodium salt
Use: Emulsifying and stiffening agent.
• **SODIUM STEARYL FUMARATE,** N.F.
XVIII.
Use: Pharmaceutic aid (tablet lubricant).
SODIUM STIBOGLUCONATE. B.A.N.
Sodium salt of a pentavalent antimony
derivative of gluconic acid.
Use: Treatment of leishmaniasis.
SODIUM SUCCINATE.
Use: Alkalinize urine & awaken patients
following barbiturate anesthesia.
SODIUM SULAMYD Ophthalmic Oint.
10% Sterile. (Schering) Sulfacetamide
sodium 10%, methylparaben, propylparaben, benzalkonium Cl, sorbitan
monolaurate, water. Tube 0.125 oz.
Use: Anti-infective, ophthalmic.
SODIUM SULAMYD Ophthalmic Soln.
10% Sterile. (Schering) Sulfacetamide
sodium 10%, methylcellulose 0.5%,
sodium thiosulfate 0.31%, methylparaben, propylparaben. Bot. 5 ml. Box
25s. 15 ml. Box 1s.
Use: Anti-infective, ophthalmic.
SODIUM SULAMYD Ophthalmic Soln.
30% Sterile. (Schering) Sulfacetamide
sodium 30%, sodium thiosulfate 0.15%,

methylparaben, propylparaben as
preservative. Bot. 15 ml. Box 1s.
Use: Anti-infective, ophthalmic.
SODIUM SULFABROMOMETHAZINE.
Sodium N^1-(5-Bromo-4,6-dimethyl-2-
pyrimidinyl) sulfanilamide.
Use: Antibacterial.
SODIUM SULFACETAMIDE.
See: Sulfacetamide Sodium Preps.
(Various Mfr.).
SODIUM SULFADIAZINE.
See: Sulfadiazine Sodium Preps. (Various Mfr.).
SODIUM SULFAMERAZINE.
See: Sulfamerazine Sodium Preps.
(Various Mfr.).
SODIUM SULFAPYRIDINE.
See: Sulfapyridine Sodium Pow. (Pfaltz
& Bauer).
• **SODIUM SULFATE,** U.S.P. XXIII. Inj.,
U.S.P. XXIII.
Use: Cathartic.
• **SODIUM SULFATE S 35.** USAN
Use: Radioactive agent.
SODIUM SULFATHIAZOLE.
Use: Antibacterial.
See: Sulfathiazole Sodium, Inj. (Various
Mfr.).
SODIUM SULFOACETATE. W/Sodium
alkyl aryl polyether sulfonate, docusate
sodium, kerohydric, sulfur, salicylic acid,
hexachlorophene.
See: Sebulex, Liq., Cream (Westwood).
SODIUM SULFOBROMOPHTHALEIN.
Sulfobromophthalein Sodium, U.S.P.
XXII.
Use: Diagnostic aid (hepatic function
determination).
SODIUM SULFOCYANATE.
See: Sodium Thiocyanate. (Various
Mfr.).
SODIUM SULFOXONE. Sulfoxone Sodium, U.S.P. XXIII. Disodium sulfonyl-
bis(p-phenyleneimino)dimethanesul-
fonate.
See: Diasone Sodium, Tab. (Abbott).
SODIUM SURAMIN.
See: Suramin Sodium.
**SODIUM TAUROCHOLATE, A BILE
SALT.**
See: Bile Salts.
W/Phenolphthalein, cascara sagrada extract, sodium glycocholate, aloin.
See: Oxiphen, Tab. (Webcon).
SODIUM TETRADECYL SULFATE.
Use: Bleeding esophageal varices. [Orphan drug]
See: Sotradecol, Inj. (Elkins-Sinn).
**SODIUM TETRAIODOPHENOLPH-
THALEIN.**

See: Iodophthalein Sodium (Various Mfr.).

SODIUM THIACETPHENARSAMIDE.
The trivalent organic arsenical p-[bis-(carboxymethylmercapto)-arsino] benzamide. Ceparsolate Sodium (Abbott).

SODIUM THIAMYLAL FOR INJECTION.
Thiamylal Sodium For Injection, U.S.P. XXIII.
Use: General anesthetic.
See: Surital, Inj. (Parke-Davis).

SODIUM THIOCYANATE. Sodium Sulfocyanate. Sodium Rhodanide.

SODIUM THIOPENTAL.
See: Thiopental Sodium, U.S.P. XXIII.

SODIUM THIOSALICYLATE.
See: Rexolate, Vial (Hyrex).
Thiolate (Hickam; Pharmex).
Th-Sal, Vial (Foy).

• **SODIUM THIOSULFATE,** U.S.P. XXIII.
Inj., U.S.P. XXIII. Sodium hyposulfite. "Hypo." Thiosulfuric acid, disodium salt, pentahydrate. Disodium thiosulfate pentahydrate.
Use: For argyria, cyanide and iodine poisoning, arsphenamine reactions; prevention of spread of ringworm of feet.
W/Salicylic acid, hydrocortisone acetate, alcohol.
See: Komed HC, Lot. (Barnes-Hind).
W/Salicylic acid, isopropyl alcohol.
See: Tinver, Lot. (Barnes-Hind).
W/Salicylic acid, resorcinol, alcohol.
See: Mild Komed, Lot. (Barnes-Hind).
Komed, Lot. (Barnes-Hind).
W/Sodium nitrite, amyl nitrite.
See: Cyanide Antidote Pkg. (Lilly).

SODIUM L-THYROXINE.
See: Letter, Tab. (Armour).
Levoid, Inj., Tab. (Nutrition Control).
Roxstan, Tab. (Reid-Rowell).
Synthroid, Tab., Inj. (Flint).

SODIUM TOLBUTAMIDE. Tolbutamide Sodium, U.S.P. XXIII.
Use: Diagnostic aid (diabetes).

SODIUM TRICLOFOS. Sodium trichloroethylphosphate.
Use: Sedative, hypnotic.

• **SODIUM TRIMETAPHOSPHATE.** USAN.
Use: Pharmaceutic aid.

SODIUM TYROPANOATE. B.A.N. Sodium 3-butyramido-α-ethyl-2,4,6-triiodohydrocinnamate. Radiopaque.
Use: Cholecystographic agent.

SODIUM VINBARBITAL INJECTION.
Use: Sedative.

SODIUM WARFARIN. Warfarin Sodium, U.S.P. XXIII.
Use: Anticoagulant.

SOD-LATE 10. (Schlicksup) Sodium salicylate 10 gr/Tab. Bot. 1000s.
Use: Analgesic.

SODOL COMPOUND. (Major) Carisoprodol 200 mg, aspirin 325 mg/Tab. Bot. 100s, 500s.
Use: Skeletal muscle relaxant.

SOFARIN. (Lemmon) Warfarin sodium 2 mg in 100s. 2.5 mg in 100s, or 5 mg/Tab. Bot. 100s, 1000s.
Use: Anticoagulant.

SOFCAPS. (Alton) Docusate sodium 100 mg or 250 mg/Cap. Bot. 100s, 1000s.
Use: Laxative.

SOFENOL 5. (C & M Pharmacal) Moisturizing lotion formulation. Bot. 8 oz.
Use: Emollient.

SOFLENS ENZYMATIC CONTACT LENS CLEANER. (Allergan) Papain, sodium Cl, sodium carbonate, sodium borate, edetate disodium/Tab. Vial 12s, 24s, 48s, Refill 24s, 36s.
Use: Soft contact lens care.

SOF/PRO CLEAN SA. (Sherman) Hypertonic solution: salt buffers, copolymers of ethylene and propylene oxide, octylphenoxypolyethoxyethanol, lauryl sulfate salt of imidazoline, sodium bisulfate 0.1%, sorbic acid 0.1%, trisodium EDTA 0.25%, thimerosal free. Bot. 30 ml.
Use: Soft contact lens care.

SOF/PRO-CLEAN. (Sherman) Buffered, hypertonic solution with thimerosal 0.004%, EDTA 0.1%, ethylene and propylene oxide, octylphenoxypolyethoxyethanol, lauryl sulfate salt of imidazoline. Bot. 30 ml.
Use: Soft contact lens care.

SOFT MATE COMFORT DROPS FOR SENSITIVE EYES. (Pilkington Barnes-Hind) Isotonic, buffered, potassium sorbate 0.13%, EDTA 0.1%. Drop. Bot. 15 ml.
Use: Soft contact lens care.

SOFT MATE CONSEPT 1. (Pilkington Barnes-Hind) Hydrogen peroxide 3% w/polyoxyl 40 stearate, sodium stannate, sodium nitrate, phosphate buffer, thimerasol free. 240 ml.
Use: Soft contact lens care.

SOFT MATE CONSEPT 2. (Pilkington Barnes-Hind) Isotonic solution of sodium thiosulfate 0.5%, NaCl, borate buffers. Lens case. 240 ml or 360 ml, aerosol 360 ml.
Use: Soft contact lens care.

SOFT MATE DAILY CLEANING FOR SENSITIVE EYES. (Pilkington Barnes-Hind) Isotonic solution w/NaCl, octylphe-

noxy (oxyethylene) ethanol hydrox-yethylcellulose w/potassium sorbate 0.13%, EDTA 0.2%. Soln. Bot. 1 or 30 ml.
Use: Soft contact lens care.
SOFT MATE DAILY CLEANING SOLUTION. (Pilkington Barnes-Hind) Sterile aqueous isotonic solution w/sodium Cl, octylphenoxy (oxyethylene) ethanol, hydroxyethylcellulose, thimerosal 0.004%, edetate disodium 0.2%. Bot. 30 ml.
Use: Soft contact lens care.
SOFT MATE DAILY CLEANING SOLUTION II. (Pilkington Barnes-Hind) Sterile aqueous isotonic solution w/sodium Cl, octylphenoxyl (oxyethylene) ethanol, hydoxyethylcellulose, potassium sorbate 0.13%, edetate disodium 0.2%. Bot. 0.5 oz, 8 oz.
Use: Soft contact lens care.
SOFT MATE DISINFECTING SOLUTION. (Pilkington Barnes-Hind) Sterile, aqueous, isotonic solution w/sodium Cl, povidone, octylphenoxy (oxyethylene) ethanol, chlorhexidine gluconate 0.005%, edetate disodium 0.1%. Thimerosal free. Bot. 8 oz.
Use: Soft contact lens care.
SOFT MATE DISINFECTION AND STORAGE SOLUTION. (Pilkington Barnes-Hind) Sterile aqueous isotonic solution w/sodium Cl, povidone, octylphenoxl (oxyethylene) ethanol with a borate buffer, thimerosal 0.001%, edetate disodium 0.1%, chlorhexidine gluconate 0.005%. Bot. 8 oz.
Use: Soft contact lens care.
SOFT MATE ENZYME PLUS CLEANER. (Pilkington Barnes-Hind) Subtilisin, poloxamer 338, povidone, citric acid, potassium bicarbonate, sodium carbonate, sodium benzoate. Tab. Pkg. 8s.
Use: Soft contact lens care.
SOFT MATE LENS DROPS. (Pilkington Barnes-Hind) Sterile aqueous isotonic solution w/sodium Cl, potassium sorbate 0.13%, edetate disodium 0.025%. Thimerosal free. Bot. 2 oz.
Use: Soft contact lens care.
SOFT MATE PRESERVATIVE-FREE SALINE SOLUTION. (Pilkington Barnes-Hind) Sterile aqueous isotonic solution w/sodium Cl, borate buffer. Contains no preservatives. Bot. 0.5 oz, 30 single use.
Use: Soft contact lens care.
SOFT MATE PROTEIN REMOVER SOLUTION. (Pilkington Barnes-Hind) Sterile aqueous solution buffered with borates. Preservative free. Single use

vials, 8 ml each. In 4s, 8s, 12s.
Use: Soft contact lens care.
SOFT MATE PS COMFORT DROPS. (Pilkington Barnes-Hind) Sterile aqueous isotonic solution w/potassium sorbate 0.13%, edetate disodium 0.1%. Bot. 15 ml.
Use: Contact lens care.
SOFT MATE PS DAILY CLEANING SOLUTION. (Pilkington Barnes-Hind) Sterile aqueous isotonic solution w/sodium Cl, octylphenoxy (oxyethylene) ethanol, hydroxyethyl cellulose, potassium sorbate 0.13%, edetate disodium 0.2%. Bot. 30 ml.
Use: Soft contact lens care.
SOFT MATE PS SALINE SOLUTION. (Pilkington Barnes-Hind) Sterile aqueous isotonic solution w/sodium Cl, potassium sorbate 0.13%, edetate disodium 0.025%. Bot. 8 oz, 12 oz.
Use: Soft contact lens care.
SOFT MATE RINSING SOLUTION. (Pilkington Barnes-Hind) Sterile aqueous isotonic solution w/sodium Cl, thimerosal 0.001%, edetate disodium 0.1%, chlorhexidine gluconate 0.005%. Bot. 8 oz.
Use: Soft contact lens care.
SOFT MATE SALINE FOR SENSITIVE EYES. (Pilkington Barnes-Hind) Isotonic, sorbic acid 0.1%, EDTA 0.1%, NaCl, borate buffer. Bot. 360 (2s) or 480 ml.
Use: Soft contact lens care.
SOFT MATE SALINE PRESERVATIVE-FREE. (Pilkington Barnes-Hind) Sodium Cl w/borate buffer. Soln. Bot. 15 ml.
Use: Soft contact lens care.
SOFT MATE SALINE SOLUTION. (Pilkington Barnes-Hind) Sterile aqueous isotonic solution of sodium Cl. Preservative free. Bot. 8 oz, 12 oz.
Use: Soft contact lens care.
SOFT MATE SOFT LENS CLEANERS. (Pilkington Barnes-Hind) Kit containing: Soft Mate daily cleaning solution II (4 oz.); soft mate weekly cleaning solution (1.2 oz.); Hydra-Mat II cleaning and storage unit.
Use: Soft contact lens care.
SOFT'N SOOTHE. (Ascher) Benzocaine, menthol, moisturizers. Tube 50 Gm.
Use: Local anesthetic.
SOFT RINSE 135. (Professional Supplies) Salt tablets for normal saline solution 135 mg/Tab. In 365s with Bot. 15 ml.
Use: Soft contact lens care.
SOFT RINSE 250. (Soft Rinse Corp.) Salt tablets for normal saline solution 250 mg/Tab. In 200s, with Bot. 27.7 ml.

Use: Soft contact lens care.

SOLANEED. (Hanlon) Vitamin A 25,000 units/Cap. Bot. 100s.
Use: Vitamin A supplement.

SOLAPSONE. B.A.N. Tetrasodium salt of bis-[4-(3-phenyl-1,3-disulfopropylamino)phenyl]sulfone.
Use: Antileprotic.
See: Solasulfone (I.N.N.).

SOLAQUIN. (Elder) Hydroquinone 2%, ethyl dihydroxypropyl PABA 5%, dioxybenzone 3%, oxybenzone 2%. Tube oz.
Use: Skin bleaching agent with sunscreen.

SOLAQUIN FORTE CREAM. (Elder) Hydroquinone 4%, ethyl dihydroxypropyl PABA 5%, dioxybenzone 3%, oxybenzone 2% in a vanishing cream base. Tube 0.5 oz, 1 oz.
Use: Skin bleaching agent with sunscreen.

SOLAQUIN FORTE GEL. (Elder) Hydroquinone 4%, ethyl dihydroxypropyl PABA 5%, dioxybenzone 3%, oxybenzone 2%. Tube 0.5 oz, 1 oz.
Use: Skin bleaching agent with sunscreen.

SOLARCAINE. (Plough).
Cream: Benzocaine 1%, triclosan. Tube oz. **Lot.:** Benzocaine 0.5%, triclosan. Bot. 3 oz, 6 oz. **Spray (aerosol):** Benzocaine 20%, triclosan 0.13%, isopropyl alcohol 35%. Can 3 oz, 5 oz.
Use: Local anesthetic.

SOLAR CREAM. (Doak) PABA, titanium dioxide, magnesium stearate in a flesh-colored, water-repellent base. Tube oz.
Use: Sunscreen.

SOLARGENTUM.
See: Mild silver protein (Various Mfr.).

SOLAR SHIELD 15 SPF. (Akorn) Ethyl-hexyl-p-methoxy-cinnamate 7.5%, oxybenzone in a moisturizing base 5%, PABA free, waterproof. Lot. Bot. 120 ml.
Use: Sunscreen.

SOLAR SHIELD 30 SPF. (Akorn) Ethyl-hexyl-p-methoxycinnamate 7.5%, oxybenzone 6%, 2-ethylhexyl salicylate 5%, 3-diphenylacrylate 7.5%, 2-ethylhexyl-2-cyano-3 in a moisturizing base, PABA free, waterproof. Lot. Bot. 120 ml.
Use: Sunscreen.

SOLATENE. (Roche) Beta-carotene 30 mg/cap. Bot. 100s.
Use: Reduce photosensitivity in patients with erythropoietic protoporphyria (EPP).

SOLBAR PF CREAM 50 SPF. (Person & Covey) Oxybenzone, octyl methoxycinnamate, octocrylene, PABA free, water-

proof. Cream. 120 Gm.
Use: Sunscreen.

SOLBAR PF LIQUID. (Person & Covey) Octyl methoxycinnamate 7.5%, oxybenzone 6%, SD alcohol 40 76%, PABA free. SPF 30. Liq. 120 ml.
Use: Sunscreen.

SOLBAR PF 15 CREAM. (Person & Covey) Octyl methoxycinnamate 7.5%, oxybenzone 5%. Bot. 1 oz, 4 oz.
Use: Sunscreen.

SOLBAR PF 50. (Person & Covey) Oxybenzone, octyl methoxycinnamate, octocrylene, PABA free. Waterproof. Cream 120 ml.
Use: Sunscreen.

SOLBAR PF PABA FREE 15. (Person & Covey) Oxybenzone 5%, octyl methoxycinnamate 7.5%. Sunscreen SPF 15. Tube 2.5 oz.
Use: Sunscreen.

SOLBAR PLUS 15. (Person & Covey) Padimate 6%, oxybenzone 4%, dioxybenzone 2%. Tube 1 oz, 4 oz.
Use: Sunscreen.

SOLEX A15 CLEAR LOTION SUNSCREEN. (Dermol) SPF 15. Octyl dimethyl PABA 5%, benzophenone 33%, SD alcohol. Lot. Bot. 120 ml.
Use: Sunscreen.

SOLFOTON. (ECR Pharm.) Phenobarbital 16 mg/Tab. or Cap. Bot. 100s, 500s.
Use: Sedative/hypnotic.

SOLFOTON S/C TABS. (Poythress) Phenobarbital 16 mg/SC Tab. Bot. 100s.
Use: Sedative/hypnotic.

SOLGANAL. (Schering) Aurothioglucose 50 mg/ml in sesame oil. Vial 10 ml; Box 1s.
Use: I.M., gold therapy, antiarthritic.

SOLIWAX. Docusate Sodium, U.S.P. XXIII. Docusate Sodium, Solasulfone (I.N.N.).

SOLPADEINE TABLETS. (Sanofi Winthrop) Paracetamol.
Use: Analgesic.

SOLTICE QUICK-RUB. (Chattem) Methyl salicylate, camphor, menthol, eucalyptol. Cream. Bot. 1.33 oz, 3.75 oz.
Use: External analgesic.

SOLU-BARB 0.25 TABLETS. (Forest Pharm.) Phenobarbital 0.25 gr/Tab. Bot. 24s.
Use: Sedative/hypnotic.

SOLU-CORTEF. (Upjohn) **100 mg:** Hydrocortisone sodium succinate, w/benzyl alcohol. Plain vial, 5s, 25s. 100 mg/2 ml Mix-O-Vial **250 mg:** Hydrocortisone sodium succinate, benzyl alcohol. Mix-O-Vial 2 ml, 5s, 25s. 25-Pack, 25s, 50s,

etc. **500 mg:** Hydrocortisone sodium succinate, benzyl alcohol. Mix-O-Vial, 5s, 25s. **1000 mg:** Hydrocortisone sodium succinate, benzyl alcohol. Mix-O-Vial, 5s, 25s.
Use: Corticosteroid.

SOLU-EZE. (Forest) Hydroxyquinoline 0.12%, carbitol acetate 12.10%. Bot. 3 oz.

SOLU-MEDROL. (Upjohn) **40 mg:** Methylprednisolone sodium succinate, benzyl alcohol. Univial 1 ml. **125 mg:** Methylprednisolone sodium succinate, benzyl alcohol. Act-O-Vial 2 ml, 5s, 25s. 25-Pack, 25s, 50s etc. **500 mg:** Methylprednisolone sodium succinate, benzyl alcohol. Vial 8 ml, vials w/diluent 8 ml. **1000 mg:** Methylprednisolone sodium succinate, benzyl alcohol. Vial 16 ml, vial w/diluent 16 ml. **2000 mg:** Methylprednisolone sodium succinate powder for injection, benzyl alcohol. Vial 30.6 ml, vial w/diluent 30.6 ml.
Use: Corticosteroid.

SOLUMOL. (C & M Pharmacal) Petrolatum, mineral oil, cetyl-stearyl alcohol, sodium lauryl sulfate, glycerin, propylene glycol, sorbic acid, purified water. Jar lb.
Use: Ointment base.

SOLU-PRED. (Kenyon) Prednisolone sodium phosphate equivalent to prednisolone phosphate 20 mg, niacinamide 25 mg, disodium edetate 0.5 mg, sodium bisulfite 1 mg, phenol 5 mg/ml. Vial 10 ml.
Use: Corticosteroid.

SOLUREX. (Hyrex) Dexamethasone sodium phosphate 4 mg/ml. W/methyl and propyl parabens, sodium bisulfite. Vial 5 ml, 10 ml, 30 ml.
Use: Corticosteroid.

SOLUREX L. A. (Hyrex) Dexamethasone acetate 8 mg/ml w/polysorbate 80, carboxymethylcellulose, sodium bisulfite, EDTA, benzyl alcohol. Susp. Vial 5 ml.
Use: Corticosteroid.

SOLUVITE CT W/FLUORIDE. (Pharmics) Vitamins A 2500 IU, D 400 IU, B_1 1.05 mg, B_2 1.2 mg, B_6 1.05 mg, B_{12} 4.5 mcg, C 60 mg, niacin 13.5 mg, E 15 IU, fluoride 1 mg, folic acid 0.3 mg/Tab. Bot. 100s, 1000s.
Use: Vitamin/mineral supplement.

SOLUVITE-F DROPS. (Pharmics) Vitamins A 1500 IU, D 400 IU, C 35 mg, fluoride 0.25 mg/0.6 ml. Bot. 57 ml.
Use: Vitamin/mineral supplement.

SOLVENT-G. (Syosset) Alcohol 47.5%, laureth-4, isopropyl alcohol 4%, propylene glycol. Lot. Bot. 50 ml.
Use: Lotion base.

SOLVISYN-A. (Towne) Water soluble vitamin A 10,000 units, 25,000 units or 50,000 units/Cap. Bot. 100s, 1000s.
Use: Vitamin A supplement.

•**SOLYPERTINE TARTRATE.** USAN. 7- 2-[4-(o-Methoxy-phenyl)-1-piperazinyl]ethyl 5H-1,3-dioxolo[4,5-f]in-dole tartrate.
Use: Antiadrenergic.

SOMA. (Wallace) Carisoprodol 350 mg/Tab. Bot. 100s, 500s, UD 500s.
Use: Skeletal muscle relaxant.

SOMA COMPOUND TABS. (Wallace) Carisoprodol 200 mg, aspirin 325 mg/Tab. Bot. 100s, 500s, UD 500s.
Use: Skeletal muscle relaxant combination.

SOMA COMPOUND W/CODEINE. (Wallace) Carisoprodol 200 mg, aspirin 325 mg, codeine phosphate 16 mg/Tab. Bot. 100s.
Use: Skeletal relaxant combination.

SOMAGARD. (Roberts Pharm)
See: DESLORELIN.

•**SOMANTADINE HYDROCHORIDE.** USAN.
Use: Antiviral.

SOMATOSTATIN.
Use: Digestive aid. [Orphan drug]
See: Zecnil.

•**SOMATREM.** USAN.
Use: Growth hormone.
See: Protropin, Inj. (Genentech).

•**SOMATROPIN.** USAN. Growth hormone derived from the anterior pituitary gland.
Use: Growth stimulant. [Orphan drug]
See: Humatrope, Inj. (Lilly). Nutropin, Inj. (Genentech).

SOMINEX. (SK-Beecham) Diphenhydramine HCl 25 mg/Tab. Blister pack 16s, 32s, 72s.
Use: Sleep aid.

SOMINEX CAPLETS. (SK-Beecham) Diphenhydramine HCl 50 mg. Tab. Blister pack 8s, 16s, 32s.
Use: Sleep aid.

SOMINEX PAIN RELIEF FORMULA. (SK-Beecham) Diphenhydramine HCl 25 mg, acetaminophen 500 mg/Tab. Blister pack 16s. Bot. 32s.
Use: Sleep aid, analgesic.

SONACIDE. (Wyeth-Ayerst) Potentiated acid glutaraldehyde. Bot. 1 gal, 5 gal.
Use: Sterilizing & disinfecting.

SONDRATE ELIXIR. (Kenyon) Chloral hydrate 1.6 Gm/fl oz. Bot. 4 oz, pt, gal.
Use: Sedative/hypnotic.

SONEKAP. (Eastwood) Cap. Bot. 100s.

SONERYL.

See: Butethal (Various Mfr.).

SOOTHADERM. (Pharmakon Labs)
Pyrilamine maleate 2.07 mg, benzocaine 2.08 mg, zinc oxide 41.35 mg/ml,
camphor, menthol. Lot. Bot. 118 ml.
Use: Antihistamine, local anesthetic.

SOOTHE. (Alcon) Tetrahydrozoline
0.05%, benzalkonium Cl 0.004%, adsorbobase. Bot. 15 ml.
Use: Decongestant, ophthalmic.

SOOTHE. (Walgreen) Bismuth subsalicylate 100 mg/Tsp. Bot. 9 oz.
Use: Antidiarrheal.

SOOTHERS THROAT DROPS. (Warner-
Lambert) Menthol 2 mg, corn syrup,
honey, sugar. Tartrazine in orange flavor.
Loz. Pkg. 10s.
Use: Mouth and throat product.

SOQUETTE. (Barnes-Hind) Polyvinyl alcohol w/benzalkonium Cl 0.01%, EDTA
0.2%. Bot. 4 fl oz.
Use: Hard contact lens care.

SORBASE COUGH SYRUP. (Fort David)
Dextromethorphan HBr 10 mg, guaifenesin 100 mg/5 ml in sorbitol base. Bot. 4
oz, pt, gal.
Use: Antitussive, expectorant.

• **SORBIC ACID,** N.F. XVIII.
Use: Preservative (antimicrobial).

SORBIDE T.D. (Mayrand) Isosorbide dinitrate 40 mg/TR Cap. Bot. 100s.
Use: Antianginal.

SORBIDE NITRATE. B.A.N. 1,4:3,6-Dian-
hydrosorbitol 2,5-dinitrate. Isosorbide
Dinitrate (I.N.N.).
Use: Coronary vasodilator.

SORBIDON HYDRATE. (Gordon) Water-
in-oil ointment. Jar 2 oz, 0.5 oz, 1 lb, 5 lb.
Use: Emollient.

SORBIMACROGOL OLEATE 300.
See: Polysorbate 80.

• **SORBINIL.** USAN.
Use: Enzyme inhibitor.

• **SORBITAN MONOLAURATE,** N.F. XVIII.
Mixture of laurate esters of sorbitol and
its anhydrides.
Use: Surface-active agent, emulsifying
agent.
See: Span 20 (ICI U.S.).

• **SORBITAN MONOOLEATE,** N.F. XVIII.
Mixture of oleate esters of sorbitol and
its anhydrides.
Use: Surface-active agent.
See: Span 80 (ICI U.S.).

**SORBITAN MONOOLEATE POLY-
OXYETHYLENE DERIVATIVES.**
See: Polysorbate 80, N.F. XVIII.

• **SORBITAN MONOPALMITATE,** N.F. XVI-
II. Mixture of palmitate esters of sorbitol
and its anhydrides.

Use: Surface-active agent.
See: Span 40 (ICI U.S.).

• **SORBITAN MONOSTEARATE,** N.F. XVI-
II. Mixture of stearate esters of sorbitol
and its anhydrides.
Use: Surface-active agent.
See: Span 60 (ICI U.S.).

• **SORBITAN SESQUIOLEATE.** USAN.
Sorbitan mono-oleate and sorbitan di-
oleate.
Use: Surfactant.
See: Arlacel C (ICI U.S.).

• **SORBITAN TRIOLEATE.** USAN.
Use: Surfactant.
See: Span 85 (ICI U.S.).

• **SORBITAN TRISTEARATE.** USAN.
See: Span 65 (ICI U.S.).
Use: Pharmaceutic aid (surfactant).

SORBITANS.
See: Polysorbate 80, U.S.P.

SORBI-TINIC-F. (Ortega) Vitamins B_1 10
mg, B_6 5 mg, B_{12} 25 mcg, folic acid
0.333 mg, iron 12 mg, l-lysine HCl 100
mg, sorbitol, sucrose. Liq. Bot. pt. gal.
Use: Vitamin supplement.

• **SORBITOL,** N.F. XVIII. Solution, U.S.P.
XXIII.
Use: Diuretic, dehydrating agent,
humectant, pharmaceutic aid (sweet-
ening agent, tablet excipient).
See: Sorbo (ICI U.S.).
W/Homatropine methylbromide.
See: Probilagol Liq. (Purdue Frederick).
W/Mannitol.
See: Sorbitol-mannitol Irrigation (Ab-
bott).

SORBITOL-MANNITOL. (Abbott) Mannitol 0.54 Gm, sorbitol/100 ml 2.7 Gm.
1500 ml, 3000 ml.
Use: Genitourinary irrigant.

SORBITON. (Kenyon) Vitamin B_{12} 5 mcg,
folic acid 0.1 mg, ferrous fumarate 100
mg, D-sorbitol 500 mg/Tab. Bot. 100s,
1000s.
Use: Vitamin/mineral supplement.

SORBITRATE. (ICI Pharma) Isosorbide
dinitrate. **Tab.:** 5 mg Bot. 100s, 500s,
UD 100s; 10 mg Bot. 500s, UD 100s; 20
mg, 30 mg/Bot. 100s, UD 100s. **SA
Tab.:** 40 mg Bot. 100s, UD 100s; **Sublingual Tab.:** 2.5 mg, 5 mg, 10 mg Bot.
100s, UD 100s. **Chew. Tab.:** 5 mg Bot.
100s, 500s, UD 100s. 10 mg Bot. 100s,
500s, UD 100s.
Use: Antianginal.

SORBITRATE SA. (ICI Pharma) Isosorbide dinitrite, oral 40 mg/SR Tab. Bot.
100s, UD 100s.
Use: Antianginal agent.

SORBO. (ICI Americas) Sorbitol Solution,

U.S.P. XXIII.
SORBSAN. (Dow B. Hickman) Calcium alginate fiber 2″ × 2″, 3″ × 3″, 4″ × 4″, 4″ × 8″. 1s. Wound packing fibers-calcium alginate fiber ¼″ × 12″. 1s.
Use: Wound dressing.
SORBUTUSS. (Dalin) Dextromethorphan HBr 10 mg, guaifenesin 100 mg, ipecac fluid extract 0.05 min, potassium citrate 85 mg, citric acid 35 mg/5 ml. Bot. 3 oz, pt.
Use: Antitussive, expectorant combination.
SORDINOL. Clopenthixol, B.A.N.
Use: Tranquilizer.
SORETHYTAN (20) MONO-OLEATE.
See: Polysorbate 80 (Various Mfr.).
• **SORIVUDINE.** USAN.
Use: Antiviral.
SOSEGON SOLUTION. (Sanofi Winthrop) Pentazocine.
Use: Analgesic.
SOSEGON SUSPENSION. (Sanofi Winthrop) Pentazocine.
Use: Analgesic.
SOSEGON TABLETS. (Sanofi Winthrop) Pentazocine.
Use: Analgesic.
SOSS-10. (Hauck) Sodium sulfacetamide 10%. Soln. Bot. 15 ml
Use: Ophthalmic.
SOTALOL. B.A.N. (±) 4′ (1 Hydroxy 2 isopropylaminoethyl)methanesulfonanilide.
Use: Beta adrenergic blocking agent.
See: Betapace.
• **SOTALOL HYDROCHLORIDE.** USAN. 4′-[1-Hydroxy-2-(isopropylamino)-ethyl]methanesulfonanilide hydrochloride. Under study.
Use: Beta-adrenergic blocking agent. [Orphan drug]
• **SOTERENOL HYDROCHLORIDE.** USAN.
Use: Adrenergic (bronchodilator).
SOTRADECOL. (Elkins-Sinn) Sodium tetradecyl sulfate 1% or 3%. Inj. Dosette amp. 2 ml.
Use: Sclerosing agent.
SOXA-FORTE. (Vita Elixir) Sulfisoxazole 0.5 Gm, phenazopyridine 50 mg/Tab.
Use: Anti-infective.
SOXA TABLETS. (Vita Elixir) Sulfisoxazole 0.5 Gm/Tab. Bot. 100s, 1000s.
Use: Anti-infective.
SOYALAC. (Loma Linda) Infant formula based on an extract from whole soybeans containing all essential nutrients. **Ready to Serve Liq.:** Can 32 fl oz. **Double Strength Conc.:** Can 13 fl oz. **Pow.:**

Can 14 oz.
Use: Nutritional supplement.
SOYALAC-i. (Loma Linda) Soy protein isolate infant formula containing no corn derivatives and a negligible amount of soy carbohydrates. Contains all essential nutrients in various forms. **Ready to Serve Liq.:** Can 32 fl oz. **Double Strength Conc.:** Can 13 fl oz.
Use: Nutritional supplement.
SOYA LECITHIN. Soybean extract. 100s.
Use: Phosphorus therapy.
See: Neo-Vadrin (Scherer).
SOYBEAN LECITHIN.
W/Safflower oil, choline bitartrate, whole liver, inositol, methionine, natural tocopherols, vitamins B_6, B_{12}, panthenol.
See: Nutricol, Cap., Vial (Nutrition Control).
• **SOYBEAN OIL,** U.S.P. XXIII.
Use: Pharmaceutic necessity.
SPABELIN No. 1. (Arcum) Phenobarbital 15 mg, belladonna powdered extract ⅛ gr/Tab. Bot. 100s, 1000s.
Use: Sedative/hypnotic.
SPABELIN NO. 2. (Arcum) Phenobarbital 30 mg, belladonna powdered extract ⅛ gr/Tab. Bot. 100s, 1000s.
Use: Sedative/hypnotic.
SPABELIN ELIXIR. (Arcum) Hyoscyamine sulfate 81 mcg, atropine sulfate 15 mcg, scopolamine HBr 5 mcg, phenobarbital 16.2 mg/5 ml. Bot. 16 oz, gal.
Use: Anticholinergic/antispasmodic, sedative/hypnotic.
SPAN 20. (ICI Americas) Sorbitan Monolaurate, N.F. XVIII.
SPAN 40. (ICI Americas) Sorbitan Monopalmitate, N.F. XVIII.
SPAN 60. (ICI Americas) Sorbitan Monostearate, N.F. XVIII.
SPAN 65. (ICI Americas) Sorbitan tristearate. Mixture of stearate esters of sorbitol and its anhydrides.
Use: Surface active agent.
SPAN 80. (ICI Americas) Sorbitan Monooleate, N.F. XVIII.
SPAN 85. (ICI Americas) Sorbitan trioleate. Mixture of oleate esters of sorbitol and its anhydrides.
Use: Surface-active agent.
SPAN C. (Freeda) Citrus bioflavonoids 300 mg, rutin 50 mg, vitamin C 200 mg/Tab. Bot. 100s, 250s, 500s.
Use: Vitamin supplement.
SPAN FF. (Metro Med) Ferrous fumarate 325 mg/Cap. Bot. 60s, 500s.
Use: Iron supplement.
SPAN PD. (Metro Med) Phentermine HCl

37.5 mg/Cap. Bot. 100s.
Use: Anorexiant.

SPAN-RD. (Metro Med) d-Methamphetamine HCl 12 mg, dl-methamphetamine HCl 6 mg, butabarbital 30 mg/Tab. Bot. 100s, 1000s.
Use: Amphetamine, sedative/hypnotic.

SPANTUSS LIQUID. (Aroo) Dextromethorphan HBr 15 mg, chlorpheniramine maleate 4 mg, phenylephrine HCl 5 mg, acetaminophen 120 mg/5 ml. Bot. 4 oz, pt.
Use: Antitussive, antihistamine, decongestant, analgesic.

•**SPARFLOXACIN.** USAN.
Use: Antibacterial.

•**SPARFOSATE SODIUM.** USAN.
Use: Antineoplastic.

SPARINE. (Wyeth-Ayerst) Promazine HCl 25 mg, 50 mg or 100 mg/Tab. Bot. 50s.
Use: Antipsychotic.

SPARKLES EFFERVESCENT GRANULES. (Lafayette) Sodium bicarbonate 2000 mg, citric acid 1500 mg, simethicone. Bot. UD 50s.
Use: Antacid.

SPARKLES GRANULES. (Lafayette) Effervescent granules 4 Gm/Packet or 6 Gm/Packet. Each 6 Gm produces 500 ml of carbon dioxide gas. Ctn. 25 packets. Pkg. 2 Ctn.
Use: Carbon dioxide production as an aid during air contrast stomach examinations.

SPARKLES TABLETS. (Lafayette) Effervescent tablets. Each 4.3 Gm of tablets produces 250 ml of carbon dioxide gas. Tab. Bot. 43 Gm (10 doses).
Use: Carbon dioxide production as an aid during air contrast stomach examination.

•**SPARSOMYCIN.** USAN.
Use: Antineoplastic.

•**SPARTEINE SULFATE.** USAN.
Use: Oxytocic.
W/Sodium Cl.
See: Tocosamine sulfate, Amp. (Trent).

SPASMATOL. (Pharmed) Homatropine MBr 3 mg, pentobarbital 12 mg, mephobarbital 8 mg/Tab. Bot. 100s, 1000s.
Use: Anticholinergic/antispasmodic, sedative/hypnotic.

SPASMED. (Jenkins) Hyoscyamine HBr 0.1037 mg, atropine sulfate 0.0194 mg, hyoscine HBr 0.0065 mg, tri-bar (1/3 each sodium butabarbital, sodium pentobarbital, sodium phenobarbital) 16.2 mg/Tab. or 5 ml **Tab.:** Bot. 1000s. **Elix.:** Bot. 4 oz, pt, gal. Alcohol 15%.

Use: Sedative/hypnotic, anticholinergic/antispasmodic.

SPASMED JR. (Jenkins) Homatropine methylbromide 1/96 gr, phenobarbital sodium gr, lactose, special mint flavor/Tab. Bot. 100s.
Use: Sedative/hypnotic.

SPASMID. (Dalin) Methscopolamine nitrate 2.5 mg, phenobarbital 8 mg/Tab. or 5 ml. **Elix.:** Bot. 4 oz, pt. **Tab.:** Bot. 50s, 100s.
Use: Anticholinergic/antispasmodic.

SPASMODINE. (Noyes) Alcohol 4%, emulsion of infused oils lobelia, stillingia, cajeput, lavender, cassia, eucalyptol. Mixture 3 oz, pt, gal.
Use: Expectorant.

SPASMOJECT. (Mayrand) Dicyclomine HCl 10 mg/ml. Vial 10 ml.
Use: Anticholinergic/antispasmodic.

SPASMOLIN. (Richlyn) Phenobarbital 16.2 mg, hyoscyamine sulfate 0.1037 mg, atropine sulfate 0.0194 mg, hyoscine HBr 0.0065 mg/Tab. Bot. 1000s.
Use: Sedative/hypnotic, anticholinergic/antispasmodic.

SPASMOLYTIC AGENTS.
See: Antispasmodics.

SPASMOPHEN. (Lannett) Phenobarbital 15 mg, hyoscyamine sulfate 0.1037 mg, atropine sulfate 0.0194 mg, hyoscine HBr 0.1037 mg/Tab. or 5 ml. **Tab.:** Bot. 1000s. **Liq.:** Bot. pt, gal.
Use: Sedative/hypnotic, anticholinergic/antispasmodic.

SPASNO-LIX. (Freeport) Phenobarbital 16.2 mg, hyoscyamine sulfate 0.1037 mg, atropine sulfate 0.0194 mg, hyoscine HBr 0.0065 mg, alcohol 21-23%/5 ml. Bot. 4 oz.
Use: Sedative/hypnotic, anticholinergic/antispasmodic.

SPASODIL. (Rand) Ethaverine HCl 50 mg and 100 mg/Tab. Bot. 100s, 1000s.
Use: Peripheral vasodilator.

SPASQUID. (Geneva Generics) Atropine sulfate 0.0194 mg, scopolamine HBr 0.0065 mg, hyoscyamine HBr 0.1037 mg, phenobarbital 16.2 mg/5 ml, alcohol 23%. Elix. Bot. pt, gal.
Use: Anticholinergic/antispasmodic, sedative/hypnotic.

SPASTIL. (Kenyon) Propantheline Br 15 mg/Tab. Bot. 100s, 1000s.
Use: Anticholinergic/antispasmodic.

SPASTYL. (Pharmex) Dicyclomine HCl 10 mg/ml. Vial 10 ml.
Use: Anticholinergic/antispasmodic.

S.P.B. TABLET. (Sheryl) Therapeutic B

complex formula with ascorbic acid 300 mg/Tab. Bot. 100s.
Use: Vitamin supplement.
SPD. (A.P.C.) Methyl salicylate, methyl nicotinate, dipropylene glycol salicylate, oleoresin capsicum, camphor, menthol. Cream Bot. 4 oz, Tube 1.5 oz.
Use: External analgesic.
•**SPEARMINT,** N.F. XVIII.
Use: Flavor.
•**SPEARMINT OIL,** N.F. XVIII.
Use: Flavor.
SPECIAL FORMULA OINTMENT "RF". (Lannett) Zinc oxide 10%, boric acid 4%, starch 10%, camphor 1%, menthol 0.5% in a petrolatum-aquaphor base. Jar lb.
Use: Dermatological.
SPECIAL SHAMPOO. (Del-Ray) Non medicated shampoo.
Use: Cleansing shampoo.
SPECTAZOLE. (Ortho) Econazole nitrate 1% in a water miscible base. Tube 15 Gm, 30 Gm, 85 Gm.
Use: Antifungal, topical.
SPECTINOMYCIN. Formerly Actinospectocin. An antibiotic isolated from broth cultures of *Streptomyces spectabilis.*
Use: Antibacterial.
See: Trobicin, Vial, Amp. (Upjohn).
•**SPECTINOMYCIN HYDROCHLORIDE, STERILE,** U.S.P. XXIII. For Susp., U.S.P. XXIII. An antibiotic produced by *Streptomyces spectabilis.*
Use: Antibacterial.
SPECTRA 360. (Parker) Salt-free electrode gel. Tube 8 oz.
Use: T.E.N.S. application, ECG pediatric, and long-term procedures.
SPECTROBID POWDER FOR ORAL SUSPENSION. (Roerig) Bacampicillin powder 125 mg/5 ml. Bot. 70 ml, 100 ml, 140 ml, 200 ml.
Use: Antibacterial; penicillin.
SPECTROBID TABLETS. (Roerig) Bacampicillin HCl 400 mg/Tab. Bot. 100s.
Use: Antibacterial; penicillin.
SPECTRO-BIOTIC. (A.P.C.) Bacitracin 400 units, neomycin sulfate 5 mg, polymyxin B sulfate 5000 units/Gm. Oint. 0.5 oz, 1 oz.
Use: Anti-infective, topical.
SPECTROCIN PLUS. (Numark Labs.) Polymyxin B sulfate 5000 units/Gm or ml, neomycin 3.5 mg/Gm or ml, bacitracin 400 units/Gm or ml, lidocaine 5 mg, mineral oil, white petrolatum. Oint. Tube 15 Gm, 30 Gm.
Use: Topical anti-infectives.
SPECTRO-JEL. (Recsei) Soap free. Methylcellulose, carboxypolymethylene,

cetyl alcohol, sorbitan mono-oleate, fumed silica, triethanolamine stearate, glycol polysiloxane, propylene glycol, glycerin, isopropyl alcohol 5%. Bot. 4 oz, pts, gal.
Use: Skin cleanser.
SPEC-T SORE THROAT ANESTHETIC LOZENGES. (Apothecon) Benzocaine 10 mg/Loz. Box 10s.
Use: Local anesthetic.
SPEC-T SORE THROAT/COUGH SUPPRESSANT LOZENGES. (Apothecon) Benzocaine 10 mg, dextromethorphan HBr 10 mg w/tartrazine.
Use: Local anesthetic, antitussive.
SPEC-T SORE THROAT/DECONGESTANT LOZENGES. (Apothecon) Benzocaine 10 mg, phenylephrine HCl 5 mg, phenylpropanolamine HCl 10.5 mg w/tartrazine. Loz. Pkg. 10s.
Use: Local anesthetic, decongestant.
SPERMACETI.
Use: Stiffening agent; pharmaceutic necessity for cold cream.
SPERMINE. Diaminopropyltetramethylene.
SPERTI OINTMENT. (Whitehall) Live yeast cell derivative supplying 2000 units skin respiratory factor/Gm w/shark liver oil 3%, phenylmercuric nitrate 1:10,000. Tube oz.
Use: Healing ointment.
SPHERULIN. (Berkeley Biologicals) Coccidioidin: 1:100 equivalent, vial 1 ml, 5 ml, 1:10 equivalent, Vial 0.5 ml.
Use: Skin test.
SPIDER-BITE ANTIVENIN.
See: Antivenin Crotalidae and Micrurus, U.S.P. XXIII.
SPIDER-MAN CHILDREN'S CHEWABLE VITAMIN. (Nature's Bounty) Vitamins A 2500 IU, D 400 IU, E 15 mg, B_1 1.05 mg, B_2 1.2 mg, B_3 13.5 mg, B_6 1.05 mg, B_{12} 4.5 mcg, C 60 mg, folic acid 0.3 mg/Tab., xylitol, sorbitol. Bot. 75s, 130s.
Use: Vitamin supplement.
•**SPIPERONE.** USAN. 8-[3-(p-Fluorobenzoyl)-propyl]-1-phenyl-1,3,8-triazaspiro-[4.5]decan-4-one.
Use: Tranquilizer.
•**SPIRAMYCIN.** USAN. Antibiotic substance from cultures of *Streptomyces ambofaciens.*
Use: Antibiotic.
•**SPIRAPRIL HYDROCHLORIDE.** USAN.
Use: ACE inhibitor.
SPIRILENE. B.A.N. 8-[4-(4-Fluorophenyl)pent-3-enyl]-1-phenyl-1,3,8-triazaspiro[4,5]decan-4-one.
Use: Tranquilizer.

SPIROBARBITAL SODIUM. 1-Ethyl-2,4-dimethyl-8-thio-7,9-diazaspiro[4.5]decane-6,8,10-trione sodium salt.

• **SPIROGERMANIUM HYDROCHLORIDE.** USAN.
Use: Antineoplastic.

• **SPIROMUSTINE.** USAN. Formerly spirohydantoin mustard.
Use: Antineoplastic.

SPIRONAZIDE. (Schein) Spironolactone 25 mg, hydrochlorothiazide 25 mg/Tab. Bot. 100s, 1000s, UD 100s.
Use: Diuretic combination.

• **SPIRONOLACTONE,** U.S.P. XXIII. Tab., U.S.P. XXIII. 17-Hydroxy-7α-mercapto-3-oxo-17α-pregn-4-ene-21-carboxylic acid a-lactone 7-acetate: 3-(3-oxo-7 α-acetylthio-17β-hydroxy-4-androsten-17 α-yl) propionic acid a-lactone.
Use: Diuretic.
See: Aldactone, Tab. (Searle).
W/Hydrochlorothiazide.
See: Aldactazide, Tab. (Searle).

SPIRONOLACTONE W/HYDROCHLOROTHIAZIDE. (Various Mfr.) Spironactone 25 mg, hydrochlorothiazide 25 mg. Tab. Bot. 30s, 60s, 100s, 250s, 500s, 1000s, UD 32s, 100s.
Use: Diuretic combination.

SPIROPITAN. (Janssen) Spiperone.
Use: Antipsychotic.

• **SPIROPLATIN.** USAN.
Use: Antineoplastic.

SPIROTRIAZINE HCl. 2,4-Diamino-5(p-chlorophenyl)-9-methyl-1,3,5-triazaspiro [5.5]undeca-1,3-diene HCl.
Use: Anthelmintic.

• **SPIROXASONE.** USAN.
Use: Diuretic.

SPIROZIDE. (Rugby) Spironolactone 25 mg, hydrochlorothiazide 25 mg/Tab. Bot. 100s, 500s, 1000s.
Use: Diuretic combination.

SPL-SEROLOGIC TYPES I AND III. (Delmont Labs) Staphylococcus aureus 120 to 180 million units , staphylococcus bacteriophage plaque forming units 100 to 1000 million/ml. Inj. Amp. 1 ml, Vial 10 ml.
Use: Anti-infective.

• **SPONGE, ABSORBABLE GELATIN,** U.S.P. XXIII.
Use: Local hemostatic.

SPORANOX. (Janssen) Itraconazole 100 mg, sucrose. Cap. Bot. 30s, UD 30s.
Use: Antifungal.

SPORTSCREME. (Thompson) Triethanolamine salicylate 10% in a nongreasy base. Cream. 37.5 Gm, 90 Gm.
Use: External analgesic.

SPORTS SPRAY EXTRA STRENGTH. (Mentholatum) Methyl salicylate 35%, menthol 10%, camphor 5%, alcohol 58%, isobutane. Spray. 90 ml.
Use: Rub/liniment.

SPRAY SKIN PROTECTANT. (Morton) Isopropyl alcohol, polyvinylpyrolidone, vinyl alcohol, plasticizer & propellant Aerosol can 6 oz.
Use: Protective skin coating.

SPRAY-U-THIN. (Caprice Greystoke) Phenylpropanolamine HCl 6.58 mg, sorbitol, saccharin. Spray. Bot. 44 ml.
Use: Nonprescription diet aid.

SPREADING FACTOR.
See: Hyaluronidase (Various Mfr.).

• **SPRODIAMIDE.** USAN.
Use: Imaging aid.

SPRX-105. (Reid-Provident) Phendimetrazine tartrate 105 mg/Cap. S.R. Bot. 28s, 500s.
Use: Anorexiant.

SPS. (Carolina Medical Prod. Co.) Sodium polystyrene sulfonate 15 Gm, sorbitol solution 21.5 ml, alcohol 0.18 ml/60 ml. Susp. Bot. 60 ml, 120 ml.
Use: Potassium-removing resin.

S-P-T. (Fleming) Pork thyroid, desiccated 1 gr, 2 gr, 3 gr, 5 gr/Cap. Bot. 100s, 1000s.
Use: Hypothyroidism.

SRC EXPECTORANT. (Edwards) Hydrocodone bitartrate 5 mg, pseudoephedrine HCl 60 mg, guaifenesin 200 mg w/alcohol 12.5%. Bot. pt.
Use: Antitussive, decongestant, expectorant.

SSD AF. (Boots) Sulver sulfadiazine 1% in a cream base containing white petrolatum, stearyl alcohol, isopropyl myristate, sorbitan monooleate, polyoxyl 40 stearate, sodium hydroxide, propylene glycol, methylparaben 3%. Cream. 50 Gm, 400 Gm, 1000 Gm.
Use: Burn preparation.

SSD CREAM. (Boots) Silver sulfadiazine cream 1%. Jar 50 g, 85 g, 400 g, 1000 g. Tube 25 g.
Use: Burn preparation.

SSKI. (Upsher-Smith) Potassium iodide 300 mg/0.3 ml. Soln. Dropper Bot. 1 oz, 8 oz.
Use: Expectorant.

S-SPAS. (Southern States) Pentobarbital 16.2 mg, atropine sulfate 0.0194 mg, hyoscyamine sulfate 0.1037 mg, hyoscine HBr 0.0065 mg/Tab. or 5 ml **Liq.:** Bot. pt. **Tab.:** Bot. 100s, 1000s.
Use: Sedative/hypnotic, anticholinergic/antispasmodic.

ST1-RTA IMMUNOTOXIN.
Use: Leukemia, graft-v-host disease in
bone marrow transplants. [Orphan
drug]
S.T. 37. (Beecham Products) Hexylresor-
cinol 0.1% in glycerin aqueous soln. Bot.
5.5 oz, 12 oz.
Use: Antiseptic, topical.
STADOL. (Bristol) Butorphanol tartrate 1
mg/ml. Vial 1 ml. 2 mg/ml. Vial 1 ml, 2
ml, 10 ml.
Use: Analgesic.
STAFTABS. (Modern) Fine bone flour
containing calcium, phosphorus, iron, io-
dine, vitamin D, magnesium/Tab. Bot.
85s, 160s.
Use: Vitamin/mineral supplement.
STAINLESS IODIZED OINTMENT. (Day-
Baldwin) Jar lb.
**STAINLESS IODIZED OINTMENT WITH
METHYL SALICYLATE 5%.** (Day-Bald-
win) Jar lb.
• **STALLIMYCIN HYDROCHLORIDE.**
USAN.
Use: Antibacterial.
STAMOIST E. (Huckaby) Pseu-
doephedrine HCl 120 mg, guaifenesin
500 mg. SR Tab. Bot. 100s.
Use: Decongestant, expectorant.
STAMOIST LA. (Huckaby) Phenyl-
propanolamine HCl 75 mg, guaifenesin
400 mg. SR Tab. Bot. 100s.
Use: Decongestant, expectorant.
STAMYL TABLETS. (Sanofi Winthrop)
Pancreatin.
Use: Digestive aid.
• **STANNOUS CHLORIDE.** USAN.
Use: Pharmaceutic aid.
• **STANNOUS FLUORIDE,** U.S.P. XXIII.
Gel, U.S.P. XXIII. Tin fluoride.
Use: Dental caries prophylactic.
STANNOUS FLUORIDE. (City Chem.)
Stannous fluoride. Bot. 4 oz, lb.
Use: Dental caries preventative.
• **STANNOUS PYROPHOSPHATE.** USAN.
Use: Diagnostic aid (bone imaging).
• **STANNOUS SULFUR COLLOID.** USAN.
Use: Diagnostic aid (bone, liver, and
spleen imaging).
STANOLONE. B.A.N. Androstanolone, di-
hydrotestosterone, androstane-17(β)-ol-
3-one. 17 β-Hydroxy-5 α-androstan-3-
one.
See: Anabolic steroid.
• **STANOZOLOL,** U.S.P. XXIII. Tab., U.S.P.
XXIII. 17 β-Hydroxy-17 α-methylan-
drostano[3,2-c] pyrazole. 17-Methyl-
2'H-5 α-androst-2-eno(3,2-c)pyrazol-17
β-ol. Formerly Androstanazole.
Use: Anabolic agent (androgen).

See: Stromba.
Winstrol Tab. (Sanofi Winthrop).
STAPHAGE LYSATE (SPL). (Delmont)
Phage-lysed staphylococci 120-180 mil-
lion/ml Amp. 1 ml, package 10s for inj.;
multidose Vial 10 ml for other methods
of administration.
Use: Anti-infective.
STAPHCILLIN. (Bristol) Methicillin sodi-
um w/3 mEq sodium/Gm, 1 Gm/Vial.
Vial 1 Gm, 4 Gm, 6 Gm; Piggyback Vial.
1 Gm, 4 Gm.
Use: Antibacterial; penicillin.
STAPHYLOCOCCUS TEST.
See: Isocult for Staphylococcus Aureus
(Smith Kline Diagnostics).
• **STARCH,** N.F. XVIII.
Use: Dusting powder; tablet disinte-
grant.
See: Mexsana, Pow. (Plough).
STARCH GLYCERITE.
Use: Emollient.
• **STARCH, PREGELATINIZED,** N.F. XVIII.
Use: Pharmaceutic aid (tablet excipi
ent).
• **STARCH, TOPICAL,** U.S.P. XXIII.
Use: Dusting powder.
STAR-OPTIC EYE WASH. (Stellar) Ster-
ile, isotonic, buffered solution containing
sodium Cl, sodium phosphate mono-
and dibasic, EDTA, benzalkonium Cl.
Drop. Bot. 120 ml.
Use: Ophthalmic.
STAR-OTIC. (Star) Burrows soln. 10%,
acetic acid 1%, boric acid 1%. Drop bot.
15 ml.
Use: Otic preparation.
STATICIN 1.5%. (Westwood) Ery-
thromycin 15 mg/ml, alcohol 55%,
propylene glycol, laureth-4, fragrance.
Soln. Bot. 60 ml.
Use: Anti-acne.
• **STATOLON.** USAN. Antiviral agent de-
rived from *Penicillium stoloniferum.*
Use: Antiviral agent.
STATOMIN MALEATE II. (Bowman)
Chlorpheniramine maleate 2 mg, aceta-
minophen 324 mg, caffeine 32 mg/Tab.
Bot. 1000s.
Use: Antihistamine, analgesic
**STATROL STERILE OPHTHALMIC
OINTMENT.** (Alcon) Polymyxin B sul-
fate 10,000 units, neomycin 3.5 mg/Gm.
Tube 3.5 Gm.
Use: Anti-infective, ophthalmic.
STATUSS EXPECTORANT. (Huckaby)
Phenylpropanolamine HCl 12.5 mg,
dextromethorphan HBr 10 mg, guaifen-
esin 100 mg, alcohol 5%. Liq. Bot. 480
ml.

Use: Decongestant, antitussive, expectorant.

STATUSS GREEN. (Huckaby) Phenylpropanolamine HCl 3.3 mg, phenylephrine HCl 5 mg, pheniramine maleate 3.3 mg, pyrilamine maleate 3.3 mg, hydrocodone bitartrate 1.67 mg/5 ml, alcohol 5%. Liq. Bot. 480 ml.
Use: Decongestant, antihistamine, antitussive.

• **STAVUDINE.** USAN.
Use: Antiviral.
See: Zerit, Cap. (Bristol-Myers Squibb).

STA-WAKE DEXTABS. (Approved) Caffeine 1.5 gr, dextrose 3 gr/Tab. Bot. 36s, 1000s.
Use: CNS stimulant.

STAY-ALERT. (Edward J. Moore) Caffeine 250 mg/Cap. Bot. 12s, 18s.
Use: CNS stimulant.

STAY AWAKE CAPSULES. (Whiteworth) Caffeine 250 mg/Cap. Bot. 30s.
Use: CNS Stimulant.

STAY-BRITE. (Sherman) EDTA 0.25%, benzalkonium Cl 0.01%. Spray 30 ml.
Use: Hard contact lens care.

STAYMINS. (Stayner) Vitamins A 5000 IU, D 500 IU, B_1 1.5 mg, B_2 1.5 mg, niacinamide 10 mg, B_6 0.5 mg, C 50 mg, B_{12} 2 mcg/5 ml. Bot. 16 oz.
Use: Vitamin supplement.

STAYMINS TABLETS. (Stayner) Vitamins A 5000 IU, D 500 IU, E 1 IU B_1 2.5 mg, B_2 2.5 mg, B_6 0.5 mg, B_{12} 2 mcg, C 50 mg, calcium pantothenate 5 mg, niacinamide 20 mg, inositol 10 mg, choline bitartrate 10 mg/Tab. Bot. 100s, 1000s.
Use: Vitamin/mineral supplement.

STAY MOIST LIP CONDITIONER. Padimate O, oxybenzone, aloe vera, vitamin E, tropical fruit flavor. SPF 15. Lip Balm: 48 g.
Use: Emollient.

STAYNERAL TABLETS. (Stayner) Vitamins A 5000 IU, D 500 IU, E 5 IU, B_1 5 mg, B_2 5 mg, B_6 1 mg, C 100 mg, B_{12} 2 mcg, niacinamide 25 mg, calcium pantothenate 5 mg, calcium 50 mg, phosphorus 40 mg, iron 10 mg, manganese 0.5 mg, zinc 0.1 mg, magnesium 0.5 mg, iodine 0.2 mg, copper 0.1 mg/Tab. Bot. 100s, 1000s.
Use: Vitamin/mineral supplement.

STAY TRIM. (Schering-Plough) Phenylpropanolamine. **Gum:** 8.33 mg. Pkg. 20s. **Mints:** 12.5 mg. Pkg. 36s.
Use: Diet aid.

STAY-WET. (Sherman) Polyvinyl alcohol, hydroxyethylcellulose, povidone, sodium Cl, potassium Cl, sodium carbonate,

benzalkonium Cl 0.01%, EDTA 0.025%. Soln. Bot. 30 ml.
Use: Hard contact lens care.

STAY-WET 3. (Sherman) Sodium and potassium Cl salts containing polyvinyl pyrrolidone, polyvinyl alcohol, hydroxyethyl cellulose, sodium bisulfate 0.02%, pure benzyl alcohol 0.1%, sorbic acid 0.05%, trisodium edetate 0.1%. Soln. 30 ml.
Use: Ophthalmic.

STAY-WET REWETTING. (Sherman) Polyvinyl alcohol, hydroxyethylcellulose, povidone, NaCl, KCl, sodium carbonate, benzalkonium Cl 0.01%, EDTA 0.025%.
Use: Ophthalmic.

STAY-WET 3 WETTING. (Sherman) Polyvinyl alcohol, hydroxyethylcellulose, povidone, sodium Cl, potassium Cl, sodium carbonate, benzalkonium Cl 0.01%, EDTA 0.025%. Soln. 30 ml.
Use: Ophthalmic.

STAZE. (Commerce) Karaya gum. Tube 1.75 oz, 3.5 oz.
Use: Denture adhesive.

S-T CORT CREAM. (Scot-Tussin) Hydrocortisone 0.5%, water washable base, parabens. 120 Gm.
Use: Corticosteroid.

S-T CORT LOTION. (Scot-Tussin) Hydrocortisone 0.5%, water washable, lanolin alcohol, mineral oil base. 60 ml, 120 ml.
Use: Corticosteroid.

STEAPSIN.
W/Oxidized bile acids, ox bile, homatropine methylbromide.
See: Oxacholin, Tab. (Philips Roxane).

• **STEARIC ACID,** N.F. XVIII. Purified, N.F. XVIII. Octadecanoic acid.
Use: Pharm aid (emulsion adjunct, tablet lubricant).

• **STEARYL ALCOHOL,** N.F. XVIII.
Use: Pharm aid (emulsion adjunct).

• **STEFFIMYCIN.** USAN.
Use: Antibacterial, antiviral.

STELAZINE. (SK-Beecham) Trifluoperazine HCl. **Tab.:** 1 mg, 2 mg, 5 mg, 10 mg. Bot. 100s, 1000s, UD 100s. **Vial:** 10 ml (2 mg/ml) Box 1s, 20s. **Oral Conc.:** (10 mg/ml) Bot. 2 fl oz. Ctn. 12s.
Use: Antipsychotic.

• **STENOBOLONE ACETATE.** USAN. 17-beta-Hydroxy-2-methyl-5-alpha-androst-1-en-3-one acetate.
Use: Inj. anabolic.

STEP 2. (GenDerm) Benzyl alcohol, cetyl alcohol, formic acid 8%, glyceryl stearate, PEG-100 stearate, polyquaterium-10. Creme rinse. 60 ml.

Use: Nit removal system.
STERAJECT. (Mayrand) Prednisolone acetate 25 mg or 50 mg/ml. Vial 10 ml.
Use: Corticosteroid.
STERAPRED DS. (Mayrand) Prednisone 10 mg/Tab. Uni-pak 21s.
Use: Corticosteroid.
STERAPRED-UNIPAK. (Mayrand) Prednisone 5 mg/Tab. Dosepak 21 tab.
Use: Corticosteroid.
STERCULIA GUM.
See: Karaya Gum (Various Mfr.).
W/Vitamin B₁.
See: Imbicoll W/Vitamin B₁ (Upjohn).
STERICOL. (Alton) Isopropyl alcohol 91%. Bot. 16 oz, 32 oz, gal.
Use: Antibacterial, topical anti-infective.
• **STERILE AUROTHIOGLUCOSE SUSPENSION,** U.S.P. XXIII. Authothioglucose Injection. Gold thioglucose. Gold, (I-thio-D-glucopyranosato)-. (I-Thio-D-glucopyranosato) gold.
Use: Antirheumatic.
See: Solganal, Vial (Schering).
• **STERILE ERYTHROMYCIN GLUCEPTATE,** U.S.P. XXIII. Erythromycin monoglucoheptonate (salt). Erythromycin glucoheptonate (1:1) (salt).
Use: Antibacterial.
STERILE LENS LUBRICANT. (Blairex) Isotonic w/borate buffer system, sodium Cl, hydroxypropyl methylcellulose, glycerin, sorbic acid 0.25%, EDTA 0.1%, thimerosol free. Soln. 15 ml.
Use: Ophthalmic.
STERILE SALINE. (Bausch & Lomb) Sodium Cl, borate buffer, EDTA, thimerosal free. Soln. 60 ml.
Use: Ophthalmic.
STERILE THIOPENTAL SODIUM.
Thiopental sodium, U.S.P. XXIII.
See: Pentothal Sodium, Amp. (Abbott).
STERILE WATER FOR IRRIGATION.
(Various Mfr.) 0.45% or 0.9%. Soln. Bot. 150 ml, 250 ml, 500 ml, 1000 ml, 1500 ml, 2000 ml, 4000 ml.
Use: Genitourinary irrigant.
STERINAIL. (Dr. Nordyke's Labs) Undecylenic acid, tolnaftate, propylene glycol, acetone, acetic acid, propionic acid, benzyl alcohol, eucalyptol and benzyl acetate, *Steri-Scrub* (mineral oil, glyceryl stearate, propylene glycol, lanolin alcohol, calcium carbonate, propylene glycol monostearate, triethanolamine, sodium hypochlorite, parabens, DMDM hydantoin, diazolidinyl urea). *Steri-Brush* included.
Use: Antifungal agent.
STERI-UNNA BOOT. (Pedinol) Glycerin,

gum acacia, zinc oxide, white petrolatum, amylum in an oil base. 10 Yds. × 3.5 in. sterilized bandage.
Use: Treatment of leg ulcers, varicosities, sprains, strains & to reduce swelling after surgery.
STEROLOX. (Kenyon) Benzethonium Cl, benzoic acid, salicylic acid, thymol, menthol, isopropyl alcohol 50%. Bot. 2 oz, pt, gal.
S-T FORTE 2 LIQUID. (Scot-Tussin) Chlorpheniramine maleate 2 mg, hydrocodone bitartrate 2.5 mg, 99.7% glycerin, menthol, parabens. Alcohol and dye free. Bot. Pt. or gal.
Use: Antihistamine, antitussive.
S-T FORTE SUGAR FREE LIQUID.
(Scot-Tussin) Hydrocodone bitartrate 2.5 mg, phenylephrine HCl 5 mg, phenylpropanolamine HCl 5 mg, pheniramine maleate 13.33 mg, guaifenesin 80 mg/5 ml w/alcohol 5%. Bot. 4 oz, 8 oz, pt, gal.
Use: Antitussive, decongestant, antihistamine, expectorant.
S-T FORTE SYRUP. (Scot-Tussin) Hydrocodone bitartrate 2.5 mg, phenylephrine HCl 5 mg, phenylpropanolamine HCl 5 mg, pheniramine maleate 13.33 mg, guaifenesin 80 mg/5 ml, w/alcohol 5%. Bot. 4 oz, 8 oz, pt. gal.
Use: Antitussive, decongestant, antihistamine, expectorant.
STIBAMINE GLUCOSIDE. B.A.N. Sodium 4- glucosylaminophenylstibonate.
Use: Treatment of leishmaniasis.
STIBOCAPTATE. B.A.N. Antimony(III) sodium meso-2, 3- dimercaptosuccinate.
Use: Treatment of schistosomiasis.
STILBAMIDINE. B.A.N. 4, 4'-Diamidinostilbene.
Use: Treatment of trypanosomiasis.
STILBAMIDINE ISETHIONATE. 2-Hydroxyethane-sulfonic acid compound with 4, 4'-stilbenedicarboxamidine.
Use: Antiprotozoal.
• **STILBAZIUM IODIDE.** USAN. 1-Ethyl-2, 6-bis(p-1-pyrrolidinyl-styryl)-pyridinium iodide.
Use: Anthelmintic.
See: Monopar.
STILBESTROL.
See: Diethylstilbestrol, U.S.P. XXIII. (Various Mfr.).
STILBESTRONATE.
See: Diethylstilbestrol Dipropionate (Various Mfr.).
STILBOESTROL.
See: Diethylstilbestrol (Various Mfr.).

STILBOESTROL DP.
See: Diethylstilbestrol Dipropionate
(Various Mfr.).
STILLMAN'S. (Stillman) Cream Jar. ⁷/₈
oz, oz, Cream Bella Aurora oz.
• STILONIUM IODIDE. USAN.
Use: Antispasmodic.
STILPHOSTROL. (Miles Pharm) Diethyl-
stilbestrol diphosphate. Amp. (250 mg/5
ml as sodium salt) 5 ml. Box 20s. Tab.
50 mg, Bot. 50s.
Use: Antineoplastic agent.
STILRONATE.
See: Diethylstilbestrol Dipropionate
(Various Mfr.).
STIMATE. (Armour) Desmopressin ac-
etate 1.5 mg/ml. Nasal spray. Vial 2.5
ml.
Use: Posterior pituitary hormone.
STIMURUB. (Otis Clapp) Menthol, methyl
salicylate, oleo resin of capsicum, in
greaseless base. Tube 36 × 0.25 oz, 1
oz, Jar. 16 oz.
Use: External analgesic.
STING-EZE. (Wisconsin) Bot. 0.5 oz.
Use: Antihistamine, topical.
STINGING INSECT ANTIGEN NO. 108.
Combined antigens of bumblebee, hon-
eybee, wasp, hornet, yellow jacket. Vial
3.5 ml.
Use: Allergenic extract.
STING-KILL. (MiLance) Benzocaine
18.9%, menthol 0.9%. Swab 14 ml, 0.5
ml (5s).
Use: Local anesthetic.
STIRIMAZOLE. B.A.N. 2-(4-Car-
boxystyryl)-5-nitro-1-vinylimidazole.
Use: Treatment of amebiasis, trichomo-
niasis, and trypanosomiasis.
• STIRIPENTOL. USAN.
Use: Anticonvulsant.
ST. JOSEPH ADULT CHEWABLE AS-
PIRIN. (Schering-Plough) Aspirin 81
mg, saccharin. Chew. Tab. Bot. 36s.
Use: Salicylate analgesic.
ST. JOSEPH ASPIRIN FOR ADULTS.
(Plough) Aspirin 5 gr/Tab. Bot. 36s,
100s, 200s.
Use: Salicylate analgesic.
ST. JOSEPH ASPIRIN-FREE COLD FOR
CHILDREN. (Schering-Plough) Phenyl-
propanolamine HCl 3.125 mg, aceta-
minophen 80 mg, fruit flavor. Chew. tab.
Bot. 30s.
Use: Pediatric decongestant combina-
tion.
ST. JOSEPH ASPIRIN-FREE ELIXIR FOR
CHILDREN. (Plough) Acetaminophen
160 mg/5 ml. Alcohol Free. Bot. 2 oz,
4oz.

Use: Analgesic.
ST. JOSEPH ASPIRIN-FREE FOR CHIL-
DREN CHEWABLE. (Plough) Aceta-
minophen 80 mg, fruit flavor. Tab. Bot.
30s.
Use: Analgesic.
ST. JOSEPH ASPIRIN-FREE INFANT
DROPS (Plough) Acetaminophen 100
mg/ml/0.8 ml dropper. Aspirin and sugar
free. Bot. 0.5 oz.
Use: Aanalgesic.
ST. JOSEPH ASPIRIN-FREE TABLETS
FOR CHILDREN. (Plough) Aceta-
minophen 80 mg/Tab. Bot. 30s.
Use: Analgesic.
ST. JOSEPH COLD TABLETS FOR CHIL-
DREN. (Plough) Aspirin 81 mg, phenyl-
propanolamine HCl 3.125 mg/Tab. Bot.
30s.
Use: Analgesic, decongestant.
ST. JOSEPH COUGH SUPPRESSANT.
(Schering-Plough) Dextromethorphan
HBr 7.5 mg/5 ml, alcohol free, sucrose,
cherry flavor. Liq. Bot. 60 ml, 120 ml.
Use: Nonnarcotic antitussive.
ST. JOSEPH COUGH SYRUP FOR CHIL-
DREN. (Plough) Dextromethorphan
HBr 7.5 mg/5 ml. Bot. 2 oz, 4 oz.
Use: Antitussive.
STOMAL. (Foy) Phenobarbital 16.2 mg,
hyoscyamine sulfate 0.1037 mg, at-
ropine sulfate 0.0194 mg, scopolamine
HBr 0.0065 mg/Tab. Bot. 1000s.
Use: Sedative/hypnotic, anticholiner-
gic/antispasmodic.
STOOL SOFTENER. (Amlab) Docusate
sodium 100 mg, 250 mg/Cap. Bot. 100s.
Use: Laxative.
STOOL SOFTENER. (Weeks & Leo) Do-
cusate sodium 100 mg, 250 mg/Cap.
Bot. 30s, 100s. Calcium docusate 240
mg/Cap. Bot. 100s.
Use: Laxative.
STOP. (Oral-B) Stannous fluoride 0.4%.
Tube 2 oz.
Use: Dental caries preventative.
STOPAYNE CAPSULES. (Springbok)
Codeine phosphate 30 mg, aceta-
minophen 357 mg/Cap. Bot. 100s, 500s,
UD 100s.
Use: Antitussive, analgesic.
STOPAYNE SYRUP. (Springbok) Aceta-
minophen 120 mg, codeine phosphate
12 mg/5 ml. Bot. 4 oz, 16 oz.
Use: Analgesic, antitussive.
STOP-ZIT. (Purepac) Denatonium ben-
zoate in a clear nail polish base. Bot.
0.75 oz.
Use: Thumbsucking-nail biting deter-
rent.

• **STORAX,** U.S.P. XXIII.
Use: Pharmaceutic necessity for Compound Benzoin Tincture.

STOVARSOL.
Use: Trichomonas vaginalis vaginitis, amebiasis, Vincent's angina.
See: Acetarsone, Tab.

STREMA. (Foy) Quinine sulfate 260 mg/Cap. Bot. 100s, 500s, 1000s.
Use: Antimalarial.

STREN-TAB. (Barth's) Vitamins C 300 mg, B_1 10 mg, B_2 10 mg, niacin 33 mg, B_6 2 mg, pantothenic acid 20 mg, B_{12} 4 mcg/Tab. Bot. 100s, 300s, 500s.
Use: Vitamin supplement.

STREPTASE. (Astra) Streptokinase I.V. infusion. Ctn. Vial 10s. 250,000 IU/Vial 6.5 ml; 750,000 IU/Vial 6.5 ml.
Use: Thrombolytic enzyme.

STREPTOCOCCI.
W/*Haemophilus influenzae, Neisseria catarrhalis, Klebsiella pneumoniae, staphylocci, pneumococci,* killed.
See: Mixed Vaccine No. 4 W-H. Influenzae (Lilly).

STREPTOCOCCI VACCINE, KILLED.
W/*Neisseria catarrhalis, Klebsiella pneumoniae, Diplococcus pneumoniae, staphylococci.*
See: Combined Vaccine No. 4 w/Catarrhalis (Lilly).

STREPTOCOCCUS IMMUNE GLOBULIN GROUP B.
Use: Immunization in neonates. [Orphan drug]

STREPTODORNASE. B.A.N. An enzyme obtained from cultures of various strains of *Streptococcus hemolyticus.*
See: Streptokinase.

STREPTODUOCIN. B.A.N. A mix. of equal parts of streptomycin & dihydrostreptomycin sulfates.
Use: Antibiotic.

STREPTOHYDRAZID. Streptoclidenelsonicotinyl hydrazine sulfate. Streptonicozid, B.A.N. Streptomycin. isoniazid.
Use: Tuberculosis treatment.

STREPTOKINASE. B.A.N. An enzyme obtained from cultures of various strains of *Streptococcus hemolyticus.*
See: Kabikinase.
Streptase, Inj. (Astra).

STREPTOLYSIN O TEST. (Laboratory Diagnostics) Reagent 6 × 10 ml, buffer 6 40 ml, Control Serum, 6 10 ml or Kit.
Use: Diagnosis of "Group A" Streptococcal infections.

STREPTOMYCIN CALCIUM CHLORIDE.

Streptomycin Calcium Chloride Complex.

STREPTOMYCIN ISONIAZID.
See: Streptohydrazid.

• **STREPTOMYCIN SULFATE INJECTION,** U.S.P. XXIII. Sterile. U.S.P. XXIII. (Various Mfr.).
Use: Antibacterial (tuberculostatic).
W/Dihydrostreptomycin sulfate.
See: Streptoduocin, Inj. (Various Mfr.).

STREPTOMYCYLIDENE ISONICOTINYL HYDRAZINE SULFATE.
See: Streptohydrazid.

STREPTONASE B. (Wampole) Tube test for determination of streptococcal infection by serum DNase-B antibodies. Kit 1.
Use: In vitro diagnostic aid.

• **STREPTONICOZID.** USAN. Streptomycylidene isonicotinyl hydrazine sulfate.
Use: Antibiotic.
See: Streptohydrazid.

• **STREPTONIGRIN.** USAN. Antibiotic isolated from both filtrates of *Streptomyces flocculus.* 5-Amino-6-(7-amino-5, 8-dihydro-6-methoxy-5, 8-dioxo-2-quinolyl)-4-(2-hydroxy-3, 4-dimethoxyphenyl)-3-methylpicolinic acid.
Use: Antineoplastic agent.
See: Nigrin (Pfizer).

STREPTOVARICIN. An antibiotic composed of several related components derived from cultures of *Streptomyces variabilis.* Dalacin (Upjohn).

• **STREPTOZOCIN.** USAN.
Use: Antineoplastic.
See: Zanosar, Powder (Upjohn).

STREPTOZYME. (Wampole) Rapid hemagglutination slide test for the qualitative detection and quantitative determination of streptococcal extracellular antigens in serum, plasma and peripheral blood. Kit 15s, 50s, 150s.
Use: An aid in the diagnosis of *Streptococcal A* sequelae.

STRESS "1000". (Nature's Bounty) Vitamins E 22 mg, B_1 15 mg, B_2 15 mg, B_3 100 mg, B_5 20 mg, B_6 5 mg, B_{12} 12 mcg, C 1000 mg/Tab. Bot. 60s.
Use: Vitamin supplement.

STRESS-BEE CAPSULES. (Rugby) Vitamins B_1 10 mg, B_2 10 mg, B_3 100 mg, B_5 20 mg, B_6 2 mg, B_{12} 6 mcg, C 300 mg/Cap. Bot. 100s.
Use: Vitamin supplement.

STRESSCAPS. (Lederle) Vitamins B_1 10 mg, B_2 10 mg, niacinamide 100 mg, C 300 mg, B_6 2 mg, B_{12} 6 mcg, calcium pantothenate 20 mg/Cap. Bot. 100s.
Use: Vitamin supplement.

STRESS FORMULA. (Various Mfr.) Vita-

mins E 30 mg, B_1 15 mg, B_2 15 mg, B_3 100 mg, B_5 20 mg, B_6 5 mg, B_{12} 12 mcg, C 600 mg, folic acid 0.4 mg, biotin 45 mcg/Cap., Tab. **Cap.**: Bot. 60s, 100s, 1000s. **Tab.**: Bot. 30s, 60s, 100s, 250s, 300s, 400s, 1000s, UD 100s.
Use: Vitamin supplement.

STRESS FORMULA 600 (Halsey)
Use: Vitamin supplement.

STRESS FORMULA 600 W/IRON.
(Halsey).
Use: Vitamin supplement.

STRESS FORMULA 600 PLUS IRON.
(Schein) Iron 27 mg, vitamins E 30 IU, B_1 15 mg, B_2 15 mg, B_3 100 mg, B_5 20 mg, B_6 5 mg, B_{12} 12 mcg, C 600 mg, folic acid 0.4 mg, biotin 45 mcg/Tab. Bot. 60s, 250s.
Use: Vitamin supplement.

STRESS FORMULA 600 PLUS ZINC.
(Schein) Vitamins E 30 mg, B_1 20 mg, B_2 10 mg, B_3 100 mg, B_5 25 mg, B_6 5 mg, B_{12} 12 mcg, C 600 mg, folic acid 0.4 mg, zinc 23.9 mg, Cu, Mg, biotin 45 mcg/Tab. Bot. 60s, 250s.
Use: Vitamin/mineral supplement.

STRESS FORMULA 600 W/ZINC.
(Halsey).
Use: Dietary supplement.

STRESS FORMULA "605". (Nature's Bounty) Vitamins E 30 mg, B_1 15 mg, B_2 15 mg, B_3 100 mg, B_5 20 mg, B_6 5 mg, B_{12} 12 mcg, C 605 mg, folic acid 0.4 mg, biotin 45 mg/Tab. Bot. 60s.
Use: Vitamin supplement.

STRESS FORMULA "605" WITH IRON.
(Nature's Bounty) Iron 27 mg, vitamins E 30 mg, B_1 15 mg, B_2 15 mg, B_3 100 mg, B_5 20 mg, B_6 5 mg, B_{12} 12 mcg, C 605 mg, folic acid 0.4 mg, biotin 45 mg/Tab. Bot. 60s.
Use: Vitamin supplement.

STRESS FORMULA "605" WITH ZINC.
(Nature's Bounty) Vitamins E 30 mg, B_1 20 mg, B_2 10 mg, B_3 100 mg, B_5 25 mg, B_6 5 mg, B_{12} 12 mcg, C 605 mg, folic acid 0.4 mg, zinc 23.9 mg, copper, biotin 45 mcg/Tab. Bot. 60s.
Use: Vitamin/mineral supplement.

STRESS FORMULA VITAMINS. (Various Mfr.) Vitamins E 30 mg, B_1 15 mg, B_2 15 mg, B_3 100 mg, B_5 20 mg, B_6 5 mg, B_{12} 12 mcg, C 600 mg, folic acid 0.4 mg, biotin 45 mcg. Cap. Bot. 100s/Tab. Bot. 60s, 100s, 250s, 300s, 400s, 600s.
Use: Vitamin supplement.

STRESS FORMULA WITH IRON. (Nature's Bounty) Vitamin C 500 mg, B_1 10 mg, B_2 10 mg, B_3 100 mg, B_5 20 mg, B_6 5 mg, B_{12} 12 mcg, E 30 IU, iron 27 mg,

folic acid 0.4 mg, biotin 45 mcg. Tab. Bot. 60s
Use: Iron with vitamin supplement.

STRESS FORMULA WITH ZINC.
(Towne) Vitamins E 45 IU, C 600 mg, folic acid 400 mcg, B_1 20 mg, B_2 10 mg, niacinamide 100 mg, B_6 10 mg, B_{12} 25 mcg, biotin 40 mcg, pantothenic acid 25 mg, copper 3 mg, zinc 23.9 mg/Tab. Bot. 60s.
Use: Dietary supplement.

STRESSTABS ADVANCED FORMULA.
(Lederle) Vitamins E 30 mg, B_1 15 mg, B_2 10 mg, B_3 100 mg, B_5 20 mg, B_6 5 mg, B_{12} 12 mcg, C 500 mg, folic acid 0.4 mg, biotin 45 mcg/Tab. Bot. 60s. (Formerly called Stresstabs 600 Advanced Formula).
Use: Vitamin supplement.

STRESSTABS + ZINC. (Lederle) Vitamins E 30 mg, B_1 15 mg, B_2 10 mg, B_3 100 mg, B_5 20 mg, B_6 5 mg, B_{12} 12 mcg, C 500 mg, folic acid 0.4 mg, zinc 23.9 mg, copper, biotin 45 mcg/Tab. Bot. 60s.
Use: Vitamin/mineral supplement.

STRESSTABS 600. (Lederle) Vitamins B_1 15 mg, B_2 10 mg, B_6 5 mg, B_{12} 12 mcg, C 600 mg, niacinamide 100 mg, vitamin E 30 IU, biotin 45 mcg, folic acid 400 mcg, calcium pantothenate 20 mg/Tab. Bot. 30s, 60s. UD 10 × 10s.
Use: Multivitamin.

STRESSTABS 600 ADVANCED FORMULA. (Lederle) Vitamins E 30 mg, B_1 15 mg, B_2 10 mg, B_3 100 mg, B_5 20 mg, B_6 5 mg, B_{12} 12 mcg, C 600 mg, folic acid 0.4 mg, biotin 45 mcg/Tab. Bot. 30s, 60s, UD 100s.
Use: Multivitamin.

STRESSTABS 600 WITH IRON TABLETS. (Lederle) Ferrous fumerate 27 mg, vitamins E 30 IU, B_1 15 mg, B_2 15 mg, B_3 100 mg, B_5 20 mg, B_6 5 mg, B_{12} 12 mcg, C 600 mg, folic acid 0.4 mg, biotin 45 mcg/Tab. Bot. 30s, 60s.
Use: Multivitamin with iron.

STRESSTABS 600 WITH ZINC. (Lederle) Vitamins B_1 15 mg, B_2 10 mg, B_3 100 mg, B_5 20 mg, B_6 5 mg, B_{12} 12 mcg, C 600 mg, E 30 IU, folic acid 0.4 mg, biotin 45 mcg, Cu, zinc 23.9 mg/Tab. Bot. 30s, 60s.
Use: Multivitamin with zinc.

STRESSTEIN. (Sandoz Nutrition) Maltodextrin, medium chain triglycerides, L-leucine, soybean oil, L-isoleucine, L-valine, L-glutamic acid, L-arginine, L-lysine acetate, L-alanine, L-threonine, L-phenylalanine, L-asparticacid, L-histidine, L-methionine, glycine, polyglycerol

esters of fatty acids, L-serine, L-proline, sodium Cl, L-tryptophan, L-cysteine, sodium citrate, vitamins and minerals. Powder 3.4 oz. packets.
Use: High protein, branched chain enriched tube feeding.

STRI-DEX ANTIBACTERIAL CLEANSING. (Sterling Health) Triclosan 1%, glycerin, acetylated lanolin alcohol, EDTA. Bar: 27 g.
Use: Anti-acne.

STRI-DEX B.P. (Glenbrook) Benzoyl peroxide 10%. in greaseless, vanishing cream base.
Use: Anti-acne.

STRI-DEX CLEAR. (Sterling Health) Salicylic acid 2%, SD alcohol 9.3%, EDTA. Gel: 30 g.
Use: Anti-acne.

STRIDEX FACE WASH. (Sterling Health) Triclosan 1%, glycerin, EDTA, alcohol free. Soln.: 237 ml.
Use: Anti-acne.

STRI-DEX LOTION. (Glenbrook) Salicylic acid 0.5%, alcohol 28%, sulfonated alkyl benzenes, citric acid, sodium carbonate, simethicone, water. Bot. 4 oz.
Use: Anti-acne.

STRI-DEX MAXIMUM STRENGTH PADS. (Glenbrook) Salicylic acid 2%, SD alcohol 44%, citric acid.
Use: Anti-acne.

STRI-DEX REGULAR STRENGTH PADS. (Glenbrook) Salicylic acid 0.5%, SD alcohol 28%, citric acid. In 42s, 75s.
Use: Anti-acne.

STROMBA AMPULES. (Sanofi Winthrop) Stanozolol.
Use: Anabolic steroid.

STRONG IODINE TINCTURE. (Various Mfr.) Iodine 7%, potassium iodide 5%, alcohol 83%. Soln. Bot. 500 ml, 4000 ml.
Use: Antiseptic and germicide.

STRONTIUM BROMIDE. Cryst. or Granule, Bot. 0.25 lb, 1 lb. Amp. 1 Gm./10 ml
Use: Sedative & antiepileptic.
W/Bromides of sodium, potassium, ammonium.
See: Lanabrom, Elix. (Lannett).

• **STRONTIUM CHLORIDE Sr 85.** USAN.
Use: Radioactive agent.

• **STRONTIUM CHLORIDE Sr 89.** USAN.
Use: Radioactive agent.

STRONTIUM CHLORIDE Sr89.
Use: Radioactive agent.
See: Metastron, Inj. (Medi-Physics/Amersham).

STRONTIUM LACTATE TRIHYDRATE.

• **STRONTIUM NITRATE Sr 85.** USAN.
Use: Radioactive agent.

STRONTIUM SR 85 INJECTION.
Use: Diagnostic aid (bone scanning).

STROPHANTHIN. K-strophanthin.

STROPHEN. (Kenyon) Prednisone 0.75 mg, salicylamide 5 gr, alum. hydroxide gel 75 mg, vitamin C 20 mg/Tab. Bot. 100s, 1000s.
Use: Arthritis.

STROVITE PLUS TABLETS. (Everett) Vitamins A 5000 IU, E 30 mg, B_1 20 mg, B_2 20 mg, B_3 100 mg, B_5 25 mg, B_6 25 mg, B_{12} 50 mcg, C 500 mg, iron 27 mg, zinc 22.5 mg, biotin 150 mcg, Cr, Cu, Mg, Mn. Bot. 100s.
Use: Vitamin supplement.

STROVITE TABLETS. (Everett) Vitamins B_1 15 mg, B_2 15 mg, B_3 100 mg, B_5 18 mg, B_6 4 mg, B_{12} 5 mcg, C 500 mg, folic acid 0.5 mg. Bot. 100s.
Use: Vitamin supplement.

STUART FORMULA. (Stuart) Vitamins A 5000 IU, B_1 1.5 mg, B_2 1.7 mg niacin 20 mg, B_6 2 mg, B_{12} 6 mcg, C 60 mg, D 400 IU, E 15 IU, iron 18 mg, phosphate 125 mg, folic acid 0.4 mg, Ca, I, Mg, P/Tab. Bot. 100s, 250s.
Use: Dietary vitamin & mineral supplement.

STUARTINIC. (Stuart) Vitamins B_{12} 25 mcg, B_1 6 mg, B_2 6 mg, niacinamide 20 mg, B_5 10 mg, calcium pantothenate 10 mg, B_6 1 mg, C 525 mg, iron 100 mg/Tab. Bot. 60s.
Use: Hematinic; iron deficiency.

STUARTNATAL PLUS. (Wyeth-Ayerst) Vitamins A 4000 IU, D 400 IU, E 11 mg, C 120 mg, B_1 1.5 mg, B_2 3 mg, B_3 20 mg, B_6 10 mg, B_{12} 12 mcg, calcium 200 mg, folic acid 1 mg, iron 65 mg, zinc 25 mg, copper 2 mg. Tab. Bot. 100s.
Use: Vitamin, mineral supplement in pregnancy and lactation.

STUARTNATAL 1 + 1. (Stuart) Vitamins A 4000 IU, B_1 1.5 mg, B_2 3 mg, niacin 20 mg, B_6 10 mg, B_{12} 12 mcg, C 120 mg, D 400 IU, E 11 mg, folic acid 1 mg, calcium 200 mg, iron 65 mg, zinc 25 mg, copper 2 mg/Tab. Bot. 100s, 500s.
Use: Vitamin, mineral supplement in pregnancy and lactation.

STUART PRENATAL. (Stuart) Vitamins A 4000 IU, B_1 1.5 mg, B_2 1.7 mg, B_6 2.6 mg, B_{12} 4 mcg, C 100 mg, D 400 IU, E 11 mg, niacin 18 mg, iron 60 mg, calcium 200 mg, copper 2 mg, zinc 25 mg, folic acid 0.8 mg/Tab. Bot. 100s.
Use: Vitamin & mineral supplement in pregnancy & lactation.

STULEX. (Bowman) Docusate sodium 250 mg/Tab. Bot. 100s, 1000s.

Use: Fecal softener.

STYPT-AID. (Pharmakon Labs) Benzocaine 28.71 mg, methylbenzethonium HCl 9.95 mg, aluminum Cl hexahydrate 55.43 mg, ethyl alcohol 70.97%/ml in a glycerine, menthol base. Spray. In 60 ml.
Use: Topical local anesthetic.

ƆTYPTIRENAL.
See: Epinephrine (Various Mfr.).

STYPTO-CAINE SOLUTION. (Pedinol) Hydroxyquinoline sulfate, tetracaine HCl, aluminum Cl, aqueous glycol base. Bot. 2 oz.
Use: Hemostatic solution.

STYRAMATE. B.A.N. 1-Phenyl-1,2-ethanediol 2-carbamate. β-Hydroxyphenethyl carbamate. 2-Hydroxy-2-phenylethyl carbamate.
Use: Skeletal muscle relaxant.

STYRENE POLYMER, SULFONATED, SODIUM SALT. Sodium Polystyrene Sulfonate, U.S.P. XXIII.

STYRONATE RESINS. Ammonium and potassium salts of sulfonated styrene polymers.
Use: Conditions requiring sodium restriction.

SUBLIMAZE. (Janssen) Fentanyl 0.05 mg as citrate/ml. Amp. 10 ml, 20 ml Pkg. 2s, 5s.
Use: Analgesic, anesthetic agent.

SUBY'S SOLUTION G. (Various Mfr.) Citric acid 3.24 Gm, sodium carbonate 0.43 Gm, magnesium oxide 0.38 Gm/100 ml. Soln. Bot. 1000 ml.
Use: Genitourinary irrigant.

• **SUCCIMER.** USAN.
Use: Diagnostic aid; cystine kidney stones, mercury and lead poisoning [Orphan drug]
See: Chemet (Johnson & Johnson).

SUCCINATES.
See: Calcium succinate.
Sodium succinate.
Succinic acid.

SUCCINCHLORIMIDE. N-Chlorosuccinimide.

SUCCINIC ACID.
W/9-Aminoacridine undecylenate, N-myristyl-3-hydroxybutylamine hydrochloride, methylbenzethonium Cl.
See: Cenasert, Tab. (Central).

• **SUCCINYLCHOLINE CHLORIDE,** U.S.P. XXIII. Inj., Sterile, U.S.P. XXIII. Ethanaminium, 2,2'-[(1,4-dioxo-1,4-butanediyl)bis(oxy)]bis-N,NN-tri-methyl-, dichlo- ride. Choline Cl succinate (2:1).
Use: Skeletal muscle relaxant.
See: Anectine Cl, Amp. (Burroughs Wellcome).

Quelicin, Amp., Additive Syringes, Fliptop & Pintop Vials (Abbott).
Sucostrin, Amp., Vial (Squibb Marsam).

SUCCINYLSULFATHIAZOLE. 4'-(2-Thiazolysulfamoyl).
Use: Intestinal antibacterial.

SUCCUS CINERARIA MARITIMA. (Walker Pharmaceutic) Aqueous and glycerin solution of senecio, compositae, hamamelis water and boric acid. Soln./Bot. 7 ml.
Use: Ophthalmic.

SUCOSTRIN. (Apothecon) Succinylcholine Cl 20 mg/ml Inj. Vial 10 ml.
Use: Depolarizing neuromuscular blocking agent.

SUCOSTRIN CHLORIDE. (Squibb-Marsam) Succinylcholine Cl 20 mg/ml w/methylparaben 0.1%, propylparaben 0.01%. Vial 10 ml; High potency 100 mg/ml. Vial 10 ml.
Use: Muscle relaxant.

• **SUCRALFATE,** U.S.P. 23, Tab., U.S.P. 23. Beta-D-fructofuranosyl-alpha-D-glucopyranoside octakis (hydrogen sulfate) aluminum hydroxide complex.
Use: Duodenal ulcer therapy; oral complications of chemotherapy [Orphan drug]
See: Carafate, Tab., Susp. (Marion Merrell Dow).

SUCRALOX. B.A.N. A polymerized complex of sucrose and aluminum hydroxide.
Use: Treatment of gastric hyperacidity.

SUCRASE (YEAST-DERIVED).
Use: Treatment of congenital sucrase-isomaltase deficiency. [Orphan drug]
See: Sacarasa.

SUCRETS CHILDREN'S SORE THROAT LOZENGES. (SK-Beecham) Dyclonine HCl 1.2 mg/Lozenge. Cherry flavor. Tin 24s.
Use: Sore throat treatment for children 3 years and over.

SUCRETS COLD DECONGESTANT LOZENGE. (SK-Beecham) Phenylpropanolamine HCl 25 mg/Lozenge. Box 24s.
Use: Decongestant.

SUCRETS COUGH CONTROL LOZENGE. (SK-Beecham) Dextromethorphan HBr 5 mg/Lozenge. Tin 24s.
Use: Antitussive.

SUCRETS MAXIMUM STRENGTH SORE THROAT LOZENGES. (SK-Beecham) Dyclonine HCl 3 mg/Lozenge. Tin 24s, 48s, 55s.

Use: Temporary relief of minor sore throat, pain and mouth irritation.

SUCRETS MAXIMUM STRENGTH SORE THROAT SPRAY & GARGLE. (SK-Beecham) Dyclonine HCl 0.1%, alcohol 10%, sorbitol. Spray Bot. 6 oz, 12 oz. Gargle Bot. 12 oz.
Use: Temporary relief of minor sore throat pain and mouth irritation.

SUCRETS SORE THROAT LOZENGE. (SK-Beecham) Hexylresorcinol 2.4 mg/Loz. **Regular:** Tin 24s, 48s. **Mentholated:** Tin 24s.
Use: Minor throat, pain and mouth irritation.

SUCRETS WINTERGREEN. (SK-Beecham) Dyclonine HCl 0.1%, alcohol 10%, sorbitol. Spray bot. 90 ml.
Use: Temporary relief of minor sore throat pain and mouth irritation.

• **SUCROSE,** N.F. XVIII. Compressible, Confectioners, N.F. XVIII. Saccharose. Sugar, α-D-Glucopyranoside, β-D-fructo-furanosyl-.
Use: I.V.; diuretic & dehydrating agent; pharm. aid (sweetening agent).

• **SUCROSE OCTAACETATE,** N.F. XVIII.
Use: Alcohol denaturant.

SUDAFED CHILDREN'S LIQUID. (Burroughs Wellcome) Pseudoephedrine HCl 30 mg/5 ml. Bot. 4 oz, pt.
Use: Nasal decongestant.

SUDAFED 12 HOUR CAPSULES. (Burroughs Wellcome) Pseudoephedrine HCl 120 mg/Sustained Action Cap. Box 10s, 20s, 40s.
Use: Nasal or eustachian tube congestion.

SUDAFED COLD & COUGH LIQUID CAPS. (Burroughs Wellcome) Dextromethorphan HBr 10 mg, pseudoephedrine HCl 30 mg, acetaminophen 250 mg, guaifenesin 100 mg. Pkg. 10s, 20s.
Use: Analgesic, decongestant, antitussive, expectorant.

SUDAFED COUGH SYRUP. (Burroughs Wellcome) Pseudoephedrine HCl 15 mg, dextromethorphan HBr 5 mg, guaifenesin 100 mg w/alcohol 2.4%. Bot. 4 oz.
Use: Cough treatment.

SUDAFED PLUS. (Burroughs Wellcome) **Tab.:** Pseudoephedrine HCl 60 mg, chlorpheniramine maleate 4 mg/Tab. Box 24s, 48s. **Syrup:** Pseudoephedrine HCl 30 mg, chlorpheniramine maleate 2 mg. Bot. 4 oz.
Use: Sinus & upper respiratory tract decongestant.

SUDAFED, SEVERE COLD FORMULA MAXIMUM STRENGTH. (Burroughs Wellcome) Pseudoephedrine HCl 30 mg, dextromethorphan HBr 15 mg, acetaminophen 500 mg/Tab. Pkg. 10s, 20s.
Use: Decongestant, antitussive, analgesic.

SUDAFED SINUS MAXIMUM STRENGTH. (Burroughs Wellcome) Pseudoephedrine HCl 30 mg, acetaminophen 500 mg. Caplets: In 24s.
Use: Decongestant, analgesic.

SUDAFED TABLETS. (Burroughs Wellcome) Pseudoephedrine HCL 30 mg or 60 mg/Tab. **30 mg:** Box 24s, 48s. Bot. 100s, 1000s. **60 mg:** Bot. 100s, 1000s.
Use: Nasal decongestant.

SUDANYL. (Dover) Pseudoephedrine HCl/Tab. Sugar, lactose and salt free. UD Box 500s.
Use: Decongestant.

SUDDEN TAN LOTION. (Plough) Padimate O, dihydroxyacetone, Bot. 4 oz.
Use: Artificial tanning agent, ultraviolet sunscreen, moisturizer.

SUDEX. (Atley) Pseudoephedrine HCl 120 mg, guaifenesin 600 mg. SR Tab.: 100s.
Use: Decongestant, antitussive.

• **SUDOXICAM.** USAN. 4-Hydroxy-2-methyl-N-thiazol-2-yl-2H-1,2-benzoth iazine-3-carboxamide 1,1-dioxide.
Use: Anti-inflammatory.

SUDRIN. (Bowman) Pseudoephedrine HCl 30 mg/Tab. Bot. 100s, 1000s.
Use: Nasal decongestant.

SUFENTA. (Janssen) Sufentanil citrate 50 mcg/ml. Amps. 1 ml, 2 ml, 5 ml.
Use: Analgesic, anesthetic agent.

• **SUFENTANIL.** USAN.
Use: Analgesic.

• **SUFENTANIL CITRATE.** USAN.
Use: Narcotic analgesic.
See: Sufenta (Janssen).

• **SUFOTIDINE.** USAN.
Use: Antagonist (to histamine H_2 receptors).

SUFREX. (Janssen) Ketanserin tartrate.
Use: Serotonin antagonist.

• **SUGAR, COMPRESSIBLE,** U.S.P. XXIII.
Use: Pharmaceutic aid (sweetening agent, tablet excipient).

• **SUGAR, CONFECTIONER'S,** N.F. XII.
Use: Pharmaceutic aid (sweetening agent; tablet excipient).

• **SUGAR SPHERES,** N.F. XVIII.
Use: Pharmaceutic aid (sweetening agent).

SULAMYD SODIUM.

Use: Ophthalmic sulfonamide.
See: Sodium Sulamyd, Ophth. Soln.
(Schering).
• **SULAZEPAM.** USAN. 7-Chloro-1,3-dihy-
dro-1-methyl-5-phenyl-2H-1,4-benzodi-
azepine-2-thione.
Use: Tranquilizer (minor).
SULAZO. (Freeport) Sulfisoxazole 500
mg, phenylazodiaminopyridine HCl 50
mg/Tab. Bot. 1000s.
Use: Urinary tract infections complicat-
ed by pain.
• **SULBACTAM BENZATHINE.** USAN.
Use: Synergistic
(penicillin/cephalosporin).
• **SULBACTAM PIVOXIL.** USAN.
Use: Inhibitor, synergist
(penicillin/cephalosporin).
• **SULBACTAM SODIUM.** USAN.
Use: Inhibitor (beta-lactamase), syner-
gist (penicillin/cephalosporin).
**SULBACTAM SODIUM/AMPICILLIN
SODIUM.**
Use: Penicillin.
See: Unasyn (Roerig).
• **SULCONAZOLE NITRATE.** U.S.P. XXIII.
USAN.
Use: Antifungal.
See: Exelderm (Westwood).
SULF-10. (Iolab Pharmaceutic) Sodium
sulfacetamide 10%. Bot. 15 ml; Drop-
perette 1 ml. Box 12s.
Use: External bacterial eye infections.
SULF-15. (Iolab) Sodium sulfacetamide
15%. Soln. Bot. 5 ml, 15 ml.
Use: External bacterial eye infection.
SULFA-10 OPHTHALMIC. (Maurry) Sodi-
um sulfacetamide 10%, hydroxyethylcel-
lulose, sodium borate, boric acid, disodi-
um edetate, sodium metabisulfite, sodi-
um thiosulfate 0.2%, chlorobutanol
0.2%, methyl paraben 0.015%. Bot. 15
ml.
Use: Antibacterial.
• **SULFABENZ.** USAN.
Use: Antibacterial, coccidiostat.
• **SULFABENZAMIDE,** U.S.P. XXIII. Ben-
zamide, N-[(4-aminophenyl) sulfonyl]-N-
Sulfanilylbenzamide. Sulfanilylbenza-
mide, N' benzoylsulfanilamide.
See: Sultrin, Vag. Tab., Cream (Ortho).
SULFABROMETHAZINE SODIUM.
Use: Antibacterial.
SULFACARBAMIDE (I.N.N.). Sulphau-
rea, B.A.N.
SULFACET. (Dermik).
See: Sulfacetamide.
• **SULFACETAMIDE,** U.S.P. XXIII. Ac-
etamide, N-[(4-aminophenyl) sulfonyl]-
N-Sulfanilylacetamine. N-acetylsulfanil-
amide.
Use: Antibacterial.
See: Isopto-Cetamide, Ophth. Soln. (Al-
con).
SULFACETAMIDE W/COMBINATIONS.
See: Acet-Dia-Mer Sulfonamides.
Cetapred, Oint. (Alcon).
Chero-Trisulfa (V), Susp. (Vita Elixir).
Sulf-10, Ophth. Soln. (CooperVision).
Sultrin, Tab., Cream (Ortho).
Triurisul, Tab. (Sheryl).
Uridium, Tab. (Pharmex).
Urotrol, Tab. (Mills).
• **SULFACETAMIDE SODIUM,** U.S.P. XXI-
II. Ophth. Oint., Ophth. Soln., U.S.P.
XXIII. Acetamide, N-[(4-
aminophenyl)sulfonyl]-,monosodium
salt, monohydrate. N-Sulfanilylac-
etamide monosodium salt monohydrate.
(Various Mfr.) **Soln.: 10% or 15%:** Bot. 2
ml, 15 ml; **30%:** Bot. 15 ml. **Oint.:** 10%
Tube 3.5 g.
Use: Antibacterial (ophthalmic).
See: AK-Sulf, Preps. (Akorn).
Bleph 10, Liquifilm (Allergan).
Cetamide, Ophth. Oint. (Alcon).
Isopto Cetamide, Ophth. Soln. (Alcon).
Ocusulf-10, Ophth. Soln. (Optopics).
Sebizon Lotion (Schering).
Sodium Sulamyd Ophthalmic Oint-
ment 30% (Schering).
Sulf-10, Drops (Maurry).
Sulf-10, Soln., Drops (Iolab).
Sulf-15, Ophth. Soln. (Iolab).
W/Fluorometholone.
See: FML-S Susp. (Allergan).
W/Methylcellulose.
See: Sodium Sulamyd Ophth. Soln.
10% (Schering).
W/Phenylephrine HCl, methylparaben,
propylparaben.
See: Vasosulf, Liq. (Iolab).
W/Prednisolone.
See: Cetapred Ophthalmic Ointment
(Alcon).
Vasocidin, Soln. (CooperVision).
W/Prednisolone acetate.
See: Blephamide S.O.P., Ophth. Oint.
and Susp. (Allergan).
Metimyd, Ophth. Oint. and Susp.
(Schering).
W/Prednisolone, methylcellulose.
See: Isopto Cetapred, Susp. (Alcon).
W/Prednisolone acetate, phenylephrine.
See: Blephamide Liquifilm, Ophth.
Susp. (Allergan).
Tri-Ophtho, Ophth. Drops (Maurry).
W/Prednisolone phosphate.
See: Optimyd Soln., Sterile (Schering).
W/Prednisolone sodium phosphate,

phenylephrine, sulfacetamide sodium.
Vasocidin, Ophth. Soln. (Iolab).
W/Sulfur.
See: Novacet, Lot. (Genderm).
Sulfacet-R, Lot. (Dermik).
• **SULFACETAMIDE SODIUM AND PRED-
NISOLONE ACETATE OPHTHALMIC
OINTMENT,** U.S.P. XXIII.
Use: Antibiotic, anti-inflammatory.
See: AK-Cide (Akorn).
Blephamide S.O.P. (Allergan).
Cetapred (Alcon).
Metimyd (Schering).
Predsulfair (Pharmafair).
Sulphrin (Bausch & Lomb).
Vasocidin (Iolab Pharm).
**SULFACETAMIDE SODIUM AND PRED-
NISOLONE SODIUM PHOSPHATE.**
(Schein) Sulfacetamide sodium 10%,
prednisolone sodium phosphate 0.25%,
thimerosal 0.1 mg/ml, EDTA, boric acid.
Soln. 5 ml, 10 ml.
Use: Ophthalmic antibiotic, anti-inflam-
matory.
**SULFACETAMIDE, SULFADIAZINE, &
SULFAMERAZINE ORAL SUSPEN-
SION.**
See: Acet-Dia-Mer-Sulfonamides.
SULFACET-R LOTION. (Dermik) Sodium
sulfacetamide 10%, sulfur 5%, in flesh-
tinted base. Bot. 25 Gm.
Use: Treatment of acne and seborrheic
dermatitis.
SULFACHLORPYRIDAZINE. B.A.N. N^1-
(6-chloro-3-pyridazinyl) sulfanilamide
SULFADIASULFONE SODIUM. Aceto-
sulfone sodium.
• **SULFADIAZINE,** U.S.P. XXIII.; Tab.,
U.S.P. XXIII. 2-Sulfanilamidopyridine,
N'-2-pyrimidinylsulfanilamide. Benzene-
sulfonamide, 4-amino-N-2-pyrimidinyl-.
(Stanley Pharm) 500 mg. Tab. Bot.
100s.
Use: Anti-infective. [Orphan drug]
SULFADIAZINE COMBINATIONS.
See: Acet-Dia-Mer-Sulfonamides. (Vari-
ous Mfr.).
Chemozine, Tab., Susp. (Tennessee
Pharmaceutic).
Chero-Trisulfa, Susp. (Vita Elixir).
Dia-Mer-Sulfonamides (Various Mfr.).
Dia-Mer-Thia-Sulfonamide (Various
Mfr.).
Lantrisul, Tab., Susp. (Lannett).
Meth-Dia-Mer-Sulfonamides (Various
Mfr.).
Silvadene (Marion).
Sulfajen, Cream. (Jenkins).
Terfonyl, Liq., Tab. (Squibb).
Triosulf, Tab. (Jenkins).

Triple Sulfa, Tab. (Various Mfr.).
SULFADIAZINE AND SULFAMERAZINE.
Citrasulfas.
See: Dia-Mer-Sulfonamides.
• **SULFADIAZINE SODIUM,** U.S.P. XXIII.
Sterile Inj., U.S.P. XXIII. Benzenesulfon-
amide, 4-amino-N-2-pyrimidinyl-,
monosodium salt. N^{1-2}-Pyrimidinylsul-
fanilamide monosodium salt.
Use: Anti-infective.
W/Sod. bicarbonate.
(Pitman-Moore)—Tab. 5 gr, Bot. 1000s;
2.5 gr, Bot. 100s, 500s, 1000s.
**SULFADIAZINE, SULFAMERAZINE &
SULFACETAMIDE SUSPENSION.**
See: Acet-Dia-Mer-Sulfonamides.
Coco Diazine (Lilly).
SULFADIMETHOXINE. Sulphadi-
methoxine, B.A.N. N'-(2,6-Dimethoxy-4-
pyrimidinyl) sulfanilamide.
Use: Anti-infective.
SULFADIMETINE. N^1-(2-6-Dimethyl 4-
pyrimidyl) sulfanilamide. Sulfisomidine.
Elkosin (Ciba).
SULFADIMIDINE.
See: Sulfamethazine.
SULFADINE.
See: Sulfadimidine.
Sulfamethazine.
Sulfapyridine, Tab. (Various Mfr.).
• **SULFADOXINE,** U.S.P. XXIII. N^1-(5,6-
dimethoxy-4-pyrimidinyl) sulfanilamide.
4-(4-Aminobenzene-sulfonamido)-5,6-
dimethoxypyrimidine. Fanasil Fanzil
(Roche).
Use: Anti-infective.
W/Pyrimethamine.
See: Fansidar, Tab. (Roche).
• **SULFADOXINE AND PYRIMETHAMINE
TABLETS,** U.S.P. XXIII.
Use: Anti-infective, antimalarial.
SULFAETHIDOLE. Sulphaethicole,
B.A.N. Sulfaethylthiadiazole. N^1-(5-eth-
yl-1,3,4-thiadiazol-2-yl) sulfanilamide.
Sulfaethylthiadiazole. Sethadil.
Use: Anti-infective.
SULFAETHYLTHIADIAZOLE.
See: Sulfaethidole.
SULFAFURAZOLE. B.A.N. 5-(4-
Aminobenzene-sul-phonamido)-3,4-di-
methylisoxazole. Gantrisin. Sulphafura-
zole. Sulfisoxazole.
SULFAGUANIDINE. (N-Guanylsulfanil-
amide; Abiguanil; Ganidan; Guamide).
Use: G.I. tract infections.
W/Sulfamethazine, sulfamerazine & sulfa-
diazine.
See: Quadetts, Tab. (Elder).
Quad-Ramoid, Susp. (Elder).
SULFAIR 15. (Pharmafair) Sodium sul-

facetamide 15%. Soln. Bot. 15 ml.
Use: Ophthalmic sulfonamide.
SULFAJEN CREAM. (Jenkins) Sulfamerazine 0.167 Gm, sulfadiazine 0.167 Gm, sulfamethazine 0.167 Gm/5 ml. Bot. 3 oz, 4 oz, gal.
Use: Triple sulfonamide therapy.
SULFALAX CALCIUM. (Major) Docusate calcium 240 mg/Cap. Bot. 500s.
Use: Laxative.
• **SULFALENE.** USAN. N'-(3-Methoxypyrazinyl) sulfanilamide. Sulfametopyrazine, B.A.N.
Use: Anti-infective.
• **SULFAMERAZINE,** U.S.P. XXIII. Tab., U.S.P. XXIII. Benzenesulfonamide, 4-amino-N-(4-methyl-2- pyrimidinyl)-. N^1-(4-Methyl-2-pyrimidinyl)-sulfanilamide. (Sumedine).
Use: Infections caused by susceptible bacteria.
SULFAMERAZINE COMBINATIONS.
Use: Anti-infective.
See: Chemozine Tab., Susp. (Tennessee Pharmaceutic).
Chero-Trisulfa-V, Susp. (Vita Elixir).
Terfonyl, Liq., Tab. (Squibb).
Triple Sulfa, Tab. (Various Mfr.).
SULFAMERAZINE SODIUM.
Use: Anti-infective.
SULFAMERAZINE & SULFADIAZINE.
See: Dia-Mer-Sulfonamides.
SULFAMERAZINE, SULFADIAZINE & SULFAMETHAZINE.
Use: Anti-infective.
See: Meth-Dia-Mer-Sulfonamides.
SULFAMERAZINE, SULFADIAZINE & SULFATHIAZOLE.
Use: Anti-infective.
See: Dia-Mer-Thia-Sulfonamides.
• **SULFAMETHAZINE,** U.S.P. XXIII, Granulated, U.S.P. 23. Benzenesulfonamide, 4-amino-N-(4,6-dimethyl-2- pyrimidinyl)-. 4,6-Dimethyl-2-sulfanilamidopyrimidine. NI-(4,6-Dimethyl-2-pyrimidinyl)sulfanilamide.
Use: Anti-infective.
See: Neotrizine, Susp., Tab. (Lilly).
W/Sulfacetamide, sulfadiazine, sulfamerazine.
See: Sulfa-Plex, Vaginal Cream (Reid-Rowell).
W/Sulfadiazine, sulfamerazine.
See: Lantrisul, Tab., Susp. (Lannett).
Sulfaloid, Susp. (Westerfield).
Terfonyl, Liq., Tab. (Squibb).
Triple Sulfa, Tab. (Various Mfr.).
• **SULFAMETHIZOLE,** U.S.P. XXIII. Oral Susp., Tab., U.S.P. XXIII. N'-(5/Methyl-1,3,4-thiadiazole-2-yl)-sulfanilamide. Methisul, Mizol, Uolueosil. Sulphamethizole.
Use: Anti-infective.
See: Bursul, Tab. (Burlington).
Microsul, Tab. (Star).
Proklar-M, Liq., Tab. (Westerfield).
Sulfasol, Tab. (Hyrex-Key).
Sulfurine, Tab. (TableRock).
Thiosulfil, Forte, Tab. (Wyeth-Ayerst).
Urifon, Tab. (Amid).
SULFAMETHIZOLE W/COMBINATIONS.
Use: Anti-infective.
See: Microsul-A, Tab. (Star).
Thiosulfil-A, Tab. (Wyeth-Ayerst).
Thiosulfil-A Forte, Tab. (Wyeth-Ayerst).
Triurisul, Tab. (Sheryl).
Urobiotic, Cap. (Pfizer).
Urotrol, Tab. (Mills).
SULFAMETHOPRIM. (Par Pharm) Sulfamethoxazole 400 mg, trimethoprim 80 mg/Tab. Bot. 100s, 500s.
Use: Anti-infective.
• **SULFAMETHOXAZOLE,** U.S.P. XXIII. Oral Susp., Tab., U.S.P. XXIII. Sulphamethoxazole, Methyl sulfanilamidoisoxazole. 5-Methyl-3-sulfanilamido-isoxazole. N'-(5-methyl-3-isoxazolyl) sulfanilamide.
Use: Anti-infective.
See: Gantanol, Prep. (Roche).
W/Trimethoprim.
See: Bactrim, Prods. (Roche).
Septra, Tab. (Burroughs Wellcome).
Septra DS, Tab. (Burroughs Wellcome).
SULFAMETHOXAZOLE AND PHENAZOPYRIDINE HCI.
Use: Urinary antibacterial.
See: Azo-Gantanol, Tab. (Roche).
• **SULFAMETHOXAZOLE AND TRIMETHOPRIM FOR INJECTION CONCENTRATE,** U.S.P. XXIII.
Use: Urinary antibacterial.
• **SULFAMETHOXAZOLE AND TRIMETHOPRIM ORAL SUSPENSION,** U.S.P. XXIII.
Use: Urinary antibacterial.
• **SULFAMETHOXAZOLE AND TRIMETHOPRIM TABLETS,** U.S.P. XXIII.
Use: Urinary antibacterial.
SULFAMETHOXAZOLE/TRIMETHOPRIM DS. (Various Mfr.) Trimethoprim 160 mg, sulfamethoxazole 800 mg. Tab, double strength. Bot. 20s, 100s, 500s.
Use: Miscellaneous anti-infective.
SULFAMETHOXYDIAZINE. Sulfameter.
Use: Anti-infective.

SULFAMETHOXYPYRIDAZINE, B.A.N.
N^1-(6-Methoxy-3-pyridazinyl) sulfanil-
amide. 3-(4-Aminobenzenesulfonami-
do)-6-methoxypyridazine.
Use: Anti-infective.
SULFAMETHOXYPYRIDAZINE ACETYL.
Use: Anti-infective.
SULFAMETHYLTHIADIAZOLE.
Use: Anti-infective.
See: Sulfamethizole Preps.
SULFAMETIN. N^1-(5-Methoxy-2-pyrim-
idinyl)sulfanilamide. (Formerly sul-
famethoxydiazine).
Use: Anti-infective.
SULFAMETOPYRAZINE. B.A.N. 2-(4-
Aminoben-zenesulfonamido)-3-
methoxypyrazine.
Use: Anti-infective.
See: Sulfalene (I.N.N.).
SULFAMEZANTHENE.
Use: Anti-infective.
See: Sulfamethazine.
SULFAMIDE SUSPENSION. (Rugby)
Prednisolone acetate 0.5%, sodium sul-
facetamide, hydroxypropyl methylcellu-
lose, polysorbate 80, sodium thiosulfate,
benzalkonium Cl 0.01%. Susp. Bot. 5
and 15 ml.
Use: Ophthalmic corticosteroid, sulfon-
amide.
• **SULFAMONOMETHOXINE.** USAN. N^1-
(6-methoxy-4-pyrimidinyl) sulfanilamide.
Use: Anti-infective.
• **SULFAMOXOLE.** USAN. N'-(4,5-di-
methyl-2-oxa-zolyl) sulfanilamide.
Use: Anti-infective.
p-SULFAMOYLBENZYLAMINE HCl.
Sulfbenzamide.
SULFAMYLON CREAM. (Dow B. Hickam) Mafenide acetate equivalent to 85
mg of base/Gm. w/cetyl alcohol, stearyl
alcohol, cetyl esters wax, polyoxyl 40
stearate, polyoxyl 8 stearate, glycerin,
water w/methylparaben and propyl-
paraben, sodium metabisulfite, edetate
disodium. Tube 2 oz, 4 oz. Can 14.5 oz.
Use: Adjunctive therapy in second and
third-degree burns.
SULFANILAMIDE. p-Aminobenzene sul-
fonamide.
Use: Anti-infective.
SULFANILAMIDE. (Various Mfr.) Sulfanil-
amide 15%. Vaginal Cream. Tube 120 g
with applicator.
Use: Anti-infective, vaginal.
SULFANILAMIDE COMBINATIONS.
Use: Anti-infective.
See: AVC/Dienestrol Cream, Supp.
(Merrell Dow).
AVC, Cream, Supp. (Marion Merrell

Dow).
D.I.T.I. Cream (Kenyon).
K.D.C. Vaginal Cream (Kenyon).
Par Cream (Parmed).
Vagacreme, Cream (Delta).
Vagisan Creme (Sandia).
Vagisul, Creme (Sheryl).
Vagitrol, Cream, Supp. (Lemmon).
2-SULFANILAMIDOPYRIDINE. Sulfadi-
azine, U.S.P. XXIII.
Use: Anti-infective.
• **SULFANILATE ZINC.** USAN.
Use: Anti-infective.
N-SULFANILYLACETAMIDE.
Use: Anti-infective.
See: Sulfacetamide, Tab. (Various Mfr.).
SULFANILYLBENZAMIDE.
Use: Anti-infective.
See: Sulfabenzamide.
• **SULFANITRAN.** USAN. 4'-[(p-Nitro-
phenyl) sulfamoyl]- acetanilide.
Use: Anti-infective.
SULFAPHENAZOLE. Sulphaphenzaole,
B.A.N. N'-(1-phenyl-5-pyrazolyl) sul-
fanilamide. 5-(4-Aminobenzene-
sulphonamido)-1-phenylpyrazole.
See: Orisulf (Ciba).
• **SULFAPYRIDINE,** U.S.P. XXIII. Tab.,
U.S.P. XXIII. Benzenesulfonamide, 4-
amino-N-2-pyridinyl-. 2-Sulfanilamidopy-
ridine. N'-2-Pyridylsulfanilamide. (Pfaltz
& Bauer) Pow., Bot. 1 lb.
Use: Dermatitic herpetiformis suppres-
sant. [Orphan drug]
SULFARSPHENAMINE. Disodium-[ar-
senobis[6-hydroxy-m-phenylene)imi-
no]]-dimethanesulfonate.
• **SULFASALAZINE,** U.S.P. XXIII. Tab.,
U.S.P. XXIII. 5-[[p-(2-Pyridylsulfamoyl)-
phenyl]azo]salicylic acid. 4-Hydroxy-4'-
(2-pyridylsulfamoyl)azobenzene-3-car-
boxylic acid. Sulphasalazine, B.A.N.
(Lederle) Tab. 0.5 Gm. Bot. 500s.
Use: Anti-infective.
See: Azulfidine, Tab., Susp. (Pharma-
cia).
Salazopyrin.
Salicylazosulfapyridine.
Salazopyrin.
S.A.S.-50, Tab. (Reid-Rowell).
S.A.S.P., Tab. (Zenith).
Sulcolon, Tab. (Lederle).
Sulfapyridine (I.N.N.).
• **SULFASOMIZOLE.** USAN. 5-(4-
Aminobenzenesulfonamido)-3-
methylisothiazole. N'-(3-methyliso-thia-
zolyl)sulfanilamide.
Use: Anti-infective sulfonamide.
See: Bidizole.
SULFASYMASINE. N'-(4,6-Diethyl-S-tri-

azin-2-yl) sulfanilamide.
Use: Anti-infective sulfonamide.
SULFA-TER-TABLETS. (A.P.C.) Trisul-
fapyrimidines, U.S.P. Bot. 1000s.
• **SULFATHIAZOLE,** U.S.P. XXIII. Ben-
zenesulfonamide, 4-amino-N-2-thia-
zolyl.
Use: Anti-infective
W/Chlorophyllin.
See: Thiaphyll Cr. (Lannett).
SULFATHIAZOLE COMBINATIONS.
See: Sultrin, Tab. & Cream (Ortho).
SULFATHIAZOLE CARBAMIDE.
See: Otosmosan, Liq. (Wyeth-Ayerst).
**SULFATHIAZOLE, SULFACETAMIDE,
AND SULFABENZAMIDE VAGINAL
CREAM.**
See: Dayto Sulf (Dayton).
Triple Sulfa Vaginal Cream.
**SULFATHIAZOLE, SULFACETAMIDE,
AND SULFABENZAMIDE VAGINAL
TABLETS.**
See: Triple Sulfa Vaginal Tablets.
SULFATRIM. (Various Mfr.) **Susp.:**
Trimethoprim 40 mg, sulfamethoxazole
200 mg/5 ml Susp. Bot. 480 ml **Tab.:**
Trimethoprim 80 mg, sulfamethoxazole
400 mg/Tab. Bot. 100s, 500s.
Use: Sulfonamide anti-infective.
SULFATRIM DS TABS. (Goldline)
Trimethoprim 800 mg, sulfamethoxazole
160 mg/Tab. Bot. 100s, 500s.
Use: Anti-infective.
SULFATRIM SS TABS. (Goldline)
Trimethoprim 400 mg, sulfamethoxazole
80 mg/Tab. Bot. 100s.
Use: Anti-infective.
SULFA-TRIP. (Major) Sulfathiazole
3.42%, sulfacetamide 2.86%, sulfaben-
zamide 3.7%, urea 0.64%. Cream. In
82.5 Gm.
Use: Vaginal sulfonamide anti-infective.
SULFA TRIPLE NO. 2. (Richlyn) Sulfadi-
azine 162 mg, sulfamerizine 162 mg,
sulfamethazine 162 mg/Tab. Bot. 1000s.
Use: Anti-infective.
• **SULFAZAMET.** USAN. N′-(3-Methyl-1-
phenylpyrazol-5-yl) sulfanilamide.
Use: Anti-infective.
See: Vesulong (Ciba).
SULFHYDRYL ION.
See: Hydrosulphosol (Lientz).
• **SULFINALOL HYDROCHLORIDE.**
USAN.
Use: Antihypertensive.
• **SULFINPYRAZONE,** U.S.P. XXIII. Caps.,
Tab., U.S.P. XXIII. 1,2-Diphenyl-4-[2-
(phenylsulphinyl)ethyl][pyrazolidine-3,5-
dione. 1,2-Diphenyl-4-(2-phenylsulfinyl-
ethyl-3,5-pyrazolidinedione. Sulphin-

pyrazone, B.A.N.
Use: Uricosuric.
See: Anturane, Tab., Cap. (Ciba).
SULFISOMIDINE. Sulfadimetine. Sulpha-
somidine, B.A.N.
• **SULFISOXAZOLE,** U.S.P. XXIII. Tab.,
U.S.P. XXIII. N′-(3,4-Dimethyl-5-isoxa-
zolyl)oulfaniamide.
Use: Anti-infective sulfa, treatment of
urinary infections.
See: Gantrisin Preps. (Roche).
Soxa, Tab. (Vita Elixir).
Sulfisoxazole, Tab. (Purepac).
Sulfium, Ophthalmic, Soln., Oint. (Al-
con).
Sulfizin, Tab. (Reid-Rowell).
Velmatrol, Tab. (Kenyon).
W/Aminoacridine HCl, allantoin.
See: Vagilia, Cream (Lemmon).
W/Phenazopyridine.
See: Azo-Gantrisin, Tab. (Roche).
Azo-Soxazole, Tab. (Quality Gener-
ics).
Azo-Sulfisoxazole, Tab. (Richlyn; Cen-
tury).
Azo-Urizole, Tab. (Jenkins).
W/Phenylazodiaminopyridine HCl.
See: Azo-Sulfizin (Solvay).
Velmatrol-A Tab. (Kenyon).
• **SULFISOXAZOLE, ACETYL,** U.S.P.
XXIII. Oral Susp., U.S.P. XXIII. Ac-
etamide, N-(4-amino-phenyl)sulfonyl-N-
(3,4-dimethyl-5-isoxazolyl)-. N-(3,4-Di-
methyl-5-isoxazolyl)-N-sulfanilylac-
etamide.
Use: Anti-infective.
W/Erythromycin Ethylsuccinate.
See: Pediazol, Susp. (Ross).
SULFISOXAZOLE DIETHANOLAMINE.
Sulfisoxazole Diolamine.
• **SULFISOXAZOLE DIOLAMINE.** U.S.P.
XXIII. Inj., Ophth. Oint, Ophth. Soln.,
U.S.P. XXIII. 2,2′-Iminodiethanol salt of
N¹-(3,4-Dimethyl-5-isoxazolyl)sulfanil-
amide compound with 2,2-iminodi-
ethanol(1:1). Gantrisin diolamine.
Use: Anti-infective.
See: Gantrisin, Ophth. Soln. & Oint.
(Roche).
**SULFOAM MEDICATED ANTIDAN-
DRUFF SHAMPOO.** (Bradley) Sulfur
2% with cleansers & conditioners. Bot. 4
oz, 8 oz, 15.5 oz.
Use: Control dandruff.
• **SULFOBROMOPHTHALEIN SODIUM,**
U.S.P. XXII. Inj., U.S.P. XXII.
Use: Liver function test.
SULFOCARBOLATES. Salts of Phenol-
sulfonic Acid, Usually Ca, Na, K, Cu, Zn.
SULFOCYANATE.

See: Potassium Thiocyanate.
SULFO-GANIC. (Marcen) Thioglycerol 20 mg, sodium citrate 5 mg, phenol 0.5%, benzyl alcohol 0.5%/ml. Vial 10 ml, 30 ml.
Use: I.M., adjunctive treatment in arthritides due to sulfur metabolism disorders or deficiencies.
SULFOGUAIACOL.
See: Pot. Guaiacolsulfonate.
SULFOIL. (C & M Pharmacal) Sulfonated castor oil, water. Bot. pt, Gal.
Use: Soap free cleanser for skin and hair.
SULFOLAX CALCIUM. (Major) Docusate calcium 240 mg/Cap. Bot. 100s.
Use: Stool softener.
SULFO-LO. (Whorton) Sublimed sulfur, freshly precipitated polysulfides of zinc, potassium, sulfate, and calamine in aqueous-alcoholic suspension. **Lotion:** Bot. 4 oz, 8 oz, **Soap:** 3 oz.
Use: Treatment of acne.
•**SULFOMYXIN.** USAN.
Use: Anti-infective.
SULFONAMIDE, DOUBLES.
See: Dia Mer Sulfonamides.
SULFONAMIDE PREPS.
See: Acet-Dia-Mer (Various Mfr.).
Dayto Sulf, Vag. cream (Dayton).
Dia-Mer Sulfonamides (Various Mfr.).
Dia-Mer-Thia (Various Mfr.).
Gyne-Sulf, Vag. cream (G & W).
Meth-Dia-Mer, Preps. (Various Mfr.).
Sultrin Triple Sulfa, Vag. cream, Tab. (Ortho).
Triple Sulfa, Vag. cream (Various Mfr.).
Trysul, Vag. cream (Savage).
V.V.S., Vag. cream (Econo Med).
SULFONAMIDES, QUADRUPLE.
See: Quadetts, Tab. (Elder).
Quad-Ramoid, Susp. (Elder).
SULFONAMIDES, TRIPLE.
See: Acet-Dia-Mer Sulfonamides.
Dia-Mer-Thia Sulfonamides.
Meth-Dia-Mer Sulfonamides.
SULFONES.
See: Avlosulfon, Tab. (Wyeth-Ayerst).
Dapsone.
Diasone, Enterabs (Abbott).
Glucosulfone Sodium.
Promacetin, Tab. (Parke-Davis).
SULFONETHYLMETHANE. 2,2-Bis-(ethylsulfonyl)butane.
SULFONITHOCHOLYLGLYCINE.
See: S.L.C.G., Kit (Abbott).
SULFONMETHANE. 2,2-Bis(ethylsulfonyl)propane.
SULFONPHTHAL.
See: Phenolsulfonphthalein, Prep. (Var-

ious Mfr.).
•**SULFONTEROL HYDROCHLORIDE.** USAN.
Use: Bronchodilator.
SULFONYLUREAS.
See: Diabinese, Tab. (Pfizer).
Dymelor, Tab. (Lilly).
Orinase, Tab., Vial (Upjohn).
Tolinase, Tab. (Upjohn).
SULFORCIN LOTION. (Owen) Sulfur 5%, resorcinol 2%, alcohol 11.65%, methylparaben. Bot. 4 oz.
Use: For acne, seborrheic dermatitis & oily skin conditions.
SULFORMETHOXINE. Name used for Sulfadoxine.
SULFORTHOMIDINE. Name used for Sulfadoxine.
SULFOSALICYLATE W/METHENAMINE.
See: Hexalet, Tab. (Webcon).
SULFOSALICYLIC ACID. Salicylsulphonic acid.
•**SULFOXONE SODIUM,** U.S.P. XXII. Tab., U.S.P. XXII.
SULFOXYL REGULAR. (Stiefel) Benzoyl peroxide 5%, sulfur 2% Bot. 2 oz.
Use: Anti-acne.
SULFOXYL STRONG. (Stiefel) Benzoyl peroxide 10%, sulfur 5% Bot. 2 oz.
Use: Anti-acne.
SULFUR-8 HAIR & SCALP CONDITIONER. (Plough) Sulfur 2%, menthol 1%, triclosan 0.1%. Jar 2 oz, 4 oz, 8 oz.
Use: Antiseborrheic.
SULFUR-8 LIGHT FORMULA HAIR & SCALP CONDITIONER. (Plough) Sulfur, triclosan, menthol. Jar 2 oz, 4 oz.
Use: Antiseborrheic.
SULFUR-8 SHAMPOO. (Plough) Triclosan 0.2%. Bot. 6.85 oz, 10.85 oz.
Use: Antiseborrheic.
SULFUR, ANTIARTHRITIC.
See: Thiocyl, Amp. (Torigian).
•**SULFURATED LIME TOPICAL SOLUTION,** U.S.P. XXIII. Vleminckx Lotion.
Use: Scabicide, parasiticide.
SULFUR COMBINATIONS.
See: Aonavoon, Bar (Cooper).
Acne-Aid, Cream, Lot. (Stiefel).
Acnederm, Liq. (Lannett).
Akne Oral Kapsulets, Cap. (Alto).
Acnomel, Cake, Cream (SK-Beecham).
Acno, Soln., Lot. (Cummins).
Acnotex, Liq. (C&M Pharmaceutic).
Akne, Drying Lot. (Alto).
Antrocol, Tab., Cap. (Poythress).
Aracain Rectal Oint. (Commerce).
Bensulfoid, Cream (E.C. Robins/Poythress).

Clearasil, Stick (Vicks).
Epi-clear, Lotion (Squibb).
Exzit, Preps. (Miles Pharm).
Fomac, Cream (Dermik).
Fostex, Liq. Cream, Bar (Westwood).
Fostex, Cream, Liq. (Westwood).
Fostex CM, Cream (Westwood).
Fostril, Cream (Westwood).
Furol Cream (Torch).
Hydro Surco, Lot. (Almo).
Klaron, Lot. (Dermik).
Liquimat, Liq. (Owen).
Lotio-P (Alto).
Neutrogena Disposables (Neutrogena).
Pernox, Lot. (Westwood).
pHisoDan, Liq. (Sanofi Winthrop).
Postacne, Lot. (Dermik).
Pragmatar, Oint. (Menley & James).
Proseca, Liq. (Westwood).
Rezamid, Lot. (Summers).
Sastid Soap (Stiefel).
Sebaveen, Shampoo (Cooper).
Sebulex Shampoo, Liq. (Westwood).
Sulfacet-R, Lot. (Dermik).
Sulfo-lo, Lot. (Wharton).
Sulforcin, Pow., Lot. (Owen).
Sulfur-8, Prods. (Plough).
Sulpho-Lac, Cream (Bradley/Kenwood).
Teenac, Cream (Elder).
Vanseb, Cream (Herbert).
Vanseb-T Tar Shampoo (Herbert).
Xerac, Oint. (Person & Covey).
• **SULFUR DIOXIDE,** N.F. XVIII.
Use: Antixodant, pharmaceutic aid.
• **SULFUR OINTMENT,** U.S.P. XXIII.
Use: Scabicide, parasiticide.
• **SULFUR, PRECIPITATED,** U.S.P. XXIII.
Use: Scabicide; parasiticide.
See: Bensulfoid, Pow., Lot. (Poythress).
Epi-Clear, Lot. (Squibb).
Ramsdell's Sulfur Cream (Fougera).
SAStid Soap, Bar (Stiefel).
Sulfur Soap (Steifel Labs).
SULFUR, SALICYL DIASPORAL.
(Doak).
See: Diasporal, Cream (Doak).
SULFUR SOAP. (Stiefel) Precipitated sulfur 10%. Cake 4.1 oz.
Use: Anti-acne.
• **SULFUR, SUBLIMED,** U.S.P. XXIII. Flowers of Sulfur.
Use: Parasiticide, scabicide.
SULFUR, TOPICAL.
See: Thylox, Liq., Soap (Dent).
• **SULFURIC ACID,** N.F. XVIII.
Use: Pharmaceutic aid (acidifying agent).
SULFURINE. (Table Rock) Sulfamethi-

zole 0.5 Gm/Tab. Bot. 100s & 500s.
Use: Treatment of urinary infections.
SULGLYCOTIDE. B.A.N. The sulfuric polyester of a glycopeptide isolated from pig duodenum.
Use: Treatment of peptic ulcer.
• **SULINDAC,** U.S.P. XXIII. Tab., U.S.P. XXIII.
Use: Anti-inflammatory.
See: Clinoril Tab. (Merck & Co.).
• **SULISOBENZONE.** USAN. 5-Benzoyl-4-hydroxy-2-methoxybenzenesulfonic acid.
Use: Sunscreen agent.
See: Uval Lotion (Dorsey).
Uvinul MS-40 (General Aniline & Film).
• **SULMARIN.** USAN.
Use: Hemostatic.
SULNAC. (NMC Labs) Sulfathiazol 3.42%, sulfacetamide 2.86%, sulfabenzamide 3.7%, urea 0.64% in cream base. Tube 2.75 oz.
Use: Anti-infective.
• **SULNIDAZOLE.** USAN.
Use: Antiprotozoal.
SULOCARBILATE. 2-Hydroxyethyl-p-sulfamylcarbanilate.
• **SULOCTIDIL.** USAN.
Use: Vasodilator.
• **SULOPENEM.** USAN.
Use: Antibacterial.
• **SULOXIFEN OXALATE.** USAN.
Use: Bronchodilator.
SULOXYBENZONE. 4-p-Anisoyl-3-hydroxybenzene sulfonic acid. 2-Hydroxy-4'-methoxy-5-sulfoben-zophenone. Cyasorb UV 284 (Lederle).
SULPHABENZIDE.
See: Sulfabenzamide.
SULPHALOXIC ACID. B.A.N. 4'-[(Hydroxymethylcarbamoyl)sulfamoyl]phthalanilic acid.
See: Enteromide calcium salt.
SULPHAMETHOXYDIAZINE. B.A.N. 2-p-Aminobenzenesulphonamido-5-methoxypyrimidine, 5-Methoxy-2-sulphanilamidopyrimidine Durenate.
SULPHAMOPRINE. B.A.N. 2-(4-Aminobenzenesul-fonamido)-4,6-dimethoxypyrimidine.
SULPHAMOXOLE. B.A.N. 2-(4-Aminobenzenesul-fonamido)-4,5-dimethyloxazole.
SULPHAN BLUE. B.A.N. Sodium 4-(4-diethylaminobenzylidene)cyclohexa-2,5-dienylidenediethylammonium-α-benzene-2,4-disulfonate.
Use: Investigation of the cardiovascular system.
See: Blue VRS.

Disulphine Blue VNS.

SULPHAPROXYLINE. B.A.N. N^1-(4-Iso-propoxyben-zoyl)-4-aminobenzenesul-fonamide.

SULPHASOMIDINE. B.A.N.4-(4-Aminobenzenesul-fonamido)-2,6-di-methylpyrimidine.
See: Sulfisomidine (I.N.N.).
Elkosin.

SULPHATHIOUREA. B.A.N. 4-Aminobenzenesulfonylthiourea.

SULPHATOLAMIDE. B.A.N. 4-Aminobenzenesul-phonylthiourea salt of α-amino-p-toluenesulfonamide.

SULPHAUREA. B.A N 4-Aminobenze-sulfonylurea.
See: Sulfacarbamide (I.N.N.).

SULPHO-LAC. (Bradley/Kenwood) Sulfur 5%. Cream. Tube 30 g, 52.5 g.
Use: Anti-acne.

SULPHO-LAC ACNE MEDICATION. (Bradley/Kenwood) Sulfur 5%, zinc sul-fate 27%, Vleminckx's Soln. 53%. Cream. Tube 28.35 g.
Use: Treatment of acne vulgaris.

SULPHO-LAC SOAP. (Bradley) Sulfur 5%, trisodium HEDTA, casamine OTB in soap base. Bar 3 oz.
Use: Anti-acne action.

SULPHOMYXIN. Penta-(N-sulphomethyl) polymyxin B.

SULPHOMYXIN SODIUM. B.A.N. A mix-ture of sulfomethylated polymyxin B and sodium bisulfite.
Use: Anti-infective.

SULPHRIN OINTMENT. (Bausch & Lomb) Prednisolone acetate 0.5%, sodi-um sulfacetamide 10%. Tube 3.5 g.
Use: Steroid/sulfonamide combination, ophthalmic.

SULPIK. (Durel) Sulfur 5%, salicylic acid 3%, in Duromantel cream.
Use: Superficial tinea infections, sebor-rheic dermatitis.

SULPIK T. (Durel) Sulfur 5%, salicylic acid 3%, LCD (coal tar solution) 3%. In Duromantel Cream.
Use: Superficial tinea, infections, non-exudative forms of seborrheic dermati-tis.

• **SULPIRIDE.** USAN. (1) N-[(1-ethyl-2-pyrrolidinyl)methyl]-5-sulfamoyl-o-anisamide; (2) N-[(Ethyl-1-pyrrolidinyl-2)-methyl]methoxy-2-sulfamoyl-5-ben-za-mide. Dogmatyl (Laboratories Delagrange, France).
Use: Antidepressant.

• **SULPROSTONE.** USAN.
Use: Prostaglandin.

SUL-RAY ACNE CREAM. (Last) Sulfur 2% in cream base. Jars 1.75 oz, 6.75 oz, 20 oz.
Use: Anti-acne.

SUL-RAY ALOE VERA ANALGESIC RUB. (Last) Camphor 3.1 %, menthol 1.25%. Bot. 4 oz, 8 oz.
Use: Pain relieving lotion, external anal-gesic.

SUL-RAY ALOE VERA SKIN PROTEC-TANT CREAM. (Last) Zinc oxide 1%, al-lantoin 0.5%. Jar 1 oz.
Use: Skin protectant cream.

SUL-RAY SHAMPOO. (Last) Sulfur shampoo 2%. Bot. 8 oz.
Use: Medicated shampoo for dandruff.

SUL-RAY SOAP. (Last) Sulfur soap. Bar 3 oz.
Use: Anti-acne.

• **SULTAMICILLIN.** USAN.
Use: Anti-infective.

• **SULTHIAME.** USAN. Formerly Sulpheny-tame. p-(Tetrahydro-2H-1,2-thiazin-2-yl)-benzenesulfonamide-S,S-dioxide.
Use: Anticonvulsant.

SULTRIN TRIPLE SULFA VAGINAL TABLETS. (Ortho) Sulfathiazole 172.5 mg, sulfacetamide 143.75 mg, sulfaben-zamide 184 mg/Vag. Tab. Pkg. 20s w/applicat.
Use: Treatment of *H. vaginalis* (Gard-nerella) vaginitis.

SULTRIN TRIPLE SULFA CREAM. (Or-tho) Sulfathiazole 3.42%, sulfacetamide 2.86%, sulfabenzamide 3.7%, urea 0.64%. Tube 78 Gm. with measured dose applicator.
Use: Treatment of *H. vaginalis* (Gard-nerella) vaginitis.

SUL-TRIO MM. (Kay) Sulfadiazine 167 mg, sulfamethazine 167 mg, sulfamer-azine 167 mg/Tab. Bot. 1000s.

• **SULUKAST.** USAN.
Use: Antiasthmatic.

SULVESOR LOTION. (Durel) Sulfur 2%, resorcinol 1%, neocalamine, talc, titani-um dioxide, alcohol 34%. 2 oz, 4 oz, gal.
Use: Antifungal, antibacterial, keratolyt-ic antiseborrheic.

SUMACAL POWDER. (Biosearch) CHO 95 Gm, 380 Cal., Na 100 mg, Chloride 210 mg, K < 39 mg, Ca 20 mg/100 Gm. Pwd. In 400 Gm.
Use: Glucose polymer.

• **SUMAROTENE.** USAN.

• **SUMATRIPTAN SUCCINATE.** USAN.
Use: Antimigraine.
See: Imitrex.

SUMMER'S EVE DISPOSABLE DOUCHE. (Fleet) Single or twin 4.5 oz. disposable units . Regular, herbal, vine-

gar & water, white flowers, hint of musk, post-menstrual.
Use: Cleansing douche.
SUMMER'S EVE MEDICATED DISPOS-ABLE DOUCHE. (Fleet) Contains povidone-iodide. Single or twin 4.5 oz. disposable units.
Use: Temporary relief of minor vaginal irritation and itching.
SUMYCIN. (Apothecon) Tetracycline HCl. **Cap.** 250 mg/Cap. Bot. 100s, 1000s. Unimatic 100s; 500 mg/Cap. Bot. 100s, 500s. Unimatic 100s. **Tab.** 250 mg/Tab. Bot. 100s, 1000s; 500 mg/Tab. Bot. 100s, 500s.
Use: Anti-infective.
SUNBURN REMEDY.
See: Solarcaine, Prods. (Plough).
• **SUNCILLIN SODIUM.** USAN. 3,3-Dimethyl-7-oxo-6-[2-phenyl-D-2-(sulfoamino)acetamido]-4-thia-1-azabicyclo[3.2.0]heptane-2-carboxylic acid disodium salt.
Use: Anti-infective.
SUNDOWN. (Johnson & Johnson) A series of products marketed under the Sundown name including: **Moderate** (SPF 4) Padimate O, oxybenzone. **Extra** (SPF 6) Oxybenzone, Padimate O. **Maximal** (SPF 8) Oxybenzone, Padimate O. **Ultra** (SPF 15, 30) oxybenzone, Padimate O, Octyl Methoxycinnamate.
Use: Prevention of sunburn (sunscreen).
SUNDOWN SPORT SUNBLOCK. (Johnson & Johnson) Titanium dioxide, zinc oxide. Waterproof. PABA free. SPF 15. Lot. 90 ml.
Use: Sunscreen.
SUNDOWN SUNBLOCK CREAM ULTRA SPF 24. (Johnson & Johnson) Padimate O, oxybenzone.
Use: Sunscreen.
SUNDOWN SUNBLOCK STICK SPF 15. (Johnson & Johnson) Octyl dimethyl PABA, oxybenzone. Stick 0.35 oz.
Use: Prevention of sunburn.
SUNDOWN SUNBLOCK STICK SPF 20. (Johnson & Johnson) Octyl dimethyl PABA, octyl methoxycinnamate, oxybenzone and titanium dioxide.
Use: Sunscreen.
SUNDOWN SUNBLOCK ULTRA LOTION 30 SPF. (Johnson & Johnson) Octyl methoxycinnamate, octyl salicylate, oxybenzone, titanium dioxide, cetyl alcohol, PABA free, waterproof. Lot. Bot. 120 ml.
Use: Sunscreen.
SUNDOWN SUNBLOCK ULTRA SPF 20. (Johnson & Johnson) Octyl dimethyl

PABA, octyl methoxycinnamate, oxybenzone, titanium dioxide.
Use: Sunscreen.
SUNDOWN SUNSCREEN STICK SPF 8. (Johnson & Johnson) Octyl Dimethyl PABA, oxybenzone. Stick 0.35 oz.
Use: Prevention of sunburn.
SUNDOWN SUNSCREEN ULTRA. (Johnson & Johnson) Octyl methoxycinnamate, octyl salicylate, oxybenzone, titanium dioxide, stearyl alcohol, cetyl alcohol, PABA free, waterproof. SPF 15. Cream. Tube 60 Gm.
Use: Sunscreen.
SUNICE. (Citroleum) Allantoin 0.25%, menthol 0.25%, methyl salicylate 10%/Cream. 3 oz.
Use: Burn remedy.
SUNKIST MULTIVITAMINS COMPLETE, CHILDREN'S. (Ciba) Iron 18 mg, vitamin A 5000 IU, D_3 400 IU, E 30 IU, B_1 1.5 mg, B_2 1.7 mg, B_3 20 mg, B_5 10 mg, B_6 2 mg, B_{12} 6 mcg, C 60 mg, folic acid 400 mcg, Ca 100 mg, Cu, I, K, Mg, Mn, P, zinc 10 mg, biotin 40 mcg, K_1 10 mcg, sorbitol, aspartame, phenylalanine, tartrazine. Chew. Tab. Bot. 60s.
Use: Vitamin-mineral supplement.
SUNKIST MULTIVITAMINS + EXTRA C, CHILDREN'S. (Ciba) Vitamin A 2500 IU, E 15 IU, D_3 400 IU, B_1 1.05 mg, B_2 1.2 mg, B_3 13.5 mg, B_6 1.05 mg, B_{12} 4.5 mcg, C 250 mg, folic acid 0.3 mg, vitamin K_1 5 mcg, sorbitol, aspartame, phenylalanine, tartrazine. Chew. Tab. Bot. 60s.
Use: Vitamin supplement.
SUNKIST MULTIVITAMINS + IRON, CHILDREN'S. (Ciba) Iron 15 mg, vitamin A 2500 IU, E 15 IU, D_3 400 IU, E 30 IU, B_1 1.05 mg, B_2 1.2 mg, B_3 13.5 mg, B_6 1.05 mg, B_{12} 4.5 mcg, C 60 mg, folic acid 0.3 mg, K_1 5 mcg, sorbitol, aspartame, phenylalanine, tartrazine. Chew. Tab. Bot. 60s.
Use: Vitamin with Iron supplement.
SUNKIST VITAMIN C. (Ciba) Vitamin C (as ascorbic acid) 500 mg. Capl. Bot. 60s.
Use: Vitamin supplement.
SUNKIST VITAMIN C. (Ciba) Vitamin C (as ascorbic acid) 60 mg, sorbitol, sucrose, lactose. Chew. Tab. Pkg. 11s.
Use: Vitamin supplement.
SUNKIST VITAMIN C. (Ciba) Vitamin C (as sodium ascorbate and ascorbic acid) 250 mg or 500 mg, fructose, sorbitol, sucrose, lactose. Chew. Tab. Bot. 60s.
Use: Vitamin supplement.
SUNSHINE CHEWABLE TABLETS. (Fib-

ertone) Iron 5 mg, vitamins A 5000 IU, D 400 IU, E 67 mg, B_1 15 mg, B_2 15 mg, B_3 25 mg, B_5 20 mg, B_6 15 mg, B_{12} 15 mcg, C 150 mg, folic acid 0.1 mg, Ca, Cu, Mn, Zn, K, iodide, biotin, betaine, PABA, choline bitartrate, inositol, lecithin, hesperidin, rutin, bioflavonoids, sorbitol, aspartame, citrus flavor/Tab. Bot. 60s.
Use: Vitamin/mineral supplement.

SUNSTICK. (Rydell) Lip and face protectant containing digalloyl trioleate 2.5% in emollient base. Plas. swivel container 0.14 oz.
Use: Prevention & relief of chapping and sunburning of lips.

SUPAC. (Mission) Acetaminophen 160 mg, aspirin 230 mg, caffeine 33 mg, calcium gluconate 60 mg/Tab. Filmstrips 24s, Bot. 100s, 1000s.
Use: Analgesic.

SUPER AFKO-HIST. (APC) Chlorpheniramine maleate 2 mg, aspirin 230 mg, phenacetin 160 mg, caffeine 32 mg/Tab. Bot. 1000s.
Use: Antihistamine, analgesic, antipyretic.

SUPER AYTINAL TABLETS. (Walgreen) Vitamins A 7,000 IU, B_1 5 mg, B_2 5 mg, B_5 10 mg, B_6 3 mg, B_{12} 9 mcg, C 90 mg, pantothenic acid 10 mg, D 400 IU, E 30 IU, niacin 30 mg, biotin 55 mcg, folic acid 0.4 mg, iron 30 mg, calcium 162 mg, P 125 mg, iodine 150 mcg, copper 3 mg, manganese 7.5 mg, magnesium 100 mg, potassium 7.7 mg, zinc 24 mg, Cl 7 mg, chromium 15 mcg, selenium 15 mcg, molybdenum 50 mcg, choline bitartrate 1000 mcg, inositol 1000 mcg, PABA 1000 mcg, rutin 1000 mcg, yeast 12 mg. Bot. 50s, 100s, 365s.
Use: Multiple vitamins with minerals.

SUPER-B. (Towne) Vitamins B_1 50 mg, B_2 20 mg, B_6 5 mg, B_{12} 15 mcg, C 300 mg, liver desic. 100 mg, dried yeast 100 mg, niacinamide 25 mg, Ca pantothenate 5 mg, iron 10 mg/Captab. Bot. 50s, 100s, 150s, 250s.

SUPER B KAPSULES. (Pharmex) High potency Vitamins B. Cap. Bot. 50s, 100s.

SUPER C-1000. (Pharmex) Vitamins C 1000 mg/Tab. Bot. 100s.

SUPER CALICAPS M-Z. (Nion) Calcium 1200 mg, magnesium 400 mg, zinc 15 mg, Vitamins A 5000 IU, Vitamins D 400 IU, selenium 15 mcg/3 Tabs. Bot. 90s.
Use: Vitamin supplement.

SUPER CALCIUM 1200. (Schiff) Calcium carbonate 1512 mg (600 mg

calcium)/Cap. Bot. 60s, 120s.
Use: Calcium supplement.

SUPER CITRO CEE. (Marlyn) Lemon bioflavonoids 500 mg, rutin 50 mg, ascorbic acid 500 mg, rosehips powder. 500 mg. Tab. Bot. 50s, 100s, 200s.
Use: Vitamin supplement.

SUPER COMPLEX C-500. (Approved Pharmaceutic) Citrus hesperidin complex 25 mg, citrus bioflavonoid complex 100 mg, rutin 50 mg, ascorbic acid 500 mg, rose hips 100 mg, acerola, green pepper & black currant concentrate, sodium free. Tab. Bot. 100s.
Use: Vitamin supplement.

SUPER D. (Upjohn) Vitamins A 10,000 IU, D 400 IU/Perle. Bot. 100s.
Use: Vitamin A & D therapy.

SUPERDOPHILUS. (Natren) *Lactobacillus acidophilus* strain DDS-1. 2 billion/Gm Pow. 37.5 g, 75 g, 135 g.
Use: Antidiarrheal.

SUPER D PERLES. (Upjohn) Vitamins A 10,000 IU, D 400 IU/Cap. Bot. 100s.
Use: Vitamins A and D.

SUPER EPA. (Advanced Nutritional Tech.) Omega-3 polyunsaturated fatty acids 1200 mg/Cap. containing EPA 360 mg, DHA 240 mg. Bot. 60s, 90s.
Use: Nutritional supplement.

SUPEREPA 2000. (Advanced Nutritional) EPA 663 mg, DHA 312 mg, vitamin E 20 IU. Cap. Bot. 30s, 60s, 90s.
Use: Fish oil.

SUPERE-PECT. (Barth's) Alpha tocopherol 400 IU, apple pectin 100 mg/Cap. Bot. 50s, 100s, 250s.
Use: Vitamin E supplement.

SUPER HYDRAMIN PROTEIN POWDER. (Nion) Protein 41%, carbohydrate 21.8%, fat 1% in powder form. Cans 1 lb.
Use: Vitamin supplement.

SUPERINONE. Tyloxapol.
See: Triton WR-1339 (Rohm & Haas).

SUPER NUTRI-VITES. (Faraday) Vitamins A 36,000 IU, D 400 IU, B_1 25 mg, B_2 25 mg, B_6 50 mg, B_{12} 50 mcg, niacinamide 50 mg, Ca pantothenate 12.5 mg, choline bitartrate 150 mg, inositol 150 mg, betaine HCl 25 mg, PABA 15 mg, glutamic acid 25 mg, desic. liver 50 mg, C 150 mg, E 12.5 IU, Mn gluconate 6.15 mg, bone meal 162 mg, Fe gluconate 50 mg, Cu gluconate 0.25 mg, Zn gluconate 2.2 mg, K iodide 0.1 mg, Ca 53.3 mg, P 24.3 mg, Mg gluconate 7.2 mg/Protein Coated Tab. Bot. 60s, 100s.

SUPEROXIDE DISMUTASE.

Use: Protection of donor organ tissue. [Orphan drug]

SUPER PLENAMINS MULTIPLE VITAMINS AND MINERALS. (Rexall) Vitamins A 8000 IU, D_2 400 IU, Vitamins B_1 2.5 mg, B_2 2.5 mg, C 75 mg, niacinamide 20 mg, B_6 1 mg, B_{12} 3 mcg, biotin 20 mcg, E 10 IU, pantothenic acid 3 mg, liver conc. 100 mg, iron 30 mg, calcium 75 mg, phosphorus 58 mg, iodine 0.15 mg, copper 0.75 mg, manganese 1.25 mg, magnesium 10 mg, zinc 1 mg/Tab. Bot. 36s, 72s, 144s, 288s, 365s.
Use: Multivitamin with minerals.

SUPER POLI-GRIP/WERNET'S CREAM. (Block) Carboxymethylcellulose gum, ethylene oxide polymer, petrolatum-mineral oil base. Tube 0.7, 1.4, 2.4 oz.
Use: Denture adhesive cream.

SUPER QUINTS-50. (Freeda) Vitamins B_1 50 mg, B_2 50 mg, B_3 50 mg, B_5 50 mg, B_6 50 mg, B_{12} 50 mcg, folic acid 0.4 mg, PABA 30 mg, d-biotin 50 mcg, inositol 50 mg. Tab. Bot. 100s, 250s, 500s.
Use: Vitamin supplement.

SUPER SHADE SPF-25. (Plough) Ethylhexyl p-methoxycinnamate, padimate 0 oxybenzone, SPF-25. Bot. 4 fl. oz.
Use: Ultraviolet sunscreen.

SUPER SHADE SUNBLOCK STICK SPF-25. (Plough) Ethylhexyl p-methoxycinnamate, oxybenzone, padimate 0 in stick, SPF-25. Tube 0.43 oz.
Use: Ultra violet sunblock.

SUPER STRESS. (Towne) Vitamins C 600 mg, E 30 IU B_1 15 mg, B_2 15 mg, niacin 100 mg, B_6 5 mg, B_{12} 12 mcg, pantothenic acid 20 mg/Tab. Bot. 60s.
Use: Vitamin supplement.

SUPER THERA 46. (Faraday) Vitamin A 36,000 IU, essential vitamins, minerals, amino acids w/nutrient factors, digestive enzymes, B_{12} 25 mcg/Tab. Bot. 100s.

SUPER TROCHE. (Weeks & Leo) Benzocaine 5 mg, cetalkonium Cl 1 mg/Lozenge. Bot. 15s, 30s.
Use: Relief of minor sore throat & irritation.

SUPER TROCHE PLUS. (Weeks & Leo) Benzocaine 10 mg, cetalkonium Cl. 2 mg/Loz. Bot. 12s.
Use: Relief of minor sore throat & irritation.

SUPER-T WITH ZINC. (Towne) Vitamins A 10,000 IU, D 400 IU, E 15 IU, C 200 mg, B_1 10 mg, B_2 10 mg, B_6 5 mg, B_{12} 6 mcg, niacinamide 50 mg, iron 18 mg, iodine 0.1 mg, copper 2 mg, manganese 1 mg, zinc 15 mg/Cap. Bot. 130s.

Use: Vitamin supplement.

SUPERVIM TABLETS. (U.S. Ethicals) Vitamins and minerals. Bot. 100s.
Use: Multiple vitamin/mineral supplement.

SUPER WERNET'S POWDER. (Block) Carboxymethylcellulose gum, ethylene oxide polymer. Bot. 0.63, 1.75, 3.55 oz.
Use: Denture adhesive.

SUPLENA. (Ross) A vanilla flavored liquid containing 29.6 g protein, 252.5 g carbohydrates, 95 g fat per liter. With appropriate vitamins and minerals. Cans 240 ml.
Use: Enteral nutritional therapy for people with renal conditions.

SUPLICAL. (Parke-Davis Prods) Calcium 600 mg/Square. Bot. 30s, 60s.
Use: Calcium supplement.

SUPPAP-120. (Raway) Acetaminophen 120 mg/Supp. 12s, 50s, 100s, 500s, 1000s.
Use: Analgesic.

SUPPAP-650. (Raway) Acetaminophen 650 mg/Supp. 50s, 100s, 500s, 1000s.
Use: Analgesic.

SUPPORT-500. (Doral) Vitamins A 12,500 IU, D 50 IU, B_1 10 mg, B_2 5 mg, niacinamide 25 mg, B_6 2 mg, calcium pantothenate 10 mg, C 500 mg, E 50 IU, magnesium sulfate 70 mg, manganese sulfate 4 mg, zinc 80 mg/Cap.
Use: Vitamin/mineral supplement.

SUPPRELIN. (Roberts) Histrelin acetate 200 mcg, 300 mcg or 600 mcg/ml. Vials 0.6 ml.
Use: Precocious puberty.

SUPPRESS. (Ferndale) Dextromethorphan HBr 7.5 mg/Loz. 1000s.
Use: Nonnarcotic antitussive.

SUPRA MIN. (Towne) Vitamins A 10,000 IU, D 400 IU, E 30 IU, C 250 mg, folic acid 0.4 mg, B_1 10 mg, B_2 10 mg, niacin 100 mg, B_6 5 mg, B_{12} 6 mcg, pantothenic acid 20 mg, iodine 150 mcg, iron 100 mg, magnesium 2 mg, copper 20 mg, manganese 1.25 mg/Tab. Bot. 130s.
Use: Vitamin supplement.

SUPRANE. (Anaquest) Desflurane. 240 ml. Bot.
Use: General anesthetic.

SUPRARENAL. Dried, partially defatted and powdered adrenal gland of cattle, sheep or swine.

SUPRAX. (Lederle) Cefixime **Tab.:** 200 mg, Bot. 100s or 400 mg, 50s, 100s. **Pow.:** (strawberry flavor) 100 mg/5 ml. 50 ml, 100 ml.
Use: Cephalosporin/related antibiotic.

SUPRAZINE TABS. (Major) Trifluoperazine 1 mg/Tab. Bot 100s, 250s, 1000s; 2 mg/Tab. Bot. 100s, 250s, 1000s, UD 100s; 5 mg/Tab. Bot. 100s, 250s, 1000s; 10 mg/Tab. Bot. 100s, 250s, 1000s.
Use: Tranquilizer.

SUPRINS. (Towne) Vitamins A palmitate 10,000 IU, D 400 IU, B_1 10 mg, B_2 10 mg, B_6 5 mg, B_{12} 6 mcg, C 250 mg, calcium pantothenate 20 mg, niacinamide 100 mg, biotin 25 mcg, vitamins E 15 IU, calcium 103 mg, phosphorous 80 mg, iron 10 mg, iodine 0.1 mg, copper 1.0 mg, zinc 20 mg, mangnese 1.25 mg/Captab. Bot. 100s.

SUPROCLONE. USAN.
Use: Sedative.

SUPROFEN.
Use: Nonsteroidal anti-inflammatory agent.
See: Profenal (Alcon).

SURAMIN SODIUM. Hexa-Sodium bis-(m-amino-benzoyl-m-amino-p-methyl-benzoyl-1-naph-thylamino-4,6,8-trisulfonate) carbamide. (Bayer 205; Germanin).

SURBEX FILMTAB. (Abbott) Thiamine mononitrate 6 mg, B_2 6 mg, nicotinamide 30 mg, B_6 2.5 mg, calcium pantothenate 10 mg, vitamins B_{12} 5 mcg/Filmtab. Bot. 100s.
Use: Vitamins B-complex therapy.
W/Vitamins C. (Abbott) Same as Surbex Filmtab, except vitamins C 250 mg/Filmtab. Bot. 100s, 500s.

SURBEX-T FILMTAB. (Abbott) Vitamins B_1 15 mg, B_2 10 mg, niacinamide 100 mg, B_6 5 mg, B_{12} 10 mcg, calcium pantothenate 20 mg, C 500 mg/Filmtab. Bot. 100s, UD 100s.
Use: Vitamin deficiencies.

SURBEX WITH C FILMTABS. (Abbott) Vitamins B_1 6 mg, B_2 6 mg, B_3 30 mg, B_3 30 mg, B_5 10 mg, B_6 2.5 mg, B_{12} 5 mg, C 500 mg/Film coated. Tab. Bot. 100s, 480s.
Use: Vitamin supplement.

SURBEX-750 WITH IRON. (Abbott) Vitamins B_1 15 mg, B_2 15 mg, B_6 25 mg, B_{12} 12 mcg, C 750 mg, calcium pantothenate 20 mg, E 30 IU, niacinamide 100 mg, iron 27 mg, folic acid 0.4 mg/Tab. Bot. 50s.
Use: Vitamin & mineral supplement.

SURBEX-750 WITH ZINC. (Abbott) B_1 15 mg, B_2 15 mg, B_6 20 mg, B_{12} 12 mcg, C 750 mg, E 30 IU, pantothenic acid 20 mg, niacin 100 mg, folic acid 0.4 mg, zinc 22.5 mg/Tab. Bot. 50s.
Use: Vitamin & mineral supplement.

SURBU-GEN-T. (Goldline) Vitamins B_1 15 mg, B_2 10 mg, B_3 100 mg, B_5 20 mg, B_6 5 mg, B_{12} 10 mcg, C 500 mg/Tab. Bot. 100s.
Use: Multivitamin.

SURECELL CHLAMYDIA TEST. (Kodak) Monoclonal antibody-based ELISA (enzyme linked immunosorbent assay) to detect lipopolysaccharide antigen from the cell wall of *Chlamydia trachomatis psittaci.* Kit 10s, 25s, 100s.
Use: Diagnostic aid.

SURECELL HCG-URINE TEST. (Kodak) Polyclonal/monoclonal antibody sandwich-based ELISA to detect human chorionic gonadotropin in urine. Kit 10s, 25s, 100s.
Use: Diagnostic aid.

SURECELL HERPES (HSV) TEST. (Kodak) Monoclonal antibody-based ELISA to detect HSV 1 & 2 antigens from lesions. Kit 10s, 25s.
Use: Diagnostic aid.

SURECELL STREP A TEST. (Kodak) ELISA to detect Group A streptococci. Kit 10s, 25s, 100s.
Use: Diagnostic aid.

SURELAC. (Caraco) 3000 FCC lactase units, sorbitol or mannitol. Chew. Tab. Bot. 60s.
Use: Enteral nutritional supplement.

SURFACE-ACTIVE AGENTS.
See: Antiseptics, Surface-Active.

SURFACE ACTIVE EXTRACT OF SALINE LAVAGE OF BOVINE LUNGS.
Use: Respiratory failure in preterm infants. [Orphan drug]

SURFACTANT, NATURAL LUNG.
Use: Surfactant replacement therapy in neonatal respiratory distress syndrome.
See: Survanta (Ross Laboratories).

SURFACTANT, SYNTHETIC LUNG.
Use: Surfactant replacement therapy in neonatal respiratory distress syndrome.
See: Exosurf Neonatal (Burroughs Wellcome).

SURFAK. (Hoechst) Docusate calcium 50 mg or 240 mg/Cap. 50 mg Bot. 30s, 100s; 240 mg Bot. 30s, 100s, 500s. UD Pack 100s.

•**SURFILCON A.** USAN.
Use: Hydrophilic contact lens material.

SURFOL POST IMMERSION BATH OIL. (Stiefel) Mineral oil, isopropyl myristate, isostearic acid, PEG-40, sorbitan peroleate. Bot. 8 oz.
Use: Post-Immersion bath oil for dry skin.

• **SURFOMER.** USAN.
Use: Hypolipidemic.

SURGASOAP. (Wade) Castile vegetable oils. Bot. qt., gal.
Use: Surgical soap.

SURGEL. (Ulmer) Sodium carboxymethylcellulose, propylene glycol, glycerin, phenylmercuric nitrate. Gel. 120 ml, 240 ml, pt., gal.
Use: Patient lubricant.

SURGEL LIQUID. (Ulmer) Patient lubricant fluid. Bot. 4 oz, 8 oz, gal.

• **SURGIBONE.** USAN. Bone and cartilage obtained from bovine embryos and young calves.
Use: Prosthetic aid (internal bone splint).
See: Unilab Surgibone (Unilab).

SURGICAL SIMPLEX P. (Howmedica) Methyl methacrylate 20 ml poly 6.7 Gm, methyl methacrylate-styrene copolymer 33.3 Gm. **Powd.** 40 Gm. **Liq.** 20 ml.
Use: Bone cement.

SURGICAL SIMPLEX P RADIOPAQUE. (Howmedica) Methyl methacrylate 20 ml, poly 6 Gm, methyl methacrylate-styrene copolymer 30 Gm. **Powd.** 40 Gm. **Liq.** 20 ml.
Use: Bone cement.

• **SURGICAL SUTURE, ABSORBABLE,** U.S.P. XXIII.
Use: Surgical aid.

• **SURGICAL SUTURE, NONAB-SORBABLE,** U.S.P. XXIII.
Use: Surgical aid.

SURGICEL. (Johnson & Johnson) Sterile absorbable knitted fabric prepared by controlled oxidation of regenerated cellulose. Sterile strips 2″ × 14″, 4″8″, 2″3″, 0.5″2″.
Use: Absorbable hemostat.

SURGIDINE. (Continental) Iodine 0.8% in iodine complex. Germicide. Bot. 8 oz, gal. Foot operated dispenser 8 oz, gal.
Use: Antiseptic.

SURGI-KLEEN. (Sween) Bot. 2 oz, 8 oz, 16 oz, 21 oz, gal., 5 gal., 30 gal., 55 gal.
Use: Skin cleanser and shampoo.

SURGILUBE. (Day-Baldwin) Sterile-bacteriostatic. Foilpac: 3 Gm, 5 Gm, Tube: 5 Gm, 2 oz, 4.5 oz.
Use: Surgical lubricant.

SURGILUBE. (Fougera) Sterile surgical lubricant. Foilpac 5 Gm.; Tube 5 Gm, 2 oz, 4.25 oz.
Use: Sterile surgical lubricant.

• **SURICAINIDE MALEATE.** USAN.
Use: Cardiac depressant (antiarrhythmic).

SURIN OINTMENT. (McKesson) Tube 1.25 oz.

SURITAL SODIUM. (Parke-Davis) Thiamylal sodium. **Steri-Vial:** 1 Gm, 25s; 5 Gm, 10s; 10 Gm, 10s.
Use: Short-acting anesthetic.

• **SURITOZOLE.** USAN.
Use: Antidepressant.

SURMONTIL. (Wyeth-Ayerst) Trimipramine maleate 25 mg, 50 mg or 100 mg/Cap. Bot. 100s. Redipaks.
Use: Antidepressant.

SUROFENE. Hexachlorophene.

• **SURONACRINE MALEATE.** USAN.
Use: Cholinergic, cholinesterase inhibitor.

SURVANTA. (Ross) Beractant 25 mg/ml. Inj. Vial 8 ml.
Use: Lung surfactant.

SUSANO. (Blue Cross) Phenobarbital 0.25 gr, hyoscyamine sulfate 0.1037 mg, atropine sulfate 0.0194 mg, scopolamine HBr 0.0065 mg/Tab. Bot. 1000s.
Use: Sedative, antispasmodic.

SUSANO ELIXIR. (Blue Cross) Phenobarbital 0.25 gr, hyoscyamine sulfate 0.1037 mg, atropine sulfate 0.0194 mg, scopolamine HBr 0.0065 mg/5 ml. Bot. 16 oz, gal.
Use: Sedative, antispasmodic.

SUSPEN. (Circle) Penicillin V potassium 250 mg/5 ml. Bot. 100 ml.
Use: Anti-infective.

SUS-PHRINE INJECTION. (Forest) Epinephrine 1:200 Amp. 0.3 ml, 12s, 25s. Multiple Dose Vial 5 ml, 1s.
Use: Bronchial asthma.

SUS SCROFA LINNE var DOMESTICUS. W/Proteolytic enzyme, autolyzed.
See: Saromide Injection, Vial (Saron).

SUSTACAL BASIC. (Mead Johnson Nutrition) A vanilla, strawberry or chocolate flavored liquid containing 36.6 g protein, 34.6 g fat, 145.8 g carbohydrate, 833 mg Na, 1583 mg K/L. 1.04 Cal/ml, with appropriate vitamin and mineral levels to meet 100% of the US RDA's. Liq. Can 240 ml.
Use: Enteral nutritional supplement.

SUSTACAL HC. (Mead Johnson Nutrition) High calorie nutritionally complete food. Protein 16%, fat 34%, carbohydrate 50%. Cans 8 oz. Vanilla, chocolate or eggnog.
Use: Complete, concentrated oral nutrition.

SUSTACAL PLUS. (Mead Johnson Nutrition) A vanilla, eggnog or chocolate flavored liquid containing 61 g protein, 58 g fat, 190 g carbohydrate, 15.2 mg Fe,

850 mg Na, 1480 mg K, 1520 cal/L, with appropriate vitamin and mineral levels to meet 100% of the US RDAs. Liq. Bot. 237 ml, 960 ml.
Use: High protein, nutritionally complete, oral nutritional supplement, lactose free.

SUSTACAL POWDER. (Mead Johnson Nutrition) Caloric distribution and nutritional value when added to milk are similar to that of Sustacal liquid except lactose. Contains vanilla: Pow. 1.9 oz. packets 4's, 1 lb. can; Chocolate 1.9 oz. packets 4's.
Use: High protein, nutritionally complete, oral nutritional supplement.

SUSTACAL PUDDING. (Mead Johnson Nutrition) Ready-to-eat fortified pudding containing at least 15% of the US RDA's for protein, vitamins and minerals, in a 240 calorie serving. As a % of the calories, protein 11%, fat 36%, carbohydrate 53%. Flavors: chocolate, vanilla, and butterscotch. Tins, 5 oz, 110 oz.
Use: Complete nutritional supplement to help increase patient acceptance of nutritional support.

SUSTAGEN. (Mead Johnson Nutrition) High calorie, high protein supplement containing as a % of the calories, 24% protein, 8% fat, 68% carbohydrate. Contains all known essential vitamins and minerals. Prepared from nonfat milk, corn syrup solids, powdered whole milk, calcium caseinate, and dextrose. Vanilla: Can 1 lb, 5 lb. Chocolate: Can 1 lb.
Use: Complete nutrient, nutritional supplement.

SUSTAIRE. (Pfizer Laboratories) Theophylline 100 mg, 300 mg/Sust. Released Tab. Bot. 100s.
Use: Long acting relief of reversible bronchospasm.

•**SUTILAINS,** U.S.P. XXIII. Oint., U.S.P. XXIII.
Proteolytic enzymes.
Use: Debriding agent.
See: Travase, Oint. (Flint).

SUVAPLEX TABLET. (Tennessee Pharmaceutic) Vitamins A 5000 IU, D 500 IU, B_1 2.5 mg, B_2 2.5 mg, B_6 0.5 mg, B_{12} 1 mcg, C 37.5 mg, Ca pantothenate 5 mg, niacinamide 20 mg, folic acid 0.1 mg/Tab. Bot. 100s.
Use: Vitamin supplement.

SUXAMETHONIUM BROMIDE. B.A.N. Bis-2-di-methylaminoethyl succinate bismethobromide 00'-Succinyldi-(2-oxyethyltrimethylammonium bromide).
Use: Neuromuscular blocking agent.

SUXAMETHONIUM CHLORIDE, B.A.N.
See: Succinylcholine Chloride.

•**SUXEMERID SULFATE.** USAN. Bis-(1,2,2,6,6-pentamethyl-4-piperidyl)succinate sulfate.
Use: Antitussive.

SUXETHONIUM BROMIDE. B.A.N. 00'-Succinyldi-[(2-oxyethyl)ethyldimethylammonium bromide].
Use: Neuromuscular blocking agent.

SWAMP ROOT. Compound of various organic roots in an alcohol base.
Use: Diuretic to the kidney.

SWEEN-A-PEEL. (Sween) Wafer 4×4. Box 5s, 20s; Sheets 1212. Box 2s, 12s.
Use: Wafer skin protectant.

SWEEN CREAM. (Sween) Vitamin A and D cream. Tube 0.5 oz, 2 oz, 5 oz. Jar 2 oz, 9 oz.
Use: Skin treatment.

SWEEN KIND LOTION. (Sween) Bot. 21 oz, gal.
Use: Lotion skin cleaner.

SWEEN PREP. (Sween) Dox wipes 54s. Dab-o-matic 2 oz. Spray top 4 oz.
Use: Medicated skin barrier.

SWEEN SOFT TOUCH. (Sween) Bot. 2 oz, 16 oz, 21 oz, 32 oz, 1 gal., 5 gal.
Use: Medicated, antimicrobial lotion skin cleanser.

SWEETA. (Squibb Mark) Saccharin sodium and sorbitol. Bot. 24 ml, 2 oz, 4 oz.
Use: Sweetening Agent.

SWEETASTE. (Purepac) Saccharin 0.25 gr, 0.5 gr, 1 gr./Tab. w/Sodium bicarbonate. Bot. 1000s.
Use: Sugar substitute.

SWEETENING AGENTS.
See: Ril-Sweet (Plough).
Saccharin, Preps. (Various Mfr.).
Sucaryl, Preps. (Abbott).
Sweetaste, Tab. (Purepac).

SWIM EAR. (Fougera) 2.75% boric acid in isopropyl alcohol. Bot. 1 oz.
Use: Prevention of external otitis.

SWISS KRISS. (Modern) Senna leaves, herbs. Coarse cut mixture. Can 1.5 oz, 3.25 oz, Tab. 24s, 120s, 250s.
Use: Laxative.

SYLLACT. (Wallace) Psyllium seed husks 3.3 g/tsp., saccharin. Pow. Bot. 11 oz.
Use: Orally, laxative.

SYLLAMALT. (Wallace) Malt soup extract 4 Gm, psyllium seed husks 3 Gm, calories/rounded tsp 13. Pow. 300 Gm.
Use: Laxative.

SYMADINE. (Solvay) Amantadine HCl. 100 mg Cap. In 100s.
Use: Antiviral agent, treatment of

Parkinson's disease, treatment of drug-induced extrapyramidal symptoms.
- **SYMCLOSENE.** USAN. Trichloroisocyanuric acid.
  Use: Local anti-infective.
- **SYMETINE HCl.** USAN. 4,4'-(Ethylenedioxy)-bis-[N-hexyl-N-methylbenzylamine dihydrochloride].
  Use: Anti-amebic.

SYMMETREL. (DuPont) Amantadine HCl. **Cap.:** 100 mg/Cap. Bot. 100s, 500s, UD 100s. **Syr.:** 50 mg/5 ml. Bot. pt.
Use: Antiviral agent, treatment of Parkinson's disease, treatment of drug induced extrapyramidal symptoms.

SYMPATHOLYTIC AGENTS.
See: Adrenergic-Blocking Agents.
D.H.E. 45, Amp. (Sandoz).
Dibenzyline, Cap. (SK-Beecham).
Dihydroergotamine.
Ergotamine Tartrate.
Gynergen, Amp., Tab. (Sandoz).

SYMPATHOMIMETIC AGENTS.
See: Adrenalin (Parke-Davis).
Adrenergic agents.
Aerolate Sr. & Jr., Cap. (Fleming).
Aerolone Cpd. (Lilly).
Afrin, Preps. (Schering).
Miles Diagnosticec, Enseal, Pulvule (Lilly).
Aramine, Amp., Vial (Merck & Co.).
Arlidin HCl, Tab. (Rhone-Poulenc Rorer).
Brethine, Amp., Tab (Geigy).
Bronkephrine, Amp., (Sanofi Winthrop).
Bronkometer (Sanofi Winthrop).
Bronkosol Soln. (Sanofi Winthrop).
Delcobese, Tab. (Delco).
Demazin, Tab., Syr. (Schering).
Desoxyn, Gradumet, Tab. (Abbott).
Dexamyl Tab. (SK-Beecham).
Dexedrine, Elix., Spansule, Tab. (SK-Beecham).
D-Feda, Cap., Liq. (Dooner).
Didrex, Liq., Tab. (Upjohn).
Dipivefrin HCl, Soln. (Schein).
Duovent, Tab. (Riker).
Ectasule Minus Sr. & Jr., Cap. (Fleming).
Ectasule III, Cap. (Fleming).
Ephedrine preps.
Epinephrine salts.
Extendryl, Cap., Syr., Tab. (Fleming).
Fedrazil, Tab. (Burroughs Wellcome).
Fiogesic, Tab. (Sandoz).
Histabid, Cap. (Glaxo).
Isoephedrine HCl.

Isuprel HCl, Preps. (Sanofi Winthrop).
Levophed Bitartrate, Amp. (Sanofi Winthrop).
Metaproterenol Sulfate (Various Mfr.).
Napril, Cap. (Marion).
Neo-Synephrine HCl, Preps. (Sanofi Winthrop).
Nolamine, Tab. (Carnrick).
Norisodrine Sulfate, Soln. (Abbott).
Obedrin-LA, Tab. (Beecham Labs).
Obetrol, Tab. (Obetrol).
Orthoxine, Orthoxine & Aminophylline (Upjohn).
Orthoxine HCl, Tab., Syr. (Upjohn).
Otrivin, Soln., Spray (Geigy).
Phenylephrine HCl, Preps.
Phenylpropanolamine HCl.
Pseudoephedrine HCl, Syr., Tab.
Rondec DSC & T (Ross).
Slo-Fedrin & Slo-Fedrin A(Dooner).
Sudafed, Tab., Syr. (Burroughs Wellcome).
Triaminic, Prep. (Dorsey).
Triaminicol, Syr. (Dorsey).
Tussagesic, Susp., Tab. (Dorsey).
Tussaminic, Tab. (Dorsey).
Ursinus, Tab. (Dorsey).
Vasoxyl HCl, Amp., Vial (Burroughs Wellcome).
Wyamine Sulfate, Amp., Vial (Wyeth-Ayerst).

SYNA-CLEAR. (Pruvo) Decongestant plus Vitamins C. 25 mg/Tab. Bot. 12s, 30s.
Use: Decongestant.

SYNACORT. (Syntex) Hydrocortisone cream. **1%:** Tube 15 Gm, 30 Gm, 60 Gm. **2.5%:** Tube 30 Gm.
Use: Topical steroid.

SYNALAR. (Syntex) Fluocinolone acetonide. **Cream: 0.01%** Tube 15 Gm, 30 Gm, 45 Gm, 60 Gm, 120 Gm. Jar 425 Gm. **0.025%** Tube 15 Gm, 30 Gm, 60 Gm, 120 Gm. Jar 425 Gm. **Oint.: 0.025%:** Tube 15 Gm, 30 Gm, 60 Gm, 120 Gm. Jar 425 Gm. **Soln. 0.01%:** Bot. 20 ml, 60 ml.
Use: Topical steroid.

SYNALAR-HP CREAM. (Syntex) Fluocinolone acetonide 0.2% in water-washable aqueous base. Tube 12 Gm.
Use: Topical steroid.

SYNALGOS-DC CAPSULES. (Wyeth-Ayerst) Dihydrocodeine bitartrate 16 mg, aspirin 356.4 mg, caffeine 30 mg/Cap. Bot. 100s, 500s.
Use: Analgesic, relaxant.

SYNAPP-R.(Blue Cross) Acetaminophen 325 mg, phenylpropanolamine HCl 25 mg, phenyltoloxamine citrate 22 mg/Tab.

Bot. 40s.
Use: Analgesic, decongestant.
SYNAREL. (Syntex) Nafarelin acetate 2 mg/ ml (as nafarelin base). Nasal solution. Bottle 10 ml with metered pump spray.
Use: Treatment of endometriosis.
SYNATUSS-ONE. (Freeport) Guaifenesin 100 mg, dextromethorphan HBr. 15 mg, alcohol 1.4%/5 ml. Bot. 4 oz.
Use: Antitussive.
SYNCAINE.
See: Procaine Hydrochloride, Inj., Tab. (Various Mfr.).
SYNCORT.
See: Desoxycorticosterone Acetate, Inj., Pellets (Various Mfr.).
SYNCORTYL.
See: Desoxycorticosterone Acetate, Inj., Pellets (Various Mfr.).
SYNDOLOR CAPSULES. (Knight) Bot. 100s, 1000s.
Use: Analgesic.
SYNEMOL. (Syntex) Fluocinolone acetonide 0.025% in water-washable aqueous emollient base. Tube 15 Gm, 30 Gm, 60 Gm, 120 Gm.
Use: Topical steroid.
SYNEPHRICOL. (Sanofi Winthrop) Paracetamol.
Use: Cold treatment.
SYNKONIN.
See: Hydrocodone (Various Mfr.).
SYNOPHYLATE. (Central) Theophylline sodium glycinate. **Elix.**: Theophylline 165 mg/15 ml w/alcohol 20%. Bot. pt, gal. **Tab.**: Theophylline 165 mg/Tab. Bot. 100s, 1000s.
Use: Anti-asthmatic.
SYNOPHYLATE-GG. (Central) Theophylline sodium glycinate 300 mg, guaifenesin 100 mg. **Syr.** 10% alcohol, pt, gal. **Tabs.** Bot. 100s.
Use: Symptomatic treatment of bronchial asthma.
SYNTHALOIDS. (Buffington) Benzocaine, calcium-iodine complex/Lozenge. Salt free. Bot. 100s, 1000s. Unit boxes 8s, 16s. Box 24s. Dispens-A-Kit 500s. Aidpaks 100s. Medipaks 200s.
Use: Sore throat relief.
SYNTHETIC LUNG SURFACTANT.
See: Exosurf Neonatal (Burroughs Wellcome).
SYNTHOESTRIN.
See: Diethylstilbestrol, Preps. (Various Mfr.).
SYNTHROID. (Boots) Sodium levothyroxine 25 mcg, 50 mcg, 75 mcg, 100 mcg, 125 mcg, 150 mcg, 200 mcg, 300

mcg/Tab. Bot. 100s, 1000s.
Use: Thyroid deficiencies.
SYNTHROID. (Boots) Levothyroxine sodium (T^4; L-thyroxine) 0.088 mg, 0.112 mg or 0.175 mg/Tab. Bot. 100s.
Use: Thyroid hormone.
SYNTHROID INJECTION. (Boots) Lyophilized sodium levothyroxine 500 mcg/vial. (100 mcg/ml when reconstituted.) Vial 10 ml.
Use: Thyroid deficiency; myxedema coma.
SYNTOCINON AMPULS. (Sandoz) A sterile aqueous sol. of synthetic oxytocin w/chlorobutanol 0.5%, alcohol 0.61%. Amp. (10 IU/ml) 1 ml.
Use: Induction, stimulation or management of labor and for prevention and control of postpartum hemorrhage.
SYNTOCINON NASAL SPRAY. (Sandoz) Syn. oxytocin 40 IU/ml w/exsic. sodium phosphate, citric acid, sodium Cl, glycerine, sorbitol, methyl & propylparaben, chlorobutanol 0.05% and Purified Water U.S.P. q.s. Squeeze bottle 2 ml & 5 ml.
Use: Initial milk let-down.
SYPHILIS (FTA-ABS) FLUORO KIT. (Clinical Sciences).
Use: Test for syphilis.
SYPRINE. (Merck & Co.) Trientine HCl 250 mg/Cap. Bot. 100s.
Use: Chelating agent.
SYRACOL. (Hauck) Phenylpropanolamine HCl 12.5 mg, dextromethorphan 7.5 mg Liq. 60 and 120 ml.
Use: Decongestant, antitussive.
SYRAJEN. (Jenkins) Codeine phosphate 10.9 mg, chlorpheniramine maleate 2 mg, pot. guaiacolsulfonate 44 mg, citric acid 60 mg, sodium citrate 197 mg/5 ml. Bot. 4 oz, gal.
Use: Expectorant.
SYROSINGOPINE. B.A.N. 4-Ethoxy-carbonyl-3,5-dimethoxybenzoic acid ester of methyl reserpate. Methyl 18β Hydroxy-11-17α-dimethoxy-3β, 20α-yohimban-16β-carboxylate-4-Hydroxy-3,5-dimethoxybenzoate Ethyl Carbonate (Ester). Methyl O-(4-ethoxycarbonyloxy-3,5-dimethoxybenzoyl)reserpate.
Use: Hypotensive.
SYROXINE TABS. (Major) Sodium levothyroxine 0.1 mg, 0.2 mg, or 0.3 mg/Tab. Bot. 100s, 250s, 1000s, UD 100s. (3 mg 1000s.).
Use: Thyroid deficiencies.
SYRPALTA. (Emerson) Syr. containing comb. of fruit flavors. Bot. 1 pt, 1 gal.
Use: Vehicle for masking drug taste.

• **SYRUP,** N.F. XVIII.
Use: Flavored vehicle.
SYRVITE. (Various Mfr.) Vitamins A 2500
IU, D 400 IU, E 15 mg, B₁ 1.05 mg, B₂
1.2 mg, B₃ 13.5 mg, B₆ 1.05 mg, B₁₂ 4.5
mcg, C 60 mg/5 ml Liq. Bot. pt, gal.
Use: Vitamin supplement.

T

T-3 RIABEAD. (Abbott Diagnostics) Test
kit 50s, 100s.
Use: Radioimmunoassay for qualitative
measurement of total circulating
serum liothyronine.
**T4 ENDONUCLEASE V, LIPOSOME EN-
CAPSULATED.**
Use: Xeroderma pigmentosum. [Or-
phan drug]
T-4 RIA (PEG). (Abbott Diagnostics) Di-
agnostic kit 50s, 100s, 500s.
Use: For quantitative measurement of
total circulating serum thyroxine.
T4, SOLUBLE, HUMAN RECOMBINANT.
(Biogen) Phase I/II HIV.
Use: Antiviral.
TA. (Wampole-Zeus) Anti-thyroid antibod-
ies by IFA. Test 48s.
Use: A useful tool in identifying two thy-
roid autoantibodies in a single test.
TABASYN. (Freeport) Chlorpheniramine
maleate 2 mg, phenylephrine HCl 10
mg, acetaminophen 5 gr, salicylamide 5
gr/Tab. Bot. 1000s.
Use: Antihistamine, decongestant, anal-
gesic.
TABAZONE TABS. (Major) Oxyphenbu-
tazone 100 mg/Tab. Bot. 100s.
Use: Antirheumatic agent.
TABRON FILMSEAL TABLETS. (Parke-
Davis) Ferrous fumarate 304.2 mg (rep-
resenting elemental iron 100 mg), do-
cusate sodium 50 mg, vitamins E 30 IU,
B₁ 6 mg, B₂ 6 mg, niacinamide 30 mg,
B₅ 10 mg, B₆ 5 mg, C 500 mg, folic acid
1 mg, B₁₂ 25 mcg/Filmseal Tab. Bot.
100s. UD pkg. 100s.
Use: Vitamin/mineral supplement.
TAC-3. (Herbert). Triamcinolone ace-
tonide 3 mg/ml. Susp. Vial 5 ml.
Use: Corticosteroid.
TAC-40. (Parnell) Triamcinolone ace-
tonide 40 mg/ml. Inj. Susp. Vial 5 ml.
Use: Corticosteroid.
TACARYL. (Westwood) Methdilazine HCl
Tab.: 8 mg/Tab. Bot. 100s. **Syr.:** 4 mg/5
ml. Bot. 16 oz.
Use: Antipruritic.

TACARYL CHEWABLE TAB. (West-
wood) Methdilazine 3.6 mg/Tab. Bot.
100s.
Use: Antipruritic.
TACE. (Marion Merrell Dow) Chlorotri-
anisene 12 mg, 25 mg, 72 mg/Cap. (12
mg) Bot. 28s, 100s, 500s; (25 mg) Bot.
60s. (72 mg) Pkg. 48s.
Use: Estrogen therapy.
TACHYSTEROL.
See: Dihydrotachysterol, Tab. (Philips
Roxane).
TACITIN. (Ciba) Under study. Benzocta-
mine, B.A.N.
• **TACLAMINE HYDROCHLORIDE.** USAN.
Use: Tranquilizer (minor).
TA CREAM. (C & M Pharmacal) Triamci-
nolone acetonide 0.025% or 0.05%. Jar
2 oz., 8 oz., 1 lb.
Use: Topical anti-inflammatory.
TACRINE. B.A.N. 9-Amino-1,2,3,4-
tetrahydroacridine.
Use: CNS stimulant.
See: Cognex, Cap. (Parke-Davis).
• **TACROLIMUS.** USAN.
Use: Immunosuppressant.
TAGAMET. (SK-Beecham) Cimetidine
FC Tab.: 200 mg Bot. 100s. **300 mg**
Bot. 100s, UD 100s. **400 mg** Bot. 60s,
UD 100s. **800 mg** Bot. 30s, UD 100s.
Liq.: 300 mg (as HCl)/5 ml 2.8% alco-
hol./Bot. 240 ml, UD 5 ml (10s). **Inj.: 300
mg** (as HCl)/2 ml with 10 mg phenol in
an aqueous solution./Vials. 2 ml, 8
ml/Disp. syringe. **300 mg** (as HCl) in 50
ml 0.9% sodium chloride. SD Viaflex
Plus container.
Use: Anti-ulcer agent.
TALACEN. (Sanofi Winthrop) Penta-
zocine HCl 25 mg, acetaminophen 650
mg/Caplet. Bot. 100s. UD 250s. (10 ×
25s).
Use: Analgesic.
• **TALAMPICILLIN HYDROCHLORIDE.**
USAN.
Use: Antibacterial.
• **TALC,** U.S.P. XXIII. A native hydrous
magnesium silicate.
Use: Dusting powder, pharmaceutical
aid.
• **TALERANOL.** USAN.
Use: Enzyme inhibitor.
• **TALISOMYCIN.** USAN.
Use: Antineoplastic.
• **TALMETACIN.** USAN.
Use: Analgesic, antipyretic, anti-inflam-
matory.
• **TALNIFLUMATE.** USAN.
Use: Anti-inflammatory, analgesic.
TALOIN. (Adria) Methylbenzethonium

chloride, zinc oxide, calamine, eucalyptol in a water-repellent base. Oint.: Tube 2 oz.
Use: Skin protectant & antiseptic.
•**TALOPRAM HYDROCHLORIDE.** USAN.
Use: Potentiator (catecholamine).
•**TALOSALATE.** USAN.
Use: Analgesic, anti-inflammatory.
TALOXIMINE. B.A.N. 4-(2-Dimethylaminoethoxy)-1,2-dihydro-1-hydroxyiminophthalazine.
Use: Respiratory stimulant.
TALWIN COMPOUND. (Sanofi Winthrop) Pentazocine HCl 12.5 mg, asprin 325 mg/Tab. Bot. 100s.
Use: Analgesic.
TALWIN INJECTION. (Sanofi Winthrop) Pentazocine lactate injection. 30 mg/ml. **Vials.** 10 ml. **Uni-Amps.** 1, 1.5, 2 ml. **Uni-Nest amps.** 1 ml, 2 ml. **Carpujects.** 1, 1.5, 2 ml.
Use: Analgesic.
TALWIN NX. (Sanofi Winthrop) Pentazocine HCl 50 mg, naloxone 0.5 mg/Tab. Bot. 100s. UD 250s.
Use: Narcotic analgesic.
TAMBOCOR. (3M Pharm) Flecainide acetate 50 mg or 150 mg/Tab. Bot. 100s, UD 100s.
Use: Antiarrhythmic agent.
TAMBOCOR. (Riker) Flecainide acetate 100 mg/Tab. Bot. 100s.
Use: Antiarrhythmic.
•**TAMETRALINE HYDROCHLORIDE.** USAN.
Use: Antidepressant.
TAMINE S.R. (Geneva Generics) Phenylpropanolamine HCl 15 mg, phenylephrine HCl 15 mg, brompheniramine maleate 12 mg. Sugar coated./Tab. Bot. 100s, 1000s.
Use: Antihistamine, decongestant.
TAMOXIFEN. (Barr) Tamoxifen citrate 10 mg. Tab. Bot. 60s, 250s.
Use: Antineoplastic agent.
•**TAMOXIFEN CITRATE,** U.S.P. XXIII. Tab., U.S.P. XXIII. (Z)-(4-(1,2-diphenyl-1-butenyl) phenoxy)-N,N-dimethylethanamine 2-hydroxy-1,2,3-propanetricarboxylate (1:1).
Use: Treatment of mammary carcinoma, anti-estrogen.
See: Nolvadex, Tab. (Zeneca).
    Tamoxifen, Tab. (Barr).
•**TAMPRAMINE FUMARATE.** USAN.
Use: Antidepressant.
TAMP-R-TEL. (Wyeth-Ayerst) A tamper-resistant package for narcotic drugs which includes the following:
Codeine phosphate 30 mg, 60 mg/1 ml.

Hydromorphone HCl 1 mg, 2 mg, 3 mg, 4 mg/Tubex.
Meperidine HCl 25 mg/ml and **Promethazine HCl** 25 mg/ml 2 ml.
Meperidine HCl 25 mg/1 ml, 50 mg/1 ml, 75 mg/1 ml, 100 mg/1 ml.
Morphine Sulfate 2mg, 4mg, 8 mg, 10 mg, 15 mg/1 ml.
Pentobarbital, Sodium 100 mg/2 ml.
Phenobarbital, Sodium 30 mg, 60 mg, 130 mg/1 ml.
Secobarbital, Sodium 100 mg/2 ml.
•**TAMSULOSIN HYDROCHORIDE.** USAN.
Use: Benign Prostotic Hypertrophy.
TANAC LIQUID. (Commerce) Benzalkonium Cl 0.12%, benzocaine 10%, tannic acid 6%. Saccharin. Bot. 0.3 oz., 0.5 oz.
Use: Mouth sores, cold sores, fever blisters.
TANAC ROLL-ON. (Commerce) Tannic acid 6%, benzalkonium Cl 0.12%, benzocaine 5%. Bot. 0.3 oz.
Use: Cold sores, fever blister, cracked lips.
TANAC STICK. (Commerce) Benzocaine 7.5%, tannic acid 6%, octyl dimethyl PABA 0.75%, allantoin 0.2%, benzalkonium Cl. 7.5%. Saccharin. Stick 0.1 oz.
Use: Cold sores, fever blisters, dry lips.
TANADEX. (Commerce) Tannic acid 2.86%, phenol 1.05%, benzocaine 0.47%. Bot. 3 oz.
Use: Throat gargle.
TAN-A-DYNE. (Archer-Taylor) Tannic acid compound w/iodine. Bot. 4 oz., pt., gal.
Use: Swab and gargle concentrate.
TANBISMUTH.
See: Bismuth Tannate.
•**TANDAMINE HYDROCHLORIDE.** USAN.
Use: Antidepressant.
•**TANNIC ACID.** U.S.P. XXIII. Gallotannic acid. Glycerite. Tannin.
Use: 1 to 20% solution as an astringent.
See: Amertan, Oint. (Lilly).
    Zilactin Medicated, Gel (Zila Pharm.).
W/Benzocaine, benzyl alcohol, diisobutylphenoxyethoxyethyl dimethyl benzyl ammonium chloride.
See: Kankex, Liq. (Edward J. Moore).
W/Benzocaine, phenol, thymol iodide, ephedrine HCl, zinc oxide, peru balsam.
See: Hemocaine, Oint. (Hauck).
W/Bisacodyl.
See: Clysodrast, Packet (Barnes-Hind).
W/Boric acid, salicylic acid, isopropyl alcohol.
See: Sal Dex Boro, Liq. (Scrip).

W/Chlorobutanol, isopropyl alcohol.
See: Outgro, Soln. (Whitehall).

W/Cyanocobalamin, zinc acetate, glutathione, phenol.
See: Depinar, Amp. (Armour).

W/Merthiolate.
See: Amertan, Oint. (Lilly).

W/Salicylic acid, boric acid.
See: Tan-Bor-Sal, Liq. (Gordon).

TANNIC SPRAY. (Gebauer) Tannic acid 4.5%, chlorobutanol 1.3%, menthol less than 1%, benzocaine less than 1%, propylene glycol 33%, ethanol 60%. Bot. 2 oz. & 4 oz.
Use: Relief of sunburn and other minor burns.

TANORAL. (Pharmed) Phenyepherine tannate 25 mg, chlorpheniramine tannate 8 mg, pyrilamine tannate 25 mg/Tab. Bot. 100s.
Use: Upper respiratory combination.

TANPHETAMIN.
See: Dextroamphetamine tannate.

TAO. (Roerig) Troleandomycin equivalent to 250 mg oleandomycin/Cap. Bot. 100s.
Use: Antibiotic therapy.

TAPAL AMPULS. (Sanofi Winthrop) Dipyrone.
Use: Analgesic, antipyretic, anti-inflammatory.

TAPAL TABLETS. (Sanofi Winthrop) Dipyrone.
Use: Analgesic, antipyretic, anti-inflammatory.

TAPAR TABLETS. (Warner-Chilcott) Acetaminophen 325 mg/Tab. Bot. 100s.
Use: Analgesic.

TAPAZOLE. (Lilly) Methimazole. 1-methyl-2-mercaptoimidazole. 5 mg or 10 mg/Tab. Bot. 100s.
Use: Hyperthyroidism.

• **TAPE, ADHESIVE,** U.S.P. XXIII.
Use: Surgical aid.

TA-POFF. (Ulmer) Adhesive tape remover. Bot. 1 pt. Aerosol. Can 6 oz.

TAPULINE. (Wesley) Activated attapulgite 600 mg, pectin 60 mg, homatropine methylbromide 0.5 mg/Chew. Tab. Bot. 100s, 1000s.
Use: Diarrhea.

TAR.
See: Coal Tar, Preps.

TAR DISTILLATE. (Doak) Decolorized fractional distillate of crude coal tar. Each ml equiv. to 1 Gm whole crude coal tar. Bot. 2 oz., 16 oz.
Use: Active ingredient for dermatologic preparations.

TARLENE LOTION. (Medco Lab) Refined crude coal tar, salicylic acid, propylene glycol. Plastic Applicator Bot. 2 oz.
Use: Seborrheic dermatitis.

TARNPHILIC. (Medco Lab) Coal tar 1%, polysorbate 0.5% in aquaphilic base. Jar 16 oz.
Use: Treatment of psoriasis, eczema, contact dermatitis.

TARPASTE. (Doak) Coal tar distilled 5% in zinc paste. Tube 1 oz, Jar 4 oz, w/Hydrocortisone 0.5%. Tube 1 oz.
Use: Dermatitis.

TAR-QUIN-HC. (Jenkins) Hydrocortisone 0.5%, liquor carbonis detergens 3.0%, clioquinol 1.0%. Oint. Tube 0.5 oz.

TARSUM SHAMPOO/GEL. (Summers) Coal tar 10%, salicylic acid 5% in shampoo base. Bot. 4 oz.
Use: Dermatologic, shampoo for treatment of psoriasis, seborrheic dermatitis, chronic eczema and dermatitis of scalp.

TARTAR EMETIC.
See: Antimony Potassium Tartrate, U.S.P.

• **TARTARIC ACID,** N.F. XVIII.
Use: Buffer.

TASHAN, Skin Cream. (Block) Vitamin A palmitate, D_2, D-panthenol, Vit. E. Tube 1 oz.

TASTE FUNCTION TEST, ACCUSENS T. (Westport Pharmaceuticals) Tastant 60 ml. Kit. 15 Bot.
Use: In vitro diagnostic aid.

TAUROCHOLIC ACID.
W/Pancreatin, pepsin.
See: Enzymet, Tabs. (Westerfield).

TAUROLIN. B.A.N. 4,4′-Methylenedi(tetrahydro-1,2,4-thiadiazine-1-dioxide).
Use: Antibacterial.

TAUROPHYLLIN. (Vale) Ext. ox bile 32.4 mg, phenolphthalein 32.4 mg, ext. cascara sagrada 32.4 mg/Tab. Bot. 100s, 1000s, 5000s.

TAURULTAM. B.A.N. Tetrahydro-1,2,4-thiadiazine 1,1-dioxide.
Use: Antibacterial; antifungal.

TA-VERM. (Table Rock) Piperazine citrate 100 mg/ml Syr. Bot. 1 pt., 1 gal. Tabs. 500 mg Bot. 100s, 500s.
Use: Anthelmintic.

TAVILEN PLUS. (Table Rock) Liver solution 1 Gm, ferric pyrophosphate soluble 500 mg, vitamins B_1 6 mg, B_2 7.2 mg, B_6 3 mg, B_{12} 24 mcg, panthenol 3 mg, niacinamide 60 mg, l-lysine HCl 300 mg, 5% alcohol/ml. Bot. 16 oz., 1 gal.
Use: Hematinic.

TAVIST. (Sandoz) Clemastine fumarate

2.68 mg/Tab. Bot. 100s.
Use: Antihistamine.
TAVIST SYRUP. (Sandoz) Clemastine fumarate 0.67 mg/5 ml. Bot. 4 oz.
Use: Relief of symptoms of allergic rhinitis.
TAVIST-1 TABLETS. (Sandoz) Clemastine fumarate 1.34 mg/Tab. Bot. 100s.
Use: Antihistamine.
TAVIST-D. (Sandoz) Clemastine fumarate 1.34 mg, phenylpropanolamine HCl 75 mg/Tab. Bot. 100s.
Use: Antihistamine, decongestant.
TAXOL. (Bristol-Myers Squibb) Paclitaxel. 30 mg/5 ml. Inj. Single-dose vial.
Use: Antineoplastic.
• **TAZADOLENE SUCCINATE.** USAN.
Use: Analgesic.
TAZICEF INJECTION. (Abbott) Ceftazidime. Vial: 1 Gm/20 ml, 2 Gm/60 ml or 6 Gm/100 ml. Piggyback: 1 Gm/100 ml or 2 Gm/100 ml. I.M. or I.V. Pharmacy Bulk: 6 Gm/100 ml.
Use: Antibacterial; cephalosporin.
TAZIDIME. (Lilly) Ceftazidime dry powder. 500 mg/10 ml Traypak 25s; 1 Gm/20 ml Traypak 10s; 1 Gm/100 ml; 2 Gm/50 ml Traypack 10s; 2 Gm/100 ml Traypack 10s; 6 Gm/100 ml Traypak 6s. ADD-Vantage Vials 1 Gm or 2 Gm Traypak 10s.
Use: Antibacterial, cephalosporin.
• **TAZIFYLLINE HYDROCHLORIDE.** USAN.
Use: Antihistamine.
• **TAZOLOL HYDROCHLORIDE.** USAN.
Use: Cardiotonic.
TBA-PRED. (Keene) Prednisolone tebutate 10 mg/ml Susp. Vial 10 ml.
Use: Corticosteroid for intra-articular and soft tissue injection.
TC SUSPENSION. (Rhone-Poulenc Rorer) Aluminum hydroxide 600 mg, magnesium hydroxide 300 mg/5 ml, sorbitol, sodium 0.8 mg Liq. In UD 15 ml, 30 ml (100s).
Use: Antacid.
T-CORT. (Torch) Triamcinolone acetonide micronized powder. Bot. 1 Gm, 10 Gm.
Use: Extemporaneous prescription compounding.
T/DERM TAR EMOLLIENT. (Neutrogena) Neutar solubized coal tar extract 5% in oil base. Bot. 4 oz.
Use: Antipsoriatic; antipruritic.
T-DRY. (Jones Medical) Pseudoephedrine HCl 120 mg, chlorpheniramine maleate 12 mg/Cap. S.R. Bot. 100s.
Use: Antihistamine, decongestant.

T-DRY JR. (Jones Medical) Pseudoephedrine HCl 60 mg, chlorpheniramine maleate 4 mg/Cap. S.R. Bot. 100s.
Use: Antihistamine, decongestant.
TDx CORTISOL. (Abbott Diagnostics) Fluorescence polarization immunoassay for the quantitative determination of cortisol in serum, plasma, or urine.
Use: Diagnostic aid.
TDx THYROXINE. (Abbott Diagnostics) Automated assay for quantitation of unsaturated thyroxine binding sites in serum or plasma.
Use: Diagnostic aid.
TDx TOTAL ESTRIOL. (Abbott Diagnostics) Fluorescence polarization immunoassay for the quantitative determination of total estriol in serum, plasma, or urine.
Use: Diagnostic aid.
TDx TOTAL T3. (Abbott Diagnostics) Automated assay for quantitation of total circulating triiodothyronine (T3) in serum or plasma.
Use: Diagnostic aid.
TDx T-UPTAKE. (Abbott Diagnostics) Automated assay for the determination of thyroxine binding capacity in serum or plasma.
Use: Diagnostic aid.
TEAR AID. (Ketchum) Vial 15 ml.
Use: Decongestant-emollient.
TEAR DROP. (Parmed) Benzalkonium Cl 0.01%, polyvinyl alcohol, NaCl, EDTA. Soln. Drop. bot. 15 ml.
Use: Artificial tears.
TEARGARD. (Medtech) Hydroxyethylcellulose in a hypertonic base, sorbic acid 0.25%, EDTA 0.1%. Soln. Bot. 15 ml.
Use: Ophthalmic.
TEARGEN. (Goldline) Benzalkonium Cl 0.01%, EDTA, NaCl. Soln. Bot. 15 ml.
Use: Artificial tears solution.
TEARGEN II. (Goldline) Hydroxypropyl methylcellulose 0.3%, dextran 70 0.1%, benzalkonium Cl 0.01%, EDTA 0.05%. Bot. 15 ml.
Use: Artificial tears solution.
TEARISOL. (Iolab) An isotonic buffered aqueous sol. of hydroxypropyl methylcellulose 0.5%, edetate disodium 0.01%, benzalkonium chloride 0.01%, boric acid, sodium carbonate, potassium chloride. Bot. 15 ml.
Use: Artificial tears in many eye conditions.
TEARS NATURALE. (Alcon) Duasorb water soluble polymeric system, benzalkonium chloride 0.01%, disodium ede-

tate 0.05%. Droptainer 15 ml, 30 ml.
Use: Artificial tear & lubricant for ocular
irritation & dry eyes.

TEARS NATURALE II. (Alcon) Sterile isotonic solution of Duosorb water soluble
polymeric system, edetate disodium
0.1% w/Polyquad 0.001% as preservative. Droptainer 15 ml, 30 ml.
Use: Artificial tear, lubricant for ocular irritation and dry eyes.

TEARS NATURALE FREE. (Alcon) Hydroxypropyl methylcellulose 2910 0.3%,
dextran 70 0.1%, NaCl, KCl, sodium borate. Soln. Single-use containers 0.6 ml.
Use: Artificial tears.

TEARS PLUS. (Allergan) Polyvinyl alcohol, povidone. Bot. 0.5 oz., 1 oz.
Use: Artificial tears solution.

TEARS RENEWED OINTMENT. (Akorn)
White petrolatum, light mineral oil. Oph-
th. Tube 3.5 g.
Use: Ophthalmic.

TEARS RENEWED SOLUTION. (Akorn)
Dextran 70, sodium chloride, hydroxypropyl methylcellulose, benzalkonium
chloride 0.01%, EDTA 0.05%. Soln. Bot.
15 ml.
Use: Artificial tears solution.

TEA TREE OIL. (Metabolic Prod.) Aus-
tralian oil of Melaleuca alternifolia 100%
pure. Bot. 1 oz, 4 oz, 8 oz, 16 oz. **Cream**
Bot. 8 oz. **Oint.** Tube 1 oz, 3 oz.
Use: Antiseptic, antifungal.

TEBAMIDE. (G & W) Trimethobenzamide
HCl 100 mg/Supp. In 10s.
Use: Antiemetic, antivertigo.

• **TEBUFELONE.** USAN.
Use: Analgesic, anti-inflammatory.

• **TEBUQUINE.** USAN.
Use: Antimalarial.

T.E.C. (Invenex) Zinc 1 mg, copper 0.4
mg, chromium. 4.0 mcg, manganese 0.1
mg. Vial 10 ml.
Use: Trace element additives for TPN
therapy.

• **TECELEUKIN.** USAN.
Use: Immunostimulant. [Orphan drug]

TECHENESCAN MAA. Aggregated albu-
min (human).
Use: Preparation of Tc 99m Aggregated
Albumin (Human).

TECHNEPLEX. (Squibb) Technetium Tc
99m penetate kit. 10 vials/kit.
Use: Radiodiagnostic.

**TECHNETIUM 99m-IRON-ASCORBATE-
DTPA.**
See: Renotec (Squibb).

• **TECHNETIUM Tc-99m ALBUMIN AG-
GREGATED INJECTION,** U.S.P. XXIII.
Use: Diagnostic aid (lung imaging).

• **TECHNETIUM Tc-99m ALBUMIN COL-
LOID INJECTION,** U.S.P. XXIII.
Use: Diagnostic aid (lung imaging).

• **TECHNETIUM Tc-99m ALBUMIN INJEC-
TION,** U.S.P. XXIII.
Use: Radioactive agent.

**TECHNETIUM Tc-99m ANTIMELANOMA
MURINE MONOCLONAL ANTIBODY.**
Use: Diagnostic aid. [Orphan drug]

• **TECHNETIUM Tc 99m DISOFENIN IN-
JECTION,** U.S.P. XXIII.
Use: Radioactive agent; diagnostic aid
(hepatobiliary function determination).

• **TECHNETIUM Tc-99m ETIDRONATE IN-
JECTION,** U.S.P. XXIII.
Use: Radioactive agent.

• **TECHNETIUM Tc-99m FERPENTETATE
INJECTION,** U.S.P. XXII.
Use: Radioactive agent.

• **TECHNETIUM Tc-99m FURIFOSMIN.**
USAN.
Use: Radiodiagnostic.

**TECHNETIUM Tc-99m GENERATOR SO-
LUTION.** (New England Nuclear)
Pertechnetate sodium Tc 99 m.
Use: Radiodiagnostic.

• **TECHNETIUM Tc-99m GLUCEPATE IN-
JECTION.** USAN.
Use: Radioactive agent.

• **TECHNETIUM Tc-99m LIDOFENIN IN-
JECTION.** U.S.P. XXIII.
Use: Radioactive agent.

• **TECHNETIUM Tc-99m MEDRONATE IN-
JECTION,** U.S.P. XXIII.
Use: Diagnostic aid (skeletal imaging),
radioactive agent.
See: Macrotec, Inj. (Squibb).

**TECHNETIUM Tc-99m MURINE MONO-
CLONAL ANTIBODY TO hCG.**
Use: Diagnostic aid. [Orphan drug]

**TECHNETIUM Tc-99m MURINE MONO-
CLONAL ANTIBODY TO HUMAN AFP.**
Use: Diagnostic aid. [Orphan drug]

**TECHNETIUM Tc-99m MURINE MONO-
CLONAL ANTIBODY (IgG2a) TO BCE.**
Use: Diagnostic aid. [Orphan drug]

• **TECHNETIUM Tc-99m OXIDRONATE IN-
JECTION,** U.S.P. XXIII.
Use: Diagnostic aid (skeletal imaging),
radioactive agent.

• **TECHNETIUM Tc-99m PENTETATE IN-
JECTION,** U.S.P. XXIII.
Use: Radioactive agent.

• **TECHNETIUM Tc-99m PYROPHOS-
PHATE INJECTION,** U.S.P. XXIII.
Use: Radioactive agent.

• **TECHNETIUM Tc-99m (Pyro- and trime-
tra-) PHOSPHATES INJECTION,**
U.S.P. XXIII.

Use: Radioactive agent.
• **TECHNETIUM Tc-99m SIBOROXIME.** USAN.
Use: Diagnostic aid, radioactive agent.
• **TECHNETIUM Tc-99m SODIUM INJECTION,** U.S.P. XXIII.
Use: Radioactive agent.
• **TECHNETIUM Tc-99m SUCCIMER INJECTION,** U.S.P. XXIII.
Use: Radioactive agent.
TECHNETIUM Tc-99m SULFUR COLLOID KIT.
Use: Radioactive agent.
See: Tesuloid (Squibb).
• **TECHNETIUM Tc-99m SULFUR COLLOID INJECTION,** U.S.P. XXIII.
Use: Diagnostic aid (liver scanning).
TECLOSINE. Under study.
Use: Amebicide.
TECLOTHIAZIDE. B.A.N. 6-Chloro-3,4-dihydro-3-trichloromethyl-1,2,4-benzothiadiazine-7-sulfonamide 1,1-dioxide.
Use: Diuretic.
• **TECLOZAN.** USAN. N,N'-(p-Phenylenedimethylene)-bis]2,2-dichloro-N-(2-ethoxy-ethyl)-acetamide].
Use: Amebicide.
See: Falmonox (Sanofi Winthrop).
TECNU POISON OAK-N-IVY. (Tec Labs) Deodorized mineral spirits, propylene glycol, polyethylene glycol, octylphenoxy-polyethoxyethanol, mixed fatty acid soap. Liq. Bot. 118.3 ml, 355 ml.
Use: Topical poison ivy treatment.
• **TECOGALAN SODIUM.** USAN.
Use: Antineoplastic adjunct
TEDRAL. (Parke-Davis) **Tab.:** Theophylline 118 mg, ephedrine HCl 24 mg, phenobarbital 8 mg/Tab. Bot. 24s, 100s, 1000s. UD 100s. **Susp. (Pediatric):** Theophylline 65 mg, ephedrine HCl 12 mg, phenobarbital 4 mg/5 ml. Bot. 8 oz.
Use: Anti-asthmatic.
TEDRAL ELIXIR. (Parke-Davis) Theophylline 32.5 mg, ephedrine HCl 6 mg, phenobarbital 2 mg/5 ml. Alcohol 15%. Pediatric. Bot. pt.
Use: Anti-asthmatic.
TEDRAL-SA. (Parke-Davis) Theophylline 180 mg, ephedrine HCl 48 mg, phenobarbital 25 mg/S.A. Tab. Bot. 100s, 1000s.
Use: Anti-asthmatic.
TEDRIGEN. (Goldline) Theophylline 130 mg, ephedrine HCl 24 mg, phenobarbital 8 mg/Tab. Bot. 100s, 1000s.
Use: Anti-asthmatic.
TEEBACIN. (CMC) Sod. p-aminosalicy-

late **Tab.** 0.5 Gm Bot. 1000s. **Pow.** Bot. lb.
Use: Antituberculosis agent.
TEEBACONIN. (CMC) Isoniazid 50, 100, 300 mg/Tab. Bot. 100s, 1000s.
Use: Antituberculosis agent.
TEEBACONIN W/Vit. B₆. (CMC) Isoniazid 100 mg, 10 mg pyridoxine HCl/Tab. Bot. 100s, 500s, 1000s. Isoniazid 300 mg, 30 mg pyridoxine HCl/Tab. Bot. 100s and 1000s.
Use: Antituberculosis agent.
TEEN MIDOL. (Glenbrook) Acetaminophen 400 mg, pamabrom 25 mg. Cap. Bot. 16s.
Use: Nonnarcotic analgesic combination.
TEEV. (Keene) Estradiol valerate 4 mg, testosterone enanthate 90 mg/ml Inj. Vial 10 ml.
Use: Estrogen/androgen.
• **TEFLURANE.** USAN. 2-Bromo-1,1,1,2-tetrafluoroethane.
Use: General inhalation anesthetic.
TEGACID.
See: Glyceryl monostearate.
• **TEGAFUR.** USAN. (Mead Johnson).
Use: Antineoplastic.
TEGAMIDE. (G&W) Trimethobenzamide HCl 100 mg, or 200 mg/ Supp. Boxes 10s, 50s.
Use: Control of nausea and vomiting.
TEGISON. (Roche) Etretinate 10 mg or 25 mg/Cap. Prescription Paks 30s.
Use: Antipsoriatic.
TEGOPEN. (Bristol) Cloxacillin sodium 250 mg/Cap. Bot. 100s. 500 mg/Cap. Bot. 100s. Granules for Soln. 125 mg/5 ml. Bot. 100 ml, 200 ml.
Use: Antibacterial; penicillin.
TEGRETOL. (Geigy) Carbamazepine **Tab.:** 200 mg. Bot. 100s, 1000s. UD 100s. **Chew. Tab.:** 100 mg/Tab. Bot. 100s. UD 100s; **Susp.:** 100 mg/5 ml, sorbitol. Bot. 450 ml.
Use: Anticonvulsant.
TEGRIN CREAM. (Block) Allantoin 2%, coal tar ext. 5% in cream base. Tube 2 oz., 4.4 oz.
Use: Antipsoriatic.
TEGRIN-LT. (Block) Pyrethrins 0.33%, piperonyl butoxide (technical) 3.15%. Shampoo/Conditioner. Bot. 118 ml available w/wo 142 g insecticide spray.
Use: Pediculicides.
TEGRIN MEDICATED. (Block) **Lot.:** Crude coal tar 5%, allantoin 1.7%. Lot. 180 ml. **Shampoo:** Crude coal tar 7%, sodium lauryl sulfate, ammonium lauryl sulfate, alcohol 6.4%. Cream 110 ml.

Use: Antiseborrheic.

**TEGRIN MEDICATED EXTRA CONDI-
TIONING.** (Block) Coal tar solution 7%,
alcohol 6.4%. Shampoo. Bot. 110 ml,
198 ml.
Use: Antiseborrheic.

T.E.H. COMPOUND. (Various Mfr.) Theophylline 130 mg, ephedrine sulfate 25
mg, hydroxyzine HCl 10 mg/Tab. Bot.
100s, 500s.
Use: Anti-asthmatic.

• **TEICOPLANIN.** USAN.
Use: Antibacterial.

TELACHLOR. (Major) Chlorpheniramine
maleate 8 or 12 mg/Cap. S.R. Bot. 100s,
250s, 1000s.
Use: Antihistamine.

TELACHLOR TD CAPS. (Major) Chlorpheniramine maleate 8 mg or 12
mg/T.D. Tab. Bot. 1000s.
Use: Antihistamine.

**TELDRIN MAXIMUM STRENGTH CAP-
SULES.**(SK-Beecham) Chlorpheniramine maleate 12 mg/Spansule. Pkg.
12s, 24s, 48s.
Use: Allergy relief.

TELDRIN TABLETS. (SK-Beecham)
Chlorpheniramine maleate 4 mg/Tab.
Use: Relief from hay fever and allergy
symptoms.

TELEFON. (Kenyon) Ferrous sulfate 150
mg/Cap. Bot. 100s, 1000s.
Use: Iron supplement.

TELEPAQUE. (Sanofi Winthrop) Iopanoic
acid. 0.5 Gm/Tab. Bot. 30s and 150s.
Use: Radiopaque agent.

TELINE. (Hauck) Tetracycline 250
mg/Cap. Bot. 100s, 1000s.
Use: Tetracycline.

TELINE-500. (Hauck) Tetracycline 500
mg/Cap. Bot. 100s, 1000s.
Use: Tetracycline.

TELODRON. (Norden) Chlorpheniramine
maleate.
Use: Antihistamine.

• **TELOXANTRONE HYDROCHLORIDE.**
USAN.
Use: Antineoplastic.

• **TELUDIPINE HYDROCHLORIDE.**
USAN.
Use: Antihypertensive; calcium channel
antagonist.

TEM. Tretamine, B.A.N.
See: Triethylenemelamine, Tab. (Lederle).

• **TEMAFLOXCIN HYDROCHLORIDE.**
USAN.

TEMARIL. (Herbert) Trimeprazine tartrate. **Tab.** Trimeprazine tartrate 2.5
mg/Tab. Bot. 100s, 1000s. Single Unit

Pak 100s. **Syr.** 2.5 mg/5 ml w/alcohol
5.7%. Bot. 4 oz. **Spansule** 5 mg Bot.
50s, Single Unit Pak, 100s.
Use: Antipruritic.

**TEMARIL SUSTAINED RELEASE SPAN-
SULES.** (Herbert) Trimeprazine tartrate
5 mg/Sustained Release Cap. Bot. 50s.
UD 100s.
Use: Treatment of pruritic symptoms in
urticaria.

TEMARIL SYRUP. (Herbert)
Trimeprazine tartrate 2.5 mg/5 ml. Bot. 4
oz.
Use: Treatment of pruritic symptoms in
urticaria.

TEMARIL TABLETS. (Herbert)
Trimeprazine tartrate 2.5 mg/Tab. Bot.
100s, 1000s. UD 100s.
Use: Treatment of pruritic symptoms in
urticaria.

• **TEMATROPIUM METHYLSULFATE.**
USAN.
Use: Anticholinergic.

TEMAZ. (Quantum). 15 mg temazepam.
30 mg temazepam. Capsules: In 100s,
500s and 1000s.
Use: Sedative/Hypnotic.

• **TEMAZEPAM.** USAN. 7-Chloro-1,3-dihy-
dro-3-hydroxy-1-methyl-5-phenyl-2H-
1,4-benzodiazepin- 2-one.
Use: Minor tranquilizer.
See: Restoril, Cap. (Sandoz).

• **TEMEFOS.** USAN.
Use: Ectoparasiticide.

• **TEMELASTINE.** USAN.
Use: Antihistamine.

TEMETAN. (Nevin) Acetaminophen 324
mg/Tab. Bot. 100s, 500s. Elixir (324
mg/5 ml) Bot. pt.
Use: Analgesic.

• **TEMOCAPRIL HYDROCHLORIDE.**
USAN.
Use: Antihypertensive.

• **TEMOCILLIN.** USAN.
Use: Antibacterial.

• **TEMODOX.** USAN.
Use: Growth stimulant.

TEMOVATE CREAM. (Glaxo Derm.) Clobetasol propionate 0.05%. Tube 15 Gm,
30 Gm, 45 Gm.
Use: Corticosteroid, topical.

TEMOVATE OINTMENT. (Glaxo Derm.)
Clobetasol propionate 0.05%. Tube 15
Gm, 30 Gm; 45 Gm.
Use: Corticosteroid, topical.

TEMOVATE SCALP. (Glaxo Derm.)
Oint.: Clobetasol propionate 0.05%,
white petro base. 15 Gm, 30 Gm, 45
Gm. **Cream:** Clobetasol propionate
0.03%, 15 Gm, 30 Gm, 45 Gm. **Scalp**

application: Clobetasol propionate 0.05%, carbomer 934 P. 25 ml, 50 ml.
Use: Corticosteroid, topical.

TEMPO. (Thompson Medical) Calcium carbonate 414 mg, aluminum hydroxide 133 mg, magnesium hydroxide 81 mg, simethicone 20 mg. Chew. Tab. Bot. 10s, 30s, 60s.
Use: Antacid, antiflatulent.

TEMPORARY INTRACANALICULAR COLLAGEN IMPLANT. (Eagle Vision) In 0.2 mm, 0.3 mm, 0.4 mm. Box 12s.
Use: Collagen implant, ophthalmic.

TEMPRA. (Mead Johnson Nutrition) Acetaminophen. **Drops:** Grape flavor. 80 mg/0.8 ml. Bot. w/dropper 15 ml. **Red syrup:** Cherry flavor. 160 mg/5 ml. Bot. 4 oz. **Tab.:** 80 mg/Chewable Grape flavor Tab. Bot 30s. 160 mg/Chewable Grape flavor Tab. Bot. 30s.
Use: Relief of fever and pain.

TENCET CAPSULES. (Hauck) Formerly G-I Capsules. Acetaminophen 500 mg, butalbital 50 mg, caffeine 40 mg. Cap. Bot. 100s, UD 1000s.
Use: Analgesic, sedative/hypnotic.

TENCON. (Inter. Ethical Labs) Acetaminophen 650 mg, butalbital 50 mg. Cap. Bot. 100s.
Use: Nonnarcotic analgesic combination.

TENEX. (Robins) Guanfacine HCl 1 mg/Tab. Bot. 100s, 500s. UD 100s.
Use: Antihypertensive.

• **TENIDAP.** USAN.
Use: Anti-inflammatory.

• **TENIPOSIDE.** USAN.
Use: Antineoplastic. [Orphan drug]
See: Vumon (Bristol Myers Oncology)

TEN-K. (Geigy) Potassium Cl 750 mg (10 mEq)/Controlled Release Cap. Bot. 100s, 500s. UD, blister pak 100s.
Use: Potassium supplement.

TENOL. (Vortech) Acetaminophen 325 mg/Tab. Bot. 1000s.
Use: Analgesic

TENOL LIQUID. (Vortech) Acetaminophen 120 mg, NAPA alcohol 7%/5 ml. Bot. 3 oz., 4 oz., Gal.
Use: Analgesic.

TENOL-PLUS. (Vortech) Acetaminophen 250 mg, aspirin 250 mg, caffeine 65 mg/Tab. Bot. 1000s.
Use: Analgesic.

TENORETIC TABLETS. (Zeneca) **50 mg:** Atenolol 50 mg, Chlorthalidone 25 mg/Tab. Bot. 100s. **100 mg:** Atenolol 100 mg, Chlorthalidone 25 mg/Tab Bot. 100s.
Use: Antihypertensive, diuretic.

TENORMIN. (ICI Pharma) **Oral:** Atenolol 50 mg or 100 mg/Tab. Bot. 100s. UD 100s. **Parenteral:** 5 mg/10 ml. Amp. 10 ml.
Use: Treatment of hypertension and angina with a cardioselective, hydrophilic beta blocker.

• **TENOXICAM.** USAN.
Use: Anti-inflammatory.

TENSEZE. (A.P.C.) Phenyltoloxamine citrate 88 mg, salicylamide 130 mg/Cap. Bot. 10s.
Use: Nervous tension.

TENSILON. (ICN Pharm.) Edrophonium chloride. **Vial:** 10 mg/ml, w/phenol 0.45%, sodium sulfite 0.2% 10 ml. **Amp.** 10 mg/ml, w/sodium sulfite 0.2%. 1 ml.
Use: Differential diagnosis of myasthenia gravis.

TENSIVE CONDUCTIVE ADHESIVE GEL. (Parker) Non-flammable conductive adhesive electrode gel, eliminates tape and tape irritation. Tube 60 Gm.
Use: For TENS, EMS, EMG, EEG and other electromedical procedures.

TENSOCAINE TABLETS. (Sanofi Winthrop) Acetaminophen.
Use: Analgesic, antipyretic.

TENSOLATE. (Apco) Phenobarbital 0.25 gr, hyoscyamine sulfate 0.1037 mg, atropine sulfate 0.0194 mg, hyoscine HBr 0.0065 mg/Tab. Bot. 100s.
Use: Antispasmodic sedative, for visceral spasm.

TENSOLAX TABLETS. (Sanofi Winthrop) Chlormezanone.
Use: Analgesic, muscle relaxant.

TENSOPIN. (Apco) Phenobarbital 0.25 gr, homatropine methylbromide 2.5 mg/Tab. Bot. 100s.
Use: Antispasmodic.

TENTRATE. (Tennessee Pharm.) Pentaerythritol tetranitrate 20 mg/Tab. Bot. 100s, 1000s.
Use: Anorexiant.

TENUATE. (Lakeside) Diethylpropion HCl 25 mg/Tab. Bot. 100s.
Use: Anorexiant.

TENUATE DOSPAN. (Lakeside) Diethylpropion HCl 75 mg/CR Tab. Bot. 100s, 250s.
Use: Anorexiant.

T.E.P. (Geneva) Phenobarbital 8 mg, theophylline 130 mg, ephedrine HCl 24 mg/Tab. Bot. 100s.
Use: Antiasthmatic combination.

TEPANIL. (Riker) Diethylpropion HCl. Tab. 25 mg. Bot. 100s.
Use: Anorexiant.

TEPANIL TEN-TAB. (Riker) Diethylpropion 75 mg/Tab. Bot. 30s, 100s, 250s.

Use: Anorexiant.
- **TEPOXALIN.** USAN.
- **TEPROTIDE.** USAN.
  Use: Enzyme-inhibitor (angiotensin-converting).
TEQUINOL SODIUM. Name used for Actinoquinol Sodium.
TERALASE. W/Pancreatin, polysorbate-80.
  See: Digolase, Cap. (Boyle).
TERAZOL 3. (Ortho) **Cream, Vaginal:** Terconazole 0.8%. Tube 20 g with applicator. **Vaginal Supp.:** Terconazole 80 mg. Pks. 3s with applicator.
  Use: Vaginal antifungal.
TERAZOL 7. (Ortho) Terconazole 0.4% Cream. In 45 Gm.
  Use: Vaginal antifungal.
- **TERAZOSIN HYDROCHLORIDE.** USAN. (1) Piperazine, 1-(4-amino-6,7-dimethoxy-2-quinazolinyl)-4-[(tetrahydro-2-furanyl)carbonyl]-, monohydrochloride, dihydrate; (2) 1-(4-Amino-6,7-dimethoxy-2-quinazolinyl)-4-(tetrahydro-2-furoyl)piperazine monohydrochloride dihydrate.
  Use: Antihypertensive.
  See: Hytrin, Tab. (Abbott and Burroughs Wellcome).
- **TERBINAFINE.** USAN.
  Use: Antifungal.
  See: Lamisil.
- **TERBUTALINE SULFATE,** U.S.P. XXIII. Inhalation Aerosol, Inj., Tab., U.S.P. XXII. a-[(tert-Butylamino)methyl]-3,5-dihydroxybenzyl alcohol sulfate.
  Use: Bronchodilator.
  See: Brethine, Amp., Tab. (Geigy).
TERCODRYL. (Approved) Codeine phos. ¾ gr, pyrilamine maleate 25 mg/fl. oz. Bot. 4 oz.
  Use: Antihistamine.
- **TERCONAZOLE.** USAN. Triaconazole.
  Use: Antifungal.
  See: Terazol 3, Vag. Cream, Supp. (Ortho).
  Terazol 7, Vag. Cream. (Ortho).
- **TERFENADINE.** USAN. U.S.P. XXIII.
  Use: Antihistamine.
  See: Seldane, Tab. (Marion Merrell Dow).
TERG-A-ZYME. (Alconox) Alconox with enzyme action. Box 4 lb. Ctn. 9×4 lb., 25 lb., 50 lb., 100 lb., 300 lb.
  Use: Biodegradeable detergent and wetting agent.
TERIDOL JR. (Approved) Terpin hydrate, cocillana, potassium guaiacolsulfonate, ammonium chloride. Bot. 3 oz.
  Use: Expectorant.

TERIPARATIDE.
  Use: Diagnostic aid, thyroid function. [Orphan drug]
  See: Parathar.
- **TERIPARATIDE ACETATE.** USAN.
  Use: Diagnostic aid (hypocalcemia).
TERLIPRESSIN.
  Use: Treatment of bleeding esophageal varices. [Orphan drug]
  See: Glypressin.
- **TERODILINE HYDROCHLORIDE.** USAN.
  Use: Vasodilator (coronary).
- **TEROXALENE HYDROCHLORIDE.** USAN 1-(3-Chloro-p-tolyl)-4-[6-(p-tertpentylphenoxy)-hexyl] piperazine hydrochloride.
  Use: Antischistosomal.
- **TEROXIRONE.** USAN.
  Use: Antineoplastic.
TERPACOF. (Jenkins) Codeine phosphate 10 mg, terpin hydrate 88 mg/5 ml. Bot. 3 oz., gal.
  Use: Cough sedative and expectorant.
TERPATE. (Geneva) Pentaerythritol tetranitrate 10 mg, 20 mg/Tab. Bot. 100s.
TERPEX JR. (Approved) d-Methorphan 25 mg, terpin hydrate, pot. guaiacolsulfonate, cocillana, ammonium chloride. Bot. 4 oz.
  Use: Children's cough syrup.
TERPHAN ELIXIR. (Vale) Terpin hydrate 85 mg, dextromethorphan hydrobromide 10 mg/5 ml w/alcohol 40% Bot. Gal.
  Use: Sedative.
- **TERPIN HYDRATE,** U.S.P. XXIII. Elixir, with Codeine Elixir, U.S.P. XXIII. cis-p-Menthane-1,8-diol hydrate. Cryst. & Pow., Pkg. 0.25 lb., 4 oz., 1 lb.
  Use: Expectorant for chronic cough.
  See: Creoterp (Jenkins).
  Terp, Liq. (Scrip).
TERPIN HYDRATE W/COMBINATIONS.
  See: Histogesic, Tab. (Century).
  Prunicodeine, Liq. (Lilly).
  W/Dextromethorphan, phenylpropanolamine HCl, pheniramine maleate, pyrilamine maleate.
  See: Tussaminic, Tab. (Dorsey).
  W/Dextromethorphan, phenylpropanolamine HCl, pheniramine maleate, pyrilamine maleate, acetaminophen.
  See: Chexit, Tab. (Dorsey).
  Tussagesic, Tab., Liq. (Dorsey).
- **TERPIN HYDRATE AND DEXTROMETHORPHAN HYDROBROMIDE ELIXIR,** U.S.P. XXIII.
  Use: Expectorant, antitussive.

See: Dicodethal, Elix. (Lannett).

TERRA-CORTRIL. (Roerig) Hydrocortisone 15 mg, oxytetracycline HCl 5 mg/ml. Ophth. Susp. Bot. w/dropper 5 ml.
Use: Corticosteroid, anti-infective, ophthalmic.

TERRAMYCIN. (Pfizer Laboratories) Oxytetracycline. **Cap.:** HCl salt 250 mg. Bot. 100s, 500s. **Oint., Ophth.:** Ocytetracycline HCl 5 mg, polymyxin B sulfate 1 mg/Gm. Tube 3.75 Gm. **Oint., Topical:** Oxytetracycline HCl 100 mg, polymyxin B sulfate 10,000 units/Gm. Tube 0.5 oz., 1 oz. **Pow. Topical:** Oxytetracycline HCl 30 mg, polymyxin B sulfate 10,000 units/Gm Bot. 28.4 Gm. **Tab., Oral:** Oxytetracycline HCl 250 mg/Tab. Bot. 100s. **Tab., Vaginal:** Oxytetracycline HCl 100 mg, polymyxin B sulfate 100,000 units/Tab. Box 10s.
Use: Anti-infective.

TERRAMYCIN CAPSULES. (Pfizer Laboratories) Oxytetracycline HCl 250 mg/Cap. Bot. 100s, 500s.
Use: Antibacterial.

TERRAMYCIN TOPICAL OINTMENT. (Leeming) Oxytetracycline HCl 30 mg, polymyxin B sulfate 10,000 units/Gm. Tube 0.5 oz, 1 oz. Ctn. 12's.
Use: Anti-infective, external.

TERRAMYCIN W/POLYMYXIN B OINTMENT. (Roerig) Polymyxin B sulfate 10,000 units/Gm or ml, oxytetracycline HCl 5 mg/Gm, white and liquid petrolatum base. Oint. Tube 3.75 Gm.
Use: Ophthalmic.

TERRAMYCIN TOPICAL POWDER WITH POLYMYXIN B SULFATE. (Leeming) Oxytetracycline HCl 30 mg, polymyxin B sulfate 10,000 units/Gm. Bot. oz.
Use: Anti-infective, external.

TERSAVID. N^1-pivaloyl-N^2-benzyl-hydrazine.
Use: Monoamine oxidase inhibitor.

TERTIARY AMYL ALCOHOL.
See: Amylene Hydrate. (Various Mfr.).

TESAMONE. (Dunhall) Testosterone aqueous suspension.
'25' (25 mg/ml) Amp.10 ml.
'50' (50 mg/ml) Amp. 10 ml.
'100' (100 mg/ml) Amp. 10 ml.
Use: Androgen therapy.

• **TESICAM.** USAN. 4'-Chloro-1,2,3,4-tetrahydro-1,3-dioxo-4-isoquinolinecarboxanilide.
Use: Anti-inflammatory.

• **TESIMIDE.** USAN.
Use: Anti-inflammatory.

TESLAC. (Squibb Mark) Testolactone 50

mg/Tab. Bot. 100s.
Use: Antineoplastic agent.

TESOGEN. (Sig) Testosterone 25 mg, estrone 2mg/ml. Vial 10 ml.
Use: Androgen.

TESOGEN L.A. (Sig) Testosterone enanthate 180 mg, 90 mg, 50 mg, estradiol valerate 8 mg, 4 mg and 2 mg respectively/ml. Vial 10 ml.
Use: Androgen/estrogen therapy.

TESONE. (Sig) Testosterone 25 mg, 50 mg, 100 mg/ml. Vial 10 ml.
Use: Androgen hormonal therapy.

TESONE L.A. (Sig) Testosterone enanthate 200 mg/ml. Vial 10 ml.
Use: Androgen.

TESPA.
Use: Alkylating agent.
See: Thiotepa (Lederle).

TESSALON PERLES. (Forest Pharm.) Benzonatate 100 mg/Cap. Bot. 100s.
Use: Antitussive.

TESTAMONE. (Dunhall) Testosterone 100 mg/ml. Inj. Vial 10 ml.
Use: Androgen.

TESTANATE No. 1. (Kenyon) Testosterone enanthate 100 mg, lipophilic Soln. 200 mg/ml. Vial 10 ml.
Use: Androgen.

TESTANATE No. 2. (Kenyon) Testosterone enanthate 90 mg, estradiol valerate 4 mg/ml. Vial 10 ml.
Use: Androgen.

TESTANATE No. 3. (Kenyon) Testosterone enanthate 180 mg, estradiol valerate 8 mg/ml. Vial 10 ml.
Use: Androgen.

TESTANDRO. (Redur) Testosterone (in aqueous solution) 100 mg/ml. Inj. vial 10 ml.
Use: Androgen.

TES-TAPE. (Lilly) Diagnostic test for glucose in urine. Glucose oxidase, glucose peroxidase, orthotolidine. Single Pkg. 100 tests.
Use: Diagnostic agent.

TEST-ESTRO CYPIONATES. (Rugby) Estradiol cypionate 2 mg, testosterone cypionate 50 mg/ml. Inj. Vial 10 ml.
Use: Estrogen/androgen.

TESTEX. (Pasadena Research) Testosterone propionate in sesame oil 50 mg, 100 mg/ml. Vial 10 ml.
Use: Androgen.

TESTODERM. (Alza) Testosterone 10 mg or 15 mg per 40 or 60 cm^2, respectively. Transdermal system. Box 30s.
Use: Treatment of hypogonadism, androgen.

TESTOJECT. (Mayrand) Testosterone

cypionate 100 mg/ml. Vial 10 ml.
Use: Androgenic hormone.
TESTOJECT-50. (Mayrand) Testosterone
50 mg/ml. Vial 10 ml.
Use: Androgenic hormone.
TESTOJECT-LA. (Mayrand) Testos-
terone cypionate 200 mg/ml in oil. Vial
10 ml.
Use: Androgen.
• **TESTOLACTONE,** U.S.P. XXII. Sterile
Suspension, Tab., U.S.P. XXII. 13-Hy-
droxy-3-oxo-13, 17-secoandrosta-1,4-
dien-17oic acid-8-lactone.
Use: Antineoplastic agent.
See: Teslac, Vial, Tab. (Squibb Mark).
TESTOLIN. (Pasadena Research)
Testosterone suspension 25 mg, 50 mg,
100 mg/ml. Vial 10 ml 25 mg/ml. Vial 30
ml.
Use: Androgen.
TESTOPEL. (Bartor Pharmacal) Testos-
terone 75 mg, stearic acid 0.2 mg,
polyvinylpyrrolidone 2 mg/pellet. 1 pel-
let/vial.
Use: Androgen.
• **TESTOSTERONE,** U.S.P. XXIII. Pellets,
Sterile Susp., U.S.P. XXII. 17 β-Hydrox-
yandrost-4-en-3-one.
Use: Androgen.
See: Android-T, Vial (Brown).
Androlan, Vial (Lannett).
Andronaq, Aq. Susp., Vial (Central).
Depotest, Vial (Hyrex).
Dura-Testrone, Vial (Pharmex).
Homogene-S, Inj., Vial (Spanner).
Malotrone Aqueous Injection (Bluco).
Neo-Hombreol-F, Aq. Susp., Vial
(Organon).
Tesone, Inj. (Sig).
Testoderm, Transdermal patch (Alza).
Testolin, Vial (Pasadena Research).
Testopel (Bartor Pharmacal).
Testrone, Vial (Pharmex).
TESTOSTERONE AQUEOUS. (Various
Mfr.) Testosterone (in aqueous suspen-
sion) 25 mg, 50 mg or 100 per ml/Inj.
Vial 10 ml, 30 ml.
Use: Androgen, parenteral.
See: Histerone 100, Inj.
(Roberts/Hauck).
Tesamone, Inj. (Dunhall).
Testandro, Inj. (Redur Co.).
TESTOSTERONE W/COMBINATIONS.
See: Andesterone, Vial (Lincoln).
Angen, Vial (Davis & Sly).
Depo-Testadiol, Vial (Upjohn).
Glutest, Vial (Brown).
Terogen, Vial (Pasadena Research).
Tesogen, Inj. (Sig).
Testrone, Vial (Pharmex).

Vi-Testrogen, Vial (Pharmex).
**TESTOSTERONE CYCLOPENTANE
PROPIONATE.** Testosterone Cypi-
onate, U.S.P. XXIII.
• **TESTOSTERONE CYPIONATE,** U.S.P.
XXIII. Inj., U.S.P. XXIII. 17-β-Hydroxyan-
drost-4-en-3-one cy- clopentanepropi-
onate. Androst-4-en-3-one, 17-(3-cy-
clopentyl-1-oxopropoxy)-, (17β- Iestos-
terone cyclopentanepropionate).
(Various Mfr.) 100 mg/ml or 200 mg/ml.
Inj. Vial 10 ml.
Use: Androgen.
See: Andro-Cyp 100, Inj. (Keene).
Andro-Cyp 200, Inj. (Keene).
depAndro, Inj. (Forest).
Depo-Testosterone, Inj. (Upjohn).
Dep-Test, Inj. (Sig).
Depotest, Vial (Hyrex).
D-Test 100, 200, Inj. (Burgin-Arden).
Durandro, Inj. (Ascher).
Duratest, Inj. (Roberts Hauck).
Testoject, Vial (Mayrand).
W/Combinations.
See: D-Diol, Inj. (Burgin-Arden).
Depotestogen, Vial (Hyrex).
Depo-Testadiol, Soln. (Upjohn).
Duo-Cyp (Keene).
Duracrine, Inj. (Ascher).
Menoject-L.A. Vial (Kay).
T.E. Ionate P.A., Inj. (Reid-Rowell).
Testadiate-Depo, Vial (Kay).
• **TESTOSTERONE ENANTHATE,** U.S.P.
XXIII. Inj., U.S.P. XXIII. Androst-4-en-3-
one, 17-(1-oxoheptyl)- oxy-(17β)-.
Testosterone heptanoate. 17β-Hydrox-
yandrost-4-en-3-one heptanoate. (Vari-
ous Mfr.) 100 mg/ml or 200 mg/ml. Inj.
Vial 10 ml.
Use: Androgen.
See: Andryl, Inj. (Keene).
Andropository-200, Inj. (Rugby).
Arderone 100, 200, Inj. (Burgin-Ar-
den).
Delatest, Inj. (Dunhall).
Delatestryl, Inj., Vial (Squibb).
Dura-Testrone, Vial (Pharmex).
Everone 200 mg, Vial (Hyrex).
Tesone L. A., Inj. (Sig).
Testate, Inj. (Savage).
Testrin-P.A., Inj. (Pasadena Re-
search).
W/Chlorobutanol.
See: Anthatest, Vial (Kay).
Andro L.A. 200, Inj. (Forest).
Delatestryl, Inj. (Gynex).
Durathate-200, Inj. (Roberts Hauck).
Everone 200, Inj. (Hyrex).
W/Estradiol valerate.
See: Ardiol 90/4, 180/8, Inj. (Burgin-Ar-

den).
Deladumone, Vial (Squibb Mark).
Delatestadiol, Vial (Dunhall).
Ditate, Ditate DS, Vial (Savage).
Duoval-P.A., Inj. (Reid-Rowell).
Repose-TE. (Paddock).
Teev, Preps. (Keene).
Testanate No. 2 & 3, Vial (Kenyon).
Valertest, Amp., Vial (Hyrex).
TESTOSTERONE HEPTANOATE.
Use: Androgen.
See: Testosterone enanthate.
• **TESTOSTERONE KETOLAURATE.**
USAN. Testosterone 3-oxodode-
canoate.
Use: Androgen.
TESTOSTERONE OINTMENT 2%.
Use: Vulvar dystrophies. [Orphan drug]
• **TESTOSTERONE PHENYLACETATE.**
USAN. Perandren phenylacetate.
Use: Androgen.
TESTOSTERONE PROPIONATE. (Vari-
ous Mfr.) Testosterone propionate (in oil)
100 mg por ml. Inj. Vial 10 ml.
Use: Androgen, parenteral.
TESTOSTERONE SUBLINGUAL.
Use: Delay of growth and puberty in
boys. [Orphan drug]
TESTRED. (ICN) Methyltestosterone 10
mg/Cap. Bot. 100s.
Use: Androgen therapy.
TESTRED CYPIONATE.
Use: Androgen hormone inhibitor.
See: Proscar (Merck & Co.).
TESTRED CYPIONATE 200. (ICN)
Testosterone cypionate 200 mg/ml. Vial
10 ml.
Use: Androgen therapy.
TESTRIN-P.A. (Pasadena Research)
Testosterone enanthate 200 mg, in
sesame oil with chlorobutanol/ml. Vial
10 ml.
Use: Androgen.
TESTRONE. (Pharmex) Testosterone 25
mg, estrone 2 mg/ml. Vial 10 ml.
Use: I.M.; androgen therapy.
TESTURIA. (Wyeth-Ayerst) Combination
kit containing 5 × 20 sterile dip strips
and 5 × 20 culture trays of trypticase
soy agar.
Use: Diagnostic aid.
TESULOID. (Squibb) Technetium Tc 99m
sulfur colloid. 5 vials/kit.
Use: Radiodiagnostic.
• **TETANUS ANTITOXIN,** U.S.P. XXIII.
Use: Passive immunizing agent.
See: Homo-Tet, Vial, Syringe (Savage).
**TETANUS AND DIPHTHERIA TOXOIDS
ADSORBED FOR ADULT USE,** U.S.P.
XXIII.

Use: Active immunizing agent for per-
sons over 7 yrs. old.
Generic Products:
(Squibb/Connaught) Vial 5 ml for I.M.
use.
(Lederle) Vial 5 ml.
**TETANUS-DIPHTHERIA TOXOIDS AD-
SORBED, ALUMINUM PHOSPHATE
ADSORBED.** (Wyeth-Ayerst) Vial 5 ml,
Tubex 0.5 ml.
Use: Agent for immunization.
TETANUS, DIPTHERIA & PERTUSSIS.
Use: Toxoid.
See: Diptheria and Tetanus Toxoids and
Pertussis Vaccine (Connaught).
Tri-Immunol (Lederle).
**TETANUS AND DIPHTHERIA TOXOIDS
ADSORBED PUROGENATED.** (Leder-
le) Adult Lederject disposable syringe 10
× 0.5 ml. Vial 5 ml New package.
Use: Agent for immunization.
• **TETANUS IMMUNE GLOBULIN,** U.S.P.
XXIII. (Hyland) Gamma globulin fraction
of the plasma of persons who have been
hyperimmunized with tetanus toxoid,
16.5%. Vial 250 u.
Use: Prophylaxis of injured, against
tetanus (passive immunizing agent).
See: Gamulin-T, Vial (Marion Merrell
Dow).
Homo-Tet Vial, 1 ml (Savage).
Hu-Tet, Vial (Hyland).
Hyper-Tet Injection Vial, 250 u. (Cut-
ter).
Immu-Tetanus, Vial, Disp. Syr. (Parke-
Davis).
T-I-Gammagee, Disp. Syr. (Merck &
Co.).
**TETANUS IMMUNE GLOBULIN,
HUMAN,** (Wyeth-Ayerst) 250 u./Tubex,
1 ml Dissolved in glycine 0.3 M; contains
thimerosal 0.01%.
See: Ar-Tet, Syringe, Vial (Armour).
• **TETANUS TOXOID,** U.S.P. XXIII.
(Squibb/Connaught)—Vial 7.5 ml for
I.M. or S.C. use.
(Lederle)—Vial 0.5 ml, 5 ml.
(Wyeth-Ayerst)—Vial 7.5 ml Tubex 0.5
ml.
Use: Active immunizing agent against
tetanus.
• **TETANUS TOXOID, ADSORBED,** U.S.P.
XXIII. (Serums and Vaccines of Ameri-
ca) 20 Lf purified tetanus toxoid, 0.01%
thimerosal as preservative/ml. Box 2
ampuls of 0.5 ml. Vial 5 ml, 7.5 ml, 0.5
ml. Amp. for booster injection.
(Squibb/Connaught) Vial 5 ml for I.M.
use.
(Lederle)—Vial 5 ml Steri-Dose sy-

ringe 0.5 ml 10s.
(Wyeth-Ayerst)—Vial 5 ml Tubex 0.5 ml.
Use: Active immunizing agent against tetanus.
TETANUS TOXOID ADSORBED PURO-GENATED. (Lederle) Vial 5 ml. Lederject disposable syringe 0.5 ml. Box 10s, 100s.
Use: Agent for immunization.
TETANUS TOXOID, ALUM PRECIPITAT-ED.
Use: Agent for immunization.
See: (Cutter)—Vial 5 ml.
(Lilly)—Vial 1 ml, 5 ml. Hyporets 0.5 ml 10s, 100s.
(Merck & Co.)—Vial 5 ml.
• **TETANUS TOXOID, ALUMINUM PHOS-PHATE ADSORBED.** U.S.P. XXIII.
Use: Active immunizing agent.
See: (Lederle) Vial 5 ml 10s. Lederject Disp. Syr. 10 × 0.5 ml.
(Wyeth-Ayerst) Vial 5 ml Tubex 0.5 ml.
TETANUS TOXOID, FLUID PURO-GENATED.
(Lederle)—Vial 7.5 ml Lederject disposable syringe.
0.5 ml. Box 10s, 100s.
Use: Agent for immunization.
TETANUS TOXOID PURIFIED, FLUID.
(Wyeth-Ayerst)—Vial 7.5 ml, Tubex 0.5 ml.
Use: Agent for immunization.
TETIOTHALEIN SODIUM.
See: Iodophthalein Sodium. (Var. Mfr.).
TETRABEAD. (Abbott Diagnostics) Solid phase radioimmunoassay for the quantitative measurement of total circulating serum thyroxine.
TETRABEAD-125. (Abbott Diagnostics) T-3 uptake radioassay for the measurement of thyroid function by indirectly determining the degree of saturation of serum thyroxine binding globulin (TBG).
TETRABENAZINE. B.A.N. 1,3,4,6,7,11b-Hexahydro-3-isobutyl-9, 10-dimethoxy-benzo[a] quinolizin-2-one.
Use: Tranquilizer.
• **TETRACAINE,** U.S.P. XXIII. Oint., Ophth. Oint., Inj., U.S.P. XXIII. 2-Dimethyl-laminoethyl p-butyl-aminobenzoate.
Use: Local anesthetic.
• **TETRACAINE AND MENTHOL OINT-MENT,** U.S.P. XXIII.
Use: Local anesthetic.
• **TETRACAINE HYDROCHLORIDE,**
U.S.P. XXIII. Cream, Inj., Ophth. Soln., Topical Soln., Sterile, U.S.P. XXIII. 2-(Di-methyl-amino)-ethyl p-(butylamino)-ben-zoate HCl. Benzoic acid, 4-(butylamino)-

, 2-(dimethylamino)ethyl ester, monohy-drochloride. (Various Mfr.) 0.5% Soln. Bot. 1 ml, 2 ml, 15 ml.
Use: Local anesthetic, topical anesthetic, spinal anesthetic.
See: Bristacycline, Cap. (Bristol). Pontocaine Hydrochloride Prods. (Sanofi Winthrop).
W/Benzocaine, butyl aminobenzoate.
See: Cetacaine, Liq., Oint., Spray (Cetylite).
W/Hexachlorophene, dimethyl polysilox-ane, methyl salicylate, pyrilamine maleate, zinc oxide.
W/Isocaine, benzalkonium Cl.
See: Isotraine Oint. (Philips Roxane).
TETRACAINE HYDROCHLORIDE 0.5%.
(Alcon) 0.5%/1 ml Drop-Tainer, Ophth. 15 ml Steri-Unit, 2 ml (Cooper Vision) Dropperettes 1 ml in 10s.
Use: Local anesthetic, ophthalmic.
TETRACAP. (Circle) Tetracycline HCl 250 mg/Cap. Bot. 100s.
Use: Antibacterial; tetracycline.
TETRACHLORETHYLENE, U.S.P. XXI. Cap., U.S.P. XXI. Perchlorethylene, tetrachlorethylene.
Use: Anthelmintic (hookworms and some trematodes).
TETRACLOR. (Kenyon) Tetracycline HCl 250 mg/Cap. Bot. 100s, 1000s.
Use: Antibacterial; tetracycline.
TETRACLOR-L. (Kenyon) Tetracycline HCl 125 mg/5 ml. Bot. pt.
Use: Antibacterial; tetracycline.
TETRACON. (Professional Pharmacal) Tetrahydrozoline HCl 0.5 mg, disodium edetate 1.0 mg, boric acid 12 mg, ben-zalkonium Cl. 0.1 mg, sodium Cl. 2.2 mg, sodium borate 0.5 mg/ml w/water. Liq. Bot. 15 ml.
Use: Minor eye irritation.
TETRACOSACTIDE. (I.N.N.) Tetracosac-trin, B.A.N.
TETRACOSACTRIN. B.A.N. β^{1-24}-Corti-cotrophin.
Use: Corticotrophic peptide.
See: Cortrosyn.
Cosyntropin.
Synacthen.
Tetracosactide (I.N.N.).
• **TETRACYCLINE,** U.S.P. XXIII. Boluses, Oral Susp., U.S.P. XXIII. 4-(Dimethyl-lamino)-1,4,4a, 5,5a,6,11,12a-octahy-dro-3,-6,10,12,12a-penta hy- droxy-6-methyl-1,11-dioxo-2-naphthacenecar-boxamide.
Use: Antibiotic.
See: Sumycin, Syrup (Squibb).
W/N-acetyl-para-amino-phenol, phenyl-

toloxamine citrate.
Use: Antibacterial; anti-amebic; antirick-
ettsial.
See: Paltet, Cap. (Hauck).
Tetrex, Bid Cap., Cap., Vial (Bristol).
**TETRACYCLINE AND AMPHOTERICIN
B,** U.S.P. XXI. Cap., Oral Susp., U.S.P.
XXI.
• **TETRACYCLINE HYDROCHLORIDE,**
U.S.P. XXIII. Cap., Inj., Oint., Ophth
Oint., Soluble Powder, Topical Soln.,
Ophth. Susp., Sterile, Tab., U.S.P. XXIII.
Use: Antibiotic.
See: Achromycin, Preps. (Storz/Leder-
le)
Bicycline, Caps. (Knight).
Centet 250, Tab. (Central).
Cyclopar, Cap. (Parke-Davis).
G-Mycin, Cap. & Syr. (Coast).
Maso-Cycline, Cap. (Mason).
Panmycin, Cap. (Upjohn).
Scotrex, Caps. (Scott/Cord).
Sumycin, Cap., Tab., Syr. (Squibb
Mark).
Tetracap 250, Cap. (Circle).
Tetraclor, Tetraclor-L, Cap., Liq. (Keny-
on).
Tetracyn, Cap. (Pfizer Laboratories).
Tetralan "250", "500", Cap. (Lannett).
Tetram, Cap., Syr. (Dunhall).
Tetramax, Cap. (Rand).
Topicycline, Liq. (Proctor & Gamble).
Trexin, Cap. (A.V.P. Pharm.).
W/Citric Acid.
See: Achromycin V, Cap., Drop, Susp.,
Syr. (Lederle).
W/Nystatin.
See: Comycin, Cap. (Upjohn).
• **TETRACYCLINE HYDROCHLORIDE
AND NYSTATIN CAPSULES,** U.S.P.
XXIII.
Use: Antibiotic, antifungal.
See: Comycin, Cap. (Upjohn)
• **TETRACYCLINE ORAL SUSPENSION,**
U.S.P. XXIII.
Use: Antibiotic.
See: Brand names under Tetracycline.
TETRACYN. (Pfizer Laboratories) Tetra-
cycline HCl. 250 mg or 500 mg/Cap. **250
mg:** Cap. Bot. 1000s. **500 mg:** Bot.
100s.
Use: Antibacterial, tetracycline.
TETRADECYL SULFATE, SODIUM.
Use: Sclerosing agent.
See: Sotradecol (Elkins-Sinn).
**TETRAETHYLAMMONIUM BROMIDE
(TEAB).**
Use: Diagnostic & therapeutic agent in
peripheral vascular disorders. Diag-
nostic in hypertension.

TETRAETHYLAMMONIUM CHLORIDE.
Use: Ganglionic blocking agent.
TETRAETHYLTHIURAM DISULFIDE.
See: Disulfiram.
• **TETRAFILCON A.** USAN.
Use: Contact lens material.
TETRAHYDROAMINOACRIDINE.
Use: A cholinergic agent for Alzheimer's
disease.
See: Cognex (Warner-Lambert).
**TETRAHYDROPHENOBARBITAL CAL-
CIUM.**
See: Cyclobarbital Calcium, Prep.
TETRAHYDROXYQUINONE. Name
used for Tetroquinone.
TETRAHYDROZOLINE. B.A.N. 2-
(1,2,3,4-Tetrahydro-1-naphthyl)-2-imida-
zoline.
Use: Vasoconstrictor.
• **TETRAHYDROZOLINE HYDROCHLO-
RIDE,** U.S.P. XXIII. Nasal Soln., Ophth.
Soln. U.S.P. XXIII. 2-(1,2,3,4-Tetrahy-
dro-1-naphthyl)-2-imidazoline HCl. (Vari-
ous Mfr.) 0.05% Soln. Bot. 15 ml, 30 ml.
Use: Adrenergic (vasoconstrictor).
See: Collyrium Fresh Eye Drops
(Wyeth Ayerst).
Eysine, Soln., (Akorn).
Mallazine Eye Drops (Roberts Hauck).
Murine Plus (Abbott).
Optigene 3, Soln. (Pfeiffer).
Soothe, Soln., (Alcon).
Tetrasine, Soln., (Optopics).
Tyzine, Soln. (Key).
Visine, Soln. (Leeming).
**TETRAIODOPHENOLPHTHALEIN SODI-
UM.**
See: Iodophthalein Sodium.
TETRAIODOPHTHALEIN SODIUM.
See: Iodophthalein Sodium.
TETRALAN. (Lannett) Tetracycline HCl
125 mg/5 ml oral susp, cherry flavor.
Syr. Bot. 480 ml.
Use: Antibacterial, tetracycline.
TETRALAN "250". (Lannett) Tetracycline
HCl 250 mg/Cap. Bot. 100s, 1000s.
Use: Antibacterial, tetracycline.
TETRALAN "500". (Lannett) Tetracycline
HCl 500 mg/Cap. Bot. 100s, 1000s.
Use: Antibacterial, tetracycline.
TETRAM. (Dunhall) Tetracycline 250
mg/Cap. Bot. 100s.
Use: Antibiotic, tetracycline.
TETRAMAX. (Rand) Tetracycline HCl
250 mg/Cap. Bot. 100s, 1000s.
Use: Antibacterial, tetracycline.
**TETRAMETHYLENE DIMETHANESUL-
FONATE.**
See: Busulfan, U.S.P. XXIII.
TETRAMETHYLTHIURAM DISULFIDE.

Thiram.
Use: Anti-infective, antifungal.
See: Rezifilm, Aerosol (Squibb).
• **TETRAMISOLE HYDROCHLORIDE.**
USAN. ±2,3,5,6-Tetrahydro-6-phenylimi-
dazo [2,1-b]-thiazole HCl.
Use: Anthelmintic.
See: Ripercol (American Cyanamid).
TETRANEED. (Hanlon) Pentaerythritol
tetranitrate 80 mg/Time Cap. Bot. 100s.
Use: Antianginal agent.
TETRANTOIN. 7,8-Benzo-1,3-diaza-
spiro(4,5)-decane-2,4-dione. 3',4-Dihy-
drospiro-[imidazolidine-4,2(1H)-naph-
thalene]-2,5-dione.
Use: Anticonvulsant.
TETRASINE. (Optopics) Tetrahydrozoline
HCl 0.05%, benzalkonium chloride,
EDTA. Bot. 15 ml, 22.5 ml.
Use: Ophthalmic vasoconstrictor/mydri-
atic.
TETRASINE EXTRA. (Optopics) Polyeth-
ylene glycol 400 1%, tetrahydrozoline
HCl 0.05%, benzalkonium chloride,
EDTA. Bot. 15 ml.
Use: Ophthalmic vasoconstrictor/mydri-
atic.
TETRATAB. (Freeport) Pentaerythritol
tetranitrate 10 mg/Tab. Bot. 1000s.
Use: Management, prophylaxis and
treatment of angina attacks.
TETRATAB NO. 1. (Freeport) Pentaery-
thritol tetranitrate 20 mg/Tab. Bot.
1000s.
Use: Management, prophylaxis, & treat-
ment of angina attacks.
TETRAZYME. (Abbott Diagnostics) Test
kit 100s, 500s.
Use: Enzyme immunoassay for quanti-
tative measurement of total circulating
serum thyroxine (free and protein
bound).
• **TETROFOSMIN.** USAN.
Use: Diagnostic aid.
• **TETROQUINONE.** USAN. Tetrahydroxy-
p-benzoquinone.
Use: Treat keloids, keratolytic (sys-
temic).
See: Kelox (Elder).
• **TETROXOPRIM.** USAN.
Use: Antibacterial.
• **TETRYDAMINE.** USAN. 4,5,6,7-Tetrahy-
dro-2-methyl-3-(methylamino)-tetrahy-
droindazole.
Use: Analgesic, anti-inflammatory.
TETRYZOLINE (I.N.N.). Tetrahydrozoline,
B.A.N.
TETTERINE. (Shuptrine) Oint.: Antifungal
agents in green petrolatum base. Tin
oz.; Antifungal agents in white petroleum

base. Tube oz. **Powder:** Fungicide, ger-
micide formula powder for heat and dia-
per rash. Can 2.25 oz. **Soap:** Bar 3.25
oz.
Use: Treatment ringworm, athlete's
foot, diaper rash and other skin condi-
tions.
TEXACORT SCALP LOTION. (GenDerm
Co.) Hydrocortisone 1%, alcohol 33%.
Lipid free. Dropper Bot. 1 fl. oz.
Use: Corticosteroid.
T-FLUORIDE. (Tennessee) Sodium fluo-
ride 2.21 mg/Tab. Bot. 100s, 1000s.
Use: Dental caries preventative.
TG.
Use: Antineoplastic.
See: Thioguanine (Burroughs Well-
come).
T/GEL SCALP SOLUTION. (Neutrogena)
Neutar coal tar extract 2%, salicyclic
acid 2%. Bot. 2 oz.
Use: Antipsoriatic, antiseborrheic.
T/GEL THERAPEUTIC CONDITIONER.
(Neutrogena) Neutar coal tar extract
1.5% in oil free conditioner base. Bot.
1.4 oz.
Use: Antipsoriatic, antiseborrheic.
T/GEL THERAPEUTIC SHAMPOO.
(Neutrogena) Neutar coal tar extract 2%
in mild shampoo base. Bot. 4.4 oz., 8.5
oz.
Use: Antipsoriatic, antiseborrheic.
T-GEN SUPPOSITORIES. (Goldline)
Trimethobenzamide HCl 100 mg/Pedi-
atric Supp. or 200 mg/Adult Supp. Box
10s, 50s.
Use: Anticholinergic.
T-GESIC CAPSULE. (T.E. Williams) Hy-
drocodone bitartrate 5 mg, aceta-
minophen 325 mg, caffeine 40 mg, bu-
talbital 30 mg/Cap. Bot. 100s.
Use: Narcotic analgesic combination,
sedative/hypnotic.
• **THALIDOMIDE.** USAN. a-(N-Phthalimi-
do)glutarimide. 2-Phthalimidoglutarim-
ide.
Use: Hypnotic, sedative; anti-infective
[Orphan drug]
THALITONE. (Boehringer Ingelheim)
Chlorthalidone 25 mg/Tab. Bot. 100s.
Use: Diuretic.
• **THALLOUS CHLORIDE TL-201 INJEC-
TION,** U.S.P. XXIII.
Use: Diagnostic aid (radioactive agent).
THAM-E. (Abbott) Tromethamine 36 Gm,
sodium Cl. 30 mEq/L, potassium Cl. 5
mEq/L, chloride 35 mEq/L. Total osmo-
larity 367 mOsm/L. Single dose contain-
er 150 ml .
Use: Parenteral nutritional supplement.

THAM SOLUTION. (Abbott) Tromethamine 18 Gm, acetic acid 2.5 Gm Single-dose container.
Use: Parenteral nutritional supplement.

THC.
Use: Antiemetic/antivertigo agent.
See: Marinol (Roxane).

THEAMIN. Monoethanolamine salt of theophylline.
See: Monotheamin, Supp. (Lilly).
W/Amobarbital.
See: Monotheamin and Amytal, Pulvule (Lilly).

THEBACON. B.A.N. O^6-Acetyl-O^3-methyl-D^6-morphine.
Use: Narcotic analgesic; cough suppressant.

THEDRAZOL. (Kenyon) Pentylenetetrazol 100 mg, nicotinic acid 50 mg/Tab. Bot. 100s, 1000s.
Use: Antihypertensive.

THEDRAZOL-L. (Kenyon) Pentylenetetrazol 100 mg, niacin 50 mg/5 ml. Bot. 4 oz, pt, gal.
Use: Antihypertensive.

THEELIN AQUEOUS SUSPENSION. (Parke Davis) A suspension of estrone in isotonic sodium chloride solution for I.M. adm. Steri-Vial: 2 mg (20,000 IU)/ml. Vial 10 ml.
Use: Estrogen.

THENALIDINE. B.A.N. 1 Methyl 4 N (2 thenyl)-anilinopiperidine.
Use: Antihistamine.

THENALIDINE TARTRATE. 1-Methyl-4-(N-2-thenylanilino) piperidine tartrate.
Use: Antihistamine; antipruritic.

• **THENIUM CLOSYLATE.** USAN. N,N-Dimethyl, N2-phenoxy-ethyl-N-2-thenylammonium p-chloroben- zenesulfonate.
Use: Canine hookworm.
See: Bancari (Burroughs Wellcome).

THENYLDIAMINE. B.A.N. 2-(N-2-Pyridyl-N-2-thenyl-amino)ethyldimethylamine.
Use: Antihistamine.

THENYLDIAMINE HYDROCHLORIDE. 2-[(2-Dimethylaminoethyl)-3-thenyl-amino] pyridine HCl, thenyldramine chloride. Dethylandiomine.
Use: Antihistamine.

THENYLPYRAMINE.
See: Methapyrilene Hydrochloride, Preps.

THEO-24. (Whitby) Theophylline anhydrous 100 mg, 200 mg, or 300 mg/Controlled-Release Cap. 100 mg Bot. 100s. UD 100s; 200 mg Bot. 100s, 500s. UD 100s; 300 mg Bot. 100s, 500s. UD 100s.
Use: Bronchodilator, anti-asthmatic.

THEOBID DURACAP. (Ross) Theophylline anhydrous 260 mg/TR Cap. Bot. 60s, 500s.
Use: Bronchodilator, anti-asthmatic.

THEOBID JR DURACAP. (Ross) Anhydrous theophylline 130 mg/TR Cap. Bot 60s.
Use: Bronchodilator, anti-asthmatic.

THEOBROMA OIL. Cocoa Butter, N.F. XVIII.
Use: Suppository base.

THEOBROMINE WITH PHENOBARBITAL COMBINATIONS.
See: Harbolin, Tab. (Arcum).
Theocardone, Tab. (Lemmon).
T.P. KI, Tab. (Wendt-Bristol).

THEOBROMINE CALCIUM GLUCONATE.
(Bates)—Tab., Bot. 100s, 1000s. Also available w/phenobarbital.
(Grant)—Tab., Bot. 100s, 500s, 1000s.

THEOBROMINE SODIUM ACETATE. Theobromine calcium salt mixture with calcium salicylate.
Use: Diuretic; smooth muscle relaxant.

THEOBROMINE SODIUM SALICYLATE.
See: Doan's Pills (Purex).
W/Cal. lactate, Phenobarbital.
See: Theolaphen, Tab. (Elder).

THEOCHRON. (Various Mfr.) Theophylline anhydrous 100 mg, 200 mg, 300 mg. ER Tab. 100s, 500s, 1000s.
Use: Bronchodilator.

THEOCHRON. (Forest Labs) Theophylline 200 mg/Tab. T.R. Bot. 100s, 500s, 1000s. 300 mg/Tab. T.R. Bot. 100s, 500s.
Use: Antiasthmatic.

THEOCLEAR 80 SYRUP. (Central) Theophylline 80 mg/15 ml. Bot. Pt., Gal.
Use: Bronchodilator.

THEOCLEAR L.A.-130. (Central) Theophylline 130 mg/Cenule. Bot. 100s.
Use: Bronchodilator.

THEOCLEAR L.A.-260. (Central) Theophylline 260 mg/Cenule Bot. 100s, 1000s.
Use: Bronchodilator.

THEOCOLATE. (My-K Labs) Theophylline 150 mg, guaifenesin 90 mg/15 ml Liq. Bot. pt., gal.
Use: Antiasthmatic.

THEODRENALINE. B.A.N. 7-[2-(3,4,β-Trihydroxyphenethylamino)ethyl] theophylline.
Use: Analeptic.

THEODRINE. (Rugby) Theophylline 130 mg, ephedrine HCl 24 mg, phenobarbital 8 mg/Tab. Bot. 100s, 1000s.
Use: Antiasthmatic combination.

THEO-DUR. (Schering) Theophylline 450

mg/Tab. S.R. Bot. 100s, UD 100s.
Use: Bronchodilator.
THEO-DUR SPRINKLE. (Key) Theo-phylline 50 mg, 75 mg, 125 mg or 200 mg/SA Cap. Bot. 100s.
Use: Bronchodilator.
THEO-DUR TABLETS. (Key) Theo-phylline 100 mg, 200 mg or 300 mg/CA Tab. Bot. 100s, 500s, 1000s, 5000s. UD 100s.
Use: Bronchodilator.
• **THEOFIBRATE.** USAN.
Use: Antihyperlipoproteinemic.
THEO-G CAPSULES. (Dixon-Shane) Theophylline 150 mg, guaifenesin 90 mg. Bot. 100s, 1000s.
Use: Antiasthmatic combination.
THEOGEN. (Sig) Conjugated estrogens 2 mg/ml. Vial 10 ml, 30 ml.
Use: Estrogen.
THEOGEN I.P. (Sig) Estrone 2 mg, potas-sium estrone sulfate 1 mg/ml. Vial 10 ml.
Use: Estrogen.
THEOLAIR. (Riker) Theophylline 125, 250 mg/Tab. Box 100s, 250s as foil strip 10s. Bot. 100s.
Use: Bronchodilator.
THEOLAIR LIQUID. (Riker) Theophylline 80 mg/15 ml. Bot. pt.
Use: Bronchodilator.
THEOLAIR-SR 200. (Riker) Theophylline 200 mg/Tab. (slow release). Bot. 100s. Box 100s as foil strip 10s.
Use: Bronchodilator.
THEOLAIR-SR 250. (Riker) Theophylline 250 mg/Tab. (slow release). Bot. 100s, 250s.
Use: Bronchodilator.
THEOLAIR-SR 300. (Riker) Theophylline 300 mg/Tab. (slow release). Bot. 100s. Box 100s as foil strip 10s.
Use: Bronchodilator.
THEOLAIR-SR 500. (Riker) Theophylline 500 mg/Tab. (slow release). Bot. 100s, 250s.
Use: Bronchodilator.
THEOLATE LIQUID. (Goldline) Theo-phylline, glyceryl guaiacolate. Bot. pt. gal.
Use: Antiasthmatic combination.
THEOMAX DF SYRUP. (Goldline) Theo-phylline 32.5 mg, ephedrine sulfate 6.25 mg, hydroxyzine HCl 2.5 mg/5 ml. Bot. pt. gal.
Use: Antiasthmatic combination.
THEO-ORGANIDIN. (Wallace) Theo-phylline anhydrous 120 mg, iodinated glycerol 30 mg/15 ml w/alcohol 15%, saccharin. Bot. pt., gal.
Use: Antiasthmatic combination.

THEOPHENYLLIN. (H.L. Moore) Theo-phylline 130 mg, ephedrine HCl 24 mg, phenobarbital 8 mg/Tab. Bot. 1000s.
Use: Antiasthmatic combination.
THEOPHYL-SR. (McNeil Pharm) Theo-phylline 125 mg. Bot. 100s.
Use: Bronchodilator.
• **THEOPHYLLINE,** Cap., U.S.P. XXIII. Tab., U.S.P. XXIII. Extended release cap., U.S.P. XXIII. 1,3-Dimethylxanthine. 1H-Purine-2,6-dione,3,-7-dihydro-1,3-di-methyl-, monohydrate.
Use: Coronary vasodilator & diuretic; pharm necessity for Aminophylline In-jection.
See: Accurbron, Liq. (Marion Merrell Dow).
Aerolate, Cap., Elix. (Fleming).
Aquaphyllin, Syr. (Ferndale).
Bronkodyl, Cap. (Sanofi Winthrop).
Duraphyl, Tab. (McNeil Pharm).
Elixicon, Susp. (Berlex).
Elixophyllin, Elix., Cap. (Berlex).
Elixophyllin SR, Cap. (Berlex).
Lanophyllin, Elix. (Lannett).
Lodrane, Cap. (Poythress).
Optiphyllin, Elix. (Fougera).
Oralphyllin, Liq. (Consol. Midland).
Quibron-T Dividose, Tab. (Bristol).
Quibron-T/SR Dividose, Tab. (Bristol).
Slo-bid, Caps. (Rhone-Poulenc Ror-er).
Slo-Phyllin, Cap., Syr., Tab. (Dooner).
Somophyllin, Cap. (Fisons).
Sustaire, Tab. (Pfizer Laboratories)
Theo-II, Elix. (Fleming).
Theobid, Cap. (Ross).
Theobid Jr, Cap. (Ross).
Theochron, ER Tab. (Various Mfr.)
Theoclear 80, Liq. (Central).
Theoclear L.A., Cenule (Central).
Theo-Dur, Tab. (Key).
Theophylline Extended Release, ER Tab. (Sidmark).
Theolair, Tab., Liq. (Riker).
Theolair SR, Tab. (Riker).
Theospan, Cap. (Laser).
Theostat, Prods. (Laser).
Theovent Long-Acting, Cap. (Scher-ing).
Theo-X, CR Tab. (Carnrick).
THEOPHYLLINE. (Various Mfr.) 100 mg, 125 mg, 200 mg, 300 mg. ER Cap. Bot. 100s.
Use: Bronchodilator.
THEOPHYLLINE, 8-CHLORO, DIPHEN-HYDRAMINE. Dimenhydrinate, U.S.P. XXIII.
See: Dramamine, Prep. (Searle).
THEOPHYLLINE AMINOISOBUTANOL.

Theophylline w/2-amino-2-methyl-1-propanol.
See: Butaphyllamine (Var. Mfr.).
THEOPHYLLINE-CALCIUM SALICYLATE.
W/Ephedrine HCl, phenobarbital, pot. iodide.
See: Quadrinal, Tab., Susp. (Knoll).
W/Phenobarbital, ephedrine HCl, guaifenesin.
See: Verequad, Tab., Susp. (Knoll).
W/Potassium iodide.
See: Theokin, Tab., Elix. (Knoll).
THEOPHYLLINE CHOLINE SALT.
See: Choledyl, Tab., Elix. (Parke-Davis).
• **THEOPHYLLINE, EPHEDRINE HYDROCHLORIDE, AND PHENOBARBITAL TABLETS,** U.S.P. XXIII.
Use: Bronchodilator, sedative.
THEOPHYLLINE ETHYLENEDIAMINE.
See: Aminophylline, Prep., (Var. Mfr.).
THEOPHYLLINE EXTENDED-RELEASE.
(Sidmak) Theophylline anhydrous 450 mg, lactose (SL 518). Tab. Bot. 100s, 250s, 500s.
Use: Bronchodilator.
• **THEOPHYLLINE EXTENDED-RELEASE CAPSULES.** U.S.P. XXIII.
THEOPHYLLINE W/COMBINATIONS.
See: Asma-lief, Tab., Susp. (Quality Generics).
B.A. Prods. (Federal).
Bronkaid, Tab. (Brew).
Co-Xan, Liq. (Central).
Elixophyllin-Kl, Elix. (Berlex).
Liquophylline, Liq. (Paddock).
Marax DF, Syr. (Roerig).
Mersaphyllin, Vial (Pharmex).
Quibron, Cap., Liq.(Bristol).
Quibron-300, Cap. (Bristol).
Quibron Plus, Cap. (Bristol).
Slo-Phyllin Gg, Cap., Syr. (Dooner).
Synophylate, Liq. (Central).
Tedral SA, Tab. (Parke-Davis).
Theocol, Cap., Liq. (Quality Generics).
Theofenal, Tab. (Cumberland).
Theolair Plus, Tab., Liq. (Riker).
Theo-Organidin, Elix. (Wampole).
• **THEOPHYLLINE AND GUAIFENESIN CAPSULES,** U.S.P. XXIII.
Use: Smooth muscle relaxant, expectorant.
THEOPHYLLINE AND GUAIFENESIN ORAL SOLUTION, U.S.P. XXIII.
Use: Smooth muscle relaxant, expectorant.
THEOPHYLLINE KI. (Various Mfr.) Theophylline 80 mg, potassium iodide 130 mg, alcohol. Elix. pt. gal.

Use: Antiasthmatic combination.
THEOPHYLLINE OLAMINE. Theophylline compound with 2-amino-ethanol (1:1).
Use: Smooth muscle relaxant.
THEOPHYLLINE WITH PHENOBARBITAL COMBINATIONS.
See: Asma-Lief, Tab., Susp. (Quality Generics).
Bronkolixir, Elix. (Sanofi Winthrop).
Bronkotab, Tab. (Sanofi Winthrop).
Ceepa, Tab. (Geneva).
THEOPHYLLINE REAGENT STRIPS.
(Miles Diagnostic) Seralyzer reagent strip. Bot. 25s.
Use: A quantitative strip test for theophylline in serum or plasma.
• **THEOPHYLLINE SODIUM GLYCINATE,** U.S.P. XXIII. Elixir, Tab., U.S.P. XXIII.
Use: Smooth muscle relaxant.
See: Synophylate, Elix., Tab. (Central).
Theofort, Elix. (Federal Pharm.).
W/Guaifenesin.
See: Asbron G, Tab., Elix. (Dorsey).
Synophylate-GG, Tab., Syr. (Central).
W/Phenobarbital.
See: Synophylate w/Phenobarbital, Tab. (Central).
W/Potassium iodide.
See: TSG-Kl, Elix. (Elder).
W/Potassium iodide, ephedrine HCl, codeine phosphate.
See: TSG Croup Liquid. (Elder).
W/Racephedrine & phenobarbital.
See: Synophedal, Tab. (Central).
THEO-R-GEN. (Goldline) Theophylline 120 mg, iodinated glycerol 30 mg/15 ml, alcohol 15%. Elix. Bot. 480 ml.
Use: Antiasthmatic combination.
THEO-SAV. (Savage) Theophylline 100 mg/Tab. Bot. 100s. 200 mg or 300 mg/Tab. Bot. 100s, 500s, 1000s.
Use: Bronchodilator.
THEOSPAN-SR 130. (Laser) Theophylline anhydrous 130 mg/Cap. Bot. 100s, 1000s.
Use: Bronchodilator.
THEOSPAN-SR 260. (Laser) Theophylline anhydrous 260 mg/Cap. Bot. 100s, 1000s.
Use: Bronchodilator.
THEOSTAT 80 SYRUP. (Laser) Theophylline anhydrous 80 mg/15 ml. Bot. Pt., Gal.
Use: Bronchodilator.
THEOTAL. (Major) Theophylline 125 mg, ephedrine HCl 25 mg, phenobarbital 8 mg, lactose. Tab. Bot. 1000s.
Use: Antiasthmatic combination.
THEO-TIME. (Major) Theophylline 100

mg, 200 mg, and 300 mg/Tab. T.R. Bot. 100s, 500s.
Use: Bronchodilator.

THEO-TIME SR TABS. (Major) Theophylline 100 mg, 200 mg, or 300 mg/S.R. Tab. Bot. 100s, 500s.
Use: Bronchodilator.

THEOVENT LONG ACTING. (Schoring) Theophylline anhydrous 125 mg or 250 mg/Cap. Bot. 100s.
Use: Bronchodilator.

THEO-X. (Carnrick) Theophylline anhydrous 100 mg, 200 mg or 300 mg/Tab. Dye free, lactose. Bot. 100s, 500s, 1000s.
Use: Bronchodilator.

THERA BATH. (Walgreen) Mineral oil 90%. Bot. 16 oz.
Use: Emollient.

THERA BATH WITH VITAMIN E. (Walgreen) Mineral oil 91%, Vit E 2000 IU/16 oz.
Use: Emollient.

THERABID. (Mission) Vitamins C 500 mg, B_1 15 mg, B_2 10 mg, niacinamide 100 mg, calcium pantothenate 20 mg, B_6 10 mg, B_{12} 5 mcg, A 5,000 IU, D 200 IU, E 30 mg/Tab. Bot. 100s.
Use: Vitamin supplement.

THERABLOAT. (Norden) Poloxalene.

THERABRAND. (Approved) Vitamins A 25,000 IU, D 1000 IU, B_1 10 mg, B_2 10 mg, niacinamide 100 mg, C 200 mg, B_6 5 mg, calcium pantothenate 20 mg, B_{12} 5 mcg/Cap. Bot. 100s, 1000s.
Use: Vitamin supplement.

THERABRAND-M. (Approved) Vitamins A 25,000 IU, D 1000 IU, C 200 mg, B_1 10 mg, B_2 10 mg, B_6 5 mg, niacinamide 100 mg, calcium pantothenate 20 mg, E 5 IU, B_{12} 5 mcg, iodine 0.15 mg, iron 15 mg, copper 1 mg, calcium 125 mg, manganese 1 mg, magnesium 6 mg, zinc 1.5 mg/Cap. Bot. 100s, 1000s.
Use: Vitamin/mineral supplement.

THERAC. (C & M Pharmacal) Colloidal sulfur 4.0%, salicylic acid 2.35% in lotion base. Bot. 2 oz.
Use: Anti-acne.

THERACAP. (Arcum) Vitamins A 10,000 IU, D 400 IU, B_1 10 mg, B_2 5 mg, niacinamide 150 mg, C 150 mg/Cap. Bot. 100s, 1000s.
Use: Vitamin supplement.

THERA-COMBEX H-P. (Parke-Davis Prods) Vitamins C 500 mg, B_1 25 mg, B_2 15 mg, B_{12} 5 mcg, niacinamide 100 mg, panthenol 20 mg/Cap. Bot. 100s.
Use: Vitamin supplement.

THERACYS. (Connaught) BCG Live 27 mg (3.4 x 10 CFU)/ vial. Freeze-dried suspension for reconstitution. Vials with diluent (1 ml/vial).
Use: Antineoplastic agent.

THERAFLU, FLU AND COLD MEDICINE. (Sandoz) Pseudoephedrine HCl 60 mg, chlorpheniramine maleate 4 mg, acetaminophon 650 mg, sucrose, lemon fla vor. Pow. Pks. 6.
Use: Upper respiratory combination.

THERAFLU, FLU COLD & COUGH MEDICINE. (Sandoz) Pseudoephedrine HCl 60 mg, chlorpheniramine maleate 4 mg, dextromethorphan HBr 20 mg, acetaminophen 650 mg, sucrose, lemon flavor. Pow. Pks. 6s.
Use: Decongestant, antihistamine, antitussive.

THERA-FLU NON-DROWSY FORMULA, MAXIMUM STRENGTH. (Sandoz) Pseudoephedrine HCl 30 mg, dextromethorphan HBr 15 mg, acetaminophen 500 mg. Capl. Pkg. 12s.
Use: Decongestant, antitussive.

THERA-FLUR. (Colgate-Hoyt) Fluoride 0.5% (from sod. fluoride 1.1%). pH 4.5. Gel-Drops. Bot. 24 and 60 ml.
Use: Dental caries preventative.

THERA-FLUR-N. (Colgate-Hoyt) Neutral sodium fluoride 1.1% Bot. 24 ml, 60 ml.
Use: Dental caries preventative.

THERAFORTIS. (General Vitamin) Vitamins A 12,500 IU, D 1000 IU, B_1 5 mg, B_2 5 mg, B_6 1 mg, B_{12} 3 mcg, niacinamide 50 mg, pantothenic acid salt 10 mg, C 150 mg, folic acid 0.5 mg/Cap. Bot. 100s, 1000s.
Use: Vitamin supplement.

THERAGENERIX. (Goldline) Vitamins A 5500 IU, D 400 IU, E 30 mg, B_1 3 mg, B_2 3.4 mg, B_3 30 mg, B_5 10 mg, B_6 3 mg, B_{12} 9 mcg, C 120 mg, folic acid 0.4 mg, biotin 15 mcg, betacarotene 2500 IU. Tab. Bot. 130s, 1000s.
Use: Vitamin supplement.

THERAGENERIX-H. (Goldline) Iron 66.7 mg, vitamins A 8333 IU, D 133 IU, E 5 IU, B_1 3.3 mg, B_2 3.3 mg, B_3 33.3 mg, B_5 11.7 mg, B_6 3.3 mg, B_{12} 50 mcg, C 100 mg, folic acid 0.33 mg, Cu, Mg/Tab. Bot. 100s, 1000s.
Use: Vitamin/mineral supplement.

THERAGENERIX-M. (Goldline) Iron 27 mg, vitamins A 5000 IU, D 400 IU, E 30 mg, B_1 3 mg, B_2 3.4 mg, B_3 30 mg, B_5 10 mg, B_6 3 mg, B_{12} 9 mcg, C 120 mg, folic acid 0.4 mg, Ca, Cl, Cr, Cu, I, K, biotin 15 mcg, Mg, Mn, Mo, P, Se, zinc 15 mg, beta carotene 2500 IU. Tab. Bot. 130s, 1000s.

Use: Vitamin/mineral supplement w/iron.

THERA-GESIC. (Mission) Methylsalicylate, menthol. Balm. In 90 Gm, 150 Gm.
Use: External analgesic.

THERAGRAN.(Squibb) Vitamins A 5,500 IU, C 120 mg, B_1 3 mg, B_2 3.4 mg, niacin 30 mg, B_6 3 mg, B_{12} 9 mcg, D 400 IU pantothenic acid 10 mg, folic acid 0.4 mg, biotin 15.5 mcg/Tab. Bot. 30s, 60s, 100s. 180s, 1000s. Unimatic 100s.
Use: Vitamin supplement.

THERAGRAN JR. WITH IRON. (Squibb) Iron 18 mg, vitamins A 5000 IU, D 400 IU, E 30 mg, B_1 1.5 mg, B_2 1.7 mg, B_3 20 mg, B_6 2 mg, B_{12} 6 mcg, C 60 mg, folic acid 0.4 mg w/tartrazine/Tab. Bot. 75s.
Use: Vitamin/mineral supplement.

THERAGRAN HEMATINIC. (Squibb) Iron 66.7 IU, vitamins A 8,333 IU, D 133 IU, E 5 IU, B_1 3.3 mg, B_2 3.3 mg, B_3 33.3 mg, B_5 11.7 mg, B_6 3.3 mg, B_{12} 50 mcg, C 100 mg, folic acid 0.33 mg, Cu, Mg, w/tartrazine, sodium bisulfite/Tab. Bot. 90s.
Use: Vitamin/mineral supplement.

THERAGRAN-M. (Squibb) Vitamins A 5,500 IU, D 400 IU, C 120 mg, B_1 3 mg, B_2 3.4 mg, niacinamide 30 mg, calcium pantothenate 10 mg, B_6 3 mg, E 30 IU, B_{12} 9 mcg, Ca, iodine 150 mcg, iron 27 mg, magnesium 100 mg, copper 2 mg, zinc 22.5 mg, manganese 7.5 mg, folic acid 0.4 mg, biotin 15 mcg, chromium 15 mcg, selenium 10 mcg, molybdenum 15 mcg, potassium 7.5 mg/Tab. Bot. 30s, 60s, 100s, 180s, 1000s, Unimatic 100s.
Use: Vitamin/mineral supplement.

THERAGRAN STRESS FORMULA. (Squibb) Iron 27 mg, vitamins E 30 IU, B_1 15 mg, B_2 15 mg, B_3 100 mg, B_5 20 mg, B_6 5 mg, B_{12} 12 mcg, C 600 mg, folic acid 0.4 mg, biotin 45 mcg/Tab. Bot. 75s.
Use: Vitamin/mineral supplement.

THERA-HIST. (Major) Pseudoephedrine HCl 60 mg, chlorpheniramine maleate 4 mg, acetaminophen 500 mg, sucrose. Pow. Pks. 6.
Use: Upper respiratory combination.

THERA H TABS. (Major) Bot. 100s, 250s.
Use: Vitamin/mineral supplement.

THERA-M. (Various Mfr.) Vitamins A 5000 IU, beta carotene 1250 IU, B_1 3 mg, B_2 3.4 mg, B_3 30 mg, B_5 10 mg, B_6 3 mg, B_{12} 9 mcg, C 90 mg, D 400 IU, E 30 IU, iron 27 mg, folic acid 0.4 mg, biotin 35 mcg, P, Ca, Cu, Cr, Se, Mo, K, Cl, I, Mg, Mn, zinc 15 mg. Tab. Bot. 1000s.

Use: Vitamin/mineral supplement.

THERAMIN. (Arcum) Vit. A 10,000 IU, D 400IU, B_1 10 mg, B_2 5 mg, niacinamide 100 mg, B_6 5 mg, B_{12} 10 mcg, C 150 mg, cal. pantothenate 15 mg, calcium 103.6 mg, iodine 0.1 mg, iron 15 mg, potassium 80 mg, magnesium 6 mg/Tab. Bot. 30s, 100s, 1000s.
Use: Vitamin/mineral supplement.

THERAMINE EXPECTORANT LIQUID. (Barre-National) Phenylpropanolamine HCl 12.5 mg, guaifenesin 100 mg, alcohol 5%. Bot. 473 ml.
Use: Decongestant, expectorant.

THERA MULTI-VITAMIN. (Major) Vitamins A 10,000 IU/5 ml, D 400 IU/5 ml, B_1 0.5 mg/5 ml, B_2 10 mg/5 ml, B_3 100 mg/5 ml, B_5 21.4 mg/5 ml, B_6 4.1 mg, B_{12} 5 mcg/5 ml, C 200 mg/5 ml, sugar. Liq. Bot. 120 ml.
Use: Vitamin supplement.

THERAMYCIN Z. (Medicis) Erythromycin 20 mg/ml, alcohol 86%, hydroxypropyl cellulose, zinc acetate, propylene glycol, lauramide DEA. Topical Soln. 60 ml.
Use: Anti-acne.

THERANEED. (Hanlon) Vitamins A 16,000 IU, B_1 10 mg, B_2 10 mg, B_6 2 mg, C 300 mg, calcium pantothenate 10 mg, niacinamide 10 mg, B_{12} 10 mcg/Cap. Bot. 100s.
Use: Vitamin supplement.

THERAPALS. (Faraday) Vitamins A 25,000 IU, D 400 IU, B_1 10 mg, B_2 5 mg, niacinamide 150 mg, B_5 0.5 mg, E 5 IU, C 150 mg, B_{12} 10 mcg, calcium 103 mg, cobalt 0.1 mg, copper 1 mg, potassium 0.15 mg, magnesium 6 mg, manganese 1 mg, molybdenum 0.2 mg, phosphorous 80 mg, potassium 5 mg, zinc 1.2 mg/Tab. Bot. 100s, 250s, 1000s.
Use: Vitamin/mineral supplement.

THERAPEUTIC B COMPLEX WITH VITAMIN C. (Upsher-Smith) Vitamins B_1 15 mg, B_2 10.2 mg, B_3 50 mg, B_5 10 mg, B_6 5 mg, C 300 mg. Cap. Bot. 100s.
Use: Vitamin supplement.

THERAPEUTIC MINERAL ICE. (Bristol-Myers Products) Menthol 2%, ammonium hydroxide, carbomer 934, cupric sulfate, isopropyl alcohol, magnesium sulfate, thymol. Gel. Tube 105 Gm, 240 Gm, 480 Gm.
Use: Rub/liniment.

THERAPEUTIC V & M. (Whiteworth) Vitamins A 10,000 IU, D 400 IU, B_1 10 mg, B_2 10 mg, B_6 5 mg, B_{12} 5 mcg, niacinamide 100 mg, calcium pantothenate 20 mg, C 200 mg, E 15 IU, iodine 0.15 mg, iron 12 mg, copper 2 mg, man-

ganese 1 mg, magnesium 60 mg, zinc 1.5 mg/Tab.
Use: Vitamin/mineral supplement.
THERAPEUTIC VITAMIN CAPSULES.
(Lannett) Vitamins A 25,000 IU, D 1000 IU, B_1 10 mg, B_2 5 mg, niacinamide 150 mg, C 150 mg/Cap. Bot. 100s, 500s, 1000s. Tab. Bot. 1000s.
Use: Vitamin supplement.
THERAPEUTIC VITAMIN CAPSULES AND TABLETS—IMPROVED FORMULA. (Lannett) Vitamins A 25,000 IU, D 1000 IU, thiamine mononitrate 12.5 mg, B_2 12.5 mg, niacinamide 100 mg, B_6 5 mg, B_{12} 5 mcg, calcium pantothenate 25 mg, C 200 mg/Cap. **Cap.:** 100s, 500s, 1000s. **Tab.:** Bot. 1000s.
Use: Vitamin supplement.
THERAPEUTIC VITAMIN FORMULA W/MINERALS. (Towne) Vitamins A palmitate 10,000 IU, D 400 IU, B_1 15 mg, B_2 10 mg, B_6 5 mg, B_{12} 12 mcg, C 200 mg, niacinamide 100 mg, calcium pantothenate 20 mg, E 15 IU, calcium 103 mg, iron 10 mg, manganese 1 mg, potassium 5 mg, zinc 1.5 mg, magnesium 6 mg/Cap. Bot. 30s, 60s, 100s, 250s.
Use: Vitamin/mineral supplement.
THERAPEUTIC VITAMIN FORMULA W/MINERALS. (Towne) Vitamins A palmitate 25,000 IU, D 1000 IU, B_1 10 mg, B_2 5 mg, B_6 1 mg, B_{12} 5 mcg, C 150 mg, niacinamide 100 mg, calcium 103 mg, phosphorus 80 mg, iron 10 mg, iodine 0.1 mg, manganese 1 mg, potassium 5 mg, copper 1 mg, zinc 1.4 mg, magnesium 5.5 mg/Cap. Bot. 100s, 1000s.
Use: Vitamin/mineral supplement.
THERAPHON. (Approved) Vitamins A 25,000 IU, D 1000 IU, B_1 10 mg, B_2 5 mg, C 150 mg, niacinamide 150 mg/Cap. Bot. 100s, 1000s.
Use: Vitamin supplement.
THERAPLEX. (Kenyon) Vitamins A 25,000 IU, D 1000 IU, B_1 10 mg, B_2 10 mg, niacinamide 150 mg, B_{12} 5 mcg/Tab. Bot. 100s, 1000s.
Use: Vitamin supplement.
THERAPLEX-PLUS. (Kenyon) Vitamins A palmitate 25,000 IU, D 1000 IU, B_1 10 mg, B_2 5 mg, B_6 1 mg, B_{12} 5 mcg, C 150 mg, niacinamide 100 mg, dicalcium phosphate 360 mg, calcium 106 mg, phosphorus 82 mg, ferrous sulfate 34 mg, manganese sulfate 3 mg, potassium sulfate 11 mg, zinc sulfate 3.9 mg, magnesium sulfate 40 mg/Cap. Bot. 100s, 1000s.

Use: Vitamin/mineral supplement.
THERAPLEX T. (Medicis) Coal tar 1%, benzyl alcohol. Shampoo. Bot. 240 ml.
Use: Antiseborrheic product.
THERAPLEX Z. (Medicis) Pyrithione zinc 1%. Shampoo. Bot. 240 ml.
Use: Antiseborrheic product.
THERAVEE HEMATINIC VITAMIN. (Vangard) Vitamins A 2.5 mg, D 3.3 mcg, thiamine 3.3 mg, riboflavin 3.3 mg, pyridoxine HCl 3.3 mg, niacinamide 33.3 mg, calcium pantothenate 11.7 mg, E 5 mg, copper 0.67 mg, magnesium 41.7 mg, iron 66.7 mg, B_{12} 50 mcg, folic acid 0.33 mcg, C 100 mg/Tab. Bot. 100s. UD 10×10s.
Use: Vitamin/mineral supplement.
THERAVEE M VITAMIN. (Vangard) Vitamin A 3 mg, D 10 mcg, E 15 mg, C 200 mg, thiamine 10.3 mg, riboflavin 10 mg, niacin 100 mg, B_6 4.1 mg, B_{12} 5 mcg, pantothenic acid 18.4 mg, iodine 150 mcg, iron 12 mg, magnesium 65 mg, copper 2 mg, zinc 1.5 mg, manganese 1 mg/Tab. Bot. 100s, 1000s. UD 10×10s.
Use: Vitamin/mineral supplement.
THERAVEE VITAMIN. (Vangard) Vitamins A 10,000 IU, D 400 IU, E 14 IU, C 200 mg, thiamine 10.3 mg, riboflavin 10 mg, niacin 100 mg, B_6 4 .1 mg, B_{12} 5 mcg, pantothenic acid 18.4 mg/Tab. Bot. 100s. UD Pkg. 250s.
Use: Vitamin supplement.
THERAVILAN CAPSULES. (Lannett) Vitamins A 25,000 IU, D 1000 IU, B_1 10 mg, B_2 5 mg, B_6 1 mg, C 150 mg, B_{12} 5 mcg, niacinamide 100 mg, dicalcium phosphate anhyd. 360 mg, ferrous sulfate dried 34 mg, potassium iodide 0.133 mg, manganese sulfate dried 3 mg, cobalt sulfate 0.49 mg, potassium sulfate 11 mg, sodium molybdate 0.45 mg, copper sulfate monohydrate 2.8 mg, zinc sulfate dried 3.9 mg, magnesium sulfate dried 40 mg/Cap. or Tab. **Cap.:** Bot. 100s, 500s, 1000s. **Tab.:** Bot. 100s, 1000s.
Use: Vitamin/mineral supplement.
THERAVIM M. (Geneva Generics) Iron 27 mg, vitamins A 5500 IU, D 400 IU, E 30 mg, B_1 3 mg, B_2 3.4 mg, B_3 30 mg, B_5 10 mg, B_6 3 mg, B_{12} 9 mcg, C 120 mg, folic acid 0.4 mg, Cl, Cr, Cu, I, K, Mg, Mn, Mo, Se, zinc 15 mg, biotin 15 mcg/Tab. Bot. 100s, 1000s.
Use: Vitamin/mineral supplement.
THEREMS. (Rugby) Vitamins A 5500 IU, D 400 IU, E 30 mg, B_1 3 mg, B_2 3.4 mg, B_3 30 mg, B_5 10 mg, B_6 3 mg, B_{12} 9 mcg, C 120 mg, folic acid 0.4 mg, biotin

15 mcg/Tab. Bot. 130s, 1000s.
Use: Vitamin supplement.

THEREMS-M. (Rugby) Iron 27 mg, vitamins A 5500 IU, D 400 IU, E 30 mg, B$_1$ 3 mg, B$_2$ 3.4 mg, B$_3$ 30 mg, B$_5$ 10 mg, B$_6$ 3 mg, B$_{12}$ 9 mcg, C 120 mg, folic acid 0.4 mg, Cl, Cr, Cu, I, K, Mg, Mn, Mo, Se, zinc 15 mg, biotin 15 mcg/Tab. Bot. 90s, 100s, 1000s.
Use: Vitamin supplement.

THEREVAC. (Bowman) Docusate potassium 283 mg, benzocaine 20 mg/Tube capsule w/soft soap in PEG 400 and glycerin base. Unit 4 ml, packages 4s, 12s, 50s.
Use: Disposable enema.

THEREVAC PLUS. (Jones Medical) Docusate sodium 283 mg, benzocaine 20 mg in a base of soft soap, PEG 400, glycerin/Cap. 3.9 Gm Jar 30s. Disposable enema.
Use: Laxative.

THEREVAC-SB. (Jones Medical) Docusate sodium 283 mg in a base of soft soap, PEG 400, glycerin/Cap. 3.9 Gm Bot. 30s. Disposable enema.
Use: Laxative.

THEREX NO. 1. (Blue Cross) Vit A 10,000 IU, D 400 IU, E 15 IU, C 200 mg, B$_1$ 10 mg, B$_2$ 10 mg, niacinamide 100 mg, B$_6$ 5 mg, B$_{12}$ 5 mcg, calcium pantothenate 20 mg/Tab. Bot. 100s.
Use: High potency vitamin supplement for adults.

THEREX AND ZINC. (Blue Cross).
Use: Dietary supplement.

THEREX-M. (Blue Cross) Vitamins A 10,000 IU, D 400 IU, E 15 IU, C 200 mg, B$_1$ 10 mg, B$_2$ 10 mg, niacinamide 100 mg, B$_6$ 5 mg, B$_{12}$ 5 mcg, calcium pantothenate 20 mg, iodine 150 mcg, iron 12 mg, Mg 65 mg, Cu 2 mg, zinc 1.5 mg, Mn 1 mg/Tab. Bot. 100s.
Use: Vitamin and mineral supplement.

THEREX-Z. (Blue Cross) Vitamins A 10,000 IU, D 400 IU, E 15 IU, C 200 mg, B$_1$ 10 mg, B$_2$ 10 mg, niacinamide 100 mg, B$_{12}$ 5 mcg, B$_6$ 5 mg, Ca pantothenate 20 mg, iodine 150 mcg, Cu 2 mg, iron 12 mg, Zn 22.5 mg/Tab. Bot. 100s.
Use: Vitamin, mineral supplement.

THERMA-KOOL. (Nortech) Compresses in following sizes: 3″ × 5″, 4″ 9″, 8.5″ 10.5″.
Use: Cold or hot compress.

THERMAZENE. (Sherwood) Silver sulfadiazine 1% in white pet. Cream. In 50, 400 and 1000 Gm.
Use: Treatment of second, third degree burns.

THERMODENT. (Mentholatum) Strontium Cl. 10%. Tubes.
Use: Toothpaste for sensitive teeth.

THERMOLENE. (Lannett) Sodium chloride 7 gr, dextrose 3 gr, Vitamins B$_1$ 1 mg/Tab. Bot. 1000s.
Use: Fluid/electrolyte replacement.

THERMOLOID. (Mills) Thyroid 1 gr, 2 gr, 3 gr, 4 gr, 5 gr/Tab. Bot. 100s.
Use: Thyroid hormone.

THEROAL. (Vangard) Theophylline 24 mg, ephedrine HCl 24 mg, phenobarbital 8 mg/Tab. Bot. 100s, 1000s.
Use: Antiasthmatic combination.

THEROXIDE WASH. (Medicis) Benzoyl peroxide 10%. Liq. 120 ml.
Use: Anti-acne.

THEXFORTE. (Lee) Vitamins B$_1$ 25 mg, B$_2$ 15 mg, B$_3$ 100 mg, B$_5$ 10 mg, B$_6$ 5 mg, C 500 mg. Cap. Bot. 75s.
Use: Vitamin supplement.

THIA. (Sig) Thiamine HCl 100 mg/ml. Vial 30 ml.
Use: Thiamine supplement.

• **THIABENDAZOLE,** U.S.P. XXIII. Oral Susp., Tab. U.S.P. XXIII. 1H-Benzimidazole,2-(4-thiazolyl)-2-(4-Thiazolyl)-benzimidazole.
Use: Anthelmintic.
See: Mintezol, Tab., Susp. (Merck & Co.).

THIACETARSAMIDE SODIUM. Sodium mercaptoacetate S,S-diester with p-carbamoyldithiobenzenearsonous acid.
Use: Antitrichomonal.

THIACETAZONE, B.A.N. p-Acetylaminobenzaldehyde thiosemicarbamazone.
Use: Treatment of tuberculosis and leprosy.

THIA-DIA-MER-SULFONAMIDES. Sulfadiazine w/sulfamerazine & sulfathiazole.
See: Trionamide, Tab. (O'Neal).

THIAHEP INJECTION. (Lannett) Liver ext. (derived from 10 U.S.P. Units injectable) 100 mg, liver ext. (derived from 10 U.S.P. Units crude liver) 100 mg, iron peptonate 20 mg, niacinamide 50 mg, pyridoxine HCl 0.3 mg, riboflavin 3 mg/2 ml multiple dose Vial 300 ml.

THIALBARBITAL.
See: Kemithal.

THIALBARBITONE. B.A.N. 5-Allyl-5-(cyclohex-2-enyl)-2-thiobarbituric acid.
Use: Anesthetic.

THIAMAZOLE (I.N.N.). Methimazole, B.A.N.

THIAMBUTOSINE. B.A.N. 1-(4-Butoxyphenyl)-3-(4-dimethylaminophenyl)thiourea.

Use: Treatment of leprosy.
• **THIAMINE HYDROCHLORIDE,** U.S.P. XXIII. Elixir, Inj., Tab., U.S.P. XXIII. 3-[(4-amino-2-methyl-5-pyrimidinyl)-methyl]-5-(2-hydroxyethyl)-4-methyl-, chloride, monohydrochloride. Aneurine HCl, thiamine chloride, Vitamins B₁ HCl. Thiazolium,
Use: Enzyme co-factor vitamin.
See: Apatate (Kenwood).
Betalin S, Amp., Elixir, Tab. (Lilly).
Thia, Vial (Sig).
• **THIAMINE MONONITRATE,** U.S.P. XXIII. Elixir, U.S.P. XXIII. Thiazolium, 3-[(4-amino-2-methyl-5-pyrimidinyl)-methyl]-5-(2-hydroxyethyl)-4-methyl-, nitrate (salt). (Various Mfr.) Thiamine nitrate.
Use: Enzyme co-factor vitamin.
W/Sodium salicylate, colchicine.
See: Sodsylate, Tab. (Durst).
• **THIAMIPRINE.** USAN. 2-Amino-6-[(1-methyl-4-nitroimidazol-5-yl)thio] purine.
Use: Antileukemic.
• **THIAMPHENICOL.** USAN.
Use: Antibacterial.
• **THIAMYLAL,** U.S.P. XXIII.
• **THIAMYLAL SODIUM, FOR INJECTION,** U.S.P. XXIII. Sodium 5-allyl-5-(1-methylbutyl)-2-thiobarbiturate.
Use: Anesthetic (systemic).
See: Surital Sodium, Prep. (Parke-Davis).
THIAPHYLL CREAM. (Lannett) Sulfathiazole 5%, chlorophyllin 1%. Jar 4 oz. & 1 lb.
Use: Wound healing agent.
• **THIAZESIM.** USAN. 5-(2-Dimethylaminoethyl) 2,3-dihydro-2-phenyl-1,5-benzothiazepin-4-one.
Use: Antidepressant.
THIAZESIM HCl. 5-[2-(Dimethylamino)-ethyl]-2,3- dihydro-2-phenylbenzo-1,5-thiazepin-4-(5H)-one hydrochloride.
Use: Antidepressant.
• **THIAZINAMINIUM CHLORIDE.** USAN.
Use: Anti-allergic.
THIETHANOMELAMINE.
See: Tretamine, B.A.N.
THIETHYLENE THIOPHOSPHORAMIDE.
See: Thiotepa, B.A.N.
• **THIETHYLPERAZINE.** USAN. 2-Ethyl-thio-10-[3-(4-methylpiperazin-1-yl)propyl]phenothiazine.
Use: Central nervous system depressant.
See: Torecan.
THIETHYLPERAZINE MALEATE,U.S.P. XXI. Inj., Suppos., Tab., U.S.P. XXI. Torecan, 2-Ethyl-mercapto-10-[3′-(1″-methyl-piperazinyl-4″propyl-1″]phenoth-

iazine maleate. 2-(Ethylthio)-10-[3-(4-methyl-1-piperazinyl)propyl]phenothiazine maleate (1:2).
Use: Antiemetic.
See: Norzine, Inj., Supp., Tab. (Purdue Frederick).
Torecan, Amp., Supp., Tab.
(Boehringer Ingelheim).
THIHEXINOL METHYLBROMIDE. alpha-Dithienyl-(4-dimethylamino-cyclohexyl)-carbinolmethbromide. [4-(Hydroxydi-2-thienylmethyl)cyclohexyl] trime- thylammonium Bromide.
Use: Anticholinergic.
• **THIMERFONATE SODIUM.** USAN. Ethyl(hydrogen p-mercaptobenzenesulfonato)mercury sodium salt; Sodium p-[(ethylmercuri)-thio] benzenesulfonate. Sulfo-Merthiolate (Lilly).
Use: Topical anti-infective.
• **THIMEROSAL,** U.S.P. XXIII. Topical Aerosol, Topical Soln., Tr., U.S.P. XXIII. Sod. Ethylmercurithiosalicylate. Sodium Ethyl (Sodium o-mercaptobenzoate)mercury.
Use: Local anti-infective; pharmaceutical aid (preservative).
See: Aeroaid, Aerosol (Aeroceuticals). Merphol Tincture 1:1000, Liq.(Bowman).
Mersol, Liq. (Century).
Merthiolate, Prep. (Lilly).
THIOCARBANIDIN. Under study.
Use: Tuberculosis.
THIOCARLIDE. B.A.N. 1,3-Di-(4-isopentyloxyphenyl)thiourea.
Use: Treatment of tuberculosis.
THIOCYANATE SODIUM. Sodium thiocyanate.
Use: Hypotensive.
THIODINONE. Name used for Nifuratel.
THIODIPHENYLAMINE.
See: Phenothiazine.
THIOFURADENE. 1[(5-Nitrofurfurylidene)-amino]-2-imidazolidinethione.
THIOGLYCEROL.
W/Sod. citrate, phenol, benzyl alcohol.
See: Sulfo-ganic, Vial (Marcen).
• **THIOGUANINE,**U.S.P. XXIII. Tab. U.S.P. XXIII. 6H-Purine-6-thione,2-amino-1,7-dihydro-.2-Amino-purine-6-thiol, hemihydrate. Tabloid (Burroughs Wellcome) 40 mg, Bot. 25s.
Use: Antineoplastic agent.
THIOHEXAMIDE. N-(p-Methyl-mercaptophenylsulfonyl)-N′-cyclohexylurea.
Use: Blood sugar lowering compound.
THIOISONICOTINAMIDE. Under study.
Use: Antituberculosis drug.
THIOLA. (Mission). Tiopronin 100 mg.

Tablets: In 100s.
Use: Kidney stone prevantative.
THIOMERSAL. B.A.N. Sodium salt of(2-carboxyphenylthio)ethylmercury.
Sodium ethylmercurithiosalicylate.
Thimerosal.
Thiomersalate.
Use: Antiseptic; preservative.
See: Merthiolate.
THIOMESTERONE. B.A.N. 1α,7α-Bis-(acetylthio)-17β-hydroxy-17α-methylandrost-4-en-3-one.
Use: Anabolic steroid.
THIOPENTAL SODIUM. (IMS) Thiopental sodium 20 mg/ml or 25 mg/ml. Pow. for Inj. **20 mg/ml:** 400 mg *Min-I-Mix* vial w/ injector; **25 mg/ml:** 250 or 500 mg *Min-I-Mix* vials w/ injector; 500 mg, 1 g, 2.5 g, 5 g, 10 g kits.
Use: General anesthetic.
• **THIOPENTAL SODIUM,** U.S.P. XXIII. Inj., U.S.P. XXIII. Sodium5-ethyl-5-(1-methylbutyl)-2-thiobarbiturate. Thiopentone sodium.
Use: Anesthetic (intravenous), anticonvulsant.
See: Pentothal Sodium, Amp. (Abbott).
THIOPHOSPHORAMIDE.
See: ThioTepa, Vial (Lederle).
THIOPROPAZATE. B.A.N. 10-[3-[4-(2-Acetoxy-ethyl)piperazin-1-yl]propyl]-2-chlorophenothiazine.
Use: Tranquilizer.
THIOPROPAZATE HYDROCHLORIDE.
2-Chloro-10-[3-[(2-acetoxyethyl)-4-piperazinyl]-propyl]phenothiazine dihydrochloride.4-[3-(2-Chlorophenothiazine-10-yl)propyl]-1-piperazine ethanol Acetate Dihydrochloride.
Use: Tranquilizer.
THIOPROPERAZINE. B.A.N. 2-Dimethylsulfamoyl-10-[3-(4-methylpiperazin-1-yl)propyl]phenothiazine.
Use: Tranquilizer; antiemetic.
THIOPROPERAZINE MESYLATE. N,N-Dimethyl-10-[3-(4-methyl-1-piperazinyl)propyl] phenothiazine-2-sulfonamide dimethanesulfonate.
Use: Central depressant; antiemetic.
• **THIORIDAZINE,** U.S.P. XXIII. Oral Susp., U.S.P. XXIII. 10-[2-(1-Methyl-2-piperidyl)ethyl]-2-methylthiopheno- thiazine.
Use: Tranquilizer, sedative.
See: Mellaril, Susp. (Sandoz).
• **THIORIDAZINE HCl,** U.S.P. XXIII. Oral Soln., Tab., U.S.P. XXIII. 10-[-2-(1-Methyl-2-piperidyl)-ethyl]-2- (methylthio) phenothiazine hydrochloride. 10H-Phenothiazine, 10-[2-(1-methyl-2-

piperidinyl)-ethyl]-2-(methylthio)-, monohydrochloride.
Use: Tranquilizer.
See: Mellaril, Tabs., Soln. (Sandoz).
THIORIDAZINE HCL CONCENTRATE.
(Various Mfr.) Thioridazine HCl **30 mg/ml.** Bot. 120 ml. **100 mg/ml.** Bot 120 ml, 3.4 ml (UD 100s).
Use: Antipsychotic agent.
THIORIDAZINE HYDROCHLORIDE INTENSOL ORAL SOLUTION. (Roxane) Thioridazine HCl oral concentrated soln. 30 mg/ml or 100 mg/ml. Bot. 120 ml w/calibrated dropper.
Use: Antipsychotic agent.
• **THIOSALAN.** USAN. 3,4',5-Tribromo-2-mercaptobenzanilide. Under study.
Use: Germicide, disinfectant.
THIOSALICYLIC ACID SALT.
• **THIOTEPA,** U.S.P. XXIII. For Inj., U.S.P. XXIII. Thiophosphoramide. N, Tris(1-Aziridinyl) phosphine sulfide. (Lederle) Triethylenethiophosphoramide 15 mg/Vial.
Use: Antineoplastic.
THIOTEPA. (Lederle) The ethylenimine-type N, N; N''-Triethylene thiophosphoramide. Powder for reconstitution: Thiotepa powder 15 mg, sodium chloride 80 mg, sodium bicarbonate 50 mg/Vial. Vial 15 mg.
Use: Antineoplastic agent.
• **THIOTHIXENE,** U.S.P. XXIII. Cap., U.S.P. XXIII. N,N,-Dimethyl-9-(3-(4-methyl-1-piperazinyl)propylidene)thioxanthene-2-sulfonamide. As HCl salt.
Use: Psychotherapeutic agent.
See: Navane, Cap., Vial (Roerig).
Navane Concentrate Solution (Roerig).
• **THIOTHIXENE HCl,** U.S.P. XXIII. Inj., Oral Soln., U.S.P. XXIII.
Use: Antipsychotic.
See: Navane Hydrochloride (Pfizer).
THIOTHIXENE HCl INTENSOL. (Roxane) Thiothixene HCl 5 mg/ml. Soln. Bot. 30 ml, 120 ml with dropper.
Use: Antipsychotic agent.
THIOURACIL. 2-Thiouracil.
Use: Treatment of hyperthyroidism, angina pectoris, congestive heart failure.
THIOUREA. (City Chem.) Pow., Bot., lb.
Use: Antithyroid agent.
THIOXANTHENES.
See: Chlorprothixine (Taractan Roche).
Navane (Roerig).
Thiothixine (Various Mfr.).
THIOXANTHENE DERIVATIVE.
See: Taractan, Prep. (Roche).

THIOXOLONE. B.A.N. 6-Hydroxy-1,3-benzoxathiol-2-one.
Use: Keratolytic agent.

THIPHENAMIL. F.D.A. S-[2-(Diethylamino)-ethyl]-diphenylthioacetate.

• **THIPHENCILLIN POTASSIUM.** USAN.
(1) Potassium 3,3-dimethyl-7-oxo-6-[2-(phenylthio)acetamido]-4-thia-1-azabicyclo[3.2.0] heptane-2-carboxylate; (2) Potassium 6-(phenylmercaptoacetamido)penicillanate.
Use: Antibacterial.

THIPYRI-12. (Sig) Vitamins B_1 1000 mg, B_6 1000 mg, cyanocobalamin (B_{12}) 10,000 mcg, sod. chloride 0.5%, sod. bisulfite 0.1%, benzyl alcohol (as preservative) 0.9%. Univial 10 ml.

• **THIRAM.** USAN. Bis(dimethylthiocarbamoyl) disulfide.
Use: Antifungal.

THIXO-FLUR TOPICAL GEL. (Hoyt) Acidulated phosphate sodium fluoride in gel base 1.2%. Bot. 32 oz. 8 oz., 4 oz.
Use: Dental caries prevention.

• **THONZONIUM BROMIDE,** U.S.P. XXII.
Hexadecyl [2-[(p-methoxybenzyl)-2-pyrimidinylamino]ethyl]dimethylammonium bromide.
Use: Detergent.
W/Colistin base, neomycin base, hydrocortisone acetate, polysorbate 80, acetic acid, sodium acetate.
See: Coly-Mycin-S, Otic, Liq. (Warner-Chilcott).
W/Isoproterenol.
See: Nebair, Aerosol (Warner-Chilcott).
W/Neomycin sulfate, gramicidin, thonzylamine HCl, phenylephrine HCl.
See: Biomydrin, Spray, Drops (Warner-Chilcott).

THONZYLAMINE. B.A.N. 2-[N-p-Anisyl-N-(pyrimidin-2-yl)amino]ethyldimethylamine.
Use: Antihistamine.

THONZYLAMINE HYDROCHLORIDE.
2[[2-(Dimethylamino)ethyl](p-methoxybenzyl)amino]pyrimidine monohydrochloride.
Use: Antihistamine.

THORAZINE. (SK-Beecham) Chlorpromazine HCl, **Tab.:** (10, 25, 50, 100, 200 mg) Bot. 100s, 1000s. Single unit pkg. 100s.
Amp.: (25 mg w/ascorbic acid 2 mg, sodium bisulfite 1 mg, sodium sulfite 1 mg, NaCl 6 mg/1 ml), 1 ml, 2 ml. Box 10s, 100s, 500s. Vial: 10 ml. Box 1s, 20s, 100s.
Spansule: 30, 75, 150 & 200 mg Bot. 50s, 100s (S.U.P.), 500s. 300 mg Bot.

50s, 100s (S.U.P.).
Syr.: (10 mg/5 ml) Bot. 4 oz.
Supp.: Chlorpromazine base, w/glycerin, glyceryl monopalmitate, glyceryl monostearate, hydrogenated coconut oil fatty acids, hydrogenated palm kernel oil fatty acids. (25, 100 mg) Box 12.
Conc.: (30 mg/ml) Bot. 4 oz. in Ctn. 36s., 1 gal. (100 mg/ml) Bot. 8 oz.
Use: Antiemetic. Neuropsychiatric disorders.

THORETS. (Buffington) Benzocaine lozenge. Dispens-A-Kits 500s. Sugar, lactose and salt free.
Use: Sore throat relief.

THOR-PROM TABS. (Major) Chlorpromazine 10 mg, 25 mg, 50 mg, or 100 mg Tab. Bot. 100s, 1000s; 200 mg/Tab. Bot. 250s, 1000s.
Use: Antiemetic, neuropsychiatric disorders.

THOR SYRUP. (Towne) Dextromethorphan HBr 90 mg, pyrilamine maleate 22.5 mg, phenylephrine HCl 10 mg, ephedrine sulfate 15mg, sod. citrate 325 mg, ammon. chloride 650 mg, guaifenesin 50 mg,/fl. oz. Bot. 4 oz.
Use: Antitussive, antihistamine, decongestant, expectorant.

• **THOZALINONE.** USAN. 2-Dimethylamino-5-phenyl-2-oxazolin-4-one.
Use: Antidepressant.
See: Stimsen (Lederle).

THREAMINE DM. (Various Mfr.) Phenylpropanolamine HCl 12.5 mg, chlorpheniramine maleate 2 mg, dextromethorphan HBr 10 mg/5 ml Syr. Bot. pt., gal.
Use: Antihistamine, decongestant, antitussive.

THREE-AMINE TD. (Vitarine) Phenylpropanolamine HBr 50 mg, pheniramine maleate 25 mg, pyrilamine maleate 25 mg/Time Rel. Cap.
Use: Antihistamine and decongestant.

• **THREONINE.** U.S.P. XXIII. $C_4H_9NO_3$ as L-threonine.
Use: Amino acid, antispasmodic. [Orphan drug]
See: Threostat.

THREONINE. (Various Mfr.) Threonine 500 mg. **Capsules:** In 60s and 100s. **Tablets:** In 100s and 250s.
Use: Oral nutritional supplements.

THREOSTAT. (Tyson)
Use: Antispasmodic.
See: Threonine.

THROAT DISCS. (SK-Beecham) Capsicum, peppermint, anise, cubeb, glycyrrhiza, linseed. Box 60s.
Use: Minor throat irritations.

THROAT-EZE. (Faraday) Cetylpyridinium chloride 1:3000, cetyl dimethyl benzyl ammonium chloride 1:3000, benzocaine 10 mg/Wafer. Loz., foil wrapped. Vial 15.
Use: Anesthetic lozenge.

THROMBATE III.
See: ANTITHROMBIN III HUMAN.

•**THROMBIN,** U.S.P. XXIII. Thrombin, topical, mammalian origin.
(Parke-Davis)—Thrombin, Topical (Bovine).
(Upjohn)—Vial (1000u.) 30 ml.
Use: Local hemostatic.

THROMBINAR. (Jones Medical) Thrombin topical. Vial 1000, 5000, 10,000, 50,000 U.S. Standard Units.
Use: hemostat.

THROMBOGEN. (Johnson & Johnson) Thrombin 1000, 5000, 10,000, 20,000 vial, isotonic saline diluent and transfer needle (except 1000 unit vial). Pow. Spray kit 10,000, 20,000 unit w/isotonic saline diluent.
Use: Hemostatic, topical.

THROMBOLYTIC ENZYMES.
See: Abbokinaise (Abbott).
Abbokinase Open-Cath (Abbott).

THROMBOPLASTIN.
Use: Diagnostic aid (prothrombin estimation).

THROMBOSTAT. (Parke-Davis) Prothrombin is activated by tissue thromboplastin in the presence of calcium chloride. **1000 U.S. (N.I.H.) units.** Vial 10 ml. **5000 U.S. units.** Vial 10 ml and 5 ml diluent. **10,000 U.S. units.** Vial 20 ml and 10 ml diluent. **20,000 U.S. units.** Vial 30 ml and 20 ml diluent.
Use: Local hemostatic.

THURFYL NICOTINATE. B.A.N. Tetrahydrofurfuryl nicotinate. Trafuril.
Use: Topical vasodilator.

THYCAL. (Mills) Thermoloid (thyroid) 2 gr, iodized calcium 2 gr, peptone 1 gr/Tab. Bot. 1000s.

THYLOX. (C.S. Dent) Medicated bar soap w/absorbable sulfur. Bar 3.4 oz.
Use: Cleansing aid.

•**THYMOL,** N.F. XVIII. Phenol, 5-methyl-2-(1-methylethyl)- p-Cymen-3-ol. (Var. Mfr.) 0.25 lb., 1 lb.
Use: Antifungal, anti-infective local anesthetic, antitussive, nasal decongestant.
See: Vicks Regular & Wild Cherry Medicated Cough Drops (Vicks).
Vicks Vaporub, Oint. (Vicks).
W/Combinations.
See: Listerine Antiseptic, Soln. (Warner-Lambert).

THYMOL IODIDE.
Use: Antifungal; anti-infective.

THYMOSIN ALPHA-1.
Use: Adjunctive treatment of hepatitis B. [Orphan drug]

THYMOXAMINE. B.A.N. 4-(2-Dimethylamino-ethoxy)-5-isopropyl-2-methylphenyl acetate. Moxisylyte (I.N.N.) Opilon [hydrochloride].
Use: Peripheral vasodilator.

THYODATIL. Name used for Nifuratel.

THYPINONE. (Abbott Diagnostics) Protirelin 500 mcg/1 ml Amp.
Use: Adjunctive agent in the diagnostic assessment of thyroid function.

THYRAR. (Rhone-Poulenc Rorer) Bovine thyroid preparation 0.5 gr, 1 gr, 2 gr/Tab. Bot. 100s.
Use: Hypothyroid states.

THYRO-BLOCK. (Wallace) Potassium iodide 130 mg/Tab. In 14s.
Use: Thyroid drug.

THYROBROM. (Mills) Brominated thyroid. Tab. or S.C. Tab. (1 gr, 2 gr, 3 gr, 4 gr) Bot. 1000s.
Use: Thyroid therapy.

•**THYROID,** U.S.P. XXIII. Tab., U.S.P. XXIII.
Use: Thyroid hormone.
See: Arco Thyroid, Tab. (Arco).
Armour Thyroid, Tab. (Rhone-Poulenc Rorer).
Delcoid, Tab. (Delco).
Marion Thyroid, Tab. (Marion).
S-P-T., Cap. (Fleming).
Thermoloid, Tab. (Mills).
Thyrocrine, Tab. (Lemmon).

THYROID BROMINATED.
See: Thyrobrom, Tab. (Mills).

THYROID COMBINATIONS.
See: Henydin, Prep. (Arcum).
Thycal, Tab. (Mills).

THYROID DESICCATED.
Use: Thyroid hormone.
See: Armour Thyroid (Rhone-Poulenc Rorer).
S-P-T (Fleming).
Thyrar (Rhone-Poulenc Rorer).
Thyroid Strong (Jones Medical).
Thyroid USP (Various Mfr.).

THYROID DIAGNOSTIC AIDS.
Use: In vivo diagnostic aid.
See: Relefact TRH (Hoechst-Roussel).
Sodium Iodide I 123 (Mallinckrodt Diagnostics).
Thypinone (Abbott).
Thytropar (Armour).

THYROID HORMONES.
See: Liothyronine Sod.
Thyroxin (Various Mfr.).

THYROID PREPARATIONS.
See: Proloid, Tab. (Parke-Davis).
Thyrar, Tab. (Rhone-Poulenc Rorer).
Thyrobrom, Tab. (Mills).
Thyroxin, Prep. (Var. Mfr.).
THYROID STIMULATING HORMONE (TSH).
Use: Adjunct in diagnosis of thyroid cancer. [Orphan drug]
THYROID STRONG. (Jones Medical) Thyroid desiccated 30 mg, 60 mg, 120 mg/Tab. Bot. 100s, 1000s; 30 mg, 120 mg, 180 mg Tab. Bot. 100s; 60 mg/sugar coated. Tab. Bot. 100s, 1000s.
Use: Thyroid hormone.
THYROLAR. (Forest) Liotrix. 0.25 gr/Tab. Bot. 100s; 0.5 gr, 1 gr, 2 gr, 3 gr/Tab. Bot. 100s, 1000s.
Use: Thyroid hormone.
• **THYROMEDAN HYDROCHLORIDE.** USAN. 2-(Die- thylamino)ethyl [3,5-diiodo-4-(3-iodo-4-methoxy-phenoxy) phenyl] acetate hydrochloride.
Use: Thyromimetic.
THYROPROPIC ACID. 4-(4-Hydroxy-3-iodophenoxy)-3,5-diiodohydrocinnamic acid. Triopron (Warner Chilcott).
Use: Anticholesteremic.
THYROTROPHIN. B.A.N. Thyrotrophic hormone. Thytropar; Thytrophin.
THYROTROPIC HORMONE.
Use: In vivo diagnostic aid.
See: Thytropar (Armour).
THYROTROPIC PRINCIPLE OF BOVINE ANTERIOR PITUITARY GLANDS.
See: Thytropar, Vial (Armour Labs.).
THYROTROPIN.
Use: In vivo diagnostic aid.
See: Thytropar (Armour).
THYROTROPIN-RELEASING HORMONE.
Use: In vivo diagnostic aid.
See: Relefact TRH (Hoechst-Roussell). Thypinone (Abbott).
• **THYROXINE I-125.** USAN.
Use: Radioactive agent.
• **THYROXINE I-131.** USAN.
Use: Radioactive agent.
THYROZYME-II A. (Abbott Diagnostics) T-4 diagnostic kit. 100 & 500 test units.
Use: Quantitative measurement of unsaturated thyroxine binding globulin in serum.
THYTROPAR. (Armour) Thyrotropin from bovine anterior pituitary glands. Thyrotropin, B.A.N. Vial 10 IU.
Use: Thyroid myxedema due to pituitary insufficiency.
TIACRILAST. USAN.
Use: Anti-allergic.

• **TIAMENIDINE HYDROCHLORIDE.** USAN.
Use: Antihypertensive.
• **TIAMULIN.** USAN.
Use: Antibacterial.
• **TIAMULIN FUMARATE.** USAN.
Use: Antibacterial.
• **TIAPAMIL HYDROCHLORIDE.** USAN.
Use: Antagonist (to calcium).
• **TIARAMIDE HYDROCHLORIDE.** USAN.
Use: Anti-asthmatic.
• **TIAZOFURIN.** USAN.
Use: Antineoplastic.
• **TIAZURIL.** USAN.
Use: Coccidiostat.
TI-BABY NATURAL. (Fischer) Titanium dioxide 5%. SPF 16. Lot. Bot. 120 ml.
Use: Sunscreen.
• **TIBENELAST SODIUM.** USAN.
• **TIBOLONE.** USAN. (1) 17-Hydroxy-7α-methyl-19-nor-17α-pregn-5(10)-en-20-yn-3-one; (2) 17α-Ethynyl-17-hydroxy-7α-methyl-5 (10)-estren-3-one.
Use: Anabolic.
• **TIBRIC ACID.** USAN. 2-Chloro-5-(cis-3,5-dimethylpiperidinosulfonyl)benzoic acid.
Use: Treatment of hyperlipemia.
• **TIBROFAN.** USAN. 4,4',5-Tribromo-2-thiophenecarboxanilide. Under study.
Use: Disinfectant.
• **TICABESONE PROPIONATE.** USAN.
Use: Glucocorticoid.
TICAR. (Beecham Labs) Ticarcillin disodium. 1 Gm, 3 Gm, 6 Gm/Vial in 10s. Piggyback Vials 3 Gm in 10s. Bulk Pharmacy Pkg. 20 Gm in 10s. Bulk Pharmacy Pkg. 30 Gm/Vial, 10s. ADD-Vantage 3 Gm Pkg. 10s.
Use: Antibiotic.
• **TICARBODINE,** USAN. α,α,α-Trifluoro-2,6-dimethylthio-1-piperidinecarboxy-m-toluidide. 2,6-Dimethylpiperidino-3'-(trifluoromethyl)thioformanilide.
Use: Anthelmintic.
• **TICARCILLIN CRESYL SODIUM.** USAN.
Use: Antibacterial.
• **TICARCILLIN DISODIUM, STERILE,** U.S.P. XXIII. 6-[2-Carboxy-2-(3-thienyl)-acetamido]penicillanic acid.
Use: Antibiotic.
See: Ticar, inj. (Beecham Labs.).
• **TICARCILLIN DISODIUM AND CLAVULANATE POTASSIUM, STERILE,** U.S.P. XXII.
Use: Antibiotic, inhibitor (β-lactamase).
TICE BCG VACCINE. (Organon) BCG. Intravesical 50 mg/2 ml amps. Freeze-dried suspension for reconstitution.
Use: Antineoplastic.

• **TICLATONE.** USAN. 6-Chloro-1,2-benzisothiazolin-3-one.
Use: Antibacterial, antifungal.

TICLID. (Syntex) Ticlopidine 250 mg/Tab. Bot. 30s, 100s.
Use: Antiplatelet agent.

• **TICLOPIDINE HYDROCHLORIDE.** USAN.
Use: Inhibitor (platelet).

TICON. (Hauck) Trimethobenzamide HCl 100 mg per ml/Inj. Vial 20 ml.
Use: Antiemetic/antivertigo agent.

• **TICONAZOLE.** U.S.P. XXIII.
Use: Vaginal antifungal.
See: Vagistat-1, Oint. (Bristol-Myers Squibb).

• **TICRYNAFEN.** USAN.
Use: Diuretic, uricosuric, antihypertensive.

TIDEX. (Allison) Dextroamphetamine sulfate, 5 mg/Tab. Bot. 100s, 1000s.
Use: Obesity control.

TIDEXSOL TABLETS. (Sanofi Winthrop) Acetaminophen.
Use: Analgesic, antipyretic.

TIEMONIUM IODIDE. B.A.N. 4-[3-Hydroxy-3-phenyl-3-(2-thienyl)propyl]-4-methylmorpholinium iodide.
Use: Antispasmodic; anticholinergic.

• **TIFURAC SODIUM.** USAN.
Use: Analgesic.

TIGAN. (Beecham Labs) Trimethobenzamide hydrochloride. **Cap.** 100 mg Bot. 100s, 250 mg Bot. 100s. **Amp.** (100 mg/ml) 2 ml. Box 10s. Vial 20 ml **Supp.** 200 mg Box 10s, 50s. **Pediatric Supp.** 100 mg Box 10s.
Use: Nausea and vomiting.

• **TIGEMONAM PICHOLINE.** USAN.

• **TIGESTOL.** USAN. (1) 19-Nor-17α-pregn-5(10)-en-20-yn-17-ol; (2) 17-α-Ethynyl-5(10)-estren-17-ol. Under study.
Use: Progestin.

TIGLOIDINE. B.A.N. Tiglyl-pseudotropeine. Tiglyssin [hydrobromide]
Use: Treatment of the Parkinsonian syndrome.

TIGO. (Burlington) Polymyxin B sulfate 5,000 u., zinc bacitracin 400 u., neomycin sulfate 5 mg/Gm Oint. Tube 0.5 oz.
Use: Triple antibiotic.

TIHIST-DP. (Vita Elixir) d-methorphan HBr 10 mg, pyrilamine maleate 16 mg, sodium citrate 3.3 gr/5 ml.
Use: Cough syrup.

TIHIST NASAL DROPS. (Vita Elixir) Pyril-

amine maleate 0.1%, phenylephrine HCl 0.25%, sodium bisulfite 0.2%, methylparaben 0.02%, propylparaben 0.01%/30 ml.
Use: Nasal decongestant.

TIJA TABLETS. (Vita Elixir) Oxytetracycline HCl 250 mg/Tab.
Use: Antibiotic.

TIJA SYRUP. (Vita Elixir) Oxytetracycline HCl 125 mg/5 ml.
Use: Antibiotic.

TILADE. (Fisons) Nedocromil sodium. 1.75 mg per actuation. Aerosol/Can. 16.2 Gm with mouthpiece.
Use: Respiratory inhalant (anti-inflammatory).

• **TILETAMINE HCl,** USAN. 2-(Ethylamino)-2-(2-thienyl)cyclohexanone HCl.
Use: Anesthetic; anticonvulsant.

TILIDATE. B.A.N. Ethyl 2-dimethylamino-1-phenylcyclohex-3-ene-1-carboxylate.
Use: Analgesic.

• **TILIDINE HCl.** USAN. (±)-Ethyl trans-2-(dime-thylamino)-1-phenyl-3-cyclohexene-1-carboxylate HCl.
Use: Analgesic.

TI-LITE. (Fischer) Ethylhexyl p methoxycinnamate 7.5%, titanium dioxide 2%, cetyl alcohol, phenethyl alcohol, parabens, EDTA. Cream 60 g.
Use: Sunscreen.

• **TILMICOSIN PHOSPHATE.** USAN.
Use: Antibacterial agent (veterinary).

• **TILOMISOLE.** USAN.
Use: Immunoregulator.

• **TILORONE HCl.** USAN. 2,7-Bis[2-(diethylamino)ethoxy]fluoren-9-one dihydrochloride.
Use: Antiviral.

• **TILUDRONATE DISODIUM.** USAN.
Use: Paget's disease, osteoporosis.

TIMED REDUCING AIDS-CAFFEINE FREE. (Weeks & Leo) Phenylpropanolamine HCl 75 mg/T.R. Cap. Bot. 28s, 56s.
Use: Reducing aid.

• **TIMEFURONE.** USAN.
Use: Anti-atherosclerotic.

TIMENTIN. (Beecham Labs) Ticarcillin disodium 3 Gm, clavulanic acid (as potassium salt) 0.1 Gm. Vials 3.1 Gm, Box 10s. Piggyback Vials 3.1 Gm, Box 10s.
Use: Antibacterial.

• **TIMOBESONE ACETATE.** USAN.
Use: Adrenocortical steroid (topical).

TIMOLIDE. (Merck & Co.) Timolol maleate 10 mg, hydrochlorothiazide 25 mg/Tab. Bot. 100s.
Use: Antihypertensive.

• **TIMOLOL.** USAN.
Use: Anti-adrenergic (beta-receptor).
• **TIMOLOL MALEATE,** U.S.P. XXIII. Ophth. Soln., Tab., U.S.P. XXIII. (S)-1-[(1, 1-dimethylethyl) amino]-3-[[4-(4 morpholinyl)-1,2,5-thiadiazol-3-yl]oxy]-2-propanol, (Z)-butenedioate (1:1) salt.
Use: Treatment of chronic open angle, aphakic and secondary glaucoma, antihypertensive, prevention of recurrent M.I.
See: Blocadren, Tab. (Merck & Co.)
Timoptic, Oph. (Merck & Co.).
Timoptic In Ocudose, Oph. (Merck & Co.).
• **TIMOLOL MALEATE AND HYDROCHLOROTHIAZIDE TABLETS,** U.S.P. XXIII.
Use: Antihypertensive.
See: Timolide,Tab. (Merck & Co.).
TIMOPTIC. (Merck & Co.) Timolol maleate 0.25% and 0.5% solution. Ocumeter Ophthalmic Dispenser 2.5 ml, 5 ml, 10 ml, 15 ml.
Use: Beta-adrenergic blocking agent.
TIMOPTIC IN OCUDOSE. (Merck & Co.) Timolol maleate 0.25% or 0.5%. Preservative-free in sterile occudose ophthalmic UD dispenser.
Use: Beta-adrenergic blocking agent.
TIMOPTIC-XE. (Merck) Timolol maleate 0.25% or 0.5%. Gel. Tube 2.5 ml, 5 ml.
Use: Beta-adrenergic blocking agent.
• **TINABINOL.** USAN.
Use: Antihypertensive.
TINACTIN. (Schering) **Soln. 1%:** Tolnaftate (10 mg/ml) w/butylated hydroxytoluene, in nonaqueous homogeneous PEG 400. Plastic squeeze bot. 10 ml.
Cream 1%: Tolnaftate (10 mg/Gm) in homogeneous, nonaqueous vehicle of PEG-400, propylene glycol, carboxypolymethylene, monoamylamine, titanium dioxide and butylated hydroxytoluene. Tube 15 Gm, 30 Gm, UD 0.7 Gm. **Powder 1%:** Tolnaftate w/corn starch, talc. Plastic container 45 Gm, 90 Gm. **Powd. Aerosol 1%:** Tolnaftate w/butylated hydroxytoluene, talc. polyethylene-polypropylene glycol monobutyl ether and inert propellant of isobutane. Spray can 100 Gm. **Liq. Aerosol 1%:** Tolnaftate w/butylated hydroxytoluene, polyethylene-polyproplyene glycol monobutyl ether, 36% alcohol, and inert propellant of isobutane. Spray can 120 ml.
Use: Topical fungicidal agent.
TINASTAT. (Vita Elixir) Sodium hyposulfite, benzethonium Cl./2 oz.
Use: Keratolytic lotion.
TINAVAL POWDER. (Vale) Tolnaftate 1%. Bot. 45 Gm.
Use: Antifungal for jock itch, athlete's foot.
TINDAL. (Schering) Acetophenazine maleate 20 mg/Tab. Bot. 100s.
Use: Tranquilizer.
TINE TEST, OLD TUBERCULIN, Rosenthal. (Lederle).
See: Tuberculin Tine Test (Lederle).
TINE TEST, PURIFIED PROTEIN DERIVATIVE. (Lederle).
See: Tuberculin Tine Test (Lederle).
TIN FLUORIDE. Stannous Fluoride, U.S.P. XXIII.
TING. (Pharmacraft) **Cream:** Benzoic acid, boric acid, zinc oxide, zinc stearate, alcohol 18.7%. Tube 0.9 oz., 1.8 oz. **Powder:** Boric acid, benzoic acid, zinc stearate, zinc oxide. Can 2.5 oz. **Spray Powder:** Total undecylenate 19% as undecylenic acid and zinc undecylenate. Can 2.5 oz.
Use: Fungus infections, athlete's foot.
• **TINIDAZOLE.** USAN. 1-[2-(Ethylsulfonyl)-ethyl]-2- methyl-5-nitroimidazole.
Use: Antiprotozoal.
See: Fasigyn (Pfizer).
Simplotan (Pfizer).
TINSET. (Janssen) Oxatomide.
Use: Anti-allergenic, anti-asthmatic.
TINVER LOTION. (Barnes-Hind) Sodium thiosulfate 25%, salicylic acid 1%, isopropyl alcohol 10%, propylene glycol, menthol, disodium edetate, colloidal alumina. Bot. 4 oz., 6 oz.
Use: Specific for tinea versicolor.
• **TINZAPARIN SODIUM.** USAN.
Use: Anticoagulant; antithrombotic.
• **TIOCONAZOLE,** U.S.P. XXIII.
Use: Antifungal.
See: Vagistat (Fujisawa SmithKline)
• **TIODAZOSIN.** USAN.
Use: Antihypertensive.
• **TIODONIUM CHLORIDE.** USAN.
Use: Antibacterial.
• **TIOPERIDONE HYDROCHLORIDE.** USAN.
Use: Antipsychotic.
• **TIOPINAC.** USAN.
Use: Anti-inflammatory, analgesic.
TIOPRONIN.
Use: Homozygous cystinuria. [Orphan drug]
See: Thiola (Mission).
• **TIOSPIRONE HYDROCHLORIDE.** USAN.
• **TIOTIDINE.** USAN.

Use: Antagonist.
• **TIOXIDAZOLE.** USAN.
Use: Anthelmintic.
• **TIPENTOSIN HYDROCHLORIDE.**
USAN.
Use: Antihypertensive.
TIPRAMINE TABS. (Major) Imipramine
10 mg/Tab. Bot. 250s; 25 mg or 50
mg/Tab. Bot. 250s, 1000s.
Use: Antidepressant.
• **TIPREDANE.** USAN.
Use: Adrenocortical steroid (topical).
TIPRENOLOL. B.A.N. 3-Isopropylamino-
1-[2-(methylthio)phenoxy]propan-2-ol.
Use: Beta-adrenergic receptor blocking
agent.
• **TIPRENOLOL HCl.** USAN. (±)-1-(Iso-
propylamino) 3 [o-(methylthio)-phe-
noxy]-2-propanol HCl.
Use: Anti-adrenergic (β-receptor).
• **TIPRINAST MEGLUMIDE.** USAN. A
Mead Johnson investigative drug.
Use: Anti-allergenic agent.
• **TIPROPIDIL HYDROCHLORIDE.** USAN.
Use: Vasodilator.
• **TIQUESIDE.** USAN.
Use: Cholesterol absorption inhibitor.
• **TIQUINAMIDE HYDROCHLORIDE.**
USAN.
Use: Anticholinergic.
• **TIRAPAZAMINE.** USAN.
Use: Antineoplastic.
TIRATRICOL.
Use: Antineoplastic. [Orphan drug]
TIREND. (SK-Beecham) Caffeine 100
mg/Tab. Bot. 12s, 25s, 50s.
Use: Stimulant.
TIRILAZAD MESYLATE. USAN.
Use: Inhibitor, lipid peroxidation.
• **TI-SCREEN.** (Fischer) **Gel:** SPF 20+, eth-
ylhexyl p-methoxycinnamate 7.5%, oxy-
benzone 5%, 2-ethylhexyl salicylate 5%,
SD alcohol 40 71%. 120 g; **Lip Balm:**
SPF 8+, ethylhexyl p-methoxycinna-
mate 7.5%, oxybenzone 5%, petrolatum. 4.5 g; **Lot.: SPF 8:** Ethylhexyl p-
methoxycinnamate 6%, oxybenzone
2%. Bot. 120 ml; **SPF 15:** Ethylhexyl p-
methoxycinnamate 7.5%, oxybenzone
5%. Bot. 120 ml; **SPF 30:** Octyl
methoxycinnamate 7.5%, octyl salicylate 5%, oxybenzone 6%, octocrylene
7.5%. Bot. 120 ml.
Use: Sunscreen.
TI-SCREEN NATURAL. (Fischer) Titanium dioxide 5%. Lot. Bot. 120 ml.
Use: Sunscreen.
TISIT. (Pfeiffer) Pyrethrins 0.3%, piperonyl butoxide technical 3%, petroleum
distillate 1.2%, benzyl alcohol 2.4%.

Shampoo. Bot. 118 ml.
Use: Treatment of lice.
TISOL. (Parnell) Benzyl alcohol 1%, men-
thol 0.04%, isotonic sodium chloride
0.9%, *Mucoprotective Factor* yerba san-
ta, cetyl pyridinium chloride, poloxamer,
sorbitol, EDTA. Soln. Bot. 237 ml.
Use: Temporary relief of minor sore
throat pain and irritation.
**TISSUE FIXATIVE AND WASH SOLU-
TION.** (Wampole-Zeus) A modified
Michel's tissue fixative and buffered
wash solution.
Use: To facilitate the transport and pro-
cessing of fresh tissue biopsies.
**TISSUE PLASMINOGEN ACTIVATOR,
RECOMBINANT.**
See: Activase (Gentech).
TISSUE RESPIRATORY FACTOR (TRF).
(International Hormone) RSF, SRF,
LYCD, PCO, Procytoxid marketed as
2000 units. Supplied as bulk liquid con-
centrate.
Use: Promotion of cellular oxidation.
TIS-U-SOL. (Travenol) Pentalyte irriga-
tion containing NaCl 800 mg, KCl 40 mg,
magnesium sulfate 20 mg, sodium
phosphate 8.75 mg, and 6.25 mg
monobasic potassium phosphate per
100 ml. Bot. 250 ml, 1000 ml.
Use: Physiologic irrigating solution.
TITAN. (Pilkington Barnes-Hind) Benza-
lkonium chloride, EDTA, nonionic clean-
er buffers. Bot. oz.
Use: Hard contact lens cleaning solu-
tion.
• **TITANIUM DIOXIDE,** U.S.P. XXIII.
Use: Solar ray protectant.
TITICUM RIPENS.
W/Oxyquinoline sulfate, charcoal.
See: Triticoll, Tabs. (Western Re-
search).
TITRALAC. (3M Pharm.) Calcium car-
bonate 420 mg, saccharin, sodium 0.3
mg. Chew. Tab. Bot. 40s, 100s, 1000s.
Use: Gastric antacid.
**TITRALAC EXTRA STRENGTH
TABLETS.** (3M Pharm.) Calcium car-
bonate 750 mg, saccharin, sodium 0.6
mg. Chew. Tab. Bot. 100s.
Use: Antacid.
TITRALAC PLUS LIQUID. (3M Personal
Health Care) Calcium carbonate 500
mg, simethicone 20 mg, saccharin, sor-
bitol, sodium 0.15 mg. Bot. 360 ml.
Use: Antacid.
TITRALAC PLUS TABLETS. (3M
Pharm.) Calcium carbonate 420 mg,
simethicone 21 mg, saccharin, sodium
1.1 mg. Chew. Tab. Bot. 100s.

Use: Antacid.
•**TIXANOX.** USAN.
Use: Anti-allergic.
•**TIXOCORTOL PIVALATE.** USAN.
Use: Anti-inflammatory (topical).
TIZANIDINE HCL.
Use: Antispasmodic.
See: Zanaflex.
•**TIZANIDINE HYDROCHLORIDE.** USAN.
Use: Antispasmodic. [Orphan drug]
T-KOFF. (T.E. Williams) Phenyl-propanolamine HCl 20 mg, phenyle-phrine HCl 20 mg, chlorpheniramine maleate 5 mg, codeine phosphate 10 mg/5 ml Syr. Bot. 480 ml Grape flavor.
Use: Antihistamine, decongestant, anti-tussive.
T-LYMPHOTROPIC VIRUS TYPE III GP 160 ANTIGENS.
Use: Treatment for AIDS. [Orphan drug]
See: Vaxsyn HIV-1.
TMP-SMZ.
Use: Anti-infective.
See: Proloprim (Burroughs Wellcome).
Trimethoprim (Various Mfr.).
Trimpex (Roche).
TOBRADES SUSPENSION. (Alcon) Dex-amethasone 0.1%, tobraycin 0.3%, thimerisol 0.001%, alcohol 0.5%, propy-lene glycol, polyoxyethylene, poly-oxypropylene. 2.5 ml, 5 ml.
Use: Ophthalmic.
TOBRADEX. (Alcon). 0.3% tobramycin and 0.1% dexamethasone. Suspension: In 2.5 ml or 5 ml.
Use: Corticosteroid, anti-infective, oph-thalmic.
TOBRADEX, OINTMENT. (Alcon Labs) Dexamethasone 0.1%, tobramycin 0.3%, chlorobutanol 0.5%, mineral oil, white petrolatum. Ophthalmic 3.5 Gm.
Use: Corticosteroid antibacterial, oph-thalmic.
•**TOBRAMYCIN,** U.S.P. XXIII. Opth. Oint., Ophth. Soln., U.S.P. XXIII. An antibiotic obtained from cultures of *Streptomyces tenebrarius.*
Use: Antibiotic.
See: Tobrex, Soln., Oint. (Alcon).
TOBRAMYCIN. (Bausch & Lomb) To-bramycin 0.3%, benzalkonium Cl 0.01%, boric acid. Soln. 5 ml.
Use: Ophthalmic antibiotic.
•**TOBRAMYCIN AND DEXAMETHASONE OPHTHALMIC OINT., U.S.P.** U.S.P. XXIII.
Use: Antibiotic.
TOBRAMYCIN SULFATE. (Various Mfr.) Tobramycin sulfate 40 mg/ml. Inj. Sy-ringes: 1.5 ml, 2 ml. Vial 2 ml. Pediatric

inj. 10 mg/ml. Vial 2 ml.
Use: Aminoglycoside, parenteral.
•**TOBRAMYCIN SULFATE,** U.S.P. XXIII. inj., U.S.P. XXIII.
Use: Antibiotic.
See: Nebcin, Amp., Hyporet. (Lilly).
TOBREX OPHTHALMIC OINTMENT. (Alcon) Tobramycin 0.3% in sterile oint-ment base. Tube 3.5 Gm.
Use: External ophthalmic bacterial in-fections.
TOBREX SOLUTION. (Alcon) To-bramycin 0.3%. ophthalmic solution. Bot. 5 ml w/dropper.
Use: Topical ophthalmic anti-infective.
•**TOCAINIDE.** USAN.
Use: Antiarrhythmic, cardiac depres-sant.
See: Tonocard, Tab. (Merck & Co.).
•**TOCAINIDE HYDROCHLORIDE,** U.S.P. XXIII. Tab., U.S.P. XXIII.
Use: Antiarrhythmic, cardiac depres-sant.
•**TOCAMPHYL.** USAN. 1-p, α-Dimethyl-benzyl camphorate 1:1 salt with 2,2′-iminodiethanol.
Use: Choleretic.
See: Gallogen, Tab. (Beecham-Mas-sengill).
TOCOPHEROL-DL-ALPHA. Vitamin E, U.S.P. XXIII. 5,7,8-Trimethyltocol, alpha-Tocopherol, dl-alpha-tocopherol, Vita-mins E, wheat germ oil. dl-2,5,7,8-Tetramethyl-2-(4′,8,12-trimethyltridecyl)-6-chromanol.
Cap. & Tab.:
Denamone, Cap. (3 min., 10 min.) wheat germ oil (Vio-Bin).
Ecofrol, Cap. (O'Neal).
Eprolin, Gelseal (Lilly).
Epsilan M, Cap. (Warren-Teed).
Lib-E, Cap. (AVP).
Oint.:
Myopone (Drug Prods.).
Sol.:
Aquasol E, Soln. (USV Pharm.).
•**TOCOPHEROLS EXCIPIENT,** N.F. XVIII.
•**TOCOPHERSOLAN.** USAN. (+)-α-Toco-pheryl polyethylene glycol 1000 succi-nate.
Use: Vitamin E supplement.
TOCOPHERYL ACETATE-d-ALPHA. Vit-amin E, U.S.P. XXIII.
See: Aquasol E, Prods. (USV Labs.).
Epsilan-M, Cap. (Warren-Teed).
Lib-E-400, Cap. (AVP).
Tocopher, Cap. (Quality Generics).
Tokols, Cap. (Ulmer).
Vitamins E. (Var. Mfr.).
TOCOPHERYL ACETATES, CONC. D-

ALPHA. Vitamin E, U.S.P. XXIII. d-alpha-Toco-pheryl acetate.
Use: Treatment of habitual & threatened abortion.
TOCOPHERYL ACID SUCCINATED D-ALPHA. Vitamin E, U.S.P. XXIII.
See: E-Ferol Succinate, Tab., Cap. (Forest).
Vitamins E (Various Mfr.).
TOCOSAMINE. (Trent) Sparteine sulfate 150 mg, sod. chl. 4.5 mg/ml. Amps. 1 ml. Box 12s, 100s.
Use: I.M. Oxytocic.
TODAY VAGINAL CONTRACEPTIVE SPONGE. (VLI) Nonoxynol-9, citric, sorbic, benzoic acid, sodium dihydrogen, citrate, sodium metabisulfite, polyurethane foam sponge. 3s, 6s, and 12s.
Use: Contraceptive.
TODRAZOLINE. B.A.N. Ethyl 3-phthalazin 1 ylcarbazate. Binazine.
Use: Antihypertensive.
TOFENACIN. D.A.N. N-Methyl-2-(2-methyl-benzhydryloxy)ethylamine. Elamol hydrochloride.
Use: Treatment of the Parkinsonian syndrome.
• **TOFENACIN HCl.** USAN. N-Methyl-2-[(o-methyl-α-phenyl-benzyl)oxy]-ethylamine HCl.
Use: Anticholinergic.
TOFRANAZINE. (Geigy) Combination of imipramine and promazine. Pending release.
TOFRANIL. (Geigy) Imipramine HCl. **Tab.** 10 mg Bot. 100s, 1000s; 25 mg & 50 mg. Bot. 100s, 1000s. UD 100s. Gy-Pak 100s, 1 unit (12×100); 6 units (72100). **Amps.** 25 mg/2 ml w/ascorbic acid 2 mg, sod. bisulfite 1 mg, sod. sulfite 1 mg and 2 ml amps.
Use: Antidepressant, anti-enuretic.
TOFRANIL-PM. (Geigy) Imipramine pamoate 75 mg, 100 mg , 125 mg or 150 mg/Cap. Bot. 30s, 100s. 75 mg/Cap. Bot. 1000s. UD 75 mg and 150 mg in 100s.
Use: Antidepressant.
TOLAMIDE TABS. (Major) Tolazamide 100 mg/Tab. Bot. 100s, 250s; 250 mg/Tab. 200s, 500s; 500 mg/Tab. Bot. 100s, 500s.
Use: Hypoglycemic agent.
• **TOLAMOLOL.** USAN. 4-[2-(2-Hydroxy-3-o-tolyloxypropylamino)ethoxy]benzamide.
Use: Beta-adrenergic receptor blocking agent, coronary vasodilator, antiarrhythmic.

• **TOLAZAMIDE,** U.S.P. XXIII. Tabs., U.S.P. XXIII. (Upjohn) 1-(Hexahydro-1-azepinyl)-3-(p-tolylsulfonyl) urea. 1-Perhydroazepin-1-yl-3-toluene-p-sul- phonylurea. Tolanase. Benzenesulfonamide, N-[[(hexahydro-1H-azepin-1-yl)amino]carbonyl]-4-methyl-. 1-(Hexahydro-1H-azepin-1-yl)-3-(p-tolylsulfonyl) urea.
Use: Hypoglycemic agent.
See: Ronase, Tab. (Reid-Rowell) Tolinase, Tab. (Upjohn).
• **TOLAZOLINE HYDROCHLORIDE,** U.S.P. XXII. Inj., Tab., U.S.P. XXII. Benzazoline HCl, 2-Benzyl-2- imidazoline HCl. VasImid, Vasodil.
Use: Anti-adrenergic, vasodilator (peripheral).
See: Priscoline, Prep. (Ciba). Tazol, Tab. (Durst). Toloxan, Tab. (Kenyon).
• **TOLBUTAMIDE,** U.S.P. XXIII. Tab. U.S.P. XXIII. N-Butyl-N'-toluene-p-sulfonylurea. Benzenesulfonamide, N-[(butylamino)carbonyl]-4-methyl-. 1-Butyl-3-(p-tolylsulfonyl)urea.
Use: Hypoglycemic.
See: Orinase, Prep. (Upjohn).
• **TOLBUTAMIDE SODIUM, STERILE,** U.S.P. XXIII.
Use: Diagnostic aid (diabetes).
See: Orinase Diagnostic (Upjohn).
• **TOLCAPONE.** USAN.
Use: Antiparkinsonian agent.
• **TOLCICLATE.** USAN.
Use: Antifungal.
TOLECTIN 200. (McNeil Pharm) Tolmetin sodium 200 mg/Tab. Bot. 100s.
Use: Nonsteroidal anti-inflammatory agent.
TOLECTIN 600. (McNeil Pharm) Tolmetin sodium 600 mg/Tab. Bot. 100s.
Use: Nonsteroidal anti-inflammatory agent.
TOLECTIN DS. (McNeil Pharm) Tolmetin sodium 400 mg/Cap Bot. 100s, 500s, UD 100s.
Use: Nonsteroidal anti-inflammatory agent.
TOLEREX. (Procter & Gamble) Protein 20.6 Gm, carbohydrate 226.3 Gm, fat 1.45 Gm, sodium 468 mg, potassium 1172 mg, mOsm/Kg H_2O 550, cal/ml 1, vitamins A, B_1, B_2, B_3, B_5, B_6, B_{12}, C, D, E, K, folic acid, biotin, choline, Ca, P, I, Fe, Mg, Cu, Zn, Mn, Se, Mo, Cr. Assorted flavors Pow. Pkts. 80 Gm.
Use: Vitamin/mineral supplement.
• **TOLFAMIDE.** USAN.

Use: Enzyme Inhibitor.

TOLFRINIC. (Ascher) Ferrous fumarate 200 mg, Vitamins B_{12} 25 mcg, Vitamins C 100 mg/Tab. Bot. 100s.
Use: Hemopoietic.

• **TOLGABIDE.** USAN.
Use: Anti-epileptic (control of abnormal movements).

• **TOLIMIDONE.** USAN.
Use: Anti-ulcerative.

TOLINASE. (Upjohn) Tolazamide. **100 mg/Tab.** 100s. **250 mg/Tab.** Bot. 100s. UD 100s. **500 mg/Tab.** 100s.
Use: Hypoglycemic agent.

• **TOLINDATE.** USAN.
Use: Antifungal.
See: Dalnate (USV Pharm.).

• **TOLIODIUM CHLORIDE.** USAN.
Use: Food additive.

• **TOLMETIN.** USAN.
Use: Anti-inflammatory.

• **TOLMETIN SODIUM,** U.S.P. XXIII. Cap., Tab., U.S.P. XXIII. Sodium 1-Methyl-5-p-toluoylpyrrole-2-acetic acid. (Various Mfr.) **Tab.:** 200 mg. Bot. 100s; 600 mg. Bot. 100s, 500s, 1000s; **Cap.:** 400 mg. Bot. 100s, 500s, 1000s.
Use: Anti-inflammatory.
See: Tolectin, Tab. (McNeil).
Tolectin DS, Cap. (McNeil).

• **TOLNAFTATE,** U.S.P. XXIII. Topical Aerosol Powder, Cream, Gel, Powder, Topical Soln., U.S.P. XXIII. o-2-Naphthyl m,N-dimethyl-thiocarbanilate. Naphthiomate-T; Tinaderm. Carbamothoic acid, methyl(3-methylphenyl)-, 0-2-naphthalenyl ester.
Use: Topical antifungal agent.
See: Absorbine Antifungal, Cream (W.F. Young).
Aftate, Prods. (Plough).
Tinactin, Soln., Cream, Pow., Pow. Aer. (Schering).

• **TOLOFOCON A.** USAN.
Use: Contact lens material (hydrophobic).

TOLONIUM CHLORIDE. 3-Amino-7-dimethyl-amino-2-methyl-phenazathionium. Blutene Chloride.

TOLOXAN. (Kenyon) Tolazoline HCl 25 mg/Tab. Bot. 100s, 1000s.

TOLOXYCHLORINAL. 1,1'-[[(o-Tolyloxy)-methyl]ethylenedioxy]bis[2,2,2-trichloro-ethanol].1,1-[3-o-Tolyloxypropylenedioxy]bis (2,2,2-trichloroethanol). Propoxychlorinol.
Use: Sedative.

TOLPENTAMIDE. B.A.N. 1-Cyclopentyl-3-toluene-p-sulfonylurea.
Use: Hypoglycemic agent.

TOLPERISONE. B.A.N. 2-Methyl-3-piperidino-1-p-tolylpropan-1-one. Mydocalm.
Use: Muscle relaxant.

TOLPIPRAZOLE. B.A.N. 5-Methyl-3-[2-(4-m-tolylpiperazin-1-yl)ethyl]pyrazole.
Use: Tranquilizer.

• **TOLPOVIDONE I-131.** USAN.[oo]-(p-lodobenzyl)-poly[1-(2-oxo-1-pyrrolidinyl)ethylene]-[131]I.
Use: Differential diagnosis of source of hypoalbuminemia.
See: Raovin (Abbott).

TOLPRONINE. B.A.N. 1-(1,2,3,6-Tetrahydro-1-pyridyl)-3-o-tolyloxypropan-2-ol. Proponesin [hydrochloride]
Use: Analgesic.

TOLPROPAMINE. B.A.N. NN-Dimethyl-3-phenyl-3-p-tolylpropylamine. Tylagel [hydrochloride]
Use: Antipruritic.

• **TOLPYRRAMIDE.** USAN. N-p-tolylsulfonyl-1-pyrrolidinecarboxamide. 1-Tetramethylene-3-p-tolysulfonylurea.
Use: Oral hypoglycemic.

• **TOLRESTAT.** USAN.
Use: Inhibitor (aldose reductase).

• **TOLTRAZURIL.** USAN.

• **TOLU BALSAM,** U.S.P. XXIII.
Use: Pharm. necessity for Compound Benzoin Tincture, expectorant.
See: Vicks Regular & Wild Cherry Medicated Cough Drops (Vicks).

• **TOLU BALSAM SYRUP,** N.F. XVII. (Lilly) Bot. 16 fl. oz.
Use: Vehicle.

• **TOLU BALSAM TINCTURE,** N.F. XVII.
Use: Flavor.

TOLUIDINE BLUE O CHLORIDE.
See: Blutene Chloride.

TOLU-SED (No Sugar). (Scherer) Codeine phosphate 10 mg, guaifenesin 100 mg/5 ml w/alcohol 10%. Bot. 4 oz., pt.
Use: Temporary relief of coughs due to colds, and minor throat irritations.

TOLU-SED DM (No Sugar). (Scherer) d-Methorphan HBr 10 mg, guaifenesin 100 mg/5 ml w/alcohol 10%. Bot. 4 oz., pt.
Use: Temporary relief of cough due to the common cold.

TOLYCAINE. B.A.N. Methyl 2-diethylaminoacetamido-m-toluate. Baycain [hydrochloride]
Use: Local anesthetic.

TOMOCAT. (Lafayette) CT barium sulfate 1.5% w/v. Case of 24 Bot.
Use: Mark alimentary tract during CT scans.

TOMOCAT 1000. (Lafayette) Barium sulfate suspension concentrate 5% w/v/Bot. for dilution to 1.5% w/v at time of use. Bot. 225 ml w/1000 ml dilution Bot. Case 24 Bot. and 2 Dilution Bot.
Use: Radiopaque medium used to mark the GI tract during CT scans.
• **TOMOXETINE HYDROCHLORIDE.** USAN.
Use: Antidepressant.
TONAVITE-M ELIXIR. (Goldline) Bot. 12 oz., pt., gal.
Use: Dietary supplement.
• **TONAZOCIN MESYLATE.** USAN.
Use: Analgesic.
TONBEC TABLETS. (A.V.P.) Vitamins B_1 15 mg, B_2 10 mg, B_6 5 mg, nicotinamide 50 mg, Ca pantothenate 10 mg, ascorbic acid 300 mg/Tab. Bot. 60s.
Use: Therapeutic Vitamin B and C supplement.
TONECOL. (A.V.P.) Promethazine w/expectorant and vasoconstrictor. Bot. pt.
Use: Cough medicine.
TONECOL COUGH SYRUP. (A.V.P.) Dextromethorphan HBr 10 mg, phenylephrine HCl 5 mg, chlorpheniramine maleate 1 mg, sodium citrate 15 mg, guaifenesin 25 mg/5 ml w/alcohol 7%. Bot. 1 pt.
Use: Treatment of cold symptoms, expectorant.
TONELAX TABLETS. (A.V.P.) Danthron 75 mg, calcium pantothenate 25 mg/Tab. Bot. 100s, 1000s.
Use: Peristaltic stimulant, laxative.
TONO-B PEDIATRIC. (Vale) Iron 5 mg, thiamine HCl 0.167 mg, riboflavin 0.133 mg/Tab. Bot. 1000s.
Use: Multivitamin.
TONOCARD. (Merck & Co.) Tocainide HCl 400 mg and 600 mg/Tab. Bot. 100s. UD 100s.
Use: Antiarrhythmic.
TONOJUG 2000. (Lafayette) Barium sulfate powder 1200 Gm for suspension to make 2000 ml. Bot. 2000 Gm Case: 8 Bot.
Use: Radiopaque contrast medium for use during x-ray examination of the GI tract.
TONOPAQUE ORAL BARIUM. (Lafayette) Barium sulfate powder 180 Gm for suspension. Bot. 180 Gm Case 24s.
Use: Radiopaque contrast medium for use during x-ray examination of the GI tract.
TOOTHACHE RELIEF-3 IN 1. (C.S. Dent) Toothache gum, toothache drops, benzocaine lotion.
Use: Treatment of toothache.
TOP BRASS ZP-11. (Revlon) Zinc pyrithione 0.5% in cream base.
Use: Anti-dandruff hairdress.
TOPEX. (Vicks Prods) Benzoyl peroxide 10%. Bot. oz.
Use: Acne clearing lotion.
TOP-FORM. (Hoyt) Topical formfitting gel applicators. Disposable trays for topical fluoride office treatments, plus permanent trays for topical fluoride home self treatments. Box 100s.
Use: Topical fluoride applications in home or office.
TOPIC. (Syntex) 5% benzyl alcohol in greaseless gel base containing camphor, menthol, w/30% isopropyl alcohol. Tube 2 oz.
Use: Antipruritic.
TOPICAL ANESTHETICS, MISCELLANEOUS.
See: Ethyl Chloride (Gebauer).
    Flouri-Methane (Gebauer).
    Fluro-Ethyl (Gebauer).
TOPICAL FLUORIDE. (Pacemaker). Acidulated phosphate fluoride. Flavors: orange, bubblegum, lime, raspberry, grape, cinnamon. Liq. Bot. 4 oz., pt.
TOPICORT CREAM. (Hoechst) Desoximetasone 0.25% emollient cream consisting of isopropyl myristate, cetyl stearyl alcohol, white petrolatum, mineral oil, lanolin alcohol and purified water. Tubes 15 Gm, 60 Gm, 120 Gm.
Use: Synthetic corticosteroid for relief of dermatoses.
TOPICORT GEL. (Hoechst) Desoximetasone 0.05% in gel base. 20% alcohol. Tube 15 Gm, 60 Gm.
Use: Synthetic corticosteroid for relief of dermatoses.
TOPICORT LP CREAM. (Hoechst) Desoximetasone 0.05%. Tubes 15 Gm, 60 Gm.
Use: Synthetic corticosteroid for relief of dermatoses.
TOPICORT OINTMENT. (Hoechst) Desoximetasone 0.25% in ointment base. Tube 15 Gm, 60 Gm.
Use: Synthetic corticosteroid for relief of dermatoses.
TOPICYCLINE. (Procter & Gamble) Tetracycline HCl 2.2 mg/ml w/4-epitetracycline HCl, sodium bisulfite. Bot. 70 ml w/diluent.
Use: Topical treatment of acne vulgaris.
TOPIMAX. (R. W. Johnson Res)
See: TOPIRAMATE.
• **TOPIRAMATE.** USAN.

Use: Anticonvulsant. [Orphan drug]
See: Topimax.
TOPOCAINE.
See: Surfacaine (Lilly).
• **TOPOTECAN HYDROCHLORIDE.**
USAN.
Use: Antineoplastic.
TOPROL XL. (Astra) Metoprolol succinate 47.5 mg, 95 mg or 190 mg/ER Tab.
Bot. 100s.
Use: Antihypertensive.
• **TOPTERONE.** USAN.
Use: Anti-androgen.
TOPY.
Use: Vaccine, viral.
See: Orimune (Lederle).
• **TOQUIZINE.** USAN.
Use: Anticholinergic.
TORADOL. (Syntex) Ketorolac tromethamine 15 mg/ ml and 30 mg/ ml.
Injection. 15 mg/ml in 1 ml and 2 ml Cartrix syringes, 30 mg/ml in 1 ml Cartrix syringes. Alcohol 10%.
Use: Nonsteroidal anti-inflammatory agent.
TORECAN. (Boehringer Ingelheim) Thiethylperazine. **Tab.** 10 mg w/Tartrazine.
Bot. 100s. **Amp.** 10 mg/2 ml (w/sod.
metabisulfite 0.5 mg, ascorbic acid 2 mg, sorbitol 40 mg, q.s. carbon dioxide).
Supp. 10 mg (w/cocoa butter) Box 12s.
Use: Antiemetic and antinauseant.
TOREMIFENE.
Use: Antineoplastic. [Orphan drug]
See: Estrinex.
• **TOREMIFENE CITRATE.** USAN.
TORGANIC-DM. (Major) Dextromethorphan HBr 10 mg, iodinated glycerol 30 mg/5 ml Liq. Bot. 473 ml. Alcohol free.
Use: Antitussive, expectorant.
TORNALATE. (Dura) Bitolterol mesylate 0.2%, alcohol 25%, propylene glycol.
Soln. for inhalation. Bot. 10 ml, 30 ml, 60 ml.
Use: Bronchodilator for bronchial asthma and reversible bronchospasms.
TORNALATE INHALER. (Sanofi Winthrop) Bitolterol mesylate metered inhaler. Bot. 16.4 Gm w/oral inhaler. Refill 16.4 Gm.
Use: Bronchodilator for bronchial asthma and reversible bronchospasms.
TORNALATE TABLETS. (Sanofi Winthrop) Bitolterol mesylate.
Use: Bronchodilator.
TORSEMIDE.
Use: Diuretic.
See: Demadex, Tab., Inj. (Boehringer Mannheim)
TORULA YEAST, DRIED, Obtained by

growing *Candida (torulopsis) utilis* yeast on wood pulp wastes (Nutritional Labs.)
Conc. 100 lb. drums.
Use: Natural source of protein & Vitamin B-complex vitamins.
• **TOSIFEN.** USAN.
Use: Anti-anginal.
TOTACILLIN. (Beecham Labs) Ampicillin trihydrate equivalent to: **Cap.** 250 mg/Cap. Bot. 500s. 500 mg/Cap. Bot. 500s. **Susp.:** 125 mg/5 ml. Bot. 100 ml, 150 ml, 200 ml; 250 mg/5 ml. Bot. 100 ml, 200 ml.
TOTACILLIN-N. (Beecham Labs) Ampicillin sodium 250 mg, 500 mg, 1 Gm, 2 Gm/Vial in 10s; Piggyback Vials 500 mg, 1 Gm, 2 Gm, in 25s; Bulk pharm. pkg. 10 Gm in 25s.
Use: Antibiotic.
TOTAL. (Allergan) Polyvinyl alcohol, edetate disodium and benzalkonium chloride in a sterile, buffered, isotonic solution. Bot: 2 fl. oz., 4 fl. oz.
Use: Hard contact lens all purpose solution.
TOTAL ECLIPSE COOLING ALCOHOL.
(Dorsey) Padimate O, oxybenzone, glyceryl PABA, alcohol 77%. SPF 15.
Lot. Bot. 120 ml.
Use: Sunscreen.
TOTAL ECLIPSE MOISTURIZING.
(Dorsey) Padimate O, oxybenzone, octyl salicylate. Moisturizing base. SPF 15.
Lot. Bot. 120 ml.
Use: Sunscreen.
TOTAL ECLIPSE OIL & ACNE PRONE SKIN SUNSCREEN. (Eclipse) Padimate O, oxybenzone, glyceryl PABA, alcohol 77%. SPF 15. Lot. Bot. 120 ml.
Use: Sunscreen.
TOTAL SOLUTION. (Allergan) Isotonic, buffered soln. of polyvinyl alcohol, benzalkonium chloride, EDTA. Soln. Bot. 60 ml, 120 ml.
Use: Ophthalmic.
TOTAQUINE, Alkaloids from Cinchona bark, 7% to 12% quinine anhydrous, 70% to 80% total alkaloids (cinchonidine, cinchonine, quinidine & quinine).
TOTOMYCIN HYDROCHLORIDE. Tetracycline, U.S.P. XXIII.
TOURO EX. (Dartmouth Pharm.) Guaifenesin 600 mg. SR Capl. Bot. 100s.
Use: Expectorant.
TOURO LA. (Dartmouth) Pseudoephedrine HCl 10 mg, guaifenesin 400 mg. Capl. Bot. 100s.
Use: Decongestant, expectorant.
• **TOXIN, DIPHTHERIA FOR SCHICK TEST,** U.S.P. XXIII.

Use: Diagnostic aid (dermal reactivity indicator).

TOXO. (Wampole-Zeus) *Toxoplasma* antibody test system. Tests 120s.
Use: An IFA test system for the detection of antibodies to Toxoplasma gondii.

TOXOIDS.
See: Antigens International. (Connaught).
Diptheria Toxoid Absorbed (Pediatric).
Diphtherial and Tetanus Toxoids and Pertussis Vaccine (Connaught).
Lederle
Sclavo
Squibb/Connaught
Tri-Immunol (Lederle).
Wyeth

• **TOXOID, DIPHTHERIA,** U.S.P. XXIII.
Use: Immunizing agent (active).
See: Diphtheria Toxoid, Aluminum Hydroxide, Adsorbed.

TOXOID MIXTURE.
See: Tri-Solgen, Vial (Lilly)

• **TOXOID, TETANUS ADSORBED,** U.S.P. XXIII.
Use: Immunizing agent (active).

TOXOPLASMOSIS TEST.
Use: In Vitro diagnostic aid.
See: TPM Test (Wampole).

T-PA.
Use: Tissue plasminogen activator.
See: Activase (Gentech).

T-PHYL. (Purdue Frederick) Theophylline 200 mg/Tab. Bot. 100s.
Use: Bronchodilator.

T.P.L. TROCHES. (Kasdenol) Triamite. Loz. 5 Gm 15s.
Use: Mouth and throat preparation.

TPM-TEST. (Wampole) Indirect hemagglutination test for the qualitative and quantitative determination of antibodies to *Toxoplasma gondii* in serum. Kit 120s,
Use: An aid in the diagnosis of toxoplasmosis.

TPN ELECTROLYTES. (Abbott Hospital Prods) Multiple electrolyte additive: 321 mg sodium chloride, 331 mg calcium chloride, 1491 mg potassium chloride, 508 mg magnesium chloride, 2420 mg sodium acetate; 20 ml in 50 ml fliptop or pintop Vial or 20 ml Univ. Add. Syr.
Use: Provides electrolytes during total parenteral nutrition.

TPN ELECTROLYTES II. (Abbott). Na 15 mEq/L, K 18 mEq/L, Ca 4.5 mEq/L, Mg 5 mEq/L, Cl 35 mEq/L, Acetate 7.5 mEq/L. In 20 ml fill in 50 ml fliptop and pintop Vials and 20 ml fill Syringes.
Use: Intravenous nutritional therapy.

TPN ELECTROLYTES III. Na 25 Eq/L, K 40.6 mEq/L, Ca 5 mEq/L, Mg 8 mEq/L, Cl 33.5 mEq/L, Acetate 40.6 mEq/L, Gluconate 5 mEq/L. In 20 ml fill in 50 ml fliptop and pintop Vials and 20 ml fill Syringes.
Use: Intravenous nutritional therapy.

TP TROCHES. (Edward J. Moore) Triamite. Jars 500s, Box 15s.
Use: Temporary relief of minor sore throat & mouth.

• **TRACAZOLATE.** USAN.
Use: Sedative.

TRACE. (Lorvic) Erythrosine conc. soln. Squeeze Bot. 30 ml, 60 ml Dispenser Packets 200s.
Use: Plaque dye sol.

TRACE 28 LIQUID. (Lorvic) D & C Red No. 28 in aqueous soln. Bot. 30 ml, 60 ml.
Use: Diagnostic aid to disclose dental plaque.

TRACE 28 TABLETS. (Lorvic) D & C Red No. 28. Tablets Box 30s, 180s, 700s.
Use: Disclosing dental plaque.

TRACELYTE. (Lyphomed) A combination of electrolytes and trace elements additive. Vial 20 ml.
Use: Electrolyte and trace element replenishment.

TRACELYTE-II. (Lyphomed) A combination of electrolytes and trace elements additive. Vial 20 ml.
Use: Electrolyte and trace element replenishment.

TRACELYTE-II WITH DOUBLE ELECTROLYTES. (Lyphomed) Combination of electrolytes and trace elements additive. Vial 40 ml.
Use: Electrolyte and trace element replenisher.

TRACELYTE WITH DOUBLE ELECTROLYTES. (Lyphomed) A combination of electrolytes and trace elements additive. Vial 40 ml.
Use: Electrolyte and trace element replenisher.

TRACEPLEX. (Enzyme Process) Iron 30 mg, iodine 0.1 mg, copper 0.5 mg, magnesium 40 mg, zinc 10 mg, B_{12} 5 mcg/4 Tabs. Bot. 100s, 250s.
Use: Mineral supplement.

TRACER BG. (Boehringer Mannheim) Reagent strips. Kit. 25s, 50s.
Use: In vitro diagnostic aid.

TRACRIUM INJECTION. (Burroughs Wellcome) Atracurium besylate 10 mg/ml Amp. 5 ml. Box 10s; 10 ml MDV. Box 10s.
Use: Surgical muscle relaxant.

TRAC TABS 2X. (Hyrex) Atropine sulfate 0.06 mg, hyoscyamine 0.03 mg, methenamine 120 mg, methylene blue 6 mg, phenyl salicylate 30 mg, benzoic acid 7.5 mg/Tab. Bot. 100s, 1000s.
Use: Urinary tract infections.
• **TRAGACANTH,** N.F. XVIII.
Use: Pharmaceutical aid (suspending agent).
TRAL FILMTAB. (Abbott) Hexocyclium methylsulfate 25 mg/Tab. Bot. 100s.
Use: Anticholinergic agent for treatment of peptic ulcer.
• **TRALONIDE.** USAN.
Use: Glucocorticoid.
• **TRAMADOL HYDROCHLORIDE.** USAN.
Use: Analgesic.
• **TRAMAZOLINE,** USAN. 2-[(5,6,7,8-Tetrahydro-1-naphthyl)amino]-2-imidazoline.
Use: Adrenergic.
TRANCIN. Fluphenazine.
Use: To treat anxiety and tension.
TRANCOGESICO TABLETS. (Sanofi Winthrop) Dipyrone, chlormezanone.
Use: Analgesic, antipyretic, muscle relaxant.
TRANCOPAL. (Sanofi Pharm) Chlormezanone 100 mg w/saccharin/Cap. Bot. 100s. 200 mg/Cap. Bot. 100s, 1000s.
Use: Relaxant and tranquilizer for mild anxiety and tension states.
TRANDATE HCT. (Allen & Hanburys) **Tablets:** Labetalol 100 mg, 200 mg or 300 mg, all w/25 mg hydrochlorothiazide. In 100s.
Use: Antihypertensive with diuretic.
TRANDATE INJECTION. (Allen & Hanburys) Labetalol HCl 5 mg/ml Amp. 1 ml. Box 1s. Vial 20 ml, 40 ml. Box 1s. Prefilled Syringes 4 ml, 8 ml.
Use: Antihypertensive.
TRANDATE TABLETS. (Allen & Hanburys) Labetalol HCl 100 mg, 200 mg or 300 mg/Tab. Bot. 100s, 500s. UD 100s.
Use: Antihypertensive.
• **TRANEXAMIC ACID.** USAN.
Use: Hemostatic for hemophiliacs. [Orphan drug]
See: Cyclokapron, Tab., Inj. (KabiVitrum).
• **TRANILAST.** USAN.
Use: Anti-asthmatic.
TRANQUILIZERS.
See: A-poxide, Cap. (Abbott).
Atarax, Prep. (Roerig).
Centrax, Cap. (Parke-Davis).
Compazine, Prep. (SK-Beecham).
Equanil, Tab. (Wyeth-Ayerst).
Fenarol, Tab. (Sanofi Winthrop).
Haldol, Tab., Inj., Conc. Soln. (McNeil).
Harmonyl, Tab. (Abbott).
Librium, Cap., Inj. (Roche).
Loxitane, Prod. (Lederle).
Mellaril, Tab., Soln. (Sandoz).
Meprobamate (Various Mfr.).
Miltown, Prep. (Wallace).
Permitil, Prep. (Schering).
Proketazine Maleate, Prep. (Wyeth-Ayerst).
Prolixin, Prep. (Squibb).
Sparine HCl, Prep. (Wyeth-Ayerst).
Stelazine, Prep. (SK-Beecham).
Taractan, Prep. (Roche).
Thorazine HCl, Prep. (SK-Beecham).
Tindal, Tab. (Schering).
Trancopal, Cap. (Sanofi Pharm).
Tranxene, Cap. (Abbott).
Trilafon, Prep. (Schering).
Ultran, Prep. (Lilly).
Valium, Prep. (Roche).
Vesprin, Prep. (Squibb).
Vistaril, Prep. (Pfizer).
TRANQUILS CAPSULES. (Blue Cross) Pyrilamine maleate 25 mg/Cap. Bot. 30s.
Use: Night-time sleep aid.
TRANQUILS TABLETS. (Blue Cross) Acetaminophen 300 mg, pyrilamine maleate 25 mg/Tab. Bot. 30s.
Use: Analgesic & nighttime sleep aid.
• **TRANSCAINIDE.** USAN.
Use: Antiarrhythmic, cardiac depressant.
TRANSCLOMIPHENE. (E)-2-[p-(2-Chloro-1, 2-di- phenylvinyl) phenoxy] triethylamine.
TRANSDERM-NITRO. (Ciba) Nitroglycerin 2.5 mg, 5 mg, 10 mg or 15 mg. **2.5 mg:** 2.5 mg/24 hr. Pkg. 30s. **5 mg:** 5 mg/24 hr. Pkg. 30s. **10 mg:** 10 mg/24 hr. Pkg. 30s. **15 mg:** 15 mg/24 hr. Pkg. 30s.
Use: Prevention and treatment of angina pectoris due to coronary artery disease.
TRANSDERMSCOP. (Ciba) Scopolamine 0.5 mg per 2-unit blister pkg. (programmed delivery over 3-day period).
Use: Antiemetic/antivertigo agent.
TRANSFORMING GROWTH FACTOR-BETA 2. (Celtrix)
Use: Treatment of macular holes. [Orphan drug]
TRANS-PLANTAR. (Tsumura Medical) Salicylic acid 15%, 20 mm patches, 25s. Securing tapes, cleaning file.
Use: Treatment of verruca plantaris.
TRANSTHYRETIN EIA. (Abbott Diagnos-

tics) Test kits 100s.
Use: Enzyme immunoassay for the quantitative determination of transthyretin in human serum or plasma.

TRANS-VER-SAL. (Minnetonka Medical) Salicylic acid 15%/Transdermal patch. 6 mm., 12 mm. in 40s.
Use: Keratolytic.

TRANXENE CAPSULES. (Abbott) Clorazepate dipotassium 3.75 mg, 7.5 mg or 15 mg/Cap. UD 100s.
Use: Minor tranquilizer.

TRANXENE-SD. (Abbott) Clorazepate dipotassium 22.5 mg/Tab. Bot. 100s.
Use: Minor tranquilizer.

TRANXENE-SD HALF STRENGTH TABLETS. (Abbott) Clorazepate dipotassium 11.25 mg/Tab. Bot. 100s.
Use: Minor tranquilizer.

TRANXENE T-TAB TABLETS. (Abbott) Clorazepate dipotassium tab. 3.75 mg, 7.5 mg or 15 mg/Tab. Bot. 100s, 500s.
Use: Minor tranquilizer.

TRANYLCYPROMINE. B.A.N. (±)trans-2-Phenylcyclopropylamine. Parnate (sulfate).
Use: Monoamine oxidase inhibitor; antidepressant.

TRANYLCYPROMINE SULFATE, U.S.P. XXI. Tab., U.S.P. XXI. Trans-dl-2-phenylcyclopropylamine sulfate (±)-trans-2-phenylcyclopropylamine sulfate (2:1).
Use: Antidepressant.
See: Parnate, Tab. (SK-Beecham).

TRAPENS. (Mills) Triticum 4 gr, oxyquinoline sulf. $^1/_{20}$ gr, pow. charcoal 0.5 gr/Tab. Bot. 100s.

TRASICOR. (Ciba) Oxprenolol HCl, B.A.N.

TRASYLOL. (Miles) Aprotinin 1.4 mg/ml. Inj. Vial 100 ml, 200 ml.
Use: Antihemophilic product.

TRAUMACAL. (Mead Johnson Nutrition) Nutritionally complete formula for traumatized patients. Cans 8 oz. Vanilla flavor.
Use: Specific for nitrogen and energy needs in a limited volume for multiple trauma and major burns.

T-RAU TABLET. (Tennessee Pharm.) Rauwolfia serpentina 50 mg or 100 mg/Tab. Bot. 100s, 1000s.
Use: Hypotensive, tranquilizer.

TRAVAMULSION 10% INTRAVENOUS FAT EMULSION. 1.1 kcal/ml 270 mOsm/liter. Bot. 500 ml.
Use: Parenteral nutrition.

TRAVAMULSION 20% INTRAVENOUS FAT EMULSION. (Travenol) 2.0 kcal/ml

300 mOsm/liter. Bot. 500 ml.
Use: Parenteral nutrition.

TRAVASE. (Flint) Proteolytic enzyme ointment, from bacillus subtilis; 82,000 casein units of proteolytic activity/Gm. Tube 14.2 Gm.
Use: Debriding agent.

TRAVASOL. (Travenol) Crystalline L-Amino acids injection 5.5%, 8.5% (with or without electrolytes). IV Bot. 500 ml, 1000 ml, 2000 ml.
Use: Parenteral nutrition.

TRAVASOL 3.5% M INJECTION WITH ELECTROLYTE #45. (Travenol) Crystalline L-Amino acids 3.5% Soln. Bot. I.V. 500 ml, 1000 ml.
Use: Parenteral nutrition.

TRAVASOL 3.5% W/ELECTROLYTES. (Clintec) Amino acid concentration 3.5%, nitrogen 0.591 Gm/100 ml, 500 ml, 1000 ml.
Use: Intravenous nutritional therapy.

TRAVASOL 10%. (Travenol) Crystalline L-amino acids injection 10%. Dot. 200 ml, 500 ml, 1000 ml, 2000 ml.
Use: Parenteral nutrition.

TRAVASORB HEPATIC DIET. (Travenol) 378 kcal/Pkt. 6 pkt./Carton.
Use: Enteral nutrition.

TRAVASORB HN PEPTIDE DIET. (Travenol) High nitrogen defined peptide 333 kcal/Pkt. 6 pkt/Carton.
Use: Enteral nutrition.

TRAVSORB MCT LIQUID DIET. (Travenol) Digestible protein medium chain triglyceride diet. 89 Gm packets.
Use: Enteral nutrition.

TRAVASORB MCT POWDER DIET. (Travenol) Digestible protein medium chain triglyceride diet 400 kcal/Pkt. 6 pkt./Carton.
Use: Enteral nutrition.

TRAVASORB RENAL DIET. (Travenol) 467 kcal/Pkt. 6 pkt/Carton. 112 Gm packets.
Use: Enteral nutrition.

TRAVASORB STANDARD DIET. (Travenol) Defined peptide diet, 333 kcal/pkt. 6 packets/Carton.
Use: Enteral nutrition.

TRAVASORB STD. (Clintec Nutrition) Enzymatically hydrolyzed lactalbum 10 Gm, glucose oligosaccharides 63.3 Gm, MCT (fractioned coconut oil) 4.5 Gm, sunflower oil 4.5 Gm, sodium 307 mg, potassium 390 mg, mOsm/560 Kg, H_2O, cal 333.3/ml, vitamins A, B_1, B_2, B_3, B_5, B_6, B_{12}, C, D, E, K, Ca, Cl, Cu, Fe, I, Mg, Mn, P, Zn. Gluten free. Pow. Pkts. 83.3 Gm.

Use: Enteral nutritional therapy.

TRAVASORB WHOLE PROTEIN LIQUID DIET. (Travenol) Lactose free complete nutrition 250 kcal/Can. Cans 8 oz.
Use: Enteral nutritional supplement.

TRAVEL AIDS. (Faraday) Dimenhydrinate 50 mg/Tab. Bot. 30s.
Use: Antiemetic/antivertigo agent.

TRAVEL-EZE. (Approved) Pyrilamine maleate 25 mg, hyoscine hydrobromide 0.325 mg/Tab. Pkg. 20s.
Use: Antiemetic/antivertigo agent.

TRAVEL SICKNESS. (Walgreen) Dimenhydrinate 50 mg/Tab. Bot. 24s.
Use: Antiemetic/antivertigo agent.

TRAVELTABS. (Geneva) Dimenhydrinate 50 mg/Tab. Bot. 100s.
Use: Antiemetic/antivertigo agent.

TRAVERT. (Travenol) Invert sugar injection. 10% in water or saline. Plastic Bot. 500 ml, 1000 ml.
W/electrolyte No. 2 Bot. 500 ml, 1000 ml,
W/electrolyte No. 4 Bot. 250, 500 ml Soln. (10%).
Use: Fluid/electrolyte replacement.

5% TRAVERT AND ELECTROLYTE NO. 2. (Baxter) Invert sugar 50 Gm/L, calories 196 Cal/L, sodium 56 mEq/L, potassium 25 mEq/L, magnesium 6 mEq/L, chloride 56 mEq/L, phosphate 12.5 mEq/L, lactate 25 mEq/L, osmolarity 449 mOsm/L. 1000 ml.
Use: Intravenous nutritional therapy.

10% TRAVERT AND ELECTROLYTE NO. 2. (Baxter) Invert sugar 100 Gm/L, calories 384 Cal/L, sodium 56 mEq/L, potassium 25 mEq/L, magnesium 6 mEq/L, chloride 56 mEq/L, phosphate 12.5 mEq/L, lactate 25 mEq/L, osmolarity 726 mOsm/L. 1000 ml.
Use: Intravenous nutritional therapy.

• **TRAZODONE HYDROCHLORIDE,** USAN. 2-[3-[4-(m-Chlorophenyl)-1-piperazinyl]propyl]-1,2,4-triazolo[4,3-a]pyridin-3(2H)-one monohydrochloride.
Use: Antidepressant.
See: Desyrel, Tab. (Mead Johnson).

• **TREBENZOMINE HYDROCHLORIDE.** USAN.
Use: Antidepressant.

TRECATOR S.C. (Wyeth-Ayerst) Ethionamide. 2-Ethyl thioisonicotinamide. 250 mg/Tab. Bot. 100s.
Use: Antitubercular agent.

• **TRELOXINATE.** USAN.
Use: Antihyperlipoproteinemic.

TRENDAR (Whitehall) Ibuprofen 200 mg/Tab. Bot. 20s, 40s.
Use: Menstrual pain.

TRENTAL TABLETS. (Hoechst) Pentoxifylline 400 mg/Controlled Release Tab. Bot. 100s. UD 100s.
Use: Oral hemorrheologic agent for peripheral vascular disease.

TREO. (Biopharm Labs) **SPF 8:** Octocrylene, octyl methoxycinnamate, benzophenone-3, octyl salicylate, isostearyl alcohol, diazolidinyl urea, propylparabens, citronella oil 0.05% (as insect repellant). Lot. Bot. 118 ml. **SPF 15:** Octocrylene, octyl methoxycinnamate, benzophenone-3, octyl salicylate, isostearyl alcohol, diazolidinyl urea, propylparabens, citronella oil 0.05% (as insect repellant). Lot. Bot. 118 ml. **SPF 30:** Octocrylene, octyl methoxycinnamate, benzophenone-3, octyl salicylate, isostearyl alcohol, diazolidinyl urea, propylparabens, citronella oil 0.05% (as insect repellant). Lot. Bot. 118 ml.
Use: Sunscreen.

TREOSULFAN. B.A.N. L-Threitol 1,4-dimethane-sul-phonate.

TREOSULFAN.
Use: Antineoplastic. [Orphan drug]
See: Ovastat.

• **TREPIPAM MALEATE.** USAN.
Use: Sedative.

• **TRESTOLONE ACETATE.** USAN.
Use: Antineoplastic, androgen.

TRETAMINE. B.A.N. 2,4,6-Tri(aziridin-1-yl)-1,3,5-triazine. Triethanomelamine; Triethylene Melamine; TEM.
Use: Antineoplastic agent.

TRETHINIUM TOSYLATE. B.A.N. 2-Ethyl-1,2,3,4-tetrahydro-2-methylisoquinolinium toluene-p-sulfonate.
Use: Hypotensive.

TRETHOCANOIC ACID. 3-Hydroxy-3,7,11-trimethyldodecanoic acid.
Use: Anticholesteremic.

• **TRETINOIN,** U.S.P. XXIII. Cream, Gel, Topical Soln., U.S.P. XXIII. 3,7-Dimethyl-9-(2,6,6-trimethylcyclohex-1-enyl)nona-2,4,6,8-all-transtetraenoicacid. All trans-Retinoic acid. Vitamins A acid.
Use: Keratolytic. [Orphan drug]
See: Retin-A, Cream, Gel, Soln. (Ortho).

TRETINOIN LF, IV. (Argus)
Use: Antineoplastic. [Orphan drug]

TREXAN TABLETS. (DuPont) Naltrexone HCl 50 mg/Tab. Bot. 50s.
Use: Opioid antagonist.

TREXIN. (A.V.P.) Tetracycline HCl 250 mg/Cap. Bot. 100s.
Use: Antibiotic.

TRIAC. (Vitarine) Triprolidine HCl 2.5 mg, pseudoephedrine HCl 60 mg/Tab. Bot.

100s, 1000s.
Use: Antihistamine, decongestant.
TRIACET CREAM. (Lemmon) Triamcinolone acetonide 0.1%. Tube 15 Gm, 80 Gm.
Use: Topical anti-inflammatory steroid.
• **TRIACETIN,** U.S.P. XXIII. Glyceryl triacetate.
Use: Topical antifungal.
See: Enzactin, Preps. (Wyeth-Ayerst).
Fungacetin, Oint. (Blair).
TRIACETYLOLEANDOMYCIN. Troleandomycin.
Use: Antibiotic.
TRIACIN C. (Various Mfr.) Pseudoephedrine HCl 30 mg, triprolidine HCl 1.25 mg, codeine phosphate 10 mg/5 ml, alcohol 4.3%. Syr. Bot. pt., gal.
Use: Antihistamine, decongestant, antitussive.
TRIACT LIQUID. (Sanofi Winthrop) Aluminum, magnesium hydroxide, simethicone.
Use: Antacid, antiflatulent.
TRIACT TABLETS. (Sanofi Winthrop) Aluminum, magnesium hydroxide, simethicone.
Use: Antacid, antiflatulent.
TRIAD. (UAD) Butalbital 50 mg, acetaminophen 325 mg, caffeine 40 mg. Cap. Bot. 100s.
Use: Nonnarcotic analgesic combination.
TRIAFED WITH CODEINE SYRUP. (Schein) Pseudoephedrine HCl 30 mg, triprolidine HCl 1.25 mg, codeine phosphate 10 mg. Bot. 473 ml.
Use: Decongestant, antihistamine, antitussive.
• **TRIAFUNGIN.** USAN.
Use: Antifungal.
TRIALODINE. (Quantum) Trazodone HCl 50 and 100 mg/Tab. Bot. 100s, 500s, 1000s.
Use: Antidepressant.
TRIAM-A. (Hyrex) Triamcinolone acetonide 40 mg/ml. Inj. Vial 5 ml.
Use: Adrenal cortical steroid.
• **TRIAMCINOLONE,** U.S.P. XXIII. Tabs., U.S.P. XXIII. 9-Alpha fluoro-16-alpha hydroxy-prednisolone. 9-Fluoro-11β, 16α,17,21-tetrahydroxypregna-1,4-diene-3, 20-dione.
Use: Adrenocortical steroid (anti-inflammatory).
See: Aristocort, Tab., Syr. (Lederle).
Aristoderm, Foam (Lederle).
Aristospan, Parenteral (Lederle).
Kenacort, Tab., Syr. (Squibb Mark).
SK-Triamcinolone, Tab. (SK-

Beecham).
• **TRIAMCINOLONE ACETONIDE,** U.S.P. XXIII. Topical Aerosol, Cream, Oint., Dental Paste, Lotion, Sterile Susp., U.S.P. XXIII. 9-α-fluoro-16-α-17-α-isopropylidenedioxy-D hydrocortisone. Pregna-1,4-diene-3,20-dione,8-fluoro-11,21-dihydroxy-16-17-[(1-methylethylidene)bis(oxy)]-,(11β,16α)-. 9-Fluoro-11β,16α,17,21-tetrahydroxypregna-1,4-diene-3,20-dione cyclic 16,17-acetal with acetone. (Various Mfr.) **Cream: 0.025%, 0.1%:** Tube 15 g, 80 g, 454 g; **0.5%:** 15 g. **Lot.:** 0.025% or 0.1%. Bot. 60 ml. **Oint.: 0.025%, 0.1%:** Tube 15 g, 80 g, 454 g; **0.5%:** Tube 15 g.
Use: Glucocorticoid, topical anti-inflammatory.
See: Aristocort, Cream, Oint (Fujisawa).
Aristoderm Foam (Lederle).
Aristogel, Gel (Lederle).
Delta-Tritex, Cream, Oint. (Dermol).
Flutex, Cream, Oint. (Syosset).
Kenalog Preps. (Westwood-Squibb).
Kenonel, Cream (Marnel).
Tramacin, Cream (Johnson & Johnson).
Triacet, Cream (Lemmon).
Triderm, Cream (Del-Ray).
Tri-Kort, Inj. (Keene).
W/Neomycin, gramicidin, Nystatin.
See: Mycolog, Preps. (Squibb).
• **TRIAMCINOLONE ACETONIDE SODIUM PHOSPHATE.** USAN.
Use: Glucocorticoid
• **TRIAMCINOLONE DIACETATE,** U.S.P. XXIII. Sterile Susp., Syrup, U.S.P. XXIII. 9-Alpha-fluoro-16-alpha-hydroxyprednisolone diacetate. 9-Fluoro-11β, 16α, 17,21-tetrahydroxy-pregna-1,4-diene-3,20-dione-16,21-diacetate.
Use: Glucocorticoid.
See: Amcort, Inj. (Keene).
Aristocort Diacetate Forte (Lederle).
Aristocort Diacetate Intralesional, Inj. (Lederle).
Kenacort, Syr. (Squibb Mark).
Tracilon, Susp. (Savage).
Triam-Forte, Inj. (Hyrex).
• **TRIAMCINOLONE HEXACETONIDE,** U.S.P. XXIII. Sterile Susp., U.S.P. XXIII. 9-Fluoro-11β,16αtetra hyroxypregna-1,-4-diene-3,20-dione cyclic 16, 17-acetal with acetone, 21-(3,3-dimethylbutyrate).
Use: Injectable glucocorticoid.
See: Aristospan, Prep. (Lederle).
TRIAM-FORTE. (Hyrex) Triamcinolone diacetate 40 mg/ml. Vial 5 ml.
Use: Adrenocortical steroid therapy.
TRIAMINIC. (Dorsey) Pyrilamine maleate

25 mg, pheniramine maleate 25 mg,
phenylpropanolamine HCl 50
mg/Timed-release Tab. Bot. 100s, 250s.
Use: Antihistamine, decongestant.
W/Dormethan, terpin hydrate.
See: Tussaminic, Tab. (Dorsey).
TRIAMINIC-12 TABLETS. (Dorsey)
Phenylpropanolamine HCl 75 mq, chlor-
pheniramine maleate 12 mg/S.R. Tab.
Pkg. 10s, 20s.
Use: Decongestant, antihistamine.
TRIAMINIC ALLERGY TABLETS.
(Dorsey) Phenylpropanolamine HCl 25
mg, chlorpheniramine maleate 4
mg/Tab. Blister pk. 24s.
Use: Decongestant, antihistamine.
**TRIAMINIC AM DECONGESTANT FOR-
MULA.** (Sandoz) Pseudoephedrine HCl
15 mg/5 ml, sorbitol, sucrose, orange
flavor, alcohol and dye free. Syr. 118 ml,
237 ml.
Use: Decongestant.
**TRIAMINIC AM COUGH AND DECON-
GESTANT FORMULA.** (Sandoz) Pseu-
doephedrine HCl 15 mg, dextromethor-
phan HBr 7.5 mg/5 ml, sorbitol, sucrose,
orange flavor, alcohol and dye free. Liq.
118 ml, 237 ml.
Use: Decongestant, antitussive.
TRIAMINIC CHEWABLES. (Sandoz Con-
sumer) Phenylpropanolamine HCl 6.25
mg, chlorpheniramine maleate 0.5
mg/Tab. Blister pkg. 24s.
Use: Chewable decongestant and anti-
histamine for children.
TRIAMINIC COLD SYRUP. (Dorsey)
Phenylpropanolamine HCl 12.5 mg,
chlorpheniramine maleate 2 mg/5 ml.
Bot. 4 oz., 8 oz. W/sorbitol.
Use: Decongestant, antihistamine.
TRIAMINIC COLD TABLETS. (Dorsey)
Phenylpropanolamine HCl 12.5 mg,
chlorpheniramine maleate 2 mg/Tab.
Blister pkg. 24s.
Use: Decongestant, antihistamine.
TRIAMINIC-DM SYRUP. (Sandoz)
Phenylpropanolamine HCl 6.25 mg,
dextromethorphan HBr 5 mg, sorbitol,
sucrose. Alcohol free. Bot. 120 ml, 240
ml.
Use: Decongestant, antitussive.
TRIAMINIC EXPECTORANT. (Dorsey)
Phenylpropanolamine HCl 12.5 mg,
guaifenesin 100 mg/5 ml w/alcohol 5%,
saccharin, sorbitol. Bot. 4 oz., 8 oz.
Use: Decongestant-expectorant.
**TRIAMINIC EXPECTORANT
W/CODEINE.** (Sandoz) Phenyl-
propanolamine HCl 12.5 mg, codeine
phosphate 10 mg, guaifenesin 100 mg/5

ml w/alcohol 5%, saccharin, sorbitol. Liq.
Bot. pt.
Use: Decongestant, antitussive, expectorant.
TRIAMINIC EXPECTORANT DH. (Sandoz) Guaifenesin 100 mg, phenylpropanolamine HCl 12.5 mg, pheniramine maleate 6.25 mq, pyrilamine
maleate 6.25 mg, hydrocodone bitartrate 1.67 mg/10 ml w/alcohol 5%, saccharin, sorbitol. Bot. pt.
Use: Expectorant, decongestant, antihistamine, antitussive.
TRIAMINIC NITE LIGHT LIQUID. (Sandoz). 15 mg pseudoephedrine, 1 mg
chlorpheniramine maleate, 7.5 mg dextromethorphan HBr. 120 and 240 ml.
Use: Decongestant, antihistamine, antitussive.
TRIAMINIC ORAL INFANT DROPS.
(Dorsey) Phenylpropanolamine HCl 20
mg, pheniramine maleate 10 mg, pyrilamine maleate 10 mg/ml. Dropper bot.
15 ml.
Use: Decongestant and antihistamine
action.
**TRIAMINIC SORE THROAT FORMULA
LIQUID.** (Sandoz) Pseudoephedrine
HCl 15 mg, dextromethorphan HBr 7.5
mg, acetaminophen 160 mg, EDTA, sucrose, alcohol free. Bot. 240 ml.
Use: Decongestant, antitussive, analgesic.
TRIAMINIC SYRUP. (Sandoz) Phenylpropanolamine HCl 12.5 mg, chlorpheniramine maleate 2 mg, sorbitol, sucrose,
alcohol free. Bot. 150 ml.
Use: Upper respiratory combination.
TRIAMINIC TR TABLETS. (Dorsey)
Phenylpropanolamine HCl 50 mg,
pheniramine maleate 25 mg, pyrilamine
maleate 25 mg/T.R. Tab. 100s, 250s.
Use: Decongestant, antihistamine.
TRIAMINICIN TABLETS. (Sandoz Consumer) Phenylpropanolamine HCl 25
mg, acetaminophen 650 mg, chlorpheniramine maleate 4 mg/Tab. Pkg. 12s,
24s, 48s, 100s. Industrial pkg. 200 × 1s.
Use: Decongestant, analgesic, antihistamine.
**TRIAMINICOL MULTI SYMPTOM COLD
SYRUP.** (Dorsey) Phenyl-
propanolamine HCl 12.5 mg, chlorpheniramine maleate 2 mg, dextromethorphan HBr 10 mg/5 ml (cough syr.), saccharin, sorbitol. Bot. 4 oz., 8 oz.
Use: Decongestant, antihistamine, antitussive.
**TRIAMINICOL MULTI-SYMPTOM COLD
TABLET.** (Sandoz Consumer) Phenyl-

propanolamine HCl 12.5 mg, chlorpheniramine maleate 2 mg, dextromethorphan HBr 10 mg/Tab. Blister pkg. 24s.
Use: Decongestant, antitussive, antihistamine.

TRIAMINICOL MULTI-SYMPTOM RELIEF. (Sandoz) Phenylpropanolamine HCl 6.25 mg, chlorpheniramine maleate 1 mg, dextromethorphan HBr 5 mg/5 ml. Liq. Bot. 120 ml.
Use: Pediatric antitussive, decongestant, antihistamine.

TRIAMINILONE-16,17-ACETONIDE.
See: Triamcinolone acetonide.

TRIAMOLONE 40. (Forest) Triamcinolone diacetate 40 mg/ml. Vial 5 ml.

TRIAMONIDE 40. (Forest) Triamcinolone acetonide 40 mg/ml. Vial 5 ml.

• **TRIAMPYZINE SULFATE.** USAN. 2-(Dimethylamino)-3,5,6-trimethylpyrazine sulfate.
Use: Anticholinergic.

• **TRIAMTERENE.** U.S.P. XXIII. Caps., U.S.P. XXIII. 2,4,7-Triamino-6-phenylpteridine. 2,4,7-Pteridinetriamine,6-phenyl-Dytac.
Use: Diuretic.
See: Dyrenium, Cap. (SK-Beecham).

TRIAMTERENE/HYDROCHLOROTHIAZIDE. (Various Mfr.) **Cap.:** Triamterene 50 mg, hydrochlorothiazide 25 mg. Bot. 100s, 1000s. **Tab.;** Triamterene 37.5 mg, hydrochlorothiazide 25 mg. Bot. 100s, 500s, 1000s; Triamterene 75 mg, hydrochlorothiazide 50 mg. Bot. 100s, 250s, 500s, 1000s.
Use: Diuretic combination.

• **TRIAMTERENE AND HYDROCHLOROTHIAZIDE CAPSULES.** U.S.P. XXIII.
Use: Diuretic.
See: Dyazide, Cap. (SK-Beecham).

TRIANIDE. (Seatrace) Triamcinolone acetonide 40 mg/ml. Vial 5 ml.
Use: Corticosteroid.

TRIAPRIN. (Dunhall) Acetaminophen 325 mg, butalbital 50 mg/Caps. Bot. 100s, 500c.
Use: Analgesic, sedative.

TRI-AQUA. (Pfeiffer) Caffeine 100 mg, extracts of buchu, uva ursi, zea, triticum/Tab. Bot. 50s, 100s.
Use: Diuretic.

TRIASYN B. (Lannett) Vitamins B_1 2 mg, B_2 3 mg, B_3 20 mg/Cap. Bot. 500s, 100s. Tab. Bot. 1000s.
Use: B vitamin combination.

TRIATROPHENE. (Lannett) Magnesium trisilicate 7.5 gr, phenobarbital 1/8 gr, atropine sulfate gr/Tab. Bot. 1000s.

Use: G.I. sedative.

TRIAVIL. (Merck & Co.) Perphenazine 4 mg, amitriptyline HCl 10 mg/salmon-colored Tab.; perphenazine 2 mg, amitriptyline HCl 25 mg/orange Tab.; perphenazine 4 mg, amitriptyline 25 mg/yellow Tab.; perphenazine 2 mg, amitriptyline HCl 10 mg/blue Tab. Bot. 100s, 500s. UD 100s. Perphenazine 4 mg, amitryptyline 50 mg/orange Tab. Bot. 60s, 100s. UD 100s.
Use: Tranquilizer, antidepressant.

TRI-A-VITE F. (Major) F 0.5 mg, Vitamins A 1500 IU, 400 IU, C 35 mg/ml Drops. Bot. 50 ml.
Use: Multivitamin.

TRIAZIQUONE. B.A.N. Tri(aziridin-1-yl)-1,4-benzoquinone. Trenimon.
Use: Antineoplastic agent.

• **TRIAZOLAM,** U.S.P. XXIII. Tab., U.S.P. XXIII.
Use: Sedative, hypnotic.
See: Halcion, Tab. (Upjohn).

TRIAZOLAM. (Various Mfr.) 0.125 mg, 0.25 mg. Tab. Bot. 500s, UD 100s, unit-of-use 100s.
Use: Sedative.

TRIBAN. (Great Southern) Trimethobenzamido HCl 200 mg, benzocaine 2%. Supp. Pkg. 10s, 50s.
Use: Treatment for nausea and vomiting.

TRIBAN, PEDIATRIC. (Great Southern) Trimethobenzamide HCl 100 mg, benzocaine 2%. Supp. Pkg. 10s.
Use: Treatment for nausea and vomiting.

• **TRIBENOSIDE.** USAN. Ethyl 3,5,6-tri-O-benzyl-D-glucofuranoside. Glyvenol. Not available in U.S.
Use: Venoprotective agent.

TRI-BIOCIN. (Approved) Bacitracin 400 u., polymyxin B sulfate 5000 u., neomycin 5 mg/Gm Tube 0.5 oz.
Use: Topical antibiotic.

TRIBIOTIC PLUS. (Thompson) Polymyx in B sulfate 5000 units, neomycin sulfate (equivalent to 3.5 mg neomycin base), bacitracin 500 units, lidocaine 40 mg/g, lanolin, light mineral oil, petrolatum. Oint. Tube 28.35 g.
Use: Topical anti-infective.

TRIBROMOETHANOL. 2,2,2-Tribromoethanol.
Use: Anesthetic (inhalation).

TRIBROMOMETHANE. Bromoform.

• **TRIBROMSALAN.** USAN. 3,4′,5-Tribromosalicylanilide. Hilomid.
Use: Germicide, disinfectant.
See: Diaphene (or ASC-4) (Stecker).

Tuasol 100 (Marion Merrell Dow).

TRICALCIUM PHOSPHATE.
Use: Minerals and electrolytes, oral.
See: Posture (Whitehall).
• **TRICETAMIDE.** USAN. 3,4,5-Trimethoxy-
benzoylglycine diethylamide.
Use: Sedative.
TRI-CHLOR. (Gordon) Trichloracetic acid
80%. Bot. 15 ml.
Use: Topical, as a caustic verruca
cauterant.
TRICHLORAN.
See: Trichloroethylene.
TRICHLOREX. (Lannett) Trichlormethi-
azide 4 mg/Tab. Bot. 100s, 1000s.
Use: Thiazides and related diuretics.
• **TRICHLORMETHIAZIDE,** U.S.P. XXIII.
Tab., U.S.P. XXIII. 3-Dichloromethyl-6-
chloro-7-sulfamyl-3,4-dihydro-1,2,4-
benzothiadiazine-1,1-dioxide. 6-Chloro-
3-(dichloromethyl)-3,4-dihydro-2H-
1,2,4-benzothiadiazine-7-sulfonamide-1,
1-Dioxide.
Use: Diuretic; antihypertensive.
See: Aquex, Tab. (Lannett).
Metahydrin, Tab. (Marion Merrell
Dow).
Naqua, Tab. (Schering).
W/Reserpine.
See: Metatensin, Tab. (Marion Merrell
Dow).
Naquival, Tab. (Schering).
TRICHLORMETHINE (I.N.N.).
See: Trimustine, B.A.N.
TRICHLOROACETIC ACID, U.S.P. XXI.
Acetic acid, trichloro.
Use: Topical, as a caustic.
TRICHLOROBUTYL ALCOHOL.
See: Chlorobutanol.
TRICHLOROCARBANILIDE. W/Salicylic
acid, sulfur.
• **TRICHLOROMONOFLUOROMETHANE,**
N.F. XVII.
Use: Aerosol propellant.
TRICHOLINE CITRATE.
See: Choline citrate.
TRICHOMONAS TEST.
See: Isocult for *Trichomonas vaginalis.*
(SmithKline Diagnostics).
TRICHOTINE. (Reed & Carnrick) **Pow.:**
Sodium lauryl sulf., sod. perborate, chlo-
ride, aromatics. Pkg. 5, 20 oz. **Liq.:**
Sodium lauryl sulfate, sodium borate,
ethyl alcohol 8%, aromatics. Bot. 4 oz., 8
oz.
Use: Vaginal douche.
• **TRICIRIBINE PHOSPHATE.** USAN.
Use: Antineoplastic.
• **TRICITRATES ORAL SOLUTION,** U.S.P.
XXIII.

TRICLOBISONIUM. Triburon, Oint.
(Roche).
TRICLOBISONIUM CHLORIDE. Hexam-
ethylenebis[dimethyl[1-methyl-3-(2,2,6-
tri-methylcyclohexyl)propyl]-ammonium]
Dichloride.
Use: Topical anti-infective.
• **TRICLOCARBAN.** USAN. 3,4,4'-
Trichloro- carbanilide.
Use: Germicide, disinfectant.
See: Artra Beauty Ban (Plough).
W/Clofulcarban.
See: Safeguard Bar Soap, (P & G).
• **TRICLOFENOL PIPERAZINE.** USAN.
Piperazine (1:2) with (2,4,5-trichlorophe-
nol).
Use: Anthelmintic (nematodes).
TRICLOFOS. B.A.N. 2,2,2-Trichloroethyl
dihydrogen phosphate. Tricloryl (mono-
sodium salt).
Use: Hypnotic.
• **TRICLONIDE.** USAN.
Use: Anti-inflammatory.
• **TRICLOSAN.** USAN. 5-Chloro-2-(2,4-
dichlorophenoxy)phenol.
Use: Antibacterial.
See: Ambi 10, Bar (Kiwi Brands).
Clearasil Daily Face Wash (Procter &
Gamble).
Clearasil Soap (Procter & Gamble).
Oxy ResiDon't, Liq. (SK-Beecham).
TRICODENE COUGH AND COLD. (Pfeif-
fer) Pyrilamine maleate 12.5 mg,
codeine phosphate 8.2 mg, menthol,
honey, glucose, sucrose. Liq. Bot. 120
ml.
Use: Narcotic antitussive combination.
TRICODENE FORTE. (Pfeiffer) Phenyl-
propanolamine HCl 12.5 mg, chlorpheniramine maleate 2 mg, dextromethorphan HBr 10 mg/5 ml Liq. Bot. 120 ml.
Use: Antihistamine, decongestant, antitussive.
TRICODENE LIQUID. (Pfeiffer) Chlorpheniramine maleate 0.5 mg, dextromethorphan HBr 10 mg, ammonium
Cl 90 mg, sodium citrate, sorbitol, man-
nitol/5 ml Liq. Bot. 120 ml.
Use: Antihistamine, antitussive, expectorant.
TRICODENE NN. (Pfeiffer) Phenylpropanolamine HCl 12.5 mg, chlorpheniramine maleate 2 mg, dextromethorphan HBr 10 mg/5 ml. Syr. Bot. 120 ml.
Use: Antihistamine, decongestant, antitussive, expectorant.
**TRICODENE PEDIATRIC COUGH &
COLD LIQUID.** (Pfeiffer) Phenylpropanolamine HCl 12.5 mg, Dextromethorphan HBr 10 mg/5 ml Liq. 120

ml.
Use: Decongestant, antitussive.

TRICODENE SUGAR FREE. (Pfeiffer) Chlorpheniramine maleate, dextromethorphan HBr 10 mg, menthol, saccharin, sorbitol, alcohol free. Liq. 120 ml.
Use: Cough preparation.

TRICODENE SYRUP. (Pfeiffer) Pyrilamine maleate 4.17 mg, codeine phosphate 8.1 mg, terpin hydrate, menthol/5 ml Syr. Bot. 120 ml.
Use: Antihistamine, antitussive, expectorant.

TRICOM. (Nutripharm) Pseudoephedrine HCl 60 mg, chlorpheniramine mleate 4 mg, acetaminophen 650 mg, sucrose, dye free. Tab. Bot. 100s.
Use: Upper respiratory combination.

TRICOMINE. (Major) Pseudoephedrine HCl 60 mg, carbinoxamine maleate 4 mg, dextromethorphan HBr 15 mg/ 5 ml, alcohol 5%. Expec. Bot. 120 ml.
Use: Antihistamine, decongestant, antitussive.

TRICOSAL. (URL) Choline magnesium trisalicylate 500 mg, 750 mg/Tab. Bot. 100s.
Use: Salicylate.

TRICYCLAMOL CHLORIDE, B.A.N. 1-(3-Cyclohexyl-3-hydroxy-3-phenylpropyl)-1-methylpyrroidinium chloride. Elorine Chloride; Lergine.
Use: Anticholinergic.

TRICYLATATE HCl. 1-Methyl-3-pyrrolidylmethyl benzilate HCl.

TRIDERM CREAM. (Del-Ray) Triamcinolone acetonide 0.1%. Tube 30 g, 90 g.
Use: Glucocortcoid.

TRIDESILON CREAM. (Miles Pharm) Desonide 0.05% in vehicle buffered to the pH range of normal skin w/glycerin, methyl paraben, sodium lauryl sulfate, aluminum sulfate, calcium acetate, cetyl stearyl alcohol, synthetic bees-wax, white petrolatum, mineral oil. Tube 15 Gm, 60 Gm.
Use: Corticosteroid therapy.

TRIDESILON OTIC. (Miles Pharm) Desonide 0.05%, acetic acid 2% in vehicle. Bot. 10 ml.
Use: Otitis externa treatment.

TRIDEX TAB., TIMED TRIDEX CAP., TIMED TRIDEX JR. CAP. (Fellows) Changed to Daro Tab., Daro Timed Cap., Daro Jr. Timed Cap.

• **TRIDIHEXETHYL CHLORIDE,** U.S.P. XXII. Inj., Tab., U.S.P. XXII. (3-Cyclohexyl-3-hydroxy-3-phenylpropyl)-tri-ethylammonium chloride.

Use: Anticholinergic.
W/Meprobamate.
  See: Milpath, Tab. (Wallace).
  Pathibamate, Tab. (Lederle).
W/Phenobarbital.
  See: Pathilon w/Phenobarbital Tab., Cap. (Lederle).

TRIDIL 0.5 mg/ml. (Du Pont) Nitroglycerin 0.5 mg/ml w/alcohol 10%, water for injection, buffered with sodium phosphate. Amp. 10 ml. Box 20s.
Use: Vasodilator; anti-anginal, hypotensive.

TRIDIL 5 mg/ml. (Du Pont) Nitroglycerin 5 mg/ml w/alcohol 30%, propylene glycol 30%, water for injection. Amp. 5 ml, 10 ml. Vial 5 ml, 10 ml, 20 ml. Box 20s. Special administration set w/10 ml Amp.
Use: Vasodilator; anti-anginal, hypotensive.

TRIDIONE. (Abbott) Trimethadione. (Troxidone). Cap. 300 mg, Bot. 100s. Dulcet Tab. 150 mg, Bot. 100s. Soln. 1.2 Gm/fl. oz., Bot. 1 pt.
Use: Anti-epileptic.

TRIDRATE BOWEL EVACUANT KIT. (Mallinckrodt) Magnesium citrate soln. 300 ml, bisacodyl 5 mg/Tab. (3s), bisacodyl 10 mg/Supp. (1). Kit.
Use: Laxative.

• **TRIENTINE HYDROCHLORIDE.** USAN.
Use: Wilson's disease therapy adjunct. [Orphan drug]
  See: Cuprid, Cap, (Merck & Co.).

TRIETHANOLAMINE,
  See: Trolamine, N.F. XVIII.

TRIETHANOLAMINE POLYPEPTIDE OLEATE CONDENSATE.
  See: Cerumenex, Drops (Purdue Frederick).

TRIETHANOLAMINE SALICYLATE.
  See: Aspercreme, Cream (Thompson).
  Aspergel, Oint. (LaCrosse).
  Myoflex, Cream (Warren-Teed).

TRIETHANOLAMINE TRINITRATE BIPHOSPHATE. Trolnitrate Phosphate.

• **TRIETHYL CITRATE,** N.F. XVIII.

TRIETHYLENEMELAMINE. Tretamine TEM. 2,4,6-Tris(1-aziridinyl)-5-triazine.
Use: Antineoplastic.

TRIETHYLENETHIOPHOSPHORAMIDE.
  See: Thiotepa (Lederle).

TRIFED. (Geneva Generics) Pseudoephedrine HCl 60 mg, triprolidine HCl 2.5 mg/Tab. Bot. 100s, 1000s.
Use: Decongestant, antihistamine.

TRIFED-C. (Geneva Generics) Pseudoephedrine HCl 30 mg, triprolidine HCl 1.25 mg, codeine phosphate 10 mg/5 ml, alcohol 4.3%. Syr. Bot. pt., gal.

Use: Antihistamine, decongestant, antitussive.

• **TRIFENAGREL.** USAN.
Use: Antithrombotic.

• **TRIFLOCIN.** USAN. 4-(α,α,α-Trifluoro-m-toluidino) nicotinic acid.
Use: Diuretic.

• **TRIFLUBAZAM.** USAN.
Use: Tranquilizer.

• **TRIFLUMIDATE.** USAN. Ethyl m-benzoyl-N-[(trifluoromethyl)sulfonyl]carbanilate.
Use: Anti-inflammatory.

TRIFLUOPERAZINE. B.A.N. 10-[3-(4-Methyl-piperazin-1-yl)propyl]-2-trifluoromethylphenothiazine.
Use: Tranquilizer, antiemetic.

• **TRIFLUOPERAZINE HCl,** U.S.P. XXIII. Inj., Syrup, Tab., U.S.P. XXIII. 10-[3-(1-Methyl-4-piperazinyl)- propyl]-2-trifluoromethyl phenothiazine HCl. 10-(3-(4-Methyl-1-piperazinyl)propyl)-2-(trifluoromethyl)phenothiazine dihydrochloride.
Use: Tranquilizer, sedative, antipsychotic.
See: Stelazine Inj., Liq., Tab. (SK-Beecham).

N-TRIFLUOROACETYLADRIAMYCIN-14-VALERATE (Anthra Pharm)
Use: Antineoplastic. [Orphan drug]

TRIFLUOROTHYMIDINE.
Use: Ophthalmic.
See: Viroptic (Burroughs Wellcome).

• **TRIFLUPERIDOL.** USAN.
Use: Antipsychotic.

• **TRIFLUPROMAZINE,** U.S.P. XXIII. Oral Susp., XXII.
Use: Tranquilizer, antipsychotic agent.

• **TRIFLUPROMAZINE HCl,** U.S.P. XXIII. Inj., Tab., U.S.P. XXIII. 10-[3-(3-Di-methylamino)propyl]-2-(tri-fluoromethyl)phenothiazine HCl. Fluopromazine, B.A.N.
Use: Tranquilizer, antipsychotic agent.
See: Vesprin Prods. (Princeton).

• **TRIFLURIDINE.** USAN.
Use: Antiviral used to treat herpes simplex eye infections.
See: Viroptic Ophthalmic Soln., (Burroughs Wellcome).

TRIGELAMINE. (Edward J. Moore) Pyrilamine maleate, pheniramine maleate, chlorpheniramine maleate, benzalkonium Cl, menthol. Tube. 1.25 oz.
Use: Triple antihistamine gel.

TRIGESIC. (Squibb Mark) Acetyl-p-aminophenol 125 mg, aspirin 230 mg, caffeine 30 mg/Tab. Bot. 100s.
Use: Analgesic.

TRIGLYCERIDES, MEDIUM CHAIN.
Use: Enteral nutritional therapy.

See: MCT (Mead Johnson Nutritionals).

TRIGLYCERIDE REAGENT STRIP. (Miles Diagnostic) Seralyzer reagent strip. Bot. 25s.
Use: A quantitative strip test for triglycerides in serum or plasma.

TRI-GRAIN. (Pharmex) Isometheptene tartrate. **Inj.:** 100 mg/ml. Vial 10 ml **Tab.:** Bot. 24s, 100s.

TRIHEMIC-600. (Lederle) Vitamins C 600 mg, B_{12} 25 mcg, intrinsic factor conc. 75 mg, folic acid 1 mg, Vitamins E 30 IU, ferrous fumarate 115 mg, dioctyl sod. succinate 50 mg/Tab. Bot. 30s, 500s.
Use: Anemias.

TRIHEXANE. (Rugby) Trihexyphenidyl 2 mg/Tab. Bot. 100s, 1000s.
Use: Anticholinergic, antiparkinson agent.

TRIHEXIDYL. (Schein) Trihexyphenidyl 2 mg/Tab. Bot. 100s, 1000s.
Use: Anticholinergic, antiparkinson agent.

TRIHEXY-2. (Geneva Generics) Trihexyphenidyl 2 mg/Tab. Bot. 100s, 1000s.
Use: Anticholinergic, antiparkinson agent.

TRIHEXY-5. (Geneva Generics) Trihexyphenidyl 5 mg/Tab. Bot. 100s, 1000s.
Use: Anticholinergic, antiparkinson agent.

• **TRIHEXYPHENIDYL HYDROCHLORIDE,** U.S.P. XXIII. Elix., Extended-release Cap., Tab. U.S.P. XXIII. α-Cyclohexyl-α-phenyl-1-piperidinepropanol HCl. 1-Piperidine-propanol, α-cyclohexyl-α-phenyl-, HCl. Benzhexol, B.A.N.
Use: Anticholinergic, antiparkinsonian.
See: Artane, Elixir & Tab. (Lederle).

TRI-HISTIN. (Recsei) **25 mg Tab.:** Pyrilamine maleate 10 mg, chlorpheniramine maleate 1 mg. **50 mg Tab.:** Pyrilamine maleate 20 mg, methapyrilene HCl 15 mg, chlorpheniramine maleate 2 mg. **100 mg S.A. Cap.:** Pyrilamine maleate 40 mg, pheniramine maleate 25 mg. **Expectorant:** Pyrilamine maleate 5 mg, chlorpheniramine maleate 0.5 mg, guaifenesin 20 mg, phenyl-propanolamine 7.5 mg, phenylephrine HCl 2.5 mg, sod. citrate 100 mg/5 ml. Bot. pt. gal. **Liquid:** Pyrilamine maleate 5 mg, chlorpheniramine maleate 0.5 mg/5 ml. Bot. pt. gal. **Tab.:** Bot. 100s, 500s, 1000s. 50 mg Bot. 1000s. **Cap.:** Bot. 100s, 500s, 1000s.
Use: Triple antihistamine therapy.
W/Benzyl alcohol, chlorobutanol & iso-

propyl alcohol.
See: Derma-Pax, Liq. (Recsei).
W/Codeine phosphate, guaifenesin,
phenylpropanolamine, phenylephrine
HCl, sodium citrate.
See: Trihista-Cod., Liq. (Recsei).
W/Ephedrine HCl, aminophylline, mepho-
barbital.
See: Asmasan, Tab. (Recsei).
TRI-HYDROSERPINE. (Rugby) Hy-
drochlorothiazide 15 mg, reserpine 0.1
mg, hydralazine HCl 25 mg. Tab. Bot.
100s, 1000s.
Use: Antihypertensive combination.
TRIHYDROXYESTRINE. Trihydrox-
yestrin.
TRIHYDROXYETHYLAMINE. Tri-
ethanolamine.
TRI-IMMUNOL. (Lederle) Diphtheria &
tetanus toxoids & pertussis vaccine
combined, aluminum phosphate-ad-
sorbed purogenated. Vial 7.5 ml.
Use: I.M., Immunization.
TRIIODOMETHANE.
See: Iodoform. (Various Mfr.).
TRI-K. (Century) Potassium acetate 0.5
Gm, potassium bicarbonate 0.5 Gm,
potassium citrate 0.5 Gm/fl. oz. Saccha-
rin. Bot. pt., gal.
Use: Potassium supplement.
• **TRIKATES ORAL SOLUTION,** U.S.P.
XXIII.
Use: Potassium deficiency.
TRI-KORT. (Keene) Triamcinalone ace-
tonide suspension 40 mg/ml. Vial 5 ml.
Use: Anti-inflammatory.
TRILAFON. (Schering) Perphenazine.
Tab.: 2, 4, 8 & 16 mg. Bot. 100s, 500s.
Inj.: 5 mg/ml, w/disodium citrate 24.6
mg, sod. bisulfite 2 mg, and water for in-
jection/ml. Amp. 1 ml **Repetabs:** 8 mg.
Bot. 100s. **Concentrate:** 16 mg/5 ml.
Bot. 4 oz. w/dropper.
Use: Tranquilizer.
TRILAX. (Drug Industries) Docusate sodi-
um 200 mg, yellow phenolphthalein 30
mg, dehydrocholic acid 20 mg/Cap. Bot.
100s, 500s.
Use: Laxative, fecal softener, choleretic.
TRI-LEVLEN 21 TABLETS. (Berlex).
　Group 1: Levonorgestrel 0.050 mg,
　ethinyl estradiol 0.030 mg/ Tab.
　Group 2: Levonorgestrel 0.075 mg,
　ethinyl estradiol 0.040 mg/ Tab.
　Group 3: Levonorgestrel 0.125 mg,
　ethinyl estradiol 0.030 mg/ Tab. Slide-
　case 21s. Box 3s.
Use: Oral contraceptive triphasic regi-
men.
TRI-LEVLEN 28 TABLETS. (Berlex).

　Group 1: Levonorgestrel 0.050 mg,
　ethinyl estradiol 0.030 mg/ Tab.
　Group 2: Levonorgestrel 0.075 mg,
　ethinyl estradiol 0.040 mg/ Tab.
　Group 3: Levonorgestrel 0.125 mg,
　ethinyl estradiol 0.030 mg/ Tab.
　Group 4: Inert tablets. Slidecase 28s.
　Box 3s.
Use: Oral contraceptive, triphasic regi-
men.
TRILISATE LIQUID. (Purdue Frederick)
Choline magnesium trisalicylate from
choline salicylate 293 mg, magnesium
salicylate 362 mg/ tsp. to provide 500
mg salicylate/tsp. Bot. 8 oz.
Use: Non-steroidal anti-inflammatory,
anti-arthritic.
TRILISATE TABLETS. (Purdue Frederick) Choline magnesium trisalicylate.
500 mg/Tab. of salicylate from choline
salicylate 293 mg, magnesium salicylate
362 mg/Tab. Bot. 100s. **750 mg/Tab.** of
salicylate from choline salicylate 400 mg
and magnesium salicylate 544 mg Bot.
100s. 1000 mg/Tab. of salicylate from
choline salicylate 587 mg, magnesium
salicylate 725 mg Bot. 60s.
Use: Non-steroidal anti-inflammatory,
anti-arthritic, analgesic.
TRILOG. (Hauck) Triamcinolone acetonide 40 mg/ml. Vial 5 ml.
Use: Steroid therapy.
TRILONE. (Century) Triamcinalone diac-
etate susp. Amp. 10 ml.
Use: Corticosteroid.
TRILONE. (Hauck) Triamcinolone diac-
etate 40 mg/ml. Vial 5 ml.
Use: Steroid therapy.
• **TRILOSTANE.** USAN.
Use: Adrenocortical suppressant.
See: Modrastane, Cap. (Winthdrop-
Breon).
TRIMAHIST ELIXIR. (Tennessee Pharm.)
Phenylephrine HCl 5 mg, prophenpyri-
damine maleate 12.5 mg, l-menthol 1
mg, alcohol 5%/5 ml. Bot. pt., gal.
Use: Antihistamine.
TRIMAX GEL. (Sanofi Winthrop) Alu-
minum, magnesium hydroxide, sime-
thicone.
Use: Antacid, antiflatulent.
TRIMAX TABLET. (Sanofi Winthrop) Alu-
minum, magnesium hydroxide, sime-
thicone.
Use: Antacid, antiflatulent.
TRIMAZIDE. (Major) **Capsules:**
Trimethobenazamide 250 mg/Cap. Bot.
100s. **Suppositories:** 100 mg and 200
mg/Supp. 10s.
Use: Treatment of nausea and vomiting.

TRIMAZINOL. α-p-[(4,6-Diaminos-triazin-2-yl)-aminol]-methyl benzyl alcohol.
Use: Anti-inflammatory agent.
• **TRIMAZOSIN HYDROCHLORIDE.**
USAN.
Use: Antihypertensive.
TRIMEDINE. (Trimen) Phenylephrine HCl 5 mg, chlorpheniramine maleate 1 mg, dextromethorphan HBr 15 mg/5 ml, sorbitol. Liq. Bot. pt., gal.
Use: Antihistamine, decongestant, antitussive.
TRIMEPERIDINE. B.A.N. 1,2,5-Trimethyl-4-phenyl-4-piperidyl propionate.
Use: Narcotic analgesic.
TRIMEPRAZINE. B.A.N. 10-(3-Dimethylamino-2- methylpropyl)phenothiazine. Alimemazine (I.N.N.) Vallergan.
Use: Tranquilizer; antihistamine.
TRIMEPRAZINE TARTRATE, U.S.P. XXII. Syrup, Tab., U.S.P. XXIII. (±)-10-(3-Dimethylamino-2-methylpro-pyl)-phenothiazine tartrate (2:1) 10H-Phenothiazine-10-propanamine N,N,β-trimethyl-2,3-dihydrox- ybutanedioate (2:1).
Use: Antipruritic.
See: Temaril, Prods. (Herbert).
TRIMETAMIDE. Trimethamide.
TRIMETAPHAN CAMSYLATE. B.A.N. 1,3-Dibenzyldecahydro-2-oxoimidazo[4,5-c]thieno[1,2-a]-thiolium(+)-camphor-10-sulfonate.
Use: Hypotensive.
TRIMETAZIDINE. B.A.N. 1-(2,3,4-Trimethoxybenzyl)piperazine.
Use: Vasodilator.
• **TRIMETHADIONE,** U.S.P. XXIII. Cap., Oral Soln., Tab., U.S.P. XXIII. 3,5,5-Trimethyl-2,4-oxazolidinedione.
Use: Anticonvulsant.
See: Tridione, Prep. (Abbott).
TRIMETHADIONE (I.N.N.). Troxidone, B.A.N.
TRIMETHAMIDE. N-[(2-Amino-6-methyl-3-pyridyl)methyl]3,4,5-trimethoxybenzamide.
Use: Antihypertensive agent.
TRIMETHAPHAN CAMPHOR SULFONATE. Trimethaphan Camsylate, U.S.P. XXIII.
• **TRIMETHAPHAN CAMSYLATE,** U.S.P. XXIII. Inj., U.S.P. XXIII. d-3,4-(1′,3-Dibenzyl-2-ketoimidazolido)-1,2-trimethylenethiophanium d-camphorsulfonate. Trimethaphan camphorsulfonate. (+)-1,3-Dibenzyldecahydro-2-oxoimidazo[4,5-c]thieno-[1,2-α]-thiolium 2-oxo-10-bornanesulfonate.
Use: Antihypertensive.
See: Arfonad, Amp. (Roche).

TRIMETHIDINIUM METHOSULFATE, B.A.N. d-(N-methyl-N-(gamma-trimethyl-ammonium-propyl))-1-methyl-8,8-di-methyl-3-azabicyclo-(3,2,1) octane dimethosulfate. 1,3,8,8-Tetram-ethyl-3-(3-(trimethylammonio)propyl)-3-azoniabicyclo(3.2.1)octane. Tab.
Use: Antihypertensive.
• **TRIMETHOBENZAMIDE HCl,** U.S.P. XXIII. Cap., Inj., U.S.P. XXIII. N-p-[2-(Dimethylamino) ethoxy]-benzyl -3,4,5-trimethoxybenzamide HCl.
Use: Antiemetic.
See: Tegamide, Suppos. (G & W). Tigan, Preps. (Beecham Labs.).
TRIMETHOBENZAMIDE HYDROCHLORIDE AND BENZOCAINE SUPPOSITORIES.
Use: Antiemetic.
See: Pediatric Triban (Great Southern). Triban (Great Southern).
• **TRIMETHOPRIM,** U.S.P. XXIII. Tab., U.S.P. XXIII. 2,4-Diamino-5-(3,4,5-trimethoxybenzyl)pyrimidine. Syraprim.
Use: Antibacterial agent.
See: Proloprim, Tab. (Burroughs Wellcome).
Trimpex, Tab. (Roche).
W/Polymyxin B Sulfate.
See: Polytrim Ophth. Soln. (Allergan).
W/Sulfamethoxazole.
See: Bactrim, Oral Susp., Ped. Susp., Tab. (Roche).
Septra, Tab. (Burroughs Wellcome).
Septra DS, Tab. (Burroughs Wellcome).
• **TRIMETHOPRIM SULFATE.** USAN.
Use: Antibacterial.
TRIMETHYLENE. Cyclopropane, U.S.P. XXIII.
• **TRIMETOZINE.** USAN.
Use: Sedative.
• **TRIMETREXATE.** USAN.
Use: Antineoplastic.
See: Neutrexin, Vial (US Bioscience).
TRIMETREXATE GLUCURONATE.
Use: Antineoplastic. [Orphan drug]
TRIMINOL. (Rugby) Phenyl-propanolamine HCl 12.5 mg, chlorpheniramine maleate 2 mg, dextromethorphan HBr 10 mg/5 ml Syr. Bot. 120 ml.
Use: Antihistamine, decongestant, antitussive.
• **TRIMIPRAMINE.** USAN. 5-[3-(Dimethylamino)-2-methylpropyl]-10,11-dihydro-5H-dibenz[b,f]-aze-pine.
Use: Antidepressant.
• **TRIMIPRAMINE MALEATE.** USAN. 5-[3-(Di-methylamino)-2-methylpropyl]-10,11-dihydro-5H-dibenz [b,f]azepine

maleate (1:1). (Various Mfr.) 25 mg, 50 mg or 100 mg. Cap. Bot. 100s, UD 100s.
Use: Antidepressant.
See: Surmontil (Wyeth-Ayerst).

TRIMIXIN. (Hance) Bacitracin 200 u., polymyxin B sulfate 4000 u., neomycin sulfate 3 mg/Gm Oint., Tube 0.5 oz.
Use: Topically, antibiotic therapy.

• **TRIMOPROSTIL.** USAN.
Use: Gastric antisecretory.

TRIMO-SAN. (Milex) Oxyquinoline sulfate, sodium lauryl sulfate 0.0084%, boric acid 1.0%, borax 0.70%. Tube 4 oz. w/boilable nylon jel Jector; 4 oz. refill tube.
Use: Restore and maintain vaginal acidity.

TRIMOX. (Squibb Mark) **Cap.:** Amoxicillin trihydrate 250 mg/Cap. Bot. 100s, 500s; 500 mg/Cap. Bot. 50s, 500s. UD 100s.
Oral Susp.: 125 mg/5 ml. Bot. 80 ml, 100 ml, 150 ml, Unimatic Bot. 5 ml, Ctn. 4 × 25s; 250 mg/5 ml. Bot. 80 ml, 100 ml, 150 ml, Unimatic Bot. 5 ml, Ctn. 4 × 25s.
Use: Antibiotic.

• **TRIMOXAMINE HYDROCHLORIDE.** USAN. α-Allyl-3,4,5-trimethoxy-N-methylphenethylamine HCl.
Use: Antihypertensive.

TRIMPEX. (Roche) Trimethoprim 100 mg/Tab. Bot. 100s; Tel-E-Dose 100s.
Use: Treatment of initial episodes of uncomplicated urinary tract infections.

TRIM-QWIK. (O'Connor) Powder based meal food supplement. Can 10 oz.
Use: Meal replacement.

TRIMSTAT. (Laser) Phendimetrazine tartrate 35 mg/Tab. Bot. 100s, 1000s.
Use: Anorexiant.

TRIM SULF D/S. (Metro Med) Sulfamethoxazole 800 mg, trimethoprim 160 mg/Tab. Bot. 100s, 500s.
Use: Antibacterial agent for urinary infections.

TRIM SULF S/S. (Metro Med) Sulfamethoxazole 400 mg, trimethoprim 80 mg/Tab. Bot. 100s, 500s.
Use: Antibacterial agent for urinary infections.

TRIM-SULFA.
Use: Anti-infective combination.
See: Proloprim (Burroughs Wellcome).
Trimethoprim (Various Mfr.).
Trimpex (Roche).

TRIMUSTINE. B.A.N. Tri-(2-chloroethyl)amine. Trichlomethine (I.N.N.) Trillekamin hydrochloride.
Use: Antineoplastic agent.

TRINALIN REPETABS. (Schering) Azata-

dine maleate 1 mg, pseudoephedrine sulfate 120 mg/Tab. Bot. 100s.
Use: Long-acting antihistamine, decongestant.

TRIND. (Mead Johnson Nutrition) Phenylpropanolamine HCl 12.5 mg, chlorpheniramine maleate 2 mg/5 ml w/alcohol 5%, sorbitol. Bot. 5 oz.
Use: Decongestant, antihistamine.

TRI-NEFRIN EXTRA STRENGTH. (Pfeiffer) Phenylpropanolamine HCl 25 mg, chlorpheniramine maleate 4 mg/Tab. in 24s, 50s.
Use: Antihistamine, decongestant.

TRINIAD. (Kasar) Isoniazid 300 mg/Tab. Bot. 30s, 100s, 1000s.
Use: Antituberculosis agent.

TRINIAD PLUS 30. (Kasar) Isoniazid 300 mg, pyridoxine HCl 30 mg/Tab. Bot. 30s, 100s, 1000s.
Use: Anti-tuberculosis agent.

TRINITRIN TABLETS.
See: Nitroglycerin Tablets, U.S.P. XXIII.

TRINITROPHENOL. Picric acid. 2,4,6-Trinitrophenol.
See: Picric Acid (Various Mfr.).

TRI-NORINYL. (Syntex) Norethindrone 1 mg with ethinyl estradiol 0.035 mg/Tab. Norethindrone 0.5 mg with ethinyl estradiol 0.035 mg/Tab. 21 & 28 day. (7 inert tabs) Wallette.
Use: Oral contraceptive.

TRINOTIC. (Forest Pharm.) Secobarbital 65 mg, amobarbital 40 mg, phenobarbital 25 mg/Tab. Bot. 1000s.
Use: Hypnotic.

TRINSICON. (Whitby) Liver-stomach concentrate 240 mg, iron 110 mg, vitamin C 75 mg, folic acid 0.5 mg, activity equivalent B_{12} 15 mcg. Cap. Bot. 60s, 500s, UD 100s.
Use: Iron w/vitamin B_{12} and intrinsic factor.

TRINSICON M. (Whitby) Formerly listed by Russ.

TRIO-BAR. (Jenkins) Butabarbital sod. 33⅓%, phenobarbital sod. 33%, phenobarbital sod. 33%. Total barbiturates 0.25 gr, gr or 1.5 gr/Tab. Bot. 1000s.
Use: Sedative.

TRIOBEAD-125. (Abbott Diagnostics) T3 diagnostic kit. Test units 50s, 100s, 500s.
Use: T3 uptake radioassay for the measurement of thyroid fuction by indirectly determining the degree of saturation of serum thyroxine binding globulin (TBG).

TRIOCIL.
See: Hexetidine.

TRIOFED SYRUP. (Various Mfr.) Pseu-
doephedrine HCl 30 mg, triprolidine HCl
1.25 mg/5 ml Syr. Bot. 120 ml, pt., gal.
Use: Antihistamine, decongestant.
• **TRIOLEIN I-125.** USAN.
Use: Radioactive agent.
• **TRIOLEIN I-131.** USAN.
Use: Radioactive agent.
TRIOSTAT. (SK Beecham) Liothyronine
10 mcg/ml w/anhydrous citric acid
0.175, ammonia 2.19 mg/ml, alcohol
6.8%. Vial 1 ml.
Use: Treatment of myxedema
coma/precoma.
TRIOSULFON DMM. (CMC) Tab. Bot.
100s, 250s, 1000s.
TRIOTANN. (Duramed) Phenylephrine
tannate 25 mg, chlorpheniramine tan-
nate 8 mg, pyrilamine tannate 25
mg/Tab. Bot. 100s, 500s.
Use: Upper respiratory combination.
TRIOTANN PEDIATRIC. (Various Mfr.)
Phenylephrine tannate 5 mg, chlor-
pheniramine tannate 2 mg, pyrilamine
tannate 12.5 mg, saccharin, sucrose.
Susp. pt.
Use: Upper respiratory combination.
TRI-OTIC. (Pharmics) Chloroxylenol 1
mg, pramoxine HCl 10 mg, hydrocorti-
sone 10 mg/ml. Drops. Vial 10 ml.
Use: Otic preparation.
TRIOXANE.
See: Trioxymethylene (Various Mfr.).
• **TRIOXIFEN MESYLATE.** USAN.
Use: Anti-estrogen.
• **TRIOXSALEN,** U.S.P. XXIII. Tab., U.S.P.
XXIII. 6-Hydroxy-β,2,7-trimethyl-5-ben-
zofuranacrylic acid,δ-lactone; 4,5,-8-
trimethylpsoralen. 2,5,9-Trimethyl-7H-
furo-(3,2-g)(1)benzopyran-7-one. 7H-
Furo[3,2-g][1]-benzopyran-7-one,
2,5,9-trimethyl-.
Use: Pigmenting and phototherapeutic
agent.
See: Trisoralen, Tab. (Elder).
TRIOXYMETHYLENE. Name is incorrect-
ly used to denote paraformaldehyde in
some pharmaceuticals.
See: Paraformaldehyde (Various Mfr.).
W/Sod. oleate, triethanolamine, docusate
sodium, stearic acid & aluminum silicate.
See: Cooper Creme (Whittaker).
TRI-PAIN. (Ferndale) Acetaminophen
162 mg, aspirin 162 mg, salicylamide
162 mg, caffeine 16.2 mg/Tab. Bot.
100s.
Use: Analgesic, antipyretic, anti-inflam-
matory.
• **TRIPAMIDE.** USAN.
Use: Antihypertensive, diuretic.

TRIPARANOL. B.A.N. 2-(p-
Chlorophenyl)-1-[p-[2-
(diethylamino)ethoxy]phenyl]-1-p-
tolylethanol.
Use: Blood lipid lowering agent.
TRIPELENNAMINE. B.A.N. 2-(N-Benzyl-
N-2-pyridyl)ethyldimethylamine.
Use: Antihistamine.
See: Pyribenzamine citrate or hy-
drochloride. (Geigy).
• **TRIPELENNAMINE CITRATE,** U.S.P.
XXIII. Elixir, U.S.P. XXIII. 2-(Benzyl[2-di-
methylamino-ethyl]-amino) pyridine di-
hydrogen citrate. 1,2-Ethanediamine,
N,N-dimethyl-N'-(phenylmethyl)-N-2-
pyridinyl-,2-hydroxy-1,2,3-propanetricar-
boxylate (1:1).
Use: Antihistamine.
• **TRIPELENNAMINE HYDROCHLORIDE,**
U.S.P. XXIII. Tab. U.S.P. XXIII.
Use: Antihistamine.
See: Pyribenzamine hydrochloride,
Preps. (Geigy).
TRIPHASIL-21. (Wyeth-Ayerst) Three
drug phases in 21 day cycle: **Phase I:** 6
brown tab. Levonorgestrel 0.050 mg,
ethinyl estradiol 0.030 mg/Tab. **Phase II:**
5 white tab. Levonorgestrel 0.075 mg,
ethinyl estradiol 0.040 mg/Tab. **Phase
III:** 10 yellow tab. Levonorgestrel 0.125
mg, ethinyl estradiol 0.030 mg/Tab.
Use: Oral contraceptive.
TRIPHASIL-28.(Wyeth-Ayerst) Three drug
phases and one inert phase in 28 day
cycle: **Phase I:** 6 brown tab. Levonorgestrel 0.050 mg, ethinyl estradiol
0.030 mg/Tab. **Phase II:** 5 white tab.
Levonorgestrel 0.075/mg, ethinyl estradiol 0.040 mg Tab. **Phase III:** 10 yellow
tab. Levonorgestrel 0.125 mg,
ethinylestradiol 0.030 mg/Tab. **Phase
IV:** 7 inert green tablets.
Use: Oral contraceptive.
TRI-PHEN-CHLOR. (Rugby) Phenylpropanolamine HCl 20 mg, phenylephrine HCl 5 mg, chlorpheniramine
maleate 2.5 mg, phenyltoloxamine citrate 7.5 mg/5 ml Syr. Bot. pt., gal.
Use: Antihistamine, decongestant.
**TRI-PHEN-CHLOR TABS, TIMED RE-
LEASED.** (Rugby) Phenyl-
propanolamine HCl 40 mg, phenylephrine HCl 10 mg, chlorpheniramine
maleate 5 mg, pheyltoloxamine citrate
15 mg. 1000s.
Use: Upper respiratory combination.
TRI-PHEN-CHLOR PEDIATRIC. (Rugby)
Phenylpropanolamine HCl 5 mg,
phenylephrine HCl 1.25 mg, chlorpheniramine maleate 0.5 mg, phenyltoloxam-

ine citrate 2 mg. Bot. w/drop 30 ml.
Use: Upper respiratory combination.
TRIPHENYL. (Rugby) Phenyl-
propanolamine HCl 12.5 mg, Chlor-
pheniramine maleate 2 mg/5 ml, alcohol
free. Syr. Bot. 120 ml, pt.
Use: Antihistamine, decongestant.
TRIPHENYL EXPECTORANT. (Rugby)
Phenylpropanolamine HCl 12.5 mg,
guaifenesin 100 mg/5 ml, alcohol 5%.
Expec. Bot. 120 ml, pt., gal.
Use: Decongestant, expectorant.
TRIPHENYLMETHANE DYES.
See: Fuchsin.
Methylrosaniline Chloride.
TRIPHENYL T.D. (Rugby) Phenyl-
propanolamine HCl 50 mg, pyrilamine
maleate 25 mg, pheniramine maleate 25
mg/Tab. Bot. 100s, 1000s.
Use: Antihistamine, decongestant.
TRIPHENYLTETRAZOLIUM CHLORIDE.
TTC.
See: Uroscreen (Pfizer).
**TRIPIPERAZINE DICITITRATE, HY-
DROUS.**
See: Piperazine Citrate, U.S.P. XXIII.
TRIPLE ANTIBIOTIC OPHTHALMICS.
(Rugby) Polymyxin B sulfate 5000
units/Gm or ml, neomycin sulfate 5
mg/Gm or ml, bacitracin 400 units. Oint.
3.5 Gm.
Use: Ophthalmic.
TRIPLE ANTIBIOTIC W/HC. (Various
Mfr.) Hydrocortisone 1%, neomycin sul-
fate = neomycin base 0.35%, bacitracin
zinc 400 units, polymyxin B sulfate/g
10,000.
Use: Ophthalmic.
TRIPLE BARBITURATE ELIXIR. (CMC)
Phenobarbital 0.25 gr, butabarbital ⅛ gr,
pentobarbital gr/5 ml. Bot. pt., gal.
Use: Pediatric sedative.
**TRIPLE BROMIDES, EFFERVESCENT
TABLETS.**
W/Phenobarbital.
See: Palagren, Liq. (Westerfield).
TRIPLE DYE. (Kerr) Gentian violet,
proflavine, hemisulfate, brilliant green in
water. Dispensing Bot. 15 ml. Single
Use Dispos-A-Swab 0.65 ml. Box 10s.
Case 10×50 Box.
Use: Umbilical area antiseptic.
TRIPLE DYE. (Xttrium) Brilliant green
2.29 mg, proflavine hemisulfate 1.14
mg, gentian violet 2.29 mg/ml. Bot. 30
ml.
Use: Umbilical area disinfectant.
TRIPLE-GEN SUSPENSION. (Goldline)
Hydrocortisone 1%, neomycin sulfate
0.35%, polymyxin B sulfate 10,000

units/ml, benzalkonium chloride, cetyl alcohol, glyceryl monostearate, polyoxyl
40 stearate, propylene glycol, mineral
oil. Bot. 7.5 ml.
Use: Ophthalmic corticosteroid, anti-in-
fective.
TRIPLEN. (Interstate) Tripelennamine
HCl 50 mg/Tab. Bot. 100s, 1000s.
Use: Antihistamine.
TRIPLE PASTE. (Torch) Burow's soln. 1
part, absorption base 2 parts, Lassar's
zinc oxide paste 3 parts. Jar 2 oz., 1 lb.
Use: Antieczematic, diaper rash prod-
uct.
TRIPLE SULFA No. 2.(Kenyon) Sulfadi-
azine 167 mg, sulfamethazine 167 mg,
sulfamerazine 167 mg/Tab. Bot. 100s.
(Kenyon) Bot. 100s, 1000s.
Use: Antibacterial, sulfonamide.
TRIPLE SULFA TABLETS. (Century;
Stanlabs) Sulfadiazine 2.5 gr, sulfamer-
azine 2.5 gr, sulfamethazine 2.5 gr/Tab.
Bot. 100s, 1000s.
Use: Antibacterial, sulfonamide.
• **TRIPLE SULFA VAGINAL CREAM.**
U.S.P. XXIII. (Various Mfr.)
Use: Antibacterial.
• **TRIPLE SULFA VAGINAL TABLETS.**
U.S.P. XXIII.
Use: Antibacterial.
TRIPLE SULFOID. (Vale) Sulfadiazine
167 mg, sulfamerazine 167 mg, sul-
famethazine 167 mg/5 ml or Tab. **Liq.:**
Bot. pt., 2 oz. 12s. **Tab.:** Bot. 100s,
1000s.
Use: Antibacterial, sulfonamide.
TRIPLE SULFONAMIDE. Dia-Mer-Thia
Sulfonamides. Meth-Dia-Mer Sulfon-
amides.
Use: Antibacterial, sulfonamide.
TRIPLE VITA. (My-K Labs) Vitamins A
1500 IU, D 400 IU, C 35 mg/ml, alcohol
free. Drops. Bot. 50 ml.
Use: Vitamin supplement.
TRIPLE VITA-FLOR. (My-K Labs) Fluo-
ride 0.5 mg, vitamins A 1500 IU, D 400
IU, C 35 mg/ml, alcohol free. Drops. Bot.
50 ml.
Use: Dental caries preventative, vitamin
supplement.
TRIPLE VITAMINS W/FLUORIDE. (Ma-
jor) Vitamin A 2500 IU, D 400 IU, C 60
mg, fluoride 1 mg/Chew. Tab. Bot. 100s.
Use: Vitamin supplement.
TRIPLEVITE W/FLUORIDE. (Geneva)
Flouride 0.25 mg/ml, vitamins A 1500 IU,
D 400 IU, C 35 mg, alcohol free. Drop.
Bot. 50 ml.
Use: Dental caries preventative, vitamin
supplement.

TRIPLEVITE W/FLUORIDE. (Geneva)
Flouride 0.5 mg/ml, vitamins A 1500 IU,
D 400 IU, C 35 mg/ml, alcohol free,
cherry flavor. Drop. Bot. 50 ml.
Use: Dental caries preventative, vitamin
supplement.

TRIPLE X. (Youngs Drug) Pyrethrins
0.3%, piperonyl butoxide 3.0%, petroleum distillate 1.2%, benzyl alcohol 2.4%.
Bot. 2 oz, 4 oz.
Use: Pediculocide.

TRIPODRINE. (Danbury) Pseudoephedrine HCl 60 mg, triprolidine HCl
2.5 mg/Tab. Bot. 100s, UD 100s.
Use: Decongestant, antihistamine.

TRIPOSED SYRUP. (Blue Cross) Triprolidine HCl 1.25 mg, pseudoephedrine HCl
30 mg/5 ml. Bot. 120 ml, 240 ml, pt, gal.
Use: Antihistamine, decongestant.

TRIPOSED TABLETS. (Blue Cross)
Triprolidine HCl 2.5 mg, pseudoephedrine HCl 60 mg/Tab. Bot. 100s,
1000s.
Use: Antihistamine, decongestant.

TRIPOTASSIUM CITRATE.
See: Potassium Citrate, U.S.P. XXIII.

• **TRIPROLIDINE HCl,** U.S.P. XXIII. Syrup,
Tab., U.S.P. XXIII. Trans 1-4-
methylphenyl)-1-(2-pyridyl)-3-pyr- rolidino-prop-1-ene HCl. Trans-2-[3-(1-pyrrolidinyl)-1-(p-tolyl)-propenyl]pyri-dine hydrochloride.
(E)-2-(3-(1-Pyrrolidinyl)-1-p-
tolypropenyl)pyridine monohydrochloride monohydrate.
Use: Antihistiminic.
See: Actidil, Syr. (Burroughs Wellcome).
W/Codeine phosphate, pseudoephedrine
HCl, guaifenesin.
See: Actifed-C Syr. (Burroughs Wellcome).

**TRIPROLIDINE AND PSEUDOEPHEDRINE HYDROCHLORIDE
SYRUP.** U.S.P. XXIII.
Use: Antihistamine, decongestant.
See: Actifed, Syr. (Burroughs Wellcome).

**TRIPROLIDINE AND PSEUDOEPHEDRINE HYDROCHLORIDE
TABLETS,** U.S.P. XXIII.
Use: Antihistamine, decongestant.
See: Actifed, Tab., (Burroughs Wellcome).
Atridine, Tab. (Interstate).
Sudahist, Tab. (Upsher-Smith).
Suda-Prol, Tab., Cap. (Quality Generics).
Triphed, Tab. (Lemmon).
Triphedrine, Tab. (Redford).

TRIPTIFED. (Weeks & Leo) Triprolidine
HCl 2.5 mg, pseudoephedrine HCl 60
mg/Tab. Bot. 36s, 100s.
Use: Antihistamine, decongestant.

TRIPTONE CAPLETS. (Commerce) Dimenhydrinate 50 mg/Tab. Bot. 12s.
Use: Antiemetic/antivertigo agent.

• **TRIPTORELIN.** USAN.
Use: Antineoplastic.

TRIPTORELIN PAMOATE.
Use: Antineoplastic. [Orphan drug]

TRISACCHARIDES A AND B.
Use: Hemolytic disease of the newborn.
[Orphan drug]

TRISOL. (Buffington) Borax, sodium Cl,
boric acid. Irrigator Bot. oz, 4 oz.
Use: Artificial tear solution.

TRISORALEN. (ICN Pharm) Trioxsalen 5
mg/Tab. Tartrazine. Bot. 28s, 100s.
Use: Psoralen.

TRI-STATIN. (Rugby) Triamcinolone acetonide 0.1%, neomycin sulfate 0.25%,
gramicidin 0.25 mg, nystatin 100,000
units/Gm Crm. In 15, 30, 60, 120 and
480 Gm.
Use: Topical corticosteroid, anti-infective.

TRI-STATIN II. (Rugby) Triamcinolone
acetonide 0.1%, 100,000 units nystatin
per Gm, white petrolatum, parabens.
Cream. Tube 15 Gm, 30 Gm, 60 Gm,
120 Gm, 480 Gm.
Use: Corticosteroid, antifungal combination.

TRISTOJECT. (Mayrand) Triamcinolone
diacetate 40 mg/ml. Vial 5 ml.
Use: Corticosteroid.

TRISULFAPYRIDMINES.
Use: Sulfonamide.
See: Triple Sulfa No. 2 (Rugby).

• **TRISULFAPYRIMIDINES.** Oral Susp.,
Tab., U.S.P. XXIII.
Use: Antibacterial.
See: Meth-Dia-Mer Sulfonamides (Various Mfr.).
Neotrizine, Prep. (Lilly).
Terfonyl, Liq., Tab. (Squibb Mark).

TRITANE. (Econo-Rx) Brompheniramine
maleate 2 mg, guaifenesin 100 mg,
phenylephrine HCl 5 mg, phenylpropanolamine HCl 5 mg, alcohol
3.5%/5 ml. Bot. Gal.
Use: Antihistamine, expectorant, decongestant.

TRITANE DC. (Econo-Rx) Brompheniramine maleate 2 mg, guaifenesin 100
mg, phenylephrine HCl 5 mg, phenylpropanolamine HCl 5 mg, alcohol 3.5%,
codeine phosphate 10 mg/5 ml. Bot.
Gal.

Use: Antihistamine, expectorant, decongestant, antitussive.

TRI-TANNATE. (Rugby) Phenylephrine tannate 25 mg, chlorpheniramine tannate, pyrilamine tannate 25 mg. Tab. Bot. 100s, 250s.
Use: Upper respiratory combination.

TRI-TANNATE PEDIATRIC. (Rugby) Phenylephrine tannate 5 mg, chlorpheniramine tannate 2 mg, pyrilamine tannate 12.5 mg, saccharin, sucrose. Susp. Bot. 473 ml.
Use: Upper respiratory combination.

TRI-TANNATE PLUS PEDIATRIC SUSPENSION. (Rugby) Phenylephrine tannate 5 mg, ephedrine tannate 5 mg, chlorpheniramine tannate 4 mg, carbetapentane tannate 30 mg/5ml. Bot. 480 ml.
Use: Decongestant, antitussive, antihistamine.

• **TRITIATED WATER.** USAN.
Use: Radioactive agent.
See: Tritiotope (Squibb).

TRI-TINIC. (Vortech) Liver desic. 75 mg, stomach 75 mg, Vitamins B_{12} 15 mcg, Fe 110 mg, folic acid 1 mg, ascorbic acid 75 mg/Cap. Bot. 100s
Use: Hematinic.

TRITUSSIN COUGH SYRUP. (Towne) Pyrilamine maleate 40 mg, pheniramine maleate 20 mg, citric acid 100 mg, codeine phosphate 58 mg/fl. oz. w/menthol and glycerin in flavored base. Bot. 4 oz.
Use: Antihistamine, expectorant, antitussive.

TRIURISUL. (Sheryl) Sulfacetamide 250 mg, sulfamethizole 250 mg, phenazopyridine HCl 50 mg/Tab. Bot. 100s.
Use: Urinary antiseptic-analgesic.

TRIVA DOUCHE POWDER. (Boyle) Alkyl aryl sulfonate 35%, sod. sulfate 52.5%, oxyquinoline sulfate 2%, lactose 9.67%, disodium ethylene hydrated silica, EDTA .33%. Packet 3 Gm, 24s.
Use: Douche for trichomonal and monilial infections.

TRI-VERT. (T.E. Williams) Dimenhydrinate 25 mg, niacin 50 mg, pentylenetetrazol 25 mg/Cap. Bot. 100s.
Use: Motion sickness treatment.

TRI-VI-FLOR 0.25 mg DROPS. (Mead Johnson Nutrition) Fluoride 0.25 mg, Vitamins A 1500 IU, D 400 IU, C 35 mg/1.0 ml Drop. Bot. 50 ml.
Use: Caries prophylaxis, dietary supplement.

TRI-VI-FLOR 0.25 mg WITH IRON DROPS. (Mead Johnson Nutrition) Fluoride 0.25 mg, Vitamins A. 1500 IU, D. 400 IU, C 35 mg, iron 10 mg/1.0 ml Drop. Bot. 50 ml.
Use: Caries prophylaxis, dietary supplement with iron.

TRI-VI-FLOR 0.5 mg DROPS. (Mead Johnson Nutrition) Fluoride 0.5 mg, Vitamins A 1500 IU, D 400 IU, C 35 mg/1.0 ml. Bot. 50 ml.
Use: Caries prophylaxis and diet supplementation.

TRI-VI-FLOR 1.0 mg CHEWABLE TABLETS. (Mead Johnson Nutrition) Fluoride 1 mg, Vitamins A 2500 IU, D 400IU, Vitamins C 60 mg/Tab. Bot. 100s, 1000s.
Use: Carries prophylaxis and diet supplementation.

TRI-VI-SOL DROPS. (Mead Johnson Nutrition) Vitamin A 1500 IU, D 400 IU, C 35 mg/1.0 ml Drops. Bot. 30, 50 ml with calibrated "Safti-dropper.
Use: Vitamin A, C and D supplement.

TRI-VI-SOL WITH IRON DROPS. (Mead Johnson Nutrition) Vitamins A 1500 IU, C 35 mg, D 400 IU, iron 10 mg/1.0 ml. Bot. 50 ml.
Use: Vitamin A, C and D with iron supplement.

TRI-VITAMIN WITH FLUORIDE. (Rugby) F 0.5 mg, Vitamins A 1500 IU, D 400 IU, C 35 mg/ml Drops. Bot. 50 ml.
Use: Multivitamin.

TRI-VITE. (Foy) Thiamine HCl 100 mg, pyridoxine HCl 100 mg, cyanocobalamine 1000 mcg/ml. Vial 10 ml.
Use: B vitamin therapy.

TROBICIN. (Upjohn) Spectinomycin HCl equivalent to spectinomycin activity: **2 Gm/Vial** w/Ampule of diluent containing bacteriostatic water for injection 3.2 ml, benzyl alcohol 0.945% in ampule. **4 Gm/Vial** w/Ampule of diluent containing bacteriostatic water for injection 6.2 ml, benzyl alcohol 0.945%.
Use: Treatment of gonorrhea.

TROCAL. (Hauck) Dextromethorphan HBr 7.5 mg, guaifenesin 50 mg/Loz. In 500s.
Use: Antitussive, expectorant.

• **TROCLOSENE POTASSIUM.** USAN. (1) 1,3-Dichloro-s-triazine-2,4,6 (1H,3H,5H)trione potassium salt; (2) Potassium dichloroisocyanurate.
Use: Topical anti-infective.

• **TROLAMINE,** N.F. XVIII. 2,2″,2″-Nitrilotriethanol Ethanol, 2,2′,2″-nitrilotris-. Triethanolamine.
Use: Pharmaceutic aid (alkalinizing agent).

W/Ortho-iodobenzoic.
See: Progonasyl (Saron).
• **TROLEANDOMYCIN,** U.S.P. XXII Cap.,
Oral Susp., U.S.P. XXII. Triacetyloleandomycin.
Use: Antibiotic; steroid-requiring asthma [Orphan drug]
See: Tao (Roerig).
TROLNITRATE PHOSPHATE, B.A.N.
Di[tri-(2-nitratoethyl)ammonium]hydrogen phosphate. Praenitrona.
Use: Vasodilator.
See: Nitretamin (Squibb).
TROMAL. Butacetin. 4'-tert-Butoxyacetanilide.
Use: Analgesic, antidepressant agent.
TROMETAMOL. B.A.N. 2-Amino-2-hydroxymethyl-propane-1,3-diol.
Tromethamine, Talatrol, Trizma.
Use: Treatment of gastric hyperacidity.
• **TROMETHAMINE,** U.S.P. XXIII. For Inj.,
U.S.P. XXIII. 2-Amino-2(hydroxymethyl)-1,3-propanediol. Trometamol, B.A.N.
Use: Alkalinizer.
TRONOLANE CREAM. (Ross) Pramoxine HCl 1% in cream base. Tubes oz, 2
oz.
Use: Anorectal preparation.
TRONOLANE SUPPOSITORIES. (Ross)
Pramoxine 1% as pramoxine and
pramoxine HCl in a lubricating suppository base. Pkg. 10s, 20s.
Use: Anorectal preparation.
TROPAMINE +. (NeuroGenesis/Matrix)
Vitamins D 250 mg, L-phenylalanine, L-tyrosine 150 mg, L-glutamine 50 mg, B$_1$
1.67 mg, B$_2$ 2.5 mg, B$_3$ 16.7 mg, B$_5$ 15
mg, B$_6$ 3.3 mg, B$_{12}$ 5 mcg, folic acid
0.067 mg, C 100 mg, calcium 25 mg,
chromiun 0.01 mg, iron 1.5 mg, magnesium 25 mg, zinc 5 mg, yeast and
preservative free. Cap. Bot. 42s, 180s.
Use: Oral nutritional supplement.
• **TROPANSERIN HYDROCHLORIDE.**
USAN.
Use: Seratonin receptor antagonist
(specific in migraine).
TROPHAMINE INJECTION. (Kendall McGaw) Nitrogen 4.65 Gm, amino acids 30
Gm, protein 29 Gm/500 ml. Bot 500 ml
IV infusion.
Use: Nutritional support.
TROPH-IRON. (SK-Beecham) Vitamins
B$_{12}$ 25 mcg, B$_1$ 10 mg, iron 20 mg/5 ml.
Saccharin. Bot. 4 fl. oz.
Use: For Vitamin B$_1$, B$_{12}$ and iron deficiencies.
TROPHITE. (SK-Beecham) Vitamin B$_{12}$
25 mcg, B$_1$ 10 mg/5 ml or Tab. **Elixir:**
Bot. 4 oz., **Tab.:**Bot. 50s.

Use: For deficiencies of vitamins B$_1$ and
B$_{12}$.
TROPICACYL. (Akorn) Tropicamide solution 0.5%. In 15 ml, 1% tropicamide. 2
ml, 15 ml.
Use: Mydriatic, cycloplegic.
TROPICAL BLEND. (Schering-Plough) A
series of products is marketed under the
Tropical Blend name including: Hawaii
Blend Oil SPF 2 (Bot. 8 oz.); Hawaii
Blend Lotion SPF 2 (Bot. 8 oz.); Rio
Blend Oil SPF 2 (Bot. 8 oz.); Rio Blend
Lotion SPF 2 (Bot. 8 oz.); Jamaica Blend
Oil SPF 2 (Bot. 8 oz.); Jamaica Blend
Lotion SPF 2 (Bot. 8 oz.). All contain homosalate in various oil and lotion bases.
Use: Ultraviolet sunscreen.
TROPICAL BLEND DARK TANNING.
(Schering-Plough) **SPF 2:** Homosalate.
Oil: Bot. 180 ml, 240 ml; **Lot.:** Bot. 240
ml. **SPF 4: Lot.:** Ethylhexyl p-methoxycinnamate, oxybenzone. Bot.
240 ml; **Oil:** Padimate O, oxybenzone.
Bot. 240 ml.
Use: Sunscreen.
TROPICAL BLEND DRY OIL. (Schering-Plough) Homosalate, oxybenzone. Oil
Bot. 180 ml.
Use: Sunscreen.
TROPICAL BLEND TAN MAGNIFIER.
(Schering-Plough) Triethanolmine salicylate. Oil Bot. 240 ml.
Use: Sunscreen.
• **TROPICAMIDE,** U.S.P. XXIII. Ophth.
Soln., U.S.P. XXIII. N-Ethyl-2-phenyl-N-(4-pyridylmethyl)hydracrylamide. Benzeneacetamide, N-ethyl-α-(hydroxymethyl)-N-(4-pyridinylmethyl)-. Formerly Bis-Tropamide. (Various Mfr.) 0.5%,
1%. Soln. Bot. 15 ml.
Use: Anticholinergic, ophthalmic.
See: Mydriacyl, Drops. (Alcon).
Opticyl, Soln. (Optopics).
Tropicacyl, Soln. (Akorn).
TROPIGLINE. B.A.N. Tiglytropeine.
Use: Treatment of the Parkinsonian
syndrome.
**TROPINE BENZOHYDRYL ESTER
METHANE-SULFONATE.** (also named
benztropine methane-sulfonate).
• **TROSPECTOMYCIN SULFATE.** USAN.
Use: Antibacterial.
TROVIT. (Sig) Vitamins B$_2$ 0.3 mg, B$_6$ 1
mg, choline Cl 25 mg, panthenol 2 mg,
dl-methionine 10 mg, inositol 20 mg,
niacinamide 50 mg, Vitamins B$_{12}$ 10
mg/ml. Vial 30 ml.
Use: B-complex deficiency.
TROXERUTIN. B.A.N. 3',4,7-Tri-[0-(2-hydroxyethyl)]rutin.

Use: Treatment of venous disorders.

TROXIDONE. B.A.N. 3,5,5-Trimethyloxazolidine-2,4-dione.
Use: Anticonvulsant.
See: Trimethadione (I.N.N.) Tridione.

TROXONIUM TOSYLATE. B.A.N. Triethyl-2-(3:4:5-trimethoxybenzoyloxy)ethylammonium toxylate (Tosylic acid is the trivial name for p-toluenesulfonic acid).
Use: Hypotensive.

TROXYPYRROLIUM TOSYLATE. B.A.N. N-Ethyl-N-2-(3:4:5-trimethyoxybenzoyloxy)-ethyl-pyrrolidinium toxylate (Tosylic acid is the trivial name for p-toluenesulphonic acid).
Use: Hypotensive.

TRUPHYLLINE. (G & W) Aminophylline 250 mg/Supp. (equiv. to theophylline 198 mg) In UD 10s, 25s.
Use: Antiasthmatic.

TRYMEGEN. (Medco Supply) Chlorpheniramine maleate 4 mg/Tab. Bot. 1000s.
Use: Antihistamine.

TRYNISIN COLD SYRUP. (Halsey) Bot. 4 oz., 8 oz.
Use: Antihistamine.

TRYPARSAMIDE. Monosodium N-(Carbamyl-methyl)arsanilate.

• **TRYPSIN, CRYSTALLIZED,** U.S.P. XXIII. For Inhalation Aerosol, U.S.P. XXIII.
Use: Proteolytic enzyme.
W/Castor oil.
See: Granulex (Hickam).
W/Chymotrypsin.
See: Chymolase, Tab. (Warren-Teed).
Orenzyme, Tab. (Marion Merrell Dow).

TRYPTACIN. (Arther Inc.) L-tryptophan 500 and 1000 mg/Tab. Bot. 100s, 250s and UD 100s.
Use: Vitamin supplement.

TRYPTIZOL HYDROCHLORIDE. Amitriptyline HCl, U.S.P XXII.

• **TRYPTOPHAN,** U.S.P. XXIII. $C_{11}H_{12}N_2O_2$ as L-tryptophan.
Use: Amino acid.

TRYSUL. (Savage) Sulfathiazole 3.42%, sulfacetamide 2.86%, sulfabenzamide 3.70%, urea 0.64%. Tube 78 Gm.
Use: Anti-infective, vaginal.

T/SCALP. (Neutrogena) Hydrocortisone 1%. Liq. Bot. 60 ml, 105 ml.
Use: Topical corticosteroid, antipruritic.

TSDA.
Use: Antineoplastic.
See: Thiotepa (Lederle).

T-SERP TABLET. (Tennessee Pharm.) Reserpine alkaloid 0.25 mg/Tab. Bot. 100s, 1000s.
Use: Antihypertensive.

T-STAT. (Westwood) Erythromycin 20 mg/ml w/alcohol 71.2%. Bot. 60 ml; Pads, disposable premoistened 60s.
Use: Anti-acne.

TTC. Triphenyltetrazolium Chloride.
See: Uroscreen, Tube (Pfizer).

• **TUAMINOHEPTANE,** U.S.P. XXII. Inhalant, U.S.P. XXII.
Use: Adrenergic.

• **TUBERCULIN.** U.S.P. XXIII.
Use: Diagnostic aid (dermal reactivity indicator).
See: Aplisol (Parke-Davis) Aplitest (Parke-Davis).

TUBERCULIN, MONO-VACC TEST. (Lincoln) Mono-Vacc test is a sterile, disposable multiple puncture scarifier with liquid Old Tuberculin on the points. Box 25 tests.
Use: Diagnostic aid.

TUBERCULIN, OLD MONOVACC TEST. (Lederle) 5 TU activity test. Soln. of Old Tuberculin containing acacia 7%, lactose 0.5%. Test. Kits 25s, 100s, 250s.
Use: Diagnostic aid.

TUBERCULIN, OLD TINE TEST. (Lederle) 5 TY activity per test. Soln. of Old Tuberculin, containing acacia 7%, lactose 8.5%. Test. Kits 25s, 100s, 250s.
Use: Diagnostic aid.

TUBERCULIN PURIFIED PROTEIN DERIVATIVE. (Squibb/Connaught) A concentrated solution for multiple puncture testing. Vial 1 ml.
Use: For screening tuberculin activity.
See: Tubersol, Inj. (Squibb/Connaught).

TUBERCULIN TESTS.
Use: Diagnostic aid.
See: Aplisol (Parke-Davis).
Aplitest (Parke-Davis).
Sclavo Test-PPD (Sclavo).
Tine Test PPD (Lederle).
Tuberculin, Old Mono Vacc Test (Merieux).
Tuberculin, Old, Tine Test (Lederle).
Tubersol (Squibb/Connaught)

TUBERCULIN TINE TEST. (Lederle) **Old Tuberculin (OT):** Each disposable test unit consists of a stainless steel disc, with four tines (or prongs) 2 millimeters long, attached to a plastic handle. The tines have been dip-dried with antigenic material. The entire unit is sterilized by ethylene oxide gas. The test has been standardized by comparative studies, utilizing 0.05 mg US Standard Old Tuberculin (5 International Units) or 0.0001 mg US Standard (5 International Units) by the Mantoux technique. The reliability appears to be comparable to the stan-

dard Mantoux. Tests in a jar 25s. Package 100s. Bin Package 250s. **Purified Protein Derivative (PPD):** Equivalent to or more potent than 5 TU PPD Mantoux test. Tests in a jar 25s. Package 100s.
Use: Diagnostic aid.

TUBERCULOSIS VACCINE.
Use: Vaccine, bacterial.
See: TICE BCG (Organon).

TUBERLATE. (Heun) Sod. p-aminosalicylate 12 gr, succinic acid 4 gr/Tab. Bot. 500s.
Use: Tuberculosis treatment.

TUBERSOL. (Squibb/Connaught) Tuberculin purified protein derivative (Mantoux) 1 TU, 5 TU, or 250 TU. In 1 and 5 ml vials.
Use: For the detection of tuberculosis infection.

TUBEX. (Wyeth-Ayerst) The following drugs are available in various Tubex sizes:
Ativan
Bicillin C-R
Bicillin C-R 900/300
Bicillin Long-Acting
Codeine Phosphate
Cyanocobalamin
Digoxin
Dimenhydrinate
Diphenhydramine HCl
Diphtheria and Tetanus Toxoids Adsorbed
  (Pediatric)
Epinephrine
Furosemide
Heparin Flush Kits
Heparin Lock Flush
Heparin Sodium Solution
Hydromorphone HCl
Hydroxyzine HCl
Influenza Virus Vaccine, Trivalent
Mepergan
Meperidine HCl
Morphine Sulfate
Naloxone Injection
Naloxone Injection, Neonatal
Oxytocin
Pentobarbital Sodium
Phenergan
Phenobarbital Sodium
Prochlorperazine Edisylate
Secobarbital Sodium
Sodium Chloride, Bacteriostatic
Sparine HCl
Tetanus and Diphtheria Toxoids Adsorbed (Adult)
Tetanus Immune Globulin (Human).
Tetanus Toxoid Alum. Phos. Ad.
Tetanus Toxoid, Fluid
Thiamine Hydrochloride
Wycillin

TUBOCURARINE CHLORIDE. U.S.P. XXIII. Inj., U.S.P. XXIII. Tubocuraranium, 7',12-dihydroxy-6,6-dimethoxy-2,2,2-trimethyl-, chloride, hydrochloride, pentahydrate. d-Tubocurarine chloride.
  Metubine Iodide (Lilly) 3 mg./ml. Amp. 10 ml.
  (Abbott) 3 mg./ml. in 10 ml. fliptop vials; 15 mg in 5 ml Abboject Syringe.
Use: Skeletal muscle relaxant.

TUBOCURARINE CHLORIDE, DIMETHYL. Dimethyl ether of d-tubocurarine chloride.

TUBOCURARINE CHLORIDE HYDROCHLORIDE PENTAHYDRATE. Tubocurarine Chloride, U.S.P. XXIII.

TUBOCURARINE IODIDE, DIMETHYL. Dimethyl ether of d-tubocurarine iodide.
Use: Skeletal muscle relaxant.
See: Metubine, Vial (Lilly).

• **TUBULOZOLE HYDROCHLORIDE.** USAN.
Use: Antineoplastic.

TUCKS. (Parke-Davis Prods) Pads saturated with solution of witch hazel 50%, glycerin 10%, methylparaben 0.1%, benzalkonium Cl 0.003%. Jar 40s, 100s.
Use: Proctologic & dermatologic disorders.

TUCKS OINTMENT AND CREAM.
(Parke-Davis Prods) Witch hazel 50% in cream or ointment base. Tube 40 Gm w/rectal applicator.
Use: Astringent.

TUCKS TAKE-ALONGS. (Parke-Davis Prods) Non-woven wipes saturated with solution of witch hazel 50%, glycerine 10% w/purified water, methylparaben 0.1%, benzalkonium chloride 0.003%. Box 12s.
Use: Anorectal preparation.

TUINAL. (Lilly) Equal parts Seconal Sod. & Amytal Sod. Pulvule **100 mg** Bot. 100s; **200 mg** Bot. 100s.
Use: Sedative/hypnotic.

TUMOR NECROSIS FACTOR-BINDING PROTEIN I AND II. (Serono)
Use: Treatment of AIDS. [Orphan drug]

TUMS. (SK-Beecham) Calcium carbonate 500 mg/Tab. Available in peppermint and assorted flavors in various package sizes. Rolls of 12 singles, 3-roll wraps. Bot. 75s, 150s.
Use: Antacid.

TUMS 500. (SK-Beecham) Calcium carbonate 1250 mg (500 mg calcium), sucrose, sodium < 4 mg. Chew. tab. Bot. 60s.

Use: Calcium supplement.
TUMS E-X EXTRA STRENGTH. (SK-Beecham) Calcium carbonate 750 mg, wintergreen or fruit flavors. 12s, 48s, 96s.
Use: Antacid.
TUMS PLUS. (SK-Beecham) Calcium carbonate 500 mg, (elemental calcium 200 mg), simethicone 20 mg, sucrose, sodium ≤ 2 mg, assorted fruit and mint flavors. Tab. Bot. 48s.
Use: Antacid.
TUMS ULTRA. (SK-Beecham) Calcium carbonate 1000 mg. Chew. tab. Bot. 36s, 72s.
Use: Calcium supplement.
TUR-BI-KAL NASAL DROPS. (Emerson) Phenylephrine HCl in a saline solution. Dropper Bot. oz., 12s.
Use: Nasal decongestant.
TURBILIXIR. (Burlington) Chlorpheniramine maleate 2 mg, phenylephrine HCl 5 mg, phonylpropanolamine HCl 5 mg/5 ml. Bot. Pts., gal.
Use: Antihistamine, decongestant.
TURBINAIRE.
See: Decadron Phosphate, Preps. (Merck & Co.).
TURBINAIRE DECADRON PHOSPHATE. (Merck & Co.) Each metered spray delivers dexamethasone sodium phosphate equivalent to ~ dexamethasone 84 mcg (170 sprays per cartridge), alcohol 2%. Aerosol. 12.6 Gm w/adapter or 12.6 Gm refill.
Use: Intranasal steroid.
TURBISPAN LEISURECAPS. (Burlington) Chlorpheniramine maleate 12 mg, 1-phenylephrine HCl 15 mg, phenylpropanolamine HCl 15 mg/Sus. Rel. Cap. Bot. 30s.
Use: Antihistamine, decongestant.
TURGASEPT AEROSOL. (Wyeth-Ayerst) Ethyl alcohol 44.25%, essential oils 0.90%, n alkyl (50% C-14, 40% C-12, 10% C-16) dimethyl benzylammonium Cl 0.33%, o-phenylphenol 0.25% w/propellant. Spray can 11.5 oz. in bouquet, fresh lemon, leather, citrus blossom scents.
Use: Spray disinfectant, air deodorant.
TURPENTINE OIL W/COMBINATIONS.
See: Sloan's Liniment, Liq. (Warner-Lambert).
TUSILAN. Dextromethorphan HBr.
TUSQUELIN. (Circle) Dextromethorphan HBr 15 mg, chlorpheniramine maleate 2 mg, phenylpropanolamine 5 mg, phenylephrine HCl 5 mg, fl. ext. ipecac 0.17 min., potassium guaiacolsulfonate

44 mg/5 ml. Alcohol 5%. Syrup, pt.
Use: Antitussive w/expectorant; antihistamine.
TUSSABAR. (Tennessee) Acetaminophen 400 mg, salicylamide 500 mg, potassium guaiacolsulfonate 120 mg, pyrilamine maleate 30 mg, ammonium chloride 500 mg, sodium citrate 500 mg, phenylephrine HCl 30 mg/oz. Bot. pt., gal.
Use: Analgesic, antipyretic, decongestant and expectorant.
TUSSABID. (Ion) Guaifenesin 200 mg, dextromethorphan HBr 30 mg/Cap. Bot. 24s, 100s.
Use: Cough relief.
TUSSACOL. (Jenkins) Dextromethorphan HBr 7.5 mg, pyrilamine maleate 8.0 mg, phenylephrine HCl 5.0 mg, acetaminophen 100.0 mg, guaifenesin 50 mg/Tab. Bot. 1000s.
Use: Antitussive, antihistamine, decongestant, analgesic, expectorant.
TUSSAFED DROPS. (Everett) Carbinoxamine maleate 2 mg, pseodoephedrine HCl 25 mg, dextromethorphan HBr 4 mg/1 ml. Bot. 30 ml with calibrated dropper.
Use: Antihistamine, decongestant, antitussive.
TUSSAFED SYRUP. (Everett) Dextromethorphan HBr 15 mg, pseudoephedrine HCl 60 mg, carbinoxamine maleate 4 mg/5 ml. Bot. 4 oz., 16 oz.
Use: Antitussive, decongestant, antihistamine.
TUSSAHIST. (Defco) Codeine phosphate 10 mg, phenylpropanolamine HCl 12.5 mg, chlorpheniramine maleate 2 mg, pyrilamine maleate 7.5 mg, guaifenesin 100 mg/5 ml. Bot. 4 oz. pt, gal.
Use: Antitussive, decongestant, antihistamine, expectorant.
TUSS ALLERGINE MODIFIED T.D. (Rugby) Phenylpropanolamine HCl 75 mg, caramiphen edisylate 40 mg/Cap. T.R. Bot. 100s, 500s, 1000s.
Use: Decongestant, antitussive.
TUSSAFIN EXPECTORANT LIQUID. (Rugby) Pseudoephedrine HCl 60 mg, hydrocodone bitartrate 5 mg, guaifenesin 200 mg, alcohol 2.5%. Bot. 480 ml.
Use: Decongestant, antitussive, expectorant.
TUSSANIL. (Misemer) Chlorpheniramine maleate 4 mg, phenylephrine HCl 10 mg/5 ml w/alcohol 5%. Bot. pt.
Use: Antihistamine, decongestant.
TUSSANIL DH. (Misemer) Phenyl-

propanolamine HCl 25 mg, guaifenesin 100 mg, hydrocodone bitartrate 1.66 mg, salicylamide 300 mg/Tab. In 100s.
Use: Decongestant, expectorant, antitussive, analgesic.

TUSSANIL DH SYRUP. (Misemer) Phenylephrine HCl 10 mg, chlorpheniramine maleate 4 mg hydrocodono bitartrate 2.5 mg/5 ml w/alcohol 5%. Bot. pt.
Use: Decongestant, antihistamine, antitussive.

TUSSANIL EXPECTORANT SYRUP. (Misemer) Hydrocodone bitartrate 2.5 mg, phenylephrine HCl 10 mg, guaifenesin 100 mg/5 ml w/alcohol 5%. Bot. pt.
Use: Antitussive, decongestant, expectorant.

TUSSANOL. (Tyler) Pyrilamine maleate ¾ gr, codeine phosphate 1 gr, ammonium chloride 7.5 gr, sodium citrate 5 gr, menthol gr/fl. oz. Bot. 4 fl. oz, pt, gal.
Use: Antihistamine, antitussive, expectorant.

TUSSANOL with EPHEDRINE. (Tyler) Ephedrine sulfate 2 gr, pyrilamine maleate ¾ gr, codeine phosphate 1 gr, ammonium chloride 7.5 gr, sodium citrate 5 gr, menthol gr/30 ml. Bot. 16 fl. oz.
Use: Bronchodilator, antihistamine, antitussive, expectorant.

TUSSAR-2 SYRUP. (Rhone-Poulenc Rorer) Codeine phosphate 10 mg, guaifenesin 100 mg, pseudoephedrine HCl 30 mg/5ml, alcohol 2.5%. Bot. 473 ml.
Use: Antitussive, expectorant, decongestant.

TUSSAR DM. (Rhone-Poulenc Rorer) Dextromethorphan HBr 15 mg, chlorpheniramine maleate 2 mg, phenylephrine HCl 5 mg/5 ml w/methylparaben 0.1% Bot. 4 oz., pt.
Use: Antitussive, antihistamine, expectorant.

TUSSAR SF. (Rhone-Poulenc Rorer) Codeine phosphate 10 mg, guaifenesin 100 mg, pseudoephedrine HCl 30 mg/5 ml, alcohol 2.5%. Bot. 120 ml, 473 ml.
Use: Antitussive, decongestant, expectorant.

TUSS-DM. (Hyrex) Dextromethorphan HBr (10 mg), guaifenesin 200 mg, dye free. Tab. Bot. 100s, 1000s.
Use: Antitussive, expectorant.

TUSSEX COUGH. (Various Mfr.) Phenylephrine HCl 5 mg, dextromethorphan HBr 10 mg, guaifenesin 100 mg/5 ml Syr. Bot. 120 ml, gal.
Use: Decongestant, antitussive, expectorant.

TUSS-GENADE MODIFIED CAPS. (Goldline) Phenylpropanolamine HCl 75 mg, caramiphen edisylate 40 mg. Bot. 100s, 1000s.
Use: Decongestant, antitussive.

TUSSGEN EXPECTORANT. (Goldline) Bot. pt, gal.
Use: Expectorant.

TUSSGEN LIQUID. (Goldline) Pseudoephedrine HCl 60 mg, hydrocodone bitartrate 5 mg/5 ml. Bot. 100s, 1000s.
Use: Decongestant, antitussive.

TUSSIDRAM. (Dram) Dextromethorphan 10 mg, phenylpropanolamine 12.5 mg, guaifenesin 50 mg, chlorpheniramine maleate 2 mg/5 ml. Bot. pt.
Use: Antitussive, decongestant, expectorant, antihistamine.

TUSSIGON. (Daniels) Hydrocodone bitartrate 5 mg, homatropine methylbromide 1.5 mg/Tab. Bot. 100s, 500s.
Use: Antitussive, anticholinergic/antispasmodic.

TUSSIONEX. (Pennwalt) Hydrocodone (as polistirex) 10 mg, chlorpheniramine 8 mg. Liq. Bot. 473 ml and 900 ml.
Use: Antitussive, antihistamine.

TUSSI-ORGANIDIN DM LIQUID. (Wallace) Dextromethorphan HBr 10 mg, Organidin 30 mg/5 ml Saccharin, sorbitol. Bot. pt., gal.
Use: Antitussive, expectorant.

TUSSI-ORGANIDIN LIQUID. (Wallace) Codeine phosphate 10 mg; Organidin 30 mg/5 ml. Saccharin, sorbitol. Bot. pt., gal.
Use: Antitussive, expectorant.

TUSSIREX. (Scot-Tussin) Phenylephrine HCl 4.2 mg, pheniramine maleate 13.3 mg, codeine phosphate 10 mg, sodium citrate 83.3 mg, sodium salicylate 83.3 mg, caffeine citrate 25 mg/5 ml Syr. Bot. 120 and 240 ml, pt, gal.
Use: Decongestant, antihistamine, antitussive, expectorant.

TUSSIREX SUGAR FREE LIQUID. (Scot-Tussin) Codeine phosphate 10 mg, pheniramine maleate 13.33 mg, phenylephrine HCl 4.17 mg, sodium citrate 83.33 mg, sodium salicylate 83.33 mg, caffeine citrate 25 mg/5 ml. Bot. 120 ml, pt. gal.
Use: Antitussive, antihistamine, decongestant, expectorant, salicylate analgesic.

TUSS-LA. (Hyrex) Pseudoephedrine HCl 120 mg, guaifenesin 500 mg/L.A. Tab. Bot. 100s.
Use: Decongestant, expectorant.

TUSSO-DM. (Everett) Dextromethorphan HBr 10 mg, iodianted glycerol 30 mg, alcohol free. Liq. Bot. 473 ml.
Use: Cough preparation.

TUSSOGEST. (Major) Phenylpropanolamine HCl 75 mg, caramiphen edisylate 40 mg/Cap. T.R. Bot. 100s, 500s, 1000s.
Use: Decongestant, antitussive.

TUSS-ORNADE LIQUID. (SK-Beecham) Caramiphen edisylate 6.7 mg, phenylpropanolamine HCl 12.5 mg/5 ml w/alcohol 5%. Bot. pt.
Use: Antitussive, decongestant.

TUSS-ORNADE SPANSULE. (SK-Beecham) Caramiphen edisylate 40 mg, phenylpropanolamine HCl 75 mg/Cap. Bot. 50s, 500s.
Use: Antitussive, decongestant.

TUSSTAT EXPECTORANT. (Century) Diphenhydramine HCl 80 mg, ammonium chloride 12 gr, sodium citrate 5 gr, monthol 1/10 gr, alcohol 5%/oz. Bot. 4 fl. oz, pt, gal.
Use: Antihistamine, expectorant.

• **TUVIRUMAB.** USAN.
Use: Antiviral.

TVC-2 DANDRUFF SHAMPOO. (Dermol) Zinc pyrithione 2%. Bot. 120 ml.
Use: Antiseborrheic.

T-VITES. (Freeda) Vitamins B_1 25 mg, B_2 25 mg, B_3 150 mg, B_5 25 mg, B_6 25 mg, C 100 mg, biotin 30 mcg, PABA 30 mg, K, Mg, Mn, Zn 20 mg/Tab. Bot. 100s.
Use: Vitamin/mineral supplement.

TWEEN 20, 40, 60, 80. (ICI Americas) Polysorbates, N.F. XVIII.
Use: Surface active agents.

12 HOUR ANTIHISTAMINE NASAL DECONGESTANT. (URL) Pseudoephedrine sulfate 120 mg, dexbrompheniramine maleate 6 mg, sugar, sucrose. SR Tab. Bot. 10s.
Use: Decongestant and antihistamine.

12 HOUR COLD CAPSULES. (Nature's Bounty) Phenylpropanolamine HCl 75 mg, chlorpheniramine maleate 4 mg/Cap. In 10s.
Use: Decongestant, antihistamine.

TWICE-A-DAY. (Major). Oxymetazoline 0.05%. Solution: In 15 and 30 ml.
Use: Decongestant.

TWILITE. (Pfeiffer) Diphenhydramine HCl 50 mg. Tab. 20s.
Use: Sleep aid.

TWIN-K LIQUID. (Boots) Potassium ions 20 mEq./15 ml. Bot. pt.
Use: Treatment of hypokalemia.

2-TONE DISCLOSING SOLUTION. (Lorvic) Dropper Bot. 2 oz.

Use: Disclosing solution.

2-24. (Walgreen) Belladonna alkaloids 0.2 mg, phenylpropanolamine HCl 50 mg, chlorpheniramine maleate 4 mg/Cap. Bot. 10s.
Use: Anticholinergic/antispasmodic, decongestant, antihistamine.

TWO-CAL HN HIGH NITROGEN LIQUID NUTRITION. (Ross) High nitrogen liquid nutrition (2 calories/ml). 1900 calories (1 quart) provide 100% US RDA for vitamins and minerals for adults and children over 4 yrs. Can 8 fl. oz.
Use: Enteral nutritional supplement.

TWO-DYNE CAPSULES. (Hyrex) Butalbital 50 mg, caffeine 40 mg, aceta minophen 325 mg/Cap. Bot. 100s, 1000s.
Use: Sedative/hypnotic, analgesic.

TY-CAPLETS. (Major) Acetaminophen 500 mg/Tab. Bot. 100s.
Use: Analgesic.

TY-CAPS. (Major) Acetaminophen 500 mg/Cap. Bot. 100s, 1000s, UD 100c.
Use: Analgesic.

TYCODENE SUGAR FREE. (Pfeiffer) Chlorpheniramine maleate 2 mg, dextromethorphan HBr 10 mg, menthol, saccharin, sorbitol, alcohol free. Liq. Bot. 120 ml.
Use: Antihistamine, antitussive.

TY-COLD TABLETS. (Major) 30 mg pseudoephedrine, 2 mg chlorpheniramine maleate, 15 mg dextromethorphan HBr, 325 mg acetaminophen. 24s.
Use: Decongestant, antihistamine, antitussive, analgesic.

TYFORMIN. B.A.N. 4-Guanidinobutyramide.
Use: Oral hypoglycemic agent.

TYLENOL CHILDREN'S. (McNeil-CPC) Acetaminophen 160mg/5 ml. Susp. Bot. 60 ml.
Use: Analgesic.

TYLENOL CHILDREN'S CHEWABLE TABLETS. (McNeil Prods) Acetaminophen 80 mg/Tab. Bot. 30s, 48s. Blisters 2s. Hospital pack 250 × 1.
Use: Analgesic.

TYLENOL CHILDREN'S ELIXIR. (McNeil Prods) Acetaminophen 160 mg/5 ml. Bot. 2 oz., 4 oz., pt. UD 100 × 5 ml, 100 × 10 ml.
Use: Analgesic.

TYLENOL COLD. (McNeil-CPC) Pseudoephedrine HCl 30 mg, chlorpheniramine maleate 2 mg, dextromethorphan HBr 15 mg, acetaminophen 325 mg, Tab. Cap. Bot. 24s, 50s.
Use: Decongestant, antihistamine, anti-

tussive, analgesic.

TYLENOL COLD EFFERVESCENT. (Mc-
Neil-CPC) Phenylpropanolamine HCl
12.5 mg, chlorpheniramine maleate 2
mg, acetaminophen 32.5 mg, saccharin,
sorbitol, sodium 525 mg, orange flavor.
Tab. Bot. 20s, 36s.
Use: Decongestant, antihistamine,
analgesic.

TYLENOL COLD & FLU MEDICATION.
(McNeil-CPC) Pseudoephedrine HCl 60
mg, chlorpheniramine maleate 4 mg,
dextromethorphan HBr, acetaminophen
650 mg, aspartame, sucrose, phenylalanine 11 mg, lemon flavor. Pow. Pks. 6s,
12s.
Use: Decongestant, antihistamine,
analgesic.

**TYLENOL COLD & FLU NO DROWSI-
NESS.** (McNeil-CPC) Acetaminophen
650 mg, pseudoephedrine HCl 60 mg,
dextromethorphan HBr per packet 30
mg, aspartame (as phenylalanine 11
mg), sucrose, lemon flavor. Pow. 6s,
12s.
Use: Decongestant, antihistamine,
analgesic.

TYLENOL COLD LIQUID, CHILDREN'S.
(McNeil-CPC) Pseudoephedrine 15 mg,
chlorpheniramine maleate 1 mg, acetaminophen 160 mg, sorbitol, sucrose, alcohol free, grape flavor. Liq. Bot. 120 ml.
Use: Pediatric decongestant, antihistamine, analgesic.

**TYLENOL COLD MULTISYMPTOM
PLUS COUGH, CHILDREN'S.** (McNeil-
CPC) Acetaminophen 160 mg, dextro-
morphan HBr 5 mg, chlorpheniramine
maleate 1 mg, pseudoephedrine 15
mg/5 ml. Liq. Bot. 120 ml.
Use: Pediatric decongestant, antihistamine, antitussive.

TYLENOL COLD NIGHT TIME. (McNeil-
CPC) Pseudoephedrine HCl 10 mg,
diphenhydramine HCl 8.3 mg, acetaminophen 108.3 mg/5 ml, alcohol 10%,
sucrose, cherry flavor. Liq. Bot. 150 ml.
Use: Decongestant, antihistamine, antitussive.

**TYLENOL COLD TABLETS, CHIL-
DRNE'S.** (McNeil-CPC) Pseudoephedrine HCl 7.5 mg, chlorpheniramine maleate 0.5 mg, acetaminophen
80 mg, aspartame, sucrose, phenylalanine 4 mg. Grape flavor. Chew. Tab. Bot.
24s.
Use: Decongestant, antihistamine,
analgesic.

TYLENOL COUGH. (McNeil-CPC) Dextromethorphan HBr, acetaminophen 250

mg, saccharin, sorbitol, sucrose. Liq.
Bot. 120 ml.
Use: Antitussive, analgesic.

TYLENOL COUGH W/DECONGESTANT.
(McNeil-CPC) Pseudoephedrine HCl 15
mg, dextromethorphan HBr 7.5 mg, acetaminophen 250 mg, alcohol 10%, saccharin, sobitol, sucrose. Liq. Bot. 120 ml,
240 ml.
Use: Decongestant, antitussive, analgesic.

TYLENOL ELIXIR, CHILDREN'S. (Mc-
Neil-CPC) Acetaminophen 160 mg/5ml.
Elix. Bot. 60 mg, 120 ml.
Use: Analgesic.

TYLENOL EXTRA-STRENGTH. (McNeil
Prods) Acetaminophen 500 mg/Tab. or
Caplet. **Tab.:** Bot. 30s, 60s, 100s, 200s.
Caplets: Bot. 24s, 50s, 100s, 175s.
Use: Analgesic.

**TYLENOL EXTRA-STRENGTH ADULT
LIQUID.** (McNeil Prods) Acetaminophen 1000 mg/30 ml w/alcohol
8.5%. Bot. 8 oz. Hosp. 8 oz.
Use: Analgesic.

**TYLENOL EXTRA STRENGTH
CAPLETS.** (McNeil-CPC) Acetaminophen 500 mg/Capl. Bot. 24s, 50s,
100s, 175s.
Use: Anaglesic.

**TYLENOL EXTRA STRENGTH GEL-
CAP.** (McNeil-CPC) Acetaminophen
500 mg/Gelcap. Bot. 24s, 50s, 100s.
Use: Analgesic.

**TYLENOL EXTRA STRENGTH
GELTABS.** (McNeil-CPC) Acetaminophen 500 mg. Tab. Bot. 24s, 50s,
100s.
Use: Analgesic.

TYLENOL INFANTS' DROPS. (McNeil
Prods) Acetaminophen 80 mg/0.8 ml.
Bot. w/dropper 7.5 ml, 15 ml.
Use: Analgesic.

**TYLENOL JUNIOR STRENGTH SWAL-
LOWABLE TABLETS.** (McNeil Prods)
160 mg/Tab. Box. 30s. Hosp. 250 × 1.
Use: Analgesic.

**TYLENOL MAXIMUM-STRENGTH AL-
LERGY SINUS.** (McNeil-CPC) Pseudoephedrine HCl 30 mg, chlorpheniramine maleate 2 mg, acetaminophen
500 mg, Capl. Bot. 24s, 50s. Gelcap.
Bot. 20s, 40s.
Use: Upper respiratory combination.

**TYLENOL MAXIMUM STRENGTH SINUS
MEDICATION.** (McNeil Prods) Aceta-
minophen 500 mg, pseudoephedrine
HCl 30 mg/Tab. or Caplet. **Tab.:** Bot.
24s, 50s. **Caplet:** Bot. 24s, 50s.
Use: Analgesic, decongestant.

TYLENOL NO DROWSINESS COLD. (McNeil-CPC) Pseudoephedrine HCl 30 g, dextromethorphan HBr 15 mg, acetaminophen 325 mg. Cap. Bot. 24s, 50s.
Use: Decongestant, antitussive, analgesic.

TYLENOL PM, EXTRA STRENGTH. (McNeil-CPC) Acetaminophen 500 mg, diphenhydramine 25 mg. Tab. Cap. Bot. 24s, 50s.
Use: Analgesic.

TYLENOL REGULAR STRENGTH. (McNeil Prods) Acetaminophen 325 mg/Tab. or Caplet. **Tab.:** Tin 12s. Vial 12s. Bot. 24s, 50s, 100s, 200s. **Caplet:** Bot. 24s, 50s.
Use: Analgesic.

TYLENOL WITH CODEINE. (McNeil Pharm) **Tab.:** Acetaminophen 300 mg with codeine phosphate. **No. 2:** codeine phosphate 15 mg Bot. 100s, 500s. UD 20 × 25s.
Use: Narcotic antipyretic.

TYLENOL WITH CODEINE ELIXIR. (McNeil Pharm) Acetaminophen 120 mg, codeine phosphate 12 mg/5 ml w/alcohol 7%. Bot. 4 oz., pt. UD Cups 10 × 5 ml, 10 × 15 ml.
Use: Narcotic analgesic combination.

TYLOSTERONE. (Lilly) Diethylstilbestrol 0.25 mg, methyltestosterone 5 mg/Tab. Bot. 100s.
Use: Estrogen, androgen combination.

TYLOX. (McNeil Pharm) Oxycodone HCl 5 mg, acetaminophen 500 mg/Cap. Bot. 100s UD 4 × 25s.
Use: Narcotic analgesic.

TYLOXAPOL.
Use: Ophthalmic.
See: Enuclene (Alcon).

TYMAZOLINE. B.A.N. 2-(5-Isopropyl-2-methylphenoxymethyl)-2-imidazoline. Pernazene hydrochloride.
Use: Vasoconstrictor.

TYMPAGESIC. (Adria) Phenylephrine HCl 0.25%, antipyrine 5%, benzocaine 5%, in propylene glycol. Liq. Bot. w/dropper 13 ml.
Use: Antihistamine & analgesic ear drops.

TY-PAP. (Major) **Elix.:** Acetaminophen 160 mg/5 ml. Bot. pt., gal. **Supp.:** Acetaminophen 120 mg, 650 mg In 12s.
Use: Analgesic, antipyretic.

•**TYPHOID VACCINE,** U.S.P. XXIII. (Wyeth-Ayerst)—Vial 5 ml, 10 ml, 20 ml.
Use: Active immunizing agent.

TYREX-2. (Ross) Protein 30 g, fat 15.5 g, carbohydrates 30 g, Fe 13 mg, Na 880 mg, K 1370 mg, Cal 410/100 g. With ap-

propriate vitamins and minerals. Phenylalanine and tyrosine free. Pow. Can 325 g.
Use: Enteral nutritional supplement.

TYRODONE. (Major) Hydrocodone bitartrate 5 mg, pseudoephedrine HCl 60 mg/5 ml, alcohol 5%. Liq. Bot. 473 ml.
Use: Decongestant, antitussive.

TYRO-LOZ. (Kenyon) Tyrothricin 2 mg, benzocaine 5 mg/Loz. Bot. 100s, 1000s.
Use: Sore throat.

TYROMEX-1. (Ross) Protein 15 g, fat 23.9 g, carbohydrates 46.3 g, linoleic acid 1800 mg, Fe 9 mg, Na 190 mg, K 675 mg, Cal 480/100 g. With appropriate vitamins and minerals. Phenylalanine, tyrosine and methionine free. Pow. Can 350 g.
Use: Enteral nutritional supplement.

•**TYROPANOATE SODIUM,** U.S.P. XXIII. Cap., U.S.P. XXIII. Sodium 3-butyramido-α-ethyl-2,4,6-triiodohydrocinnamate.
Use: Diagnostic aid.
See: Bilopaque (Sanofi Winthrop).

TYROPAQUE CAPS. (Sanofi Winthrop) Tyropanoate sodium.
Use: Oral cholecystographic medium.

•**TYROSINE,** U.S.P. XXIII. L-Tyrosine.
Use: Amino acid.

TYROSINE HYDROXYLASE INHIBITOR.
Use: Antihypertensive.
See: Demser (Merck & Co.).

TYROSUM SKIN CLEANSER. (Summers) Isopropanol 50%, polysorbate 80 2%, and acetone 10%. Bot. 4 oz., 1 pt. Towlettes 24s, 50s.
Use: Skin cleaner for acne and oily skin.

•**TYROTHRICIN,** U.S.P. XXIII. Spray. Soln., Troches: An antibiotic from *Bacillus brevis.* Tyrodac; Tyroderm.
Use: Antibacterial.

TY-TABS. (Major) Acetaminophen with codeine #2, #3, #4. Bot. 100s, 500s, 1000s.
Use: Narcotic analgesic combination.

TY-TABS, CHILDREN'S. (Major) Acetaminophen 80 mg/Tab. Bot. 30s, 100s.
Use: Analgesic, antipyretic.

TY-TABS EXTRA STRENGTH. (Major) Acetaminophen 500 mg/Tab. Bot. 100s, 1000s.
Use: Analgesic, antipyretic.

TYZINE NASAL SOLUTION. (Key) Tetrahydrozoline HCl 0.1%. Bot. pt., oz.
Use: Nasal decongestant.

TYZINE NASAL SPRAY. (Key) Tetrahydrozoline HCl 0.1%. Bot. 0.5 oz.
Use: Nasal decongestant.

TYZINE PEDIATRIC NASAL DROPS. (Key) Tetrahydrozoline HCl 0.05%. Bot.

0.5 oz.
Use: Nasal decongestant.

U

UAA. (Econo Med) Methenamine 40.8 mg, phenyl salicylate 18.1 mg, methylene blue 5.4 mg, benzoic acid 4.5 mg, atropine sulfate 0.03 mg, hyoscyamine 0.03 mg/Tab. Bot. 100s, 1000s.
Use: Urinary anti-infective.
UAD CREAM. (UAD) Clioquinol 3%, hydrocortisone 1%, ceresin, glyceryl oleate, propylene glycol, parabens, mineral oil, pramoxine HCl. 15 Gm.
Use: Corticosteroid combination.
UAD LOTION. (UAD) Clioquinol 0.75%, hydrocortisone 0.25%, cetyl alcohol, glyceryl stearate, lanolin, parabens, mineral oil, pramoxine HCl, propylene glycol. 20 ml.
Use: Corticosteroid combination.
UAD OTIC, (UAD) Hydrocortisone 1%, neomycin sulfate 5 mg, polymyxin B sulfate 10,000 units per ml, thimersol 0.01%, cetyl alcohol, propylene glycol, polysorbate 80. Susp. 10 ml w/dropper.
Use: Otic preparation.
UBT. (NMS) For detection of blood in the urine.
Use: Diagnostic aid.
UCEPHAN. (Kendall-McGaw) Sodium benzoate 10%, sodium phenylacetate 10% (10 Gm/100 ml). Liq. Bot. 100 ml.
Use: For urea cycle enzymopathies.
UCG-BETA SLIDE MONOCLONAL II. (Wampole) Two-minute latex agglutination inhibition slide test for the qualitative detection of B-hCG/hCG (sensitivity 0.5 IU hCG/ml) in urine. Kit 50s, 100s, 300s.
Use: Diagnostic aid.
UCG-BETA STAT. (Wampole) One-hour passive hemagglutination inhibition tube test for the qualitative detection and quantitative determination of B-hCG/hCG (sensitivity 0.2 IU hCG/ml) in urine. Kit 50s, 300s.
Use: Diagnostic aid.
UCG-LYPHOTEST. (Wampole) One-hour passive hemagglutination inhibition tube test for the qualitative or quantitative determination of human chorionic gonadotropin (sensitivity 0.5-1 IU hCG/ml) in urine. Kit 10s, 50s, 300s.
Use: Diagnostic aid.
UCG-SLIDE TEST. (Wampole) Rapid latex agglutination inhibition slide test for the qualitative detection of human chorionic gonadotropin (Sensitivity: 2 IU hCG/ml) in urine. Kit 30s, 100s, 300s, 1000s.
Use: Diagnostic aid.
UCG-TEST. (Wampole) Two-hour hemagglutination inhibition tube test for the determination of human chorionic gonadotropin (sensitivity 0.5 IU hCG/ml undiluted specimen. 1.5 IU hCG/ml 1:3 diluted specimen) in urine and serum. Kit 10s, 25s, 100s, 300s.
Use: Diagnostic aid.
UCG-TITRATION SET. (Wampole) A two-hour hemagglutination inhibition tube test for the determination of human chorionic gonadotropin (Sensitivity 1 IU hCG/ml) in urine or serum. Kit 45s.
Use: Diagnostic aid.
U-CORT. (Thames) Hydrocortisone acetate 1%, water washable, EDTA, sodium bisulfate. Cream. 30, 120 Gm.
Use: Corticosteroid, topical.
ULCERIN P TABLETS. (Sanofi Winthrop) Aluminum hydroxide.
Use: Antacid.
ULCERIN TABLETS. (Sanofi Winthrop) Aluminum hydroxide.
Use: Antacid.
ULCER THERAPY.
See: Antacids.
Anticholinergic Agents.
•**ULDAZEPAM.** USAN.
Use: Sedative.
ULR-LA. (Geneva) Phenylpropanolamine HCl 75 mg, guaifenesin 400 mg. Tab. Bot. 100s.
Use: Decongestant, expectorant.
ULTRA B50. (Nature's Bounty) Vitamins B_1 50 mg, B_2 50 mg, B_3 50 mg, B_5 50 mg, B_6 50 mg, B_{12} 50 mcg, folic acid 0.1 mg, PABA 50 mg, inositol 50 mg, biotin 50 mcg, choline 50 mg, lecithin 50 mg/Tab. Bot. 60s, 180s.
Use: Vitamin supplement.
ULTRA B100. (Nature's Bounty) Vitamins B_1 100 mg, B_2 100 mg, B_3 100 mg, B_5 100 mg, B_6 100 mg, B_{12} 100 mcg, folic acid 0.1 mg, PABA 100 mg, inositol 100 mg, biotin 100 mcg, choline bitartrate 100 mg/TR Tab. Bot. 50s.
Use: Vitamin supplement.
ULTRABEX. (Approved) Vitamins B_1 20 mg, C 50 mg, B_2 2 mg, B_6 0.5 mg, niacinamide 35 mg, calcium pantothenate 0.5 mg, wheat germ oil 30 mg, B_{12} 20 mcg, liver desiccated 150 mg, iron 11.58 mg, calcium 29 mg, phosphorus 23 mg, dicalcium phosphate 100 mg, magnesium 1.11 mg, manganese 1.3 mg, potassium 2.24 mg, zinc 0.68 mg, choline 25 mg, inositol 25 mg, pepsin

32.5 mg, diastase 32.5 mg, hesperidin 25 mg, biotin 20 mcg, hydrolyzed yeast 81.25 mg, protein digest 47.04 mg, amino acids 34.21 mg/Cap. Bot. 50s, 100s, 1000s.
Use: Vitamin/mineral supplement.

ULTRACAL. (Mead Johnson Nutritional) Protein 44 Gm, carbohydrate 123 Gm, fat 45 Gm, Na 930 mg, K 1610 mg, mOsm 310 kg H_2O, cal. 1.06/ml, vitamins A B_1, B_2, B_3, B_5, B_6, B_{12}, C, D, E, K, folic acid, choline, biotin, Ca, P, I, Fe, Mg, Cu, Zn, Mn, Cl, Se, Cr, Mo. Liq. Can. 8 oz.
Use: Enteral nutritional therapy.

ULTRA CAP. (Weeks & Leo) Acetaminophen 300 mg, guaifenesin 100 mg, chlorpheniramine maleate 4 mg, phenylephrine HCl 10 mg, dextromethorphan HBr 6 mg/Cap. Vial 18s.
Use: Analgesic, expectorant, antihistamine, decongestant, antitussive.

ULTRA-CARE. (Allergan) **Disinfecting Soln.:** Hydrogen peroxide 3%, sodium stannate, sodium nitrate, phosphate buffer. Bot. 360 ml; **Neutralizer Tab.:** Catalase, hydroxypropyl methylcellulose, buffering agents. Pkg. 36s w/ cup.
Use: Soft contact lens care.

ULTRACEF. (Bristol Labs) **Cap.:** Cefadroxil monohydrate 500 mg. Bot. 50s, 100s, UD 100s. **Tab.:** 1 Gm. Bot. 24s, UD 100s. **Pow. for oral susp.:** 125 mg/ml or 250 mg/5 ml. Bot. 50 ml, 100 ml.
Use: Antibacterial, cephalosporin.

ULTRACORTINOL. (Ciba) Agent to suppress overactive adrenal glands. Pending release.

ULTRA-DERM BATH OIL. (Baker/Cummins) Bot. 8 oz.
Use: Emollient.

ULTRA-DERM MOISTURIZER. (Baker/Cummins) Bot. 8 oz.
Use: Emollient.

ULTRA-FREEDA. (Freeda) Vitamins A 3333 IU, D 133 IU, E 66.7 mg, B_1 16.7 mg, B_2 16.7 mg, B_3 33 mg, B_5 33 mg, B_6 16.7 mg, B_{12} 33 mcg, C 333 mg, iron 0.27 mg, calcium 66.7 mg, zinc 7.5 mg, choline 33 mg, inositol 33 mg, beta carotene 833 IU, bioflavonoids 33 mg, PABA 16.7 mg, biotin 100 mcg, Cr, I, K, Mg, Mn, Mo, Se. Tab. Bot. 90s, 180s, 270s.
Use: Vitamin/mineral supplement.

ULTRA-FREEDA IRON FREE. (Freeda) Vitamins A 3,333 IU, D 133 IU, E 66.7$_2$ mg, B_1 16.7 mg, B_2 16.7 mg, B_3 33 mg, B_5 33 ng, B_6 16.7 mg, B_{12} 33 mcg, C

333 mg, FA 0.27 mg, Ca 66.7 mg, Zn 7.5 mg, choline 33 mg, inositol 33 mg, betacarotene 833 IU, bioflavonoids 33 mg, PABA 16.7 mg, biotin 100 mcg, Cr, I, K, Mg, Mn, Mo, Se. Tab. Bot. 90s, 180s, 270s.
Use: Geriatric supplements w/multivitamins and minerals.

ULTRAGESIC. (Stewart-Jackson) Acetaminophen 500 mg, hydrocodone bitartrate 5 mg/Cap. Bot. 100s.
Use: Narcotic analgesic combination.

ULTRALAN. (Elan) Protein 60 g, fat 50 g, carbohydrates 202 g, Na 1.035 g, K 1.755 g/L. Lactose free. With appropriate vitamins and minerals. Liq. In 1000 ml New Pak systems with and without ColorCheck.
Use: Enteral nutritional supplement.

ULTRALENTE INSULIN.
See: Iletin (Lilly).

ULTRALENTE U. (Novo Nordisk) Insulin zinc suspension, extended 100 units/ml, beef. Inj. Vial 10 ml.
Use: Antidiabetic agent.

ULTRA MIDE 25. (Baker/Cummins) Bot. 8 oz.
Use: Emollient.

ULTRAPEN POTASSIUM SALT.
See: Propicillin, B.A.N.

ULTRAPRED. (Horizon) Prednisolone acetate 1%. Susp. Bot. 5 ml.
Use: Corticosteroid, ophthalmic.

ULTRASONE. (Gordon) Ultrasonic contact cream. Bot. qt, gal. Plastic Bot. 8 oz.
Use: Ultrasonic contact cream.

ULTRA TEARS. (Alcon) Hydroxypropyl methylcellulose 1%, benzalkonium Cl 0.01%/15 ml. Drop-tainer disp. 15 ml.
Use: Artificial tears.

ULTRAVATE. (Westwood Squibb) Halobetasol propionate.
Use: Corticosteroid, topical.

ULTRA VITAMIN A & D. (Nature's Bounty) Vitamins A 25,000 IU, D 1000 IU. Tab. Bot. 100s.
Use: Vitamin A & D combination.

ULTRAVITA TIME. (Nature's Bounty) Fe 5.8 mg, vitamins A 10,000 IU, D 400 IU, E 10.3 mg, B_1 25 mg, B_2 25 mg, B_3 50 mg, B_5 12.5 mg, B_6 15 mg, B_{12} 50 mcg, C 150 mg, FA 0.4 mg, Ca, Cu, I, Mg, Mn, P, Zn, biotin, PABA, choline bitartrate, betaine, rutin, inositol, bioflavonoids, desiccated liver, bone meal, lecithin. Tab. Bot. 50s, 100s.
Use: Multivitamin w/iron and other minerals.

ULTRAZYME ENZYMATIC CLEANER. (Allergan) Subtilisin A, effervescing,

buffering and tableting agents for dilution in hydrogen peroxide 3%. Tab. Pkg. 5s, 10s, 20s.
Use: Soft contact lens care.
ULTRUM. (Towne) Vitamins A 5000 IU, E 30 IU, C 90 mg, folic acid 400 mcg, B$_1$ 2.25 mg, B$_2$ 2.6 mg, niacinamide 20 mg, B$_6$ 3 mg, B$_{12}$ 9 mcg, biotin 45 mcg, D 400 IU, pantothenic acid 10 mg, calcium 162 mg, phosphorus 125 mg, iodine 150 mcg, iron 27 mg, magnesium 100 mg, copper 3 mg, manganese 7.5 mg, potassium 7.5 mg, zinc 22.5 mg/Tab. Bot. 100s.
Use: Vitamin/mineral supplement.
ULTRUM WITH SELENIUM. (Towne) Vitamins A 5000 IU, E 30 IU, C 90 mg, folic acid 2.25 mg, B$_1$ 2.25 mg, B$_2$ 2.6 mg, niacinamide 20 mg, B$_6$ 3 mg, B$_{12}$ 9 mcg, D 400 IU, biotin 45 mcg, pantothenic acid 10 mg, calcium 162 mg, phosphorus 125 mg, iodine 150 mcg, iron 27 mg, magnesium 100 mg, copper 3 mg, manganese 7.5 mg, potassium 7.7 mg, chloride 7 mg, molybdenum 15 mcg, selenium 15 mcg, zinc 22.5 mg/Tab. Bot. 130s.
Use: Vitamin/mineral supplement.
UNASYN. (Roerig) Ampicillin sodium 1 Gm, sulbactam sodium 0.5 Gm, ampicillin sodium 2 Gm, sulbactam sodium 1 Gm. Pow. for inj. Vial, piggyback vial.
Use: Antibacterial, penicillin.
10-UNDECENOIC ACID. Undecylenic Acid, U.S.P. XXIII.
Use: Antifungal, external.
10-UNDECENOIC ACID, ZINC (2+) SALT. Zinc Undecylenate, U.S.P. XXIII.
Use: Antifungal, external.
UNDECOYLIUM CHLORIDE-IODINE. 1-[[(2-Hydroxyethyl) carbamoyl]methyl]-pyridimium Cl alka-noates compound with I$_2$ (1:1). Virac, Preps. (Ruson).
Use: Anti-infective, external.
• **UNDECYLENIC ACID,** U.S.P. XXIII. Compound Oint. U.S.P. XXIII. 10-Undecenoic acid. (Lannett) Cap. 0.44 Gm, Bot. 100s, 500s, 1000s.
Use: Topical antifungal.
See: Desenex, Preps (Ciba).
W/Benzethonium Cl, benzalkonium Cl, tannic acid, isopropyl alcohol.
See: Tulvex, Liq. (Commerce).
W/Dichlorophene.
See: Fungicidal Talc (Gordon).
Onychomycetin, Liq. (Gordon).
W/Salicylic acid.
See: Sal-Dex, Liq. (Scrip).
W/Salicylic acid, benzoic acid, sulfur, dichlorophene.

See: Fungicidal, Oint. (Gordon).
W/Salicylic acid, dichlorophene, hexachlorophene.
See: Podiaspray, Aerosol Pow. (Dalin).
W/Sodium propionate, sodium caprylate, propionic acid, salicylic acid, copper undecylenate.
See: Verdefam, Soln. (Texas).
W/Zinc undecylenate.
See: Cruex Cream, Spray Pow. (Pharmacraft)
Desenex, Preps. (Pharmacraft).
Ting, Aerosol (Pharmacraft).
Undoguent, Cream (Torch).
UNDECYLENIC ACID SALTS. Calcium, copper, zinc.
UNDELENIC OINTMENT. (Gordon) Undecylenic acid 5%, zinc undecylenate 20%. Jar oz, lb.
Use: Antifungal, external.
UNDELENIC TINCTURE. (Gordon) Undecylenic acid 10%, chloroxylenol 0.5%. Brush Bot. oz. Bot. pt.
Use: Antifungal, external.
UNDEX CREAM. (Durel) Undecylenic acid 5%, zinc undecylenate 5% in duromantel cream.
Use: Antifungal, external.
UNDOGUENT. (Torch) Undecylenic acid 5%, zinc undecylenate 20% in a nongreasy, water-washable cream base. Jar 2 oz, lb.
Use: Antifungal, external.
UNDULANT FEVER DIAGNOSIS. Brucella Abortus Antigen. Brucellergen.
UNGUENTINE AEROSOL SPRAY. (Mentholatum) Alcohol 0.33 gm/oz, isobutane, menthol. Bot. 90 ml.
Use: Minor skin irritations.
UNGUENTINE OINTMENT "ORIGINAL FORMULA.". (Mentholatum) Phenol 1% in ointment base. Tube oz.
Use: Minor skin irritations.
UNGUENTINE PLUS FIRST AID CREAM. (Mentholatum) Parachlorometaxylenol 2%, lidocaine HCl 2%, phenol 0.5% in a moisturizing cream base. Tube ½ oz, 1 oz, 2 oz.
Use: Minor skin irritations.
UNGUENTINE SPRAY. (Mentholatum) Benzocaine, alcohol. Can 5 oz.
Use: Minor skin irritations.
UNGUENTUM BOSSI. (Doak) Ammoniated mercury 5%, hexamethylene tetramine sulfosalicylic acid 2%, tar distillate "Doak" 5%, Doak oil 40%, nonionic emulsifiers 5%, unguentum "Doak" 48%. Tube 2 oz. Jar 16 oz.
Use: Antipsoriatic.
UNI-ACE. (URL) Acetaminophen 100 mg

per ml. Alcohol free. Fruit flavor. Liq. Bot. 15 ml with dropper.
Use: Pain reliever.

UNIAD. (Kasar) Isoniazid 100 mg/Tab. Bot. 100s, 1000s.
Use: Antituberculous agent.

UNIAD-PLUS. (Kasar) Isoniazid 100 mg, pyridoxine HCl 5 mg or 10 mg/Tab. Bot. 1000s.
Use: Antituberculous agent.

UNIBASE. (Parke-Davis) Water-absorbing oint. base. Jar lb.
Use: Ointment base.

UNI-BENT COUGH. (URL) Diphenhydramine HCl 12.5 mg/5 ml, alcohol 5%. Syr. Bot 118 ml.
Use: Antitussive.

UNICAP. (Upjohn) Vitamins A 5000 IU, D 400 IU, E 16.5 mg, C 60 mg, folic acid 400 mcg, B_1 1.5 mg, B_2 1.7 mg, niacin 20 mg, B_6 2 mg, B_{12} 6 mcg, tartrazine/Tab. or Cap. **Tab.:** Bot. 90s, 120s. **Cap.:** Bot. 90s, 120s, 240s, 1000s.
Use: Vitamin supplement.

UNICAP JUNIOR CHEWABLE. (Upjohn) Vitamins A 5000 IU, D 400 IU, E 15 IU, C 60 mg, folic acid 400 mcg, B_1 1.5 mg, B_2 1.7 mg, niacin 20 mg, B_6 2 mg, B_{12} 6 mcg/Tab. Bot. 90s, 120s.
Use: Vitamin supplement.

UNICAP M. (Upjohn) Vitamins A 5000 IU, D 400 IU, E 33 mg, C 60 mg, folic acid 400 mcg, B_1 1.5 mg, B_2 1.7 mg, niacin 20 mg, B_6 2 mg, B_{12} 6 mcg, pantothenic acid 10 mg, iodine 150 mcg, iron 18 mg, copper 2 mg, zinc 15 mg, calcium 60 mg, phosphorus 45 mg, manganese 1 mg, potassium 5 mg, tartrazine/Tab. Bot. 30s, 90s, 180s, 500s.
Use: Vitamin/mineral supplement.

UNICAP PLUS IRON. (Upjohn) Vitamins A 5000 IU, D 400 IU, E 16.5 mg, C 60 mg, folic acid 400 mcg, B_1 1.5 mg, B_2 1.7 mg, niacin 20 mg, B_6 2 mg, B_{12} 6 mcg, pantothenic acid 10 mg, iron 18 mg/Tab. Bot. 90s.
Use: Vitamin/mineral supplement.

UNICAP SENIOR. (Upjohn) Vitamins A 5000 IU, D 200 IU, E 16.5 mg, C 60 mg, folic acid 400 mcg, B_1 1.2 mg, B_2 1.4 mg, niacin 16 mg, B_6 2.2 mg, B_{12} 3 mcg, pantothenic acid 10 mg, iodine 150 mcg, iron 10 mg, copper 2 mg, zinc 15 mg, calcium 100 mg, phosphorus 77 mg, magnesium 30 mg, manganese 1 mg, potassium 5 mg/Tab. Bot. 90s.
Use: Vitamin/mineral supplement.

UNICAP T. (Upjohn) Vitamins A 5000 IU, D 400 IU, E 33 mg, C 500 mg, folic acid

400 mcg, B_1 10 mg, B_2 10 mg, niacin 100 mg, B_6 6 mg, B_{12} 18 mcg, pantothenic acid 25 mg, iodine 150 mcg, iron 18 mg, copper 2 mg, zinc 15 mg, manganese 1 mg, potassium 5 mg, selenium 10 mcg/Tab. Bot. 60s, 500s.
Use: Vitamin/mineral supplement.

UNICOMPLEX-M. (Rugby) Iron 18 mg, vitamins A 5000 IU, D 400 IU, E 15 mg, B_1 1.5 mg, B_2 1.7 mg, B_3 20 mg, B_5 10 mg, B_6 2 mg, B_{12} 6 mcg, C 60 mg, folic acid 0.4 mg, Ca, Cu, I, K, Mn, Zn/Tab. Bot. 90s, 1000s.
Use: Vitamin/mineral supplement.

UNICOMPLEX-T WITH MINERALS. (Rugby) Iron 10 mg, vitamins A 5000 IU, D 400 IU, E 15 mg, B_1 10 mg, B_2 10 mg, B_3 100 mg, B_5 20 mg, B_6 2 mg, B_{12} 4 mcg, C 300 mg, folic acid 0.4 mg, Ca, Cu, I, K, Mg, Mn/Tab. Bot. 60s, 1000s.
Use: Vitamin/mineral supplement.

UNICOMPLEX T&M. (Rugby) Iron 10 mg, vitamins A 5000 IU, D 400 IU, E 15 mg, B_1 10 mg, B_2 10 mg, D_3 100 mg, B_3 20 mg, B_6 2 mg, B_{12} 4 mcg, C 300 mg, FA 0.4 mg, Ca, Cu, I, K, Mg, Mn. Tab. Bot. 60s.
Use: Vitamin/mineral supplement.

UNI-DECON. (URL) Phenylpropanolamine HCl 40 mg, phenylephrine HCl 10 mg, chlorpheniramine maleate 5 mg, phenyltoloxamine citrate 15 mg/Tab. Bot. 100s, 500s and 1000s.
Use: Decongestant and antihistamine.

UNIFIBER. (Dow B. Hickam) Powdered cellulose 3 Gm per tbsp. < 4 calories per serving. Corn syrup solids, xanthan gum. Pow. Bot. 454 Gm.
Use: Laxatives.

• **UNIFOCON A.** USAN.
Use: Contact lens material.

UNILAX. (B.F. Ascher) Docusate 230 mg, phenolphthalein 130 mg. Sorbitol. Cap. Bot. 15s, 20s, 60s.
Use: Laxative combination.

UNIPEN. (Wyeth-Ayerst) Sodium nafcillin. **Cap.:** 250 mg. Bot. 100s, Redipak 100s. **Tab.:** 500 mg. Bot. 50s, Cap. and Tab. buffered w/calcium carbonate. **Vial:** Vial 2 Gm, Piggyback Vial 2 Gm, Bulk vial 10 Gm. **Oral Soln.** 250 mg/5 ml w/alcohol 2%. Bot. to make 100 ml.
Use: Antibacterial, penicillin.

UNIPHYL TABLETS. (Purdue Frederick) Theophylline 200 mg or 400 mg/Controlled-release Tab. **200 mg:** Bot. 60s, 100s, UD 100s. **400 mg:** Bot. 60s, 100s, 500s, UD 100s.
Use: Bronchodilator.

UNIPRES. (Solvay) Hydralazine HCl 25

mg, hydrochlorothiazide 15 mg, reserpine 0.1 mg/Tab. Bot. 100s, 1000s.
Use: Antihypertensive.

UNISOL. (Alcon) Buffered isotonic solution with sodium Cl, boric acid, sodium borate. Bot. 15 ml.
Use: Soft contact lens care.

UNISOL 4 STERILE SALINE (Alcon) Buffered isotonic solution with sodium Cl, boric acid, sodium borate. Bot. 120 ml.
Use: Soft contact lens care.

UNISOL PLUS. (Alcon) Buffered isotonic solution w/ NaCl, boric acid, sodium borate. Aerosol 240 ml or 360 ml.
Use: Soft contact lens care.

UNISOM NIGHTTIME SLEEP-AID. (Pfizer) Doxylamine succcinate 25 mg/Tab. Blister 8s, 16s, 32s, 48s.
Use: Sleep aid.

UNISOM WITH PAIN RELIEF. (Pfizer) Acetaminophen 650 mg, diphenhydramine HCl 50 mg/Tab. Blister 16s.
Use: Analgesic, sleep aid.

UNITROL. (Republic Drug) Phenylpropanolamine HCl 75 mg/TR Cap. Pkg. 28s.
Use: Diet aid.

UNI-TUSSIN DM. (URL) Dextromethorphan HBr 10 mg, guaifenesin 100 mg/5 ml. Syr. Bot.118 ml.
Use: Antitussive, expectorant.

UNI-TUSSIN SYRUP. (United Research Laboratories) Dextromethorphan HBr 15 mg, guaifenesin 100 mg, alcohol 1.4%. Bot. 120 ml.
Use: Antitussive, expectorant.

UNIVERSAL ANTIDOTE.
See: Res-Q (Boyle).

UNNA'S BOOT.
See: Zinc Gelatin, U.S.P. XXIII.

UNPROCO CAPSULES. (Solvay) Dextromethorphan HBr 30 mg, guaifenesin 200 mg/Cap. Bot. 100s.
Use: Antitussive, expectorant.

UNSATURATED ACIDS.
See: Fatty acids, unsaturated; fats, unsaturated.

UPLEX. (Arcum) Vitamins A 5000 IU, D 400 IU, B_1 3 mg, B_2 3 mg, B_6 1 mg, B_{12} 2.5 mcg, nicotinamide 20 mg, calcium pantothenate 5 mg, C 50 mg/Cap. Bot. 100s, 1000s.
Use: Vitamin supplement.

UPLEX NO. 2. (Arcum) Vitamins A palmitate 10,000 IU, D 400 IU, B_1 5 mg, B_2 5 mg, C 100 mg, B_6 2 mg, B_{12} 3 mcg, E 2.5 IU, niacinamide 25 mg, calcium pantothenate 5 mg/Cap. Bot. 100s, 1000s.
Use: Vitamin supplement.

URABETH TABS. (Major) Bethanechol 5 mg, 10 mg, 25 mg or 50 mg/Tab. **5 mg:** Bot. 100s. **10 mg:** Bot. 250s. **25 mg:** Bot. 250s, 1000s. **50 mg:** Bot. 100s, UD 100s.
Use: Urinary tract product.

URACID. (Wesley) dl-Methionine 0.2 Gm/Cap. Bot. 100s, 1000s.
Use: Diaper rash product.

• **URACIL MUSTARD,** U.S.P. XXII. Cap., U.S.P. XXII. 5-[Bis(2-Chloroethyl)amino]uracil. (Upjohn) 1 mg/Cap. Bot. 50s.
Use: Antineoplastic.

URADAL.
See: Carbromal (Various Mfr.)

URAMUSTINE. B.A.N. 5-Di-(2-chloroethyl) aminouracil.
Use: Antineoplastic agent.

URAPINE TABS. (Major) Bot. 1000s.
Use: Urinary analgesic.

URDEX. (Pharmex) Phenylpropanolamine 12.5 mg, atropine sulfate 0.2 mg, chlorpheniramine 5 mg/ml. Vial 10 ml.
Use: Decongestant, anticholinergic/antispasmodic, antihistamine.

• **UREA,** U.S.P. XXIII. Sterile U.S.P. XXIII. Carbamide.
Use: Topically for dry skin; diuretic.
See: Aquacare, Cream, Lot. (Herbert).
Aquacare-HP, Cream, Lot. (Herbert).
Artra Ashy Skin, Cream (Schering-Plough).
Calmurid, Cream (Pharmacia).
Carmol, Cream (Ingram).
Carmol Ten, Lot. (Ingram).
Elaqua 10% or 20%, Cream (Elder).
Gormel, Cream (Gordon).
Nutraplus, Cream, Lot. (Owen).
Rea-lo, Lot. (Whorton).
W/Benzocaine, benzyl alcohol, p-chloro-m-xylenol, propyleneglycol.
See: 20-Cain Burn Relief (Alto).
W/Hydrocortisone acetate.
See: Carmol-HC, Cream (Ingram).
W/Glycerin.
See: Kerid Ear Drops, Liq. (Blair).
W/Sulfur colloidal, red mercuric sulfide.
See: Teenac, Cream, Oint. (Elder).
W/Zinc oxide, sulfur, salicylic acid, benzalkonium Cl, isopropyl alcohol.
See: Akne Drying Lotion

UREA PEROXIDE.
See: Cankaid (Becton Dickinson).
Gly-Oxide Liquid (Marion).
Oragel Brace-aid Rinse (Commerce).
Proxigel (Reed & Carnrick). (Alto).

UREACIN-10 LOTION. (Pedinol) Urea 10%. Bot. 8 oz.

Use: Emollient.
UREACIN-20 CREME. (Pedinol) Urea 20%. Jar 2.5 oz.
Use: Emollient.
UREACIN-40 CREME. (Pedinol) Urea 40%. Jar oz.
Use: Treatment of nail destruction and dissolution.
UREAPHIL. (Abbott Hospital Prods) Sterile urea 40 Gm, citric acid 1 mg/150 ml. Bot. 150 ml.
Use: Osmotic diuretic.
URECHOLINE. (Merck & Co.) Bethanechol Cl. **Inj.:** 5 mg/ml Vial 1 ml, 6s. **Tab.:** 5 mg, 10 mg, 25 mg or 50 mg. Bot. 100s, UD 100s.
Use: Urinary tract product.
• **UREDEPA.** USAN. Ethyl[bis(1-aziridinyl)-phos-phinyl]carbamate.
Use: Antineoplastic.
See: Avinar (Armour).
• **UREDOFOS.** USAN.
Use: Anthelmintic.
See: Sansalid (Beecham).
p-UREIDOBENZENEARSONIC ACID.
See: Carbarsone, U.S.P. XXIII.
URELIEF. (Rocky Mtn.) Methenamine 2 gr, salol 0.5 gr, methylene blue 1/10 gr, benzoic acid gr, hyoscyamine sulfate gr, atropine sulfate gr/Tab. Bot. 100s.
Use: Urinary anti-infective.
URESE. (Roerig)
See: Benzthianide.
URETHAN. Ethyl Carbamate, Ethyl Urethan, Urethane.
Use: Antineoplastic agent.
UREX TABLETS. (Riker) Methenamine hippurate 1 Gm/Tab. Bot. 100s, 500s.
Use: Urinary anti-infective.
U.R.I. (Sig) Atropine sulfate 0.2 mg, chlorpheniramine maleate 5 mg, phenylpropanolamine HCl 12.5 mg/ml. Vial 10 ml.
Use: Anticholinergic/antispasmodic, antihistamine, decongestant.
URIC ACID REAGENT STRIPS. (Miles Diagnostic) Seralyzer reagent strip. For uric acid in serum or plasma. Bot. 25s.
Use: Diagnostic aid.
URICOSURIC AGENTS.
See: Anturane, Tab., Cap. (Geigy). Benemid, Tab. (Merck & Co.). ColBenemid, Tab. (Merck & Co.).
URICULT. (Medical Technology) Urine culture test to detect bacteria and identify uropathogens. Bot. 10s.
Use: Diagnostic aid.
URIDINE, 2-DEOXY-5-IODO-. Idoxuridine, U.S.P. XXIII.
URIDIUM. (Ferndale; Pharmex) Phenylazodiamine pyridine HCl 75 mg, sulfacetamide 250 mg/Tab. Bot. 30s, 100s, 1000s. (Ferndale) 100s.
Use: Urinary anti-infective.
URIDON MODIFIED. (Rugby) Methenamine 40.8 mg, phenylsalicylate 18.1 mg, atropine sulfate 0.03 mg, hyoscyamine 0.03 mg, benzoic acid 4.5 mg, methylene blue 5.4 mg/Tab. Bot. 100s, 1000s.
Use: Urinary anti-infective.
URIFON-FORTE. (T.E. Williams) Sulfamethizole 450 mg, phenazopyridine HCl 50 mg/Cap. Bot. 100s, 1000s.
Use: Urinary anti-infective.
URIGEN. (Fellows) Calcium mandelate 0.2 Gm, methenamine 0.2 Gm, phenazopyridine HCl 50 mg, sodium phosphate 80 mg/Cap. Bot. 100s, 1000s.
Use: Urinary anti-infective.
URIMAR-T. (Marnel) Methenamine 81.6 mg, sodium biphosphate 40.8 mg, phenyl salicylate 30.2 mg, methylene blue 10.8 mg, hyoscyamine sulfate 0.12 mg. Tab. Bot. 100s.
Use: Urinary anti-infective.
URINARY ANTISEPTIC #2. (Vitarine) Atropine sulfate 0.03 mg, hyoscyamine 0.03 mg, methenamine 40.8 mg, methylene blue 5.4 mg, phenylsalicylate 18.1 mg, benzoic acid 4.5 mg/Tab. Bot. 100s, 1000s.
Use: Urinary anti-infective.
URINARY ANTISEPTIC #2 S.C.T. (Lemmon) Atropine sulfate 0.03 mg, hyoscyamine sulfate 0.03 mg, methenamine 40.8 mg, methylene blue 5.4 mg, phenyl salicylate 18.1 mg, benzoic acid 4.5 mg/Tab. Bot. 100s, 1000s.
Use: Urinary anti-infective.
URINARY ANTISEPTIC #3 S.C.T. (Lemmon) Atropine sulfate 0.06 mg, hyoscyamine sulfate 0.03 mg, methenamine 120 mg, methylene blue 6 mg, phenyl salicylate 30 mg, benzoic acid 7.5 mg/Tab. Bot. 100s, 1000s.
Use: Urinary anti-infective.
URINE.
See: Diagnostic agents.
URINE GLUCOSE TESTS.
See: Biotel Diabetes (Biotel). Clinitest Tablets (Miles Diagnostic). Chemstrip uG Strips (Boehringer Mannheim). Clinistix Strips (Miles Diagnostic). Dialstix Strips (Miles Diagnostic). Test Tape (Lilly).
URINE SUGAR TEST.
See: Clinistix (Miles Diagnostic).

URINE TESTS MISC.
See: Nitrazine Paper (Apothecon).
Phenistix Reagent Strips (Miles Diagnostic).
URIN-TEK. (Miles Diagnostic) Tubes,
plastic caps, adhesive labels, collection
cups, and disposable tube holder. Package 100×5
URISAN-P. (Sandia) Atropine sulfate 0.03
mg, hyoscyamine 0.03 mg, gelsemium
6.1 mg, methenamine 40.8 mg, salol
18.1 mg, benzoic acid 4.5 mg, methylene blue 5.4 mg, phenylazodiaminopyridine HCl 100 mg/Tab. Bot. 100s, 1000s.
Use: Urinary anti-infective.
URISED. (PolyMedica) Atropine sulfate
0.03 mg, hyoscyamine 0.03 mg,
methenamine 40.8 mg, methylene blue
5.4 mg, benzoic acid 4.5 mg, phenyl salicylate 18.1 mg/Tab. Bot. 100s, 500s,
1000s.
Use: Urinary anti-infective.
URISEDAMINE. (PolyMedica)
Methenamine mandelate 500 mg, l-
hyoscyamine 0.15 mg/Tab. Bot. 100s.
Use: Urinary anti-infective.
URISPAS. (SK-Beecham) Flavoxate HCl
100 mg/Tab. Bot. 100s, UD 100s.
Use: Urinary antispasmodic.
URISTIX 4 REAGENT STRIPS. (Miles Diagnostic) Urinalysis reagent strip test for
glucose, protein, nitrite, leukocytes. Bot.
100s.
Use: Diagnostic aid.
URISTIX REAGENT STRIPS. (Miles Diagnostic) Urinalysis reagent strip test for
protein and glucose. Bot. 100s.
Use: Diagnostic aid.
URI-TET. (American Urologicals) Oxytetracycline HCl 250 mg/Cap. Bot. 100s,
1000s.
Use: Antibacterial, tetracycline.
URITIN. (Richlyn) Methenamine 40.8 mg,
atropine sulfate 0.03 mg, hyoscyamine
sulfate 0.03 mg, salol 18.1 mg, benzoic
acid 4.5 mg, methylene blue 5.4 mg,
gelsemium 6.1 mg/Tab. Bot. 1000s.
Use: Urinary anti-infective.
URITIN FORMULA. (Vangard) Atropine
sulfate 0.03 mg, hyoscyamine 0.03 mg,
methenamine 40.8 mg, methylene blue
5.4 mg, phenyl salicylate 18.1 mg, benzoic acid 4.5 mg/Tab. Bot. 1000s.
Use: Urinary anti-infective.
URITROL. (Kenyon) Atropine sulfate 0.03
mg, hyoscyamine 0.03 mg, gelsemium
6.1 mg, methenamine 40.8 mg, salol
18.1 mg, benzoic acid 4.5 mg, methylene blue 5.4 mg/Tab. Bot. 100s, 1000s.
Double Strength Tab. Bot. 100s, 1000s.

Use: Urinary anti-infective.
URIZOLE. (Jenkins) Sulfisoxazole 7.7
gr/Tab. Bot. 1000s.
Use: Antibacterial, sulfonamide.
UROBAK. (Shionogi) Sulfamethoxazole
500 mg/Tab. Bot. 100s, 1000s.
Use: Antibacterial, sulfonamide.
UROBIOTIC. (Roerig) Oxytetracycline as
the HCl equivalent to oxytetracycline
250 mg, sulfamethizole 250 mg,
phenazopyridine HCl 50 mg/Cap. Bot.
50s, UD pack Box 100s.
Use: Urinary anti-infective.
UROBIOTIC-250. (Roerig) Oxytetracy-
cline (as HCl) 250 mg, sulfamethizole
250 mg, phenazopyridine HCl 50
mg/Cap. Bot. 50s, UD 100s.
Use: Urinary anti-infective.
UROCIT-K. (Mission) Potassium citrate
540 mg: Tab. Bot. 100s; **10 mEq:** Tab.
Bot. 100s.
Use: Urinary tract product.
URODINE. (Kenyon) Phenylazodi-
aminopyridine HCl 100 mg/Tab. Bot.
100s, 1000s.
Use: Urinary analgesic.
URODINE. (Robinson) Phenylazodi-
aminopyridine HCl 1.5 gr/Tab. Bot. 100s,
1000s.
Use: Urinary analgesic.
• **UROFOLLITROPIN.** USAN.
Use: Hormone (follicle-stimulating). In-
duction of ovulation in patients with
polycystic ovary disease. [Orphan
drug]
See: Metrodin, Inj. (Serono).
UROGASTRONE.
Use: Corneal transplant surgery. [Or-
phan drug]
UROGESIC. (Edwards) Phenazopyridine
HCl 100 mg, hyoscyamine HBr 0.12 mg,
atropine sulfate 0.08 mg, scopolamine
HBr 0.003 mg/Tab. Bot. 100s, 500s.
Use: Urinary analgesic.
UROGESIC BLUE. (Edwards)
Methenamine 81.6 mg, sodium biphos-
phate 40.8 mg, phenyl salicylate 36.2
mg, methylene blue 10.8 mg,
hyoscyamine (as sulfate) 0.12 mg. Tab.
Bot. 100s.
Use: Urinary anti-infective.
UROGRAPHY AGENTS.
See: Diodrast.
Iodohippurate Sodium, Inj.
Iodopyracet.
Iodopyracet Compound.
Methiodal, Inj.
Renografin (Squibb).
Renovist (Squibb).
Renovue (Squibb).

Sodium Acetrizoate, Inj.
Sodium Iodomethamate, Inj.
• **UROKINASE.** USAN. Plasminogen activator isolated from human kidney tissue.
Use: Plasminogen activator.
URO-KP-NEUTRAL.(Star) Sodium (as dibasic sodium phosphate) 1361 mg, potassium 298.6 mg, phosphorus (as dibasic potassium phosphate) 1037 mg/6 Tab. Bot. 100s.
Use: Phosphorus supplement.
UROLENE BLUE. (Star) Methylene blue 65 mg/Tab. Bot. 100s, 1000s.
Use: Urinary anti-infective.
UROLOGIC SOL G. (Abbott Hospital Prods) Bot. 1000 ml.
Use: Irrigating solution.
See: Thiosulfil, Preps. (Wyeth-Ayerst).
URO-MAG. (Blaine) Magnesium oxide 140 mg/Cap. Bot. 100s, 1000s.
Use: Antacid.
URONAL.
See: Barbital (Various Mfr.).
URO-PHOSPHATE. (Poythress) Sodium biphosphate 500 mg, methenamine 300 mg/Film Coated Tab. Bot. 100s, 1000s.
Use: Urinary anti-infective.
UROPLUS DS. (Shionogi) Trimethoprim 160 mg, sulfamethoxazole 800 mg/Tab. Bot. 100s, 500s.
Use: Anti-infective.
UROPLUS SS. (Shionogi) Trimethoprim 80 mg, sulfamethoxazole 800 mg/Tab. Bot. 100s, 500s.
Use: Anti-infective.
UROQID-ACID. (Beach) Methenamine mandelate 350 mg, sodium acid phosphate 200 mg/Tab. Bot. 100s, 500s.
Use: Urinary anti-infective.
UROQID-ACID NO. 2. (Beach) Methenamine mandelate 500 mg, sodium acid phosphate 500 mg/Tab. Bot. 100s, 500s.
Use: Urinary anti-infective.
UROTROL. (Mills) Sulfacetamide 250 mg, sulfamethizole 250 mg, phenazopyridine HCl 50 mg/Tab. Bot. 100s.
Use: Urinary anti-infective.
UROTROPIN NEW. Methenamine Anhydromethylene Citrate (Various Mfr.).
UROVIST CYSTO. (Berlex) Diatrizoate meglumine 300 mg, edetate calcium disodium 0.05 mg/ml. Dilution bot. 500 ml w/300 ml soln.
Use: Radiopaque agent.
UROVIST CYSTO PEDIATRIC. (Berlex) Diatrizoate meglumine 300 mg, edetate calcium disodium 0.1 mg/ml. Dilution bot. 300 ml w/100 ml soln.
Use: Radiopaque agent.

UROVIST MEGLUMINE DIU/CT. (Berlex) Diatrizoate meglumine 300 mg, edetate calcium disodium 0.05 mg/ml. Bot. 300 ml, Ctn. 10s.
Use: Radiopaque agent.
UROVIST SODIUM 300. (Berlex) Diatrizoate sodium 500 mg, edetate calcium disodium 0.1 mg/ml. Vial 50 ml, Box 10s.
Use: Radiopaque agent.
URSINUS INLAY-TABS. (Sandoz Consumer) Pseudoephedrine HCl 30 mg, aspirin 325 mg/Tab. Bot. 24s, 100s.
Use: Decongestant, salicylate analgesic.
URSODEOXYCHOLIC ACID.
Use: Primary biliary cirrhosis. [Orphan drug]
URSODIOL. Ursodeoxycholic acid.
Use: Gallstone solubilizing agent. [Orphan drug]
See: Actigall (Ciba).
URSULFADINE NO. 1. (Kenyon) Phenylazodiaminopyridine HCl 50 mg, sulfacetamide 250 mg/Tab. Bot. 100s, 1000s.
Use: Urinary anti-infective.
UTICORT CREAM. (Parke-Davis) Betamethasone benzoate 0.025%. Tube 15 Gm, 60 Gm.
Use: Corticosteroid.
UTICORT GEL. (Parke-Davis) Betamethasone benzoate 0.025% in solubilized gel base. Tube 15 Gm, 60 Gm.
Use: Corticosteroid.
UTICORT LOTION. (Parke-Davis) Betamethasone benzoate 0.025%. Bot. 15 ml, 60 ml.
Use: Corticosteroid.
UTIMOX. (Parke-Davis) Amoxicillin trihydrate. **Cap.:** 250 mg Bot. 100s, 500s, UD 100s; 500 mg Bot. 100s, UD 100s; **Oral susp.:** 125 mg or 250 mg/5 ml Bot. 80 ml, 100 ml, 150 ml, 200 ml.
Use: Antibacterial, penicillin.
U-TRAN. (Scruggs) Atropine sulfate 0.03 mg, hyoscyamine 0.03 mg, methenamine 40.8 mg, benzoic acid 4.5 mg, salol 18.1 mg, methylene blue 5.4 mg/Tab. Bot. 100s, 1000s.
Use: Urinary anti-infective.
U-TRI SPECIAL FORMULA OINTMENT. (U-Tri) Oint. Jar 4 oz, 7 oz.
Use: External analgesic.
UVADEX. (Therakos, Inc.)
See: 8-METHOXSALEN.
UVALERAL.
See: Bromisovalum.
UVASAL POWDER. (Sanofi Winthrop) Sodium bicarbonate, tartaric acid.
Use: Antacid.
UVA URSI. Leaves. (Sherwood Labs.)

Fluidextract. Bot. pt, gal.
UVIBAN. Sodium Actinoquinol.
Use: Treatment of flash burns (oph-
thalmic).
UVINUL MS-40. (General Aniline & Film)
See: Sulisobenzone.

V

VACCINE, MUMPS. Mumps Virus Vac-
cine Live, U.S.P. XXIII.
Agent for immunization.
• **VACCINE, PERTUSSIS.** Pertussis Vac-
cine, U.S.P. XXIII.
Use: Active immunizing agent.
• **VACCINE, PERTUSSIS, ADSORBED.**
Pertussis Vaccine Adsorbed, U.S.P.
XXIII.
Use: Active immunizing agent.
See: Pertussis Vaccine, Aluminum Hy-
droxide Adsorbed.
**VACCINE, PERTUSSIS, ALUM PRECIPI-
TATED.**
Use: Agent for immunization.
See: Pertussis Vaccine, Alum Precipi-
tated (Various Mfr.).
• **VACCINE, POLIOMYELITIS.** Poliovirus
Vaccine Inactivated, U.S.P. XXIII.
Use: Active immunizing agent.
• **VACCINE, RABIES (DUCK EMBRYO),**
Rabies Vaccine U.S.P. XXIII.
Use: Active immunizing agent.
• **VACCINE, SMALLPOX.** Smallpox Vac-
cine, U.S.P. XXIII.
Use: Active immunizing agent.
VACCINE, WHOOPING COUGH. Pertus-
sis Vaccine, U.S.P. XXIII.
Use: Active immunizing agent.
• **VACCINIA IMMUNE GLOBULIN,** U.S.P.
XXIII. (Hyland) Gamma globulin fraction
of serum of healthy adults recently im-
munized w/vaccinia virus 16.5%. Vial 5
ml.
Use: Prevention or modification of
smallpox or vaccinia infections; pas-
sive immunizing agent.
VACOCIN. Under study.
Use: Antibiotic.
VADEMIN-Z. (Hauck) Vitamin A 12,500
IU, D 50 IU, E 50 mg, B_1 10 mg, B_2 5
mg, B_3 25 mg, B_5 10 mg, B_6 2 mg, C 150
mg, zinc 20 mg, Mg, Mn/Cap. Bot. 60s,
500s.
Use: Vitamin/mineral supplement.
VAGILLA TRIPLE SULFA. (Lemmon)
Sulfathiazole 3.42%, sulfacetamide
2.86%, sulfabenzamide 3.7%, urea
0.64% in cream base. Tube 78 Gm.
Use: Anti-infective, vaginal.

VAGINEX CREME. (Schmid) Benzo-
caine, resorcinol in cream base.
Use: Vaginal preparation.
VAGISAN CREME. (Sandia) Sulfanilamide 15%, 9-aminoacridine HCl 0.2%,
allantoin 1.5% in a dispersible base.
Tube 4 oz w/applicator.
Use: Anti-infective, vaginal.
VAGISEC. (Schmid) Polyoxyethylene
nonyl phenol, sodium ethylene diamine
tetraacetate, docusate sodium. Plastic
Bot. 4 oz. Liq. Packette 12s.
Use: Vaginal preparation.
VAGISEC PLUS SUPPOSITORIES.
(Schmid) Polyoxyethylene nonyl phenol
5.25 mg, sodium edetate 0.66 mg, do-
cusate sodium 0.07 mg, 9-aminoacri-
dine HCl 6 mg, in a polyethylene glycol
base w/glycerin, citric acid. Box 28s.
Use: Vaginal preparation.
VAGISIL. (Combe) Creme. Benzocaine
and resorcin with lanolin alcohol,
parabens, trisodium HEDTA, mineral oil
and sodium sulfite. 30, 60 g.
Use: Vaginal preparation.
VAGISTAT-1. (Bristol-Myers Squibb) Tio-
conazole 6.5%. Vaginal oint. Prefilled
applicator 4.6 Gm.
Use: Antifungal, vaginal.
VAGISUL CREME. (Sheryl) Sulfanilamide
15%, aminoacridine 0.2%, allantoin
1.5%. Tube 4 oz.
Use: Anti-infective, vaginal.
VALACET. (Vale) Hyoscyamus 10.8 mg,
aspirin 259.2 mg, caffeine anhydrous
16.2 mg, gelsemium extract 0.6 mg/Tab.
or Cap. Bot. 100s, 1000s, 5000s.
Use: Anticholinergic/antispasmodic,
salicylate analgesic.
• **VALACYCLOVIR HYDROCHLORDIDE.**
USAN.
Use: Antiviral agent.
VALERGEN. (Hyrex) Estradiol valerate
10 mg, 20 mg or 40 mg/ml. Vial 10 ml.
Use: Estrogen.
VALERIAN. (Lilly) Tincture, alcohol 68%.
Bot. 4 fl oz, 16 fl oz.
W/Phenobarbital, passiflora, hyoscyamus.
See: Aluro, Tab. (Foy).
VALERTEST. (Hyrex) **No. 1:** Estradiol
valerate 4 mg, testosterone enanthate
90 mg/ml. Vial 10 ml. **No. 2:** Double
strength. Vial 10 ml. Amp. 2 ml, 10s.
Use: Estrogen, androgen combination.
VALETHAMATE BROMIDE. 2-Diethyl-
laminoethyl 3-methyl-2-phenylvalerate
methylbromide. Di-ethyl(2-hydrox-
yethyl)methyl-ammonium bromide 3-
methyl-2-phenylvalerate. Murel.
Use: Anticholinergic.

VALIHIST TABLETS. (Otis Clapp) Phenylephrine 5 mg, acetaminophen 325 mg, chlorpheniramine maleate 2 mg, caffeine 45 mg/Tab. Bot. 500s. *Use:* Decongestant, analgesic, antihistamine.

• **VALINE, U.S.P. XXIII.** $C_5H_{11}NO_2$ **as L-valine.**
Use: Amino acid.

VALISONE. (Schering) Betamethasone valerate. **Cream:** 1 mg/Gm Hydrophilic cream of water, mineral oil, petrolatum, polyethylene glycol 1000 monocetyl ether, cetostearyl alcohol, monobasic sodium phosphate, phosphoric acid, 4-chloro-m-cresol as preservative. Tube 15 Gm, 45 Gm, 110 Gm. Jar 430 Gm. **Oint.:** 1 mg/Gm Base of liquid and white petrolatum and hydrogenated lanolin. Tube 15 Gm, 45 Gm. **Lot.:** 1 mg/Gm w/isopropyl alcohol 47.5%, water slightly thickened w/carboxy vinyl polymer, pH adjusted w/sodium hydroxide. Bot. 20 ml, 60 ml. **Reduced Strength Cream 0.01%:** Hydrophilic cream of water, mineral oil, petrolatum, polyethylene glycol 1000 monocetyl ether, cetostearyl alcohol, monobasic sodium phosphate, phosphoric acid, 4-chloro-m-cresol as preservative. Tube 15 Gm, 60 Gm.
Use: Corticosteroid.

VALIUM INJECTABLE. (Roche) Diazepam 5 mg/ml, propylene glycol 40%, ethyl alcohol 10%, sodium benzoate, benzoic acid 5%, benzyl alcohol 1.5%. Amp. 2 ml, 10s. Vial 10 ml, Box 10s. Tel-E-Ject (Disposable syringe) 2 ml, Box 10s.
Use: Antianxiety agent.

VALIUM TABLETS. (Roche) Diazepam 2 mg, 5 mg or 10 mg/Tab. Bot. 100s, 500s, Tel-E-Dose 100s (10×10), (425) RPN (Reverse Numbered Packages), Prescription Pak 50s.
Use: Antianxiety agent.

VALLERGINE.
See: Promethazine HCl, U.S.P. XXIII.

VALNAC CREAM. (NMC Labs) Betamethasone valerate 0.1%. Cream Tube 15 Gm, 45 Gm.
Use: Corticosteroid.

VALNAC OINTMENT. (NMC Labs) Betamethasone valerate 0.1%. Oint. Tube 15 Gm, 45 Gm.
Use: Corticosteroid.

• **VALNOCTAMIDE.** USAN.
Use: Tranquilizer.

VALORIN. (Otis Clapp) Acetaminophen 325 mg/Tab. Sugar, caffeine, lactose and salt free. Safety pack 500s, Aidpack 100s.
Use: Analgesic.

VALORIN EXTRA. (Otis Clapp) Acetaminophen 500 mg/Tab. Sugar, caffeine, lactose and salt free. Safety pack 500s, Aidpack 100s.
Use: Analgesic.

VALORIN SUPER. (Otis Clapp) Acetaminophen 500 mg/Tab. w/caffeine. Sugar, salt, lactose free. Safety pack 500s.
Use: Analgesic.

VALPIPAMATE METHYLSULFATE.
See: Pentapiperide Methylsulfate.

• **VALPROATE SODIUM.** USAN.
Use: Anticonvulsant.

• **VALPROIC ACID, U.S.P. XXIII.** Cap., Syr., U.S.P. XXIII. 2-Propylpentanoic acid.
Use: Anticonvulsant.
See: Depakene, Cap., Liq. (Abbott). Myproic Acid Syr. (PBI).

VALRELEASE. (Roche) Diazepam 15 mg/SR Cap. Bot. 100s, Prescription Pak 30s.
Use: Antianxioty agent.

VALUPHED. (H.L. Moore) Pseudoephedrine HCl 60 mg, triprolidine HCl 2.5 mg/Tab. Pkg. 24s.
Use: Decongestant, antihistamine.

VAMATE. (Major) Hydroxyzine pamoate 50 mg/Cap. Bot. 100s, 250s, 500s, UD 100s.
Use: Antianxiety agent.

VANADRYX TR. (Vangard) Dexbrompheniramine maleate 6 mg, psuedoephedrine sulfate 120 mg/Tab. Bot. 100s, 500s.
Use: Antihistamine, decongestant.

VANCENASE AQ NASAL. (Schering) Beclomethasone dipropionate monohydrate 0.042%. Bot. 25 Gm with metering atomizing pump and nasal adapter.
Use: Intranasal steroid.

VANCENASE NASAL INHALER. (Schering) Metered-dose aerosol unit containing beclomethasone dipropionate in propellants. Each actuation delivers 42 mcg. Canister 16.8 Gm w/nasal adapter.
Use: Intranasal steroid.

VANCERIL INHALER. (Schering) Metered-dose aerosol unit of beclomethasone dipropionate in propellants. Each actuation delivers 42 mcg of beclomethasone dipropionate. Canister 16.8 Gm w/oral adapter. Box 1s.
Use: Respiratory inhalant.

VANCOCIN IV. (Lilly) Vancomycin HCl 500 mg/Vial. 1s; 1 Gm/Vial. 10s; ADD-Vantage 500 mg or 1 Gm/Vial. 1s.
Use: Anti-infective.

VANCOCIN CAPSULES. (Lilly) Van-

comycin HCl 125 mg or 250 mg/Pulvule. Bot. 10s, 20s.
Use: Anti-infective.

VANCOCIN ORAL. (Lilly) Vancomycin HCl for oral soln. Traypak 1 Gm, Container 10 Gm.
Use: Anti-infective.

VANCOLED INJECTION. (Lederle) Vancomycin HCl equivalent to vancomycin 500 mg/10 ml reconstituted soln. Vial 10 ml.
Use: Anti-infective.

• **VANCOMYCIN HCl**, U.S.P. XXIII. Cap., For Oral Soln., Sterile, U.S.P. XXIII. An antibiotic from *Streptomyces orientalis.*
Use: (I.V.) Gram-positive (staph.) infection; antibacterial.
See: Vancocin, Prods. (Lilly).
Vancoled, Vial (Lederle).

VANCOR INTRAVENOUS. (Adria) Vancomycin HCl 500 mg or 1 Gm. Pow. for inj. Vials.
Use: (I.V.) Gram-positive (staph.) infection, anti-bacterial.

VANEX EXPECTORANT LIQUID. (Abana) Pseudoephedrine HCl 30 mg, hydrocodone bitartrate 2.5 mg, guaifenesin 100 mg, alcohol 5%, glucose, saccharin, sorbitol, sucrose, tartrazine. Tropical fruit punch flavor. Liq. Bot. 473 ml.
Use: Decongestant, antitussive, expectorant.

VANEX-FORTE. (Abana) Phenylpropanolamine HCl 50 mg, phenylephrine HCl 10 mg, chlorpheniramine maleate 4 mg, pyrilamine maleate 25 mg, lactose, sugar. Cap. Bot. 100s, 250s.
Use: Decongestant, antihistamine.

VANEX-HD. (Abana) Phenylephrine HCl 5 mg, chlorpheniramine maleate 2 mg, hydrocodone bitartrate 1.67 mg. Liq. Bot. Pt. gal.
Use: Decongestant, expectorant.

VANEX-LA. (Abana) Phenylpropanolamine HCl 75 mg, guaifenesin 400 mg. Tab. Bot. 100s, 500s.
Use: Cough preparation.

VANICREAM. (Pharmaceutical Specialties) Oil in water vanishing cream containing white petrolatum, cetearyl alcohol, ceteareth-20, sorbitol, propylene glycol, simethicone, glyceryl monostearate, polyethylene glycol monostearate, sorbic acid. Oint. lb.
Use: Ointment base.

• **VANILLA**, N.F. XVII. Tinct. N.F. XVII.
Use: Pharmaceutic aid (flavor).

VANILLAL.
See: Ethyl Vanillin.

• **VANILLIN**, N.F. XVIII. 4-Hydroxy-3-methoxy-ben- zaldehyde.
Use: Pharmaceutic aid (flavor).

VANIROME.
See: Ethyl Vanillin.

VANODONNAL TIMECAPS. (Drug Industries) Phenobarbital 50 mg, atropine sulfate 0.0582 mg, hyoscyamine sulfate 0.311 mg, hyoscine hydrobromide 0.0195 mg/SR Cap. Bot. 100s.
Use: Sedative/hypnotic, anticholinergic/antispasmodic.

VANOXIDE. (Dermik) Benzoyl peroxide 5%, propylene glycol, hydroxyethyl cellulose, FD & C color, cholesterol-sterol, cetyl alcohol, propylene glycol stearate, polysorbate 20, lanolin alcohol, propylparaben, decyl oleate, purcelline oil syn., antioxidants, vegetable oil, methylparaben, tetrasodium EDTA, buffers, cyclohexanediamine tetraacetic acid, calcium phosphate, silicone emulsion, silica. Bot. 25 Gm, 50 Gm.
Use: Anti-acne.

VANOXIDE-HC. (Dermik) Hydrocortisone alcohol 0.5%, benzoyl peroxide 5%/25 Gm in lotion w/same ingredients as Vanoxide. Bot. 25 Gm.
Use: Anti-acne.

VANQUISH. (Glenbrook) Aspirin 227 mg, acetaminophen 194 mg, caffeine 33 mg, dried aluminum hydroxide gel 25 mg, magnesium hydroxide 50 mg/Tab. Capsule shaped tablets. Bot. 15s, 30s, 60s, 100s.
Use: Salicylate analgesic combination, antacid.

VANSEB DANDRUFF SHAMPOO. (Herbert) Sulfur 2%, salicylic acid 1%, surfactants, protein. **Cream:** Tube 3 oz. **Lot.:** Bot. 4 oz.
Use: Antidandruff, antiseborrheic.

VANSEB-T TAR DANDRUFF SHAMPOO. (Herbert) Sulfur 2%, salicylic acid 1%, coal tar solution 5%, surfactants, protein. **Cream:** Tube 3 oz. **Lot.:** Bot. 4 oz.
Use: Antidandruff, antiseborrheic.

VANSIL. (Pfizer Laboratories) Oxamniquine 250 mg/Cap. Bot. 24s.
Use: Anthelmintic.

VANTIN. (Upjohn) Cefpodoxime proxetil, lactose. **Tab.:** 100 mg/Bot. 20s, 100s, UD 100s; 200 mg/Bot. 20s, 100s, UD 100s; **Gran. for Susp.:** 50 mg/5 ml/Bot. 100 ml; 100 mg/5 ml. Bot. 100 ml.
Use: Antibiotic.

• **VAPIPROST HYDROCHLORIDE.** USAN.
Use: Platelet aggregation inhibitor.

VAPOCET TABLETS. (Major) Hydrocodone 5 mg, acetaminophen 500 mg/Tab. Bot. 100s.
Use: Narcotic analgesic combination.

VAPONEFRIN SOLUTION. (Fisons) A 2.25% solution of bioassayed racemic epinephrine as HCl, chlorobutanol 0.5%. Vial 7.5 ml, 15 ml, 30 ml.
Use: Bronchodilator.

VAPORIZER IN A BOTTLE. (O'Connor) Wick dispensed medicated vapors.
Use: Cough, cold, sinus, hayfever treatment.

VAPOR LEMON SUCRETS. (SK-Beecham) Dyclonine HCl 2 mg, sucrose. Loz. Pkg. 24s.
Use: Mouth and throat product.

VAPORUB. (Vicks).
See: Vicks Vaporub (Vicks).

VAPOSTEAM. (Vicks).
See: Vicks Vaposteam (Vicks).

• **VAPREOTIDE.** USAN.
Use: Antineoplastic.

VARICELLA-ZOSTER IgG IFA TEST SYSTEM. (Wampole-Zeus) Test for the qualitative or semi-qualitative detection of VZ IgG antibody in human serum. Test kit 100s.
Use: Diagnostic aid.

• **VARICELLA-ZOSTER IMMUNE GLOBULIN**, U.S.P. XXIII. A sterile buffered solution of the globulin fraction of human plasma containing 99% immunoglobulin G with traces of immunoglobulins A and M. It is derived from adult human plasma selected for high titers of varicella-zoster antibiodies.
Use: Passive immunizing agent.

VARICELLA ZOSTER IMMUNE GLOBULIN, HUMAN. (Massachusetts Public Health Biologic Labs) Varicella-zoster virus antibody 125 units/ ≤ 2.5 ml. Vial, single dose.
Use: Immune serum.

VARI-FLAVORS. (Ross) Flavor packets to provide flavor variety for patients on liquid diets. Dextrose, artificial flavor, artificial color. Packet 1 Gm, Ctn. 24s.
Use: Liquid nutrition flavoring aid.

VARIPLEX-C. (Nature's Bounty) Vitamins B_1 15 mg, B_2 10 mg, B_3 100 mg, B_5 20 mg, B_6 5 mg, B_{12} 10 mcg, C 500 mg/Tab. Bot. 100s.
Use: Vitamin supplement.

VARITOL. (Kenyon) Atropine sulfate 0.03 mg, hyoscyamine 0.03 mg, gelsemium 6.1 mg, methenamine 40.8 mg, salol 18.1 mg, benzoic acid 4.5 mg, methylene blue 5.4 mg/Tab. Bot. 100s, 1000s.
Use: Urinary anti-infective.

VARITOL-D.S. (Kenyon) Atropine sulfate 0.06 mg, hyoscyamine 0.06 mg, gelsemium 12.2 mg, methenamine 81.6 mg, salol 36.2 mg, benzoic acid 9 mg, methylene blue 10.8 mg/Tab. Bot. 100s, 1000s.
Use: Urinary anti-infective.

VASCOR. (McNeil) Bepridil HCl, 200 mg, 300 mg or 400 mg/Tab. Bot. 30s, UD 100s.
Use: Antianginal.

VASCORAY. (Mallinckrodt) Iothalamate meglumine 52%, iothalamate sodium 26% (40% iodine). Vial 50 ml. Bot. 100 ml, 150 ml, 200 ml.
Use: Radiopaque agent.

VASCUNITOL. (Apco) Mannitol hexanitrate 0.5 gr/Tab. Bot. 100s.
Use: Vasodilator.

VASCUSED. (Apco) Mannitol hexanitrate 0.5 gr, phenobarbital 0.25 gr/Tab. Bot. 100s.
Use: Vasodilator.

VASELINE DERMATOLOGY FORMULA CREAM. (Chesebrough-Pond's) Petrolatum, mineral oil, dimethicone. Jar 3 oz, 5.25 oz.
Use: Emollient.

VASELINE DERMATOLOGY FORMULA LOTION. (Chesebrough-Pond's) Petrolatum, mineral oil, dimethicone. Bot. 5.5 oz, 11 oz, 16 oz.
Use: Emollient.

VASELINE FIRST AID CARBOLATED PETROLEUM JELLY. (Chesebrough-Pond's) Petrolatum, chloroxylenol. Plastic Jar 1.75 oz, 3.75 oz. Plastic Tube 1 oz, 2.5 oz.
Use: Medicated antibacterial.

VASELINE INTENSIVE CARE ACTIVE SPORT. (Chesebrough-Pond's) Ethylhexyl p-methoxycinnamate, oxybenzone. PABA free. **SPF 8:** Lot. Bot. 120 ml; **SPF 15:** Lot. Bot. 120 ml.
Use: Sunscreen.

VASELINE INTENSIVE CARE BABY SPF 15. (Chesebrough Pond's) Titanium dioxide. PABA free. Waterproof. Lot. Bot. 120 ml.
Use: Sunscreen.

VASELINE INTENSIVE CARE BABY SPF 30. (Chesebrough Pond's) Ethylhexyl p-methoxycinnamate, oxybenzone, 2-ethylhexyl salicylate, titanium dioxide, C12-15 alkyl benzoate, glycerin, aloe vera gel, vitamin E, cetyl alcohol, parabens, EDTA. Lot. Bot. 118 ml.
Use: Sunscreen.

VASELINE INTENSIVE CARE BLOCKOUT SPF 30. (Chesebrough Pond's)

Ethylhexyl p-methoxycinnamate, oxybenzone, 2-ethylhexyl salicylate, titanium dioxide. Waterproof. Lot. Bot. 120 ml.
Use: Sunscreen.

VASELINE INTENSIVE CARE BLOCKOUT SPF 40+. (Chesebrough Pond's) Padimate, ethylhexyl p-methoxycinnamate, oxybenzone, 2-ethylhexyl salicylate, titanium dioxide. Waterproof. Lot. Bot. 120 ml.
Use: Sunscreen.

VASELINE INTENSIVE CARE MOISTURIZING SUNSCREEN. (Chesebrough Pond's) Ethylhexyl p-methoxycinnamate, oxybenzone, C12-15 alkyl octanoate, glycerin, aloe vera gel, cetyl alcohol, petrolatum, vitamin E, parabens, EDTA. **SPF8, SPF4:** Lot. Bot. 117 ml.
Use: Sunscreen.

VASELINE INTENSIVE CARE NO BURN NO BITE SPF 15. (Chesebrough Pond's) Ethylhexyl p-methoxycinnamate, oxybenzone. PABA free. Waterproof. Lot. Bot. 180 ml.
Use: Sunscreen.

VASELINE INTENSIVE CARE SPORT SUNBLOCK. (Chesebrough Pond's) Ethylhexyl p-methoxycinnamate, oxybenzone, C12-15 alkyl benzoate, aloe vera gel, vitamin E, EDTA. Lot. Bot. 118 ml.
Use: Sunscreen.

VASELINE INTENSIVE CARE SUNBLOCK. (Chesebrough Pond's) Ethylhexyl p-methoxycinnamate, oxybenzone, 2-ethylhexyl salicylate. PABA free. Waterproof. **SPF 4:** Lot. Bot. 180 ml; **SPF 8:** Lot. Bot. 120 ml, 180 ml; **SPF 15:** Lot. Bot. 120 ml, 180 ml; **SPF 25:** Lot. Bot. 120 ml, 180 ml.
Use: Sunscreen.

VASELINE INTENSIVE CARE ULTRA VIOLET DAILY DEFENSE. (Chesebrough Pond's) Ethylhexyl p-methoxycinnamate, oxybenzone, vitamin E, cetyl alcohol, acetylated lanolin alcohol, parabens, EDTA. **SPF 15** Lot. Bot. 118 ml.
Use: Sunscreen.

VASELINE PURE PETROLEUM JELLY SKIN PROTECTANT. (Chesebrough-Pond's) White petrolatum. Tube 1 oz, 2.5 oz. Jar 1.75 oz, 3.75 oz, 7.75 oz, 13 oz.
Use: Protectant for minor skin irritations.

VASERETIC. (Merck Sharp & Dohme) Enalapril maleate 10 mg, hydrochlorothiazide 25 mg/Tab. Bot. 100s.

Use: Antihypertensive.

VASIMID.
See: Tolazoline HCl, U.S.P. XXIII.

VASOACTIVE INTESTINAL POLYPEPTIDE. (Research Triangle)
Use: Treatment of acute esophageal food impaction. [Orphan drug]

VASOCIDIN OPHTHALMIC OINTMENT. (Iolab) Prednisolone acetate 5 mg, sulfacetamide sodium 100 mg/Gm. Tube 3.5 Gm.
Use: Corticosteroid, anti-infective.

VASOCIDIN OPHTHALMIC SOLUTION. (Iolab) Prednisolone sodium phosphate 0.25% (equivalent to prednisolone phosphate 0.23%), sulfacetamide sodium 10%, thimerosal 0.01%. Plastic dropper-tip squeeze bot. 5 ml, 10 ml.
Use: Corticosteroid, anti-infective.

VASOCLEAR. (Iolab) Naphazoline HCl 0.02% in Lipiden polymeric vehicle, benzalkonium Cl 0.01%. Bot. 15 ml.
Use: Vasoconstrictor/mydriatic.

VASOCLEAR A. (Iolab) Naphazoline HCl 0.02%, zinc sulfate 0.25%, polyvinyl alcohol 0.25%. Bot. 15 ml.
Use: Vasoconstrictor/mydriatic.

VASOCON-A OPHTHALMIC SOLUTION. (Iolab) Naphazoline HCl 0.05%, antazoline phosphate 0.5%. Plastic squeeze bot. w/dropper tip 15 ml.
Use: Vasoconstrictor/mydriatic.

VASOCON REGULAR. (Iolab) Naphazoline HCl 0.1%. Bot. plastic squeeze w/dropper tip 15 ml.
Use: Vasoconstrictor/mydriatic.

VASOCONSTRICTOR.
See: Epinephrine Preps.

VASODERM. (Taro) Fluocinonide 0.05%, anhydrous glycerin base. Cream. Tube 15 Gm, 30 Gm, 60 Gm.
Use: Topical corticosteroid.

VASODERM-E. (Taro) Fluocinonide 0.05%, emollient mineral oil and white petrolatum base. Cream. Tube 15 Gm, 30 Gm, 60 Gm, 120 Gm.
Use: Topical corticosteroid.

VASODILAN. (Mead Johnson) Isoxsuprine HCl 10 mg or 20 mg/Tab. **10 mg:** Bot. 100s, 1000s, UD 100s. **20 mg:** Bot. 100s, 500s, 1000s, UD 100s.
Use: Peripheral vasodilator.

VASODILATORS.
See: Amyl Nitrite.
    Apresoline, Tab., Amp. (Ciba).
    Arlidin, Tab. (USV).
    Cardilate, Tab. (Burroughs Wellcome).
    Cyclospasmol, Tab., Cap. (Wyeth).
    Erythrityl Tetranitrate, Tab.
    Glyceryl Trinitrate Preps.

Isordil, Tab. (Wyeth).
Kortrate, Cap. (Amid).
Mannitol Hexanitrate.
Metamine, Tab. (Pfizer).
Nisane, Elix. (Amid).
Nitroglycerin.
Pentritol, Cap., Tempule (Armour).
Peritrate, Tab. (Parke-Davis).
Sodium Nitrate.
Sorbitrate, Tab. (Stuart).
Vasodilan, Tab., Amp. (Mead Johnson).
VASODILATORS, CORONARY.
See: Glyceryl Trinitrate, Preps. (Various Mfr.).
Isordil, Tab. (Wyeth).
Khellin (Various Mfr.).
Papaverine, Inj., Tab. (Various Mfr.).
Pentaerythritol Tetranitrate, Tab.
Peritrate, Tab. (Parke-Davis).
Roniacol Elix., Tab. (Roche).
Sorbitrate, Tab. (Stuart).
VASOFLO. (Hauck) Papaverine HCl 150 mg/Cap. Bot 100s.
Use: Peripheral vasodilator.
VASOLATE. (Parmed) Pentaerythritol tetranitrate 30 mg/Cap. Bot. 100s, 1000s.
Use: Antanginal.
VASOLATE-80. (Parmed) Pentaerythritol tetranitrate 80 mg/Cap. Bot. 100s, 1000s.
Use: Antianginal.
VASOMIDE TABLETS. (Lannett) Niacin 50 mg, salicylamide 300 mg, ascorbic acid 15 mg, vitamins B$_1$ 3 mg, dl-desoxyephedrine HCl 2.5 mg, B$_{12}$ 3 mcg/Tab. Bot. 100s, 1000s.
VASOMINIC-T.D. (A.V.P.) Phenylpropanolamine HCl 40 mg, chlorpheniramine maleate 5 mg, phenylephrine HCl 10 mg, phenyltoloxamine citrate 15 mg/TR Tab. Bot. 100s.
Use: Decongestant, antihistamine.
• **VASOPRESSIN INJECTION,** U.S.P. XXIII. beta-Hypophamine. Posterior pituitary pressor hormone.
Use: Posterior pituitary hormone (antidiuretic).
See: Pitressin, Amp. (Parke-Davis).
VASOSULF. (Iolab) Sulfacetamide sodium 15%, phenylephrine HCl 0.125%. Bot. 5 ml, 15 ml.
Use: Anti-infective, decongestant (ophthalmic).
VASOTEC. (Merck Sharp & Dohme) Enalapril maleate 2.5 mg, 5 mg, 10 mg or 20 mg/Tab. Bot. 100s, UD 100s.
Use: Antihypertensive.
VASOTEC I.V. (Merck Sharp & Dohme)

Enalaprilat 1.25 mg/ml. Inj. Vial 2 ml.
Use: Antihypertensive.
VASOTHERM INJ. (Pharmex) Niacin as sodium salt 100 mg, benzyl alcohol 1.5%/ml. Vial 30 ml.
Use: Vasodilator.
VASOTUS LIQUID. (Sheryl) Codeine phosphate ¹⁄₆ gr, phenylephrine HCl, prophenpyridamine maleate. Liq. Bot. pt.
Use: Antitussive, decongestant, antihistamine.
VASOXYL. (Burroughs Wellcome) Methoxamine HCl 0.1%. Inj. 20 mg/ml.
Use: Vasopressor used in shock.
VA-TRO-NOL. (Vicks).
See: Vicks Va-Tro-Nol (Vicks).
VAXSYN HIV-1. (Microgenesys)
See: T-LYMPHOTROPIC VIRTUS TYPE III GP 160 ANTIGENS.
VAZOSAN. (Sandia) Papaverine HCl 150 mg/Tab. Bot. 100s, 1000s.
Use: Peripheral vasodilator.
VCF. (Apothecus) Contraceptive film: nonoxynol-9 28%, glycerin and polyvinyl alcohol. Pkg. 3s, 6s, 12s.
Use: Spermicide.
V-CILLIN-K. (Lilly) Penicillin V potassium 125 mg, 250 mg or 500 mg/Tab. **125 mg:** Bot. 100s. **250 mg:** Bot. 100s, 500s. **500 mg:** Bot. 24s, 100s, 500s.
Use: Antibacterial, penicillin.
V-CILLIN-K FOR ORAL SOLUTION. (Lilly) Penicillin V potassium 125 mg or 250 mg/5 ml. **125 mg:** Bot. 100 ml, 150 ml, 200 ml, UD 5 ml. **250 mg:** Bot. 100 ml, 150 ml, 200 ml.
Use: Antibacterial, penicillin.
V-DEC-M. (Seatrace) Pseudoephedrine HCl 120 mg, guaifenesin 500 mg/SR Tab. Bot. 100s.
Use: Decongestant, expectorant.
VDRL ANTIGEN. (Laboratory Diagnostics) VDRL antigen with buffered saline. Blood test in diagnosis of syphillis. **Vial:** Sufficient for 500 tests. **Amp.:** 10 × 0.5 ml sufficient for 500 tests.
Use: Diagnostic aid.
VDRL SLIDE TEST. (Laboratory Diagnostics) VDRL antigen. Slide flocculation and spinal fluid test for syphilis. Vial 5 ml Complete kit, reactive control, nonreactive control, 5 ml.
Use: Diagnostic aid.
VE-400. (Western Research) Vitamin E 400 IU/Cap. Bot. 1008s.
Use: Vitamin E supplement.
• **VECURONIUM BROMIDE.** USAN.
Use: Blocking agent (neuromuscular).
VEETIDS. (Squibb) Penicillin-V potassi-

um. **Soln.:** 125 mg or 250 mg/5 ml Bot.
100 ml, 200 ml. **Tab.:** 250 mg or 500 mg.
Bot. 100s, 1000s, Unimatic 100s.
Use: Antibacterial, penicillin.
VEETIDS '500'. (Squibb) Penicillin V
potassium 500 mg/Tab. Bot. 100s,
1000s, UD 100s.
Use: Antibacterial, penicillin.
• **VEGETABLE OIL, HYDROGENATED,**
U.S.P. XXIII.
Use: Pharmaceutic aid (tablet lubri-
cant).
VEHICLE/N AND VEHICLE/N MILD.
(Neutrogena) Topical vehicle system for
compounding. Appliderm Applicator Bot.
oz.
Use: Extemporaneous compounding.
VELACYCLINE. N-Pyrrolidinomethyl
tetracycline.
Use: Antibacterial, tetracycline.
VELBAN. (Lilly) Extract from Vinca rosea
Linn. Vinblastine sulfate, lyophilized. Vial
10 mg/10 ml. Box 1s.
Use: Antineoplastic agent.
VELMATROL. (Kenyon) Sulfisoxazole
500 mg/Tab. Bot. 100s, 1000s.
Use: Antibacterial, sulfonamide.
VELMATROL-A. (Kenyon) Sulfisoxazole
500 mg, phenylazodiaminopyridine HCl
50 mg/Tab. Bot. 100s, 1000s.
Use: Urinary anti-infective.
VELOSEF. (Squibb) Cephradine. **Oral
Susp.:** 125 mg or 250 mg/5 ml. Bot. 100
ml, 200 ml. **Cap.:** 250 mg or 500 mg Bot.
24s, 100s, UD Unimatic 100s. **Inj.:**
(w/anhydrous sodium carbonate. Sodium equivalent to 136 mg/Gm of cephra-
dine) 250 mg, 500 mg, 1 Gm or 2
Gm/vial. 2 Gm vial is sodium free for in-
fusion. Bot. 200 ml.
Use: Antibacterial, cephalosporin.
VELOSULIN HUMAN. (Novo Nordisk)
Human insulin injection 100 IU/ml, Vial
10 ml.
Use: Antidiabetic agent.
VELTANE. (Lannett) Brompheniramine
maleate 4 mg/Tab. Bot. 1000s.
Use: Antihistamine.
VELTAP. (Lannett) Brompheniramine
maleate 4 mg, phenylephrine HCl 5 mg,
phenylpropanolamine HCl 5 mg, alcohol
3%/5 ml. Bot. pt, gal.
Use: Antihistamine, decongestant.
VELTAP LANATABS. (Lannett) Phenyl-
propanolamine HCl 15 mg, phenyle-
phrine HCl 15 mg, brompheniramine
maleate 12 mg. Tab. Bot. 100s, 500s,
1000s.
Use: Decongestant, antihistamine.
VELVACHOL. (Owen) Hydrophilic oint-

ment base petrolatum, mineral oil, cetyl
alcohol, cholesterol, parabens, stearyl
alcohol, purified water, sodium lauryl sul-
fate. Jar lb.
Use: Hydrophilic ointment base.
VELVEDERM CLEANSER. (Torch) Sul-
fonated detergent with a stable emulsion
of vegetable oil. Lot. Bot. 8 oz.
Use: Cleanser.
VELVEDERM-HANDORA NORMALIZER.
(Torch) Glycerin, fatty alcohols, fatty acid
in hydrophilic base w/pH of 5.0 to 5.5.
Cream. Jar 4 oz, 8 oz. Lot. Bot. 8 oz.
Use: Emollient.
VELVEDERM MOISTURIZER. (Torch)
Mineral oil, emulsifiers, fatty alcohol,
propylene glycol, hydroxymethylcellu-
lose, water. Bot. 4 oz.
Use: Emollient.
VENESETIC.
See: Amobarbital Sodium, Preps. (Vari-
ous Mfr.).
VENETHENE. No mfr. listed.
VENLAFAXINE.
Use: Antidepressant.
See: Effexor, Tab. (Wyeth-Ayerst).
VENOGLOBULIN-I. (Alpha Therapeutic)
Immune Globulin Intravenous (IGIV).
Pow. for Inj. Vial 2.5 Gm, 5 Gm.
Use: Immune serum.
VENOGLOBULIN-S. (Alpha Therapeutic)
Immune globulin IV (human) 5%. Sol-
vent detergent treated. Inj. 50, 100, 200
ml w/sterile IV administration set.
Use: Immune serum.
VENOMIL. (Hollister-Stier) Diagnostic 1
mcg/ml, Maintenance 100 mcg/ml. Indi-
vidual patient kit.
Use: Allergenic extract.
VENSTAT. (Seatrace) Brompheniramine
maleate 10 mg/ml. Vial 10 ml.
Use: Antihistamine.
VENTOLIN INHALATION AEROSOL.
(Allen& Hanburys) Albuterol 90 mcg/ac-
tuation. Aerosol canister 17 Gm contain-
ing 200 metered inhalations. Canister 17
Gm w/oral adapter. Refill canister 17
Gm.
Use: Bronchodilator.
VENTOLIN INHALATION SOLUTION.
(Allen & Hanburys) Albuterol sulfate 5
mg/ml. Bot. 20 ml w/calibrated dropper.
Use: Bronchodilator.
VENTOLIN NEBULES. (Allen & Han-
burys) Albuterol sulfate 0.083%, sulfuric
acid. Soln. for inhalation. In 3 ml unit
dose nebules.
Use: Bronchodilators.
VENTOLIN ROTACAPS. (Allen & Han-
burys) Microfine albuterol 200 mg. Cap.

for inhalation. Bot. UD 96s, Hosp. UD 24s. For use with the Rotahaler inhalation device.
Use: Bronchodilator.

VENTOLIN SYRUP. (Allen & Hanburys) Albuterol sulfate 2 mg/5 ml. Bot. pt.
Use: Bronchodilator.

VENTOLIN TABLETS. (Allen & Hanburys) Albuterol sulfate 2 mg or 4 mg/Tab. Bot. 100s, 500s.
Use: Bronchodilator.

VEPESID. (Bristol-Myers/Bristol Oncology) Etoposide. **Vial:** 100 mg/Vial. **Cap.:** 50 mg/Cap. Bot.20s.
Use: Antineoplastic agent.

VERACOLATE. (Numark) Phenolphthalein 0.5 gr, capsicum oleoresin 0.05 min, cascara extract 1 gr/Tab. Bot. 100s.
Use: Laxative.

VERACTIL. Methotrimeprazine, B.A.N.

• **VERADOLINE HYDROCHLORIDE.** USAN.
Use: Analgesic.

• **VERAPAMIL.** USAN. 5-[3,4-(Dimethoxyphenethyl)methylamino]-2-(3,4-dimethoxyphenyl)-2-isopropylvaleronitrile. Isoptin. Cordilox HCl.
Use: Coronary vasodilator.

• **VERAPAMIL HYDROCHLORIDE.** USAN.
Use: Antianginal, cardiac depressant (antiarrhythmic).
See: Calan, Tab. (Searle).
Calan SR, Capl. (Searle).
Isoptin, Tab. Inj. (Knoce).
Verelan, SR Cap. (Lederle).

VERAPAMIL HCl. (Zenith) 180 mg. SR Tab. Bot. 100s, 500s.
Use: Antianginal, cardiac depressant (antiarrhythmic).

VERATRUM ALBA.
See: Protoveratrines A and B (Various Mfr.).

VERAZEPTOL. (Femco) Chlorothymol, eucalyptol, menthol, phenol, boric acid, zinc sulfate. Pow. Bot. 3 oz, 6 oz, 10 oz.
Use: Vaginal preparation.

VERAZIDE. B.A.N. 2'-Veratrylideneisonicotino hydrazide.
Use: Treatment of tuberculosis.

VERAZINC. (Forest) Zinc sulfate 220 mg/Cap. Bot. 100s, 1000s.
Use: Zinc supplement.

VERCYTE. (Abbott) Pipobroman 25 mg/Tab. Bot. 100s.
Use: Antineoplastic agent.

VERELAN. (Lederle) Verapamil HCl 120, 240 mg/SR Cap. Bot. 100s.
Use: Antihypertensive.

VERGO OINT. (Daywell) Calcium pantothenate 8%, ascorbic acid 2%, starch.

Tube 0.5 oz.
Use: Keratolytic.

VERGON. (Marnel) Meclizine HCl 30 mg. Cap. Bot. 100s.
Use: Antiemetic/Antivertigo agent.

• **VERILOPAM HYDROCHLORIDE.** USAN.
Use: Analgesic.

VERIN. (Hauck) Aspirin (Acetylsalicylic Acid; ASA) 650 mg/TR Tab. Bot. 100s.
Use: Salicylate analgesic.

• **VERLUKAST.** USAN.
Use: Antiasthmatic.

VERMICIDE. (Pharmex) Tube 2 oz.
Use: Pediculicide.

VERMOX. (Janssen) Mebendazole 100 mg/Tab. Box 12s.
Use: Anthelmintic.

VERNACEL. (Professional Pharmacal) Prophenpyridamine maleate 0.5%, phenylephrine HCl ⅛% in a methylcellulose solution. Plastic Bot. 15 ml, 30 ml.
Use: Antihistamine, decongestant, ophthalmic.

VERNAMYCINS. Under study.
Use: Antibiotic.

VERNOLEPIN. A sesquiterpene dilactone. Under study.
Use: Against Walker carcinosarcoma 256

• **VEROFYLLINE.** USAN.
Use: Bronchodilator, antiasthmatic.

VERONAL SODIUM.
See: Barbital Sodium (Various Mfr.).

VERR-CANTH. (C & M Pharmacal) Cantharidin 0.7%, penederm 0.5%. Bot. 7.5 ml.
Use: Keratolytic.

VERREX. (C & M Pharmacal) Salicylic acid 30%, podophyllin 10%. Bot. 7.5 ml w/applicator tip.
Use: Keratolytic.

VERRUSOL. (Palisades) Salicylic acid 30%, podophyllum 5%, cantharidin in an adherent film-forming vehicle of penederm (octylphenylpolyethylene glycol) 1%, ethylcellulose, cellosolve, collodion, castor oil, acetone. Liq. Bot. 75 ml.
Use: Keratolytic combination.

VERSACAPS. (Seatrace) Pseudoephedrine HCl 60 mg, guaifenesin 300 mg/Cap. Bot. 100s.
Use: Decongestant, expectorant.

VERSAL. (Suppositoria) Bismuth subgallate, balsam peru, zinc oxide, benzyl benzoate/Supp. Box 12s, 100s, 1000s.
Use: Anorectal preparation.

VERSA-QUAT. (Ulmer) Quaternary ammonium one-step cleaner-disinfectant-sanitizer-fungicide-virucide for general housekeeping. Bot. gal.

Use: Cleanser, disinfectant.

VERSED. (Roche) Midazolam HCl 1 mg or 5 mg/ml, sodium Cl 0.8%, disodium edetate 0.01%, benzyl alcohol 1%. **1 mg/ml:** Vial 2 ml, 5 ml, 10 ml. Box 10s. **5 mg/ml:** Vial 1 ml, 2 ml, 5 ml, 10 ml. Box 10s. Disposable Syringe 2 ml Box 10s.
Use: General anesthetic.

VERSENATE, CALCIUM DISODIUM.
See: Calcium Disodium Versenate, Amp. (Riker).

VERSENATE DISODIUM.
See: Disodium Versenate, Amp. (Riker).

VERSIDYNE. Methopholine. 1-(p-Chlorophenethyl)-2-methyl-6,7-dimethoxy-1,2,3,4-tetrahydroisoquinoline.
Use: Analgesic.

VERSTRAN. (Parke-Davis) Prazepam.
Use: Antianxiety agent.
See: Centrax, Tab. (Parke-Davis).

VERTAB. (UAD) Dimenhydrinate 50 mg. Tab. Bot. 100s.
Use: Anticholinergic.

• **VERTEPORFIN.** USAN.
Use: Antineoplastic.

VERUKAN-20. (Syosset) Salicylic acid 16.7%, lactic acid in flexible collodione 16.7%. Bot. 15 ml.
Use: Keratolytic.

VERV ALERTNESS CAPSULES. (APC) Caffeine 200 mg/Cap. Vial 15s.
Use: Analeptic.

• **VESNARINONE.** USAN.
Use: Cardiotonic.

V-GAN. (Hauck) Promethazine HCl 25 mg or 50 mg/ml. Vial 10 ml.
Use: Antiemetic, antihistamine.

VIACAPS. (Manne) Vitamins A (soluble) 45,000 IU, C 500 mg/Cap. Bot. 60s, 120s, 1000s.
Use: Vitamin supplement.

VIBESATE. Polvinate 9.3%, molrosinol 3.1% with propellant.

VIBRAMYCIN. (Pfizer Laboratories) Doxycycline. **Cap.:** 50 mg Bot. 50s, UD pak 100s, X-Pack (10 Cap.) 5s; 100 mg Bot. 50s, 500s; UD pak 100s, V-Pak (5 Cap) 5s, Nine-Pak 10s. **Pediatric Oral Susp.:** 25 mg/5 ml. Bot. 2 oz. **Syr.:** 50 mg/5 ml. Bot. oz, pt.
Use: Antibacterial, tetracycline.

VIBRAMYCIN IV. (Roerig) Doxycycline (as hyclate) 200 mg. Powder for Inj. Vial.
Use: Antibacterial, tetracycline.

VIBRA-TABS. (Pfizer Laboratories) Doxycycline hyclate 100 mg/Tab. Bot. 50s, 500s, UD Pack 100s.
Use: Antibacterial, tetracycline.

VICAM IV. (Keene) Vitamins B_1 50 mg,

B_2 5 mg, B_{12} 1000 mcg, B_6 5 mg, dexpanthenol 6 mg, niacinamide 125 mg, C 50 mg/ml, benzyl alcohol 1% as preservative in water for injection. Vial multiple dose.
Use: Parenteral nutritional supplement.

VICAM INJECTION. (Keene) Vitamins B_1 50 mg, B_2 5 mg, B_6 125 mg, B_3 6 mg, B_6 5 mg, B_{12} 1000 mcg, C 50 mg/ml. Inj. Vial 10 ml.
Use: Vitamin supplement.

VICEF. (Drug Industries) Thiamine HCl 10 mg, pyridoxine HCl 10 mg, B_{12} 50 mcg, C 100 mg, E 100 IU, niacinamide 25 mg, folic acid 1.5 mg, ferrous fumarate 45 mg/2 Cap. Bot. 100s.
Use: Vitamin/mineral supplement.

VICKS CHILDREN'S CHLORASEPTIC. (Richardson-Vicks) Phenol 0.5%, saccharin, sorbitol. Spray. Bot. 180 ml.
Use: Antiseptic, anesthetic.

VICKS CHILDREN'S NYQUIL NIGHTTIME COLD/COUGH LIQUID. (Richardson-Vicks) Pseudoephedrine HCl 10 mg, dextromethorphan HBr 5 mg, chlorpheniramine maleate 0.67 mg/5 ml, alcohol free. Bot. 120 ml, 240 ml.
Use: Decongestant, antihistamine, antitussive.

VICKS COUGH DROPS. (Vicks) Menthol. **Menthol flavor:** Benzyl alcohol, camphor, corn syrup, eucalyptus oil, sucrose, thynol. **Cherry flavor:** Corn syrup, sucrose, citric acid. Box 14. Bag 30.

VICKS DAYQUIL ALLERGY RELIEF 4 HOUR. (Richardson-Vicks) Phenylpropanolamine HCl 25 mg, brompheniramine maleate 4 mg. Tab. Pkg. 24s.
Use: Decongestant, antitussive.

VICKS DAYQUIL ALLERGY RELIEF 12 HOUR. (Richardson-Vicks) Phenylpropanolamine HCl 75 mg, brompheniramine maleate 12 mg. Tab. Pkg. 12s, 24s.
Use: Decongestant, antitussive.

VICKS DAYQUIL LIQUICAPS. (Richardson-Vicks) Dextromethorphan HBr 10 mg, pseudoephedrine HCl 30 mg, acetaminophen 250 mg, guaifenesin 100 mg. Softgel Cap. Pkg. 12s, 20s.
Use: Analgesic, decongestant, antitussive, expectorant.

VICKS DAYQUIL LIQUID. (Vicks) Pseudoephedrine HCl 60 mg, guaifenesin 200 mg, acetaminophen 650 mg, dextromethorphan HBr 20 mg/30 ml. Bot. 6 oz.

VICKS DAYQUIL SINUS PRESSURE & CONGESTION RELIEF. (Richardson-

Vicks) Phenylpropanolamine HCl 25 mg, guaifenesin 200 mg. Cap. Pkg. 12s, 24s.
Use: Decongestant, expectorant.
VICKS DAYQUIL SINUS PRESSURE & PAIN RELIEF. (Richardson-Vicks) Pseudoephedrine HCl 30 mg, acetaminophen 500 mg. Cap. Pkg. 24s.
Use: Decongestant.
VICKS DRY HACKING COUGH. (Vicks) Dextromethorphan HBr 30 mg/10ml, alcohol 10%, invert sugar. Liq. Bot. 4 oz, 8 oz w/ *Vicks Accutip* Dispenser
VICKS 44 NON-DROWSY COLD & COUGH LIQUICAPS. (Richardson-Vicks) Dextromethorphan HBr 30 mg, pseudoephedrine HCl 60 mg. Cap. Pkg. 10s
Use: Decongestant, antitussive.
VICKS 44D COUGH & DECONGESTANT LIQUID. (Richardson-Vicks) Pseudoephedrine HCl 20 mg., dextromethorphan HBr 10 mg/5 ml, alcohol 10% saccharin, cucrose. Bot. 120 ml, 240 ml.
Use: Decongestant, antitussive.
VICKS 44D DRY HACKING COUGH & HEAD CONGESTANT, PEDIATRIC. (Richardson-Vicks) Dextromethorphan HBr 15 mg/15 ml, pseudoephedrine HCl 30 mg, alcohol free, sorbitol, sucrose, cherry flavor. Liq. Bot. 120 ml with *Vicks Accutip* Dispenser.
VICKS 44D PEDIATRIC COUGH & DECONGESTANT LIQUID. (Richardson-Vicks) Pseudoephedrine HCl 10 mg, dextromethorphan HBr 5 mg/5 ml, alcohol free. Bot. 120 ml.
Use: Decongestant, antitussive.
VICKS 44E LIQUID. (Richardson-Vicks) Dextromethorphan HBr 20 mg, guaifenesin 200 mg.
VICKS 44E PEDIATRIC LIQUID. (Richardson-Vicks) Dextromethorphan HBr 10 mg, guaifenesin 100 mg, sorbitol, sucrose. Alcohol free. Bot. 120 ml w/ *Vicks Accutip* Dispenser.
Use: Pediatric nonnarcotic antitussive w/expectorant.
VICKS 44M COUGH, COLD & FLU LIQUID. (Vicks) Dextromethorphan HBr 30 mg, pseudoephedrine HCl 60 mg, chlorpheniramine maleate 4 mg, acetaminophen 650 mg/20 ml, alcohol 10%. Bot. 4 oz, 8 oz, with *Vicks Accutip* Dispenser.
Use: Antitussive, decongestant, expectorant, analgesic.
VICKS 44M COLD, FLU & COUGH LIQUICAPS. (Richardson-Vicks) Dextromethorphan HBr 10 mg, pseudoephedrine HCl 30 mg, chlorpheni-

ramine maleate 2 mg, acetaminophen 250 mg. Cap. Pkg. 12s.
Use: Decongestant, antitussive, antihistamine.
VICKS NYQUIL LIQUICAPS. (Richardson-Vicks) Acetaminophen 250 mg, pseudoephedrine HCl 30 mg, dextromethorphan HBr 10 mg, doxylamine succinate 6.25 mg, glycerin. Alcohol free. Bot. 12s, 20s.
VICKS NYQUIL LIQUID MULTI-SYMPTOM COLD FLU RELIEF. (Vicks) Acetaminophen 1000 mg, doxylamine succinate 12.5 mg, pseudoephedrine HCl 60 mg, dextromethorphan HBr 30 mg/30 ml, alcohol 10%. Regular and cherry flavors. Regular contains FD&C Yellow No. 6. Bot. 6 oz, 10 oz, 14 oz.
Use: Analgesic, antihistamine, decongestant, antitussive.
VICKS SINEX. (Vicks) Phenylephrine HCl 0.5%, camphor, menthol, eucalyptol, disodium EDTA. Nasal Spray. Plastic Squeeze Bot. 0.5 oz, 1 oz.
Use: Nasal decongestant.
VICKS SINEX 12-HOUR. (Vicks) Oxymetazoline HCl 0.05%, camphor, menthol, eucalyptol, disodium EDTA. Nasal Spray. Plastic Squeeze Bot. 1 oz, 0.5 oz.
Use: Nasal decongestant.
VICKS VAPOR INHALER. (Vicks) l-Desoxyephedrine 50 mg, Special Vicks Vapors (menthol, camphor, bornyl acetate, lavender oil) Inhaler 0.007 oz (198 mg)
Use: Nasal decongestant.
VICKS VAPORUB. (Vicks) Camphor 4.7%, menthol 2.6%, eucalyptus oil 1.2%, cedarleaf oil, nutmeg oil. **ointment:** Mineral oil, petrolatum. **Cream:** Isopropyl palmitate, EDTA, glycerin, imidazolidinyl urea, cetyl alcohol, parabens, stearyl alcohol. Cream. Jar 56.7 g.
Use: Decongestant vaporizing ointment.
VICKS VAPOSTEAM. (Vicks) Eucalyptus oil 1.5%, camphor 6.2%, menthol 3.2%, alcohol 74%, cedarleaf oil, nutmeg oil. Bot. 4 oz, 8 oz.
Use: Steam medication, decongestant, antitussive.
VICKS VA-TRO-NOL. (Vicks) Ephedrine sulfate 0.5%, menthol, eucalyptol, camphor, cedarleaf oil, nutmet oil, 0.06%, thimerosal 0.001%. Drop. Bot. 0.5 oz, 1 oz.
Use: Nasal decongestant.
VICKS VITAMIN C DROPS. (Richardson-Vicks) Vitamin C 60 mg as sodium

ascorbate and absorbic acid. Orange flavor. Bag. 14s, 30s.
Use: Vitamin supplement.

VICODIN. (Knoll) Hydrocodone bitartrate 5 mg, acetaminophen 500 mg/Tab. Bot. 100s, 500s. Hospital pack 100s.
Use: Narcotic analgesic combination.

VICODIN ES. (Knoll) Hydrocodone bitartrate 7.5 mg, acetaminophen 750 mg/Tab. Bot. 100s, UD 100s.
Use: Narcotic analgesic combination.

VICODIN TUSS. (Knoll) Hydrocodone bitartrate 5 mg, guaifenesin 100 mg/5 ml, sugar free. Syrup. Bot. 480 ml.
Use: Narcotic antitussive, expectorant.

VICON-C. (Whitby) Ascorbic acid 300 mg, niacinamide 100 mg, zinc sulfate 80 mg, magnesium sulfate 70 mg, thiamine mononitrate 20 mg, d-calcium pantothenate 20 mg, B_2 10 mg, B_6 5 mg/Cap. Bot. 60s, 500s, UD 100s.
Use: Vitamin/mineral supplement.

VICON FORTE. (Russ) Vitamins A 8000 IU, E 50 IU, C 150 mg, niacinamide 25 mg, thiamine mononitrate 10 mg, d-calcium pantothenate 10 mg, B_2 5 mg, B_6 2 mg, B_{12} 10 mcg, folic acid 1 mg, zinc sulfate 80 mg, magnesium sulfate 70 mg, manganese Cl 4 mg/Cap. Bot. 60s, 500s, UD 100s.
Use: Vitamin/mineral supplement.

VICON PLUS. (Russ) Vitamins A 4000 IU, E 50 IU, C 150 mg, niacinamide 25 mg, thiamine mononitrate 10 mg, d-calcium pantothenate 10 mg, B_2 5 mg, zinc sulfate 80 mg, magnesium sulfate 70 mg, manganese Cl 4 mg, B_6 2 mg/Cap. Bot. 60s.
Use: Vitamin/mineral supplement.

VICRYL SUTURES. (Ethicon) Polyglactin 910.

VICTORS. (Vicks) Special Vicks Medication (menthol, eucalyptus oil) in a soothing Vicks sugar base. Regular or Cherry flavor drops. Stick-Pack 10s, Bag 40s.
Use: Local anesthetic.

VICTOR'S VAPOR COUGH. (Vicks) Menthol, eucalyptus oil. Loz. Pkg. 10s.
Use: Local anesthetic.

• **VIDARABINE PHOSPHATE.** USAN.
Use: Antiviral.

• **VIDARABINE, STERILE**, U.S.P. XXIII., Conc. for Inj., Ophth. Oint., U.S.P. XXIII. 9-β-D-Arabinofuranosyladenine.
Use: Antiviral.
See: Vira-A Ophthalmic, Oint. (Parke-Davis).
Vira-A, Inj. (Parke-Davis).

• **VIDARABINE SODIUM PHOSPHATE.** USAN.

Use: Antiviral.

VI-DAYLIN ADC DROPS. (Ross) Vitamins A 1500 IU, C 35 mg, D 400 IU/ml. Bot. 30 ml, 50 ml. Bot. 50 ml w/dropper.
Use: Vitamin supplement.

VI-DAYLIN ADC PLUS IRON DROPS. (Ross) Vitamins A 1500 IU, C 35 mg, D 400 IU, iron 10 mg/ml. Bot. 50 ml w/dropper.
Use: Vitamin/mineral supplement.

VI-DAYLIN CHEWABLE. (Ross) Vitamins A 2500 IU, D 400 IU, E 15 IU, C 60 mg, folic acid 0.3 mg, B_1 1.05 mg, B_2 1.2 mg, niacin 13.5 mg, B_6 1.05 mg, B_{12} 4.5 mcg/Tab. Bot. 100s.
Use: Vitamin supplement.

VI-DAYLIN/F CHEWABLE TABLETS. (Ross) Fluoride 1 mg, vitamins A 2500 IU, D 400 IU, E 15 mg, B_1 1.05 mg, B_2 1.2 mg, B_3 13.5 mg, B_6 1.05 mg, B_{12} 4.5 mg, C 60 mg, folic acid 0.3 mg, sucrose, cherry flavor. Tab. Bot. 100s.
Use: Dental caries preventative, vitamin/mineral supplement.

VI-DAYLIN CHEWABLE W/FLUORIDE. (Ross) Fluoride 1 mg, vitamins B_1 1.05 mg, B_2 1.2 mg, niacinamide 13.5 mg, B_6 1.05 mg, C 60 mg, A 2500 IU, B_{12} 4.5 mcg, E 15 IU, folic acid 0.3 mg, D 400 IU/Tab. Bot. 100s.
Use: Dental caries preventative, vitamin/mineral supplement.

VI-DAYLIN DROPS. (Ross) Vitamins A 1500 IU, D 400 IU, E 5 IU, C 35 mg, B_1 0.5 mg, B_2 0.6 mg, niacin 8 mg, B_6 0.4 mg, B_{12} 1.5 mcg/ml. Bot. 50 ml.
Use: Vitamin supplement.

VI-DAYLIN/F ADC DROPS. (Ross) Vitamins A 1500 IU, D 400 IU, C 35 mg, fluoride 0.25 mg/ml. Bot. 50 ml.
Use: Vitamin supplement, dental caries preventative.

VI-DAYLIN/F ADC PLUS IRON DROPS. (Ross) Vitamins A 1500 IU, C 35 mg, D 400 IU, iron 10 mg, fluoride 0.25 mg/ml. Bot. 50 ml.
Use: Vitamin/mineral supplement, dental caries preventative.

VI-DAYLIN/F DROPS. (Ross) Vitamins A 1500 IU, D 400 IU, E 5 IU, C 35 mg, B_1 0.5 mg, B_2 0.6 mg, niacin 8 mg, B_6 0.4 mg, fluoride 0.25 mg/ml. Bot. 50 ml.
Use: Vitamin supplement, dental caries preventative.

VI-DAYLIN/F PLUS IRON. (Ross) **Drops:** Fluoride 0.25 mg, vitamins A 1500 IU, D 400 IU, E 4.1 mg, B_1 0.5 mg, B_2 0.6 mg, B_3 8 mg, B_6 0.4 mg, C 35 mg, iron 10 mg/ml, alcohol < 0.1%. Bot. 50 ml.
Chew. Tab.: Fluoride 1 mg, vitamins A

2500 IU, D 400 IU, E 15 mg, B_1 1.05 mg, B_2 1.2 mg, B_3 13.5 mg, B_6 1.05 mg, B_{12} 4.5 mcg, C 60 mg, folic acid 0.3 mg, iron 12 mg. Bot. 100s.
Use: Dental caries preventative, vitamin/mineral supplement.

VI-DAYLIN LIQUID. (Ross) Vitamins A 2500 IU, B_1 1.05 mg, B_2 1.2 mg, B_6 1.05 mg, B_{12} 4.5 mcg, C 60 mg, D 400 IU, E 20.4 mg (as d-alpha tocopheryl acetate), niacin 13.5 mg/5 ml. Bot. 8 oz, pt.
Use: Vitamin supplement.

VI-DAYLIN MULTIVITAMIN DROPS. (Ross) Vitamins A 1500 IU/ml, D 400 IU/ml, E 4.13/mg/ml, B_1 0.5 mg/ml, B_2 0.6 mg/ml, B_3 8 mg/ml, B_6 0.4 mg/ml, B_{12} 1.5 mcg/ml, C 34 mg/ml, < 0.05% alcohol, fruit flavor. Bot. 50 ml.
Use: Vitamin supplement.

VI-DAYLIN MULTIVITAMIN LIQUID. (Ross) Vitamins A 2500 IU/5 ml, D 400 IU/5 ml, E 11 mg/5 ml, B_1 1.05 mg/5 ml, B_2 1.2 mg/5 ml, B_3 13.5 mg/5 ml, B_6 1.06 mg/5 ml, B_{12} 4.5 mcg/5 ml, C 60 mg/5 ml, < 0.05% alcohol, glucose, sucrose, lemon/orange flavor. Bot. 240, 480 ml.
Use: Vitamin supplement.

VIDAYLIN MULTIVITAMIN + IRON DROPS. (Ross) Iron 10 mg, vitamins A 1500 IU, D 400 IU, E 4.1 mg, B_1 0.5 mg, B_2 0.6 mg, B_3 8 mg, B_6 0.4 mg, C 35 mg, < 0.5% alcohol, fruit flavor. Bot. 50 ml.
Use: Vitamin/mineral supplement.

VI-DAYLIN PLUS IRON CHEWABLE. (Ross) Vitamins A 2500 IU, D 400 IU, E 15 IU, C 60 mg, folic acid 0.3 mg, B_1 1.05 mg, B_2 1.2 mg, niacin 13.5 mg, B_6 1.05 mg, B_{12} 4.5 mcg, iron 12 mg/Tab. Bot. 100s.
Use: Vitamin/mineral supplement.

VI-DAYLIN PLUS IRON DROPS. (Ross) Vitamins A 1500 IU, D 400 IU, E 5 IU, C 35 mg, B_1 0.5 mg, B_2 0.6 mg, niacin 8 mg, B_6 0.4 mg, iron 10 mg/ml. Bot. 50 ml w/dropper.
Use: Vitamin/mineral supplement.

VI-DAYLIN PLUS IRON LIQUID. (Ross) Vitamins A 2500 IU, D 400 IU, C 60 mg, E 15 IU, B_1 1.05 mg, B_2 1.2 mg, niacin 13.5 mg, B_6 1.05 mg, B_{12} 4.5 mcg, iron 10 mg/tsp. Bot. 8 oz, 16 oz.
Use: Vitamin/mineral supplement.

VIDECON. (Vita Elixir) Vitamin D 50,000 units/Cap.
Use: Vitamin D supplement.

VI-DERM SOAP. (Arthrins) Extract of Amaryllis 10%. Pkg. cake 1s. Bar 3.5 oz.
Use: Skin cleanser.

• **VIFILCON A.** USAN.

Use: Contact lens material.
• **VIFILCON B.** USAN.
Use: Contact lens material (hydrophilic).

VIFLUORINEED. (Hanlon) Vitamins A 5000 IU, D 400 IU, C 75 mg, B_1 2 mg, B_2 3 mg, niacinamide 20 mg, fluoride 1 mg/Chew. Tab. Bot. 100s.
Use: Vitamin/mineral supplement.

• **VIGABATRIN.** USAN.
Use: Anticonvulsant.

VIGEROLAN. (Lannett) Geriatric vitamin-mineral capsule with choline, inositol, methionine. Bot. 100s, 500s, 1000s.
Use: Vitamin/mineral supplement.

VIGORTOL. (Rugby) Vitamins B_1 2.5 mg, B_2 1.25 mg, B_3 25 mg, B_5 5 mg, B_6 0.5 mg, B_{12} 0.5 mcg, iron 10 mg, choline 50 mg, inositol 50 mg, zinc 1 mg, I, K, Mg, Mn/15 ml, alcohol 18%. Liq. Bot. pt, gal.
Use: Vitamin/mineral supplement.

VILEX. (Dunhall) Vitamin B_1 100 mg, riboflavin phosphate sodium 1 mg, B_6 10 mg, panthenol 5 mg, niacinamido 100 mg/ml. Amp. 30 ml.
Use: Vitamin supplement.

VILIVA. (Vita Elixir) Ferrous fumarate 3 gr.
Use: Iron supplement.

VILOXAZINE. B.A.N. 2-(2-Ethoxyphenoxymethyl)-tetrahydro-1,4-oxazine.
Use: Treatment of mental disease.
See: Vivalan hydrochloride.

• **VILOXAZINE HCL.** USAN.
Use: Antidepressant.

VIMINATE. (Various Mfr.) Vitamins B_1 2.5 mg, B_2 1.25 mg, B_3 25 mg, B_5 5 mg, B_6 0.5 mg, B_{12} 0.5 mcg, iron 7.5 mg, zinc 1 mg, choline 50 mg, inositol 50 mg, I, K, Mg, Mn/15 ml, alcohol 18%. Liq. Bot. pt, gal.
Use: Vitamin/mineral supplement.

VIMIN-CO. (Jenkins) Vitamins A 5000 IU, D 400 IU, B_1 3 mg, B_2 2.5 mg, B_6 1 mg, B_{12} 2 mcg, C 50 mg, niacinamide 20 mg, calcium 46 mg, phosphorus 35 mg, iron 13.4 mg, calcium pantothenate 2 mg, magnesium 1 mg, manganese 1.5 mg, potassium 5 mg, zinc 1.4 mg/Cap. Bot. 1000s.
Use: Vitamin/mineral supplement.

VI-MIN-FOR-ALL. (Barth's) Vitamins A 3 mg, D 10 mcg, C 120 mg, B_1 35 mg, B_{12} 15 mcg, biotin, niacin 2.33 mg, E 30 IU, B_6, pantothenic acid, calcium 375 mg, phosphorus 180 mg, iron 20 mg, iodine 0.1 mg, rutin 10 mg, hesperidin-lemon bioflavonoid complex 10 mg, choline, inositol 2.4 mg, copper 10 mcg, manganese 2 mg, zinc 110 mcg, silicone 210

mcg/Tab. Bot. 100s, 500s.
Use: Vitamin/mineral supplement.

VIMMS-38. (Approved) Vitamins A 12,500 IU, D 1200 IU, B_1 15 mg, B_2 10 mg, C 75 mg, niacinamide 30 mg, calcium pantothenate 2 mg, B_6 0.5 mg, E 5 IU, Brewer's yeast 10 mg, B_{12} 15 mcg, iron 11.58 mg, desiccated liver 15 mg, choline bitartrate 30 mg, inositol 30 mg, calcium 59 mg, phosphorus 45 mg, zinc 0.68 mg, dicalcium phosphate 200 mg, manganese 1.11 mg, magnesium 1 mg, potassium 0.68 mg, pepsin 16.5 mg, diastase 16.5 mg, yeast 40.63 mg, protein digest 23.52 mg, amino acids 34.22 mg/Cap. Bot. 50s, 100s, 1000s.
Use: Vitamin/mineral supplement.

VINACTANE SULFATE. (Ciba) Viomycin Sulfate.

• **VINAFOCON A.** USAN.
Use: Contact lens material.

VINBARBITAL. 5-Ethyl-5-(1-methyl-1-butenyl)barbituric acid.
Use: Sedative/hypnotic.

VINBARBITAL SODIUM. 5-Ethyl-5-(1-methylbut-1-enyl)-barbiturate sodium
Use: Sedative/hypnotic.

VINBARBITONE. B.A.N. 5-Ethyl-5-(1-methylbut-1- enyl)barbituric acid.
Use: Hypnotic; sedative.

VINBLASTINE SULFATE. (Lyphomed) Vinblastine sulfate 10 mg/vial. Pow. for inj.
Use: Antineoplastic agent.

• **VINBLASTINE SULFATE**, U.S.P. XXIII. Inj., Sterile, U.S.P. XXIII. Vincaleukoblastine. Alkaloid extracted from *Vinca rosea* Linn.
Use: Antineoplastic.
See: Velban, Amp., Vial (Lilly).

VINCALEUKOBLASTINE, 22-OXO-, SULFATE (1:1)(SALT). Vincristine Sulfate, U.S.P. XXIII.

VINCASAR PFS. (Adria) Vincristine sulfate 1 mg/ml. Vial 1 ml.
Use: Antineoplastic agent.

• **VINCOFOS.** USAN.
Use: Anthelmintic.

• **VINCRISTINE SULFATE**, U.S.P. XXIII. Inj., U.S.P. XXIII. (Lilly) Vincaleukoblastine, 22-oxo-,sulfate (1:1)(salt) Leurocristine. An alkaloid extracted from Vinca rosea Linn.
Use: Antineoplastic.
See: Oncovin, Amp. (Lilly).
Vincasar PFS, Vial (Adria).

• **VINDESINE.** USAN.
Use: Antineoplastic.

• **VINDESINE SULFATE.** USAN.
Use: Antineoplastic.

• **VINEPIDINE SULFATE.** USAN.
Use: Antineoplastic.

• **VINGLYCINATE SULFATE.** USAN. 4-Deacetylvincaleukoblastine 4-(N,N-dimethylglycinate) (ester) sulfate (1:1.5)(salt).
Use: Antineoplastic.

• **VINLEUROSINE SULFATE.** USAN. Sulfate salt of an alkaloid extracted from *Vinca rosea* Linn. Also see Vinblastine.
Use: Antineoplastic.

• **VINORELBINE TARTRATE.** USAN. Sulfate salt of an alkaloid extracted from *Vinca Rosea* Linn.
Use: Antineoplastic.
See: Navelbine, Inj. (Burroughs Wellcome).

• **VINPOCETINE.** USAN. Ethyl apovincamin-22-oate.
Use: Antineoplastic.

• **VINROSIDINE SULFATE.** USAN. Sulfate salt of an alkaloid extracted from *vinca rosea* Linn.
See: Vinblastine.
Use: Antineoplastic.

VINYLACETATE-POLYVINYLPYRROLIDONE.
See: Ivy-Rid Spray (Mallard).

VINYL ALCOHOL POLYMER, U.S.P. XXI-II.
See: Polyvinyl alcohol.

VINYLBITONE. B.A.N. 5-(1-Methylbutyl)-5-vinyl-barbituric acid.
Use: Hypnotic; sedative.

VINYL ETHER, U.S.P. XXI.
Use: General anesthetic (inhalation.).
See: Vinethene, Liq.

VINYZENE. Bromchlorenone.
Use: Fungicide, bactericide.

• **VINZOLIDINE SULFATE.** USAN.
Use: Antineoplastic.

VIO-BEC. (Solvay) Vitamins B_1 25 mg, B_2 25 mg, niacinamide 100 mg, calcium pantothenate 40 mg, B_6 25 mg, C 500 mg/Cap. Bot. 100s.
Use: Vitamin supplement.

VIODO HC. (NMC Labs) Iodochlorhydroxyquin 3%, hydrocortisone 1% in cream base. Tube 20 Gm.
Use: Corticosteroid, antifungal (external).

VIOFORM. (Ciba) Clioquinol. **Cream:** 3%. Tube oz. **Oint.:** 3% in petrolatum base. Tube oz.
Use: Antifungal, external.

VIOGEN-C. (Goldine) Vitamins B_1 20 mg, B_2 10 mg, B_3 100 mg, B_5 20 mg, B_6 5 mg, C 300 mg, Mg, zinc 18 mg/Cap. Bot. 60s, 500s, UD 100s.

Use: Vitamin/mineral supplement.

VIOKASE. (Robins) **Tab.:** Lipase 8000 units, protease 30,000 units, amylase 30,000 units/Tab. Bot. 100s, 500s. **Pow.:** Lipase 16,800 units, protease 70,000 units, amylase 70,000 units/0.7 Gm (0.25 tsp.).
Use: Digestive enzymes.

VIOPAN-T. (Trimen) Vitamins A 8000 IU, D 400 IU, E 30 mg, B_1 10 mg, B_2 10 mg, B_3 100 mg, B_5 5 mg, B_6 2 mg, B_{12} 6 mcg, C 200 mg, iron 15 mg, folic acid 0.4 mg, calcium 100 mg, zinc 15 mg, choline 25 mg, L-lysine 25 mg, biotin 10 mcg, Cu, I, K, Mg, Mn, phosphorus 42 mg/Tab. Bot. 100s.
Use: Vitamin/mineral supplement.

VIOSTEROL W/HALIBUT LIVER OIL. Vitamins A 50,000 IU, D 10,000 IU/Gm. (Abbott)—Bot. 5 ml, 20 ml, 50 ml. Cap.: Vitamins A 5000 IU, D 1000 IU (Ives) Cap.: Vitamins A 5000 IU, D 1700 IU.
Use: Vitamin supplement.

• **VIPROSTOL.** USAN.
Use: Hypotensive, vasodilator.

VIPRYNIUM EMBONATE. B.A.N. 6-Dimethyl-amino-2-[2-(2:5-dimethyl-1-phenyl-3-pyrrolyl)vinyl]-1-methylquinolinium embonate. (Embonic acid is adopted as the trivial name for 4:4' methylenebis-(3-hydroxymaphthalene-2-carboxylic acid). Vanquin. Pyrvinium Pamoate.
Use: Anthelmintic.

VIRA-A OPHTHALMIC. (Parke-Davis) Vidarabine 3% in a sterile inert base. Tube 3.5 Gm.
Use: Antiviral.

VIRAC. (Ruson) Undecoylium Cl-iodine. Iodine complexed with a cationic detergent. Surgical soln. Bot. 2 oz, 8 oz, 1 gal.
Use: Antiseptic.

VIRACIL. (Approved) Phenylephrine HCl 5 mg, hesperidin 50 mg, thenylene HCl 12.5 mg, pyrilamine maleate 12.5 mg, vitamin C 50 mg, salicylamide 2.5 gr, caffeine 0.5 gr, sodium salicylate 1.25 gr/Cap. Bot. 16s, 36s.
Use: Decongestant, vitamin supplement, antihistamine, analgesic.

VIRAMISOL. (Seatrace) Adenosine phosphate 25 mg/ml. Vial 10 ml.
Use: Relief of varicose vein complications.

VIRANOL. (American Dermal) Salycylic acid in collodion gel w/lactic acid, camphor, pyroxylin, ethyl alcohol, ethyl acetate. Gel 8 Gm.
Use: Treatment and removal of plantar and other common warts.

VIRAZOLE. (ICN) Ribavirin 6 Gm/Vial.
Use: Antiviral.

• **VIRGINIAMYCIN.** USAN. An antibiotic produced by Streptomyces virginie.
Use: Antibacterial.

VIRIDIUM. (Vita Elixir) Phenylazodiaminopyridine HCl 100 mg/Tab.
Use: Urinary tract product.

• **VIRIDOFULVIN.** USAN.
Use: Antifungal.

VIRILON. (Star) Methyltestosterone 10 mg/SR Cap. Bot. 100s, 1000s.
Use: Androgen.

VIROGEN HERPES SLIDE TEST. (Wampole) Latex agglutination slide test for the detection of herpes simplex virus antigens directly from lesions or cell culture. Test kit 100s.
Use: Diagnostic aid.

VIROGEN ROTATEST. (Wampole) Latex agglutination slide test for the qualitative detection of rotavirus in fecal specimens. Test kit 50s.
Use: Diagnostic aid.

VIROGEN RUBELLA MICROLATEX TEST. (Wampole) Latex agglutination microlatex test for the detection of rubella virus antibody in serum. Test kit 500s, 5000s.
Use: Diagnostic aid.

VIROGEN RUBELLA SLIDE TEST. (Wampole) Latex agglutination slide test for the detection of rubella virus antibody in serum. Test kit 100s, 500s, 5000s.
Use: Diagnostic aid.

VIROGEN RUBELLA SLIDE TEST WITH FAST TRAK SLIDES. (Wampole) Latex agglutination slide test for the detection of rubella virus antibody in serum.
Use: Diagnostic aid.

VIRO-MED TABLETS. (Whitehall) Acetaminophen 500 mg, chlorpheniramine maleate 2 mg, pseudoephedrine HCl 30 mg, dextromethorphan HBr 15 mg/Tab. Bot. 20s, 48s.
Use: Analgesic, antihistamine, decongestant, antitussive.

VIROPTIC OPHTHALMIC SOLUTION. (Burroughs Wellcome) Trifluridine 1%. Bot. 7.5 ml.
Use: Antiviral.

• **VIROXIME.** USAN.
Use: Antiviral.

VIROZYME INJECTION. (Marcen) Sodium nucleate 2.5%, phenol 0.5%, protein hydrolysate 2.5%, benzyl alcohol 0.2%. Vial 5 ml, 10 ml.
Use: Promote leukocytosis and phagocytosis.

VIRUGON. Under study. Anhydro bis-

(beta-hydroxyothyl) biguanide deriva-
tive.
Use: Treatment of influenza, mumps,
measles, chicken pox and shingles.
**VISCARIN W/IODINE, BORIC ACID,
PHENOL, CHLOROPHYLL.**
See: Triophyll, Liq. (Schaffer).
VISCOAT SOLUTION. (Alcon) Sodium
chondroitin sulfate 40 mg, sodium
hyaluronate 30 mg, sodium dihydrogen
phosphate hydrate 0.45 mg, disodium
hydrogen phosphate 2.65 mg, sodium
Cl 4.3 mg/ml. Glass syringe disposable
0.5 ml.
Use: Viscoelastic solution.
VISCUM ALBUM, EXTRACT. Visnico.
Use: Vasodilator.
VISINE. (Leeming) Tetrahydrozoline HCl
0.05%, sodium Cl, boric acid, sodium
borate, benzalkonium Cl 0.01%, disodium ethylenediamine tetraacetate 0.1%.
Dropper Bot. 0.5 oz, Plastic bot. 0.5 oz,
3/4 oz, 1 oz.
Use: Vasoconstrictor/mydriatic (ophthalmic).
VISINE AC. (Pfizer) Tetrahydrozoline HCl
0.05%, zinc sulfate 0.25%, benzalkonium Cl 0.01%, sodium Cl, boric acid,
sodium citrate, ethylenediamine tetraacetate 0.1%. Bot. 0.5 oz, 1 oz.
Use: Vasoconstrictor/mydriatic (ophthalmic).
VISINE EXTRA. (Pfizer) Polyethylene glycol 400 1%, tetrahydrozoline HCl 0.05%,
benzalkonium Cl 0.013%, boric acid,
EDTA, sodium borate. Drop Bot. 15 ml,
30 ml.
Use: Ophthalmic vasoconstrictors/my-
driatics.
VISINE L.R. (Pfizer) Oxymetazoline HCl
0.025% sodium chloride, boric acid,
sodium borate, benzalkonium chloride
0.01%, EDTA 0.1%. Soln. Bot. 15, 30 ml.
Use: Ophthalmic vasoconstrictors/my-
driatics.
VISION CARE ENZYMATIC CLEANER.
(Alcon) Highly purified pork pancreatin
to be diluted in saline solution. Tab. Pkg.
24s.
Use: Soft contact lens care.
VISKEN. (Sandoz) Pindolol 5 mg or 10
mg/Tab. Bot. 100s.
Use: Antihypertensive.
VISNADINE. B.A.N. 10-Acetoxy-9,10-di-
hydro-8,8-dimethyl-9-α-methylbutyry-
loxy-2H,8H-benzo-[1,2-b:3,4-b']dipyran-
2-one. Cardine.
Use: Coronary vasodilator.
VISTACON. (Hauck) Hydroxyzine HCl 50
mg/ml. Vial 10 ml.

Use: Antianxiety agent.
VISTAJECT 25 & 50. (Mayrand) Hydrox-
yzine HCl 25 mg or 50 mg/ml. Vial 10 ml.
Use: Antianxiety agent.
VISTAQUEL 50. (Pasadena) Hydroxyzine
HCl 50 mg/ml. Vial 10 ml.
Use: Antianxiety agent.
VISTARIL (Pfizer Laboratories) Hydrox-
yzine pamoate equivalent to hydrox-
yzine HCl. **Cap.:** 25 mg, 50 mg or 100
mg. Bot. 100s, 500s, UD 100s. **Oral
Susp.:** 25 mg/5 ml. Bot. 120 ml, pt.
Use: Antianxiety agent.
VISTARIL I.M. (Roerig) Hydroxyzine HCl.
25 mg/ml: Vial 10 ml, Box 1s. **50 mg/ml:**
Vial 10 ml, Box 1s.; Vial 1 ml, UD 25s.
100 mg/2 ml: Vial 2 ml, UD 25s.
Use: Antianxiety agent.
VISTARIL ISOJECT I.M. (Roerig) Hydrox-
yzine HCl 50 mg/ml or 100 mg/2 ml
Amp. 1 ml, 2 ml.
Use: Antianxiety agent.
VISTAZINE 50. (Keene) Hydroxyzine HCl
50 mg/ml. Vial 10 mg/ml.
Use: Antianxiety agent.
VISUAL EYES. (Optopics) Sodium Cl,
sodium phosphate mono- and dibasic,
benzalkonium Cl, EDTA. Soln. Bot. 120
ml.
Use: Ophthalmic irrigation solution.
VITA-BEE C-800. (Rugby) Vitamins E 45
mg, B_1 15 mg, B_2 17 mg, B_3 100 mg, B_5
25 mg, B_6 25 mg, B_{12} 12 mcg, C 800
mg/Tab. Bot. 60s.
Use: Vitamin supplement.
VITA-BEE W/C. (Rugby) Vitamins B_1 15
mg, B_2 10 mg, B_3 10 mg, B_5 10 mg, B_6 5
mg, C 300 mg/TR Cap. Bot. 50s, 100s.
Use: Vitamin supplement.
VITABIX. (Spanner) Vitamins B_1 100 mg,
B_2 2 mg, B_6 5 mg, B_{12} 30 mcg, niacinamide 100 mg, panthenol 10 mg/ml.
Vial 10 ml. Multiple dose vial 30 ml.
Use: Vitamin supplement.
VITA-BOB CAPSULES. (Scot-Tussin) Vit-
amins A 5000 IU, D 400 IU, E 30 mg, B_1
1.5 mg, B_2 1.7 mg, B_3 20 mg, B_6 2 mg,
B_{12} 6 mcg, C 60 mg, folic acid 0.4
mg/Cap. Bot. 100s.
Use: Vitamin supplement.
V-I TABS. (Kenyon) Vitamins A 5000 IU,
D-2 500 mg, B_1 3 mg, B_2 2.5 mg, B_6 1
mg, B_{12} 1 mg, C 50 mg, niacinamide 20
mg, calcium pantothenate 1 mg, iron 15
mg/Tab. Bot. 100s, 1000s.
Use: Vitamin/mineral supplement.
VITA-C. (Freeda) Ascorbic acid 4 Gm/tsp.
Crystals 100 Gm, 500 Gm, 1000 Gm.
Use: Vitamin C supplement.
VITACARN. (Kendall McGaw) L-Carnitine

1 Gm/10 ml. UD Box 50s, 100s.
Use: L-carnitine supplement.
VITACREST. (Nutrition) Vitamins A
25,000 IU, D 400 IU, E 10 IU, B_1 25 mg,
B_2 12 mg, B_6 10 mg, B_{12} 10 mcg, biotin
10 mcg, folic acid 0.1 mg, calcium pantothenate 25 mg, niacinamide 50 mg, inositol 25 mg, l-glutamic acid 10 mg, l-lysine HCl 20 mg, p-aminobenzoic acid 25
mg, C 250 mg, wheat germ oil 10 mg,
brewers yeast (dried) 10 mg, whole liver
desiccated 10 mg, soybean lecithin 50
mg, iron 10 mg, calcium carbonate 625
mg, copper 0.2 mg, zinc 0.2 mg, magnesium 10 mg, manganese 0.2 mg, potassium 10 mg/Cap. Bot. 100s.
Use: Vitamin/mineral supplement.
VIT-A-DROPS. (Vision Pharm.) Vitamin A
5000 IU, polysorbate 80. Bot. 10 ml, 15
ml.
Use: Ocular lubricant.
VITADYE. (Elder) FD & C yellow No. 5, D.
& C. red. No. 40, FD & C blue No. 1 dyes
and dihydroxyacetone 5%. Bot. 0.5 oz, 2
oz.
Use: Cosmetic cover for hypopigment-
ed skin.
VITA ELIXIR. (Vita Elixir) Alcohol 25%, vitamins A palmitate 5000 IU, D-2 500 IU,
iron 10 mg/45 ml w/multivitamins and
minerals.
Use: Vitamin/mineral supplement.
VITA-FERON. (Vitaline) Iron 150 mg, folic
acid 800 mcg, B_{12} 6 mcg. Tab. Bot. 90s.
Use: Iron with vitamin supplement.
VITAFOL. (Everett) Vitamins B_{12} 8.34
mcg, B_6 2 mg, ferric pyrophosphate 100
mg, folic acid 0.25 mg, niacinamide 13.3
mg/5 ml, raspberry-mint flavor. Syr. Bot.
473 ml.
Use: Iron w/vitamins.
VITAFOL. (Everett) Iron 65 mg, vitamins
A 6000 IU, D 400 IU, E 30 mg, B_1 1.1
mg, B_2 1.8 mg, B_3 15 mg, B_6 2.5 mg, B_{12}
5 mcg, C 60 mg, folic acid 1 mg, calci-
um/Tab. Bot. 100s, 1000s.
Use: Vitamin/mineral supplement.
VITAFORT. (Kessel) Vitamins A 4000 IU,
D 400 IU, E 15 IU, C 70 mg, folic acid 1
mg, B_1 2 mg, B_2 2 mg, niacinamide 20
mg, B_6 2 mg, B_{12} 5 mcg, calcium pantothenate 10 mg/Cap. Bot. 60s.
Use: Vitamin supplement.
VITA-IRON FORMULA. (Barth's) Iron 120
mg, vitamins B_1 5 mg, B_2 10 mg, C 20
mg, niacin 2 mg, B_{12} 25 mcg, lysine,
desiccated liver 200 mg, bromelain/Tab.
Bot. 100s, 500s.
Use: Vitamin/mineral supplement.
VITAJEN. (Jenkins) Vitamins B_1 12 mg,

B_2 4 mg, B_{12} 10 mcg, B_6 2 mg, calcium
pantothenate 6 mg, nicotinic acid 40
mg/fl oz. Bot. 4 oz, gal.
Use: Vitamin supplement.
VITA-KAPS FILMTABS. (Abbott) Vitamins A 5000 IU, D 400 IU, B_1 3 mg, B_2
2.5 mg, nicotinamide 20 mg, B_6 1 mg, C
50 mg, B_{12} 3 mcg/Filmtab. Bot. 100s,
1000s.
Use: Vitamin supplement.
VITAKAPS-M. (Abbott) Vitamins A 5000
IU, D 400 IU, B_1 3 mg, B_2 2.5 mg, nicotinamide 20 mg, B_6 1 mg, B_{12} 3 mcg, C
50 mg, iron 10 mg, copper 1 mg, iodine
0.15 mg, manganese 1 mg, zinc 7.5
mg/Filmtab. Bot. 100s.
Use: Vitamin/mineral supplement.
VITA-KID CHEWABLE WAFERS. (Solgar) Vitamins A 5000 IU, D 400 IU, E 8.2
mg, B_1 2 mg, B_2 2 mg, B_3 10 mg, B_6 2
mg, B_{12} 5 mg, C 100 mg, FA 0.3 mg, orange flavor. Tab. Bot. 50s.
Use: Multivitamin Supplement.
VITALAX. (Vitalax) Candy base, gumdrop
flavored. Pkg. 20s.
Use: Laxative.
VITAL B50. (Goldline) Vitamins B_1 50 mg,
B_2 50 mg, B_3 50 mg, B_5 50 mg, B_6 50
mg, B_{12} 50 mcg, folic acid 0.1 mg, biotin
50 mcg, PABA 50 mg, choline bitartrate
50 mg, inositol 50 mg, bromelain 20
mg/TR Tab. Bot 60s.
Use: Vitamin supplement.
VITALETS TABLETS. (Freeda) Iron 3.3
mg, vitamins A 5000 IU, D 400 IU, E 5
mg, B_1 2.5 mg, B_2 0.9 mg, B_3 20 mg, B_5
3 mg, B_6 2 mg, B_{12} 5 mcg, C 60 mg, biotin 25 mcg, Mn 25 mcg, Ca 25 mcg,
raspberry, orange, carob, unflavored.
Chew. Tab. Bot 100s, 250s.
Use: Multivitamin w/iron supplement.
VITAL HIGH NITROGEN. (Ross) Amino
acids, partially hydrolyzed whey, meat
and soy, hydrolyzed cornstarch, su-
crose, safflower oil, MCT mono and
diglycerides, soy lecithin, vitamins A, B_1,
B_2, B_3, B_5, B_6, B_{12}, C, D, E, K, folic acid,
biotin, choline, Ca, P, Mg, Fe, Cu, Zn,
Mn, I, Cl. Packet 80 Gm.
Use: Enteral nutritional supplement.
VITAMEL-M. (Eastwood) Liq. Bot. 16 oz.
VITAMEL WITH IRON. (Eastwood) Drops
50 ml. Chew. Tab. Bot. 100s.
• **VITAMIN A,** U.S.P. XXIII. Cap., U.S.P.
XXIII. Oleovitamin A.
Use: Anti-xerophthalmic vitamin, emol-
lient.
Amp.
Aquasol A, Preps. (USV Pharm.).
Cap.

Acon (Du Pont).
Alphalin (Lilly).
Aquasol A (USV Labs.).
Vi-Dom-A (Miles Pharm).
Cream:
Retinol (Nature's Bounty).
Oint.
Aquasol A (USV Pharm.).
Retin-A (Johnson & Johnson).
Tab.
Dispatabs (Person & Covey).
Vial
Aquasol A (USV Labs.).
VITAMIN A, ALPHALIN. (Lilly) Vitamin A
50,000 IU/Gelseal. Bot. 100s.
Use: Vitamin A supplement.
**VITAMIN A, WATER MISCIBLE, OR SOL-
UBLE.** Water miscible vitamin A.
Use: Vitamin A supplement.
VITAMIN Bc.
See: Folic Acid (Various Mfr.).
VITAMIN B1. Thiamine HCl, U.S.P. XXIII.
Use: Vitamin B_1 supplement.
VITAMIN B1 MONONITRATE. Thiamine
mononitrate.
Use: Vitamin B_1 supplement.
VITAMIN B1 & B12. (Pharmex) Vitamins
B_1 100 mg, B_{12} 1000 mcg/ml. Vial 10 ml.
Use: Vitamin supplement.
**VITAMIN B1 W/PANCREATIN, OX BILE
EXTRACT PEPSIN, GLUTAMIC ACID
HCl.**
See: Maso-Gestive, Tab. (Mason).
VITAMIN B1 W/THYROID.
See: T & T, Tab. (Mason).
• **VITAMIN B2.** Riboflavin, U.S.P. XXIII.
Use: Vitamin B_2 supplement.
• **VITAMIN B3.** Niacinamide, U.S.P. XXIII.
Nicotinamide.
Use: Vitamin B_3 supplement.
• **VITAMIN B5.** Calcium Pantothenate
U.S.P. XXIII.
Use: Vitamin B_5 supplement.
• **VITAMIN B6.** Pyridoxine HCl, U.S.P. XXIII.
Use: Vitamin B_6 supplement.
See: Hexa-Betalin, Tab. (Lilly).
Hexavibex, Vial (Parke-Davis).
VITAMIN B6 & B1. (Pharmex) Vitamins
B_6 100 mg, B_1 100 mg/ml. Vial 10 ml.
Use: Vitamin supplement.
VITAMIN B-8.
See: Adenosine phosphate.
• **VITAMIN B12.** Cyanocobalamin, U.S.P.
XXIII. Cobalamine.
See:
Cap., Tab. Redisol (Merck Sharp &
Dohme).
Vial, Amp. Bedoce (Lincoln). Berubi-
gen (Upjohn). Betalin-12 (Lilly).
Cabadon-M (Solvay). Cobadoce

Forte (Solvay). Crysto-Gel (Solvay).
Cyano-Gel, Liq. (Maurry). Dodex
(Organon). Redisol (Merck Sharp &
Dohme). Rubramin (Squibb). Ruvite
1000 (Savage). Sigamine (Sig).
Sytobex-H (Parke-Davis). Vi-Twel,
Inj. (Berlex).
W/Ferrous-sulfate, ascorbic acid, folic
acid.
See: Intrin, Cap. (Merit).
W/Folic acid, niacinamide, liver.
See: Hepfomin 500, Inj. (Keene
Pharm.).
W/Thiamine.
See: Cobalin, Vial (Ulmer).
Cyamine, Vial (Keene).
W/Thiamine, vitamin B_6.
See: Orexin, Tab. (Stuart).
VITAMIN B12. (Various Mfr.) Cyanocobal-
amin crystalline 100 mcg/ml or 1000
mcg/ml. **100 mcg/ml:** Vials 30 ml. **1000
mcg/ml:** Multidose vials 10 ml or 30 ml.
Use: Vitamin supplement.
VITAMIN B12. (Goldline) Cyanocobal-
amin crystalline 500 mcg or 1000 mcg.
Tab. Bot. 100s.
Use: Vitamin supplement.
VITAMIN B12 a & b.
See: Hydroxocobalamin (Various Mfr.).
VITAMIN B15. Pangamic acid, betaglu-
cono-dimethylaminoacetic acid.
Use: Alleged to increase oxygen supply
in blood. Not approved by FDA as a vi-
tamin or drug. Illegal to sell Vitamin
B_{15}.
VITAMIN B COMPLEX. Concentrated ex-
tract of dried brewer's yeast and extract
of corn processed w/**Clostridium ace-
tobutylicum.**
See: Becotin, Pulvules (Lilly).
Betalin Complex, Amp. (Lilly).
Savaplex, Vial (Savage).
VITAMIN B COMPLEX NO. 104. (Century) Vitamins B_1 100 mg, B_2 2 mg, B_6 2
mg, d-panthenol 10 mg, niacinamide
125 mg, benzyl alcohol 1%, gentisic acid
ethanolamide 2.5%/Vial 30 ml.
Use: Vitamin supplement.
**VITAMIN B COMPLEX, BETALIN COM-
PLEX, ELIXIR.** (Lilly) Vitamins B_1 2.7
mg, B_2 1.35 mg, B_{12} 3 mcg, B_6 0.555
mg, pantothenic acid 2.7 mg, niacinamide 6.75 mg, liver fraction 500 mg/5
ml, alcohol 17%. Bot. 16 oz.
Use: Vitamin supplement.
VITAMIN B COMPLEX W/VITAMIN C.
(Century) Vitamins B_1 25 mg, B_2 5 mg,
B_6 5 mg, niacinamide 50 mg, panthenol
5 mg, calcium 50 mg, propethylene glycol 300 10%, gentisic acid ethanolamide

2.5%, benzyl alcohol 2%/Vial 30 ml.
Use: Vitamin supplement.
**VITAMIN B COMPLEX, BETALIN COM-
PLEX CAPSULES.** (Lilly) Vitamins B_1 1
mg, B_2 2 mg, B_6 0.4 mg, pantothenic
acid 3.333 mg, niacinamide 10 mg, B_{12}
1 mcg/Pulvule. Bot. 100s.
Use: Vitamin supplement.
VITAMIN C.
See: Ascorbic Acid Preps.
VITAMIN C, CEVALIN. (Lilly) Ascorbic
acid 250 mg or 500 mg/Tab. Bot. 100s.
Use: Vitamin C supplement.
VITAMIN C W/COMBINATIONS.
See: Allbee C-800, Prods. (Robins).
Allbee with C, Cap. (Robins).
Allbee-T, Tab. (Robins).
Antiox, Cap. (Mayrand).
Anti-therm, Tab. (Scrip).
Bejectal w/Vitamin C (Abbott).
Colrex, Cap. (Solvay).
Nialexo-C, Tab. (Mallard).
Protegra Softgels, Cap. (Lederle).
Thex, Cap. (Ingram).
Thex Forte, Cap. (Ingram).
Vicon-C, Cap. (Glaxo).
Vicon Forte, Cap. (Glaxo).
Vicon Plus, Cap. (Glaxo).
Vi-Zac, Cap. (Glaxo).
Z-BEC, Tab. (Robins).
• **VITAMIN D.** Cholecalciferol, U.S.P. XXIII.
Use: Vitamin D supplement.
VITAMIN D, DELTALIN. (Lilly) Vitamin D-
2 50,000 units (1.25 mg)/Gelseal. Bot.
100s.
Use: Vitamin D supplement.
VITAMIN D, SYNTHETIC.
See: Activated 7-Dehydro-cholesterol
Calciferol.
VITAMIN D-1.
See: Dihydrotachysterol.
VITAMIN D-2. Activated ergasterol, Ergo-
calciferol.
See: Calciferol, Preps. (Various Mfr.).
Drisdol, Liq. (Winthrop Pharm).
Vlosterol (Various Mfr.).
VITAMIN D-3.
See: Activated 7-dehydrocholesterol.
Calciferol Prep. for related activity.
VITAMIN D-3-CHOLESTEROL. Com-
pound of crystalline vitamin D-3 and
cholesterol.
VITAMIN D-4.
See: Dihydrotachysterol, Preps. (Vari-
ous Mfr.).
• **VITAMIN E**, U.S.P. XXIII. Cap., U.S.P.
XXIII. It may consist of: d- or dl-alpha to-
copherol, d-or dl-alpha tocopheryl ac-
etate, d- or dl-alpha tocopheryl acid suc-
cinate, mixed tocopherols concentrate,

or d-alpha tocopheryl acetate concen-
trate.
Use: Vitamin E supplement.
See: Aquasol E (USV).
Eprolin, Gelseal (Lilly).
E-Vites, Cap. (Quality Generics).
Lactinol-E Creme (Pedinol).
Pertropin Cap. (Lannett).
Tega-E-Cream (Ortega).
Tocopher, Prod. (Quality Generics).
Tocopherol, Preps. (Various Mfr.).
Wheat Germ Oil (Various Mfr.).
VITAMIN E, EPROLIN. (Lilly) Alpha-toco-
pherol 100 units/Gelseal. Bot. 100s.
Use: Vitamin E supplement.
**VITAMIN E W/QUININE SULFATE,
NIACIN.**
See: Myodyne, Tab. (Paddock).
VITAMIN F.
See: Fats, Unsaturated.
Fatty Acids, Unsaturated.
VITAMIN G.
See: Riboflavin.
VITAMIN K.
See: Hykinone, Amp. (Abbott).
Menadiol, Sodium Diphosphate,
Preps. (Various Mfr.).
Menadione, Preps. (Various Mfr.).
Menadione Sodium Bisulfite, Preps.
(Various Mfr.).
VITAMIN K-1.
See: Phytonadione, U.S.P. XXIII.
VITAMIN K-3.
See: Menadione, U.S.P. XXIII.
VITAMIN K OXIDE. Not available, but
usually K-1 is desired.
VITAMIN M.
See: Folic Acid, U.S.P. XXIII.
**VITAMIN-MINERAL-SUPPLEMENT LIQ-
UID.** (PBI) Vitamins B_1 0.83 mg, B_2 0.42
mg, B_3 8.3 mg, B_5 1.67 mg, B_6 0.17 mg,
B_{12} 0.17 mcg, I 16.67 mcg, Fe 2.5 mg,
Mg, 0.33 mg, Zn 0.33 mg, Mn 0.33 mg,
choline 16.67 mg, alcohol 18%. Liq. Pt.
Gal.
Use: Vitamin/mineral supplement.
VITAMIN P. Citrin.
See: Bio-Flavonoid Compounds (Vari-
ous Mfr.).
Hesperidin Preps. (Various Mfr.).
Quercetin (Various Mfr.).
Rutin, Preps. (Various Mfr.).
VITAMIN T. Sesame seed factor, termite
factor.
Use: Claimed to aid proper blood coag-
ulation and promote formation of blood
platelets. Not approved by FDA as an
active vitamin.
VITAMIN U. Present in cabbage juice.
VITAMIN, MAINTENANCE FORMULA.

Soo: Stuart Formula, Tab., Liq. (Stuart).
Vi-Magna, Cap. (Lederle).

VITA-MINS. (Mills) Vitamins A 5000 IU, D 200 IU, C 30 mg, B_1 1 mg, B_2 2 mg, B_6 0.1 mg, B_{12} 1 mcg, d-calcium pantothenate 0.5 mg, niacinamide 20 mg, folic acid 0.1 mg, ferrous gluconate 25 mg, copper gluconate 5 mg, zinc gluconate 5 mg, manganese gluconate 5 mg/Tab. Bot. 100s.
Use: Vitamin/mineral supplement.

VITAMINS: STRESS FORMULA.
See: Cebefortis, Tab. (Upjohn).
Folbesyn, Tab., Vial (Lederle).
Probec-T, Tab. (Stuart).
Stresscaps, Cap. (Lederle).
Stresscaps With Iron (Lederle).
Stresscaps With Zinc (Lederle).
StressForm "605" w/ Iron, Tab. (Nature's Bounty).
Stress Formula with Iron, Tab. (Nature's Bounty).
Stresstabs-600 (Lederle).
Thera-combex Kap. (Parke-Davis).

VITAMINS W/ANTIOBESITY AGENTS.
See: Fetamin, Tab. (Mission).
Obedrin, Cap. or Tab. (Massengill).

VITAMINS W/LIVER & LIPOTROPIC AGENTS.
See: Heptuna, Cap. (Roerig).
Lederplex, Preps. (Lederle).
Livitamin, Preps. (Beecham Labs).
Metheponex, Cap. (Rawl).
Methischol, Cap. (USV Pharm.).

VITA NATAL. (Scot-Tussin) Folic acid 1 mg/Tab. Bot. 100s.
Use: Folic acid supplement.

VITANEED. (Biosearch) P-beef, Ca and Na caseinates, CHO-maltodextrin. F-partially hydrogenated soy oil, mono and diglycerides, soy lecithin. Protein 35 Gm, CHO 125 Gm, fat 40 Gm, sodium 500 mg, potassium 1250 mg/L, 1 Cal/ml, 375 mOsm/kg H_2O. Liq. Ready-to-use 250 ml.
Use: Enteral nutritional supplement.

VITAON. (Vita Elixir) Vitamin B_{12} 25 mcg, thiamine HCl 10 mg, ferric pyrophosphate 250 mg/5 ml.
Use: Vitamin supplement.

VITA-PLUS B12. (Scot-Tussin) Vitamin B_{12} 1000 mcg/ml. Inj.
Use: Vitamin B_{12} supplement.

VITA-PLUS E. (Scot-Tussin) Vitamin E 294 mg as d-alpha tocopheryl acetate/Cap.
Use: Vitamin E supplement.

VITA-PLUS G. (Scot-Tussin) Vitamins A 10,000 IU, D 400 IU, E 2 mg, B_1 5 mg, B_2 2.5 mg, B_3 40 mg, B_5 4 mg, B_6 1 mg,

B_{12} 2 mcg, C 75 mg, Iron 30 mg, calcium 75 mg, zinc 0.5 mg, choline 31.4 mg, inositol 15 mg, K, Mg, Mn, phosphorus 58 mg/Cap. Bot. 100s.
Use: Vitamin/mineral supplement.

VITA-PLUS H CAPSULES. (Scot-Tussin) Vitamins B_1 17.5 mg, B_2 8.5 mg, B_3 35 mg, B_5 5 mg, B_6 0.25 mg, B_{12} 5 mcg, iron 11.7 mg, C 60 mg, choline, inositol, dessicated liver/Cap. Bot. 100s.
Use: Vitamin/mineral supplement.

VITA-PLUS H LIQUID SUGAR FREE. (Scot-Tussin) Vitamins B_1 30 mg, l-lysine monohydrochloride 300 mg, B_{12} 75 mcg, B_6 15 mg, iron pyrophosphate soluble 100 mg/5 ml. Bot. 4 oz, 8 oz, pt, gal.
Use: Vitamin/mineral supplement.

VITA-PMS. (Bajamar) Vitamins A 2083 IU, E 16.7 IU, D_3 16.7 IU, folic acid 33 mcg, B_1 4.2 mg, B_2 4.2 mg, B_3 4.2 mg, B_5 4.2 mg, B_6 50 mg, B_{12} 10.4 mcg, biotin 10.4 mcg, choline bitartrate 52 mg, inositol 4.2 mg, PABA 4.2 mg, C 250 mg, bioflavonoid 42 mg, rutin 4.2 mg, Ca, Mg, I 21 mg, Fe, Cu 2.5 mg, Zn, Mn, K, Se, Cr 4.2 mg, 2500 NF units amylase activity, 2500 NF units protease activity, 200 NF units lipase activity, betaine acid HCl 16.7 mg. Tab. Bot. 100s.
Use: Vitamin/mineral supplement.

VITA-PMS PLUS. (Bajamar) Vitamins A 667 IU, E 16.7 IU, D_3 16.7 IU, folic acid 33 mcg, B_1 4.2 mg, B_2 4.2 mg, B_3 4.2 mg, B_5 4.2 mg, B_6 17 mg, B_{12} 10.4 mcg, biotin 10.4 mcg, choline bitartrate 52 mg, inositol 4.2 mg, PABA 4.2 mg, C 250 mg, bioflavonoid 42 mg, rutin 4.2 mg, Mg, I 21 mg, Ca 167 mg, Fe, Cu 2.5 mg, Zn, Mn, K, Se, Cr 4.2 mg, 2500 NF units amylase activity, 2500 NF units protease activity, 200 NF units lipase activity, betaine acid HCl 16.7 mg. Tab. Bot. 100s.
Use: Vitamin/mineral supplement.

VITA-RAY CREME. (Gordon) Vitamins E 3000 IU, A 200,000 IU/oz w/aloe 10%. Jar 0.5 oz, 2.5 oz.
Use: Emollient.

VITAREX. (Pasadena Research) Vitamins A 10,000 IU, D 200 IU, B_1 15 mg, B_2 10 mg, B_6 5 mg, B_{12} 5 mcg, C 250 mg, niacinamide 100 mg, calcium pantothenate 20 mg, E 15 mg, iron 15 mg, iodine 0.15 mg, calcium 50 mg, phosphorus 40 mg, copper 0.1 mg, manganese 0.1 mg, magnesium 5 mg, potassium 2 mg/Tab. Bot. 100s.
Use: Vitamin/mineral supplement.

VITA-SUP. (Kenyon) Vitamins A 12,500 IU, D 1000 IU, B_1 5 mg, B_2 2.5 mg, B_6 1 mg, B_{12} 2 mcg, C 75 mg, niacinamide 40

mg, calcium pantothenate 4 mg, E 3 IU, dicalcium phosphate 260 mg, choline bitartrate 31.4 mg, inositol 15 mg, liver protein fraction 25 mg, ferrous sulfate 102 mg, manganese sulfate 1.5 mg, potassium sulfate 4.5 mg, zinc sulfate 1.4 mg, magnesium sulfate 21.6 mg/Cap. Bot. 100s, 1000s.
Use: Vitamin/mineral supplement.

VITATONE DROPS. (Winthrop Products) Multivitamin.
Use: Dietary supplement.

VITATRUM. (Halsey).
Use: Dietary supplement.

VITAZIN. (Mesemer) Ascorbic acid 300 mg, niacinamide 100 mg, thiamine mononitrate 20 mg, d-calcium pantothenate 20 mg, riboflavin 10 mg, pyridoxine HCl 5 mg, magnesium sulfate 70 mg, zinc 25 mg/Cap. Bot. 100s.
Use: Vitamin/mineral supplement.

VITA-ZOO. (Towne) Vitamins A 2500 IU, D 400 IU, E 15 IU, C 60 mg, folic acid 0.3 mg, B_1 1.05 mg, B_2 1.2 mg, niacin 13.5 mg, B_6 1.05 mg, B_{12} 4.5 mcg/Tab. Bot. 100s.
Use: Vitamin supplement.

VITA-ZOO PLUS IRON. (Towne) Vitamins A 2500 IU, D 400 IU, E 15 IU, C 60 mg, folic acid 0.3 mg, B_1 1.05 mg, B_2 1.2 mg, niacin 13.5 mg, B_6 1.05 mg, B_{12} 4.5 mcg, iron 15 mg/Tab. Bot. 100s.
Use: Vitamin supplement.

VITEC. (Pharmaceutical Specialties) Dl-alpha tocopheryl acetate in a vanishing cream base. Cream. 120 Gm.
Use: Emollient.

VI-TESTROGEN. (Pharmex) Testosterone 10 mg, estrogenic substance (natural) 1 mg, vitamins B_1 50 mg, B_2 2 mg, B_6 5 mg, panthenol 10 mg, niacinamide 100 mg, inositol 25 mg, choline Cl 25 mg, d,l-methionine 25 mg/cc, sodium carboxymethylcellulose 0.05%, procaine HCl 1%, benzyl alcohol 2%. Vial 10 ml.
Use: Androgen, estrogen, vitamin supplement.

VITORMAINS. (Hauck) Tab. Bot. 100s.
Use: Vitamin supplement.

VITRON-C. (Ciba Consumer) Ferrous fumarate 200 mg, ascorbic acid 125 mg/Tab. Bot. 100s, 1000s.
Use: Vitamin/mineral supplement.

VITRON-C PLUS TABLETS. (Ciba Consumer) Ferrous fumarate 400 mg, vitamin C 250 mg/Tab. Bot. 30s, 100s, 500s.
Use: Vitamin/mineral supplement.

VIVACTIL. (Merck Sharp & Dohme) Protriptyline HCl 5 mg or 10 mg/Tab. **5 mg:**

Bot. 100s. **10 mg:** Bot. 100s, UD 100s.
Use: Antidepressant.

VIVA-DROPS. (Vision Pharm) Polysorbate 80, sodium Cl, EDTA, retinyl palmitate, mannitol, sodium citrate, pyruvate. Soln. Bot. 10 ml, 15 ml.
Use: Artificial tears.

VIVARIN. (Beecham Products) Caffeine alkaloid 200 mg/Tab. Blister Pk. 16s, 40s, 80s.
Use: Analeptic.

VIVIKON. (Brown) Vitamins B_1 5 mg, B_2 2 mg, B_6 10 mg, d-panthenol 5 mg, niacinamide 10 mg, procaine HCl 2%/ml. 100 ml.
Use: Vitamin supplement.

VIVONEX FLAVOR PACKETS. (Norwich Eaton) Non-nutritive flavoring for Vivonex diets when consumed orally. Orange-pineapple, lemon-lime, strawberry and vanilla. Pkg. 60s.
Use: Flavoring.

VIVONEX, STANDARD. (Norwich Eaton) Free amino acid/complete enteral nutrition. Six packets provide kilocalories 1800, available nitrogen 5.88 Gm as amino acids 37 Gm, fat 2.61 Gm, carbohydrate 407 Gm, and full day's balanced nutrition. Calorie:nitrogen ratio is 300:1. Unflavored pow. Packet 80 Gm, Pkg. 6s.
Use: Enteral nutritional supplement.

VIVONEX T.E.N. (Procter & Gamble) Free amino acid, high nitrogen/high branched chain amino acid complete enteral nutrition. Ten packets provide kilocalories 3000, available nitrogen 17 Gm, amino acids 115 Gm, fat 8.33 Gm, carbohydrate 617 Gm and full day's balanced nutrition. Calorie:nitrogen ratio is 175:1. Unflavored pow. Packet 80 Gm, Pkg. 10s.
Use: Enteral nutritional supplement.

VIVOTIF BERNA. (Berna) Typhoid vaccine (oral). *S. typhi* Ty21a (viable) 2 to 6 X 10^9 colony forming units and *S. typhi* Ty21a^2 (non-viable) 5 to 50 X 10^9 colony forming units/Cap. Single foil blister with 4 doses.
Use: Agent for immunization.

V-LAX. (Century) Psyllium mucilloid (hydrophilic) 50%, dextrose 50%. Pow. 0.25 lb, 1 lb.
Use: Laxative.

VLEMASQUE. (Dermik) Sulfurated lime topical solution 6% (Vleminck's Soln.), alcohol 7% in drying clay mask. Jar 4 oz.
Use: Anti-acne.

VM. (Last) Vitamins B_1 6 mg, B_2 4 mg, niacinamide 40 mg, iron 100 mg, calcium 188 mg phosphorus 188 mg, man-

gancac 4 mg, alcohol 12%. Bot. 10 oz.
Use: Vitamin/mineral supplement.
V-M CAPSULES. (Vale) Vitamins A, D,
B₁, B₂, B₆, C, niacinamide, Ca, Fe, calcium pantothenate, Mg, Mn, K, Zn, P/Tab.
Bot. 100s, 1000s.
Use: Vitamin/mineral supplement.
V-M TAB. (Kenyon) Vitamins A palmitate
5000 IU, D-2 500 IU, B₁ 2.5 mg, B₂ 2.5
mg, B₆ 0.5 mg, B₁₂ 1 mcg, C 50 mg,
niacinamide 15 mg, E 0.5 IU, d-calcium
pantothenate 5 mg, iron 25 mg, copper
0.375 mg, manganese 0.5 mg, zinc 0.15
mg, potassium 2.5 mg, magnesium 2.5
mg, iodine 0.05 mg/Tab. Bot. 100s,
1000s.
Use: Vitamin/mineral supplement.
• **VOLAZOCINE.** USAN. 3-(Cyclopropyl-
methyl)-1,2,3,4,5,6-hexahydro-cis-6,11-
dimethyl-2,6-methano-3-benzazocine.
Under study.
Use: Analgesic.
VOLIDAN. (British Drug House) Megestrol acetate.
VOLITANE. (Trent) Parethoxycaine 0.2%,
hexachlorophene 0.025%,
dichlorophene 0.025%. Aerosol spray
can 3 oz.
Use: Counterirritant, antiseptic.
VOLMAX TABLETS. (Muro) Albuterol su-
fate 4 mg or 8 mg. ER Tab. Bot. UD 60s.
Use: Bronchodilator.
VOLTAREN. (Geigy) Diclofenac sodium
25 mg, 50 mg, 75 mg. Tab. **25 mg:** Bot.
60s, 100s, UD 100s; **50 mg, 75 mg:** Bot.
60s, 100s, 1000s, UD 100s.
Use: Nonsteroidal anti-inflammatory
drug; analgesic.
VOLTAREN. (Ciba Vision Ophth.) Di-
clofenac sodium. 0.1% sol. Bot. 2.4, 5 ml
and dropper.
Use: Nonsteroidal anti-inflammatory
drug, ophthalmic.
VONEDRINE HYDROCHLORIDE.
Vonedrine (phenylpropylmethylamine)
HCl.
Use: Decongestant.
VONTROL. (Smith Kline & French)
Diphenidol 25 mg as HCl/Tab. Bot. 100s.
Use: Antiemetic/antivertigo agent.
• **VOROZOLE.** USAN.
Use: Antineoplastic.
VORTEL. Clorprenaline HCl.
Use: Bronchodilator.
VOSOL HC OTIC SOLUTION. (Wallace)
Propylene glycol diacetate 3%, acetic
acid 2%, benzethonium Cl 0.02%, hy-
drocortisone 1%. Bot. 10 ml.
Use: Otic preparation.
VOSOL OTIC SOLUTION. (Wallace)

Propylene glycol diacetate 3%, acetic
acid 2%, benzethonium Cl 0.02%, sodi-
um acetate 0.015%. Bot. 15 ml, 30 ml.
Use: Otic preparation.
• **VOTUMUMAB.** USAN.
Use: Monoclonal antibody.
VOXSUPRINE TABS. (Major) Isoxsuprine
HCl 10 mg or 20 mg/Tab. Bot. 100s,
250s, 1000s, UD 100s.
Use: Vasodilator.
V-TUSS EXPECTORANT. (Vangard) Hydrocodone bitartrate 5 mg, pseudoephedrine HCl 60 mg, guaifenesin
200 mg/5 ml, alcohol 12.5%.
Use: Antitussive, decongestant, expec-
torant.
VUMON. (Bristol-Myers Oncology) Teniposide 10 mg/ml. Amp. 5 ml.
Use: Antineoplastic.
V.V.S. (Econo Med) Sulfathiazole 3.42%,
sulfacetamide 2.86%, sulfabenzamide
3.7%, urea 0.64%. Cream. Tube 90 Gm
w/applicator.
Use: Vaginal preparations, anti-infective.
VYTONE CREAM. (Dermik) Hydrocortisone 1%, iodoquinol 1%, greaseless
base. Cream. Bot. 30 Gm.
Use: Corticosteroid combination, topical.
VZIG. (Varicella-zoser Immune Globulin)
Human (American Red Cross, North-
east Region) Globulin fraction of human
plasma, primarily 1 G/10% to 18% in single dose vials containing 125 units varicella-zoster virus antibody in 2.5 mg or
less. Inj.
Use: Immune serum.

W

WADE GESIC BALM. (Wade) Menthol
3%, methyl salicylate 12%, petrolatum
base. Tube oz, Jar lb.
Use: External analgesic.
WADE'S DROPS. Compound Benzoin
Tincture.
WAKESPAN. (Weeks & Leo) Caffeine
250 mg/TR Cap. Vial 15s.
Use: Analeptic.
WAL-FINATE ALLERGY TABS. (Wal-
green) Chlorpheniramine maleate 4
mg/Tab. Bot. 50s.
Use: Antihistamine.
WAL-FINATE DECONGESTANT TABS.
(Walgreen) Chlorpheniramine maleate 4
mg, pseudoephedrine sulfate 60
mg/Tab. Bot. 50s.
Use: Antihistamine, decongestant.

WAL-FORMULA COUGH SYRUP WITH d-METHORPHAN. (Walgreen) Dextromethorphan HBr 15 mg, doxylamine succinate 7.5 mg, sodium citrate 500 mg/10 ml. Bot. 6 oz, 8 oz.
Use: Antitussive, antihistamine, expectorant.

WAL-FORMULA D COUGH SYRUP. (Walgreen) Dextromethorphan HBr 20 mg, phenylpropanolamine HCl 25 mg, guaifenesin 100 mg/10 ml, alcohol 10%. Bot. 6 oz, 8 oz.
Use: Antitussive, decongestant, expectorant.

WAL-FORMULA M COUGH SYRUP. (Walgreen) Dextromethorphan HBr 30 mg, pseudoephedrine HCl 60 mg, guaifenesin 200 mg, acetaminophen 500 mg/20 ml Bot. 8 oz.
Use: Antitussive, decongestant, expectorant, analgesic.

WAL-FRIN NASAL MIST. (Walgreen) Phenylephrine HCl 0.5%, pheniramine maleate 0.2% Bot. 0.5 oz.
Use: Decongestant, antihistamine.

WALGREEN ARTIFICIAL TEARS. (Walgreen) Hydroxypropyl methylcellulose 0.5%. Bot. 0.5 oz.
Use: Artificial tear solution.

WALGREEN'S FINEST IRON TABLETS. (Walgreen) Iron 30 mg/Tab. Bot. 100s.
Use: Iron supplement.

WALGREEN'S FINEST VIT B$_6$. (Walgreen) Pyridoxine HCl 50 mg/Tab. Bot. 100s.
Use: Vitamin B$_6$ supplement.

WALGREEN SODA MINTS. (Walgreen) Sodium bicarbonate 300 mg/Tab. Bot. 100s, 200s.
Use: Antacid.

WAL-MINIC. (Walgreen) Phenylpropanolamine HCl 12.5 mg, guaifenesin 100 mg/5 ml, alcohol 5%. Bot. 6 oz, 8 oz.
Use: Decongestant, expectorant.

WAL-MINIC COLD RELIEF MEDICINE. (Walgreen) Phenylpropanolamine HCl 12.5 mg, chlorpheniramine maleate 2 mg/5 ml Bot. 6 oz, 8 oz.
Use: Decongestant, antihistamine.

WAL-MINIC DM. (Walgreen) Phenylpropanolamine HCl 12.5 mg, dextromethorphan HBr 10 mg/5 ml Bot. 6 oz, 8 oz.
Use: Decongestant, antitussive.

WAL-PHED PLUS. (Walgreen) Pseudoephedrine HCl 60 mg, chlorpheniramine maleate 4 mg/Tab. Bot. 50s.
Use: Decongestant, antihistamine.

WAL-PHED SYRUP. (Walgreen) Pseudoephedrine HCl 30 mg/5 ml. Bot. 4 oz.
Use: Decongestant.

WAL-PHED TABLETS. (Walgreen) Pseudoephedrine HCl 30 mg/Tab. Bot. 50s, 100s.
Use: Decongestant.

WAL-TAP ELIXIR. (Walgreen) Brompheniramine maleate 2 mg, phenylpropanolamine HCl 12.5 mg/5 ml. Bot. 4 oz.
Use: Antihistamine, decongestant.

WAL-TUSSIN. (Walgreen) Guaifenesin 100 mg/5 ml. Bot. 4 oz.
Use: Expectorant.

WAL-TUSSIN DM. (Walgreen) Guaifenesin 100 mg, dextromethorphan HBr 15 ml/5 ml. Bot. 4 oz, 8 oz.
Use: Expectorant, antitussive.

WAMPOLE ONE-STEP hCG. (Wampole) For in vitro detection of human chorionic gonadotropin in serum and urine. Test. In 3, 24, 96, 500 test kits.
Use: Pregnancy test.

WARFARIN. B.A.N. (Various Mtr.) Comp. 42. 3-(alpha-Acetonylbenzyl)-4-hydroxy coumarin. 4-Hydroxy-3-(3-oxo-1-phenyl-butyl)coumarin.
Use: Rodenticide, anticoagulant.
See: Coumadin.
Marevan (sodium derivative).

•**WARFARIN SODIUM,** U.S.P. XXIII. For Inj., Tab., U.S.P. XXIII 2H-1-Benzopyran-2-one, 4-hydroxy-3-(3-oxo-1-phenylbutyl)-, sodium salt. 3-(alpha-Acetonyl-benzyl)-4-hydroxycoumarin and its sodium salt athrombin.
Use: Anticoagulant.
See: Coumadin Sodium, Tab., Inj. (DuPont).
Sofarin, Tab. (Lemmon).
Panwarfin, Tab. (Abbott).

WART-AID. (Republic) Calcium pantothenate, ascorbic acid, starch. 15 Gm.
Use: Keratolytic.

WART FIX. (Last) Castor oil 100%. Bot. 0.3 fl oz.
Use: Wart removal.

WARTGON. (E.J. Moore) Castor oil. Tube 0.5 oz.
Use: Wart removal.

WART-OFF. (Leeming) Salicylic acid 17% in flexible collodion, alcohol 20.5%, ether 54.2%. Bot. 0.5 oz.
Use: Keratolytic.

•**WATER,** U.S.P. XXIII is found in the following grades of purity:
Bacteriostatic Water for Injection, U.S.P. XXIII.
Purified Water, U.S.P. XXIII.
Sterile Water For Inhalation, U.S.P.

XXIII.
Sterile Water For Injection, U.S.P.
XXIII.
Sterile Water For Irrigation, U.S.P.
XXIII.
Water, U.S.P. XXIII.
Water For Injection, U.S.P. XXIII.
Use: Pharmaceutic aid (solvent), irriga-
tion therapy, vehicle, fluid.
See: Abbott Labs. for sizes of each
available.
Upjohn for sizes available.
• **WATER O 15,** Inj., U.S.P. 23.
**WATER BABIES LITTLE LICKS BY COP-
PERTONE.** (Plough) SPF 30, ethyl-
hexyl p-methoxycinnamate, oxyben-
zone, 2-ethylhexyl salicylate, cherry fla-
vor. Tube 4.8 Gm.
Use: Sunscreen.
WATER BABIES SUNBLOCK CREAM.
(Plough) SPF 25, ethylhexyl p-
methoxycinnamate, 2-ethylhexyl salicy-
late, homosalate, oxybenzone, benzyl
alcohol. PABA free, waterproof. Cream.
Bot. 90 Gm.
Use: Sunscreen.
**WATER BABIES UVA/UVB SUNBLOCK
LOTION.** (Schering-Plough) SPF 30
ethylhexyl p-methoxycinnamate, 2-eth-
ylhexyl salicylate, homosalate, oxyben-
zone, benzyl alcohol. PABA free, water-
proof. Lot. Bot. 120 ml, 240 ml.
Use: Sunscreen.
**WATER BABIES UVA/UVB SUNBLOCK
LOTION.** (Schering-Plough) SPF 45,
ethylhexyl p-methoxycinnamate, 2-eth-
ylhexyl salicylate, otocrylene oxyben-
zone, benzyl alcohol. PABA free, water-
proof. Lot. Bot. 120 ml.
Use: Sunscreen.
**WATER BABIES UVA/UVB SUNBLOCK
LOTION.** (Schering-Plough) Ethylhexyl-
P-methoxycinnamate, oxybenzone in lo-
tion base, SPF-15. Bot. 120 ml.
Use: Sunscreen.
WATERMELON SEED EXTRACT. Citrin
(Table Rock).
WATERMELON SEED EXTRACT.
W/Phenobarbital, theobromine. Cithal
(Table Rock).
WATER-MISCIBLE VITAMIN A.
See: Acon, Cap. (DuPont).
Aquasol Vitamin A, Cap. (USV Labs.).
Vi-Dom-A, Cap. (Miles Pharm).
• **WATER O/#15.** USAN.
Use: Diagnostic aid (radioactive, vascu-
lar disorders); radioactive agent.
• **WAX, CARNAUBA,** N.F. XVIII.
Use: Pharmaceutic aid (tablet polishing
agent).

• **WAX, EMULSIFYING,** N.F. XVIII.
Use: Emulsifying agent, stiffening
agent.
• **WAX, MICROCRYSTALLINE,** N.F. XVIII.
Use: Pharmaceutic aid (stiffening
agent).
• **WAX, WHITE,** U.S.P.XVII.
Use: Pharmaceutic aid (stiffening
agent).
• **WAX, YELLOW,** N.F. XVIII.
Use: Stiffening agent.
WAXSOL. Docusate Sodium, U.S.P.
XXIII.
WAYDS. (Wayne) Docusate sodium 100
mg/Cap. Bot. 100s.
Use: Laxative.
WAYDS-PLUS CAPSULES. (Wayne) Do-
cusate w/casanthranol. Bot. 50s.
Use: Laxative.
WAYNADE T-D CAPSULES. (Wayne)
Antihistamine compound. Bot. 100s.
Use: Antihistamine.
WAYNE-E CAPSULES. (Wayne) Vitamin
E **100 IU or 200 IU/Cap.:** Bot. 1000s.
400 IU/Cap.: Bot. 100s.
Use: Vitamin E supplement.
WAYSED TABLETS. (Wayne) Bot. 100s,
1000s.
WEHDRYL. (Hauck) Diphenhydramine
HCl 50 mg/ml. Inj. Vial 10 ml.
Use: Antihistamine.
WEHGEN. (Hauck) Estrogenic substance
or estrogens (mainly estrone) 2 mg/ml,
sodium carboxymethylcellulose,
polysorbate 80, methyl and propyl
parabens. Inj. Aqueous susp. Vial 10 ml.
Use: Estrogen.
WEHLESS. (Hauck) Phendimetrazine
tartrate 35 mg/Cap. Bot. 100s.
Use: Anorexiant.
WEHLESS-105 TIMECELLES. (Hauck)
Phendimetrazine tartrate 105 mg/SA
Cap. Bot. 100s.
Use: Anorexiant.
WEHYDRYL. (Hauck) Diphenhydramine
HCl 50 mg/ml. Vial 10 ml.
Use: Antihistamine.
WELDERS EYE LOTION. (Weber) Tetra-
caine, potassium Cl, boric acid, cam-
phor, glycerin, disodium edetate, benza-
lkonium Cl as preservatives. Bot. oz.
Use: Burn preparation.
WELLBUTRIN. (Burroughs Wellcome)
Bupropion 75 mg or 100 mg/Tab. Bot.
100s.
Use: Antidepressant.
WELLCOVORIN. (Burroughs Wellcome)
Leucovorin 5 mg or 25 mg as calcium.
Tab.: 5 mg: Bot. 20s, 100s, UD 50s. **25**

mg: Bot. 25s, UD 10s. **Pow. for Inj.:** 100 mg/vial as calcium.
Use: Prophylaxis and treatment of the undesired hematopoietic effects of folic acid antagonists.
WELLDORM. Dichloralphenazone. B.A.N.
WERNET'S ADHESIVE CREAM. (Block) Carboxymethylcellulose gum, ethylene oxide polymer, petrolatum in mineral oil base. Cream. Tube 1.5 oz.
Use: Denture adhesive.
WERNET'S POWDER. (Block) Karaya gum, ethylene oxide polymer. Bot. 0.63 oz, 1.75 oz, 3.55 oz.
Use: Denture adhesive.
WES-B/C. (Western Research) Vitamins B_1 15 mg, B_2 10 mg, B_6 5 mg, niacinamide 50 mg, calcium pantothenate 10 mg, C 300 mg/Cap. Bot. 1000s.
Use: Vitamin supplement.
WESCOHEX. (West) Bot. 5 oz, pt, gal.
Use: Antibacterial skin cleanser.
WESMATIC FORTE TABLETS. (Wesley) Phenobarbital 1/8 gr, ephedrine sulfate 0.25 gr, chlorpheniramine maleate 2 mg, guaifenesin 100 mg/Tab. Bot. 100s, 1000s.
Use: Sedative/hypnotic, decongestant, antihistamine, expectorant.
WESTCORT CREAM. (Westwood-Squibb) Hydrocortisone valerate 0.2% in a hydrophilic base with white petrolatum. Tube 15 Gm, 45 Gm, 60 Gm, 120 Gm.
Use: Corticosteroid, topical.
WESTCORT OINTMENT. (Westwood-Squibb) Hydrocortisone valerate 0.2% in hydrophilic base with white petrolatum, mineral oil. Tube 15 Gm, 45 Gm, 60 Gm.
Use: Corticosteroid, topical.
WESTHROID. (Western Research) Thyroid 0.5 gr, 1 gr, 2 gr, 3 gr or 4 gr/Tab.; 5 gr/SC Tab. Handicount 28s (36 bags of 28s).
Use: Thyroid hormone.
WESTRIM. (Western Research) Phenylpropanolamine HCl 37.5 mg/Tab. Bot. 100s.
Use: Diet aid, decongestant.
WESTRIM-LA 50. (Western Research) Phenylpropanolamine HCl 50 mg/TR Cap. Bot. 1000s.
Use: Diet aid, decongestant.
WESTRIM-LA 75. (Western Research) Phenylpropanolamine HCl 75 mg/TR Cap. Bot. 1000s.
Use: Diet aid, decongestant.
WESVITE. (Western Research) Vitamins B_1 10 mg, B_2 5 mg, B_6 2 mg, pantothenic acid 10 mg, niacinamide 30 mg,

B_{12} 3 mcg, C 100 mg, E 5 IU, A 10,000 IU, D 400 IU, iron 15 mg, copper 1 mg, iodine 0.15 mg, manganese 1 mg, zinc 1.5 mg/Tab. Bot. 1000s.
Use: Vitamin/mineral supplement.
WET-N-SOAK. (Allergan) Borate buffered. WSL 0.006%, hydroxyethylcellulose. Soln. Bot. 15 ml.
Use: Hard contact lens care.
WET-N-SOAK PLUS. (Allergan). Polyvinyl alcohol, edetate disodium, benzalkonium Cl 0.003%. Soln. Bot. 120 ml, 180 ml.
Use: Contact lens care.
WETTING SOLUTION. (Pilkington Barnes Hind) Polyvinyl alcohol, benzalkonium Cl 0.004%, EDTA 0.02%. Soln. Bot. 60 ml.
Use: Hard contact lens care.
WETTING AND SOAKING. (Pilkington Barnes Hind) Buffered, isotonic. Chlorhexidine gluconate 0.005%, EDTA 0.002%, NaCl, octylphenoxy (oxyethylene) ethanol, povidone, polyvinyl alcohol, propylene glycol, hydroxyethylcellulose. Soln. Bot. 120 ml.
Use: Hard contact lens care.
WETTING AND SOAKING SOLUTION. (Bausch & Lomb) Polyvinyl alcohol, hydroxethyl cellulose w/chlorhexidine gluconate and EDTA. Soln. Bot. 120 ml.
Use: Disinfecting/wetting/soaking solution.
WHEAT GERM OIL. (Viobin) **Liq.:** Bot. 4 oz, 8 oz, pt, qt. **Cap.: 3 min.** Bot. 100s, 400s; **6 min.** Bot. 100s, 225s, 400s; **20 min.** Bot. 100s.
Use: Vitamin E supplement.
WHEAT GERM OIL. (Various Mfr.).
See: Natural Wheat Germ Oil, Cap., Oint. (Spirt).
Natural Viobin Wheat Germ Oil, Liq. (Spirt).
Tocopherol Preps. (Various Mfr.).
Use: Vitamin E supplement.
WHEAT GERM OIL CONCENTRATE. (Thurston) Perles. 6 min. Bot. 100s.
Use: Heart disorders, heart muscle fatigue.
WHIRL-SOL. (Sween) Moisturizing bath additive. Bot. 2 oz, 8 oz, 16 oz, 21 oz, gal, 5 gal, 30 gal, 55 gal.
Use: Emollient.
WHITE IODINE. (Pharmex) Bot. 0.5 oz.
• **WHITE LOTION,** U.S.P. XXIII. Lotio Alba.
Use: Astringent, topical protectant.
See: Lotioblanc, Lot. (Arnar-Stone).
• **WHITE OINTMENT,** U.S.P. XXIII.
Use: Pharmaceutic aid (oleaginous ointment base).

WHITE PRECIPITATE.
See: Ammoniated Mercury, U.S.P. XXIII.
WHITFIELD'S OINTMENT. (Various Mfr.)
Benzoic acid 6%, salicylic acid 3%.
Use: Anti-infective, external.
WHITSPHILL. (Torch) Salicylic acid 6%,
benzoic acid 12% in hydrophilic vehicle.
Jar 2 oz, lb. Also available in half
strength.
Use: Anti-infective, external.
WHOOPING COUGH VACCINE.
See: Pertussis Vaccine, U.S.P. XXIII.
WHORTON'S CALAMINE LOTION.
(Whorton) Calamine, zinc oxide, glycerin
(U.S.P. strength) in carboxymethylcellu-
lose lotion vehicle. Bot. 4 oz, gal.
Use: Minor skin irritations.
WHORTON'S SKIN CARE CREAM.
(Whorton) 5 oz, 16 oz.
WIBI LOTION. (Owen) Purified water, SD
alcohol 40, glycerin, PEG-4, PEG-6-32
stearate, PEG-6-32, glycol stearate, car-
bomer 940, PEG-75, methylparaben,
propylparaben, triethanolamine, men-
thol, fragrance. Bot. 8 oz, 16 oz.
Use: Emollient.
**WIDOW SPIDER SPECIES ANTIVENIN
(LATRODECTUS MACTANS).** An-
tivenin, Lactrodectus mactans, U.S.P.
XXIII.
Use: Passive immunizing agent.
WIGRAINE. (Organon) Ergotamine tar-
trate 1 mg, caffeine 100 mg/Tab. or
Supp. **Tab.:** Box 20s, 100s. **Supp.:** Box
12s.
Use: Agent for migraine.
WILD CHERRY.
Use: Flavored vehicle.
WILPOWR. (Foy) Phentermine HCl 30
mg/Cap. Bot. 100s, 500s, 1000s.
Use: Anorexiant.
WILPOR-CLEAR. (Foy) Phentermine HCl
30 mg/Cap. Bot. 1000s.
Use: Anorexiant.
WINSTROL. (Sanofi Winthrop)
Stanozolol 2 mg/Tab. Bot. 100s.
Use: Anabolic steroid.
WINTERGREEN OINTMENT. (Wiscon-
sin) Bot. 2 oz, lb.
Use: External analgesic.
WINTERGREEN SUCRETS. (SK-
Beecham) Dyclonine HCl 0.1%, alcohol
10%, sorbitol. Spray. Bot. 90 ml.
Use: Mouth, throat product.
WITCH HAZEL. (Various Mfr.) Ham-
mamelis water (Witch Hazel). Bot. 120
ml, 240 ml, 280 ml, 480 ml, 960 ml, gal.
Use: Astringent.
WITHIN. (Miles) Vitamins A 5000 IU, E 30
IU, C 60 mg, folic acid 0.4 mg, B_1 1.5

mg, B_2 1.7 mg, niacin 20 mg, B_6 2 mg,
B_{12} 6 mcg, pantothenic acid 10 mg, D
400 IU, iron 27 mg, calcium 450 mg, zinc
15 mg/Tab. Bot. 60s, 100s.
Use: Vitamin/mineral supplement.
WNS SUPPOSITORIES. (Sanofi
Winthrop) Sulfamylon HCl.
Use: Anorectal preparation.
WONDERFUL DREAM SALVE. (Kondon)
Phenylmercuric nitrate 1:5000, oils of
tar, turpentine, olive and linseed oil,
rosin, burgundy pitch, camphor.
WONDER ICE. (Pedinol) Menthol in a
specially formulated base. Gel. Tube
113 Gm.
Use: Liniment.
WONDRA. (Procter & Gamble) Petrolatum, lanolin acid, glycerin, stearyl alco-
hol, cyclomethicone, EDTA, hydrogenat-
ed vegetable glycerides phosphate,
cetyl alcohol, isopropyl palmitate, stearic
acid, PEG-100 stearate, carbomer-934,
dimethicone, titanium dioxide, imidazo-
lidinyl urea, parabens. Lot. Bot. 180 ml,
300 ml, 450 ml.
Use: Emollient.
WOOD CHARCOAL TABLETS. (Cowley)
5 gr or 10 gr/Tab. Bot. 1000s.
WOOD CREOSOTE.
See: Creosote (Various Mfr.).
WOOL FAT. Lanolin, Anhydrous.
W/W-ANTI-SPAS. (Whiteworth) Antispas-
modic compound Bot. 16 oz.
Use: Antispasmodic.
W/W-BROMINE. (Whiteworth)
Brompheniramine. Elix. Bot. 16 oz, gal.
Use: Expectorant.
W/W-BROMINE DS. (Whiteworth)
Brompheniramine DC. Bot. 16 oz.
Use: Expectorant.
W/W-FED LIQUID. (Whiteworth) Triproli-
dine, pseudoephedrine. Syr. Bot. 16 oz,
gal.
Use: Antihistamine, decongestant.
W/W-FED TABLETS. (Whiteworth)
Triprolidine, pseudoephedrine. Tab. Bot.
100s, 1000s.
Use: Antihistamine, decongestant.
W/W FED w/C. (Whiteworth) Triprolidine,
pseudoephedrine, codeine. Bot. 16 oz,
gal.
Use: Antihistamine, decongestant, anti-
tussive.
W/W HISTINE DH. (Whiteworth) Phenyl-
histine DH. Elix. Bot. 16 oz.
Use: Antihistamine.
W/W-HISTINE ELIXIR. (Whiteworth)
Phenylhistine. Elix. Bot. 16 oz.
Use: Antihistamine.
W/W-HISTINE EXPECTORANT. (White-

worth) Phenylhistine expectorant. Bot. 16 oz.
Use: Antihistamine.
WYAMINE SULFATE INJECTION.
(Wyeth-Ayerst) Mephentermine sulfate 15 mg or 30 mg, methylparaben 1.8 mg, propylparaben 0.2 mg/ml. Vial 10 ml. Amp. 2 ml.
Use: Vasopressor.
WYANOIDS. (Wyeth-Ayerst) Ephedrine sulfate 3 mg, belladonna extract 15 mg, boric acid, zinc oxide, bismuth oxyiodide and subcarbonate, balsam peru, beeswax, cocoa butter/Supp. Box 12s.
Use: Anorectal preparation.
WYDASE LYOPHILIZED. (Wyeth-Ayerst) Hyaluronidase. Vial 150 units/ml or 1500 units/10 ml with lactose and thimerosal.
Use: Hyaluronidase.
WYDASE STABILIZED SOLUTION.
(Wyeth-Ayerst) Hyaluronidase 150 units in sterile saline soln. with sodium Cl, EDTA, thimerosal. Vial 1 ml, 10 ml.
Use: Hyaluronidase.
WYGESIC. (Wyeth-Ayerst) Propoxyphene HCl 65 mg, acetaminophen 650 mg/Tab. Bot. 100s, 500s, Redipak 100s.
Use: Narcotic analgesic combination.
WYMOX. (Wyeth-Ayerst) Amoxicillin as trihydrate. **Cap.:** 250 mg Bot. 100s, 500s; 500 mg Bot. 50s, 500s. **Oral Susp.:** 125 mg/5 ml Bot. to make 80 ml, 100 ml, 150 ml; 250 mg/5 ml Bot. to make 80 ml, 100 ml, 150 ml.
Use: Antibacterial, penicillin.
WYOVIN HYDROCHLORIDE. Dicyclomine. B.A.N.
WYTENSIN. (Wyeth-Ayerst) Guanabenz acetate. **4 mg/Tab.:** Bot. 100s, 500s, Redipak 100s. **8 mg/Tab.:** Bot. 100s. **16 mg/Tab.:** Bot. 100s.
Use: Antihypertensive.

X

• **XAMOTEROL.** USAN.
Use: Cardiac stimulant.
XAMOTEROL FUMARATE. USAN.
Use: Cardiac stimulant.
XANAX. (Upjohn) Alprazolam 0.25 mg, 0.5 mg, 1 mg or 2 mg. Tab. **0.25 mg, 0.5 mg, 2 mg:** Bot. 100s, 500s, UD 100s. Visipack 4 × 25s. **1 mg:** Bot. 30s, 90s, 100s, 500s, UD 100s.
Use: Antianxiety agent.
• **XANOMELINE.** USAN.
Use: cholinergic agonist.
• **XANOXATE SODIUM.** USAN.

Use: Bronchodilator.
• **XANTHAN GUM,** N.F. XVIII.
Use: Suspending agent.
XANTHINE DERIVATIVES.
See: Caffeine.
Theobromine.
Theophylline.
• **XANTHINOL NIACINATE.** USAN. 7-{2-Hydroxy-3-[(2-hydroxyethyl))methylamino]-propyl theophylline compound with nicotinic acid.
Use: Vasodilator (peripheral).
See: Complamex.
Complamin.
XANTHIOL HCl. 4-[3-(2-Chlorothioxanthene-9-yl)-propyl]-1-pipera zine-propanol dihydrochloride.
Use: Antinauseant.
See: Daxid (Roerig).
XANTHOCILLIN. B.A.N. Antibiotics obtained from the mycelium of *Penicillium notatum* (Xanthocillin X is 2:3-Diisocyano1:4-di(p-hydroxyphenyl)buta-1:3-diene).
XANTHOTOXIN. Methoxsalen.
X-DRIN. (Pharmex) **Cap.:** Bot. 72s. **Pellet:** Bot. 144s. **Tab.:** Bot. 21s, 90s.
Use: Dietary.
• **XENBUCIN.** USAN.
Use: Antihypercholesteremic.
• **XENON Xe 127,** U.S.P. XXIII.
Use: Radioactive agent.
• **XENON Xe 133,** U.S.P. XXIII.
Use: Radioactive agent.
XENTHIORATE HCl. 2-Diethylaminoethyl-2(4-bi-phenylyl)thiobutyrate HCl.
XENYSALATE. B.A.N. 2-Diethylaminoethyl 3-phenylsalicylate. Sebaclen is the hydrochloride.
Use: Treatment of seborrhea.
XERAC AC. (Person & Covey) Aluminum Cl hexahydrate 6.25% in anhydrous ethanol 96%. Bot 35 ml, 60 ml.
Use: Anti-acne.
XERODERM LOTION. (Dermol Pharm.) Mineral oil, acetylate lanolin alcohol, cetyl alcohol, glycerin, triethanolamine, parabens, imidazolidinyl urea. Lot. Bot. 267 ml.
Use: Emollient.
XEROFORM OINTMENT 3%.
(City) Pow. 0.25 lb, 1 lb.
(Consolidated) Jar 1 lb, 5 lb.
XERO-LUBE. (Scherer) Monobasic potassium phosphate, dibasic potassium phosphate, magnesium Cl, potassium Cl, calcium Cl, sodium Cl, sodium fluoride, sorbitol soln., sodium carboxymethylcellulose, methylparaben.

Bot. 6 oz.
Use: Mouth and throat product.
- **XILOBAM.** USAN.
  Use: Relaxant (muscle).
- **XIPAMIDE.** USAN.
  Use: Antihypertensive, diuretic.
- **XORPHANOL MESYLATE.** USAN.
  Use: Analgesic.

X-PREP BOWEL EVACUANT KIT-1.
(Purdue Frederick) Kit contains Senokot S tab., X-Prep liquid, Rectolax supp.
Use: Laxative.

X-PREP BOWEL EVACUANT KIT-2.
(Purdue Frederick) Kit contains citralax granules, X-Prep liquid, Rectolax supp.
Use: Laxative.

X-PREP LIQUID. (Gray) Senna extract with alcohol 7%, sucrose 50 Gm. Bot. 2.5 oz.
Use: Laxative.

X-RAY CONTRAST MEDIA.
See: Iodine Products, Diagnostic.

X-SEB PLUS. (Baker Cummins) Pyrithionic zinc 1%, salicylic acid 2%. Shampoo. Bot. 120 ml.
Use: Antiseborrheic combination.

X-SEB SHAMPOO. (Baker/Cummins) Salicylic acid 4%, coal tar soln. 10% in a blend of surface-active agents. Bot. 4 oz.
Use: Antiseborrheic.

X-SEB T. (Baker/Cummins) Coal tar soln. 10%, salicylic acid 4%. Bot. 4 oz.
Use: Antiseborrheic.

X-SEP T PLUS. (Baker Cummins) Coal tar solution 10%, salicylic acid, menthol 1%. Shampoo. Bot. 120 ml.
Use: Antiseborrheic combination.

XTRACARE. (Sween) Bot. 2 oz, 4 oz, 8 oz, 21 oz, gal.
Use: Emollient.

XTRA-VITES. (Barth's) Vitamins A 10,000 IU, D 400 IU, C 150 mg, B_1 5 mg, B_2 1 mg, niacin 3.33 mg, pantothenic acid 183 mcg, B_6 250 mcg, B_{12} 215 mg, E 15 IU, rutin 20 mg, citrus bioflavonoid complex 15 mg, choline 6.67 mg, inositol 10 mg, folic acid 50 mcg, biotin, aminobenzoic acid/Tab. Bot. 30s, 90s, 180s, 360s.
Use: Vitamin supplement.

X-TROZINE CAPSULES. (Rexar) Phendimetrazine tartrate 35 mg/Cap. Bot. 1000s.
Use: Anorexiant.

X-TROZINE S.R. CAPSULES. (Rexar) Phendimetrazine tartrate 105 mg/SR Cap. Bot. 100s, 200s, 1000s.
Use: Anorexiant.

X-TROZINE TABLETS. (Rexar) Phendimetrazine tartrate 35 mg/Tab.

Bot. 1000c.
Use: Anorexiant.
- **XYLAMIDINE TOSYLATE.** USAN. N-[2-(m-Methoxyphenoxy)propyl]-2-m-tolylacetamidine mono-p-toluenesulfonate hemihydrate.
  Use: Antiserotonin.
- **XYLAZINE HYDROCHLORIDE.** USAN.
  Use: Analgesic, relaxant (muscle).
- **XYLITOL,** N.F. XVIII.

XYLOCAINE HYDROCHLORIDE. (Astra) Lidocaine HCl. **Amp.:** (1%): 2 ml, 5 ml, 30 ml; w/epinephrine 1:200,000 30 ml. (1.5%): 20 ml; w/epinephrine 1:200,000 30 ml. (2%): 2 ml, 10 ml; w/epinephrine 1:200,000 20 ml. (4%): 5 ml. **Multi-dose Vial:** (0.5%): 50 ml; w/epinephrine 1:200,000 50 ml. (1%): 20 ml, 50 ml; w/epinephrine 1:100,000 20 ml, 50 ml. (2%): 20 ml, 50 ml; w/epinephrine 1:100,000 20 ml, 50 ml. **Single-dose Vial:** (1%): 30 ml. (1.5%) 20 ml; w/epinephrine 1:200,000 10 ml, 30 ml. (2%) w/epinephrine 1:200,000 20 ml.
Use: Local anesthetic.

XYLOCAINE HYDROCHLORIDE FOR CARDIAC ARRHYTHMIA. (Astra) **Intravenous:** Lidocaine 2%. Amp 5 ml, disp. syringe 5 ml. Continuous infusion 1 Gm/25 ml Vial; 2 Gm/50 ml Vial. Prefilled syringe 100 mg/5 ml, 12s. Continuous infusion prefilled syringe 1 Gm, 2 Gm. **Intramuscular:** Amp. 10%, 5 ml.
Use: Local anesthetic.

XYLOCAINE HYDROCHLORIDE 4% SOLUTION. (Astra) Topical use. Bot. 50 ml.
Use: Local anesthetic.

XYLOCAINE HYDROCHLORIDE FOR SPINAL ANESTHESIA. (Astra) Lidocaine HCl 1.5% or 5%, glucose 7.5%, sodium hydroxide to adjust pH. Specific gravity 1.028-1.034. Amp. 2 ml. Box 10s.
Use: Local anesthetic.

XYLOCAINE HYDROCHLORIDE W/DEXTROSE. (Astra) Lidocaine HCl 1.5%, dextrose 7.5%. Inj. Amps. 2 ml.
Use: Local anesthetic, injectable.

XYLOCAINE HYDROCHLORIDE W/EPINEPHRINE. (Astra) Lidocaine HCl 2% w/epinephrine 1:200,000. Amps w/sodium metabisulfate 20 ml. Inj. Single dose vials w/sodium metabisulfate. 20 ml.
Use: Local anesthetic, injectable.

XYLOCAINE HYDROCHLORIDE W/GLUCOSE. (Astra) Lidocaine HCl 5%, glucose 7.5%. Inj. Amp. 2 ml.
Use: Local anesthetic, injectable.

XYLOCAINE JELLY. (Astra) Lidocaine HCl 2% in sodium carboxymethylcellu-

lose with parabens. Tube 30 ml.
Use: Local anesthetic.
XYLOCAINE OINTMENT. (Astra) Lido-
caine base 5%. Tube 3.5 Gm, 35 Gm.
Ointment base of polyethylene glycols
and propylene glycol.
Use: Local anesthetic.
XYLOCAINE VISCOUS. (Astra) Lido-
caine HCl 2%, sodium carboxymethyl-
cellulose, parabens. Bot. 20 ml (25s),
100 ml, 450 ml.
Use: Local anesthetic.
• **XYLOFILCON A.** USAN.
Use: Contact lens material.
• **XYLOMETAZOLINE HCl,** U.S.P. XXIII.
Nasal Soln., U.S.P. XXIII. 2-(4-tert-Butyl-
2,6-dimethyl benzyl)-2- imidazoline HCl.
Use: Adrenergic (vasoconstrictor).
See: Isohalent L.A., Liq. (Elder).
Long Acting Neo-Synephrine, Prods.
(Winthrop Consumer Products).
Otrivin Spray (Geigy).
Rhinall L.A., Liq. (First Texas).
Sine-Off, Spray (Menley & James).
Vicks Sinex Long Acting, Nasal Spray
(Vicks).
XYLO-PFAN. (Adria) Xylose 25 Gm/Bot.
Use: Diagnostic aid.
**XYLOPHAN D-XYLOSE TOLERANCE
TEST.** (Pfanstiehl) D-xylose 25 Gm/UD
bot.
Use: Diagnostic aid.
• **XYLOSE,** U.S.P. XXIII.
Use: Diagnostic aid (intestinal function
determination).

Y

YAGER'S LINIMENT. (Yager) Oil of tur-
pentine and camphor w/clove oil fra-
grance, emulsifier, emollient, ammonium
oleate (less than 0.5% free ammonia)
penetrant base.
Use: Rubefacient.
YATREN.
See: Chiniofon, Tab.
YDP LICE SPRAY. (Youngs Drug) Syn-
thetic pyrethroid in aerosoln. Can 5 oz.
Use: Pediculicide for inanimate objects.
YEAST ADENYLIC ACID. An isomer of
adenosine 5-monophosphate, has been
found inactive.
See: Adenosine 5-Monophosphate,
Preps. for active compounds.
YEAST, DRIED.
Use: Protein and vitamin B Complex
source.
YEAST TABLETS, DRIED.
Use: Supplementary source of B com-

plex vitamins.
See: Brewer's Yeast, Tab.
YEAST, TORULA.
See: Torula Yeast.
YEAST W/IRON.
See: Natural Super Iron Yeast Powder
(Spirt) (Pharmex) Bot. 200s.
YEAST-X. (C.B. Fleet) **Supp.:** Pulsatilla
28x. Pkg. 12s; **Pow.:** Cornstarch, zinc
oxide, benzethonium chloride. 196 g.
Use: Vaginal preparation.
YELETS. (Freeda) Iron 60 mg, vitamins A
10,000 IU, D 400 IU, E 10 IU, B_1 10 mg,
B_2 10 mg, B_3 25 mg, B_5 10 mg, B_6 10
mg, B_{12} 10 mcg, C 100 mg, folic acid 0.1
mg, PABA, lysine, glutamic acid, Ca, I,
Mg, Mn/Tab. Bot. 100s, 250s, 500s.
Use: Vitamin/mineral supplement.
YELLOW ENZYME.
See: Riboflavin (Various Mfr.).
• **YELLOW FERRIC OXIDE,** N.F. XVIII.
Use: Pharmaceutic aid (color).
• **YELLOW FEVER VACCINE,** U.S.P. XXIII.
Use: Active immunizing agent.
See: YF-VAX, Inj. (Squibb/Connaught).
YELLOW MERCURIC OXIDE 1%. (Vari-
ous Mfr.) Oint. Tube 3.5, 3.75, 30 Gm.
Use: Antiseptic preparation.
YELLOW MERCURIC OXIDE 2%. (Vari-
ous Mfr.) Oint. Tube 3.5, 3.75, 30 Gm.
Use: Antiseptic preparation.
See: Stye, Oint. (Del Pharm).
• **YELLOW OINTMENT,** U.S.P. XXIII.
Use: Pharmaceutic aid (ointment base).
• **YELLOW WAX,** N.F. XVIII.
Use: Pharmaceutic aid (stiffening
agent).
YF-VAX. (Squibb/Connaught) Yellow
fever vaccine. Vial 1 dose, 5 dose with
diluent.
Use: Agent for immunization.
YOCON. (Palisades) Yohimbine HCl 5.4
mg/Tab. Bot. 100s, 1000s.
Use: Impotence.
YODORA DEODORANT CREAM. (SK-
Beecham) Jar 2 oz.
Use: Deodorant.
YODOXIN. (Glenwood) Iodoquinol 210
mg or 650 mg/Tab. Bot. 100s, 1000s.
Pow. Bot. 25 Gm.
Use: Amebicide.
YOHIMBINE HCl. Indolalkylamine alka-
loid. Available as 5.4 mg tab. under the
tradenames Aphrodyne (Star), Dayto
Himbin (Dayton), Yocon (Palisades) and
Yohimex (Kramer).
**Yohimbine has no FDA sanctioned in-
dications.**
W/Methyltestosterone, nux vomica extract.
See: Climactic, Tab. (Burgin-Arden)

YOHIMEX. (Kramer) Yohimbine HCl 5.4 mg/Tab. Bot. 100s.
Use: Impotence.

YOMESAN. (Farbenfabriken Bayer) Niclosamide. B.A.N. Under study.
Use: Anthelmintic.

YOUR CHOICE NON-PRESERVED SALINE SOLUTION. (Amcon) Buffered isotonic soln. w/ NaCl, boric acid, sodium borate. Bot. 360 ml.
Use: Soft contact lens care.

YOUR CHOICE STERILE PRESERVED SALINE SOLUTION. (Amcon) Isotonic. Sorbic acid 0.1%, EDTA, NaCl, boric buffer. Bot. 60 ml or 360 ml.
Use: Soft contact lens care.

• **YTTERBIUM Yb 169 PENTETATE INJECTION,** U.S.P. XXII.
Use: Radioactive agent.

YUTOPAR. (Astra) Ritodrine HCl. **Tab.:** 10 mg Bot. 60s, UD 100s. **Inj.:** 10 mg/ml, Amp. 5 ml; 15 mg/ml, vial 10 ml, syringe 10 ml.
Use: Uterine relaxant.

Z

• **ZACOPRIDE HYDROCHLORIDE.** USAN.
Use: Antiemetic, stimulant (peristaltic).

ZALCITABINE.
Use: AIDS [Orphan drug]

• **ZALOSPIRONE HYDROCHLORIDE.** USAN.
Use: Anxiolytic.

• **ZALTIDINE HYDROCHLORIDE.** USAN.
Use: Antagonist to histamine H_2 receptors.

ZANAFLEX. (Athena)
See: TIZANIDINE HCl.

• **ZANKIREN HYDROCHLORIDE.** USAN.
Use: Antihypertensive.

ZANOSAR. (Upjohn) Streptozocin sterile pow. 100 mg/ml. Vial 1 Gm.
Use: Antineoplastic agent.

• **ZANOTERONE.** USAN.
Use: Aniandrogen (androgen receptor blocker).

ZANTAC INJECTION. (Glaxo and Roche) Ranitidine 25 mg HCl/ml. Vial 2 ml, 10 ml, 40 ml, syringe 2 ml.
Use: Histamine H_2 antagonist.

ZANTAC INJECTION PREMIXED. (Glaxo and Roche) Ranitidine 0.5 mg as HCl/ml. 100 ml single-dose flexible plastic container.
Use: Histamine H_2 antagonist.

ZANTAC SYRUP. (Glaxo and Roche) Ranitidine 15 mg as HCl/ml, alcohol 7.5%. Bot. pt.
Use: Histamine H_2 antagonist.

ZANTAC TABLETS. (Glaxo and Roche) Ranitidine 150 mg or 300 mg as HCl/Tab. **150 mg:** Bot. 60s, 100s, UD 100s. **300 mg:** Bot. 30s, UD 100s.
Use: Histamine H_2 antagonist.

ZANTINE. (Metro Med) Dipyridamole 25 mg, 50 mg or 75 mg/Tab. Bot. 1000s.
Use: Coronary vasodilator.

ZANTRYL. (Ion) Phentermine HCl 30 mg/SR Cap. Bot. 100s.
Use: Anorexiant.

ZARONTIN. (Parke-Davis) Ethosuximide. **Cap.:** 250 mg. Bot. 100s. **Syr.:** 250 mg/5 ml. Bot. pt.
Use: Anticonvulsant.

ZAROXOLYN. (Pennwalt) Metolazone 2.5 mg, 5 mg or 10 mg/Tab. Bot. 100s, 500s, 1000s, UD 100s.
Use: Diuretic.

ZARTAN. (Dartmouth) Cephalexin monohydrate 500 mg. Cap. Bot. 100s.
Use: Cephalosporin.

• **ZATOSETRON MALEATE.** USAN.
Use: Antimigraine.

Z-BEC. (Robins) Vitamins E 45 mg, C 600 mg, B_1 15 mg, B_2 10.2 mg, B_3 100 mg, B_6 10 mg, B_{12} 6 mcg, pantothenic acid 25 mg, zinc 22.5 mg/Tab. Bot. 60s, 100s, 500s.
Use: Vitamin/mineral supplement.

ZBT BABY. (Glenwood) Talc, mineral oil, magnesium stearate, propylene glycol, BHT. Pow. 120 Gm.
Use: Diaper rash product.

ZEASORB-AF POWDER. (Stiefel) Miconazole nitrate 2%. Can 2.5 oz.
Use: Antifungal, external.

ZEASORB POWDER. (Stiefel) Talc, microporous cellulose, supersorb carbohydrate acrylic copolymer. Sifter-top Can 2.5 oz, 8 oz.
Use: Moisture absorbent.

ZEBETA. (Lederle) Bisoprolol fumarate. **5 mg:** Tab/Bot. 14s, 30s, 100s, 500s, 1000s, UD 10s, **10 mg:** Tab/Bot. 14s, 30s, 100s, 500s, 1000s, UD 10s.
Use: Beta adrenergic blocker

ZECAPS. (Everett) Vitamin E 200 mg, zinc 9.6 mg as gluconate/Cap. Bot. 60s.
Use: Vitamin/mineral supplement.

ZECNIL. (Ferring)
See: SOMATOSTATIN.

ZEFAZONE. (Upjohn) Cefmetazole sodium 1 Gm or 2 Gm/vial. Pow. for inj.
Use: Anti-infective.

ZEIN, N.F. XVIII.

ZEMALO. (Barre) Sulfur, zinc oxide, camphor, titanium oxide. Bot. 4 oz, pt, gal.

Use: Minor skin irritations.

ZENATE. (Reid-Rowell) Vitamins A 5000 IU, D 400 IU, E 30 mg, C 80 mg, folic acid 1 mg, thiamine 3 mg, riboflavin 3 mg, niacin 20 mg, B_6 10 mg, B_{12} 12 mcg, calcium 300 mg, iodine 175 mcg, iron 65 mg, magnesium 100 mg, zinc 20 mg/Tab. Bot. 100s.
Use: Vitamin/mineral supplement.

ZENATE PRENATAL TABLETS. (Solvay) Formerly distributed by Reid-Rowell. Ca 300 mg, Fe 65 mg, vitamins A 5000 IU, D 400 IU, E 30 mg, B_1 3 mg, B_2 3 mg, B_3 20 mg, B_6 10 mg, B_{12} 12 mcg, C 80 mg, FA 1 mg, I, Mg, Zn 20 mg. Cap. Bot. 100s.
Use: Multivitamin w/calcium and iron.
Use: Vitamin/mineral supplement.

• **ZENAZOCINE MESYLATE.** USAN.
Use: Analgesic.

ZENDIUM. (Oral-B) Sodium fluoride 0.22%. Tube 0.9 oz, 2.3 oz.
Use: Dental caries preventative.

• **ZENIPLATIN.** USAN.
Use: Antineoplastic.

ZEPHIRAN. (Winthrop Pharm) **Aqueous soln.:** Benzalkonium Cl 1:750. Bot. 240 ml, gal. **Disinfectant concentrate:** 17% in 120 ml, gal. **Tincture:** 1:750 in gal. **Tincture spray:** 1:750 in 30 Gm, 180 Gm, gal.
Use: Antiseptic, germicide.

ZEPHIRAN TOWELETTES. (Winthrop Pharm) Moist paper towels with soln. of zephiran Cl 1:750. Box 20s, 100s, 1000s.
Use: Antiseptic, germicide.

ZEPHREX TABLETS. (Bock) Pseudoephedrine HCl 60 mg, guaifenesin 400 mg/SR Tab. Bot. 100s.
Use: Decongestant, expectorant.

ZEPHREX-LA TABLETS. (Bock) Pseudoephedrine HCl 120 mg, guaifenesin 600 mg/Tab. Bot. 100s.
Use: Decongestant, expectorant.

ZEPINE. (Foy) Reserpine alkaloid 0.25 mg/Tab. Bot. 100s, 500s, 1000s.
Use: Antihypertensive.

• **ZERANOL.** USAN. (1) (3S, 7X)-3,4,5,6,7,8,9,10,11,12- Decahydro-7, 14, 16-trihydroxy-3-methyl-1H-2-benzoxacyclotetradecin-1-one; (2) (6X, 10S)-6-(6,-10-dihyroxyundecyl)-β-resorcylic acid lactone.
Use: Anabolic.

ZERIT. (Bristol-Myers Squibb) Stavudine 15 mg, 20 mg, 30 mg, 40 mg/Cap.
Use: HIV treatment.

ZESTORETIC. (ICI Pharma) Lisinopril 20 mg, hydrochlorothiazide 12.5 mg or

lisinopril 20 mg, hydrochlorothiazide 25 mg/Tab. Bot. 100s.
Use: Antihypertensive combination.

ZESTRIL. (Stuart) Lisinopril 5 mg, 10 mg or 20 mg/Tab. Bot. 100s, UD 100s.
Use: Antihypertensive.

ZETAR EMULSION. (Dermik) Colloidal whole coal tar 30% (300 mg/ml) in polysorbates. Bot. 6 oz.
Use: Antiseborrheic.

ZETAR SHAMPOO. (Dermik) Colloidal whole coal tar 1% in a shampoo. Bot. 6 oz.
Use: Antiseborrheic.

ZETRAN. (Hauck) Diazepam 5 mg/ml. Inj. Vial 10 ml.
Use: Antianxiety agent.

Z-GEN. (Goldline) Vitamins E 45 mg, B_1 15 mg, B_2 10.2 mg, B_3 100 mg, B_5 25 mg, B_6 10 mg, B_{12} 6 mcg, C 600 mg, zinc 22.5 mg/Tab. Bot. 60s, 100s.
Use: Vitamin/mineral supplement.

ZIAC. (Lederle) Bisoprolol fumarate 2.5 mg, 5 mg or 10 mg; hydrochlorothiazide 6.25 mg. Tab. **2.5 mg or 5 mg:** Bot. 30s, 100s. **10 mg:** Bot. 30s.
Use: Antihypertensive.

• **ZIDOMETACIN.** USAN.
Use: Anti-inflammatory.

• **ZIDOVUDINE.** USAN. (Formerly azidothymidine, AZT).
Use: Antiviral for management of certain AIDS and other serious HIV infections. [Orphan drug]
See: Retrovir, Cap. (Burroughs Wellcome).

• **ZIFROSILONE.** USAN.
Use: Acetylcholinesterase inhibitor.

ZILACTIN-L. (Zila) Lidocaine 2.5%, alcohol 79.3%. Liq. Bot. 7.5 ml.
Use: Local anesthetic, topical.

ZILACTIN MEDICATED GEL. (Zila) Tannic acid 7%, suspended in alcohol 80.8%. Tube 0.25 oz.
Use: Treatment of cold sores.

ZILADENT. (Zila) Benzocaine 6%, alcohol 74.9%. Gel. Tube. 7.5 Gm and single packs.
Use: Local anesthetic.

• **ZILANTEL.** USAN.
Use: Anthelmintic.

• **ZILEUTON.** USAN.
Use: Inhibitor (5-lipoxygenase).

ZIMCO. (Sterwin) Vanillin.

• **ZIMELDINE HYDROCHLORIDE.** USAN.
Use: Antidepressant.

ZINACEF. (Glaxo Pharmaceuticals) Cefuroxime 750 mg, 1.5 Gm or 7.5 Gm as sodium for parenteral administration. **750 mg:** Tray 25s. Infusion Pack Tray

10s. **1.5 Gm:** Tray 25s. Infusion Pack Tray 10s. **7.5 Gm:** Pharmacy Bulk Pkg. Tray 6s.
Use: Anti-infective, cefalosporin.
ZINCATE. (Paddock) Zinc sulfate 220 mg/Cap. Bot. 100s, 500s, 1000s.
Use: Emetic, astringent.
ZINC-220 (Alto) Zinc sulfate 220 mg/Cap. Bot. 100s, 1000s, UD 100s.
Use: Zinc supplement.
•**ZINC ACETATE,** U.S.P. XXIII. Acetic acid, zinc salt, dihydrate.
Use: Pharmaceutic necessity for Zinc-Eugenol Cement; Wilson's disease [Orphan drug]
ZINCA-PAK. (SoloPak) Zinc 1 mg or 5 mg/ml. Inj. **1 mg:** Vial 10 ml, 30 ml. **5 mg:** Vial 5 ml.
Use: Parenteral nutritional supplement.
ZINCATE. (Paddock) Zinc sulfate 220 mg (elemental zinc 50 mg)/Cap. Bot. 100s, 1000s.
Use: Zinc supplement.
ZINC BACITRACIN. Bacitracin Zinc, U.S.P. XXIII.
Use: Antibiotic.
•**ZINC CHLORIDE,** U.S.P. XXIII. Inj., U.S.P. XXIII.
Use: Astringent, desensitizer for dentin, replacement therapy.
W/Formaldehyde.
See: Forma Zincol Concentrate (Ingram).
•**ZINC CHLORIDE Zn 65.** USAN.
Use: Radioactive agent.
ZINC-EUGENOL CEMENT, U.S.P. XXI.
Use: Dental protectant.
ZINCFRIN. (Alcon) Zinc sulfate 0.25%, phenylephrine HCl 0.12% in buffered soln. Droptainer 15 ml.
Use: Astringent, decongestant, ophthalmic.
ZINC GELATIN, U.S.P. XXI. Zinc gelatin boot. Unna's Boot.
Use: Topical protectant.
ZINC GELATIN IMPREGNATED GAUZE, U.S.P. XXI.
Use: Topical protectant.
ZINC-GLENWOOD. (Glenwood) Zinc Sulfate 220 mg/Cap. Bot. 100s.
Use: Zinc supplement.
•**ZINC GLUCONATE,** U.S.P. XXIII.
Use: Supplement (trace mineral).
ZINCHLORUNDESAL. Zincundesal.
ZINC INSULIN.
See: Insulin Zinc, Preps. (Various Mfr.).
ZINCON SHAMPOO. (Lederle) Pyrithione zinc 1%, sodium methyl cocoyltaurate, sodium Cl, magnesium aluminum silicate, sodium cocoyl isethionate, glu-

taral, water w/pH adjusted. Bot. 4 oz, 8 oz.
Use: Antiseborrheic.
•**ZINC OXIDE,** U.S.P. XXIII. Flowers of zinc.
Use: Mild astringent and antiseptic in skin diseases.
See: Calamine Preps.
W/Combinations.
See: Akne, Drying Lot. (Alto).
Almophen, Oint. (Bowman).
Anecal, Cream (Lannett).
Anocaine, Supp. (Mallard).
Anugesic, Oint., Supp. (Parke-Davis).
Anulan, Vial (Lannett).
Anusol, Oint., Supp. (Parke-Davis).
Anusol-HC, Supp. (Parke-Davis).
Aracain Rectal Oint., Supp. (Commerce).
Biscolan, Supp. (Lannett).
Bonate, Supp. (Suppositoria).
Calamatum, Preps. (Blair).
Cala-Zinc-Ol, Liq. (Emerson).
Caldesene, Oint. (Pharmacraft).
Caleate HC Cream, Oint. (Elder).
Caloxol, Oint. (Bowman).
CZO, Lot. (Elder).
Dereq Medicone HC, Supp. (Medicone).
Dermatrol, Oint. (Gordon).
Desitin, Oint. (Leeming).
Diaprex, Oint. (Moss, Belle).
Doctient, Supp. (Suppositoria).
Elder Diaper Rash Oint. (Elder).
Epinephricaine, Oint. (Upjohn).
Ergophene, Oint. (Upjohn).
Hemocaine, Oint. (Mallard).
Hemorrhoidal Oint. (Towne).
Hydro Surco, Lot. (Alma).
Ladd's Paste (Paddock).
Lanaburn, Oint. (Lannett).
Lasan, Oint. (Stiefel).
Medicated Powder (Johnson & Johnson).
Medicated Foot Powder (Upjohn).
Mexsana, Pow. (Plough).
Nullo Foot Cream (DePree).
Obtundia Calamine Cream (Otis Clapp).
Pazo, Oint., Supp. (Bristol-Myers).
Petrozin Compound Oint. (Bowman).
Pile-Gon, Oint. (E.J. Moore).
PZM Oint. (Wendt-Bristol).
Rectal Medicone HC, Supp. (Medicone).
RVPaque, Oint. (Elder).
Saratoga, Oint. (Blair).
Schamberg, Lot. (Paddock).
Sebasorb, Lot. (Summer).
Supertah, Oint. (Purdue Frederick).

Taloin, Tube (Warren-Teed).
Ting, Cream, Pow. (Pharmacraft).
Unguentine Oint. "Original Formula"
 (Norwich-Eaton).
Versal, Supp. (Suppositoria).
Wyanoids, Preps. (Wyeth-Ayerst).
Xylocaine Supp. (Astra).
Zinc Boric Lotion, Liq. (Emerson).
• **ZINC OXIDE OINTMENT,** U.S.P. XXIII.
 (Norwich Eaton) Tube 1 oz, 2.25 oz.
 Use: Protective coating for minor skin ir-
 ritations.
• **ZINC OXIDE PASTE,** U.S.P. XXIII.
 Use: Topical protectant, astringent.
• **ZINC OXIDE AND SALICYLIC ACID
 PASTE,** U.S.P. XXIII.
 Use: Topical protectant, astringent.
 ZINC PHENOLSULFONATE.
 Use: Astringent.
W/Belladonna leaf extract, kaolin, pectin,
 sodium carboxymethylcellulose.
 See: Gelcomul, Liq. (Commerce).
W/Bismuth subgallate, kaolin, pectin, opi-
 um pow
 See: Diastay,Tab. (Elder).
W/Bismuth subsalicylate, salol, methyl sal-
 icylate.
 See: Pepto-Bismol, Liq. (Norwich
 Eaton).
W/Kaolin, pectin.
 See: Pectocel, Liq. (Lilly).
W/Opium pow., bismuth subgallate, pectin,
 kaolin.
 See: Bismuth, Pectin & Paregoric (Lem
 mon).
 ZINC PYRITHIONE. Bis-[1-hydroxy-
 2(1H)-pyridinethionato] zinc.
 Use: Bactericide, fungicide, antisebor-
 rheic.
 See: Breck One, Shampoo (Breck).
 TVC-2 Dandruff Shampoo (Dermol).
 Zincon, Shampoo (Lederle).
 ZP-11, Liq. (Revlon).
• **ZINC STEARATE,** U.S.P. XXIII. Octade-
 canoic acid, zinc salt.
 Use: Dusting powder.
W/Combinations.
 See: Ting, Cream, Pow. (Pharmacraft).
 ZINC SULFANILATE. Zinc sulfanilate
 tetrahydrate. Nizin, Op-Isophrin-Z, Op-
 Isophrin-Z-M (Broemmel).
 Use: Antibacterial.
 ZINC SULFATE. (Various Mfr.) Zinc 1
 mg/ml (as sulfate 4.39 mg). Inj. Vial 10,
 30 ml.
 Use: Intravenous nutritional therapy.
• **ZINC SULFATE,** U.S.P. XXIII. Inj., Ophth.
 Soln. U.S.P. XXIII. Sulfuric acid, zinc salt
 (1:1), heptahydrate.
 Use: Astringent (ophthalmic).

See: Eye-Sed, Soln. (Scherer).
 Op-Thal-Zin Ophth. (Alcon).
 Scrip-Zinc, Cap. (Scrip).
 Zinc-Glenwood, Cap. (Glenwood).
 Zin-Cora, Cap. (Elder).
W/Boric acid, phenylephrine HCl.
 See: Phenylzin Drops, Ophth. Soln.
 (Smith, Miller & Patch).
W/Calcium lactate.
 See: Zinc-220, Cap. (Alto).
W/Menthol, methyl salicylate, alum, boric
 acid, oxyquinoline citrate.
 See: Maso pH Powder (Mason).
W/Phenylephrine HCl, polyvinyl alcohol.
 See: Prefrin-Z, Liquifilm (Allergan).
W/Piperocaine HCl, boric acid, potassium
 Cl.
 See: M-Z Drops (Smith, Miller & Patch).
W/Sodium Cl.
 See: Bromidrosis Crystals (Gordon).
W/Sulfur, hexachlorophene.
 See: Acnederm, Lot. (Lannett).
W/Vitamins.
 See: Noovicapc TR, Cap. (Scherer).
 Vicon-C, Cap. (Glaxo).
 Vicon Forte, Cap. (Glaxo).
 Vicon Plus, Cap. (Glaxo).
 Vl-Zac, Cap. (Glaxo).
 7-Rec, Tab. (Robins).
 ZINC SULFATE. (Various Mfr.) Zinc 5
 mg/ml (as sulfate 21.95 mg). Inj. Vial 5,
 10 ml.
 Use: Intravenous nutritional therapy.
 ZINC SULFIDE, LOTION.
 See: White Lotion, U.S.P.
 ZINC SULFOCARBOLATE.
W/Aluminum hydroxide, pectin, kaolin, bis-
 muth subsalicylate, salol.
 See: Wescola Antidiarrheal-Stomach
 Upset (Western Research).
 ZINC TRACE METAL ADDITIVE. (IMS)
 Zinc 4 mg/ml. Inj. Vial. 10 ml.
 Use: Parenteral nutritional supplement.
 ZINCUNDESAL.
 See: Zinchlorundesal.
 ZINC-10-UNDECENOATE.
 See: Zinc Undecylenate, U.S.P. XXIII.
• **ZINC UNDECYLENATE,** U.S.P. XXIII. 10-
 Undecenoic acid, zinc (2+) salt. Zinc 10-
 undecenoate. (Various Mfr.).
 Use: Antifungal.
W/Benzocaine, hexachlorophene.
 See: Fung-O-Spray (Scrip).
W/Benzocaine, undecylenic acid, menthol.
 See: Decyl-Cream LBS (Scrip).
W/Caprylic acid, sodium propionate.
 See: Deso-Cream (Quality Generics).
 Deso-Talc, Foot Pow. (Quality Gener-
 ics).
W/Undecylenic acid.

See: Cruex Cream, Spray Pow. (Phar-
macraft).
Desenex, Prods. (Pharmacraft).
Ting, Aerosol (Pharmacraft).
Quinsana, Med. Oint. (Mennen).
• **ZINDOTRINE.** USAN.
  Use: Bronchodilator.
• **ZINOCANAZOLE HYDROCHLORIDE.**
  USAN.
  Use: Antifungal.
• **ZINOSTATIN.** USAN.
  Use: Antineoplastic.
• **ZINTEROL HYDROCHLORIDE.** USAN.
  Use: Bronchodilator.
• **ZINVIROXIME.** USAN.
  Use: Antiviral.
ZIRADRYL LOTION. (Parke-Davis
Prods) Benadryl HCl 2%, zinc oxide 2%,
alcohol 2%. Bot. 6 oz.
  Use: Antihistamine-containing prepara-
tion, external.
ZIRCONIUM CARBONATE OR OXIDE.
See: Dermaneed, Lot. (Hanlon).
W/Benzocaine, menthol, camphor.
See: Rhulicream, Oint. (Lederle).
W/Benzocaine, menthol, camphor,
calamine, pyrilamine maleate.
See: Ivarest, Cream (Carbisulphoil).
W/Benzocaine, menthol, camphor,
calamine, isopropyl alcohol.
See: Rhulispray, Aerosol (Lederle).
W/Parethoxycaine, calamine.
See: Zotox, Spray, Oint. (Commerce).
ZITHROMAX. (Pfizer) Azithromycin (as
dihydrate) 250 mg, lactose. Cap. Bot.
50s, UD 50s, Z-Pak 6s.
  Use: Antibiotic.
ZNG. (Western Research) Zinc gluconate
35 mg/Tab. Handicount 28s (36 bags of
28 tab.).
  Use: Zinc supplement.
ZNP BAR. (Stiefel) Zinc pyrithione 2%.
Bar 4.2 oz.
  Use: Antiseborrheic.
Zn-PLUS PROTEIN. (Miller) Zinc in a
zinc-protein complex made with isolated
soy protein 15 mg/Tab. Bot. 100s.
  Use: Zinc supplement.
ZOCOR. (MSD) Simvastatin w/lactose **5
mg Tab.** Bot. 60s, 90s, UD 100s. **10 mg
Tab.** Bot. 60s, 90s, UD 100s, 1000s,
10,000s. **20 mg Tab.** Bot. 60s, 1000s,
10,000s. **40 mg Tab.** Bot. 60s.
  Use: Antihyperlipidemic agent.
ZODEAC-100. (Econo Med) Iron 60 mg,
vitamins A 8000 IU, D 400 IU, E 30 IU,
B_1 1.7 mg, B_2 2 mg, B_3 20 mg, B_5 11 mg,
B_6 4 mg, B_{12} 8 mcg, C 120 mg, folic acid
1 mg, biotin 300 mcg, Ca, Cu, I, K, Mg,
Zn. Bot. 100s.

Use: Vitamin/mineral supplement.
• **ZOFENOPRIL CALCIUM.** USAN.
  Use: Enzyme inhibitor (angiotensin-
converting).
• **ZOFENOPRILAT ARGININE.** USAN.
  Use: Antihypertensive.
ZOFRAN. (Cerenex) Ondansetron HCl
Tab.: 4 mg, 8 mg Bot. 30s, UD 100s, 1 x
3 UD pack. **Inj.:** 2 mg/ml. Vial 20 ml.
  Use: Antiemetic (cancer chemothera-
py).
ZOLADEX. (Zeneca) Goserelin acetate
3.6 mg. Implant. Syringes.
  Use: LHRH agonist.
• **ZOLAMINE HCl.** USAN. 2-[[2-(Dimethyl-
lamino)ethyl]-(p-methoxybenzyl)-
amino]thiazole monohydrochloride.
  Use: Antihistamine, local anesthetic.
W/Eucupin dihydrochloride.
See: Otodyne, Soln. (Schering).
• **ZOLAZEPAM HYDROCHLORIDE.**
  USAN.
  Use: Sedative.
• **ZOLERTINE HYDROCHLORIDE.** USAN.
  1-Phenyl-4-[2-(1H-tetrazol-5-
yl)ethyl]piperazine HCl.
  Use: Antiadrenergic, vasodilator.
ZOLICEF. (Apothecon) Cefazolin 500
mg. Pow. for inj. Vial 10 ml.
  Use: Antibacterial, cephalosporin.
• **ZOLIMOMAB ARITOX.** USAN.
  Use: Monoclonal antibody (anti-T lym-
phocyte).
ZOLOFT. (Roerig) Sertraline 50 mg, 100
mg/Tab. Bot. 50s.
  Use: Antidepressant.
• **ZOLPIDEM TARTRATE.** USAN.
  Use: Hypnotic, sedative.
  See: Ambien.
ZOMEPIRAC SODIUM, U.S.P. XXI. Tab.,
U.S.P. XXI. Sodium 5-(4-chlorobenzoyl)-
1, 4-dimethyl-1H-pyrrole-2-acetate dihy-
drate.
  Use: Non-steroidal, anti-inflammatory,
analgesic agent.
• **ZOMETAPINE.** USAN.
  Use: Antidepressant.
ZONE-A FORTE. (UAD) Hydrocortisone
2.5%, pramoxine HCl in a hydrophilic
base containing stearic acid 1%, forlan-
L, glycerin, triethanolamine, polyoxyl-40-
stearate, diisopropyl adipate, providone,
silicone fluid-200. Paraben free. Lot.
Bot. 60 ml.
  Use: Corticosteroid combination, topi-
cal.
ZONE-A LOTION. (UAD Labs) Hydrocor-
tisone acetate 1%, pramoxine HCl 1%.
Bot. 2 oz.
  Use: Corticosteroid, local anesthetic.

- **ZONICLEZOLE HYDROCHLORIDE.**
  USAN.
  Use: Anticonvulsant.
- **ZONISAMIDE.** USAN.
  Use: Anticonvulsant.
  ZONITE LIQUID DOUCHE CONCEN-TRATE. (SK-Beecham) Benzalkonium Cl 0.1%, propylene glycol, menthol, thymol, EDTA in buffered soln. Bot. 8 fl oz, 12 fl oz.
  Use: Vaginal preparation.
  ZONIUM CHLORIDE. (Lannett) Benzalkonium Cl 12.8%, 17% or 50%. Bot. pt, gal. 12.8%, 17%; also Bot. 4 oz. Also as 1:1,000, Bot. pt, gal.
  Use: Antiseptic.
- **ZOPOLRESTAT.** USAN.
  Use: Antidiabetic.
- **ZORBAMYCIN.** USAN.
  Use: Antibacterial.
  ZORPRIN. (Boots) Aspirin 800 mg/SR Tab. Bot. 100s.
  Use: Salicylate analgesic.
- **ZORUBICIN HYDROCHLORIDE.** USAN.
  Use: Antineoplastic.
  ZOSTRIX. (GenDerm) Capsaicin 0.025%. Cream 45 Gm.
  Use: External analgesic.
  ZOSTRIX-HP. (GenDerm) Formerly called Axsain, formerly marketed by Galen.
  ZOSYN. (Lederle) Piperacillin sodium/tazobactam sodium 2 g/0.25 g, 3 g/0.375 g, 4 g/0.5 g vials.
  Use: Antibiotics, penicillins.
  ZOVIRAX. (Burroughs Wellcome) **Tab.:** Acyclovir 400 mg, 800 mg. Bot. 100s. **Susp.:** Acyclovir 200 mg/5 ml, methylparaben 0.1%, propylparaben 0.02%, sorbital, banana flavor. Bot. 473 ml.
  Use: Antiviral agent.
  ZOVIRAX CAPSULES. (Burroughs Wellcome) Acyclovir 200 mg/Cap. Bot. 100s, UD 100s.
  Use: Antiviral.
  ZOVIRAX OINTMENT 5%. (Burroughs Wellcome) Acyclovir 50 mg/Gm. Tube 15 Gm.
  Use: Antiviral, external.
  ZOVIRAX STERILE POWDER. (Burroughs Wellcome) Acyclovir sodium 500 mg/Vial. Vial 10 ml.
  Use: Antiviral.
  ZOXAZOLAMINE. B.A.N. 2-Amino-5-chlorobenzoxazole. Flexin.
  Use: Skeletal muscle relaxant, uricosuric.

Z-PRO-C. (Person & Covey) Zinc sulfate 200 mg (elemental zinc 45 mg), ascorbic acid 100 mg/Tab. Bot. 100s.
Use: Vitamin/mineral supplement.
Z-TEC. (Seatrace) Iron equivalent 50 mg/ml from iron dextran complex. Vial 10 ml.
Use: Iron supplement.
- **ZUCAPSAICIN.** USAN.
  Use: Topical analgesic.
- **ZUCLOMIPHENE.** USAN. Transclomiphene.
  ZURINOL. (Major) Allopurinol. **100 mg/Tab.:** Bot. 100s, 500s, 1000s, UD 100s. **300 mg/Tab.:** Bot. 100s, 500s, UD 100s.
  Use: Agent for gout.
  ZYDERM I. (Collagen Corp.) Highly purified bovine dermal collagen 35 mg/ml implant. Sterile syringe 0.1 ml, 0.5 ml, 1 ml, 2 ml.
  Use: Collagen implant.
  ZYDERM II. (Collagen Corp.) Highly purified bovine dermal collagen 65 mg/ml implant. Syringe 0.75 ml.
  Use: Collagen implant.
  ZYDONE. (DuPont) Hydrocodone bitartrate 5 mg, acetaminophen 500 mg/Cap. Bot. 100s.
  Use: Narcotic analgesic combination.
  ZYLOPRIM. (Burroughs Wellcome) Allopurinol. **100 mg/Tab.:** Bot. 100s, 1000s, UD 100s; **300 mg/Tab.:** Bot. 30s, 100s, 500s, UD 100s.
  Use: Agent for gout.
  ZYMACAP. (Upjohn) Vitamins A 5000 IU, D 400 IU, E 15 mg, C 90 mg, folic acid 400 mcg, B_1 2.25 mg, B_2 2.6 mg, niacin 30 mg, B_6 3 mg, B_{12} 9 mcg, pantothenic acid 15 mg/Cap. Bot. 90s, 240s.
  Use: Vitamin supplement.
  ZYMASE. (Organon) Lipase 12,000 units, protease 24,000 units, amylase 24,000 units. Cap. Bot. 100s.
  Use: Digestive enzyme.
  ZYMENOL. (Houser) Mineral oil 50%, yeast, cellulose gum, sorbitol, saccharin. Bot. 14 oz.
  Use: Laxative.
  ZYNOXUN OINTMENT. (Alton) Tube 5 oz. Jar lb.
  Use: Protective ointment.
  ZYPAN TABLETS. (Standard Process) Pancreatin 1.5 Gm, pepsin (1:3000) 1.5 Gm, betaine HCl 2.75 Gm, ammonium Cl 0.15 Gm/Tab. Bot. 100s.

Reference
Information

Common Abbreviations

Word	Abbreviation	Meaning
ana	$\overline{aa}$, aa	of each
ante cibum	a.c.	before meals or food
ad	ad	to, up to
aurio dextra	a.d.	right ear
ad libitum	ad lib.	at pleasure
aurio laeva	a.l.	left ear
ante meridiem	A.M.	morning
aqua	aq.	water
aqua destillata	aq. dest.	distilled water
aurio sinister	a.s.	left ear
aures utrae	a.u.	each ear
bis in die	b.i.d.	twice daily
bowel movement	b.m.	bowel movement
blood pressure	b.p.	blood pressure
cong	c.	a gallon
cum	$\overline{c}$	with
capsula	caps.	capsule
	cc.	cubic centimeter
compositus	comp.	compound
dies	d.	day
dilue	dil.	dilute
dispensa	disp.	dispense
divide	div.	divide
dentur tales doses	d.t.d.	give of such a dose
elixir	el.	elixir
	e.m.p.	as directed
et	et	and
	ex aq.	in water
fac, fiat, fiant	f., ft.	make, let be made
Food and Drug Administration	FDA	Food and Drug Administration
gramma	Gm., g.	gram
granum	gr.	grain
gutta	gtt.	a drop
hora	h.	hour
hora somni	h.s., hor. som.	at bedtime
	i.m., I.M	intramuscular
	i.v.	intravenous
liquor	liq.	a liquor, solution
	mcg.	microgram
	mg.	milligram
	ml.	milliliter
misce	M.	mix
more dictor	m. dict.	as directed
mixtura	mixt.	a mixture
National Formulary	N.F.	National Formulary
numerus	no.	number
nocturnal	noc.	in the night
non repetatur	non. rep.	do not repeat, no refills
octarius	O, Oct.	a pint
oculus dexter	o.d.	right eye
oculus laevus	o.l.	left eye
oculus sinister	o.s.	left eye
oculo uterque	o.u.	each eye
post cibos	p.c., post. cib.	after meals
post meridiem	P.M.	afternoon or evening
per os	p.o.	by mouth

Word	Abbreviation	Meaning
pro re nata	p.r.n.	as needed
pulvis	pulv.	a powder
quoque alternis die	q.a.d.	every other day
	q.d.	every day
quiaque hora	q.h.	every hour
quater in die	q.i.d.	four times a day
	q.o.d.	every other day
quantum sufficiat	q.s.	a sufficient quantity
	q.s. ad	a sufficient quantity to make
quam volueris	q.v.	as much as you wish
recipe	Rx	take, a recipe
repetatur	rep.	let it be repeated
sine	s̄, s	without
secundum artem	s.a.	according to art
sataratus	sat.	saturated
signa	Sig.	label, or let it be printed
solutio	sol.	solution
	solv.	dissolve
semis	s̄s̄., ss	one-half
si opus sit	s.o.s.	if there is need
statim	stat.	at once, immediately
suppositorium	supp.	suppository
syrupus	syr.	syrup
tabella	tab.	tablet
	tal.	such
	tal. dos.	such doses
ter in die	t.i.d.	three times a day
tincture	tr., tinct.	tincture
tritura	trit.	triturate
	tsp.	teaspoonful
unguentum	ung.	ointment
United States Adopted Names	USAN	official adopted names
United States Pharmacopeia	U.S.P.	United States Pharmacopeia
ut dictum	ut. dict.	as directed
while awake	w.a.	while awake

[NOTE: *The listing of commonly used abbreviations is included as an aid in interpreting medical orders.]

Common Systems of Weight and Measure*

METRIC SYSTEM

Metric Weight

1 microgram†	μg (mcg)	=	0.000,001	g
1 milligram	mg	=	0.001	g
1 centigram	cg	=	0.01	g
1 decigram	dg	=	0.1	g
1 gram	g	=	1.0	g
1 dekagram	Dg	=	10.0	g
1 hectogram	Hg	=	100.0	g
1 kilogram	Kg	=	1000.0	g

Metric Liquid Measure

1 microliter	μl	=	0.000,001	L
1 milliliter	ml	=	0.001	L
1 centiliter	cl	=	0.01	L
1 deciliter	dl	=	0.1	L
1 liter	L	=	1.0	L
1 dekaliter	Dl	=	10.0	L
1 hectoliter	Hl	=	100.0	L
1 kiloliter	Kl	=	1000.0	L

APOTHECARY SYSTEM

Apothecary Weight

1 grain‡	gr	=	1 gr		
1 scruple	℈	=	20 gr		
1 dram	ℨ	=	60 gr	=	3℈
1 ounce	℥	=	480 gr	=	8ℨ
1 pound	℔	=	5760 gr	=	12℥

Apothecary Liquid Measure

1 minim	♏	=	1 ♏		
1 fluidram	fℨ	=	60 ♏		
1 fluidounce	fℨ	=	480 ♏	=	8 fℨ
1 pint	pt	=	7680 ♏	=	16 fℨ
1 quart	qt	=	15630 ♏	=	32 fℨ
1 gallon	gal	=	61440 ♏	=	8 ptℨ

AVOIRDUPOIS SYSTEM

Avoirdupois Weight

1 ounce = 1 oz	=	437.5 grains (gr)			
1 pound = 1 lb	=	16 ounces (oz)	=	7000 grains (gr)	

*The listing of common systems of weight and measure is included to aid the practitioner in calculating dosages.

†Note: The abbreviation μg or mcg is used for microgram in pharmacy rather than gamma (γ) as in biology.

‡Note: The grain in each of the above systems has the same value, and thus serves as a basis for the interconversion of the other units.

Approximate
Practical Equivalents*

Weight Equivalents

1 grain	= 1 gr	=	64.8	milligrams
1 gram	= 1 Gm or g	=	15.432	grains
1 kilogram	= 1 Kg	=	2.20	pounds avoirdupois (lb)
1 ounce avoirdupois	= 1 oz	=	28.35	grams
1 ounce apothecary	= 1 ℥	=	31.1	grams
1 pound avoirdupois	= 1 lb	—	454.	grams

Measure Equivalents

1 milliliter	— 1 ml	—	16.23	minims (m)
1 fluidram†	= 1 f℥	=	3.4	ml
1 teaspoonful	= 1 tsp	=	5.00	ml
1 tablespoonful	— 1 tbs or tbsp	=	15.	ml
1 fluidounce	= 1 f℥	=	29.57	ml
1 wineglassful	= 2 f℥	=	60.	ml
1 teacupful	= 4 f℥	=	120.	ml
1 tumblerful	= 8 f℥	=	240.	ml
1 pint	= 1 pt or O or Oct	=	473.	ml
1 liter	= 1 L	=	33.8	fluidounces (f℥)
1 gallon	= 1 gal or C or Cong	=	3785.	ml

*The listing of approximate practical equivalents is included to aid the practitioner in calculating and converting dosages among the various systems.

†Note: On prescription a fluidram is assumed to contain a teaspoonful which is 5 ml.

International System of Units

The *Système international d'unités* (International System of Units) or *SI* is a modernized version of the metric system. The primary goal of the conversion to SI units is to revise the present confused measurement system and to improve test-result communications. The SI has 7 basic units from which other units are derived:

Base Units of SI		
Physical Quantity	Base Unit	SI Symbol
length	meter	m
mass	kilogram	kg
time	second	s
amount of substance	mole	mol
thermodynamic temperature	kelvin	K
electric current	ampere	A
luminous intensity	candela	cd

Combinations of these base units can express any property although, for simplicity, special names are given to some of these derived units.

Representative Derived Units		
Derived Unit	Name and Symbol	Derivation from Base Units
area	square meter	m^2
volume	cubic meter	m^3
force	newton (N)	$kg \cdot m \cdot s^{-2}$
pressure	pascal (Pa)	$kg \cdot m^{-1} \cdot s^{-2}$ (N/m²)
work, energy	joule (J)	$kg \cdot m^2 \cdot s^{-2}$ (N·m)
mass density	kilogram per cubic meter	kg/m^3
frequency	hertz (Hz)	s^{-1}
temperature	degree Celsius (°C)	°C = °K -273.15
concentration		
mass	kilogram/liter	kg/L
substance	mole/liter	mol/L
molality	mole/kilogram	mol/kg
density	kilogram/liter	kg/L

Prefixes to the base unit are used in this system to form decimal multiples and submultiples. The preferred multiples and submultiples listed below change the quantity by increments of 10^3 or 10^{-3}. The exceptions to these recommended factors are outlined by the rectangle.

Prefixes and Symbols for Decimal Multiples and Submultiples		
Factor	Prefix	Symbol
10^{18}	exa	E
10^{15}	peta	P
10^{12}	tera	T
10^{9}	giga	G
10^{6}	mega	M
10^{3}	kilo	k
10^{2}	hecto	h
10^{1}	deka	da
10^{-1}	deci	d
10^{-2}	centi	c
10^{-3}	milli	m
10^{-6}	micro	μ
10^{-9}	nano	n
10^{-12}	pico	p
10^{-15}	femto	f
10^{-18}	atto	a

To convert drug concentrations to or from SI units:

Conversion factor (CF) $= \dfrac{1000}{\text{mol wt}}$

Conversion *to* SI units: $\mu g/ml \times CF = \mu mol/L$

Conversion *from* SI units: $\mu mol/L \div CF = \mu g/ml$

Normal Laboratory Values

In the following tables, normal reference values for commonly requested laboratory tests are listed in traditional units and in SI units. The tables are a guideline only. Values are method dependent and "normal values" may vary between laboratories.

Blood, Plasma or Serum		
	Reference Value	
Determination	Conventional Units	SI Units
Ammonia	10-80 µg/dl	5-50 µmol/L
Amylase	≤30 U/L	≤30 U/L
Antinuclear antibodies	negative at 1:8 dilution of serum	
Bilirubin: direct	≤ 0.2 mg/dl	≤ 4 µmol/L
total	0.1-1 mg/dl	2 18 µmol/L
Calcitonin, male	0-14 pg/ml	0-4.1 pmol/L
female	0-28 pg/ml	0-8.2 pmol/L
medullary carcinoma	> 100 pg/ml	> 29.3 pmol/L
Calcium[1]	8.8-10.3 mg/dl	2.2-2.6 mmol/L
Carbon dioxide content	22-28 mEq/L	22-28 mmol/L
Chloride	95-105 mEq/L	95-105 mmol/L
Coagulation screen:		
Bleeding time	3-9.5 min	180-570 sec
Prothrombin time	< 2 sec from control	< 2 sec from control
Partial thromboplastin time (activated)	25-38 sec	25-38 sec
Copper, total	70-140 µg/dl	11-22 µmol/L
Corticotropin (ACTH)	20-100 pg/ml	4-22 pmol/L
Cortisol: 8 am	5-25 µg/dl	0.14-0.69 µmol/L
8 pm	< 10 µg/dl	< 0.28 µmol/L
4 hr ACTH test	30-46 µg/dl	0.83-1.24 µmol/L
Overnight suppression test	< 5 µg/dl	< 0.14 µmol/L
Creatine phosphokinase, total (CK, CPK)	≤ 130 U/L	≤ 130 U/L
Creatine phosphokinase isoenzymes	CK-MB = ≤ 5% total CK	≤ 0.05
Creatinine	0.6-1.2 mg/dl	50-110 µmol/L
Follicle stimulating hormone (FSH), female	2-15 mIU/ml	2-15 IU/L
peak production	20-50 mIU/ml	20-50 IU/L
male	1-10 mIU/ml	1-10 IU/L
Glucose, fasting	70-110 mg/dl	3.9-6.1 mmol/L
Hematologic tests:		
Hematocrit (Hct), female	33%-43%	0.33-0.43
male	39%-49%	0.39-0.49
Hemoglobin (Hb), female	11.5-15.5 g/dl	115-155 g/L
male	14-18 g/dl	140-180 g/L
Leukocyte count (WBC)	3200-9800/mm³	3.2-9.8 x 10⁹/L
Erythrocyte count (RBC), female	3.5-5 million/mm³	3.5-5 x 10¹²/L
male	4.3-5.9 million/mm³	4.3-5.9 x 10¹²/L
Mean corpuscular volume (MCV)	76-100 µm³/cell	76-100 fl/cell
Mean corpuscular hemoglobin (MCH)	27-33 pg/RBC	27-33 pg/RBC
Mean corpuscular hemoglobin concentration (MCHC)	33-37 g/dl	330-370 g/L

[1] Slightly higher in children.   (Table continued on following page)

Blood, Plasma or Serum (Cont.)		
	Reference Value	
Determination	**Conventional Units**	**SI Units**
Hematologic tests (cont.):		
Erythrocyte sedimentation rate		
(sedrate, ESR): female	≤ 30 mm/hr	≤ 30 mm/hr
male	≤ 20 mm/hr	≤ 20 mm/hr
Erythrocyte enzymes:		
Glucose-6-phosphate dehydrogenase		
(G6PD)	5-15 U/g Hb	5-15 U/g Hb
Pyruvate kinase	13-17 U/g Hb	13-17 U/g Hb
Ferritin (serum): Iron deficiency	0-12 ng/ml	0-4.8 nmol/L
Borderline	13-20 ng/ml	5.2-8 nmol/L
Iron excess	> 400 ng/L	> 160 nmol/L
Folic acid: normal	> 3.3 ng/ml	> 7.3 nmol/L
borderline	2.5-3.2 ng/ml	5.75-7.39 nmol/L
Platelet count	150,000-450,000/mm³	150-450 x 10⁹/L
Vitamin B₁₂: normal	205-876 pg/ml	150-674 pmol/L
borderline	140-204 pg/ml	102.6-149 pmol/L
Iron		
female	60-160 μg/dl	11-29 μmol/L
male	80-180 μg/dl	14-32 μmol/L
Iron binding capacity	250-460 μg/dl	45-82 μmol/L
Lactic acid	0.5-2.2 mmol/L	0.5-2.2 mmol/L
Lactic dehydrogenase	50-150 U/L	50-150 U/L
Lead	≤ 50 μg/dl	≤ 2.4 μmol/L
Lipids: Cholesterol		
< 29 yr	< 200 mg/dl	< 5.2 mmol/L
30-39 yr	< 225 mg/dl	< 5.85 mmol/L
40-49 yr	< 245 mg/dl	< 6.35 mmol/L
> 50 yr	< 265 mg/dl	< 6.85 mmol/L
Triglycerides	40-150 mg/dl	0.4-1.5 g/L
LDL	50-190 mg/dl	1.3-4.9 mmol/L
HDL		
female	30-90 mg/dl	0.8-2.35 mmol/L
male	30-70 mg/dl	0.8-1.8 mmol/L
Magnesium	1.8-3 mEq/L	0.8-1.2 mmol/L
Osmolality	280-296 mOsm/kg water	280-296 mmol/kg
Oxygen saturation (arterial)	96%-100%	0.96-1
PCO₂, Arterial	35-45 mm Hg	4.7-6 kPa
pH, Arterial	7.35-7.45	7.35-7.45
PO₂, Arterial: breathing room air[1]	75-100 mm Hg	10-13.3 kPa
on 100% O₂	> 500 mm Hg	
Phosphatase (acid), total:	≤ 3 King-Armstrong units/dl	≤ 5.5 U/L
	≤ 3 Bodansky units/dl	≤ 16.1 U/L
Phosphatase (alkaline)[2]	30-120 U/L	30-120 U/L
Phosphorus, inorganic[3]	2.5-5 mg/dl	0.8-1.6 mmol/L
Potassium	3.5-5 mEq/L	3.5-5 mmol/L

[1] Age dependent.
[2] Infants and adolescents up to 104 U/L.
[3] Infants in the first year up to 6 mg/dl.

Blood, Plasma or Serum (Cont.)		
	Reference Value	
Determination	Conventional Units	SI Units
Progesterone		
Follicular phase	$<$ 2 ng/ml	$<$ 6 nmol/L
Luteal phase	2-20 ng/ml	6-64 nmol/L
Prolactin	2-15 ng/ml	0.08-6 nmol/L
Protein: Total	6-8 g/dl	60-80 g/L
Albumin	4-6 g/dl	40-60 g/L
Globulin	2.3-3.5 g/dl	23-35 g/L
Rheumatoid factor	$<$ 60 IU/ml	
Sodium	135-147 mEq/L	135-147 mmol/L
Testosterone, female	$<$ 0.6 ng/ml	$<$ 2 nmol/L
male	4-8 ng/ml	14-28 nmol/L
Thyroid Hormone Function Tests:		
Thyroid-stimulating hormone (TSH)	0.5-5 μU/ml	0.5-5 arb unit
Thyroxine-binding globulin capacity	15-25 μg T_4/dl	193-322 nmol/L
Total triiodothyronine (T_3)	75-220 ng/dl	1.2-3.4 nmol/L
Total thyroxine by RIA (T_4)	4-12 μg/dl	52-154 nmol/L
T_3 resin uptake	25%-35%	0.25-0.35
Transaminase, AST (aspartate aminotransferase, SGOT)	$\leq$ 35 U/L	$\leq$ 35 U/L
Transaminase, ALT (alanine aminotransferase, SGPT)	$\leq$ 35 U/L	$\leq$ 35 U/L
Urea nitrogen (BUN)	8-18 mg/dl	3-6.5 mmol/L
Uric acid	2-7 mg/dl	120-420 μmol/L
Vitamin A	0.15-0.6 μg/ml	0.5-2.1 μmol/L
Zinc	75-120 μg/dl	11.5-10.5 μmol/L

URINE				
	Reference Value			
Determination	Conventional Units		SI Units	
Catecholamines: Epinephrine	$<$ 20 μg/day		$<$ 109 nmol/day	
Norepinephrine	$<$ 100 μg/day		$<$ 590 nmol/day	
Creatinine	15-25 mg/kg/day		0.13-0.22 mmol/kg/day	
Potassium[1]	25-125 mEq/day		25-125 mmol/day	
Protein, quantitative	$<$ 150 mg/day		$<$ 0.15 g/day	
Sodium[1]	40-220 mEq/day		40-220 mmol/day	

Steroids:		(mg/day)		(μmol/day)	
	Age (yrs)	male	female	male	female
17-Ketosteroids	10	1-4	1-4	3-14	3-14
	20	6-21	4-16	21-73	14-56
	30	8-26	4-14	28-90	14-49
	50	5-18	3-9	17-62	10-31
	70	2-10	1-7	7-35	3-24
17-Hydroxycorticosteroids (as cortisol),					
female		2-8 mg/day		5-25 μmol/day	
male		3-10 mg/day		10-30 μmol/day	

[1] Varies with intake.

DRUG LEVELS†		
	Reference Value	
Drug Determination	**Conventional Units**	**SI Units**
Aminoglycosides (peak levels)		
Amikacin	16-32 µg/ml	nd
Gentamicin	4-8 µg/ml	nd
Kanamycin	15-40 µg/ml	nd
Netilmicin	6-10 µg/ml	nd
Streptomycin	20-30 µg/ml	nd
Tobramycin	4-8 µg/ml	nd
Antiarrhythmics		
Amiodarone	0.5-2.5 µg/ml	nd
Bretylium	0.5-1.5 µg/ml	nd
Digitoxin	9-25 µg/L	11.8-32.8 nmol/L
Digoxin	0.5-2.2 ng/ml	0.6-2.8 nmol/L
Disopyramide	2-8 µg/ml	6-18 µmol/L
Flecainide	0.2-1 µg/ml	nd
Lidocaine	1.5-6 µg/ml	4.5-21.5 µmol/L
Mexiletine	0.5-2 µg/ml	nd
Phenytoin	10-20 µg/ml	40-80 µmol/L
Procainamide	4-8 µg/ml	17-34 µmol/L
Propranolol	50-200 ng/ml	190-770 nmol/L
Quinidine	2-6 µg/ml	4.6-9.2 µmol/L
Tocainide	4-10 µg/ml	nd
Verapamil	0.08-0.3 µg/ml	nd
Anticonvulsants		
Carbamazepine	4-12 µg/ml	17-51 µmol/L
Phenobarbital	15-40 µg/ml	65-172 µmol/L
Phenytoin	10-20 µg/ml	40-80 µmol/L
Primidone	5-12 µg/ml	25-46 µmol/L
Valproic acid	50-100 µg/ml	350-7000 µmol/L
Antidepressants		
Amitriptyline	110-250 ng/ml	nd
Amoxapine	200-500 ng/ml	nd
Bupropion	25-100 ng/ml	nd
Clomipramine	80-100 ng/ml	nd
Desipramine	125-300 ng/ml	nd
Imipramine	200-350 ng/ml	nd
Maprotiline	200-300 ng/ml	nd
Nortriptyline	50-150 ng/ml	nd
Protriptyline	100-200 ng/ml	nd
Antipsychotics		
Chlorpromazine	30-500 ng/ml	nd
Fluphenazine	0.13-2.8 ng/ml	nd
Haloperidol	5-20 ng/ml	nd
Perphenazine	0.8-1.2 ng/ml	nd
Thiothixene	2-57 ng/ml	nd
Miscellaneous		
Amantadine	300 ng/ml	nd
Amrinone	3.7 µg/ml	nd
Chloramphenicol	10-20 µg/ml	31-62 µmol/L
Cyclosporine[1]	250-800 ng/ml (whole blood, RIA)	nd
	50-300 ng/ml (plasma, RIA)	nd
Ethanol[2]	0 mg/dl	0 mmol/L
Hydralazine	100 ng/ml	nd
Lithium	0.5-1.5 mEq/L	0.5-1.5 mmol/L
Salicylate	100-200 mg/L	724-1448 µmol/L
Sulfonamide	5-15 mg/dl	nd
Terbutaline	0.5-4.1 ng/ml	nd
Theophylline	10-20 µg/ml	55-110 µmol/L
Vancomycin (peak)	30-40 ng/ml	nd

† The values given are generally accepted as desirable for achieving therapeutic effect without toxicity for most patients. However, exceptions are not uncommon.
[1] 24 hour trough values. [2] Toxic: 50-100 mg/dl (10.9-21.7 mmol/L). nd – No data available.

Trademark Glossary

Many companies use trademarks to identify specific dosage forms or unique packaging materials. The following list is provided as a guide to the interpretation of these descriptions.

Abbo-Pac (Abbott)
Unit dose package

Accu-Pak (Ciba)
Unit dose blister pack

Act-O-Vial (Upjohn)
Vial system

ADD-Vantage (Abbott)
Sterile dissolution system for admixture

ADT (Upjohn)
Alternate day therapy

Arm-A-Med (Armour)
Single-dose plastic vial

Arm-A-Vial (Armour)
Single-dose plastic vial

Aspirol (Lilly)
Crushable ampule for inhalation

Back-Pack (MSD)
Unit-of-use package

bidCAP (Bristol Labs)
Double strength capsule

Bristoject (Bristol Labs)
Unit dose syringe

Caplet (Various)
Capsule shaped tablet

Carpuject (Winthrop Pharm.)
Cartridge needle unit

Chronosule (Schering)
Sustained action capsule

Chronotab (Schering)
Sustained action tablet

Clinipak (Wyeth-Ayerst)
Unit dose package

ControlPak (Sandoz)
Unit dose rolls, tamper resistant

Delcap (Ortho)
Unit dispensing cap

Detecto-Seal (Winthrop Pharm.)
Tamper resistant parenteral package

Dialpak (Ortho)
Compliance package

Dis-Co Pack (Robins)
Unit dose package

Disket (Lilly)
Dispersible tablet

Dispenserpak (Burroughs Wellcome)
Unit-of-use package

Dispertab (Abbott)
Particles in tablet

Dispette (Lederle)
Disposable pipette

Divide-Tab (Abbott)
Scored tablet

Dividose (Mead Johnson)
Tablet, bisected/trisected

D·Lay (Lemmon)
Timed release tablet

Dosette (Elkins-Sinn)
Single dose ampule or vial

Dosepak (Upjohn)
Unit of use package

Drop Dose (Burroughs Wellcome)
Ophthalmic dropper dispenser

Drop-Tainer (Alcon)
Ophthalmic dropper dispenser

Dulcet (Abbott)
Chewable tablet

Dura-Tab (Berlex)
Sustained release tablet

Enduret (Boehringer Ingelheim)
Prolonged action tablet

Enseal (Lilly)
Enteric coated tablet

EN-tabs (Pharmacia)
Enteric coated tablet

Extencap (Robins)
Controlled release capsule

Extentab (Robins)
Continuous release tablet

Filmlok (Squibb)
Veneer coated tablet

Filmseal (Parke-Davis)
Film coated tablet

Filmtab (Abbott)
Film coated tablet

Flo-Pack (Burroughs Wellcome)
Vial for preparation of IV drips

Gelseal (Lilly)
Soft gelatin capsule

Gradumet (Abbott)
Controlled release tablet

Gy-Pak (Geigy)
Unit-of-issue package

Gyrocap (Rhone-Poulenc Rorer)
Timed release capsule

Hyporet (Lilly)
Unit dose syringe

Identi-Dose (Lilly)
Unit dose package

Infatab (Parke-Davis)
Chewable pediatric tablet

Inject-all (Bristol Labs)
Prefilled disposable dilution syringe

Inlay-Tabs (Dorsey/Sandoz)
Inlaid tablets

Isoject (Pfizer)
Unit dose syringe

Kapseal (Parke-Davis)
Banded (sealed) capsule

Kronocap (Ferndale)
Sustained release capsule

Lederject (Lederle)
Disposable syringe

Liquitab (Mission)
Chewable tablet

Memorette (Syntex)
Compliance package

Mix-O-Vial (Upjohn)
Two compartment vial

Mono-Drop (Winthrop Pharm.)
Ophthalmic plastic dropper

Ocumeter (MSD)
Ophthalmic dropper dispenser

Ovoid (Winthrop Pharm.)
Sugar coated tablet

Perle (Forest)
Soft gelatin capsule

Pilpak (Wyeth-Ayerst)
Compliance pack

Plateau CAP (Marion Merrell Dow)
Controlled release capsule

Pulvule (Lilly)
Bullet-shaped capsule

Rediject (Organon)
Unit dose syringe

Redipak (Wyeth-Ayerst)
Unit dose or unit-of-issue package

Redi Vial (Lilly)
Dual compartment vial

Repetabs (Schering)
Extended-release tablet

Rescue Pak (Burroughs Wellcome)
Unit dose packaging

Respihaler (MSD)
Aerosol for inhalation

Robicap (Robins)
Capsule

Robitab (Robins)
Tablet

SandoPak (Sandoz)
Unit dose blister package

Sani-Pak (Hauck)
Sanitary dispensing box

Secule (Wyeth-Ayerst)
Single dose vial

Sequels (Lederle)
Sustained release capsule or tablet

SigPak (Sandoz)
Unit-of-use package

Snap Tabs (Sandoz)
Tablet with facilitated bisect

Softab (Stuart)
Chewable tablet

Solvet (Lilly)
Soluble tablet

Spansule (SmithKline Beecham)
Sustained release capsule

Stat-Pak (Adria)
Unit dose package

Steri-Dose (Parke-Davis)
Unit dose syringe

Steri-Vial (Parke-Davis)
Ampule

Supprette (Webcon)
Suppository

Supule (Lemmon)
Suppository

Tabloid (Burroughs Wellcome)
Branded tablet (with raised lettering)

Tamp-R-Tel (Wyeth-Ayerst)
Tubex, tamper resistant

Tel-E-Amp (Roche)
Single dose amp

Tel-E-Dose (Roche)
Unit dose strip package

Tel-E-Ject (Roche)
Unit dose syringe

Tel-E-Pack (Roche)
Packaging system

Tel-E-Vial (Roche)
Single dose vial

Tembid (Wyeth-Ayerst)
Sustained action capsule

Tempule (Armour)
Timed release capsule or tablet

Ten-Tab (3M Pharmaceuticals
Controlled release tablet

Thera-Ject (SmithKline Beecham)
Unit dose syringe

Tiltab (SmithKline Beecham)
Tablet shape

Timecap (Schwarz Pharma Kremers Urban)
Sustained release capsule

Timecelle (Hauck)
Timed release capsule

Timespan (Roche)
Timed release tablet

Titradose (Wyeth-Ayerst)
Scored tablet

Traypak (Lilly)
Multivial carton

Tubex (Wyeth-Ayerst)
Cartridge-needle unit

Turbinaire (MSD)
Aerosol for nasal inhalation

UDIP (Marion Merrell Dow)
Unit dose indentification pak

U-Ject (Upjohn)
Disposable syringe

Uni-Amp (Winthrop Pharm.)
Single dose ampule

Unimatic (Squibb)
Unit dose syringe

Uni-nest (Winthrop Pharm.)
Ampule

UNI-Rx (Marion Merrell Dow)
Unit dose packages and containers

Unisert (Upsher-Smith)
Suppository

Vaporole (Burroughs Wellcome)
Crushable ampule for inhalation

Visipak (Upjohn)
Reverse numbered pack

Wyseal (Wyeth-Ayerst)
Film coated tablet

Glossary

Abduction—the act of drawing away from a center.

Abstergent—a cleansing application or medicine.

Acaricide—an agent lethal to mites.

Achlorhydria—the absence of hydrochloric acid from gastric secretions.

Acidifier, systemic—a drug used to lower internal body pH in patients with systemic alkalosis.

Acidifier, urinary—a drug used to lower the pH of the urine.

Acidosis—an accumulation of acid in the body.

Acne—an inflammatory disease of the skin accompanied by the eruption of papules or pustules.

Addison's Disease—a condition caused by adrenal gland destruction.

Adduction—the act of drawing toward a center.

Adenitis—a gland or lymph node inflammation.

Adjuvant—an ingredient added to a prescription which complements or accentuates the action of the primary agent.

Adrenergic—a sypathomimetic drug that activates organs innervated by the sympathetic branch of the autonomic nervous system.

Adrenocorticotropic Hormone—an anterior pituitary hormone that stimulates and regulates secretion of the adrenocortical steroids.

Adrenocortical steroid, anti-inflammatory—an adrenal cortex hormone that participates in regulation of organic metabolism and inhibits the inflammatory response to stress; a glucocorticoid.

Adrenocortical steroid, salt regulating—an adrenal cortex hormone that maintains sodium-potassium electrolyte balance by stimulating and regulating sodium retention and potassium excretion by the kidneys.

Adsorbent—an agent that binds chemicals to its surface; it is useful in reducing the free availability of toxic chemicals.

Alkalizer, systemic—a drug that raises internal body pH in patients with systemic acidosis.

Allergen—a specific substance that causes an unwanted reaction in the body.

Amblyopia—pertaining to a dimness of vision.

Amebiasis—an infection with a pathogenic amoeba.

Amenorrhea—an abnormal discontinuation of the menses.

Amphiarthrosis—a joint in which the surfaces are connected by discs of fibrocartilage.

Anabolic—an agent that promotes conversion of simple substance into more complex compounds; a constructive process for the organism.

Analeptic—a potent central nervous system stimulant used to maintain vital functions during severe central nervous system depression.

Analgesic—a drug that selectively suppresses pain perception without inducing unconsciousness.

Ancyclostomiasis—the presence of hookworms in the intestine.

Androgen—a hormone that stimulates and maintains male secondary sex characteristics.

Anemia—a deficiency of red blood cells.

Anesthetic, general—a drug that eliminates pain perception by inducing unconsciousness.

Anesthetic, local—a drug that eliminates pain perception in a limited area by local action on sensory nerves; a topical anesthetic.

Angina pectoris—a sharp chest pain starting in the heart, often spreading down the left arm. A symptom of coronary disease.

Angiography—an X-ray of the blood vessels.

Anhydrotic—a drug that checks perspiration flow systemically; an antidiaphoretic.

Anodyne—a drug which acts on the sensory nervous system, either centrally or peripherally, to produce relief from pain.

Anorexiant—a drug that suppresses appetite, usually secondary to central stimulation of mood.

Anorexigenic—an agent promoting a dislike or aversion to food.

Antacid—a drug that neutralizes excess gastric acid locally.

Anthelmintic—a drug that kills or inhibits worm infestations such as pinworms and tapeworms (nematodes, cestodes, trematodes).

Antiadrenergic—a drug that prevents response to sympathetic nervous system stimulation and adrenergic drugs; a sympatholytic or sympathoplegic drug.

Antiamebic—a drug that kills or inhibits the pathogenic protozoan *Entamoeba histolytica,* the causative agent of amebic dysentery.

Antianemic—a drug that stimulates the production of erythrocytes in normal size, number and hemoglobin content; useful in treating anemias.

Antiasthmatic—an agent that relieves the symptoms of asthma.

Antibacterial—a drug that kills or inhibits pathogenic bacteria, the causative agents of many systemic gastrointestinal and superficial infections.

Antibiotic—an agent produced by or derived from living cells of molds, bacteria or other plants, which destroy or inhibit the growth of microbes.

Anticholesteremic—a drug that lowers blood cholesterol levels.

Anticholinergic—a drug that prevents response to parasympathetic nervous system stimulation and cholinergic drugs; a parasympatholytic or parasympathoplegic drug.

Anticoagulant—a drug that inhibits clotting of circulating blood or prevents clotting of collected blood.

Anticonvulsant—a drug that selectively prevents epileptic seizures; a central depressant used to arrest convulsions by inducing unconsciousness.

Antidepressant—a psychotherapeutic drug that induces mood elevation, useful in treating depressive neuroses and psychoses.

Antidiabetic—a drug used to prevent the development of diabetes.

Antidote—a drug that prevents or counteracts the effects of poisons or drug overdoses, by adsorption in the gastrointestinal tract (general antidotes) or by specific systemic action (specific antidotes).

Antieczematic—a topical drug that aids in the control of exudative inflammatory skin lesions.

Antiemetic—a drug that prevents vomiting, especially that of systemic origin.

Anti-fibrinolytic—an agent (drug) that inhibits liquifaction of fibrin.

Antifilarial—a drug that kills or inhibits pathogenic filarial worms of the superfamily *Filarioidea,* the causative agents of diseases such as loaiasis.

Antiflatulant—an agent inhibiting the excessive formation of gas in the stomach or intestines.

Antifungal—a drug that kills or inhibits pathogenic fungi, the causative agents of systemic, gastrointestinal, and superficial infections.

Antihemophilic—a blood derivative containing the clotting factors absent in the hereditary disease hemophilia.

Antihistaminic—a drug that prevents response to histamine, including histamine released by allergic reactions.

Antihypercholesterolemic—a drug that lowers blood cholesterol levels, especially elevated levels sometimes associated with cardiovascular disease.

Antihypertensive—a drug that lowers blood pressure, especially diastolic blood pressure in hypertensive patients.

Anti-infective, local—a drug that kills a variety of pathogenic microorganisms and is suitable for sterilizing the skin or wounds.

Anti-inflammatory—a drug which counteracts or suppresses inflammation, and produces suppression of the pain, heat, redness and swelling of inflammation.

Antileishmanial—a drug that kills or inhibits pathogenic protozoa of the genus *Leishmania,* the causative agents of diseases such as kala-azar.

Antileprotic—an agent which fights leprosy, a generally chronic skin disease.

Antilipemic—an agent reducing the amount of circulating lipids.

Antimalarial—a drug that kills or inhibits the causative agents of malaria.

Antimetabolite—a substance that competes with or replaces a certain metabolite.

Antimethemoglobinemic—a drug that reduces non-functional methemoglobin (Fe^{+++}) to normal hemoglobin (Fe^{++}).
normal hemoglobin (Fe^{++}).

Antimycotic—an agent inhibiting the growth of fungi.

Antinauseant—a drug that suppresses nausea, especially that due to motion sickness.

Antineoplastic—a drug that is selectively toxic to rapidly multiplying cells and is useful in destroying malignant tumors.

Antioxidant—an agent used to reduce decay or transformation of a material from oxidation.

Antiperiodic—a drug that modifies or prevents the return of malarial fever; an antimalarial.

Antiperistaltic—a drug that inhibits intestinal motility, especially for the treatment of diarrhea.

Antipruritic—a drug that prevents or relieves itching.

Antipyretic—a drug employed to reduce fever temperature of the body; a febrifuge.

Antirheumatic—a drug that alleviates inflammatory symptoms of arthritis and related connective tissue diseases.

Antirickettsial—a drug that kills or inhibits pathogenic microorganisms of the genus Rickettsia, the causative agents of diseases such as typhus (e.g. Chloramphenicol USP).

Antischistosomal—a drug that kills or inhibits pathogenic flukes of the genus *Schistosoma,* the causative agents of schistosomiasis.

Antiseborrheic—a drug that aids in the control of seborrheic dermatitis ("dandruff").

Antiseptic—a substance that will inhibit the growth and development of microorganisms without necessarily destroying them.

Antisialagogue—a drug which diminishes the flow of saliva.

Antispasmodic—an agent used to quiet the spasms of voluntary and involuntary muscles; a calmative or antihysteric.

Anti-syphilitic—a remedy used in the treatment of syphilis.

Antitoxin—a biological drug containing antibodies against the toxic principles of a pathogenic microorganism, used for passive immunization against the associated disease.

Antitrichomonal—a drug that kills or inhibits the pathogenic protozoan *Trichomonas vaginalis,* the causative agent of trichomonal vaginitis.

Antitrypanosomal—a drug that kills or inhibits pathogenic protozoa of the genus *Trypanosoma,* the causative agents of diseases such as West African trypanosomiasis.

Antitussive—a drug that suppresses coughing.

Antivenin—a biological drug containing antibodies against the venom of a poisonous animal; an antidote for a venomous bite.

Anxiety—a feeling of apprehension, uncertainty and fear.

Aperient—a mild laxative.

Aphasia—the inability to use and/or understand written and spoken words, due to damage of cortical speech centers.

Aphonia—a whisper voice due to disease of the larynx or its innervation.

Apnea—the absence of breathing.

Areola—a pigmented ring on the skin.

Arsenical—having to do with arsenic.

Arteriosclerosis—a hardening of the arteries.

Arthritis—an inflammation of a joint.

Ascariasis—a condition caused by roundworms in the intestine.

Ascaricide—an agent that kills roundworms of the genus *Ascaris*.

Aspergillus—a fungi genus including many types of molds.

Astasia—the ability to stand up without help.

Asthma—a disease characterized by recurring breathing difficulty due to bronchial muscle constriction.

Astringent—a mild protein precipitant suitable for local application to toughen, shrink, blanch, wrinkle and harden tissue, diminish secretions and coagulate blood.

Ataractic—an agent having a quieting, tranquilizing effect.

Ataxia—incoordination, especially of gait.

Atheroma—a fatty granular degeneration of an artery wall.

Atrophy—a wasting away.

Avitaminosis—a disease caused by lack of one or more vitamins in the diet.

Axilla—armpit.

Bacteriostatic—an agent that inhibits the growth of bacteria.

Basedow's disease—a form of hyperthyroidism, also known as Grave's disease and Parry's disease.

Biliary Colic—a sharp pain in the upper right side of the abdomen due to a gallstone impaction.

Bilirubin—a bile pigment.

Biliuria—the presence of bile in the urine.

Blood Calcium Regulator—a drug that maintains the blood level of ionic calcium, especially by regulating its metabolic disposition elsewhere.

Blood Volume Supporter—an intravenous solution whose solutes are retained in the vascular system to supplement the osmotic activity of plasma proteins.

Bradycardia—a slow heart rate.

Bright's Disease—a disease of the kidneys, including the presence of edema and excessive urine protein formation.

Bromidrosis—foul smelling perspiration.

Bronchitis—an inflammation of the bronchi.

Bronchodilator—a drug which can dilate the lumina of air passages of the lungs.

Bruit—an arterial sound audible with a stethoscope.

Buerger's Disease—a thromboangiitis obliterans inflammation of the walls and surrounding tissue of the veins and arteries.

Bursitis—an inflammation of the bursa.

Callus—a hard bonelike material developing around a fractured bone.

Calmative—a sedative.

Candidiasis—an infection by the yeastlike organism *Candida albicans*.

Carbonic Anhydrase Inhibitor—an enzyme inhibitor, the therapeutic effects of which are diuresis and reduced formation of intraocular fluid.

Carcinoma—a malignant growth.

Cardiac Depressant—a drug that depresses myocardial function so as to supress rhythmic irregularities characterized by fast rate; an antiarrhythmic.

Cardiac Stimulant—a drug that increases the contractile force of the myocardium, especially in weakened conditions such as congestive heart failure; a cardiotonic.

Cardiopathy—a disease of the heart.

Caries—decay of the teeth.

Carminative—an aromatic or pungent drug that mildly irritates the gastrointestinal tract and is useful in the treatment of flatulence and colic. Peppermint Water is a common carminative.

Caruncle—a small fleshy projection on the skin.

Cathartic—a drug that promotes defecation, usually by enhancing peristalsis or by softening or lubricating the feces.

Caudal—pertains to the distal end or tail.

Caustic—a topical drug that destroys tissue on contact and is suitable for removal of abnormal skin growths.

Central Depressant—a drug that reduces the functional state of the central nervous system and with increasing dosage induces sedation, hypnosis, and general anesthesia; respiration is depressed.

Central Stimulant—a drug that increases the functional state of the central nervous system and with increasing dosage induces restlessness, insomnia, disorientation, and convulsions; respiration is stimulated.

Cerebral—pertaining to the brain.

Cerumen—earwax.

Chloasma—skin discoloration.

Cholagogue—a drug that stimulates the emptying of the gallbladder and the flow of bile into the duodenum.

Cholecystitis—an inflammation of the gallbladder.

Cholecystokinetic—an agent that promotes emptying of the gallbladder.

Cholelithiasis—the presence of calculi (stones) in the gallbladder.

Choleretic—a drug that increases the production and secretion of dilute bile by the liver.

Chorea—a disorder, usually of childhood, characterized by uncontrolled spasmotic muscle movements; sometimes referred to as St. Vitus' dance.

Chymotrypsin—a proteinase in the gastrointestinal tract; its proposed use has been the treatment of edema and inflammation.

Claudication—limping.

Climacteric—a time period in women just preceding termination of the reproductive processes.

Clonus—a spasm in which rigidity and relaxation succeed each other.

Coagulant—a drug that replaces a deficient blood factor necessary for coagulation; clotting factor.

Coccidiostat—a drug used in the treatment of coccidal (protozoal) infections in animals, especially birds; used in veterinary medicine.

Colitis—an inflammation of the colon.

Colloid—a disperse system of particles larger than those of true solutions but smaller than those of suspensions (1 to 100 millimicrons in size).

Collyrium—an eyewash.

Colostomy—the surgical formation of a more or less permanent opening into the colon.

Corticoid—a term applied to hormones of the adrenal cortex or any substance, natural or synthetic, having similar activity.

Corticosteroid—a steroid produced by the adrenal cortex.

Coryza—a headcold.

Counterirritant—an agent (irritant) which causes irritation of the part to which it is applied, and draws blood away from a deep seated area.

Cranial—pertaining to the skull.

Crepitation—the grating of a joint.

Cryptitis—an inflammation of a follicle or glandular tubule, usually in the rectum.

Cryptococcus—a genus of fungi which does not produce spores, but reproduces by budding.

Cryptorchidism—the failure of one or both testes to descend.

Cutaneous—pertaining to the skin.

Cyanosis—a blue or purple skin discoloration due to oxygen deficiency.

Cycloplegia—the loss of accommodation.

Cyclopegic—a drug which paralyzes accommodation of the eye.

Cystitis—an inflammation of the bladder.

Cystourethography—the examination by x-ray of the bladder and urethra.

Cytostasis—a slowing of the movement of blood cells at an inflamed area, sometimes causing capillary blockage.

Debridement—the cutting away of dead or excess skin from a wound.

Decongestant—a drug which reduces congestion caused by an accumulation of blood.

Decubitus—the patient's position in bed; the act of lying down.

Demulcent—an agent used generally internally to sooth and protect mucous membranes.

Dermatitis—an inflammation of the skin.

Dermatomycosis—lesions or eruptions caused by fungi on the skin.

Detergent—an emulsifying agent useful for cleansing wounds and ulcers as well as the skin.

Dextrocardia—when the heart is located on the right side of the chest.

Diagnostic Aid—a drug used to determine the functional state of a body organ or the presence of a disease.

Diaphoretic—a drug used to increase perspiration; a hydroticorsudorfice.

Diarrhea—an abnormal frequency and fluidity of stools.

Digestive Enzyme—an enzyme that promotes digestion by supplementing the naturally occurring counterpart.

Digitalization—the administration of digitalis to obtain a desired tissue level of drug.

Diplopia—double vision.

Disinfectant—an agent that destroys pathogenic microorganisms on contact and is suitable for sterilizing inanimate objects.

Distal—farthest from a point of reference.

Diuretic—a drug that promotes renal excretion of electrolytes and water, thereby increasing urine volume.

Dysarthria—difficulty in speech articulation.

Dysmenorrhea—pertaining to painful menstruation.

Dysphagia—difficulty in swallowing.

Dyspnea—difficult breathing.

Eobolic—a drug used to stimulate the gravid uterus to the expulsion of the fetus, or to cause uterine contraction; an oxytocic.

Eclampsia—a toxic disorder occurring late in pregnancy involving hypertension, weight gain, edema and renal dysfunction.

Ectasia—pertaining to distension or stretching.

Ectopic—out of place; not in normal position.

Eczema—an inflammatory disease of the skin with infiltrations, watery discharge, scales and crust.

Effervescent—bubbling; sparkling; giving off gas bubbles.

Embolus—a blood clot in the blood stream lodged in a vessel, thus obstructing circulation.

Emetic—a drug that induces vomiting, either locally by gastrointestinal irritation or systemically by stimulation of receptors in the central nervous system.

Emollient—a topical drug, especially an oil or fat, used to soften the skin and make it more pliable.

Endometrium—the uterine mucous membrane.

Enteralgia—an intestinal pain.

Enterobiasis—a pinworm infestation.

Enuresis—involuntary urination, as in bedwetting.

Epidermis—the outermost layer of the skin.

Episiotomy—a surgical incision of the vulva when deemed necessary during childbirth.

Epistaxis—a nosebleed.

Erythema—redness.

Erythrocyte—a red blood cell.

Escharotic—corrosive.

Estrogen—a hormone that stimulates and maintains female secondary sex characteristics and functions in the menstrual cycle to promote uterine gland proliferation.

Etiology—the cause of a disease.

Euphoria—an exaggerated feeling of well being.

Eutonic—having normal muscular tone.

Exfoliation—a scaling of the skin.

Exophthalmos—a protrusion of the eyeballs.

Expectorant—a drug that increases secretion of respiratory tract fluid, thereby lowering its viscosity and cough-inducing irritancy and promoting its ejection.

Extension—the movement of a joint to move 2 body parts away from each other.

Exteroceptors—receptors on the exterior of the body.

Fasciculations—the visible twitching movements of muscle bundles.

Fibroid—a tumor of fibrous tissue, resembling fibers.

Filariasis—the condition of having round worm parasites reproducing in the body tissues.

Fistula—an abnormal opening leading from a body cavity to the outside of the body or to another cavity.

Flexion—the movement of a joint in which 2 moveable parts are brought toward each other.

Fungistatic—inhibiting the growth of fungi.

Furunculosis—a condition marked by the presence of boils.

Gallop Rhythm—a heart condition where 3 separate beats are heard instead of 2.

Gastralgia—a stomach pain.

Gastritis—inflammation of the stomach lining.

Gastrocele—a hernial protrusion of the stomach.

Gastrodynia—pain in the stomach, a stomach ache.

Geriatrics—a branch of medicine which treats problems peculiar to old age.

Germicidal—an agent that is destructive to pathogenic microorganisms.

Gingivitis—an inflammation of the gums.

Glaucoma—a disease of the eye evidenced by an increase in intraocular pressure and resulting in hardness of the eye, atrophy of the retina and eventual blindness.

Glossitis—an inflammation of the tongue.

Glucocorticoid—a corticoid which increases gluconeogenesis, thereby raising the concentration of liver glycogen and blood sugar.

Glycosuria—an abnormal quantity of glucose in the urine.

Gout—a disorder which is characterized by a high uric acid level and sudden onset of recurrent arthritis.

Granulation—the formation of small round fleshy granules on a wound in the healing process.

Hematemesis—the vomiting of blood.

Hematinic—a drug that promotes hemoglobin formation by supplying a factor essential for its synthesis.

Hemiplegia—a condition in which one side of the body is paralyzed.

Hematopoietic—a drug that stimulates formation of blood cells, especially by supplying deficient vitamins.

Hemoptysis—expectoration of blood.

Histoplasmosis—a lung infection caused by the inhalation of fungus spores, often resulting in pneumonitis.

Hodgkin's Disease—a disease marked by chronic lymph node enlargement sometimes including spleen and liver enlargement.

Hydrocholeresis—putting out a thinner, more watery bile.

Hypercholesterolemia—the condition of having an abnormally large amount of cholesterol in the body cells.

Hemorrhage—copious bleeding.

Hemostatic—a locally acting drug that arrests hemorrhage by promoting clot formation or by serving as a mechanical matrix for a clot.

Hepatitis—an inflammation of the liver.

Hyperemia—an excess of blood in any part of the body.

Hyperesthesia—an increase in sensations.

Hyperglycemic—a drug that elevates blood glucose level, especially for the treatment of hypoglycemic states.

Hypertension—blood pressure above the normally accepted limits, high blood pressure.

Hypertriglyceridemia—an increased level of triglycerides in the blood.

Hypnotic—a central depressant which, with suitable dosage, induces sleep.

Hypodermoclysis—a subcutaneous injection with a solution.

Hypoesthesia—a diminished sensation of touch.

Hypoglycemic—a drug that promotes glucose metabolism and lowers blood glucose level, useful in the control of diabetes mellitus.

Hypokalemia—an abnormally small concentration of potassium ions in the blood.

Hyposensitize—to reduce the sensitivity to an agent, referring to allergies.

Hypotensive—a drug which diminishes tension or pressure, to lower blood pressure.

Ichthyosis—an inherited skin disease characterized by dryness and scales.

Idiopathic—denoting a disease of unknown cause.

Ileostomy—the establishment of an opening from the ileum to the outside of the body.

Immune Serum—a biological drug containing antibodies for a pathogenic microorganism, useful for passive immunization against the associated disease.

Immunizing Agent, active—an antigenic preparation (toxoid or vaccine) used to induce formation of specific antibodies against a pathogenic microorganism, which provides delayed but permanent protection against the associated disease.

Immunizing Agent, passive—a biological preparation (antitoxin, antivenin or immune serum) containing specific antibodies against a pathogenic microorganism, which provides immediate but temporary protection against the associated disease.

Impetigo—an inflammatory skin infection with isolated pustules.

Insulin—one of the hormones that regulate carbohydrate metabolism, used as replacement therapy in diabetes mellitus.

Inversion—a turning inward.

Irrigating solution—a solution for washing body surfaces and/or various body cavities.

Isoniazid—a compound effective in tuberculosis treatment.

Keratitis—an inflammation of the cornea.

Keratolytic—a topical drug that softens the superficial keratin-containing layer of the skin to promote exfoliation.

Lacrimal—pertaining to tears.

Laxative—a gentle purgative medicine; a mild cathartic.

Leishmaniasis—a number of types of infections transmitted by sand flies.

Leucocytopenia—a decrease in the number of white cells.

Leucocytosis—an increased white cell count.

Leukoderma—an absence of pigment from the skin.

Libido—sexual desire or creative energy.

Leucocyte—a white blood cell.

Lipoma—a fatty tumor.

Lipotropic—a drug, especially one supplementing a dietary factor, that prevents the abnormal accumulation of fat in the liver.

Lochia—a vaginal discharge of mucus, blood and tissue after childbirth.

Lues—a plague; specifically syphilis.

Macrocyte—a large red blood cell.

Malaise—a general feeling of illness.

Melasma—a darkening of the skin.

Melena—black feces or black vomit from altered blood in the higher GI tract.

Meninges—the membranes covering the brain and spinal cord.

Metastasis—the shifting of a disease or its symptoms from one part of the body to another.

Mastitis—an inflammation of the breast.

Miotics—agents which constrict the pupil of the eye; a myotic.

Moniliasis—an infection with any of the species of monilia types of fungi *(Candida)*.

Mucolytic—an agent that can destroy or dissolve mucous membrane secretions.

Myalgia—a pain in the muscles.

Myasthenia Gravis—a chronic progressive muscular weakness caused by myoneural conduction, usually spreading from the face and throat.

Myelocyte—an immature white blood cell in the bone marrow.

Myelogenous—originating in bone marrow.

Myoclonus—involuntary, sudden and rapid unpredictable jerks; faster than chorea.

Mydriatic—a drug that dilates the pupil of the eye, usually by anticholinergic or adrenergic mechanism.

Myoneural—pertaining to muscle and nerve.

Myopia—nearsightedness.

Narcotic—a drug that produces insensibility or stupor; a class of drug regulated by law.

Neonatal—pertaining to the first four weeks of life.

Neoplasm—an abnormal tissue growing more rapidly than usual showing a lack of structural organization.

Nephritis—an inflammation of the kidney.

Nephrosclerosis—a hardening of the kidney tissue.

Neuralgia—a pain extending along the course of one or more of the nerves.

Neurasthenia—nervous prostration.

Neuroglia—the supporting elements of the nervous system.

Neuroleptic—a substance that acts on the nervous system.

Neurosis—a functional disorder of the nervous system.

Nocturia—urination at night.

Normocytic—pertaining to anemia due to some defect in the blood-forming tissues.

Nuchal—the nape of the neck.

Nystagmus—a rhythmic oscillation of the eyes.

Oleaginous—oily or greasy.

Omphalitis—an inflammation of the navel in a newborn.

Onychomycosis—a ringworm or fungus infection of the nails.

Ophthalmic—pertaining to the eye.

Oral—pertaining to the mouth.

Orthopnea—a discomfort in breathing in any but the upright sitting or standing positions.

Ossification—a formation of, or conversion to, bone.

Osteomyelitis—an inflammation of the marrow of the bone.

Osteoporosis—a reduction in bone quantity; skeletal atrophy.

Otalgia—pain in the ear; an earache.

Otitis—inflammation of the ear.

Otomycosis—an ear infection caused by fungus.

Otorrhea—a discharge from the ear.

Oxytocic—a drug that selectively stimulates uterine motility and is useful in obstetrics, especially in the control of postpartum hemorrhage.

Palpitations—an awareness of one's heart action.

Paget's Disease—a disease characterized by lesions around the nipple and areola found in elderly women.

Pallor—the lack of the normal red color imparted to the skin by the blood of the superficial vessels.

Parasympatholytic—See Anticholinergic.

Parasympathomimetic—See Cholinergic.

Parenteral—pertaining to the administration of a drug by means other than through the alimentary canal; subcutaneous, intramuscular or intravenous administration of drug.

Parkinsonism—a group of neurological disorders marked by hypokinesia, tremor, and muscular rigidity.

Paroxysm—a sudden recurrence or intensification of symptoms.

Pathogenic—giving origin to disease.

Pediatric—pertaining to children's diseases.

Pediculicide—an insecticide suitable for eradicating louse infestations in humans (pediculosis).

Pediculosis—an infestation with lice.

Pellagra—characterized by GI disturbances, mental disorders, and skin redness and scaling due to niacin deficiency.

Pernicious—particularly dangerous or harmful.

Phlebitis—an inflammation of a vein.

Pleurisy—an inflammation of the membrane surrounding the lungs and the thoracic cavity.

Pneumonia—an infection of the lungs.

Poikilocytosis—a condition in which pointed or irregularly shaped red blood cells are found in the blood.

Polydipsia—excessive thirst.

Posology—the science of dosage.

Posterior Pituitary Hormone(s)—a multifunctional hormone with oxytocic-milk ejection, and antidiuretic-vasopressor fractions.

Progestin—a hormone that functions in the menstrual cycle and during pregnancy to promote uterine gland secretion and to reduce uterine motility.

Pronation—the act of turning the palm downward or backward.

Prophylactic—a remedy that tends to prevent disease.

Protectant—a topical drug that remains on the skin and serves as a physical barrier to the environment.

Proteolytic Enzyme—an enzyme used to liquefy fibrinous or purulent exudates.

Psoriasis—an inflammatory skin disease accompanied with itching.

Psychotherapeutic—a drug that selectively affects the central nervous system to alter emotional state. See Antidepressant; Tranquilizer.

Ptosis—a drooping or sagging of the muscle.

Pulmonary—pertaining to the lungs.

Purulent—containing or forming pus.

Pyelitis—a local inflammation of renal and pelvic cells due to bacterial infection.

Pylorospasm—a spasmodic muscle contraction of the pyloric portion of the stomach.

Pyoderma—any skin discharge characterized by pus formation.

Radiopaque Medium—a diagnostic drug, opaque to X rays, whose retention in a body organ or cavity makes X-ray visualization possible.

Raynaud's Phenomenon—spasms of the digital arteries with blanching and numbness of the fingers, usually with another disease.

Reflex Stimulant—a mild irritant suitable for application to the nasopharynx to induce reflex respiratory stimulation.

Rheumatoid—a condition resembling rheumatism.

Rhinitis—an inflammation of the mucous membrane of the nose.

Rubefacient—a topical drug that induces mild skin irritation with erythema, sometimes used to relieve the discomfort of deep-seated inflammation.

Rubeola—a synonym popularly used for both measles and rubella.

Saprophytic—getting nourishment from dead material.

Sarcoma—a malignant tumor derived from connective tissue.

Scabicide—an insecticide suitable for the eradication of itch mite infestations in humans (scabies).

Schistosomacide—an agent which destroys schistosomes; destructive to the trematodic parasites or flukes.

Schistosomiasis—an infection with *Schistosoma haematobium* involving the urinary tract and causing cystitis and hematuria.

Scintillation—a visual sensation manifested by an emission of sparks.

Sclerosing Agent—an irritant suitable for injection into varicose veins to induce their fibrosis and obliteration.

Scotomata—an area of varying size and shape within the visual field in which vision is absent or depressed.

Seborrhea—a condition arising from an excess secretion of sebum.

Sebum—the fatty secretions of sebaceous glands.

Sedative—a central depressant which, in suitable dosage, induces mild relaxation useful in treating tension.

Sinusitis—an inflammation of a sinus.

Skeletal Muscle Relaxant—a drug that inhibits contraction of voluntary muscles, usually by interfering with their innervation.

Smooth Muscle Relaxant—a drug that inhibits

contraction of involuntary (e.g., visceral) muscles, usually by action upon their contractile elements.

Sociopath—a psychopathic person who, due to his unaccepted attitudes, is badly adjusted to society.

Spasmolytic—an agent that relieves spasms and involuntary contraction of a muscle; an antispasmodic.

Sputum—mucous spit from the mouth.

Stenosis—the narrowing of the lumen of a blood vessel.

Stomachic—a drug which is used to stimulate the appetite and gastric secretion.

Stomatitis—an inflammation of the mouth.

Subcutaneous—under the skin.

Sudorific—causing perspiration.

Superacidity—an increase of the normal acidity of the gastric secretion; hyperacidity.

Supination—the act of turning the palm forward or upward.

Suppressant—a drug useful in the control, rather than the cure, of a disease.

Surfactant—a surface active agent that decreases the surface tension between two miscible liquids; used to prepare emulsions, act as a cleansing agent, etc.

Synarthrosis (fibrous joint)—a joint in which the bony elements are united by continuous fibrous tissue.

Syncope—fainting.

Synovia—clear fluid which lubricates the joints; joint oil.

Systole—the ventricular contraction phase of a heartbeat.

Tachycardia—a rapid contraction rate of the heart.

Taeniacide—an agent used to kill tapeworms.

Taeniafuge—agent to expel tapeworms.

Therapeutic—a treatment of disease.

Thoracic—pertaining to the chest.

Thyroid Hormone—a drug containing one or more of the iodinated amino acids that stimulate and regulate the metabolic rate and functional state of body tissues.

Thyroid Inhibitor—drug that reduces excessive thyroid hormone production, usually by blocking hormone synthesis.

Tics—a repetitive twitching of muscles, often in the face and upper trunk.

Tinea—a fungal infection of the skin.

Tonic—an agent used to stimulate the restoration of tone to muscle tissue.

Tonometry—the measurement of tension in some part of the body.

Topical—the local external application of a drug to a particular place.

Toxoid—a modified bacterial toxin, less toxic than the original form, used to induce active immunity to bacterial pathogens.

Tranquilizer—a psychotherapeutic drug that induces emotional repose without significant sedation, useful in treating certain neuroses and psychoses.

Tremors—involuntary rhythmic tremulous movements.

Trichomoniasis—an infestation with parasitic flagellate protozoa of the genus *Trichomonas*.

Trypanosomiasis—a disease caused by protozoan flagellates in the blood.

Uricosuric—drug that promotes renal uric acid excretion; used to treat gout.

Urolithiasis—a condition marked by the formation of stones in the urinary tract.

Urticaria—a rash of hives generally of systemic origin.

Vaccine—preparation of live attenuated or dead pathogenic microorganisms, used to induce active immunity.

Vasoconstrictor—an adrenergic drug used locally in the nose to constrict blood vessels and reduce tissue congestion.

Vasodilator—a drug that relaxes vascular smooth muscles, especially for the purpose of improving peripheral or coronary blood flow.

Vasopressor—an adrenergic drug used systemically to constrict blood vessels and raise blood pressure.

Verruca—a wart.

Vertigo—illusion of movement.

Vesicant—an agent which, when applied to the skin causes blistering and the formation of vesicles; an epispastic.

Visceral—pertaining to the internal organs.

Vitamin—an organic chemical essential in small amounts for normal body metabolism, used therapeutically to supplement the naturally occurring counterpart in foods.

Container Requirements for U.S.P. XXIII Drugs

Legend:

WC	= well closed container	TP	= tamper-proof
T	= tight container	In	= inert atmosphere
LR	= light resistant container	U	= unit dose
+	= controlled temperature	S	= separate ingredient
P	= plastic specified		packaging before mixing
G	= glass specified	A	= pressurized container
C	= collapsible tubes	OT	= Ophthalmic Tube
S/M	= Single Dose/Multi Dose	SC	= Radioactive Shielding
H	= Reduced Moisture	R	= Remote from fire
SP	= Special consideration	F	= Avoid Freezing
WP	= Well Filled Container	Ox	= Protect from Oxidation

a	= Tablets	g	= Ointment	m	= Vaginal	t	= Gel/Jelly
b	= Capsules	h	= Lotion	n	= Lozenges	v	= Otic
c	= Solution	i	= Suppository	o	= Powder	w	= Intraocular solution
d	= Syrup	j	= Suspension	p	= Enema	x	= Veterinary use
e	= Elixir	k	= Ophthalmic	r	= Inhalation	y	= Emulsion
f	= Cream	l	= Aerosol	s	= Nasal	z	= Tincture

Drug (Dosage Form)	WC	T	LR	Drug (Dosage Form)	WC	T	LR
Acepromazine	$X^{o\,a}$		$X^{o\,a}$	Acyclovir		X^{o}	
Acetaminophen	$X^{i\,t}$	$X^{a\,b\,c\,e}$		Albendazole	X^{o}		
Acetaminophen Oral		$X^{e\,j}$		Albuterol	$X^{o\,a}$		$X^{o\,a}$
Acetaminophen & Aspirin				Albuterol Sulfate	X^{o}		X^{o}
(tab)		X		Alcohol		R	
Acetaminophen, Aspirin &				Alcohol, Dehydrated		R	
Caffeine	X^{a}	X^{b}		Alcohol, Rubbing		R	
Acetaminophen &				Alclometasone			
Caffeine		$X^{a\,b}$		Dipropionate		$C^{f\,g}$	
Acetaminophen &				Allopurinol (tab)	X		
Codeine Phosphate	$X^{a\,b}$	$X^{a\,b}$		Alprazolam	X^{o}	X^{a}	X^{a}
Acetaminophen and				Alum	X		
Codeine Phosphate				Ammonium Alum	X		
Oral	$X^{c\,j}$	$X^{c\,j}$		Potassium Alum	X		
Acetaminophen &				Alumina & Magnesia	X^{a}	$X^{j\,+}$	
Diphenhydramine				Alumina & Magnesium			
Citrate (tab)		X		Carbonate		X^{a}	$X^{j\,+}$
Acetaminophen for				Alumina and Magnesium			
Effervescent Oral Soln.		X		Carbonate and			
Acetaminophen and				Magnesium Oxide (tab)		X	
Pseudoephedrine HCl		X^{a}		Alumina & Magnesium			
Acetohydroxamic Acid				Trisilicate		$X^{j\,+\,a}$	
(tab)		$X^{a\,o\,+}$		Alumina, Magnesia,			
Acetazolamide (tab)	X			Calcium Carbonate,			
Acetic Acid Otic Soln.		X		Simethicone (tab)		X	
Acetohexamide (tab)	X			Alumina, Magnesia &			
Acetophenazine Maleate	$X^{a\,o}$	$X^{a\,o}$		Simethicone Oral		$X^{j\,+}$	
Acetylcysteine (soln)	S/M (IN)			Aluminum Acetate			
Acetylcysteine &				Topical Soln.		X	
Isoproterenol HCl				Aluminum Carbonate			
Inhalation Soln.	G/P			Gel, Basic	$X^{a\,b}$	X^{+}	
Acrisorcin (cream)	C			Aluminum Hydroxide Gel	$X^{a\,b}$	$X^{j\,+}$	

*The listing of container requirements for Compendial drugs is included as an aid to the practitioner in storing and dispensing.

Drug (Dosage Form)	WC	T	LR
Aluminum Phosphate Gel	X^a	X$^{j\,+}$	
Aluminum Subacetate Topical Soln.		X	
Amantadine HCl		X$^{b\,d}$	
Amdinonide		X$^{f\,g}$	
Amikacin Sulfate		X^o	
Amiloride HCl (tab)	X		
Amiloride HCl & Hydrochlorothiazide (tab)	X		
Aminobenzoic Acid		X$^{t\,c}$	X$^{t\,c}$
Aminobenzoate Potassium	X$^{b\,a}$	X^c	
Aminocaproic Acid		X$^{a\,d}$	
Aminoglutethimide (tab)	X		X
Aminophylline	X$^{i\,+}$	X^a	
Aminophylline, Oral		X^c	
Aminosalicylate Sodium (tab)		X$^+$	X$^+$
Aminosalicylic Acid(tab)		X$^+$	X$^+$
Amitriptyline HCl (tab)	X		
Aromatic Ammonia Spirit		X$^+$	X$^+$
Ammonium Chloride Delayed Release (tab)		X	
Amobarbital (tab)	X		
Amobarbital Sodium (cap)		X	
Amodiaquine		X	
Amodiaquine HCl (tab)		X	
Amoxapine		X^o	
Amoxicillin		X$^{a\,b\,+}$	
Amoxicillin for Oral Susp.		X$^+$	
Amoxicillin Oral Susp.	M$^+$		
Amoxicillin & Clavulanate Potassium		X$^{h\,+\,a}$	
Amoxicillin & Clavulanate Potassium for Oral Susp.		X$^+$	
Amphetamine Sulfate (tab)		X	
Amphotericin B	X^h	C$^{f\,g}$	
Ampicillin (all dosage forms)		X	
Ampicillin Boluses		X^x	
Ampicillin Soluble Powder		X^x	
Ampicillin & Probenecid (cap)		X	
Ampicillin & Probenecid for Oral Susp.		U	
Amprolium (all dosage forms)		X	
Amyl Nitrate (inhalant)		UG$^+$	UG$^+$
Anileridine HCl (tab)		X	
Anthralin		X$^{f\,g\,+}$	X$^{f\,g\,+}$
Antimony Sodium Tartrate		X	
Antipyrine & Benzocaine Otic Soln.			X
Antipyrine, Benzocaine & Phenylephrine HCl Otic Soln.		X	X
Apomorphine HCl (tab)		X	
Apraclonidine HCl		X^o	X^o
Apraclonidine Ophthalmic		X^c	X^c
Ascorbic Acid		X$^{a\,c}$	X$^{a\,c}$
Calcium Ascorbate		X^o	X^o
Aspirin	X$^{i\,+}$	X$^{a\,b}$	
Aspirin, Buffered		X^a	
Aspirin, Delayed Release		X$^{a\,b}$	
Aspirin, Effervescent Tablets for Oral Soln.		X	
Aspirin, Extended Release (tab)		X	
Aspirin, Alumina & Magnesia (tab)		X	
Aspirin, Alumina & Magnesium Oxide (tab)		X	
Aspirin, Caffeine & Dihydrocodeine (cap)		X	
Aspirin & Codeine Phosphate (tab)	X		X
Aspirin, Codeine Phosphate, Alumina & Magnesia (tab)	X		X
Aspirin, Codeine Phosphate & Caffeine	X$^{a\,h}$		
Atropine Sulfate	X^a	C$^{k\,g}$	
Attapulgite, Activated	X		
Attapulgite, Colloidal Activated	X		
Azaperone	X^o		
Azatadine Maleate (tab)	X		
Azathioprine (tab)			X
Azithromycin	X^b	X^o	
Aztreonam		X^o	
Bacampicillin HCl (tab)		X	
Bacampicillin HCl for Oral Susp.		X	
Bacitracin (ointment)	X$^{g\,+}$	COT$^{k\,+}$	
Bacitracin & Polymyxin B Sulfate, Topical		A$^{l\,+}$	
Bacitracin Methylene Disalicylate, Soluble	X^x	X$^{o\,x}$	
Bacitracin Zinc Soluble Powder		X^x	
Bacitracin Zinc	X$^{g\,+}$		
Bacitracin Zinc & Polymyxin B Sulfate (ointment)	X	COT^k	X
Baclofen	X^a	X^o	
Barium Sulfate	X^j		
Beclomethasone Dipropionate	X		
Belladonna Extract (tab)		X	X
Belladonna (tincture)		X$^+$	X$^+$

Drug (Dosage Form)	WC	T	LR
Bendroflumethiazide (tab)		X	
Benoxinate HCl Ophthalmic Soln.		X	
Benzethonium Chloride		$X^{c\ z}$	$X^{c\ z}$
Benzocaine		$X^{f\ g\ +}$	$X^{f\ g\ +}$
Benzocaine Otic Soln.		X^{+}	X^{+}
Benzocaine, Topical		$X^{c\ l\ +}$	$X^{c\ +}$
Benzocane, Butamben, and Tetracaine HCl Topical	$A^{l\ +}$	F^{c}	
Benzocaine, Butamben, and Tetracaine HCl		$F^{g\ t}$	
Benzoic & Salicylic Acid (oint.)	X^{+}		
Benzoin Tincture Compound		X^{+}	X^{+}
Benzonatate (cap)		X	X
Benzoyl Peroxide		$X^{h\ t}$	
Benzthiazide (tab)		X	
Benztropine Mesylate (tab)	X		
Benzyl Alcohol		X	X
Benzyl Benzoate (lot)		X	X
Benzylpenicilloyl Polylysine Concentrate			X
Beta Carotene (cap)		X	X
Betaine HCl	X		
Betamethasone	$X^{a\ d}$	C^{f}	
Betamethasone Benzoate (gel)		XC	
Betamethasone Dipropionate	XC^{g}	$X^{h\ i}$	C^{f}
Betamethasone Valerate	$C^{f\ g}$	$X^{f\ g}$	X^{h}
Betaxolol HCl		$X^{o\ a}$	
Betaxolol HCl Ophthalmic		X^{c}	
Bethanechol Chloride (tab)	X		
Biotin		X^{o}	
Biperiden HCl (tab)	X		
Bisacodyl	$X^{a\ i\ +}$		
Bismuth Subgallate		X^{o}	X^{o}
Bismuth, Milk of	X^{+}		
Bromodiphenhydramine HCl		X^{b}	X^{e}
Bromocriptine Mesylate		$X^{a\ o\ +}$	$X^{a\ o\ +}$
Brompheniramine Maleate	X^{e}	X^{a}	X^{e}
Brompheniramine Maleate & Pseudoephedrine Sulfate Syrup	X		X
Bumetanide		$X^{a\ o}$	$X^{a\ o}$
Busulfan (tab)	X		
Butalbital, Acetaminophen & Caffeine		$X^{a\ b}$	
Butalbital, Aspirin, Caffeine and Codeine Phosphate		X^{b}	X^{b}
Butabarbital & Aspirin (tab)		X	
Butamben	X		
Butoconazole Nitrate	X^{o}	$C^{f\ +}$	X^{o}
Calamine (lot)		X	
Calamine, Phenolated (lot)		X	
Calciferol (cap)		X	X
Calcium Acetate		X	
Calcium Carbonate	$X^{a\ o}$		
Calcium Carbonate Oral Susp.		X^{t}	
Calcium Carbonate & Magnesia (tab)	X		
Calcium & Magnesium Carbonates (tab)	X		
Calcium Carbonate, Magnesia & Simethicone (tab)	X		
Calcium Citrate	X^{o}		
Calcium Glubionate		$X^{d\ +}$	
Calcium Gluconate (tab)	X		
Calcium Hydroxide Topical Soln.		X	
Calcium Lactate (tab)	X		
Calcium Lactobionate	X^{o}		
Calcium Pantothenate (tab)		X	
Calcium Phosphate, dibasic (tab)	X		
Calcium Undecylenate	X^{o}		
Camphor Spirit		X	
Candicidin	$XT^{g\ +}$	$X^{m\ +}$	
Captopril		$X^{o\ a}$	
Carbachol Soln.		$X^{k\ w\ +}$	
Carbamazepine (tab)	GH		
Carbamazepine Oral	$F^{j\ +}$		$F^{j\ +}$
Carbamide Peroxide		$X^{o\ +}$	$X^{o\ +}$
Carbamide Peroxide Topical Soln.		X^{+}	X^{+}
Carbenicillin Indanyl Sodium (tab)	X		
Carbidopa & Levodopa (tab)	X		X
Carbinoxamine Maleate (tab)		X	X
Carbol-Fuchsin Topical Soln.		X	X
Carbomer 910		X	
Carbomer 934		X	
Carbomer 934a		X	
Carbomer 940		X	
Carbomer 1341		X	
Carboxymethylcellulose Sodium Paste	X^{+}		
Carboxymethylcellulose Sodium (tab)		X	
Carisoprodol	X^{a}	X^{o}	
Carisoprodol & Aspirin (tab)	X		

Drug (Dosage Form)	WC	T	LR
Carisoprodol, Aspirin & Codeine Phosphate (tab)	X		
Carphenazine Maleate Oral Soln.		X	X
Casanthranol		X^{o+}	X^{o+}
Cascara (tab)		X	
Cascara, Aromatic Fluidextract		X$^+$	X$^+$
Cascara Sagrada Extract		X$^+$	X$^+$
Cascara Sagrada Fluidextract		X$^+$	X$^+$
Castor Oil		X$^{b\ y\ +}$	
Castor Oil Aromatic		X	
Cefaclor		X^b	
Cefaclor for Oral Susp.		X	
Cefadroxil		X$^{a\ b}$	
Cefadroxil for Oral Susp.		X	
Cefixime		X$^{a\ o}$	
Cefixime for Oral Susp.		X^j	
Cefoperazone Sodium		X^o	
Cefotaxime Sodium		X^e	
Cefoxitin Sodium		X^o	
Cefpiramide		X^o	
Cefprozil		X$^{o\ a}$	
Cefrozil for Oral		X^j	
Ceftazidime		X^o	
Cefuroxime Axetil	X^a	X^o	
Cefuroxime Sodium		X^o	
Cellulose, Microcrystalline		X	
Cellulose, Microcrystalline & Carboxymethyl-cellulose Sodium		X	
Cellulose Sodium Phosphate	X		
Cephalexin		X$^{a\ b}$	
Cephalexin for Oral Susp.		X	
Cephalexin HCl		X^o	
Cephalothin Sodium		X^o	
Cephradine		X$^{a\ b\ j}$	
Cetylpyridinium Chloride	X^n	X^c	
Charcoal, Activated	X		
Chloral Hydrate		X^b	X^d
Chlorambucil (tab)	X		X
Chloramphenicol (all dosage forms)		X	
Chloramphenicol Ophthalmic		CTP$^{c\ g\ +}$	
Chloramphenicol Palmitate Oral Susp.		X	X
Chloramphenicol & Hydrocortisone Acetate for Ophthalmic Susp.		X	
Chloramphenicol & Polymyxin B Sulfate Ophthalmic Oint.		COT	
Chloramphenicol, Polymyxin B Sulfate & Hydrocortisone Acetate Ophthalmic Oint.		COT	
Chloramphenicol & Polymyxin B Sulfate Ophthalmic Oint.		COT	
Chloramphenicol & Prednisolone Ophthalmic Oint.		COT	
Chlordiazepoxide (tab)		X	X
Chlordiazepoxide & Amitriptyline HCl (tab)		X	X
Chlordiazepoxide HCl (cap)		X	X
Chlordiazepoxide HCl & Clidinium Bromide (cap)		X	X
Chloroquine Phosphate (tab)	X		
Chlorothiazide (tab)	X		
Chlorothiazide Oral Susp.		X	
Chlorotrianisene	H^{b+}	X^o	
Chloroxylenol	X^o		
Chlorpheniramine Maleate		X$^{a\ d}$	X^d
Chlorpheniramine Maleate Extended-Release		X	
Chlorpromazine HCl	X^a	X^d	X^a
Chlorpromazine HCl Oral Concentrate		X	X
Chlorpromazine HCl (supp)	X$^+$		X$^+$
Chlorpropamide (tab)	X		
Chlorprothixene (tab)	X		X
Chlorprothixene Oral Susp.		X	X
Chlortetracycline HCl	C^g	X$^{a\ b}$	C^{g}X$^{a\ h}$
Chlortetracycline & Sulfamethazine Soluble Pow.		X^x	X^x
Chlortetracycline HCl Ophthalmic Oint.		COT	
Chlortetracycline HCl Soluble Pow.		X^x	X^x
Chlorthalidone (tab)	X		
Chlorzoxazone (tab)		X	
Cholestyramine Oral Susp.		X	
Chymotrypsin for Ophthalmic Soln.		UG$^+$	
Ciclopirox Olamine Cream	C$^+$		
Ciclopirox Olamine Topical		X^j	
Cimetidine		X$^{a\ o\ +}$	X$^{a\ o\ +}$
Ciprofloxacin		X^o	X^o
Ciprofloxacin HCl	X^a	X^o	X^o
Ciprofloxacin Soln.		RT^k	X^k
Cinoxacin (cap)	X		
Cinoxate Lotion		X	X
Cisplatin		X^o	X^o
Clavulanate Potassium		X	

Drug (Dosage Form)	WC	T	LR	Drug (Dosage Form)	WC	T	LR
Clemastine Fumarate (tab)	X			Cyanocobalamin Co-57	X^b	X^c	X^b c
Clindinium Bromide (cap)		X	X	Cyanocobalamin Co-60	X^b	U^c	X^b c
Clindamycin HCl (cap)		X		Cyclacillin (tab)		X	
Clindamycin Palmitate HCl Oral Soln.		X		Cyclacillin for Oral Susp.		X	
Clindamycin Phosphate		X^o t		Cyclizine HCl (tab)		X	X
Clindamycin Phosphate, Topical		X^c j		Cyclobenzaprine HCl (tab)	X		
Clioquinol (Iodochlorhydroxyquin)	X^o	C^f g	C^f g	Beta Cyclodextrin	X^o		
Compound Clioquinol Topical		X^o		Cyclopentolate HCl Ophthalmic Soln.		X^+	
Clioquinol & Hydrocortisone		XC^f g	X^f g	Cyclophosphamide		X^a o +	
Clocortolone Pivalate		C^f	C^f	Cycloserine HCl (tab)	X		
Clofazime	X^b	X^o +	X^o +	Cyclosporine		X^o b	X^o
Clofibrate (cap)	X		X	Cyclosporine Oral Soln.		X	
Clomiphene Citrate (tab)	X		X	Cyclothiazide	X^a o		
Clonazepam		X^a +	X^a +	Cyproheptadine HCl	X^a	X^d	
Clonidine HCl (tab)	X			Danazol (cap)	X		
Clonidine HCl & Chlorthalidone (tab)	X			Dapsone (tab)	X		X
Clorazepate Dipotassium		In^o	In^o	Decoquinate Powder/ Premix		X	
Clorsulon	X^o			Dehydrocholic Acid (tab)	X		
Clotrimazole	X^m	X^c h +	X^c +	Demecarium Bromide Ophthalmic Soln.		X	X
Clotrimazole (cream)		C^+		Demeclocycline HCl		X^a b	X^a b
Clotrimazole & Betamethasone Dipropionate (cream)		XC		Demeclocycline HCl & Nystatin		X^a b	X^a b
Cloxacillin Benzathine		X^o x		Demeclocycline Oral Susp.		X	X
Cloxacillin Sodium (cap)		X		Desipramine HCl		X^a b	
Coal Tar		X^c g		Desoximetasone	C^f g t +	C^f t +	C^f
Cocaine HCl Tablets for Topical Soln.	X			Desoxycorticosterone Acetate Pellets		U	
Cod Liver Oil		In		Dexamethasone	X^a	X^e k C^t +	
Codeine Phosphate (tab)	X		X	Dexamethasone Sodium Phosphate		C^f X^r t	C^k
Codeine Sulfate (tab)	X			Dexchlorpheniramine Maleate		X^a d	X^d
Colchicine (tab)	X		X	Dextroamphetamine Sulfate	X^a	X^e b	X^e
Colestipol HCl for Oral Susp.		XU		Dextromethorphan HBr (syr)		X	X
Colistin Sulfate for Oral Susp.		X	X	Diatrizoate Meglumine & Diatrizoate Sodium Soln.		X	X
Colistin & Neomycin Sulfates & Hydrocortisone Acetate Otic Susp.		X		Diatrizoate Sodium Soln.		X	X
Collodion		X		Diazepam		X^a b	X^a b
Collodion, Flexible		X^+		Diazepam Extended Release (cap)		X	X
Colloidal Oatmeal	X			Diazoxide (cap)	X	X	
Copper Gluconate	X^o			Diazoxide Oral Susp.		X	X
Cortisone Acetate (tab)	X			Dibucaine		XC^f g	XC^f g
Cromolyn Sodium Inhalation		S/M		Dichlorphenamide	X^a o		
Cromolyn Sodium Soln.		X^s	X^s	Dicloxacillin Sodium (cap)	X		
Cromolyn Sodium Ophthalmic		S/M^o	S/M^o	Dicloxacillin Sodium for Oral Susp.		X	
Croscarmellose Sodium		X		Dicumarol (tab)	X		
Crotamiton(cream)		C	X	Dicyclomine HCl	X^a b	X^d	
				Dienestrol (cream)		C	
				Diethylcarbamazine Citrate (tab)		X	
				Diethylpropion HCl (tab)	X		

Drug (Dosage Form)	WC	T	LR
Diethylstilbestrol (tab)	X		
Diethyltoluamide Topical Soln.		X	
Diflorasone Diacetate		C^{fg+}	C^{fg+}
Diflunisal (tab)	X		
Digitalis		X^{ab}	
Digitoxin (tab)	X		
Digoxin		X^{ae+}	
Dihydrocodeine Bitartrate		X^o	
Dihydrostreptomycin Sulfate (Boluses)		X^x	
Dihydrotachysterol	X^{ab}		X^{ab}
Dihydrotachysterol Oral Soln.		X	X
Dihydroxyaluminum Aminoacetate (tab)	X		
Dihydroxyaluminum Aminoacetate Magma	X$^+$		
Dihydroxyaluminum Sodium Carbonate (tab)	X$^+$		
Diltiazem HCl		X^{ao}	X^{ao}
Dimenhydrinate	X^a	X^d	
Dimethyl Sulfoxide		X$^+$	X$^+$
Dinoprost Tromethamine (tab)		X	
Dioxybenzone & Oxybenzone (cream)		X	
Diperodon (ointment)		X	
Diphemanil Methylsulfate (tab)		X	
Diphenhydramine & Pseudoephedrine (cap)		X	
Diphenhydramine HCl		X^b	X^e
Diphenhydramine Citrate		X	X
Diphenoxylate HCl & Atropine Sulfate (tab)	X		X
Diphenoxylate HCl & Atropine Sulfate Oral Soln.		X	X
Diphylline	X	X^{ac}	
Dipivefrin HCl		X^{ko}	X^{ko}
Dipyridamole (tab)		X	X
Disopyramide Phosphate (cap)	X		
Disopyramide Phosphate Extended-Release (cap)	X		
Disulfiram (tab)		X	X
Docusate Calcium (cap)		X$^+$	
Docusate Potassium (cap)		X$^+$	
Docusate Sodium	X^a	X^{b+dc}	X^d
Doxepin HCl (cap)	X		
Doxepin HCl Oral Soln.		X	X
Doxycycline		X^o	X^b
Doxycycline for Oral Susp.		X	X
Doxycycline Calcium Oral Susp.		X	X

Drug (Dosage Form)	WC	T	LR
Doxycycline Hyclate		X^{ab}	X^{ab}
Doxycycline Hyclate Delayed-Release (cap)		X	X
Doxylamine Succinate	X^a	X^d	X^{ad}
Dronabinol		In^{o+}	In^{o+}
Dusting Powder, Absorbable	X		
Dyclonine HCl Topical Soln.		X	X
Dyclonine HCl (gel)		P/G	G
Dydrogesterone (tab)	X		
Dyphylline Elixir		X	
Dyphylline & Guaifenesin		X^{ac}	
Echothiophate Iodide for Ophthalmic Soln.		G$^+$	
Econazole Nitrate	X^o		X^o
Enalapril Maleate	X^{ao}		
Enalaprilat	X^o		
Ephedrine Sulfate	X^a	X^{bds}	X^{bds}
Ephedrine Sulfate & Phenobarbital (cap)	X		
Epinephrine		X^{krs}	X^{krs}
Epinephrine Bitartrate		X^k	X^k
Epinephrine Bitartrate Inhalation Aerosol	X	X	
Epinephrine Inhalation Aerosol		X	X
Epinephryl Borate Ophthalmic Soln.		X	X
Ergocalciferol		X^{ab}	X^{ab}
Ergocalciferol Oral Soln.		X	X
Ergoloid Mesylates (tab)		X	X
Ergoloid Mesylates Oral Soln.		X^I	X$^+$
Ergonovine Maleate (tab)	X		
Ergotamine Tartrate (tab)	X		
Ergotamine Tartrate Inhalation Aerosol		X	X
Ergotamine Tartrate & Caffeine	X^a	X^{i+}	X^a
Erythrityl Tetranitrate (tab)		X$^+$	
Erythrityl Tetranitrate, Diluted		X$^+$	
Erythromycin (tab)		X	
Erythromycin Delayed-Release		X^{ab}	
Erythromycin (oint)		CX$^+$	
Erythromycin Ophthalmic		COT^g	
Erythromycin Pledgets		X	
Erythromycin Topical		X^{ct}	
Erythromycin & Benzoyl Peroxide Topical		SX^t	
Erythromycin Estolate		X^{abj}	
Erythromycin Estolate for Oral Soln.		X	

Drug (Dosage Form)	WC	T	LR
Erythromycin Estolate Oral Susp.		X[+]	
Erythromycin Estolate & Sulfisoxazole Acetyl Oral		X[j]	
Erythromycin Ethylsuccinate (tab)		X	
Erythromycin Ethylsuccinate Oral Susp.	X		
Erythromycin Ethylsuccinate for Oral Susp.		X	
Erythromycin Ethylsuccinate & Sulfisoxazole Acetyl for Oral Susp.	X		
Erythromycin Stearate (tab)		X	
Erythromycin Stearate for Oral Susp.		X	
Erythrosine Sodium		X[a c]	X[a c]
Estradiol (cream)		C[m]	
Estradiol (tab)		X	X
Estrogens, Conjugated (tab)	X		
Estrogens, Esterified (tab)	X		
Estropipate	X[a]	C[m f]	
Ethacrynic Acid (tab)	X		
Ethambutol HCl (tab)	X		
Ethchlorvynol (cap)		X	X
Ether		R[+]	R[+]
Ethinamate (cap)		X	
Ethinyl Estradiol (tab)	X		
Ethionamide (tab)	X		
Ethopropazine HCl (tab)	X	X	
Ethosuximide (cap)		X	
Ethotoin		X[a o]	
Ethylcellulose Aqueous Dispersion		X[+]	
Ethynodiol Diacetate & Ethinyl Estradiol (tab)	X		
Ethynodiol Diacetate & Mestranol (tab)	X		
Etidronate Disodium (tab)		X	
Eucatropine HCl Ophthalmic Soln.		X	
Eugenol	X	X	
Famotidine	X[a o]		X[a o]
Fenoprofen Calcium	X[a b]		
Fentanyl Citrate		X[o]	
Ferrous Fumarate (tab)		X	
Ferrous Gluconate		X[a b e]	X[a b e]
Ferrous Sulfate		X[a c d]	X[c]
Floxuridine		X[o]	X[o]
Flucytosine (cap)		X	X
Fluhydrocortisone Acetate (tab)	X		
Flumethasone Pivalate (cream)		C	

Drug (Dosage Form)	WC	T	LR
Flunisolide Nasal Soln.		X[+]	X[+]
Fluocinolone Acetonide		C[f g]	
Fluocinolone Acetate Topical Soln.		X	
Fluocinonide	C[f g t]		
Fluorescein Sodium & Benoxinate HCl Ophthalmic		X[c]	X[c]
Fluorescein Sodium & Proparacaine HCl Ophthalmic		G[+]	G[+]
Fluorometholone (cream)		C	
Fluorometholone Ophthalmic Susp.		X	
Fluorouracil		XT[c f +]	
Fluoxymesterone (tab)	X		X
Fluphenazine Decanoate		X[o]	X[o]
Fluphenazine HCl		X[a e]	X[a e]
Fluphenazine HCl Oral Soln.		X	X
Flurandrenolide		X[f g h]	X[f g h]
Flurandrenolide (tab)	X[+]		
Flurazepam HCl (cap)		X	X
Flurbiprofen	X[a]	X[o]	
Flurbiprofen Sodium		X[o]	
Flurbiprofen Sodium Ophthalmic Soln.		X	
Folic Acid (tab)	X		
Formaldehyde Soln.		X[+]	
Furazolidone		X[j +]	X[j +]
Furosemide (tab)	X		X
Gauze (all)	X		
Gemfibrozil		X[a b]	
Gentamicin Sulfate		X[d]C[f g]	
Gentamicin Sulfate Ophthalmic		COT[g]	
Gentamicin & Prednisolone Acetate Ophthalmic		OT[g +]	X[j]
Gentian Violet		X[c]C[f t]	
Glipizide		X[o]	
Gluconolactone	X[o]		
Glutaral Concentrate		X[+]	X[+]
Glutethimide	X[a b]		
Glycerin Oral Solution		X	
Glycerin Suppository	X[+]		
Glycerin Ophthalmic Soln.		TPG/P	X
Glycopyrrolate (tab)	X		
Gold Sodium Thiomalate		X[o]	X[o]
Green Soap Tincture	X		
Griseofulvin		X[a b]	
Griseofulvin Oral Susp.	X		
Griseofulvin, Ultramicrosize (tab)	X		
Guaifenesin		X[a b d]	
Guanabenz Acetate		X[a o]	X[a o]
Guanadrel Sulfate	X[o]	X[a]	X[a]
Guanethidine Monosulfate (tab)	X		

Drug (Dosage Form)	WC	T	LR
Halazepan	X^a o		
Halazone Tablets for Soln.		X	X
Halcinonide	X^a f g		
Haloperidol (tab)		X	X
Haloperidol Oral Soln.		X	X
Haloprogin		X^+ f	X^f
Haloprogin Topical Soln.		X^+	X^f
Halothane		G^+	X^+
Heparin Sodium		X^o +	
Hetacillin (tab)		X	
Hetacillin for Oral Susp.		X	
Hetacillin Potassium		X^b	X^a x
Hetacillin Potassium Oral Susp.		X	
Hexachlorophene Cleansing Emulsion		X	X
Hexachlorophene Liquid Soap		X	X
Hexylcaine HCl Topical Soln.		X	
Hexylresorcinol		X^n	X^o
Homatropine Hydrobromide Ophthalmic Soln.		X	
Homatropine Methylbromide (tab)		X	X
Hydralazine HCl (tab)		X	X
Hydrochlorothiazide (tab)	X		
Hydrocodone Bitartrate (tab)		X	X
Hydrocodone Bitartrate and Acetaminophen		X^a	X^a
Hydrocortisone (Cortisol)	X^a g	X^f h p t	
Hydrocortisone Acetate	X^f g	X^h	
Hydrocortisone Acetate Ophthalmic		X	
Hydrocortisone Butyrate	X^f o		
Hydrocortisone Cypionate Oral Susp.		X	X
Hydrocortisone Valerate (cream)	X		
Hydrocortisone & Acetic Acid Otic Soln.		X	X
Hydroflumethiazide (tab)		X	
Hydrogen Peroxide Concentrate	SP^+		
Hydrogen Peroxide Topical Soln.		X^+	X^+
Hydromorphone HCl (tab)		X	X
Hydroquinone (cream)	X		X
Hydroquinone Topical Soln.		X	X
Hydroxyamphetamine HBr Ophthalmic Soln.		X	X
Hydroxychloroquine Sulfate (tab)		X	X
Hydroxypropyl Cellulose Ocular System		U^+	
Hydroxypropyl Methylcellulose Ophthalmic Soln.		X	
Hydroxyurea (cap)		X	
Hydroxyzine HCl		X^a d	X^d
Hydroxyzine Pamoate (cap)	X		
Hydroxyzine Pamoate Oral Susp.		X	X
Hyoscyamine (tab)	X		X
Hyoscyamine Sulfate (tab)		X	X
Hyoscyamine Sulfate Oral Soln.		X^i	X^+
Ibuprofen (tab)	X		
Ichthammol (ointment)		C^+	
Idoxuridine Ophthalmic	C^g t	X^c	X^c
Ifosfamide		X^o +	
Imipramine HCl (tab)		X	
Indapamide	X^o a		
Indium In^111 Oxyquinoline		U^c +	
Indomethacin (cap)	X^b i +		
Indomethacin Extended-Release (cap)	X		
Indomethacin Oral		X^j	X^j
Indomethacin Sodium	X^o		X^u
Insulin		X^+	X
Insulin Human		X^+	X
Iocetamic Acid (tab)		X	
Iodide, Sodium, I-123, I-125, I-131 (cap)	X		
Iodine (all Soln. & Tinct.)		X^+	X^+
Iodoquinol (tab)	X		
Iohexol	X^o		X^o
Iopamidol	X^o		X^o
Iopanoic Acid (tab)		X	X
Ipecac Syrup		X^+	
Iopodate Calcium for Oral Susp.	X		
Iopodate Sodium (cap)		X	
Isocarboxazide (tab)	X		X
Isoetharine Inhalation Soln.		WF	Ox
Isoetharine Mesylate Inhalation Aerosol			X
Isoflurophate Ophthalmic		C^g	
Isoniazid	X^a	X^d	X^a d
Isopropamide Iodide (tab)	X		
Isopropyl Alcohol (all)		X^+	
Isoproterenol Inhalation Soln.		WF	Ox
Isoproterenol HCl	X^a	X^a r l	X^a r l
Isoproterenol HCl & Phenylephrine Bitartrate Inhalation Aerosol		X	X

Drug (Dosage Form)	WC	T	LR	Drug (Dosage Form)	WC	T	LR
Isoproterenol Sulfate Inhalation		WF$^{c\,l}$	Ox$^{c\,l}$	Lithium Citrate (syr)		X	
Isosorbide Concentrate		X	X	Loperamide HCl (cap)	X		
Isosorbide Dinitrate (tab)	X			Lorazepam		X$^{a\,o}$	X$^{a\,o}$
Isosorbide Dinitrate Chewable (tab)	X			Loxapine (cap)		X	
Isosorbide Dinitrate, Diluted		X		Loxapine Succinate		X^o	
Isosorbide Dinitrate, Extended-Release	X$^{a\,b}$			Lypressin Nasal Soln		P	
Isosorbide Dinitrate, Sublingual (tab)	X			Mafenide Acetate (cream)		X$^+$	X$^+$
Isosorbide Oral Soln.	X			Magaldrate	X^a	X^j	
Isotretinoin		I$^{m\,o}$	X^o	Magaldrate & Simethicone (tab)	X		
Isoxsuprine HCl (tab)		X		Magaldrate & Simethicone Oral Susp.		X$^+$	
Kanamycin Sulfate (cap)		X		Magnesia (tab)	X		
Ketoconazole (tab)	X			Magnesium Carbonate & Sodium Bicarbonate for Oral Susp.		X	
Labetolol HCl		X$^{o\,a\,t}$	X$^{o\,a\,t}$	Magnesium Citrate Oral Soln.		SP$^+$	
Lactic Acid		X		Magnesium Gluconate	X$^{a\,o}$		
Lactulose (syr/conc)		X$^+$		Magnesium Hydroxide Paste		X	
Modified Lanolin		X$^+$ (Rust proof)		Magnesium Oxide	X$^{a\,b}$		
Lanolin, Anhydrous	X$^+$			Magnesium Salicylate (tab)		X	
Levamisole HCl	X$^{a\,o}$		X^o	Magnesium Trisilicate (tab)	X		
Levobunolol HCl	X^o			Malathion		X^{o}G^h	X^o
Levobunolol HCl Ophthalmic Soln.		X		Maltitol		X^c	
Levocarnitine		X^o		Maltodextrin	H$^+$	H$^+$	
Levocarnitine, Oral Soln.		X		Manganese Carbonate	X^o		
Levodopa		X$^{a\,b\,+}$	X$^{a\,b\,+}$	Maprotiline HCl (tab)	X		
Levonorgestrel (tab)	X		X	Mazindol (tab)		X$^+$	
Levonorgestrel & Ethinyl Estradiol (tab)	X			Mebendazol (tab)	X		
Levopropoxyphene Napsylate (tab)		X	X	Mebrofenin		X^o	
Levopropoxyphene Napsylate Oral Susp.		X$^+$	X$^+$	Mecamylamine HCl	X^a	X^o	
Levorphanol Tartrate (tab)	X			Mechlorethamine HCl		X	X
Levothyroxine Sodium (tab)		X	X	Meclizine HCl (tab)	X		
Levothyroxine Sodium Oral		X^o	X^o	Meclocycline Sulfosalicylate Cream		X	X
Lidocaine		X$^{g\,l}$		Meclofenamate Sodium (cap)		X	X
Lidocaine Oral Topical Soln.		X		Medroxyprogesterone Acetate (tab)	X		
Lidocaine HCl Oral Topical Soln.		X		Medrysone Ophthalmic Susp.		X	X
Lidocaine Topical Soln.		X		Mefenamic Acid		X$^{b\,o}$	X^o
Lidocaine HCl Jelly		X		Megestrol Acetate (tab)	X		
Lime		X		Melphalan (tab)	X		
Lincomycin HCl		X$^{b\,d}$		Menadiol Sodium Diphosphate (tab)	X		X
Lindane		X$^{f\,h}$		Menotropins		G$^{o\,+}$	
Lindane Shampoo		X		Mepenzolate Bromide	X^a	X$^{d\,o}$	X^d
Liothyronine Sodium (tab)		X		Meperidine HCl	X^a	X^d	X$^{a\,d}$
Liotrix (tab)		X		Mephenytoin (tab)	X		
Lisinopril	X$^{a\,o}$			Mephobarbital (tab)	X		
Lithium Carbonate	X$^{a\,b}$			Meprobamate (tab)	X		
Lithium Carbonate Extended-Release (tab)	X			Meprobamate Oral Susp.		X	
				Mercaptopurine (tab)	X		

Drug (Dosage Form)	WC	T	LR
Mercury, Ammoniated (oint.)	X	C[k]	X
Mesoridazine Besylate (tab)	X		X
Mesoridazine Besylate Oral Soln.		X[+]	X[+]
Metaproterenol Sulfate	X[a]	X[o,l,d]	X[o,d,l,a]
Metaproterenol Sulfate Soln.		WF[1]	Ox[1]
Metaraminol Bitartrate	X[o]		
Methacycline HCl (cap)		X	X
Methacycline HCl Oral Susp.		X	X
Methadone HCl (tab)	X		
Methadone HCl Oral Concentrate		X[+]	X[+]
Methadone HCl Oral Soln.		X[+]	X[+]
Methamphetamine	X[a,o]		X[a,o]
Methamphetamine HCl (pow)		X	X
Methantheline Bromide (tab)	X		
Metharbital (tab)		X	
Methazolamide (tab)	X		
Methdilazine (tab)		X	X
Methdilazine HCl		X[a,d]	X[a,d]
Methenamine	X[a]	X[e]	
Methenamine & Monobasic Sodium Phosphate (tab)		X	
Methenamine Hippurate (tab)	X		
Methenamine Mandelate (tab)	X		
Methenamine Mandelate for Oral Soln.	X[c]	X[j]	
Methimazole (tab)	X		X
Methocarbamol (tab)		X	
Methotrexate (tab)	X		
Methoxsalen (cap)		X	X
Methoxsalen Topical Soln.		X	X
Methscopolamine Bromide (tab)		X	
Methsuximide (cap)		X	
Methyclothiazide (tab)	X		
Methylbenzethonium Chloride	X[e]	X[h]C[g]	
Methylbenzethonium Chloride Topical		X[o]	
Methylcellulose	X[a]	X[k,+]	
Methylcellulose Oral Soln.		X[+]	X[+]
Methyldopa (tab)	X		
Methyldopa Oral Susp.		X[+]	X[+]
Methyldopa & Chlorothiazide (tab)	X		
Methyldopa & Hydrochlorothiazide (tab)	X		

Drug (Dosage Form)	WC	T	LR
Methylergonovine Maleate (tab)		X	X
Methylphenidate HCl (tab)		X	
Methylphenidate HCl Extended-Release (tab)		X	
Methylprednisolone (tab)		X	
Methylprednisolone Acetate	X[p]	XC[f]	X[f]
Methyltestosterone	X[a,b]		
Methyprylon		X[a,b]	X[a,b]
Methysergide Maleate (tab)		X	
Metoclopramide HCl		X[a,o]	X[a,o]
Metoclopramide Oral Soln.		F[+]	F[+]
Metolazone		X[a,o]	X[a,o]
Metoprolol Tartrate (tab)		X	X
Metoprolol Tartrate & Hydrochlorothiazide (tab)		X	X
Metronidazole	X[a]	CP[t,+]	X[a]
Metyrapone (tab)		X[+]	X[+]
Metyrosine (cap)	X		
Mexiletine HCl		X[b,o]	
Miconazole Nitrate		X[m,i] C[f]	
Miconazole Nitrate, Topical	X[o]		
Mineral Oil		X[p,y]	
Mineral Oil, Light, Topical		X	
Minocycline HCl		X[a,b]	X[a,b]
Minocycline HCl Oral Susp.		X	X
Minoxidil	X[o]	X[a]	
Mitotane (tab)		X	X
Mitoxantrone HCl		X[o]	
Monobenzene (cream)		X[+]	
Molindone HCl		X[a,o]	X[a,o]
Mupirocin	XC[g]	X[o]	
Nadolol	X[o]	X[a]	
Nadolol & Bendroflumethiazide (tab)		X	
Nafcillin Sodium		X[a,b]	X[a]
Nafcillin Sodium for Oral Soln.		X	
Nalidixic Acid (tab)		X	
Nalidixic Acid Oral Susp.		X	
Nandrolone Phenpropionate		X[o]	X[o]
Naphazoline HCl Soln.		X[k,s]	X[k,s]
Naproxen (tab)	X		
Naproxen Oral		X[j,+]	X[j,+]
Naproxen Sodium (tab)	X		
Natamycin Ophthalmic Susp.		TP	
Neomycin Sulfate	X[f,g,+]	X[a,c,+]	X[c,+]
Neomycin Sulfate Ophthalmic Oint.		COT[+]	

Drug (Dosage Form)	WC	T	LR
Neomycin Sulfate & Bacitracin		X^{g+}	X^{g+}
Neomycin Sulfate & Bacitracin Zinc	XC^g		
Neomycin Sulfate & Dexamethasone Sodium Phosphate		X^f	
Neomycin Sulfate & Dexamethasone Sodium Phosphate Ophthalmic	X^{c+}	COT^g	X^{c+}
Neomycin Sulfate & Fluocinolone Acetonide	XC^f		
Neomycin Sulfate & Fluorometholone	CX^g		
Neomycin Sulfate & Flurandrenolide		CX^{fgh}	X^{fgh}
Neomycin Sulfate & Gramicidin	CX^g		
Neomycin Sulfate & Hydrocortisone	CX^{fg}		
Neomycin Sulfate & Hydrocortisone Otic Susp.	X	X	
Neomycin Sulfate & Hydrocortisone Acetate	CX^{fgh}		
Neomycin Sulfate & Hydrocortisone Acetate Ophthalmic		$X^j COT^g$	
Neomycin Sulfate & Methylprednisolone Acetate		CX^f	X^f
Neomycin Sulfate & Prednisolone Acetate Ophthalmic		$COTX^j$	X^h
Neomycin Sulfate & Prednisolone Sodium Phosphate Ophthalmic Oint.		COT	
Neomycin Sulfate, Sulfacetamide Sodium & Prednisolone Acetate, Ophthalmic		COT^g	
Neomycin Sulfate & Triamcinolone Acetonide	XCT^f		
Neomycin Sulfate & Triamcinolone Acetonide Ophthalmic Oint.		COT	
Neomycin & Polymyxin B Sulfates Ophthalmic	COT^{g+}		X^{c+}
Neomycin & Polymyxin B Sulfate & Bacitracin Zinc	CX^g	CX^g	X^{g+}
Neomycin & Polymyxin B Sulfate & Bacitracin Zinc & Hydrocortisone Acetate Ophthalmic Oint.		COT	

Drug (Dosage Form)	WC	T	LR
Neomycin & Polymyxin B Sulfate & Bacitracin Zinc & Hydrocortisone Acetate Oint.	CX^+		
Neomycin & Polymyxin B Sulfates, Bacitracin & Lidocaine		X^{g+}	
Neomycin & Polymyxin B Sulfates, Bacitracin Zinc & Hydrocortisone Acetate Ointment	X^{gk+}		
Neomycin & Polymyxin B Sulfate & Hydrocortisone Otic Soln.		X	X
Neomycin & Polymyxin B Sulfates & Dexamethasone Ophthalmic	COT^gX^j	X^j	
Neomycin & Polymyxin B Sulfate & Gramicidin	CX^f		
Neomycin & Polymyxin B Sulfate & Gramicidin Ophthalmic Soln.		X	
Neomycin & Polymyxin B Sulfates, Gramicidin & Hydrocortisone Acetate Cream	X		
Neomycin & Polymyxin B Sulfates & Hydrocortisone Susp.		TP^{kv}	X^{kv}
Neomycin & Polymyxin B Sulfate & Hydrocortisone Soln.		TP^{kv}	X^{kv}
Neomycin & Polymyxin B Sulfates & Hydrocortisone Acetate Ophthalmic Susp.		X	
Neomycin & Polymyxin B Sulfates & Prednisolone Acetate Ophthalmic Susp.		X	
Neostigmine Bromide	X^{ao}		
Neostigmine Methylsalicylate	X^o		
Niacin (tab)	X		
Niacinamide (tab)	X		
Nifedipine (cap)	X^+	X^+	
Nitrofurantoin	X^{abj}	X^{abj}	
Nitrofurazone	X^{fg}	X^{fg}	
Nitrofurazone Topical Soln.	X	X	
Nitroglycerin	G^{a+}	X^g	
Nitromersol Topical Soln.	X	X	
Nizatidine	X^{bo+}	X^{bo+}	
Nonoxynol 9	X		
Norethindrone (tab)	X		
Norethindrone & Ethinyl Estradiol (tab)	X		
Norethindrone & Mestranol (tab)	X		

Drug (Dosage Form)	WC	T	LR
Norethindrone Acetate (tab)	X		
Norethindrone Acetate & Ethinyl Estradiol (tab)	X		
Norfloxacin	X^a	X^o	X^o
Norgestrel (tab)	X		
Norgestrel & Ethinyl Estradiol (tab)	X		
Nortriptyline HCl		X^{ac}	X^c
Novobiocin Calcium Oral Susp.		X	X
Nylidrin HCl (tab)	X		
Nystatin	X^{g+}	X^{ah+n}	X^{ah+n}
Nystatin Cream		XC$^+$	
Nystatin for Oral Susp.	X		
Nystatin Oral Susp.		X	X
Nystatin Vaginal		X^{ai+}	X^{ai+}
Nystatin & Clioquinol Ointment		XC$^+$	
Nystatin & Iodoquinol (Iodochlorhydroxyquin)		X^g	X^{g+}
Nystatin, Neomycin Sulfate, Gramicidin & Triamcinolone Acetonide		X^{fg}	
Nystatin, Neomycin Sulfate, Thiostrepton, and Triamcinolone Acetonide		X^{fg}	
Nystatin & Triamcinolone Acetonide		X^{fg}	
Ointment, White and/or Yellow	X		
Oleovitamin A & D (cap)		X	X
Ophthalmic Oint., Bland Lubricating	OT^g		
Opium Powder	X		
Opium Tincture		X$^+$	X$^+$
Oxacillin Sodium (cap)		X$^+$	
Oxacillin Sodium for Oral Soln.		X$^+$	
Oxamniquine (cap)		X	
Oxandrolone (tab)		X	X
Oxazepam (tab/cap)	X^{ab}		
Oxprenolol HCl	X^o	X^a	X^a
Oxprenolol Extended-Release (tab)		X	X
Oxtriphylline	X^{eo}		
Oxtriphylline Delayed-Release (tab)		X	
Oxtriphylline Extended-Release (tab)		X	
Oxybutynin Chloride	X^o	X^{ad}	X^{ad}
Oxycodone (tab)		X	X
Oxycodone & Acetaminophen		X^{ab}	X^{ab}
Oxycodone & Aspirin (tab)		X	X
Oxycodone HCl		X^o	
Oxycodone HCl Oral Soln.		X	X
Oxycodone Terephthalate		X^o	

Drug (Dosage Form)	WC	T	LR
Oxymetazoline HCl Soln.		X^{ks}	
Oxymetholone (tab)	X		
Oxymorphone HCl Suppositories	X$^+$		
Oxyphenbutazone (tab)		X	
Oxyphencyclimine HCl (tab)		X	
Oxytetracycline (tab)		X	X
Oxytetracycline Calcium Oral Susp.		X	X
Oxytetracycline HCl (cap)		X	X
Oxytetracycline & Nystatin (cap)		X	X
Oxytetracycline & Nystatin for Oral Susp.		X$^+$	X$^+$
Oxytetracycline HCl & Hydrocortisone Ointment	X		X
Oxytetracycline HCl & Hydrocortisone Acetate Ophthalmic Susp.		X	X
Oxytetracycline & Phenazopyridine Hydrochlorides & Sulfamethizole (cap)		X	X
Oxytetracycline HCl & Polymyxin B Sulfate	X^{gom}		X^q
Oxytetracycline HCl & Polymyxin B Ophthalmic Oint.		COT	
Pancreatin		X^{ab+}	
Pancrelipase		X^{ab+}	
Papain Tablets for Topical Soln.		X$^+$	X$^+$
Papaverine HCl (tab)		X	
Parachlorophenol Camphorated		X	X
Paramethadione (cap)		X	
Paramethadione Oral Soln.		X	X
Paramethasone Acetate (tab)	X		
Paregoric		X$^+$	X$^+$
Pargyline HCl (tab)	X		
Paromomycin Sulfate		X^{bd}	
Pectin	X		
Penicillamine		X^{ab}	
Penicillin G Benzathine (tab)		X	
Penicillin G Benzathine Oral Susp.		X	
Penicillin G Potassium (tab)		X	
Penicillin G Potassium Tablets for Oral Soln.		X	
Penicillin G Procaine, Neomycin & Polymyxin B Sulfates & Hydrocortisone Acetate Topical Susp.	X		

Drug (Dosage Form)	WC	T	LR
Penicillin V (tab)		X	
Penicillin V for Oral Susp.	X		
Penicillin V Benzathine	X[l+]		
Penicillin V Benzathine, Oral Susp.	X[+]		
Penicillin V Potassium (tab)	X		
Penicillin V Potassium for Oral Soln.	X		
Pentaerythritol Tetranitrate (tab)		X	
Pentazocine HCl (tab)		X	X
Pentazocine HCl & Aspirin(tab)		X	X
Pentazocine & Naloxone HCl (tab)		X	X
Pentetic Acid	X[o]		
Pentobarbital Elixir		X	
Pentobarbital Sodium (cap)		X	
Peppermint Spirit		X	
Perphenazine	X[d]	X[a]	X[a d]
Perphenazine Oral Soln.	X		X
Perphenazine & Amitriptyline HCl (tab)	X		
Phenacemide (tab)	X		
Phenazopyridine HCl (tab)		X	
Phendimetrazine Tartrate	X[a]	X[b]	
Phenelzine Sulfate (tab)		X[+]	X[+]
Phenindione (tab)	X		
Phenmetrazine HCl (tab)		X	
Phenobarbital	X[a]	X[e]	X[e]
Phenol		X	X
Phenol, Liquefied		X	X
Phenolphthalein (tab)		X	
Phenoxybenzamine HCl	X[ob]		
Phenprocoumon (tab)	X		
Phensuximide (cap)		X	
Phentermine HCl		X[a b]	
Phenylbutazone		X[a b]	
Phenylephrine HCl Soln.		X[k s]	X[k s]
Phenylephrine HCl Nasal Jelly		X	
Phenylpropanolamine HCl Extended-Release		X[a b]	X[a b]
Phenytoin (tab)	X		
Phenytoin Oral Susp.		X[+]	
Phenytoin Sodium, Extended (cap)		X	
Phenytoin Sodium, Prompt (cap)		X	
Physostigmine Salicylate Ophthalmic Soln.		X	X
Physostigmine Sulfate Ophthalmic Ointment		COT	
Phytonadione (tab)	X		X
Pilocarpine HCl Ophthalmic Soln.		X	
Pilocarpine Nitrate Ophthalmic Soln.		X	X
Pimozide		X[a o]	X[a o]
Pindolol	X[a o]		X[a o]
Piperacetazine (tab)	X		X
Piperazine Citrate		X[a d]	
Pipobroman (tab)	X		
Piroxicam		X[h o]	X[h o]
Podophyllum Resin		X[o]	X[o]
Podophyllum Resin Topical Soln.		X	X
Polycarbophil		X[o]	
PEG 3350 & Electrolytes for Oral Soln.		X	
Polyethylene Oxide		X	X
Polymyxin B Sulfate & Bacitracin Zinc Topical	X[o]	A[l t]	
Polymyxin B Sulfate & Hydrocortisone Otic Soln.		X	X
Polythiazide (tab)		X	X
Potassium Bicarbonate Effervescent Tabs for Oral Soln.		X[+]	
Potassium Bicarbonate & Potassium Chloride for Effervescent Oral Soln.		X[+ a o]	
Potassium & Sodium Bicarbonate & Citric Acid Effervescent for Oral Soln. (tab)		X	X
Potassium Carbonate	X[o]		
Potassium Chloride Oral Soln.		X	
Potassium Chloride for Oral Soln.		X	
Potassium Chloride Extended-Release		X[a b +]	
Potassium Chloride, Potassium Bicarbonate, & Potassium Citrate Effervescent Tablets for Oral Soln.		X[+]	
Potassium Citrate & Citric Acid Oral Soln.		X	
Potassium Gluconate		X[a e]	X[e]
Potassium Gluconate & Potassium Chloride for Oral Soln.	X		
Potassium Gluconate & Potassium Chloride Oral		X	
Potassium Gluconate & Potassium Citrate Oral Soln.	X		
Potassium Gluconate, Potassium Citrate & Ammonium Chloride, Oral Soln.		X	
Potassium Iodide (tab)		X	

Drug (Dosage Form)	WC	T	LR
Potassium Iodide Oral Soln.		X	X
Povidone Iodide Topical Soln.		X[+]	
Povidone-Iodine Oint.		X	
Povidone-Iodine Cleansing Soln.		X	
Pralidoxime Chloride (tab)	X		
Pramoxine HCl		X[f t]C[t]	
Prazepam		X[a b]	X[a b]
Praziquantel	X[o]	X[a]	X[o]
Prazosin HCl (cap)	X		X
Prednisolone	X[a]	X[c d f]	X[d]
Prednisolone Acetate Ophthalmic Susp.		X	
Prednisolone Sodium Phosphate Ophthalmic Soln.		X	X
Prednisone	X[a]	X[d]	
Prednisone Oral Soln.		X	
Primaquine Phosphate (tab)	X		X
Primidone (tab)	X		
Primidone Oral Susp.		X	X
Probenecid (tab)	X		
Probenecid & Colchicine (tab)	X		X
Probucol	X		X
Procainamide HCl		X[a b]	
Procainamide HCl Extended Release (tab)	X		
Procarbazine HCl		X[bo]	X[bo]
Prochlorperazine Edisylate Oral Soln.		X	X
Prochlorperazine Edisylate Syr.		X	X
Prochlorperazine Maleate (tab)	X		X
Prochlorperazine Suppositories		X	
Procyclidine HCl (tab)		X[+]	
Promazine HCl		X[a c d]	X[a c d]
Promethazine HCl		X[a d i +]	X[a d i +]
Propantheline Bromide (tab)	X		
Proparacaine HCl Ophthalmic Soln.		X	X
Propiomazine HCl		X[o]	X[o]
Propoxyphene HCl (cap)	X		
Propoxyphene HCl & Acetaminophen (tab)	X		
Propoxyphene HCl, Aspirin & Caffeine (cap)		X[+]	
Propoxyphene Napsylate		X[a o]	
Propoxyphene Napsylate Oral Susp.		X	X
Propoxyphene Napsylate & Acetaminophen (tab)		X[+]	
Propoxyphene Napsylate & Aspirin (tab)		X	
Propranolol HCl (tab)	X		
Propranolol HCl Extended-Release (cap)		X	
Propranolol HCl & Hydrochlorothiazide (tab)		X	
Propranolol HCl & Hydrochlorothiazide Extended-Release (cap)		X	
Propylene Glycol		X	
Propylhexedrine Inhalant		X[+]	
Propylthiouracil (tab)	X		
Protamine Sulfate		X[+]	X[+]
Protriptyline HCl (tab)		X	
Pseuodephedrine HCl		X[a d]	X[d]
Psyllium Hydrophilic Mucilloid for Oral Susp.		X	
Pyrantel Pamoate Oral Susp.		X	X
Pyrazinamide (tab)	X		
Pyrethrum Extract		X	X
Pyridostigmine Bromide		X[a d]	X[d]
Pyridoxine HCl (tab)	X		
Pyrilamine Maleate (tab)	X		
Pyrimethamine (tab)		X	X
Pyroxylin			SP
Pyrvinium Pamoate		X[a j]	X[a j]
Quinacrine HCl (tab)		X	
Quinestrol (tab)	X		
Quinethazone (tab)		X	
Quinidine Gluconate Extended-Release	X[a o]		X[a o]
Quinidine Sulfate	X[a]	X[b]	X[a b]
Quinidine Sulfate Extended-Release (tab)	X		X
Quinine Sulfate	X[a]	X[b]	
Racepinephrine		X[o]	X[o]
Racepinephrine Soln.		X[r +]	X[r +]
Ranitidine HCl		X[a o]	X[a o]
Ranitidine Oral Soln.		X[+]	X[+]
Rauwolfia Serpentina (tab)		X	X
Oral Rehydration Salts		SX[a +]	
Reserpine		X[a e]	X[a e]
Reserpine & Chlorothiazide (tab)		X	X
Reserpine & Hydrochlorothiazide (tab)		X	X
Reserpine, Hydralazine & Hydrochlorothiazide (tab)		X	X
Resorcinol, Compound (oint)		X[+]	
Resorcinol & Sulfur (lot)	X		
Ribavirin		X[o]	

Drug (Dosage Form)	WC	T	LR
Ribavirin for Inhalation Soln.		H[+]	
Riboflavin (tab)	X	X	
Rifampin (cap)	X[+]	X[+]	
Rifampin & Isoniazid (cap)	X[i]	X[i]	
Ritodrine HCl (tab)	X[+]		
Rose Water Oint.	X	X	
Saccharin Sodium	X[a]	X[c]	
Safflower Oil	X	X	
Salicylamide		X[o]	
Salicylic Acid Collodion		X[+]	
Salicylic Acid Gel		XC[+]	
Salicylic Acid Plaster	X[+]		
Salicylic Acid Topical Foam	X		
Salsalate	X[oab]		
Scopolamine HBr Ophthalmic	X[c]C[g]		
Scopolamine HBr (tab)	X	X	
Secobarbital Elixir	X		
Secobarbital Sodium (cap)	X		
Secobarbital Sodium & Amobarbital (cap)	X		
Selenious Acid		X	
Selenium Sulfide Lotion		X	
Senna Syrup		X[+]	
Sennosides (tab)	X		
Silver Nitrate Ophthalmic Soln.		X	X
Silver Nitrate, Toughened		X	X
Silver Sulfadiazine	X[o]	CT[f]	
Simethicone	X[a]	X[y]	
Simethicone Oral Susp.		X	X
Sodium Acetate Soln.		X	
Sodium Bicarbonate	X[ao]		
Sodium Chloride	X[a]	C[k]	
Sodium Chloride & Dextrose (tab)	X		
Sodium Citrate & Citric Acid Oral Soln.		X	
Sodium Fluoride (tab)		X	
Sodium Fluoride Oral Soln.		XP	
Sodium Fluoride & Phosphoric Acid		P[t]	
Sodium Fluoride & Phosphoric Acid Topical Soln.		P	
Sodium Gluconate	X[o]		
Sodium Lactate Soln.		X	
Sodium Phosphate	X[p]		
Sodium Phosphates Oral Soln.		X	
Sodium Polystyrene Sulfonate Susp.	X[+]		
Sodium Salicylate (tab)	X		
Sorbitol Soln.		X	
Spironolactone (tab)		X	X
Spironolactone & Hydrochlorothiazide		X[a]	X[o]
Squalane		X	
Stannous Fluoride Gel	X		
Stanozolol (tab)		X	X
Topical Starch	X		
Sufentanil Citrate	X[o]		
Sulconazole Nitrate	X[o]		X[o]
Sulfacetamide Sodium Ophthalmic	COT[g]	X[c+]	X[c+]
Sulfacetamide Sodium & Prednisolone Acetate Ophthalmic	CTP[g]	TP[j]	
Sulfadiazine (tab)	X		X
Silver Sulfadiazine		SC[f]	X[f]
Sulfadoxine & Pyrimethamine (tab)	X		X
Sulfamerazine (tab)	X		
Sulfamethizole (tab)	X		
Sulfamethizole Oral Susp.		X	X
Sulfamethoxazole (tab)	X		X
Sulfamethoxazole Oral Susp.		X	X
Sulfamethoxazole & Trimethoprim	X		
Sulfamethoxazole & Trimethoprim Oral Susp.		X	X
Sulfapyridine (tab)	X		X
Sulfasalazine (tab)	X		
Sulfathiazole, Sulfacetamide & Sulfabenzamide Vaginal	C[f]X[a]		X[af]
Sulfinpyrazone	X[ab]		
Sulfisoxazole (tab)	X		X
Sulfisoxazole Acetyl Oral Susp.		X	X
Sulfisoxazole Diolamine Ophthalmic		C[g]X[c]	X[c]
Sulfoxone Sodium (tab)		X	X
Sulfur Ointment	X[+]		
Sulindac (tab)	X		
Suprofen	X[o]		
Suprofen Ophthalmic	X[c]		
Sutilains Ointment	CX[+]		
Talbutal (tab)	X		
Talc	X		
Tamoxifen Citrate (tab)	X		X
Tape, Adhesive	X[+]		
Temazepam	X[bo]		X[bo]
Terbutaline (tab)		X[+]	
Terfenadine	X[ao]		X[ao]
Terpin Hydrate Elixir	X		
Terpin Hydrate & Codeine Elixir		X	
Terpin Hydrate & Dextromethorphan HBr Elixir		X	

Drug (Dosage Form)	WC	T	LR	Drug (Dosage Form)	WC	T	LR
Testolactone (tab)		X		Thyroglobulin (tab)		X	
Tetracaine Oint.		C		Thyroid (tab)		X	
Tetracaine Ophthalmic Oint.		C		Ticarcillin Monosodium		X^o	
Tetracaine & Menthol Oint.		C		Timolol Maleate Ophthalmic Soln.		X	
Tetracaine HCl		C^f		Timolol Maleate (tab)	X		X
Tetracaine HCl Topical Soln.		X	X	Timolol Maleate & Hydrochlorothiazide (tab)	X		X
Tetracaine HCl Ophthalmic Soln.		X	X	Tioconazole		$X^{a f o}$	
Tetracycline Boluses		X^x		Tobramycin Ophthalmic		$X^c COT^g$	
Tetracycline HCl Ophthalmic	COT^g			Tobramycin & Dexamethasone Ophthalmic		$X^l C^g$	
Tetracycline HCl Soluble Pow.		X^x		Tobramycin & Fluorometholone Acetate Ophthalmic		X^c	
Tetracycline HCl & Novobiocin Sodium (tab)		X^x		Tobranycin Sulfate	X^o		
Tetracycline Phosphate Complex & Novobiocin Sodium (cap)		X^x		Tocainide HCl	$X^{a o}$		
Tetracycline Oral Susp.		X	X	Tolazamide (tab)		X	
Tetracycline HCl (tab/cap/Ophthalmic Susp/topical soln)		X	X	Tolazoline HCl (tab)	X		
Tetracycline HCl & Nystatin (cap)		X	X	Tolbutamide (tab)	X		
Tetracycline Phosphate Complex (cap)		X	X	Tolmetin Sodium	X^a	X^b	
Tetrahydrozoline HCl Soln.		$X^{k s}$		Tolnaftate		$X^{f o t}$	
Theophylline	$X^{a h}$			Tolnaftate Topical		$X^{l c o +}$	
Theophylline Extended Release (cap)	X			Tolu Balsam		X^+	
Theophylline, Ephedrine HCl & Phenobarbital (tab)	X			Trazodone HCl		X^n	X^o
Theophylline & Guaifenesin		$X^{b c}$		Trazodone (tab)		X^a	X^a
Theophylline Sodium Glycinate	X^a	X^e		Tretinoin		$C^f X^c$	$X^{c f t}$
Thiabendazole (tab)		X		Triamcinolone (tab)	X		
Thiabendazole Oral Susp.		X		Triamcinolone Acetonide	X^g	$X^{f h}$	
Thiamine HCl		$X^{a e}$	$X^{a e}$	Triamcinolone Acetonide Dental Paste		X	
Thiamine Mononitrate Elixir		X	X	Triamcinolone Acetonide Topical		$X^{i +}$	
Thiamylal	X^o			Triamcinolone Diacetate (syr)		X	X
Thiethylperazine Maleate		$X^{a i o +}$	$X^{a i o +}$	Triamterene (cap)		X	X
Thimerosol, Topical		$X^{c l +}$	$X^{c l +}$	Triamterene & Hydrochlorothiazide		$X^{a b}$	$X^{a b}$
Thimerosal, Tincture		X^+	X^+	Triazolam (tab)		X	X
Thioguanine (tab)	X			Trichlormethiazide (tab)		X	
Thioridazine, Oral		$X^{c j +}$	$X^{c j +}$	Tricitrates Oral Soln		X	
Thioridazine HCl (tab)		X	X	Tridihexethyl (tab)	X		
Thiostrepton		X^o		Trientine HCl		$X^{a o +}$	In^o
Thiothixene (cap)	X		X	Trifluoperazine HCl	X^a	X^d	$X^{a d}$
Thiothixene HCl Oral Soln.		X	X	Triflupromazine Oral Susp.		X	X
				Triflupromazine HCl (tab)	X		X
				Trihexyphenidyl HCl		$X^{a c}$	
				Trihexyphenidyl HCl Extended-Release (cap)		X	
				Trikates Oral (soln)		X	X
				Trimeprazine Tartrate	X^a	X^d	$X^{a d}$
				Trimethadione		$X^{a b c +}$	
				Trimethobenzamide HCl (cap)	X		

Drug (Dosage Form)	WC	T	LR	Drug (Dosage Form)	WC	T	LR
Trimethoprim (tab)		X	X	Vancomycin HCl (cap)		X	
Trioxsalen (tab)	X		X	Vancomycin HCl for Oral Soln.		X	
Tripelennamine HCl (tab)	X			Verapamil HCl (tab)		X	X
Tripelennamine Citrate Elixir		X	X	Vidarabine Ophthalmic Ointment		COT[+]	
Triprolidine HCl		X[u d]	X[u d]	Vinblastine Sulfate		X[+]	X[+]
Triprolidine & Pseudoephedrine Hydrochlorides		X[a d]	X[a d]	Vincristine Sulfate		X[+]	X[+]
				Vitamin A (cap)		X	X
Trisulfapyrimidines (tab)	X			Vitamin E (cap)		X	X
Trisulfapyrimidines Oral Susp.		X[+]		Vitamin E Preparation		In	X
Troleandomycin (cap)		X		Oil-Soluble Vitamines	X[a b]	X[a b]	
Troleandomycin Oral Susp.		X[+]		Water-Soluble Vitamin	X[a b]	X[a b]	
Tropicamide Ophthalmic Soln.		X[+]		Warfarin Sodium (tab)		X	
Tuaminoheptane Inhalant		X[+]		Water, purified		X	
Tyropanoate Sodium (cap)		X	X	White Lotion		X	
Undecylenic Acid, Compound Ointment		X[+]		Xylometazoline HCl Nasal Soln.		X	X
Uracil Mustard (cap)		X		Xylose		X[+]	
Valproic Acid	GP°X[b d +]			Zinc Gluconate	X[a o]		
				Zinc Oxide (oint/paste)	X[+]		
				Zinc Oxide & Salicylic Acid Paste	X		
				Zinc Sulfate Ophthalmic Soln.		X	

Provided by Dr. Kenneth S. Alexander, Associate Professor of Pharmacy, College of Pharmacy, University of Toledo.
The listing of container requirements for Compendial drugs is included as an aid to the practitioner in storing and dispensing.

Container and Storage Requirements for Sterile U.S.P. XXIII Drugs

*Legend:

I	= Containers for sterile solids as described under injections	D	=	Type II or III Glass Depending on Final Soln. pH
N	= Intact Flexible Container Meeting The General Requirements	IN	=	Inert atmosphere
S	= Single dose	M	=	Protect from moisture
M	= Multiple dose	LR	=	Light Resistant
U	= Unspecified	L	=	Protect From Light
P	= Plastic	R	=	Refrigerator (2°–8°C)
A	= Type I glass	F	=	Freezer (−4°C)
B	= Type II glass	H	=	Protect from Heat
C	= Type III glass	RT	=	Controlled Room Temperature
Sy	= Syringe	TP	=	Tamper-Proof
O	= Original Package	W	=	Transparent
T	= Avoid Toxic Substances	SC	=	Radioactive Shielding
SS	= Stated Size Limitation	Tr	=	To Prevent Adsorption
X	= Colorless	WC	=	Well Closed

Drugs	Container	Glass Type	Storage Conditions
Acepromazine Maleate Inj.	S,M	A	L
Acetazolamide Sodium, Sterile	I	C	
Acetic Acid Irrigation	S,P	A,B	
Acetylcysteine Solution	S,M	A,P	O_2 excluded
Acetylcholine for Ophthalmic Soln.	I		
Dehydrated Alcohol Inj.	S	A	
Alcohol and Dextrose Inj.	S	A,B	
Alphaprodine HCl Inj.	S,M	A	
Alprostadil Inj.	S	A	R
Amdinocillin, Sterile	I		
Amikacin Sulfate Inj.	S,M	A,C	
Aminoacetic Acid Irrigation	S	A,B	
Aminocaproic Acid Inj.	S,M	A	
Aminohippurate Sodium Inj.	S,M	A	
Aminophylline Inj.	S	A	CO_2 excluded
Amitriptyline HCl Inj.	S,M	A	
Ammonia N 13 Inj.	S,M		SC
Ammonium Chloride Inj.	S,M	A,B	
Ammonium Molybdate Inj.	S,M	A,B	
Amobarbital Sodium, Sterile	I	D	
Amoxicillin, Sterile	I		
Amphotericin B for Inj.	I		R,L
Ampicillin, Sterile	I		
Ampicillin Sodium, Sterile	I		R,L
Ampicillin Sodium and Sulbactam Sodium, Sterile	I		
Anileridine Inj.	S,M	A	L
Anticoagulant Citrate Dextrose Solution	S,M,P	A,B	
Anticoagulant Citrate Phosphate Dextrose Adenine Solution	S,P	A,B	X,W

*The listing of container and storage requirements for sterile Compendial drugs is included as an aid to the practitioner in storing and dispensing.

Drugs	Container	Glass Type	Storage Conditions
Anticoagulant Sodium Citrate Soln.	S	A,B	
Anticoagulant Heparin Soln.	S,P	A,B	
Antihemophilic Factor			R
Antihemophilic Factor, Cryoprecipitated			F (−18°C)
Antirabies Serum	U		R
Antivenin (Latrodectus mectans)	S		H
Antivenin (Crotalidae) Polyvalent	S		H
Antivenin (Micrurus fulvius)	S		H
Arginine HCl Inj.	S	B	
Ascorbic Acid Inj.	S	A,B	LR
Atropine Sulfate Inj.	S,M	A	
Aurothioglucose Susp., Sterile	S,M	A	L
Azaperone Inj.	S, M	A	L
Azathioprine Sodium for Inj.	I	C	RT
Azlocillin Sodium, Sterile	I		
Aztreonam for Inj.	I		
Aztreonam, Sterile	I		
Bacitracin, Sterile	I	D	R
Bacitracin Zinc, Sterile	I		R(cool place)
BCG Vaccine	U	A	R
Benztropine Mesylate Inj.	S,M	A	
Benzylpenicilloyl Polylysine Inj.	S,M	A	R
Betamethasone Sodium Phosphate Inj.	S,M	A	
Betamethasone Sodium Phosphate and Betamethasone Acetate (Susp.), Sterile	M	A	
Bethanechol Chloride Inj.	S	A	
Biological Indicator for Dry Heat Sterilization, Paper Strip	O		L,H,M,T
Biological Indicator for Ethylene Oxide Sterilization, Paper Strip	O		L,H,M,T
Biological Indicator for Steam Sterilization, Paper Strip	O		L,H,M,T
Biperiden Lactate Inj.	S	A	L
Bleomycin Sulfate, Sterile	I	B	
Blood Grouping Serums (All)	U		R
Botulism Antitoxin	S		R
Brompheniramine Maleate Inj.	S,M	A	L
Bumetanide Inj.	S,M	A	L
Bupivacaine HCl Inj.	S,M	A	
Bupivacaine and Epinephrine Inj.	S,M	A	L
Bupivacaine in Dextrose Inj.	S	A	
Butorphanol Tartrate Inj.	S,M	A	L
Caffeine and Sodium Benzoate Inj.	S	A	
Calcium Chloride Inj.	S	A	
Calcium Gluceptate Inj.	S	A,B	
Calcium Gluconate Inj.	S	A	
Calcium Levulinate Inj.	S	A	
Capreomycin Sulfate, Sterile	I	B	R
Carbenicillin Disodium, Sterile	I	D	
Carboprost Tromethamine Inj.	S,M	A	R
Cefamandole Naftate for Inj.	I	D	
Cefamandole Sodium, Sterile	I		
Cefamandole Sodium for Inj.	I		
Cefazolin Sodium, Sterile	I	B	
Cefazolin Sodium Inj.	I		F
Cefanocid Sodium, Sterile	I		
Cefmenoxime for Inj.	I		

Drugs	Container	Glass Type	Storage Conditions
Cefmenoxime HCl, Sterile	I		
Cefmetazole Sodium, Sterile	I		
Cefoperazone Sodium, Sterile	I		
Cefoperazone Sodium Inj.	I		F
Cefotaxime Sodium, Sterile	I	B	
Cefotaxime Sodium Inj.	S,M		F
Cefotetan Disodium, Sterile	I		
Ceforanide for Inj.	I		
Cefotiam for Injj.	I	C	
Cefotiam HCl, Sterile	I	C	
Cefoxitin Sodium, Sterile	I	B	
Cefoxitin Sodium Inj.	I		F
Cefpiramide for Inj.	I		
Ceftazidime Inj.	I		F
Ceftazidime for Inj.	I		L
Ceftazidime, Sterile	I		L
Ceftizoxime Sodium Inj.	I		F
Ceftizoxime Sodium, Sterile	I		
Ceftriaxone Sodium Inj.	I		
Ceftriaxone Sodium, Sterile	I		F
Cefuroxime Sodium Inj.	I		F
Cefuroxime Sodium, Sterile	I		
Cellulose Oxidized (all)	I		L,R
Cephalothin Sodium Inj.	I		F
Cephapirin Sodium, Sterile	I	D	
Cephradine, Sterile	I		
Cephradine for Inj.	I		
Chloramphenicol Inj.	S,M		
Chloramphenicol, Sterile	I		
Chloramphenicol Sodium Succinate, Sterile	I	B	
Chlordiazepoxide HCl, Sterile	I	B	L
Chloroprocaine HCl Inj.	S,M	A	
Chloroquine HCl Inj.	S	A	
Chlorothiazide Sodium for Inj.	I	C	
Chlorpheniramine Maleate Inj.	S,M	A	L
Chlorpromazine HCl Inj.	S,M	A	L
Chlorprothixene Inj.	S		L
Chlortetracycline HCl, Sterile	I		L
Cholera Vaccine	U		R
Sodium Chromate Cr51 Inj.	S,M		
Chromic Chloride Inj.	S,M	A,B	
Cilastatin Sodium, Sterile	I	C	R
Cisplatin for Inj.	I		
Citric Acid, Magnesium Oxide Sodium Carbonate Irrigation	S	A,B	
Clavulanate Potassium, Sterile	I		
Clindamycin Phosphate, Sterile	I	D	
Clindamycin Phosphate Inj.	S,M	A,P	
Cloxacillin Benzathine, Sterile	U(tight)		
Cloxacillin Sodium, Sterile	U(tight)		
Cloxacillin Sodium Intramammary Infusion	Sy		TP
Coccidioidin			R
Codeine Phosphate Inj.	S,M	A	L
Colchicine Inj.	S	A	L
Colistimethate Sodium, Sterile	I	D	
Corticotropin Inj.	S,M	A	R
Corticotropin for Inj.	I	B	

Drugs	Container	Glass Type	Storage Conditions
Corticotropin Inj., Repository	S,M	A	
Corticotropin Zinc Hydroxide, (Susp.), Sterile	S,M	A	RT
Cortisone Acetate Susp., Sterile	S,M	A	
Cromolyn Sodium Inhalation	S(double-ended ampule)	A,B,P	
Cupric Chloride Inj.	S,M	A,B	
Cupric Sulfate Inj.	S,M	A,B	
Cyanocobalamin Inj.	S,M	A	LR
Cyclophosphamide for Inj.	I		RT
Cyclosporin Concentrate for Inj.	S,M		
Cyclizine Lactate Inj.	S	A	
Cyclophosphamide for Inj.	I	B	RT
Cysteine HCl Inj.	S,M	A	
Cytarabine, Sterile	I	B	
Dacarbazine for Inj.	S,M, or I	A	L
Dactinomycin for Inj.	I	B	LR
Daunorubicin HCl for Inj.	I	B	LR
Deslanoside Inj.	S	A	
Dexamethasone Acetate Suspension, Sterile	S,M	A	
Dextrose Inj.	S	A,B,P	
Dextrose and Sodium Chloride Inj.	S	A,B,P	
Diatrizoate Meglumine Inj.	S,M	A,C	L
Diatrizoate Meglumine and Diatrizoate Sodium Inj.	S	A,C	L
Diatrizoate Sodium Inj.	S,M	A,C	L
Diazepam Inj.	S,M	A	L
Diazoxide Inj.	S	A	L
Dibucaine HCl Inj.	S,M	A	L
Dicloxacillin Sodium, Sterile	I	D	
Dicyclomine HCl Inj.	S,M	A	
Diethylstilbestrol Inj.	S,M	A	LR
Digitoxin Inj.	S	A	Avoid excessive heat
Digitoxin Inj.	S,M	A	L
Digoxin Inj.	S	A	LR,H
Dihydroergotamine Mesylate Inj.	S	A	avoid heat
Dihydroergotamine Mesylate, Heparin Sodium and Lidocaine HCl Inj.	S,M	A	
Dihydrostreptomycin Sulfate, Sterile	I		
Dimenhydrinate Inj.	S,M	A,C	
Dimercaprol Inj.	S,M	A,C	
Dimethyl Sulfate Irrigation	S		RT,L
Dinoprost Tromethamine Inj.	S,M	A	
Diphenhydramine HCl Inj.	S,M	A	L
Diphtheria Antitoxin	U		R
Diphtheria Toxoid	U		R
Diphtheria Toxoid Adsorbed	U		R
Diphtheria and Tetanus Toxoids/Adsorbed	U		R
Diphtheria and Tetanus Toxoids and Pertussis Vaccine/Adsorbed	U		R
Dobutamine HCl for Inj.	I	B	RT
Dopamine HCl Inj.	S	A	
Dopamine HCl and Dextrose Inj.	S	A,B	
Doxapram HCl Inj.	S,M	A	
Doxorubicin HCl Inj.	S,M	A	LR,R (not to exceed 250 ml if multidose)
Doxorubicin HCl for Inj.	I	B	(Not to exceed 250 ml if multidose)

Drugs	Container	Glass Type	Storage Conditions
Doxorubicin HCl for Inj.	I		
Doxycycline Hyclate for Inj.	I	B	L
Doxycycline Hyclate, Sterile	I		L
Droperidol Inj.	S,M	A	L
Dyphylline Inj.	S,M	A	RT,L
Edetate Calcium Disodium Inj.	S	A	
Edetate Disodium Inj.	S	A	
Edrophonium Chloride Inj.	S,M	A	
Electrolytes Inj. (Type 1), Multiple	S	A,B,P	
Electrolytes Inj. (Type 2), Multiple	S	A,B,P	
Electrolytes and Dextrose Inj. (Type 1), Multiple	S	A,B,P	
Electrolytes and Dextrose Inj. (Type 2), Multiple	S	A,B,P	
Electrolytes and Dextrose Inj. (Type 3), Multiple	S	A,B,P	
Electrolytes and Dextrose Inj. (Type 4), Multiple	S	A,B,P	
Electrolytes and Invert Sugar Inj. (Type 1), Multiple	S	A,B,P	
Electrolytes and Invert Sugar Inj. (Type 2), Multiple	S	A,B,P	
Electrolytes and Invert Sugar Inj. (Type 3), Multiple	S	A,B,P	
Elements Inj., Trace	S,M	A,B	
Emetine HCl Inj.	S	A	LR
Ephedrine Sulfate Inj.	S,M	A	LR
Epinephrine Bitartrate for Ophthalmic Soln.	I		
Epinephrine Inj.	S,M	A	LR
Epinephrine Oil Susp., Sterile	S	A,C	LR
Ergonovine Maleate Inj.	S	A	LR,R
Ergotamine Tartrate Inj.	S	A	LR
Erythromycin Ethylsuccinate Inj.	S,M	A	
Erythromycin Ethylsuccinate, Sterile	I		
Erythromycin Gluceptate, Sterile	I	D	
Erythromycin Lactobionate, Sterile	I		
Erythromycin Lactobionate for Inj.	I	D	
Estradiol Cypionate Inj.	S,M	A	LR
Estradiol Suspension, Sterile	S,M	A	
Estradiol Valerate Inj.	S,M	A,C	LR
Estrone Inj.	S,M	A	
Estrone Suspension, Sterile	S,M	A	
Ethacrynate Sodium for Inj.	I	D	
Ethiodized Oil Inj.	S,M		LR
Ethylnorepinephrine HCl Inj.	S,M	A	LR
Evans Blue Inj.	S	A	
Fentanyl Citrate Inj.	S	A	L
Ferrous Citrate Fe 59 Inj.	S,M		L (discard after 2 weeks when reconstituted)
Floxuridine, Sterile	M	A	
Fludeoxyglucose F18 Inj.	S,M		SC
Fluorescein Sodium Inj.	S	A	
Fluorouracil Inj.	S	A	RT,L
Fluphenazine Decanoate	S, M	A	L
Fluphenazine Enanthate Inj.	S,M	A,C	L
Fluphenazine HCl Inj.	S,M	A	L
Folic Acid Inj.	S,M	A	

Drugs	Container	Class Type	Storage Conditions
Fructose Inj.	S	A,B	
Fructose and Sodium Chloride Inj.	S	A,B	
Furosemide Inj.	S,M	A	LR
Gallamine Triethiodide Inj.	S,M	A	L
Gallium Citrate Ga67 Inj.	S,M		
Gallium Citrate Ga67 Inj., Sterile	I	D	
Gentamicin Sulfate Inj.	S,M	A	
Globulin Serum, Anti-Human	U		R
Glucagon for Inj. w/solvent	I/S,M		
Glycine Irrigation	S	A,B	
Glycopyrrolate Inj.	S,M	A	
Gold Sodium Thiomalate Inj.	S,M	A	L
Gonadotropin Chorionic for Inj.	I	D	
Haloperidol Inj.	S,M	A	L
Heparin Calcium Inj.	S,M	A	R
Heparin Lock Flush Soln.	S,M	A	
Heparin Sodium Inj.	S,M	A	
Hepatitis B Virus Vaccine Inactivated	U		R
Hetacillin Potassium, Sterile	I		
Histamine Phosphate Inj.	S,M	A	L
Hyaluronidase for Inj.	I	A,C	RT
Hyaluronidase Inj.	S,M	A	R
Hydralazine HCl Inj.	S,M	A	
Hydrocortisone (Cortisol) Suspension, Sterile	S,M	A	
Hydrocortisone (Cortisol) Acetate Suspension, Sterile	S,M	A	
Hydrocortisone (Cortisol) Sodium Phosphate Inj.	I	C	
Hydrocortisone (Cortisol) Sodium Succinate for Inj.	I	C	
Hydromorphone HCl Inj.	S,M	A	L
Hydroxyocobalamin Inj.	S,M	A	L
Hydroxyprogesterone Caproate Inj.	S,M	A,C	
Hydroxystilbamidine Isethionate, Sterile	I	D	LR
Hydroxyzine HCl Inj.	S,M		L
Hyoscyamine Sulfate Inj.	S,M	A	
Imipenem, Sterile	I		R
Imipramine HCl Inj.	S	A	LR
Indigotindisulfonate Sodium Inj.	S	A	LR
Indium In-III Pentetate Inj.	S		
Indocyanine Green, Sterile	I	B	
Indomethacin Sodium, Sterile	I	C	
Insulin Inj.	M		R
Isophane Insulin Suspension	M		R
Insulin Zinc Suspension	M		R
Insulin Zinc Suspension, Extended	M		R
Insulin Zinc Suspension, Prompt	M		R
Insulin Suspension, Protamine Zinc	M		R
Insulin Human Inj.	M		R
Insulin and Sodium Chloride Inj.	S	A,B	
Iodinated I-125 Albumin Inj.	S,M		R
Iodinated I-131 Albumin Inj.	U		
Iodinated I-131 Albumin Aggregated Inj.	S,M		R
Iodohippurate Sodium I 123 Inj.	S,M		SC
Iodohippurate Sodium I-131 Inj.	S,M		
Rose Bengal Sodium I-131 Inj.			
Iodipamide Inj.	S	A	L

Drugs	Container	Glass Type	Storage Conditions
Iodipamide Meglumine Inj.	S	A,C	
Iohexol Inj. (Intravascular/Intrathecal)	S	A	L
Iopamidol Inj. (Intravascular/Intrathecal)	S	A	L
Iophendylate Inj.	S	A	
Iothalamate Meglumine Inj.	S	A	L
Iothalamate Meglumine and Sodium Iothalamate Inj.	S	A	L
Iothalamate Sodium Inj.	S	A	L
Iron Dextran Inj.	S,M	A,B	
Iron Sorbitex Inj.	S	A	
Isoniazid Inj.	S,M	A	L
Isoproterenol HCl Inj.	S	A	L
Isoxsuprine HCl Inj.	S,M	A	
Kanamycin Sulfate, Sterile	I		
Kanamycin Sulfate Inj.	S,M	A,C	
Ketamine HCl Inj.	S,M	A	L,H
Labetolol HCl Inj.	S,M(60ml max)	A	R,RT,L
Leucovorin Calcium Inj.	S	A	LR
Levorphanol Tartrate Inj.	S,M	A	
Lidocaine HCl, Sterile	I		
Lidocaine HCl Inj.	S,M	A	
Lidocaine HCl and Dextrose Inj.	S	A,B	
Lidocaine HCl and Epinephrine Inj.	S,M	A	LR
Lincomycin HCl, Sterile	I		
Lincomycin HCl Inj.	S,M	A	
Lorazepam Inj.	S,M	A	L
Magnesium Sulfate	S,M	A	
Manganese Chloride Inj.	S,M	A,B	
Manganese Sulfate Inj.	S,M	A,B	
Mannitol Inj.	S	A,R,P	
Mannitol and Sodium Chloride Inj.	U	D	
Measles Virus Vaccine Live	S,M		LR,R
Measles and Mumps Virus Vaccine, Live	S,M		LR,R
Measles, Mumps and Rubella Virus Vaccine, Live	S,M		LR,R
Measles and Rubella Virus Vaccine, Live	S,M		LR,R
Mechlorethamine HCl for Inj.	I	B	
Medroxyprogesterone Acetate Susp., Sterile	S,M	A	
Menadiol Sodium Diphosphate Inj.	S	A	LR
Menadione Inj.	S,M	A	
Meningococcal Polysaccharide Vaccine (Group A)	M		R
Meningococcal Polysaccharide Vaccine (Group C)	M		R
Meningococcal Polysaccharide Vaccine (Groups A and C combined)	M		R
Menotropins for Inj.	S,M	A	
Meperidine HCl Inj.	S,M	A	
Mephentermine Sulfate Inj.	S,M	A	
Mepivacaine HCl Inj.	S,M	A	
Mepivacaine HCl and Levonordefrin Inj.	S,M	A	
Meprobamate Inj.	S	A	
Meprylcaine HCl and Epinephrine Inj.	S	A	L

Drugs	Container	Glass Type	Storage Conditions
Mesoridazine Besylate Inj.	S	A	L
Metaraminol Bitartrate Inj.	S,M	A	L
Methadone HCl Inj.	S,M	A	LR
Methantheline Bromide, Sterile	I	D	
Methicillin Sodium, Sterile	I		RT
Methicillin Sodium for Inj.	I		L,RT
Methocarbamol Inj.	S	A	
Methohexital Sodium for Inj.	I	C	
Methotrexate Sodium for Inj.	I		L
Methotrexate Sodium Inj.	S,M	A	L
Methotrimeprazine Inj.	S,M	A	L
Methoxamine HCl Inj.	S,M	A	L
Methydopate HCl Inj.	S	A	
Methylene Blue Inj.	S	A	
Methylergonovine Maleate Inj.	S	A	LR
Methylprednisolone Acetate Susp., Sterile	S,M	A	
Methylprednisolone Sodium Succinate for Inj.	I	C	
Metoclopramide Inj.	S,M	A	LR(no antioxidant)
Metocurine Iodide Inj.	S,M	A	
Metoprolol Tartrate Inj.	S	A,B	L
Metronidazole Inj.	S,P	A,B	L
Mezlocillin Sodium, Sterile	I		
Miconazole Inj.	S	A	RT
Minocycline HCl, Sterile	I		L
Mitomycin for Inj.	I	D	L
Mitoxantrone for Inj. Conc.	S	A	
Morphine Sulfate Inj.	S,M	A	L
Morphine Sulfate Inj. (Preservative Free)	S	A	L
Morrhuate Sodium Inj.	S,M	A	
Moxalactam Disodium for Inj.	I		
Mumps Virus Vaccine Live	S,M		LR,R
Nafcillin Sodium, Sterile	I		
Nafcillin Sodium Inj.	I		F
Nafcillin Sodium for Inj.	I	D	
Nalorphine HCl Inj.	S,M	A	
Naloxone HCl Inj.	S,M	A	
Nandrolone Decanoate Inj.	S,M	A	L
Nandrolone Phenpropionate Inj.	S,M	A	L
Neomycin Sulfate, Sterile	I		
Neostigmine Methylsulfate Inj.	S,M		L
Netilmicin Sulfate Inj.	S,M	A	
Niacin Inj.	S,M	A	
Niacinamide Inj.	S,M	A	
Nitroglycerin Inj.	S,M	A,B	
Norepinephrine Bitartrate Inj.	S	A	LR
Novobiocin Sod. Intramammary Infusion	Sy		WC
Nylidrin HCl Inj.	S,M	A	
Orphenadrine Citrate Inj.	S,M	A	L
Oxacillin Sodium Inj.	I		F
Oxacillin Sodium for Inj.	I	D	RT
Oxacillin Sodium, Sterile	I		
Oxymorphone HCl Inj.	S,M	A	L
Oxytetracycline, Sterile	I		L
Oxytetracycline Inj.	S,M		L
Oxytetracycline HCl for Inj.	I	B	L
Oxytetracycline HCl, Sterile	I		L

Drugs	Container	Glass Type	Storage Conditions
Papaverine HCl Inj.	S,M	A	
Penicillin G Benzathine, Sterile	I		
Penicillin G Benzathine Susp., Sterile	S,M	A,B	R
Penicillin G Benzathine and Penicillin G Procaine Susp., Sterile	S,M	A,C	
Penicillin G Potassium for Inj.	I	D	
Penicillin G Potassium, Sterile	I	D	
Penicillin G Procaine, Sterile	I		
Penicillin G Procaine for Susp., Sterile	S,M	A,C	
Penicillin G Procaine Susp., Sterile	S,M	A,C	R
Penicillin G Procaine Intramammary Infusion	Sy(well closed)		
Penicillin G Procaine w/Aluminum Stearate Susp., Sterile	S,M	A,C	
Penicillin G Procaine and Dihydrostreptomycin Sulfate Susp., Sterile	S,M(tight)		
Penicillin G Procaine Dihydrostreptomycin Sulfate Intramammary Infusion	Sy(well closed)		
Penicillin G Procaine, Dihydrostreptomycin Sulfate & Prednisolone Susp., Sterile	S,M(tight)		
Penicillin G Procaine, Dihydrostreptomycin Sulfate, Chlorpheniramine Maleate, and Dexamethasone Susp., Sterile	S,M(tight)		R
Penicillin G Sodium for Inj.	I	D	
Penicillin G Sodium for Inj.	I		
Penicillin G Sodium, Sterile	I	D	
Pentazocine Lactate Inj.	S,M	A	
Pentobarbital Sodium Inj.	S,M	A	
Perphenazine Inj.	S,M	A	L
Pertussis Vaccine	U		R
Pertussis Vaccine Adsorbed	U		R
Phenobarbital Sodium, Sterile	I	D	
Phenobarbital Sodium Inj.	I	D	
Phentolamine Mesylate for Inj.	I	B	
Phenylephrine HCl Inj.	S,M	A	L
Phenytoin Sodium Inj.	S,M	A	RT
Phosphate P^{32} Chromic Susp.	S,M		
Phosphate P^{32} Sodium Soln.	S,M	Tr	
Physostigmine Salicylate Inj.	S	A	L
Phytonadione Inj.	S,M	A	L
Pilocarpine Ocular System	S		R
Piperacillin Sodium, Sterile	I		
Plicamycin for Inj.	I	D	L
Poliovirus Vaccine Inactivated	U		R
Polymyxin B Sulfate, Sterile	I	D	L
Posterior Pituitary Inj.	S,M	A	
Potassium Acetate Inj.	S,M	A,B	
Potassium Chloride for Inj. Conc.	S,M	A,B	
Potassium Chloride in Dextrose Inj.	S	A,B,P	
Potassium Chloride in Dextrose and Sodium Chloride Inj.	S	A,B,P	
Potassium Chloride in Lactated Ringers and Dextrose Inj.	S	A,B,P	

Drugs	Container	Glass Type	Storage Conditions
Potassium Chloride in Sodium Chloride Inj.	S	A,B,P	
Potassium Phosphates Inj.	S,M	A	
Pralidoxone Chloride, Sterile	I	B	
Prednisolone Acetate Susp., Sterile	S,M	A	
Prednisolone Sodium Phosphate Inj.	O,M	A	L
Prednisolone Sodium Succinate for Inj.	I	D	
Prednisolone Tebutate Susp., Sterile	S,M	A	
Prilocaine HCl Inj.	S,M	A	
Prilocaine & Epinephrine Inj.	S,M	A	L
Procainamide HCl Inj.	S,M	A	
Procaine HCl Inj.	S,M	A,B	
Procaine HCl, Sterile	I	D	
Procaine HCl and Epinephrine Inj.	S,M	A,B	LR
Procaine and Phenylephrine HCl Inj.	S,M	A	
Procaine HCl, Tetracycline HCl and Levonordefrin Inj.	S,M	A	
Prochlorperazine Edisylate Inj.	S,M	A	L
Progesterone Inj.	S,M	A,C	
Progesterone Susp., Sterile	S,M	A	
Progesterone Intrauterine Contraceptive Sys.	S		
Promazine HCl Inj.	S,M	A	L
Promethazine HCl Inj.	S,M	A	L
Propantheline Bromide, Sterile	S	D	
Propiomazine HCl Inj.	S	A	RT,L
Propoxycaine HCl, Procaine HCl and Levonordefrin Inj.	SA		
Propoxycaine HCl, Procaine HCl and Norepinephrine Bitartrate Inj.	S,M	A	
Propranolol HCl Inj.	S	A	LR
Propyliodone Oil Susp., Sterile	S	D	LR
Protamine Sulfate Inj.	S	A	R
Protamine Sulfate for Inj.	I	D	
Protein Hydrolysate Inj.	S	A,B	H
Pyridostigmine Bromide Inj.	S	A	L
Pyridoxine HCl Inj.	S,M	A	L
Quinidine Gluconate Inj.	S,M	A	
Rabies Immune Globin	U		R
Rabies Vaccine	U		R
Ranitidine Inj.	S,M	I	LR,RT
Ranitidine in Sodium Chloride Inj.	N		LR,R/RT
Reserpine Inj.	S	A	LR
Riboflavin Inj.	S,M	A	LR
Rifampin for Inj.	I		
Ringer's Inj.	S	A,B,P	
Ringer's and Dextrose Inj.	S	A,B,P	
Ringer's Inj., Lactated	S	A,B,P	
Ringer's and Dextrose Inj., Lactated	S	A,B,P	
Ringer's and Dextrose Inj., Half-Strength Lactated	S	A,B,P	
Ringer's and Dextrose Inj., Modified Lactated	S	A,B,P	
Ritodrine HCl Inj.	S	A	RT
Rolitetracycline for Inj.	I	B	L
Rolitetracycline, Sterile	I		L

Drugs	Container	Glass Type	Storage Conditions
Rubella Virus Vaccine Live	S,M		LR,R
Rubella and Mumps Virus Vaccine Live	S,M		LR,R
Scopolamine Hydrobromide Inj.	S,M	A	LR
Secobarbital Sodium, Sterile	I	D	
Secobarbital Sodium Inj.	S,M	A	L,R
Selenious Acid Inj.	S,M	A,B	
Selenomethionine Se75 Inj.	U		R
Sisomicin Sulfate Inj.	S,M	A	
Smallpox Vaccine	U		R
Sodium Acetate Inj.	S	A	
Sodium Bicarbonate Inj.	S	A	
Sodium Chloride Inhalation Soln.	S		
Sodium Chloride Inj.	S	A,B	
Sodium Chloride Inj., Bacteriostatic	S,M	A,B	
Sodium Lactate Inj.	S	A,B	
Sodium Nitrate Inj.	S	A	
Sodium Nitroprusside, Sterile	I	D	L
Sodium Pertechnetate Tc99m Inj.	S,M		R
Sodium Phosphates Inj.	S,M	A	
Sodium Sulfate Inj.	S	A	
Sodium Thiosulfate Inj.	S	A	
Spectinomycin HCl, Sterile	I		
Spectinomycin HCl for Suspension, Sterile	I		
Streptomycin Sulfate, Sterile	I	D	
Streptomycin Sulfate Inj.	S,M	A	
Succinylcholine Chloride, Sterile	I	D	
Succinylcholine Chloride Inj.	S,M	A,B	R
Sufentanil Citrate Inj.	S, M	A	
Invert Sugar Inj	S,P	A,B	
Sulbactam Sodium, Sterile	I		
Sulfadiazine Sodium Inj.	S	A	LR
Sulfamethoxazole & Trimethoprim Concentrate for Inj.	S,M	A	L
Sulfisoxazole Diolamine Inj.	S,M	A	L
Sulfobromophthalein Sodium Inj.	S	A	
Technetium Tc99m Albumin Inj.	S,M		R
Technetium Tc99m Albumin Aggregated Inj.	S,M		R
Technetium Tc99m Albumin Colloid Inj.	S,M		R
Technetium Tc99m Disofenin Inj.	S,M		In
Technetium Tc99m Etiodonate Inj.	S,M		
Technetium Tc99m Ferpentate Inj.	S,M		R,I
Technetium Tc99m Gluceptate Inj.	S,M		R
Technetium Tc99m Lidofenin Inj.	S,M		R
Technetium Tc99m Medronate Inj.	S,M		
Technetium Tc99m Oxidronate Inj.	S,M		
Technetium Tc99m Penetate Inj.	S,M		R
Technetium Tc99m Pyrophosphate Inj.	S,M		R
Technetium Tc99m (Pyro- and trimeta-) Phosphates Inj.	U	D	
Technetium Tc99m Succimer Inj.	S		RT,L
Technetium Tc99m Sulfur Colloid Inj.	S,M		
Terbutaline Sulfate Inj.	S	A	L,RT
Testolactone Susp., Sterile	S,M	A	
Testosterone Pellets	S		
Testosterone Susp., Sterile	S,M	A	
Testosterone Cypionate Inj.	S,M	A	L
Testosterone Enanthate Inj.	S,M	A	

Drugs	Container	Glass Type	Storage Conditions
Testosterone Propionate Inj.	S,M	A	
Tetanus Antitoxin	U		R
Tetanus Immune Globulin	U		R
Tetanus Toxoid	U		R
Tetanus Toxoid Adsorbed	U		R
Tetanus and Diphtheria Toxoids Adsorbed (for adult use)	U		R
Tetracaine HCl, Sterile	I	A	
Tetracaine HCl Inj.	S,M	A	R,L
Tetracaine HCl in Dextrose Inj.	S,M(up to 100 ml)	A	R,L,RT(tray for 12 months)
Tetracycline HCl, Sterile	I		L
Tetracycline HCl for Inj.	I	B	L
Tetracycline Phosphate Complex for Inj.	I		L
Tetracycline Phosphate Complex for Inj.	I	B	L
Tetracycline Phosphate Complex, Sterile	I		L
Thallous Chloride Tl201 Inj.	S,M		
Theophylline in Dextrose Inj.	S	A,B,P	
Thiamine HCl Inj.	S,M	A	L
Thiamylal Sodium for Inj.	I	C	
Thiethylperazine Maleate Inj.	S	A	L
Thiopental Sodium for Inj.	I	C	
Thiotepa for Inj.	I	D	R,L
Thiothixene HCl Inj.	S	A	L
Thiothixene HCl for Inj.	I		LR
Ticarcillin Disodium, Sterile	I	D	
Ticarcillin Disodium & Clavulanate Potassium, Sterile	I		
Ticarcillin Disodium & Clavulanate Potassium, Inj.	I		F
Tobramycin Sulfate, Sterile	I		
Tobramycin Sulfate Inj.	S,M	A,P	
Tolazoline HCl Inj.	S,M	A	
Tolbutamide Sodium, Sterile	I	D	
Triamcinolone Diacetate Susp., Sterile	S,M	A	
Triamcinolone Hexacetonide Susp., Sterile	S,M	A	
Tridihexethyl Chloride Inj.	S	A	
Trifluoperazine HCl Inj.	M	A	L
Trifluopromazine HCl Inj.	S,M	A	L
Trimethaphan Camsylate Inj.	S,M	A	R
Trimethobenzamide HCl Inj.	S,M	A	
Tromethamine for Inj.	I	C	
Tubocurarine Chloride Inj.	S,M		
Typhoid Vaccine	U		R
Urea, Sterile	I	D	
Vaccinia Immune Globulin	U		R
Vancomycin HCl, Sterile	I	B	
Vancomycin HCl for Inj.	I		
Varicella-Zoster Immune Globulin	U		R
Vasopressin Inj.	S,M	A	
Verapamil (HCl) Inj.	S	A	LR
Vidarabine Concentrate for Inj.	S,M	A	
Vinblastine Sulfate, Sterile	I	D	R
Vincristine Sulfate Inj.	U	U	L,R
Vincristine Sulfate for Inj.	U		L,R

Warfarin Sodium for Inj.	I	D	LR
Water for Inhalation, Sterile	S		
Water for Inj., Bacteriostatic	S,M	A,B	
Water for Inj., Sterile	S	A,B,P	SS
Water for Irrigation, Sterile	S	A,B	
Xenon Xe 127	S (leakproof stoppers)		RT,SC
Xenon Xe 133	S (leakproof stoppers)		RT,SC
Xenon Xe 133 Inj.	S (totally filled)		RT,SC
Yellow Fever Vaccine	U (nitrogen filled		R
Ytterbium Yb 169 Pentetate Inj.	ampuls®)		RT
Zinc Chloride Inj.	S		
Zinc Sulfate Inj.	S,M	A,B	
	S,M		

Provided by Dr. Kenneth S. Alexander, Associate Professor of Pharmacy, College of Pharmacy, University of Toledo.
*The listing of container and storage requirements for sterile Compendial drugs is included as an aid to the practitioner in storing and dispensing.

Oral Dosage Forms That Should Not Be Crushed

Drug Product	Manufacturer	Dosage Form	Reason/Comments
Accutane	Roche	Capsule	Mucous membrane irritant
Acutrim	Ciba	Tablet	Slow release
Adalat-CC	Miles	Tablet	Slow release
Aerolate SR, JR, III	Fleming & Co.	Capsule	Slow release* (i)
Anaplex SR	Medi-Plex	Capsule	Slow release
Afrinol Repetabs	Schering	Tablet	Slow release
Allerest 12-Hour	Ciba-Geigy Consumer Products	Caplet	Slow release
Anaplex SR	Medi-Plex	Capsule	Slow release
Ansaid	Upjohn	Tablet	Taste (c)
Artane Sequels	Lederle	Capsule	Slow release* (i)
Arthritis Bayer TR	Glenbrook	Capsule	Slow release
ASA Enseals	Lilly	Tablet	Enteric-coated
Asacol	Procter & Gamble Pharmaceuticals	Tablet	Slow release
Asbron G Inlay	Sandoz	Tablet	Multiple compressed tablet (i)
Aspirin Delayed-Release	Upsher-Smith Labs	Tablet	Enteric-coated
Atrohist Plus	Adams	Tablet	Slow release
Atrohist Sprinkle	Adams	Capsule	Slow release*
Azulfidine Entabs	Pharmacia Labs	Tablet	Enteric-coated
Baros	Lafayette	Tablet	Effervescent tablet(d)
Betachron E-R	Inwood	Capsule	Slow release
Betapen-VK	Apothecon	Tablet	Taste (c)
Biphetamine	Fisons	Capsule	Slow release
Bisacodyl	Various	Tablet	Enteric-coated (a)
Bisco-Lax	Raway	Tablet	Enteric-coated (a)
Bontril-SR	Carnrick	Capsule	Slow release
Breonesin	Sanofi Winthrop	Capsule	Liquid filled (b)
Brexin L.A.	Savage	Capsule	Slow release
Bromfed	Muro	Capsule	Slow release (i)
Bromfed PD	Muro	Capsule	Slow release (i)
Calan SR	Searle	Tablet	Slow release (h)
Cama Arthritis Pain Reliever	Sandoz Consumer	Tablet	Multiple compressed tablet
Carbiset-TR	Nutripharm	Tablet	Slow release
Cardizem	Marion-Merrell Dow	Tablet	Slow release
Cardizem CD	Marion-Merrell Dow	Capsule	Slow release*
Cardizem SR	Marion-Merrell Dow	Tablet	Slow release*
Carter's Little Pills	Carter-Wallace	Tablet	Enteric-coated
Cefal Filmtab	Abbott	Tablet	Enteric-coated
Charcoal Plus	Kramer	Tablet	Enteric-coated
Chloral Hydrate	Various	Capsule	Liquid in capsule (i)
Chlorphedrine SR	Goldline	Capsule	Slow release
Chlorpheniramine Maleate Time Release	Various	Capsule	Slow release
Chlor-Trimeton 12 hour Allergy	Schering	Tablet	Slow release (i)
Choledyl SA	Parke-Davis	Tablet	Slow release (i)
Chromagen	Savage	Capsule	Taste (e)
Cipro	Miles	Tablet	Taste (c)
Cleocin	Upjohn	Capsule	Taste (c)(i)

The listing of oral dosage forms that should not be crushed is included as an aid to the practitioner in dispensing drugs and consulting with patients.

Drug Product	Manufacturer	Dosage Form	Reason/Comments
Codimal-LA	Central	Capsule	Slow release
Codimal-LA Half	Central	Capsule	Slow release
Colace	Roberts Pharmaceutical	Capsule	Taste (c)
Comhist-LA	Roberts Pharmaceutical	Capsule	Slow release*
Compazine Spansule	SmithKline Beecham	Capsule	Slow release
Congess SR, JR	Fleming & Co.	Capsule	Slow release
Contac	SmithKline Beecham	Capsule	Slow release*
Cotazym-S	Organon	Capsule	Enteric-coated*
Creon	Solvay	Capsule	Enteric-coated*
Creon 10 Minimicropheres	Solvay	Capsule	Enteric-coated*
Creon 25	Solvay	Capsule	Enteric-coated*
Dallergy	Laser	Capsule	Slow release (i)(h)
Dallergy - D	Laser	Capsule	Slow release
Dallergy - JR	Laser	Capsule	Slow release
Deconamine-SR	Berlex	Capsule	Slow release (i)
Deconsal II	Adams	Tablet	Slow release
Deconsal Sprinkle	Adams	Capsule	Slow release*
Demazine Repetabs	Schering	Tablet	Slow release (i)
Depakene	Abbott	Capsule	Slow release-mucous membrane irritant (i)
Depakote	Abbott	Tablet	Enteric coated
Desoxyn Gradumets	Abbott	Tablet	Slow release
Desyrel	Mead Johnson	Tablet	Taste (c)
Dexatrim Max Strength	Thompson	Tablet	Slow release
Dexedrine Spansule	SmithKline Beecham	Capsule	Slow release
Diamox Sequels	Lederle	Capsule	Slow release
Dilacor-XR	Rhone-Poulenc Rorer	Capsule	Slow release
Dilatrate-SR	Reed & Carnrick	Capsule	Slow release
Dimetane Extentab	Robins	Tablet	Slow release (i)
Disobrom	Geneva	Tablet	Slow release
Disophrol Chronotab	Schering	Tablet	Slow release
Dital	UAD	Capsule	Slow release
Docusate	Upsher-Smith	Capsule	Liquid filled (b)
Docusate with Casanthranol	Upsher-Smith	Capsule	Liquid filled (b)
Donnatal Extentab	Robins	Tablet	Slow release (i)
Donnazyme	Robins	Tablet	Enteric-coated
Doxidan Liquigels	Upjohn	Capsule	Liquid filled (b)
Drisdol	Sanofi Winthrop	Capsule	Liquid filled (b)
Drixoral	Schering	Tablet	Slow release (i)
Drixoral Sinus	Schering	Tablet	Slow release*
Dulcolax	Ciba-Geigy	Tablet	Enteric-coated (a)
Dura-Vent	Dura	Tablet	Slow release
Dura-Vent/A	Dura	Capsule	Slow release
Dura-Vent/DA	Dura	Tablet	Slow release
Dura-Tap/PD	Dura	Capsule	Slow release
Duratuss	Whitby	Tablet	Slow release (h)
Easprin	Parke-Davis	Tablet	Enteric-coated
Ecotrin	SmithKline Beecham	Tablet	Enteric-coated
E.E.S. 400	Various	Tablet	Enteric-coated (i)
Efidac 124	Ciba	Tablet	Slow release
Elixophyllin SR	Forest	Capsule	Slow release* (i)
E-Mycin	Boots	Tablet	Enteric-coated
Endafed	UAD	Capsule	Slow release
Entex LA	Procter & Gamble Pharmaceuticals	Tablet	Slow release (i)
Entex PSE	Procter & Gamble Pharmaceuticals	Tablet	Slow release (i)
Entozyme	Robins	Tablet	Enteric-coated

Drug Product	Manufacturer	Dosage Form	Reason/Comments
Equanil	Wyeth-Ayerst	Tablet	Taste (c)
Ergostat	Parke-Davis	Tablet	Sublingual form (g)
Eryc	Parke-Davis	Capsule	Enteric-coated*
Ery-tab	Abbott	Tablet	Enteric-coated
Erythrocin Stearate	Various	Tablet	Enteric-coated
Erythromycin Base	Various	Tablet	Enteric-coated
Eskalith CR	SmithKline Beecham	Tablet	Slow release
Fedahist Timecaps	Schwarz Pharma	Capsule	Slow release (i)
Feldene	Pfizer	Capsule	Mucous membrane irritant
Fenesin	Dura	Tablet	Slow release
Feocyte	Dunhall	Tablet	Slow release
Feosol	SmithKline Beecham	Tablet	Enteric-coated (i)
Feosol Spansule	SmithKline Beecham	Capsule	Slow release* (i)
Feratab	Upsher-Smith	Tablet	Enteric-coated (i)
Fergon	Sanofi Winthrop	Tablet	May cause excessive GI upset
Fero-Grad 500 mg	Abbott	Tablet	Slow release
Fero-Gradumet	Abbott	Tablet	Slow release
Ferralet SR	Mission	Tablet	Slow release
Ferrous Gluconate	Upsher-Smith	Tablet	Film-coated
Feverall Sprinkle Caps	Upsher-Smith	Capsule	Taste* (j)
Fumatinic	Laser	Capsule	Slow release
Gastrocrom	Fisons	Capsule	Dissolve in water (k)
Geocillin	Roerig	Tablet	Taste
Glucotrol XL	Pratt	Tablet	Sustained Release
Gris-Peg	Allergan, Herbert	Tablet	Crushing may precipitate (l)
Guaifed	Muro	Capsule	Slow release
Guaifed-PD	Muro	Capsule	Slow release
Guaimax-D	Central	Tablet	Slow release
Halfprin	Kramer	Tablet	Enteric coated
Humabid DM	Adams	Tablet	Slow release
Humabid DM Sprinkle	Adams	Capsule	Slow release*
Humabid LA	Adams	Tablet	Slow release
Humabid Sprinkle	Adams	Capsule	Slow release*
Hydergine LC	Sandoz	Capsule	Liquid in capsule (i)
Hydergine Sublingual	Sandoz	Tablet	Sublingual form (i)
Hytakerol	Sanofi	Capsule	Liquid-filled (b) (i)
Iberet	Abbott	Tablet	Slow release (i)
Iberet-500	Abbott	Tablet	Slow release (i)
Ilotycin	Dista	Tablet	Enteric-coated
Imdur	Key	Tablet	Slow release (h)
Inderal-LA	Wyeth-Ayerst	Capsule	Slow release
Inderide-LA	Wyeth-Ayerst	Capsule	Slow release
Indocin SR	MSD	Capsule	Slow release* (i)
Ionamin	Fisons	Capsule	Slow release
Isoclor Timesule	Ciba-Geigy Consumer Products	Capsule	Slow release (i)
Isoptin SR	Knoll	Tablet	Slow release
Isordil Sublingual	Wyeth-Ayerst	Tablet	Sublingual form (g)
Isordil Tembid	Wyeth-Ayerst	Tablet	Slow release
Isosorbide Dinitrate Sublingual	Various	Tablet	Sublingual form (g)
Isosorbide Dinitrate SR	Various	Tablet	Slow release
Isuprel Glossets	Sanofi Winthrop	Tablet	Sublingual route (g)
Kaon-CL 6.7 mEq	Savage	Tablet	Slow release (i)
Kaon-CL 10	Adria	Tablet	Slow release (i)
K-Dur	Key	Tablet	Slow release (h)
Klor-Con	Upsher-Smith	Tablet	Slow release (i)

Drug Product	Manufacturer	Dosage Form	Reason/Comments
Klor-Con/EF	Upsher-Smith	Tablet	Effervescent tablet (d) (i)
Klorvess	Sandoz	Tablet	Effervescent tablet (d) (i)
Klotrix	Mead Johnson	Tablet	Slow release (i)
K-Lyte	Mead Johnson	Tablet	Effervescent tablet (d)
K-Lyte CL	Mead Johnson	Tablet	Effervescent tablet (d)
K + 10	Alra	Tablet	Slow release (i)
K + Care	Alra	Tablet	Effervescent tablet (d) (i)
K-Tab	Abbott	Tablet	Slow release (i)
Levsinex Timecaps	Schwarz Pharma	Capsule	Slow release
Macrobid	Procter & Gamble Pharmaceuticals	Capsule	Slow release
Meprospan	Wallace	Capsule	Slow release*
Mestinon Timespan	ICN	Tablet	Slow release (i)
MI-Cebrin	Dista	Tablet	Enteric-coated
MI-Cebrin T	Dista	Tablet	Enteric-coated
Micro-K	Robins	Capsule	Slow release* (i)
Motrin	Upjohn	Tablet	Taste (c)(i)
Motrin IB	Upjohn	Tablet	Taste (c)(i)
Motrin IB-sinus	Upjohn	Caplet	Taste (c)(i)
MS Contin	Purdue Frederick	Tablet	Slow release (i)
MSC Triaminic	Sandoz	Tablet	Enteric-coated
Naldecon	Bristol	Tablet	Slow release (i)
Nasabid	Abana	Capsule	Slow release
Nasatab	Medi-Plex	Tablet	Slow release
Nico 400	Jones Medical	Capsule	Slow release
Nicobid	Rhone-Poulenc Roror	Capsule	Slow release
Nitro-Bid	Marion-Merrell Dow	Capsule	Slow release*
Nitrocine Timecaps	Schwarz Pharma	Capsule	Slow release*
Nitroglyn	Kenwood	Capsule	Slow release*
Nitrostat	Parke-Davis	Tablet	Sublingual route (g)
Nitrong	Rhone-Poulenc Rorer	Tablet	Sublingual route (g)
Nolamine	Carnrick	Tablet	Slow release
Nolex LA	Carnrick	Tablet	Slow release
Norflex	3M Pharmaceuticals	Tablet	Slow release
Norpace CR	Searle	Capsule	Slow release
Novafed	Marion-Merrell Dow	Capsule	Slow release
Novafed A	Marion-Merrell Dow	Capsule	Slow release
Optilets 500 Filmtab	Abbott	Tablet	Enteric-coated
Optilets M 500 Filmtab	Abbott	Tablet	Enteric-coated
Oragrafin	Squibb	Capsule	Liquid in cap.
Ordrine Sr	Vitarine	Capsule	Sustained release
Oramorph SR	Roxane	Tablet	Slow release (i)
Ornade Spansule	SmithKline Beecham	Capsule	Slow release
Oruvail	Wyeth-Ayerst	Capsule	Slow release
Pabalate	Robins	Tablet	Enteric-coated
Pabalate SF	Robins	Tablet	Enteric-coated
Pancrease	McNeil	Capsule	Enteric-coated*
Pancrease MT	McNeil	Capsule	Enteric-coated*
Panmycin	Upjohn	Capsule	Taste
Papaverine Sustained Action	Various	Capsule	Slow release
Pathilon Sequels	Lederle	Capsule	Slow release*
Pavabid Plateau	Marion-Merrell Dow	Capsule	Slow release*
PBZ-SR	Geigy	Tablet	Slow release (i)
Pentasa	Marion-Merrell Dow	Capsule	Slow release
Perdiem	Rhone-Poulenc Rorer	Granules	Wax-coated
Peritrate SA	Parke-Davis	Tablet	Slow release (h)
Permitil Chronotab	Schering	Tablet	Slow release (i)
Phazyme	Reed & Carnrick	Tablet	Slow release

Drug Product	Manufacturer	Dosage Form	Reason/Comments
Phazyme 95	Reed & Carnrick	Tablet	Slow release
Phenergan	Wyeth-Ayerst	Tablet	Taste (c) (i)
Phyllocontin	Purdue Frederick	Tablet	Slow release
Plendil	MSD	Tablet	Slow release
Pneumonist	ECR Pharm	Tablet	Slow release (i)
Polaramine Repetabs	Schering	Tablet	Slow release (i)
Prelu-2	Boehringer Ingelheim	Capsule	Slow release
Prilosec	MSD	Capsule	Slow release
Pro-Banthine	Schiapparelli Searle	Tablet	Taste
Procainamide HCl S.R.	Various	Tablet	Slow release
Procan SR	Parke-Davis	Tablet	Slow release
Procardia	Pfizer	Capsule	Delays absorption (b) (e)
Procardia XL	Pfizer	Tablet	Slow release, AUC is unaffected
Pronestyl-SR	Bristol-Myers Squibb	Tablet	Slow release
Proventil Repetabs	Schering	Tablet	Slow release (i)
Prozac	Dista	Capsule	Slow release
Quadra-Hist	Schein	Tablet	Slow release
Quibron-T/SR	Bristol-Myers Squibb	Tablet	Slow release (i)
Quinaglute Dura-Tabs	Berlex	Tablet	Slow release
Quinalan Lanatabs	Lannett	Tablet	Slow release
Quinalan S.R.	Lannett	Tablet	Slow release
Quinidex Extentabs	Robins	Tablet	Slow release
Respaire S.R.	Laser	Capsule	Slow release
Respbid	Boehringer Ingelheim	Tablet	Slow release
Ritalin-SR	Ciba	Tablet	Slow release
Robimycin Robitab	Robins	Tablet	Enteric-coated
Rondec-TR	Ross	Tablet	Slow release (i)
Roxanol-SR	Roxane	Tablet	Slow release (i)
Ru-Tuss	Boots	Tablet	Slow release
Ru-Tuss DE	Boots	Tablet	Slow release
Seldane-D	Marion-Merrell Dow	Tablet	Slow release
Sinemet CR	DuPont Pharm	Tablet	Slow release (h)
Singlet	Marion-Merrell Dow	Tablet	Slow release
Slo-Bid Gyrocaps	Rhone-Poulenc Rorer	Capsule	Slow release*
Slo-Niacin	Upsher Smith	Tablet	Slow release
Slo-Phyllin GG	Rhone-Poulenc Rorer	Capsule	Slow release (i)
Slo-Phyllin Gyrocaps	Rhone-Poulenc Rorer	Capsule	Slow release* (i)
Slow-FE	Ciba Consumer	Tablet	Slow release (i)
Slow-K	Summit	Tablet	Slow release (i)
Slow-Mag	Searle	Tablet	Slow release
Sorbitrate S.A.	ICI Pharma	Tablet	Slow release
Sorbitrate Sublingual	ICI Pharma	Tablet	Sublingual route
Sparine	Wyeth-Ayerst	Tablet	Taste (c)
S-P-T	Fleming	Capsule	Liquid gelatin susp.
Stamoist E	Huckaby	Tablet	Slow release
Stamoist LA	Huckaby	Tablet	Slow release
Sudafed 12 hour	Burroughs Wellcome	Caplet	Slow release (i)
Surfak Liquigels	Upjohn	Capsule	Liquid filled (b)
Tavist-D	Sandoz	Tablet	Multiple compressed tablet
Teldrin	SmithKline Beecham	Capsule	Slow release*
Temaril Spansules	Allergan, Herbert	Capsule	Slow release (i)
Tepanil Ten-Tab	3M Pharmaceuticals	Tablet	Slow release
Tessalon Perles	Forest	Capsule	Slow release
Theo-24	Searle	Tablet	Slow release (i)
Theobid	Russ	Capsule	Slow release* (i)
Theobid Jr.	Russ	Capsule	Slow release* (i)
Theoclear-LA	Central	Capsule	Slow release (i)

Drug Product	Manufacturer	Dosage Form	Reason/Comments
Theochron	Various	Tablet	Slow release
Theo-Dur	Key	Tablet	Slow release (i)(h)
Theo-Dur Sprinkle	Key	Capsule	Slow release* (i)
Theo-Sav	Savage	Tablet	Slow release (h)
Theolair-SR	3M Pharmaceuticals	Tablet	Slow release (i)
Theovent	Schering	Capsule	Slow release (i)
Theox	Carnrick	Tablet	Slow release
Therapy Bayer	Glenbrook	Caplet	Enteric-coated
Thorazine Spansule	SmithKline Beecham	Capsule	Slow release
Toprol XL	Astra	Tablet	Slow release (h)
T-Phyl	Purdue Frederick	Tablet	Slow release
Trental	Hoechst-Roussel	Tablet	Slow release
Triaminic	Sandoz	Tablet	Enteric-coated (i)
Triaminic-12	Sandoz	Tablet	Slow release (i)
Trilafon Repetabs	Schering	Tablet	Slow release (i)
Trinalin Repetabs	Key	Tablet	Slow release
Touro A & H	Dartmouth	Capsule	Slow release*
Touro Ex	Dartmouth	Tablet	Slow release (h)
Touro LA	Dartmouth	Tablet	Slow release (h)
Tuss-LA	Hyrex	Tablet	Slow release
Tuss-Ornade Spansule	SmithKline Beecham	Capsule	Slow release
ULR-LA	Geneva	Tablet	Slow release
Unicap	Upjohn	Capsule	Liquid filled (b)
Uniphyl	Purdue Frederick	Tablet	Slow release
Valrelease	Roche	Capsule	Slow release
Vantin	Upjohn	Tablet	Taste (c)(i)
Verelan	Lederle	Capsule	Slow release*
Volmax	Muro	Tablet	Slow release (i)
Wellbutrin	Burroughs Wellcome	Tablet	Anesthetize mucous membrane
Wyamycin-S	Wyeth-Ayerst	Tablet	Slow release
Wygesic	Wyeth-Ayerst	Tablet	Taste
Zephrex LA	Central	Tablet	Slow release
ZORprin	Boots	Tablet	Slow release
Zymase	Organon	Capsule	Enteric-coated

The listing is included to alert the health care practitioner about oral dosage forms that should not be crushed, and to serve as an aid in consulting with patients. Reprinted from Mitchell, John F: Hospital Pharmacy 20: 310, 1985 and revised by John F. Mitchell, Pharm. D. and Kathleen S. Pawlicki, M.S.

*Capsule may be opened and the contents taken without crushing or chewing; soft food such as applesauce or pudding may facilitate administration; contents may generally be administered via nasogastric tube using an appropriate fluid such as cherry syrup.

(a) Antacids and/or milk may prematurely dissolve the coating of the tablet.

(b) Capsule may be opened and the liquid contents removed for administration.

(c) The taste of the product in a liquid form would likely be unacceptable to the patient; administration via nasogastric tube should be acceptable.

(d) Effervescent tablets must be dissolved in the amount of diluent recommended by the manufacturer.

(e) If the liquid capsule is crushed or the contents expressed, the active ingredient will be, in part, absorbed sublingually.

(f) Acid contents of the stomach may prematurely activate the ingredients.

(g) Tablets are made to disintegrate under the tongue.

(h) Tablet is scored.

(i) Liquid dosage forms of the product are available; however, dose, frequency of administration and manufacturers may differ from that of the solid dosage form.

(j) Capsule contents intended to be placed in a teaspoonful of water or soft food.

(k) Contents may be dissolved in water for administration.

(l) Crushing may result in precipitation of larger particles.

Pharmaceutical Company Labeler Code Index

0000
Carnation

0002
Lilly, Eli, & Co.

0003
Convatec Div. E. R. Squibb Co.

0003
Princeton Pharmaceutical
Div. E. R. Squibb Co.

0003
Squibb Mark
Div. E. R. Squibb Co.

0003
Squibb Marsam
Div. E. R. Squibb Co.

0003
Squibb-Novo
Div. E. R. Squibb Co.

0004
Roche Laboratories

0005
Lederle Laboratories,
    Davis & Geck, American Cyanamid Co.

0006
Merck Sharp & Dohme

0007
Smith Kline & French Laboratories

0008
Wyeth Laboratories
See: Wyeth-Ayerst Laboratories

0009
Upjohn Company, The

0011
Hynson, Westcott & Dunning Inc.

0013
Adria Laboratories, Inc.
Div. of Erbamont Inc.

0014
Searle & Co.

0015
Apothecon

0016
Pharmacia Laboratories

0017
Wampole Laboratories

0019
Mallinckrodt Pharmaceuticals Div.

0021
Reed & Carnrick

0023
Herbert Laboratories
Allergan Pharmaceuticals, Inc.

0024
Sanofi Winthrop Laboratories

0025
Searle Laboratories

0026
Miles Pharmaceuticals

0028
Geigy Pharmaceuticals

0029
Beecham Laboratories

0031
Robins, A.H., Company

0032
Solvay

0033
Syntex Laboratories, Inc.

0034
Purdue Frederick Co., The

0037
Wallace Laboratories

0038
Stuart Pharmaceuticals

0039
Hoechst-Roussel Pharmaceuticals, Inc.

0041
Oral-B Laboratories, Inc.

0043
Sandoz Pharmaceutical Corp.

0044
Knoll Pharmaceutical Co.

0045
McNeil Labs

0046
Wyeth-Ayerst Laboratories

0047
Warner/Chilcott Laboratories

0048
Boots Pharmaceuticals, Inc.

0049
Roerig

0052
Organon Inc.

0053
Armour Pharmaceutical Co.

0054
Roxane Laboratories, Inc.

0056
DuPont Pharmaceuticals

0058
Iolab Pharmaceuticals

0062
Ortho Pharmaceutical Corporation

0065
Alcon Laboratories, Inc.

0066
Dermik Laboratories, Inc.

0067
Rorer, William H., Inc.

0068
SKB Consumer Healthcare

0068
Merrell Dow Pharmaceuticals

0069
Pfizer Laboratories

0070
Arcola Laboratories

0071
Parke, Davis & Co.

0072
Westwood Pharmaceuticals, Inc.

0074
Abbott Laboratories
Murine Company
Ross Laboratories

0075
Rhone-Poulenc Rorer Pharm Inc.

0076
Star Pharmaceuticals, Inc.

0078
Sandoz Pharmaceuticals

The "Pharmaceutical Company Labeler Code Index" is presented to aid the practitioner in the identification of drug products. In this section the codes are listed in numerical order. Additionally, the pharmaceutical labeler codes are also listed with the alphabetical listing of Pharmaceutical Manufacturers and/or Drug Distributors.

0081
Burroughs Wellcome Co.

0083
CIBA Pharmaceutical Company

0085
Schering Corporation

0086
Carnrick Laboratories

0087
Mead Johnson & Company

0088
SKB Consumer Healthcare

0089
3M Pharmaceutical

0089
3M Personal Care Products

0091
Kremers-Urban Co.

0093
Lemmon Company

0094
DuPont Merck Pharmaceutical Co.

0095
E.C.R. Pharmaceuticals

0096
Person & Covey, Inc.

0098
Kirkman Laboratories, Inc.

0116
Xttrium Laboratories, Inc.

0118
Hollister-Stier Laboratories

0122
Rexall Group

0126
Colgate-Hoyt Laboratories

0127
Ulmer Pharmacal Co.

0128
SKB Consumer Healthcare

0131
The Central Pharmacal Co.

0132
Fleet, C. B., Co., Inc.

0137
Johnson & Johnson
Dermatological Division

0140
Roche Products, Inc.

0143
West-ward, Inc.

0145
Stiefel Laboratories, Inc.

0147
Camall Company

0149
Procter & Gamble Pharmaceuticals

0152
Gray Pharmaceutical Company

0154
Blair Laboratories, Inc.

0161
Cutter Laboratories, Inc.

0164
Carter Products

0165
Blaine Co., Inc.

0168
Fougera, E. & Co., Inc.

0172
Zenith Laboratories, Inc.

0173
Glaxo Inc.

0178
Mission Pharmacal Co.

0182
Generix Drug Sales Co., Inc.

0185
Eon Labs Manufacturing, Inc.

0186
Astra Pharmaceutical Products, Inc.

0187
ICN Pharmaceuticals

0192
Miles Laboratories, Inc.

0193
Miles Inc.

0195
Rhone-Poulenc Rorer

0196
Rachelle Laboratories

0197
Ex-Lax Inc.

0212
Sandoz Nutrition

0217
Dunhall Pharmaceuticals, Inc.

0222
Boyle & Co.

0224
Konsyl Pharmaceuticals

0225
Ascher, B.F., & Co., Inc.

0228
Purepac Pharmaceutical Co.

0234
Schmid Laboratories

0235
Fisons Consumer Health

0245
Upsher-SmithLaboratories, Inc.

0249
Geriatric Pharmaceutical Corp.

0252
JMI-Canton

0256
Fleming & Company

0258
Inwood Laboratories, Inc.

0259
Mayrand Incorporated

0261
Drug Industries Co., Inc.

0263
Rystan Co., Inc.

0268
Center Laboratories, Inc.

0273
Lorvic Corp., The

0274
Scherer Laboratories,Inc.

0275
Arco Pharmaceuticals, Inc.

0276
Misemer Pharmaceuticals, Inc.

0277
Laser, Inc.

0281
Savage Laboratories

0283
Beutlich, Inc.

0288
Fluoritab Corp.

0299
Owen Laboratories

0314
Hyrex Pharmaceuticals

0316
Del-Ray Laboratories, Inc.

0317
Whorton Pharmaceuticals, Inc.

0327
Guardian Chemical Corp.

0348
Medtech Laboratories

0349
Parmed Pharmaceuticals, Inc.

0362
Novocol Chemical Mfg. Co., Inc.

0374
Lyne Laboratories

0377
Pal-Pak, Inc.

0386
Gebauer Chemical Co.

0394
Mericon Industries, Inc.

0395
Humco Laboratory, Inc.

0396
Milex Products, Inc.

0398
C & M Pharmacal, Inc.

0418
Pasadena Research Laboratories, Inc.

0421
Fielding Co., The

0436
Century Pharmaceuticals, Inc.

0451
Muro Pharmacal Labs., Inc.

0454
Lexis Laboratories

0456
Forest Pharmaceuticals, Inc.

0463
C.O. Truxton, Inc.

0466
Macsil, Inc.

0469
LyphoMed

0472
Barre National, Inc.

0477
Rexar Pharmaceuticals

0482
Bradley/Kenwood Laboratories

0485
Edwards Pharmacal Co.

0486
Beach Pharmaceuticals

0487
Nephron Corporation

0494
Foy Laboratories, Inc.

0496
Ferndale Laboratories, Inc.

0514
Dow B. Hickam, Inc.

0516
Glenwood Laboratories, Inc.

0517
American Regent

0521
Chesebrough-Pond's Inc.

0527
Lannett Co., Inc.

0534
Health & Medical Techniques

0535
Gilbert Laboratories

0536
Rugby Laboratories

0539
American Urologicals, Inc.

0551
Seatrace Co., The

0555
Barr Laboratories, Inc.

0563
Bock Pharmacal Company

0573
Whitehall Labs.

0574
Paddock Laboratories

0575
Baker Norton Pharmaceutical, Inc.

0576
Medical Prods. Panamericana, Inc.

0585
Fisons Corporation

0588
Keene Pharmaceuticals, Inc.

0590
DuPont Pharmaceuticals Div.

0597
Boehringer Ingelheim Ltd.

0598
Triage Pharmaceuticals

0615
Vangard Laboratories

0619
Walker Pharmacal Co.

0641
Elkins-Sinn, Inc.

0642
Everett Laboratories, Inc.

0659
Circle Pharmaceuticals, Inc.

0689
Daniels Pharmaceuticals

0697
Delco Chemical Co., Inc.

0698
Grafton Pharmaceutical Co.

0701
My-K Laboratories

0713
G & W Laboratories, Inc.

0729
Fidelity Halsom

0731
Alto Pharmaceuticals, Inc.

0741
Walker Corp. & Co., Inc.

0766
SKB Consumer Healthcare

0777
Dista Products Co.

0781
Geneva Generics

0785
UAD Laboratories, Inc.

0814
Interstate Drug Exchange

0832
Pharmaceutical Basics, Inc.
Pennex Pharmaceuticals Inc.

0837
Columbia Laboratories, Inc.

0839
Moore, H. L., Drug Exchange, Inc.

0879
Halsey Drug Co., Inc.

0884
Pedinol Pharmacal, Inc.

0904
Major Pharmaceutical Corp.

0917
Wesley Pharmacal Co., Inc.

0938
Davis and Geck

0944
Baxter Hyland

0995
Pfipharmecs
See: Pfizer

10038
Ambix Laboratories, Inc.

10223
Cetylite Industries, Inc.

10244
Otis Clapp & Son, Inc.
Buffington Division
Cross Division

10310
Del Laboratories, Inc.

10651
Lavoptik Co., Inc.

10706
Manne, Kenneth A., Co.

10712
Marlyn Company, Inc.

10797
Oakhurst Company

10812
Neutrogena Corp.

10952
Recsei Laboratories

10956
Reese Chemical Co.

10961
Requa

11086
Summers Laboratories, Inc.

11089
Superior Chemical International, Inc.
McGregor & Co.

11290
Thompson Medical Co., Inc.

11299
Torch Laboratories, Inc.

11311
Trimen Laboratories, Inc.

11370
Warner-Lambert Company

11414
Willen Drug Co.

11444
Young, W. F. Inc.

11509
Combe Inc.

11588
DEP Corporation

11808
Ion Laboratories, Inc.

11940
Medco Lab. Inc.

11980
Allergan America

12120
Wisconsin Pharmacal Co., Inc.

12136
Bird Corporation

12547
Warner-Lambert Co.

12758
Mason Pharmaceuticals, Inc.

12843
Sterling Laboratories

12939
Marlop Pharmaceuticals, Inc.

16500
Miles Laboratories

19810
Bristol-Myers Products

22200
Mennen Co.

23900
Vicks Health Care

25866
Vicks Pharmacy Products
Div. of Richardson-Vicks Inc.

37000
Procter and Gamble

38083
Campbell Laboratories, Inc.

41383
AK Pharma, Inc.

41701
Inagra

42021
Sclavo, Inc.

43797
Mallard Medical Products

44081
Med-Corp, Inc.

44087
Serono Laboratories, Inc.

45800
SKB Consumer Healthcare

46500
Rydelle Laboratories

48017
Hermal Pharmaceutical Labs.

48532
Delmont Laboratories Inc.

48663
Unimed Co.

49281
Connaught/Squibb Inc.

49447
Chattem Consumer Products
Div. of Chattem, Inc.

49692
SKB Consumer Healthcare

50361
Merieux Institute, Inc.

50383
Health Care Products

50419
Berlex Laboratories

50445
Novo/Nordisk Pharmaceuticals, Inc.

50474
Whitby Pharmaceuticals, Inc.

51201
American Dermal Corp.

53100
SKB Consumer Healthcare

53169
Boehringer Mannheim Pharm.

55390
Bedford Laboratories

58579
Hogil Pharmaceutical Copr.

59012
Pratt Pharmaceuticals

59512
Healthline Laboratories, Inc.

59702
Atley Pharmaceuticals, Inc.

60575
Respa Pharmaceuticals, Inc.

76660
Richardson-Vicks, Inc.

93312
Trask Industries, Inc.

00089
3M Personal Care Products
3M Center, Bldg. 225-4W-02
St. Paul, MN 55144-1000
612-733-1110

00089
3M Pharmaceutical
3M Center, Bldg. 275-3W-01
St. Paul, MN 55144-1000
612-736-4930

A.L. Labs
One Executive Dr., POB 1399
Ft. Lee, NJ 07024
201-947-7774

41383
AKPharma, Inc.
P.O. Box 111
Pleasantville, NJ 08232
609-645-5100

ALK Laboratories, Inc.
132 Research Dr.
Milford, CT 06460
203-949-2727

12463
Abana Pharmaceuticals, Inc.
P.O. Box 360388
Birmingham, AL 35236
205-988-4588

00074
Abbott Diagnostics
Customer Support Cnt. Dept 94P
Abbott Park, IL 60064
800-323-9100

00074
Abbott Hospital Products
1 Abbott Park Rd. D39b AP30
Abbott Park, IL 60064-3500
708-937-6100

00074
Abbott Laboratories
1 Abbott Park Rd. D422 AP6A
Abbott Park, IL 60064-3500
708-937-6100

Academic Pharmaceuticals, Inc.
25720 Saunders Road North
Lake Forest, IL 60045

Acme United Corporation
75 Kings Highway Cutoff
Fairfield, CT 06430
203-332-7330

53014
Adams Laboratories
14801 Sovereign Road
Ft. Worth, TX 76155-2645
817-545-7791

Adolphs
Van den Berg, 75 Merritt Blvd.
Trumbull, CT 06611
203-381-3500

00013
Adria Laboratories
P.O. Box 16529
Columbus, OH 43216-6529
614-764-8100

Advanced Care Products
Route 202, P.O. Box 610
Raritan, NJ 08869
908-218-8625

10888
Advanced Nutrit. Tech. Inc.
P.O. Box 3225
Elizabeth, NJ 07207
201-354-2740

17478
Akorn, Inc.
100 Akorn Drive
Abita Springs, LA 70420
504-893-9300

00065
Alcon Laboratories, Inc.
6201 South Freeway
Ft. Worth, TX 76134
817-293-0450

00173
Allen & Hanburys
5 Moore Drive
Research Triangle Pk NC 27709
919-248-2100

00299
Allercreme
P.O. Box 6600
Ft. Worth, TX 76115
817-293-0450

11980
Allergan Americana
2525 DuPont Dr., POB 19534
Irvine, CA 92713-9534
714-752-4500

00023
Allergan Herbert
2525 DuPont Drive
Irvine, CA 92715-9534
800-347-4500

00023
Allergan Pharmaceuticals
2525 DuPont Drive PO Box 19534
Irvine, CA 92713-9534
714-752-4500

54569
Allscrips
1033 Butterfield Rd.
Vernon Hills, IL 60061
708-680-3515

Alpha 1 Biomedicals, Inc.
6903 Rockledge Drive
Bethesda, MD 20817
301-564-4400

49669
Alpha Therapeutic Corp.
5555 Valley Blvd.
Los Angeles, CA 90032
213-225-2221

51641
Alra Laboratories, Inc.
3850 Clearview Court
Gurnee, IL 60031
708-244-9440

00731
Alto Pharmaceuticals, Inc.
P.O. Box 1910
Land O'Lakes, FL 34639-1910
813-949-7464

72959
Alva Laboratories
6625 Avondale Ave.
Chicago, IL 60631
312-792-0200

17314
Alza Corporation
950 Page Mill Road
Palo Alto, CA 94303-0802
415-496-5000

10038
Ambix Laboratories, Inc.
210 Orchard Street
East Rutherford, NJ 07073
201-939-2200

90605
Amcon Laboratories
40 N. Rock Hill Rd.
St. Louis, MO 63119
314-961-5758

89709
Amcon Laboratories
40 N. Rock Hill Rd.
St. Louis, MO 63119
314-961-5758

53443
Americal Pharmaceutical Inc.
1340 N. Jefferson St.
Anaheim, CA 92807
714-579-7545

51201
American Dermal Corp.
51 Apple Tree Ln P.O. Box 900
Plumsteadville, PA 18949-0900
610-454-8000

57506
American Drug Industries, Inc.
5810 S. Perry Ave.
Chicago, IL 60621
312-667-7070

52769
American Red Cross
Washington, DC 20006
202-639-3347

00517
American Regent
1 Luitpold Dr.
Shirley, NY 11967
516-924-4000

50349
American Therapeutics, Inc.
83 Carlough Rd.
Bohemia, NY 11716
516-563-1830

00539
American Urologicals, Inc.
7881 Hollywood Blvd. Suite 4
Pembroke Pines, FL 33024
305-932-2830

55513
Amgen, Inc.
1840 Dehavilland Dr.
Thousand Oaks, CA 91320-1789
805-499-5725

52152
Amide Pharmaceuticals, Inc.
101 E. Main Street
Little Falls, NJ 07424
201-890-1440

53926
Amsco Scientific
1002 Lufkin Road PO Box 747
Apex, NC 27502
800-388-5155

Amswiss Scientific, Inc.
2170 Broadway, Suite 1200
New York, NY 10024

10019
Anaquest
110 Allen Rd.
Liberty Corner, NJ 07938
908-647-9200

Andrulis Research Corporation
11800 Baltimore Ave.
Beltsville, MD 20705
301-419-2400

Anthra Pharmaceuticals, Inc.
19 Carson Road
Princeton, NJ 08540

Apothecary Products, Inc.
11531 Rupp Drive
Burnsville, MN 55337
612-890-1940

00003
Apothecon
P.O. Box 4500
Princeton, NJ 08543-4500
609-897-2111

00015
Apothecon
P.O. Box 4500
Princeton, NJ 08543-4500
609-897-2111

48723
Apothecus, Inc.
132 South Street
Oyster Bay, NY 11771
516-624-8200

Applied Genetics
205 Buffalo Avenue
Freeport, NY 11520
516-868-9026

Applied Medical Research
1600 Hayes Street
Nashville, TN 37203

00275
Arco Pharmaceuticals, Inc.
90 Orville Drive
Bohemia, NY 11716
516-567-9500

00070
Arcola Laboratories
500 Arcola Road
Collegeville, PA 19426-0107
215-454-8000

Argus Pharmaceuticals, Inc.
6400 Research Forest Drive
The Woodlands, TX 77381

00053
Armour Pharmaceutical
500 Arcola Rd. P.O. Box 1200
Collegeville, PA 19426-0107
800-727-6737

48558
Arther, Inc.
P.O. Box 1455
W. Caldwell, NJ 07007
201-226-5288

00186
Astra Pharmaceutical Products
50 Otis Street
Westborough, MA 01581
508-366-1100

59075
Athena Neurosciences, Inc.
800 F Gateway Blvd.
South San Francisco CA 94080
415-877-0900

59702
Atley Pharmaceuticals, Inc.
340 S. Richardson Road Ste. 1
Ashland, VA 23005
804-550-1979

Autoimmune, Inc.
128 Spring Street
Lexington, MA 02173
617-860-0710

Axion Pharmaceuticals
395 Oyster Point Blvd. Ste.405
South San Francisco, CA 94080

00225
B. F. Ascher and Company
15501 W. 109th St.
Lenexa, KS 66215
913-888-1880

44184
Bajamar Chemical Co. Inc.
9609 Dielman Rock Island
St. Louis, MO 63132
314-997-3414

58174
Baker Cummins Dermatologicals
1950 Swarthmore Ave.
Lakewood, NJ 08701
908-905-5200

10106
J.T. Baker, Inc.
222 Red School Lane
Phillipsburg, NJ 08865
908-859-2151

00575
Baker Norton Pharm. Inc.
8800 N.W. 36th St.
Miami, FL 33178-2404
305-590-2282

00304
J.J. Balan, Inc.
5725 Foster Ave.
Brooklyn, NY 11234
718-251-8663

00555
Barr Laboratories, Inc.
2 Quaker Road
Pomona, NY 01970
914-362-1100

00472
Barre-National, Inc.
333 Cassell Drive Suite 3500
Baltimore, MD 21224
410-558-7250

58887
Basel Pharmaceuticals
556 Morris Avenue
Summit, NJ 07901
908-277-5000

10119
Bausch & Lomb
1400 N. Goodman St. PO Box 450
Rochester, NY 14692-0450
716-338-6000

24208
Bausch & Lomb
8500 Hidden River Parkway
Tampa, FL 33637
813-975-7700

57782
Bausch & Lomb Pharmaceutical
Tampa, FL 33637

10119
Bausch and Lomb Consumer
1400 N. Goodman St. PO Box 450
Rochester, NY 14692-0450
716-338-6000

10119
Bausch and Lomb Pharm.
8500 Hidden River Parkway
Tampa, FL 33637
813-975-7700

00338
Baxter Healthcare Corporation
Route 120 and Wilson Road
Round Lake, IL 60073
800-933-0303

47679
Baxter Healthcare Corporation
Route 120 and Wilson Road
Round Lake, IL 60073
800-933-0303

00944
Baxter Hyland
550 North Brand Blvd.
Glendale, CA 91203
818-956-3200

00486
Beach Pharmaceuticals
P.O. Box 128
Conestee, SC 29636
803-277-7282

31280
Becton Dickinson & Company
One Becton Drive
Franklin Lakes, NJ 07417-1881
201-847-6800

55390
Bedford Laboratories
300 Northfield Road
Bedford, OH 44146
216-232-3320

Behringwerke Aktiengesellschaft
500 Arcola Road, P.O. Box 1200
Collegeville, PA 19426-0107

10356
Beiersdorf, Inc.
P.O. Box 5529
S. Norwalk, CT 06856-5529
203-853-8008

38697
Berkeley Biologicals
2840 Eighth St.
Berkeley, CA 94710-2707
510-843-6846

50419
Berlex Laboratories, Inc.
300 Fairfield Rd.
Wayne, NJ 07470-2095
201-694-4100

58337
Berna Products Corporation
4216 Ponce De Leon Blvd.
Coral Gables, FL 33146
305-443-2900

54274
Best Generics
19589 N.E. 10th Avenue
North Miami Beach, FL 33179-3501

00283
Beutlich, Inc.
1541 Shields Dr.
Waukegan, IL 60085
708-473-1100

53191
Bio-Tech
P.O. Box 1992
Fayetteville, AR 72702
501-443-9148

Bio-Technology General Corp.
70 Wood Ave. South
Iselin, NJ 08830
908-632-8800

Bio-Technology General Corporation
1250 Broadway 20th Floor
New York, NY 10001

59527
BioDevelopment Corporation
8180 Greensboro Dr. Suite 1000
McLean, VA 22102

BioGenex Laboratories
4600 Norris Canyon Rd Ste. 400
San Ramon, CA 94583
510-275-0550

00332
Biocraft Laboratories, Inc.
18-01 River Road
Fair Lawn, NJ 07410
800-631-0165

Biocryst Pharmaceuticals, Inc.
2190 Parkway Lake Drive
Birmingham, AL 35244

Biofilm Inc.
P.O. Box 965302
Marietta, GA 30066
404-565-6078

Biogen
14 Cambridge Center
Cambridge, MA 02142
617-864-8900

Biomedical Frontiers, Inc.
1095 10th Avenue S.E.
Minneapolis, MN 55414
612-378-0228

Biomerica, Inc.
1533 Monrovia Avenue
Newport Beach, CA 92663
714-645-2111

Biomune Systems, Incorporated
40 East South Temple, Ste. 310
Salt Lake City, UT 84111

Biopure Corporation
68 Harrison Avenue
Boston, MA 02111

52311
Biosearch Medical Products
P.O. Box 1700
Somerville, NJ 08876
908-722-5000

20699
Biotel Corporation
366 Madison Avenue #1506
New York, NY 10017
800-445-4551

50289
Birchwood Laboratories, Inc.
7900 Fuller Rd.
Eden Prairie, MN 53344
800-328-6156

12136
Bird Corporation
1100 Bird Center Dr.
Palm Springs, CA 92262
619-778-7200

00165
Blaine Company, Inc.
1465 Jamike Lane
Erlanger, KY 41018-1878
606-283-9437

00154
Blair Laboratories
100 Connecticut Ave.
Norwalk, CT 06850-3590
203-853-0123

50486
Blairex Labs., Inc.
P.O. Box 2127
Columbus, IN 47202-2127
812-378-1864

10157
Blistex, Inc.
1800 Swift Drive
Oak Brook, IL 60521
708-571-2870

10158
Block Drug Company, Inc.
257 Cornelison Ave.
Jersey City, NJ 07302
201-434-3000

10160
Bluco Inc./Med. Discnt. Outlet
14849 W. McNichols
Detroit, MI 48235
313-273-0322

00563
Bock Pharmacal Company
P.O. Box 419056
St. Louis, MO 63141-9056
314-579-0770

00597
Boehringer Ingelheim, Inc.
900 Ridgebury Road
Ridgefield, CT 06877
203-798-9988

50924
Boehringer Mannheim Diags.
9115 Hague Rd. P.O. Box 50100
Indianapolis, IN 46250-0100
800-428-5074

53169
Boehringer Mannheim Pharm.
101 Orchard Ridge Dr.
Gaithersburg, MD 20878
301-216-3545

44437
Bolan Pharmaceutical, Inc.
P.O. Box 230
Hurst, TX 76053
817-268-6110

00524
Boots Pharmaceuticals, Inc.
300 Tri-State Internat. Center
Lincolnshire, IL 60069-4415
708-405-7400

00048
Boots Pharmaceuticals, Inc.
300 Tri-State Internat. Center
Lincolnshire, IL 60069-4415
708-405-7400

00222
Boyle and Company Pharm.
1030 S. Arroyo Parkway
Pasadena, CA 91105
818-441-0284

00482
Bradley/Kenwood Laboratories
383 Rt. 46 W.
Fairfield, NJ 07006-2402
201-882-1505

52268
Braintree Laboratories, Inc.
60 Columbian, P.O. Box 361
Braintree, MA 02184
617-843-2202

72363
Brimms Inc.
425 Fillmore Ave.
Tonawanda, NY 14150
716-694-7100

19810
Bristol-Myers Oncology Div.
P.O. Box 4500
Princeton, NJ 08543
609-897-2000

62443
Cal-White Mineral Company
7700 SE Beaverton Hillside Hwy
Portland, OR 97225
503-884-0687

70526
Carme, Inc.
84 Galli
Novato, CA 94949
415-382-4000

19810
Bristol-Myers Products
345 Park Ave. 4th Floor
New York, NY 10154
800-468-7746

55559
Calgon Vestal Laboratories
P.O. Box 147
St. Louis, MO 63166-0147
314-535-1810

00000
Carnation
800 North Brand Blvd
Glendale, ca 91203
818-549-6000

00087
Bristol-Myers Squibb
P.O. Box 4000
Princeton, NJ 08543-4000
609-252-4000

California Dept. Health Service
2151 Berkeley Way
Berkeley, CA 94704

00086
Carnrick Laboratories, Inc.
65 Horse Hill Road
Cedar Knolls, NJ 07927
201-267-2670

Britannia Pharmaceuticals
Forum Hs Brighton Rd. Redhil
Surrey, UK RH 1 6YS

00147
Camall Company, Inc.
P.O. Box 307
Romeo, MI 48065-0307
313-752-9683

46287
Carolina Medical Products
P.O. Box 147
Farmville, NC 27828
919-753-7111

00081
Burroughs Wellcome Co.
3030 Cornwallis Road
Research Triangle Pk NC 27709
919-248-3000

Cambridge Neuroscience, Inc.
1 Kendall Square Bldg. 700
Cambridge, MA 02139
617-225-0600

Carrington Labs
1300 E. Rochelle Blvd.
Irving, TX 75062
214-518-1300

00398
C & M Pharmacal, Inc.
1721 Maple Lane
Hazel Park, MI 48030-1215
313-548-7846

38083
Campbell Laboratories
P.O. Box 639
Deerfield Beach, FL 33443
305-570-9834

00164
Carter Products
Half Acre Road, P.O. Box 1001
Cranbury, NJ 08512-0181
609-655-6000

00132
C. B. Fleet Co., Inc.
4615 Murray Place
Lynchburg, VA 24506
804-528-4000

Capmed USA
P.O. Box 14
Bryn Mawr, PA 19010

Cav-Con, Inc.
55 Knollwood Road
Farmington, CT 06032

00463
C. O. Truxton Inc.
P.O. Box 1594
Camden, NJ 08101
609-365-4118

59046
Caprice-Greystoke
1259 Activity Drive
Vista, CA 92083
619-598-9300

Cavitation-Control Technology
55 Knollwood Road
Farmington, CT 06032
203-673-0507

57664
Caraco Pharmaceutical Lab.,Ltd
1150 Elijah McCoy Drive
Detroit, MI 48202
313-871-8400

Celgene Corporation
7 Powder Horn Drive
Warren, NJ 07059

10486
C. S. Dent & Co. Division
317 E. Eighth St.
Cincinnati, OH 45202
513-241-1677

Cell Pathways, Inc.
1700 Broadway, Ste. 2000
Denver, CO 80290

88395
J. R. Carlson Laboratories
15 College Drive
Arlington Heights, IL 60004-1985
708-255-1600

CTRC Research Foundation
11812 Becket Street
Potomac, MD 20854

Cell Technology
1668 Valtec Lane
Boulder, CO 80301
303-790-0587

Cellegy Pharmaceuticals, Inc.
371 Bel Marin Keys, Ste. 210
Novato, CA 94949

Celtrix Pharmaceuticals, Inc.
3055 Patrick Henry Drive
Santa Clara, CA 95054

00556
H.R. Cenci Labs., Inc.
1420 E Street,PO Box 12524
Fresno, CA 93778-2524
209-237-3346

00268
Center Laboratories
35 Channel Drive
Port Washington, NY 11050
516-767-1800

Centers for Disease Control
1600 Clifton Rd,Mail Stop D-09
Atlanta, GA 30000
404-639-3670

Centocor Inc.
200 Great Valley Parkway
Malvern, PA 19355
215 296-4488

00131
Central Pharmaceuticals, Inc.
120 E. Third Street POB 328
Seymour, IN 47274-9985
812-522-3915

00436
Century Pharmaceuticals, Inc.
10377 Hague Road
Indianapolis, IN 46256-3399
317-849-4210

Cephalon, Inc.
145 Brandywine Parkway
West Chester, PA 19380
215-344-0200

00173
Cerenex Pharmaceuticals
Five Moore Drive
Research Triangle PK NC 27709
919-248-2100

10223
Cetylite Industries, Inc.
PO Box 90006 9051 River Road
Pennsauken, NJ 08110
609-665-6111

54429
Chase Laboratories
280 Chestnut Street
Newark, NJ 07105-1598
201-589-8181

49447
Chattem Consumer Products
1715 W. 38th Street
Chattanooga, TN 37409
615-821-4571

Chembiomed, LTD.
P.O. Box 8050
Edmonton, AB T6H4NP

52489
Chemi-Tech Laboratories
74-80 Marine Street
Farmingdale, NY 11735

00521
Chesebrough-Pond's, Inc.
33 Benedict Place
Greenwich, CT 06830
203-661-2000

Chiesi Pharmaceuticals, Inc.
150 Danbury Road
Ridgefield, CT 06877

53905
Chiron Corporation
4560 Horton Street
Emeryville, CA 94608
510-420-3300

Chiron IntraOptics
9342 Jeronimo Road
Irvine, CA 92718-1903
714-768-4690

Chugai-Upjohn, Inc.
6133 North River Rd. Ste. 800
Rosemont, IL 60018

00083
Ciba Consumer Pharmaceuticals
Mack WoodBridge II 581 Main St
WoodBridge, NJ 07095
908-602-6600

00346
Ciba Vision Corporation
11460 Johns Creek Parkway
Duluth, GA 30136
404-476-3937

00083
Ciba-Geigy Pharmaceuticals
556 Morris Avenue
Summit, NJ 07901
908-277-5000

00725
Circa Pharmaceuticals, Inc.
33 Ralph Avenue
Copiague, NY 11726-0030
516-842-8383

00659
Circle Pharmaceuticals, Inc.
10377 Hague Road
Indianapolis, IN 46256
317 475 1921

City Chemical Corporation
132 W. 22nd Street
New York, NY 10011
201 653 6000

45802
Clay-Park Labs, Inc.
1700 Bathgate Ave.
Bronx, NY 10457
212-901-2800

00338
Clintec Nutrition
Three Parkway North Suite 500
Deerfield, IL 60015
708-317-2800

Cocensys, Inc.
213 Technology Drive
Irvine, CA 92718
714-453-0131

00126
Colgate-Hoyt
1 Colgate Way
Canton, MA 02021
617-821-2880

Colgate-Palmolive Co.
300 Park Avenue
New York, NY 10022
212-310-2000

Collagen Corporation
2500 Faber Place
Palo Alto, CA 94303
415-856-0200

00837
Columbia Laboratories, Inc.
2665 S. Bayshore Dr. PH 2B
Miami, FL 33133
800-749-1919

21406
Columbia Laboratories, Inc.
4000 Hollywood Blvd.,3rd Fl So
Hollywood, FL 33021-4000
800-749-1919

11509
Combe Incorporated
1101 Westchester Ave.
White Plains, NY 10604
914-694-5454

49281
Connaught Laboratories, Inc.
Route 611, P.O. Box 187
Swiftwater, PA 18370-0187
800-822-2463

11793
Connaught Labs
Route 611, P.O. Box 187
Swiftwater, PA 18370-0187
800-822-2463

00223
Consolidated Midland Corp.
195 E. Main St.
Brewster, NY 10509
914-279-6108

34044
Continental Consumer Products
770 Forest Suite B
Birmingham, MI 48009
800-542-5903

33130
Continental Quest Research
220 W. Carmel Drive
Carmel, IN 46032
800-451-5773

00003
ConvaTec Research/Development
P.O. Box 5254
Princeton, NJ 08543-5254
908-359-9200

00961
Cook-Waite Laboratories, Inc.
90 Park Avenue
New York, NY 10016
212-907-2000

Cooper Biomedical, Inc.
One Technology Court
Malvern, PA 19355
215-219-6300

Cooper Development Company
455 East Middlefield Road
Mountain View, CA 94043
415-969-9030

54027
Cooper Pharmaceuticals
155 Webster Street Suite D
Hanover, MA 02339
617-871-3991

59426
CooperVision
930-A Calle Negocio
San Clemente, CA 92673
714-366-8692

38245
Copley Pharmaceutical, Inc.
25 John Road
Canton, MA 02021
617-821-6111

Cord Labs, See Geneva

Coulter Corporation
11800 SW 147 Ave PO Box 169015
Miami, FL 33116-9015
305-380-3800

01020
Cumberland Packing Corp.
35 Old Ridgefield Rd, POB 7688
Willton, CT 06897
203-762-7227

55326
Curatek (Ltd. Partnership)
1965 Pratt Boulevard
Elk Grove Village, IL 60007
708-806-7680

00161
Cutter Bio., See Miles Inc.

00161
Cutter Medical, See Miles Inc.

54799
Cynacon/OCuSOFT
P.O. Box 429
Richmond, TX 77406-0429
800-233-5469

CytRx
150 Technology Parkway
Norcross, GA 30092
404-368-9500

Cytel Corporation
3525 John Hopkins Court
San Diego, CA 92121
619-552-3000

Cytogen
600 College Road East
Princeton, NJ 08540
609-987-8200

11588
DEP Corporation
2101 East Via Arado
Rancho Dominguez, CA 90220
310-604-0777

55994
Dakryon Pharmaceuticals
2579 S. Loop Suite # 8
Lubbock, TX 79423-1400
806-745-2872

55425
Dal-Med Pharmaceuticals
5701 N. Pine Island Road
Tamarac, Fl 33321
800-543-9151

00591
Danbury Pharmacal
PO Box 990, 12 Stoneleigh Ave.
Carmel, NY 10512
914-225-1700

00689
Daniels Pharmaceuticals, Inc.
2517 25th Avenue North
St. Petersburg, FL 33713-3918
813-323-5151

Darby Pharmaceuticals, Inc.
100 Banks Avenue
Rockville Centre, NY 11570

58869
Dartmouth Pharmaceuticals
19 Whaler's Way
North Dartmouth, MA 02747
508-636-5553

00938
Davis and Geck
One Cyanamid Plaza
Wayne, NJ 07470
201-831-2000

52041
Dayton Laboratories,Inc.
3307 NW 74th Ave.
Miami, FL 33122
305-594-0988

00744
Daywell Laboratories Corp.
78 Unquowa Place
Fairfield, CT 06430
203-255-3154

Degussa Corporation
65 Challenger Road
Ridgefield Park, NJ 07660
201-641-6100

10310
Del Pharmaceuticals, Inc.
565 Broad Hollow Road
Farmingdale, NY 11735
516-293-7070

00316
Del-Ray Laboratory, Inc.
22 20th Avenue N.W.
Birmingham, AL 35215
205-853-8217

48532
Delmont Laboratories, Inc.
P.O. Box 269
Swarthmore, PA 19081
215-543-3365

00295
Denison Laboratories, Inc.
60 Dunnell Ln. PO Box 1305
Pawtucket, RI 02862
401-723-5500

00066
Dermik Laboratories, Inc.
500 Arcola Rd., P.O. Box 1200
Collegeville, PA 19426-0107
215-454-8000

50744
Dermol Pharmaceuticals, Inc.
3807 Roswell Road
Marietta, GA 30062
404-977-7779

17271
Deseret Medical, Inc.
See Becton Dickinson

49502
Dey Laboratories, Inc.
2751 Napa Valley Corporate Dr.
Napa,, CA 94558
707-224-3200

10331
E. E. Dickinson Co.
2 Enterprise Dr.
Shelton, CT 06484
203-929-1197

Discovery Exp. & Devel., Inc.
29949 SR 54 West
Wesley Chapel, FL 33543
813-973-7200

00777
Dista Products Co.
Lilly Corp. Center
Indianapolis, IN 46285
317-276-4000

Dixon & Williams Pharma.
43 Old Wood Road
Bernardsville, NJ 07924
908-766-3558

17236
Dixon-Shane Inc.
256 Geiger Road
Philadelphia, PA 19115
215-673-7770

25358
Donell DerMedex
342 Madison Ave. Suite 1422
New York, NY 10173
212-697-3800

00514
Dow B. Hickam, Inc.
P.O. Box 2006
Sugarland, TX 77487
713-240-1000

13723
Dr. Nordyke Footcare Products
1650 Palma Drive Suite 102
Ventura, CA 93003
805-650-8333

00261
Drug Industries Co.
3237 Hilton Road
Ferndale, MI 48220
313-547-3784

00094
DuPont Merck Pharmaceutical Co
See DuPont Pharm

00056
DuPont Pharm.
Wilmington, DE 19880-0027
800-441-7516

00590
DuPont Pharma
P.O. Box 363
Manati, PR 00674
800-441-7516

00217
Dunhall Pharmaceuticals, Inc.
P.O. Box 100
Gravette, AR 72736
501-787-5232

51479
Dura Pharmaceuticals
5880 Pacific Center Blvd.
San Diego, CA 92121-4202
619-457-2553

51285
Duramed Pharmaceuticals
5040 Lester Road
Cincinnati, OH 45213
513-731-9900

55516
Dyna Pharm, Inc.
P.O. Box 2141
Del Mar, CA 92014-2141
619-792-9523

00095
E.C.R. Pharmaceuticals
3911 Deep Rock Rd.
Richmond, VA 23233
804-527-1950

EM Industries, Inc.
5 Skyline Drive
Hawthorne, NY 10532
914-592-4660

EM Pharmaceuticals
5 Skyline Drive
Hawthorne, NY 10532
914-592-4660

59911
ESI Pharma Inc.
PO Box 41502
Philadelphia, PA 19101
215-688-4400

Eagle Vision, Inc.
6263 Poplar Avenue Ste. 650
Memphis, TN 38119
901-682-9400

Eastman Pharmaceuticals
90 Park Ave.
New York, NY 10016
716-724-4000

Eaton Medical Corporation
2288 Dunn Ave.
Memphis, TN 38114
901-744-8024

19458
Eckerd Drug Company
P.O. Box 4689
Clearwater, FL 34618
813-397-7461

00803
Eclipse
100 Robins Road
Lynchburg, VA 24506
804-846-7161

38130
Econo Med Pharmaceuticals
4305 Sartin Rd.
Burlington, NC 27217-7522
919-226-1091

00485
Edwards Pharmaceuticals Inc.
111 Mulberry St.
Ripley, MS 38663
601-837-8182

55806
Effcon Labs Inc.
P.O. Box 71206
Marietta, GA 30007-1206
800-722-2428

Elan Corporation
1300 Gould Drive
Gainesville, GA 30504
404-534-8239

00641
Elkins-Sinn, Inc.
PO Box 8299
Philadelphia, PA 19101
215-688-4400

57665
Enzon, Inc.
40 Kingsbridge Road
Piscataway, NJ 08854-3998
908-980-4500

00185
Eon Labs Manufacturing, Inc.
227-15 North Conduit Ave.
Laurelton, NY 11413
718-276-8600

58177
Ethex Corporation
10888 Metro Court
St. Louis, MO 63043-2413
314-567-3307

Ethicon Inc.
Route 22 West, PO Box 151
Somerville, NJ 08876-0151
908-218-0707

54686
Ethitek Pharmaceuticals
7701 North Austin
Skokie, IL 60077
708-675-6611

00642
Everett Laboratories, Inc.
71 Glenwood Place
East Orange, NJ 07017
201-674-8455

Evreka
600 Montgomery Street
San Francisco, CA 94111
415-627-2040

Farmacon, Inc.
90 Grove St., Ste. 109
Ridgefield, CT 06877-4118
203-431-9989

99766
Faulding USA
200 Elmora Avenue
Elizabeth, NJ 07207
800-526-6978

00496
Ferndale Laboratories, Inc.
780 W. Eight Mile Road
Ferndale, MI 48220-1218
313-548-0900

55566
Ferring Laboratories, Inc.
400 Rella Blvd., Suite# 201
Suffern, NY 10901
914-368-7900

31795
Fibertone Co.
14851 N. Scottsdale Rd.
Scottsdale, AZ 85254
800-462-7596

00729
Fidelity Halsom
1330 Farr Drive at Stanley
Dayton, OH 45404
800-356-3065

Fidia Pharmaceutical
1401 I Street, N.W.
Washington, DC 20005
202-371-9898

00421
The Fielding Company
94 Weldon Parkway
Maryland Heights, MO 63043
314-567-5462

51687
Fischer Pharmaceuticals Inc.
3 Autry, Suite B
Irvine, CA 92718
408-747-1760

Fiske Industries
339 N. Main St.
New City, NY 10956
914-634-5099

00235
Fisons Consumer Health
P.O. Box 1710
Rochester, NY 14603
716-475-9000

00585
Fisons Corp.
P. O. Box 1710
Rochester, NY 14603
716-475-9000

54323
Flanders Incorporated
P.O. Box 39143
Charleston, SC 29407-9143
803-571-3363

00256
Fleming & Co.
1600 Fenpark Drive
Fenton, MO 63026-2918
314-343-8200

00288
Fluoritab Corp.
P.O. Box 507
Temperance, MI 48182-0507
313-847-3985

00456
Forest Pharmaceutical, Inc.
13622 Lakefront Drive
St. Louis, MO 63045
314-344-8870

00535
Forest Pharmaceutical, Inc.
13622 Lakefront Drive
St. Louis, MO 63045
314-344-8870

00168
E. Fougera and Co.
60 Baylis Road
Melville, NY 11747
516-454-6996

00494
Foy Laboratories
906 Penn Ave.
Wyomissing, PA 19610
215-678-9460

Free Radical Sciences, Inc.
245 First Street
Cambridge, MA 02142
617-374-1200

10432
Freeda Vitamins, Inc.
36 E. 41st St.
New York, NY 10017-6203
212-685-4980

Fuisz Technologies, Ltd.
3810 Concorde Pkwy., Ste. 100
Chantilly, VA 22021
703-803-3260

57317
Fujisawa SmithKline Corp.
3 Parkway North Center
Deerfield, IL 60015-2548
708-317-0600

00713
G & W Laboratories
111 Coolidge Street
South Plainfield, NJ 07080
908-753-2000

Galagen, Incorporated
4001 Lexington Avenue North
Arden Hills, MN 55126-2998
612-481-2105

00299
Galderma Laboratories, Inc.
P.O. Box 331329
Ft. Worth, TX 76163
817-263-2600

57284
Galen Pharma Inc.
See GenDerm

51552
Gallipot Inc.
2020 Silver Bell Road
St. Paul, MN 55122
612-681-9517

00254
Gambro Inc.
1185 Oak Street
Lakewood, CO 80215
800-525-2623

57844
Gate Pharmaceuticals
650 Cathill Road
Sellersville, PA 18960
800-292-4283

00386
Gebauer Company
9410 St. Catherine Ave.
Cleveland, OH 44104
216-271-5252

00028
Geigy Pharmaceuticals
556 Morris Avenue
Summit, NJ 07901
908-277-5000

Gencon
6116 N. Central Expy. 200
Dallas, TX 75206
214-373-4665

52761
GenDerm Corporation
600 Knightsbridge Parkway
Lincolnshire, IL 60069-3657
708-634-7373

50242
Genentech, Inc.
460 Point San Bruno Blvd.
South San Francisco, CA 94080
415-225-1000

50272
General Generics, Inc.
P.O. Box 510
Oxford, MS 38655
601-234-0130

52584
General Inj. & Vac., Inc.
U.S. Highway 52/P.O. Box 9
Bastian, VA 24314-0009
703-688-4121

00918
General Medical Corp.
8741 Landmark Road
Richmond, VA 23261
804-264-7500

00302
Genetco, Inc.
711 Union Parkway
Ronkonkoma, NY 11779
516-585-1000

Genetic Therapy, Inc.
938 Copper Road
Gaithersburg, MD 20878
301-590-2626

00781
Geneva Pharmaceuticals
2599 W. Midway Blvd., POB 469
Broomfield, CO 80038-0469
800-525-8747

35470
Gen-King
80-25 Cornish Ave.
Elmhurst, NY 11373
718-478-8800

58468
Genzyme Corporation
One Kendall Square
Cambridge, MA 02139
617-252-7500

00249
Geriatric Pharmaceutical Corp.
P.O. Box 99
Butler, WI 53007
414-272-2552

59366
Glades Pharmaceuticals
255 Alhambra Circle #1000
Coral Gables, FL 33134
305-567-1319

00173
Glaxo, Inc.
Five Moore Drive
Research Triangle Pk NC 27709
919-248-2100

00516
Glenwood, Inc.
83 N. Summit St.
Tenafly, NJ 07670
201-569-0050

Glycomed, Inc.
860 Atlantic Avenue
Alameda, CA 94501
510-523-5555

00182
Goldline Laboratories, Inc.
1900 W. Commercial Blvd.
Ft. Lauderdale, FL 33309
305-491-4002

74684
Goody's Manufacturing Corp.
436 Salt Street
Winston-Salem, NC 27108
910-723-1831

10481
Gordon Laboratories
6801 Ludlow Street
Upper Darby, PA 19082-1694
215-734-2011

12165
Graham Field
400 Rabro Drive East
Hauppauge, NY 11788
516-582-5900

00152
Gray Pharmaceutical Co.
100 Connecticut Ave.
Norwalk, CT 06856
203-853-0123

51301
Great Southern Laboratories
10863 Rockley Road
Houston, TX 77099
713-530-3077

22840
Greer Laboratories, Inc.
P.O. Box 800
Lenoir, NC 28645-0800
704-754-5327

00327
Guardian Laboratories
230 Marcus Blvd.
Hauppauge, NY 11788
516-273-0900

Gulf Bio-Systems, Inc.
1415 Michigan St.
Adrian, MI 49221-3445
214-386-0442

54396
Gynex Pharmaceuticals, Inc.
1175 Corporate Woods Parkway
Vernon Hills, IL 60061
708-913-1144

54765
GynoPharma Laboratories
50 Division Street
Somerville, NJ 08876
908-725-3100

HDC Corporation
2109 O'Toole Ave.
San Jose, CA 95131
408-954-1909

HEM Research
1617 John F. Kennedy Blvd.
Philadelphia, PA 19103
215-988-0080

HEM Research
1617 John F. Kennedy Blvd.
Philadelphia, PA 19103
215-988-0080

00879
Halsey Drug Company
1827 Pacific Street
Brooklyn, NY 11233
718-467-7500

60322
Hamilton Pharma, Inc.
3401 Hillview Ave.
Palo Alto, CA 94304
415-855-5050

Hannan Ophthalmic Mktg. Services, I
163 Meetinghouse Road
Duxbury, MA 02332

51432
Harber Pharmaceutical Co.
350 Meadowlands Pkwy.
Secaucus, NJ 07094
201-348-3700

00534
Health & Medical Techniques,
See Graham Field

50383
Health Care Products
369 Bayview Ave
Amityville, NY 11701
516-789-8455

51662
Healthfirst Corporation
22316 70th Ave. W. #A
Mountlake Terrace, WA 98043
206-771-5733

59512
Healthline Laboratories, Inc.
835 Potts Avenue
Green Bay, WI 54304
414-497-3322

00586
Heather Drug Company, Inc.
1 Fellowship Road
Cherry Hill, NJ 08003
609-424-3663

Helena Laboratories
P.O. Box 752
Beaumont, TX 77704-0752
409-842-3714

Hemacare Corporation
4954 Van Nuys Boulevard
Sherman Oaks, CA 91403
818-986-3883

48017
Hermal Pharmaceutical Labs
163 Delaware Ave
Delmar, NY 12054
518-475-0175

28105
Hill Dermaceuticals, Inc.
P.O. Box 149283
Orlando, FL 32814-9283
407-896-8280

17808
Himmel Pharmaceuticals Inc.
P.O. Box 5479
Lake Worth, FL 33466 5479
407-585-0070

50673
Hirsch Industries, Inc
4912 West Broad Street
Richmond, VA 23230-0964
804-355-4500

Hiscia
CH-4144, Arlesheim Kirshweg
Switzerland
4106172-2323

00039
Hoechst-Roussel Pharm., Inc.
Route 202-206 P.O. Box 2500
Somerville, NJ 08876-1258
908-231-2000

58573
Hogil Pharmaceutical Corp.
1 Byram Brook Place
Armonk, NY 10504
914-273-9666

47992
Holles Laboratories, Inc.
30 Forest Notch
Cohasset, MA 02025-1198
617-383-0741

00118
Hollister-Stier
P.O. Box 3145
Spokane, WA 99220-3153
509-489-5656

59229
Horus Therapeutics Inc.
2320 Brighton-Henrietta Town
Rochester, NY 14623
716-292-4820

58407
Huckaby Pharmacal, Inc.
104 E. Main St.
LaGrange, KY 40031
502-222-4700

25077
The Hudson Corporation
90 Orville Drive
Bohemia, NY 11716
516-567-9500

00395
Humco Holding Group, Inc.
P.O. Box 2550
Texarkana, TX 75504
903-793-3174

Hybritech
P.O. Box 269006
San Diego, CA 92196-9006
619 455 6700

00011
Hynson, Westcott & Dunning
PO Box 243, 250 Schilling Cir
Cockeysville, MD 21030
410-771-0100

00314
Hyrex Pharmaceuticals
P.O. Box 18385
Memphis, TN 38181-0385
901-794-9050

51244
I.C.P. Pharmaceuticals
P.O. Box 294
Cudahy, WI 53110
414-521-4647

00548
I.M.S. Ltd.
1886 Santa Anita Ave.
South El Monte, CA 91733
818-913-4660

00163
ICN Pharmaceuticals, Inc.
3300 Hyland Avenue
Costa Mesa, CA 92626
714-545-0100

00187
ICN Pharmaceuticals, Inc.
3300 Hyland Avenue
Costa Mesa, CA 92626
714-545-0100

IDEC Pharmaceuticals
11099 N. Torrey Pines Rd. #160
La Jolla, CA 92037
619-458-0600

11808
ION Laboratories, Inc.
7431 Pebble Drive
Ft. Worth, TX 76118
817-589-7257

IOP Incorporated
3100 Airway Avenue Suite 106
Costa Mesa, CA 92626
714-549-1185

54921
IPR Pharmaceuticals, Inc.
P.O.Box 6000
Carolina, PR 00984
800-477-6385

Iatric Corporation
2330 S. Industrial Park Drive
Tempe, AZ 85282-1893
602-966-7248

Immucell Corporation
56 Evergreen Dr.
Portland, ME 04103
207-878-2770

00205
Immunex Corporation

58406
Immunex Corporation
51 University St.
Seattle, WA 98101
206-587-0430

Immuno Clinical Research Corp.
155 East 56th Street
New York, NY 10022
212-759-3521

54129
Immuno U.S., Inc.
1200 Parkdale Rd.
Rochester, MI 48307-1744
313-652-7872

Immunobiology Research Inst.
Route ££ East, P.O. Box 000
Annandale, NJ 08801-0999
908-730-1700

ImmunoGen
148 Sidney Street
Cambridge, MA 02139
617-661-9312

Immunomedics
300 American Road
Morris Plains, NJ 07950
201-605-8200

Immunomedics, Inc.
150 Mt. Bethel Road
Warren, NJ 07059

Immunotherapeutics
3505 Riverview Circle
Morehead, MN 56560
701-232-9575

Imreg
144 Elk Place, Suite 1400
New Orleans, LA 70112
504-523-2875

41701
Inagra
4366 Glendale-Milford Road
Cincinnati, OH 45242
513-554-6200

Infusaid, Inc.
1400 Providence Highway
Norwood, MA 02062
617-769-8330

18686
InnoVisions, Inc.
6065 Frantz Rd., Ste. 202
Dublin, OH 43017
614-766-5477

Interchem Corporation
120 Rt. 17 North Ste. 115
Paramus, NJ 07652

Interfalk U.S. Inc.
25 Margaret
Plattsburgh, NY 12901

Interferon Sciences
783 Jersey Avenue
New Brunswick, NJ 08901
908-249-3250

11584
International Ethical Labs
Reparto Metropolitano
Rio Piedras, PR 00921
809-765-3510

00665
International Laboratories
901 Sawyer Road
Marietta, GA 30062
404-578-5583

Interneuron Pharmaceuticals
1 Ledgemont Ctr. 99 Hayden Ave
Lexington, MA 02173
617-861-8444

Interpro
P.O. Box 1823
Haverhill, MA 01831
508-373-2438

00814
Interstate Drug Exchange
1500 New Horizons Blvd.
Amityville, NY 11701-1130
516-957-8300

Intramed
102 Tremont Way
Augusta, GA 30907

52189
Invamed Incorporated
12 Dwight Place
Fairfield, NJ 07006
201-575-3303

00258
Inwood Laboratories
300 Prospect Street
Inwood, NY 11696
516-371-1155

00058
Iolab Pharmaceuticals
500 Iolab Drive
Claremont, CA 91711
909-624-2020

50914
Iso Tex Diagnostics, Inc.
P.O. Box 909
Friendswood, TX 77546
713-482-1231

00252
JMI-Canton Pharmaceuticals Inc
119 Schroyer Ave. S.W.
Canton, OH 44702
216-456-2873

49938
Jacobus Pharmaceutical Co.
37 Cleveland Lane
Princeton, NJ 08540
609-921-7447

50458
Janssen Pharmaceutical, Inc.
P.O. Box 200
Titusville, NJ 08560-0200
609-730-2000

00137
Johnson & Johnson
Grandview Rd.
Skillman, NJ 08558-9418
908-524-0400

56091
Johnson & Johnson Medical Inc.
P.O. Box 130
Arlington, TX 76004-0130
800-433-5009

52604
Jones Medical Industries
P.O. Box 46903
St. Louis, MO 63146-6903
314-432-7557

KLI Corp
1119 Third Avenue S.W.
Carmel, IN 46032
317-846-7452

00601
KabiVitrum, Inc.
160 Industrial Drive
Franklin,, OH 45005
800-526-5224

00588
Keene Pharmaceuticals Inc.
P.O. Box 7
Keene, TX 76059-0007
817-645-8083

28851
Kendall Health Care Products
15 Hampshire St
Mansfield, MA 02048
508-261-8000

00085
Key Pharmaceuticals
Galloping Hill Road
Kenilworth, NJ 07033
908-298-4000

55299
Kingswood Laboratories, Inc.
10375 Hague Rd.
Indianapolis, IN 46256
317-849-9513

58223
Kirkman Sales Co., Inc.
P.O. Box 1009
Wilsonville, OR 97070-1009
503-694-1600

00098
Kirkman Sales Company
P.O. Box 1009
Wilsonville, OR 97070
503-694-1600

31600
Kiwi Brands, Inc.
447 Old Swede Rd.
Douglassville, PA 19518-1239
215-385-9322

00044
Knoll Pharmaceuticals
30 N. Jefferson Rd.
Whippany, NJ 07981
201-887-8300

00224
Konsyl Pharmaceuticals
4200 South Hulen, Suite 513
Ft. Worth, TX 76109
817-763-8011

55505
Kramer Laboratories, Inc.
8778 S.W. 8th Street
Miami, FL 33174-9990
305-223-1287

LTR Pharmaceuticals, Inc.
145 Sakonnet Blvd.
Narragansett, RI 02882

41383
Lactaid Inc.
P.O. Box 111
Pleasantville, NJ 08232

59081
Lafayette Pharmaceuticals Inc.
P.O. Box 4499
Lafayette, IN 47903-4499
317-447-3129

00527
The Lannett Co., Inc.
9000 State Road
Philadelphia, PA 19136
215-333-9000

00277
Laser, Inc.
P.O. Box 905, 2000 N.Main St.
Crown Point, IN 46307
219-663-1165

10651
Lavoptik Co., Inc.
661 Woctorn Avo. N.
St. Paul, MN 55103
612-489-1351

00005
Lederle Laboratories
North Middletown Road
Pearl River, NY 10965-1299
914-732-5000

53124
Lederle-Praxis Biologicals
North Middletown Road
Pearl River, NY 10965
716-272-7000

23558
Lee Pharmaceuticals
1444 Santa Anita Blvd.
South Elmonte, CA 91733
800-950-5337

25332
Legere Pharmaceuticals, Inc.
7326 E. Evans Rd.
Scottsdale, AZ 85260
602-991-4033

19200
Lehn & Fink
225 Summit Avenue
Montvale, NJ 07645
201-573-5700

Leiner Health Products
1845 W. 205th Street
Torrance, CA 90501
310-328-9610

Leiras Pharmaceuticals, Inc.
2345 Waukegan Road, Ste N-135
Bonnockburn, IL 60015
none

00093
Lemmon Company
650 Cathill Road
Sellersville, PA 18960
215-256-8400

Lenti-Chemico Pharmaceuticals
500 Frank W. Burr Blvd.
Teaneck, NJ 07666
201-836-1196

00454
Lexis Laboratories
P.O. Box 202887
Austin, TX 78720
512-328-8484

Life's Finest
P.O. Box 30
Clearwater, FL 33518-5610
813-536-7650

Ligand Pharmaceuticals, Inc.
9393 Towne Centre Drive
San Diego, CA 92121
619-535-3900

00002
Eli Lilly and Co.
Lilly Corp. Center
Indianapolis, IN 46285
317-276-2000

Lincoln Diagnostics
P.O. Box 1128
Decatur, IL 62525
217-877-2531

Liposome Company
One Research Way
Princeton, NJ 08540
609-452-7060

Loma Linda Foods,
See Nutricia, Inc.

00273
Lorvic Corporation
8810 Frost Ave.
St. Louis, MO 63134-1095
011 601 7111

00374
Lyne Laboratories
260 Tosca Drive
Stoughton, MA 02072
617-344-4676

00469
Lyphomed
3 Parkway North
Deerfield, IL 60015-2548
708-317-8800

58607
ME Pharmaceuticals, Inc.
2800 Southeast Parkway
Richmond, IN 47375
800-637-4276

58063
MGI Pharma, Inc.
9900 Bren Road East Ste. 300E
Minneapolis, MN 55343-9667
800-562-5580

00466
Macsil, Inc.
P.O. Box 29276
Philadelphia, PA 19125-0976
215-739-7300

00904
Major Pharmaceuticals
1640 W. Fulton
Chicago, IL 60612
312-666-9600

43797
Mallard Medical Products
645 Hembree Pkwy. Ste. D
Roswell, GA 30076
404-410-0888

00019
Mallinckrodt Medical, Inc.
675 McDonnell Blvd., POB 5840
St. Louis, MO 63134
314-895-2000

10706
Manne Company
P.O. Box 825
Johns Island, SC 29457
800-517-0228

00088
Marion Merrell Dow, Inc.

00068
Marion Merrell Dow, Inc.
P. O. Box 9627
Kansas City, MO 64134
800-362-7466

Marlin Industries
P.O. Box 560
Grover City, CA 93483-0560
805-473-2743

12939
Marlop Pharmaceuticals, Inc.
5704 Mosholu Ave., P.O. Box536
Bronx, NY 10471
800-345-7192

10712
Marlyn Company, Inc.
14851 N. Scottsdale Road
Scottsdale, AZ 85254
800-462-7596

00682
Marnel Pharmaceuticals, Inc.
206 Luke Dr.
Lafayette, LA 70506
318-232-1396

00209
Marsam Pharmaceuticals Inc.
P.O. Box 1022
Cherry Hill, NJ 08034
609-424-5600

52555
Martec Pharmaceutical, Inc.
P.O. Box 33510
Kansas City, MO 64120-3510
816-241-4144

11845
Mason Distributors, Inc.
5105 N.W. 159th Street
Hialeah, FL 33014-6370
305-624-5557

12758
Mason Pharmaceuticals, Inc.
4425 Jamboree, Suite 250
Newport Beach, CA 92660
714-851-6860

14362
Mass. Public Health Bio. Lab.
305 South Street
Jamaica Plains, MA 02130
617-522-3700

Matrix Laboratories
1430 O'Brian Drive, Suite G
Menlo Park, CA 94025
415-326-6100

00259
Mayrand, Inc.
915 Bridge St.
Winston-Salem, NC 27101
919-725-2019

00264
McGaw, Inc.
ASC2 P.O. Box 19791
Irvine, CA 92713-9791
714-660-2000

11089
McGregor Pharmaceuticals, Inc.
8420 Ulmenton Road #305
Largo, FL 34641
813-530-4361

49072
McGuff Company, Inc.
3617 W. MacArthur Blvd. #507
Santa Ana, CA 92704
800-854-7220

50185
McHenry Laboratories Inc.
118 N. Wells-Lee Bldg.
Edna,, TX 77957
512-782-5438

00045
McNeil Consumer Products Co.
Mail Stop 278, Camp Hill Rd.
Ft. Washington, PA 19034-2292
215-233-7000

00045
McNeil Pharmaceutical
P.O.Box 300
Raritan, NJ 08869-0602
800-542-5365

00087
Mead Johnson Laboratories
P.O. Box 4500
Princeton, NJ 08543-4500
609-897-2000

00087
Mead Johnson Nutritionals
2404 Pennsylvania Street
Evansville, IN 47721
812-426-6000

Medac GmbH c/o Princeton Reg. Assoc
65 South Main Street
Pennington, NJ 08534
609-951-9596

Medarex
12 Commerce Avenue
West Lebanon, NH 03784
603-298-8456

MedChem
232 W. Cummings Park
Woburn, MA 01801
617 938 9328

Medclone, Inc.
2435 Military Avenue
Los Angeles, CA 90064

11940
Medco Lab, Inc.
P.O. Box 864
Sioux City, IA 51102-0864
712-255-8770

Medco Research
8455 Beverly Blvd.
Los Angeles, CA 90048
213-966-4148

44081
Med-Corp
5001 Spring Valley Road
Dallas, TX 75244-3910
214-385-7214

45565
Med-Derm Pharmaceuticals
P.O. Box 5193
Kingsport, TN 37663
615-477-3991

Medea Research Laboratories
200 Wilson Street
Port Jefferson, NY 11776
516-331-7718

Medi Aid Corporation
8250 S. Akron Street Suite 205
Englewood, CO 80155
303-790-1655

17156
Medi-Physics, Inc.
2636 So. Clearbrook Dr.
Arlington Heights, Il 60005
800-322-6334

59010
Medi-Plex Pharm. Inc.
3714 Alliance Dr. Ste. 302
Greensboro, NC 27407
919-299-1026

00576
Medical Products Panamericana
647 West Flagler Street
Miami, FL 33130
305-545-6524

Medical Technology Corporation
71 Veronica Avenue, PO Box 218
Somerset, NJ 08875-0218
908-246-3366

99207
Medicis Dermatologicals, Inc.
100 East 42nd St., 15th Floor
New York, NY 10017-5613
212-599-2000

Medimmune, Inc.
35 West Watkins Mill Road
Gaithersburg, MD 20878
301-417-0033

Medimorphics
245 East 6th Street
St. Paul, MN 55101
612-224-2800

00348
Medtech Laboratories, Inc.
3510 N. Lake Creek, POB 1108
Jackson, WY 83011-1108
307-733-1680

75137
Medtech Laboratories, Inc.
3510 N. Lake Creek, POB 1108
Jackson, Wy 83011-1108
800-433-4908

58281
Medtronic
800 53rd Ave. N.E.
Minneapolis, Mn 55421
612-572-5000

87900
Menley & James Labs, Inc.
100 Tournament Drive
Horsham, PA 19044
215-441-6500

22200
Mennen Company
Hanover Avenue
Morristown, NJ 07962-1928
201-631-9000

10742
Mentholatum Co., Inc.
1360 Niagara St.
Buffalo, NY 14213
716-882-7660

00006
Merck & Co.
WP 38M-2
West Point, PA 19486
215-652-5000

16837
J & J Merck Consumer Pharm.
Camp Hill Road
Ft. Washington, PA 19034
215-233-7000

Merck Sharpe & Dohme
See Merck & Co.

00394
Mericon Industries, Inc.
8819 N. Pioneer Road
Peoria, IL 61615
309-693-2150

50361
Merieux Institute, Inc.
See Connaught

30727
Merit Pharmaceuticals
2611 San Fernando Road
Los Angeles, CA 90065
213-227-4831

Michigan Department of Health
PO Box 30035
Lansing, MI 48909
517-335-8000

46672
Mikart, Inc.
2090 Marietta Blvd., N.W.
Atlanta, GA 30318
404-351-4510

32954
MiLance Laboratories, Inc.
P.O. Box 39
Maplewood, NJ 07040

52836
Milance Laboratories, Inc.
P.O. Box 368
Millington, NJ 07946
908-580-1591

00026
Miles Inc.
400 Morgan Lane
West Haven, CT 06516
203-937-2000

00193
Miles Inc.
1127 Myrtle St. P.O. Box 3100
Elkhart, IN 46514
219-264-8487

16500
Miles, Inc.
1127 Myrtle Street, POB 340
Elkhart, IN 46515-0340
219-264-8111

00192
Miles, Inc.
1127 Myrtle Street, POB 340
Elkhart, IN 46515-0340
219-264-8111

00396
Milex Products, Inc.
5915 Northwest Highway
Chicago, IL 60631-1032
312-631-6484

17204
Miller Pharmacal Group, Inc.
245 W. Roosevelt Road
West Chicago, IL 60185-0279
708-231-3632

53118
Millgood Laboratories, Inc.
250 D Arizona Ave., POB 170159
Atlanta, GA 30317
404-377-6538

00276
Misemer Pharmaceuticals, Inc.
4553 S. Campbell
Springfield, MO 65810-5918
417-881-0660

00178
Mission Pharmacal Company
P.O. Box 1676
San Antonio, TX 78296-1676
210-650-3273

Monoclonal Antibodies
See Quidel Corporation

Montgomery Medical Ventures
600 Montgomery St.
San Francisco, CA 94111

00839
H.L. Moore Drug Exchange, Inc.
389 John Downey Dr.
New Britain, CT 06050
203-826-3600

Morton Salt
100N. Riverside Plaza, 27th Fl
Chicago, IL 60606-1597
312-807-2000

Murdock Pharmaceuticals, Inc.
1400 Mountain Springs Parkway
Springvale, UT 84663
801-489-1505

00451
Muro Pharmaceutical, Inc.
890 East Street
Tewksbury, MA 01876-9987
508-851-5981

00150
Murray Drug Corporation
415 S. 4th Street
Murray, KY 42071
502-753-6654

53489
Mutual Pharmaceutical Co.,Inc.
1100 Orthodox Street
Philadelphia, PA 19124
215-288-6500

00378
Mylan Pharmaceuticals
P.O. Box 4310
Morgantown, WV 26505
304-599-2595

72559
NCI Medical Foods
5801 Ayala Avenue
Irwindale, CA 91706
818-812-3393

23317
NMC Laboratories
70-36 83rd Street
Glendale, NY 11385
718-326-1500

NPDC-AS101, Inc.
783 Jersey Avenue
New Brunswick, NJ 08901
716-636-9096

05745
Nastech Pharmaceutical Co.,Inc
1 Shields Dr., Route 2, Box 30
Bennington, VT 05201
800-526-6698

National Patent Medical
P.O. Box 419
Dayville, CT 06241
800-243-1172

74312
Nature's Bounty, Inc.
105 Orville Drive
Bohemia, NY 11716
516-567-9500

Neorx Corporation
410 West Harrison
Seattle, WA 98119
206-281-7001

00487
Nephron Pharmaceuticals Corp.
4121 SW 34th Street
Orlando, FL 32811-6458
407-246-1389

NeuroGenesis/Matrix Tech. Inc.
100 Louisiana Suite 600
Houston, TX 77002
800-345-8912

10812
Neutrogena Corporation
5760 W. 96th Street
Los Angeles, CA 90045
310-642-1150

70501
Neutrogena Corporation
5760 W. 96th St.
Los Angeles, CA 90045-5595
310-642-1150

Neutron Technology Corporation
877 Main Street
Boise, ID 83702
208-345-3460

New World Trading Corp.
P.O. Box 952
DeBary, FL 32713
407-668-7520

Newport Pharmaceuticals
140 Columbia
Laguna Hills, CA 92656-1459
714-362-1330

59016
Niche Pharmaceuticals, Inc.
200 N. Oak St. P.O. Box 449
Roanoke, TX 76262
807-491-2770

12934
Nion Corporation
15501 First Street
Irwindale, CA 91706
818-969-1932

51801
Nomax, Inc.
40 North Rock Hill Road
St. Louis, MO 63119
314-961-2500

10118
Norstar Consumer Products, Inc
206 Pegasus Avenue
Northvale, NJ 07647
201-784-8155

North American Biologicals, Inc.
16500 NW 15th Avenue
Miami, FL 33169
305-625-5303

50732
H.N. Norton, Co.
9205 Slack Road
Shreveport, LA 71106
318-688-4800

Nova Pharmaceutical
6200 Freeport Centre
Baltimore, MD 21224
301-558-7000

Novaferon Labs
2658 Patton Road
Roseville, MN 55713

00169
Novo Nordisk
100 Overlook Center, Ste. 200
Princeton,, NJ 08540
800-727-6500

00003
Novo/Nordisk Pharm., Inc.
100 Overlook Center, Ste. 200
Princeton, NJ 08540
800-727-0500

50445
Novo/Nordisk Pharm., Inc.
100 Overlook Center, Ste 200
Princeton, NJ 08540
800 727 6500

00362
Novocol Chemical Mfr. Co.
P.O. Box 11926
Wilmington, DE 19850
302-328-1102

55953
Novopharm USA Inc.
165 E. Commerce, Suite 100/200
Schaumburg, IL 60173-5326
708-882-4200

55499
Numark Laboratories, Inc.
P.O. Box 6321
Edison, NJ 08818
800-338-8079

34999
Nutraloric
350 N. Lantana, Unit G1
Camarillo, CA 93010
805-388-2811

41470
Nutricia Inc.
11503 Pierce Street
Riverside, CA 92505
714-687-7800

51081
Nutripharm Laboratories, Inc.
8 Bartles Corner Road Ste. 101
Flemington, NJ 08822
908-806-8954

O.P.R. Development, LP
1501 Wakarusa Drive
Lawrence, KS 66047

51660
OHM Laboratories, Inc.
PO Box 279
Franklin Park, NJ 08823
908-297-3030

ONY
1576 Sweet Home Road
Amherst, NY 14228
716-636-9096

10797
Oakhurst Company
3000 Hempstead Turnpike
Levittown, NY 11756
516-731-5380

Obetrol Pharmaceuticals
See Rexar

55515
Oclassen Pharmaceuticals, Inc.
100 Pelican Way
San Rafael, CA 94901
415-258-4500

51944
Ocumed, Inc.
119 Harrison Avenue
Roseland, NJ 07068
201-226-2330

12622
Olin Corporation
120 Long Ridge Road
Stamford, CT 06904-1355
203-356-2000

Omex International Inc.
6001 Savoy Ste. 110
Houston, TX 77036
713-975-8325

Oncotherapeutics, Inc.
1002 EastPark Blvd.
Cranbury, NJ 08512
609-655-5300

Ophidian Pharmaceuticals, Inc.
2800 South Fish Hatchery Road
Madison, WI 537 I I
608-271-0878

Optikem International, Inc.
2172 S. Jason Street
Denver, CO 80223
303-936-1137

50520
Optimox Corporation
2720 Monterey, Suite 406
Torrance, CA 90503
310-618-9370

52238
Optopics Laboratories, Corp.
32 Main Street, P.O. Box 210
Fairton, NJ 08320-0210

00041
Oral-B Laboratories, Inc.
1 Lagoon Drive
Redwood City, CA 94065
415-961-8130

Organon Teknika Corp.
100 Akzo Avenue
Durham, NC 27704
919-620-2000

00052
Organon, Inc.
375 Mt. Pleasant Ave.
West Orange, NJ 07052
201-325-4500

Orphan Medical
13911 Ridgedale Drive
Minnetonka, MN 55305
612-541-1868

59676
Ortho Biotech Inc.
700 US Highway 202 POB 670
Raritan, NJ 08869-0670
800-325-7504

00062
Ortho Dermatologic
Route 202, P.O. Box 300
Raritan, NJ 08869-0602
908-218-6000

00062
Ortho Diagnostic Systems
Route 202
Raritan, NJ 08869
908-218-1300

00062
Ortho Pharmaceutical Corp.
Route 202, P.O. Box 600
Raritan, NJ 08869
908-218-6000

10244
Otis Clapp & Son, Inc.
115 Shawmut Road
Canton, MA 02021-9160
617-821-5400

59148
Otsuka America Pharmctl.,Inc.
2440 Research Blvd.
Rockville, MD 98101
206-682-5300

00574
Paddock Laboratories
3101 Louisiana Ave. North
Minneapolis, MN 55427
612-546-4676

00377
Pal-Pak, Inc.
1201 Liberty Street, POB 299
Allentown, PA 18105
215-433-7579

53159
Palisades Pharmaceuticals Inc.
64 N. Summit St.
Tenafly, NJ 07670
201-569-8502

49884
Par Pharmaceuticals
One Ram Ridge Road
Spring Valley, NY 10977
914-425-7100

00071
Parke-Davis
201 Tabor Road
Morris Plains, NJ 07950

00071
Parke-Davis Consumer Products
201 Tabor Road
Morris Plains, NJ 07950
201-540-2000

00349
Parmed Pharmaceuticals, Inc.
4220 Hyde Park Blvd.
Niagara Falls, NY 14305
716-284-5666

50930
Parnell Pharmaceuticals, Inc.
Larkspur Landing Circle
Larkspur, CA 94939
415-461-4900

10865
Parthenon Company, Inc.
3311 W. 2400 South
Salt Lake City, UT 84119
801-972-5184

00418
Pasadena Research Labs
P.O. Box 5136
San Clemente, CA 92674-5136
714-492-4030

Pediatric Pharmaceuticals
718 Bradford Avenue
Westfield, NJ 07090
908-225-0989

00884
Pedinol Pharmacal, Inc.
30 Banfi Plaza North
Farmingdale, NY 11735
516-293-9500

10974
Pegasus Medical, Inc.
1 Technology Dr Bldg 1C Ste525
Irvine, CA 92718-2325
714-753-9055

00832
Pennex Pharmaceutical Inc.
6451 West Main Street
Morton Grove, IL 60053
708-967-5600

00426
Pennex Pharmaceuticals
6451 Main Street
Morton Grove, IL 60053
708-967-5617

Permeable Technologies, Inc.
712 Ginesi Drive
Morganville, NJ 07751
908-972-8585

00096
Person and Covey, Inc.
616 Allen Ave, PO Box 25018
Glendale, CA 91221-5018
818-240-1030

00927
Pfeiffer Company
43-45 N. Washington, POB 100
Wilkes Barre, PA 18701
717-826-9000

00995
Pfipharmecs, see Pfizer

71300
Pfizer Inc. Cons. Hlthcr. Div.
235 E. 42nd Street
New York, NY 10017
212-573-3131

00069 00663
Pfizer Laboratories
235 E. 42nd Street
New York, NY 10017-5755
212-573-2422

58197
Pharmacel Laboratory Inc.
203 South Coolidge Avenue
Tampa, FL 33609
813-289-2750

21659
Pharmacetical Labs, Inc.
1229 W. Corporate Dr.
Arlington, TX 76006
817-633-1461

00121
Pharmaceutical Associates, Inc
P.O. Box 128
Conestee, SC 29636
803-277-7282

00832
Pharmaceutical Basics, Inc.
301 South Cheroke St.
Denver, CO 80223
303-733-7207

51655
Pharmaceutical Corporation
12348 Hancock Street
Carmel, IN 46032
317-573-8000

45334
Pharmaceutical Specialties Inc
P.O. Box 729
Rochester, MN 55903-0729
507-288-8500

Pharmachemie U.S.A., Incorp.
P.O.Box 145
Oradell, NJ 07049
201-265-1942

00016
Pharmacia Inc.
PO box 16529
Columbus, OH 43216-6529
614-764-8100

PharmaControl
661 Palisade Ave.,P.O. Box 931
Englewood Cliffs, NJ 07632
201-567-9004

00462
Pharmaderm Div. of Altana Inc.
See E. Fougera

55422
Pharmakon Laboratorless, Inc.
6050 Jet Port Industrial Blvd.
Tampa, FL 33634
813-886-3216

Pharmaquest Corporation
4470 Redwood Highway St. 101
San Rafael, CA 94903
415-491-6460

Pharmatec
County Rd 2054, P.O. Box 730
Alachua, FL 32615
904-462-1210

39822
Pharma Tek, Inc.
P.O. Box 1920
Huntington, NY 11743-0568
516-757-5522

Pharmavene, Inc.
35 West Watkins Mill Road
Gaithersburg, MD 20878
301-417-0033

Pharmedic Company
417 Harvester Court
Wheeling, IL 60090
708-215-6603

00813
Pharmics, Incorporated
P.O. Box 27554
Salt Lake City, UT 84127
801-972-4138

00077
Pilkington Barnes Hind
810 Kifer Road
Sunnyvale, CA 94086-5200
619-277-9873

60104
Pioneer Pharmaceuticals, Inc.
209 40th Street
Irvington, NJ 07111
201-372-6200

Plexus Pharmaceuticals, Inc.
8122 Datapoint Dr., Ste. 600
San Antonio, TX 78229

41100
Plough, Inc.
110 Allen Rd
Liberty Corner, NJ 07938
908-604-1995

00998
PolyMedica Industries
2 Constitution Way
Woburn, MA 01801
617-933-2020

47144
Polymer Technology Corporation
100 Research Drive
Wilmington, MA 01887
800-343-1445

Polymer Technology Intern'l
1595 NW Gilman Blvd., Suite 17
Issaquah, WA 98027
206-391-2650

55688
Porton Product Limited
30401 Agoura Road
Agoura Hills, CA 91301
818-879-2200

59012
Pratt Pharmaceuticals
235 E. 42nd Street
New York, NY 10017-5755
212-573-2323

Precision-Cosmet
500 Iolab Drive
Claremont, CA 91711
800-423-1871

Premier Inc.
Greenwich Office Park One
Greenwich, CT 06831
203-622-5800

00684
Primedics Laboratories
15524 S. Broadway
Gardenia, CA 90248
213-770-3005

00003
Princeton Pharm. Products
P.O. Box 4000
New Brunswick, NJ 08543-4000
609-252-4000

00149
Procter & Gamble Pharm.
P.O. Box 191
Norwich, NY 13815-0191
607-335-2111

37000
The Procter and Gamble Co.
P.O. Box 5544
Cincinnati, OH 45202
513-983-1100

Professional Supplies, Inc.
See SoftRinse Corporation

00034
Purdue Frederick Co.
100 Connecticut Ave.
Norwalk, CT 06856
203-853-0123

00228
Purepac Pharmaceutical Co.
200 Elmora Ave.
Elizabeth, NJ 07207
908-527-9100

QLT Phototherapeutics, Inc.
401 North Middletown Road
Pearl River, NY 10965

51309
Quad Pharmaceuticals, Inc.
6340 LaPas Trail
Indianapolis, IN, 46268
317-299-6611

00603
Qualitest Products, Inc.
1231 Jordan Road
Huntsville, AL 35811
205-859-4011

52446
Qualitest Products, Inc.
1236 Jordan Road
Huntsville, AL 35811
205-859-4011

12225
Quality Formulations, Inc.
P.O. Box 827
Zachary, LA 70791-0827
504-654-6880

52273
Quantum Pharmics, Ltd.
26 Edison Street
Amityville, NY 11701
516-842-4200

Quidel Corporation
10165 McKellar Court
San Diego, CA 92121
619-552-1100

54391
R & D Laboratories, Inc.
4204 Glencoe Avenue
Marina Del Rey, CA 90292-5612
310-305-8053

R & R Registrations
P.O. Box 262079
San Diega, CA 92196-2069
619-586-0751

54807
R.I.D. Inc.
525 Mednik Avenue
Los Angeles, CA 90022
213-268-0635

RH Pharmaceuticals, Inc.
104 Chancellor Matheson Rd.
Winnipeg,, R3T 2N2
204-989-6850

00196
Rachelle Laboratories, Inc.
P.O. Box 187
Culver, IN 46511
219-842-3305

30103
Randob Laboratories, Ltd.
P.O. Box 440
Cornwall, NY 12518
914-699-3131

00686
Raway Pharmacal, Inc.
15 Granit Road
Accord, NY 12404-0047
914-626-8133

12496
Reckitt & Colman
1901 Huguenot Rd. Ste. 110
Richmond, VA 23235
804-379-1090

10952
Recsei Laboratories
330 S. Kellogg Bldg. M
Goleta, CA 93117-3875
805-964-2912

53506
Redi-Med, Inc.
801-N N Blacklawn Rd. POB 1407
Conyers, GA 30207
404-929-0961

48028
Redi-Products Labs, Inc.
P.O. Box 126
Prichard, WV 25555
304-486-5656

00021
Reed & Carnrick
257 Cornelison Ave.
Jersey City, NJ 07302
908-981-0070

10956
Reese Chemical Co.
10617 Frank Ave.
Cleveland, OH 44106
216-231-6441

00102
Regal Laboratories
1925 Enterprise Parkway
Twinsburg, OH 44087
216-425-9811

Regeneron Pharmaceuticals, Inc
777 Old Saw Mill River Road
Tarrytown, NY 10591-6707
914-347-7000

10960
Republic Drug Company
P.O. Box 186
Buffalo, NY 14216
716-874-5060

10961
Requa, Inc.
1 Seneca Place, P.O. Box 4008
Greenwich, CT 06830
203-869-2445

00433
Research Industries Corp.
6864 S. 300 West
Midvale, UT 84047
801-562-0200

Research Triangle Pharm.
4364 So. Alston Ave.
Durham, NC 27713
919-544-4029

60575
Respa Pharmaceuticals, Inc.
P.O. Box 88222
Carol Stream, IL 60188
708-462-9986

00122
Rexall Group
4031 N.E. 12th Terrace
Ft. Lauderdale, FL 33334
800-255-7399

00478
Rexar Pharmacal Corp.
396 Rockaway Ave.,P.O. Box 397
Valley Stream, NY 11582
516-561-7662

00477
Rexar Pharmaceuticals
396 Rockaway Ave, P.O. Box 397
Valley Stream, NY 11582
516-561-7662

00195
Rhone-Poulenc Rorer
500 Virginia Drive
Ft. Washington, PA 19034
215-628-6000

00067, 00075
Rhone-Poulenc Rorer Pharm Inc.
500 Arcola Rd/P.O. Box 1200
Collegeville, PA 19426-0107
215-454-8000

Ribi Immunochem Research, Inc.
553 Old Corvallis Road
Hamilton, MT 59840-3131
406-363-6214

76660
Richardson-Vicks, Inc.
PO Box 599
Cincinnati, OH 45202
513-983-1100

12071
Richie Pharmacal Co., Inc.
197 State Avenue P.O. Box 460
Glasgow, KY 42141
800-626-0250

00115
Richlyn Laboratories, Inc.
Castor & Kensington Avenues
Philadelphia, PA 19124
215-289-2220

59441
Roberts Hauck Pharmaceuticals
6 Industrial Way West
Eatontown, NJ 07724
800-828-2088

54092
Roberts Pharmaceuticals
6 Industrial Way West
Eatontown, NJ 07724
908-389-1182

00031
A. H. Robins Company, Inc.
P.O. Box 8299
Philadelphia, PA 19101-1245
215-688-4400

00031
A.H. Robins Cons. Prod. Div.
Five Giralda Farms
Madison, NJ 07940-0871
201-660-5500

00004
Roche Dermatologics Prod.
340 Kingsland Streeet
Nutley, NJ 07110-1199
800-526-6367

00004
Roche Laboratories
340 Kingsland Street
Nutley, NJ 07110-1199
800-526-6367

00140
Roche Products, Inc.
340 Kingsland Street
Nutley, NJ 07110-1199
800-526-6367

00049
J.B. Roerig Division
235 E. 42nd St.
New York, NY 10017
212-573-2187

00074
Ross Laboratories
6480 Busch Blvd.
Columbus, OH 43229
614-624-3333

00054
Roxane Laboratories, Inc.
P.O. Box 16532
Columbus, OH 43216-6532
614-276-4000

51075
Royce Laboratories, Inc.
16600 N.W. 54 Avenue
Miami, FL 33014
305-624-1500

00536
Rugby Labs., Inc.
898 Orlando Ave.
West Hempstead, NY 11552
516-536-8565

46500
Rydelle Laboratories
1525 Howe Street
Racine, WI 53403-5011
414-631-2000

00263
Rystan Company, Inc.
P.O. Box 214
Little Falls, NJ 07424-0214
201-256-3737

S.C. Johnson & Son, Inc.
1525 Howe Street
Racine, WI 53403
414-631-2000

97692
S.G. Labs., Incorporated
500 North Broadway
Jericho, NY 11753
516-822-2900

00905
SCS Pharmaceuticals
P.O. Box 5110
Chicago, IL 60680
708-470-6576

00068, 00088, 00128, 00766, 45800,
49692, 53100
SKB Consumer Healthcare
P.O. Box 1467
Pittsburgh, PA 15230
412-928-1000

00212
Sandoz Nutrition
5320 W. 23rd Street
Minneapolis, MN 55440
612-925-2100

00043
Sandoz Pharmaceutical Corp.
59 Route 10
East Hanover, NJ 07936
201-503-7500

00078
Sandoz Pharmaceuticals
Route 10
East Hanover, NJ 07936
201-503-7500

51353
The Sanitube Company
19 Concord Street
S. Norwalk, CT 06854
203-853-7856

00024
Sanofi Winthrop Pharm.
90 Park Avenue
New York, NY 10016
212-907-2000

00281
Savage Laboratories
60 Baylis Road
Melville, NY 11747-2006
516-454-9071

58914
Scandipharm, Inc.
22 Inverness Cntr Pkwy # 310
Birmingham, AL 35242
800-950-8085

11012
Oshaffer Laboratories
1058 North Allen Ave.
Pasadena, CA 91104
818-798-8644

00364
Schein Pharmaceutical, Inc.
Mt. Ebo Corporate Park Rte. 22
Brewster, NY 10509
914-278-3723

00274
Scherer Laboratories, Inc.
16200 N. Dallas Pkwy, Ste 165
Dallas, TX 75248
800-858-9888

00085
Schering-Plough Corporation
110 Allen Road
Liberty Corner, NJ 07938
908-604-1995

00085
Schering-Plough Corporation
2000 Galloping Hill Road
Kenilworth, NJ 07033
908-298-4000

Schiff Products
P.O. Box 26708
Salt Lake City, UT 84126
801-975-1166

00234
Schmid Products Co.
P.O. Box 4703
Sarasota, FL 34230-4703
800-827-0987

Scholl, Inc.
3030 Jackson, P.O. Box 377
Memphis, TN 38151
901-320-2011

00091
Schwarz Pharma Kremers Urban
5600 W. County Line
Mequon, WI 53092
414-238-5484

Scios Nova Inc.
2450 Bayshore Parkway
Mountain View, CA 94043
415-966-1550

42021
Sclavo, Inc.
5 Mansard Court
Wayne, NJ 07470
201-696-8300

00372
Scot-Tussin Pharmacal Co., Inc
50 Clemence Street, Box 8217
Cranston, RI 02920-0217
800-638-7268

00444
Scrip, Inc.
101 South St.
Peoria, IL 61602-1986
309-674-3488

00014
G.D. Searle & Company
5200 Old Orchard Road
Skokie, IL 60077
708-982-7000

00025
G.D. Searle & Company
5200 Old Orchard Road
Skokie, IL 60077
708-982-7000

00551
The Seatrace Company
P.O. Box 363
Gadsden, AL 35902-0363
205-442-5023

50694
Seres Laboratories
3331 Industrial Drive, POB 470
Santa Rosa, CA 95401
707-526-4526

44087
Serono Laboratories, Inc.
100 Longwater Circle
Norwell, MA 02061
617-982-9000

49731
Sherman Pharmaceuticals, Inc.
P.O. Box 1377
Mandeville, LA 70470-1377
504-893-0007

08881
Sherwood Medical
1915 Olive Street
St. Louis, MO 63103
314-621-7788

08884
Sherwood Medical
1915 Olive Street
St. Louis, MO 63103

45809
Shionogi USA
3848 Carson Street #206
Torrance, CA 90503
310-540-1161

50111
Sidmak Laboratories, Inc.
P.O. Box 371
East Hanover, NJ 07936
201-386-5566

54482
Sigma-Tau Pharmaceuticals
200 Orchard Ridge Drive
Gaithersburg, MD 20878
301-948-1041

54838
Silarx Pharmaceuticals, Inc.
15 West Street
Spring Valley, NY 10977
914-352-4020

39769
Smith & Nephew SoloPak
1845 Tonne Road
Elk Grove Village, IL 60007-5125
708-806-0080

08026
Smith + Nephew United
P. O. Box 1970
Largo, FL 34649
800-876-1261

00007, 00029, 00108
SmithKline Beecham Pharm.
P.O. Box 7929
Philadelphia, PA 19103
215-751-4000

00978
SmithKline Diagnostics
225 Baypoint Parkway
San Jose, CA 95134-1622
800-877-6242

47631
SoftRinse Corporation
2411 Third Street South
Wisconsin Rapids, WI 54494
715-423-4801

33984
Solgar Company, Inc.
410 Ocean Ave.
Lynbrook, NY 11563
516-599-2442

00032
Solvay
901 Sawyer Road
Marietta, GA 30062-2224
404-578-9000

39506
Somerset Pharmaceuticals
777 S Harbour Island Blvd #880
Tampa, FL 33602
813-223-7677

Sparta Pharmaceuticals
P.O. Box 13288
Resrch Triang Pk, NC 27709
919-361-3461

Spectra Pharmaceuticals
See Cooper Pharmaceuticals

38137
Spectrum Chemical Mfg. Corp.
14422 S. San Pedro Street
Gardena, CA 90248-9985
800-772-8786

00537
Spencer Mead, Inc.
100 Banks Avenue
Rockville Center, NY 11570
800-645-3737

Sphinx Pharmaceutical Corp.
P.O. Box 52330
Durham, NC 27717
919-489-0909

00003
Squibb
P.O. Box 1022
Cherry Hill, NJ 08034
609-424-5600

00003
Squibb Diagnostic Division
P.O. Box 4500
Princeton, NJ 08543-4500
609-897-2000

00003
E.R. Squibb & Sons, Inc.
P.O. Box 4000
Princeton, NJ 08543-4000
609-252-4000

53385
Standard Drug Company
P.O. Box 710
Riverton, IL 62561
217-629-9884

00076
Star Pharmaceuticals, Inc.
1990 N.W. 44th Street
Pompano Beach, FL 33064-1278
305-971-9704

51318
Stellar Pharmacal Corp.
1990 N.W. 44th Street
Pompano Beach, FL 33064
800-845-7827

00402
Steris Laboratories, Inc.
620 N. 51st Avenue
Phoenix, AZ 85043
602-278-1400

12843
Sterling Health
90 Park Avenue 5th Floor
New York, NY 10016
212-907-2000

00024
Sterling Winthrop
90 Park Avenue
New York, NY 10016
212-907-2000

00145
Stiefel Laboratories, Inc.
Route 145
Oak Hill, NY 12422-9603
518-239-6901

89223
Stockhausen Inc.
2408 Doyle Street
Greensboro, NC 27406
800-334-0242

57706
Storz Ophthalmics
3365 Tree Court Industrial
St. Louis, MO 63122-6694
314-225-7365

Storz Ophthalmics
3365 Tree Court Industrial
St. Louis, MO 63122-6694
314-225-7600

58980
Stratus Pharmaceuticals, Inc.
P.O. Box 4632
Miami, FL 33265
800-442-7882

00038
Stuart Pharmaceuticals
Concord Pike and New Murphy Rd
Wilmington, DE 19897
302-886-2231

11086
Summers Laboratories, Inc.
103 G.P. Clement Dr.
Collegeville, PA 19426
610-454-1471

57267
Summit Pharmaceuticals
556 Morris Avenue
Summit, NJ 07901
908-277-5000

11704
Survival Technology, Inc.
2275 Research Blvd.
Rockville, MD 20850
301-926-1800

Syncom Pharmaceuticals, Inc.
155 Passaic Avenue
Fairfield, NJ 07004

Synergen, Inc.
1885 33rd Street
Boulder, CO 80301
303-938-6200

00033
Syntex Laboratories
3401 Hillview Ave.
Palo Alto, CA 94304
415-855-5050

Syntex-Synergen Neuroscience
1885 33rd Street
Boulder, CO 80301
303-442-1926

47854
Syosset Laboratories Co., Inc.
150 Fileen Way
Syosset, NY 11791
516-921-6306

Syva Company
929 Queensbridge
St. Louis, MO 63021
314-391-5374

51189
T.E. Williams Pharmaceuticals
P.O. Box 312
Divide, CO 80814-0312
719-687-8770

T/I Pharmaceuticals, Inc.
See Fischer Pharmaceuticals

TNI Pharmaceuticals
5105 N. Pearl Street
Schiller Park, IL 60176
708-678-3067

Tag Pharmaceuticals
P.O. Box 904
Sellersville, PA 18960
215-723-5544

Tambrands, Incorporated
777 Westchester Ave
White Plains, NY 10604
914-696-6060

74586
Tanning Research Labs., Inc.
1190 U.S. 1 North
Ormond Beach, FL 32174
904-677-9559

00300
Tap Pharmaceuticals
2355 Waukegan Rd.
Deerfield, IL 60015
800-621-1020

51672
Taro Pharmaceuticals U.S.A,Inc
Six Skyline Drive
Hawthorne, NY 10532-9998
914-345-9001

83926
Tec Laboratories Inc.
615 Water Ave. S.E. PO Box1958
Albany, OR 97321-0512
503-926-4577

Telluride Pharm. Corp.
140 Flanders Drive
Hillsborough, NJ 08876-4656
908-359-1375

49158
Thames Pharmacal Co., Inc.
2100 Fifth Avenue
Ronkonkoma, NY 11779-6906
516-737-1155

Therakos, Incorporated
201 Brandywine Parkway
West Chester, PA 19380
610-430-7900

Therapeutic Antibodies Inc.
1500 21st Ave. So., Ste 310
Nashville, TN 37212
615-327-1027

11290
Thompson Medical Co.
222 Lakeview Ave.
West Palm Beach, FL 33401
407-820-9900

11926
Thompson Medical Co.
222 Lakeview Ave.
West Palm Beach, FL 33401
407-820-9900

11299
Torch Laboratories, Inc.
P.O. Box 248
Reistertown, MD 21136
301-363-6350

93312
Trask Industries, Inc.
163 Farrell St.
Somerset, NJ 08873
908-214-9267

00598
Triage Pharmaceuticals
1643 E. Genesee St.
Syracuse, NY 13210
315-478-6303

11311
Trimen Laboratories, Inc.
80-26th Street
Pittsburgh, PA 15222
412-261-0339

53020
Trinity Technologies Inc.
28510 Hayes
Roseville, MI 48066
313-778-5630

Triton Bioscience
See Berlex

79511
Triton Consumer Products, Inc.
561 West Golf
Arlington Heights, IL 60005
708-228-7650

Tsumura Medical
1000 Valley Park Drive
Shakopee, MN 55379
612-496-4700

53335
Tyson & Associates, Inc.
12832 Chadron Ave.
Hawthorne, CA 90250-5525
310-676-1080

00785
UAD Laboratories, Inc.
P.O. Box 10587 8339 Hwy. 18
Jackson, MS 39289-0587
601-372-7773

UCB Pharmaceuticals, Inc.
P.O. Box 4410
Hampton, VA 23664-0410
804-851-4618

51079
UDL Laboratories, Inc.
P.O. Box 10319
Rockford, IL 61131-3019
815-282-1201

58178
US Bioscience
100 Front Street, Suite 400
West Conshohocken, PA 19428
800-447-3969

US Packaging Corp. Medical Div
506 Clay Street
LaPorte, IN 46350
219-362-9782

52747
US Pharmaceutical Corp.
2401 C Mellon Court
Decatur, GA 30035
404-987-4745

Ueno Fine Chemicals Industry
31, Koraibashi 2-chome
Osaka 541, Japan
06-203-0761

00127
Ulmer Pharmacal Co.
2440 Fernbrook Lane
Plymouth, MN 55447-9987
612-559-0601

Unimed
2150 E. Blake Cook Road
Buffalo Grove, IL 60089
708-541-2525

41785
Unimed
2150 E. Lake Cook Road
Buffalo Grove, IL 60089
800-541-3492

00677
United Research Laboratories
3600 Meadow Lane, P.O. Box 8546
Bensalem, PA 19020-8546
215-638-2626

48663
Unitek Corporation
2724 South Peck Road
Monrovia, CA 91016
818-445-7960

Univax Biologics
12280 Wilkins Avenue
Rockville, MD 20852
301-770-3099

00009
The Upjohn Company
7000 Portage Road
Kalamazoo, MI 49001
616-323-4000

00245
Upsher-Smith Labs., Inc.
14905-23rd Ave. N.
Minneapolis, MN 55447
612-473-4412

53258
VHA Supply Company
300 Decker Drive, POB 160909
Irving, TX 75016
214-650-4444

54627
ValMed, Inc.
203 Southwest Cutoff
Northboro, MA 01532
800-477-0487

00615
Vangard Labs., Inc.
PO Box 1268
Glasgow, KY 42142-1268
502-651-6188

17022
Veratex Corp.
1304 E. Maple Road, POB 4031
Troy,, MI 48007
313-588-2970

Vertex Pharmaceuticals, Inc.
40 Allston Street
Cambridge, MA 02139-4211
617-576-3111

23900
Vicks Health Care Products
11370 Reed Hartman Hwy
Cincinnati, OH 45241
513-983-1100

25866
Vicks Pharmacy Products
One Far Mill Crossing
Shelton, CT 06484
203-929-2500

Viratek
3300 Hyland Avenue
Costa Mesa, CA 92627
714-540-1866

54891
Vision Pharmaceuticals, Inc.
P.O. Box 400
Mitchell, SD 57301-0400
605-996-3356

49727
Vita-Rx Corporation
P.O. Box 8229
Columbus, GA 31908
706-568-1881

54022
Vitaline Corporation
385 Williamson Way
Ashland, OR 97520
503-482-9231

00298
Vortech Pharmaceuticals
6851 Chase Rd. P.O. Box 189
Dearborn, MI 48121
313-584-4088

59196
WE Pharmaceuticals, Inc.
P.O. Box 1142
Ramona, CA 92065
619-788-9155

WTD, Incorporated
8819 No. Pioneer Road
Peoria, IL 61615
309-693-2150

00619
Walker Pharmacal Company
4200 Laclede Ave.
St. Louis, MO 63108
314-533-9600

00741
Walker, Corp and Co., Inc.
P.O. Box 1320
Syracuse, NY 13201
315-463-4511

00037
Wallace Laboratories
Halfacre Road
Cranbury, NJ 08512
609-655-6000

00017
Wampole Laboratories
Half Acre Road, POB 1001
Cranbury, NJ 08515-0181
609-655-6000

00047
Warner Chilcott Laboratories
201 Tabor Road
Morris Plains, NJ 07950
201-540-2000

11370, 12546
Warner-Lambert Cons. Hlth Prod
170 Tabor Road
Morris Plains, NJ 07950
201-540-2000

12547
Warner Wellcome
See Warner-Lambert Conc. Hlth. Prod.

52544
Watson Laboratories
132-A Business Center Drive
Corona, CA 91720
909-270-1400

Wendt Laboratories
P.O. Box 128
Belle Plaine, MN 56011
800-328-5890

00917
Wesley Pharmacal Co., Inc.
114 Railroad Drive
Ivyland, PA 18974
215-953-1680

59591
West Point Pharma
WP 38M-2
West Point, PA 19486
215-661-5000

50893
Westport Pharmaceuticals, Inc.
1 Turkey Hill Road S.
Westport, CT 06880
203-226-0622

00143
West-Ward, Inc.
465 Industrial Way West
Eatontown, NJ 07724
908-542-1191

00072
Westwood Pharmaceuticals
100 Forest Avenue
Buffalo, NY 14213
716-887-3400

00003
Westwood Squibb Pharmaceutical
100 Forest Avenue
Buffalo, NY 14213
716-887-3400

50474
Whitby Pharmaceuticals, Inc.
1211 Sherwood Ave.
Richmond, VA 23261-5054
804-254-4400

00573
Whitehall Laboratories
Five Giralda Farms
Madison, NJ 07940-0871
201-660-5500

00317
Whorton Pharmaceuticals, Inc.
4202 Gary Ave.
Fairfield, AL 35064
205-786-2584

12120
Wisconsin Pharmacal Co.
N. 168 W. 22223 Main Street
Jackson, WI 53037
414-677-4121

11428
Wonderful Dream Salve Corp.
20441 Eastwood Dr.
Harper Woods, MI 48225
313-543-2556

00008
Wyeth-Ayerst Laboratories
P.O. Box 8299
Philadelphia, PA 19101
215-688-4400

50962
Xactdose, Inc.
722 Progressive Lane
South Beloit, IL 61080
815-624-8523

Xoma
2910 Seventh Street
Berkeley, CA 94710
510-644-1170

00116
Xttrium Laboratories, Inc.
415 West Pershing Road
Chicago, IL 60609
312-268-5800

60077
Young Dental
13705 Shoreline Court East
Earth City, MO 63045
314-344-0010

11444
W. F. Young, Inc.
111 Lyman Street
Springfield, MA 01102
413-737-0201

00310
Zeneca Inc.
Concord Pike and Murphy Road
Wilmington, DE 19897
302-886-3000

00172
Zenith Laboratories, Inc.
140 Legrand Avenue
Northvale, NJ 07647
201-767-1700

05128
Zila Pharmaceuticals, Inc.
5227 N. 7th Street
Phoenix, AZ 85014-2817
602-266-6700

Zymogenetics, Inc.
1201 Eastlake Ave. E.
Seattle, WA 98102
206-547-8080

Notes

Notes

Notes

Notes

ISBN 0-932686-32-X

90000